Textbook of Diagnostic Microbiology

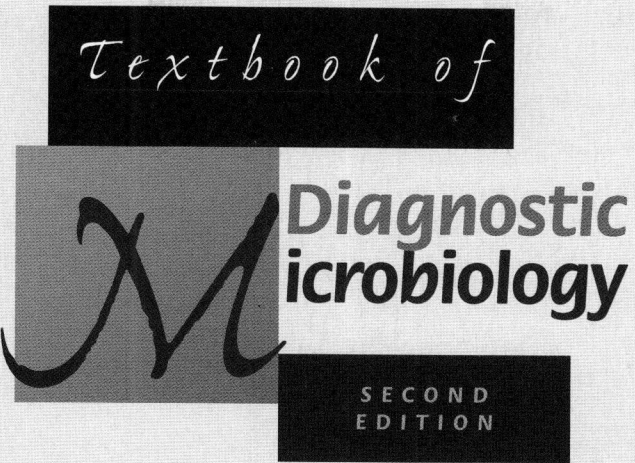

Textbook of Diagnostic Microbiology

SECOND EDITION

Edited by

Connie R. Mahon, MS, MT(ASCP), CLS
Associate Professor and Undergraduate Program Director
Department of Clinical Laboratory Sciences
The University of Texas Health Science Center at San Antonio
San Antonio, Texas

George Manuselis, MA, MT(ASCP)
Emeritus Faculty
Medical Technology Division
The Ohio State University
Columbus, Ohio

Adjunct Professor
Wayne College
The University of Akron
Orville, Ohio

with 600 color illustrations

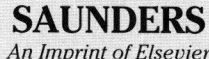

SAUNDERS
An Imprint of Elsevier

SAUNDERS
An Imprint of Elsevier

The Curtis Center
Independence Square West
Philadelphia, Pennsylvania 19106

Acquisitions Editor: Karen Fabiano
Developmental Editor: Sarahlynn Lester
Project Manager: Linda McKinley
Production Editors: Cathy Comer, Kristin Hebberd, and René Spencer Saller
Design: Judi Lang
Cover Design: Liz Rudder

Library of Congress Cataloging in Publication Data

Textbook of diagnostic microbiology / edited by Connie R. Mahon,
George Manuselis.—2nd ed.

p.   cm.

Includes bibliographical references and index.

ISBN 0–7216–7917–X

1. Diagnostic microbiology.   I. Mahon, Connie.   II. Manuselis, George.
   [DNLM: 1. Microbiological Techniques.   QW 25 T355 2000]

QR67.T49 2000   616'.01—dc21

99-462321

TEXTBOOK OF DIAGNOSTIC MICROBIOLOGY   ISBN 0–7216–7917–X

Permissions may be sought directly from Elsevier's Health Sciences Rights Department in Philadelphia, USA: phone: (+1)215-238-7869, fax: (+1)215-238-2239, email: healthpermissions@elsevier.com. You may also complete your request on-line via the Elsevier Science homepage (http://www.elsevier.com), by selecting 'Customer Support' and then 'Obtaining Permissions'.

Printed in China

Last digit is print number: 9   8   7   6   5   4

Contributors

Shirley Adams, MS, CLS(NCA), CLDir
Peripheral Laboratory Supervisor
Anderson Area Medical Center
Anderson, South Carolina

Gerald L. Alderson, MD, DDS
Associate Professor of Pathology
The University of Texas Health Science Center
   at San Antonio
Medical Director, Clinical Virology Laboratory
   and Immunology Laboratory
University Hospital
Chief, Pathology and Laboratory Medicine Service
Audie L. Murphy Memorial Veterans Hospital
San Antonio, Texas

Gerald Andrews, PhD
Lieutenant Colonel, United States Army
Chief, Microbiology and Immunology
Department of Pathology
Landstuhl Regional Medical Center
Landstuhl, Germany

Leona W. Ayers, MD
Director
Ohio Department of Health
Columbus, Ohio

Jean Barnishan, BS, M(ASCP)
Clinical Instructor, School of Allied Medicine
Senior Medical Technologist
University Hospitals
The Ohio State University
Columbus, Ohio

Amy M. Carnahan, MS, M(ASCP), SM(ASCP)
Senior Research Scientist
Division of Hospital Epidemiology
University of Maryland School of Medicine
Baltimore, Maryland

Mary Castiglia, PharmD
Assistant Professor of Clinical Pharmacy
School of Pharmacy
Robert C. Byrd Health Science Center
West Virginia University
Morgantown, West Virginia

James L. Cook, MD
Chief of Infectious Diseases
University of Illinois Medical Center Chicago
Department of Medicine
College of Medicine
Chicago, Illinois

David W. Craft, PhD
Lieutenant Colonel, United States Army
Laboratory Director, Infectious Disease Laboratories
Walter Reed Army Medical Center
Washington, DC

Vee E. Davison, MS, PhD
Academy of Learning in Retirement
Branch of the University of Texas
San Antonio, Texas

Kirk M. Doing, PhD
Director, Clinical Microbiology
Affiliated Laboratory Inc.
Associate Faculty
Department of Microbiology, Biochemistry,
   and Molecular Biology
University of Maine
Orono, Maine

Janet Duben-Engelkirk, EdD, MT(ASCP), CLS
Program Director
Clinical Laboratory Science
Scott & White Memorial Hospital
Temple, Texas

Denise F. Dunbar, BA, M(ASCP)
Section Chief, Mycobacteriology/Mycology Section
Bureau of Laboratories
Texas Department of Health
Austin, Texas

Janice Eisenstadt, DO
Fellow, Department of Pathology
Section of Clinical Microbiology
Cleveland Clinic Foundation
Cleveland, Ohio
Staff Physician, Department of Internal Medicine
Infectious Disease Section
Sinai Hospital of Detroit
Detroit, Michigan

Paul G. Engelkirk, PhD, MT(ASCP)
Faculty
Department of Science
Central Texas College
Killeen, Texas

Annette W. Fothergill, MBA, MT(ASCP), CLS
Supervisor
Fungus Testing Laboratory
Department of Pathology
The University of Texas Health Science Center
    at San Antonio
San Antonio, Texas

Susan M. Gibson, BA, M(ASCP)
Supervisor (Retired), Bacteriology/Mycology Branch
Bureau of Laboratories
Texas Department of Health
Austin, Texas

Larry J. Goodman, MD
Associate Professor of Medicine and Associate Dean
Medical Student Programs, Rush Medical College
Attending Physician, Section of Infectious Disease
Rush-Presbyterian-St. Luke's Medical Center
Chicago, Illinois

Margaret Gregory, BS, MT(ASCP)
Clinical Faculty, Medical Technologist, and
    Laboratory Safety Officer
School of Allied Medical Professions
University Hospitals
The Ohio State University
Columbus, Ohio

James T. Griffith, PhD, CLS
Chancellor, Professor, and Chair
Department of Medical Laboratory Science
University of Massachusetts-Dartmouth
North Dartmouth, Massachusetts

Gerri S. Hall, PhD
Associate Professor
Microbiology
Department of Clinical Pathology
The Cleveland Clinic
Cleveland, Ohio

Patricia K. Hargrave, PhD, CLS(NCA), MT(ASCP)
Assistant Professor
Department of Medical Technology
University of Kansas Medical Center
Kansas City, Kansas

James L. Harris, PhD
Training Coordinator
Bureau of Laboratories
Texas Department of Health
Austin, Texas

Janet A. Hindler, MCLS, MT(ASCP)
Senior Specialist
Department of Pathology and Laboratory Medicine
    Microbiology Laboratory
University of California at Los Angeles
Los Angeles, California

Ronald H. Holton, PhD
Assistant Professor
Department of Clinical Laboratory Sciences
University of Mississippi Medical Center
Jackson, Mississippi

James H. Jorgensen, PhD
Professor
Department of Pathology
The University of Texas Health Science Center
    at San Antonio
San Antonio, Texas

Raymond L. Kaplan, PhD
Clinical Associate Professor, The College of Health
    Sciences
Georgia State University
Technical Manager, Microbiology
SmithKline Beecham Clinical Laboratories
Atlanta, Georgia

Susan L. Koletar, MD
Assistant Professor
Internal Medicine
University Hospitals
Columbus, Ohio

Boo H. Kwa, PhD
Associate Professor, College of Public Health
University of South Florida
Tampa, Florida

Hal S. Larsen, PhD, MT(ASCP), CLS
Professor and Chair
Department of Clinical Laboratory Science
School of Allied Health
Texas Tech University Health Sciences Center
Lubbock, Texas

Karen S. Long, MS, CLS
Assistant Professor
Medical Technology Program
West Virginia University
Morgantown, West Virginia

Connie R. Mahon, MS, MT(ASCP), CLS
Associate Professor and Undergraduate Program
  Director
Department of Clinical Laboratory Sciences
The University of Texas Health Science Center
  at San Antonio
San Antonio, Texas

George Manuselis, MA, MT(ASCP)
Emeritus Faculty
Medical Technology Division
The Ohio State University
Columbus, Ohio
Adjunct Professor
Wayne College
The University of Akron
Orville, Ohio

Mario J. Marcon, PhD
Clinical Associate Professor of Pediatrics
  and Pathology
The Ohio State University College of Medicine
Director, Clinical Microbiology/Virology Laboratories
Columbus Children's Hospital
Columbus, Ohio

David P. Marmaduke, MD
Dahl-Chase Pathology Associates
Bangor, Maine
Adjunct Professor
Department of Microbiology, Biochemistry,
  and Molecular Biology
University of Maine
Orono, Maine

Frederic J. Marsik, PhD, ABMM
Clinical Microbiology Consultant
Food and Drug Administration
Rockville, Maryland

Jeffrey P. Massey, DrPH, MT(ASCP)
Chief, Molecular Epidemiology Unit
Michigan Department of Public Health
Lansing, Michigan

Deanna A. McGough, BS, MT, SM(ASCP), RM, SM(AAM)
Instructor, Department of Pathology
Administrative Director, Fungus Testing Laboratory
Department of Pathology
The University of Texas Health Science Center
  at San Antonio
San Antonio, Texas

Darlene Miller, MA, MT(ASCP)
Director of Microbiology
Bascom Palmer Eye Institute
University of Miami
Miami, Florida

Denise Miller, MS, MT(ASCP)
Staff Medical Technologist
University Hospital
San Antonio, Texas

William F. Nauschuetz, PhD
Lieutenant Colonel, Medical Service Corps, United
  States Army
Chief, Microbiology and Immunology
Department of Pathology and Area Laboratory
  Services
Brooke Army Medical Center
Fort Sam Houston, Texas

Vinnie Pawar, PhD, MT(ASCP)
Microbiological Associates
Rockville, Maryland

Michael A. Pentella, BS, MS
Clinical Microbiologist
Lakeland Regional Medical Center
Lakeland, Florida

Richard B. Prior, PhD
Associate Professor
The Ohio State University College of Medicine
Columbus, Ohio

Thomas Pulchalski, MS, MT(ASCP)
Clinical Instructor, School of Allied Medical
   Professions
The Ohio State University
Senior Medical Technologist
The Ohio State University Medical Center
Columbus, Ohio

Merrily Rausch, BS, MT(ASCP)
Clinical Faculty
School of Allied Medical Professions
Supervisor
Clinical Microbiology
University Hospitals
The Ohio State University
Columbus, Ohio

Joy G. Remley, BS, MT(ASCP), SM
Clinical Faculty
School of Allied Medical Professions
Senior Medical Technologist
University Hospitals
The Ohio State University
Columbus, Ohio

Alonza S. Romo, BS, MBA
Evening Supervisor
Metropolitan Hospital
San Antonio, Texas

Sharon S. Rowland, PhD, MT(ASCP)
Assistant Professor, Department of Medical
   and Research Technology
University of Maryland School of Medicine
Baltimore, Maryland

Leonard H. Schleicher, Jr., MS, MT(ASCP)
Section Chief, Clinical Microbiology Laboratory
Grant Medical Center
Columbus, Ohio

Patricia M. Simone, MD
Deputy Branch Chief, Program Services Branch
Division of Tuberculosis Elimination
Centers for Disease Control and Prevention
Atlanta, Georgia

Raymond A. Smego, Jr., MD
Professor and Chair
Department of Infectious Diseases & Tropical
   Medicine
University of Wit Waters Rand Medical School
Johannesburg, Republic of South Africa

Linda A. Smith, PhD, CLS(NCA)
Professor and Graduate Programs Director
Department of Clinical Laboratory Sciences
The University of Texas Health Science Center
   at San Antonio
San Antonio, Texas

Deanna A. Sutton, MT(ASCP), SM(ASCP), RM
Instructor
Fungus Testing Laboratory
Department of Pathology
The University of Texas Health Science Center
   at San Antonio
San Antonio, Texas

John G. Thomas, PhD
Professor
Department of Pathology
Director
Medical Research Laboratory
West Virginia University Hospitals
Morgantown, West Virginia

Sherry Trevino, MPH, MT(ASCP), CLS(NCA)
Core I Microbiology Supervisor
Wilford Hall Medical Center
Lackland Air Force Base, Texas

Ronald R. Trudel, MS, PhD
Associate Professor of Medical Laboratory Science
University of Massachusetts-Dartmouth
North Dartmouth, Massachusetts

James L. Vossler, MS, MT(ASCP)SM, CLS(NCA)
Assistant Professor, Department of Clinical
   Laboratory Science
College of Health Professions
State University of New York Health Science Center
   at Syracuse
Syracuse, New York

A. Christian Whelen, PhD, ABMMM
Lieutenant Colonel, United States Army
Chief, Department of Parasitology
Division of Experimental Therapeutics
Walter Reed Army Institute of Research
Washington, DC
Adjunct Associate Professor of Pathology
The George Washington University School of Medicine
   and Health Sciences
Washington, DC

Robert G. Whiddon, PhD
Quality Assurance Director
Virus Reference Laboratory
San Antonio, Texas

To my husband, Dan; my daughter, Kathleen; and my son, Sean Patrick,

for their love, understanding, and encouragement

CRM

To my daughters, Kristina and Shellie; my parents, Katherine and George;

my sisters, Libby and Helen; and my brother, Demetrious

GM

Preface

Since the initial conception, organization, and publication of the 1st edition of the *Textbook of Diagnostic Microbiology,* clinical microbiology has changed dramatically. New pathogens and infectious diseases continue to be recognized and to plague society. The resurgence of "classic" pathogens, which many healthcare professionals once believed would be eradicated, has been noted. These infectious agents seem likely to follow us well into the new millennium. Microorganisms that previously were treated empirically have expanded their scope of infections and become more virulent and resistant to antimicrobials. In many instances the advent of new diagnostic procedures, treatment modalities, and instrumentation methods has influenced changes in the epidemiology of infectious diseases.

Nevertheless, the 2nd edition of the *Textbook of Diagnostic Microbiology* has maintained the characteristics that originally attracted clinical laboratory science and clinical laboratory technician students, entry-level clinical laboratory practitioners, microbiologists, and educators. This edition has kept its building-block approach and student-friendly tradition. It was written to help students and professionals navigate the maze of background theoretical concepts, identification schemas, diagnostic characteristics, biochemical reactions, and isolation techniques to produce clinically relevant results. The *Textbook of Diagnostic Microbiology* has continued to rely on the "organ system" approach to microbiology and the bench technologist's perception of isolating, identifying, and performing antimicrobial susceptibilities of microorganisms. New tables, flow charts, and featured illustrations have been added to reinforce learning. In addition to the learning objectives listed at the beginning of each chapter, key terms and opening case studies have been added. At the end of each chapter, readers will find learning assessment questions to reinforce comprehension and understanding of important concepts.

The textbook is divided into three parts. Part I presents basic principles and concepts of diagnostic microbiology, which provide students with a firm theoretical foundation. Part II highlights methods for the identification of significant isolates. Part III focuses on the clinical and laboratory diagnoses of infectious diseases at various body sites. Because the goal of the *Textbook of Diagnostic Microbiology* is to provide a strong foundation for students, entry-level practitioners, and other healthcare professionals, organisms discussed are limited to those that are medically important and commonly encountered.

The *Textbook of Diagnostic Microbiology* contains a number of other significant features. Chapter 4 presents general guidelines for the establishment of a comprehensive Continuous Quality Improvement Program, a distinctive feature of this textbook. Another quality assurance issue discussed within this chapter is the section on "Putting the Laboratory to the Test," which describes the principles of clinical sensitivity and specificity and their applications in the determination of the predictive values of laboratory tests. Understanding the usefulness of predictive values is important for the appropriate use of tests and the interpretation of laboratory results. Chapter 3 provides an update on the emerging resistance of several bacterial species and describes the principles of and procedures in antimicrobial susceptibility.

Although recovery of etiologic agents in cultures has remained the "gold standard" in microbiology to determine the probable cause of an infectious disease, rapid diagnostic tests, including molecular probes, have expanded during the last several years. Therefore Chapter 5 has been revised and expanded to include the lastest clinical applications of PCR (polymerase chain reaction) testing and probe technology. Chapters 8 and 9 still play vital roles in the textbook. These two chapters help students and practitioners who may have difficulty recognizing bacterial morphology on direct smear preparations, as well colonial morphology on primary culture plates, develop these skills through the use of color photomicrographs of stained direct smear and culture from clinical samples. These chapters also illustrate how microscopic and colonial morphology of organisms can aid in the initial identification of the bacterial isolate.

In the 2nd edition, Part I continues to be the "backbone" of the *Textbook of Diagnostic Microbiology,* whereas Part II emphasizes the laboratory identification of etiologic agents. Chapters in this section describe organisms by taxonomic groups. Although diseases caused by the organisms are discussed and the opening case scenarios describe illnesses, the emphasis is on the characteristics and methods used to recover and identify each group of organisms. Many tables summarize the major features of organisms, and schematic networks are used to show relationships and differences between similar or closely related species. Photographs are used generously to show the characteristics of particular organisms. Chapters devoted to anaerobic species, medically important fungi, parasites, and viruses affirm the significance of these agents. Newly recognized parasitic agents are presented in Chapter 24, whereas Chapter 25 describes emerging viral pathogens.

The organ system approach to diagnostic microbiology provides an opportunity for students and other readers to "pull things together." In Part III each chapter begins with the anatomic considerations of the organ system to be discussed and the role of the usual flora found at this particular site in the pathogenesis of disease. It is important for students to become comfortable with their knowledge of the usual inhabitants at a body site before they can recognize the significance of the opportunistic infectious agents they most likely would encounter. The chapters in Part III include case studies to enhance problem-solving and critical thinking skills. The case histories describe the clinical and laboratory findings associated with the patients, allowing students opportunities to correlate these observations with possible etiologic agents. In most cases the cause of the illness is not disclosed in the case history; rather, it is revealed elsewhere in the chapter to give students time to think the case through.

The expertise of the contributors, full-color photographs and photomicrographs, engaging and easy-to-follow design, learning assessment questions, opening case scenarios, and lists of key terms all strengthen the building-block approach used in the *Textbook of Diagnostic Microbiology* for students and healthcare professionals. This edition of the *Textbook of Diagnostic Microbiology* has maintained its tradition as a user-friendly textbook designed to facilitate and enhance learning.

Connie R. Mahon
George Manuselis

Acknowledgements

We are grateful to the contributing authors of both editions and to many other individuals who have made significant suggestions and invaluable comments on ways to improve this edition. Many thanks to our friends and colleagues, Bill Nauschuetz, Chris Whelen, David Craft, Ron Holton, Robert Whiddon, and Linda Canas for their critical review of the previous edition. Our appreciation also goes to Peggy D. Wilson, Maureta Ott, Richard Brust, Authur Weeks, Marilyn Solomon, and Darlene Spurgeon.

Connie R. Mahon
George Manuselis

Contents

PART I

Introduction to Clinical Microbiology   1

1 Bacterial Cell Structure, Physiology, Metabolism, and Genetics   2
George Manuselis, Connie R. Mahon

Significance   4
Classification   4
  Taxonomy   4
  Nomenclature   5
  Classification by Phenotypic and Genotypic
    Characteristics   5
  Classification by Cellular Type: Prokaryotes,
    Eukaryotes, and Archaeobacteria   5
Comparison of Eukaryotic and Prokaryotic Cell
  Structure   7
  Eukaryotic Cell Structure   7
  Prokaryotic Cell Structure   7
Bacterial Morphology   10
  Microscopic Shapes   10
  Common Stains Used for Microscopic
    Visualization   11
Microbial Growth and Nutrition   13
  Nutritional Requirements for Growth   14
  Environmental Factors Influencing Growth   14
  Bacterial Growth   15
Bacterial Biochemistry and Metabolism   16
  Metabolism   16
  Fermentation and Respiration   16
  Biochemical Pathways from Glucose to
    Pyruvic Acid   17
  Anaerobic Utilization of Pyruvic Acid
    (Fermentation)   18
  Aerobic Utilization of Pyruvate
    (Oxidation)   19
  Carbohydrate Utilization and Lactose
    Fermentation   19

Bacterial Genetics   20
  Terminology   20
  Genetic Elements and Alterations   21
  Mechanisms of Gene Transfer   21

2 Control of Microorganisms   25

A. Disinfection and Sterilization   25
  Connie R. Mahon

Sterilization Versus Disinfection   26
Factors that Influence the Degree of Killing   27
  Types of Organisms   27
  Number of Organisms   27
  Concentration of Disinfecting Agent   27
  Organic Soil Present   27
  Nature of Surface to Be Disinfected   28
Methods of Disinfection and Sterilization   28
  Physical Methods   28
  Chemical Methods   30

B. Microbiology Laboratory Safety   34
  Margaret Gregory

General Safety Principles   35
  Safety Program for the Microbiology
    Laboratory   35
Handling of Biologic Hazards   35
  Major Sources of Biologic Hazards   35
  OSHA Regulations for Blood-Borne
    Pathogens   39
Disposal of Infectious Waste   41
Chemical Safety   41
  Employee Right-to-Know   41
  Material Safety Data Sheets   41
  Hazardous Chemicals Inventory   46
  Laboratory Safety for Hazardous
    Chemicals   46
Hazardous Waste Reduction   47
Fire Safety   47
  Thermal Injuries   47
Electrical Safety   48

Miscellanous Safety Considerations   48
   Back Safety   48
   Storage of Gases   48
   First Aid Training   48
   Immunizations   49
Safety Training   49

3 Concepts in Antimicrobial Therapy   52

A. Antimicrobial Mechanisms of Action   52
   Susan L. Koletar

Effects on Cell Wall Integrity   54
   β-Lactam Antibacterial Agents   55
   β-Lactamase Inhibitors   56
   Other Antimicrobial Agents Whose Primary
      Site of Action Is the Cell Wall   57
Interruption of Cell Membrane Structure
   and Function   57
Inhibition of Protein Synthesis   57
Inhibition of Essential Metabolites   58
Interference with Nucleic Acid Metabolism   59
Resistance to Antibacterial Agents   59

B. Procedures in Antimicrobial Susceptibility Testing   62
   Janet A. Hindler, James H. Jorgensen

Reasons and Indications for Performing
   Antimicrobial Susceptibility Tests   64
   Factors to Consider When Determining
      Whether Testing Is Warranted   64
Selecting Antimicrobial Agents for Testing
   and Reporting   65
   Selection of Test Batteries   65
   Reporting of Susceptibility Test Results   65
Traditional Antimicrobial Susceptibility Test
   Methods   67
   Inoculum Preparation and Use of McFarland
      Standards   67
   Dilution Methods   69
   Disk Diffusion Testing   73
   Modified Methods for Testing Slow-Growing
      or Fastidious Bacteria   77
   Additional Organism and Antimicrobial Agent
      Testing Concerns   81
Automated Antimicrobial Susceptibility Test
   Methods   84
   Principles of Technologies Used   84
   Currently Available Automated Systems   85
   Nonautomated Antimicrobial Susceptibility
      Test Method: E Test   87
Interpretation of In Vitro Antimicrobial
   Susceptibility Test Results   88
Methods of Detecting Antimicrobial-Inactivating
   Enzymes   89
   β-Lactamase Tests   89

Quality Control of Antimicrobial Susceptibility
   Tests   90
Selecting an Antimicrobial Susceptibility Test
   Method   93

C. Special Antimicrobial Susceptibility Tests   97
   Janet A. Hindler

Minimum Bactericidal Concentration (MBC)
   Test   98
   Controlling Test Variables   100
   Interpretation Concerns   100
Time-Kill Assays   100
Synergy Tests   100
Serum Bactericidal Test   102
Molecular Probes for Identifying Determinants
   of Antimicrobial Resistance   103
Measurement of Antimicrobial Agents in Serum
   and Body Fluids   103
   Biologic Assays   103
   Immunoassays   103
   Chromatographic Assays   104

4 Performance Improvement in the Microbiology Laboratory   105

A. Quality Issues in Clinical Microbiology   105
   Merrily Rausch

General Guidelines for Establishing Quality
   Control   107
   Temperatures   107
   Thermometer Calibration   108
   Equipment QC   108
   Reagent QC   112
   Antimicrobial Susceptibility QC   112
   Personnel Competency   112
   Use of Stock Cultures   114
   QC Manual   114
Performance Improvement (PI)   116
   Mission Statement   116
   Indicators of PI: Process Versus Outcome   116
   Establishing Performance Monitors   116
   Problem/Action Form   116
   The Customer Concept   117
   Fixing the Process   117
   Benchmarking   117
   Commercially Purchased Monitors   118

B. Putting the Laboratory Test to the Test   121
   Frederic J. Marsik

Analytical Analysis of Tests   121
   Analytical (Technical) Sensitivity   122
   Analytical (Technical) Specificity   122
   Accuracy   122
Clinical Analysis of Tests   122
   Clinical (Diagnostic) Sensitivity   122
   Clinical (Diagnostic) Specificity   122

Operational Analysis of Tests   123
   Incidence of Disease   123
   Prevalence of Disease   123
   Predictive Values of Tests   123
   Efficiency of Tests   125
   Other Concepts   125
Choosing a Laboratory Method   125
Test Validation   127

5 Emergent Technologies   129

A. Direct Microbial Antigen Detection   129
David W. Craft

Historical Perspective   131
Antigen Detection Methods   133
   Precipitin Tests   133
   Particle Agglutination   135
   Immunofluorescent Assays   139
   Enzyme Immunoassays   141
   Optical Immunoassays   145
   Other Immunoassays   145
Current Clinical Applications   145
   Respiratory Tract Infections   145
   Meningitis and Sepsis   149
   Gastrointestinal Tract Infections   149
   Sexually Transmitted Diseases   150
   Blood-Borne and Body Fluid-Borne
     Diseases   151
Future Applications   151

B. Serologic Diagnosis of Infectious Diseases   154
Ronald H. Holton

Immune Response to Infectious Agents   156
   Host Resistance to Infection   156
   Nature of the Immune Response to Infectious
     Agents   158
   Antigens and Antibodies   159
   Primary and Secondary Antibody
     Responses   161
Interpreting Serologic Test Data   162
   Acute and Convalescent Antibody Titers   162
   Antibody Specificity and Cross-Reactivity   162
   False-Negative and False-Positive Serologic
     Test Results   163
   Value of Serologic Tests   164
Antibody Detection Methods
  and Applications   165
   Particle Agglutination Assays   165
   Precipitation Assays   167
   Complement Fixation Test   168
   Neutralization Tests   170
   Microscope-Assisted Labeled-Reagent
     Techniques   171
   Enzyme-Linked Immunosorbent Assay
     and Related Techniques   173
   Western Blotting   175

Use of Serologic Testing in Specific Diseases   177
   Serologic Testing of Syphilis   177
   Serologic Testing for Streptococcal
     Infections   177
   Serologic Testing of Toxoplasmosis   178
   Serologic Testing of Important Viral
     Diseases   178
   Serologic Diagnosis of Fungal Infection   180

**C. Rapid Methods and Automation in the Microbiology
   Laboratory   182**
David W. Craft

The Term *Rapid*   183
Microscopic Methods for Rapid Detection   183
Rapid Biochemical Tests Performed on Isolated
  Colonies   184
Identification Systems Relying Upon
  Carbohydrate Utilization or Chromogenic
  Substrates   184
   Principles of Identification   184
   Manual Rapid Tests   185
   Automated Rapid Tests   188
   Evaluation of Rapid Methods   189

D. Molecular Applications in the Clinical Laboratory   191
Gerri S. Hall

Hybridization Formats   192
   Probe Labels   193
   Probe Target   194
Applications for Probe Technology   194
   Probes for Culture Confirmation   194
   Probes for Rapid Diagnosis of Infectious
     Diseases   195
   Amplification   199
   Detection of the Amplicon   200
Clinical Applications of Amplification   204
   Technical Considerations for Implementation
     of Amplification   205
   Measures to Control Contamination   205
   Commercially Available Amplification
     Systems   205
   Detection of *Mycobacterium tuberculosis*   207
   Other Available Assays   207

6 Host-Parasite Interaction   211

A. Indigenous Microbial Flora   211
Hal S. Larsen

Flora   212
   Origin of Microbial Flora   212
   Characteristics of Indigenous Microbial
     Flora   212
Usual Flora at Different Body Sites   213
   Usual Flora of the Skin   213
   Usual Flora of the Mouth   213
   Usual Flora of the Respiratory Tract   214
   Usual Flora of the Gastrointestinal Tract   214
   Usual Flora of the Genitourinary Tract   215

B. Pathogenesis of Infection   218
  Hal S. Larsen

Pathogenicity   219
  Pathogens   219
  Opportunistic Pathogens   219
Virulence   220
Host Resistance Factors   220
  Physical Barriers   220
  Cleansing Mechanisms   221
  Antimicrobial Substances   222
  Indigenous Microbial Flora   222
  Phagocytosis   222
  Inflammation   224
  Immune Responses   226
Infectious Agent Factors   227
  Adherence   227
  Proliferation   227
  Tissue Damage   228
  Invasion   228
  Dissemination   228
Routes of Transmission   230
  Airborne Transmission   230
  Transmission by Food and Water   231
  Close Contact   232
  Cuts and Bites   232
  Arthropods   232
  Zoonoses   232
Epidemiology   233
  Definitions   233
  Surveillance and Reporting   234

7 General Concepts in Specimen Collection
   and Handling   237
   Merrily Rausch, Joy G. Remley

Basic Principles of Specimen Collection   239
  Appropriate Collection Techniques   239
Patient Education and Preparation   240
  Patient Education: Patient-Collected
    Samples   240
  Patient or Site Preparation   241
Preservation, Storage, and Transport
  of Specimens   242
  Use of Preservatives   242
  Use of Anticoagulants   242
  Use of Holding and Transport Media   243
  Unprotected Specimens   243
  Storage of Specimens   243
  Mailing Etiologic Agents   244
Safety   245
  Protection of the Specimen Transporter   245
  Protection of the Specimen Processor   245
Labeling and Rejection of Specimens   245
  Requisitions   245
  Unacceptable Specimens   247

Processing of Clinical Samples for Optimal
  Organism Recovery   247
  Prioritization During Processing   247
  Gross Examination of Specimens   248
  Direct Examination Techniques   248
  Primary Inoculation of Routine
    Specimens   250
  Processing Nonroutine Specimens   255

8 Microscopic Examination of Infected
   Materials   261
   Leona W. Ayers

Preparation of Samples   263
  Smears from Swabs   263
  Smears from Thick Liquids or Semisolids   263
  Smears from Thick, Granular, or Mucoid
    Materials   264
  Smears from Thin Fluids   265
  Cytocentrifuge Preparations   265
Stains   266
Microscopes   266
Terminology for Direct Examinations   271
Examination of Prepared Material   273
  Characterization of Background
    Materials   273
  Search for Microorganisms   274
  Evaluation of Choice of Antibiotic   275
  Direct Examination Summary   275
  Initiation of Special Handling for Unsuspected
    or Special Pathogens   275
Grading or Classifying Materials   275
  Contaminating Materials   276
  Local Materials   276
  Purulence   277
  Mixed Materials   277
Reports of Direct Examinations   277
Examples of Sample Observations
  and Reports   278
Quality Control in Direct Microscopic
  Interpretations   278
Direct Examination Showing Local and
  Contaminating Materials   282
Direct Examination in Common Bacterial
  Infections   284
Direct Examination in Gram-Positive Bacillary
  Infections   286
Direct Examination in Uncommon Gram-Positive
  Bacilli   288
Direct Examination in Gram-Positive Bacilli
  with Filaments and Branches   290
Direct Examination in Selected Gram-Negative
  Bacterial Infections   292
Direct Examination in Selected Gram-Negative
  Bacillary Infections   294

Direct Examination in Polymicrobial
  Infections   298
Direct Examination in Fungal Infections   300
Direct Examination in Parasitic Infections   304
Direct Examination in Viral Infections   308

**9 Use of Colonial Morphology for the
Presumptive Identification
of Microorganisms   311**
George Manuselis

Importance of Colonial Morphology as a
  Diagnostic Tool   313
Initial Observation and Interpretation
  of Cultures   313
Gross Colony Characteristics Used
  to Differentiate and Presumptively Identify
  Microorganisms   316
    Hemolysis   316
    Size   317
    Form or Margin   317
    Elevation   317
    Density   319
    Color   319
    Consistency   319
    Pigment   319
    Odor   319
Colonies with Multiple Characteristics   321
Growth of Organisms in Liquid Media   321

PART II

**Laboratory Identification
of Significant Isolates   327**

10 Staphylococci   329
Hal S. Larsen, Connie R. Mahon

General Characteristics   330
Clinically Significant Species   332
    Staphylococcus aureus   332
    Staphylococcus epidermidis   335
    Staphylococcus saprophyticus   335
    Other Coagulase-Negative Staphylococci   335
Laboratory Diagnosis   335
    Specimen Collection and Handling   335
    Microscopic Examination   335
    Isolation and Identification   336
Antimicrobial Susceptibility   341
Methicillin-Resistant Staphylococci   341

11 *Streptococcaceae*   345
Hal S. Larsen

Streptococcus and *Enterococcus:* General
  Characteristics   347
    Cell Wall Structure   347
    Classification   347
    Noncultural Identification   356
Clinically Significant Streptococci and their
  Associated Diseases   358
    Streptococcus pyogenes (Group A
      Streptococci)   358
    Streptococcus agalactiae (Group B
      Streptococci)   361
    Other Groups   362
    Enterococcus   364
    Streptococcus pneumoniae   364
    Viridans Streptococci   367
    Nutritionally Variant Streptococci   368
Streptococcus-like Oganisms   368
    Aerococcus   369
    Leuconostoc   369
    Pediococcus   369
    Gemella   370

**12 *Corynebacterium* and Other
Non–Spore-Forming Gram-Positive
Rods   373**
Hal S. Larsen

Corynebacterium   375
    General Characteristics   375
    Corynebacterium diphtheriae   375
    Other Corynebacteria   380
    Arcanobacterium   381
    Rhodococcus   381
    Undesignated CDC Coryneform Groups   381
    Rothia dentocariosa   381
Listeria monocytogenes   382
    General Characteristics   382
    Physiology   382
    Virulence Factors   382
    Clinical Infections   382
    Laboratory Diagnosis   383
Erysipelothrix rhusiopathiae   385
    General Characteristics   385
    Clinical Infections   385
    Laboratory Diagnosis   385

13 Aerobic Gram-Positive Bacilli   389
Hal S. Larsen

Bacillus   390
    General Characteristics   390
    Bacillus anthracis   392

Other *Bacillus* Species   394
Aerobic Actinomycetes   395
Nocardia Species   396
Other Actinomycetes   399

14 *Neisseria* Species and *Moraxella catarrhalis*   401

Karen S. Long, John G. Thomas, Jean Barnishan

General Characteristics   404
Pathogenic *Neisseria* Species   404
Neisseria gonorrhoeae   404
Neisseria meningitidis   415
Moraxella catarrhalis   417
Nonpathogenic *Neisseria* Species   418
Identification   418
Neisseria polysaccharea   418
Neisseria cinerea   421
Kingella denitrificans   421
Neisseria lactamica   421
Neisseria mucosa   422
Neisseria sicca   422
Neisseria subflava   422
Neisseria flavescens   422
Neisseria elongata   422
Neisseria weaveri   422

15 *Haemophilus* and Other Fastidious Gram-Negative Rods   425

A. *Haemophilus* Species, Hacek Group *Pasteurella*, *Brucella*, and *Francisella* Species   425
George Manuselis, Jean Barnishan

Haemophilus Species   426
General Characteristics   426
Haemophilus influenzae   428
Infections Associated with Other *Haemophilus* Species   429
Laboratory Diagnosis   430
Treatment   434
HACEK Group and *Capnocytophaga* Species   436
Haemophilus aphrophilus   436
Actinobacillus actinomycetemcomitans   436
Cardiobacterium hominis   438
Eikenella corrodens   439
Kingella Species   439
Capnocytophaga Species   440
Pasteurella Species   441
General Characteristics   441
Pasteurella multocida   441
Brucella Species   443
General Characteristics   443
Francisella Species   444
Francisella tularensis   444

B. *Legionella* Species   447
A. Christian Whelen

Epidemiology   448
Clinical Infections   448
Legionnaires' Disease   448
Pontiac Fever   449
Laboratory Diagnosis   449
Specimen Collection and Handling   449
Direct Microscopic Examination   449
DNA Probe   451
Culture and Identification   451
Urine Antigen Test   453
Serology   454
Antimicrobial Susceptibility   455

C. *Bordetella*   457
A. Christian Whelen

General Characteristics   457
Epidemiology   457
Virulence Factors   458
Clinical Infections   458
Laboratory Diagnosis   458
Specimen Collection and Transport   458
Direct Fluorescent Antibody Test   459
Nucleic Acid Detection   459
Culture and Identification   459
Serology   460
Antimicrobial Susceptibility   461

16 *Enterobacteriaceae*   463

Connie R. Mahon, George Manuselis

General Characteristics   465
Microscopic and Colonial Morphology   465
Classification   465
Virulence and Antigenic Factors   465
Clinical Significance   465
Opportunistic Members of the Family Enterobacteriaceae and Associated Infections   468
Escherichia coli   468
Other Escherichia Species   473
Klebsiella, Enterobacter, Serratia, and Hafnia Species   473
Proteus, Morganella, and Providencia Species   477
Edwardsiella Species   478
Erwinia and Pectobacterium Species   478
Citrobacter Species   478
Primary Intestinal Pathogens and Related Human Infections   479
Salmonella Species   479
Shigella Species   484

Yersinia Species   486
New Genera and Biotypes   488
Laboratory Diagnosis   490
Specimen Collection and Transport   490
Isolation and Identification   490
Biochemical Principles and Reactions on
Conventional Media   496
Lactose Fermentation and Utilization of
Carbohydrates   496
Glucose Metabolism and Its Metabolic
Products   498
Screening Stool Cultures for Pathogens   506
Serologic Grouping   508
Salmonella Species   508
Shigella Species   508

**17 *Vibrio, Aeromonas, Plesiomonas,*
and *Campylobacter* Species   515**
Amy M. Carnahan, Gerald Andrews

Vibrio   516
General Characteristics   517
Vibrio cholerae   519
Vibrio parahaemolyticus   520
Vibrio vulnificus   521
Vibrio alginolyticus   521
Laboratory Diagnosis   521
Antimicrobial Susceptibility   524
Aeromonas   524
General Characteristics   524
Clinical Infection   525
Laboratory Diagnosis   526
Antimicrobial Susceptibility   526
Plesiomonas   528
Epidemiology   528
General Characteristics   529
Clinical Infections   529
Laboratory Diagnosis   529
Antimicrobial Susceptibility   530
Campylobacter and *Campylobacter*-like
Species   530
Epidemiology   530
General Characteristics   532
Clinical Infection   532
Laboratory Diagnosis   532
Antimicrobial Susceptibility   536

**18 Nonfermenting Gram-Negative Bacilli
and Miscellaneous Gram-Negative
Rods   539**
Gerri S. Hall

General Characteristics of Nonfermenters   540
Clinical Infections   541
Biochemical Characteristics   541

Initial Clues to Nonfermenters   542
Identification Methods   543
Most Commonly Encountered Nonfermentative
Organisms   547
The Pseudomonads   547
Stenotrophomonas maltophilia   549
Acinetobacter Species   549
Other Pseudomonads   550
Pseudomonads and Other Nonfermenters
Whose Names Have Been Changed   551
Miscellaneous Nonfermenting Gram-Negative
Bacilli   554
Nonfermenters with Peritrichous Flagellation
554
Nonmotile Gram-Negative Bacilli   556
Other Gram-Negative Nonfermenters   559

19 Anaerobes of Clinical Importance   565
Paul G. Engelkirk, Janet Duben-Engelkirk

Important Concepts in Anaerobic
Bacteriology   567
Anaerobes Defined   567
Why Are They Anaerobes?   568
Where Anaerobes Are Found   568
Anaerobes at Specific Anatomic Sites   569
Factors that Predispose Patients to Anaerobic
Infections   571
Indications of Anaerobe Involvement
in Human Disease   571
Specimen Selection, Collection, Transport,
and Processing   573
Specimen Quality   573
Specimen Transport and Processing   573
Processing Clinical Samples for Maximum
Recovery of Anaerobic Pathogens   575
Procedures for Identifying Anaerobic
Isolates   583
Preliminary Procedures   583
Identification of Anaerobic Isolates   587
Frequently Encountered Anaerobes and their
Associated Diseases   594
Gram-Positive Spore-Forming Anaerobic
Bacilli   594
Gram-Positive Non–Spore-Forming Anaerobic
Bacilli   599
Anaerobic Gram-Negative Bacilli   606
Anaerobic Cocci   611
Susceptibility and β-Lactamase Testing   618
Anaerobe Resistance to Antimicrobial
Agents   618
Susceptibility Testing of Anaerobes   619
Problems in Susceptibility Testing of
Anaerobic Isolates   620
Susceptibility Testing Options   620

Quality-Assurance Considerations Pertaining to Susceptibility Testing   620
β-Lactamase Testing   620
Treating Anaerobe-Associated Diseases   621

20 **The Spirochetes   623**
A. Christian Whelen

Leptospires   625
General Characteristics   625
Virulence Factors and Pathogenicity   625
Clinical Infections   625
Laboratory Diagnosis   626
Treatment and Prevention   626
Borreliae   626
General Characteristics   626
Borrelia recurrentis and Other Borreliae   627
Borrelia burgdorferi   628
Treponemes   628
General Characteristics   629
Clinical Infections   629
Other Treponemal Diseases   631

21 *Chlamydia, Mycoplasma,* and *Ureaplasma* **Species   635**

A. Chlamydia Species   635
John G. Thomas, Karen S. Long

General Characteristics   636
Chlamydia pneumoniae   639
Clinical Infections   639
Laboratory Diagnosis   640
Chlamydia trachomatis   642
Clinical Infections   642
Laboratory Diagnosis   644
Culture   646
Nonculture, Nonamplified   647
Nonculture, Amplified   647
Results Reporting   649
Chlamydia psittaci   649

B. *Mycoplasma* and *Ureaplasma* Species   652
John G. Thomas, Karen S. Long

General Characteristics   653
Clinical Infections   655
Mycoplasma pneumoniae   655
Mycoplasma hominis and *Ureaplasma urealyticum*   656
Emerging *Mycoplasma* Pathogens   657
Laboratory Diagnosis   658
Specimen Collection and Transport   658
Culture   658
Serologic Diagnosis   663
Antimicrobial Susceptibility   663
Interpretation of Laboratory Results   663

22 *Mycobacterium tuberculosis* and Other Nontuberculous Mycobacteria   667
James L. Vossler

General Characteristics   670
Safety Considerations   671
Personnel Safety   671
Proper Ventilation   671
Proper Use of Biologic Safety Cabinet   671
Use of Proper Disinfectant   671
Other Precautions   672
Specimen Collection and Processing   672
Sputum and Other Respiratory Secretions   672
Gastric Aspirates and Washings   673
Urine   673
Stool   674
Blood   674
Tissue and Other Body Fluids   674
Digestion and Decontamination of Specimens   674
Decontamination and Digestion Agents   675
Concentration   677
Staining for Acid-Fast Bacteria   677
Examination and Interpretation of Smears   677
Culture Media and Isolation Methods   677
Egg-Based Media   678
Serum- or Agar-Based Media   678
Liquid Media   679
Other Culture Media for Recovery of Mycobacteria   680
Isolator Lysis-Centrifugation System   681
Identification   681
Laboratory Levels or Extents of Service   681
Identification of Mycobacteria   682
Biochemical Identification   682
Chromatography   689
Amplification for *Mycobacterium tuberculosis*   690
Serology   691
Susceptibility of *Mycobacterium tuberculosis*   691
Mycobacterium tuberculosis Complex   692
Mycobacterium tuberculosis   692
Mycobacterium bovis   695
Nontuberculous Mycobacteria: Clinical Significance and Differentiation   696
Mycobacterium avium Complex   696
Mycobacterium kansasii   697
Mycobacterium fortuitum-chelonei Complex   698
Mycobacterium marinum   699
Mycobacterium scrofulaceum   699

Mycobacterium xenopi   700
Mycobacterium szulgai   701
Mycobacterium malmoense   701
Mycobacterium simiae   701
Mycobacterium ulcerans   702
Mycobacterium haemophilum   702
Mycobacterium gordonae   702
Mycobacterium asiaticum   702
Mycobacterium thermoresistibile   703
Mycobacterium terrae-triviale Complex   703
Mycobacterium nonchromogenicum   703
Mycobacterium flavescens   703
Mycobacterium smegmatis   703
Mycobacterium phlei   704
Mycobacterium vaccae   704
Mycobacterium gastri   704
Mycobacterium paratuberculosis   704
Mycobacterium genavense   704
Mycobacterium leprae   704

23 Medically Significant Fungi   709

Linda A. Smith, Annette W. Fothergill,
Deanna A. Sutton, James L. Harris

General Characteristics   711
   Yeasts versus Molds   711
   Septate versus Sparsely Septate   712
   Hyaline versus Dematiaceous   712
   Dimorphism   713
   Reproduction   713
Taxonomy   714
   Zygomycota   714
   Ascomycota   714
   Basidiomycota   714
   Fungi Imperfecti   714
Clinical Sites of Infection   715
   Superficial Mycoses   715
   Cutaneous Mycoses   715
   Subcutaneous Mycoses   715
   Systemic Mycoses   716
Specimen Collecting, Handling,
   and Transport   716
   Hair   716
   Skin   716
   Nails   716
   Blood and Bone Marrow   717
   Cerebrospinal Fluid   717
   Abscess Fluid and Wound Exudates   717
   Respiratory Specimens   717
   Urogenital and Fecal Specimens   717
Methods of Identifying Fungal Agents   717
   Direct Microscopic Examination
      of Specimens   717
   Culture   718

Beginning the Identification   719
   Gross Examination of the Culture   719
   Microscopic Examination for Fungal
      Structures   721
Safety Issues   722
Agents of Superficial Mycoses   722
   Malassezia furfur   722
   Piedraia hortae   723
   Trichosporon beigelli   723
   Phaeoannellomyces werneckii   724
Agents of Dermatophytoses   724
   Epidemiology   724
   Clinical Infections   724
   Treatment   726
   Commonly Encountered Dermatophytes   726
   Laboratory Diagnosis   728
Agents of Subcutaneous Mycoses   729
   Sporotrichosis   729
   Chromoblastomycosis   730
   Eumycotic Mycetoma   731
   Subcutaneous Phaeohyphomycosis   733
Agents of Systemic Mycoses   734
   Blastomyces dermatitidis   735
   Histoplasma capsulatum var. *capsulatum*   737
   Coccidioides immitis   740
   Paracoccidioides brasiliensis   741
Agents of Opportunistic Fungal Infections:
   the Saprobes   742
Agents of Yeast Infections   748
   General Characteristics   748
   Clinically Significant Yeast Species   748
   Methods of Yeast Identification   749

24 Diagnostic Parasitology   755

Linda A. Smith

General Concepts in Parasitology Laboratory
   Methods   757
   Fecal Specimens   757
   Other Specimens Examined for Intestinal
      Parasites   761
   Examination of Specimens for Blood
      and Tissue Parasites   762
   Immunologic Diagnosis   763
   Quality Assurance in the Parasitology
      Laboratory   763
Medically Important Parasitic Agents   764
   Protozoa   764
   Apicomplexa   783
   Microsporidia   799
   Helminths   800

25 Clinical Virology   833

William F. Nauschuetz

Viruses   834
   Structure   834
   Taxonomy   835
Laboratory Diagnosis of Viral Infections   835
   Specimen Collection and Transport   835
   Appropriate Specimens for Maximum
      Recovery   837
   Methods in Diagnostic Virology   837
Cell Culture for Viral Isolation   840
   Cytopathic Effect on Cell Cultures
      for Presumptive Identification of Viral
      Agents   840
   Centrifugation-Enhanced Shell Vial
      Culture   842
Respiratory Viruses   842
   Influenza Viruses   842
   Parainfluenza Viruses   843
   Respiratory Syncytial Virus   844
   Adenoviruses   844
   Rhinoviruses   845
   Coronaviruses   845
Exanthemas   845
   Mumps   845
   Measles (Rubeola)   845
   Rubella   846
   Hand, Foot, and Mouth Disease   846
   Parvovirus B19   847
Immunodeficiency Viruses: Human
   Immunodeficiency Virus Type 1   847
Central Nervous System Viruses:
   Enteroviruses   849
Agents of Gastrointestinal Infections   850
   Rotaviruses   850
   Norwalk and Norwalk-Like Agents   850
   Enteric Adenoviruses   851
   Other Viruses   851
Arboviruses   851
   Family Bunyaviridae   852
   Family Togaviridae   853
   Family Flaviviridae   853
   Family Reoviridae   854
   Laboratory Diagnosis of Arboviral
      Infections   855
Family Arenaviridae   855
Genus *Hantavirus*   856
Family Filoviridae   857
Rabies   858
Human Papillomaviruses   859
Hepatitis Viruses   859
   Hepatitis A   859
   Hepatitis B   861
   Hepatitis D (Delta Hepatitis)   862
   Hepatitis C   864
   Hepatitis E   864
Herpesviruses   866
   Herpes Simplex Virus   866
   Human Cytomegalovirus   868
   Epstein-Barr Virus   868
   Varicella-Zoster Virus   870
   Human Herpesvirus 6   870
   Human Herpesvirus 7   870
   Human Herpesvirus 8   870
Antiviral Therapy   871
   Absorption   871
   Penetration   872
   Uncoating   872
   Eclipse/Synthesis   872
   Maturation/Release   872

Part III

**Laboratory Diagnosis of Infectious
Diseases: an Organ System
Approach to Diagnostic
Microbiology   875**

**26 Upper and Lower Respiratory Tract
Infections   877**

James L. Cook

General Concepts of Infectious Diseases
   of the Respiratory Tract   879
   The Role of Normal Flora   879
   The Immune Status of the Host   880
   Seasonal and Community Trends
      in Infections   882
   Empiric Antimicrobial Therapy   882
Anatomic Characterization of the Respiratory
   Tract   883
   Anatomy of the Respiratory Tract   883
   Barriers to Infection   883
Virulence Factors of Pathogenic Organisms   884
   Adherence   884
   Toxin Elaboration   884
   Evasion of Host Defenses   884
Upper Respiratory Tract Infections   885
   Pharyngitis   885
   Sinusitis   887
   Otitis Media   891
   Epiglottitis   892
   Pertussis   894
Lower Respiratory Tract Infections   895
   Bronchitis and Bronchiolitis   896
   Acute Pneumonia   899
   Aspiration Pneumonia   904

Chronic Pneumonia   907
Empyema   911
Opportunistic Infections of the Respiratory
Tract   912
Granulocytopenic Patients   912
Patients with Defects in Cellular
Immunity   913
Patients with Defects in Humoral
Immunity   914
Diagnosis   914

27 **Skin and Soft-Tissue Infections   919**
Raymond A. Smego, Jr.

Skin and Skin Structures   920
Anatomy of the Skin   920
Usual Skin Flora   921
Clinical Infections   921
Bacterial Skin Infections   921
Cutaneous Infections Caused by Miscellaneous
Agents   931
Spirochetal Infections   931
Mycoplasmal Infections   932
Viral Skin Diseases   933
Fungal Skin Infections   936
Parasitic Skin Infections   940

28 **Gastrointestinal Infections and Food
Poisoning   945**
Connie R. Mahon, George Manuselis

General Concepts in Evaluating Gastrointestinal
Infections and Food Poisoning   946
Anatomic Considerations   947
The Role of the Usual Flora   948
A Practical Approach to Diagnosis of the Patient
with Diarrhea   949
History   949
Physical Examination   950
Laboratory Studies   950
Pathogenic Mechanisms and Clinical
Presentations of Acute Diarrhea   950
Enterotoxin-Mediated Diarrhea   950
Diarrhea Mediated by Invasion of Bowel
Mucosal Surface   951
Diarrhea Mediated by Invasion of Full Bowel
Thickness with Lymphatic Spread   952
Common Bacterial, Viral, and Parasitic
Gastrointestinal Infections and Their
Agents   952
Bacterial Agents   953
Viral Agents   958
Parasitic Agents   958
Complications of Diarrheal Infections   960
Newly Recognized Agents of Acute Diarrhea   960
Agents of Food Poisoning   961

Laboratory Diagnosis of Gastrointestinal
Pathogens   963
Specimen Collection and Handling   963
Direct Microscopic Examination   963
Culture   963
Treatment of Diarrhea   967

29 **Infections of the Central Nervous
System   973**
Kirk M. Doing, David P. Marmaduke

General Concepts Related to Infections of the
Central Nervous System   975
Anatomic Organization   975
Cerebrospinal Fluid Characteristics   976
Host-Pathogen Relationships   976
Infections of the Central Nervous System   977
Bacterial Infections   977
Brain Abscesses   981
Spirochetal Infections   982
Fungal Meningitis   982
Viral Infections   984
Parasitic Infections   988
Laboratory Diagnosis of Central Nervous System
Infections   990
Specimen Collection: Lumbar Puncture   990
Laboratory Evaluation   991

30 **Bacteremia   997**
Sherry Trevino, Connie R. Mahon

General Concepts Related to Bacteremic
Infections   999
Bacteremia Versus Septicemia   999
Forms of Bacteremia   999
Bacteremic Episodes   999
Other Conditions   999
Epidemiology   999
Risk Factors   1000
Pathogenesis   1000
Sources of Bacteremic Spread   1000
Clinical Signs and Symptoms   1001
Complications   1002
Laboratory Diagnosis   1002
Specimen Collection   1002
Blood Culture Methods   1003
Treatment   1007

31 **Urinary Tract Infections   1011**
John G. Thomas

Overview   1012
The Urinary System   1013
Epidemiology and Risk Factors   1014
Age   1014

Clinical Signs and Symptoms   1016
Etiology of Urinary Tract Infections   1018
  Pathogenesis of Urinary Tract
  Infections   1018
  Etiologic Agents of Urinary Tract
  Infections   1018
Laboratory Diagnosis   1021
  Significance of Colony Counts: A Historical
  Background   1021
  Specimen Collection   1022
  Additives   1024
  Specimen Transport   1024
Microbial Detection   1024
  Specimen Screening: Rapid, Nonculture
  Methodologies   1024
  Rejection Criteria   1027
  Culture for Etiologic Agents of Urinary Tract
  Infections   1027
Interpretation of Results   1028
Susceptibility Reporting   1031
  UTI Antibiograms   1031

32 Sexually Transmitted Diseases   1033
William F. Nauschuetz

Common Exudative Sexually Transmitted
  Infections   1035
  Gonorrhea   1035
  Genital Chlamydiosis   1037
  Bacterial Vaginosis   1038
Common Ulcerative Sexually Transmitted
  Infections   1039
  Syphilis   1039
  Chancroid   1041
  Genital Herpes   1042

**33 Infections in Special Patient
Populations   1045**
James T. Griffith

Malignancy   1047
  Decrease in Humoral and Cellular Immune
  Response   1047
  Granulocytopenia   1048
  Decrease in Leukocyte Function   1048
  Infections in Neutropenic Patients   1048
  Infections in Cancer Patients   1048
  Infections in Patients with Hodgkin's
  Disease   1049
Burns and Surgery   1049
Antimicrobial Therapy   1050
Organ Transplantation   1050
Aging   1050

34 Zoonotic and Rickettsial Infections   1053
William F. Nauschuetz, Robert G. Whiddon

Zoonotic Infections Transmitted by Scratches
  and Bites   1056
  Plague   1056
  Lyme Borreliosis   1058
  Pasteurellosis   1060
  Erysipeloid   1062
  Capnocytophaga canimorsus Infection
    (Formerly CDC Group DF-2)   1063
  Bacillary and Spirillary Rat-Bite Fevers   1064
Zoonotic Infections Transmitted by Direct
  Contact or Inhalation   1065
  Anthrax   1065
  Tularemia   1068
  Brucellosis   1070
  Leptospirosis   1073
The Rickettsiae   1074
  Rickettsia   1075
  Ehrlichiosis   1078

35 Ocular Infections   1083
Darlene Miller

Ocular Structures   1084
  Conjunctiva   1084
  Lids   1085
  Cornea   1085
  Sclera   1086
  Orbit   1086
  Lacrimal Apparatus   1086
  Anterior Chamber   1086
  Vitreous Chamber   1086
  Uveal Tract   1086
  Retina   1086
Pathogenesis of Ocular Infections   1086
Usual Ocular Flora   1088
Infections of the Conjunctivae
  (Conjunctivitis)   1089
  Bacteria   1089
  Viruses   1091
  Rickettsia   1092
  Fungi   1092
  Parasites   1092
Infections of the Lids (Blepharitis)   1093
  Bacteria   1093
  Viruses   1094
  Fungi   1094
  Parasites   1094
Infections of the Cornea (Keratitis)   1094
  Bacteria   1094
  Viruses   1095
  Fungi   1097
  Parasites   1097

Infections of the Sclera and Episclera (Scleritis and Episcleritis)   1098
Infections of the Orbit (Preseptal and Orbital Cellulitis)   1098
Infections of the Lacrimal Apparatus   1100
Infections of the Intraocular Chambers (Endophthalmitis)   1101
    Bacteria   1101
Infections of the Uveal Tract (Uveitis)   1102
Infections of the Retina (Retinitis)   1102
    Viruses   1103
    Parasites   1103
Scleral Buckle Infections   1103
Ocular Manifestations in Patients with Human Immunodeficiency Virus   1104
Laboratory Diagnosis of Ocular Infections   1104
    Specimen Collection   1104
    Direct Smear Examination   1105
    Culture   1107
    Special Procedures for Recovering Ocular Pathogens   1109
    Special Culture Techniques   1109
Ocular Therapy   1111

Appendixes   1115

Appendix A   1117
Patricia K. Hargrave, Shirley Adams

Selected Bacteriologic Culture Media

Appendix B   1141
Patricia K. Hargrave, Shirley Adams

Selected Mycology Media, Fluids, and Stains

Appendix C   1145

Nomenclature Changes for the Enterobacteriaceae and Nonfermentative Bacilli

Appendix D   1147

Answers to Learning Assessment Questions

Index   1167

PART I

Introduction to Clinical Microbiology

Bacterial Cell Structure, Physiology, Metabolism, and Genetics

George Manuselis, Connie R. Mahon

SIGNIFICANCE

CLASSIFICATION
  Taxonomy
  Nomenclature
  Classification by Phenotypic and Genotypic
    Characteristics
  Classification by Cellular Type: Prokaryotes,
    Eukaryotes, and Archaeobacteria

COMPARISON OF EUKARYOTIC AND
PROKARYOTIC CELL STRUCTURE
  Eukaryotic Cell Structure
    Cytoplasmic structures
    Cell envelope structures
  Prokaryotic Cell Structure
    Cytoplasmic structures
    Cell envelope structures

BACTERIAL MORPHOLOGY
  Microscopic Shapes
  Common Stains Used for Microscopic Visualization
    Gram stain
    Acid-fast stains
    Acridine orange
    Methylene blue
    Lactophenol cotton blue
    Calcofluor white
    India ink

MICROBIAL GROWTH AND NUTRITION
  Nutritional Requirements for Growth
    Types of growth media

Environmental Factors Influencing Growth
Bacterial Growth
  Generation time
  Growth curve
  Determination of cell numbers

BACTERIAL BIOCHEMISTRY AND METABOLISM
  Metabolism
  Fermentation and Respiration
  Biochemical Pathways from Glucose
    to Pyruvic Acid
  Anaerobic Utilization of Pyruvic Acid
    (Fermentation)
  Aerobic Utilization of Pyruvate (Oxidation)
  Carbohydrate Utilization and Lactose Fermentation

BACTERIAL GENETICS
  Terminology
  Genetic Elements and Alterations
    The bacterial genome
    Extrachromosomal elements
    Mobile genetic elements
    Mutations
    Genetic recombination
  Mechanisms of Gene Transfer
    Transformation
    Transduction
    Conjugation
    Restriction enzymes

OBJECTIVES

1. Describe microbial classification (taxonomy), and accurately apply the rules of scientific nomenclature for bacterial names.

2. List and define five methods used by epidemiologists to subdivide bacterial species.

3. Differentiate among prokaryotic, eukaryotic, and archaeobacterial cell types.

4. Compare and contrast prokaryotic and eukaryotic cytoplasmic and cell envelope structures and functions.

5. Describe the cell walls of gram-positive and gram-negative bacteria. Explain the Gram stain reaction of each cell wall type. Describe two other bacterial cell wall types, and give microbial examples of each.

6. Explain the use of the following stains in the diagnostic microbiology laboratory: Gram stain, acid-fast stains (Ziehl-Neelsen, Kinyoun, auramine-rhodamine), acridine orange, methylene blue, calcofluor white, lactophenol cotton blue, and India ink.

7. List the nutritional and environmental requirements for bacterial growth, and define the categories of media used for culturing bacteria in the laboratory.

8. Define the atmospheric requirements of obligate aerobes, microaerophiles, facultative anaerobes, obligate anaerobes, and capnophilic bacteria.

9. Describe the stages in the growth of bacterial cells.

10. Describe the importance of microbial metabolism in clinical microbiology.

11. Differentiate between fermentation and oxidation (respiration).

12. Name and compare three biochemical pathways that bacteria use to convert glucose to pyruvate.

13. Identify and compare the two types of fermentation that explain positive results with the methyl red or Voges-Proskauer test.

14. Define the following genetic terms: *genotype, phenotype, constitutive, inducible, replication, transcription, translation, genome, chromosome, plasmids, IS element, transposon, point mutations, frame-shift mutations,* and *recombination.*

15. Discuss the development and transfer of antibiotic resistance in bacteria.

16. Differentiate among the mechanisms of transformation, transduction, and conjugation in the transfer of genetic material from one bacterium to another.

17. Define the terms *bacteriophage, lytic phage, lysogeny,* and *temperate phage.*

18. Define *restriction endonuclease enzyme,* and explain the use of such enzymes in the clinical microbiology laboratory.

KEY TERMS

Family	Capsule	Obligate aerobes	Plasmids
Genus	Flagella	Obligate anaerobes	Transformation
Species	Fimbrae	Facultative anaerobes	Transduction
Prokaryote	Pleomorphic	Capnophilic	Bacteriophage
Eukaryotes	Autotrophs	Microaerophilic	Lysogeny
Archaeobacteria	Heterotrophs	Fermentation	Temperate
Pathogenic bacteria	Selective media	Respiration	Conjugation
Gram positive	Differential media	Phenotype	Restriction enzyme
Gram negative	Transport media		

CASE STUDY

A 4-year-old female child had the presenting symptoms of redness, burning, and light sensitivity in both eyes. She also complained of her eyelids sticking together because of the exudative discharge present. A Gram stain of the conjunctival exudate showed gram-positive intracellular diplococci. The Gram stain of the stock staphylococci (gram-positive) and *Escherichia coli* (gram-negative) showed gram-positive reactions for both organisms on review of the quality control slides. The technologist repeated the Gram stain procedure on the exudate and the quality control organisms.

In this chapter the basic concepts of bacterial cell structure, physiology, metabolism, and genetics are reviewed. Common stains used to visualize microorganisms microscopically also are presented. The reader is made aware of the practical importance of each topic to diagnostic microbiologists in their efforts to culture, identify, and characterize the microbes that cause disease in humans. As presented in the opening case study, proper characterization of the bacterial cells in human samples is critical in the correct identification of the infecting organism.

SIGNIFICANCE

Microbial inhabitants have evolved to survive in a variety of ecologic niches and growth habitats. Some grow rapidly, some slowly. Some can replicate with a minimal number of nutrients present, whereas others require enriched nutrients to survive. Variation exists in atmospheric growth conditions, temperature requirements, and cell structure. This diversity is also found in the microorganisms that inhabit the human body as normal flora, as opportunistic pathogens, or as true pathogens. Each microbe has its own unique physiology and metabolic pathways that allow it to survive in its particular habitat. One of the main roles of a diagnostic or clinical microbiologist is to isolate, identify, and analyze the bacteria that cause disease in humans. Knowledge of microbial structure and physiology is extremely important to clinical microbiologists in three areas:

- Culture of organisms from patient specimens
- Classification and identification of organisms after they have been isolated
- Prediction and interpretation of antimicrobial susceptibility patterns

Understanding the growth requirements of a particular bacterium enables the microbiologist to select the correct media for primary culture and optimize the chance of isolating the pathogen. Determination of staining characteristics, based on differences in cell wall structure, is the first step in bacterial classification. Metabolic biochemical differences between organisms form the basis for most bacterial identification systems in use today. The cell structure and biochemical pathways of an organism determine its susceptibility to various antibiotics.

The ability of microorganisms to change rapidly, acquire new genes, and undergo mutations presents continual challenges to diagnostic microbiologists as they isolate and characterize the microorganisms associated with humans.

CLASSIFICATION

Taxonomy

Taxonomy refers to the classification and grouping of organisms. It is based on genotypic (genetic) and phenotypic (observable) similarities and differences. The formal levels of bacterial classification, in successively smaller subsets, are kingdom, division, class, order, family, tribe, genus, and species, Bacteria have been placed in a kingdom separate from the animal and plant kingdoms, Prokaryotae. The kingdom Prokaryotae includes unicellular organisms such as bacteria, fungi, protozoa, and algae. Diagnostic microbiologists traditionally emphasize placement of bacterial species into three categories: the **family** (similar to a human "clan"), a **genus** (equivalent to a human last name), and a **species** epithet (equivalent to a human first name). For example,

Staphylococcus (genus) *aureus* (species epithet) belongs to the Micrococcaceae family.

Nomenclature

Nomenclature provides naming assignments for each organism. The following standard rules for denoting bacterial names are used in this book. The family name is capitalized and has an *-aceae* ending (e.g., Micrococcaceae). The genus name is capitalized and followed by the species name, which begins with a lowercase letter; both the genus and species should be *italicized* in print but underlined in the script (e.g., *Staphylococcus aureus* or Staphylococcus aureus). Often, the genus name is abbreviated by using the first letter of the genus followed by a period and the species epithet (name) (e.g., *S. aureus*). The genus name followed by the word *species* (e.g., *Staphylococcus* species) may be used to refer to the genus as a whole. Species abbreviated *sp.* (singular) or *spp.* (plural) is used when the species is not specified. When bacteria are referred to as a group, their names are neither capitalized nor underlined (e.g., staphylococci). The plural of *genus* is *genera* (e.g., there are many genera with the Enterobacteriaceae family).

Classification by Phenotypic and Genotypic Characteristics

The traditional method of placing an organism into a particular genus and species is based on the similarity of all members in a number of phenotypic characteristics. In the diagnostic microbiology laboratory, this is accomplished by testing each bacterial culture for a variety of metabolic characteristics and comparing the results with those listed in established charts. In many rapid identification systems, a numeric taxonomy is used, in which phenotypic characteristics are assigned a numeric value and the derived number indicates the genus and species of the bacterium.

Epidemiologists constantly seek means of further subdividing bacterial species to follow the spread of bacterial infections. Species may be subdivided into subspecies, based on phenotypic differences (abbreviated *subsp.*); serovarieties, based on serologic differences (abbreviated *serovar*); or biovarieties, based on biochemical test result differences (abbreviated *biovar*). Phage typing (based on susceptibility to specific bacterial phages) has also been used for this purpose. Epidemiologists also find a molecular method termed *RFLP (restriction fragment length polymorphism) analysis* very useful for determining differences among strains. In this method the DNA is cut by enzymes known as *restriction endonucleases,* and the patterns of the resulting DNA fragment lengths are compared.

Current technology has allowed the analysis of genetic relatedness (DNA and RNA structure and homology) for taxonomic purposes. The analysis of ribosomal RNA (rRNA) has proved particularly useful for this purpose. The information obtained from these studies has resulted in the reclassification of some bacteria.

Classification by Cellular Type: Prokaryotes, Eukaryotes, and Archaeobacteria

Another method of classifying organisms is by cell organization. It is now recognized that organisms fall into three distinct groups based on type of cell organization and function: the **prokaryotes,** the **eukaryotes,** and the most recently identified, **archaeobacteria.** Bacteria are prokaryotic, whereas fungi, algae, protozoa, animal cells, and plant cells are eukaryotic in nature. The archaeobacterial cell type appears to be more closely related to eukaryotic cells than to prokaryotic cells and is found in microorganisms that grow under extreme environmental conditions. The structure of the cell envelope and enzymes of archaeobacteria allows them to survive under stressful conditions. Because archaeobacteria are not encountered in clinical microbiology, they are not discussed further in this chapter.

In general, the interior organization of eukaryotic cells is more complex than that of prokaryotic cells (Figure 1-1). The eukaryotic cell is usually larger and contains membrane-encased organelles or compartments that serve various functions; the prokaryotic cell is noncompartmentalized. Differences also exist in the processes of DNA synthesis, protein synthesis, and cell envelope synthesis and structure. Table 1-1 compares some of the characteristics of eukaryotic and prokaryotic cells.

Pathogenic bacteria are prokaryotic cells that infect eukaryotic hosts. Targeting antibiotic ac-

Figure 1-1 _____

Comparison of prokaryotic and eukaryotic cell organization and structures. **A,** Diagram of a prokaryotic bacterial cell. Note the location of the cell wall *(CW)*, the cell membrane *(CM)*, the nuclear region (nucleoid) free in the cytoplasm *(N)*, and the ribosomes located in the cytoplasm *(R).* Other structures that may be present are pili or fimbriae *(P)*, capsules or slime layers *(C)*, and flagella *(F).* **B,** Diagram of a eukaryotic cell. Note the presence of the plasma membrane (PM), nuclear membrane *(NM)* surrounding the nucleus *(N)*, which contains a nucleolus *(NC)*, mitochondria *(M)*, ribosomes attached to the rough endoplasmic reticulum *(RER)*, the smooth endoplasmic reticulum *(SER)*, vacuole *(V)*, and storage granules *(G).*

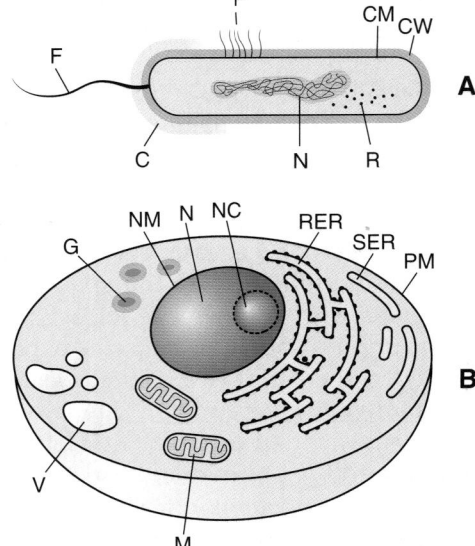

TABLE 1-1 _____

Comparison of Eukaryotic and Prokaryotic Cell Organization

Characteristic	Eukaryote	Prokaryote
Genetic material		
Location	Contained within a membrane-bound nucleus inside the cell	Free in the cytoplasm attached to a structure called a *mesosome* located in the cell membrane
Form	Multiple chromosomes, which are surrounded by basic proteins called *histones*	A single circular piece of DNA
Replication	By mitosis and meiosis	By binary fission
Extrachromosomal DNA	In mitochondria	Plasmids, small circular pieces of DNA containing accessory information, may be present in the cytoplasm
Protein production		
Site	Rough endoplasmic reticulum, a membrane covered with ribosomes, where protein is made	No endoplasmic reticulum; ribosomes—free in the cytoplasm or attached to the cell membrane
	Smooth endoplasmic reticulum or Golgi complex, where secreted proteins are packaged and transported to the cell surface	
Ribosomes	80S in size, consisting of a 60S and a 40S subunit	70S in size, consisting of a 50S and a 30S subunit
Energy production site	Within membrane-bound mitochondria	Electron transport chain located in the cell membrane; no mitochondria present
Intracellular organelles (lysosomes)	Contain hydrolytic enzymes	Not present
Cell envelope		
Plasma membrane	Lipoprotein membrane; regulates transport	Lipoprotein membrane; regulates transport
Cell wall	Usually absent except for fungi, which contain chitin in the cell wall	Present; imparts rigidity; see text for types

tion against unique prokaryotic structures and functions inhibits bacterial growth without harming eukaryotic host cells. This is one reason that pharmaceutical companies have been so successful in developing effective antibiotics against bacterial pathogens but have been less successful in finding drugs effective against parasites, medically important fungi, and viruses, which are eukaryotic like their human hosts.

COMPARISON OF EUKARYOTIC AND PROKARYOTIC CELL STRUCTURE

Eukaryotic Cell Structure

The following structures are associated with eukaryotic cells. In the diagnostic microbiology laboratory the eukaryotic cell type occurs in medically important fungi and in parasites.

Cytoplasmic structures

The nucleus of the eukaryotic cell contains the DNA of the cell in the form of discrete chromosomes, which are covered with basic proteins called *histones.* The number of chromosomes in the nucleus varies according to the particular organism. A rounded refractile body called a *nucleolus* is also located within the nucleus. The nucleolus is the site of ribosomal RNA synthesis. The nucleus is bounded by a bilayered lipoprotein nuclear membrane.

The endoplasmic reticulum is a system of membranes that occur throughout the cytoplasm. It is found in two forms. The rough endoplasmic reticulum is covered with ribosomes and is the site of protein synthesis. The smooth endoplasmic reticulum, or Golgi apparatus, is the site where secreted proteins are packaged for export to the exterior of the cell.

Eukaryotic ribosomes, where protein synthesis occurs, are 80S in size and dissociate into two subunits, 60S and 40S. They are attached to the rough endoplasmic reticulum.

Eukaryotic cells contain several membrane-enclosed organelles. Mitochondria are the main sites of energy production. They contain their own DNA and the electron transport system that produces energy for cell functions. Lysosomes contain hydrolytic enzymes for degradation of macromolecues and microorganisms within the cell. Peroxisomes contain protective enzymes that break down hydrogen peroxide and other peroxides generated within the cell. Chloroplasts, found in plant cells, are the sites of photosynthesis.

Cell envelope structures

PLASMA MEMBRANE

The plasma membrane is a bilayered lipoprotein membrane that encircles the cell cytoplasm and regulates transport of macromolecules into and out of the cell. The presence of sterols is a trait of eukaryotic cell membranes.

CELL WALL

The function of a cell wall is to provide rigidity and strength to the exterior of the cell. *Most eukaryotic cells do not have cell walls.* Fungi, however, have cell walls principally made of polysaccharides such as chitin, mannan, and glucan. Chitin is a distinct component of fungal cell walls.

MOTILITY ORGANELLES

Cilia are short projections (3-10 μm), usually numerous, that extend from the surface and are used for locomotion. They are found in certain protozoa and in ciliated epithelial cells of the respiratory tract. Flagella are longer projections (>150 μm) used for locomotion by cells such as spermatozoa. The basal body, or kinetosome, is a small structure located at the base of cilia or flagella, where microtubule proteins involved in movement originate.

Prokaryotic Cell Structure

The bacterial cell is smaller and less compartmentalized than a eukaryotic cell. A variety of structures are, however, unique to prokaryotic cells.

Cytoplasmic structures

Bacteria do not contain a membrane-bound nucleus. Their DNA consists of a single circular chromosome. This appears as a diffuse nucleoid or chromatin body (nuclear body), which is attached to a mesosome, a saclike structure in the cell membrane.

Bacterial ribosomes are found free in the cytoplasm and attached to the cytoplasmic membrane. They are 70S in size and dissociate into two subunits, 50S and 30S in size.

Stained bacteria sometimes reveal the presence of granules in the cytoplasm (cytoplasmic granules). These granules are storage deposits and may consist of polysaccharides such as

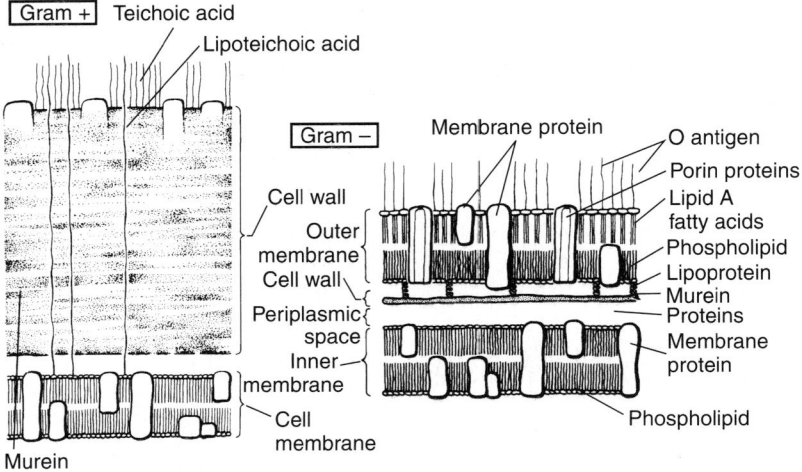

Figure 1-2

The cell envelope structure of a gram-positive *(left)* and a gram-negative *(right)* bacterium. (From Schaechter M, Medoff G, Eisenstein BI: *Mechanisms of microbial disease,* ed 2, Baltimore, 1993, Williams & Wilkins.)

glycogen, lipids such as poly-β-hydroxybutyrate, or polyphosphates.

Certain genera, such as *Bacillus* and *Clostridium,* produce endospores in response to harsh environmental conditions. The spores occur as highly refractile bodies in the cell. Spores are visualized microscopically as unstained areas in a cell with the use of traditional bacterial stains or specific spore stains. The size, shape, and interior location of the spore can be used as identifying characteristics.

Cell envelope structures

The cell envelope consists of the membrane and structures surrounding the cytoplasm. In bacteria, these are the cell membrane and the cell wall. Some species also produce capsules and slime layers.

PLASMA MEMBRANE (CELL MEMBRANE)

The cell membrane is a lipoprotein membrane that surrounds the cytoplasm. It is made of phospholipids and proteins but does not contain sterols, unlike eukaryotic plasma membranes (except for *Mycoplasma*). The plasma membrane regulates transport across the membrane, acts as an osmotic barrier (prokaryotes have a high osmotic pressure inside the cell), and is the location of the electron transport chain, where energy is generated.

CELL WALL

The cell wall of prokaryotes is a rigid structure that maintains the shape of the cell and prevents bursting of the cell from the high osmotic pressure inside it. There are several different types of cell wall structures in bacteria, which have traditionally been categorized according to their staining characteristics. The two major types of cell walls are the **gram-positive** and the **gram-negative** types (Figure 1-2). In addition, some mycobacteria have an acid fast cell wall, and mycoplasmas have no cell wall.

Gram-positive cell wall The gram-positive cell wall is composed of a very thick protective peptidoglycan (murein) layer. Because the peptidoglycan layer is the principal component of the gram-positive cell wall, many antibiotics effective against gram-positive organisms (such as penicillin) act by preventing synthesis of peptidoglycan. Gram-negative bacteria, which have a thinner layer of peptidoglycan and a different cell wall structure, are less affected by these antibiotics.

The peptidoglycan or murein layer consists of

glycan (polysaccharide) chains of alternating *N*-acetyl-D-glucosamine (NAG) and *N*-acetyl-D-muramic acid (NAM) (Figure 1-3). Short peptides, each consisting of four amino acid residues, are attached to a carboxyl group on each NAM residue. The chains are then cross-linked to form a thick network via a peptide bridge (varying in number of peptides) connected to the tetrapeptides on the NAM.

Other components of the gram-positive cell wall that penetrate to the exterior of the cell are teichoic acid (anchored to the peptidoglycan) and lipoteichoic acid (anchored to the plasma membrane). These two components are unique to the gram-positive cell wall (see Figure 1-2). Other antigenic polysaccharides may be present on the surface of the peptidoglycan layer.

Acid-fast cell wall Certain genera (*Mycobacterium* and *Nocardia*) have a gram-positive cell wall structure but, in addition, contain a waxy layer of glycolipids and fatty acids (mycolic acid) bound to the exterior of the cell wall. This makes *Mycobacterium* species difficult to stain with the Gram stain. The mycobacteria and nocardiae can be stained with an acid-fast stain, in which the bacteria are stained with carbolfuchsin, followed by acid-alcohol as a decolorizer. Other bacteria are decolorized by acid-alcohol, whereas mycobacteria and nocardiae retain the stain. They have therefore been designated *acid-fast bacteria*.

Gram-negative cell wall The cell wall of gram-negative microorganisms is composed of two layers. The inner peptidoglycan layer is much thinner than in gram-positive cell walls. Outside the peptidoglycan layer is an additional outer membrane unique to the gram-negative cell wall. The outer membrane contains proteins, phospholipids, and lipopolysaccharide (LPS) (see Figure 1-2). LPS contains three regions: an antigenic O–specific polysaccharide, a core polysaccharide, and an inner lipid A (also called endotoxin). The lipid A moiety is responsible for producing fever and shock conditions in patients infected with gram-negative bacteria. The outer membrane functions in the following ways:

- It acts as a barrier to hydrophobic compounds and harmful substances.

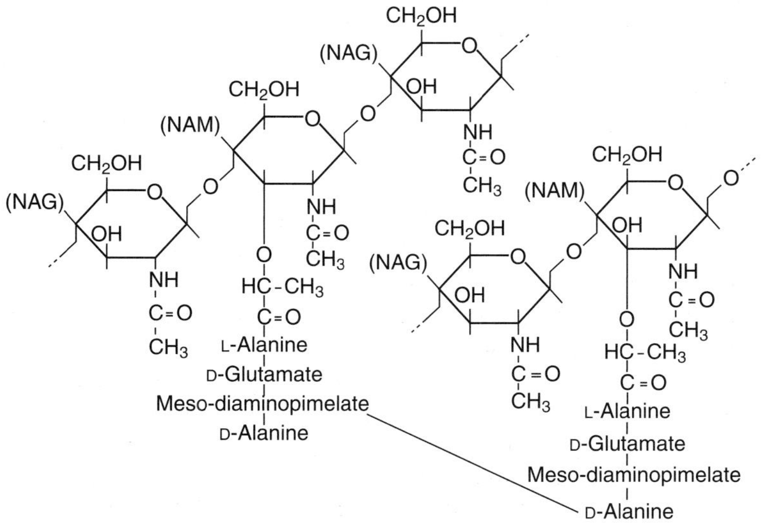

Figure 1-3

A diagram that demonstrates the structure of the peptidoglycan layer in the cell wall of *E. coli*. NAG, *N*-acetyl-D-glucosamine; NAM, *N*-acetyl-D-muramic acid. The amino acids in the cross-linking tetrapeptides may vary among species. (From Neidhardt FC, Ingraham M, Schaechter M: *Physiology of bacterial cell: a molecular approach,* Sunderland, Mass, 1990, Sinauer Associates.)

- It acts as a sieve, allowing water-soluble molecules to enter through protein-lined channels called porins.
- It provides attachment sites that enhance attachment to host cells.

Between the outer membrane and the inner membrane, and encompassing the thin peptidoglycan layer, is an area referred to as the *periplasmic space*. Within the periplasmic space is a gel-like matrix containing nutrient-binding proteins and degradative and detoxifying enzymes.

Absence of cell wall Prokaryotes that belong to the *Mycoplasma* and *Ureaplasma* genera are unique in that they lack a cell wall and contain sterols in their cell membranes. Because they lack the rigidity of the cell wall, they are seen in a variety of shapes microscopically. Gram-positive and gram-negative cells can lose their cell walls and grow as L-forms in media supplemented with serum or sugar to prevent osmotic rupture of the cell membrane.

SURFACE POLYMERS

A variety of pathogenic bacteria produce a discrete organized covering termed a ***capsule.*** Capsules are usually made of polysaccharide polymers, although they may also be made of polypeptides. Capsules act as virulence factors in helping the pathogen evade phagocytosis. During identification of certain bacteria by serologic typing, capsules sometimes must be removed in order to detect the somatic (cell wall) antigens present underneath them. Capsule removal is accomplished by boiling a suspension of the microorganism. *Salmonella typhi* must have its capsular (Vi) antigen removed in order for the technologist to observe agglutination with *Salmonella* somatic (O) antisera. The capsule does not ordinarily stain with use of common laboratory stains, such as Gram or India ink. Instead, it appears as a clear area ("halo-like") between or surrounding the stained organism and the stained background material in a direct smear from a clinical specimen.

Slime layers are similar to capsules but are more diffuse layers surrounding the cell. They also are made of polysaccharides and serve either to inhibit phagocytosis or, in some cases, to aid in adherence to host tissue or synthetic implants.

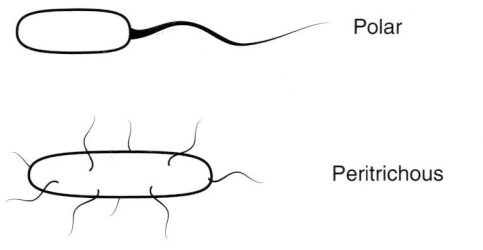

Figure 1-4 _____

Diagram of flagellar arrangements that occur in bacteria.

CELL APPENDAGES

The flagellum is the organ of locomotion. **Flagella** are exterior protein filaments that rotate and cause bacteria to be motile. Bacterial species vary in their possession of flagella from none (nonmotile) to many (Figure 1-4). Flagella that extend from one end of the bacterium are polar. Polar flagella may occur singly at one or both ends or multiply in tufts. Flagella that occur on all sides of the bacterium are peritrichous. The number and arrangement of flagella are sometimes used for identification purposes. Flagella can be visualized microscopically with special flagellum stains.

Pili (also known as **fimbriae**) are hairlike protein structures that aid in attachment to surfaces. Specialized pili known as *sex pili* are involved in bacterial conjugation and gene exchange. Bacterial pathogens often have adherence pili that allow them to attach to specific eukaryotic host cell surfaces. The proteins within pili that aid in attachment are called *adhesins*.

BACTERIAL MORPHOLOGY

Microscopic Shapes

Bacteria vary in size from 0.4 to 2 μm. They occur in three basic shapes (Figure 1-5):

- Cocci (spherical)
- Bacilli (rod-shaped)
- Spirochetes (helical)

Individual bacteria may form characteristic groupings. Cocci may occur singly, in pairs (diplococci), in chains (streptococci), or in clusters (staphylococci). Bacilli may vary greatly in size and length from very short coccobacilli to long filamentous rods. The ends may be square or rounded. Bacilli with tapered, pointed ends are termed *fusiform*. Some bacilli are curved. When a species varies in size and shape within a pure culture, the bacterium is **pleomorphic.** Bacilli may occur as single rods or in chains or may align themselves side by side (palisading). Spirochetes vary in length and in the number of helical turns.

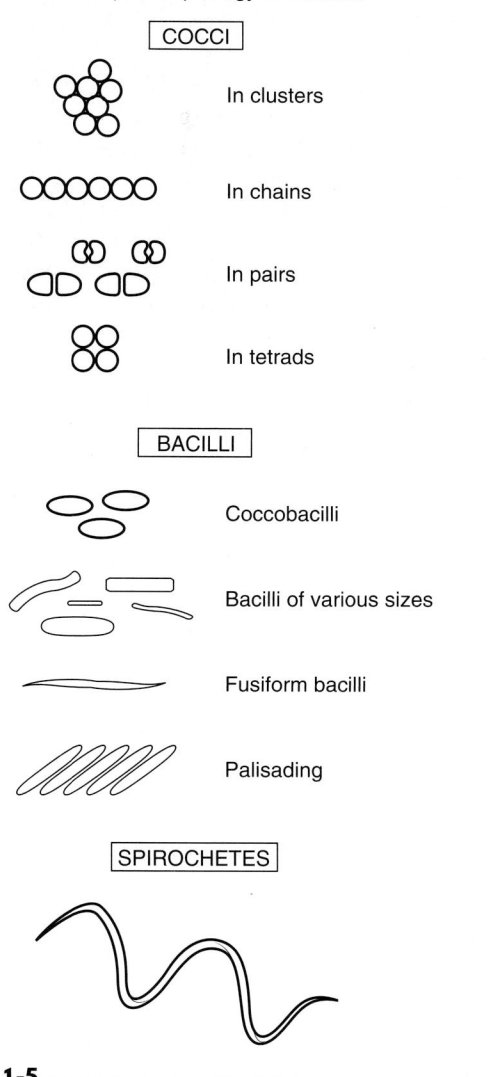

Figure 1-5

Diagram of the microscopic shapes and arrangements of bacteria.

Common Stains Used for Microscopic Visualization

Stains that impart color or fluorescence are needed to visualize bacteria under the microscope. The microscopic staining characteristics, shape, and grouping are used in the classification of microorganisms (Figure 1-6).

Gram stain

The Gram stain in the most commonly used stain in the clinical microbiology laboratory. It places bacteria into one of the two groups: gram-positive (purple) or gram-negative (pink) (see Figure 1-6, *A* and *B*). As mentioned previously, the cell wall structure determines the Gram-staining characteristics of a species. The Gram stain consists of four components: crystal violet (the primary stain), iodine (the mordant or fixative), acetone alcohol (the decolorizer), and safranin (the counterstain). The bacteria are initially stained purple by the crystal violet, which is bound to the cell wall with the aid of iodine. When alcohol is applied to bacteria with a gram-negative type of cell wall structure, the crystal violet washes out of the cells, which then take up the pink counterstain, safranin. Gram-negative bacteria therefore appear pink under the light microscope. Bacteria with a gram-positive cell wall retain the primary crystal violet stain during alcohol treatment and therefore remain purple. As presented in the case study at the beginning of the chapter, review of quality control slides is important in the detection of errors in the performance of the Gram stain procedure.

Acid-fast stains

Acid-fast stains are used to stain bacteria that have a high lipid and wax content in their cell walls and do not stain well with traditional bacterial stains. Carbolfuchsin (a red dye) is used as the primary stain (see Figure 1-6, *C*). The cell wall is treated to allow penetration of the dye either by heat (Ziehl-Neelsen method) or by a detergent (Kinyoun method). Acidified alcohol is used as a decolorizer, and methylene blue is the counterstain. Acid-fast bacteria retain the primary stain and are red. Bacteria that are not acid-fast are blue.

Two other gram-positive genera, *Nocardia* and *Rhodococcus,* may stain acid-fast by a modified method. Acid-fast staining is used to identify a

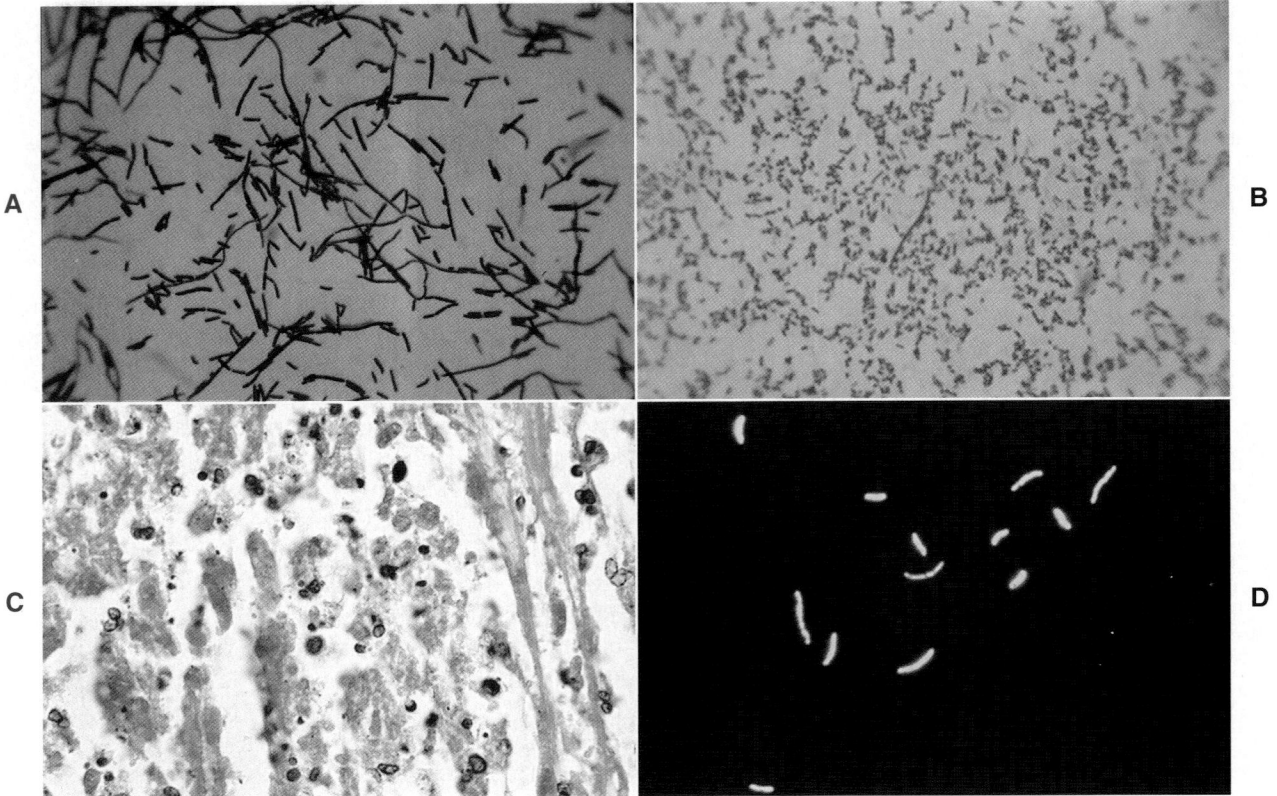

Figure 1-6

A, Gram stain of *Lactobacillus* species illustrating gram-positive bacilli, singly and in chains. A few gram-negative–staining bacilli are also present. (Courtesy Dr. Andrew G. Smith, Baltimore.) **B,** Gram stain of *Escherichia coli* illustrating short gram-negative bacilli. (Courtesy Dr. Andrew G. Smith, Baltimore.) **C,** Acid-fast stain, carbolfuschin based. A sputum smear demonstrating the presence of acid-fast *Mycobacterium* species stained by the Kinyoun or Ziehl-Neelsen carbolfuchsin method. **D,** Acid-fast stain, fluorochrome based. *Mycobacterium* species stained with the acid-fast fluorescent auramine-rhodamine stain. This stain is useful for screening for the presence of acid-fast bacteria in clinical specimens. (Courtesy Clinical Microbiology Audiovisual Study Units, Health and Education Resources, Inc., Bethesda, Md.)   *Continued*

yeast, *Saccharomyces,* and coccidian parasites, such as *Isospora belli, Cryptosporidium,* and other coccidia-like bodies. A fluorochrome (i.e., fluorescent) stain, auramine-rhodamine, has also been used to screen for acid-fast bacteria (see Figure 1-6, *D*). This stain is selective for the cell wall of acid-fast bacteria. Acid-fast bacteria appear yellow or orange under a fluorescent microscope, making them easier to find.

Acridine orange
Acridine orange is a fluorochrome dye that stains both gram-positive and gram-negative bacteria, living or dead. It binds to the nucleic acid of the cell and fluoresces as a bright orange. Acridine orange is used to locate bacteria in blood cultures and other specimens where discerning bacteria might otherwise be difficult (see Figure 1-6, *E*).

Methylene blue
Methylene blue has been traditionally used to stain *Corynebacterium diphtheriae* for observation of metachromatic granules (see Figure 1-6, *F*). It is also used as a counterstain in the acid-fast staining procedures.

Lactophenol cotton blue
Lactophenol cotton blue is used to stain the cell walls of medically important fungi grown in slide culture (see Figure 1-6, *G*).

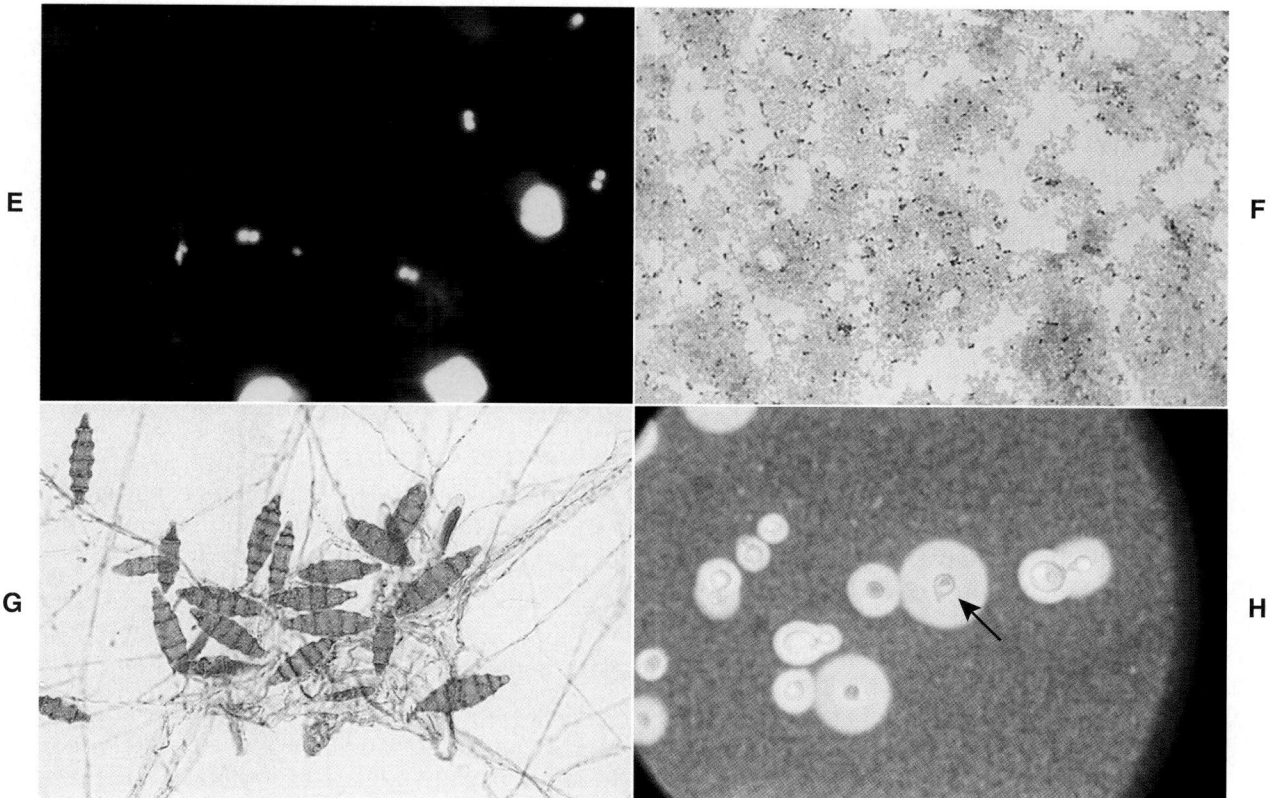

Figure 1-6, cont'd ————————————————————————————————

E, Acridine orange stain. A fluorescent stain demonstrating the presence of staphylococci in a blood culture broth. This stain is useful for detecting bacteria in situations where debris may mask the bacteria. (Courtesy Dr. John E. Peters.) **F,** Methylene blue stain. A methylene blue stain demonstrating the typical morphology of *Corynebacterium diphtheriae*. **G,** Lactophenol cotton blue stain. Lactophenol cotton blue stained–slide of macroconidia and hyphae of the fungal dermatophyte *Microsporum gypsum*. **H,** India ink. An India ink wet mount of *Cryptococcus neoformans* demonstrating the presence of a capsule *(arrow)*. (Courtesy Dr. Andrew G. Smith, Baltimore.)

Calcofluor white

Calcofluor white is a fluorochrome that binds to chitin in fungal cell walls. It fluoresces as a bright apple-green or blue-white, allowing visualization of fungal structures with a fluorescent microscope.

India ink

India ink is a negative stain used to visualize capsules surrounding certain yeasts, such as *Cryptococcus* (see Figure 1-6, *H*). The fine ink particles are excluded from the capsule, leaving a dark background and a clear capsule surrounding the yeast.

MICROBIAL GROWTH AND NUTRITION

All bacteria have three major nutritional needs for growth:

- A source of carbon (for making cellular constituents)
- A source of nitrogen (for making proteins)
- A source of energy (ATP) (for carrying out cellular functions)

Smaller amounts of molecules such as phosphate (for nucleic acids) and a variety of metals and ions (for enzymatic activity) must also be present. Although the basic building blocks required for growth are the same for all cells, bacteria vary widely in their ability to use different sources of these molecules.

Nutritional Requirements for Growth

Bacteria are classified into two basic groups according to how they meet their nutritional needs. Members of the first group, the **autotrophs** (lithotrophs), are able to grow simply, using CO_2 as the sole source of carbon, with only water and inorganic salts required in addition. Autotrophs obtain energy either photosynthetically (phototrophs) or by oxidation of inorganic compounds (chemolithotrophs). Autotrophs occur in environmental milieus.

The second group of bacteria, the **heterotrophs,** require more complex substances for growth. They require an organic source of carbon, such as glucose, and obtain energy by oxidizing or fermenting organic substances. Often, the same substance (for example, glucose) is used as both the carbon source and energy source.

All bacteria that inhabit the human body fall into the heterotrophic group. Within this group, however, nutritional needs vary greatly. Bacteria such as *Escherichia coli* and *Pseudomonas aeruginosa* can use a wide variety or organic compounds as carbon sources and therefore grow on most simple laboratory media. Other pathogenic bacteria, such as *Haemophilus influenzae* and the anaerobes, are fastidious, requiring additional metabolites such as vitamins, purines, pyrimidines, and hemoglobin supplied in the growth medium. Some pathogenic bacteria, such as *Chlamydia,* cannot be cultured on laboratory media at all and must be grown in tissue culture or detected by other means.

Types of growth media

A laboratory growth medium whose contents are simple and completely defined is termed *minimal medium.* This type of medium is not usually used in the diagnostic microbiology laboratory. Media that are more complex and made of extracts of meat or soy beans are termed *nutrient media* (e.g., nutrient broth, trypticase soy broth). A growth medium that contains added growth factors, such as blood, vitamins, and yeast extract, is referred to as *enriched* (e.g., blood agar, chocolate agar). Media containing additives that inhibit the growth of some bacteria but allow others to grow are called *selective* (e.g., MacConkey agar). Media that allow visualization of metabolic differences between groups or species of bacteria are **differential.** When a delay between collection of the specimen and culturing the specimen is necessary, a transport medium is used. A **transport medium** is a holding medium designed to preserve the viability of microorganisms in the specimen but not allow multiplication. Stuart broth and Amies and Cary-Blair transport media are common examples.

Environmental Factors Influencing Growth

Three environmental factors influence the growth rate of bacteria and must be considered when bacteria are cultured in the laboratory:

▪ pH
▪ Temperature
▪ Gaseous composition of the atmosphere

Most pathogenic bacteria grow best at a neutral pH, and diagnostic laboratory media for bacteria are usually adjusted to a final pH between 7.0 and 7.5.

Temperature influences the rate of growth of a bacterial culture. Microorganisms have been categorized according to their optimal temperature for growth. Bacteria that grow best at cold temperatures are called *psychrophiles* (optimal growth at 10° to 20° C). Bacteria that grow optimally at moderate temperatures are called *mesophiles* (optimal growth at 20° to 40° C). Bacteria that grow best at high temperatures are called *thermophiles* (optimal growth at 50° to 60° C). Psychrophiles and thermophiles are found environmentally in places such as the arctic seas and hot springs, respectively. Most bacteria that have adapted to humans are mesophiles that grow best near human body temperature (37° C). Diagnostic laboratories routinely incubate cultures for bacterial growth at 35° C. Some pathogenic species, however, prefer a lower temperature for growth; when these organisms are suspected, the specimen plate is incubated at a lower temperature. Fungal cultures are incubated at 30° C. The ability to grow at room temperature (25° C) or at an elevated temperature (42° C) is used as a diagnostic characteristic for some bacteria.

The bacteria that grow on humans vary in their atmospheric requirements for growth. Some require oxygen **(obligate aerobes).** Some cannot grow in the presence of oxygen **(obligate anaerobes).** Some can grow either with or without oxygen **(facultative anaerobes).** Many grow better when the atmosphere is enriched with extra carbon dioxide **(capnophilic).**

Air contains approximately 21% oxygen and 1% carbon dioxide. When the carbon dioxide content of an aerobic incubator is increased to 10%, the oxygen content of the incubator is lowered to approximately 18%. Obligate aerobes must have oxygen to grow; incubation in air or an aerobic incubator with 10% CO_2 present satisfies their oxygen requirement. **Microaerophilic** bacteria require a reduced level of oxygen to grow. An example of a pathogenic microaerophile is *Campylobacter,* which requires 5% to 6% oxygen. This type of atmosphere can be generated in culture jars or pouches using a commercially available microaerophilic atmosphere generating system. Obligate anaerobes must be grown in an atmosphere either devoid of oxygen or with a very reduced oxygen content. Facultative anaerobes are routinely cultured in an aerobic atmosphere because aerobic culture is easier and less expensive than anaerobic culture; an example is *E. coli.* Capnophilic bacteria require extra carbon dioxide (5% to 10%) for growth; an example is *H. influenzae.* Because many bacteria grow better in the presence of increased carbon dioxide, diagnostic microbiology laboratories often maintain their aerobic incubators at a 5% to 10% carbon dioxide level.

Bacterial Growth

Generation time

Bacteria replicate by binary fission, with one cell dividing into two cells. The time required for one cell to divide into two cells is called the *generation time* or *doubling time.* The generation time of a bacterium in culture can be as little as 20 minutes for a fast-growing bacterium such as *E. coli* or as long as 24 hours for a slow-growing bacterium such as *Mycobacterium tuberculosis.*

Growth curve

If bacteria are in a balanced growth state, with enough nutrients and no toxic products present, the increase in bacterial numbers is proportional to the increase in other bacterial properties, such as mass, protein content, and nucleic acid content. Thus measurement of any of these properties can be used as an indication of bacterial growth. When the growth of a bacterial culture is plotted during balanced growth, the resulting curve shows four phases of growth: (1) a lag phase, during which bacteria are preparing to divide, (2) a log phase, during which bacteria numbers increase logarithmically, (3) a stationary phase, in which nutrients are becoming limited and the numbers of bacteria remain constant (although viability may decrease), and (4) a death phase, when the number of nonviable bacterial cells exceeds the number of viable cells. An example of such a growth curve is shown in Figure 1-7.

Determination of cell numbers

In the diagnostic laboratory the number of bacterial cells present is determined in one of three ways:

- **Direct counting under the microscope:** This method can be used to estimate the number of bacteria present in a specimen. It does not distinguish between live and dead cells.
- **Direct plate count:** By growing dilutions of broth cultures on agar plates, one can determine the number of colony-forming units per

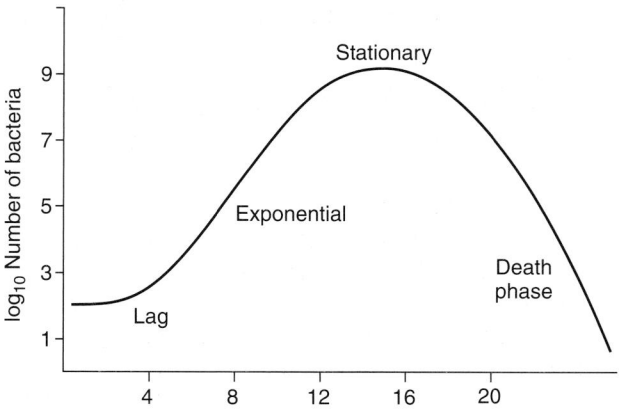

Figure 1-7 _____

The typical growth curve of a bacterial culture. (Modified from Schaechter M, Medoff G, Eisenstein BI: *Mechanisms of microbial disease,* ed 2, Baltimore, 1993, Williams & Wilkins.)

mL (CFU/mL). This provides a count of viable cells only. This method is used in determining the bacterial cell count in urine cultures.

▪ **Density measurement:** The density of a bacterial broth culture in log phase can be correlated to CFU/mL of the culture. This method is used to prepare a standard inoculum for antimicrobial susceptibility testing.

BACTERIAL BIOCHEMISTRY AND METABOLISM

Metabolism

Microbial metabolism consists of the biochemical reactions bacteria use to break down organic compounds as well as those they use to synthesize new bacterial parts from the resulting carbon skeletons. Energy for the new constructions is generated during the metabolic breakdown of the substrate.

The occurrence of all biochemical reactions in the cell depends on the presence and activity of specific enzymes. Thus metabolism can be regulated in the cell either by regulating the production of an enzyme itself (a genetic type of regulation, in which production of the enzyme can be induced or suppressed by molecules present in the cell) or by regulating the activity of the enzyme (via feedback inhibition, in which the products of the enzymatic reaction or a succeeding enzymatic reaction inhibit the activity of the enzyme).

Bacteria vary widely in their ability to use various compounds as substrates and in the end products generated. A variety of biochemical pathways exist for substrate breakdown in the microbial world, and the particular pathway used determines the end product and final pH of the medium (Figure 1-8). Microbiologists use these metabolic differences as phenotypic markers in the identification of bacteria. Diagnostic schemes analyze each unknown microorganism for (1) utilization of a variety of substrates as a carbon source, (2) production of specific end products from various substrates, and (3) production of an acid or alkaline pH in the test medium. Thus knowledge of the biochemistry and metabolism of bacteria is important in the clinical laboratory.

Fermentation and Respiration

Bacteria use biochemical pathways to catabolize (break down) carbohydrates and produce energy by two mechanisms—fermentation and respiration (commonly referred to as *oxidation*). **Fermentation** is an anaerobic process carried out by both obligate and facultative anaerobes. In fer-

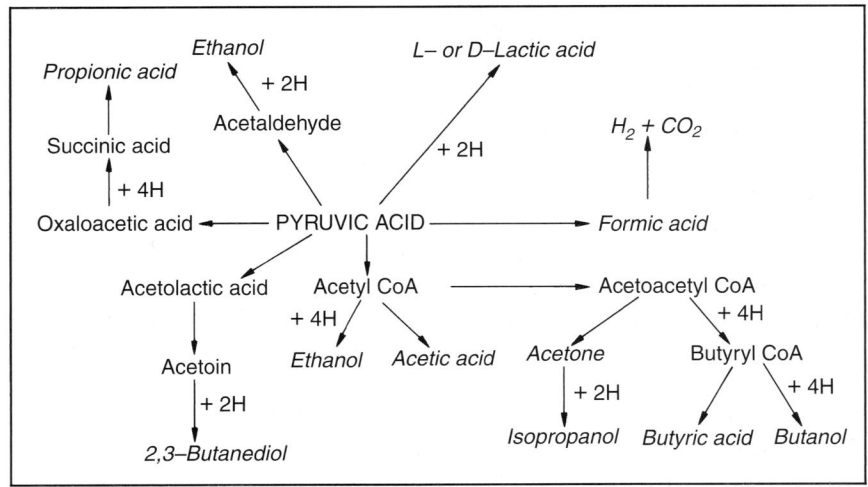

Figure 1-8

The fate of pyruvate in major fermentation pathways by microorganisms. (From Joklik WK et al: *Zinsser microbiology,* ed 20, Norwalk, Conn, 1992, Appleton & Lange.)

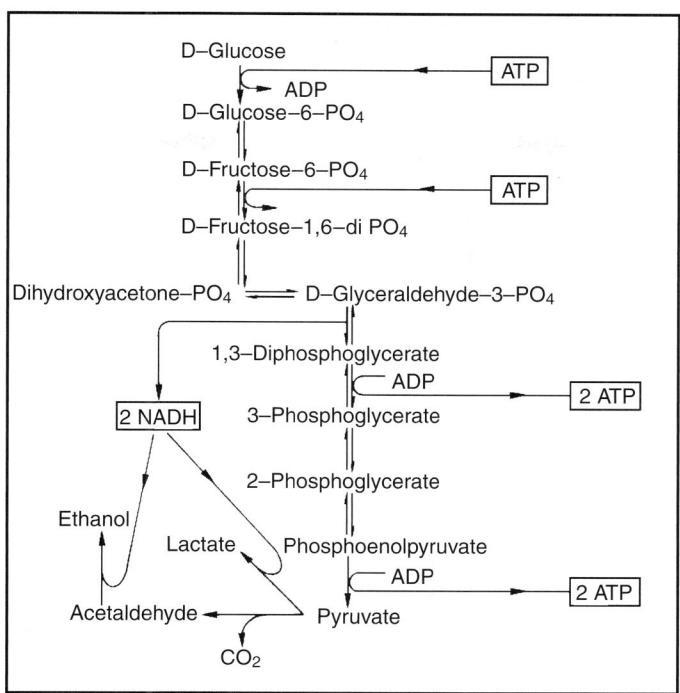

Figure 1-9

The Embden-Meyerhof-Parnas (EMP) glycolytic pathway. (From Joklik WK et al: *Zinsser microbiology,* ed 20, East Norwalk, Conn, 1992, Appleton & Lange.)

mentation the electron acceptor is an organic compound. Fermentation is less efficient in energy generation than respiration (oxidation) because the beginning substrate is not completely reduced, and therefore all the energy in the substrate is not released. When fermentation occurs, a mixture of end products (such as lactate, butyrate, ethanol, and acetoin) accumulates in the medium. Analysis of these end products is particularly useful for the identification of anaerobic bacteria. End-product determination is also used in the Voges-Proskauer (VP) and methyl red tests, two important diagnostic tests used in the identification of the Enterobacteriaceae. (The term *fermentation* is often used loosely in the diagnostic microbiology laboratory to indicate any type of utilization—fermentative or oxidative—of a carbohydrate—sugar—with the resulting production of an acid pH.)

Respiration is an efficient energy-generating process in which molecular oxygen is the final electron acceptor. Obligate aerobes and facultative anaerobes carry out aerobic respiration, in which oxygen (O_2) is the final electron acceptor. Certain anaerobes can carry out anaerobic respiration, in which inorganic forms of oxygen, such as nitrate and sulfate, act as the final electron acceptors.

Biochemical Pathways from Glucose to Pyruvic Acid

The starting carbohydrate for bacterial fermentations or oxidations is glucose. When bacteria use other sugars as a carbon source, they first convert the sugar to glucose, which is then processed by one of three pathways. These pathways are designed to generate pyruvic acid, a key three-carbon intermediate. The three major biochemical pathways bacteria use to break down glucose to pyruvic acid are as follows: (1) the Embden-Meyerhof-Parnas (EMP) glycolytic pathway (Figure 1-9), (2) the pentose phosphate pathway (Figure 1-10), and (3) the Entner-Doudoroff pathway

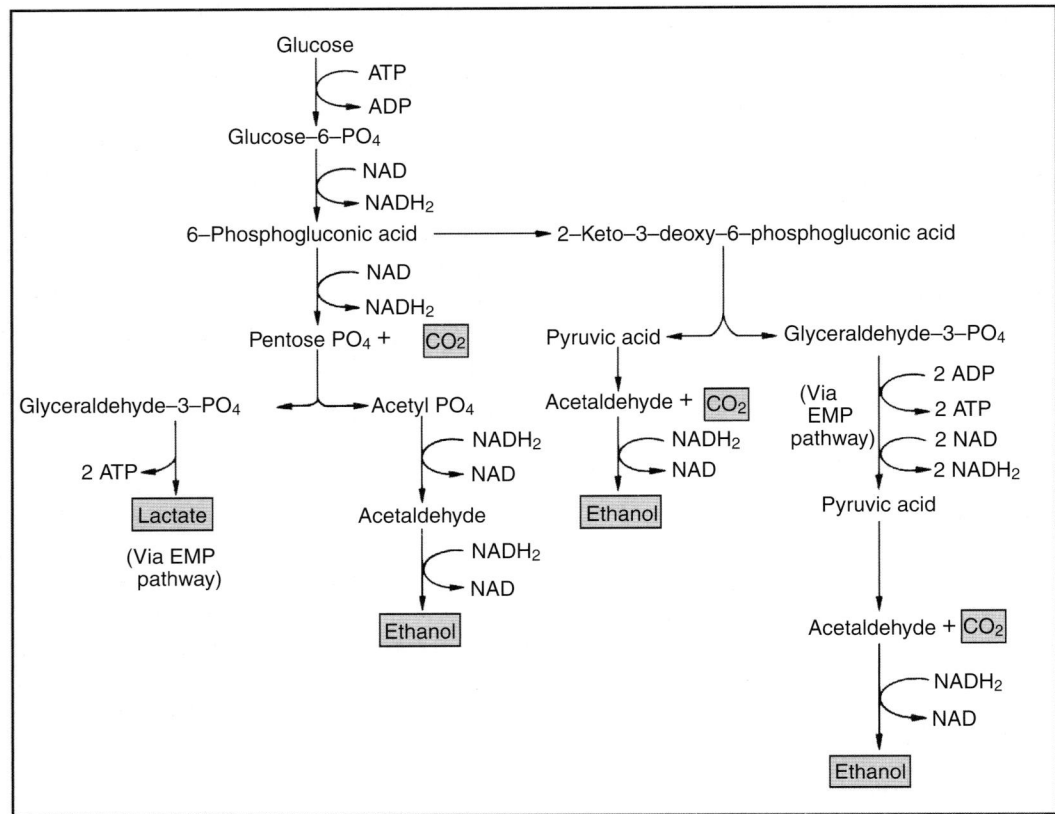

Figure 1-10

Alternative microbial pathways to the EMP pathway for glucose fermentation. The pentose phosphate pathway is on the left, and the Entner-Doudoroff pathway on the right. (From Joklik WK et al: *Zinsser microbiology,* ed 20, Norwalk, Conn, 1992, Appleton & Lange.)

(see Figure 1-10). Pyruvate can then be further processed either fermentatively or oxidatively. The three major metabolic pathways and their key characteristics are described in Box 1-1.

Anaerobic Utilization of Pyruvic Acid (Fermentation)

Pyruvic acid is a key metabolic intermediate. Bacteria process pyruvic acid further using a variety of fermentation pathways. Each pathway yields different end products, which can be analyzed and used as phenotypic markers (see Figure 1-8). Some of the fermentation pathways used by the microbes that inhabit the human body are as follows:

▪ **Alcoholic fermentation:** The major end product is ethanol. This is the pathway used by yeasts when they ferment glucose to produce ethanol.

▪ **Homolactic fermentation:** The end product is almost exclusively lactic acid. All members of the *Streptococcus* genus and many members of the *Lactobacillus* genus ferment pyruvate using this pathway.

▪ **Heterolactic fermentation:** Some lactobacilli use this mixed fermentation pathway, of which, in addition to lactic acid, the end products include CO_2, alcohols, formic acid, and acetic acid.

▪ **Propionic acid fermentation:** Propionic acid is the major end product of fermentations carried out by *Propionibacterium acnes* and some anaerobic non–spore-forming gram-positive bacilli.

▪ **Mixed acid fermentation:** Members of the genera *Escherichia, Salmonella,* and *Shigella* within the Enterobacteriaceae use this pathway for sugar fermentation and produce a number of acids as end products—lactic, acetic, succinic, and formic acids. The strong acid produced is the basis for the positive reaction on the methyl red test exhibited by these organisms.

- **Butanediol fermentation:** Members of the genera *Klebsiella, Enterobacter,* and *Serratia* within the Enterobacteriaceae use this pathway for sugar fermentation. The end products are acetoin (acetyl methyl carbinol) and 2,3-butanediol. Detection of acetoin is the basis for the positive Voges-Proskauer (VP) reaction characteristic of these microorganisms. Little acid is produced by this pathway. Thus organisms that have a positive VP reaction usually have a negative reaction on the methyl red test, and vice versa.

- **Butyric acid fermentation:** Certain obligate anaerobes, including many *Clostridium* species, *Fusobacterium,* and *Eubacterium,* produce butyric acid as their primary end product along with acetic acid, CO_2, and hydrogen.

Aerobic Utilization of Pyruvate (Oxidation)

The most important pathway for the complete oxidation of a substrate under aerobic conditions is the Krebs or TCA (tricarboxylic acid) cycle. In this cycle, pyruvate is oxidized, carbon skeletons for biosynthetic reactions are created, and the electrons donated by pyruvate are passed through an electron transport chain and used to generate energy in the form of ATP. This cycle results in the production of acid and the evolution of CO_2 (Figure 1-11).

Carbohydrate Utilization and Lactose Fermentation

The ability of microorganisms to use various "sugars" (carbohydrates) for growth is an integral part of most diagnostic identification schemes. The fermentation of the sugar is usually detected by acid production and a concomitant change of color resulting from a pH indicator present in the culture medium. In general, bacteria ferment glucose preferentially over other sugars, and therefore glucose must not be present if the ability to ferment another sugar is being tested.

One of the important steps in classifying members of the Enterobacteriaceae family is the determination of the microorganism's ability to ferment lactose. These bacteria are classified as either lactose fermenters or lactose nonfermenters. Lactose is a disaccharide consisting of one molecule of glucose and one molecule of galactose linked together by a galactoside bond. Two steps are involved in the utilization of lactose by a bacterium. The first step requires an enzyme, β-galactoside permease, for the transport of lactose across the cell wall into the bacterial cytoplasm. The second step occurs inside the cell and requires the enzyme β-galactosidase to break the galactoside bond, re-

---

Box 1-1

The Three Major Metabolic Pathways

Embden-Meyerhof-Parnas (EMP) glycolytic pathway

The major pathway in conversion of glucose to pyruvate

Generates reducing power in the form of $NADH_2$

Generates energy in the form of ATP

Anaerobic; does not require oxygen

Used by many bacteria, including all members of Enterobacteriaceae

Pentose phosphate (phosphogluconate) pathway

An alternative to EMP pathway for carbohydrate metabolism

Conversion of glucose to ribulose-5-phosphate, which is then rearranged into other 3-, 4-, 5-, 6-, and 7-carbon surgars

Provides pentoses for nucleotide synthesis

Produces glyceraldehyde-3-phosphate, which can be converted to pyruvate

Generates NADPH, which provides reducing power for biosynthetic reactions

May be used to generate ATP (yield is less than with the EMP pathway)

Used by heterolactic fermenting bacteria, such as lactobacilli, and by *Brucella abortus,* which lacks some of the enzymes required in the EMP pathway

Entner-Doudoroff pathway

Converts glucose-6-phosphate (rather than glucose) to pyruvate and glyceraldehyde phosphate, which can then be funneled into other pathways

Generates one NADPH per molecule of glucose but uses one ATP

Aerobic process used by *Pseudomonas, Alcaligenes, Enterococcus faecalis,* and other bacteria lacking certain glycolytic enzymes

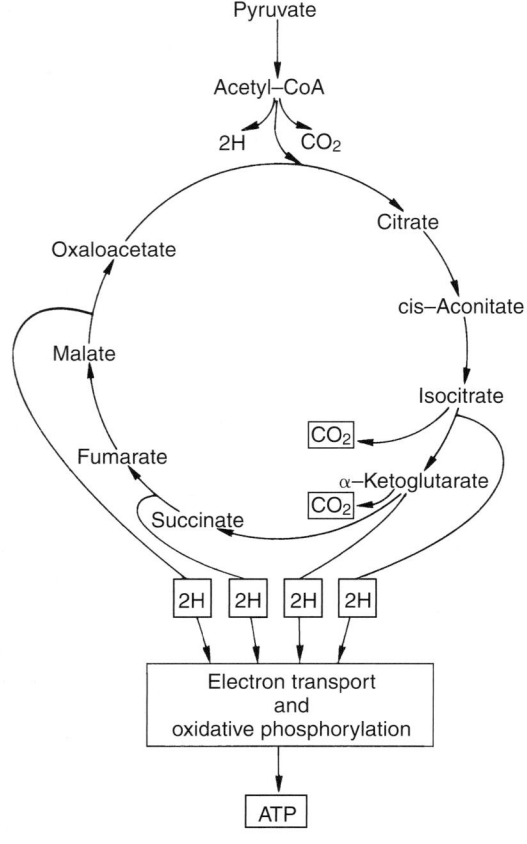

Figure 1-11 _____

The Krebs tricarboxylic acid (TCA) cycle allowing the complete oxidation of a substrate. (From Joklik WK et al: *Zinsser microbiology,* ed 20, Norwalk, Conn, 1992, Appleton & Lange.)

leasing glucose, which can then be fermented. Thus all organisms that can ferment lactose can also ferment glucose.

BACTERIAL GENETICS

Bacterial genetics is increasingly important in the diagnostic microbiology laboratory. New diagnostic tests have been developed that are based on identifying unique RNA or DNA sequences present in each bacterial species. The polymerase chain reaction (PCR) technique is a means of amplifying specific DNA sequences and thus detecting very small numbers of bacteria present in a specimen.

Genetic tests circumvent the need to culture bacteria, providing a more rapid method of identifying pathogens. Analysis of DNA structure using restriction endonuclease fragment patterns, called *RFLP,* provides a fine tool for epidemiologists.

An understanding of bacterial genetics is also necessary to understand the development and transfer of antimicrobial resistance by bacteria. The occurrence of mutations can result in a change in the expected phenotypic characteristics of an organism and provides an explanation for atypical results sometimes encountered on diagnostic biochemical tests. This section briefly reviews some of the basic terminology and concepts of bacterial genetics.

Terminology

The genotype of a cell is the genetic potential of the DNA of an organism. It includes all the characteristics that are coded for in the DNA of a bacterium and that have the potential to be expressed. Some genes are silent genes, expressed only under certain conditions. Genes that are always expressed are constitutive. Genes that are expressed only under certain conditions are inducible. The **phenotype** of a cell consists of the genetic characteristics of a cell that actually are expressed and can be observed. The ultimate aim of a cell is to produce the proteins that are responsible for cellular structure and function and to transmit the information for accomplishing this to the next generation of cells.

Information for protein synthesis is encoded in the bacterial DNA and transmitted in the chromosome to each generation. The general flow of information in a bacterial cell is from DNA (which contains the genetic information) to messenger RNA (mRNA) (which acts as a blueprint for protein construction) to the actual protein itself (made on ribosomes containing ribosomal RNA with the aid of transfer RNA, which places specific amino acids in the growing peptide chain). Replication is the duplication of chromosomal DNA for insertion into a daughter cell. Transcription is the synthesis of single-stranded RNA (with the aid of the enzyme RNA polymerase) using one strand of the DNA as a template. Translation is the actual synthesis of a specific protein from the mRNA code. The term *protein expression* also refers to the synthesis (i.e., translation) of a protein.

Genetic Elements and Alterations

The bacterial genome

The bacterial chromosome (also called the *genome*) consists of a single, closed, circular piece of double-stranded DNA that is supercoiled in order to fit inside the cell. It contains all the information needed for cell growth and replication. Genes are specific DNA sequences that code for the amino acid sequence in one protein (i.e., one gene equals one protein). In front of each gene on the DNA strand is an untranscribed area containing a promoter region, which the RNA polymerase recognizes for transcription initiation. This area may also contain regulatory regions to which molecules may attach and cause either a decrease or an increase in transcription.

Extrachromosomal elements

In addition to the genetic information encoded in the bacterial chromosome, many bacteria contain extra information on small circular pieces of DNA called **plasmids.** Genes that code for antibiotic resistance (and sometimes toxins or other virulence factors) are often located on plasmids. Antibiotic therapy selects for bacterial strains containing plasmids encoding antibiotic resistance genes; this is one reason antibiotics should not be overprescribed. The number of plasmids present in a bacterial cell may vary from one (low copy number) to hundreds (high copy number). Plasmids are located in the cytoplasm of the cell and can be replicated and passed to daughter cells just like chromosomal DNA. They may also sometimes be passed from one bacterial species to another. This is one way resistance to antibiotics is acquired.

Mobile genetic elements

Certain pieces of DNA are mobile and may jump from one place in the chromosome to another place. These are sometimes referred to as "jumping genes." The simplest mobile piece of DNA is an insertion sequence (IS) element. It is about 1000 base pairs long with inverted repeats on each end. Each IS element codes for only one gene, a transposase enzyme that allows the IS element to pop into and out of DNA. Bacterial genomes contain many IS elements. The main effect of IS elements in bacteria is that when an IS element inserts itself into the middle of a gene, it disrupts and inacti-

vates the gene. This can result in loss of an observable characteristic, such as the ability to ferment a particular sugar. Transposons are related mobile elements that contain additional genes. Transposons often carry antibiotic-resistance genes and are usually located in plasmids.

Mutations

A gene sequence must be read in the right "frame" for the correct protein to be produced. This is because every set of three bases (known as a *codon*) specifies a particular amino acid, and when the reading frame is askew, the codons are interpreted incorrectly. Mutations are changes that occur in the DNA code and result in a change in the coded protein or in the prevention of its synthesis. A mutation may be the result of a change in one nucleotide base (a point mutation) that leads to a change in a single amino acid within a protein or may be the result of insertions or deletions in the genome that lead to disruption of the gene and/or a frameshift mutation. Incomplete, inactive proteins are often the result. Spontaneous mutations occur in bacteria at a rate of about one in 10^9 cells. Mutations also occur as the result of error during DNA replication at a rate of about one in 10^7 cells. Exposure to certain chemical and physical agents can greatly increase the mutation rate.

Genetic recombination

Genetic recombination is a method by which genes are transferred or exchanged between homologous (similar) regions on two DNA molecules. This method provides a way for organisms to obtain new combinations of biochemical pathways and cope with changes in their environment.

Mechanisms of Gene Transfer

Genetic material may be transferred from one bacterium to another in three basic ways:

- Transformation
- Transduction
- Conjugation

Transformation

Transformation is the uptake and incorporation of naked DNA into a bacterial cell (Figure 1-12, *A*). Once the DNA has been taken up, it can be incor-

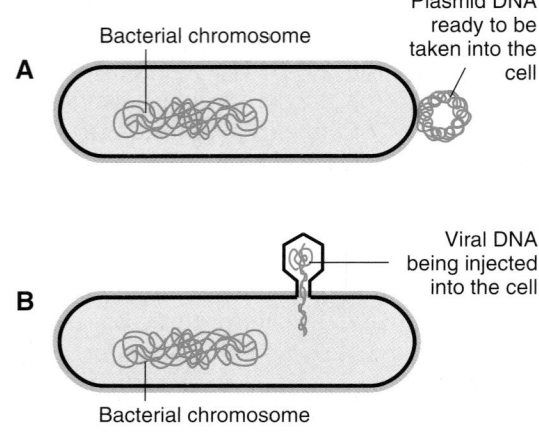

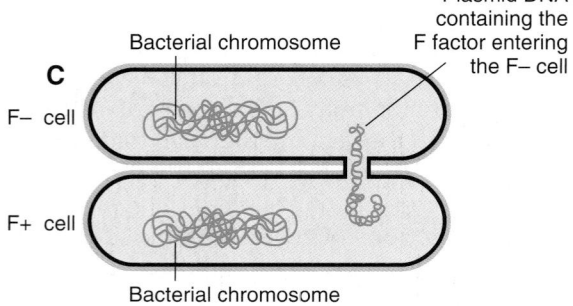

Figure 1-12

Diagram of methods of gene transfer into bacterial cells.
A, Bacterial transformation. Free or "naked" DNA is taken up
by a competent bacterial cell. After uptake the DNA may take
one of three courses: (1) it is integrated into existing bacterial genetic material, (2) it is degraded, or (3) if it is a compatible plasmid, it may replicate in the cytoplasm. **B,** Bacterial transduction. A phage injects DNA into the bacterial cell.
The phage tail combines with a receptor of the bacterial cell
wall and injects the DNA into the bacterium. One of two
courses may then be taken. In the lytic cycle, replication of
the bacterial chromosome is disrupted; phage components
are formed and assembled into phage particles. The bacterial cell is lysed, releasing mature phage. In the lysogenic cycle the phage DNA is incorporated into the bacterial genetic
material, and genes encoded on the phage DNA may be expressed from this site. At a later time the phage may be "induced," and a lytic cycle will then ensue. **C,** Bacterial conjugation. An F+ cell connects with an F− cell via sex pili. DNA
is then transferred from one cell to the other.

porated into the bacterial genome by recombination. If the DNA is a circular plasmid and the
recipient cell is compatible, the plasmid can replicate in the cytoplasm and be transferred to
daughter cells. Cells that can take up naked DNA

are referred to as being *competent.* Only a few
bacterial species, such as *Streptococcus pneumoniae, Neisseria gonorrhoeae,* and *H. influenzae,* do
this naturally. Bacteria can be made competent in
the laboratory, and transformation is the main
method used to introduce genetically manipulated plasmids into bacteria, such as *E. coli,* during cloning procedures.

Transduction

Transduction is the transfer of bacterial genes by
a bacteriophage (a bacterial virus) from one cell
to another (see Figure 1-12, *B*). A **bacteriophage**
consists of a chromosome (DNA or RNA) surrounded by a protein coat. When a phage infects
a bacterial cell, it injects its genome into the bacterial cell, leaving the protein coat outside. The
phage may then take a lytic pathway, in which the
bacteriophage DNA directs the bacterial cell to
synthesize phage DNA and phage protein and
package it into new phage particles. The bacterial
cell then lyses, releasing new phage, which can infect other bacterial cells. In some instances, the
phage DNA instead becomes incorporated into
the bacterial genome, where it is replicated along
with the bacterial chromosomal DNA; this state is
known as *lysogeny,* and the phage is referred to
as being *temperate.* During lysogeny, genes present in the phage DNA may be expressed by the
bacterial cell. An example of this in the clinical
laboratory is *Corynebacterium diphtheriae.* Strains
of *C. diphtheriae* that are lysogenized with a temperate phage carrying the gene for diphtheria
toxin cause disease. Strains lacking the phage do
not cause disease.

Under certain conditions a temperate phage can
be induced, the phage DNA is excised from the
bacterial genome, and a lytic state occurs. During
this process, adjacent bacterial genes may be excised with the phage DNA and packaged into the
new phage. The bacterial genes may then be transferred when the phage infects a new bacterium. In
the field of biotechnology, phages are often used
to insert cloned genes into bacteria for analysis.

Conjugation

Conjugation is the transfer of genetic material
from a donor bacterial strain to a recipient strain
(see Figure 1-12, *C*). It requires close contact between the two cells. In the *E. coli* system the

donor strain (F+) possesses a fertility factor (F factor) on a plasmid that carries the genes for conjugative transfer. The donor strain produces a hollow surface appendage called a sex pilus, which binds to the recipient F− cell and brings the two cells in close contact. Transfer of DNA then occurs. Both plasmids and chromosomal genes can be transferred by this method. When the F factor is integrated into the bacterial chromosome rather than a plasmid, there is a higher frequency of transfer of adjacent bacterial chromosomal genes. These strains are known as *Hfr (high-frequency) strains.*

Restriction enzymes

Bacteria have evolved a system to restrict the incorporation of foreign DNA into their genomes. Specific **restriction enzymes** are produced that cut incoming foreign DNA at specific DNA sequences. The bacteria methylate their own DNA at these same sequences so that the restriction enzymes do not cut the DNA in their own cell. Many restriction enzymes with a variety of recognition sequences have now been isolated from various microorganisms. The first three letters in the restriction endonuclease name indicate the bacterial source of the enzyme. For instance, the enzyme *Eco*RI was isolated from *E. coli,* and the enzyme *Hind*III was isolated from *H. influenzae* type d.

These enzymes are used in the field of biotechnology to create sites for insertion of new genes. In clinical microbiology, epidemiologists use restriction enzyme fragment analysis to determine whether strains of bacteria have identical restriction sites in their genomic DNA.

Bibliography

De Robertis EDP, De Robertis EMF Jr: *Cell and molecular biology,* Philadelphia, 1987, Lea & Febiger.

Holt JG et al: *Bergey's manual of determinative bacteriology,* ed 9, Baltimore, 1993, Williams & Wilkins.

Howard BJ: *Clinical and pathogenic microbiology,* ed 2, St Louis, 1994, Mosby.

Joklik WK et al, editors: *Zinsser microbiology,* ed 20, Norwalk, Conn, 1992, Appleton & Lange.

Krieg NR, Holt JG, editors: *Bergey's manual of systematic bacteriology,* vol 1, Baltimore, 1984, Williams & Wilkins.

Mims CA et al: *Medical microbiology,* London, 1993, Mosby Europe Limited.

Murry PR et al: *Medical microbiology,* St Louis, 1990, Mosby.

Neidhardt FC, Ingraham JL, Schaechter M: *Physiology of the bacterial cell,* Sunderland, Mass, 1990, Sinauer Associates.

Sadava DE: *Cell biology,* Boston, 1993, Jones & Bartlett.

Schaechter M, Medoff G, Eisenstein BI: *Mechanisms of microbial disease,* Baltimore, 1993, Williams & Wilkins.

Sneath PHA et al, editors: *Bergey's manual of systematic bacteriology,* vol 2, Baltimore, 1986, Williams & Wilkins.

Woese CR: Bacterial evolution, *Microbiol Rev* 51:221, 1987.

LEARNING ASSESSMENT

1. Explain the reason that the technologist repeated the Gram stain procedure on the exudate.

2. What may have occurred to make the results invalid?

3. Differentiate the role of the pili from that of the flagella.

4. What is the role of the capsule in the pathogenesis of infectious diseases?

5. If the technologist forgets to add the Gram's iodine to the staining procedure, what will most likely occur?

6. Why is lipopolysacchride (LPS) a significant outer-membrane structure in Gram negative bacteria?

7. What cell wall structure is responsible for allowing bacteria to resist decolorization with acetone or alcohol?

8. Why are older bacterial cells more easily decolorized than younger colonies?

9. What maintains the shape of the bacterial cell?

10. Why are spore-forming organisms more resistant than non–spore-forming species?

11. Explain the three ways in which genetic material may be transferred from one bacterium to another.

CHAPTER 2

Control of Microorganisms

A. DISINFECTION AND STERILIZATION

Connie R. Mahon

STERILIZATION VERSUS DISINFECTION

FACTORS THAT INFLUENCE THE DEGREE OF KILLING
Types of Organisms
Number of Organisms
Concentration of Disinfecting Agent
Organic Soil Present
Nature of Surface to Be Disinfected

METHODS OF DISINFECTION AND STERILIZATION
Physical Methods
Heat
Filtration
Radiation

Chemical Methods
Alcohols
Aldehydes
Halogens
Heavy metals
Detergents: quaternary ammonium compounds
Phenolics
Gases

OBJECTIVES

1. Define the following terms: *sterilization, disinfection, bacteriostatic,* and *bactericidal.*
2. Differentiate the functions and purposes of a disinfectant and an antiseptic.
3. Describe the general modes of antimicrobial action.
4. Describe the way each physical agent controls the growth of microorganisms.
5. Give the mechanism of action for each type of chemical agent commonly used in antiseptics and disinfectants.
6. Describe the different heat methods and their respective applications.

KEY TERMS

Disinfection	Antiseptic
Sterilization	Microbial load
Filtration	Moist heat
Disinfectants	Pasteurization

CASE STUDY

A 35-year-old infectious disease specialist complained of experiencing fever, chills, myalgia, and severe headache for the past several days. The patient had otherwise been healthy until 2 weeks ago, when he began to experience fatigue and felt the slightly swollen lymph nodes. The patient then recalled that he had demonstrated to his medical students and residents a culture of *Brucella melitensis* isolated from a patient's blood sample. He remembered that while handling the Petri dish without gloves, he picked up the telephone to answer a page. While talking on the telephone, he touched his mustache as he habitually does when he speaks.

Safety in the laboratory cannot be overemphasized. Moreover, quantitating the risk of working with an infectious agent is difficult. Risk to an individual increases with the frequency and level of contact with the agent, as demonstrated by the case study at the beginning of this chapter. Therefore each laboratory must develop and institute an exposure control plan that will effectively minimize the risks and overt laboratory-associated hazards to persons who may be directly or indirectly ex-

posed to them. This chapter provides information on standard disinfection and sterilization techniques and laboratory safety guidelines for both students and clinical laboratory practitioners.

This section, on disinfection and sterilization, provides a practical overview of the following topics:

- Sterilization and disinfection
- Chemical and physical methods commonly used
- Principles and application of each method

STERILIZATION VERSUS DISINFECTION

The scientific use of **disinfection** and **sterilization** methods originated over 100 years ago, when Joseph Lister introduced the concept of aseptic surgery. Since that time the implementation of effective sterilization and disinfection methods remains crucial in the control of nosocomial infections.

To fully understand the principles of disinfection and sterilization, we need to have accurate definitions of certain terms. *Sterilization* refers to the removal of all forms of life, including bacterial spores. By definition, there are no degrees of sterilization—it is an all-or-nothing process. Chemical or physical methods may be used to accomplish this form of microbial removal. *Disinfection* refers to the removal of pathogenic organisms but does not necessarily include removal of bacterial or other spores. Physical or chemical methods may be employed, but most **disinfectants** are chemical agents applied to inanimate objects. A disinfectant that is applied to living tissue is referred to as an ***antiseptic.***

FACTORS THAT INFLUENCE THE DEGREE OF KILLING

Before discussion of particular methods, a review of the factors that influence the degree of killing of organisms is important. The following factors play a significant role in the selection and implementation of the appropriate method of disinfection:

- Types of organisms
- Number of organisms present
- Concentration of disinfecting agent
- Amount of organic soil present
- Nature of surface to be disinfected

Types of Organisms
Organisms vary greatly in their ability to withstand chemical and physical treatment (Figure 2-1). This variety is due to the biochemical composition of the cells and the protective mechanism afforded by the constituents. For example, spores have coats rich in proteins, lipids, and carbohydrates as well as cores rich in dipicolinic acid and calcium, all of which offer protection to spores. Cell walls of mycobacteria are rich in lipids, which may account for their resistance to chemical and environmental stresses, particularly desiccation. By contrast, viruses containing lipid-rich envelopes are more susceptible to the effects of detergents and wetting agents.

Number of Organisms
Another factor to consider is the total number of organisms present, referred to as the ***microbial load.*** If the number of organisms is plotted against the time they are exposed to the killing agent (exposure time) logarithmically, the result is a straight line (Figure 2-2). The death curve is logarithmic. Because the microbial load is most likely composed of organisms with varying susceptibilities to killing agents, not all the organisms die at the same time. The microbial load determines the exposure time. In general, higher numbers of organisms require longer exposure times.

Concentration of Disinfecting Agent
The concentration of a disinfecting agent is also important. Agents vary substantially among manufacturers, and, consequently, manufacturers' instructions on preparation, dilution, and use must be followed very carefully. Proper concentrations of disinfecting agents ensure the inactivation of target organisms and promote safe and cost-effective practices.

Organic Soil Present
Organic soil, such as blood, mucus, and pus, affects killing activity by actually inactivating the disinfecting agent. In addition, by coating the surface to be treated, organic soil prevents full contact be-

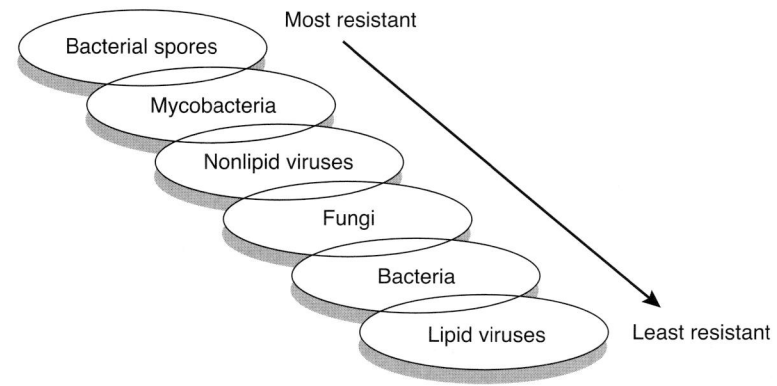

Figure 2-1

The different types of organisms and their resistance to killing agents.

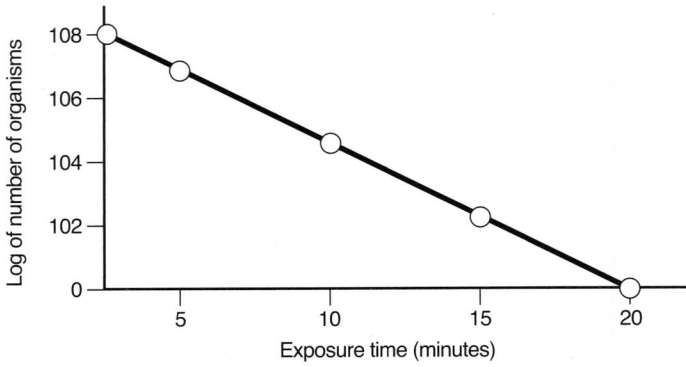

Figure 2-2

The effect of exposure time versus number of organisms.

tween object and agent. For optimal killing activity, instruments and surfaces should be cleansed of excess organic material before disinfection.

Nature of Surface to Be Disinfected

Certain medical instruments are manufactured of biomaterials that exclude the use of certain disinfection or sterilization methods because of possible damage to the instruments. An example is endoscopic instruments, which are readily damaged by the heat generated in an autoclave. Alternative methods must be used for this class of instruments.

METHODS OF DISINFECTION AND STERILIZATION

We have seen the way factors that affect the survival of microorganisms influence disinfection and sterilization. We will now look at the ways in which methods are selected. E.H. Spaulding categorized medical materials into three device classifications:

- Critical materials
- Semicritical materials
- Noncritical materials

Critical materials are those that invade sterile tissues or enter the vascular system. These materials are most likely to produce infection if contaminated and therefore require sterilization. Before semicritical materials come into contact with mucous membranes,

they require high-level disinfection agents. Noncritical materials require intermediate-level to low-level disinfection before contact with intact skin. High-level disinfectants have activity against bacterial endospores, whereas intermediate-level disinfectants have tuberculocidal activity but not sporicidal activity. Finally, low-level disinfectants have a wide range of activity against microorganisms but do not demonstrate sporicidal or tuberculocidal activity. Table 2-1 presents a summary of these principles.

Physical Methods

As mentioned earlier, sterilization and disinfection can be carried out by both physical and chemical methods. Although several physical methods are available, we will restrict our discussion to those methods most commonly used in a laboratory or hospital setting.

Heat

Because of its reliable effects, ease of use, and economy, heat is the most common method used for the elimination of microorganisms. Heat can be used in several ways. **Moist heat,** or *heat under steam pressure,* is the agent used in autoclaves. Putting steam under 1 atm of pressure or 15 psi achieves a temperature of 121° C. At this temperature, all microorganisms and their endospores are destroyed in approximately 15 minutes of exposure. The time varies somewhat according to the size of the object; the important factor is that the exposure time is sufficient for complete penetra-

TABLE 2-1

Device Classification and Methods of Effective Disinfection

Device Classification	Disinfection Method	Killing Action Against				
		Spores	Mycobacteria	Nonlipid Viruses	Fungi	Bacteria
Critical	Sterilization	+	+	+	+	+
	Steam					
	Dry heat					
	Gas					
	Chemical					
	Ionizing radiation					
Semicritical	High-level disinfection					
	2% glutaraldehyde	±	+	+	+	+
	Chlorine dioxide	±	+	+	+	+
	Wet pasteurization	−	+	+	+	+
Noncritical	Low-level disinfection:					
	Sodium hypochlorite	−	+	+	+	+
	Quaternary ammonium compounds	−	−	±	+	+
	Ethyl, isopropyl alcohol (70%-90%)	−	−	+	+	+
	Phenolics	−	±	+	+	+
	Iodophors	−	−	+	+	+

tion of the steam at the proper temperature. An added advantage of moist heat is the shorter time required for sterilization. (Heat in water is transferred more readily to a cool body than heat in air.) Moist heat is the sterilization method of choice for heat-stable objects.

Dry heat may also be used as a sterilizing agent, although it requires much longer exposure times and higher temperatures than moist heat. This method may be used for heat-stable substances that are not penetrated by moist heat, such as oils. Dry heat is commonly used to sterilize glassware.

Boiling and **pasteurization** are both methods that achieve disinfection but not sterilization; neither method eliminates spores. Boiling (100° C) kills most microorganisms in approximately 10 minutes. Pasteurization, used mostly in the food industry, eliminates food-borne pathogens as well as organisms responsible for food spoilage. It is carried out at 63° C for 30 minutes. The main advantage of pasteurization is that treatment at this temperature reduces spoilage of food without affecting its taste.

Table 2-2 summarizes the applications of heat.

TABLE 2-2

Control of Microorganisms Using Health Methods

Method	Temperature (°C)	Time Required	Applications
Boiling water (steam)	100	15 minutes	Kills microbial vegetative forms Endospores survive
Autoclave (steam under pressure)	121.6	15 minutes at 15 psi	Sterilizes and kills endospores
Pasteurization			
Batch method	63	30 minutes	Disinfects and kills milk-borne pathogens and vegetable forms, but endospores survive
Flash methods	72	15 seconds	Same, but shorter time at higher temperature
Over (dry heat)	160-180	1.5-3 hours	Sterilizes; keeps materials dry

Adapted from VanDemark PJ, Batzing BL: *The microbes: an introduction to their nature and importance,* Redwood City, Calif, 1987, Benjamin-Cummings.

Filtration

Filtration methods may be used with both liquid and air. **Filtration** of liquids is accomplished through the use of thin membrane filters composed of plastic polymers or cellulose esters. The liquid is pulled through small, mechanically introduced pores with a vacuum. Organisms larger than the size of the pores are retained. Filters with various pore sizes are available. Bacteria, yeasts, and molds are retained by pore sizes 0.45 μm and 0.80 μm, which may also allow passage of *Pseudomonas*-like organisms; therefore a 0.22-μm size is available for critical sterilizing (e.g., parenteral solutions). Membranes with pore sizes as small as 0.01 μm are capable of retaining small viruses. The most common application of filtration is in the sterilization of heat-sensitive solutions, such as vaccines and antibiotic solutions. Filtration of air is accomplished with the use of high-efficiency particulate air (HEPA) filters. These filters are able to remove microorganisms larger than 0.3 μm and are used in laboratory hoods and in rooms of immunocompromised patients.

Radiation

Radiation may be used in two forms, ionizing and nonionizing. Ionizing radiation, in the form of gamma rays or electron beams, is of short wavelength and high energy. This method of sterilization is used by the medical industry for the sterilization of disposable supplies, such as syringes, catheters, and gloves. Nonionizing radiation in the form of ultraviolet rays is of long wavelength and low energy. Because of its poor penetrability, the usefulness of nonionizing radiation is limited; it is commonly used to disinfect surfaces.

Chemical Methods

Just as physical methods are used mainly to achieve sterilization, chemical agents are used mainly as disinfectants. Some chemical agents, however, may be used to sterilize. These are known as *chemosterilizers*. All disinfectants are regulated by the U.S. Environmental Protection Agency (EPA). Chemical agents exert their killing effect by the following mechanisms:

- Reaction with components of the cytoplasmic membrane

- Denaturation of cellular proteins
- Reaction with the thiol (−SH) groups of enzymes
- Damage of RNA and DNA

The fact that agents can exert one or a combination of actions on microorganisms is important to remember. Damage to the integrity of the cytoplasmic membrane causes the cytoplasm and its contents to leak out, resulting in cell death. Denaturation of proteins effectively disrupts the metabolism of the cells. Some agents specifically react with the thiol (−SH) groups of enzymes, thereby inactivating them. Thiol groups occur usually as the amino acid cysteine. Finally, damage to RNA and DNA inhibits the replication of the organism. For ease of discussion, we group the chemical agents on the basis of chemical composition. Table 2-3 summarizes the applications of chemicals commonly used as disinfectants and antiseptics.

Alcohols

The two most effective alcohols used in hospitals for disinfection purposes are ethyl alcohol and isopropyl alcohol. Although alcohols have a wide spectrum, they are nonsporicidal. This and several other factors limit their use as disinfectants. Because their action is greatly reduced in concentrations less than 50%, alcohols should be used in concentrations between 60% and 90%. Contact time is also reduced because of their rapid evaporation and inability to penetrate organic material. Alcohols inactivate microorganisms by denaturing proteins. They are used principally as antiseptics and disinfectants for small areas, such as injection vial septa and thermometers.

Aldehydes

FORMALDEHYDE
Formaldehyde is an aldehyde generally used as formalin, a 37% aqueous solution of formaldehyde gas. Although it can be used as a chemosterilizer in high concentrations, its usefulness is limited by its adverse effects. Formaldehyde has been found to be a carcinogen, and the U.S. Occupational Safety and Health Administration (OSHA) has set worker exposure limits. In addition, it is highly irritating and is slow acting because of poor penetrability.

TABLE 2-3

Chemical Agents Commonly Used As Disinfectants and Antiseptics

Type	Agent(s)	Action(s)	Applications and Precautions
Alcohols (50%-70%)	Ethanol, isopropanol, benzyl alcohol	Denature proteins; make lipids soluble	Skin antiseptics
Aldehydes (in solution)	Formaldehyde (8%), glutaraldehyde (2%)	React with NH_2, $-SH$, and $-COOH$ groups	Disinfectants; kill endospores Toxic to humans
Halogens	Tincture of iodine (2% in 70% alcohol)	Inactivates proteins	Skin disinfectants
	Chlorine and chlorine compounds	Reacts with water to form hypochlorous acid (HClO); oxidizing agent	Used to disinfect drinking water Surface disinfectants
Heavy metals	Silver nitrate ($AgNO_3$)	Precipitates proteins	Eye drop (1% solution)
	Mercuric chloride ($HgCl_2$)	Reacts with $-SH$ groups Lyses cell membrane	Disinfectant: toxic at high concentrations
Detergents	Quaternary ammonium compounds	Disrupt cell membranes	Skin antiseptics; disinfectants
Phenolics	Phenol, carbolic acid, Lysol, hexachlorophene	Denature proteins; disrupt cell membranes	Disinfectants at high concentrations; used in soaps at low concentrations
Gases	Ethylene oxide	Alkylating agent	Sterilization of heat-sensitive objects

Adapted from VanDemark PJ, Batzing BL: *The microbes: an introduction to their nature importance,* Redwood City, Calif, 1987, Benjamin-Cummings.

GLUTARALDEHYDE

Glutaraldehyde is also an aldehyde—more precisely, a saturated five-carbon dialdehyde that has broad-spectrum activity and rapid killing action and remains active in the presence of organic matter. Glutaraldehyde is extremely susceptible to pH changes because it is active only in an alkaline environment. When used as a 2% solution, it is germicidal in approximately 10 minutes and sporicidal in 3 to 10 hours. Its killing activity is due to inactivation of DNA and RNA through alkylation of sulfhydryl and amino groups. Because it does not corrode lenses, metal, or rubber, it is the sterilizer of choice for medical equipment that is not heat-stable and therefore cannot be autoclaved and for material that cannot be gas-sterilized.

Halogens

IODINE

Iodine can be used as a disinfectant in one of two forms: tincture or iodophore. Tinctures are alcohol and iodine solutions, used mainly as antiseptics. An iodophore is a combination of iodine and a neutral polymer carrier that increases the solubility of the agent. This combination allows the slow release of

iodine. Iodophores have the added advantage of being less irritating, nonstaining, and more stable than iodine in its pure form. Iodophores may be used as antiseptics or disinfectants, depending on the concentration of free iodine. The best-known iodophore is povidone-iodine, which is mainly used as an antiseptic. Iodophores are used only as disinfectants because they are not sporicidal. Their bactericidal action is due to the oxidative effects of molecular iodine (I_2) and hypoiodic acid (HOI), both of which are found in solution.

CHLORINE AND CHLORINE COMPOUNDS

Chlorine and chlorine compounds are some of the oldest and most commonly used disinfectants. They are usually used in the form of hypochlorites, such as the liquid sodium hypochlorite (household bleach) and solid calcium hypochloride. Their killing activity is based on the oxidative effects of hypochlorous acid, formed when chloride ions are dissolved in water, on microbial enzyme systems. Hypochlorites are inexpensive and have a broad spectrum of activity; however, they are not used as sterilants because of the long exposure time required for sporicidal action and their inactivation by organic matter. Hypochlorites are corrosive, and hypochlorite solutions are greatly influenced by the pH of the surrounding medium. They are commonly used as surface disinfectants (e.g., for tabletops and CPR mannequins). Their most important use is, of course, the chlorination of water.

Heavy metals

Disinfectants containing heavy metals are now rarely used in clinical applications; they have been replaced by more effective compounds. Slowly bactericidal, the action of heavy metal disinfectants is primarily bacteriostatic. Because of the toxic effects of mercuric chloride and other mercury compounds, their use as disinfectants has declined, and they are used mainly as preservatives for paint. Silver nitrate (1% eyedrop solution) has been used as a prophylactic treatment to prevent gonococcal conjunctivitis in newborns.

Detergents: quaternary ammonium compounds

Quaternary ammonium compounds are derived by substitution of the four-valence ammonium ion with alkyl halides. They are cationic, surface-active agents, or surfactants, that work by reducing the surface tension of molecules in a liquid. Their effectiveness is reduced by hard water and soap, and they are inactivated by excess organic matter. Their bactericidal action is mediated through disruption of the cellular membrane, resulting in leakage of cell contents. Because they are not sporicidal or tuberculocidal, the use of quaternary ammonium compounds is limited to disinfection of noncritical surfaces such as bench tops and floors.

Phenolics

Phenolics are molecules of phenol (carbolic acid) that have been chemically substituted, typically by halogens, alkyl, phenyl, or benzyl groups. These groups serve to increase the bactericidal effectiveness of phenol. The most common are ortho-phenylphenol and ortho-benzyl-para-chlorophenol. Phenolics have a fairly broad bactericidal spectrum but are not sporicidal. They are stable, biodegradable, and relatively active in the presence of organic soil. Their mechanism of inactivation is disruption of cell walls, resulting in precipitation of proteins. At lower concentrations, they are able to disrupt enzyme systems. Their main use is in the disinfection of hospital, institutional, and household environments. They are also commonly found in germicidal soaps.

Gases

Ethylene oxide is the gas most commonly used for sterilization. Because it is explosive in its pure form, it is mixed with nitrogen or carbon dioxide before use. Factors such as temperature, time, and relative humidity are extremely important in determining the effectiveness of gas sterilization. The recommended concentration is 450 to 700 mg of ethylene oxide per liter of chamber space at 55° to 60° C for 2 hours. A relative humidity of 30% is optimal for the destruction of spores. The killing mechanism of ethylene oxide is the alkylation of nucleic acids in the spore and vegetative cell. Gas sterilization is widely used in hospitals for materials that cannot withstand steam sterilization. This method is also used extensively by the manufacturing industry for the sterilization of low-cost thermoplastic products.

LEARNING ASSESSMENT

1. What is the difference between sterilization and disinfection?

2. When is an antiseptic used?

3. Boiling water kills spores: true or false?

4. What method is required to effectively kill endospores?

5. Which chemical component or agent is used in soaps at low concentrations?

B. MICROBIOLOGY LABORATORY SAFETY

Margaret Gregory

GENERAL SAFETY PRINCIPLES
   Safety Program for the Microbiology Laboratory

HANDLING OF BIOLOGIC HAZARDS
   Major Sources of Biologic Hazards
      Processing of patient specimens
      Working with actively growing cultures
   OSHA Regulations for Blood-Borne Pathogens

DISPOSAL OF INFECTIOUS WASTE

CHEMICAL SAFETY
   Employee Right-to-Know
   Material Safety Data Sheets

   Hazardous Chemicals Inventory
   Laboratory Safety for Hazardous Chemicals

HAZARDOUS WASTE REDUCTION

FIRE SAFETY
   Thermal Injuries

ELECTRICAL SAFETY

MISCELLANEOUS SAFETY CONSIDERATIONS
   Back Safety
   Storage of Gases
   First Aid Training
   Immunizations

SAFETY TRAINING

OBJECTIVES

1. Describe the safe handling, storage, and disposal of chemicals and radioactive substances.
2. Describe the major sources of biologic hazards in the microbiology laboratory.
3. Discuss the use of the different types of biologic safety cabinets.
4. Discuss the practice of universal precautions.
5. Describe the different levels of protection and when each is applied.
6. Name the common hazardous chemicals in the laboratory.
7. Describe the methods of hazardous water reduction.
8. Describe the different types of fire extinguishers and when each is used.

KEY TERMS

Blood-borne pathogen
Universal precautions
Personal protective devices
Biohazard
High-efficiency particulate air (HEPA) filters
Employee right-to-know
National Fire Protection Association (NFPA) hazard-rating diamond
Material safety data sheets (MSDSs)

The concept of laboratory safety has changed drastically in the last decade. Before 1980, safety practices in most microbiology laboratories were lax. Mouth pipetting was a widely used technique, and eating, drinking, and smoking in the laboratory, although discouraged, were common. Beginning in the early 1980s, this relaxed attitude toward safety among personnel changed dramatically. The impetus behind the change was the arrival in the United States of a previously unheard-of disease with an apparent 100% mortality rate. This disease became known as the acquired immune deficiency syndrome (AIDS). In addition to being a global calamity, AIDS initiated a major rethinking of employee risk for laboratory-acquired infections in hospitals around the country. Beginning with an emphasis on reducing the risks of biologic hazards (biohazards), safety became a priority for laboratory personnel. The attitude "What you don't know can't hurt you," common among laboratory employees, rapidly went out of date. With the passage of time, the concept of laboratory safety expanded to include chemical, radioactive, electrical, and fire hazard protection. Currently, microbiologists must pay special attention to all safety measures employed by the laboratory for their protection.

This section of Chapter 2 discusses the following topics:

- A safety program in the microbiology laboratory
- Pertinent state and federal regulations
- Procedures in handling biohazardous, chemical, radioactive wastes and materials

GENERAL SAFETY PRINCIPLES

Safety in the microbiology laboratory can be best achieved by a combination of knowledge and common sense. Knowing current safety regulations, incorporating them into safety procedures manuals, and teaching the procedures to each employee through in-service education should be the duties of an assigned safety officer. Although the provision of a safe work environment is ultimately the employer's responsibility, it cannot be achieved without the commitment of all persons in that environment to practice safe techniques for their own and their coworkers' protection.

Because microbiology laboratory personnel frequently deal with a variety of infectious agents—viral, bacterial, parasitic, and mycobacterial—laboratory-acquired infection is an obvious hazard. The case study at the beginning of this chapter illustrated a laboratory-acquired infection that could have been prevented with the use of proper precautions. There are, however, many unseen hazards that also need to be addressed to provide a comprehensive and thorough safety program.

Safety Program for the Microbiology Laboratory

The comprehensive safety program for the microbiology laboratory needs to fulfill the following:

- Address biologic hazards
- Describe the safe handling, storage, and disposal of chemicals and radioactive substances
- Clearly outline the laboratory or hospital policies for correct procedures in the event of fire, natural disasters, and even bomb threats
- Teach correct techniques for lifting and moving heavy objects and patients

This safety program needs to be ongoing and consistent with current federal and state regulations. Most important, it must be presented in a way that encourages employees to incorporate these safety practices into their daily routines and take responsibility for keeping the work environment safe.

HANDLING OF BIOLOGIC HAZARDS

Major Sources of Biologic Hazards

Biologic hazards in the microbiology lab come from two major sources: (1) processing of the patient specimens and (2) handling of the actively growing cultures of microorganisms. Either activity puts the employee at risk of potential contact with infectious agents through mucous membranes (rubbing the nose or eyes with contaminated hands, similar to the case study), inhalation of aerosols of microorganisms, accidental ingestion (putting pens or fingers into the mouth), or needle sticks. Families of microbiology personnel and persons who work in adjacent laboratories may also be at risk. Table 2-4 lists the agents most commonly associated with laboratory-acquired infections.

Many infectious agents pose a high risk to laboratory employees. *Mycobacterium tuberculosis* has long been known to cause tuberculosis in laboratory workers exposed to aerosols created in processing sputum samples. A laboratory accident involving a spill of active *M. tuberculosis,* which could easily aerosolize through the ventilation system, is

TABLE 2-4

Most Common Agents Associated With Laboratory-Acquired Infections

Agent	Disease	Route(s) of Infection	Source(s)
Hepatitis B virus	Hepatitis	Oral, percutaneous	Specimen
Coccidioides immitis	Coccidioidomycosis	Pulmonary	Culture
Bacillus anthracis	Human anthrax	Pulmonary	Culture
Brucella species	Brucellosis	Pulmonary, oral percutaneous, eye	Specimen, culture
Mycobacterium tuberculosis	Tuberculosis	Pulmonary	Specimen, culture
Francisella tularensis	Tularemia	Unbroken skin, pulmonary	Culture
Shigella species	Shigellosis	Oral	Specimen, culture

every microbiologist's nightmare. *Brucella* species and *Franciscella tularensis* are other infectious agents that can be transmitted through inhalation of aerosol created during processing or handling of specimens (e.g., blood, which may harbor these organisms) or cultures of the organism. *Coccidioides immitis,* the most infectious of all the fungi, can infect several people in a room if culture plates on which the organism is growing are not sealed with tape or are open in the absence of a biosafety hood. In the 1970s, *Bacillus anthracis* was responsible for the deaths of a laboratory worker's wife and infant, who were infected through handling his contaminated laboratory coat.

Hepatitis B virus (HBV) can be transmitted to laboratory workers through needle-stick injuries. The Centers for Disease Control and Prevention (CDC) estimate that approximately 12,000 health care workers become accidentally infected with this **blood-borne pathogen** annually. Human immunodeficiency virus (HIV) is another blood-borne pathogen that may be transmitted to laboratory personnel from contaminated specimens through a needle-stick injury or another percutaneous route. Needless to say, all these infectious agents must be handled with extreme care. Laboratory workers must follow all necessary precautions to avoid exposure and minimize risks for exposure to these infectious agents.

Processing of patient specimens

Labeling only those specimens from patients diagnosed with hepatitis or AIDS and requiring "extra precautions" for dealing with these specimens do not provide adequate protection for laboratory workers. Many patients come into emergency rooms or are admitted to the hospital with no apparent diagnosis. These patients may be in the early stages of either disease and may be asymptomatic but still contagious. Because the incidence of both hepatitis and AIDS is increasing steadily, the likelihood of exposure to one or both of these blood-borne pathogens is also increasing.

UNIVERSAL PRECAUTIONS

The CDC and the U.S. Occupational Safety and Health Administration (OSHA) jointly published recommendations entitled **"Universal Precautions,"** which, simply stated, required that blood and body fluids from *all* patients be treated as infectious material (Box 2-1).

Protective protocol varies from institution to institution. For example, The Ohio State University Hospitals Microbiology Laboratory has incorporated a three "Levels of Protection" scheme for laboratory workers (Table 2-5). The scheme relates the level of precaution or protection required of an employee to the potential risk of infection for the laboratory work station and task to be performed.

Figure 2-3 illustrates goggles, masks, and laboratory garments appropriate for use in laboratory work stations.

Working with actively growing cultures

Many of the guidelines in place for the protection of microbiology personnel against exposure to blood-borne pathogens also apply to working with cultures of microorganisms at the bench. Hands must be washed frequently and kept away from the nose, mouth, and eyes. Adhesive bandages or small finger cots should be worn directly over cuts or hangnails. Any plates growing a fungus should immedi-

Box 2-1

Universal Precautions

1. Assume that patients are infectious for HIV and other blood-borne pathogens.
2. Place every specimen of blood or body fluid in a well-constructed container with a secure lid to prevent leaking during transport.
3. Whenever processing blood and body fluid specimens, wear gloves plus a face shield (or a mask with glasses or goggles) if there is a likelihood of spattering, and wash hands when finished processing specimens.
4. Never pipette by mouth; use pipetting aids.
5. Decontaminate all laboratory work surfaces with an appropriate chemical germicide after a spill of blood or other body fluids and when work activities are completed.
6. Limit use of needles and syringes to situations for which there are no other alternatives.
7. Decontaminate contaminated materials used in laboratory tests before reprocessing or place them into appropriately labeled biohazard bags for disposal in accordance with institutional policies.
8. Always wash hands after completing laboratory activities, and remove all protective clothing before leaving the laboratory.

---

ately be sealed, and the culture should then be worked on in a biosafety cabinet. Any cultures suspected of growing other potentially aerosolized infectious agents, such as *M. tuberculosis* or *Brucella* species, should also be worked on only in a biosafety cabinet. In an effort to educate those at risk for laboratory-acquired infection, CDC publishes a booklet entitled *Classification of Etiologic Agents on the Basis of Hazard,* which contains useful information on the degree of risk of biologic agents for laboratory workers.

To provide protection in the processing of patient specimens and handling of actively growing cultures in the microbiology laboratory, a combination of environmental and engineering or equipment controls, work practices, and **personal protective devices** are implemented. An example of an engineering control is the use of a Level II **biohazard** safety cabinet for plating of all specimens. This safety cabinet sterilizes the internal air containing infectious particles by passage through a **high-efficiency particulate air (HEPA) filter.** Examples of work practices include frequent handwashing (recommended after removing gloves and before leaving the laboratory); decontamination of all work stations with a 1:10 dilution of chlorine bleach (prepared fresh weekly); no eating, drinking, or smoking in the lab; and no application of cosmetics or lip balm in the laboratory. Personal protective devices are well-fitted gloves, needle resheathing devices, non–strike-through clothes covers, and face masks and goggles (or full-face shield). Figure 2-4 shows the three levels of biologic safety cabinets.

TABLE 2-5

Three Levels of Protection

Level	Protection Required	Activities
0	Clothes covers (wraparound cloth garments or laboratory coats or disposable cover)	Handling materials and performing tasks that do not involve contact with or exposure to blood, body fluids, body secretions, or tissue (e.g., reading routine culture plates at the bench)
1	Fitted gloves and non–strike-through disposable clothes cover	Presence at any laboratory work station where closed specimens are handled; specimen receiving (e.g., entering blood culture bottles into Bactec)
2	Fitted gloves, non–strike-through disposable clothes cover, and use of certified biologic safety cabinet–Class II; a mask and eye cover and faceshield must be worn if safety cabinet is not available	Processing and planting specimens for culture and direct examination on slides; venting blood culture bottles; performing any activity that can generate aerosols

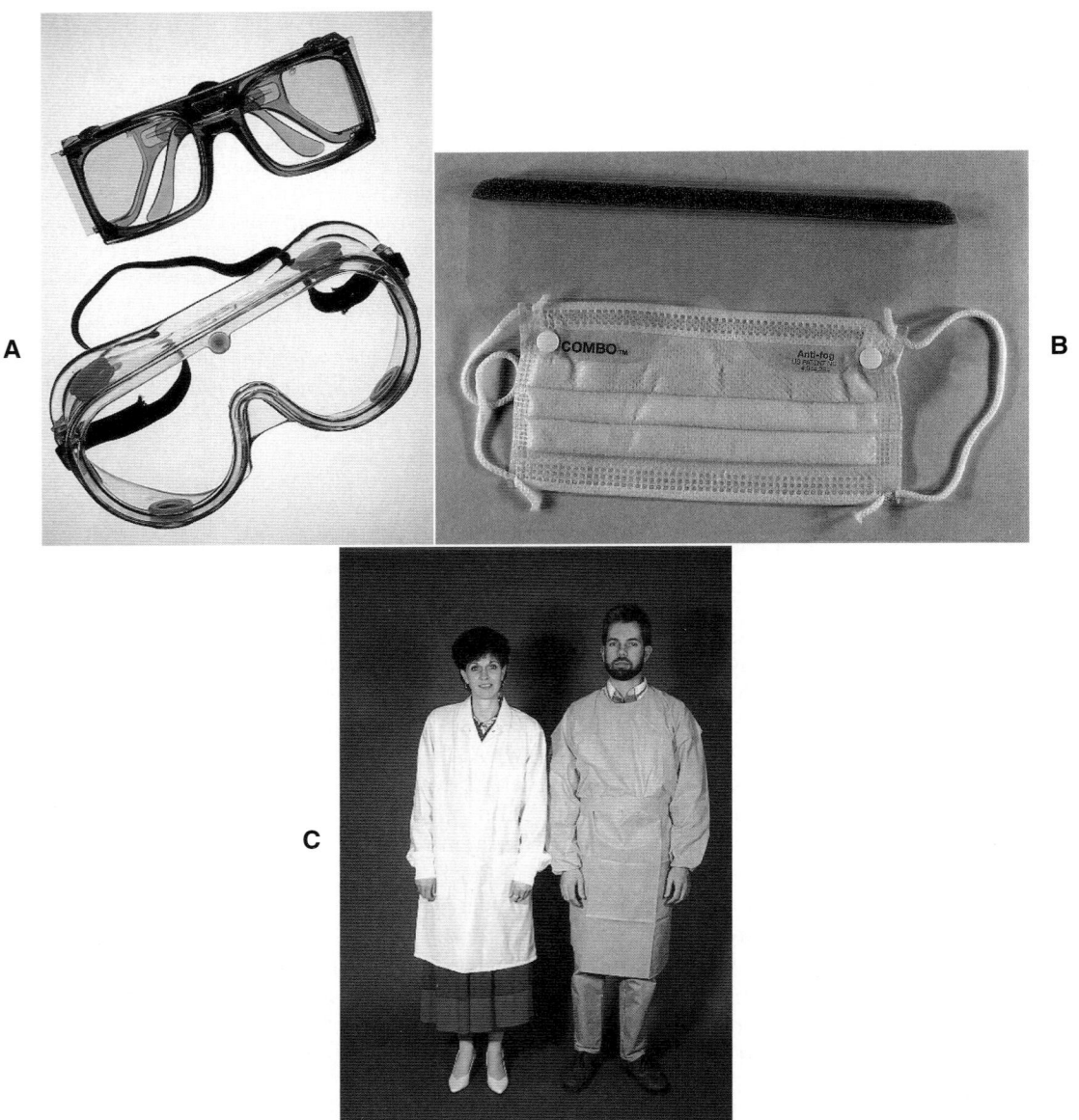

Figure 2-3

A, Eye protection used when chemical splashing could occur. **B,** Integrated eye protection and mask. **C,** Laboratory coats. The material of the white laboratory coat slows the penetration of liquids that splash or soak it. The blue coat on the right is disposable.

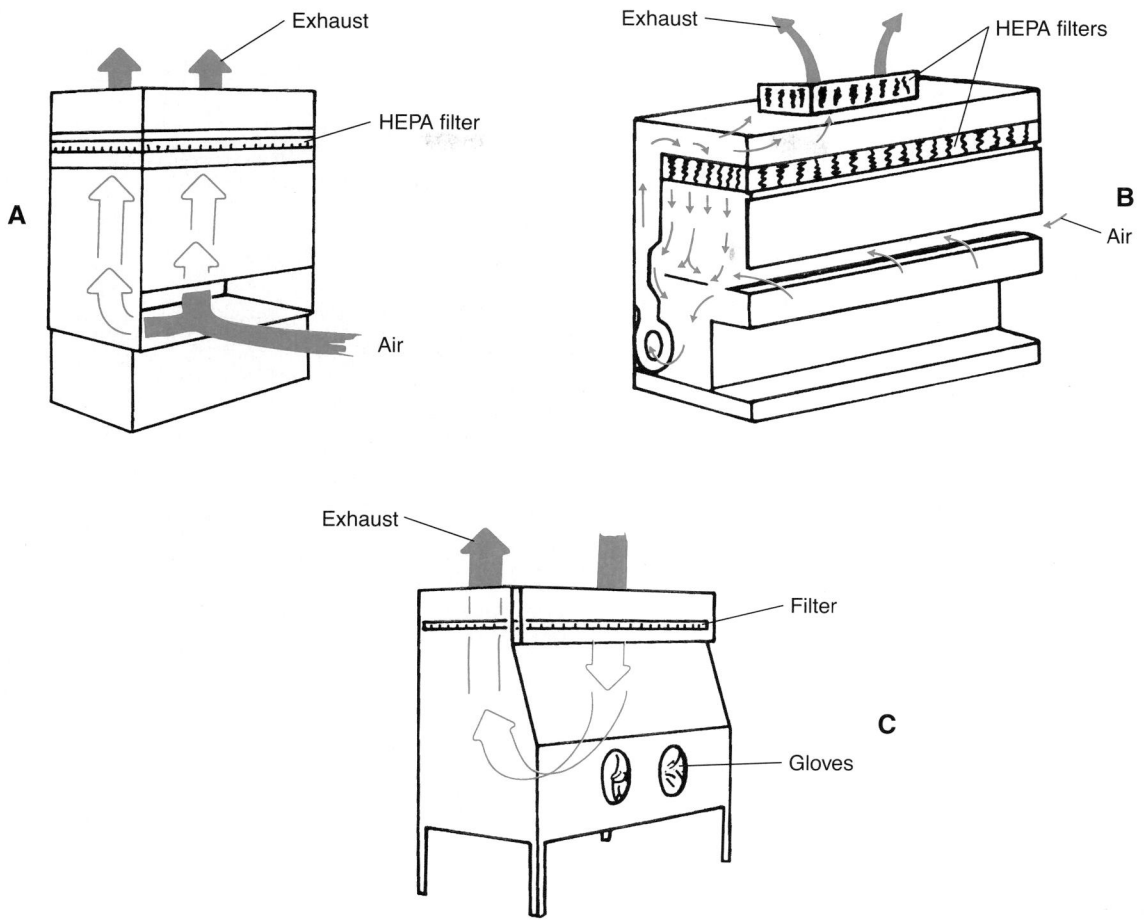

Figure 2-4 _____

A, The Class I biologic safety hood utilizes the same principle as the chemical fume hood. An exhaust fan moves the air inward through the open front. The air is uncirculated and is passed through a high-efficiency particulate air (HEPA) filter before reaching the environment. **B,** The Class II biologic safety hood is the most common in microbiology laboratories. Air is pulled inward and downward by a blower and passed up through the airflow plenum where it passes through a HEPA filter before reaching the work surface. A percentage of the remaining air is HEPA filtered before reaching the environment. **C,** The Class III biologic safety hood is a self-contained, ventilated system for highly infectious microorganisms or materials and provides the highest level of personal protection. The closed front contains attached gloves for manipulation on the work surface.

OSHA Regulations for Blood-Borne Pathogens

In 1992 the OSHA Final Rule on Blood-Borne Pathogens became effective. This document contains the following requirements:

- All personnel at risk for exposure to blood and body fluids must be identified by their employers.
- These personnel must be properly trained in the use of all personal protective devices and/or engineering controls required for their particular jobs and must receive counseling and follow-up treatment if exposure occurs.
- All employees at risk must receive annual retraining.
- All employees who work with infectious material must be offered the hepatitis B vaccination free of charge.

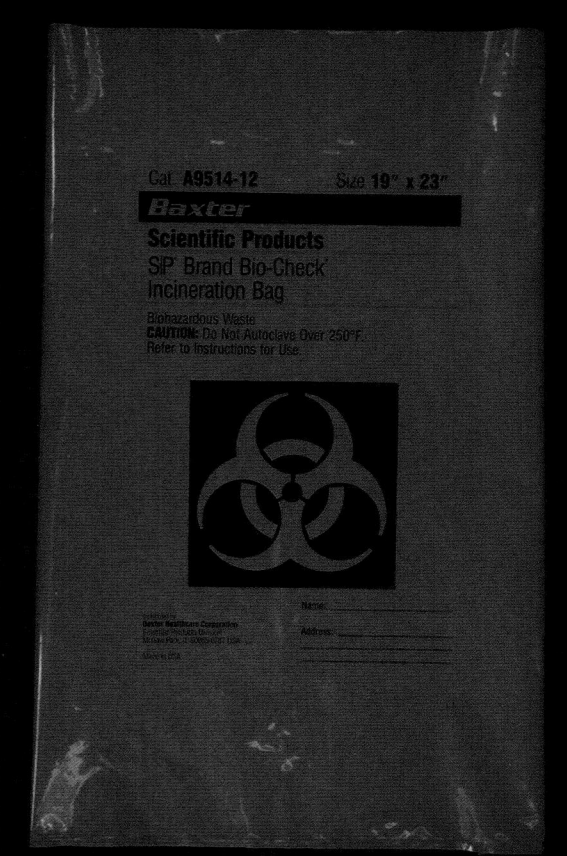

Figure 2-5 _____

Biohazard bag used to dispose of culture plates and other nonsharp contaminated materials. The bag is sealed and incinerated. In the center of the bag is the biohazard symbol.

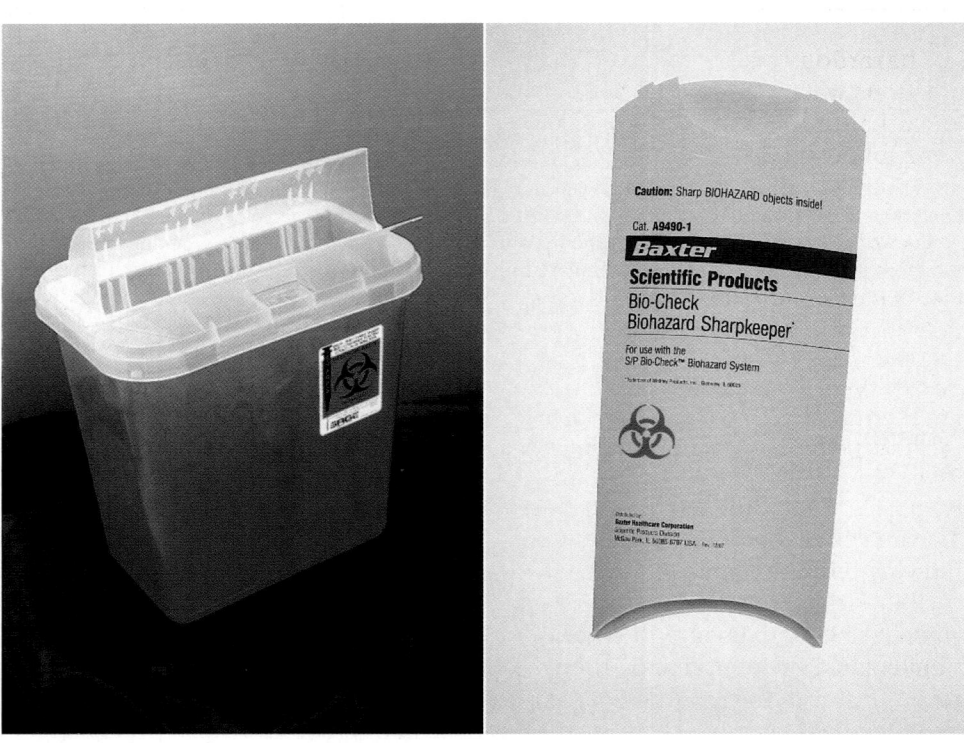

Figure 2-6 _____

Examples of biohazard containers for disposable needles, glass slides, and other sharp materials.

DISPOSAL OF INFECTIOUS WASTE

In addition to laboratory employees who work with potentially infectious material, the general public must be protected from exposure to these same materials after the laboratory or hospital has disposed of them. The surfacing of contaminated needles and other sharps along lake and ocean beaches has led to a public outcry to make hospitals accountable for their infectious waste disposal. In an effort to deal with this increasing problem, the U.S. Congress passed The Medical Wastes Tracing Act in 1988 to regulate the states of New York, New Jersey, Connecticut, and Rhode Island and Puerto Rico.

The microbiology laboratory's safety program must follow state and local regulations for the safe disposal of its infectious wastes, usually by either autoclaving or incineration. Warning signs containing the warning symbol for biohazardous materials must be placed on all biohazard wastes and material disposal containers. Figures 2-5 and 2-6 show disposal containers appropriate for contaminated and biohazardous materials.

CHEMICAL SAFETY

The scope of hazardous waste comprises more than just infectious waste. The National Committee for Clinical Laboratory Standards (NCCLS; 1986) gives the following definition of hazardous waste:

Considered in the laboratory sense, hazardous wastes are those substances which singly or in combination pose a significant present or potential threat or hazard to human health or to the environment and which singly or in combination require special handling, processing, or disposal because they are flammable, explosive, reactive, corrosive, toxic, infectious, carcinogenic, bioconcentrative-persistent in nature, potentially lethal, an irritant or a strong sensitizer.

Employee Right-to-Know

OSHA addresses employee safety with hazardous chemicals in 29 CFR 1910.1200, Hazard Communication Standard (HCS). This provides for a laboratory Chemical Hygiene Plan and a Hazard Communication, which states that all clinical laboratory personnel should have a thorough working knowledge of the hazards of the chemicals with which they come into contact, or **employee right-to-know.** All hazardous chemicals in the workplace must be identified and clearly labeled with the **National Fire Protection Association (NFPA) hazard-rating diamond,** stating risk for flammability, reactivity, and health (Figure 2-7).

Material Safety Data Sheets

Material safety data sheets (MSDSs) provided by the manufacturer for every hazardous chemical indicate the following:

- The nature of the chemical (e.g., flammable, toxic, carcinogenic)
- Precautions to take in using a chemical
- Spill clean-up procedure
- Disposal recommendations

An example of an MSDS is shown in Figure 2-8. These documents should be kept on file and
Text continued on p. 46

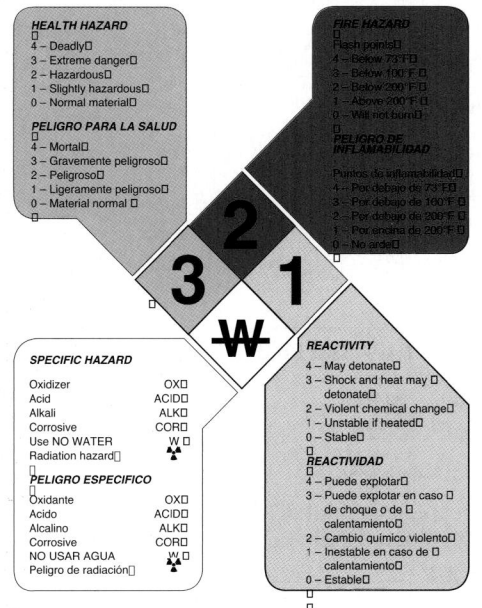

Figure 2-7

Hazardous material classification symbol. (Courtesy Lab Safety Supply, Inc., Janesville, Wis.)

MATERIAL SAFETY DATA SHEET

Material Safety Data Sheet **CHIRON RIBA (TM) HCV TEST SYSTEM SECOND GENERATION ASSAY—SUBSTRATE**	Page: 1 Rev. Date 09/19/94

Ortho Diagnostic Systems Inc.
U.S. Route 202
Raritan, NJ 08869

Telephone number: (800) 322-6374
Emergency phone number: (800) 424-9300

SECTION #1—IDENTIFICATION

Product: CHIRON RIBA (TM) HCV TEST SYSTEM SECOND GENERATION ASSAY—SUBSTRATE

Product Code: 933490

Synonyms: CHIRON RIBA HCV TEST SYS. 2ND GEN. ASSAY SUBSTRATE

This product is a component of the CHIRON RIBA (TM) HCV test system second generation assay.

SECTION #2—HAZARDOUS CHEMICAL COMPONENTS

Component: METHANOL
CAS Number: 67-56-1   Percent of mixture: 99.7%
    ACGIH TLV-TWA: 200 ppm (skin)   OSHA PEL-TWA: 200 ppm (skin)
    ACGIH TLV-STEL: 250 ppm (skin)   OSHA PEL-STEL: 200 ppm (skin)

SECTION #3—PHYSICAL DATA

Vapor pressure: not determined
Vapor density (air=1): not determined
Specific gravity: not determined
Percent volatiles: 99.7%

Appearance

Colorless liquid

Odor

Methanol (alcohol) odor

SECTION #4—FIRE FIGHTING AND EXPLOSION DATA

Flash point: 52° F
Autoignition: 725° F

Flammability class: IA

Lower explosive limit: 6%
Upper explosive limit: 36%

Figure 2-8 ——

Material safety data sheet. (Courtesy Ortho Diagnostic Systems, Inc., A Johnson & Johnson Company, Raritan, N.J.)

Material Safety Data Sheet **CHIRON RIBA (TM) HCV TEST SYSTEM SECOND GENERATION ASSAY—SUBSTRATE**	Page: 2 Rev. Date 09/19/94

SECTION #4—FIRE FIGHTING AND EXPLOSION DATA—cont'd

Fire and explosion hazards

Methanol is extremely flammable (flash point = 52° F). Its vapor may travel considerable distance to source of ignition and flash back.

Extinguishing media

Use foam, dry chemical or carbon dioxide, as suitable for the surrounding fire.

Special fire fighting instructions

Wear self-contained breathing apparatus and protective clothing that is appropriate for fighting a typical fire involving chemical materials.

SECTION #5—EXPOSURE EFFECTS AND FIRST AID

Route of exposure—inhalation

Overexposure may cause irritation of the nose and throat. Extensive inhalation may cause behavioral changes.

First aid—inhalation

Remove victim to fresh air. If necessary, get medical attention.

Route of exposure—skin

Contact may cause skin irritation.

First aid—skin

Promptly wash exposed areas thoroughly with soap and water.

Route of exposure—eyes

Contact may cause eye irritation.

First aid—eyes

Immediately flush eyes with low pressure water. Remove contact lenses to ensure a thorough flush, and continue to flush with water for at least 15 minutes. If irritation persists, get medical attention.

Route of exposure—ingestion

Ingestion may cause irritation of gastrointestinal tract. Swallowing methanol may be fatal or cause blindness and can cause behavioral changes.

First aid—ingestion

Contact a physician or the Poison Control Center.

Miscellaneous toxicological information

Carcinogenicity: NTP: No   IARC: No   OSHA: No

The health effects noted are based on the extrapolation of data on the pure product ingredients. To the best of our knowledge, no health effects have been identified for the product mixture under normal conditions of use, although the health effects of the product have not been thoroughly investigated.

Exposure to methanol can cause damage to the eyes, liver, heart, and kidneys.

Figure 2-8, cont'd ⎯⎯

For legend see opposite page.   *Continued*

Material Safety Data Sheet **CHIRON RIBA (TM) HCV TEST SYSTEM SECOND GENERATION ASSAY—SUBSTRATE**	Page: 3 Rev. Date 09/19/94

SECTION #5—EXPOSURE EFFECTS AND FIRST AID—cont'd

Miscellaneous toxicological information—cont'd

Methanol target organ data: Sense organs and special senses (optic nerve neuropathy, visual field changes); behavioral (headache); lungs, thorax, or respiration (dyspnea, other changes); gastrointestinal (nausea or vomiting). TARGET ORGANS: Eyes, kidneys.

SECTION #6—REACTIVITY AND POLYMERIZATION

Stability: stable

Incompatible materials

Methanol: acids, acid chlorides and anhydrides, oxidizing or reducing agents

Hazardous decomposition products

Not determined

Hazardous polymerization: will not occur

SECTION #7—SPILL, LEAK, AND DISPOSAL PROCEDURES

Steps to be taken in the event of spills, leaks, or release

Ventilate the area. Eliminate all sources of ignition. Cover with dry-lime, sand, or soda ash. Place in covered container. Wash spill site after material pickup is complete.

Waste disposal methods

Burn in a chemical incinerator equipped with an afterburner and scrubber, but exert extra care in igniting because methanol is highly flammable.

Dispose of in accordance with local, state, and federal regulations.

SARA Title III notifications and information

SARA Title III—Hazard classes: acute health hazard
chronic health hazard
fire hazard

SARA Title III—Section 313 supplier notification:

This product contains the following toxic chemicals subject to the reporting requirements of Section 313 of the Emergency Planning and Community Right-To-Know Act (EPCRA) of 1986 and of 40 CRF 372:

CAS #	Chemical Name	Percent of Mixture
67-56-1	METHANOL	99.7%

This information must be included on all MSDSs that are copied and distributed for this material.

Other Environmental Information

Figure 2-8, cont'd ─────────────────────

For legend see p. 42.

Material Safety Data Sheet **CHIRON RIBA (TM) HCV TEST SYSTEM SECOND GENERATION ASSAY—SUBSTRATE**	Page: 4 Rev. Date 09/19/94

SECTION #8—SPECIAL PROTECTIVE MEASURES

Ventilation

None normally required

Eye protection

Safety glasses, goggles, or full-face shield

Skin protection

Latex gloves

Respiratory protection

None normally required; dust respirator (disposable) when ventilation is inadequate

Other protection

Lab coat

Work/hygienic practices

CAUTION: This product is intended for use with human blood or blood elements. All blood components and products containing blood components should be handled and disposed as if capable of transmitting infectious agents.

SECTION #9—SPECIAL PRECAUTIONS—STORAGE AND HANDLING

Storage and handling conditions

Keep refrigerated at 2° C-8° C until use.

SECTION #10—SHIPPING INFORMATION

Proper shipping name: none required

SECTION #11—MISCELLANEOUS COMMENTS AND REFERENCE DOCUMENTATION

Primary references used in the preparation of this document:

1. Ortho Diagnostics product circular
2. OSHA Z-Table, 1910.1000 (revised final rule)
3. ACGIH threshold limit values and biological exposure indices (1991-1992)
4. Methanol MSDS (Sigma Chemical Co., 4/17/90)

N/A = not applicable   ~ = approximately equal to

DISCLAIMER OF EXPRESSED AND IMPLIED WARRANTIES

Although reasonable care has been taken in the preparation of this document, we extend no warranties and make no representations as to the accuracy or completeness of the information contained therein and assume no responsibility regarding the suitability of this information for the user's intended purposes or for the consequences of its use. Each individual should make a determination as to the suitability of the information for their particular purpose(s).

Ortho Diagnostic Systems Inc.

Figure 2-8, cont'd ——

For legend see p. 42.

made available to every employee. Some of the more common hazardous chemicals that can be found in the microbiology laboratory are listed in Box 2-2.

Hazardous Chemicals Inventory

The laboratory must maintain a current inventory of hazardous chemicals, which must be updated annually, and the MSDSs for those particular chemicals. The following four sources should be consulted in preparing an inventory:

- 29 CFR Part 1910, Subpart Z, Toxic and Hazardous Substances, OSHA
- National Toxicology Program Annual Report on Carcinogens
- International Agency for Cancer Research Monographs
- Manufacturers' material safety data sheets

Laboratory Safety for Hazardous Chemicals

Fume hoods must be provided to prevent inhalation of fumes. Such a hood may be vented to the outside or may be a tabletop model with charcoal filters attached that can be periodically replaced. Personal protective devices, such as fume masks, gloves, aprons, and eyewear, must be used in the

WARNING SIGNS AND SYMBOLS	POTENTIAL DANGER
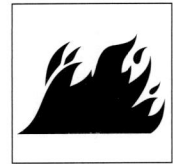	Flammable
	Toxic hazard Poisonous
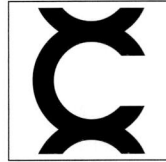	Carcinogenic Cancer-causing agent
	Corrosive Harmful to mucous membranes, skin, eyes, or tissues
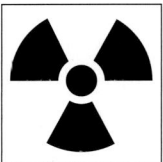	Radiation Radioactive material present

Figure 2-9 _____
Miscellaneous warning signs and symbols.

case of a large spill to protect the workers from exposure. Acid spill kits and flammable spill kits should be kept in areas where such substances are used. Warning signs and symbols, as shown in Figure 2-9, must be placed in appropriate locations. Employees must be able to recognize each of these symbols and must be knowledgeable about the danger each indicates and the proper precautions that must be observed.

Box 2-2

Hazardous Chemicals Commonly Used in the Microbiology Laboratory

Flammables
Methanol
Acetone
Ethanol

Potential or proven carcinogens
Formaldehyde
Aniline (crystal violet) stain
Auramine-rhodamine (Truant) stain

Irritants and corrosives
Hydrogen peroxide
Acids: HCl, H_2SO_4, acetic acid
NaOH

HAZARDOUS WASTE REDUCTION

The EPA has also made recommendations for hazardous waste reduction through the following methods:

- Substitute less hazardous chemicals when possible
- Develop procedures that use less of a hazardous chemical
- Recycle chemicals when possible
- Segregate infectious wastes from uncontaminated trash
- Substitute micromethodology in antibiotic susceptibility testing and identification of organisms to reduce volume of chemical reagents as well as infectious waste

FIRE SAFETY

Bunsen burners and other open-flame burners are among the biggest sources of fire hazards in the clinical microbiology laboratory. Employees must strive not to be careless or negligent in the use of this equipment. Flammable materials should never be opened near a Bunsen burner in use. Another hazard associated with Bunsen burners and other open-flame burners is the fuel. Bunsen burners use a gas. A leaking gas line may be a source of explosion or may cause illness in employees who work near the leak. If gas lines are in use, any lines that are not used daily should be connected to a burner and the gas burned for 5 minutes once a month to prevent "falling out" of the mercaptans (the odor of which alerts personnel to a possible leak). Other burners use a flammable liquid as the fuel, which is in itself a hazard. If at all possible, the use of burners should be replaced with other methods or techniques, such as fixing slides with methanol or using disposable loops. Other sources of ignition are heating elements, hot plates, and spark gaps in motors and light switches.

All personnel must be thoroughly trained in the procedure for responding to a fire emergency. Most institutions use the acronym *RACE:*

- **Rescue:** Remove anyone who is in danger. The safety of handicapped personnel (deaf or physically disabled) should be a priority.
- **Alarm:** Know where the nearest fire pull box or alarm station is located and the number to call to report the fire.
- **Contain:** Close doors to contain fire and smoke.
- **Extinguish:** Use the properly rated fire extinguisher on small fires, as described in Table 2-6. If the situation is out of control, the best course of action is to evacuate.

The fire evacuation plan must be posted, and employees should be familiar with fire exit locations and evacuation procedures. Periodic fire drills should be conducted to ensure that all personnel react quickly and efficiently in case of a real fire emergency. The drills should include both exit and nonexit procedures. Exit drills will familiarize personnel with the escape routes and location of fire doors and stairwells. Nonexit procedures alert personnel to the potential for evacuation if the fire is located elsewhere in the building. The laboratory should be kept free of clutter, and exitways should remain clear of obstructions.

Thermal Injuries

Personnel should be warned of any hot surface or situation in which the potential for burns is present. Use of long thermal gloves that extend to the shoulder is recommended when reaching into autoclaves or hot-air ovens. Signs should be posted warning employees about hot instruments or

TABLE 2-6

Classes of Fire Extinguishers

Symbol	Class	Use
Ⓐ	A	Fires in ordinary combustible materials, such as wood, cloth, paper, rubber, and many plastics; contains water or dry chemical to *cool*
Ⓑ	B	Fires in flammable liquids, gases, and greases; contains CO_2 or dry chemical to *smother*
Ⓒ	C	Fires involving electrical equipment, for which the electrical nonconductivity of the extinguishing media is important; contains CO_2 or dry chemical to *smother* without damaging the equipment

flasks that have just been sterilized. Burns may also come from extremely low temperatures found with use of liquid nitrogen or freezers that maintain temperatures below 70° C.

ELECTRICAL SAFETY

Today's microbiology laboratories contain many instruments. Each instrument must undergo regular preventive maintenance to ensure that it is functioning properly and in the best repair. Electrical cords should be checked for fraying. All cords should have grounded (three-pronged) plugs. Electrical grounding and leakage checks are required annually by the College of American Pathologists (CAP), an organization that provides accreditation to laboratories. Electrical equipment should never be placed near safety showers because of the risk of electrocution.

MISCELLANEOUS SAFETY CONSIDERATIONS

Box 2-3 summarizes general laboratory safety design, controls, and procedures.

Back Safety
The best way to care for the back is to prevent back injuries. Carrying heavy trays of culture plates, lifting heavy loads into and out of the autoclaves, and sitting or standing improperly can all contribute to back stress or injury. The following are some ways to prevent back injuries:

- Using the legs to lift, not the back
- Asking for assistance or using a cart when a load is too heavy
- Using good posture
- Staying physically fit

Storage of Gases
Flammable and nonflammable gas cylinders in use in the laboratory must be properly secured or stored and secured in vented areas.

Because a leaking pressurized gas cylinder may become a potential "missile," care must be taken to avoid accidental breakage or removal of

---

Box 2-3

Recommended Laboratory Safety Design and Practices

Engineering controls and equipment

Biosafety cabinets for processing specimens
Rigid-walled needle containers for disposal of needles
Foot pedals at sinks for "hands-off" water flow control
Automated blood culture systems in place of blind subcultures and Gram stains from blood bottles
"Closed-head" centrifuges
Fume hoods

Work practices

Frequent handwashing
No mouth pipetting
No eating, drinking, smoking, or applying of cosmetics in the laboratory
Use of carts for transporting trays of cultures
Disinfecting of work stations at end of each shift
Storage of flammables in "Flammable" storage cupboards

Personal protective devices

Gloves
Hospital-laundered lab coats
Non–strike-through clothes covers
Goggles/masks
Full-face masks
Needle resheathing devices
MSDS sheets

Environmental controls

Air flow from low-risk to high-risk areas within laboratory
Limited access to high-risk areas
Good ventilation

---

the pressure valve on top. The metal cap that protects this valve on top of the cylinder must be kept in place when the cylinder is not in use.

First Aid Training
All personnel should be trained in CPR and other life-saving first aid so that they will be able to act quickly in an emergency involving either fellow workers or patients.

Immunizations

OSHA requires that the hepatitis B vaccination be offered free of charge to all personnel who are at risk for exposure to blood-borne pathogens. Microbiology personnel working with sputum specimens or mycobacterial cultures should be screened for exposure to *M. tuberculosis* with an annual TB skin test.

| SAFETY TRAINING

To be in compliance with the OSHA standard as required by Joint Commission for the Accreditation of Healthcare Organizations (JCAHO), safety training must be documented. Training must include the following safety issues:

- **Fire:** knowledge of how and when to report fires, the location of the nearest alarm box and fire extinguishers, how to use fire extinguishers in small fires, and blocking of fire doors.
- **Hazardous materials management:** how to use material safety data sheets.
- **Proper storage of gases**
- **Blood-borne pathogens program:** appropriate practice of infection control, how to handle sharps, compliance with exposure control plan, and handling of biologic spills.

Safety training programs for microbiology personnel should be conducted annually to keep safe techniques fresh in everyone's mind. New personnel should be thoroughly trained in safety proce-dures for the department within 2 weeks of their hiring. It is a good idea to focus on one safety topic at a time and to make the training sessions enjoyable. Safety is each employee's responsibility.

Bibliography

Baron EJ, Finegold SM, editors: *Bailey & Scott's diagnostic microbiology,* ed 8, St Louis, 1990, Mosby.

Block SS, editor: *Disinfection, sterilization, and preservation,* ed 3, Philadelphia, 1983, Lea & Febiger.

Buesching W, Neff JC, Sharma HM: Infectious hazards in the clinical laboratory: a program to protect laboratory personnel, *Clin Lab Med* 9 (2):351, 1989.

Favero MS, Bond WW: Sterilization, disinfection, and antisepsis in the hospital. In Balows A, editor: *Manual of clinical microbiology,* ed 5, Washington, DC, 1991, American Society for Clinical Microbiology.

Kruse RH: *Microbiological Safety Cabinetry* (monograph). Lexington, Ky, Sept, 1981, Medico-Biological Environmental Development Institute.

National Committee for Clinical Laboratory Standards: *Proposed guidelines GP5-P: clinical laboratory hazardous waste,* Villanova, Pa, 1992, NCCLS.

Richardson JH, Barkley WE: Biological safety in the clinical laboratory. In Lennette EH et al, editors: *Manual of clinical microbiology,* ed 4, Washington, DC, 1985, American Society for Clinical Microbiology.

Rutala WA: APIC Guidelines for Selection and Use of Disinfectants, *Am J Infect Control* 18:99, 1990.

The Occupational Safety & Health Administration: Bloodborne Pathogens Standards, CFR, Washington, DC, 1991, OSHA.

Spaulding EH: Chemical disinfection and antisepsis in the hospital, *J Hosp Res* 9:5, 1972.

VanDemark PJ, Batzing BL: *The microbes: an introduction to their nature and importance,* Redwood City, Calif, 1987, Benjamin-Cummings.

LEARNING ASSESSMENT

1. By requiring their employers to offer the Hepatitis B vaccine free of charge, OSHA seeks to protect employees who are at risk for exposure to Hepatitis B: true or false?

2. Material Safety Data Sheets (MSDS) are important to employees because they contain information relating to which of the following?
   a. Blood-borne pathogens
   b. Fume hoods
   c. Chemical safety
   d. Fire extinguishers

3. Which of the following would be a correct definition of universal precautions?
   a. Wearing only gloves to handle blood and body fluids
   b. Viewing all specimens as potentially infectious and using the appropriate protective equipment
   c. Delaying testing of blood and body fluids pending results of HIV and Hepatitis B antigen testing
   d. Flagging only those specimens that come from patients who are known HIV carriers for "extra precautions"

4. What type of filter does a Class II biologic safety cabinet use to filter out infectious agents?
   a. Millipore filters
   b. HEPA filters
   c. Dust filters
   d. Charcoal filters

5. Infectious agents can enter the body through which of the following routes?
   a. Inhalation
   b. Ingestion
   c. Inoculation
   d. All of the above

Continued

LEARNING ASSESSMENT—cont'd

6. Employees can remember the steps to take in case of a fire by remembering which of the following acronyms?
   a. RUSH
   b. REST
   c. RACE
   d. RISK

7. How often must safety training for laboratory employees be conducted for compliance with OSHA regulations?
   a. Annually
   b. Quarterly
   c. At time of employment only
   d. No set requirement

8. Briefly describe the NFPA hazard-rating diamond found on all chemical containers to warn employees of potential hazards associated with that chemical.

9. Washing hands frequently, disinfecting work areas, using needle-resheathing devices, wearing gloves, and using other forms of barrier protection when handling specimens are examples of which of the following?
   a. Universal precautions
   b. Safe work habits
   c. Responsible methods of fire safety
   d. Chemical hygiene

10. List four hazardous chemicals commonly found in a microbiology laboratory.

CHAPTER 3

Concepts in Antimicrobial Therapy

A. ANTIMICROBIAL MECHANISMS OF ACTION

Susan L. Koletar

EFFECTS ON CELL WALL INTEGRITY
  β-Lactam Antibacterial Agents
  β-Lactamase Inhibitors
  Other Antimicrobial Agents Whose Primary Site
   of Action Is the Cell Wall

INTERRUPTION OF CELL MEMBRANE
  STRUCTURE AND FUNCTION

INHIBITION OF PROTEIN SYNTHESIS

INHIBITION OF ESSENTIAL METABOLITES

INTERFERENCE WITH NUCLEIC ACID
  METABOLISM

RESISTANCE TO ANTIBACTERIAL AGENTS

OBJECTIVES

1. Correlate the basic structure of microorganisms and the specific functions of individual components with the actions of antimicrobial agents.

2. Define *bacteriostatic* and *bactericidal*. Discuss the factors that can influence ultimate outcome of specific antimicrobial activity.

3. List the major sites of action for major classes of antimicrobial agents.

4. List the classic examples of antimicrobial agents that affect structural integrity; describe how β-lactam agents result in antibacterial activity.

5. List the agents whose primary mechanism of action is inhibition of protein synthesis. Differentiate between reversible and irreversible binding at the ribosomal level.

6. List the agents whose primary mechanism of action is interference with metabolic functions, including DNA synthesis, RNA synthesis, and folic acid metabolism.

7. Describe the major mechanisms by which resistance to various antimicrobial agents can occur.

KEY TERMS

Antimicrobial therapy
Antibiotic
Synthetic compounds
Semisynthetic compounds
Bacteriocidal
Bacteriostatic
Indifference
Synergy

Antagonism
β-lactam antibiotics
Penicillin-binding proteins
Macrolides
Quinolones
Resistance
Susceptibility

CASE STUDY

A 68-year-old man with known aortic valve disease came to the hospital emergency room with a 10-day history of fevers and night sweats but no skin lesions. Bacterial endocarditis was diagnosed. *Staphylococcus aureus* was isolated from three sets of blood cultures. To determine appropriate antimicrobial therapy, susceptibility testing was performed. The results showed penicillin and methicillin resistance.

Antimicrobial therapy is a broad term for the use of chemical compounds to treat diseases caused by microorganisms. ***Antibiotic*** is the term most commonly used, and although it is often used interchangeably with *antimicrobial agent*. The purest meaning of *antibiotic* is a chemical substance, produced by a microorganism, with the capacity to kill or inhibit other microorganisms. Antimicrobial agents may also be **synthetic compounds** (those that are completely manufactured or artificial) or **semisynthetic compounds** (naturally occurring substances that have been chemically altered). Whether naturally occurring or not, all antimicrobial agents are intended to destroy or inhibit disease-causing organisms. The specific activities of antimicrobial agents and their mechanisms of action are primarily dictated by the biologic characteristics of the microbe. For treating actual disease, the pharmacokinetic properties of the specific drugs (such as absorption, distribution, and excretion) are also important factors influencing the clinical utility of specific agents against specific disease-causing organisms. Potential problems include toxicity to the host and the development of resistance by the organisms.

Antimicrobial agents are generally categorized according to their targeted sites of action (Table 3-1). Basic activities are (1) interruption of the structural integrity by interfering with cell wall or cell membrane composition and (2) interruption of basic metabolic functions, such as protein synthesis, nucleic acid metabolism, and inhibition of essential metabolites (Figure 3-1). Additional characterization may be made based on whether the agent actually kills the organism **(bacteriocidal)** or whether it serves to inhibit microbial growth **(bacteriostatic).**

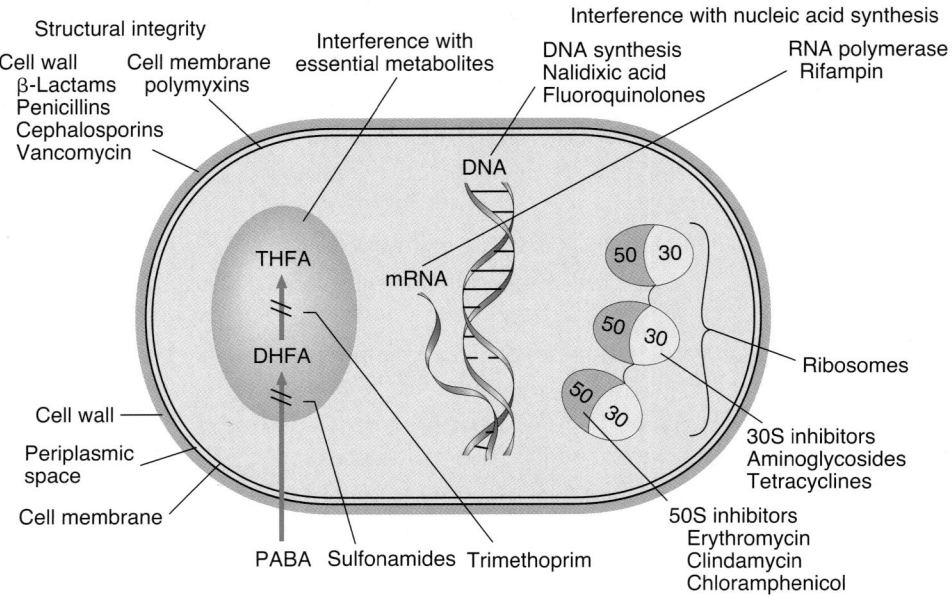

Figure 3-1

Primary sites of antibacterial action for major classes of antimicrobial agents. *THFA,* Tetrahydrofolic acid; *DHFA,* dihydrofolic acid; *PABA,* para-aminobenzoic acid.

Properties of individual drugs and their mechanisms of action are also important to consider when antimicrobial agents are to be used in combination. Combining the agents may cause twice the effect of two drugs (additive) or perhaps no effect of combination therapy **(indifference).** One potentially good effect of using more than one drug is **synergy.** This means that the combined effect is even greater than two individual effects added together, and the overall antimicrobial activity is enhanced. A potentially bad effect is **antagonism;** one drug may counteract the other so that the desired antimicrobial result is much less than would be expected.

The fact that the majority of our available antimicrobial armamentarium comprises antibacterial agents is good evidence of the way our understanding of the basic biology of specific microorganisms affects antimicrobial development. As microbiology techniques improve and we become better at determining the structure and function of other microorganisms, new classes of antimicrobials, including antifungal, antiviral, and antiparasitic agents, have also emerged.

EFFECTS ON CELL WALL INTEGRITY

For the most part, the task of protecting the bacterial cytoplasmic membrane, which is of paramount importance in bacterial survival, falls to

TABLE 3-1

Common Mechanisms of Action for Different Antimicrobial Agents

Mechanism	Class of Antimicrobials
Effects on cell wall integrity	β-Lactams
	Vancomycin
Effects on cell membrane structure and function	Polymyxins
Inhibition of protein synthesis	Aminoglycosides
	Tetracyclines
	Macrolides
	Clindamycin
	Chloramphenicol
Inhibition of essential metabolites	Sulfonamides
	Trimethoprim
Interference with nucleic acid metabolism	Rifampin
	Quinolones
	Metronidazole

the bacterial cell wall. This structure is composed primarily of a peptidoglycan layer, the synthesis of which depends, at least in part, on specific integral enzymes. Inactivating or interfering with these enzymes structurally or functionally destroys bacterial cell walls.

β-Lactam Antibacterial Agents

The group of natural and semisynthetic agents known as **β-lactam antibiotics** accounts for a sizable proportion of available antibacterial agents; it comprises the penicillins, cephalosporins, carbapenems, and monobactams (Box 3-1). Their antibacterial activity is based on the basic chemical structure that they all share, the β-lactam ring. Modifications of this basic structure (Figure 3-2) allow for varying spectra of activity, ranging from very specific and narrow to very broad and inclusive.

The final stage of peptidoglycan synthesis, the formation of peptide bonds, requires specific enzymes known as *transpeptidases.* This critical cross-linking reaction can be interrupted by the β-lactam antibiotics, which can bind with these enzymes. Because of this feature, the transpeptidases are also commonly referred to as **penicillin-binding proteins (PBPs).** A number of PBPs have been identified with varying affinity for different β-lactam agents. In addition, because distinct bacterial species have distinct types of PBPs and their β-lactam drug interactions can be quite specific, not all agents have the same effect on all organisms. For example, a monobactam agent like aztreonam, which binds primarily to PBP 3 of gram-negative aerobes, has no activity against gram-positive or anaerobic organisms because they do not possess that specific PBP. Even if an organism has a specific PBP, β-lactam agents must be able to physically reach those proteins to work. For example, oxacillin is particularly active against gram-positive organisms, such as staphylococci, because those PBPs are located at an easily accessible place on the cell wall. On the other hand, similar PBPs in gram-negative bacilli are not so easily reached, and thus oxacillin is not active against that group. In addition, penicillins and cephalosporins trigger autolytic enzymes that further enhance the destruction of the cell. The ultimate effect of the binding of such agents with a specific PBP is death of that particular bacterium.

Box 3-1

Some Common β-Lactam Antibacterial Agents

Pencillins	Cephalosporins
Penicillin G	Cephalothin
Ampicillin	Cefamandole
Methicillin	Cefoxitin
Ticarcillin	Cefotaxime
Piperacillin	Ceftazidime
	Cefepime
Monobactams	
Aztreonam	**Carbapenems**
	Meropenem
	Imipenem

The spectrum of activity of the β-lactam drugs depends on their particular structural modification (Table 3-2). Simple penicillins are particularly effective against many gram-positive and gram-negative cocci, including *Streptococcus pneumoniae, Streptococcus pyogenes, Streptococcus bovis,* viridans streptococci, *Neisseria gonorrhoeae, Neisseria meningitidis,* and *Pasteurella multocida,* as well as a number of anaerobic species such as *Clostridium* sp., *Fusobacterium sp.,* and some *Bacteroides* spp., in addition to anaerobic streptococcus–like organisms. Ampicillin has a similar spectrum, with additional activity against

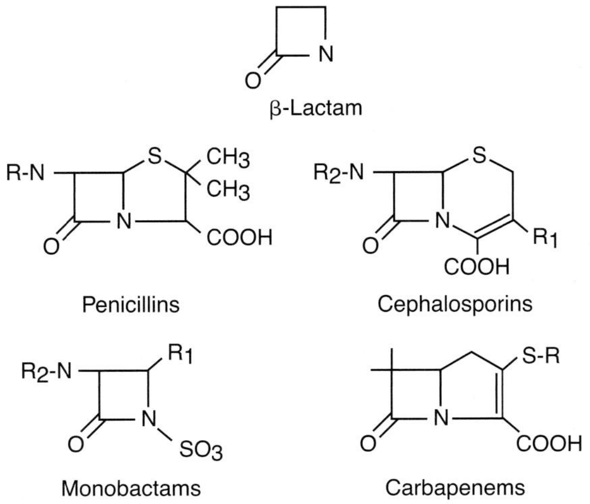

Figure 3-2

Chemical structures of major classes of β-lactam antibiotics.

enterococci, *Listeria monocytogenes,* and some gram-negative coccobacillary organisms, such as *Haemophilus influenzae* and *Haemophilus parainfluenzae, Proteus mirabilis,* and a few Enterobacteriaceae such as *Escherichia coli,* and *Salmonella* and *Shigella* species. Carboxypenicillins and ureidopenicillins have a broader gram-negative spectrum of activity, most notably among the Enterobacteriaceae and with reasonable activity against *Pseudomonas aeruginosa.*

The generally accepted scheme of classifying cephalosporins is based on their spectrum of activity and spoken of in terms of "generations" (Table 3-3). First-generation cephalosporins are characterized by their good gram-positive but relatively modest gram-negative activity. Second-generation cephalosporins generally have better

TABLE 3-3

Examples of Cephalosporins by Generation and Spectrum of Activity

Generation	Spectrum
First Cephalothin Cefazolin Cephapirin Cephradine	Staphylococci (methicillin sensitive); streptococci; few Enterobacteriaceae
Second Cefamandole Cefonicid Cefoxitin Cefotetan Cefuroxime	More Enterobacteriaceae; some β-lactamase producers, including some anaerobes
Third Cefotaxime Ceftizoxime Ceftriaxone	Many Enterobacteriaceae; many β-lactamase producers
Ceftazidime Cefoperazone Cefepime	*Pseudomonas aeruginosa*

TABLE 3-2

Clinical Utility of Different Antimicrobial Agents

Agent	Organisms Useful Against	Organisms Not Useful Against
Penicillin	Streptococci Spirochetes	Staphylococci Mycoplasmas
Oxacillin	Staphylococci*	Enterobacteriaceae
Piperacillin	*Pseudomonas aeruginosa*	Staphylococci
Cefazolin	Staphylococci*	Enterococci
Cefoxitin	Enterobacteriaceae *Bacteroides*	MRSA Enterococci
Cefotaxime	Enterobacteriaceae	*Pseudomonas aeruginosa*
Ceftazidime	*Pseudomonas aeruginosa*	Anerobes
Aztreonam	Enterobacteriaceae	Gram-positives
Imipenem	Many	*Stenotrophomonas maltophilia,* MRSA
Vancomycin	MRSA	Gram-negatives
Aminoglycosides	Gram-negatives	Gram-positives, anaerobes
Tetracyclines	*Chlamydia Rickettsia*	Enterobacteriaceae
Erythromycin	*Legionella* Mycoplasmas	Enterobacteriaceae *Haemophilus influenzae*
Clindamycin	Anaerobes	Enterobacteriaceae
Sulfonamides	Enterobacteriaceae	*Pseudomonas aeruginosa*
Quinolones	Enterobacteriaceae *Pseudomonas aeruginosa*	Gram-positives Anaerobes
Metronidazole	Anaerobes	Aerobes

MRSA, Methicillin-resistant *Staphylococcus aureus.*
*Methicillin-sensitive *Staphylococcus aureus.*

gram-negative activity as a result of their greater stability against certain β-lactamases. Third-generation cephalosporins are thought to have less activity against gram-positive organisms but improved activity against Enterobacteriaceae; a few have particular activity against *P. aeruginosa.*

The only currently available monobactam is aztreonam. Its spectrum of activity is limited to aerobic gram-negative bacilli. It has achievable inhibitory levels against *P. aeruginosa, Serratia marcescens,* and *Enterobacter* spp. Imipenem and meropenem are the two available carbapenems. This class of β-lactam antimicrobials has the broadest antimicrobial spectrum, with excellent activity against most major pathogens, including aerobic and anaerobic streptococcal species, methicillin-susceptible staphylococci, and most Enterobacteriaceae, including *Enterobacter* sp., *Citrobacter* sp., *Serratia* sp., *Acinetobacter* sp., and *P. aeruginosa.*

β-Lactamase Inhibitors

In response to exposure to β-lactam type of drugs, bacteria may produce enzymes (β-lactamases) that can hydrolyze the β-lactam ring and consequently inactivate the antimicrobial agent. One way to compensate for this potential resistance is to combine a standard β-lactam drug (e.g., ampicillin, amoxicillin, ticarcillin, piperacillin) with a β-lacatamase inhibitor, namely clavulanic acid, sulbactam, or tazobactam. These agents alone all have weak antibacterial activity, but their combination with β-lactam drugs can be synergistic. Their main purpose in such a combination, however, is to bind with and thus inactivate the β-lactamases produced by a variety of organisms, including staphylococci and many aerobic and anaerobic gram-negative bacteria. The currently available and clinically used combinations include amoxicillin/clavulanate, ticarcillin/clavulanate, ampicillin/sulbactam, and piperacillin/tazobactam.

Other Antimicrobial Agents Whose Primary Site of Action Is the Cell Wall

Another group of agents affects different aspects of peptidoglycan (cell wall) synthesis. This group includes vancomycin, bacitracin, and cycloserine. Of these, vancomycin has the most established clinical value. It affects the second stage of cell wall synthesis, before transpeptidation, by inhibiting enzymes that are vital to the continued formation of peptidoglycan. The end result is that the bacteria cannot maintain their structural integrity. Because vancomycin is a large molecule, it can cross the cell walls only of gram-positive organisms; thus its primary utility is against only those types of bacteria.

Bacitracin and cycloserine also affect continued formation of the basic structural units of the cell wall. Because their spectra of activity are relatively narrow and their toxicities relatively broad, their usefulness in the clinical arena is limited.

INTERRUPTION OF CELL MEMBRANE STRUCTURE AND FUNCTION

Two antibacterial agents are available whose primary site of action is the bacterial cell membrane. Their spectra of activity are relatively limited and their toxicities significant, making them moderately useful at best. Polymyxins interact with the phospholipids of the bacterial cell membrane and thereby alter permeability and osmotic integrity.

Their primary activity is against gram-negative bacilli, and their primary clinical utility is in the form of topical preparations. Bacitracin acts by disrupting the cytoplasmic membrane, in addition to its interference with cell wall synthesis. Its primary activity is against gram-positive organisms, and it, too, is most useful as a topical agent for superficial dermatologic infections.

INHIBITION OF PROTEIN SYNTHESIS

A number of different antimicrobial agents exert their bactericidal or bacteriostatic effects by interfering with protein synthesis at the ribosomal level. This is accomplished by binding of the agent to either the 50S or 30S ribosomal subunit, and the resultant inhibition or death of the organism depends on whether this binding is reversible or irreversible, respectively. For example, the aminoglycosides irreversibly bind to the 30S ribosomal subunit, making that integral cell structure unavailable for translation of mRNA during protein synthesis; the result is death of the cell. A secondary feature of these types of agents is that this ribosomal interaction also results in misreading of the genetic code. To be effective, aminoglycosides depend on an aerobic, energy-dependent process to reach the inside of the bacterial cell. They are especially useful in situations in which a cell wall–active agent, such as a β-lactam, is being used because of their facilitated uptake in those instances. The spectrum of activity of the aminoglycosides is primarily toward aerobic gram-negative bacilli, especially Enterobacteriaceae, *P. aeruginosa, Acinetobacter* sp., and *Providencia* sp.; they also have activity against staphylococci but should not be used as single agents to treat staphylococcal infections.

Tetracyclines are like the aminoglycosides in that they have the same site of action (30S ribosome), but their binding is reversible; consequently, their activity is bacteriostatic. Although they can enter human cells, their antimicrobial activity is enhanced by being actively concentrated in some bacteria. Tetracyclines have a broad spectrum of activity against a number of microbial species, including gram-positive and gram-negative bacteria as well as mycoplasmas.

They are particularly useful against intracellular pathogens such as chlamydiae and rickettsiae.

The **macrolides** (erythromycin, clarithromycin, azithromycin), the lincosamide (clindamycin), and chloramphenicol also inhibit bacterial protein synthesis, their primary target being the 50S ribosomal subunit. As with the tetracyclines, the binding of these drugs is reversible. Interference or actual antagonism can occur if these agents are used in combination with each other.

Erythromycin has a relatively broad spectrum of activity, including gram-positive cocci, mycoplasmas, chlamydiae, rickettsiae, and treponemes. Its gram-negative activity is marginal at best and is clearly influenced by changes in pH, with improved potency in alkalinized environments. Erythromycin is typically used in the treatment of *Legionella pneumophila* and *Mycoplasma pneumoniae*. The newer macrolides, azithromycin and clarithromycin, also have activity against these respiratory pathogens. In addition to having an otherwise similar spectrum of activity as erythromycin, a potential benefit of azithromycin and clarithromycin is the expanded in vitro spectrum that includes some gram-negative organisms, such as *Haemophilus influenzae* and *Moraxella catarrhalis*. The clinical relevance of this finding remains to be seen. The primary advantages of azithromycin and clarithromycin over erythromycin are improved pharmacokinetic properties and tolerance in terms of fewer side effects.

Clindamycin has excellent activity against aerobic gram-positive organisms, including various species of clinically important streptococci as well as methicillin-susceptible staphylococci. Its claim to fame, however, is its extremely potent anaerobic activity. Clindamycin has also been used to treat some protozoal infections, such as babesiosis, malaria, and toxoplasmosis.

Chloramphenicol also enters bacteria by an energy-requiring process. The end result of its reversible binding to the 50S ribosome is the prevention of peptide bond formation. Although its spectrum of activity is quite broad, including both gram-positive and gram-negative aerobes and anaerobes as well as a number of rickettsial species, concern about toxicities and significant drug interactions has limited the clinical usefulness of this once valuable antibiotic.

INHIBITION OF ESSENTIAL METABOLITES

Folinic acid is necessary for the synthesis of bacterial DNA. Many bacteria depend on making their own folinic acid because they are unable to take up this essential metabolite. The synthesis of folinic acid occurs as the result of modification of para-aminobenzoic acid and relies on several different enzymes (Figure 3-3). Inhibiting one or both of these enzymes essentially prevents bacterial replication.

Sulfonamides competitively inhibit the bacterial enzyme dihydropteroate synthetase, which ultimately allows for the incorporation of para-aminobenzoic acid into dihydrofolate. For optimal efficacy the bacteria must be exposed to a continued source of sulfonamide to achieve the desired result of affecting bacterial replication. The pyrimidine analog trimethoprim competi-

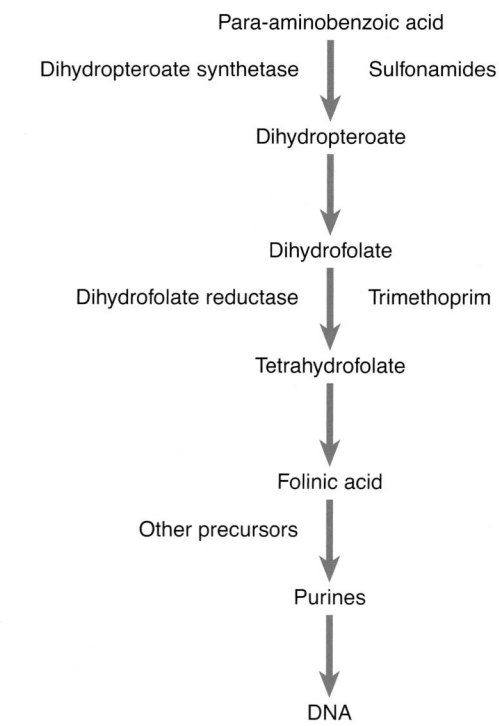

Figure 3-3

Sites of action of sulfonamides and trimethoprim and their effects on synthesis of essential amino acids and nucleic acids.

tively inhibits the enzyme dihydrofolate reductase, effectively blocking the conversion to tetrahydrofolate, a precursor of folinic and other amino acids. Because these agents act at different metabolic sites, using them in combination has a synergistic effect. The spectrum of activity of these agents, when combined in a fixed preparation, is quite broad and includes many gram-positive and gram-negative organisms, with the notable exception of *P. aeruginosa*.

INTERFERENCE WITH NUCLEIC ACID METABOLISM

Interference with either DNA or RNA metabolism can have devastating consequences for bacteria. Rifampin interferes with the production of mRNA by binding to one of the four subunits of DNA-directed RNA polymerase. As a result, transcription of the RNA chain is aborted at the initiation step. Rifampin also has a wide range of antibacterial activity, but its most noteworthy clinical application is still in the treatment of mycobacterial diseases, particularly *Mycobacterium tuberculosis*.

Two distinct categories of antimicrobial agents interfere with DNA synthesis: those that disrupt replication and those that disrupt the finished product. Nalidixic acid and the subsequent fluorinated **quinolones** interfere with DNA synthesis and result in bacterial killing by rendering an essential enzyme ineffective. This enzyme, a type II topoisomerase DNA gyrase, is responsible for supercoiling of DNA, which allows for the bacterial chromosome to be condensed to a size that is contained within the bacterium. DNA gyrase is composed of four subunits: two A proteins and two B proteins. The first fluoroquinolones (norfloxacin, ciprofloxacin, ofloxacin) primarily inhibited the A subunit, resulting in the DNA backbone being unable to align itself properly, with consequent bacterial killing. These agents were noted for their activity against gram-negative aerobes, with Enterobacteriaceae and *Haemophilus, Neisseria, Moraxella, Campylobacter, Vibrio,* and *Aeromonas* species being most susceptible. In addition, ciprofloxacin had predictable and clinically useful activity against *Pseudomonas aeruginosa*. Activity against gram-positive and anaerobic or-

ganisms, however, was often suboptimal. More recently, structural modifications of the basic fluoroquinolone molecule have expanded the spectrum to include gram-positive aerobes (sparfloxacin, levofloxacin, and trovafloxacin). Of these, trovafloxacin is distinguished by its excellent antianaerobic activity.

Metronidazole disrupts DNA by making it unstable. In its usual form, metronidazole is inactive. When it is partially reduced and incorporated into DNA, however, it disrupts nucleic acid. Only anaerobic bacteria and organisms that grow anaerobically, such as certain protozoa, have this ability for partial reduction of metronidazole; hence, the spectrum of activity is limited to those types of organisms.

RESISTANCE TO ANTIBACTERIAL AGENTS

In the face of continuing antibiotic challenge, bacteria have found several ways to adapt and thus survive. The mechanisms of **resistance** have developed in response to the mechanisms of action of antimicrobial drugs (Table 3-4).

For antimicrobial agents to have specific activity, they must somehow associate with the organism and reach a specified target site. One mechanism of resistance is to prevent access to that target by inhibiting uptake of the substance. For example, anaerobic bacteria are not equipped to ac-

TABLE 3-4

Common Mechanisms of Resistance for Different Antimicrobial Agents

Mechanism	Class of Antimicrobial
Prevent access to target	Aminoglycosides
	β-Lactams
	Tetracyclines
Modify target	Macrolides
	Quinolones
	Rifampin
	Sulfonamides
	β-Lactams
Produce inactivating enzymes	β-Lactams
	Chloramphenicol
	Aminoglycosides

tivate the electron transport system that is necessary for aminoglycosides to reach their ribosomal site of action. Consequently, anaerobes are intrinsically resistant to aminoglycosides. Decreased accumulation can also result, owing to characteristics specific to the bacteria, such as extracellular slime or altered lipopolysaccharide, or characteristics specific to the antimicrobial agent, such as size, electronic charge, and affinity for lipids. Even in specific families of microorganisms, subtle differences may result in varied patterns of **susceptibility** to a single class of antibiotics. A classic example is the decreased sensitivity of *Enterobacter cloacae* to β-lactam drugs compared with *E. coli.* The blueprints for these types of mechanisms of resistance are usually encoded on the chromosomes.

The other way to prevent access to the antimicrobial's site of action is to increase excretion of the drug. This is the primary mechanism of resistance to the tetracyclines. Organisms resistant to tetracyclines do not concentrate these drugs in the cell because of an active transport exit mechanism that does not allow intracellular accumulation. The proteins responsible for the phenomenon occur as a result of plasmid encoding.

Another important mechanism of resistance is structural or functional modification of the target site of action. Such alterations may be expressed in various ways. One such mechanism is biochemical alterations that reduce the target site's affinity for a drug. For example, in response to an enzyme, methylase, which is made from a plasmid-encoded gene in staphylococci, methylation of the 23S ribosome occurs, with the ultimate result being a modification in the 50S ribosome, the site of action of the macrolide class of antimicrobials. Along the same line of thinking, though not as clearly defined, alterations in RNA polymerase and DNA gyrase provide plausible explanations for resistance patterns seen with rifampin and the quinolones, respectively.

Other ways that the target site may be modified by the microorganism include the production of different proteins that can function like the targets but do not bind the drug or the excessive production of targets to overwhelm the drug with competitive inhibition. Bacterial resistance to sulfonamides and trimethoprim are expressed by such mechanisms. By producing different enzymes that function in an alternative pathway or by overproducing necessary synthetase and reductase enzymes, folinic acid synthesis can be achieved.

On the other hand, some organisms, such as staphylococci, can synthesize "new" proteins that maintain their usual function as transpeptidases but do not bind even stable β-lactam drugs such as methicillin. As a group, these staphylococci are known as *methicillin-resistant.* This event was presented in the case study described at the beginning of the chapter. They pose difficult problems in terms of treatment because such staphylococci do not respond well to any of the β-lactam drugs. Alterations in PBPs have also been demonstrated in other species, notably those that account for the relatively new phenomenon of penicillin resistance in pneumococci. The continued presence of β-lactam–resistant strains has reinforced the ongoing search for effective antibiotics.

One of the first-recognized ways for bacteria to resist the actions of antimicrobial agents was the production of enzymes that inactivate a drug. A number of antimicrobial agents, such as aminoglycosides and chloramphenicol, have been found to be affected by inactivating enzymes, but the classic example of this phenomenon is β-lactamase production. In response to exposure to β-lactam drugs, bacteria may produce enzymes (β-lactamases) that can hydrolyze the β-lactam ring and consequently inactivate the antimicrobial agent. This was first described as a penicillinase produced by staphylococci, and since then more than a hundred such enzymes produced by a number of bacterial species have been identified. Many of these β-lactamases are the result of plasmid encoding. Pharmacologic compensations have been based on either structural manipulation of the side chain, so that the β-lactam ring is sterically protected (such as in some of the later-generation cephalosporins), or combination of the major drugs with β-lactamase inhibitor agents.

LEARNING ASSESSMENT

1. Infections with penicillinase-producing *Staphylococcus aureus* can be treated with all the following antibiotics EXCEPT for which of the following?
   a. Cephalothin
   b. Nafcillin
   c. Vancomycin
   d. Ampicillin/sulbactam
   e. Piperacillin

2. Which of the following antibiotics affords a broad spectrum of antimicrobial coverage against aerobic and anaerobic bacteria, rickettsiae, chlamydiae, and mycoplasmas?
   a. Penicillin
   b. Vancomycin
   c. Tetracycline
   d. Metronidazole
   e. Aminoglycosides (e.g., gentamicin)

3. Which of the following antibiotics does NOT have good activity against Enterobacteriaceae?
   a. Trimethoprim-sulfamethoxazole
   b. Ciprofloxacin
   c. Cefoxitin
   d. Clindamycin
   e. Aminoglycosides

4. Which of the following antibiotics is NOT generally clinically useful for *Pseudomonas aeruginosa* infections?
   a. Trimethoprim-sulfamethoxazole
   b. Ciprofloxacin
   c. Ceftazidime
   d. Piperacillin
   e. Aminoglycosides

B. PROCEDURES IN ANTIMICROBIAL SUSCEPTIBILITY TESTING

Janet A. Hindler, James H. Jorgensen

REASONS AND INDICATIONS FOR PERFORMING ANTIMICROBIAL SUSCEPTIBILITY TESTS
  Factors to Consider When Determining Whether Testing Is Warranted
    Body site
    Presence of other bacteria and quality of specimen
    Host status

SELECTING ANTIMICROBIAL AGENTS FOR TESTING AND REPORTING
  Selection of Test Batteries
  Reporting of Susceptibility Test Results

TRADITIONAL ANTIMICROBIAL SUSCEPTIBILITY TEST METHODS
  Inoculum Preparation and Use of McFarland Standards
    Inoculum preparation
    McFarland turbidity standards
    Inoculum standardization
  Dilution Methods
    Principle
    Antimicrobial stock solutions
    Broth macrodilution (tube dilution) tests
    Broth microdilution tests
    Agar dilution tests
  Disk Diffusion Testing
    Principle
    Establishing zone diameter interpretive breakpoints
    Test performance

Modified Methods for Testing Slow-Growing or Fastidious Bacteria
    Haemophilus influenzae and *Haemophilus* spp.
    Streptococcus pneumoniae and *Streptococcus* spp.
    Neisseria gonorrhoeae and *Neisseria meningitidis*
    Anaerobes
  Additional Organism and Antimicrobial Agent Testing Concerns
    Detection of oxacillin (methicillin) resistance in staphylococci
    Enterococci
    Extended spectrum β-lactamases (ESBLs)

AUTOMATED ANTIMICROBIAL SUSCEPTIBILITY TEST METHODS
  Principles of Technologies Used
  Currently Available Automated Systems
    Automated reader devices for broth microdilution susceptibility tests
    Automated instruments that provide more rapid test results
  Nonautomated Antimicrobial Susceptibility Test Method: E Test

INTERPRETATION OF IN VITRO ANTIMICROBIAL SUSCEPTIBILITY TEST RESULTS

METHODS OF DETECTING ANTIMICROBIAL-INACTIVATING ENZYMES
  β-Lactamase Tests

QUALITY CONTROL OF ANTIMICROBIAL SUSCEPTIBILITY TESTS

SELECTING AN ANTIMICROBIAL SUSCEPTIBILITY TEST METHOD

OBJECTIVES

1. Explain the rationale behind the performance of antimicrobial susceptibility tests.
2. Describe the method for selection of specific drugs in testing and reporting.
3. Define *MIC* and the methods that are used for determination of MICs.
4. Explain how zone interpretive criteria used with the disk diffusion test are established.
5. List the variables that must be controlled when antimicrobial susceptibility tests are performed.
6. Describe test modifications for antimicrobial susceptibility testing of *Haemophilus* spp, *Streptococcus* spp (including *Streptococcus pneumoniae*), *Neisseria gonorrhoeae,* and anaerobes.
7. Explain the principles behind automated antimicrobial susceptibility test methods.
8. Discuss several commercially available antimicrobial susceptibility test systems in current use.
9. List the organisms for which β-lactamase testing is useful.
10. Describe the significance of high-level aminoglycoside resistance in enterococci.
11. Discuss QC procedures for antimicrobial susceptibility tests.
12. Describe the way in which antibiograms can be used to help verify the accuracy of results generated by testing of patient isolates.
13. Explain how to select a particular susceptibility test method for routine use.
14. Explain the meanings of *susceptible, intermediate,* and *resistant* as applied to antimicrobial susceptibility test results.
15. Discuss the predictive value of antimicrobial susceptibility test results.

KEY TERMS

National Committee for Clinical Laboratory Standards (NCCLS)
Selective reporting
McFarland turbidity standards
Minimal inhibitory concentration (MIC)
Susceptible
Intermediate
Resistant
Broth macrodilution

Tube dilution
Broth microdilution MIC testing
Breakpoint
Trailing
Skipped wells
Agar dilution
Kirby Bauer test
Zone of inhibition
Penicillinase-producing *N. gonorrhoeae* (PPNG)

Chromosomally mediated resistant *N. gonorrhoeae* (CMRNG)
Penicillinase-resistant penicillins
mecA
Heteroresistant
Methicillin-resistant *S. aureus* (MRSA)
Oxacillin screen plate
Borderline-resistant

High-level aminoglycoside resistance
E-test
Susceptible
Resistant
Intermediate
β-Lactamases
Cumulative antibiogram statistics

CASE STUDY

A physician called the microbiology laboratory supervisor to inquire about a recent wound culture with *Staphylococcus aureus*. Five days earlier, blood cultures from the patient were found to be positive with MRSA (methicillin-resistant *S. aureus*). The cultures had a typical MRSA profile in that they were also resistant to cefazolin, clindamycin, erythromycin, and penicillin. The wound culture isolate was reported as resistant to clindamycin, erythromycin, and penicillin but susceptible to cefazolin and oxacillin. Susceptibility testing on both of the isolates was done using the disk diffusion method.

The supervisor reviewed recent quality control results and the procedures documented on the worksheet for each culture. No problems were documented with regard to quality control testing over the past 2 months. When she spoke to the two technologists involved in the workups of the implicated cultures, she learned that the technologist who examined the blood culture isolate (reported as MRSA) recalled that this particular strain showed a subtle haze of growth within a zone around the oxacillin disk. This haze was visible only when the zone isolate was examined using transmitted light. The technologist who examined the disk diffusion test on the wound isolate (reported as oxacillin-susceptible) admittedly forgot to examine the oxacillin zone with transmitted light.

Fortunately, both isolates were saved. On repeat testing, both isolates demonstrated the same profile, each with a haze of growth around the oxacillin disk. The physician was called, and a corrected report was issued stating that the wound isolate was indeed MRSA.

REASONS AND INDICATIONS FOR PERFORMING ANTIMICROBIAL SUSCEPTIBILITY TESTS

Antimicrobial susceptibility tests are performed on bacteria isolated from clinical specimens if the isolate is determined to be a probable cause of the patient's infection and the susceptibility of the isolate to particular antimicrobial agents is uncertain. Susceptibility tests are not performed on bacteria that are predictably susceptible to the antimicrobial agents commonly used to treat infections caused by these bacteria. Group A β-hemolytic *Streptococcus,* for example, is not routinely tested because it is universally susceptible to penicillin, the drug of choice in treating infections caused by this bacterium. In contrast, the recommended agent for treating *Straphylococcus aureus* infections is oxacillin, and *S. aureus* may or may not be susceptible to oxacillin. Consequently, susceptibility testing is indicated for *S. aureus* isolates that are the suspected cause of an infection.

Factors to Consider When Determining Whether Testing Is Warranted

In addition to the unpredictable susceptibility profile of a potential pathogen, other important factors must be considered when determining whether antimicrobial susceptibility testing is warranted; these factors include the following:

- The body site from which the organism was isolated
- The presence of other bacteria and the quality of the specimen from which the organism was grown
- The host's status

Body site

Susceptiblity tests are not performed on bacteria that are isolated from the anatomic site of which they are normal inhabitants. For example, *Escherichia coli* is normal flora in the lower gastrointestinal tract and therefore would not be tested when isolated from stool; however, *E. coli* from a blood culture would be tested because blood should be sterile. Similarly, viridans streptococci represent normal flora in throat specimens and would not be routinely tested. Coagulase-negative staphylococci isolated from multiple blood culture bottles would be tested. Because coagulase-negative staphylococci are commonly found on skin surfaces, these organisms would not be tested when isolated from superficial wound specimens. Testing of normal flora isolates or isolates likely to represent contamination or colonization should be avoided because reporting of antimicrobial susceptibility results may encourage a physician to treat a normal condition and refrain from further investigation of the true cause of the patient's problem.

Presence of other bacteria and quality of specimen

The isolation of an organism in pure culture is less likely to represent contamination than a mixed culture. More than two species at greater that 10^5 CFU (colony-forming units) per mL isolated from urine suggests contamination, and these organisms may not require susceptibility testing; however, a pure culture of *E. coli* at greater than 10^5 CFU/mL would likely represent infection and would be tested. A few *Klebsiella pneumoniae* in the presence of many normal flora in a sputum culture may not be significant. In the absence of normal flora, however, a few colonies of this species, particularly if noted on a Gram stain of the sputum, may be significant and warrant testing of the isolates.

Host status

The host status of the patient often influences susceptibility testing decisions. Species usually viewed as normal flora may be responsible for an infection and at times may require testing in immunosuppressed patients. Additionally, in patients who are allergic to penicillin and who have a group A β-hemolytic streptococcal infection, erythromycin is the drug of choice, and β-hemolytic streptococci are occasionally resistant to this agent. Consequently, testing of erythromycin is warranted on isolates from penicillin-allergic patients whose disease is not responding to erythomycin.

SELECTING ANTIMICROBIAL AGENTS FOR TESTING AND REPORTING

Approximately 50 antimicrobial agents are available for treating bacterial infections, and many of these have comparable clinical efficacy. Each laboratory must determine the types of agents appropriate for testing against various organisms (or organism groups) in its particular setting. Laboratory workers alone should not formulate testing and reporting protocols. Representatives from the infectious diseases department, the pharmacy, and perhaps other services must provide input regarding the clinical utility of various agents in an institution. From the laboratory perspective, the limiting factor for the numbers of drugs tested is usually the number that can be practically tested with a particular method. For example, the stan-

dard disk diffusion test uses a 150-mm agar plate, which can accommodate no more than 12 disks. Depending on the format of the panel, some of the commercial antimicrobial susceptibility systems can test slightly more drugs.

The patient population must be considered in the choice of antimicrobial agents to be tested. Some agents are contraindicated in pediatric patients (e.g., quinolones, which impair cartilage development, and tetracycline, which damages developing teeth). Emphasis should be placed on testing oral agents when dealing with outpatient specimens.

Additional guidelines for developing a testing and reporting strategy are found within the **National Committee for Clinical Laboratory Standards (NCCLS)** documents for disk diffusion or MIC testing. These documents include a table ("Table 1: Suggested Groupings of US FDA-Approved Antimicrobial Agents that Should be Considered for Routine Testing and Reporting by Clinical Microbiology Laboratories") that lists primary and secondary agents appropriate for testing against various organism groups. Also listed are drugs that should be reported on urine isolates only. An example of a listing for Enterobacteriaceae is shown in Box 3-2.

Selection of Test Batteries

Generally, a laboratory will define a battery of 10 to 15 antimicrobial agents for routine testing against Enterobacteriaceae, *Pseudomonas* spp, and related nonfastidious gram-negative bacilli and another battery for gram-positive bacteria. Sometimes, a separate battery is performed for urine isolates, representing drugs appropriate for treating urinary tract infections. A supplemental battery that contains antimicrobial agents with enhanced spectra of activity is often included by laboratories that encounter a significant number of highly resistant isolates. Some may elect to establish a separate battery that contains agents specific for *Pseudomonas aeruginosa,* particularly if space is insufficient for testing a wide variety of antipseudomonal agents as part of the routine gram-negative battery.

Reporting of Susceptibility Test Results

Because the identity of the isolate is often unknown at the time the susceptibility test is performed, some drugs may be tested on an isolate

Box 3-2

Some Suggested Groupings of US FDA-Approved Antimicrobial Agents that Should Be Considered for Routine Testing and Reporting by Clinical Microbiology Laboratories for Enterobacteriaceae

Group A primary test and report

Ampicillin[a,h]
Cefazolin[a,b]
Cephalothin[a,b]
Gentamicin[a]

Group B primary test report selectively

Amikacin
Amoxicillin/clavulanic acid or ampicillin/sulbactam
Piperacillin/tazobactam
Ticarcillin/clavulanic acid
Cefamandole or cefonicid or cefuroxime
Cefepime
Cefmetazole
Cefoperazone[h]
Cefotetan
Cefoxitin
Cefotaxime[h,i,j] or ceftizoxime[h,j] or ceftriaxone[h,i,j]
Ciprofloxacin[a,h] or levofloxacin[a,h]
Imipenem or meropenem
Mezlocillin or piperacillin
Ticarcillin
Trimethoprim/sulfamethoxazole[a,h]

Group C supplemental report selectively

Aztreonam
Ceftazidime
    (Both are helpful indicators of extended
    spectrum β-lactamases.)[j]
Chloramphenicol[c,h]
Kanamycin
Netilmicin
Tetracycline[a]
Tobramycin

Group U supplemental for urine only

Carbenicillin
Cinoxacin
Lomefloxacin or norfloxacin or ofloxacin
Loracarbef
Nitrofurantoin
Sulfisoxazole
Trimethoprim

Modified from NCCLS publication M100-S9, *Performance standards for antimicrobial susceptibility testing; ninth informational supplement.* Copies of the current edition may be obtained from NCCLS, 940 West Valley Road, Suite 1400, Wayne, PA, 19087-1898.
[a]May also be appropriate for inclusion in a panel for testing of urinary tract isolates along with agents in the Group U.
[b]Cephalothin can be used to represent cephalothin, cephapirin, cephradine, cephalexin, cefaclor, and cefadroxil. Cefazolin, cefuroxime, cefpodoxime, cefprozil, and loracarbef (urinary isolates only) may be tested individually because some isolates may be susceptible to these agents when resistant to cephalothin.
[c]Not routinely reported on organisms isolated from the urinary tract.
[h]For isolates of *Salmonella* and *Shigella* spp., only ampicillin, a quinolone, and trimethoprim/sulfamethoxazole should be tested and reported routinely. In addition, chloramphenicol and a third-generation cephalosporin should be tested and reported for extraintestinal isolates of *Salmonella* spp.

[i]Should be tested and reported on isolates from cerebrospinal fluid along with agents in Group A.
[j]Strains of *Klebsiella* spp. and *E. coli* that produce extended spectrum β-lactamases (ESBLs) may be clinically resistant to therapy with penicillins, cephalosporins, or aztreonam, despite apparent in vitro susceptibility to some of these agents. Some of these strains will show zones of inhibition below the normal susceptible population but above the standard breakpoints for certain extended-spectrum cephalosporins or aztreonam; such strains may be screened for potential ESBL production by using the screening breakpoints listed in the table below. Other strains may test intermediate or resistant by standard breakpoints to one or more of these agents. In all strains with ESBLs the zone diameters should increase in the presence of clavulanic acid. For all ESBL-producing strains, the test interpretation should be reported as resistant for all penicillins, cephalosporins, and aztreonam.

that may be inappropriate for reporting. In such instances, a drug should never be indiscriminantly reported because results may be misleading. Some drugs may appear active against certain species in vitro but are inappropriate for clinical use (e.g., cephalosporins against enterococci). The final reporting decision should be made once the isolate's identity is known (sometimes a preliminary identification is sufficient), and the overall antibiogram and specimen source must be taken into consideration.

As mentioned previously, reporting protocols should be developed following discussion with infectious disease clinicians, pharmacists, and others who have clinical experience with the antimicrobial therapy practices of the particular institution. A primary objective of antimicrobial therapy is to use the least toxic, most cost-effective, and most clinically appropriate agents and to refrain from more costly, broader-spectrum agents when they are unnecessary. Physician compliance with this objective is often difficult. Sometimes all drugs tested are reported, and the mechanism of control for inappropriate prescribing is outside the laboratory's purview. Alternatively, the laboratory may assist in discouraging inappropriate antimicrobial prescribing by refraining from reporting broad-spectrum agents if narrower-spectrum agents appear useful. NCCLS provides guidance for development of such a selective-reporting or cascade-reporting protocol.

For several organism groups, NCCLS categorizes antimicrobial agents into four groups (see Box 3-2). As a general guideline, it is suggested that within a particular antimicrobial class, primary (group A) agents be reported first and that secondary (group B) agents be reported only if one of the following conditions exists:

- The isolate is resistant to the primary agents.
- The patient cannot tolerate the primary agents.
- The infection has not responded to the primary agents.
- A secondary agent would be a better clinical choice for the particular infection.

For example, a primary cephalosporin, such as cephalothin or cefazolin (first-generation cephalosporin), would be a reasonable choice for a susceptible *E. coli*, and secondary cephalosporins, such as

cefoxitin (second-generation celphalosporin) or cefotaxime (third-generation cephalosporin), would generally not be required. An exception would occur with meningitis because third-generation cephalosporins cross the blood-brain barrier much more effectively than their first-generation counterparts. Gentamicin is usually the aminoglycoside of choice for treating serious infections caused by gentamicin-susceptible *P. aeruginosa,* and tobramycin or amikacin may be considered for gentamicin-resistant isolates. Aminoglycosides are not effective for treating meningitis because they do not readily cross the blood-brain barrier.

A secondary agent may also be reported if the patient has a polymicrobial infection and a secondary (but not a primary) agent would be more likely to be effective against all pathogens present. Similarly, a secondary agent may be reported if the patient has a disseminated infection and a secondary (but not a primary) agent would be more likely to be effective at all sites.

Agents with very broad-spectrum activity (group C) may be tested and reported for the reasons listed for secondary agents. In addition, group C agents would be considered for routine testing if a particular institution encounters large numbers of isolates resistant to group A and group B agents. Finally, agents listed in group U should be reported only on isolates from urine, as these drugs are clinically ineffective in treating infections other than urinary tract infections. Examples of reports generated following a **selective reporting** protocol are shown in Table 3-5; NCCLS Table 1 (Box 3-2) was used to determine whether agents are considered primary or secondary.

TRADITIONAL ANTIMICROBIAL SUSCEPTIBILITY TEST METHODS

Inoculum Preparation and Use of McFarland Standards

Inoculum preparation

Inoculum preparation is the most important step in any susceptibility test. Inocula are prepared by adding cells from four to five isolated colonies of similar colony morphology to a broth medium and then allowing them to grow to the log phase. Four to five colonies, rather than a single colony, are selected to minimize the possibility of testing

TABLE 3-5

Examples of Antimicrobial Agents Reported Following a Selective Reporting Protocol, as Suggested in Table 1, NCCLS M100-S9. Primary Agents (Group A) Are in Plain Type and Secondary Agents (Group B) Are in Bold Type

	Drug	Result		Drug	Result
E. Coli source—urine	Ampicillin	S	*Enterobacter cloacae* source—blood	Amikacin	S
	Cephalothin	S		Ampicillin	R
	Gentamicin	S		**Ampicillin/sulbactam**	R
	Nitrofurantoin	S		**Cefoxitin**	R
	Trimethoprim/sulfamethoxazole	S		**Cefotaxime**	S
E. Coli source—urine	Ampicillin	R		Cephalothin	R
	Ampicillin/sulbactam	R		Gentamicin	R
	Cefoxitin	S		Trimethoprim/sulfamethoxazole	R
	Cephalothin	R			
	Gentamicin	S			
	Nitrofurantoin	S			
	Trimethoprim/sulfamethoxazole	R			

Modified from NCCLS publication M100-S9, *Performance standards for antimicrobial susceptibility testing; ninth informational supplement.* Copies of the current edition may be obtained from NCCLS, 940 West Valley Road, Suite 1400, Wayne, PA 19087-1898.

a colony that might have been derived from a susceptible mutant. Inocula may also be prepared directly by inoculating colonies grown overnight on an agar plate into broth or saline. This direct inoculum suspension preparation technique, which is preferred for bacteria that grow unpredictably in broth (e.g., fastidious bacteria), does not require incubation, but the use of fresh (16-24-hour) colonies is imperative.

McFarland turbidity standards

The numbers of bacteria tested must be standardized regardless of the method used. False-susceptible results may occur if too few bacteria are tested, and false-resistant results may result from the testing of too many bacteria. The most widely used method of inoculum standardization involves **McFarland turbidity standards.** McFarland standards are prepared by adding specific volumes of 1% sulfuric acid and 1.175% barium chloride to obtain a barium sulfate solution with a specific optical density. The most commonly used is the McFarland 0.5 standard, which contains 99.5 mL of 1% sulfuric acid and 0.5 mL of 1.175% barium chloride. This solution is dispensed into tubes comparable to those used for inoculum preparation, which are sealed tightly and stored in the dark at room temperature. The McFarland 0.5 standard provides a turbidity comparable to that of a bacterial suspension containing 1.5×10^8 CFU/mL. Recently, suspensions of latex particles have been used as an alternative to barium sulfate to achieve turbidity comparable to that of the McFarland standard.

Inoculum standardization

To standardize the inoculum, the inoculated broth and the McFarland 0.5 standard are vortexed thoroughly and then, under adequate lighting, the two tubes are positioned side by side against a white card containing several horizontal black lines (Figure 3-4). The turbidities are compared by looking at the black lines through the suspensions. The suspension is too dense if it is more difficult to see the lines through the inoculum suspension than through the McFarland 0.5 standard. In this case, the inoculum is diluted with additional sterile broth or saline. If the test suspension is too light, more organisms are added or the suspension is reincubated (depending on the inoculum preparation protocol) until the turbidity reaches that of the McFarland standard. The standardized inoculum suspensions should be used within 15 minutes of preparation.

An alternative to McFarland standards for the adjustment of visual turbidity involves use of a nephelometric or spectrophotometric device. Several commercially available bench-top instru-

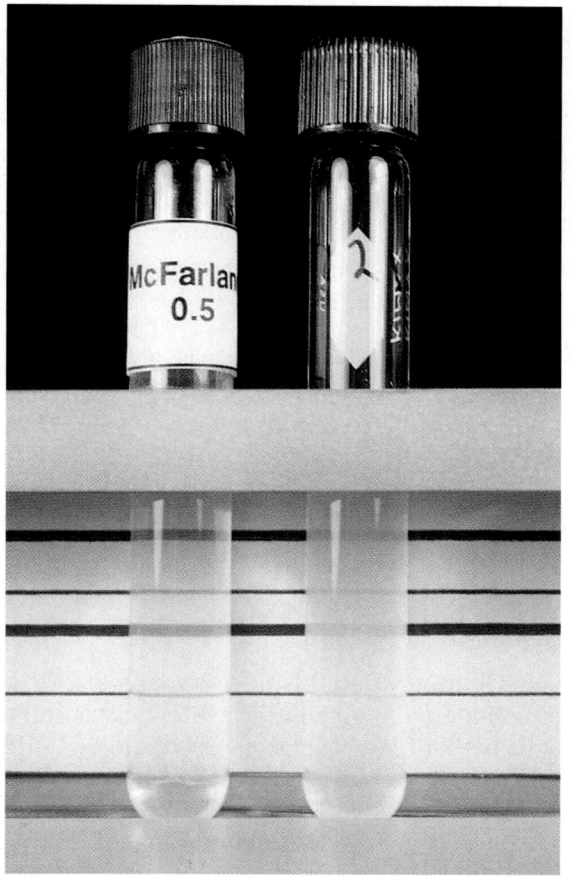

Figure 3-4 _____

The tube on the left is a McFarland 0.5 turbidity standard. The tube on the right is a test bacterial suspension that has a turbidity greater than that of the McFarland standard; it is more difficult to see the black lines through the test suspension than through the McFarland standard. Sterile saline or broth must be added to the test suspension to dilute it until the turbidity matches that of the McFarland standard.

ments are available for more objective standardization of bacterial inocula in the clinical microbiology laboratory (Figure 3-5).

Dilution Methods

Principle

Dilution antimicrobial susceptibility test methods are used to determine the **minimal inhibitory concentration (MIC),** or the lowest concentration of antimicrobial agent required to inhibit the growth of a bacterial isolate. Varying concentrations of antimicrobial agent are added to broth or agar media. Generally, serial twofold-dilution con-

centrations are tested (expressed in μg/mL), and these represent concentrations that are attainable in vivo following standard dosages for each respective antimicrobial agent. Because the concentrations attainable in vivo vary with different agents, the ranges of concentrations tested vary also. For example, concentrations above 8 μg/mL for gentamicin and tobramycin cannot be safely attained in the patient, and therefore the ranges of concentrations tested are generally 0.25 to 8.0 μg/mL. In contrast, much higher levels of the extended-spectrum penicillin ticarcillin are attainable in vivo, and a range of 4 to 128 μg/mL is commonly tested. Once the MIC is determined, the organism is interpreted as either **susceptible, intermediate,** or **resistant** to each agent with the use of a table provided in the NCCLS dilution testing document. An example is shown in Table 3-6. Note that for some antimicrobial agents, different MIC interpretive criteria exist for different organisms or organism groups. For each antimicrobial agent the MIC breakpoint separates susceptible from resistant results. Organisms with MICs at or below the breakpoint are susceptible, and those with MICs above the breakpoint are intermediate or resistant. The NCCLS documents describe the details of performing MIC tests by broth macrodilution, broth microdilution, and agar dilution.

Antimicrobial stock solutions

Antimicrobial stock solutions used in MIC tests must be prepared from reference standard an-

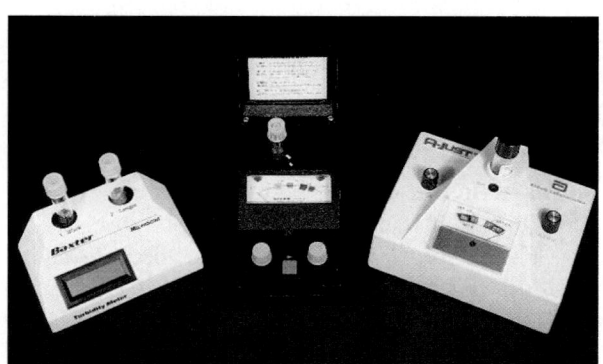

Figure 3-5 _____

Three bench-top nephelometric-type devices that can be used to standardize the turbidity of a test inoculum suspension to match that of a McFarland 0.5 (or other) turbidity standard.

TABLE 3-6

MIC Interpretive Standards (μg/mL) for Several Organism Groups

Antimicrobial Agent	Susceptible	Intermediate	Resistant
Ampicillin			
When testing Enterobacteriaceae	≤8	16	≥32
When testing staphylococci	≤0.25	—	≥0.5
When testing enterococci	≤8	—	≥16
When testing *Haemophilus* spp.	≤1	—	≥2
When testing streptococci other than *S. pneumoniae*	≤0.25	0.5-4	≥8
When testing *Listeria monocytogenes*	≤2	—	—
Gentamicin			
When testing Enterobacteriaceae	≤4	8	≥16
When testing nonEnterobacteriaceae	≤4	8	≥16
When testing staphylococci	≤4	8	≥16
Oxacillin			
When testing *S. aureus*	≤2	—	≥4
When testing coagulase-negative staphylococci	≤0.25	—	≥0.5

Modified from NCCLS publication M100-S9, *Performance standards for antimicrobial susceptiblity testing; ninth informational supplement.* Copies of the current edition may be obtained from NCCLS, 940 West Valley Road, Suite1400, Wayne, PA 19087-1898.

timicrobial powders. Details of preparation are found in the NCCLS protocols. Stock solutions and other antimicrobial solutions must be stored frozen in non–frost-free freezers. Temperatures at or below −70° C are optimal and necessary for more temperature-labile drugs such as imipenem and clavulanic acid; however −20° C storage is acceptable for some agents. Antimicrobial solutions must never be refrozen following thawing.

Broth macrodilution (tube dilution) tests

Broth dilution MIC tests performed in test tubes are referred to as *broth macrodilution* or *tube dilution* susceptibility tests. Generally, a twofold serial dilution, each containing 1 to 2 mL of antimicrobial agent, is prepared. Mueller-Hinton broth is the medium most commonly used for broth dilution MIC tests of nonfastidious bacteria. A standardized suspension of test bacteria is added to each dilution to obtain a final concentration of 5×10^5 CFU/mL. A growth control tube (broth plus inoculum) and an uninoculated control tube (broth only) are used in each test. After overnight incubation at 35° C, the MIC is determined visually as the lowest concentration that inhibits growth, as demonstrated by the absence of turbidity.

Broth macrodilution is impractical for use as a routine method when several antimicrobial agents must be tested on an isolate or if several isolates must be tested. Some laboratories use broth macrodilution when it is necessary to test drugs not included in their routine system or fastidious bacteria that require special growth media. Additionally, this method is often used when minimum bactericidal concentration (MBC) endpoints are to be subsequently determined. The MBC test is discussed later in this chapter.

Broth microdilution tests

The broth macrodilution test has been adapted to multi-well microdilution trays (Figure 3-6) for **broth microdilution MIC testing**. Polystyrene

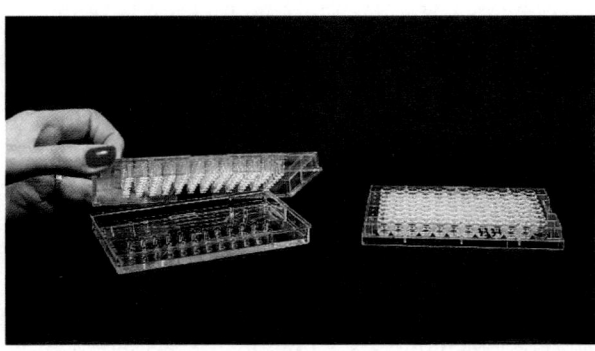

Figure 3-6

Broth microdilution MIC tray shown with inoculum reservoir trough. Diluted inoculum suspension is placed in the reservior trough. Then the prongs are dipped into the suspension, raised, and subsequently lowered into the wells of the broth microdilution MIC tray to inoculate all wells simultaneously.

trays containing between 80 and 100 wells are filled with small volumes (usually 0.1 mL) of two-fold dilution concentrations of antimicrobial agent in broth. Because of the large number of wells, several dilutions of as many as 12 to 15 antimicrobial agents can be contained on a single tray that will be subsequently inoculated with one bacterial isolate. The inoculum suspension is prepared and standardized as described previously. An intermediate dilution of this inoculum suspension is prepared in water, and a multi-pronged inoculator or other type of inoculating device is used to inoculate the wells to obtain a final concentration of approximately 1 to 5×10^5 CFU/mL (1-5×10^4 CFU per 0.1-mL well). The actual dilution factor used for preparation of the intermediate dilution depends on the volume of inoculum delivered to each well by the inoculating device. An example of this calculation is illustrated in Table 3-7. A growth control well and uninoculated control well are included on each tray. After overnight incubation at 35° C, the tray is placed on one of several types of tray-reading devices to facilitate close visual examination of each well (Figure 3-7). Provided that growth is adequate in the growth control well, the MIC for a particular agent is the lowest concentration showing no obvious growth. Growth may be noted as turbidity, a haze, or a pellet in the bottom of the well.

Some larger laboratories have dispensing devices that are used to prepare broth microdilution panels. For most laboratories, however, a practical approach to broth microdilution MIC testing involves purchasing prepared panels, either frozen or dried, from a commercial vendor. Frozen panels are thawed at room temperature before inoculation. For dried panels the dried or lyophilized drugs in the wells are reconstituted at the same time the panels are inoculated. In addition to the panels, all commercial companies sell other materials needed for testing (e.g., inoculum broths, inoculum diluents, panel inoculators, and reading devices). Usually, a variety of panels containing different drugs are available for testing various organism groups (e.g., gram-positive, gram-negative), and some panels are designed to include wells containing various biochemical reagents so that organism identification and antimicrobial susceptibility testing can be done simultaneously on a single panel. Some companies

TABLE 3-7

Example of Calculations Representing Dilution Schema for Preparation of Inocula for Broth Microdilution MIC Tests*

Step	Resulting Organism Concentration
1. Standardize suspension to McFarland 0.5	1.5×10^8 CFU/mL
2. Add 0.75 mL from step 1 to 25 mL water diluent (1:33 dilution)	4-5×10^6 CFU/mL
3. Use inoculator prong set to inoculate wells of MIC tray (each prong delivers 0.01 mL, which results in an additional 1:100 dilution)	4-5×10^4 CFU/100-μL well 4-5×10^5 CFU/mL

*Calculations shown here are based on use of inoculator prong set (each prong delivering 0.01 mL). Dilutions in Step 2 vary, depending on the number of organisms in the initial suspension and the volume delivered to each well by the inoculating device.

have automated or semiautomated devices to facilitate inoculation and reading. These are discussed in the following sections.

BREAKPOINT MIC PANELS

A variation of the standard broth microdilution MIC panel is the **breakpoint** panel, in which only one or two concentrations of each antimicrobial agent are tested on a single panel. *Breakpoint* is

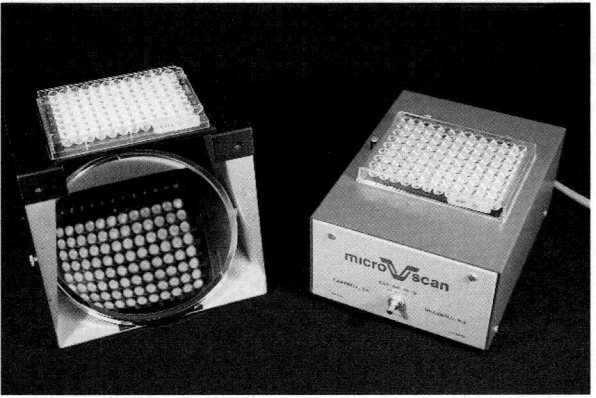

Figure 3-7

Dynatech tray-reading stand with magnifying mirror *(left)* and a light box *(right)*. Following incubation, either of these devices is used to examine growth in the broth microdilution MIC trays. A tray is placed on the Dynatech tray-reading stand, and wells are examined by looking into the magnifying mirror. A tray is placed over the hole in the light box, and light is allowed to shine through the tray to facilitate close examination of the wells.

the term applied to the concentration of an antimicrobial that can be achieved in body fluids with optimal therapy. These concentrations typically include the concentration that defines the MIC breakpoint for susceptibility and one dilution above the breakpoint. When two concentrations are tested and no growth is present in either well, the isolate is susceptible. When there is growth in the low concentration but no growth in the high concentration, the isolate has intermediate susceptibility, and a resistant isolate grows in both wells. The qualitative interpretation—*susceptible, intermediate,* or *resistant*—rather than an MIC value is generally reported. The primary advantage of breakpoint panels is that numerous drugs can be tested on a single panel (often in combination with biochemical tests). The primary disadvantage of breakpoint panels is that a precise MIC is not obtained because most results are either equal to or lower than the lowest concentration tested or greater than the highest concentration tested. Additionally, performing relevant quality control on breakpoint panels is difficult.

TRAILING AND SKIPPED WELLS

Dilution methods, particularly broth microdilution methods, sometimes produce an MIC endpoint that is not clear-cut, and growth in the wells may demonstrate trailing or skipped wells. **Trailing** involves heavy growth at lower concentrations, followed by one or more wells that show greatly reduced growth in the form of a small button or a light haze. This commonly occurs with sulfonamides, trimethoprim, and trimethoprim/sulfamethoxazole; the mode of action of the agents allows the bacterial cells to grow through several generations before inhibition. In this case, the trailing is ignored, and the endpoint is read as an 80% reduction in growth. Trailing with other drugs, however, may represent contamination and should not be ignored, unless it is known that trailing commonly occurs with the particular antimicrobial agent–organism combination.

Skipped wells involve growth at higher concentrations and no growth at one or more of the lower concentrations. This may occur as a result of contamination, improperly inoculated wells, improper concentrations of antimicrobial agent in the wells, presence of unusual resistance with the test isolate (e.g., a small resistant subpopulation), or a combination of two or more of these

factors. As with trailing, each skipped well occurrence must be evaluated individually to determine whether results are reportable. If any doubt exists with regard to the accuracy of the results, they should not be reported and the test should be repeated.

One shortcoming of the broth microdilution MIC method is its inability to produce a penicillin MIC that is consistently within the resistant range for staphylococci that are low-level β-lactamase producers. If the penicillin MIC is 0.03 μg/mL or less, the isolate may be reported as susceptible; a result 0.25 μg/mL or higher is considered resistant. An induced β-lactamase test must, however, be performed on isolates with penicillin MICs of 0.06 to 0.12 μg/mL. If the β-lactamase test result is positive, the isolate is reported as penicillin resistant; if the result is negative, the isolate is reported as penicillin susceptible.

Agar dilution tests

MIC tests can also be performed using an **agar dilution** method. Specific volumes of antimicrobial solutions are dispensed into premeasured volumes of molten and cooled agar, which is subsequently poured into standard Petri dishes. Mueller-Hinton agar is generally used for testing aerobic isolates; however, this can be supplemented with sheep's blood (to a final concentration of 5% sheep's blood) or other nutrients for testing fastidious bacteria. A series of plates, containing varying concentrations of each antimicrobial agent, and growth control plates without antimicrobial agent are prepared. The agar is allowed to solidify, and then a standard number of test bacteria (10^4 CFU for aerobes) are "spot" inoculated onto each plate using a multipronged replicating device, such as a Steer's replicator (Figure 3-8). As many as 32 different isolates can be simultaneously inoculated onto each 100-mm round Petri dish; 100-mm square plates generally accommodate 36 isolates. After overnight incubation the MIC is read as the lowest concentration of antimicrobial agent that inhibits the visible growth of the test bacterium (one or two colonies are ignored).

The shelf life of agar dilution plates is only 1 week for most antimicrobial agents because plates must be stored at 2° to 8° C, and many drugs are labile at this temperature. Because plate preparation is laborious and this procedure is practical

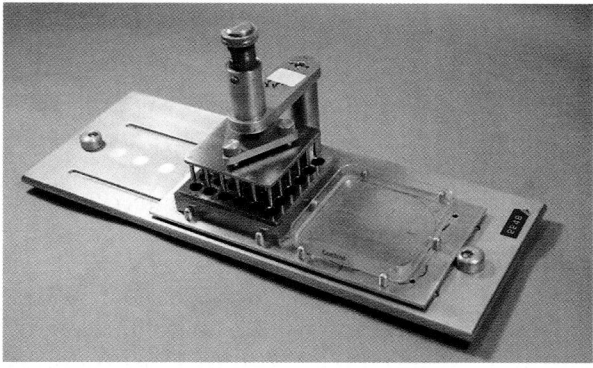

Figure 3-8

Steer's replicator. The inoculator prongs are positioned above a 36-well seed trough that contains 36 different standardized inoculum suspensions. The handle on top of the prong unit is pressed to lower the prongs into all suspensions simultaneously, and when the prongs are raised, each contains a standardized volume of inoculum. The agar plate containing a defined concentration of antimicrobial agent is positioned under the prongs (steel plate holding agar plate slides back and forth), and the prongs are carefully lowered to the agar, at which point the inocula are deposited on the agar surface. This process is repeated until all antimicrobial-containing and control agar plates (without antimicrobial agent) have been inoculated.

only if large numbers of isolates are tested, agar dilution is generally performed only in research settings, although it is currently the reference method for antimicrobial susceptibility testing of anaerobes and *N. gonorrhoeae.*

Disk Diffusion Testing
Principle
The disk diffusion test, also commonly known as the ***Bauer Kirby test,*** has been widely used in clinical laboratories since 1966, when the first standardized method was described. Briefly, a McFarland 0.5 standardized suspension of bacteria is swabbed over the surface of an agar plate, and paper disks containing single concentrations of each antimicrobial agent are placed onto the inoculated surface. After overnight incubation, the diameters of the zones produced by antimicrobial inhibition of bacterial growth are measured and the isolate is interpreted as either susceptible, intermediate, or resistant to a particular drug according to preset criteria. A photograph of an isolate of *Enterobacter aerogenes* tested by disk diffusion is shown in Figure 3-9.

Establishing zone diameter interpretive breakpoints
The disk diffusion test depends on the formation of a gradient of antimicrobial concentrations as the antimicrobial agent diffuses radially into the agar. The drug concentration decreases at increasing distances from the disk. At a critical point, the amount of drug at a specific location in the medium is unable to inhibit the growth of the test organism, and a **zone of inhibition** is formed.

The zones of inhibition are related to MICs, and it is this relationship that has been used to determine the breakpoints for interpreting a particular zone measurement as indicating that the isolate is susceptible, intermediate, or resistant. To establish breakpoints for a single agent, the first step is to determine the optimum concentration of drug to incorporate into the disk. This is done by reviewing the drug's pharmacokinetic properties (e.g., antimicrobial concentration attainable in vivo) and also some of the biochemical properties (e.g., molecular size, solubility, and diffusibility in agar). Next, a sample of 150 to 200 isolates with comparable growth rates and varying susceptibility to the agent are tested by both the standard disk diffusion test and a standard dilution MIC test, and results are plotted on a graph. For

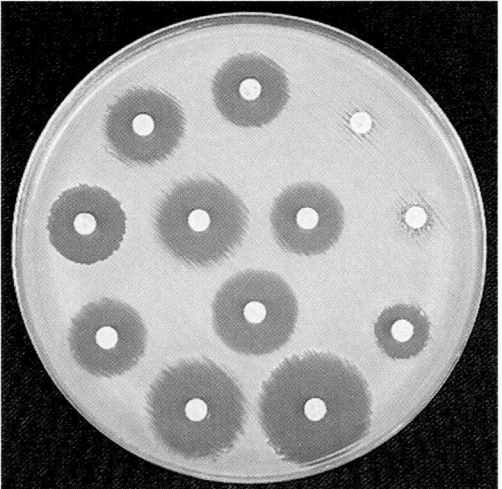

Figure 3-9

Enterobacter aerogenes tested by the disk diffusion method. Zone measurements confirm that the isolate is susceptible to all agents tested except ampicillin (at the 1 o'clock position) and cefazolin (at the 2 o'clock position). No zones are present for either of these agents.

each isolate the observed MIC value is expressed in logarithmic form (log$_2$) and plotted on the *y* axis, and the corresponding zone measurement is plotted on the *x* axis on an arithmetic scale (scattergram). A linear regression analysis is performed through the plotted points, and a line of best fit, or regression line, is drawn. The concentrations representing therapeutically achievable blood levels after standard dosing are identified.

Results of clinical treatment situations in which the MICs of the implicated organisms and therapeutic outcomes are known are examined. The distribution of the plotted points is reviewed, and efforts are made to avoid defining breakpoints that will split a population of isolates that are probably either all susceptible or all resistant. All this information is considered, and MICs defining *susceptible, intermediate,* and *resistant* are identified. These are correlated with MIC values specified on the *y* axis of the graph, and the regression line is further examined to match the MIC value to its corresponding zone diameter to obtain the zone diameter breakpoints. A generic

scattergram and regression analysis is shown in Figure 3-10.

The NCCLS and the U.S. Food and Drug Administration (FDA) are involved in developing zone interpretive criteria, and the procedure just described has been performed for every antimicrobial agent for which zone interpretive criteria exist. One concern in establishing zone interpretive criteria for some of the newer, extremely active agents, such as the fluoroquinolones, is the lack of resistant isolates to include in the analysis to provide a balanced distribution of points on the graph. This has led in some cases to define criteria for *susceptible* only; no intermediate or resistant zone interpretive criteria are specified.

Test performance
DISK STORAGE
Most clinical laboratories follow the protocol specified by the NCCLS for disk diffusion testing, and the NCCLS document contains explicit details for test performance. Only FDA-approved disks should be used; they must be stored properly to

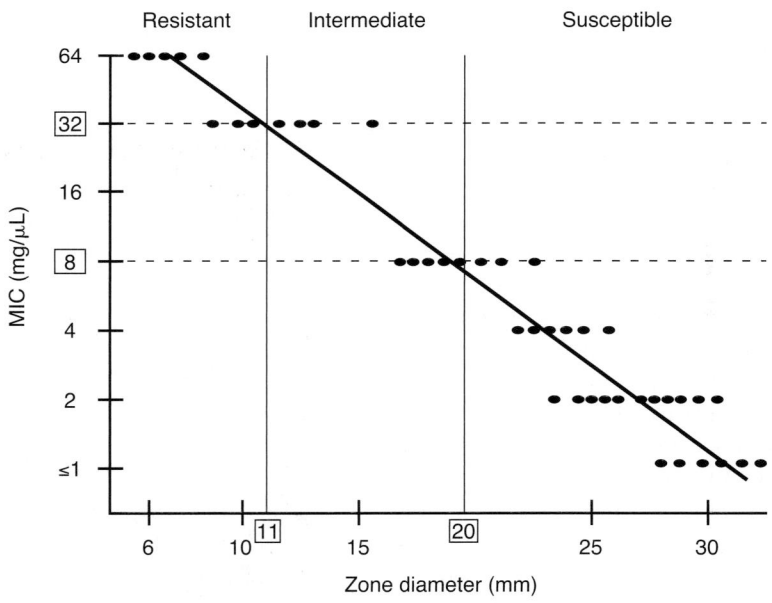

Figure 3-10

Example of a scattergram and regression analysis plot used to determine disk diffusion zone diameter interpretive breakpoints for hypothetical drug "X." Based on clinical response data, isolates with MICs ≤8.0 μg/mL are considered susceptible. As derived from this scattergram, corresponding zones ≥20 mm would be interpreted as susceptible. Isolates with MICs ≥32.0 μg/mL and zones ≤11 mm are resistant. The intermediate designation is used for isolates whose values fall between the susceptible and the resistant MICs (16 μg/mL) and zone interpretive breakpoints (12-19 mm).

ensure that the drugs maintain their potency. For long-term storage, disks are stored at $-14°$ C or below in a non–frost-free freezer. A working supply of disks can be stored in a refrigerator at $2°$ to $8°$ C for at least 1 week. Disks should always be stored in a tightly sealed container with desiccant. The container should be allowed to warm to room temperature before it is opened to prevent condensation from forming on the disks when warm room air contacts the cold containers.

INOCULATION AND INCUBATION

Inoculum suspensions are prepared using either a log-phase or direct inoculum suspension standardized to match the turbidity of a McFarland 0.5 standard, as previously described. A sterile cotton swab is dipped into the suspension, press and rotated firmly against the side of the tube to express excess liquid, and then swabbed evenly across the surface of a Mueller-Hinton agar plate. Usually, a plate 150 mm in diameter is used; it can accommodate testing of up to 12 different antimicrobial disks (placement of more than 12 disks on the plate may result in overlapping zones, which are difficult to measure and may produce erroneous results). Within 15 minutes of inoculation,

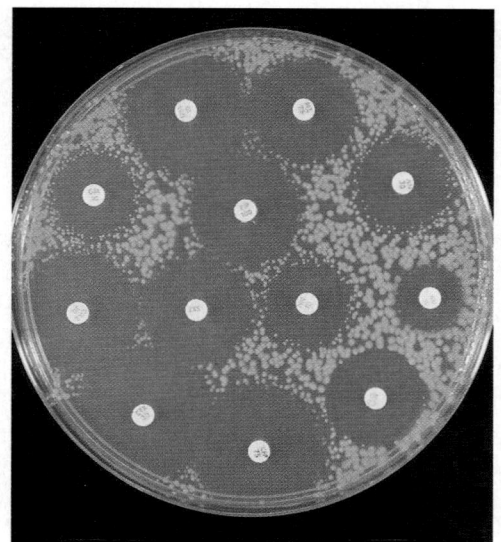

Figure 3-12 ——————————————

Escherichia coli tested by the disk diffusion method. The lawn of growth following overnight incubation shows individual colonies, representing unsatisfactory growth. The most likely explanation for the scanty growth is the use of an inoculum that either is too light or contains too many nonviable cells, resulting in larger than normal zones and potentially false susceptible results.

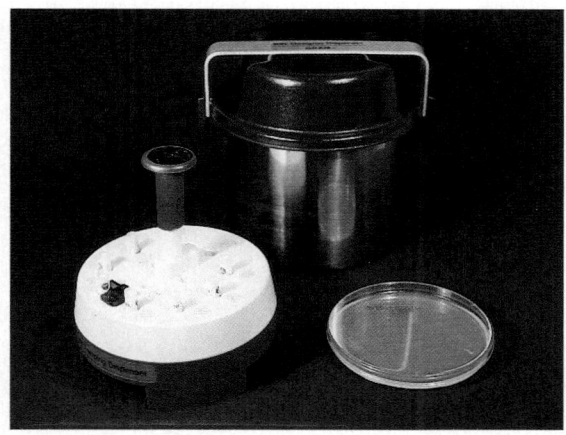

Figure 3-11 ——————————————

Cartridges containing antimicrobial susceptibility test disks are inserted into the dispenser *(left)*. The dispenser (which can hold up to 12 different cartridges of disks) is positioned over an inoculated plate, and light pressure is applied to the handle to simultaneously deposit one of each type of disk onto the plate. The tight-sealing container in the background contains a desiccant packet and is used for storage (at $2°$-$8°$ C) of the dispenser containing a working supply of disks.

the antimicrobial-containing disks are applied to the agar with a forceps for individual disks or with a multiple-disk dispenser (Figure 3-11). The disks are pressed firmly to ensure contact with the agar. Within 15 minutes of disk placement, plates are inverted and placed in a $35°$ C ambient air incubator for 16 to 18 hours. Mueller-Hinton agar containing 5% sheep's blood is used for testing streptococci that do not grow adequately on unsupplemented Mueller-Hinton agar. Although incubation in an atmosphere of increased CO_2 is recommended for testing some fastidious bacteria, this should be avoided unless the impact on the results is known. Incubation in CO_2 results in a decreased pH, which affects the activity of some antimicrobial agents.

READING PLATES AND TEST INTERPRETATION

After incubation the plate is examined to make certain the test organism has grown satisfactorily. The lawn of growth must be confluent or almost confluent, and the appearance of individual colonies is unacceptable (Figure 3-12). Provided that growth

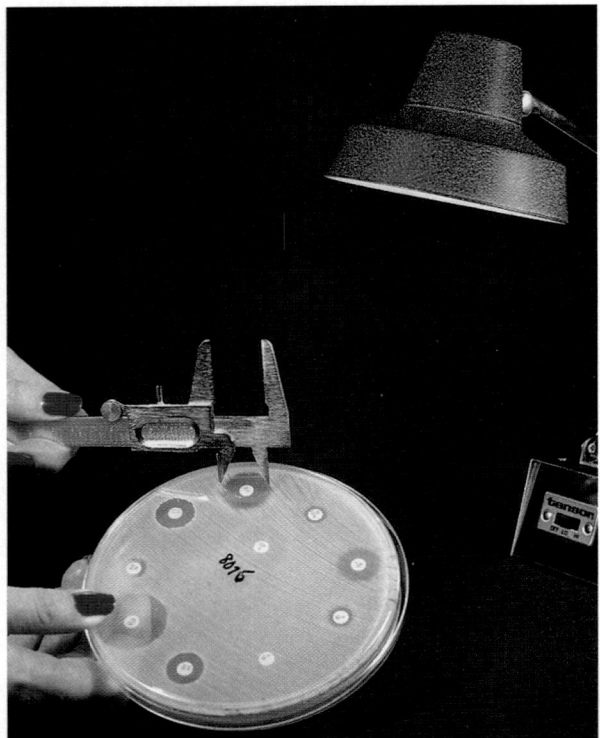

Figure 3-13

Routine disk diffusion tests are examined by placing the plate on or 2 to 3 inches above a black, nonreflecting surface. Reflected light is used to illuminate the plate.

sults or repeat testing of the subcultured colonies from within the zone suggests resistance, the isolate should be reported as resistant.

Transmitted light (plate held up to light source) (Figure 3-14) rather than reflected light must be used to examine zones for the penicillinase-resistant penicillins when testing staphylococci and for vancomycin when testing enterococci; otherwise, zone measurements may become erroneous, as described in the case study. Tests performed on media containing blood are examined from the top of the plate with the lid removed. For plates containing blood, it is important to read the zone of inhibition of growth and not the zone of inhibition of hemolysis.

Once zone measurements have been made, the millimeter reading for each antimicrobial agent is compared with that specified in the interpretive

is satisfactory, the diameter of each inhibition zone is measured using a ruler or calipers. Plates are placed on or 2 to 3 inches above a black, nonreflecting surface, and zones are examined from the back side (agar side) of the plate illuminated with reflected light (Figure 3-13). Tiny colonies at the zone edge and the swarm of growth into the zone that often occurs with swarming *Proteus* spp are ignored; the obvious zone is measured. As with dilution tests, the end point for the sulfonamides, trimethoprim, and trimethoprim/sulfamethoxazole is an 80% reduction of growth. Obvious colonies within a clear zone should not be ignored. These colonies may occur as a result of contamination; however, these colonies sometimes represent a small resistant subpopulation. When such colonies are noted, the original isolate should be retested and the colonies within the zone should be subcultured to check for contamination. If repeat testing of the original isolate produces the same re-

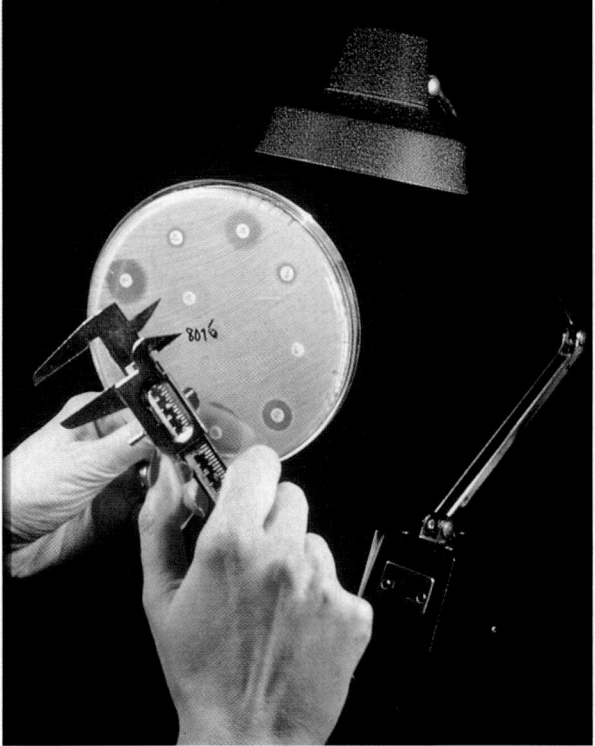

Figure 3-14

Disk diffusion tests for staphylococci with oxacillin (or methicillin or nafcillin) and enterococci with vancomycin are examined by holding the plate up to a light source (transmitted light) for zone examination. Any growth within the zone is significant.

TABLE 3-8

Zone Diameter Interpretive Standards and Equivalent Minimum Inhibitory Concentration (MIC) Breakpoints for Several Organism Groups

Antimicrobial Agent	Disk Content (µg)	Zone Diameter, nearest whole mm			Equivalent MIC Breakpoints (µg/ml)	
		Resistant	Intermediate	Susceptible	Resistant	Susceptible
Ampicillin						
When testing Enterobacteriaceae	10	≤13	14-16	≥17	≥32	≤8
When testing staphylococci	10	≤28	—	≥29	β-lactamase	≤0.1
When testing enterococci	10	≤16	—	≥17	≥16	≤8
When testing *Haemophilus* spp.	10	≤18	19-21	≥22	≥4	≤1.0
When testing streptococci other than *S. pneumoniae*	10	≤18	19-25	≥26	≥8	≤0.25
Gentamicin						
When testing Enterobacteriaceae	10	≤12	13-14	≥15	≥8	≤4
When testing nonEnterobacteriaceae	10	≤12	13-14	≥15	≥8	≤4
When testing staphylococci	10	≤12	13-14	≥15	≥8	≤4
Oxacillin						
When testing *S. aureus*	1	≤10	11-12	≥13	≥4	≤2
When testing coagulase-negative staphylococci	1	≤17	—	≥18	≥0.5	≤0.25
When testing *S. pneumoniae* for penicillin G susceptiblity	1	≤19	—	≥20	—	≤0.06

Modified from NCCLS publication M100-S9, *Performance standards for antimicrobial susceptibility testing; ninth informational supplement.* Copies of the current edition may be obtained from NCCLS, 940 West Valley Road, Suite 1400, Wayne, PA 19087-1898.

tables of the NCCLS documents, and results are interpreted as either susceptible, intermediate, or resistant. An excerpt from the chart is shown in Table 3-8. The equivalent MIC breakpoints that are used to define resistance and susceptibility are also shown. Note that as with MIC interpretive criteria, several sets of interpretive criteria may exist for some antimicrobial agents, which are specific for various organisms or organism groups.

A summary of the variables that must be carefully controlled in the performance of routine disk diffusion and broth microdilution MIC tests is listed in Table 3-9.

Modified Methods for Testing Slow-Growing or Fastidious Bacteria

Mueller-Hinton agar and broth are the standard media used for routine dilution and disk diffusion tests. These media, however, do not support the growth of all bacteria requiring antimicrobial susceptibility tests, and consequently, routine methods must be modified for testing fastidious bacteria that require supplemental nutrients, modified incubation conditions, or both.

Haemophilus influenzae and *Haemophilus* spp.

Haemophilus test medium (HTM), which consists of Mueller-Hinton agar base supplemented with X (hematin) and V (nicotinamide adenine dinucleotide or NAD) factors, has been standardized for testing *Haemophilus influenzae* and other *Haemophilus* spp. HTM broth is used for broth dilution tests, and HTM agar is used for disk diffusion tests. The test procedures for *Haemophilus* spp. are identical to those described for nonfastidious bacteria with the exception that the disk diffusion test with HTM is incubated in an atmosphere of 5% to 7% CO_2. The NCCLS has established zone diameter and MIC interpretive criteria that are unique for this genus. For some agents, such as cefotaxime, only a susceptible range is defined. Again, this is because cefotaxime-resistant *Haemophilus* spp. have not been identified, and consequently, criteria to identify such resistance

TABLE 3-9

Primary Variables that Must Be Controlled in Performance of Routine Disk Diffusion and Broth Microdilution MIC Tests

Variable	Standard	Comments
Inoculum	Disk diffusion: 1.5×10^8 CFU/mL	Use "adequate" McFarland turbidity standard (0.5 for disk diffusion)
	Microbroth dilution: 5×10^5 CFU/mL (final concentration)	When preparing direct suspensions (without incubation), do not use growth from plates >1 day old
Media		
Formulation	Mueller-Hinton	Prepare in-house purchase from reliable source
		Perform media QC to verify acceptability before use for patient tests
Ca^{++}, Mg^{++} content	25 mg/L Ca^{++}, 12.5 mg/L Mg^{++}	Increased concentrations result in decreased activity of aminoglycosides against *P. aeruginosa* and decreased activity of tetracyclines against all organisms (decreased concentrations have the opposite effect)
Thymidine content	Minimal or absent	Excessive concentrations can result in false resistance to sulfonamides and trimethoprim
pH	7.2-7.4	Decreased pH can lead to decreased activity of aminoglycosides, erythromycin, and clindamycin and increased activity of tetracyclines (increased pH has the opposite effect)
Agar depth (disk diffusion)	3-5 mm	Possibility for false susceptibility if <3 mm, or false resistance if >5 mm
Incubation		
Atmosphere	Humidified ambient air	CO_2 incubation decreases pH, which can lead to decreased activity of aminoglycosides, erythromycin, and clindamycin, and increased activity of tetracyclines
Temperature	$-35°$ C	Some MRSA may go undetected if >35° C
Length	Disk diffusion 16-18 hours	Some MRSA may go undetected if <24 hours
	Microbroth dilution: 16:20 hours	Some vancomycin-resistant enterococci may go undetected if <24 hours with disk diffusion
	(24 hours staphylococci with oxacillin* and enterococci with vancomycin and with gentamicin HLAR; 48 hours enterococci with streptomycin HLAR; 24 hours sometimes needed for fastidious bacteria)	Some HLAR (gentamicin) enterococci may go undetected if <24 hours (microbroth dilution)
		Some HLAR (streptomycin) enterococci may go undetected if <48 hours (microbroth dilution)

Modified from Hindler JA, Mann LM: Principles and practices for the laboratory guidance of antimicrobial therapy. In Tilton RC et al, editors: *Clinical laboratory medicine,* St Louis, 1992, Mosby.
HLAR, High level aminoglycoside resistance.
MRSA, methicillin-resistant *Staphylococcus aureus.*
*Includes all penicillinase-resistant penicillins (oxacillin, methicillin, nafcillin, cloxacillin, and dicloxacillin).

could not be established. Further tests, possibly in a reference laboratory, should be performed on any *Haemophilus* spp isolate that is interpreted as other than susceptible to cefotaxime. These recommendations hold true for all drugs for which only susceptible criteria are specified by NCCLS.

Ampicillin or amoxicillin is often effective in treating localized, less serious *H. influenzae* infections; however, 20% to 50% of *H. influenzae* produce a β-lactamase that inactivates these agents. β-Lactamase–producing strains can be quickly identified by using a rapid β-lactamase test. *Haemophilus influenzae* also may be resistant to ampicillin and amoxicillin because of altered penicillin-binding proteins, but this resistance occurs in less than 1.0% of clinical isolates. Because most ampicillin-resistant (amoxicillin-resistant) *H. influenzae* produce β-lactamase, and

TABLE 3-9 ━━━━━━━━━━━━━━━━━━━━━━━━━━━━━━━━━━━━━━

Primary Variables that Must Be Controlled in Performance of Routine Disk Diffusion and Broth Microdilution MIC Tests—cont'd

Variable	Standard	Comments
Antimicrobial agents		
Disks	Used disks containing appropriate FDA/NCCLS-defined concentration of drug	Check NCCLS publication or FDA package insert (accompanying disks) for specifications
	Proper storage	For long-term storage, use *non*–frost-free freezer at ≤−20° C in tightly sealed, desiccated container
		For short-term storage (at least 1 week), maintain temperature at 2°-8° C in tightly sealed, desiccated container
		Allow to warm to room temperature before opening container
	Proper placement on agar	Store 12 or fewer disks per 150-mm plate (no overlapping zones)
Solutions	Prepared from reference standard powders	Pharmacy-grade antimicrobial agents are unacceptable (they may not show antimicrobial activity in vitro)
	Proper storage	Store in *non*–frost-free freezer, optimally at ≤−70° C
		Never refreeze
End point measurement		
Disk diffusion	Reflected light (except for staphylococci and oxacillin* and for vancomycin and enterococci) and plate held against black background	Lawn must be confluent or almost confluent
		Ignore faint growth of tiny colonies at zone edge
	Zones measured from back of plate	Trimethoprim and sulfonamides—end point at ≥80% inhibition
		Ignore swarm within obvious zone for swarming *Proteus* spp.
		Retest colonies within zone (except staphylococci and oxacillin, enterococci and vancomycin)
	Transmitted light used for staphylococci and oxacillin* and for enterococci and vancomycin	Call "resistant" if *any* growth within zone (unless possibly artifactual or contaminated)
		Reproducibility is with ±2 mm
Microbroth dilution	Adequate lighting and reading device	MIC = lowest concentration that inhibits growth (turbidity, haze, or pellet)
		Sulfonamides and trimethoprim may trail (ignore trailing <2 mm buttons)
		Justify "skip wells" or repeat
		Staphylococci and penicillin—perform induced β-lactamase test if MIC is 0.06-0.12 μg/mL
		Reproducibility should be within ±1 two-fold dilution

because *H. influenzae* are often susceptible to alternative agents currently recommended, some laboratories do not routinely perform disk diffusion or MIC tests but perform only a β-lactamase test unless the isolate is from blood or CSF.

Streptococcus pneumoniae and *Streptococcus* spp.

Streptococcus pneumoniae and *Streptococcus* spp. require a more nutritious medium for antimicrobial susceptibility testing; they will not grow satisfactorily on unsupplemented Mueller-Hinton medium. Broth dilution tests are usually performed in Mueller-Hinton broth that has been supplemented with 2% to 5% lysed horse's blood. Agar dilution and disk diffusion tests are performed using Mueller-Hinton agar supplemented with 5% sheep's blood.

Penicillin remains the drug of choice for treating pneumococcal infections; however, resistance to penicillin as well as to other potentially useful agents is becoming widespread. Penicillin resistance is due to the presence of altered penicillin-binding proteins and is not enzymatically mediated. Consequently, β-lactamase testing is inappropriate for pneumococci.

The disk diffusion test can be used to screen for penicillin susceptibility in *S. pneumoniae.* An oxacillin disk (1 μg) rather than a penicillin disk must be used, however, for reliable detection of penicillin resistance. Using the standard disk diffusion procedure, an isolate is tested on Mueller-Hinton agar with 5% sheep's blood and incubated in CO_2. If the oxacillin zone of inhibition is 20 mm or larger, the isolate is reported as penicillin (not oxacillin) susceptible. If the oxacillin zone is 19 mm or smaller, a penicillin (not oxacillin) MIC test must be performed to clarify the level of resistance (Figure 3-15). Penicillin MICs of 0.06 μg/mL or less are interpreted as susceptible, of 0.12 to 1.0 μg/mL as intermediate, and 2.0 μg/mL or more as resistant. Determining the degree of penicillin resistance is important because the recommended therapy may be different for intermediate and resistant strains. It is also important to test penicillin-resistant isolates with other clinically relevant antimicrobial agents, such as cefotaxime or ceftriaxone, and perhaps erythromycin.

Accurate penicillin susceptibility results are needed for viridans streptococci isolated from the blood of patients with bacterial endocarditis. If the isolate has a penicillin MIC of 0.12 μg/mL or less, penicillin alone is often prescribed; however, higher penicillin MICs (0.25-2.0 μg/mL) suggest the need for concomitant therapy with an amino-

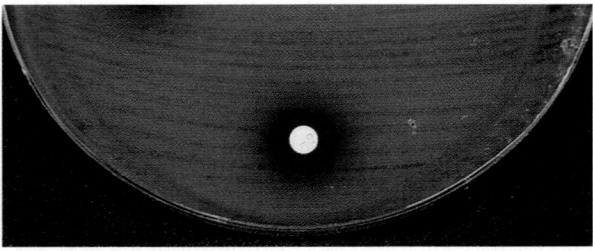

Figure 3-15 ———————————————
An oxacillin (1-μg) disk is used to screen for penicillin susceptibility in *Streptococcus pneumoniae.* If the oxacillin zone of inhibition is ≥20 mm, the isolate is reported as susceptible. If the oxacillin zone is ≤19 mm, a penicillin MIC test must be performed. The isolate pictured has an oxacillin zone of approximately 15 mm, so a penicillin MIC test must be performed.

glycoside. Isolates with penicillin MICs greater than 2.0 μg/mL are highly resistant, and for these vancomycin rather than penicillin is generally prescribed. Because of the critical nature of penicillin results, the disk test is not recommended in these situations, and dilution tests should be performed. As with *S. pneumoniae,* penicillin resistance in viridans streptococci is due to altered penicillin-binding proteins, and β-lactamase testing should not be performed on this group of organisms.

Neisseria gonorrhoeae and *Neisseria meningitidis*

GC agar base is supplemented with various nutrients for testing *Neisseria gonorrhoeae.* Dilution tests are performed using agar dilution because this species has a tendency to lyse in broth media, resulting in false-susceptible results. Disk diffusion tests are performed on the same agar, and all tests are incubated in an atmosphere containing 5% to 7% CO_2. NCCLS has specified interpretive criteria unique for this species. For several agents for which resistant isolates have not yet been encountered, only susceptible criteria are available.

Although for many years penicillin was the drug of choice for treating uncomplicated gonorrhea, the increased incidence of penicillin-resistant isolates has led to the use of ceftriaxone or a fluoroquinolone as first-line therapy. Penicillin resistance in *N. gonorrhoeae* may be due to production of a β-lactamase similar to that produced by ampicillin-resistant *H. influenzae,* and this resistance can be readily detected with a rapid β-lactamase test. β-Lactamase–producing isolates are also referred to as **penicillinase-producing** *N. gonorrhoeae,* or **PPNG.** Some *N. gonorrhoeae* are penicillin resistant due to an altered penicillin-binding protein; this resistance can be detected only with conventional dilution or disk diffusion tests. The production of altered penicillin-binding proteins is choromosomally mediated, and *N. gonorrhoeae* with altered penicillin-binding proteins are often referred to as **chromosomally mediated resistant** *N. gonorrhoeae,* or **CMRNG.** Because current therapeutic recommendations do not include penicillin and because virtually all *N. gonorrhoeae* are currently susceptible to ceftriaxone and most are susceptible to the recommended flouroquinolones, testing is rarely indicated in the routine clinical laboratory. Some laboratories continue to perform β-lactamase tests, however, and public health laboratories test multiple agents against *N. gonorrhoeae* for surveillance purposes.

Except for very rare isolates that have been shown to produce β-lactamase, *Neisseria meningitidis* remains susceptible to penicillin, the drug of choice for treating infections caused by this organism. Isolates with slightly elevated penicillin MICs have been observed, however. These have not caused major problems yet because the penicillin MICs are still below penicillin levels attainable in CSF, although they are higher than those for normally susceptible isolates. Meningococci are often resistant to sulfonamides and occasionally resistant to rifampin. Either of these agents or a fluoroquinolone is administered prophylactically to individuals in close contact with patients who have meningococcal meningitis. No standard procedures for performing either disk diffusion or MIC tests on meningococci currently exist.

Anaerobes

The reference method described by the NCCLS for testing anaerobic bacteria is an agar dilution method, and the recommended medium is supplemented Brucella blood agar. As previously mentioned, however, agar dilution is not practical for use in the routine clinical laboratory, and a broth microdilution method is more often used. The broth microdilution procedure is similar to that used for testing aerobes except for the broth. Several different broths have been used for microdilution testing of anaerobes, including Schaedler's, Brucella, West-Wilkins, brain-heart infusion, and Wilkins-Chalgren. Sometimes supplements (e.g., horse serum or lysed horse blood) are added to facilitate growth of the more fastidious species. Additionally, the number of organisms in the test inoculum is 0.5 $\log_{10}$ higher (10^6 CFU/mL) than that for testing aerobes, and trays are incubated anaerobically at 35° C for 48 hours. As with tests for aerobic bacteria, the NCCLS has defined susceptible, intermediate, and resistant criteria for interpretation of MICs for anaerobes. Additionally, several commercial companies provide broth microdilution MIC panels for testing anaerobes.

The E test, discussed in detail later, has been shown to perform satisfactorily for antimicrobial susceptibility testing of anaerobes, and this method is used in some clinical laboratories.

Additional Organism and Antimicrobial Agent Testing Concerns

Some special procedures must be employed to detect clinically significant resistance in nonfastidious bacteria.

Detection of oxacillin (methicillin) resistance in staphylococci

Oxacillin and other **penicillinase-resistant penicillins,** such as methicillin, nafcillin, cloxacillin, and dicloxacillin, constitute the drug class of choice for treating staphylococcal infections. Oxacillin is the class representative most commonly used to detect resistance in staphylococci and produces the most reliable results. When an isolate shows resistance to any of the penicillinase-resistant penicillins, however, it must be considered resistant to the entire group. Staphylococcal resistance to the penicillinase-resistant penicillins is due to the presence of a unique penicillin-binding protein (2a or 2') on the surface of resistant cells. The penicillin-binding protein, which has a low affinity for penicillinase-resistant penicillins, is encoded by the gene **mecA.** Detecting oxacillin resistance in isolates that possess the *mecA* gene may be difficult under the standard test conditions described previously, because staphylococci sometimes exhibit herteroresistance in their response to oxacillin. In **heteroresistant** strains, all cells in the test population have the genetic elements (the *mecA* gene) for oxacillin resistance, but not all the cells express this resistance. Consequently, in the susceptibility test, some cells appear resistant and some appear susceptible. If too few cells appear resistant, an oxacillin-resistant strain may go undetected.

In vitro testing conditions can be modified to enhance the expression of oxacillin resistance; they are as follows:

- Preparation of inocula using the direct inoculum suspension procedure
- Incubation of tests at temperatures no greater than 35° C
- Obtaining final test readings after a full 24 hours of incubation

▪ Supplementation of Mueller-Hinton broth or agar with 2% NaCl for dilution tests

The extended incubation allows the slower-growing resistant subpopulation sufficient time to grow to detectable numbers. In addition, test plates should always be examined very closely. For disk tests, zones of inhibition must be examined by using transmitted light (holding plate up to the light source; see Figure 3-14), and *any* growth is considered significant. A "haze" of growth within the inhibition zone for oxacillin-resistant isolates is sometimes observed (Figure 3-16).

The clinical significance of oxacillin-resistant or **methicillin-resistant *S. aureus* (MRSA)** is heightened by the fact that these isolates are usually resistant to other antistaphylococcal agents (clindamycin, erythromycin, tetracycline, and sometimes gentamicin and trimethoprim/sulfamethoxazole), with the exception of vancomycin. Sometimes, oxacillin-resistant staphylococci appear susceptible in vitro to other β-lactam agents, such as the cephalosporins; however, these are clinically ineffective. Consequently, all oxacillin-resistant staphylococci must be reported as resistant to all β-lactam agents (including cephalosporins, β-lactam/β-lactamase inhibitor combinations, and imipenem) regardless of the in vitro test results.

According to recent research, the oxacillin zone and MIC breakpoints initially described for all staphylococci are problematic for coagulase negative staphylococci. Specifically, some strains that contained *mecA* gave zones or MICs in the susceptible range. Consequently, these have been modified and separate oxacillin zone and MIC interpretive breakpoints now exist for *S. aureus* and coagulase negative staphylococci. An **oxacillin screen plate** that contains Mueller-Hinton agar supplemented with 4% NaCl and 6 μg/mL oxacillin has been used to detect oxacillin-resistant *S. aureus* (MRSA). To perform the oxacillin screen test, a McFarland 0.5 suspension is prepared as for the disk diffusion test. A swab is dipped into this suspension and streaked over an area of approximately 2 × 5 cm or deposited as a "spot" on the agar surface. After overnight incubation at 35° C *any* growth is an indication that the isolate is oxacillin resistant. This method does not reliably detect oxacillin-resistant coagulase negative staphylococci.

Some *S. aureus* strains have more subtle and less common type of oxacillin resistance that is unrelated to the presence of the *mecA* gene. The resistance mechanism in these isolates is due to either hyperproduction of β-lactamase or the presence of altered penicillin-binding proteins (not related to 2a or 2'). These strains generally have MICs right above (or zones of inhibition right below) the breakpoint for susceptibility, and they are sometimes referred to as ***borderline-resistant*** isolates. Additionally, these isolates are usually susceptible to other antistaphylococcal agents. The clinical response of isolates with borderline oxacillin resistance to penicillinase-resistant penicillins as well as to other β-lactam agents is not as well defined as the *mecA* gene–positive isolates. Isolates with borderline resistance generally do not grow on oxacillin screen plates. In 1996 the first MRSA isolate that was not susceptible to vancomycin was identified. Shortly thereafter, several similar isolates were encountered that all had vancomycin MICs of 8 μg/ml. At this time, strains of *S. aureus* organisms with reduced susceptibility to vancomycin (sometimes referred to as *GISA,* or *glycopeptide intermediate S. aureus*) are not abundant. Nevertheless, they are of great concern because vancomycin is the only agent that is consistently effective in treating serious MRSA infections.

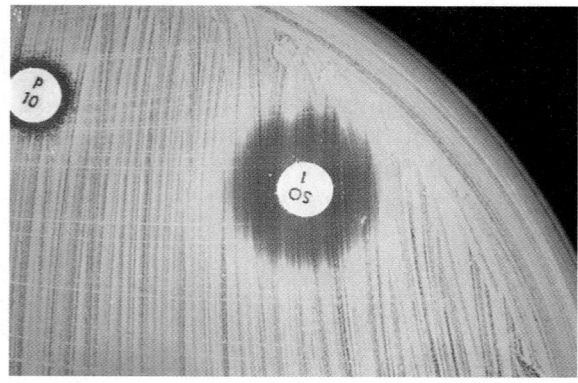

Figure 3-16 _____

The oxacillin zone for heteroresistant oxacillin-resistant *Staphylococcus aureus* often shows a haze of growth within the zone of inhibition. This haze is significant, and the isolate here is oxacillin resistant.

Enterococci

Ampicillin or penicillin is effective in treating uncomplicated enterococcal infections (e.g., urinary

TABLE 3-10

Aminoglycosides Represented When High Concentrations of Gentamicin and Streptomycin Are Tested to Determine High-Level Aminoglycoside Resistance in Enterococci

Agent Tested	Aminoglycoside(s) Represented
Gentamicin*	Gentamicin
	Amikacin
	Kanamycin
	Netilmicin
	Tobramycin
Streptomycin†	Streptomycin

*An isolate that has high-level resistance to gentamicin also has high-level resistance to the other aminoglycosides listed; enzymes that inactivate gentamicin also inactivate the other agents.
†An isolate that has high-level resistance to streptomycin has high-level resistance to this agent only (unless it also has high-level resistance to gentamicin as indicated by testing high concentrations of gentamicin).

tract infections). These cell wall–active agents are only bacteriostatic against enterococci and, when administered alone, are inadequate for treating serious infections, such as endocarditis, that require bactericidal therapy. To obtain a bactericidal effect, ampicillin or penicillin (or vancomycin in the penicillin-allergic patient) must be given in combination with an aminogylcoside—usually gentamicin and sometimes streptomycin.

DETECTION OF HIGH-LEVEL AMINOGLYCOSIDE RESISTANCE IN ENTEROCOCCI

Enterococci are inherently resistant to low concentrations of aminoglycosides, precluding their use as single agents for treatment of enterococcal infections. This low-level resistance is caused by poor drug uptake by the enterococcal cells. For isolates with low-level aminoglycoside resistance, a synergistic interaction occurs when an aminoglycoside is administered together with a cell wall–active agent such as ampicillin, penicillin, or vancomycin. Sometimes, however, enterococci develop **high-level aminoglycoside resistance,** in which the particular aminoglycoside does not demonstrate synergism with the cell wall–active agent (ampicillin, penicillin, or vancomycin). High-level aminoglycoside resistance in enterococci is usually the result of enzymatic inactivation of the drugs, and the enzymes that destroy gentamicin also destroy tobramycin, amikacin, kanamycin, and netilmicin, as shown in Table 3-10. Conse-

quently, none of these agents is used in treating infections caused by enterococci with high-level gentamicin resistance. If the isolate does not have concomitant high-level streptomycin resistance, however, streptomycin could be used, although some isolates have high-level resistance to both gentamicin and streptomycin. These latter isolates represent a significant therapeutic dilemma when encountered in serious infections, and the most appropriate strategy for treating infections caused by them has yet to be defined.

In vitro tests are used to detect high-level aminoglycoside resistance. Disk diffusion tests have been described that utilize special disks containing very high concentrations of gentamicin (120 μg/mL) or streptomycin (300 μg/mL). More commonly, routine agar or broth dilution types of tests are used. Gentamicin is tested at concentrations of 500 μg/mL and streptomycin at 2000 μg/mL (agar) or 1000 μg/mL (broth). The tests are performed as described for routine dilution tests, and growth at the high concentration indicates that the isolate has high-level resistance to the agent tested.

DETECTION OF AMPICILLIN AND PENICILLIN RESISTANCE IN ENTEROCOCCI

Ampicillin and penicillin resistance in enterococci may result from altered penicillin-binding proteins and, rarely, to β-lactamase production. Resistance caused by altered penicillin-binding proteins, which is readily detected by routine dilution and disk diffusion tests, occurs infrequently in *Enterococcus faecalis* but is common in *Enterococcus faecium*. Because of difficulties in obtaining a "resistant" result with the standard inocula used in routine dilution and disk diffusion tests, a rapid β-lactamase test is needed to identify β-lactamase–producing enterococci.

DETECTION OF VANCOMYCIN RESISTANCE IN ENTEROCOCCI

The incidence of vancomycin resistance in enterococci is increasing. Isolates that are highly resistant to vancomycin can be readily detected as vancomycin resistant when tested by conventional antimicrobial susceptibility test methods. Some isolates, however, may have a more subtle type of vancomycin resistance whereby MICs or inhibition zone measurements are just slightly above or below, respectively, the susceptible breakpoints. Hence, dilution tests must be viewed closely, and inhibition zones in disk diffusion testing must be examined using transmitted (rather than reflected) light; any growth within the zone should be considered significant. A BHI agar plate supplemented with 6 μg/ml vancomycin is useful to screen for vancomycin resistance.

The low-level vancomycin resistance appears to be inherent in the motile enterococcal species, including *Enterococcus gallinarum, Enterococcus casseliflavus,* and *Enterococcus flavescens.* These differ from true vancomycin-resistant enterococci for infection control purposes. Additionally, *Leuconostoc* spp., *Pediococcus* spp., and *Lactobacillus* spp. inherently demonstrate high-level vancomycin resistance, and these bacteria should not be confused with the morphologically similar enterococci.

Extended spectrum β-lactamases (ESBLs)

Most *Klebsiella pneumoniae, Klebsiella oxytoca,* and *E. coli* are susceptible to expanded-spectrum cephalosporins and aztreonam. However, on occasion they may produce novel β-lactamases that inactivate expanded-spectrum cephalosporins, aztreonam, and extended-spectrum penicillins. These β-lactamases are known as extended-spectrum β-lactamases or extended spectrum β-lactamases (ESBLs).

Strategies for laboratory detection of ESBL-producing *E. coli* and *Klebsiella* spp. include use of specific indicator drugs (e.g., cefpodoxime, ceftazidime, cefotaxime, ceftriaxone, aztreonam) and special screening zone or MIC breakpoints to facilitate recognition of ESBL production. Indicator drugs have been selected based on the likelihood of their being readily hydrolyzed by one of the many types of ESBLs. Once a suspect isolate is encountered, confirmatory tests can be performed. Because ESBL activity is inhibited by β-lactamase inhibitor agents such as clavulanic acid, this property forms the basis of the confirmatory tests. If the activity of either cefotaxime or ceftazidime or both is restored when tested in combination with clavulanic acid by either a disk or an MIC test, the resistance is due to ESBL production.

Resistance in ESBL-producing bacteria to various β-lactam agents is not always predicted by in vitro tests performed using standard inoculum density. For example, a confirmed ESBL-producing *Klebsiella pneumoniae* isolate may appear susceptible to cefotaxime by disk diffusion or MIC tests; however, cefotaxime is hydrolyzed at a high inoculum density and is ineffective in treating infections caused by such strains. Consequently, when an ESBL-producing isolate is identified, it should be reported as clinically resistant to all cephalosporins, penicillins, and aztreonam, despite the standard in vitro test results. The carbapenems (imipenem and meropenem) have remained active against ESBL-producing bacteria as have the cephamycins (cefoxitin and cefotetan). ESBL-producing isolates show variable susceptibility to aminoglycosides, fluoroquinolones, and trimethoprim/sulfamethoxazole, although many isolates are multiply resistant to those agents.

AUTOMATED ANTIMICROBIAL SUSCEPTIBILITY TEST METHODS

Principles of Technologies Used

The automated susceptibility testing instruments that are currently available represent a choice of several different levels of automation. Some instruments interpret growth end points of broth microdilution panels only when they are placed into an automated reader device, whereas certain other instruments provide hands-off incubation and reading functions for microdilution trays or special cards in an incubator/reader device. The instruments that offer the highest level of automation generally accomplish these tasks through the use of robotics to move the trays or cuvettes during the incubation/reading sequences in the instrument or to add reagents to certain test wells for biochemical tests.

Instruments also vary in the optical methods used for examining the test wells of the antimicrobial-containing trays or cards. Most current instruments utilize the principle of turbidimetric detection of bacterial growth in a broth medium by use of a photometer to examine the test wells. The determination of antimicrobial susceptibility based on lack of development of turbidity (suppression of growth) or, conversely, an indication of resistance based on an increase in turbidity in the presence of an antimicrobial agent is the same principle as that used when manual interpretation of growth endpoints is performed. The second means of growth detection, used by two instruments, is the detection of hydrolysis of a fluorogenic growth substrate incorporated in a special test medium. With this technology, growth is detected by a fluorometer as emission of a fluorescent signal when a microorganism consumes fluorophore-labeled substrate in the test medium.

Instruments for antimicrobial susceptibility testing may function to provide assistance in the interpretation of test results after a conventional overnight incubation period, or they may allow results to be determined in a shortened analysis period of 4 to 8 hours. Instrumentation may allow the interpretation of antimicrobial susceptibility test endpoints sooner than manual readings because of the greater sensitivity of the instruments' optical systems in the detection of subtle changes in microbial growth. All the instruments rely heavily on micropocessor-controlled functions and utilize personal computer hardware to provide final printed reports and to store and retrieve data on antimicrobial susceptibility. Most of the instruments may also be used to perform identifications of gram-negative or gram-positive bacteria and may be able to merge and print identification and antimicrobial susceptibility results into a single report.

Currently Available Automated Systems
Automated reader devices for broth microdilution susceptibility tests
Virtually every manufacturer of broth microdilution antimicrobial susceptibility testing panels offers a view box or other device to facilitate manual interpretation of results after incubation. Those products that feature freeze-dried antimicrobial panels also offer a mechanized device to simplify hydration and inoculation of trays. In addition, most manufacturers offer an instrument-assisted reader device that allows the technologist to record the results of manual readings of the panels by use of a video display screen resembling the configuration of the tray, or, alternatively by use of a touch-sensitive template that overlies the microdilution tray (e.g., Dade MicroScan Touch-SCAN, Pasco Data Management System). These reader devices facilitate data recording and provide a computer-printed report as well as long-term data storage. The personal computers included with these systems provide the capability

of data storage and retrieval for periodic generation of cumulative susceptibility profiles for various organisms that have been tested.

Automated photometers, which interpret growth patterns in panels by turbidimetric analysis, represent the next level of instrumentation available from several manufacturers; among these are the API UniScept Autoreader (BioMerieux Vitek, Hazelwood, Mo) and the Dade MicroScan AutoSCAN-4 (Dade MicroScan, Inc., West Sacramento, Calif). These instruments provide automated interpretation of the results of broth microdilution susceptibility tests after overnight incubation in a standard laboratory incubator. They are also configured with personal computers for report printing and data storage. Therefore this level of automation involves only the final, reading step of the microdilution susceptiblity panels. A published evaluation of one of these instruments has shown that the interpretation of MIC endpoints can be accomplished by the instrument with reasonable accuracy.

Automated instruments that provide more rapid test results
Only two currently available instruments are capable of generating rapid (4 to 8 hours) susceptibility test results. The Sensititre fluorogenic substrate test with AutoReader (Trek Diagnostic Systems, Inc., Westlake, Ohio) was the first system to be marketed in the United States that incorporated fluorogenic substrate hydrolysis as its method of detecting bacterial growth during an antimicrobial susceptibility test. The use of a fluorometric detection system was intended for testing of Enterobacteriaceae and some *S. aureus* using either MIC or breakpoint formats after a 5-hour or 18-hour incubation period. Problems were reported, however, with the 5-hour version during testing of *Proteus mirabilis, P. aeruginosa,* MRSA, coagulase-negative staphylococci, and enterococci. Marketing of the 5-hour version of the Sensititre has been discontinued, although the 18-hour fluorogenic substrate version of the instrument is still available.

AutoSCAN Walkaway
The Dade MicroScan AutoSCAN Walkaway (Dade Microscan, Inc., West Sacramento, Calif) consists of a large, self-contained incubator/reader unit with capacities for either 40 or 96 test panels and

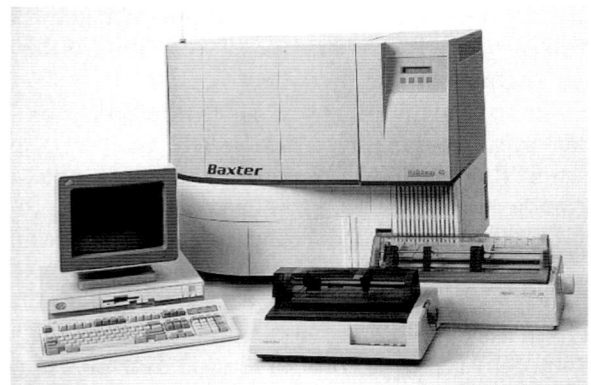

Figure 3-17 _____

AutoSCAN®—W/A or for 96 (pictured) Walkaway™ instrument. (Courtesy Dade MicroScan, Inc., West Sacramento, Calif.)

a personal computer with video display terminal and printer (Figure 3-17). The Walkaway utilizes standard-size microdilution trays, which are hydrated and inoculated with a hand-operated inoculator device, then placed in one of the positions in the incubator module. The type of test to be performed is indicated on an instrument-readable bar-code label placed on the end of each tray. The instrument then incubates the trays for the appropriate period (depending on the type of panel and organism), robotically positions the trays to add reagents if needed, and moves them under the central photometer/fluorometer station to perform the final readings of growth endpoints at the conclusion of the tests.

The Walkaway offers a choice of either overnight incubation with conventional photometric detection of turbidity for MIC or breakpoint testing of gram-positive and gram-negative bacteria or rapid (3.5-7 hours for gram-negative; 3.5-15 hours for gram-positive) readings of special MIC or breakpoint panels incorporating fluorogenic substrates. Special "combo" trays are available that allow susceptibility and organism identification in the same tray using either conventional substrates (overnight incubation) or special fluorogenic substrates that allow identification of some gram-negative bacilli in only 2 hours.

VITEK SYSTEM

The Vitek System (BioMerieux Vitek, Hazelwood, Mo) was originally designed for use in the U.S. space exploration efforts of the 1970s as an on-

board test system for spacecraft exploring other planets for life. Because of its original design intention, it was highly automated and relatively compact (Figure 3-18). Small plastic reagent cards (similar in size to a credit card) contain microliter quantities of various biochemical test media in 30 test wells for organism identification (Figure 3-19). Other cards contain various concentrations of a varity of antimicrobial agents for susceptiiblity testing. The Vitek can be configured to accommodate 30, 60, 120, or 240 cards. The susceptibility cards allow either quantitative MIC or qualitative susceptible/intermediate/resistant results for most rapidly growing gram-positive and gram-negative aerobic bacteria in a period of 4 to 10 hours.

Vitek hardware consists of a filling module for inoculation of the cards, an incubator/reader module that incorporates a carousel to hold the test cards, a robotic system to manipulate the cards, a photometer for measurement of optical density and biochemical reaction color changes in the cards, and a computer module with video display terminal and printer for viewing and printing results. Vitek also offers an information management system for storing and retrieving test data for a variety of statistical reports. The Vitek uses kinetic (every 60 minutes) measurements of growth in the presence of antimicrobial agents to provide analysis of growth curves, leading to computer algorithm–derived MIC values. The technologist can choose to have susceptibility test results printed using either qualitative (S, I, R) or quantitative (MIC) formats.

Although the fixed configuration of the Vitek cards imposes some limitations on the selection

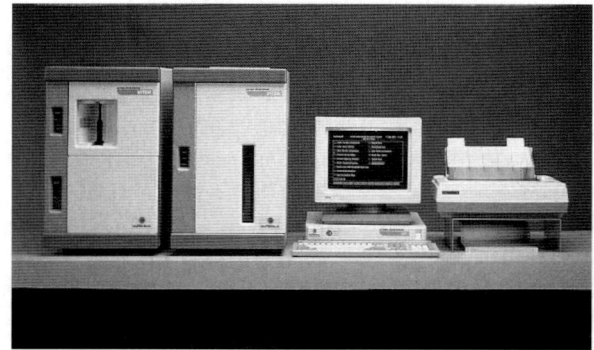

Figure 3-18 _____

Vitek instrument. (Courtesy bioMerieux Vitek, Hazelwood, Mo.)

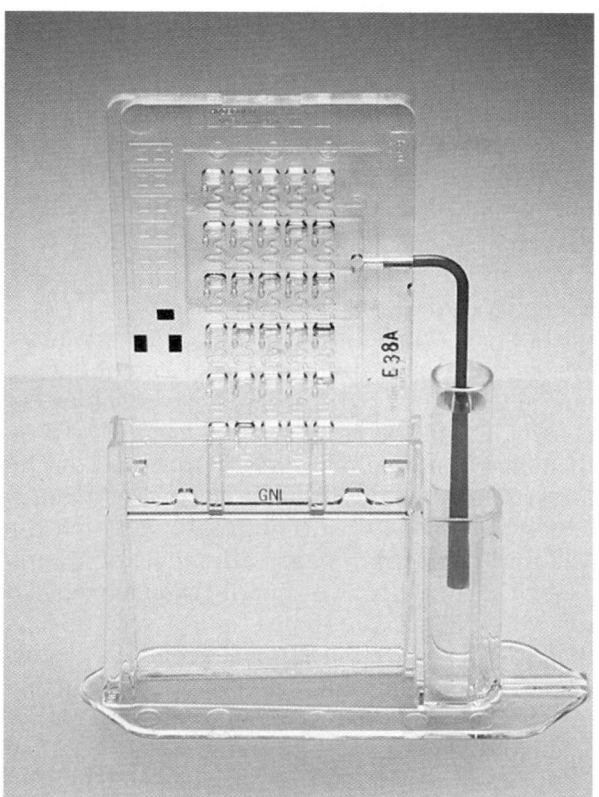

Figure 3-19 _____

Vitek test card containing dried antimicrobials connected by a transfer straw to a tube containing a standardized inoculum suspension of bacteria to be tested. These are placed into an evacuating chamber, which allows the inoculum to be transferred into the card. All wells containing varying concentrations of various antimicrobial agents are reconstituted during this inoculation process. Finally, the inoculated cards are placed into the Vitek instrument for processing.

The E test (AB Biodisk, Solna, Sweden) employs the principle of establishing an antimicrobial density gradient in an agar plate as a means of determining antimicrobial susceptibility. The E test utilizes very thin plastic test strips that are impregnated on the under surface with an antimicrobial concentration gradient and are marked on the upper surface with a concentration index or scale. The strips may be placed in a radial fashion on the surface of an agar plate that has been inoculated in a manner similar to that for a disk diffusion test. After overnight incubation the test results are read by viewing the plates from the top side with the lids removed. The antimicrobial gradient that forms in the agar around the E test strips gives rise to elliptic inhibitory areas with each strip. The MIC is determined where the growth ellipse intersects the E test strip (Figure 3-20). The E test shares with the disk diffusion test the intrinsic flexibility of drug selection and testing because selected strips are applied to the surface of test plates. The cost of E test strips is much greater than that of disks, however, and represents one of the main limitations of this product. Initial published studies have indicated that MICs determined using the E test compare favorably (within one twofold dilution interval) with those determined by conventional methods.

The E test may be especially useful for testing fastidious organisms such as *H. influenzae, S. pneumoniae,* and anaerobic bacteria. This is in part due to the fact that the strips can be placed on special enriched media or in a special incubation atmosphere (e.g., anaerobic or increased CO_2) and

of drugs for testing, Vitek offers a combination of two cards (called Flex cards) at a reduced price that are tested together; results from both cards can be merged into one report containing many different drugs. To some degree, this has solved the problem for Vitek that is inherent in all the commercial systems: inflexibility of the standard test panels. Owing in part to its aerospace design heritage, the Vitek offers one of the highest levels of automation currently available in microbiology and is a reliable, proven instrument.

Nonautomated Antimicrobial Susceptibility Test Method: E Test

A product that differs slightly in principle from the test methods described thus far is **E test.**

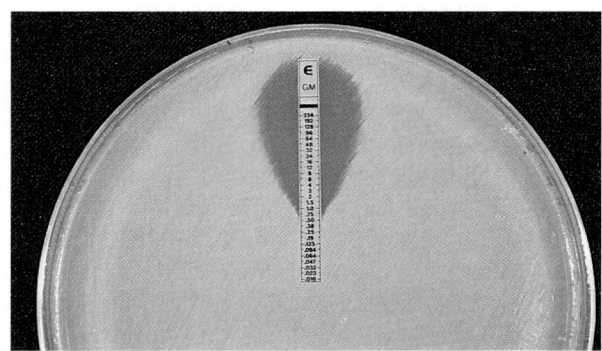

Figure 3-20 _____

Escherichia coli tested with an E test gentamicin strip. The gentamicin MIC (where the ellipse crosses the gradient) is 0.75 μg/mL.

the fact that fewer antimicrobial agents may need to be tested against fastidious organisms. Consequently, the relatively high cost of the E test strips would be minimized.

INTERPRETATION OF IN VITRO ANTIMICROBIAL SUSCEPTIBILITY TEST RESULTS

Several elements are important in performing any in vitro antimicrobial susceptibility test. This chapter has described the methodology for several types of tests. The procedural steps of each method must be followed explicitly to obtain reproducible results. A susceptibility test should never be performed using an unstandardized inoculum or a mixed culture. For that reason, direct susceptibility tests that incorporate the use of a patient's infected body fluid cannot be recommended, even to obtain a presumptive result.

The results of a susceptibility test must be interpreted in the laboratory before a report is communicated to a patient's physician. In the case of a disk diffusion test, the inhibition zone size must be interpreted using a table of values that relates the diameter of the zone to a category of susceptibility, which is sometimes related to the identity of the isolate for correct interpretation. The table used for such interpretations must represent the most up-to-date criteria that have been reviewed and accepted by the NCCLS. It is important to bear in mind that the NCCLS documents are updated frequently, usually once per year. Use of old or outdated NCCLS tables could represent a serious shortcoming in the reporting of patients' results.

The inhibition zone size and MIC interpretive criteria published by the NCCLS are established by careful analysis of three kinds of data—microbiologic data (e.g., a comparison of MICs versus zone sizes on a large number of bacterial strains), pharmacokinetic data (e.g., serum, CSF, urine, and other secretion and tissue levels of an antimicrobial agent), and results of clinical studies obtained during the phase before FDA approval and marketing of an antimicrobial agent. Thus MIC interpretive criteria are not based simply on a comparison of serum levels of an antimicrobial agent and MIC values. Zone size interpretive criteria are, however, based in large part on direct correlations of MICs and zone sizes.

Whether based on determination of an MIC or on interpretation of a disk diffusion zone size, the three categories of susceptibility currently recommended by the NCCLS should be interpreted in the same manner. If the MIC or zone size is interpreted as **susceptible** using the latest NCCLS tables, the clinical interpretation of the result is that the patient's infecting organism should respond to therapy with that antimicrobial agent using the dosage recommended normally for that type of infection and that species. Conversely, an MIC or zone size interpreted as **resistant** should not be inhibited by the normally achievable concentrations of the antimicrobial agent based on the dosages normally used with that drug. An **intermediate** result indicates that a microorganism falls into a range of susceptibility in which the MIC approaches or exceeds the level of antimicrobial agent that can ordinarily be achieved and for which clinical response is likely to be less than with a susceptible strain. Exceptions can occur if the antimicrobial agent is highly concentrated in a body fluid, such as urine, or if higher than normal doses of the antimicrobial agent can be safely administered (e.g., some penicillins and cephalosporins). At times, the intermediate result means that certain variables in the susceptibility test may not have been well controlled and the values have fallen into a "buffer zone" separating susceptible from resistant strains. Certain other specific aspects of susceptibility test reporting are detailed in the NCCLS tables, such as refraining from reporting results for antimicrobial agents that do not penetrate into the CSF on isolates from patients who have meningitis. Additionally, results for antimicrobial agents that are only useful for treating urinary tract infections must not be reported on isolates from specimens other than urine.

Lastly, no objective evidence suggests that the reporting of an MIC result is any more relevant clinically than the reporting of a category *(S, I, R)* result in the majority of infections. Perhaps the reporting of MIC results could aid a physician in selecting from among a group of similar drugs for therapy of infective endocarditis or osteomyelitis, in which therapy is likely to be protracted. For virtually all other infections, however, category results provide the clinician with the information necessary to select appropriate therapy. Only those physicians trained in infectious diseases are likely to be familiar with expected MICs for the multitude of antimicrobial agents currently available. Thus if MIC results are to be reported, the inclusion of appropriate interpretive criteria with the results is essential.

METHODS OF DETECTING ANTIMICROBIAL-INACTIVATING ENZYMES

β-Lactamase Tests

β-Lactamases are enzymes that selectively destroy β-lactam molecules by attacking the β-lactam ring component of the molecule (Figure 3-21). Production of β-lactamase is a significant mechanism contributing to β-lactam resistance in certain organisms, such as *H. influenzae, N. gonorrhoeae, Moraxella catarrhalis, Staphylococcus* spp., *Enterococcus* spp., and some *Bacteroides* spp. Simple β-lactamase tests are performed in the clinical laboratory to identify β-lactamase production in these organisms, and a positive reaction means that the β-lactam agent(s) commonly used to treat infections caused by them (primarily ampicillin, amoxicillin, and penicillin) would be ineffective. Although many other organisms, such as Enterobacteriaceae and *Pseudomonas* spp., produce a variety of different types of β-lactamases, the β-lactamase tests as currently performed in clinical laboratories cannot predict resistance to all β-lactam agents that might be considered for therapy here, and the β-lactamase test should not be used.

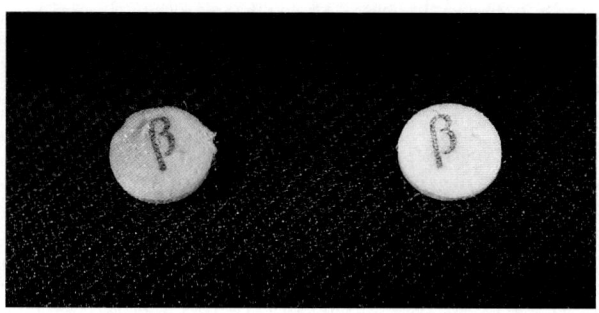

Figure 3-22

Cefinase β-lactamase disk test. Cells from several colonies of *Haemophilus influenzae* were applied to a moistened disk. This photo shows results following testing of two different isolates. Within 10 minutes, the disk on the left turned brown-red (positive), and that on the right maintained a light yellow color (negative).

Several methods may be used to detect β-lactamase production. The most commonly employed β-lactamase test utilizes the chromogenic cephalosporin nitrocefin. Cefinase disks commercially available from Becton Dickinson Microbiology Systems (Cockeysville, Md) are filter paper disks impregnated with nitrocefin. A disk is moistened, and a loopful of organisms is rubbed onto it. Within 10 minutes (or within 60 minutes for staphylococci), the area where the organisms are deposited will turn brownish red in the presence of β-lactamase–producing organisms. No color change occurs with β-lactamase–negative organisms (Figure 3-22).

The other types of β-lactamase test methods, acidimetric and iodometric, are based on the de-

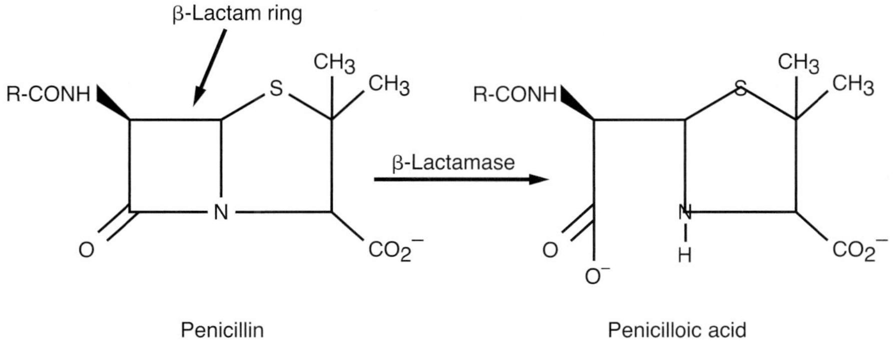

Figure 3-21

β-Lactamase hydrolyzes the β-lactam ring portion of the penicillin molecule. The hydrolysis results in the formation of penicilloic acid, which does not have antibacterial activity.

tection of penicilloic acid, which results from the action of β-lactamase on penicillin. The acidimetric method uses citrate-buffered penicillin and phenol red as a pH indicator. When colonies of a β-lactamase–positive organism are added to the solution, the penicilloic acid present results in a drop in pH, causing a color change from red to yellow. In the iodometric method a solution of phosphate-buffered penicillin and starch-iodine complex is used. With β-lactamase–positive organisms, penicilloic acid reduces iodine and prevents it from combining with starch. A positive reaction is colorless, and a negative reaction is purple.

All of the species mentioned previously in this section, except staphylococci, produce β-lactamase constitutively, meaning that the same amount of enzyme is produced regardless of exposure to an inducing agent. An inducing agent is simply a β-lactam agent that stimulates production of the enzyme. Production of β-lactamase in staphylococci is inducible, and exposure to an inducing agent (β-lactam agent) is often required in the laboratory to obtain enough of the enzyme for detection with conventional β-lactamase tests.

Testing organisms that have been exposed to an inducing agent can be accomplished by using growth from the periphery of a zone surrounding a β-lactam disk (e.g., oxacillin disk). Here, the bacteria at the zone edge have been exposed to β-lactam molecules. Alternatively, the test can be performed on bacteria growing in a well of a broth microdilution tray that contains a subinhibitory concentration (low concentration that does not inhibit visual growth) of a β-lactam agent.

The rapidity of β-lactamase tests makes them attractive. A positive reaction confirms resistance to ampicillin, amoxicillin, and penicillin, and a negative reaction indicates that the test organisms do not produce β-lactamase, although they may be resistant to these agents through an alternative mechanism. Resistance related to other mechanisms may be detected only with conventional types of dilution or disk diffusion tests. With organisms in which the rate of resistance associated with alternative mechanisms is low, such as *M. catarrhalis,* supplemental tests may not be routinely warranted in the clinical laboratory.

QUALITY CONTROL OF ANTIMICROBIAL SUSCEPTIBILITY TESTS

Quality control of antimicrobial susceptibility tests involves testing standard reference strains that have defined antimicrobial susceptibility (or resistance) to the drugs tested. It is important to use strains that represent the types of patient isolates tested in the respective laboratory. Additionally, the quality control strains should represent varying degrees of susceptibility (or resistance). Ideal quality control strains for MIC tests have what is known as *onscale MIC endpoints* for the drugs tested. An onscale end point falls within the range of concentrations tested.

The NCCLS has identified ATCC (American Type Culture Collection) strains that are useful for quality control testing (Table 3-11). The NCCLS documents also include tables that define acceptable results (zone measurements for disk diffusion tests or MICs for dilution tests) for these strains; examples are shown in the Tables 3-12 and 3-13, respectively.

The procedure followed in testing quality control reference strains must be identical to that used for testing patient isolates. If results do not fall within the defined acceptable limits, corrective action must be taken to determine the reason for the out-of-control observation before reporting of any patient results. Quality control testing is recommended each day that patient tests are performed; however, the frequency of quality control testing can be reduced to weekly if a laboratory can demonstrate acceptable proficiency in performing the test. Proficiency consists of obtaining acceptable results with each antimicrobial agent/quality control strain combination after the test performance for 30 consecutive test days. Quality control procedures must always be performed when new lots of materials are put into use, and test materials must never be used beyond their stated expiration dates.

There are other, less obvious components of a quality control program for antimicrobial susceptibility tests. Supplemental quality control strains may be periodically tested to validate acceptable performance of specific antimicrobial agent/organism combinations that may be only modestly controlled with the routine reference strains. An

TABLE 3-11

Strains Commonly Used for Quality Control of Routine Antimicrobial Susceptibility Tests

Test	QC Strain(s) Used	Comments
Antimicrobial susceptibility of gram-positive organisms	*Straphylococcus aureus* ATCC 25923 *S. aureus* ATCC 29213	β-Lactamase negative for disk diffusion tests β-Lactamase positive for MIC tests
Oxacillin salt agar screen for *S. aureus*	*S. aureus* ATCC 43300	Oxacillin resistant
Vancomycin BHI screen, synergy screen for enterococci	*Enterococcus faecalis* ATCC 29212	Susceptible to vancomycin and susceptible to high levels of gentamicin and streptomycin (synergy screen tests negative)
	E. faecalis ATCC 51299	Resistant to vancomycin and resistant to high levels of gentamicin and streptomycin (synergy screen tests positive)
Antimicrobial susceptibility of gram-negative organisms	*Escherichia coli* ATCC 25922 *Pseudomonas aeruginosa* ATCC 27853 *E. coli* ATCC 35218	 β-Lactamase positive for testing β-lactam/β-lactamase inhibitor combination agents only
Antimicrobial susceptibility of *Haemophilus* spp.	*Haemophilus influenzae* ATCC 49247 *H. influenzae* ATCC 49766 *H. influenzae* ATCC 10211	Ampicillin resistant, non–β-lactamase producing Ampicillin susceptible Used by media manufacturers to assess growth-supporting capabilities of the medium
Antimicrobial susceptibility of *Neisseria gonorrhoeae*	*N. gonorrhoeae* ATCC 49226	β-Lactamase negative
Antimicrobial susceptibility testing of *S. pneumoniae* and other streptococci	*Streptococcus pneumoniae* ATCC 49619	Penicillin-intermediate
Antimicrobial susceptibility of anaerobes	*Bacteroides fragilis* ATCC 25285 *Bacteroides thetaiotamicron* ATCC 29741 *Eubacterium lentum* ATCC 43055 *E. faecalis* ATCC 29212	
Assessment of acceptability of medium (low thymine and thymidine content) for testing sulfonamides, trimethoprim, and trimethoprim/sulfamethoxazole		

TABLE 3-12

Control Limits for Monitoring Antimicrobial Disk Susceptibility Tests—Zone Diameter (mm) Limits for Individual Tests for Nonfastidious Organisms Using Mueller-Hinton Medium Without Blood or Other Supplements

Antimicrobial Agent	Disk Content (μg)	*E. coli* ATCC 25922	*S. aureus* ATCC 25923	*P. aeruginosa* ATCC 27853	*E. coli* ATCC 35218
Ampicillin	10	16-22	27-35	—	—
Amoxicillin/clavulanic acid	20/10	19-25	28-36	—	18-22
Cefazolin	30	23-29	29-35	—	—
Gentamicin	10	19-26	19-27	16-21	—

From NCCLS publication M100-S9, *Performance standards for antimicrobial susceptibility testing; ninth informational supplement.* Copies of the current edition may be obtained from NCCLS, 940 West Valley Road, Suite 1400, Wayne, PA 19087-1898.

TABLE 3-13

Acceptable Quality Control Ranges of MICS (mg/mL) for Reference Strains

Antimicrobial Agent	*E. coli* ATCC 25922	*S. aureus* ATCC 29213	*P. aeruginosa* ATCC 27853	*E. coli* ATCC 35218
Ampicillin	2-8	0.5-2	—	—
Amoxicillin/clavulanic acid	2/1-8/4	0.12/0.06-0.5/0.25	—	4/2-16/8
Cefazolin	1-4	0.25-1	—	—
Gentamicin	0.25-1	0.12-1	0.5-2	—

From NCCLS publication M100-S9, *Performance standards for antimicrobial susceptibility testing; ninth informational supplement.* Copies of the current edition may be obtained from NCCLS, 940 West Valley Road, Suite 1400, Wayne, PA 19087-1898.

TABLE 3-14

*Examples of Typical Antibiograms for Several Gram-Negative Species**

Antimicrobial Agent	Escherichia coli	Enterobacter cloacae	Proteus mirabilis	Pseudomonas aeruginosa	Stenotrophomonas maltophilia
Amikacin	S	S	S	S	R
Ampicillin	S	R	S	R	R
Ampicillin/sulbactam	S	R	S	R	R
Cephalothin	S	R	S	R	R
Cefoxitin	S	S-R	S	R	R
Cefotaxime	S	S-R	S	S-R	R
Ceftazidime	S	S	S	S	S-R
Ciprofloxacin	S	S	S	S	R
Gentamicin	S	S	S	S	R
Imipenem	S	S	S	S	R
Piperacillin	S	S	S	S	R
Nitrofurantoin	S	S	R	R	R
Tobramycin	S	S	S	S	R
Trimethoprim/sulfamethoxazole	S	S	S	R	S

*Results indicated represent the typical response found in the majority of clinical isolates; however, these can vary significantly. *R*, Resistant; *S*, susceptible; *S-R*, variable result.

MRSA strain could be included to ensure that the test system can detect heteroresistant strains. Similarly, an ampicillin-resistant *Enterobacter cloacae* might be included to ensure that the system can detect ampicillin resistance. Supplemental quality control strains are sometimes used for troubleshooting specific problems or training new employees. Another component of a quality control program involves the inclusion of mechanisms to ensure that personnel performing testing are proficient in their tasks. Self-assessment checklists and supervisory review of reported results are examples of such mechanisms. Satisfactory performance on proficiency survey specimens and utilization of relevant testing strategies are also quality control parameters.

The most widely used supplemental quality control measure is the use of antibiograms to verify results generated on patient isolates. An antibiogram is the overall antimicrobial susceptibility profile of a bacterial isolate to a battery of antimicrobial agents. Certain species have "typical" antibiograms, which can be used to verify the identification as well as the susceptibility results generated on the isolate (Table 3-14). For example, *P. aeruginosa* is typically resistant to ampicillin, cefazolin (and other first- and second-generation cephalosporins), and trimethoprim/sulfamethoxazole; however, it is often suscepti-

ble to gentamicin (and other aminoglycosides), extended-spectrum penicillins (e.g., piperacillin), and ciprofloxacin. In contrast, *E. coli* is generally susceptible to all the aforementioned antimicrobial agents. Table 3-15 shows several atypical antibiograms suggesting the result highlighted is erroneous. When atypical antibiograms are encountered, the results must be verified. Verification procedures include the following:

- Re-examination of the disk diffusion plate, MIC tray, and other components to ensure that results were properly interpreted and that the materials were not overtly defective (e.g., empty well in tray)
- Checking previous reports to see whether the particular patient previously had an isolate with an atypical antibiogram (that was verified)
- Repeating the test, if necessary (sometimes it is necessary to repeat the identification tests as well as the antimicrobial susceptibility tests to verify the atypical results; sometimes testing with an alternative method is useful)

Accrediting agencies require hospitals to compile **cumulative antibiogram statistics** to help monitor antimicrobial resistance within the institution. Cumulative antibiograms are generated by examining the overall incidence of susceptibility

TABLE 3-15

Examples of "Problem" Antibiograms Highly Suspicious for Technical Errors

Antimicrobial Agent	*Escherichia coli**	*Enterobacter cloacae†*	*Pseudomonas aeruginosa‡*	*Stenotrophomonas maltophilia§*
Amikacin	R	S	S	R
Ampicillin	S	R	S	R
Cephalothin	S	S	R	R
Cefoxitin	S	R	R	R
Cefotaxime	S	R	S-R	R
Gentamicin	S	S	S	R
Tobramycin	S	S	S	R
Trimethoprim/sulfamethoxazole	S	S	R	R

R, Resistant; *S,* susceptible; *S-R,* variable result.

*It is very unusual for an isolate to be resistant to amikacin and susceptible to gentamicin and tobramycin because amikacin is the most active of these three aminoglycosides.

†Third-generation cephalosporins (e.g., cefotaxime) are usually more active than second-generation cephalosporins (e.g., cefoxitin), which in turn are more active than first-generation cephalosporins (e.g., cephalothin) against the Enterobacteriaceae. Consequently, this antibiogram is unusual.

‡Ampicillin does not have activity against *P. aeruginosa,* and this antibiogram is unusual.

§*S. maltophilia* shows nearly universal susceptibility to trimethoprim/sulfamethoxazole, which is the drug of choice for infections caused by this very resistant species. This antibiogram is unusual.

(or resistance) for a given antimicrobial agent/organism combination (e.g., the percentage of *E. coli* isolates that are susceptible to ampicillin). Cumulative antibiograms are compiled regularly (e.g., monthly, quarterly, or yearly depending on the institution's policies), and newly tabulated data are compared with data from previous intervals and sometimes with that of other institutions. On review of such data, an increase in the incidence of MRSA, for example, from 15% in January to 25% in February, might suggest a problem with nosocomial transmission of MRSA among patients. An investigation by infection control personnel into the reason behind such observations would be warranted.

SELECTING AN ANTIMICROBIAL SUSCEPTIBILITY TEST METHOD

Clinical microbiology laboratories can choose from among several manual or instrument-assisted methods to perform their routine antimicrobial susceptibility testing: the disk diffusion (or Kirby-Bauer) test, broth microdilution (with or without use of an instrument or growth indicator), and rapid automated instrument methods. The E test may also be useful for certain fastidious or anaerobic bacteria.

The Kirby Bauer test is becoming more popular because of its inherent flexibility and cost-effectiveness. One frequently mentioned problem with commercial microdilution or automated systems is the inflexibility of the standard antimicrobial batteries or test panels. With the current availability of more than 50 antimicrobial agents in the United States and the diversity that exists among antimicrobial agent formularies in different hospitals, it is virtually impossible for manufacturers to provide standard test panels that fit every hospital's needs. Thus the inherent flexibility of the disk diffusion test allows a laboratory to test any 12 antimicrobial agents deemed appropriate on a 150-mm Mueller-Hinton agar plate. Other assets of the disk diffusion procedure are that it is one of the best standardized tests and that its performance is continually updated by the NCCLS consensus efforts. The interpretive category results (susceptible, intermediate, resistant) of the disk diffusion test should be readily understood by all physicians who use them. The latter has not always been the case with MIC results. In fact, a survey of United States infectious disease physicians indicated that MIC results may be misinterpreted by some physicians and S, I, R category results may be preferable.

As stated previously, commercial microdilution susceptibility test products have become the most popular among U.S. clinical laboratories. Advantages of this method include its quantitative nature: that is, an MIC rather than a strict category result, the fact that MICs may be determined with some organisms for which the disk test may not be standardized, and the attraction of the computerized hardware systems available from several manufacturers. Indeed, the computerized data management systems that accompany some of these instruments are extremely useful to some laboratories, which may not possess a laboratory information system. An MIC method should not be chosen, however, on the grounds that MICs are more valuable to physicians. As stated previously, many physicians who are not infectious diseases specialists are not familiar with MIC values for the myriad of contemporary antimicrobial agents.

Another problem with automated susceptibility test instruments has been imitations of instrument quality control procedures, largely because control strains used with the systems often result in many offscale values (i.e., MIC values less than or equal to the lowest concentration or greater than the highest concentration tested by the instrument). The instruments are mechanically and optically complex devices that must function properly for reproducible test results. Each manufacturer describes routine maintenance and function checks to prevent or detect overt malfunctions. The lack of on-scale control values means, however, that the potency of antimicrobials and functioning of the instrument may not be determined with the level of precision that clinical microbiologists have come to expect with the disk diffusion susceptibility test.

When a serious mechanical failure occurs, only tests from instruments that utilize conventional microdilution trays and photometric analysis of growth patterns after overnight incubation can be completed by manual incubation and interpretation. The instrument methods that incorporate rapid test interpretation or use fluorogenic substrate analysis cannot be manually interpreted. Therefore laboratories must maintain a back-up testing procedure, such as disk diffusion or manual overnight broth microdilution testing, to avoid delays in generating patients' results.

A laboratory may perform automated antimicrobial susceptibility testing to generate test results more rapidly than can be accomplished by manual methods or to reduce the amount of labor required for susceptibility tests. Provision of important laboratory results one day sooner than by conventional methods is a logical advancement in patient care. Despite this self-evident statement, however, little objective evidence suggests that rapid susceptibility test results reduce mortality or morbidity. This situation may be due in part to the fact that physicians have come to expect antimicrobial susceptibility test results on the second day after a specimen is submitted, rather than in the afternoon of the day after submission. Thus a period of transition (and education) may be necessary for this approach to be fully accepted.

One of the previous shortcomings of rapid susceptibility testing methods has been some sacrifice in the ability to detect certain inducible or otherwise subtle antimicrobial resistance mechanisms. The instruments most notorious for such problems are no longer marketed, however, and manufacturers of the remaining instruments have made significant strides to correct earlier problems. Nevertheless, it is important to emphasize that accuracy should not be sacrificed in an effort to generate a rapid susceptibility result.

The concept that automated susceptibility instruments reduce labor requirements through greater efficiency has been overly optimistic. Obviously, the greatest savings would involve use of panels that allow antimicrobial susceptibility testing and organism identification on the same panel, but a review of previous CAP workload values for both manual and automated susceptibility test methods reveals that only minimal labor savings are provided by current instrumentation. These modest labor savings may be most meaningful to large clinical microbiology laboratories that perform large numbers of tests daily. The magnitude of the labor savings realized in clinical chemistry or hematology through automation has yet to be manifest in clinical microbiology.

In an era of cost containment, it is important to recognize that the most economical susceptibility test method currently available is the disk diffusion test. The microdilution and rapid automated instrument methods offer several direct or ancillary benefits, as described previously, but, with rare exception, they are more costly than the disk diffusion test.

Bibliography

Baker CN et al: Comparison of the E test to agar dilution, broth microdilution and agar diffusion susceptibility testing techniques by using a special challenge set of bacteria, *J Clin Microbiol* 29:533, 1991.

Bauer AW et al: Antibiotic susceptibility testing by a standardized single disk method, *Am J Clin Pathol* 45:493, 1996.

Citron DM et al: Evaluation of E test for susceptibility testing of anaerobic bacteria, *J Clin Microbiol* 29:2197, 1991.

DeLencaster H et al: Multiple mechanisms of methicillin resistance and improved methods for detection in clinical isolates of *Staphylococcus aureus, Antimicrob Agents Chemother* 35:632, 1991.

Doern GV et al: Antibiotic resistance among clinical isolates of *Haemophilus influenzae* in the United States in 1994 and 1995 and detection of β-lactamase positive strains resistant to amoxicillin-clavulanate: results of a national multicenter surveillance study, *Antimicrob Agents Chemother* 41:292, 1997.

Doern GV et al: Clinical impact of rapid in vitro susceptibility testing and bacterial identification, *J Clin Microbiol* 32:1757, 1994.

Hindler JA, Mann LM: Principles and practices for the laboratory guidance of antimicrobial therapy. In Tilton RC et al, editors: *Clinical laboratory medicine,* St Louis, 1992, Mosby.

Kaplan SL, Mason EO Jr: Management of infections due to antibiotic-resistant *Streptococcus pneumoniae, Clin Microbiol Rev* 11:628, 1999.

Klugman KP: Pneumococcal resistance to antibiotics, *Clin Microbiol Rev* 3:171, 1990.

Lorian V, editor: *Antibiotics in laboratory medicine,* ed 4, Baltimore, 1996, Williams & Wilkins.

Moellering RC Jr: Vancomycin-resistant enterococci, *Clin Infect Dis* 26:1186, 1998.

National Committee for Clinical Laboratory Standards: *Methods for antimicrobial susceptibility testing of anaerobic bacteria,* ed 4, Approved Standard M11-A3. Wayne, Penn, 1997, NCCLS.

National Committee for Clinical Laboratory Standards: *Methods of dilution antimicrobial susceptibility testing for bacteria that grow aerobically,* ed 4, Approved Standard M7-A4. Wayne, Penn, 1997, NCCLS.

National Committee for Clinical Laboratory Standards: *Performance standards for antimicrobial disk susceptibility tests,* ed 6, Approved Standard M2-A6. Wayne, Penn, 1997, NCCLS.

National Committee for Clinical Laboratory Standards: *Development of In Vitro Susceptibility Testing Criteria and Quality Control Parameters. Tentative Guideline M23-T3.* Wayne, Penn, 1998, NCCLS.

Pugliese G, Weinstein RA: *Issues and controversies in prevention and control of VRE,* Chicago, 1998, ETNA Communications.

Smith TL et al: Emergence of vancomycin resistance in *Staphylococcus aureus, N Engl J Med* 340:493, 1999.

Tenover FC, editor (section): Antimicrobial agents and susceptibility testing. In Murray P et al, editors: *Manual of clinical microbiology,* ed 6, Washington, DC, 1995, American Society for Microbiology.

LEARNING ASSESSMENT

1. Specific modifications of routine procedures are sometimes necessary to detect certain types of antimicrobial resistance. List the test modifications necessary to detect the following:
   a. Methicillin-resistant *S. aureus* (MRSA)
   b. Vancomycin-resistant enterococci
   c. ESBL-producing *Klebsiella pneumoniae*

2. For some antimicrobial agent/organism combinations, isolates may appear susceptible to certain agents in vitro even though these agents are clinically ineffective. Which agents commonly tested fall into this category for the following?
   a. MRSA
   b. ESBL-producing *Klebsiella pneumoniae*

3. Acceptable results obtained when testing the recommended quality control strains do not guarantee accurate results on all patients' isolates. What measures might be taken to ensure the accuracy of results on the patient's isolates?

C. SPECIAL ANTIMICROBIAL SUSCEPTIBILITY TESTS

Janet A. Hindler

MINIMUM BACTERICIDAL CONCENTRATION (MBC) TEST
  Controlling Test Variables
  Interpretation Concerns

TIME-KILL ASSAYS

SYNERGY TESTS

SERUM BACTERICIDAL TEST

MOLECULAR PROBES FOR IDENTIFYING DETERMINANTS OF ANTIMICROBIAL RESISTANCE

MEASUREMENT OF ANTIMICROBIAL AGENTS IN SERUM AND BODY FLUIDS
  Biologic Assays
  Immunoassays
  Chromatographic Assays

OBJECTIVES

1. Describe the MBC test, and list the indications for performing it.
2. Define *synergism, antagonism,* and *indifference* as related to testing combinations of antimicrobial agents.
3. Describe the serum bactericidal test, and list the indications for performing it.
4. Explain how molecular probes might be used to detect antimicrobial resistance.
5. Discuss methods used for measuring concentrations of antimicrobial agents in serum and body fluids, and describe when such tests are used.

KEY TERMS

Minimum inhibitory concentration (MIC)
Minimum bactericidal concentration (MBC)
MBC endpoint
Paradoxic, or Eagle, effect
Persisters

Tolerance
Time-kill assays
Synergistic
Antagonism
Indifference
Serum bactericidal test (SBT)

CASE STUDY

Viridans streptococcus was isolated from six of six blood culture bottles submitted for a patient with suspected bacterial endocarditis. The isolate was susceptible to penicillin (MIC $\leq$ 0.03 μg/ml), but the physician was concerned about the bactericidal activity of penicillin alone. The laboratory performed MBC testing and reported an MBC result of 32 μg/ml. The physician considered this information in conjunction with clinical observations of the patient and documentation in the literature of previous experiences with patients with similar conditions. This patient was continued on a therapeutic regimen of penicillin and gentamicin.

TABLE 3-16
Special Antimicrobial Susceptibility Tests

Test	Purpose
Antimicrobial level test (assay)	Measure of the amount of antimicrobial agent in serum or body fluid
Minimum bactericidal concentration (MBC) test	Measure of the lowest concentration of antimicrobial agent that kills a bacterial isolate
Serum bactericidal test (SBT)	Measure of the highest dilution or titer of a patient's serum that is inhibitory to and the highest dilution or titer that is bactericidal to the patient's own infecting bacterium
Synergy test	Measure of the susceptibility of a bacterial isolate to a combination of two antimicrobial agents
	MICs and often MBCs for each antimicrobial agent alone and in combination are determined
Time-kill assay	Measure of the rate of killing of bacteria by an antimicrobial agent as determined by examining the number of viable bacteria remaining at various intervals after exposure to the agent

Several special antimicrobial susceptibility tests are generally performed only in specialized laboratories and used in only a few defined clinical settings. They are listed in Table 3-16.

MINIMUM BACTERICIDAL CONCENTRATION (MBC) TEST

Minimum inhibitory concentration (MIC) tests identify the amount of antimicrobial agent required to inhibit the growth or multiplication of a bacterial isolate. If a concentration of antimicrobial agent that exceeds the MIC is attained at the infection site, the drug generally inhibits multiplication of the bacteria so that the patient's immune defense mechanisms are no longer overwhelmed. The immune defense mechanisms (e.g., phagocytic cells, antibody) work in concert with antimicrobial agents to eradicate infecting bacteria; for this reason, inhibitory concentrations of the drug at the infection site are generally sufficient for treating most infections.

In immunosuppressed patients, however, and in patients with serious infections such as endocarditis and osteomyelitis, the immune defense mechanisms are suboptimal. Inhibitory concentrations of the drug may not be sufficient, and obtaining bactericidal concentrations of antimicrobial agents at the infection site is important to effect a cure. For many types of infections, the bactericidal capacity of a specific antimicrobial regimen can be predicted on the basis of previous experience. For example, most β-lactam antimicrobial agents are bactericidal for *Escherichia coli,* provided that their MIC is in the susceptible range. On the other hand, the bactericidal activity of β-lactams and other cell wall–active agents (e.g., vancomycin) against *Staphylococcus aureus* is less predictable. When a serious *S. aureus* infection occurs in a patient with poor immune defense mechanisms, an in vitro determination of the amount of antimicrobial agent required to kill as well as inhibit the isolate may be helpful; the **minimum bactericidal concentration (MBC)** test can be used for this purpose. The National Committee for Clinical Laboratory Standards (NCCLS) has described several procedures for assessing bactericidal activity; however, unlike disk diffusion and MIC tests, a standardized MBC test has not been in use for a sustained period. In the past, numerous methodologic variations existed that compromised the use of the test results.

The MBC test is performed in conjunction with a broth macrodilution or broth microdilution MIC test. The antimicrobial agent concentrations that show inhibition (at and above the MIC) may or may not have killed the bacteria in the test inoculum (Figure 3-23). After the MIC determination, a 0.01-mL aliquot of each clear tube or well is subcultured to an agar medium to determine the MBC or the lowest concentration of antimicrobial agent needed to kill the test bacterium. The numbers of colonies that grow on subculture are compared with the actual number of organ-

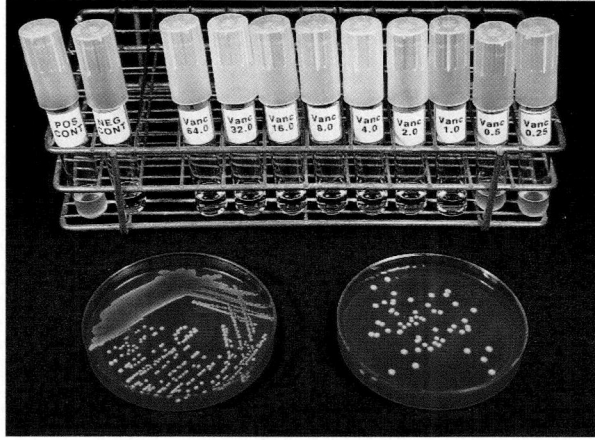

Figure 3-23 _____

Broth macrodilution test showing vancomycin and *Staphylococcus aureus*. The MIC is 1.0 µg/mL. The purity plate shows a pure culture. The colony count plate shows 53 colonies, which means that 5.3×10^5 CFU/mL bacteria were in the test tubes immediately after inoculation of the MIC test. For the colony count plate, immediately after inoculation the growth control tube was diluted 1:1000, and 0.1 mL was plated. Now, 0.01 mL will be plated from each clear tube (tubes containing 1.0 through 128 µg/mL) for the MBC determination. Because it was shown that the actual colony count in the MIC test was 5.3×10^5 CFU/mL, growth of five or fewer colonies would indicate a 3 $\log_{10}$ decrease or 99.9% killing. By definition, the concentration of drug in the respective tube would be considered bactericidal.

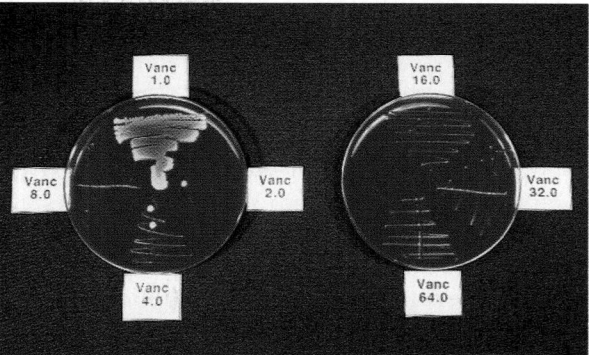

Figure 3-24 _____

Subculture plates from the MIC test of vancomycin and *Staphylococcus aureus* shown in Figure 3-23. Subcultures from tubes containing 8.0 to 128 µg/mL show no growth. Subcultures from the tubes containing 2.0 µg/mL and 4.0 µg/mL show one and two colonies, respectively, indicating >99.9% killing. More than five colonies have grown from the 1.0 µg/mL tube, so the MBC is 2.0 µg/mL.

isms inoculated into the MIC test to determine the extent of bactericidal activity at each antimicrobial concentration. If the numbers of colonies on a subculture plate total less than 0.1% of the initial inoculum (indicating ≥99.9% killing), a bactericidal effect has by definition been achieved.

As described previously, the final number of bacteria in each tube (or well) immediately after inoculation of the MIC test is approximately 5×10^5 CFU/mL (colony-forming units per mL). For the MBC test, however, an actual colony count must be performed on the test inoculum at the time the MIC test is inoculated. A small aliquot from the growth control tube or well is diluted in saline or broth to obtain a countable number of colonies; the final dilution is plated to an agar medium. Generally, a 1:1000 dilution is performed (0.01 mL from the growth control tube is diluted

in 10 mL), and 0.1 mL is spread over the surface of an agar plate. Following overnight incubation, the number of colonies that have grown on the colony count plate are noted. Because this count represents a 1:10,000 dilution, the count is multiplied by 10^4 to determine the number of bacteria in the original growth control (and antimicrobial agent) solutions. A calculation is performed to determine the number of colonies representing 99.9% of the test inoculum in the MIC test because the **MBC endpoint** is defined as the lowest concentration of antimicrobial agent that kills 99.9% of the test bacteria.

In the example shown in Figure 3-23, the actual count on the colony count plate is 53; therefore the number of bacteria in each tube of the MIC test immediately after inoculation was 5.3×10^5 CFU/mL (calculated by multiplying 53 times the dilution factor, which is 10^4). A 99.9% killing (or 0.1% survival) would be accomplished if 5 or fewer colonies grow upon subculture of each clear well or tube after reading of the MIC test (Figure 3-24). In this example, subcultures from all tubes containing 2.0 µg/mL vancomycin or more grew fewer than 5 colonies. Consequently, the MBC is 2.0 µg/mL. The 99.9% end point (or three $\log_{10}$ reduction in growth of the original inoculum) is an arbitrary value with 95% confidence limits, although its clinical relevance has not been rigorously confirmed.

Controlling Test Variables

MBC tests are subject to more technical pitfalls than MIC tests, and several variables must be rigidly controlled during MBC testing. The first involves inoculum. Because many antimicrobial agents exert a bactericidal effect only on growing cells, bacteria in the mid-logarithmic phase of growth must be used as the inoculum to prevent falsely elevated MBCs. The inoculum preparation methods described for MIC tests that use stationary phase growth are unacceptable for MBC tests.

Secondly, during inoculation for MIC tests, care must be taken to ensure that all bacteria in the test inoculum are deposited directly into the antimicrobial solution. If this is not done, bacteria may stick to the wall of the tube or well above the meniscus of the antimicrobial solution and may remain viable during incubation of the MIC portion of the test. These cells (which have not been exposed to antimicrobial agent) may then be inadvertently transferred during the subculture step, ultimately resulting in falsely elevated MBCs.

Third, the volume subcultured following reading of the MIC test must be large enough to contain sufficient inoculum but small enough to prevent carryover of large amounts of antimicrobial agent to continue to exert an antibacterial effect. Usually, 10 µL (0.01 mL) is recommended.

Interpretation Concerns

Several interpretive problems, most common with β-lactam agents, have been associated with MBC tests, and they relate to technical or biologic issues. Sometimes there are more colonies growing on subcultures at higher drug concentrations than at lower concentrations. This decreased bactericidal activity at higher concentrations is referred to as a **paradoxic, or Eagle, effect.** Sometimes, small numbers (but slightly greater than 0.1% of the test inoculum) of bacteria grow on several subculture plates **(persisters).** This may occur if some bacteria are metabolically inactive at the times of testing; however, when the persisting colonies are retested, their MICs are comparable to those orginally obtained. Finally, **tolerance** to the intrinsic bactericidal effect of an antimicrobial agent is demonstrated when the numbers of colonies growing on subculture plates exceed the 0.1 cutoff for several successive drug concentrations above the MIC. *Tolerance* is generally defined as an MBC:MIC ratio of 32 or greater. Tolerance has been associated with a defect in bacterial cellular autolytic enzymes.

TIME-KILL ASSAYS

Bactericidal activity of antimicrobial agents can also be assessed by performance of in vitro **time-kill assays.** Briefly, test bacteria in the mid-logarithmic growth phase are inoculated into several tubes of broth containing varying concentrations of antimicrobial agent and a growth control tube without drug. These tubes are incubated at 35° C. Then, small aliquots are removed at specific time intervals (e.g., at 0, 4, 8, and 24 hours), diluted to obtain countable numbers of colonies, and plated to agar for colony count determinations. The number of bacteria remaining in each sample is plotted over time to determine the rate of antimicrobial agent killing. Generally, a three or more $\log_{10}$ reduction in bacterial counts in the antimicrobial suspensions as compared with the growth control indicates an adequate bactericidal response. Because this test is quite labor intensive, it is usually performed only in research settings.

SYNERGY TESTS

Some types of infections require therapy with a combination of two or more antimicrobial agents. Enterococcal endocarditis, for example, requires use of a penicillin (or vancomycin) and an aminoglycoside for reliable killing of the organism. A broad-spectrum cephalosporin and an aminoglycoside are often prescribed for gram-negative sepsis in neutropenic patients. Goals of combination therapy are to obtain broad-spectrum coverage, enhance antibacterial activity through synergistic interactions, and minimize resistance development. For most infections requiring combination therapy, single-agent MIC results and previous experience in treating similar types of infections are sufficient to guide the selection of an antimicro-

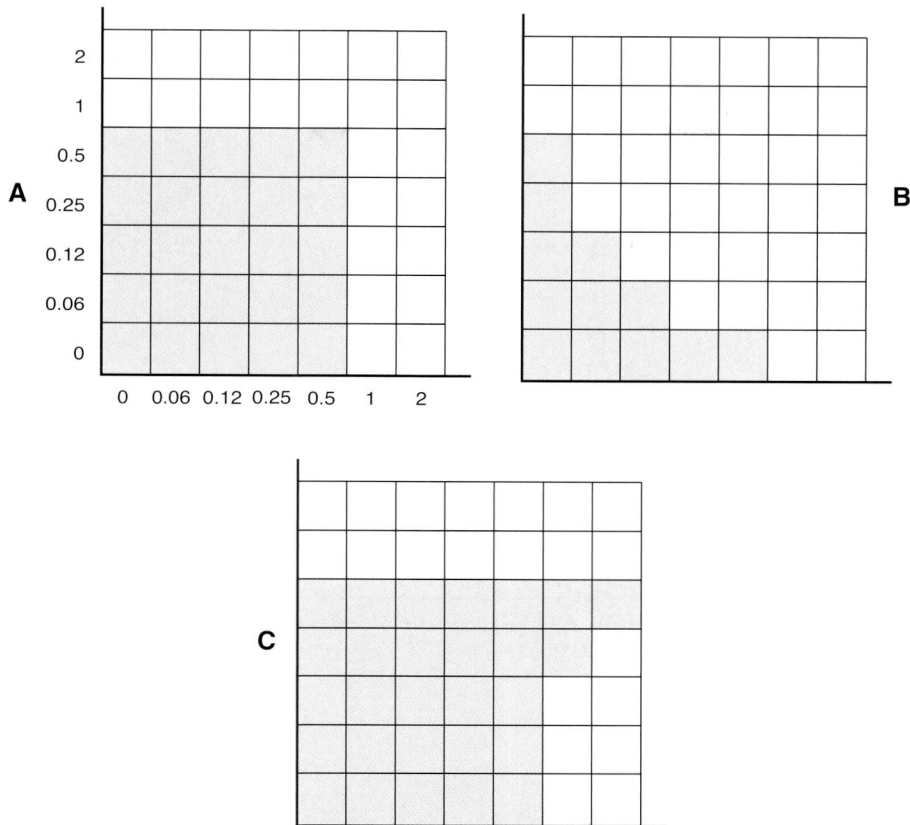

Figure 3-25

Assessment of antimicrobial combinations with the checkerboard method. Panels **A, B,** and **C** depict the results of testing combinations of two drugs (diluted in geometric twofold increments along the x and y axes; drug **A** along x axis and drug **B** along y axis). Shading indicates visible growth, and concentrations are expressed as multiples of the minimum inhibitory concentration. **A,** Indifference; **B,** synergism; **C,** antagonism. (Modified from Eliopoulos GM, Moellering RC, Jr: Antimicrobial combinations. In Lorian V, editor: *Antibiotics in laboratory medicine,* ed 4, Baltimore, 1996, Williams & Wilkins.)

bial agent. In unusual situations, however, in which the patient may not be responding to what would appear to be an adequate regimen, unusual organisms or resistance properties are encountered, or host factors preclude use of certain agents, in vitro synergy tests may be warranted.

In vitro synergy tests may be performed using a broth dilution checkerboard method or time-kill assays. The checkerboard assay is a type of two-dimensional test; all steps are performed as for single agents, but two agents are tested in each well or tube.

Checkerboard synergy tests are usually performed in broth microdilution MIC trays. A wide variety of combinations of concentrations are tested by dispensing drugs in a two-dimensional "checkerboard" format, and each drug tested in the combination is also tested by itself. A combination is **synergistic** if its antibacterial activity is significantly greater than that of the single agents—that is, when the MIC for each drug in the combination is less than or equal to one-fourth of the single-agent MICs. Conversely, **antagonism** is defined as the activity of the combination less than (and MICs are greater than) that of the single agents. In **indifference** the activity of the combination is equal to that of the single agents (Figure 3-25).

Time-kill assays can also be used to study synergistic interactions by testing a combination of drugs in a single tube and each drug individually

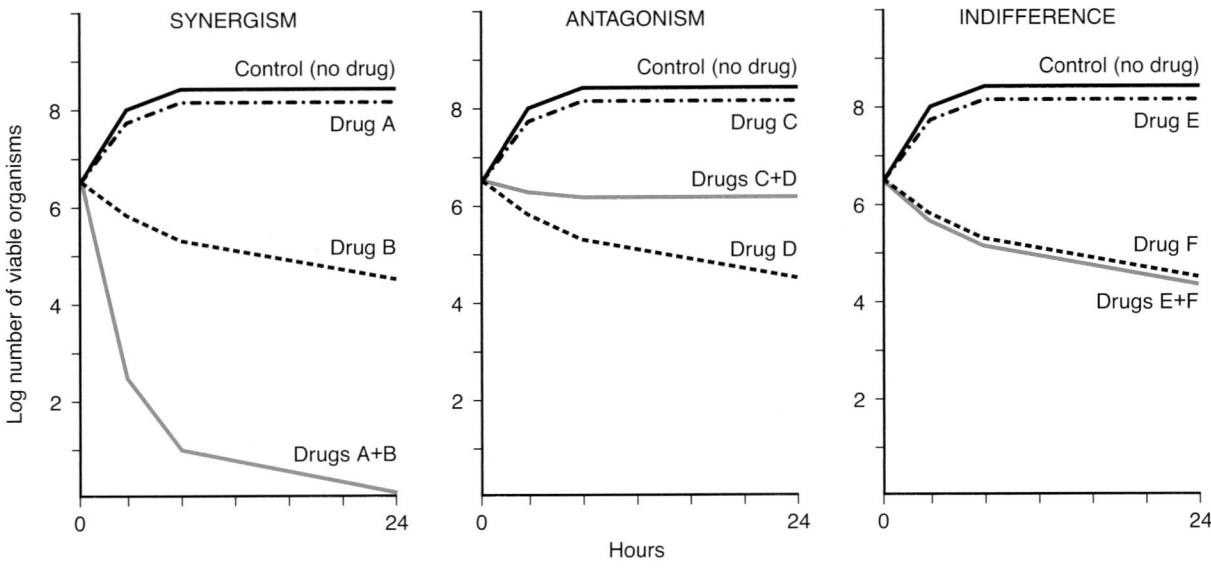

Figure 3-26

Effects of antimicrobial combinations as measured with the killing-curve method. A + B = synergism; C + D = antagonism; E + F = indifference. (Modified from Eliopoulos GM, Moellering RC, Jr: Antimicrobial combinations. In Lorian V, editor: *Antibiotics in laboratory medicine,* ed 4, Baltimore, 1996, Williams & Wilkins.)

in additional tubes. Several drug concentrations alone and in combination are usually examined. If subsequent colony counts reveal a two or more log_{10} reduction in the combination tube counts at 24 hours compared with the most active single-agent tube count, synergy has been demonstrated (Figure 3-26). A change of less than tenfold (increase or decrease) in colony counts from the combination tube compared with the most active single-agent tube represents indifference.

The NCCLS has not addressed synergy testing, and a number of methodologic variations exist.

SERUM BACTERICIDAL TEST

In the late 1940s Schlichter and MacLean described a test that measured the effectiveness with which penicillin in serum killed bacteria associated with endocarditis. This test was subsequently modified slightly and standardized; it is now referred to as the **serum bactericidal test (SBT).** NCCLS has published procedures for serum bactericidal tests, including broth macrodilution and microdilution methods. Some clinical data

available support the use of the SBT to evaluate specimens from patients with serious bacterial infections such as endocarditis, osteomyelitis, and gram-negative bacteremia.

The SBT is similar to the MIC/MBC test in that both inhibitory and bactericidal parameters are evaluated. The patient's serum and the bacterial isolate responsible for the patient's infection are required. Serial twofold dilutions of the patient's serum are prepared, and then a standardized inoculum of the patient's bacterial isolate is added to each dilution. Following overnight incubation, the tubes or wells are examined to determine the highest dilution of patient's serum that inhibits the bacteria. Subsequently, as with the MBC tests, all tubes or wells showing inhibition are subcultured to an agar medium to determine the highest dilution that kills the bacteria. All the potential technical pitfalls mentioned for the MBC test also apply to the SBT test.

SBT results relate to the amount of antimicrobial agent and any other antibacterial factors (e.g., antibody, opsonins, complement) present in the patient's serum. Timing the collection of serum is critical, and generally both trough and peak titers

TABLE 3-17

Guidelines for Obtaining Serum Specimens for the Serum Bactericidal Test and Antimicrobial Assays

Trough*	Obtain 0-30 minutes before next dose.
Peak*	Obtain either
	■ 30-60 minutes after completion of a 30-minute intravenous (IV) infusion.
	■ 60 minutes after an intramuscular (IM) injection.
	■ 90 minutes after an oral dose (varies by specific drug).

*Ideally, trough and peak specimens should be collected around the same dose.

are tested (Table 3-17). Older literature holds that a peak bactericidal titer of 1:8 or greater indicates that therapy was adequate. NCCLS states that a trough bactericidal titer of 1:32 or greater and a peak bactericidal titer of 1:64 or greater correlated with bacteriologic cure in patients with endocarditis. The NCCLS interpretive guidelines are applicable only if NCCLS methods are followed in performing the test. As with the MBC tests, technical complexity limits the widespread use of the SBT.

MOLECULAR PROBES FOR IDENTIFYING DETERMINANTS OF ANTIMICROBIAL RESISTANCE

Molecular methods are being used throughout the clinical microbiology laboratory to identify certain microorganisms. Several probes directed toward antimicrobial resistance genes have been developed; at this time, however, their use is confined to research settings. A probe directed toward the *mec* gene, which codes for oxacillin (methicillin) resistance in staphylococci, has been studied. Probes directed toward genes responsible for other resistance mechanisms (e.g., β-lactamases, aminoglycoside-modifying enzymes, tetracycline resistance factors, vancomycin resistance factors) have also been described. A concern about using probes to confirm resistance involves the ability of some bacteria to contain specific resistance genes that may not be expressed. In these cases, the clinical significance of the presence of the resistance genes is questionable. Use of molecular methods to study resistance is in its infancy, and further studies will undoubtedly elucidate the clinical correlation of various findings.

MEASUREMENT OF ANTIMICROBIAL AGENTS IN SERUM AND BODY FLUIDS

The amount of antimicrobial agent in serum or other body fluid can be measured by a variety of antimicrobial assay procedures. Antimicrobial assays are performed for those antimicrobial agents in which the therapeutic concentration is close to the toxic concentration. Assay results often lead to modification of subsequent doses to prevent accumulation of excessive drug concentrations that may be harmful to the patient. A patient's renal and hepatic status greatly influences in vivo levels of some antimicrobial agents. The antimicrobial agents with the greatest toxic risks and those most commonly monitored are the aminoglycosides, vancomycin, and chloramphenicol. For evaluation of antimicrobial levels, both trough and peak samples should be assayed as for the serum bactericidal test (see Table 3-17).

Biologic Assays

Antimicrobial assays were initially performed by a biologic assay method; bioassays are still sometimes used today when the focus is on the amount of biologically active drug present rather than the amount of "chemical" present. The bioassays utilize a specific strain of bacteria (indicator organism) that is susceptible to the drug to be assayed, and the test is performed in either broth or agar. The antibacterial activity of the patient's specimen against this bacterium is compared with that of solutions containing defined concentrations of the antimicrobial being assayed to determine the concentration in the patient's specimen through use of standard dose-response curves.

Immunoassays

Radioimmunoassay (RIA), fluorescent immunoassay, fluorescent polarization immunoassay, and enzyme immunoassay (EIA) procedures have all been used to measure antimicrobial agents in serum and other body fluids. The basic principles of these assays are similar in that they all utilize antibodies directed against the specific antimicrobial agents to be assayed. Because of the nature of these tests, they are often performed in the chemistry or therapeutic drug monitoring sections of the laboratory. Several commercial manufacturers offer various types of immunoassay kits for performing gentamicin, tobramycin, amikacin, vancomycin, and chloramphenicol assays.

Chromatographic Assays

Various chromatographic methods, including gas-liquid, thin-layer, and paper chromatography, have been used on occasion for antimicrobial assays. The most widely employed chromatographic methods, however, has been high-performance liquid chromatography (HPLC). Chromatographic methods are used primarily to measure levels of antimicrobial agents for which commercial immunoassay kits are not available. These tests are usually performed in research settings.

Bibliography

Berenbaum MC: A method for testing synergy with any number of agents, *J Infect Dis* 137:122, 1978.

Eliopoulos GM, Moellering RC: Antimicrobial combinations. In Lorian V editor: *Antibiotics in laboratory medicine,* ed 4, Baltimore, 1996, Williams & Wilkins.

Halbert DN: DNA probes for the detection of antibiotic resistance genes, *Clin Microbiol Newsletter* 10:33, 1988.

Klassen M, Edberg SC: Measurement of antibiotics in human body fluids: techniques and significance. In Lorian V, editor: *Antibiotics in laboratory medicine,* ed 4, Baltimore, 1996, Williams & Wilkins.

Moody J: Synergism tests. In Isenberg HI, editor: *Clinical microbiology procedures handbook,* Washington, DC, 1992, American Society for Microbiology.

National Committee for Clinical Laboratory Standards: *Methodology for the serum bactericidal test: tentative guideline M21-T,* Wayne, Penn, 1992, NCCLS.

National Committee for Clinical Laboratory Standards: *Methods for determining bactericidal activity of antimicrobial agents: tentative guideline M26-T,* Wayne, Penn, 1992, NCCLS.

Schlicter JG, MacLean H: A method for determining the effective therapeutic level in the treatment of subacute bacterial endocarditis with penicillin: a preliminary report, *Am Heart J* 34:209, 1947.

Swenson JM, JA Hindler, Peterson LR: Special tests for detecting antibacterial resistance. In Murray P et al: *Manual of clinical microbiology,* ed 6, Washington, DC, 1995, American Society for Microbiology.

LEARNING ASSESSMENT

1. Why is a bactericidal drug regimen necessary for treating patients with endocarditis?

2. What are some of the limitations to consider when interpreting results from MBC tests?

CHAPTER 4

Performance Improvement in the Microbiology Laboratory

A. QUALITY ISSUES IN CLINICAL MICROBIOLOGY

Merrily Rausch

GENERAL GUIDELINES FOR ESTABLISHING QUALITY CONTROL
  Temperatures
  Thermometer Calibration
  Equipment QC
  Reagent QC
  Antimicrobial Susceptibility QC

Personnel Competency
Use of Stock Cultures
QC Manual

PERFORMANCE IMPROVEMENT (PI)
  Mission Statement
  Indicators of PI: Process Versus Outcome
  Establishing Performance Monitors
  Problem/Action Form
  The Customer Concept
  Fixing the Process
  Benchmarking
  Commercially Purchased Monitors

OBJECTIVES

1. Define *quality control* (QC) as it applies in the clinical microbiology laboratory.
2. Discuss the general guidelines for establishing a QC program, describing the way to monitor equipment maintenance and performance, culture media and reagent performance, personnel competency, use of stock cultures, and the development and updating of procedure manuals.
3. Describe proper documentation and institution of appropriate corrective action.
4. Define *performance improvement (PI),* and describe in what way it differs from QC.
5. Discuss the ten-step plan for establishing quality monitors.
6. Describe the customer concept.
7. Define *benchmarking.*

KEY TERMS

Quality control
Analytical activity
Preanalytical activity
Postanalytical activity
Performance improvement (PI)
Preventive maintenance
National Committee for Clinical Laboratory Standards (NCCLS)
Proficiency testing
Competency
Clinical Laboratory Improvement Act of 1988 (CLIA)
Continuing education (CE)
Joint Commission on Accreditation of Healthcare Organizations (JCAHO)
College of American Pathologists (CAP)
Process monitors
Outcome monitors
Focused monitors
Customer concept
Cross-functional teams
Facilitator
Benchmarking
Q-Probes

CASE STUDY

A night-shift technologist received a cerebrospinal fluid (CSF) for culture and direct smear. While performing the Gram stain procedure, she was interrupted by a telephone call. Later, she finished staining the smear. Microscopic examination of the CSF showed numerous white blood cells and few Gram-negative cocci in pairs. She also noted that the quality-control stock *Staphylococcus aureus* and *Escherichia coli* appeared as gram-negative cocci and gram-negative bacilli, respectively. The technologist prepared another CSF smear and repeated the procedure.

The issue of quality in the laboratory is complex. The emphasis and the terminology have changed tremendously in recent years. Laboratories have always taken measures to control the testing performed on patient specimens. This effort has been termed **quality control;** it is defined as those measures designed to ensure the medical reliability of laboratory data. Examples are checking media and reagents with specific organisms to see whether expected results are obtained and documenting that instrumentation meets all operating parameters before it is used on patient samples.

Laboratory professionals now realize that quality control is only a small part of the issue of quality. Even when the laboratory has effectively controlled media, reagents, and instruments, the quality of the test result is poor if the specimen degraded before arriving in the laboratory but was still tested. Suppose a specimen contained the wrong patient name; again, the media can be top quality, the incubator temperature accurate, and the technologist very competent, but if the results are recorded on the wrong patient chart, quality patient care management does not exist for the intended patient.

The actual laboratory testing is called an *analytical activity.* It is now important to realize that **preanalytical, analytical,** and **postanalytical** activities all affect quality. An outcome can be interrupted or destroyed at any point in the process. Table 4-1 attempts to clarify these three stages by giving examples of each kind of activity.

TABLE 4-1

Three Stages of Activities that Affect Outcome of Laboratory Testing

Stage	Activities
Preanalytical	Test ordering
	Order transcription
	Patient preparation
	Specimen collection
	Specimen identification
	Specimen transport
Analytical	Sample testing
Postanalytical	Result transcription
	Result delivery
	Result review
	Action taken on basis of result

What has always been known as *quality control* relates only to analytical activities. *Quality assurance* was used to define those measures taken to ensure high-quality patient care. Quality assurance involves monitoring and regulating preanalytical, analytical, and postanalytical activities, and it is measured completely by patient outcome. It did not take long for managers to realize that "assurance" was probably the wrong word because we cannot actually assure the quality. The Joint Commission for the Accreditation of Healthcare Organizations (JCAHO) now uses the term ***performance improvement (PI).*** The focus changed when the terminology changed. PI is a more proactive approach that becomes the responsibility of all employees. It involves correcting whole processes instead of just pieces of processes. Any complicated, multifaceted process can always be improved.

Prevention also became a bigger emphasis than detection. Terminology continued to change. For a while, the prevalent term was *total quality management (TQM);* later, it was *continuous quality improvement (CQI). Continuous improvement* means the daily attempt to improve, even if a problem does not exist. The emphasis is still on processes, with organization-wide commitment, so quality control is actually a piece of continuous quality improvement, or performance improvement.

This section presents two major quality issues:

- Applications of quality control
- Performance improvement

GENERAL GUIDELINES FOR ESTABLISHING QUALITY CONTROL

All quality control activities that take place must be recorded to prove their existence. All record sheets must list tolerance limits, when applicable, so that the person recording the results will always know whether the value being recorded is acceptable. Corrective action must also be recorded when any measurement falls outside a tolerance limit. The responsibility for quality control may rest mainly with one person, but in reality everyone must participate for a program to be successful. A quality control program for a laboratory must include procedures for control of the following items: temperatures, equipment, media, reagents, susceptibility testing, and personnel.

Temperatures

Daily temperature checks are required on all temperature-dependent equipment:

- Incubators
- Heating blocks
- Water baths
- Refrigerators
- Freezers

Incubator and refrigerator thermometers are easier to read if they are permanently immersed in glycerol. This helps prevent temperature fluctuations when the door is opened to read the thermometer. Before use, each thermometer must be checked against a reference thermometer from the National Bureau of Standards (NBS). The most efficient method is to check a large batch of thermometers at the same time, at all temperature ranges likely to be used. A common practice in clinical microbiology is to test all thermometers at 0° C, 37° C, and 56° C. The NBS thermometer comes with certification papers that list correction factors to be used at various temperature ranges. These correction factors are applied to all values obtained on individual laboratory thermometers. Laboratories arbitrarily determine the acceptable temperature variance. For most routine work, thermometers that vary by 1° C or more from the reference thermometer are discarded.

PROCEDURE 4-1. **Thermometer Calibration Procedure**

Labeling

1. Create a calibration log sheet.

2. Etch a number on the back of each thermometer using a diamond-tipped marker.

Calibration Method

1. Place the reference thermometer and the thermometer(s) to be calibrated in an ice bath.

2. When the reference thermometer reads $0°$ C, take the reading of all thermometer(s) being calibrated, and record the readings on the log sheet.

3. Repeat steps 1 and 2 at all other applicable temperatures, such as $37°$ C and $56°$ C.

Calculation of Correction Factor

1. Correct for the difference in readings between the reference thermometer (reference temperature) and that of each thermometer being calibrated by substracting the higher reading from the lower reading. If the thermometer being calibrated reads less than the reference thermometer, assign a plus (+) sign to the result of the subtraction step. This value must be added to the thermometer reading to equal the reading that would be taken from the reference thermometer. Conversely, if the reading of the thermometer being calibrated is greater than the reference thermometer, assign a minus (−) sign to the result. This value must then be subtracted from that thermometer's reading to equal the reference value.

2. Correct for the difference between the reading of the reference thermometer and the "real" temperature, using the process just described. Add the correction factor for the reference thermometer to the correction factor calculated in step 1 for each thermometer being calibrated.

3. Determine the correction factor at each temperature for each thermometer, and record it on the log sheet for the thermometer. The log sheet should be kept for the life of the thermometer.

4. Tolerance limits are set by each laboratory, but are usually $1°$ C. Discard all thermometers that exceed the established tolerance limit.

Examples of correction factors are shown in the table below.

"Real" Temperature	Reference Temperature	Correction Factor
$0°$	$+0.1°$	$+0.1$
$37°$	$36.9°$	$+0.1$
$56°$	$55.9°$	$+0.1$

Thermometer Calibration

Thermometers are calibrated by batch on arrival to the laboratory. Procedure 4-1 outlines the calibration procedure. Once the thermometer has passed calibration and is placed in use, repeat calibration of the thermometer should not be necessary. Alternatively, thermometers already checked against an NBS thermometer can be purchased. For environmental and safety reasons, nonmercury thermometers are recommended. Mineral spirits with nontoxic red-dyed alcohol are used in place of the mercury.

Equipment QC

Equipment used in the clinical microbiology laboratory must be tested for proper performance at intervals appropriate for each piece. This may involve checking the percentage of CO_2 in an incubator daily or measuring the rpm of a centrifuge twice a year. Sometimes, frequency of testing is dictated by a regulatory agency, and other times, it is arbitrary. Table 4-2 gives examples of some laboratory equipment, the type of testing done, and the frequency of testing.

A **preventive maintenance** program must be

TABLE 4-2

Frequency of Equipment Testing

Equipment	Test Type	Frequency
Incubator	Temperature, CO_2	Daily
GasPak jar	Anaerobiasis, catalyst heated	Each use
Anerobe chamber	Anaerobiasis, humidity, temperature	Daily
Biohazard hood	Air flow (done by specialist)	Annually or any time hoods are moved
Centrifuge	RPM check	Every 6 months
Microscope	Cleaned and adjusted	Four times per year or as needed
Autoclave	Temperature	Each load
	Spore testing	Weekly
Balance	Accuracy of weights	Annually

established as an additional control measure. Preventive maintenance performed on equipment generally involves tasks such as oiling and cleaning, replacing filters, and recalibrating instruments. Keeping an instrument in top shape and functioning at the proper level will increase its lifetime and help control the quality of the results. Figure 4-1 shows an example of a preventive maintenance log sheet.

All prepared media must be quality controlled to document their performance and sterility. Records must be maintained for 2 years. The criteria are established by the **National Committee for Clinical Laboratory Standards (NCCLS)** and listed in document M22-A2. Commercial media are always tested by the manufacturer. The laboratory must obtain a statement of quality control from the manufacturer for all media the laboratory will not retest. Only certain kinds of media must be retested by the user, usually because of complexity or history of failure rate. Media that require retesting are chocolate agar, selective media for pathogenic *Neisseria,* and *Campylobacter* media. Figure 4-2 lists specialty commercial media that have been retested by the laboratory.

Media that are not quality controlled by the laboratory should still undergo daily observation for moisture, sterility, and color:

- **Moisture:** Plates should be free of moisture before use but should never show signs of drying around the edges.
- **Sterility:** Plates should be free of contaminants.

- **Color:** Blood-based plates should not show signs of hemolysis, and any other plate that deviates from the normal color should not be used.

Results of daily media observation must be recorded and must include lot numbers. Figure 4-3 shows an example of a daily media observation log, which helps ensure that good-quality media are used on all patient samples. Corrective action must be taken when a medium does not meet standards. This can be documented on a separate record known as a media failures log (Table 4-3).

When a medium does need to be quality controlled because it was prepared "in-house" (in the laboratory) or because it is complex, several basic rules must be followed:

TABLE 4-3

Media Failures Log

Date:	2/14/98
Media:	TMS slants
Lot #:	In-house preparation 2/13/98
Expiration date:	6 months from preparation
Quantity:	2 racks
Failure:	Failure to give proper reaction with *S. epidermidis; S. aureus* and other coagulase-neg. staphs are OK
Action taken:	QC repeated. *S. epidermidis* failed. Memo sent to all techs and all tubes discarded. New TMS prepared.
Technologist:	MAR

MEDIA, REAGENTS, AND SMALL EQUIPMENT	JANUARY	FEBRUARY	MARCH
MEDIA, REAGENTS:			
1. Check refrigerators and freezers for outdated material.	1/21/98 AF	2/24/98 LH	3/28/98 DS
2. Check for "received" and "opened" dating.	1/21/98 AF	2/24/98 LH	3/28/98 DS
THERMOMETERS: Calibrate by batch on arrival.			
PIPETTORS: Calibrate.			3/10/98 MS
pH METER: (Rooms 337 and 354)			
1. Clean the exterior.	1/21/98 AF	2/24/98 LH	3/28/98 DS
2. Replace water in the electrode holder.	1/21/98 AF	2/24/98 LH	3/28/98 DS
3. Check the AgCl level of the electrode.	1/21/98 AF	2/24/98 LH	3/28/98 DS
EYEWASHES: Flush.			
(Rooms 332, 337, 339, 342, 351[2], 354)	1/21/98 AF	2/24/98 LH	3/28/98 DS
STAINING SINK: Clean.	1/20/98 AF	2/24/98 LH	3/28/98 DS
GROUNDING: Check annually.			
REVIEWED BY: M Rausch Page 1 of 5			
YEAR: 1998			
Preventive maintenance is to be performed in the months highlighted for each item listed.			

Figure 4-1

Preventive maintenance log sheet.

- All media must be tested before use.
- Each medium must be tested with organisms expected to grow or give a positive reaction as well as with organisms expected either not to grow or to produce a negative reaction.
- The medium should be tested for sterility and pH.
- The organisms selected for QC should represent the most fastidious organisms for which the medium was designed.
- Testing techniques should be different for primary plating media than for biochemical or subculture media. Primary plating media should be tested with dilute suspensions of organisms, whereas biochemical media can be tested with undiluted organisms.
- QC testing should be performed according to NCCLS recommendations.
- Expiration dates must be established.

MEDIUM TESTED	MFG	LOT NUMBER	EXP. DATE	STERILITY	TEST ORGANISMS	RESULT	ACTION TAKEN	DATE	TECH
Chocolate II	BD	L3RTPO	5/23/98	OK	H. influenzae N. meningitidis	Pass	None	3/8/98	MR
GC-Lect	BD	—							
Jembec-Neiss.	BD	A 3NENC	4/3/98	OK	N. gonorrhoeae N. meningitidis S. epidermidis C. albicans E. coli	Pass	None	3/8/98	MR
Campy bld	BD	LINDHK	4/28/98	OK	C. jejuni E. coli	Pass	None	3/8/98	LM
Campy thio	BD	H4EOAJ	2/1/99	OK	C. jejuni E. coli	Pass	None	3/8/98	LM

Reviewed by: _____ Date: _____

Figure 4-2 _____

Commercial media that have been retested by the laboratory. Result = Pass/Fail.

DATE	MEDIUM	LOT NUMBER	MOISTURE	STERILITY	COLOR	COMMENT	INITIALS
3/4/99	BAP	A2RUWO	✔	✔	✔		MR
	MAC	A4RUUH	✔	✔	✔		MR
	CHOC	A4RUUX	✔	✔	✔		MR
	CNA	A1RUWB	✔	✔	✔		MR
	HE	AZRCUF	✔	✔	✔		MR
	CIN	AZNEJE	✔	✔	✔		MR
	PD	OSU PREP: 1/6/99	✔	✔	✔		MR
	GC-LECT	K3RTNZ	✔	✔	✔		MR
	SCH	A4NETG	✔	✔	✔		MR
	SCH-GV	A3NENN	✔	✔	✔		MR
	CDC ANA	AZRWAW	✔	✔	✔		MR
	SMAC	OSU PREP: 2/15/99	✔	✔	✔		MR

Figure 4-3 _____

Daily media observation log. A check in each column indicates that the medium is acceptable.

Figure 4-4 shows a log sheet used for testing media prepared in-house.

Reagent QC

With few exceptions, reagents should be tested each day of use with both positive and negative controls. Reagents that are documented to have consistent and dependable results may be tested less frequently. Some reagents may be tested more than once a day. When more than one vial of disks such as bacitracin disks is in use at the same time in large laboratories, each vial should be tested daily. This is necessary because each vial is refrigerated at night but usually left at room temperature during the day and therefore has the opportunity to degrade while in use. Examples of reagents that should undergo QC in microbiology are as listed:

- All stains
- Bacitracin
- β-Lactamase
- CAMP
- Catalase
- Coagulase
- FeCl$_3$
- Gelatin
- Germ tube
- Hippurate
- Kovács
- Nitrate
- Optochin
- Oxidase
- L-Pyroglutamyl-β-naphthylamine (PYR)
- Typing sera
- Voges-Proskauer (VP)
- X and V strips

Figure 4-5 shows a variety of testing that might be performed daily at an individual workstation.

Antimicrobial Susceptibility QC

The NCCLS provides guidelines for control of susceptibility testing. The recommended control organisms are specific strains from the American Type Culture Collection (ATCC) (Table 4-4). In addition to the organisms listed in Table 4-4, specific strains of *Haemophilus influenzae* and *Neisseria gonorrhoeae* are used to test patient isolates of these organisms.

In any susceptibility system, many variables can affect the accuracy of results, including the following:

- Antibiotic potency
- Agar depth (Kirby Bauer test)
- Evaporation (microtiter dilution)
- Cation content
- pH
- Thymidine content
- Instrument failure
- Inoculum concentration
- Temperature
- Moisture (Kirby Bauer test)
- Difficulty in determining endpoints

TABLE 4-4

Recommended Control Organisms for Susceptibility Testing

Organism	Susceptibility Test(s)
Escherichia coli, ATCC 25922	Gram-negative drugs
Escherichia coli, ATCC 35218	β-Lactamase-inhibitor drugs
Staphylococcus aureus, ATCC 25923	Gram-positive drugs—Kirby Bauer test
Staphylococcus aureus, ATCC 29213	Gram-positive drugs—minimal inhibitory concentration
Pseudomonas aeruginosa, ATCC 27853	Monitors Ca^{++}, Mg^{++} content*
Enterococcus faecalis, ATCC 29212	Monitors thymidine†

*As Ca^{++} and Mg^{++} concentrations increase, *P. aeruginosa* becomes more resistant to the aminoglycosides.
†Increases in thymidine cause false resistance to certain drugs, such as sulfonamides, trimethoprim, and trimethoprim/sulfamethoxazole.

Careful storage of degradable supplies and precision in implementation of recommended procedures are mandatory to obtain accurate and reproducible susceptibility results.

Susceptibility testing is usually conducted daily. Control organism results must be evaluated previous to determining endpoints on patient isolates. Minimal inhibitory concentration (MIC) values must be within one log dilution of the expected MIC based on NCCLS guidelines. If precision can be demonstrated with 30 consecutive days of susceptibility testing using NCCLS guidelines, QC organisms may be tested weekly instead of daily.

Personnel Competency

Even the personnel must pass quality control repeatedly, using a variety of techniques. One popular technique is **proficiency testing,** whereby

DATE	MEDIA AND LOT NUMBER	ORGANISM PLATED	QC PLATED DATE	QC READ DATE	QC PASSED/FAILED	INITIALS
3/8/99	TMA	S. aureus S. epidermidis	3/9/99	3/10/99	Pass	MR
3/8/99	Beta toxin	S. agalactiae ⊕ S. pyogenes ⊖	3/9/99	3/9/99	Pass	MR
3/8/99	PSE	E. faecalis	3/9/99	3/10/99	Pass	MR
3/8/99	TSI	P. aeruginosa C. freundii	3/9/99	3/10/99	Pass	MR

Figure 4-4

Log sheet for testing media prepared in-house.

BLOOD CULTURE WORKSTATION QUALITY CONTROL

Month _____ March _____
Year _____ 1999 _____

DATE	INITIALS	GAS PAK JAR Anaerobic	HEAT CATALYST	CHANGE DESICCANT Date (weekly)	ACRIDINE ORANGE Pos	Neg	NaDesoxy/ WELLCOGEN Pos	Neg	HEATING BLOCKS (35°- 37° C) #20	#17
1	LM	OK	✔		N	D	+	−	35°	36°
2	AD	OK	✔		N	D	+	−	35°	36°
3	AD	OK x 2	✔		N	D	N	D	35°	36°
4	MCl	OK	✔		+	−	N	D	36°	36°
5	MCl	OK	✔		N	D	N	D	35°	36°
6	LH	OK x 2	✔		N	D	N	D	35°	36°
7	AD	OK x 2	✔	✔	N	D	+	−	36°	36°
8	AD	OK x 2	✔		N	D	+	−	36°	37°
9	LH	OK	✔		N	D	+	−	36°	36°
10	AD	OK	✔		N	D	N	D	36°	36°
11	Cl	OK	✔		+	−	N	D	36°	36°
12	MG	OK	✔		+	−	+	−	36°	36°
13	DS	OK x 2	✔		N	D	N	D	36°	36°
14	DS	OK	✔	✔	N	D	N	D	36°	35°

REVIEWED BY: Mbtt
DATE: 4/4//99

Figure 4-5

Various testing methods that can be performed daily at an individual workstation. Example of a 2-week workstation quality control. *ND*, not done.

carefully designed samples are given to technologists as "unknowns" for the purpose of determining competency in identifying them. Proficiency samples may be purchased commercially or prepared internally. All tests performed on patients must be subjected to proficiency testing twice a year even if commercial proficiency testing is not available. Technologists may perform testing without knowing they are working on a proficiency sample or may clearly understand that the sample is a proficiency test. In either case, samples should not receive any "special" treatment.

Another form of personnel quality control is to prohibit all technologists from "signing out" or finalizing their own work. If each technologist's results are reviewed by another technologist, mistakes are likely to be caught before release.

Employee **competency** has always played a large role in quality. The **Clinical Laboratory Improvement Act of 1988 (CLIA)** has mandated that the competency of each employee be determined and verified upon employment. Reverification must take place annually. Proof of competency must be maintained in each employee's personnel file. A person may be qualified to prepare a slide for staining but may not be able to stain it; a person may be qualified to prepare and stain a slide but not to read or interpret the smear. As part of CLIA requirements, all tests or analyses have been assigned a complexity rating. In microbiology, all tests are either moderately complex or highly complex. Personnel must meet certain educational requirements before being permitted to perform at each level of complexity.

In addition to meeting educational requirements, a person's competency must be observed and documented for each test performed. The many agencies involved in accreditation and inspection have different requirements and interpretations of competency verification, making this a complicated task for all laboratories. An example of a competency check-off form is shown in Figure 4-6.

The requirement for ongoing **continuing education (CE)** programs for all employees is yet another form of quality control. These programs may teach theory or new techniques, present case studies, or simply provide training on new instrumentation. Documentation that all CE programs have been completed is essential. Training for new instrumentation should also be documented in the individual employee's personnel competency file.

Use of Stock Cultures

To operate a quality control program, stock cultures must be maintained by all laboratories. They are available from many sources:

- Commercial sources
- Proficiency testing isolates
- Patient isolates
- American Type Culture Collection (ATCC) organisms

When quality control testing appears to have failed, it is usually the stock culture rather than the test itself that has failed. Organisms may mutate with repeated subculturing. For best results, a stock culture should be grown in a large volume of broth, then divide among enough small freezer vials to last a year. With this technique a new vial can be removed from the freezer weekly so that organisms do not have to be continually subcultured. An organism may need to be subcultured twice after thawing to return it to a healthy state. Media selection for freezing is at the discretion of individual laboratories but should not contain sugars. If organisms utilize sugars while being maintained, the acid products that result may kill the organisms with time. Popular media choices for stock cultures are as follows:

- Schaedler broth with glycerol
- Skim milk
- Chopped meat (anaerobes)
- Tryptic soy agar deeps (at room temperature)
- Cysteine-tryptic agar (CTA) without carbohydrates

If organisms are stored in a freezer, they should be kept at $-70°$ C. Alternative storage methods include freezing in liquid nitrogen and lyophilization.

QC Manual

All rules and procedures for quality control should be available to employees at the workstation in written form in a QC manual. The manual must be reviewed and signed at least annually and revised as needed by a supervisor.

Employee name: _Carol Johnson_   Year _1998_

Demonstrates following abilities:	Work station		
	#1 Respiratory	#2 Urines	#3 O & Ps
1. Handles specimens safely during testing, storing, and discarding	✔	✔	✔
2. Prepares specimens for analysis according to laboratory policies and procedures (parasitology and special procedure areas)	—	—	✔
3. Analyzes specimens according to laboratory procedures for the workstation; knows theory and principles of the tests being performed	✔	✔	✔
4. Clearly records all work done so that another person could take over the work station	✔	✔	✔
5. Reports results accurately and in a timely manner	✔	✔	✔
6. Makes appropriate critical value and courtesy calls	✔	✔	✔
7. Consistently performs and records quality control and documents all remedial action	✔	✔	✔
8. Remedial action necessary (yes or no)	No	No	No

Remedial actions:_____

_____

_____

_____

Date remediation completed:_____

Evaluator signature _A Holbrook_   Date _2/11/98_   (Work station 1)

Evaluator signature _L Creme_   Date _6/9/98_   (Work station 2)

Evaluator signature _S Young_   Date _8/27/98_   (Work station 3)

Employee signature _Carol Johnson_   Date _8/28/98_

Figure 4-6 _____

Competency documentation.

PERFORMANCE IMPROVEMENT (PI)

Accrediting agencies such as the **Joint Commission on Accreditation of Healthcare Organizations (JCAHO)** and the **College of American Pathologists (CAP)** emphasize performance improvement (PI) in their accreditation checklists. CLIA also mandates use of written performance improvement policies in laboratories that include all three phases of testing. Every laboratory must have a plan for improvement. To improve quality effectively, *all* employees must understand the plan and take active roles.

Mission Statement

Creating a short mission statement for all employees to learn can be an effective tool for uniting everyone behind the same cause. It can be as simple as "Working Together For A Healthy America," used at The Ohio State University Medical Center, or "The Right Thing, The Right Way, The First Time, Every Time," used by Intermountain Healthcare. Putting the statement on the backs of employee identification badges is one way to focus on and emphasize the mission so that all become involved and understand that they have roles in the mission and must make PI a part of everyday life. Problems are not to be viewed as true problems but as opportunities for improvement.

Indicators of PI: Process Versus Outcome

Many types of monitors or indicators can be incorporated into a quality improvement program. Accrediting agencies generally check that a variety of types are used. Some monitors are ongoing data collections with no suspected problems. Results are compiled and evaluated routinely. This procedure establishes a trend and makes problems easy to spot as disruptions in the trend. These are often referred to as *process monitors.*

Outcome monitors are measurements of the result of a process. An example is the complications a patient experiences as the result of a process.

Other monitors may be created in response to a suspected problem. Data may be collected for a short period to resolve a specific issue. These monitors are called *focused monitors.*

Establishing Performance Monitors

The JCAHO makes recommendations as an accrediting agency for establishing performance monitors. The components of the recommendation are to *plan, design, measure, assess,* and *improve.*

- **Plan:** The plan is not expected to be a single-department approach. Rather, it should be a coordinated, organization-wide approach to improving patient outcomes that includes interdisciplinary collaborative actions.
- **Design:** Clear objectives are needed to describe a new process, component, or service.
- **Measure:** Systematic data collection is necessary either for improvements or for ongoing measurements. (See Box 4-1 for suggested measurable processes.)
- **Assess:** A review of the collected data should be systematic, interdisciplinary, and interdepartmental, using statistically based analytical tools. Internal comparisons or comparisons to similar processes in other organizations are appropriate. Guidelines for assessments might be accreditation standards, practice guidelines, or legal and regulatory requirements.
- **Improve:** Current processes or a design of new processes may need to be redesigned. Because more opportunities are usually identified than can be acted on, priorities must be established. Priorities are often based on risk, frequency, or high-volume processes.

Problem/Action Form

A simpler approach to monitoring or documenting quality issues is a problem/action form. This is

---

Box 4-1

Measureable Processes

Patient preparation
Specimen handling
   Collection
   Labeling
   Preservation
   Transportation
Communication processes
   Transfer of information
   Completeness of requisitions
   Reporting timeliness
   Report accuracy
Test appropriateness
Patient needs/expectations
Risk management activities
QC activities

TABLE 4-5
Clinical Microbiology Problem/Action Report

Date	11/15/98
Problem	A blood culture was required from a patient at the urgent care facility, but no staff member was trained to draw blood cultures. The patient had to drive from the urgent care facility to the hospital to have the blood drawn by a phlebotomist at the hospital who was trained in the appropriate techniques.
Evaluation	No employees at the urgent care facility have been trained to collect bood cultures. The same is true of the Clinic Outpatient Lab. This is the second occurrence in about 2 months.
Corrective action	Seriously ill patients should not have to travel from one facility to another to have their blood drawn. Laboratory Administration was informed of this situation.
Outcome	All outpatient sites will receive training and written instructions for the proper collection of blood for culture. Patients will no longer have to drive to the hospital for this service if they are already at an outpatient facility.

Submitted by M. Rausch
Attached documentation? No

most commonly used to document issues that are quickly resolved, but it could also be used for long-term monitor summation. The form is a brief statement consisting of the following information:

- Date
- Problem
- Evaluation
- Corrective action
- Outcome

The form may be signed by the person submitting it, and additional documentation may be attached as necessary. Table 4-5 illustrates the use of the problem/action form.

The Customer Concept

Laboratories must focus on the **customer concept.** Who are the customers and what is a customer's perception of quality? Patients are not the only customers. Anyone who looks to the laboratory for a service is a customer. Doctors, nurses, insurers, and patients are all customers. Each customer may view quality differently and may have different expectations. Laboratory workers may judge quality in terms of accuracy, whereas a physician views it

as turnaround time, the patient as compassion and relief from pain, and the insurance company as cost-effectiveness. Customer satisfaction must be surveyed to determine perceptions.

Fixing the Process

When patient outcome is less than desirable, the process must be evaluated and corrected. The focus is on the process, not on an individual. The primary rule to follow is to refrain from finger-pointing or fault-finding. Preanalytical and post-analytical activities usually take place outside the laboratory and require **cross-functional teams** to evaluate and correct the process. Department representatives can easily become defensive and territorial. Barriers to cooperation must be removed. Cross-functional teams must include a trained **facilitator.** Facilitators are most effective when they have no vested interest in the process being evaluated. The facilitator's role on the team is to use problem-solving training and experience to help the team brainstorm and stay on track. In the formation of a cross-functional team the people "in the trenches" must be represented; the team should not consist solely of supervisory personnel. If the issue is transportation of specimens, for example, the team should include, at minimum, a transporter, a specimen processor, a staff nurse, a medical student or physician representative, appropriate supervisory personnel, and a facilitator. The most accurate and meaningful brainstorming ideas usually come from the people who perform the tasks, not from those who designed the process.

When is a process fixed? It is not fixed just because the reason something went wrong is explained. It is fixed only when the problem is prevented from happening again. For example, a laboratory result was never recorded on a patient's chart. Investigation determined that the patient was transferred to another unit while the report was being generated. This explanation does not suffice to fix the problem. To fix the problem, a process must be established to ensure that charting follows every patient in a timely manner every time.

Benchmarking

A benchmark is a reference point. **Benchmarking** is seeking an industry's or profession's best practices to imitate and improve. Benchmarking was initially practiced in business and industry but has now become an important part of hospital quality management programs. It is done willingly and openly. A hospital may join a large group of other hospitals that all share operating statistics. Productivity and cost-effectiveness are two large categories commonly used in a benchmarking comparison. The best performers in a group of hospitals are highlighted. Hospitals can individually and anonymously see where they are by comparison with other hospitals' statistics, then contact the best performers to evaluate their differences. A code of conduct is followed when benchmarking that includes both ethics and etiquette. Although hospitals generally benchmark other hospitals, they will eventually incorporate lessons from other successful industries.

Commercially Purchased Monitors

The College of American Pathologists (CAP) has put together a national PI assessment program called **Q-Probes.** Laboratories throughout the country subscribe to an annual series of monitors. At least one of these monitors each year has a microbiology focus. Q-Probes have covered topics such as adequacy of sputum cultures, turnaround time for spinal fluid Gram stain results, blood culture contamination rates, and appropriateness of ordering patterns for stool specimens. The method of data collection is precisely outlined, and all worksheets and data forms are provided. Information is returned to subscribers in a manner that enables institutions to benchmark.

It has been said that quality is a journey, not a destination. There are always more things to monitor than there are people or resources to monitor them. The focus is usually on high-volume, high-risk, and problem-prone issues. One of the most important factors in a successful PI program is that it originates at the top of the organization, with the chief executive officer, and involves all employees working together. Another essential element is pointing out team successes and giving group rewards. A PI program does not materialize overnight. It takes a tremendous amount of planning, education, and resources. The process is forever changing. A nursery rhyme from *The Quality Quest* describes the process well:

> *Good, Better, Best*
> *Never let it rest,*
> *Until the good becomes better*
> *And the better becomes best.*

Bibliography

August MJ et al: *Quality control and quality assurance practices in clinical microbiology, Cumitech 3A,* Washington, DC, 1990, American Society for Microbiology.

Bartlett RC: Quality control in clinical microbiology. In Balows A et al, editors: *Manual of clinical microbiology,* ed 5, Washington, DC, 1991, American Society for Microbiology.

Clark GB: Quality assurance: an administrative means to a managerial end, *Clin Lab Manage Rev,* part I, 4:7, 1990; Part II, 4:224-252, 1990; Part III, 5:463, 1991.

Clinical Laboratory Improvement Act of 1988: Rules and regulations, Fed Reg, Feb 28, 1992.

College of American Pathologists: *Standards for laboratory accreditation,* Northfield, Ill, 1993, College of American Pathologists.

Continuous Quality Improvment: Can it work in hospitals? Panel discussion via AHA Teleconference, March 12, 1992.

Deming WE: *Quality, productivity, and competitive position,* Cambridge, Mass, 1982, MIT Center for Advanced Engineering Study.

Eisenberg HD, editor: *Clinical microbiology procedures handbook,* secs 12 and 13, Washington, DC, 1992, American Society for Microbiology.

Joint Commission on Accreditation of Healthcare Organizations: *Accreditation manual for hospitals.* Vol 1: Standards, Oakbrook Terrace, Ill, 1993, JCAHO.

Leibor W: *The quality quest,* Chicago, Ill, 1991, American Hospital Publishing.

National Committee for Clinical Laboratory Standards: *Performance standards for antimicrobial susceptibility testing,* M100-S3, Villanova, Pa, 1991, NCCLS.

National Committee for Clinical Laboratory Standards: *Performance standards for antimicrobial disk susceptibility tests,* ed 4 (Approved Standard; M2-4A), Villanova, Pa, 1990, NCCLS.

National Committee for Clinical Laboratory Standards: *Methods for dilution antimicrobial susceptibility tests for bacteria that grow aerobically,* ed 2 (Approved Standard; M7-A2), Villanova, Pa, 1990, NCCLS.

National Committee for Clinical Laboratory Standards: *Quality assurance for commercially prepared microbiological culture media,* ed 2, (Approved Standard; M22-A2), Wayne, Pa, 1996, NCCLS.

LEARNING ASSESSMENT

1. Which of the following terms refers to checking media and reagents with specific organisms to see whether expected results are obtained?
   a. Preventative maintenance
   b. Quality control
   c. Performance improvement

2. Which of the following describe the process of performance improvement?
   a. It involves only preanalytical activities
   b. It is measured by patient outcome
   c. It singles out individuals with poor performance
   d. It is enhanced by understanding customer perception

3. Which media must the laboratory subject to quality control?
   a. All media obtained from a commercial source
   b. Complex media
   c. Media with a history of failure
   d. Media made by the laboratory

4. Which of the following describes the correct way to select organisms for quality control?
   a. They should represent the most fastidious organisms for which the media was designed
   b. They should be organisms that will grow most easily
   c. They should be immediately removed from the freezer

5. Susceptibility tests must be quality controlled daily *except* when which of the following is the case?
   a. An automated system is in use
   b. Controls have been in an acceptable range for 6 months
   c. Precision is demonstrated for 30 consecutive days

Continued

LEARNING ASSESSMENT—cont'd

6. Which of the following mandates annual employee competency testing?
   a. NCCLS
   b. CLIA
   c. NBS
   d. ATCC

7. What is the term for performance improvement monitors that are created in response to a specific issue?
   a. Focused monitors
   b. Process monitors
   c. Outcome monitors

8. Who is defined as a customer in the laboratory?
   a. The patient
   b. The doctor
   c. The nurse
   d. The insurance company
   e. All of the above

B. PUTTING THE LABORATORY TEST TO THE TEST

*Frederic J. Marsik**

ANALYTICAL ANALYSIS OF TESTS
  Analytical (Technical) Sensitivity
  Analytical (Technical) Specificity
  Accuracy
CLINICAL ANALYSIS OF TESTS
  Clinical (Diagnostic) Sensitivity
  Clinical (Diagnostic) Specificity

OPERATIONAL ANALYSIS OF TESTS
  Incidence of Disease
  Prevalence of Disease
  Predictive Values of Tests
    Positive predictive value
    Negative predictive value
    Example
    Clinical applications of positive and negative
      predictive values
  Efficiency of Tests
  Other Concepts
CHOOSING A LABORATORY METHOD
TEST VALIDATION

OBJECTIVES

1. Define and differentiate *analytical sensitivity* and *specificity* and *clinical sensitivity* and *specificity*.
2. Define *prevalence* and *incidence of disease,* and discuss the importance of prevalence in computing predictive values of tests.
3. Discuss predictive values of tests, and show how they are computed.
4. Apply the concepts of predictive values of tests to several clinical examples.

KEY TERMS

Analytical sensitivity
Analytical specificity
Accuracy
Clinical (diagnostic) sensitivity
Clinical (diagnostic) specificity
Incidence
Prevalence
Positive predictive value (PPV)
Negative predictive value (NPV)
Test validation

New diagnostic tests under development in clinical microbiology are directed more toward the detection of antigens rather than toward the detection of antibodies. Although culture still remains the gold standard for diagnostic purposes, the newer, noncultural antigen detection tests offer simplicity and speed for detection of the etiologic agent. In addition, the immune status of the patient does not affect test results. These noncultural antigen detection tests are being designed for physician's office use and, as such, are easily performed by nonlaboratory personnel. Because the test results are available quickly, the physician can make an informed decision regarding patient management.

These tests can be misused, however, or their test results misinterpreted. Tests with a high sensitivity and specificity may be promoted as extremely reliable diagnostic tests. In certain clinical situations, however, such tests may not add meaningful information to the diagnosis. This section reviews the pertinent definitions related to evaluating tests and presents several clinical examples to illustrate the basic concepts.

ANALYTICAL ANALYSIS OF TESTS

The following terms relate to the actual test and are not used in the critical evaluation of a test in the

*This chapter was prepared in part by F. Marsik in his private capacity. No official support by the FDA is intended or implied.

clinical setting. *Analytical sensitivity* and *specificity* should not be confused with *clinical sensitivity* and *specificity.*

Analytical (Technical) Sensitivity

The **analytical sensitivity** of a test refers to its ability to detect a particular analyte or a small change in its concentration. *Analytical sensitivity* is usually defined at the 0.95 confidence level (±2 standard deviations) and may be referred to as the *detection limit.* In microbiology the detection limit may be correlated to the number of colonies in the culture or the lowest quantity of antigen or antibody a test can detect. For example, the enzyme immunoassay (EIA) is more sensitive than the precipitation test in detecting antibody. EIA can detect lower concentrations of antibody.

Analytical (Technical) Specificity

A test's **analytical specificity** refers to its ability *not* to react with substances other than the analyte of interest.

Accuracy

The degree of conformity of a measurement to a standard or a true value is **accuracy.** It is a measure of analytical capability. For example, with the Performance Standards for Antimicrobial Disk Susceptibility Tests, a mean value of several observations is compared with a predetermined standard value or range. If the mean (or range) of control limits found in standard tables is exceeded, a technical systematic error (variation) exists that may lead to misinterpretation of test results.

Accuracy is a function of two characteristics: precision and bias. Precision is the measure of exactness or the degree of refinement with which a test is performed. It is the dispersion of repeated observations caused by random errors. The precision (reproducibility) of a test is usually monitored by means of the range (maximum minus minimum) within sets of observations. Bias is the mean difference of test results from an accepted reference method caused by systematic errors.

Typically, precision and bias are determined by studies whereby several investigators or laboratories perform repeated testing of several specimens of known values. Then, test results are analyzed by statistical methods to determine the test's precision and bias within and among laboratories.

CLINICAL ANALYSIS OF TESTS

Clinical (Diagnostic) Sensitivity

Clinical (diagnostic) sensitivity is the proportion of positive test results obtained when a test is applied to patients known to have the disease. Thus, it is the frequency of positive test results in patients *with* the disease (true-positive results). For example, if 100 patients who have gonorrhea are tested for that disease and the test yields positive results in 95 and is negative in the other 5, then the sensitivity of the test is 95%. Five of these 100 patients had false-negative test results.

The highest clinical sensitivity is desired when a disease is serious and when false-positive results will not lead to serious clinical or economic problems. Sensitivity is expressed as a percent.

$$\frac{\text{Number of true-positive results}}{\text{Number of true-positive plus}} \times 100$$
$$\text{false-negative results}$$

The sensitivity of a particular test does not change if the test is performed correctly. The sensitivity is determined by multicenter clinical trials whereby the test results, obtained by performing the test according to a specific protocol, are compared with a gold standard. In microbiology the standard is usually culture, which in many cases is not absolute. Thus the reported sensitivity for a certain test may vary among laboratories. Evaluating new diagnostic tests is difficult because of these imperfect standards.

Clinical (Diagnostic) Specificity

Clinical (diagnostic) specificity is the proportion of negative results obtained when a test is applied to patients known to be free of the disease. Thus it is the frequency of negative test results in patients *without* the disease (true-negative results). For example, if 100 patients without gonorrhea are tested for that disease and the test yields negative results in 90 and is positive in the other 10, then the specificity of the test is 90%. Ten of these 100 patients had false-positive test results.

The highest clinical specificity is desired when the disease is serious but not treatable, when disease absence has either psychologic or public health value, or when false-positive results might cause serious clinical or economic problems. Specificity is expressed as a percent.

$$\frac{\text{Number of true-negative results}}{\text{Number of true-negatives plus}} \times 100$$
$$\text{false-positive results}$$

As with sensitivity, the specificity does not change if the test is performed correctly. The specificity is also determined by clinical trials whereby the test results are confirmed by a more definitive test or procedure.

OPERATIONAL ANALYSIS OF TESTS

Although sensitivity and specificity do not change for a given test, the prevalence of the disease and the positive and negative predictive values of a test do change. In clinical medicine these parameters are extremely important to know when evaluating a particular test result.

Incidence of Disease

Incidence is the number of new cases of a disease over a period of time (e.g., months, year) and is a measure of events. The incidence rate is most often calculated by dividing the number of infections acquired during a given period (e.g., month, year) by the population at risk for that same time. The relation between prevalence (P) and incidence (I) can be seen in the equation $P = I \times D$, where D is duration of disease from onset (diagnosis) to termination.

For chronic diseases, such as cancer, the prevalence is greater than the incidence; for acute diseases, such as gonorrhea, the prevalence is less than the incidence.

Prevalence of Disease

Prevalence is the frequency of a disease at a designated single point in time in the population being tested. For example, during influenza season the prevalence of "strep" throat in children attending daycare centers will be higher than the prevalence in children who do not attend such centers. The role prevalence plays in determining the positive and negative predictive values of a test can be seen in the formulas below. To properly interpret test results, the clinician must have an understanding or estimate of the prevalence of the disease in the population being tested. Prevalence can be estimated on the basis of clinical experience and information provided by the local and state health departments as well as information periodically provided by the Centers for Disease Control and Prevention (CDC).

Predictive Values of Tests

A test can have both a positive and a negative predictive value. The following three elements are needed to compute the positive and negative predictive values of a test:

- Sensitivity of the test
- Specificity of the test
- Prevalence of the disease being tested

Although predictive value theory has only recently been used in clinical medicine, the formulas and concepts are not new. The formulas for calculating positive and negative predictive values are commonly referred to as *Bayes theorem*, which was published posthumously in 1763.

The predictive value of a test is the probability that a positive result **(positive predictive value [PPV])** accurately indicates the presence of an analyte or a specific disease or that a negative result **(negative predictive value [NPV])** accurately indicates the absence of an analyte or a specific disease. Predictive values vary significantly with the prevalence of the disease or analyte unless the test is 100% sensitive (for NPV) or specific (for PPV).

Positive predictive value

The positive predictive value can be computed as follows:

Number of true positive results = (P) (Se):

$$PPV = \frac{(P)\,(Se)}{(P)\,(Se) + (1 - P)\,(1 - Sp)} \times 100$$

Number of true positive results plus false positive results = (P) (Se) + 1 (1 −P)(1 − Sp):
where:

PPV = positive predictive value of test
  P = prevalence of the disease being tested
 Se = sensitivity of test
 Sp = specificity of test.

Negative predictive value

The negative predictive value can be computed as follows:

Number of true negative results = $(1 - P)$ (Sp):

$$NPV = \frac{(1 - P)\,(Sp)}{(1 - P)\,(Sp) + (P)\,(1 - Se)} \times 100$$

Number of true negative plus true positive results:

where:

  NPV = negative predictive value of test
  P = prevalence of the disease being tested
  Se = sensitivity of test
  Sp = specificity of test.

Example

To illustrate the concepts of predictive values, consider a certain diagnostic test that has a sensitivity (Se) of 95% and a specificity (Sp) of 95%. In a primary care hospital where the prevalence of the disease being tested is 1%, the positive predictive value of the test is only 16%. This is calculated using the PPV equation, as follows:

$$PPV = \frac{(0.01)\,(0.95)}{(0.01)\,(0.95) + (1 - 0.01)\,(1 - 0.95)} \times 100$$
$$= 0.16 \text{ or } 16\%$$

The clinician has only a 16% certainty that a patient with a positive test result actually has the disease. If, however, the same test is used in a tertiary care hospital where the prevalence of the disease may be 50%, the positive predictive value increases to 95% (calculated using the same equation). The clinician in this case has a 95% certainty that a patient with a positive test result actually has the disease. Therefore prevalence of the disease has a great influence on the predictive value of a test.

Clinical applications of positive and negative predictive values

GROUP A STREPTOCOCCUS TESTING
OF THROAT SAMPLES

Acute pharyngitis is one of the most common conditions seen by primary care physicians. Although most of the infections are caused by viruses, 5% to 15% of cases have a bacterial etiology, usually group A β-hemolytic streptococci *(Streptococcus pyogenes)*. To test these organisms, 28 to 36 million throat cultures are performed annually in the United States.

Noncultural tests have been developed and approved for use in the private office setting to evaluate patients with acute pharyngitis for the presence of group A streptococci. The reported sensitivities and specificities of these tests vary considerably, however, ranging from the low sixties of the high nineties. Although speculative, explanations for such variations may be the difficulty in obtaining an adequate throat sample, especially in children, and the use of imperfect culture methods as standards.

Assuming that a certain test for streptococci has reported sensitivity and specificity of 90% and 98%, respectively, and that the estimated prevalence for streptococcal infection in acute pharyngitis cases is 5%, the positive and negative predictive values would be 70.3% and 99.5%, respectively. With a positive test result, approximately a 30% chance exists that the patient does not have a streptococcal infection. If the test result is negative, a greater than 99% chance exists that the patient is not infected. If the prevalence in the population being tested increases to 15%, the positive predictive value increases to 88.8%, but the negative predictive value decreases slightly, to 98.2%.

Usually, negative test results are more reliable in predicting the absence of disease than positive test results are in predicting the presence of disease. In this example, a negative result would indicate the absence of group A β-hemolytic streptococci with a high degree of certainty, and the patient could be spared the administration and cost of penicillin. Although clinical judgment is important, these tests can be helpful to clinicians in the proper evaluation and management of patients with acute pharyngitis.

DIRECT DETECTION OF *CHLAMYDIA TRACHOMATIS*
IN URETHRAL AND CERVICAL SPECIMENS

Chlamydia is the most prevalent STD in the United States, with estimates of from 3 to 10 million new cases occurring annually. Many of the individuals infected are asymptomatic, and proper diagnosis and treatment are essential to prevent the spread of this disease and associated complications.

The growth cycle of the bacterium *C. trachomatis* is unique because it is an obligate intracellular parasite that requires living cells for cultivation. Several days are necessary to obtain results, however, and the sensitivity of the culture is only about 85%. As a result, newer noncultural methods have been developed and tested. Several tests are now available for use, including tests utilizing the EIA, the immunofluorescence assay (IF), and DNA probes. Each has a considerable variance in reported sensitivities and specificities, most likely because of the nature of the organism and the imperfect culture standard to which the results are compared. In addition, each test requires specialized equipment that must be maintained and calibrated.

Table 4-6 shows the positive and negative predictive values for the IF and DNA probe tests applied directly to cervical samples in a population of patients in an obstetrics and gynecology clinic, in whom the prevalence of chlamydial cervicitis is estimated to be 5%. The sensitivities and specificities for the two tests are similar, but the positive predictive value is better for the DNA probe test. Thus patients with positive results of the DNA probe test are more likely to have chlamydial cervicitis than are those with positive results of the IF test. On the other hand, both tests identify patients with negative test results as not having chlamydial cervicitis with a high degree of certainty (99.5%).

Table 4-6 also shows the predictive values if the same tests are used in a sexually transmitted disease (STD) clinic where the prevalence of chlamydial cervicitis is estimated to be 30%. The positive predictive values increase significantly, especially for the IF test, and both tests would function well as diag-

nostic tools. The negative predictive values drop for both tests, however, to 95.8%. Thus approximately 4% of patients with negative test results could be infected with *C. trachomatis;* this rate may not be acceptable given the nature of the disease.

Efficiency of Tests

The efficiency of a test indicates the percentage of patients who are correctly classified as having disease or not having disease. The efficiency is calculated using the following equation:

$$\text{Efficiency} = \frac{(TP + TN)}{(TP + FP + RN + FN)} \times 100$$

where:
TP = number of patients with true-positive results
TN = number of patients with true-negative results
FP = number of patients with false-positive results
FN = number of patients with false-negative results.

Other Concepts

Additional concepts, such as the medical decision-making analysis of tests, "benefit-cost analysis," combination testing, and nondisease factors affecting laboratory test results, are beyond the scope of this discussion. For those wishing to examine these in detail, an excellent discussion with appropriate tables may be found in the "Statistics" chapter by Robert Galen in *Gradwohl's Clinical Laboratory Methods and Diagnosis* (see Bibliography). The tables for the positive and negative predictive values in this reference are not needed because predictive values are easy to compute using a simple hand calculator. Anyone with access to a computer can set up a spreadsheet incorporating the predictive value formulas. When the disease prevalence and test sensitivity and specificity are entered, the computer program calculates the predictive values for the specified prevalence.

CHOOSING A LABORATORY METHOD

Once an institution has made the decision to offer a new test, the next step generally is for the labo-

TABLE 4-6

Comparison of the IF and DNA Probe Tests to Detect Chlamydial Cervicitis in Patient Populations with 5% and 30% Prevalences of the Disease*

Test	Sensitivity	Specificity	5% Prevalence		30% Prevalence	
			PPV	NPV	PPV	NPV
IF probe	90.0	98.0	70.3	99.5	95.1	95.8
DNA probe	89.8	99.5	90.4	99.5	98.7	95.8

*The positive (PPV) and negative (NPV) predictive values were computed using equations (see text). All values are given in percentages.

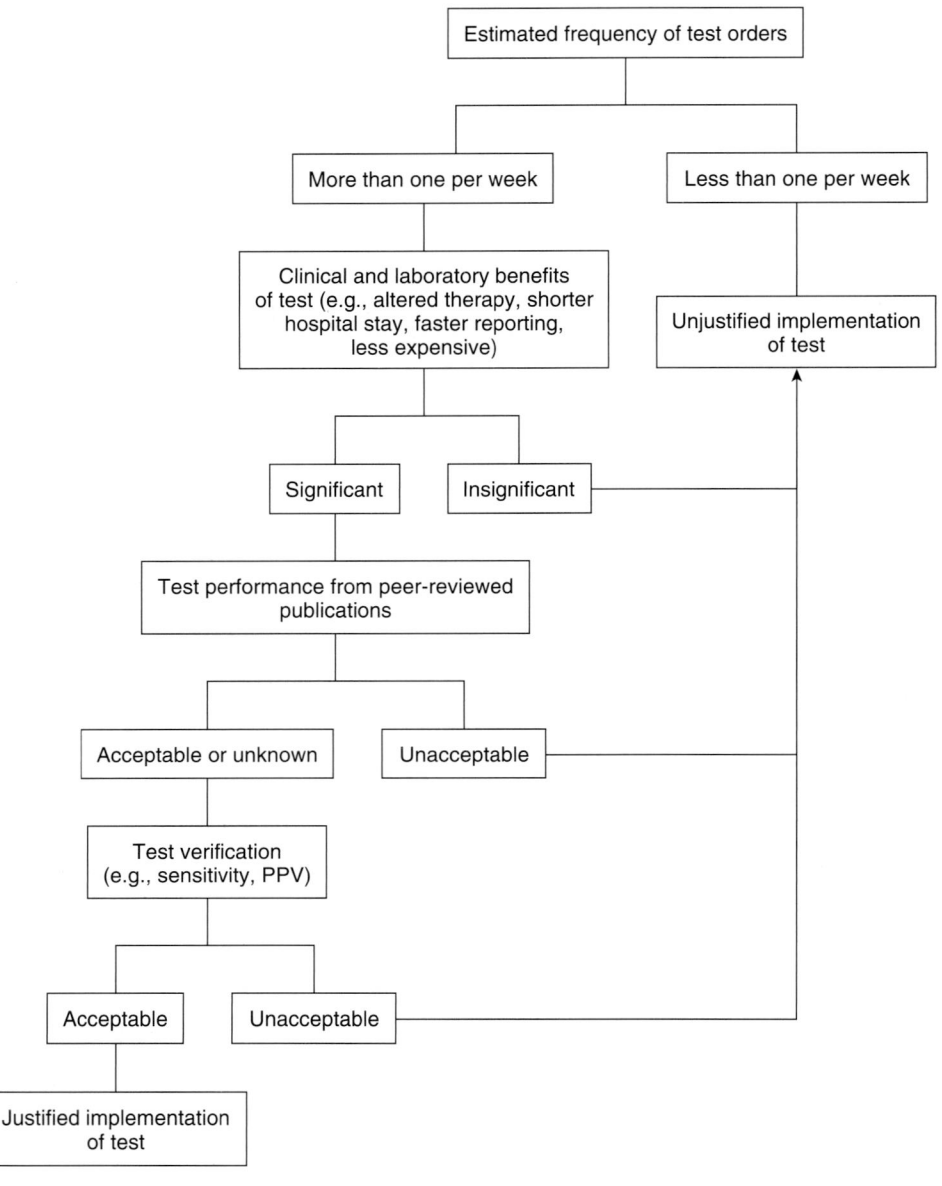

Figure 4-7

Choosing a laboratory method. (Modified from McCurdy B editor: *Verification and validation of procedures in the clinical microbiology laboratory, Cumitech 31,* Washington, DC, 1997, American Society for Microbiology.)

ratory to select the method (Figure 4-7). The following are some steps that may be followed when deciding on the method:

1. Define the purpose for which the method is used. Common purposes for tests are as follows:
   - **Screening:** Screening is used for testing large populations of patients. Generally,

screening tests have high clinical sensitivity and NPV. Positive results with such tests generally require confirmation by a more specific test.
   - **Confirmation:** Confirmation is used after obtaining a positive screening result to ensure the accuracy of the initial result. Specificity and PPV are generally the considerations for such tests.

- **Diagnosis:** Diagnosis is used for the evaluation of persons suspected of having a given disease state or characteristic.
2. Decide which type of analyte (e.g., organism, antigen, nucleic acid) is to be detected.
3. In conjunction with the end user of the test (e.g., the physician) and information from steps 1 and 2, determine the medical usefulness of the test (e.g., to improve patient care, to shorten hospital time).
4. Survey the technical and medical literature for performance claims of various methods. When reviewing the literature, confirm that the method described is actually the test to be evaluated in the laboratory.
5. Other considerations are as follows:
   - Cost
   - Practicality
   - Specimen requirements
   - Quantities of reagents and controls needed for test
   - Shelf life of reagents and controls before and after opening
   - Availability of supplies, service, technical support
   - Possible safety hazards
   - Whether the reference range is appropriate for that test and how it will be determined for that institution.
6. Perform an in-house verification. Verification of a test serves to establish that the performance parameters of the test are satisfactory.
   The result of test verification should indicate one of three possibilities:
   - The test is acceptable for routine use.
   - Further verification studies are required
   - The test is unsuitable for routine use until its performance parameters can be verified.

Test verification records must be kept for at least two years. However, it is good laboratory practice to maintain the records for as long as the test is in use.

TEST VALIDATION

Verification of a test does not provide ongoing assurance that the test is continually performing as expected. **Test validation** is the ongoing process providing information that a test is performing correctly. The components of validation are quality control, proficiency testing, verification of employee competency, and instrument calibration. The results of the validation indicate one of three possibilities:

1. The test continues to be acceptable.
2. Further investigation is warranted.
3. Immediate corrective action must be undertaken, and the test must be considered unsuitable for routine use until it can be validated.

Lot numbers and expiration dates should be documented for all reagents and materials used in the validation process. Records of validation should be kept for at least 2 years.

Validation should be done frequently enough to ensure the continual correct performance of tests. In most cases, following the manufacturer's guidelines and the requirements of the regulatory or accrediting agencies will provide this assurance.

New laboratory tests as well as old ones should always be validated. Understanding and using the concepts of predictive values and the effect of prevalence on those values is important for the proper use of a test and interpretation of the results. The development of rapid noncultural tests for the detecting of infectious diseases makes the use of these concepts even more important. A test result can no longer be considered as simply "positive" or "negative" but must be interpreted in view of the concepts presented in this discussion. When test results are interpreted properly, better patient care is achieved.

Bibliography

Galen R: Statistics. In Sonnenwirth AC, Jarett L, editors: *Gradwohl's clinical laboratory methods and diagnosis,* ed 8, St Louis, 1980, Mosby.

Gullen WH, Bearman JE: Put laboratory tests to the test! *Patient Care,* Feb 15, 1980, p 74-93.

Healthcare Financing Administration. Medicare, Medicaid, and CLIA programs: regulations implementing the Clinical Laboratory Improvement Amendments of 1988 (CLIA), *Fed Regist* 57:7002, 1992.

Ilstrup D: Statistical methods in microbiology, *Clin Micro Rev* 3:219, 1990.

Jenkins SG. Evaluation of new technology in the clinical microbiology laboratory, *Diagn Microbiol Infect Dis* 23:53, 1993.

McCurdy B, editor: *Verification and validation of procedures in the clinical microbiology laboratory, Cumitech 31.* Washington, DC, 1997, American Society for Microbiology.

National Committee for Clinical Laboratory Standards: *Specifications for immunological testing for infectious diseases: approved guideline I/LA18-A,* Wayne, Pa, 1994, NCCLS.

National Committee for Clinical Laboratory Standards: *Training verification for laboratory personnel: approved guideline GP21-A,* Wayne Pa, 1995, NCCLS.

National Committee for Clinical Laboratory Standards: *Terminology and definitions for NCCLS documents: approved guideline NRSCL8-A,* Wayne, Pa, 1998, NCCLS.

Radetsky M, Tood JK: Criteria for the evaluation of new diagnostic tests, *Pediat Infect Dis* 3:461, 1984.

Vecchio TJ: Predictive value of a single diagnostic test in unselected populations, *N Eng J Med* 274:1171, 1966.

Weigert HT, Weigert O: The impact of disease prevalence on the predictive value of laboratory tests in primary care, *J Fam Pract* 8:1199, 1979.

CHAPTER 5

Emergent Technologies

A. DIRECT MICROBIAL ANTIGEN DETECTION

David W. Craft

HISTORICAL PERSPECTIVE

ANTIGEN DETECTION METHODS
  Precipitin Tests
    Tube and agar precipitin
    Counterimmunoelectrophoresis
  Particle Agglutination
    Latex agglutination
    Staphylococcal coagglutination
    Liposome-mediated agglutination
  Immunofluorescent Assays
  Enzyme Immunoassays
    Membrane-bound EIA
  Optical Immunoassays
  Other Immunoassays

CURRENT CLINICAL APPLICATIONS
  Respiratory Tract Infections
    Streptococcal pharyngitis
    Whooping cough (pertussis)

    Legionnaires' disease
    Respiratory virus infections
    Pneumonia in immunocompromised patients
  Meningitis and Sepsis
    Bacterial meningitis and sepsis
    Cryptococcal meningitis
  Gastrointestinal Tract Infections
    Clostridium difficile: associated enteric disease
    Shiga-toxin producing *Escherichia coli*
    Campylobacter
    Viral gastroenteritis
    Giardiasis and cryptosporidiosis
  Sexually Transmitted Diseases
    Chlamydial infections
  Blood-Borne and Body Fluid-Borne Diseases
    Hepatitis B virus detection
    Human immunodeficiency virus (HIV)

FUTURE APPLICATIONS

Monoclonal antibodies are a result of the development of cell hybridoma technology (Figure 5-2). A **hybridoma** results from the ability to fuse a single plasma B cell producing an antibody of interest with a mouse myeloma cell. The myeloma cells are transformed cells and thus able to grow and divide in culture forever. The progeny of these cells, if appropriately selected, can be grown in culture or in animals and can secrete large amounts of the antibody of interest. The monoclonal antibody secreted by these cells is so named because it originates from a single B cell or clone and is thus chemically homogeneous. Monoclonal antibodies are highly specific for a single antigenic determinant and less likely to cross-react with chemically related antigens than poly-

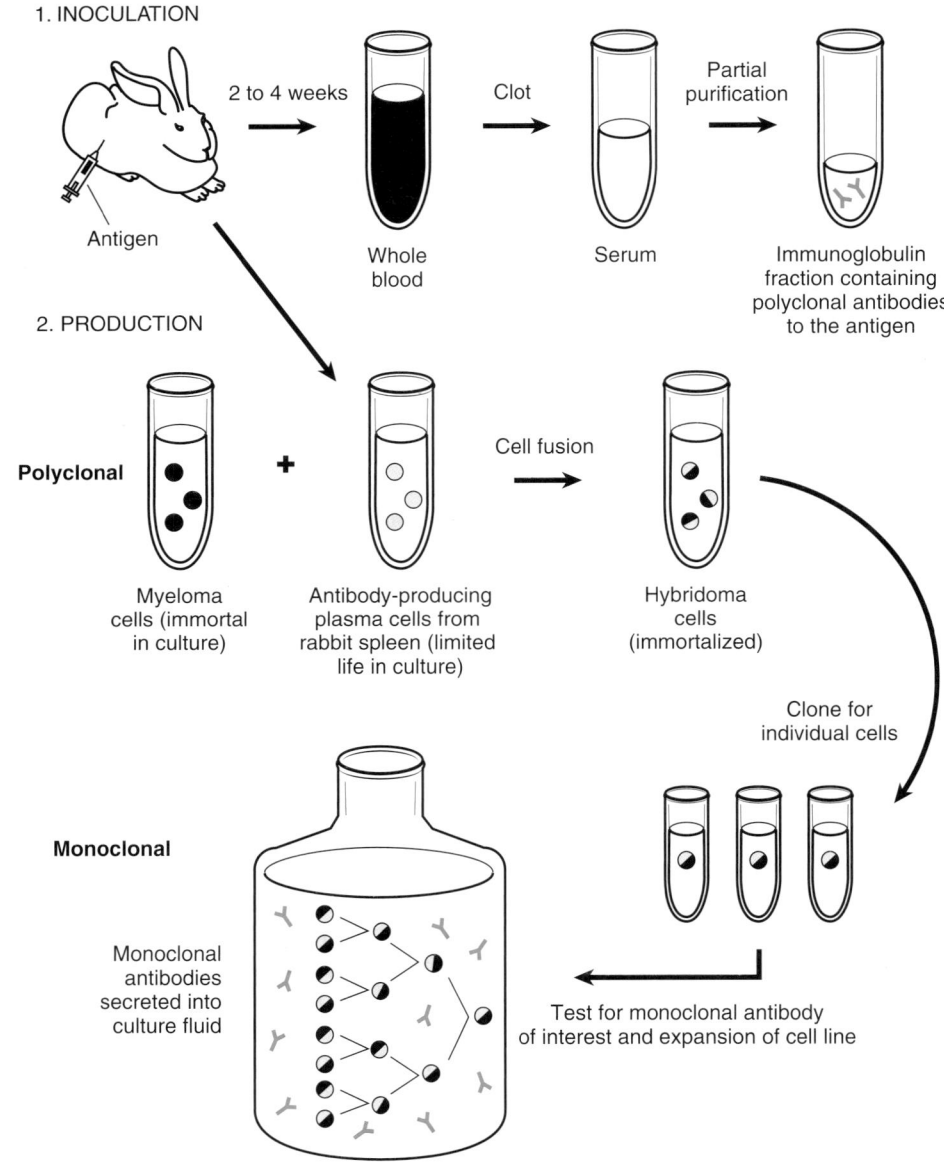

1. INOCULATION

2 to 4 weeks

Antigen

Whole blood

Clot

Serum

Partial purification

Immunoglobulin fraction containing polyclonal antibodies to the antigen

2. PRODUCTION

Polyclonal

Myeloma cells (immortal in culture)

+

Antibody-producing plasma cells from rabbit spleen (limited life in culture)

Cell fusion

Hybridoma cells (immortalized)

Clone for individual cells

Monoclonal

Monoclonal antibodies secreted into culture fluid

Test for monoclonal antibody of interest and expansion of cell line

Figure 5-2 —————————————————————————————

Preparation of polyclonal and monoclonal antibodies.

clonal antibodies, which recognize multiple antigenic determinants.

Polyclonal antibodies are commonly produced by immunizing animals with the antigen of interest and then isolating and purifying the antibody from the animal's serum. These antibodies are generally heterogeneous in nature because of the variability associated with the immune response; they may lack avidity or specificity compared with monoclonal antibodies.

Many of the methods and commercial products discussed in this chapter utilize monoclonal and polyclonal antibodies for the rapid and direct detection of bacteria, fungi, parasites, and viruses in patient specimens.

ANTIGEN DETECTION METHODS

Precipitin Tests
Tube and agar precipitin
Historically, the basic type antigen-antibody reaction is the **precipitin** reaction. This reaction is found in test systems that allow the free diffusion of soluble antigen and soluble antibody fronts toward one another. At a critical point of interface, at which the concentrations are optimal, a visible precipitate forms, which is composed of combined anti-

gens and antibodies. These reactions are most stable when performed in an agarose gel (Figure 5-3).

Antibody-antigen reactions in agarose are commonly performed in the clinical laboratory by a technique called double **immunodiffusion,** or Ouchterlony gel diffusion (Figure 5-4). In this technique, cylindrical holes or wells are cut out of an agarose gel in a small petri dish and spaced appropriately. The specimen containing the unknown soluble antigen is placed in one well, and a known antibody-containing solution is placed in an adjacent well. The antigen and antibody molecule in solution diffuse out of the wells and through the porous agarose. If antigen specific for the known antibody is present, the two components combine and produce a visible precipitin band, or line of precipitation, at a point of optimal concentration of each component. Diffusion is a slow process and is not generally amenable to rapid diagnosis. It is most commonly used to detect fungal exoantigens or serum antibodies.

Counterimmunoelectrophoresis
Counterimmunoelectrophoresis (CIE) is a modification of the principle of immunodiffusion that dramatically quickens the migration of soluble antigens and antibodies by applying an electric current. Antigen and antibody solutions are placed

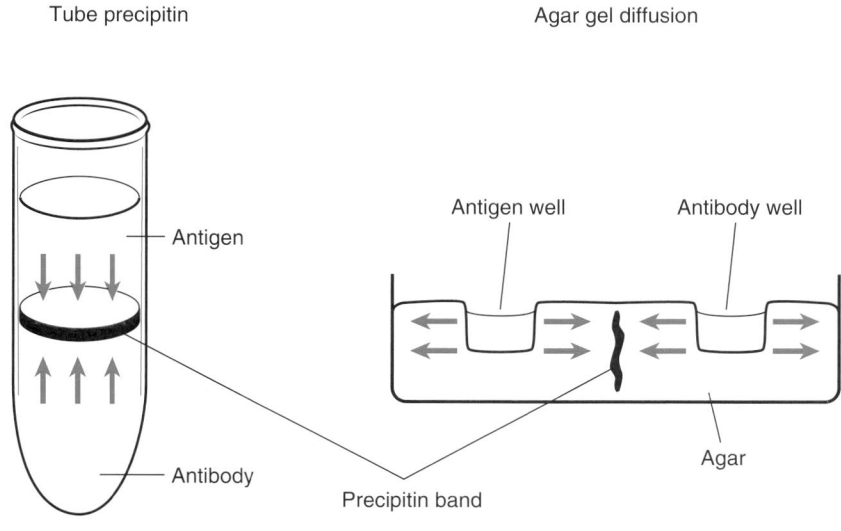

Tube precipitin

Agar gel diffusion

Figure 5-3 _____

Comparison of tube and agar gel diffusion precipitin tests.

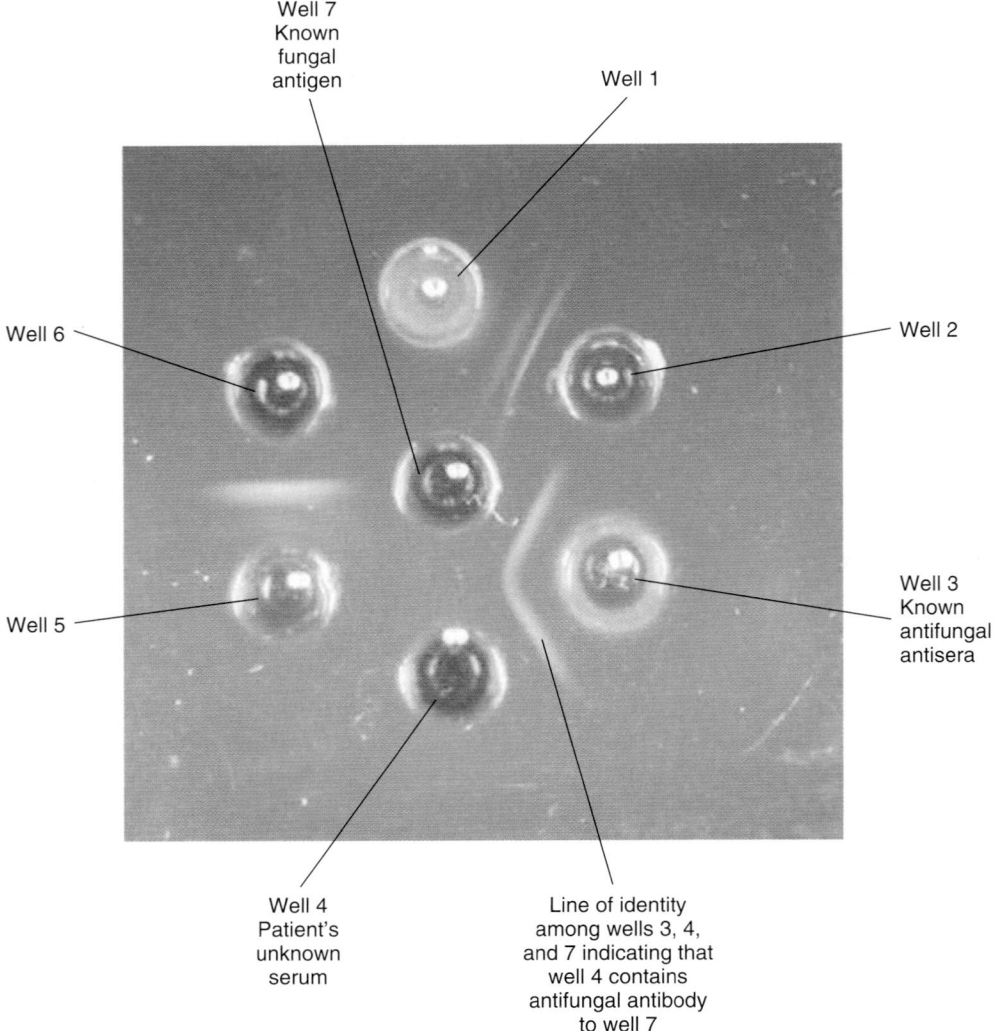

Well 7
Known
fungal
antigen

Well 1

Well 6

Well 2

Well 5

Well 3
Known
antifungal
antisera

Well 4
Patient's
unknown
serum

Line of identity
among wells 3, 4,
and 7 indicating that
well 4 contains
antifungal antibody
to well 7

Figure 5-4

Ouchterlony plate. A serum specimen containing an unknown antibody is placed in one well, a known antigen of interest is placed in an adjacent well, and a known antisera to the antigen (positive control) is placed in another adjacent well. The antigen and antibody molecules in the solution diffuse from the wells and through the porous agarose. If the unknown serum contains antibody to the known antigen, a precipitin ban forms at a point of optimal concentration of each component. This precipitin ban is called a *line of identity*.

in adjacent wells cut out of agarose supported on a glass or plastic surface. The gel is placed in an alkaline buffer–containing electrophoresis chamber, and the electric field is applied (Figure 5-5). Under the buffer conditions chosen, most microbial antigens have a net negative charge (anions) and thus migrate in the gel toward the positively charged electrode (anode). Antibody molecules, on the other hand, are very weakly negatively charged or neutral under alkaline buffer conditions. They do not migrate significantly in the charged field but rather are carried toward the negatively charged electrode (cathode) by the effect of buffer ions. This phenomenon is known as

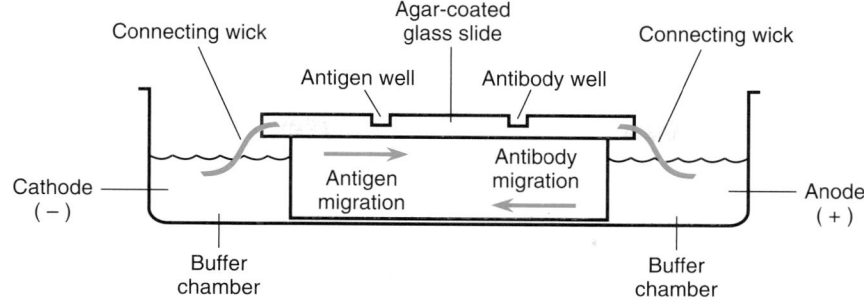

Figure 5-5 _____

Diagram of counterimmunoelectrophoresis apparatus.

electroendosmosis. If specific antigen and antibody are present, the antigen and the antibody will meet in the gel at some point of optimum proportion or equilibrium and form a visible precipitin band (Figure 5-6).

The process may occur in 1 hour or less, compared with 24 hours required for precipitin bands to form in gels by passive diffusion. Counterimmunoelectrophoretic plates are generally read immediately after electrophoresis, again after washing to remove nonspecific precipitins, and once again after overnight refrigeration to allow the specific bands to intensify.

Although very popular in the 1970s for a number of applications, CIE has been replaced by particle **agglutination** tests and immunoassays for rapid microbial antigen detection. CIE is not really a rapid method when one considers that overnight refrigeration is required. In addition, the CIE method for antigen detection is cumbersome to set up, and some antigens are not detected by standard buffer systems.

Particle Agglutination

Latex agglutination

The basic chemical principles that govern antigen-antibody interactions are the same for precipitin and agglutination reactions—with one exception. In agglutination reactions, the antigen or antibody is bound to a particulate carrier. Latex agglutination takes advantage of the fact that monoclonal or polyclonal antibody molecules can be bound to the surface of latex (polystyrene) beads. These beads are usually about 1 micron in diameter (Figure 5-7), which enhances the visible agglutination reaction.

Each bead can be charged with thousands of antibody molecules. The antibody-charged latex beads form a homogeneous milky suspension, which when mixed with a specimen containing specific antigen, results in antigen-antibody binding. However, this primary binding between antigen and antibody molecules does not produce a visible agglutination (clumping) reaction. Only if the antigen molecules contain multiple antigenic determinants, as is common for high molecular weight (HMW) polysaccharides, proteins, or microorganisms, will antigen molecules be cross-linked by the antibody-coated latex beads. It is this secondary cross-linking of antigen and antibody,

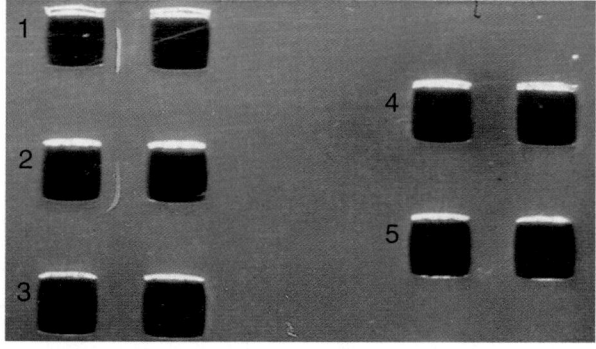

Figure 5-6 _____

Photograph showing precipitin band formation between antigen and antibody wells of a counterimmunoelectrophoresis test. Note strong (1), weak (2), and no bands.

resulting in a macromolecular lattice, that precipitates out of solution and results in a visible agglutination reaction (Figure 5-8).

Latex agglutination is generally conducted on a treated cardboard or glass slide using liquid specimen and latex volumes of about 50 ul each (Figure 5-9). The reagents are mixed thoroughly. Then the slide is rocked or rotated by hand or with a mechanical device for 2 to 3 minutes before being read using appropriate lighting and the naked eye. The reaction depends on many variables; therefore, standardization is imperative. Variables include latex particle size, avidity of antibody, type of antibody (monoclonal or polyclonal), reaction temperature, pH, ionic strength, and concentration of antigen in the specimen. Levels of detection of microbial polysaccharide or protein can be as low as 0.1 ng/ml.

The strength and rapidity of the reaction varies depending on all these test conditions and, most importantly, on the concentration of antigen in the specimen. With high antigen concentration, a maximum agglutination reaction (4+ on a 1+ to 4+ scale) may occur in only a few seconds. In the absence of specific antigen, the latex suspension remains homogeneous and milky, that is, no agglutination. Although most applications of latex agglutination use white latex beads, colored latexes are also available to enhance visual detection.

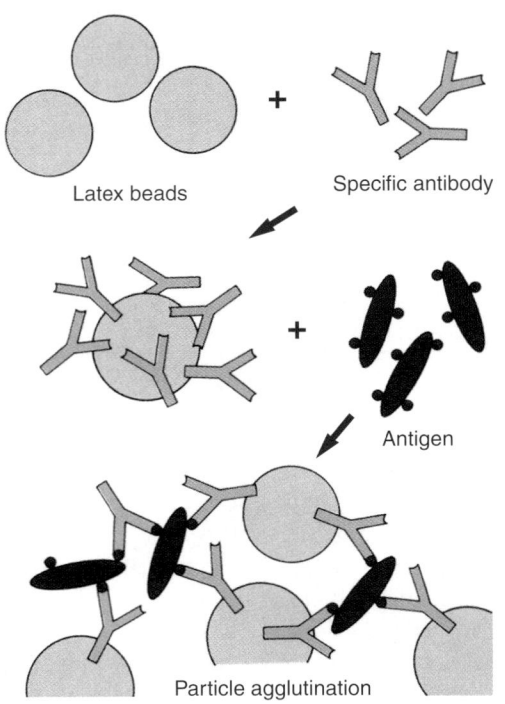

Figure 5-8 —————————————————————
Alignment of antibody molecules bound to the surface of a latex particle and latex agglutination reaction. (From Forbes B, Sahm D, Weissfeld S: *Bailey and Scott's diagnostic microbiology,* ed 10, St Louis, 1998, Mosby.)

Some important controls must accompany the test latex and patient specimen (Table 5-1). These controls include (1) a positive antigen control (a solution containing the known antigen of interest), (2) a negative antigen control (a solution not containing the antigen), and (3) a control latex suspension to detect the presence of nonspecific agglutination reactions. The control latex involves testing the patient specimen with latex beads coated with an immunoglobulin whose specificity is not directed to the test antigen. This nonimmune serum is generally obtained from the same animal species in which the specific antibody was made. A nonspecific agglutination reaction occurs when the patient's specimen reacts with both the test and the control latex. When such reactions occur, the test is uninterpretable. A positive test result requires that the test latex, but not the control latex, agglutinate the patient specimen.

A number of specimen pretreatment procedures can be used to eliminate or minimize nonspecific

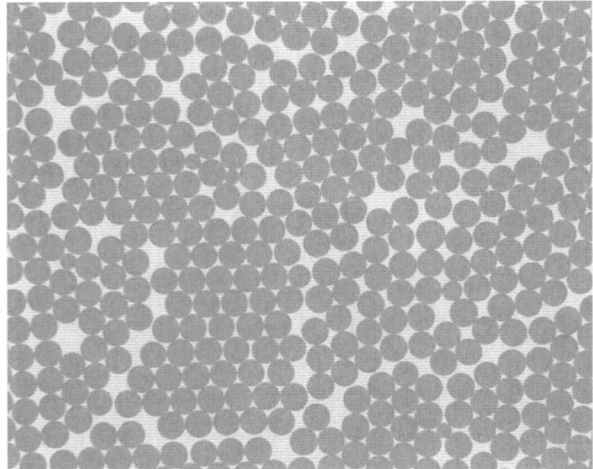

Figure 5-7 —————————————————————
Transmission electron micrograph of a latex suspension. Each latex bead is about 1 micron in diameter. (Courtesy Interfacial Dynamics Corp., Portland, Ore.)

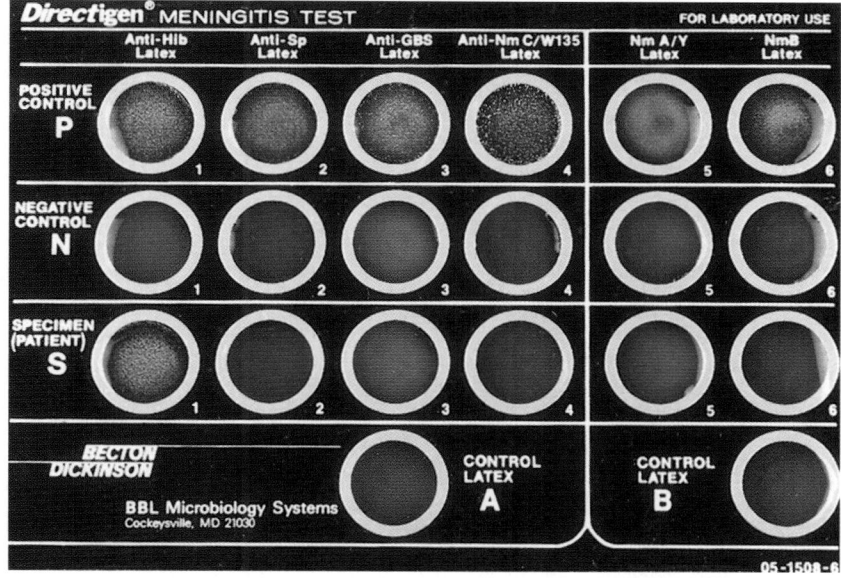

Figure 5-9

Commercial latex agglutination test slide showing reaction of controls and a patient's cerebrospinal fluid with latex reagents specific for *Haemophilus influenzae* b (Hib), *Streptococcus pneumoniae* (Sp), group B *Streptococcus* (GBS), and five different serogroups (groups C and W135, groups A and Y, and group B) of *Neisseria meningitidis* (Nm). Note the positive reactions with each test latex reagent and positive control (P), as well as the positive reaction with the patient's specimen and Hib test latex. (Courtesy Becton Dickinson and Company, Cockeysville, Md.)

agglutinations, presumably by removing or inactivating factors in the specimen responsible for these reactions. These procedures include specimen centrifugation to remove particulate material, boiling to inactivate protein constituents (acceptable when test antigen is a heat-stable polysaccharide), and passing the specimen through a membrane filter.

Specimens such as serum contain high concentrations of protein. If the antigen of interest is a heat-stable polysaccharide, it is necessary to first treat the specimen with ethylenediamine tetra-acetic acid (EDTA) or a proteolytic enzyme before heating. Otherwise the polysaccharide antigen may be trapped in the coagulated protein leading to false-negative test results. Furthermore, if the specimen is centrifuged, the polysaccharide may be completely removed from the test supernate.

Latex agglutination tests for microbial antigens, like other laboratory tests, are subject to false-negative and false-positive reactions when compared with culture. False-negative reactions (negative antigen test result, positive culture) may be

TABLE 5-1

Interpretation of Latex Agglutination Test Controls and Patient Specimens

| Reaction Number | Test Specimen | Agglutination Reaction | | Interpretation |
		Test Latex	*Control Latex*	
1	Positive antigen control	+	0	Control OK
2	Negative antigen control	0	0	Control OK
3	Patient A	+	0	Positive test
4	Patient B	0	0	Negative test
5	Patient C	+	+	Nonspecific agglutination

+, Agglutination; 0, no agglutination.

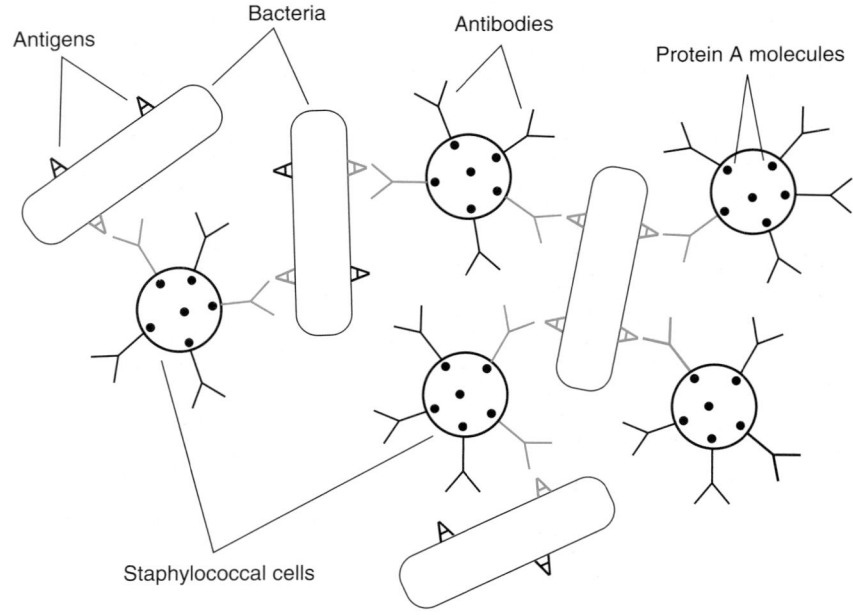

Figure 5-10

Diagram of coagglutination reaction with whole bacterial cell antigen.

due to the presence of antigen in the specimen at concentrations below the test detection limit. False-positive reactions (positive antigen test result, negative culture) are more difficult to explain; they may be due to the presence of cross-reacting antigens or nonviability of organisms in the original specimen. It is important to remember that antigen detection tests do not require viable microbes. Antibody-coated latex suspensions can agglutinate viable or nonviable organisms, microbial components such as cell wall or membrane fragments, or soluble antigen such as bacterial capsular polysaccharide. Thus an apparent false-positive latex test result may really represent a true-positive result for disease in a patient with a negative culture.

Some specimens, such as urine, may be concentrated by centrifugation or membrane filtration before testing. Filters typically hold back or exclude HMW antigenic materials while allowing water and small compounds to pass through. These concentration methods increase the sensitivity of the test.

The advantages of latex agglutination tests are the availability of good quality reagents in complete kit form, good sensitivity, relative rapidity, and ease of performance. Disadvantages include subjectivity in reading end points, nonspecific re-actions resulting from interfacing substances in clinical samples, and the fact that some tests are not as "rapid" as an ordering physician might expect. Still it is one of the most widely used antigen detection methods in the clinical laboratory. In many clinical laboratories, detection of *C. neoformans* in serum or cerebrospinal fluid (CSF), detection of bacteria causing meningitis in CSF, and identification of serogroup beta-hemolytic *Streptococcus* from culture plates are routinely performed using latex agglutination test kits.

Staphylococcal coagglutination

Similar to latex agglutination, staphylococcal co-agglutination, or simply **coagglutination,** utilizes particle-bound antibody to enhance the visibility of antigen-antibody reactions. Instead of a latex bead, intact formalin-killed *Staphylococcus aureus* cells (typically Cowan 1 strain) are utilized. The cell wall of this strain of *S. aureus* contains a large amount of protein A that has the capacity to bind antibody molecules in the Fc portion (base of the heavy immunoglobulin chain) of the IgG antibody. This leaves the antigen-binding sites of the molecule (Fab portion) available to react with specific antigens (Figures 5-10 and 5-11). It has been estimated that each staphylococcal cell has about

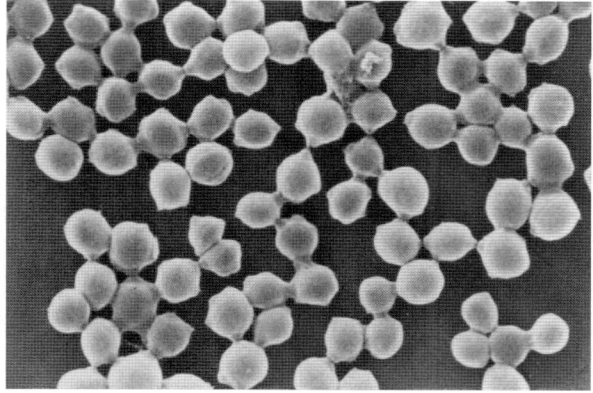

Figure 5-11

Scanning electron micrograph of a coagglutination reaction showing cross-linking of the staphylococcal cells by soluble antigen. (Courtesy Boule Diagnostics AB, Huddinge, Sweden.)

80,000 antibody binding sites. The actual number of antibody molecules bound to the staphylococcal cell is limited by stearic hindrance. Coating is sufficient, however, to render the product of clinical utility in direct antigen tests.

Most of the observations made regarding latex agglutination are also true for coagglutination. Reactions are prepared by mixing antibody-sensitized staphylococcal cells with a solution containing the antigen of interest on a slide or card (Figure 5-12). Coagglutination procedures appear more susceptible to nonspecific agglutination reactions, and thus, specimen preparation is important. This is particularly true for testing serum

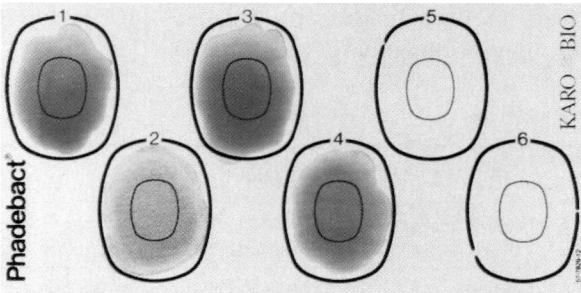

Figure 5-12

Commercial coagglutination test card showing negative *(1, 3, 4)* and positive *(2)* reactions. The blue color is an indicator dye added to make the agglutination reaction easier to read against a white background. (Courtesy Boule Diagnostics AB, Huddinge, Sweden.)

specimens, probably because staphylococcal cells may bind human IgG in test serum specimens and subsequently be agglutinated by the presence of rheumatoid factor (IgM anti-IgG) in the serum. Co-agglutination is highly specific but may be less sensitive in detecting small quantities of antigen than latex agglutination. Therefore these reagents are often used to confirm the identification of bacterial colonies on culture plates, but not for rapid antigen detection from clinical specimens.

Liposome-mediated agglutination

One of the newest developments in agglutination technology, **liposome-mediated agglutination,** involves the use of liposomes, single-lipid bilayer membranes that form closed vesicles under appropriate conditions. In their manufacture, antigen or antibody molecules may be incorporated into the surface of the membrane and thus be available for interaction with the corresponding molecule (Figure 5-13). In addition, the liposome vesicle may be constructed with a chemical dye or bioactive molecule trapped in the interior. The colored dye allows easy visual detection of lattice formation and agglutination between liposome-bound antibody and antigen. Alternatively, combining dye-containing liposomes and latex beads, both of which contain the reactive antibody on the surface, may increase the sensitivity of latex agglutination. Perhaps the greatest potential advantage of liposome technology is in its application to immunoassays other than particle agglutination that make use of the ability of the liposome to carry reactive chemicals. Liposomes have yet to reach their full potential as diagnostic reagents in the clinical laboratory. A comparison of particle agglutination methods are found in Table 5-2.

Immunofluorescent Assays

Immunofluorescent assays (FA) are a very popular method for rapid antigen detection in the clinical microbiology laboratory. When specific monoclonal or polyclonal antibodies are conjungated with fluorescent dyes (fluorochromes), they can be visualized with a fluorescent microscope. In these tests, the clinical specimen containing the unknown antigen of interest is fixed onto a glass slide with formalin, methanol, ethanol, or acetone. Fixation renders mammalian cell membranes permeable to the stains. Detection techniques may be direct or indirect. In the **direct fluorescent antibody (DFA)**

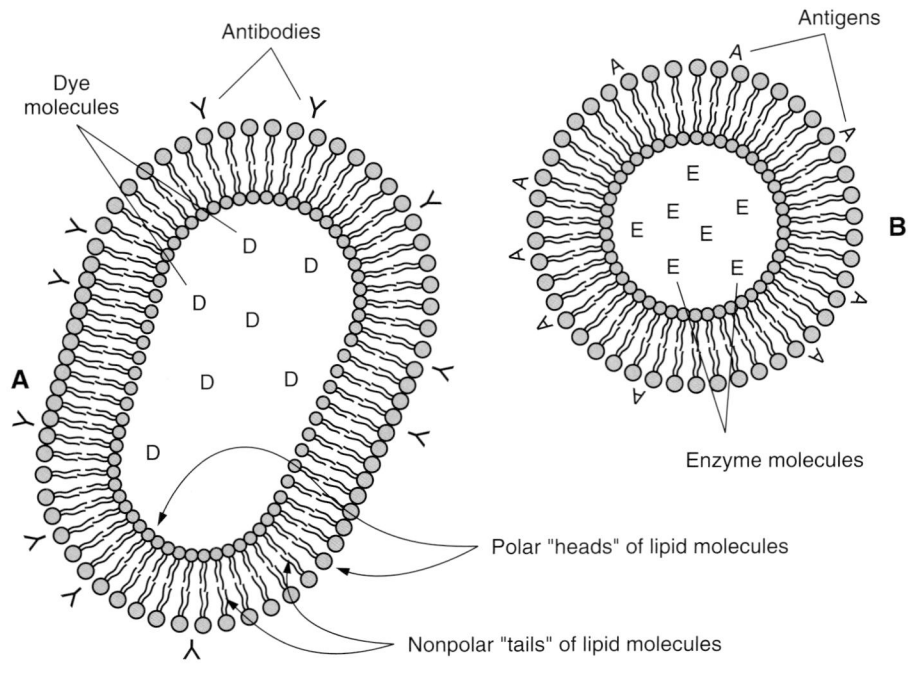

Figure 5-13

Diagram of liposome particles showing bilipid layer structure. Either antibody **(A)** or antigen **(B)** can be attached to the surface of the liposome. The interior of the liposome can carry indicator or reporter molecules (e.g., dyes, enzymes).

test, the antigen specific labeled antibody is applied to the fixed specimen, incubated, washed, and visualized using a fluorescent microscope (Figure 5-14, *A*). In the **indirect fluorescent antibody (IFA)** test, an unlabeled antigen specific antibody is applied, incubated, and washed. A second fluorochrome labeled antibody specific for the first antibody is applied, washed, and read using a fluorescent microscope (Figure 5-14, *B*). For both DFA and IFA, a counterstain is often used as a last step to quench background nonspecific fluorescence.

The microscopy utilizes an epi-illuminescent (incident) light system of vertical illumination, wavelength filters, and a dichroic mirror (Figure 5-15). The dichroic mirror allows passage of light at an excitation wavelength from the light source to the specimen. The mirror also allows passage of the emission (longer) wavelength light from the labeled source to the objective. This emitted, or excited, wavelength light appears as a bright color based on the dye used. A very popular fluorochrome is fluorescein isothiocyanate (FITC), which, when excited, emits a bright apple green fluorescence through the objective to the naked eye (Figure 5-16).

TABLE 5-2

Comparison of Particle Agglutination Methods

Agglutination Method	Particle Type	Nature of Antibody-Binding to Particle	Diagnostic Utility
Latex agglutination	Latex beads	Nonspecific absorption or chemical coupling	Most widely used agglutination method for direct detection
Staphylococcal coagglutination	Formalin-fixed staphylococci	Fc portion of antibody molecule combines with protein A on staphylococcal cell wall	Commonly used for antigenic identification of bacteria in culture
Liposome-mediated agglutination	Liposomes	Chemical coupling	Newer method; limited applications of commercial tests

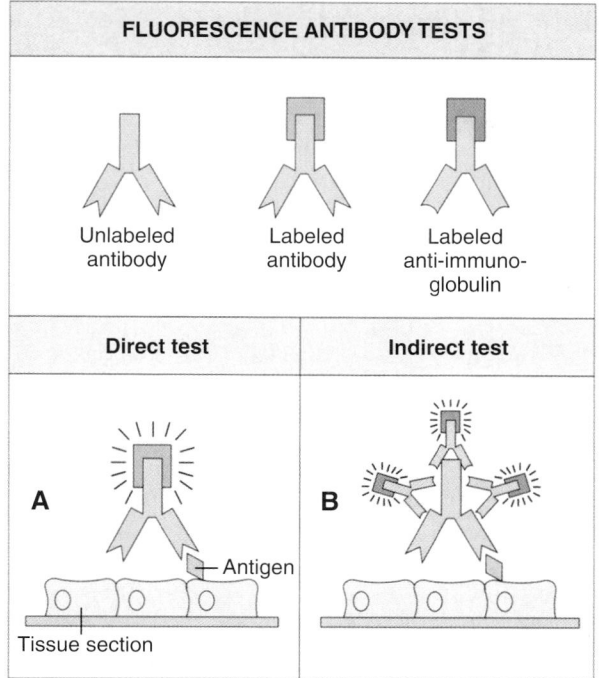

Figure 5-14 ───────────────

The fluorescence antibody test for identification of tissue antigens or their antibodies. **A,** Direct fluorescent antibody (DFA) test. The antigen specific-labeled antibody is applied to the fixed specimen, incubated, washed, and visualized with a fluorescent microscope. **B,** Indirect fluorescent antibody (IFA). A second fluorochrome-labeled antibody specific for the first unlabeled antibody is applied. (From *Medical Microbiology*, London, Mosby.)

Immunofluorescent staining allows for rapid visualization of infected tissue, cell culture, body fluids, and swab specimens. Disadvantages include the requirement for a fluorescent microscope and the significant subjective interpretation involved in reading the slides. In addition, the procedure may not be very rapid (1 to 4 hours) and is not easily amenable to automation. Finally, fluorescence fades over time. Therefore, antibodies have been conjugated to other markers besides fluorochromes. The newer colorimetric labels use enzymes, such as horseradish peroxidase, alkaline phosphatase, and avidinbiotin, to detect the presence of antigen by converting a colorless substrate into a colored end product. These products do not fade with storage and can be detected with a simple light microscope.

Fluorescent antibody tests are commonly used to detect *Bordetella pertussis, Legionella pneumophila, Chlamydia* spp., *Giardia* spp., *Cryptospo-*

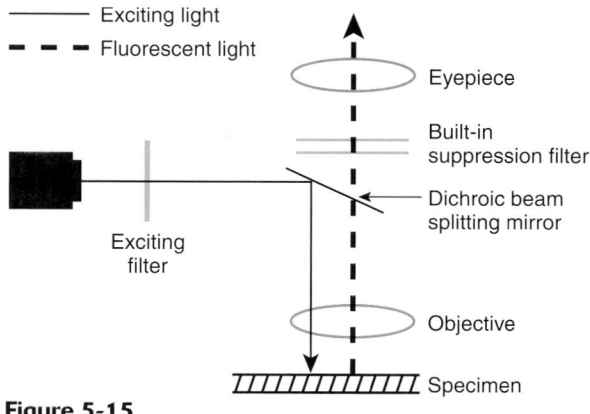

Figure 5-15 ───────────────

Light path of incident light microscope.

ridium spp., *Pneumocystis* spp., herpes simplex virus, cytomegalovirus, varicella-zoster virus, and most of the commonly isolated respiratory viruses such as parainfluenzae, influenzae, adenovirus, and respiratory syncytial virus in clinical specimens.

Enzyme Immunoassays

Enzyme immunoassay (EIA) provides an alternative to FA for detecting antigens in clinical samples. Instead of tagging an antibody with a fluorochrome, EIA depends on the fact that enzyme molecules can be conjugated to specific monoclonal or polyclonal antibodies in such a way that both enzymatic and antigen-binding activities are preserved. The enzymes used are often alka-

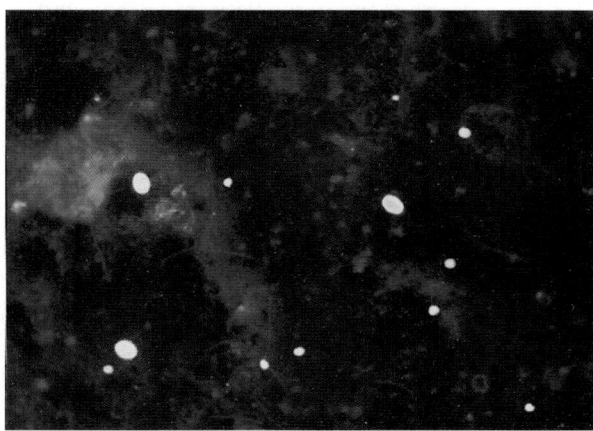

Figure 5-16 ───────────────

Direct fluorescent antibody–stained cells of *Giardia lamblia* (three larger apple-green, oval cells) and *Cryptosporidium* sp. (smaller cells) in stool. (Courtesy Meridian Diagnostics, Cincinnati, Ohio.)

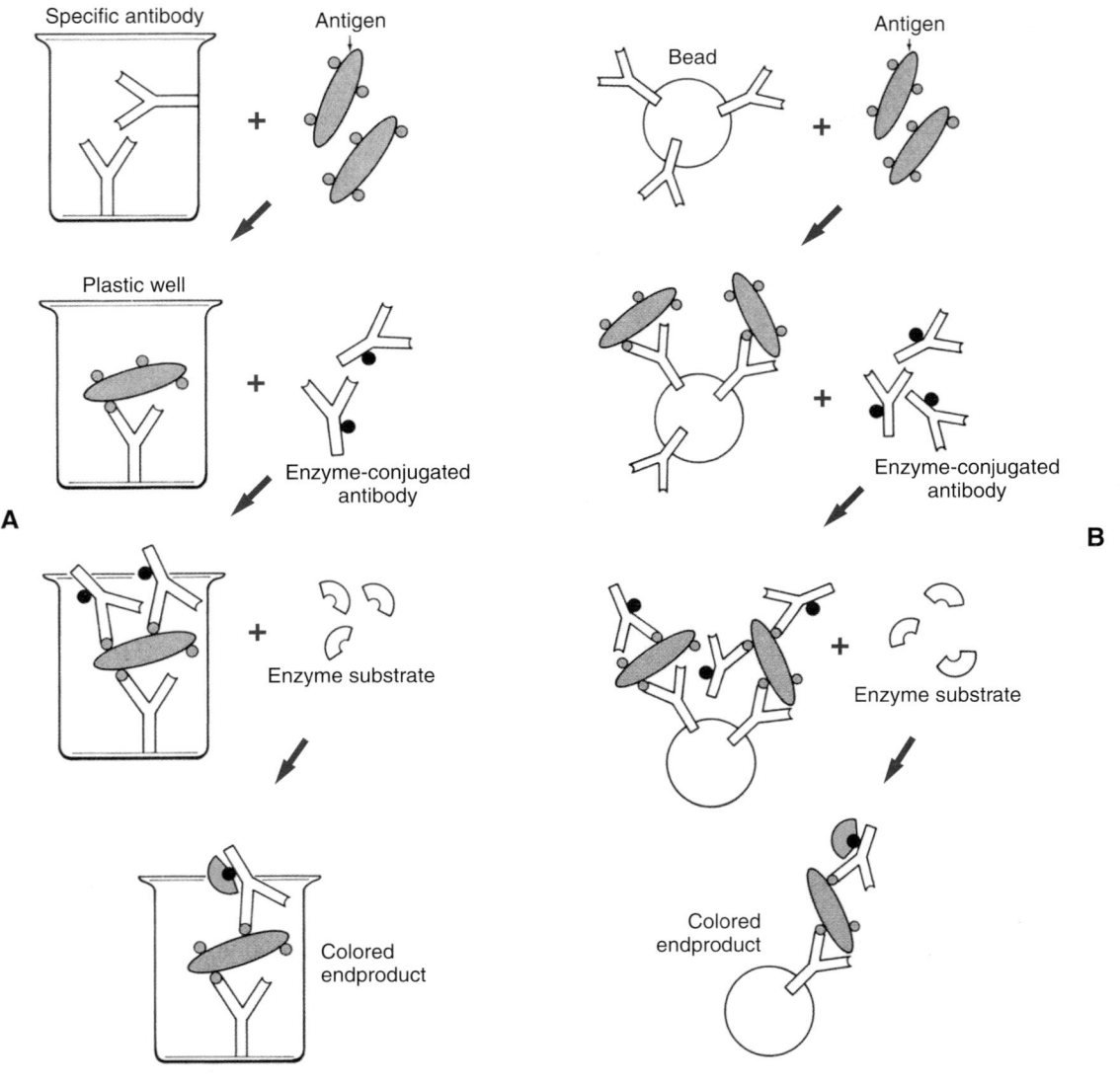

Figure 5-17

Principle of direct solid-phase immunosorbent assay (SPIA). **A,** Solid phase is microtiter well. **B,** Solid phase is bead. (From Forbes B, Sahm D, Weissfeld A: *Bailey and Scott's diagnostic microbiology,* ed 10, St Louis, 1998, Mosby.)

line phosphatase or horseradish peroxidase. When the appropriate substrate is added to the antigen-conjugated antibody complex, the enzyme catalyzes the production of a visible (colored) end product that can be quantitated spectrophotometrically. These procedures are very amenable to automation and testing large volumes of samples.

Most commercially developed EIA systems for

detection of infectious agents require physical separation of the specific antigens from nonspecific complexes found in clinical samples. Such systems are called **solid-phase immunosorbent assays (SPIA).** Separation is achieved through binding the antigen specific antibody to a solid phase or matrix. A variety of solid matrix platforms are commercially available to include individual wells of polystyrene microtiter trays (Figure 5-17 *A*), spherical plastic beads, or magnetic beads. (Figure 5-17 B). This solid matrix allows for separation, or washing, of sample and reagent to decrease nonspecific binding or background activity.

When performing an EIA, a clinical sample is first added to the solid matrix. If the antigen of interest is present in sample, it will form a stable complex with the antibody bound to the matrix. Unbound sample is removed by washing, and a second antibody specific for the antigen is added. In the *direct method,* this second antibody is conjugated to an enzyme. In the *indirect method,* a second nonconjugated antibody is added and washed; to which a third antibody specific for the second is added. The third antibody is conjugated to the enzyme and is directed against the Fc portion of the unlabeled second antibody.

In either method, once the conjugate is added and washed, a specific substrate is added. The amount of colored end product is directly proportional to the amount of enzyme-bound conjugate, and therefore, antigen present in the original clinical sample. Both methods of detection are described in a step-by-step manner in Figure 5-18.

The methods just described are often called **direct sandwich** and **indirect sandwich immunoassays.** The advantage of the indirect sandwich immunoassay is the need for only one enzyme conjugated anti-immunoglobulin antibody (third antibody) that can be used to detect a variety of antigens.

Commercial companies have produced good quality EIA kits for detection of a variety of microbial antigens. Conjugates can be inexpensively prepared, are stable for up to 6 months, and have reasonably good sensitivity in most applications. The use of microtitration plates and instrumentation for dispensing reagents, wash procedures, and automated optical reading of reactions has greatly facilitated EIA methods to allow large volumes to be batch tested (Figure 5-19). Some methods are time consuming, however, and may not be practical for low-volume labs or STAT runs. Thus they cannot always be considered rapid tests when compared with other procedures such as latex agglutination. Enzyme immunoassay kits are commonly used for rapid detection of *Chlamydia trachomatis, L. pneumophila, Clostridium difficile* toxins, *Giardia lamblia,* and *Cryptosporidium.*

A variation of enzyme labeling involves coupling

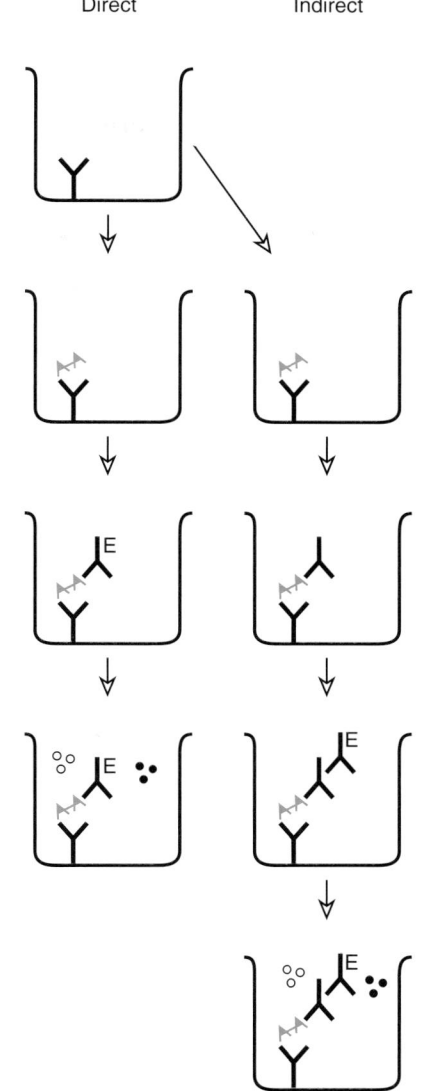

Figure 5-18

Principle of various EIA assays for antigen. Both methods (direct and indirect sandwich immunoassays) start with specific antibody bound to the solid phase. Arrows (→) separate steps in the procedures where washing of the solid phase takes place. *Y,* Antibody; ▲, antigen; *E,* enzyme; ○, enzyme substrate; ●, enzyme product.

a reactive molecule such as biotin to the primary antibody. Binding of antibody to specific antigen is then detected by reacting with enzyme-labeled streptavidin, which binds very tightly and specifically to biotin by one of four reactive sites on each

Figure 5-19 ―――――――――――――――

EIA test in microtitration tray *(top)* and strip *(bottom)* showing wells with product of enzymatic reaction before *(blue)* and after *(yellow)* addition of an acidic stop solution. (Courtesy Meridian Diagnostics, Cincinnati, Ohio.)

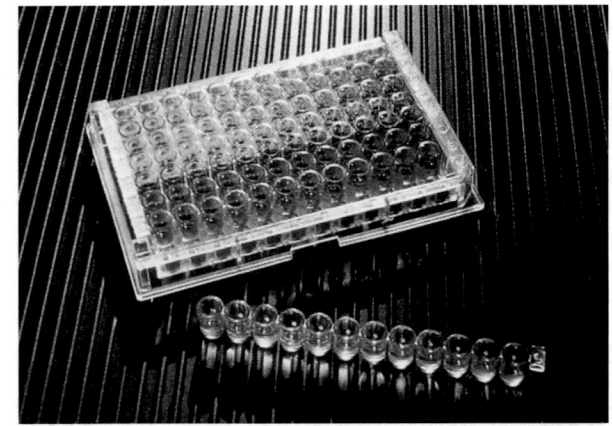

streptavidin molecule. The avidin-biotin interaction takes the place of primary antibody-secondary antibody interaction. This method tends to increase the amount of signal detected (increased sensitivity) for the following reasons: (1) Multiple biotin molecules may be bound to the primary antibody, and (2) Each avidin molecule has four reactive sites to biotin. In combination, avidin-biotin interactions allow for multiple complexes with enzyme to bind and cleave substrate.

Newer formats for EIAs are constantly being developed which have resulted in greater speed and simplicity of EIAs. The most popular method is described below.

Membrane-bound EIA

The flow-through and large surface area characteristics of nitrocellulose, nylon, or other membranes have been demonstrated to enhance the speed and sensitivity of EIA reactions. The improvements associated with **membrane-bound EIAs** are largely the result of immobilizing antibody onto the surface of porous membranes. This modification of SPIA utilizes a disposable plastic cassette consisting of the antibody-bound membrane and a small chamber to which the clinical sample can be added (Figure 5-20). An absorbent material is placed below the membrane to pull, or wick, the liquid reactants through the membrane.

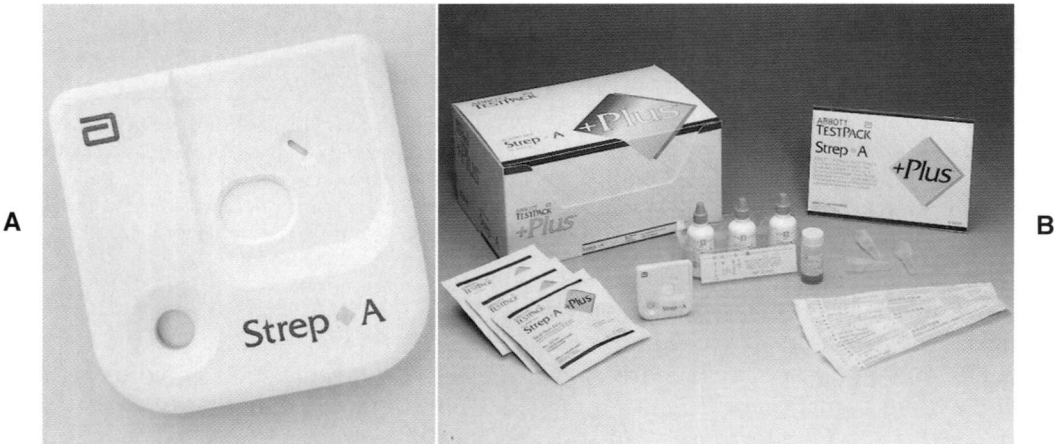

A   B

Figure 5-20 ―――

TestPack Strep A kit components **(A)** and individual cassette **(B)** of membrane-bound EIA test for group A streptococcal polysaccharide antigen. (Courtesy Abbott Laboratories.)

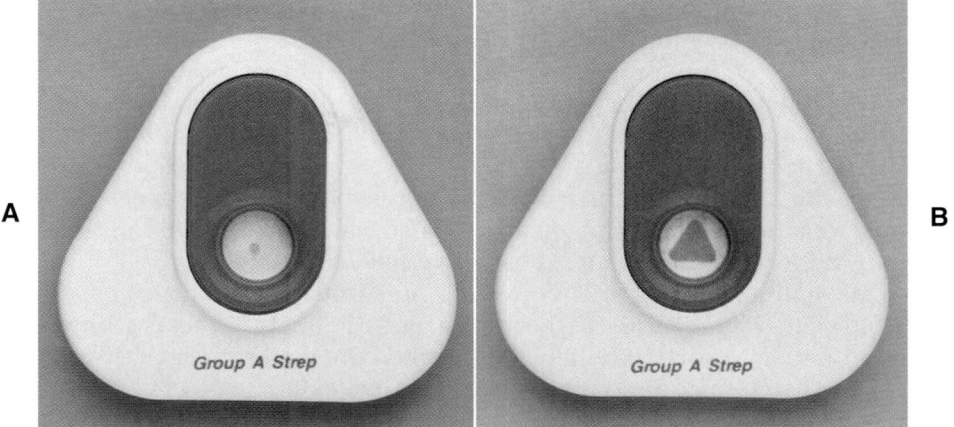

This helps to separate nonreacted components from the antigen-antibody complexes of interest bound to the membrane and thus simplify washing steps. Incubation times are also decreased because the rate of antigen binding is proportional to its concentration in solution near the membrane surface; this action increases the rate and extent of binding.

These "flow-through" EIAs have become popular because they can easily be performed as rapid single tests and because positive and negative controls can be incorporated at different sites on the same membrane used for clinical samples. Membrane-bound EIA tests are commonly used for the rapid detection of rotavirus, RSV, *C. difficile* toxins, influenza A, and group A *Streptococcus* (Figure 5-21).

Optical Immunoassays

Optical immunoassay (OIA) relies on the interaction of antigen-antibody complexes on inert surfaces. Specific antigen-antibody interaction actually alters the thickness of the reactants on the test surface. Light reflecting off the surface film containing antibody only is viewed as one color. However, when specific antigen is bound to antibody, it increases the thickness of the film. This causes the surface to appear a different color to the naked eye. An optical immunoassay is used in many laboratories to detect group A *Streptococcus* (GAS) in pediatric populations (Figure 5-22). Recently, a second OIA has been FDA approved for the detection of influenza A.

Other Immunoassays

Several other methods, including **radioimmunoassay (RIA)** and **fluorescent immunoassay (FIA),** are similar to EIA. However, radionucleotides (usually ^{125}I or ^{14}C) are substituted for enzymes in RIA and fluorochromes are substituted for enzymes in FIA. Although RIA was once the key method for antigen detection of numerous infectious agents, especially hepatitis B virus, it has largely been replaced by EIA, which does not require use of radioactive substances.

CURRENT CLINICAL APPLICATIONS

A wide variety of infectious diseases can be diagnosed using commercially available antigen detection test reagents. Some of these are listed in Table 5-3 and described here.

Respiratory Tract Infections
Streptococcal pharyngitis
One of the most widely used applications of direct antigen tests, popularized in the 1980s, is for the detection of GAS in throat swab specimens for

the diagnosis of streptococcal pharyngitis. The main advantage of rapid direct antigen testing for GAS over standard throat culture procedures is that results are available while the patient is in the physician's office. Also, antibiotic therapy can be given immediately instead of waiting 24 to 48 hours for culture results. This is more convenient for the physician and patient alike. Although antibiotic treatment is critical for prevention of post streptococcal pharyngitis syndromes such as rheumatic fever and glomerulonephritis, early antibiotic administration may shorten the illness. Early treatment may also reduce secondary infections or spread to close contacts, allowing the patient to return to work or school sooner.

Currently, more than 20 manufacturers produce diagnostic test kits for direct GAS detection. The majority of these kits use either latex agglutination or some version of solid-phase immunoassay. Both types of tests contain reagents to perform initial extraction of the group A carbohydrate antigen from the cell wall of the organism. This is most commonly achieved by exposing the sample to nitrous acid, but it can be accomplished by enzymatic digestion. Once the solubilized antigen preparation has been pH adjusted in a buffer solution, the specimen is tested according to the specific procedure of the manufacturer. A number of EIA tests have become popular, particularly those that use membrane-bound antibody to speed up the reaction and facilitate the washing procedure. Because of the colored product, they are generally easier to read than latex agglutination tests. One variation of the membrane-bound EIA for GAS uses colored, dye-filled liposomes bound to antibody as the detection reagent. As previously mentioned, a highly sensitive and specific OIA is commercially available.

Numerous studies have compared the performance of direct GAS tests with one another and against the gold standard: throat culture. A conservative estimate of the accuracy of GAS tests suggests sensitivity and specificity in the range of 60% to 80% and 90% to 95%, respectively. These values vary by manufacturer, individual performing the test, and accuracy of the throat culture procedure used for comparison. Overall, the sensitivities of the rapid GAS antigen tests are not sufficiently high to permit their use without an accompanying culture. However, studies of the OIA (Figure 5-22) suggest that its sensitivity and specificity are 90% to 95%. Even so, the best overall approach for diagnosis of streptococcal pharyngitis would be to couple a rapid direct test with a throat culture only when the direct test is negative. Positive direct test results would lead to immediate initiation of antibiotic therapy. It must be remembered that the most important rea-

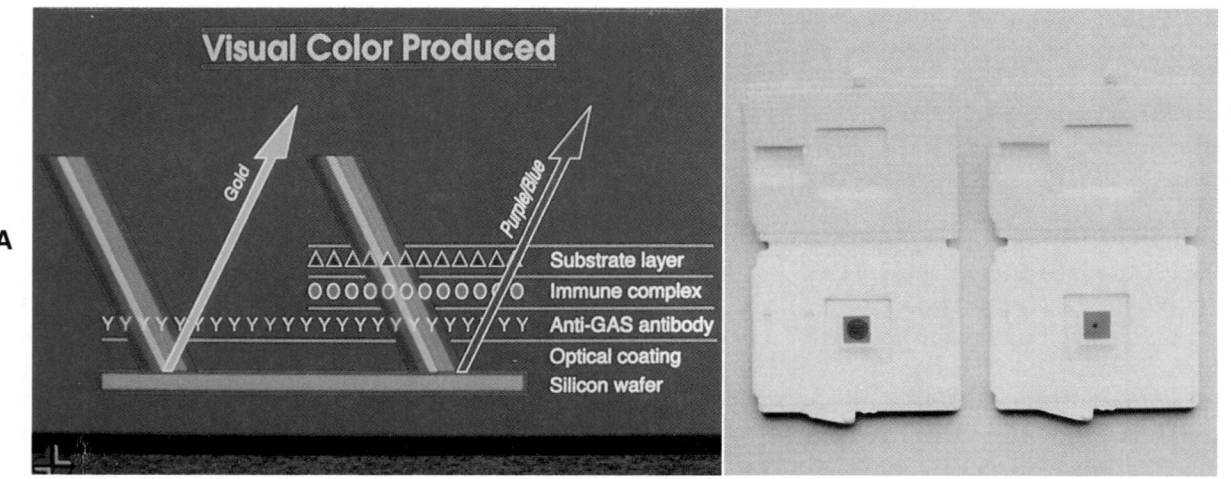

A   B

Figure 5-22

Optical ImmunoAssay (OIA™) for group A streptococcus. **A,** Principle of Biostar Strep A OIA™ test showing color change from gold to purple following attachment of immune complex containing group A streptococcal antigen. **B,** Test cassettes showing a positive reaction on the left and negative on the right. (Courtesy BioStar, Inc., Boulder, Co.)

TABLE 5-3

Some Representative Infectious Diseases and the Direct Antigen Detection Methods Commercially Available to Detect Them

Type of Infection	Test Methods
Bacterial	
Group A streptococcal pharyngitis	LA, EIA, liposome-enhanced immunoassay, OIA
Bacterial meningitis*	LA, CoA
Clostridium difficile colitis	LA, EIA
Chlamydial urethritis	EIA, FA
Pertussis	FA
Legionnaires' disease	FA, RIA
Fungal	
Cryptococcal meningitis	LA, EIA
Parasitic	
Giardiasis	FA, EIA
Cryptosporidiosis	FA, EIA
Pneumocystis pneumonia	FA
Trichomonas vaginitis	FA
Viral	
Rotavirus gastroenteritis	LA, EIA
Hepatitis B infection	EIA
Respiratory virus infection†	FA, EIA
Herpes simplex virus infection	FA, EIA
Cytomegalovirus infection	FA
AIDS	EIA

EIA, Enzyme immunoassay; *FA,* fluorescent antibody test; *LA,* latex agglutination test; *RIA,* radioimmunoassay; *OIA,* optical immunoassay.
*Includes *Haemophilus influenzae* b, *Streptococcus pneumoniae, Neisseria meningitidis,* and *Streptococcus agalactiae.*
†Includes influenza, parainfluenza, and respiratory syncytial viruses.

son for diagnosing and treating GAS pharyngitis is to prevent the nonsuppurative sequelae previously mentioned. Delay in initiation of therapy for a few days (while awaiting culture results) will not increase the patient's risk of developing such complications.

Whooping cough (pertussis)

Bordetella pertussis, the agent of whooping cough, is a slow-growing, fastidious, gram-negative coccobacilli. Recovery of the organism in culture from nasopharyngeal swabs or aspirates may take 7 to 10 days, even when selective media and optimal culture conditions are used. An FA test may be performed on smears prepared from nasopharyngeal washings or swabs. It has been reported to be positive in up to 70% of culture-positive specimens. As in any FA performed on respiratory specimens, specificity is dependent upon the expertise of a well-trained technologist. Thus, if using FA, culture must also be performed. A positive FA for *B. pertussis* may result in early initiation of therapy and isolation of the patient to prevent secondary spread of this highly contagious organism.

Legionnaires' disease

Legionella pneumophila and other *Legionella* sp. cause acute lobar pneumonia with multisystem involvement, known as legionnaires' disease. Early diagnosis and therapy are important, particularly in immunosuppressed patients. Disease may occur as community-acquired individual cases or outbreaks, and as nosocomial infections. A variety of antigen detection methods have been evaluated and compared with culture isolation. A commonly performed test is the FA on respiratory specimens. A monoclonal antibody is usually directed against *L. pneumophila* serogroup 1, whereas polyclonal antibody may include other serogroups and in some cases, other species of *Legionella*. Sensitivity of FA is approximately 70%. Specificity has been a problem with some reagents, owing to antigens shared with other gram-negative rods. A number of immunoassays have been evaluated, including an RIA for soluble urinary antigen. These assays have sensitivities in the 85% to 95% range, with even higher specificity. Most recently an EIA for urinary antigen has become commercially available with published sensitivity of 80% and specificity equal to that of RIA. The EIA test is limited to monoclonal antibody detection of *L. pneumophila* serogroup 1 only.

Respiratory virus infections

A number of respiratory viruses can be directly detected in both upper respiratory and lower respiratory specimens. Fluorescent antibody is a common technique used for detecting RSV; influenza A and B; parainfluenza 1, 2, and 3; and adenovirus. These reagents may be used for direct detection by FA or to confirm cytopathic effect in conventional tissue culture tubes or shell vials. When used for direct detection, these reagents are between 80% and 95% sensitive and 90% to 99% specific. Of particular importance, direct detection of RSV by FA or membrane-bound EIA in nasopharyngeal samples is commonly performed in the clinical laboratory (Figure 5-22). Rapid direct detection is im-portant because RSV causes serious lower respiratory tract disease (bronchiolitis and pneumonia) in young children, often requiring hospitalization. Rapid results can help in making cohorting decisions upon hospital admission. Also, it is difficult to maintain viral viability during transport and therefore can be difficult to recover in culture.

Pneumonia in immunocompromised patients

Cryptococcus neoformans, cytomegalovirus (CMV), and *Pneumocystis carinii* are important pulmonary pathogens in transplant, cancer, or AIDS patients. Those with cryptococcal pneumonia or meningitis can be quantitatively monitored for presence of antigen in serum or CSF by latex agglutination. Early CMV structural proteins can be monitored by the CMV antigenemia assay. In this procedure, buffy coats from whole blood specimens are stained by FA and the number of positive PMNs per 100,000 cells are counted. Increased numbers of fluorescently stained PMN nuclei are indicative of increased risk of developing CMV pneumonia or other end organ disease. An FA procedure for *P. carinii* is approved for use on induced sputum and bronchoscopy specimens (Figure 5-23). In patients with high probability of pneumocystis pneumonia, a negative FA on induced sputum should be followed by FA on a bronchoscopically obtained specimen. *P. carinii* culture is not widely available, making FA the only reliable method available for its detection in the clinical microbiology laboratory.

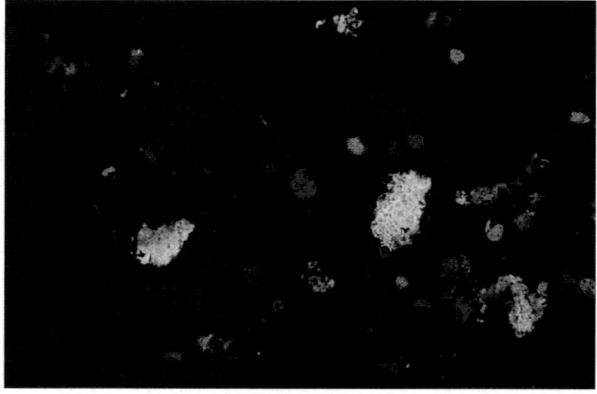

Figure 5-23 ────────────────────────
Bronchoalveolar lauage showing *Pneumocystis carinii* using fluorescent antibody test.

Meningitis and Sepsis

Bacterial meningitis and sepsis

For approximately 25 years, clinical laboratories have regularly used antigen detection testing of CSF and other body fluids to detect organisms causing bacterial meningitis. Techniques have included CIE, popular in the 1970s, EIA, and coagglutination. Today, clinical laboratories typically use latex agglutination when performing rapid antigen testing for bacterial meningitis. The bacterial agents detected in the commercially available kits include *Haemophilus influenzae* type b, *Neisseria meningitidis, Streptococcus pneumoniae,* and *Streptococcus agalactiae* (group B streptococcus). Although antibodies in each kit vary, they are all designed to detect capsular polysaccharide antigens of the organisms. When these organisms cause infection, the antigens are shed by growing bacterial cells into the body tissues and fluids. These organisms often cause bacteremia before the organism invades the central nervous system. Thus, the organism and antigens may be detected in the serum before or at the same time they are found in the CSF in cases of meningitis. Furthermore, circulating organisms and soluble antigens are trapped, degraded, and released by phagocytic cells of the liver and spleen. These products are cleared from the body by filtration in the kidney and excreted in the urine; thus urine can be examined for the presence of antigen in addition to CSF in suspected meningitis. Urine is also useful as a test specimen either alone or in addition to serum in cases of bacteremia and focal infections other than meningitis. It may be concentrated by ultrafiltration (removing water but not microbial antigens) to increase test sensitivity.

It should be mentioned that with the advent of *H. influenzae* type b vaccine, the incidence of *H. influenzae* meningitis and/or bacteremia has declined by 90%. Fortunately, no other microorganism seems to have filled this potential niche. For this reason, and others mentioned below, the utilization of antigen tests for bacterial meningitis has declined sharply.

The clinical utility of antigen tests for diagnosing meningitis varies with a number of factors, including the manufacturer of the kit, the specific organism, and the specimen type tested. In many clinical laboratories, the use of these tests is reserved for very specific diagnostic testing requirements. In most situations, the Gram stain is sufficiently sensitive to detect bacterial meningitis. However, as in the case presented, the Gram-stained direct smear was negative. The responsible organism was detected by a direct antigen test. Gram stains and/or antigen detection tests must always be performed along with appropriate culture. Most importantly, appropriate antibiotic treatment should never be withheld pending culture results in patients with negative antigen test results (unlike the situation with antigen testing for group A streptococci). The greatest clinical utility of these antigen tests probably occurs when testing specimens from patients who have received antibiotic therapy before cultures were collected and in whom the Gram stain was negative. In this situation, the likelihood of recovering the organism in culture is dramatically decreased.

Cryptococcal meningitis

The clinical utility of antigen detection for *C. neoformans,* an important fungal pathogen causing meningitis, pneumonia, and disseminated disease, is considerably different. Antigen testing of CSF, commonly performed by latex agglutination (LA), is considerably more sensitive than India ink direct examination of CSF. In addition, quantitative antigen detection, which consists of titrating CSF antigen by performing serial dilutions, is an important prognostic indicator of clinical response to antifungal therapy. An EIA test is also available for detection of *C. neoformans.*

Gastrointestinal Tract Infections

Clostridium difficile: associated enteric disease

Direct microbial detection methods have been applied to the diagnosis of bacterial, viral, and parasitic agents of gastrointestinal tract infections. *Clostridium difficile,* an anaerobic gram-positive rod, causes pseudomembranous colitis and antibiotic-associated diarrhea. These are typically hospitalized patients receiving antibiotics or other chemotherapeutic agents that alter bowel flora. The organism produces two exotoxins, toxin A and B, which are involved in pathogenesis. Toxin A functions as an enterotoxin that causes inflammation, increased vascular permeability, and fluid secretion. Toxin B is a cytotoxin that causes mucosal damage with tenfold more potency than toxin A and causes hemorrhagic colitis and cytopathic effects.

Two gold standard laboratory tests exist for *C. difficile.* One is a cell culture cytotoxicity test, which is a primary indicator of toxin B presence. The other method is culture on selective media in anaerobic conditions. Both procedures require 24 to 96 hours for final identification. A large number of EIA tests for toxin A have been evaluated. Sensitivities range from 75% to 95% or higher, and therefore negative predictive values may be close to 99%. However, with the possible emergence of toxin B producing and non–toxin A producing strains, the use of recently introduced A + B tests must be thoroughly investigated.

Shiga-toxin producing *Escherichia coli*

Food-borne outbreaks of shiga-toxin producing enterohemorrhagic *E. coli* are being reported with increased frequency. Enterohemorrhagic strains of *E. coli,* such as O157:H7 and others, secrete a verotoxin that causes endothelial injury that can result in the development of hemolytic-uremic syndrome (HUS). Rapid EIA tests are available for detection of verotoxin and/or specific enterohemorrhagic strains of *E. coli* directly from stool samples. Rapid identification may prove useful in identifying exposed individuals in an outbreak situation. Those individuals can then be carefully watched for progression to systemic disease including HUS.

Campylobacter

Campylobacter species are microaerophilic, gram-negative, curved rods, requiring incubation in a 5% O_2, 10% CO_2 and 85% N_2 atmosphere. These bacteria often take up to 72 hours to grow in culture on a selective agar medium in the microaerophilic environment. A 2-hour EIA kit is commercially available to detect antigen directly from stool specimens.

Viral gastroenteritis

The most important identifiable agents of viral gastroenteritis are human rotaviruses, enteric adenoviruses, caliciviruses, and Norwalk virus. These agents are either very difficult or impossible to grow in cell culture, and electron microscopy capabilities are rarely cost efficient in a clinical microbiology laboratory. Therefore, antigen detection methods are very important for diagnosis. Rotaviruses are the most important agents in this group for a number of reasons. They commonly infect very young infants, often in day care settings, causing vomiting and diarrhea and resulting in dehydration. Rotavirus disease can also be severe and long lasting, while gastroenteritis due to these other viruses is usually much shorter in duration. Both EIA and LA tests are available for rotavirus detection in stool specimens, EIA is generally more sensitive than LA. In either case, soluble antigen must be extracted from the particulate matter in stool before testing. This is generally accomplished by mixing the stool with extract buffer solution. At least one EIA is available for detection of enteric adenoviruses. No rapid tests for Norwalk virus or caliciviruses are commercially available.

Giardiasis and cryptosporidiosis

The classical workup for ova and parasites (O&P) requires chemical extraction, concentration, and microscopy of stool specimens. These methods are technically demanding and time consuming. In settings not including areas of endemicity for certain parasites, a number of studies have recently been published suggesting that 95% of all clinically important parasites detected are either *Giardia lamblia* or *Cryptosporidium parvum.* Direct FA and EIA kits are available for detection of soluble antigen directly from stool. Some formats include one monoclonal antibody to detect one organism, other formats include separate monoclonal antibodies for both organisms. In particular, by FA (see Figure 5-16) the difference in size between these two parasites allows the technologist to visually distinguish the two organisms using both antibodies in one procedure. Many laboratories offer these tests to screen the nonimmunocompromised outpatient population. Testing algorithms usually are set up so that only those patients with a history of travel or immunosuppression require a full O&P workup when the screen by EIA/FA is negative. Recently a membrane EIA has been FDA approved for the simultaneous detection of *G. lamblia, C. parvum,* and *Entamoeba histolytica* in stool samples.

Sexually Transmitted Diseases

Chlamydial infections

Chlamydia trachomatis, an obligate intracellular bacterium, infects the genital tract, causing urethritis, cervicitis, and other infections. In addition, neonates born to infected mothers are at risk for developing conjunctivitis and pneumonia. Although isolation in cell culture is still considered the gold standard for diagnosis, a large number of direct antigen detection assays are commercially available. Most of these assays are EIA- or FA-based. The numerous published evaluations of these products suggest moderately good sensitivity and very good specificity when they are used on symptomatic patients at high risk for infection (e.g., patients visiting a sexually transmitted disease clinic). The tests do not, however, perform as well when used in low-prevalence populations or asymptomatic patients (e.g., OB-GYN clinics). In addition, they are not approved for use in children in whom evidence of chlamydial infection subsequent to sexual abuse is being sought.

Blood-Borne and Body Fluid-Borne Diseases

Hepatitis B virus detection

Nonculture methods are the mainstays for laboratory diagnosis of both hepatitis B (HBV) and human immunodeficiency virus (HIV). Measurement of serologic response to viral antigens and direct viral antigen detection are important. For HBV, EIA methods have largely replaced RIA methods. Both hepatitis B surface antigen and hepatitis B e (capsid) antigen can generally be detected early in acute infection and may also be detected in patients who are chronically infected. These antigen tests, when performed concurrently with antibody detection tests, have important diagnostic and prognostic value in the workup of acute versus chronic disease.

Human immunodeficiency virus (HIV)

Although diagnosis of HIV infection is generally accomplished by serology, EIA for the viral p24 antigen has been used to detect active viral replication in blood. Its greatest value is in the early detection in neonates in whom serologic diagnosis is of little value because of maternal anti-HIV IgG from a seropositive mother. It is also used in screening blood in transfusion medicine or blood bank laboratories.

FUTURE APPLICATIONS

One classical immunology technique that may soon find rapid antigen detection application in the clinical microbiology laboratory is flow cytometry. Recent developments in flow cytometry analysis are utilizing multiple monoclonal antibodies attached to different sized latex beads containing various amounts of different fluorochromes in a multiplex format. These multiplex assays provide the potential to detect up to 64 different antigens in a clinical sample.

Significant progress has been made in the development and improvement of direct antigen detection tests. Yet many of these methods have not replaced, but instead are used in addition to, cultural techniques. Such applications are justifiable when patient care decisions are based on rapid antigen detection methods or when culture methods fail to isolate the organism. And of course, the importance of antigen detection for organisms that are difficult or impossible to culture ensures the diagnostic use of these technologies. Other techniques developed for similar reasons, such as nucleic acid detection in clinical samples, are discussed at length later in this chapter. The variety and quality of antigen detection reagents will most likely increase in the future. Again, laboratory scientists will have to make wise choices regarding the most cost-effective and clinically relevant use of these reagents.

Bibliography

Aldeen WE et al: Comparison of nine commercially available enzyme-linked immunosorbent assays for detection of *Giardia lamblia* in fecal specimens, *J Clin Microbiol* 36:1338, 1998.

Buck GE: Noncultural methods of detection and identification of microorganisms in clinical specimens, *Pediatr Clin North Am* 36:95, 1989.

Cook L: New assays for infectious agents replacing traditional serologic methods, *Advance for Medical Laboratory Professionals,* Dec 7, 1998, p 12.

Dean D et al: Comparison of performance and cost-effectiveness of direct fluorescent-antibody, ligase chain reaction, and PCR assays for verification of chlamydial enzyme immunoassay results for populations with a low to moderate prevalence of *Chlamydia trachomatis* infection, *J Clin Microbiol* 36:94, 1998.

Forbes BA et al, editors: Immunochemical methods used for organism detection. In *Bailey and Scott's diagnostic microbiology,* ed 10, St Louis, 1998, Mosby, p 208.

Gerna G et al: Standardization of the human cytomegalovirus antigenemia assay by means of in vitro–generated positive peripheral blood polymorphonuclear leukocytes, *J Clin Microbiol* 36:3585, 1998.

Gray LD, Fedorko DP: Laboratory diagnosis of bacterial meningitis, *Clin Microbiol Rev* 5:130, 1992.

Halsted DC: Noncultural methods for diagnosing respiratory syncytial virus infections, *Clin Microbiol Newsletter* 9:181, 1987.

Henrard DR et al: Detection of p24 antigen with and without immune complex dissociation for longitudinal monitoring of human immunodeficiency virus type 1 infection, *J Clin Microbiol* 33:72, 1995.

Hermann JE: Immunoassays for the diagnosis of infectious diseases. In Murray PR et al, editors: *Manual of clinical microbiology,* ed 6, Washington, DC, 1995, American Society for Microbiology, p 110.

Kehl KSC et al: Comparison of four different methods for detection of *Cryptosporidium* species, *J Clin Microbiol* 33:416, 1995.

Kohler RB, editor: *Antigen detection to diagnose bacterial infections,* Boca Raton, Fl, 1986, CRC Press.

Koneman EW et al, editors: *Color atlas and textbook of diagnostic microbiology,* ed 5, Philadelphia, 1997, Lippincott-Raven.

Mackenzie AMR et al: Sensitivities and specificities of Premier *E. coli* O157 and Premier EHEC enzyme immunoassays for diagnosis of infection with verotoxin (shiga-like toxin)-producing *Escherichia coli, J Clin Microbiol* 36:1608, 1998.

Needham CA et al: Streptococcal pharyngitis: impact of a high-sensitivity antigen test on physician outcome, *J Clin Microbiol* 36:3468, 1998.

Rose NR et al, editors: *Manual of clinical laboratory immunology,* ed 5, Washington, DC, 1997, American Society for Microbiology.

Whittier S et al: Evaluation of four commercially available enzyme immunoassays for laboratory diagnosis of *Clostridium difficile*–associated disease, *J Clin Microbiol* 31:2861, 1994.

Wolfson JS et al: Blinded comparison of a direct immunofluorescent monoclonal antibody staining method for identification of *Pneumocystis carinii* in induced sputum and bronchoalveolar lavage specimens of patients infected with human immunodeficiency virus, *J Clin Microbiol* 28:2136, 1989.

Woods GL, Washington JA: The clinician and the microbiology laboratory. In Mandell GL et al, editors: *Principles and practice of infectious disease,* ed 4, New York, 1995, Churchill Livingstone, p 169.

Zimmerman SK, Needham CA: Comparison of conventional stool concentration and preserved-smear methods with Merifluor *Cryptosporidium/Giardia* direct immunofluorescence assay and ProSpectT *Giardia* ED microplate assay for detection of *Giardia lamblia, J Clin Microbiol* 33:1942, 1995.

LEARNING ASSESSMENTS

1. What is avidity? How does it differ from specificity?

2. What antigenic detection methods are available in detecting infectious agents in clinical samples?

3. What are examples of clinical applications of antigen detection methods?

4. When are these methods most important?

5. What other upcoming antigen detection technology would be available to detecting infectious agents?

6. Of what does innate or natural immunity consist?

7. How does it protect the host?

8. How does it differ from acquired or specific immunity?

9. Which type of antibody indicates a primary response? A secondary response?

10. Why is it important to obtain both an acute and a convalescent sera to confirm a serologic diagnosis?

B. SEROLOGIC DIAGNOSIS OF INFECTIOUS DISEASES

Ronald H. Holton

IMMUNE RESPONSE TO INFECTIOUS AGENTS
  Host Resistance to Infection
    Immunity
    Physical and chemical barriers
    Innate or natural immunity
    Specific or acquired immunity
  Nature of the Immune Response to Infectious
  Agents
  Antigens and Antibodies
    Testing for antigen
    Characteristics of antigens
    Classification and characteristics of antibodies
  Primary and Secondary Antibody Responses

INTERPRETING SEROLOGIC TEST DATA
  Acute and Convalescent Antibody Titers
  Antibody Specificity and Cross-Reactivity
  False-Negative and False-Positive Serologic
    Test Results
  Value of Serologic Tests
    Population studies
    Immune status testing
    Congenital infections
    Infections after the newborn period

ANTIBODY DETECTION METHODS
  AND APPLICATIONS
  Particle Agglutination Assays
    Direct, natural particle agglutination
    Indirect, carrier particle agglutination
  Precipitation Assays
    Double immunodiffusion
    Counterimmunoelectrophoresis
    Flocculation
  Complement Fixation Test
  Neutralization Tests
    Viral neutralization
    Antistreptolysin-O test
    Treponema pallidum immobilization
  Microscope-Assisted Labeled-Reagent Techniques
    Indirect fluorescent antibody test
    Fluorescent antibody tests with enhanced
      sensitivity
  Enzyme-Linked Immunosorbent Assay
    and Related Techniques
    Enzyme immunoassays
    Other immunoassays
  Western Blotting

USE OF SEROLOGIC TESTING IN SPECIFIC
  DISEASES
  Serologic Testing of Syphilis
  Serologic Testing for Streptococcal Infections
  Serologic Diagnosis of Toxoplasmosis
  Serologic Diagnosis of Important Viral Diseases
  Serologic Diagnosis of Fungal Infection

OBJECTIVES

1. Describe how physical and chemical barriers protect the host from infectious agents.
2. Differentiate the dynamics of the humoral from the cell-mediated immune response.
3. Explain how both types of immune responses are used as indicators of infectious process.
4. Describe antigens. Classify and characterize the different types of antibodies.
5. Differentiate the primary from the secondary antibody response.
6. Discuss the importance of acute and convalescent antibody titers. Interpret significant results.
7. Recognize the significance of serologic tests in the following situations:
   - Population studies
   - Immune status testing
   - Congenital infections
   - Infections beyond the newborn period
8. Describe the principles and applications of each of the following serologic methods:
   - Particle agglutination assays
   - Precipitation assay
   - Complement fixation
   - Neutralization
   - Indirect FA test
   - Indirect ELISA
   - IgM antibody capture ELISA
   - Western blotting

KEY TERMS

Physical barrier
Chemical barrier
Inate immunity
Opsonization
Chemotaxis
Acquired immunity
Immunologic memory
Antibodies

Antigen
Immunogen
Immunoglobulin G
 (IgG)
Immunoglobulin M
 (IgM)
Immunoglobulin A
 (IgA)

Immunoglobulin E
 (IgE)
Primary immune
 response
Secondary, or anamnes-
 tic, immune response
Acute antibody titer

Convalescent antibody
 titer
Antibody cross-
 reactivity
False-negative serologic
 test
False-positive serologic
 test

The phenomenon of bacterial agglutination was discovered as early as 1896 and was quickly recognized as a powerful tool by bacteriologists. Not only could antisera be used to identify and differentiate bacteria but also the serum from infected patients could be tested for the ability to agglutinate a given organism. This reaction was therefore indicative of prior exposure to the organism and of the level of immune response and protection against the infectious agent.

Serologic testing describes serum tests used to identify antibodies initiated by infectious agents without the necessity of culturing the organism.

Serology is the study of these antibodies and their reaction to antigens. This type of testing has many advantages. Serologic testing is an excellent means for detecting infectious agents that are either difficult or impossible to culture. Organisms, such as viruses or some sexually transmitted agents, are difficult to culture usually because of either their specific growth requirements or previous antibiotic treatment that decreases the number of viable organisms available for growth. In addition, many organisms are not grown because of significant risk to laboratory workers. Fungi and mycobacteria, for example, take an extremely long time to grow.

Not only are serologic tests used under these conditions, but they also can and are used for prognostic information and in the monitoring of therapy (viral load testing in HIV and chronic hepatitis).

As powerful as these tests are, using serologic procedures in diagnosis has significant disadvantages. The most significant problem is that to measure the host immune response to an organism, 10 to 14 days must pass after infection and in some cases (HIV, hepatitis B and C) as much as weeks to months before antibody levels are detectable. IgM antibodies are the first to appear and measure; however, they are only present transiently. IgG antibodies, on the other hand, take much longer to appear but will persist for years and may even be present for life. Immunocompromised patients have an antibody response that may either be diminished or nonexistent, thereby impairing the ability to use any serologic procedures. Also, the antibody being detected may actually have been produced against another organism and a false-positive test is observed. Serologic tests are available to detect antigens that are detectable earlier than antibody levels; however, they are not available for as many organisms as the classic antibody tests.

The discovery of the precipitin reaction extended the concept of serologic diagnosis to include the assay of antigens and antibodies in systems involving both bacterial and nonbacterial products. Reactions and cross-reactions of antisera prepared against proteins, both animal and plant, have shown that these immune responses might be applied to the study of taxonomic relationships and even in forensics. The further understanding that immune hemolysis might actually be mediated by antierythrocyte antibodies in the presence of complement and could be titrated precisely added a new approach to the diagnosis of disease. The blood of patients could be examined for the presence of antibodies that do not agglutinate or precipitate their respective antigens but do fix complement. This serologic method could not only determine the prior exposure of the patient to a pathogen but also could be used to follow the course of the disease. The best example of this technique is the serodiagnostic complement fixation test for syphilis.

The first practical laboratory tests for newly discovered infectious agents are still generally based on serology. The types of tests available have increased dramatically during this decade, allowing the diagnosis of many new infections.

For example, three recently discovered diseases—acquired immune deficiency syndrome (AIDS), hepatitis C virus infection, and Lyme disease—are diagnosed in the laboratory most frequently with serologic tests. These three diseases are all caused by infectious agents (human immunodeficiency virus type 1, hepatitis C virus, and *Borrelia burgdorferi,* respectively) that are difficult to cultivate in routine clinical laboratories. Although currently available serologic tests for these and other agents are not perfect, significant improvements in quality and methodology of tests have been made over the past several years. Many of these improvements have resulted from advancements in preparation of antibodies and antigens of high purity. In addition, assay techniques such as immunoassays with labeled antibodies or antigens have notably improved. A wide variety of commercial kits of high quality are available. This section discusses the aspects of the immune response that are important in understanding serologic testing and reviews principles of antibody detection methods and current clinical applications. Many of these applications are based on the principles already presented in the preceding section on antigen detection.

IMMUNE RESPONSE TO INFECTIOUS AGENTS

Host Resistance to Infection
Immunity

Classically, the term *immunity* has been defined as a complex mechanism whereby the body is able to protect itself from invasion by disease-causing organisms. This mechanism, known as the immune system, consists of numerous cells and protein molecules that are responsible for recognizing and removing these foreign substances. This general definition has been broadened over the years to mean a reaction to any foreign substance, including proteins and polysaccharides, as well as invading microorganisms. Research advances over the years have dramatically increased our understanding of the basic immune response and given us an appreciation of the cellular interrelationships. The immune response can be divided into two broad categories. The first is known as innate or natural immunity with little or no specificity and the second, called adaptive or specific, which is highly specialized.

Physical and chemical barriers

The human has evolved a complex system of defense mechanisms to prevent infectious agents from gaining access to and replicating in the body. The skin and mucous membranes of the respiratory, digestive, and urogenital systems provide a **physical barrier** to penetration by many microorganisms. This is particularly evident in the keratinized outer layer of the skin. Furthermore, the secretions of the mucous membranes and the ciliated epithelial cells of the respiratory tract promote trapping and removal of microorganisms.

In addition, many body secretions provide a **chemical barrier** to infection. For example, the acidic pH of the stomach and vagina, the presence of enzymes such as *lysozyme* in saliva and tears, and oils produced by the sebaceous glands of the skin have chemical properties useful in inhibiting invasion by pathogenic microorganisms. Interestingly, the normal flora of these sites survive and contribute to the host resistance to pathogens.

Innate or natural immunity

INNATE IMMUNITY

Innate immunity, or natural immunity, consists of several components. These include (1) physical and chemical barriers such as the skin and mucous membranes; (2) blood proteins that act as mediators of infection; and (3) a cellular mechanism capable of phagocytosis (neutrophils and macrophages) and other leukocytes such as natural killer cells. This first line of defense has a limited capacity to distinguish one organism from another; however, previous exposure to a particular foreign substance is not required. Physical barriers may be as simple as the keratinized outer layer of the skin. Also, the secretions of the mucous membranes and the ciliated epithelial cells of the respiratory tract promote trapping and removal of microorganisms. In addition, many secretions provide a chemical barrier, such as the acidic pH of the stomach and vagina. Saliva and tears contain enzymes such as *lysozyme,* and the sebaceous glands of the skin contain oils capable of inhibiting invasion by pathogenic organisms. The normal flora of all of these sites is able to add another

dimension to the hosts ability to resist invading pathogens.

Once the physical and chemical barriers to infection have been penetrated, *nonspecific mechanisms of immunity* or *natural immunity* become operational. Phagocytic cells ingest and kill microorganisms, whereas activated complement components contribute to a wide variety of immunologic events, including promotion of attachment and engulfment of bacteria by neutrophils **(opsonization)** and attraction of neutrophils to sites of infection **(chemotaxis).** Collectively, these immunologic defense mechanisms, along with host tissue damage caused by the invading organisms, combine to produce an *acute inflammatory response* in the host. The importance of natural immune mechanisms rests in their rapid response to invading organisms. However, these mechanisms are effective primarily against extracellular bacterial pathogens, playing only a minor role by themselves in immunity to intracellular bacterial pathogens, viruses, and fungi.

Specific or acquired immunity

SPECIFIC IMMUNITY

Specific or **acquired immunity** is much more highly evolved and complex than innate immunity and enhances the protective mechanism of the innate or natural defense. This arm of the immune response is capable of being specific for distinct molecules; responding in particular ways to different types of foreign substances; and developing memory, which allows for a more vigorous response to repeated exposures to the same foreign invader. Lymphocytes and their products, known as *antibodies,* are the major constituents of the specific immune response. Substances that are capable of inducing the immune response are called *antigens.* Also, an interrelationship exists between the mechanisms of the innate and the specific. For instance, inflammation, a nonspecific response of the innate system, provides a signal that triggers the specific response.

The specific immune system is able to enhance the protective mechanisms of the innate system as mentioned before. For instance, the activation of complement (a component of innate immunity) by invading bacteria is further enhanced by the presence of specific antibodies (components of specific immunity) which leads to complement activation by bacteria that are not capable of complement activation alone. This activation leads to phagocytic clearance and elimination of the bacteria. Secondly, the specific immune response adds a high degree of specialization to the passive mechanisms of the innate response. The nature of the specific immune response varies according to the type of organism and is designed to eliminate it efficiently. For instance, antibodies are produced by B lymphocytes in response to blood-borne organisms and aid in their elimination. However, the response to phagocytosed antigens is primarily by T lymphocytes that produce chemicals that enhance the activities of the phagocytic cells. Most importantly, the specific response is able to remember each time it encounters a particular foreign antigen, called **immunologic memory.** Subsequent exposure to that antigen is able to stimulate an increasingly effective and specific defense. Ultimately, the specific immune response is the second line of defense and is able to significantly improve upon the first.

Lymphocytes originate in the bone marrow from *stem* and *progenitor* cells. Lymphocytes mature and take up residence in various body tissues and organs, including the thymus, lymph nodes, and spleen. They are a diverse group of cells that can be classified into two major types—*T* (thymus-derived) *cells* and *B* (bone marrow–derived) *cells*—on the basis of cell surface markers. The uniqueness of these cells lies in the presence of specific cell surface receptor molecules that recognize and bind a unique antigen, activating the cell to divide, differentiate, and secrete a number of effector substances. The millions of lymphocytes found in the body have been preengineered during embryogenesis to recognize a vast array of substances as foreign while learning which substances constitute self. Thus, the result of encounter with antigen is an expanded clone or clones of activated lymphocytes.

HUMORAL IMMUNITY

B lymphocytes play the predominant role in acquired humoral immunity. Each B cell has surface receptors that recognize only one type of antigen. After antigen binding, the B cell undergoes multiple divisions, and the resulting cells, known as *plasma cells,* actively secrete proteins known as *immunoglobulins* or **antibodies.** All of the antibody molecules derived from a single clone of B cells are of a single specificity (recognize a unique antigen), identical to the receptor molecule on the original activated B cell. These antibody molecules circulate in the blood stream and lymphatics, bathe body tissues, and are capable of binding to infectious agents or substances to aid the host in eliminating them from the body. The detection and quantification of these antibody molecules, obtained from a patient's serum, constitute the primary goal of diagnosing infectious diseases through *serologic* methods.

CELL-MEDIATED IMMUNITY

In contrast to humoral immunity, the primary effector cell in cell-mediated immunity is the T lymphocyte. The T cell does not secrete antibody molecules; however, the result of antigen binding, activation, cell division, and differentiation is the production of a number of low-molecular-weight (LMW) proteins known as *lymphokines.* Lymphocytes effect their immunologic function through direct cell-to-cell contact or through the activity of the lymphokines on other cells, such as macrophages. The measurement and diagnostic significance of cell-mediated immunity are beyond the scope of this book, and cellular immune function tests generally are not performed in microbiology or microbial serology laboratories.

Nature of the Immune Response to Infectious Agents

Although both humoral immunity and cell-mediated immunity are important in protecting the human from a wide variety of infectious agents, each contributes differently, in terms of overall importance, according to the type of pathogen and virulence mechanisms. Immunity to *extracellular* bacterial pathogens, such as *Staphylococcus aureus* and *Streptococcus pyogenes,* is mediated primarily by antibody functioning either alone (neutralization of toxins and extracellular bacterial enzymes) or with complement and neutrophils (chemotaxis and phagocytosis of bacterial cells). Immunity to *intracellular* bacterial pathogens, such as *Mycobacterium tuberculosis,* is primarily cell mediated, through the activities of T lymphocytes, lymphokines, and macrophages. If antibody is produced, it plays little role in eliminating this pathogen, because the pathogen is sequestered (hidden) intracellularly, where antibody cannot reach.

Viral infections often elicit both humoral and cell-mediated immune responses. Antibody may bind directly to and neutralize viral particles (render the virus noninfectious—unable to infect other cells) when they are found free in the blood stream or other body fluids. For example, central nervous system infection by *arboviruses* (which cause encephalitis) or by certain *enteroviruses* (which cause meningitis) may be prevented if neutralizing antibody against these organisms is present when the virus reaches the blood stream and before it enters the central nervous system. Some viruses, however, cause infections that spread by cell-to-cell transmission (herpes simplex virus, which causes cold sores); they would not be subject to the neutralizing effect of antibodies. In these cases, cell-mediated immunity plays a predominant role in eliminating the agent. Immunity to both fungal and parasitic infections is also primarily cell-mediated; antibody plays little or no role in prevention of or recovery from infection resulting from these agents.

Although antibodies may *not* have protective value for certain infectious agents, they may nonetheless have diagnostic and prognostic value in serologic tests. The remainder of this chapter focuses on humoral immunity and the detection and significance of antibodies.

Antigens and Antibodies

Testing for antigen

Antibody testing requires a certain amount of time to become positive as discussed earlier. Testing directly for the antigen produced by the organism allows the laboratory to establish a diagnosis in a much more timely fashion. This is extremely important in treatments that require the documentation of the presence of a specific organism.

A large number of infectious agents produce proteins that can be identified from almost any body fluid or surface (serum, urine, sputum, CSF, or exudates on surfaces). The tests used to detect these proteins (antigens) are very similar to those used in the detection of antibody. In an ELISA test for a protein antigen, an antibody specific to that antigen is first attached to a solid support such as a micro titer plate. The patient fluid containing the antigen is then added, followed by a second labeled antibody to the antigen for identification and quantitation. This technique produces what is known as an antibody-antigen-antibody sandwich assay. This type of direct test is widely used for known antigens. As with any type of laboratory testing, known positive and negative samples are always included to ensure that the test is working as it should. Antigen-based testing is generally considered to be less sensitive than culture; however, they are able to yield diagnostic information much sooner.

Characteristics of antigens

Antigens are relatively high-molecular-weight (HMW) substances, usually proteins or polysaccharides (less commonly, lipids or nucleic acids either alone or complexed to proteins or polysaccharides), that can combine specifically with antibody molecules. Antigens that are recognized as foreign substances by a host are said to be immunogenic (antigenic), capable of eliciting an immune response. Often, the terms **antigen** and **immunogen** are used interchangeably, but the former term really refers to the antibody-binding properties of the molecule, whereas the latter term refers to the antibody-eliciting property of the molecule.

A number of factors determine whether a chemical compound will be an effective immunogen in a given host. First and foremost, the compound must be recognized as foreign or *nonself* by the host's immune system. This is a complex event largely related to the size and structural complexity of the compound. The larger and more chemically diverse a substance, the greater the likelihood it will be recognized as foreign. In addition, the compound must be present in sufficient quantity and have ample stability to remain in the host for enough time to "expose" the immune system. It should be remembered that some large molecules, such as complex proteins, may be of sufficient diversity to contain two or more different antigenic determinants. Complex polysaccharides may also contain multiple antigenic determinants (multivalent antigen), but these are generally identical because of the repeating subunit nature of polysaccharides.

Microorganisms contain a wide array of molecules capable of eliciting an immune response in the host. Immunogenic substances may be structural or nonstructural components of the microorganism. For example, many bacteria have polysaccharide or protein *capsules* that coat the organism. Because these capsules are located on the cell surface, they are often the first antigenic determinants recognized by the host. Additional structural antigenic components are the bacterial cell wall and membrane proteins and polysaccharides. Nonstructural antigens include bacterial enzymes and toxins that may be found within the cell or released into the host tissues. Because many bacterial components are "hidden" deep within the cell, antibody responses to some of them may not develop until the cell has been partially degraded by the host's natural immunity (phagocytic cells, complement, etc.). Thus, a single infecting bacterial species might stimulate the production of a wide array of antibodies.

POLYCLONAL VS MONOCLONAL ANTIBODIES
IN SEROLOGIC TESTING

The typical immune response to a large complex antigen, such as a bacteria or a virus, results in the stimulation of many different lymphocytes with differing specificity to all of the available antigenic determinants. Most natural antigens are extremely large. Therefore, the response generated to these molecules is polyclonal, which includes multiple antibody molecules that differ in their binding affinities. Polyclonal antibody is a mixture of multiple antibody molecules derived from multiple cells against multiple antigenic determinants found on an antigen. For instance, when an animal or person is exposed to any bacteria, different antibody molecules are made to each of the numerous antigenic determinants found on the bacteria. This is the general response initiated when a patient is immunized against a particular disease-causing organism. In serologic testing, these antibodies can and are used to detect antigen in the serum of patients. The problems with this type of diverse antibody are low specificity, because the antibody contains multiple antibodies and a high level of cross-reactivity for the same reason.

The problems addressed have been minimized through the development and use of what is termed a monoclonal antibody. This antibody is derived from one cell initially, which has been exposed to one antigenic determinant. This cell then expands, divides, and produces an antibody specific to this one antigenic determinant. This type of antibody is found rarely in nature and is usually associated with some type of abnormal immune disease process. The production of this type of an-

tibody in the laboratory has become commonplace. It is used almost extensively in serologic testing, where the identification or quantitation of an antigen is the primary goal. Monoclonal antibodies are purified antibodies cloned from a single cell. They are designed to bind to a single specific antigen. George Kohler, in 1975, originated the technique for developing monoclonal antibodies in the laboratory. This hybridoma technique allows a scientist to inject a crude antigen mixture into a mouse and then select a clone producing a specific antibody against a single cell surface antigen. This process of producing a monoclonal antibody may take as long as 3 to 6 months. The actual process involves fusing a single antibody-producing lymphocyte to a myeloma cell to form a hybrid. This hybrid then proliferates to form a cell-line called a *hybridoma*.

Classification and characteristics of antibodies

Antibody molecules, found in serum and other body fluids and secretions, may be classified into one of five distinct immunoglobulin groups or classes. The classes differ from one another in several ways, including chemical structure, serum concentration, half-life, and functional activity.

Immunoglobulin G (IgG) class antibodies constitute about 70% to 75% of the total serum immunoglobulin pool. Their half-life in serum is about 3 to 4 weeks, and IgG can cross the maternal placenta to the fetus, possibly conferring some protection in both the prenatal and postnatal periods. Structurally, IgG is about a 150,000-MW protein molecule consisting of four polypeptides (two identical light chains and two identical heavy chains) bridged by several disulfide bonds (see Figure 5-1). Although the amino acid sequence of some regions of the polypeptides is nearly identical among all IgG molecules (conserved regions), one of the ends of each polypeptide is highly variable. These variable regions create two active sites for antigen binding on each IgG molecule (see Figure 5-1). Thus, IgG antibodies are said to be bivalent—capable of binding two antigen molecules.

Antibodies of the **Immunoglobulin M (IgM)** class account for 10% to 15% of serum immunoglobulins. Their half-life in serum is about 5 days, and IgM cannot cross the placenta. A developing fetus in the second or third trimester, as well as a new-

TABLE 5-4

Comparison of IgG and IgM

Property	Immunoglobulin Class	
	IgG	*IgM*
Molecular weight (daltons)	150,000	900,000
Number of 4-polypeptide subunits	1	5
Number of antigen-binding sites	2	10
Serum concentration (mg/dL)	800-1600	50-200
Percentage of total immunoglobulin	75	10
Ability to cross placenta	+	−
Half-life (days)	23-25	5-8

born, may respond to an infectious agent with an IgM antibody response. IgM antibody molecules are very large; the whole molecule has a molecular weight of about 900,000 daltons and consists of five basic subunits—each composed of two heavy chains and two light chains (similar to an IgG molecule) and linked to another polypeptide chain (J chain) by disulfide bonds (Figure 5-24). Thus, the IgM molecule has ten antigen-binding sites available. Both IgG and IgM antibodies are commonly assayed in a variety of serologic tests. The differences in size and configuration of IgG and IgM molecules result in differences in functional activity of the molecules in serologic tests (Table 5-4).

Immunoglobulin A (IgA) antibodies represent 15% to 20% of the total serum immunoglobulin pool. IgA constitutes the predominant immuno-globulin class in certain body secretions, such as saliva, tears, and intestinal secretions. Because of this association of IgA with mucosal surfaces, it provides protection against microorganisms invading at those sites. Serum IgA occurs primarily as two subunits (each similar to an IgG molecule) linked together by a J chain. When found in secretions, however, the molecule also contains a secretory component that stabilizes the molecule. Although significant increases in serum IgA may occur in association with certain infections, the function of serum IgA is unclear, and few serologic tests for the diagnosis of infectious disease are designed to specifically detect IgA antibody.

The remaining two immunoglobulin classes, IgD and IgE, are found in very low concentrations in serum (<1%). **Immunoglobulin E (IgE)** antibody levels rise during infection by a number of parasites and may play a role in eliminating these infectious agents from the host. Although total serum IgE levels may rise during parasitic infection, IgE-specific serologic tests for the diagnosis of parasitic agents have not been developed. The role of serum IgD antibodies during infection is not known.

Primary and Secondary Antibody Responses

After exposure to an infectious agent, the host's acquired humoral immunity may respond through the production of various classes of antibody directed to one or more antigens associated with the agent. If the host has *not* been previously exposed to the antigen(s), a **primary immune response,** characterized by the relatively rapid appearance of IgM antibodies, occurs. IgM antibody levels usually peak in 1 to 2 weeks, followed by a gradual decline to undetectable levels over the next few months. At the time when IgM levels have nearly peaked, IgG (and in some cases IgA) antibodies become detectable and continue to increase for about 1 month, surpassing peak IgM levels. IgG levels remain elevated for months and then decline slowly, often persisting at low but detectable levels for years (Figure 5-25).

A subsequent exposure to the same antigen elicits a **secondary** or **anamnestic immune response,** characterized by a rapid increase in IgG antibody associated with higher levels, a prolonged elevation, and a more gradual decline (see Figure 5-25).

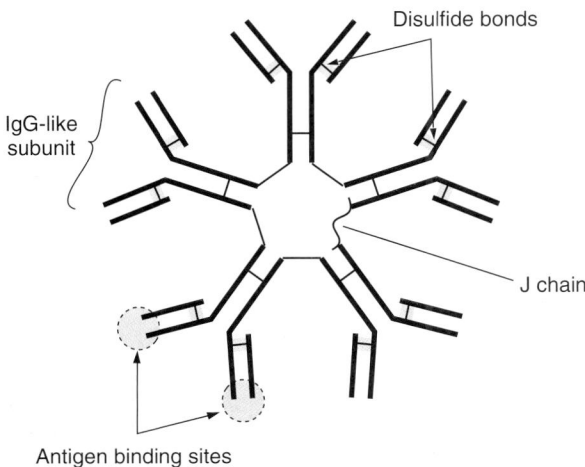

Figure 5-24

Structure of an IgM molecule.

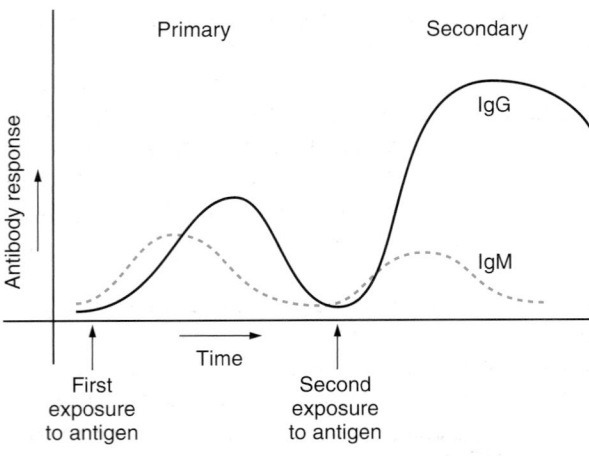

Figure 5-25

Primary and secondary antibody responses.

IgM antibody synthesis plays a minor role in a secondary immune response. Serologic tests that are designed to separately detect IgG and IgM antibodies take advantage of the differences in IgM production between a primary and a secondary immune response. Thus, a positive test result for IgM antibody is considered indicative of a primary current or very recent infection, whereas the presence of IgG antibody alone suggests a previous infection or exposure. Similarly, the presence of significant levels of IgM antibody (with or without IgG) in a newborn suggests in utero infection (IgM can be synthesized by the fetus and cannot cross the placenta), whereas IgG antibody only in the newborn is indicative of passive maternal transfer of IgG across the placenta, not in utero infection.

INTERPRETING SEROLOGIC TEST DATA

Acute and Convalescent Antibody Titers

Unless a serologic test is designed to measure IgM-specific antibody for diagnosing a current infection or is being used to determine previous infections or immunization (immune status) by testing the IgG level in a single serum specimen, serodiagnosis of an infectious disease requires measurement of IgG antibody concentration on both *acute-phase* and *convalescent-phase* serum specimens. Specific IgG antibody is usually not detected in serum col-

lected during the acute phase of the illness (within 1 week of manifestation of symptoms). A significant rise in IgG detected during the convalescent (recovery) phase (usually 2 weeks later) is diagnostic for infection and is referred to as *seroconversion*. Although seroconversion usually occurs within 2 to 3 weeks after onset of illness, it may be delayed in certain patients or types of infection.

Because some IgG antibody may already be present in a patient's acute-phase serum specimen, it is generally necessary to quantitate the concentration of antibody in both the acute-phase and convalescent-phase specimens. The concentration or *titer* of the antibody is the reciprocal of the highest serum dilution that reacts in the serologic test. Sera are generally tested as two-fold dilutions in a series of tubes. A four-fold rise (two doubling dilutions) in antibody titer between acute-phase **(acute antibody titer)** and convalescent-phase **(convalescent antibody titer)** serum specimens is considered diagnostic for a current infection. It is important that both sera be tested at the same time, because most serologic tests have an inherent variability that can alter the titer by at least two-fold. Testing the sera at the same time reduces this variability.

In practice, it is not uncommon to test a single serum specimen for IgG antibody to attempt to diagnose current or recent infection. In many cases, the presence of IgG antibody is difficult or impossible to evaluate; it may represent past infection, either clinically apparent or subclinical (without overt symptoms). In certain other cases, however, such as infections that are rare (rabies) or will have been present a relatively long time when symptoms first appear (AIDS), the presence of IgG antibody in a single serum may be diagnostic.

Antibody Specificity and Cross-Reactivity

Most antigen-antibody reactions show high specificity; that is, the antigen-binding sites on the antibody molecule react with specific antigenic determinants and not with other antigens containing different determinants. Some antigens associated with different microorganisms are closely related, however, and a host may respond by producing antibody not only to the invading organism but also to antigenically closely related organisms. These antibodies are said to *cross-react,* which may lead to misinterpretation of serologic tests. Because of this **an-**

tibody cross-reactivity, it is often best to perform a battery of serologic tests using the organisms known to show cross-reactivity and to do so on paired sera. An example of this type of testing would be a fungal battery consisting of tests for histoplasmosis, blastomycosis, and coccidioidomycosis.

False-Negative and False-Positive Serologic Test Results

An ideal serologic test should have 100% diagnostic accuracy; that is, it should be positive on all specimens from patients with infection and negative on all specimens from patients without infection by the specific agent. In practice, serologic tests, like other laboratory tests, fall short of this ideal.

A **false-negative serologic test** is defined as a negative result for a patient who really is infected. It may occur for a number of reasons. For example, a patient may *not* have an intact immune system, and therefore may not be able to respond to an antigenic stimulus. This might be the case in an individual with a congenital or acquired immunodeficiency disease or in a patient receiving either immunosuppressive therapy after organ transplantation or cancer chemotherapy. In addition, neonates may not always respond to an infectious agent because their immune systems are not fully mature. For some infections, such as Lyme disease and legionnaires' disease, antibody titers may not rise until months after acute infection, thus leading to apparent false-negative serologic test results. It is important to remember that not all individuals react the same way to antigenic stimuli, owing to the inherent genetic differences in the immune system among individuals.

A different type of false-negative result may occur in assays designed specifically to detect IgM antibody. It might be a result of competition for antigen-binding sites between IgG and IgM antibody in a serum specimen from a patient with high levels of IgG and relatively low levels of IgM (Figure 5-26). For example, IgM antibody tests are sometimes performed on the serum of a newborn to diagnose a suspected in utero infection. A newborn's serum specimen might contain maternal IgG to a specific infectious agent as well as low levels of fetal IgM. The IgG antibody molecules bind to antigen in the assay and block IgM binding, thus producing a false-negative IgM result. Most assays designed to detect IgM antibody include some ini-

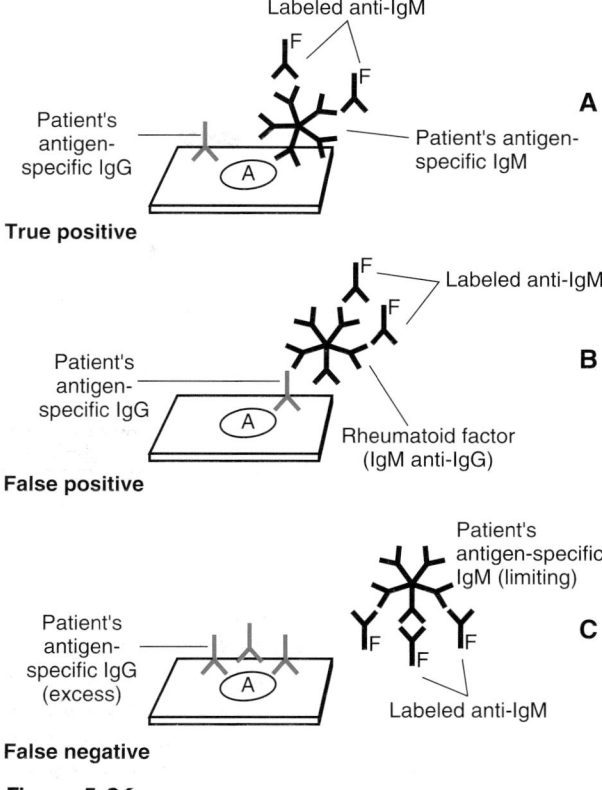

Figure 5-26 _____

Causes of false-positive and false-negative IgM assays. **A,** True-positive IgM assay. **B,** False-positive IgM assay. Rheumatoid factor (RF) binds to antigen-specific IgG and is detected with labeled anti-IgM antibody. **C,** False-negative IgM assay. Excess antigen-specific IgG inhibits antigen-specific IgM from binding.

tial procedure to physically separate IgG from IgM or to "capture" IgM in the assay and then remove IgG (discussed later in this chapter).

A **false-positive serologic test** result is a positive result for a patient who is not infected by the specific agent for which the test is designed. It might occur from the production of cross-reacting antibody, as discussed previously, or from the reactivation of a latent organism due to infection by a different organism. For example, influenza virus A infection may cause reactivation of latent cytomegalovirus (CMV) with a concomitant rise in CMV antibody. False-positive IgM antibody assays may also occur (see Figure 5-26, *B*). These are due to the presence of rheumatoid factor activity in the serum. *Rheumatoid factor* is IgM antibody (produced in some individuals) that reacts with the individual's own IgG when the IgG is bound to antigen (complexed). IgM rheumatoid factor cannot be readily differentiated from organism-specific IgM in some serologic tests. Thus, if both organism-specific IgG and rheumatoid factor (but not organism-specific IgM) are present in a patient's serum specimen, the serologic test result may be falsely positive for organism-specific IgM antibody. Finally, individuals receiving intravenous immunoglobulin, a product prepared by pooling large quantities of plasma from multiple volunteer donors, may show specific antibody to a variety of infectious agents because of passive transfer, not active infection. Laboratory personnel must be aware of this and any therapy that may be of significance in interpreting serologic test results for a specific patient specimen.

Value of Serologic Tests
Population studies
Serologic tests for a specific infectious agent or a battery of agents may be performed to determine the percentage of individuals previously exposed or infected with the agent(s) in a geographic area. This information provides investigators and public health officials with information about how widespread an infectious agent is in a given area. For example, such studies have shown that the fungus *Histoplasma capsulatum* (which causes histoplasmosis), found in soil, is widely distributed in the Ohio River Valley and that the bacterium *Borrelia correlia burgdorferi* (which causes Lyme disease), transmitted by a tick vector, is common in the upper Midwest, New England, and Middle Atlantic states. Similarly, serologic studies performed on animals that are reservoirs for human disease may alert public health officials that the disease (for example, viral encephalitis) may be active in the area and may pose a threat to humans.

Immune status testing
In several situations it may be important to determine whether an individual is immune (either through previous infection or immunization) to a specific infectious disease. For example, many state health agencies require that individuals must undergo serologic testing for syphilis before being issued a marriage license. Also, health care fa-

cilities may require prospective employees to show evidence of immunity to varicella-zoster virus (which causes chicken-pox). This is because if infected, they may transmit the virus during the incubation period (before symptoms develop) to susceptible patients. Infection with varicella-zoster in a newborn or immunosuppressed patient may be life threatening. Similarly, female employees at risk for becoming pregnant may be screened for rubella or CMV infection, both agents that may cause significant morbidity or mortality to the developing fetus if contracted during pregnancy. It is generally recommended that all women of childbearing age be tested for their rubella immune status and, if it is negative, that they be vaccinated before considering pregnancy.

An additional situation in which immune status testing might be considered is whole organ or bone marrow transplantation. Cytomegalovirus may reside latently in leukocytes of donor tissue and may cause significant disease in a nonimmune recipient. Thus, it is recommended that a CMV-negative transplant recipient receive tissue and blood products from a CMV-negative donor.

Congenital infections
Serology is often used to attempt to establish the diagnosis of congenital infection (acquired in utero) in a newborn, because some agents have the ability to cross the placenta and cause infection of the fetus. Such infections may cause only minimal symptoms in the mother during pregnancy, and thus may go undiagnosed at the time. If the mother is nonimmune, however, the infection may be significant to the fetus. The agents most commonly tested for are the TORCH agents— Toxoplasma gondii (which causes toxoplasmosis), rubella virus, CMV, and herpes simplex virus—and *Treponema pallidum* (which causes syphilis). Testing the mother's serum for IgG antibody is useless unless she was screened prenatally or early in pregnancy and found to be negative. Because the TORCH agents are common infectious agents, many individuals have antibody remaining from previous infections. Similarly, testing for IgG antibody in the newborn is of no value, because maternal IgG crosses the placenta and is present in neonatal serum. Testing for maternal IgM antibody is likewise of little value (unless infection occurred

near the time of delivery), because it may be undetectable by 1 or 2 months following infection. Thus, as previously discussed, IgM antibody detection on neonatal serum is the method of choice for serologic diagnosis of congenital infection by one of the TORCH agents.

Infections after the newborn period

Beyond the newborn period, serologic diagnosis generally requires testing paired sera to detect a four-fold rise in antibody. More and more commercial diagnostic tests are designed, however, to be performed without serial dilution (on undiluted serum or after a single serum dilution) and establishment of titers; in these cases, the determination of a single positive result suggests, but does not always prove, current infection. Generally, if serologic diagnosis of current infection on a single serum specimen is to be attempted, an IgM assay as well as an IgG-specific assay should be done. If both assays are *negative,* the patient has probably not been infected. If both assays are positive, or just IgM antibody is detected, the patient has probably been recently infected. If just IgG antibody is present, the patient has probably been infected in the past and does not have a current infection. It is very important that laboratorians completely understand all the performance characteristics of a commercial serologic test system.

ANTIBODY DETECTION METHODS AND APPLICATIONS

The earliest serologic test used serum from the patient in progressive 1:2 dilutions, which produce progressively lower amounts of antibody. The antigen from an infectious agent is added to each tube in the same amount. This antigen is often attached to some form of indicator such as latex beads or red blood cells. A positive response is reported as the highest dilution of serum showing reactivity (1:16, 1:32, etc.). This type of serial dilution method is not very precise. The difference of only one tube in dilution is not considered significant in determining the presence of a recent infection.

Many of the test methods described in the discussion of antigen detection are useful for antibody detection. These include particle agglutina-

tion tests such as latex agglutination, precipitation tests (Ouchterlony diffusion and counterimmunoelectrophoresis), enzyme immunoassays, and microscope-assisted, labeled-reagent methods. In addition, a number of methods have been developed uniquely for antibody detection. Antibody tests for a wide variety of infectious agents are available commercially (Table 5-5). All of these methods, along with specific diagnostic applications, are discussed in the remainder of this section.

Particle Agglutination Assays

Agglutinating antibodies react with antigens on the surface of microscopic particles to form visible clumps of particles. Such agglutination tests can be performed on the surface of glass slides or in test tubes. Agglutination tests can be classified as either *direct* (natural particle) or *indirect* (carrier particle) agglutination.

Direct, natural particle agglutination

Serologic tests based on direct or natural particle agglutination take advantage of antigens that are nat-

TABLE 5-5

Examples of Some Commercially Available Serologic Tests for the Diagnosis of Infectious Disease

Organisms	Serologic Test Method(s) Available
Blastomyces dermatitidis	CF, ID, EIA
Bordetella pertussis	EIA
Borrelia burgdorferi	IFA, EIA, WB, IgM cap
Cytomegalovirus	EIA, LA, IFA
Helicobacter pylori	EIA
Hepatitis virus A, B, C	EIA
Herpes simplex virus	EIA, LA, IFA
Human immunodeficiency virus types 1, 2	EIA, IFA, WB
Histoplasma capsulatum	CF, ID, EIA
Influenza virus A, B	EIA
Legionella pneumophila	IFA, EIA
Mycoplasma pneumoniae	CF, EIA, IFA
Respiratory syncytial virus	EIA
Rubella virus	EIA, IFA, HAI
Streptococcus pyogenes	NT
Toxoplasma gondii	EIA, IFA, LA
Treponema pallidum	IHA, IFA

CF, Complement fixation; *EIA,* enzyme immunoassay; *HAI,* hemagglutination inhibition; *ID,* immunodiffusion; *IFA,* indirect fluorescent antibody; *IgM cap,* IgM capture; *IHA,* indirect hemagglutination; *LA,* latex agglutination; *NT,* neutralization; *WB,* Western blot.

urally occurring on biologic cells. Most commonly, these cells are whole bacteria or erythrocytes.

WHOLE BACTERIAL CELL AGGLUTINATION

In whole bacterial cell agglutination, surface antigens that make up the bacterial cell wall or capsule function to allow cross-linking and visible agglutination of the cells in the presence of specific antibody. The so-called febrile agglutinin tests, for the detection of antibodies to *Brucella* sp., *Salmonella* sp., and *Francisella tularensis,* are based on bacterial agglutination. In some cases, an organism different from the suspected infectious agent may carry a chemically related antigen and may be more easily used in agglutination tests than the actual infectious agent. This approach is used in the Weil-Felix test to determine infection resulting from certain rickettsial agents by testing for agglutinating antibodies to various bacteria in the genus *Proteus.* Both febrile agglutinin and Weil-Felix agglutinin tests have been generally replaced in the United States by more sensitive and specific methods of diagnosis.

DIRECT HEMAGGLUTINATION

A special kind of natural particle agglutination test, known as hemagglutination, detects antibodies to naturally occurring antigens present on the surface of erythrocytes. During infection with *Mycoplasma pneumoniae,* for example, antibodies that can agglutinate human erythrocytes at 4° C but not at 37° C develop in some patients. These *cold-agglutinating antibodies,* which rise very quickly, may suggest *Mycoplasma pneumoniae* infection, but the test lacks sensitivity and specificity.

Another example of a direct hemagglutination test is the detection of heterophile antibodies in the acute stage of infectious mononucleosis (resulting from Epstein-Barr virus infection). Heterophile antibodies are antibodies developed in one mammalian species that react with surface antigens on cells of an unrelated mammalian species. In the case of infectious mononucleosis, human heterophile antibody reacts with horse, ox, and sheep erythrocytes. In the appropriate clinical setting, and when performed by the appropriate method, heterophile antibody testing is diagnostically very useful and is commonly used in clinical laboratories today. It may be performed as a tube test or, more commonly, as a slide or card agglutination test (Monospot, Ortho Diagnostics, Raritan, NJ; Mono-Test, Wampole Laboratories, Cranbury, NJ: Figure 5-27).

HEMAGGLUTINATION INHIBITION

A serologic test that has great historic significance to diagnostic serology, particularly to viral serology, is the hemagglutination inhibition (HI) test. This test takes advantage of the fact that a number of viral agents, including rubella and influenza viruses, have surface antigens that can agglutinate erythrocytes from certain mammalian species. Antibodies present in sera can bind to the virus, thus inhibiting this agglutination reaction. The hemagglutination inhibition antibody titer is the highest dilution of the patient's serum that completely inhibits agglutination of the erythrocytes by the virus. Most HI tests have been replaced by other methods for determining viral antibodies, particularly enzyme immunoassays.

Indirect, carrier particle agglutination

A variety of antigens can be passively or chemically coupled to naturally occurring particles such as erythrocytes or to synthetic particles such as latex beads. In this arrangement, the particle can then be agglutinated by specific antibody found in a patient's serum.

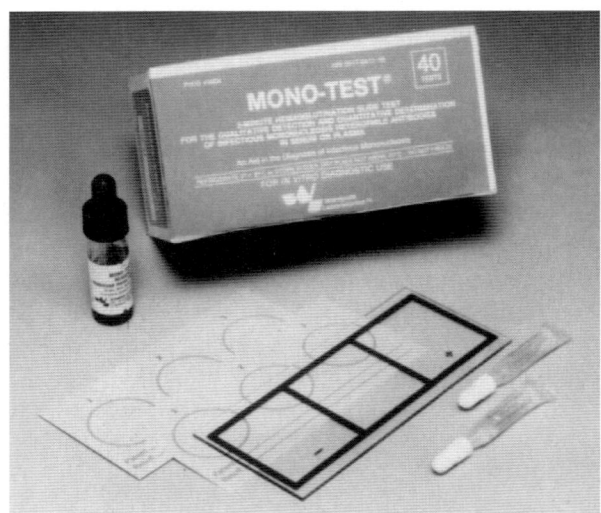

Figure 5-27

Mono-Test for the detection of heterophile antibodies produced during infectious mononucleosis. (Courtesy Wampole Laboratories, Division of Carter-Wallace, Inc., Cranbury, NJ.)

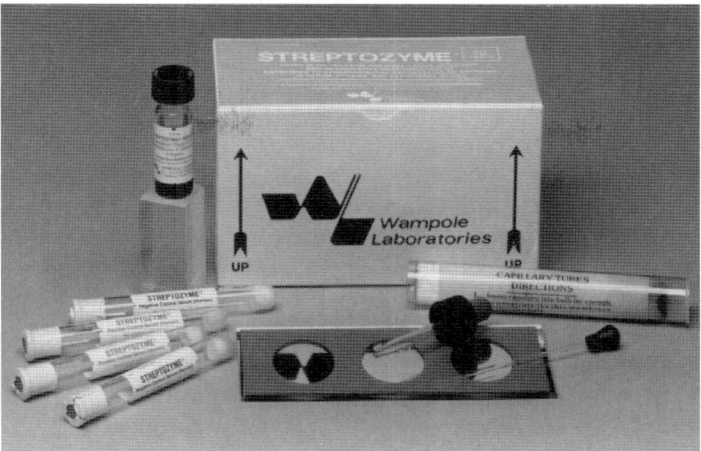

Figure 5-28

Streptozyme test for the detection of antibodies to streptococcal products. (Courtesy Wampole Laboratories, Division of Carter-Wallace, Inc., Cranbury, NJ.)

INDIRECT HEMAGGLUTINATION

In indirect or passive hemagglutination (IHA), microbial antigens are attached to erythrocytes after chemical treatment of the cells with tannic acid, chromic chloride, glutaraldehyde, or another substance that promotes cross-linking of the antigens. The sensitized cells can then be reacted with patient's serum to determine agglutinating antibody. One example of an IHA test is for the detection of antibodies to streptococcal extracellular antigens (Streptozyme, Wampole Laboratories, Cranbury, NJ). In this procedure, aldehyde-fixed sheep erythrocytes are sensitized with group A streptococcal exoantigens. When patient serum containing specific antibody is reacted with the cells on a slide, a positive agglutination reaction occurs (Figure 5-28). Another important diagnostic application for the IHA test is the microhemagglutination assay for *Treponema pallidum* (MHA-TP), the causative agent of syphilis. In this test, specific treponemal antibodies are detected using treponemal antigen-coated erythrocytes. The MHA-TP test is generally used as a second or confirmatory test in patients who have tested positive on a syphilis screening test to detect nontreponemal antibodies (VDRL, RPR; see Serologic Testing of Syphilis).

LATEX AGGLUTINATION

Latex beads, which can bind antibodies and can be used to detect microbial antigens in clinical spec-imens, can also be sensitized with antigen and used in agglutination tests to detect serum antibodies. Commercial serologic tests based on latex agglutination are available for a number of viral infections, including CMV, rubella, and infectious mononucleosis (heterophile antibody), as well as a few bacterial (streptococcal, mycoplasmal antibodies), fungal (candidal antibody), and parasitic (toxoplasmal antibody) infections.

Precipitation Assays

Unlike agglutination assays, which rely on visible clumping of sensitized, insoluble particles when antigen and antibody are cross-linked, precipitation assays rely on transforming soluble antigens and antibody into insoluble, visible products that precipitate in a limited space. Those methods with diagnostic significance for serologic tests are double immunodiffusion, counterimmunoelectrophoresis, and flocculation tests.

Double immunodiffusion

As described previously in this chapter, double or Ouchterlony immunodiffusion tests (Figure 5-4) are performed in agar or agarose gels and rely on passive diffusion of antigen and antibody. For antibody detection, a known crude or purified antigen extract of a microorganism is placed in one well of the agar plate, and patient's serum in an adjacent well. If the patient has precipitating antibodies to the antigen(s), one or more precipitin lines will develop between the wells. Because the test relies on passive diffusion of molecules, reactions may take 48 to 72 hours to develop. Double immunodiffusion is commonly used today to detect antibody to a battery of fungal pathogens, including *Histoplasma capsulatum, Blastomyces dermatitidis,* and *Coccidioides immitis.*

Counterimmunoelectrophoresis

Counterimmunoelectrophoresis (CIE) is a variation of double immunodiffusion; it adds an electric current to the gel to allow known antigens and a patient's serum containing antibodies to migrate and form precipitin bands more quickly. CIE was fully discussed earlier as it related to antigen detection. It is not commonly used for serologic diagnosis today, because more sensitive and less cumbersome methods are available.

Flocculation

Flocculation tests are a variation of precipitation tests that also have some properties of agglutination assays. In these tests, because of the chemical nature of the antigen (not a truly soluble antigen), the antigen-antibody reaction forms a macroscopically or microscopically visible clump or precipitate of fine particles that remain in suspension. The most important applications for flocculation tests in antibody detection relate to syphilis serology, and these are discussed in detail.

Following infection with *T. pallidum,* the body reacts by developing two different types of antibodies—*specific* or *treponemal* antibodies, directed against *T. pallidum* antigens, and *nonspecific* or *nontreponemal* antibodies, directed against normal host tissue. These nontreponemal antibodies are also referred to as *reagin* antibodies.

The most commonly used treponemal tests for the diagnosis of syphilis are the MHA-TP, already discussed, and the fluorescent treponemal antibody absorption test (FTA-ABS; see later in this chapter). These tests are very sensitive and specific, but they are not suited for testing (screening) large numbers of individuals, because (1) they are technically demanding and time consuming and (2) like other diagnostic tests, they would result in decreased diagnostic accuracy if applied to a large population with a disease of low prevalence. They are best suited for confirmatory testing.

Nontreponemal tests are technically easier and more rapid to perform; therefore, they are the tests of choice for syphilis screening. The most commonly used nontreponemal tests today are the VDRL (Venereal Disease Research Laboratory) and the RPR (rapid plasma reagin) tests.

The VDRL test is a microscopic flocculation test run on heat-inactivated serum and performed on glass slides. The test uses cardiolipin-lecithin-cholesterol particles as antigen and may be performed as both a qualitative and quantitative test. It may also be used to test cerebrospinal fluid to diagnose neurosyphilis and to follow titers in a newborn to diagnose congenital syphilis. Because of the extreme attention to reagent preparation and quality control required, the VDRL test is being replaced by tests like the RPR.

The RPR test is a commercially available nontreponemal test that uses cardiolipin-lecithin-cholesterol antigen with carbon particles to allow macroscopic determination of flocculation (Figure 5-29). Sera are tested (without heating) on cardboard cards. Newborn serum and cerebrospinal fluid should not be tested by this method.

Because both the VDRL and RPR tests are not specific for treponemal antigens, they are subject to false-positive results, the rate of which may be as high as 10% to 30% for all sera tested. False-positive results occur most commonly in conjunction with autoimmune disorders (lupus erythematosus, rheumatic fever), infectious diseases (infectious mononucleosis, hepatitis), in pregnancy, and in old age. It is imperative that positive VDRL or RPR test results be followed by specific confirmatory treponemal antibody tests.

Complement Fixation Test

Complement fixation (CF) tests are versatile assays that can be used for both antibody and antigen detection. They have been used for many years, particularly for antibody detection, but have gradually been replaced by more rapid and sensitive assays. CF tests are broadly applicable for a variety of infectious agents, however, and are still used in reference and public health laboratories for certain agents.

Although a discussion of the serum complement

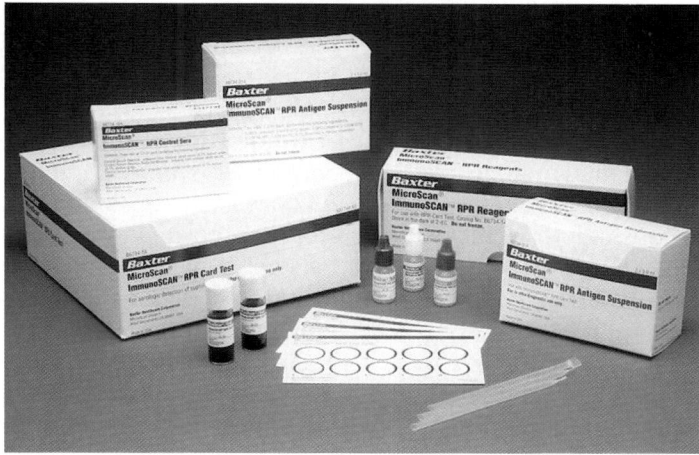

Figure 5-29

RPR card test for detection of nontreponemal antibodies. (Courtesy Baxter U.S. Distribution, Division of Baxter Healthcare, Inc., Deerfield, Ill.)

protein system is beyond the scope of this chapter, it is important to note that the system plays a vital role in a number of immunologic functions. The proteins involved in the system are usually found in an inactive form; however, once activated, the proteins become involved in a chemical cascade that involves production of enzymes with a variety of biologic activities. Activation of complement occurs by the classical pathway when specific IgG or IgM antibody combines with antigen and exposes a complement-binding site on the antibody molecule. It is the cell-lysing ability of activated complement components that is important in CF tests.

The CF test requires both an indicator system and a test system (Figure 5-30). The *indicator system* typically consists of a combination of sheep erythrocytes, rabbit antibody to sheep erythrocytes, and guinea pig complement (a menagerie of biologics). When these three components are present and active, the rabbit antibody first combines with the sheep erythrocytes, and complement is subsequently bound (fixed) to the antibody-antigen complex, resulting in activation of complement by the classical pathway; this results in cell lysis. The *test system* consists of a mixture of known antigen and the patient's serum that may or may not contain specific antibody.

The CF test is performed as a two-step procedure (see Figure 5-30). The patient's serum is seri-

ally diluted in test tubes, and each dilution is mixed with a known amount of antigen (test system). A fixed amount of complement is then added to each tube, and the mixture is incubated for a short time. Next, the sheep erythrocytes and rabbit antibody are added to each tube, and the tubes are incubated

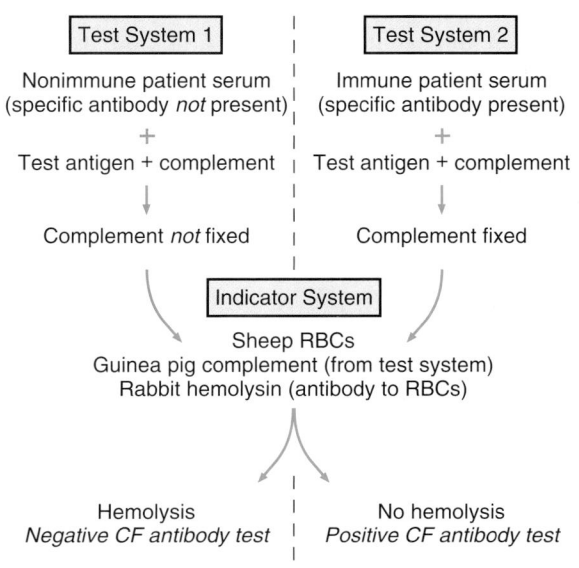

Figure 5-30

Principles of complement fixation (CF) test. *RBCs,* Red blood cells.

again (indicator system). If the patient's serum had specific antibodies to the test antigen, complement would be fixed by the test system and *not* available to lyse the erythrocytes of the indicator system. If the patient's serum did not have specific antibody to the test antigen, complement would be fixed by the indicator system, resulting in erythrocyte lysis. The CF antibody titer is considered the highest dilution of patient serum resulting in no hemolysis. It is usually read spectrophotometrically.

Neutralization Tests

Neutralization tests for antibody detection are based on the interaction of a biologically active antigen with antibodies that can block or render inactive the biologic activity of the antigen. These neutralizing antibodies may play an important role not only in serologic tests but also in functioning as protective antibodies in vivo. For example, immunity to a number of viruses depends on circulating antibodies that may neutralize, or destroy the infectivity of, viruses that reach the blood stream. Neutralization probably occurs because the antibody binds to the viral particle and blocks subsequent attachment of the virus to receptor sites on target cells. Neutralizing antibodies to viruses can be measured in vitro by the use of cell cultures. Other examples of neutralization assays are the antistreptolysin-O (ASO) neutralization test to detect antistreptococcal antibodies and the *Treponema pallidum* immobilization (TPI) test to measure antitreponemal antibodies.

Viral neutralization

In viral neutralization, a patient's serum is serially diluted, and each dilution is mixed with a standard amount of a known virus suspected of causing disease in the patient. The virus-serum mixtures are then inoculated to a series of cell culture tubes or flasks. If the patient's serum contains neutralizing antibody to the virus, the antibody will block viral infection and cytopathic effect (CPE) on the cells. The neutralizing antibody titer is the highest dilution of the patient's serum to completely block CPE. For diagnosis of current disease, acute-phase and convalescent-phase sera should be tested. Viral neutralization assays are highly sensitive and specific, but they are also technically demanding and require the use of live virus and cell culture.

They are not commonly used serologic tests today, but neutralization tests are valuable in identifying an unknown virus with known antibody.

Antistreptolysin-O test

Streptococcus pyogenes, or group A β-hemolytic streptococcus, causes a number of acute, common pyogenic (associated with pus, or neutrophil response) infections, including pharyngitis and skin infections. In addition, the organism is responsible for certain nonsuppurative (nonpyogenic) diseases, such as acute rheumatic fever and poststreptococcal glomerulonephritis, which occur weeks after the acute infectious process and are thought to be autoimmune or immune complex–mediated diseases; that is, the host develops antibodies to streptococcal components that cross-react with normal host tissue. Although the pyogenic infections are best diagnosed by isolation of the organism in culture, the nonsuppurative diseases occur at a time when the organism may no longer be present; thus, serologic diagnosis is usually performed.

The antistreptolysin-O or ASO antibody test is commonly used to demonstrate serologic response to *S. pyogenes.* This test measures the ability of a patient's serum to neutralize the erythrocyte-lysing ability of a specific streptococcal enzyme, streptolysin O. Very high titers of antistreptolysin-O antibody usually develop in most cases of rheumatic fever, but the titers and percentages of patients with poststreptococcal glomerulonephritis who develop ASO antibodies is significantly lower. Thus, when these diseases are suspected in patients who do *not* show an elevation in ASO titers, additional serologic tests directed at other streptococcal enzymes should be performed; the most valuable of these are antibody to DNase B and antibody to hyaluronidase. These latter tests are also performed as enzyme neutralization assays.

Because serodiagnosis is usually attemped late after acute infection, it may be difficult to show seroconversion in streptococcal neutralization tests. Thus, "upper limit of normal" titers have been established: these vary by patient age and geographic location. These upper limits should not discourage an attempt to show seroconversion, however. A number of screening tests, based on particle agglutination, are also available to detect antibodies to streptococcal enzymes.

Treponema pallidum immobilization

The TPI test, like the MHA-TP and FTA-ABS tests mentioned previously, is a specific treponemal antibody test. Because it requires live organisms, however, it is generally performed only in research laboratories evaluating newer treponemal tests. The TPI test measures the ability of a patient's serum to neutralize the motility (immobilize) of *T. pallidum* organisms and is read microscopically.

Microscope-Assisted Labeled-Reagent Techniques

The basic principles that were discussed in section A for the immunomicroscopic detection of antigens with labeled antibodies (fluorescent or enzymatic labels) also apply to the detection of antibodies. The most commonly used test method for this purpose is the indirect fluorescent antibody (IFA) test. This method has been used for many years and still remains the method of choice for serologic detection of a number of infectious diseases. In addition, the method can be used to differentially measure IgG and IgM antibodies. The

IFA test and some variations that increase the sensitivity of the basic technique are discussed.

Indirect fluorescent antibody test

In the basic IFA test for antibody, whole microbial cells (bacteria, fungi, protozoan parasites) or virus-infected mammalian cells are washed and then fixed at a given density to glass slides (Figure 5-31, *A*). Fixation is usually accomplished with methanol, ethanol, or acetone at room temperature or lower. The patient's serum is then serially diluted, applied to different fixed-cell preparations, and incubated for a short time (10 to 30 minutes) at 22° to 37° C in a humid environment to prevent drying; this procedure allows antigen-antibody binding to occur. The slides are then washed repeatedly with a buffered solution to remove unbound antibody, and a second, nonhuman antibody, which is fluorescein-labeled and reactive with human immunoglobulin (IgG, IgM, or total), is applied. The slides are incubated again as described, and then washed, air-dried, and viewed using a microscope fitted with a light source and fil-

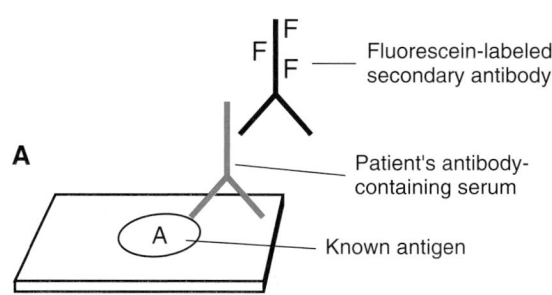

A

Fluorescein-labeled secondary antibody

Patient's antibody-containing serum

Known antigen

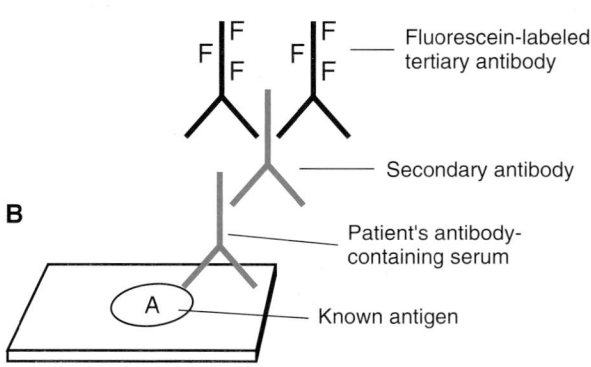

B

Fluorescein-labeled tertiary antibody

Secondary antibody

Patient's antibody-containing serum

Known antigen

Figure 5-31

Indirect fluorescence antibody **(A)** and double indirect fluorescence antibody **(B)** tests for antibody detection.

ters to excite the fluorescein (FA microscope). If specific antibody to the microbial antigen is present in the patient's serum, the antibody will bind and permit the fluorescein-labeled antibody to form secondary binding. The cells will fluoresce and be scored on a semiquantitative scale as positive (1+ to 4+) or negative. The FA titer is given as the reciprocal of the highest dilution of the patient's serum giving a minimum level of fluorescence (often at 2+ or greater).

Indirect FA tests are commonly used to detect antibody to a number of infectious agents, including the TORCH agents, Epstein-Barr virus, *Legionella pneumophila, B. burgdorferi, Rickettsia rickettsii, M. pneumoniae,* and *T. pallidum.* As mentioned previously, the detection of *T. pallidum* using the classic fluorescent treponemal antibody absorption (FTA-ABS) test is perhaps the most widely used and important application of IFA tests. This procedure uses the pathogenic Nichols strain of *T. pallidum* as test antigen and the nonpathogenic Reiter strain in a pretest absorption procedure to remove cross-reacting serum antibodies that could produce false-positive results.

Indirect FA tests are also useful in detecting IgM or IgG specific antibody, by using a fluorescein-labeled second antibody highly specific for human IgM or IgG, respectively. As discussed previously, IgM-specific assays are particularly important in several clinical settings. As with any IgM test, indirect FA for IgM is subject to false-negative results owing to excess IgG and to false-positive results owing to rheumatoid factor (IgM anti-IgG). To avoid these problems, IgG should be physically removed or functionally inactivated during IgM-specific assays.

Several methods are available for removal or inactivation of serum IgG. One of the most popular methods for physical removal of IgG uses miniature ion-exchange chromatography columns to trap IgM while allowing IgG to be washed through with a buffer solution. The IgM antibody is then collected by elution from the column with a lower-pH buffer; these columns are available commercially. Another method of removing IgG from whole serum utilizes adsorption to protein A found in the cell wall of staphylococci. Protein A binds most subclasses of human IgG, thus facilitating their removal. Yet another useful method utilizes anti–human IgG to inactivate or remove

(requires precipitation and centrifugation) IgG for IgM specific assays. This method has the additional advantage of removing rheumatoid factor, because the latter will bind to the IgG–anti-IgG complexes.

The utility of indirect FA tests is limited by a number of factors, including the labor-intensive nature of the procedures and the subjectivity of reading endpoints. The ability to visualize and evaluate reactions, however, gives a high level of certainty to the procedure. Thus, newer serologic assays are often evaluated with indirect FA procedures. Indirect FA tests are also quickly adaptable to studying serologic response to newly discovered infectious agents.

In cases in which the infectious agent does not produce enough antigen for detection in body fluids, testing the cell directly must be considered. The use of specific antibody for the infectious agent enables the detection of the agent inside the infected cells. Direct immunofluorescent techniques are the assay of choice under these conditions.

Fluorescent antibody tests with enhanced sensitivity

A number of variations of the indirect FA test have been developed. The basic objective in most of these procedures has been to increase sensitivity while maintaining specificity of the assay. One example of such a procedure is the *double indirect* FA test (see Figure 5-31, *B*). This method uses a second, unlabeled antibody to bind to microbial-specific antibody in the patient's serum. The fluorescein-labeled antibody is directed at the second antibody. The additional step amplifies the reaction, because multiple molecules of the second antibody may bind to the patient's antibody, thus providing additional binding sites for the fluorescein-labeled antibody. Another example of enhanced FA test sensitivity uses a biotin-labeled second antibody. The binding of this reagent to the patient's antibody is detected using fluorescein-labeled avidin. Each biotin molecule binds four avidin molecules, thus increasing the total amount of bound fluorescein and, ultimately, the sensitivity of the assay. These and other microscopic techniques using fluorescent as well as enzymatic labels will continue to play an important role in serologic diagnosis of infectious diseases.

Enzyme-Linked Immunosorbent Assay and Related Techniques

Today, many laboratories are using some form of ELISA testing. In this type of test, results are reported not as titer but as to how the results relate to the relative amount of signal generated by the patient's serum when compared with that of a known weakly positive serum. Results are usually reported as either relative units with a numerical reference range (5 to 20 U/mL), or as a ratio of results in the sample to the low positive control (patient 15 U/mL, control 10 U/mL, ratio 1.5). It is impossible to compare the results of serial dilution methods with those of ELISA because of the variation from test to test. There is, however, a linear relationship in each individual assay between the amount of antibody present. This means that a doubling in the result yields a two-fold rise in the amount of antibody.

Immunoassays for the detection of serum antibody are performed in a manner similar to immunoassays for microbial antigen detection, except that the roles of antigen and antibody are reversed. Most serum antibody assays are performed as solid-phase assays using antigen-coated tubes or wells. Ninety-six-well microtitration plates have become popular for this purpose because of the large number of tests that can be run and the small serum volume required. Single-test, single-

serum dilution cassettes are also available from commercial sources for the low-volume or infrequent test setting. In either case, patient antibody is bound to the microbial antigen–coated surface, and the antibody is detected using a labeled (radioactive, fluorescent, enzymatic) anti–human immunoglobulin. Enzyme immunoassays (EIAs), or more specifically, solid-phase EIAs (enzyme-linked immunosorbent assay, ELISA), are the most popular types of immunoassay in use today.

Enzyme immunoassays

Enzyme immunoassays are widely used for the serologic diagnosis of infectious diseases. They have become popular for a number of reasons. These include (1) the availability of commercial EIA kits for a large number of infectious agents; (2) the adaptability of EIA tests to automation, thus allowing more tests to be performed in shorter times; and (3) the objective interpretation of test results with colored end products that can be read spectrophotometrically. Many commercial products are tailored to suit high-volume laboratories; others are designed for single-use applications on individual patient specimens (Figure 5-32).

INDIRECT ELISA

Most EIAs used in the clinical laboratory for antibody detection are performed as indirect ELISA

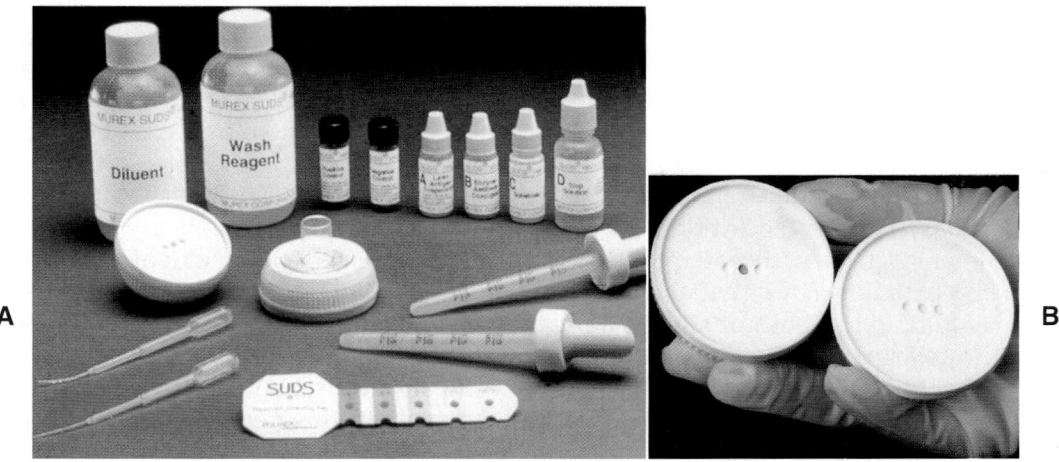

Figure 5-32

Single-use diagnostic system (SUDS®) for the detection of antibody to HIV-1 by enzyme immunoassay (EIA). **A,** Components of the test kit. **B,** Cartridges showing positive *(left)* and negative *(right)* reactions. (Courtesy Murex Corp., Norcross, GA.)

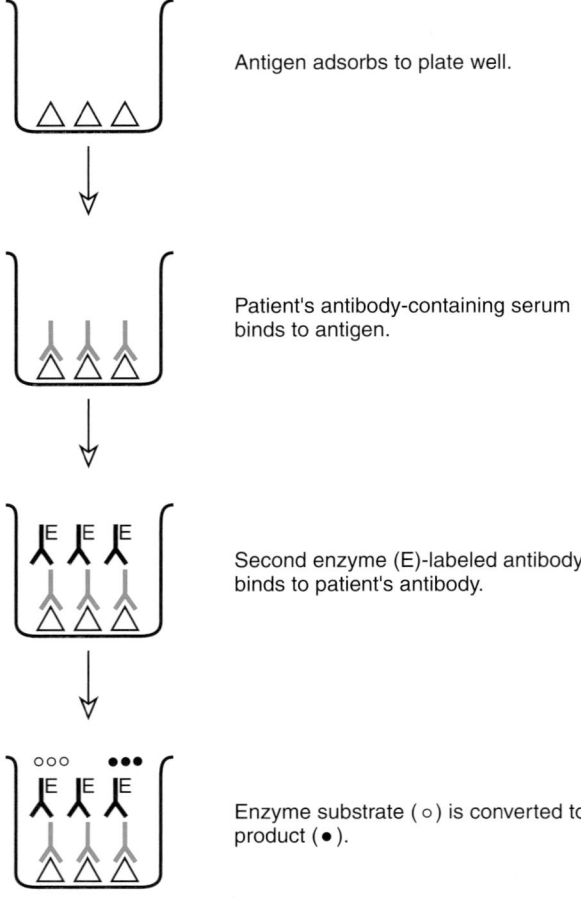

Antigen adsorbs to plate well.

Patient's antibody-containing serum binds to antigen.

Second enzyme (E)-labeled antibody binds to patient's antibody.

Enzyme substrate (○) is converted to product (●).

Figure 5-33

Principle of indirect solid-phase enzyme immunoassay (ELISA) for antibody detection.

tests (Figure 5-33). In this procedure, the antigen of interest is first attached to the solid phase. The patient's serum is then added and allowed to incubate. After a wash procedure, antibody bound to the solid phase is detected with an enzyme-labeled, anti-immunoglobulin, secondary antibody. This secondary antibody may be anti–human IgG, IgM, or a combination of both. It should be remembered, however, that ELISA tests for IgM antibody are susceptible to the same problems of false-positive and false-negative results as IFA assays for IgM. One of the methods to physically separate patient's IgG and IgM antibodies should also be employed for ELISA tests for IgM.

IgM ANTIBODY CAPTURE ELISA

One of the alternative approaches that can be used to detect IgM antibody is referred to as *IgM antibody capture ELISA* (Figure 5-34). In this procedure, the solid phase is first coated with animal antibody specific for human IgM. The patient's serum is added and incubated, and then the tube or plate is washed. At this point, IgM antibody molecules, regardless of specificity, should be bound to the solid phase, and antibodies of other immunoglobulin classes should be washed away. The next step in the IgM capture assay involves adding the antigen of interest and can be performed in one of two ways. The antigen can be directly labeled with an enzyme or can be added unlabeled. In either case, the antigen is bound to the solid phase if specific IgM antibody is present. With labeled antigen, the assay is completed by added enzyme substrate and measuring the colored product. Alternatively, unlabeled antigen bound to IgM is detected by adding a secondary enzyme-labeled antibody directed against the specific antigen, followed by addition of enzyme substrate. The amount of colored product is proportional to the amount of specific IgM captured on the solid phase.

The IgM antibody capture assay has the advantage of eliminating the need for separation of IgG that might compete with IgM and yield false-negative results. The capture assay may be susceptible to false-positive results because of IgM rheumatoid factor bound to the solid phase. Modifications of the assay can be employed to reduce the possibility of this problem. Although IgM capture assays offer several advantages, they have not become readily available from commercial sources. Indirect ELISA tests for IgM employing IgG-IgM separation steps are much more widely available.

Other immunoassays

The basic principles of immunoassays utilizing fluorochromes or radiolabels have been described earlier in the discussion of antigen detection. Fluorescent immunoassays (FIAs) for antibody detection use fluorochrome-labeled anti–human immunoglobulin to detect antigen-specific antibody bound to the solid phase. The bound fluorochrome gives a fluorescent signal that may be detected by fluorometry. The assay has the advantage of not re-

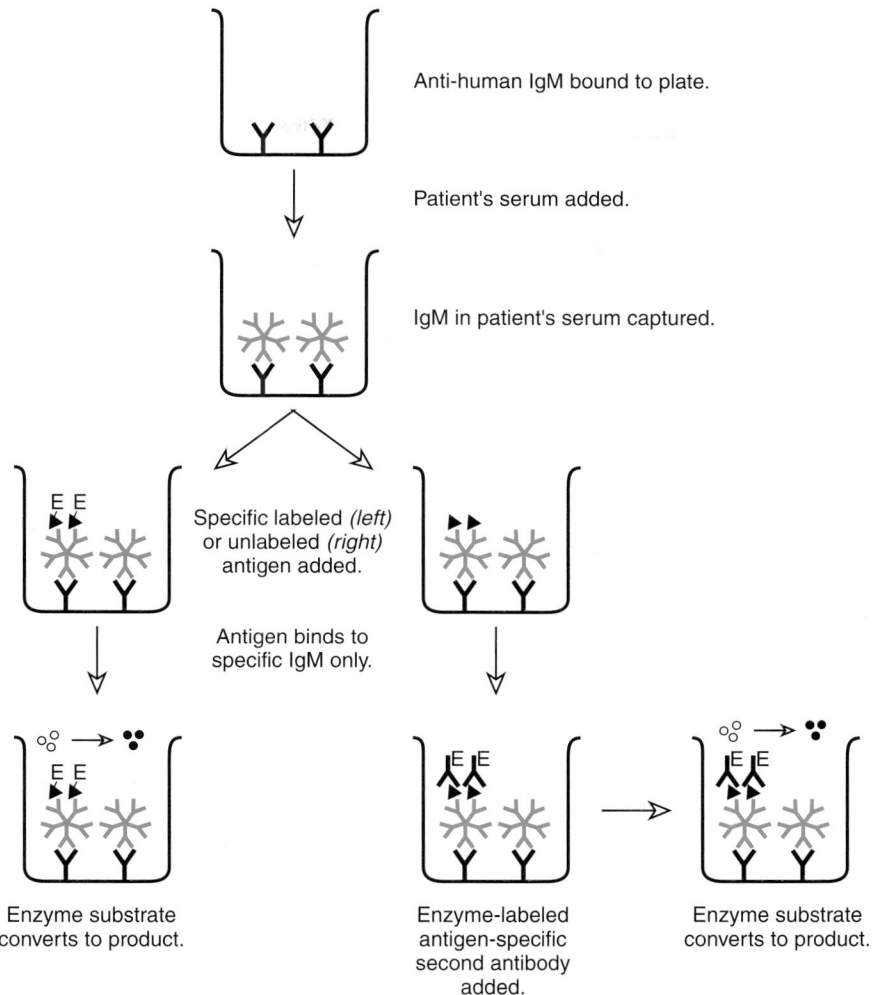

Anti-human IgM bound to plate.

Patient's serum added.

IgM in patient's serum captured.

Specific labeled *(left)* or unlabeled *(right)* antigen added.

Antigen binds to specific IgM only.

Enzyme substrate converts to product.

Enzyme-labeled antigen-specific second antibody added.

Enzyme substrate converts to product.

Figure 5-34

IgM antibody capture enzyme-linked immunosorbent assay (ELISA) using labeled antigen *(left)* or unlabeled antigen; a secondary enzyme-labeled antibody is added later *(right)*.

quiring the addition of enzyme substrate and the washing steps needed in ELISA. Some additional problems, however, are associated with FIA, and only a few commercial companies offer antibody detection tests using this assay. Similarly, radioimmunoassays (RIAs) for antibody detection, although very sensitive and specific, are not commonly available for serodiagnosis. Because of the hazards and disposal problems associated with radioisotopes, most commercial companies have replaced RIAs with EIAs.

Western Blotting

Although serologic test methods such as IFA assays and EIAs generally provide excellent sensitivity and specificity in most clinical applications, they are limited in their ability to resolve the complex antibody response occurring during infection by most microbes. Because most antigens used in these assays are crude microbial extracts, a positive result may represent an antibody response to one or to many antigens. EIA tests may be designed to detect antibody to a number of individual microbial antigens, but this requires the expensive and labor-intensive process of purifying antigens and running multiple EIAs. As an alternative, the technique of immunoblotting or Western blotting was developed. This technique allows for characterization of multiple antibodies to a microorganism by first utilizing an electrophoretic separation of the microbial antigens and transfer to a nitrocellulose membrane. Western blotting has gained importance and is extensively used to confirm antibodies to human immunodeficiency virus type 1 (HIV-1) in patients whose sera have been repeatedly reactive in EIA tests. It is also applied to serologic diagnosis of Lyme disease and other infections in which the development of antibody to a specific microbial antigen or antigens has diagnostic significance.

In the Western blotting procedure, a crude microbial antigen preparation (e.g., a partially purified virus preparation) is first heated with a detergent such as sodium dodecyl sulfate (SDS). The SDS releases individual polypeptides from complex proteins. The polypeptides are then separated according to their molecular weight by polyacrylamide gel electrophoresis with SDS (SDS-PAGE). The separated polypeptides form invisible protein "bands" in the gel. At this point, the protein bands are electrophoretically transferred to an inert filter membrane support, usually made of nitrocellulose. The nitrocellulose membrane thus becomes a solid matrix to which the separated protein antigens tightly adhere and upon which an antibody-antigen reaction can occur and be visualized—much like a microtitration plate well with an ELISA essay. A number of commercial kits for Western blotting contain nitrocellulose membrane strips on which the protein antigens of interest have already been electrophoretically separated. For analysis, the nitrocellulose membrane is immersed in a patient's serum sample (usually diluted) and allowed to incubate. Specific antibodies in the sample, if present, will bind to unique antigenic determinants in the protein bands. After incubation, the nitrocellulose membrane is thoroughly washed to removed unbound antibody, and a labeled anti–human immunoglobulin (secondary antibody) is allowed to react with the membrane. The secondary antibody is commonly labeled with an enzyme or biotin. The detection of an antigen-antibody reaction at any protein band

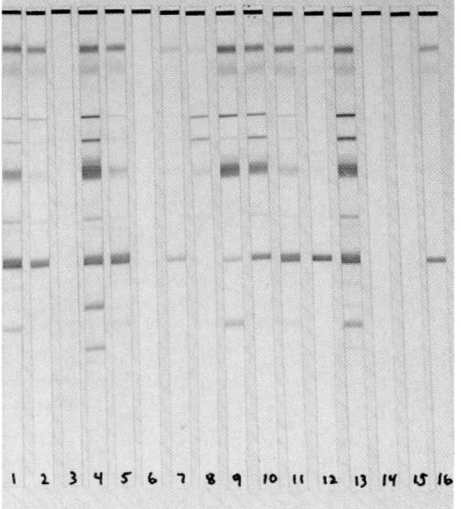

Figure 5-35 _____

Western blot for the detection of antibody to HIV-1. Strips 1 and 4 are high-positive; strips 2 and 5 are low-positive; and strips 3 and 6 are negative controls. Strips 7 through 13 and strip 16 are positive reactions of patient sera. Strips 14 and 15 are negative reactions of patient sera. Gp160 represents a viral glycoprotein with a molecular weight of 160,000 daltons; gp41 and p24 represent other viral proteins. (Coutesy Organon Tenika Corp., Durham, N.C.).

is accomplished by the addition of enzyme substrate (or enzyme-labeled strepavidin followed by enzyme substrate) and final wash (Figure 5-35).

Western blotting has added a new dimension of versatility and specificity to immunoassays. It has helped to resolve false-positive EIA results (particularly for HIV-1 infection) due to antibodies cross-reacting to other viruses, autoimmune disorders, technical error, and other, undetermined reasons. It has also helped to dissect and analyze the antibody response to individual proteins in complex mixtures. Western blotting is a procedure that must be well controlled and interpreted using strict criteria. It should also be recognized that antigens detected by other methods may not be detected by Western blotting techniques, because the polypeptide antigens are not native, intact proteins (SDS treatment denatures the proteins), and some antigens may not be transferred well to the membranes. Nevertheless, Western blotting will continue to play an important role in immunoserology of selected infectious agents.

USE OF SEROLOGIC TESTING IN SPECIFIC DISEASES

Table 5-6 lists different serologic tests commonly used in microbiology and the organisms detected by these tests.

Serologic Testing of Syphilis

Sexually transmitted diseases are some of the most common infectious diseases in the United States, second only to the common cold and influenza. The most common of these diseases are still chlamydia and herpes infections; however, it is syphilis that is the most dangerous if left undetected or untreated. *Treponema pallidum,* the spirochete that causes syphilis, may be identified from a sore, or chancre. However, the serologic testing for syphilis is the most common form of diagnosis. Two forms of testing exist for syphilis: screening tests and confirmatory tests. The Wasserman test was the first test used for the detection of syphilis by the complement fixation technique, but it is no longer used. The most common screening tests are the Venereal Disease Research Laboratories (VDRL) or the rapid plasma reagin (RPR). Confirmatory tests are the FTA-ABS and the micro-hemagglutinin (MHA).

The flocculation test for syphilis, VDRL, is named after the laboratory that developed it. The test measures a globulin complex called *reagin* that appears early in infection. If reagin is present, an aggregation occurs. The RPR test used the same VDRL antigen; however, carbon particles have been added so that the flocculation reaction can be more clearly seen on a plastic card. The VDRL and the RPR tests detect the globulin and not the spirochete itself. Therefore, a patient in the early stage of infection will not have antibodies until 3 to 4 weeks after exposure. This is a screening test that reacts to abnormal globulins. For this reason, numerous false-positives may occur with other diseases, such as malaria, malignant tumors, and some connective tissue disorders.

The confirmatory tests for a positive screen are the FTA-ABS and MHA-TP. Both of these tests detect specific antibodies to *T. pallidum.* The laboratory prepares a slide and stains it to make the antibodies appear yellow-green under an ultraviolet microscope. The MHA-TP test may be substituted for the FTA-ABS and is both easier to perform and cheaper.

Serologic Testing for Streptococcal Infections

The Streptozyme Test is a commercial product that is a more general test than either the ASO or anti-DNase-B tests. This test measures antibodies against five different streptococcal enzymes: (1) streptolysin-O, (2) deoxyribonuclease-B, (3) hyaluronidase, (4) streptokinase, and (5) nicotinamide adenine dinucleotidase. A newer test is the LINK2™ Strep A Rapid Test, which is a lateral-flow, one-step immunoassay for detection of group A streptococcal antigen directly from throat swabs.

TABLE 5-6

Summary of Serologic Tests Commonly Used in Microbiology

Test	Organism Detected
Anti-DNase-B Streptozyme test	Group A β-hemolytic streptococci—useful to measure antibodies only after acute infection
Anti-HAV	Hepatitis A virus
Anti-HCV	Hepatitis C virus—used in blood screening
CMV	Cytomegalovirus—emerging infection in pregnancy and immunosuppressed patients
Cold agglutinins	Produced by *Mycoplasma pneumoniae*—may cause atypical pneumonia
Fungus antibody tests	Histoplasmosis and Coccidoidiomycosis (confirmatory diagnosis by culture)
HBsAg	Hepatitis B virus (serum hepatitis)
Hemagglutination for amebiasis	*Entamoeba histolytica*—causative agent of amebic dysentery
HSV	Herpes simplex virus
Monospot - HAT - ASO	Epstein-Barr virus—infectious mononucleosis
Rubella titer	Rubella virus (3-day measles/German measles) extremely dangerous during pregnancy to fetus
TPM - Toxo	*Toxoplasma gondii*—protozoan causing toxoplasmosis
VDRL, RPR, FTA-ABS, MHA-TP	*Treponema pallidum*—causative agent of syphilis

This is a CLIA-waved, rapid test that has an overall accuracy of 95.8% according to the manufacturer. The test utilizes a two-site sandwich immunoassay for the detection of group A strep antigen. It consists of a membrane strip precoated with rabbit anti-group A *Streptococcus* antibody on the test band region and goat anti-rabbit antibody on the control band region. A colored rabbit anti-group A *Streptococcus* antibody-colloidal gold conjugate pad is placed at the end of the membrane. Visible, easy-to-read results are available in as little as 1 minute.

Serologic Diagnosis of Toxoplasmosis

The protozoan *Toxoplasma gondii* causes the disease toxoplasmosis (TPM or Toxo), which is found in raw or poorly cooked meat and in the feces of cats. Because cats are the host, pregnant women should be careful about handling the feces of a cat, cat litter, and especially avoid strange cats. Symptoms of the disease may be fatigue, fever, and lymph gland swelling. If passed to a fetus during pregnancy, TPM can cause severe neurologic damage and eye problems. TPM can be treated with drugs and is usually not serious in adult patients unless they are immunocompromised, as in AIDS. TPM in an immunosuppressed patient may be serious or even fatal unless treated early. IgM antibody is usually tested and infants may have an increased titer resulting from transfer of antibodies from the mother. The presence of lymphadenopathy (enlarged lymph glands) in an adult healthy patient with vague nonspecific symptoms may be suggestive of a viral infection. The patient may undergo tests for infectious mononucleosis. In contrast to infectious mononucleosis, however, is not elevated.

Serologic Diagnosis of Important Viral Diseases

Rubella *(German measles)* is normally of no significance except in pregnant women. This disease may cause a miscarriage, or it may cause congenital heart disease, cataracts, deafness, and brain damage in the unborn fetus. Therefore, it is extremely important to determine whether women who may become pregnant have an immunity to rubella. Serologic testing is generally by EIA for either IgM or IgG anti-rubella antibodies. Women who are not immune or have a low anti-body titer should be vaccinated before becoming pregnant.

The HAT (heterophile antibody titer) is one of the tests used in the diagnosis of Epstein-Barr infection, the causative agent of infectious mononucleosis. *Heterophile* is a word that refers to an affinity to more than one group or species. Humans rarely have antibodies to the RBCs of sheep. However, patients with infectious mononucleosis have been shown to develop antibodies that will agglutinate sheep RBCs. Because other factors may increase heterophile antibodies, the test is not specifically diagnostic. Other tests are therefore used to confirm active infectious mononucleosis. Tests for the Epstein-Barr nuclear antigen (EBNA) as well as for antibodies to the viral capsid antigen (VCA) are used. Either IgM or IgG antibodies can be identified by these methods.

Diagnostic kits detect infectious mononucleosis. These are generally known as spot tests and use a saline suspension of antigen derived from the RBCs of horses. Mixing of the test material with a drop of the patient's serum causes a coarse granulation if the patient has infectious mononucleosis. These tests are very rapid, specific, and sensitive for screening. However, they do not positively identify the Epstein-Barr virus. Although infectious mononucleosis is known as the *kissing disease,* its exact mode of transmission is undetermined and virus isolation by culture is not possible.

A number of different forms of hepatitis all potentially cause severe disease. Hepatitis A *(infectious hepatitis),* hepatitis B *(serum hepatitis),* and hepatitis C *(non–A non–B hepatitis)* are the most common forms diagnosed. Hepatitis B was discovered as early as 1965 and was originally named *Australian antigen,* because it was first diagnosed in an Australian man. The blood of an infected patient is infectious. The earliest laboratory test was called HAA. The test used now is for *hepatitis B surface antigen* (HBsAg). Though the virus has numerous antigens, HBsAg is highly antigenic and easy to detect. There are currently a large number of tests available for the detection of hepatitis B. These include the following tests for antigen hepatitis B core antigen (HBcAg) and hepatitis B e antigen (HBeAg). The detection of HBsAg in a patient's serum signifies that the patient is either ill with the disease or is a carrier and is potentially infectious. The laboratory can also test for antibody to the various antigens. Antibody can also be detected using Anti-HBsAg, Anti-BcAg, and Anti-HBeAg tests.

Hepatitis A is spread generally by the fecal-oral route and is often spread by food handlers and children. The tests most commonly used for detection are the Anti-HAV-IgM and Anti-HAV-IgG. A positive test of the IgM-Anti-HAV test is suggestive of acute infection, whereas a positive IgG-Anti-HAV test is indicative of past exposure. Patients diagnosed with acute infection should not be allowed to handle or prepare food for others. The disease may also be transmitted by sexual contact.

In the 1980s, a protein associated with hepatitis C virus (HCV) was cloned. This protein was then used to develop a test to detect antibodies to HCV in the blood. This was the first time that a viral genome was used to develop a serologic test without first isolating the causative agent. Research has determined that the primary agent in non–A non–B transfusion hepatitis is HCV. In 1990, the United States Food and Drug Administration approved the first test kits for the detection of HCV. It is now used in routine screening of blood. Many patients with hepatitis C virus infection may be asymptomatic. However, even asymptomatic cases can progress to chronic hepatitis and cirrhosis. Both hepatitis C and hepatitis B have been associated with the development of liver cancer. In these cases, the only clue to HCV infection may be an elevated liver enzyme known as alanine aminotransferase (ALT). For this reason, the most effective test for the diagnosis of HCV may be the use of nucleic acid probes and the polymerase chain reaction (see section D on Molecular Diagnosis).

The detection of human immunodeficiency virus (HIV) anti-HIV antibodies has generally used two main tests. The use of ELISA for screening of anti-HIV antibodies and the Western blot test for confirmation. The Western blot used electrophoresis to separate HIV proteins, which are then transferred to a membrane support for blotting. If antibodies are present in the patient, a reaction will be observed. This test is highly sensitive and specific and remains the standard confirmatory test for HIV infection. Another assay, the latex agglutination test was licensed by the FDA in 1989. This test detects HIV-1 antibodies in as little as 5 minutes. In addition, this was the first test to use a protein engineered by DNA technology. This new test does not replace the ELISA but can be used in situations where a major laboratory is not available. However, this test may be licensed for in home use in the near future. The problem with HIV infection is that antibody development has a wide variation, depending on the patient, from as little as 12 days to as much as 5 years. For this reason, other tests that identify specific HIV proteins or antigens such as P24, a core protein, or GP 41, a glycoprotein on the envelop of the virus may be preferred. Nucleic acid probes and the polymerase chain reaction may also be used in the identification of viral antigens. Cultures of HIV-1 may also be used; however, these tests are available in only a few laboratories at research institutions.

Cytomegalovirus (CMV), a herpesvirus, can be found in almost all body secretions. The virus can cross the placenta and may be transfused in blood and blood products. Most adults have been exposed to the virus and have some level of immunity. Pregnant women should be concerned about potential damage to the fetus such as cerebral malformation and necrosis of brain tissue. Patients who are immunosuppressed are highly susceptible to CMV infection. AIDS patients acquiring an acute infection with CMV may have eye damage and blindness as well as cerebral damage. The risk to healthcare workers is minimal because of the fact that healthy individuals have active immune systems. Infection from CMV is considered positive with a fourfold rise in titer between acute and convalescent patient samples. A single IgM-specific titer of more than 1:8 is evidence of an acute infection. CMV can also be detected with a DNA probe and by electron microscopy; however, both methods are extremely expensive.

Chickenpox (varicella) and shingles (herpes zoster) are both caused by the herpes zoster virus (a herpes virus). A varicella-zoster antibody screen is performed to see if the patient has immunity to the virus. Titers are of no use in determining acute infection. Testing is implemented to help curtail a possible epidemic in the clinical setting. It is very useful to know which medical staff does not have immunity to the herpes zoster virus. Staff without immunity should not take care of patients who are believed to have either shingles or chickenpox. The actual incubation period is 10 to 20 days after the initial exposure; however, the disease is infectious for 5 days before the rash appears. Patients who are immunosuppressed should be protected from anyone who has a negative titer, since they could become carriers if exposed. Disseminated herpes zoster can be fatal to any immunosuppressed patient.

Serologic Diagnosis of Fungal Infection

The laboratory can identify antibodies that occur in response to fungal disease by the use of complement fixation or immunodiffusion techniques. The primary fungi diagnosed by these means are histoplasmosis and coccidioidomycosis. Histoplasmosis is found primarily in the Ohio Valley and coccidioidiomycosis or valley fever is primarily seen in the San Jaoquin Valley of California. One fungal titer is not enough to be diagnostic, since the people who live in an endemic area may have positive serologic tests from past exposure. A fourfold rise in titer is evidence of current infection. A travel history is mandatory when fungal disease is suspected, however. Skin testing and cultures may also be used in the identification of the organism causing a systemic infection. A positive skin test does not however indicate a current infection because of antibodies from a past exposure. The conversion of a skin test from a negative to a positive is the most diagnostically significant. Skin tests should be started only after the blood is drawn for serologic testing, because the skin test itself can cause the serologic test to be falsely positive.

Two fungi found commonly in immunocompromised patients are cryptococcus and candidiasis. Cryptococcosis is a devastating systemic infection caused by the yeast *Cryptococcus neoformans*. Infection occurs initially in the lungs and rapidly disseminates to the brain and meninges. Before the advent of AIDS, disseminated cryptococcal infection occurred rarely. The number of cases of cryptococcal infection has increased significantly since the early 1980s when AIDS became the major factor for developing the disease. Traditionally the diagnosis of cryptococcosis has been based on culture of CSF or the presence of encapsulated yeast cells in India ink preparations of CSF. Antigen tests to identify these antigens (rather than antibodies) are under development as antibodies are undetectable in these patients. Latex agglutination has become the assay of choice in the diagnosis of the disease. Two such tests, CRYPTO-LEX (Trinity Laboratories, Inc.) and Crypto-LA (Wampole Laboratories) are simple and easy to use tests. The CRYPTO-LEX tests uses a mouse monoclonal anticryptococcal antibody to coat latex beads, whereas the Crypto-LA test uses a rabbit polyclonal antibody. Both tests show high sensitivity and specificity.

Bibliography

Abbas AK, Lichtman AH, Pober JS: General properties of immune responses. In *Cellular and molecular immunology*, ed 3, Philadelphia, 1997, WB Saunders, p 3.

Alois RM: *Principles of immunology and immunodiagnostics*, Philadelphia, 1988, Lea & Febiger.

Alter H et al: Detection of antibody to hepatitis C virus in prospectively followed transfusion recipients with acute and chronic non-A, non-B hepatitis, *New Engl J Med* 321:1494, 1989.

Baron EJ, Finegold SM, editors: Diagnostic immunologic principles and methods. In *Bailey and Scott's diagnostic microbiology*, ed 9, St Louis, 1994, Mosby, p 153.

Barrett J: *Textbook of immunology*, St Louis, 1988, Mosby.

Berzofsky JA, Berkower IJ, Epstein SL: Antigen-antibody interactions and monoclonal antibodies. In *Fundamental immunology*, ed 4, Philadelphia, 1999, Lippincott & Raven, p 75.

Bullock B, Rosenthal P: *Pathophysiology: adaptations and alterations in function*, ed 2, Boston, 1988, Scott, Foresman.

Cao Y et al: Virologic and immunologic characterization of long-term survivors of human immunodeficiency virus type 1 infection, *New Engl J Med* 332:201, 1988.

Chernesky MA, Ray CG, Smith TF: In Drew WL, editor: *Laboratory diagnosis of viral infections: Cumitech 15*, Washington, DC, 1982, American Society for Microbiology, p 9.

Conroy JM, Stevens RW, Hechemy KE: Enzyme immunoassay. In Balows A et al: *Manual of clinical microbiology*, ed 5, Washington, DC, 1991, American Society for Microbiology, p 87.

Coonrod JD: Immunologic diagnosis. In Hoeprich PD, Jordan MC, editors: *Infectious diseases*, ed 4, Philadelphia, 1989, JB Lippincott, p 166.

Dufour DR: Use of serologic procedures to diagnose infections. In *Clinical use of laboratory data*, Baltimore, 1998, Williams & Wilkins, p 400.

Eisen HN: Antibody-antigen reactions. In Davis BD et al, editors: *Microbiology*, ed 4, Philadelphia, 1990, JB Lippincott, p 249.

Eisen HN: Immunoglobulins and immunoglobulin genes. In Davis BD et al, editors: *Microbiology*, ed 4, Philadelphia, 1990, JB Lippincott, p 277.

Food and Drug Administration: Immune globulin–associated hepatitis C transmission, *FDA Medical Bulletin* 24:2, 1994.

Gurevich I: Hepatitis Part I. Enterically transmitted viral hepatitis: etiology, epidemiology, and prevention, *Heart and Lung* 22:370, 1993a.

Gurevich I: Hepatitis Part II. Viral hepatitis B, C, and D, *Heart and Lung*, 22:450, 1993b.

Jacobson E: Hospital hazards: how to protect yourself, *Am J Nurs* 90:48, 1990.

James K: Immunoserology of infectious diseases, *Clin Microbiol Rev* 3:132, 1990.

Kiska DL, et al: Evaluation of new monoclonal antibody-based latex agglutination test for detection of cryptococcal polysaccharide antigen in serum and cerebrospinal fluid, *J Clin Microbiol* 32:2309, 1994.

Landay A, Folds JD: Section 9: immunology. In Isenberg HD, editor: *Clinical microbiology procedures handbook,* Washington, DC, 1992, American Society for Microbiology, p 9.1.9.

Lappalainen M et al: Screening of toxoplasmosis during pregnancy, *Israel J Med Sci* 30:362, 1994.

Lederman M: Transmission of the acquired immune deficiency syndrome through heterosexual activity, *Ann Internal Med* 104:115, 1986.

Lee FK: Detection and qualitation of specific immunoglobulin responses. In Balows A et al, editors: *Manual of clinical microbiology,* ed 5, Washington, DC, 1991, American Society for Microbiology, p 105.

Marx J: Viral hepatitis, *Nursing 93,* 23:35, 1993.

Peter JB: *The use and interpretation of tests in medical laboratory immunology,* ed 5, Los Angeles, 1989, Specialty Laboratories, Inc.

Proffitt MR: Blotting techniques for the diagnosis of infectious diseases, *Clin Microbiol Newsl* 16:121, 1990.

Ravel R: *Clinical laboratory medicine,* ed 6, Chicago, 1995, Mosby.

Rose N et al, editors: *Manual of clinical immunology,* ed 4, Washington, DC, 1990, American Society for Microbiology.

Silverstein AM: The history of immunology. In *Fundamental immunology,* ed 4, Philadelphia, 1999, Lippincott & Raven, p 19.

Stepanuk KM: Congenital syphilis: are we missing infected newborns? *MCN Am J Maternal Child Health Nurs* 19:272, 1994.

Thompson KD, VanEnk RA: Changing technologies in immunodiagnosis: enzyme immunoassays versus immunofluorescence assays, *Clin Microbiol Newsl* 10:73, 1991.

Turgeon ML: *Immunology and serology in laboratory medicine,* St Louis, 1990, Mosby.

Wheat L et al: Diagnosis of disseminated histoplasmosis capsulatum in serum and urine specimens, *New Engl J Med* 314:83, 1986.

Wolach B et al: Some aspects of the humoral immunity and the phagocytic function in newborn infants, *Israel J Med Sci* 30:331, 1994.

Yolken RH: Immunoassays for the diagnosis of infectious diseases. In Wilcheck M, Bauer EA, editors: *Methods in enzymology,* vol 184, San Diego, 1990, Academic Press, p 529.

C. RAPID METHODS AND AUTOMATION IN THE MICROBIOLOGY LABORATORY

David W. Craft

THE TERM *RAPID*

MICROSCOPIC METHODS FOR RAPID DETECTION

RAPID BIOCHEMICAL TESTS PERFORMED ON ISOLATED COLONIES

IDENTIFICATION SYSTEMS RELYING UPON CARBOHYDRATE UTILIZATION OR CHROMOGENIC SUBSTRATES
Principles of Identification
Manual Rapid Tests
Automated Rapid Tests
  Vitek
  MicroScan
  Sensititre
  Pasco
Evaluation of Rapid Methods

OBJECTIVES

1. Describe the significance of rapid reporting.
2. Describe microscopic and rapid biochemical tests used for rapid detection.
3. Describe how established manual methods have been designed for the rapid identification of isolates.
4. Compare the automated methods for rapid identification of bacteria and yeasts.

KEY TERMS

Rapid method	Profile number	Vitek System	Sensititre System
Numeric codes	Chromogenic substrates	MicroScan System	Pasco

Until the late 1970s, microbiologists relied on the growth and isolation of bacteria in broth culture and agar media. Once bacteria are cultured in vitro, their biochemical or metabolic characteristics can be used for identification. Isolation of the infectious agent from clinical samples typically requires 24 to 48 hours. Identification protocols often require another 48 hours of incubation in the presence of specific carbohydrates or biochemical substrates.

Rapid diagnosis of infectious disease therefore remains a major challenge for the clinical microbiology laboratory. The clinical outcome of rapid and accurate reporting of results should directly impact patient care in two ways: early diagnosis and subsequent institution or selection of appropriate antimicrobial therapy. When these outcomes are achieved, the clinical microbiology laboratory will have a proactive, rather than retrospective, effect on patient management.

Rapid reporting also becomes increasingly important in light of today's diagnostic challenges. Newly emerging pathogens, recognition of old pathogens in different clinical settings, world travel, increasing nosocomial infections, and the prevalence of multi-drug resistant organisms all contribute to the need for the design and development of new identification capabilities.

This section generally describes the major concepts and applications of rapid methods and automation currently available for the identification of clinically significant microorganisms. Although not exhaustive, it includes the principles of most rapid identification technologies found in the clinical microbiology laboratory. Other specific identification methods are discussed in greater detail in subsequent chapters in association with specific organism descriptions.

THE TERM *RAPID*

For decades, microbiologists relied on the ability of an organism to ferment sugars, degrade amino acids, and produce unique end products for identification purposes. Diagnosis of an infectious disease has been a complex, laborious, and frequently slow process. In the late 1950s and 1960s, traditional biochemical tests became miniaturized. Smaller test tubes and molded plastic vessels were introduced. These changes made testing more convenient but did not improve turnaround times in reporting results. In the 1970s, microbiologists began to rely on computerized databases, so that numerous results could be considered simultaneously and the most statistically probable result could be regarded as the identification of the unknown organism. This development improved reliability of the results but still did not improve reporting turnaround times. In the mid to late 1970s, automated instruments for identification and susceptibility testing gradually appeared. In many laboratory settings, they shortened turnaround times, yielded greater precision, improved productivity, and provided accurate test results.

The term **rapid method** encompasses a wide variety of procedures and techniques and has been loosely applied to any procedure affording results faster than the conventional method. Rapid methods exist for microscopy, biochemical identification, antigen detection, and antibody detection. *Rapid* is a relative term used to describe time and depends on the procedures being compared. For example, a 3-hour enzyme immunoassay (EIA) method to detect *Clostridium difficile* toxin is rapid compared with a 48-hour cell culture cytotoxicity assay. On the other hand, the radiometric detection of *Mycobacterium tuberculosis* within 2 weeks is rapid compared with 6 weeks required to grow the organism on agar slants.

Microscopic procedures using common stains and fluorescent antibody to detect specific organisms are rapid methods; so are some conventional procedures used for initial differentiation or presumptive identification of certain groups of organisms. These procedures have been modified to provide immediate results that may lead to presumptive identification.

Rapid identification of clinical isolates often involves commercially packaged identification kits and fully automated instruments. These manufactured kits are usually miniaturized test systems that employ chromogenic or fluorogenic substrates to assess preformed enzymes. Reaction end points may be reached after 2 to 6 hours of incubation, although some may require an overnight incubation. The capabilities of these kits and systems vary widely. Certain systems may still require manual reading by the technologist, whereas others may utilize mechanized reading through spectrophotometry, numerical coding, and computerized databases. Some of these instruments also incubate, read, and interpret the enzymatic test results.

MICROSCOPIC METHODS FOR RAPID DETECTION

Direct microscopic examination of body fluids provides results within 15 to 30 minutes; these results are often valuable in patient management. For example, Gram stain results from a spinal fluid specimen along with blood chemistry (glucose and protein) and hematology (CBC and differential) may be critical in establishing the cause of infectious meningitis. Table 5-7 shows common stains that are used for direct smear examination of clinical samples.

TABLE 5-7

Microscopic Methods for Rapid Detection of Pathogens

Stain	Application	Expected Results	Comments
Gram stain	Provides presumptive diagnosis of bacterial pneumonia, meningitis	White blood cells (WBCs) are detected Gram stain morphology of common bacterial agents is recognized	Requires skill and experience for proper evaluation Does not include other infectious agents
Acridine orange	Useful in differentiating true organisms from artifacts, especially in blood cultures	Fluorochrome stain binds the nucleic acid of organisms Organisms show orange fluorescence against a dark background Both viable and nonviable organisms will fluoresce	Requires a fluorescent microscope
Darkfield microscopy	Direct examination of suspected primary syphilitic lesions	Motile spirochetes are visualized	Requires experience
Calcofluor white	Direct examination of spinal fluids and other body fluids for fungal elements	Yeast and fungi will show white fluorescence	Fluorescent stain that binds cell wall of fungi and yeast but not bacteria or inflammatory cells Preferred to India ink and KOH preparations
India ink	Direct smear examination of spinal fluid, blood, and urine for *Cryptococcus*	*Cryptococcus* possess a polysaccharide capsule that appears as halo against the black background	Reverse stain Capsule does not stain Requires experience to differentiate WBC from yeast
KOH 10%	Direct smear examination of skin, hair, and nails for dermatophytes	Visualizes fungal elements	KOH with gentle heating digests protein in samples to allow visualization

RAPID BIOCHEMICAL TESTS PERFORMED ON ISOLATED COLONIES

Table 5-8 summarizes the principles, modes of action, and applications of certain established manual procedures for quick presumptive differentiation between groups of organisms or presumptive identification to bacterial species. Often more than one test must be performed for a presumptive identification. These tests may also provide direction about additional tests needed for definitive identification. Further discussion of these and other similar rapid biochemical methods can be found in subsequent chapters as they apply to specific organism identification.

IDENTIFICATION SYSTEMS RELYING UPON CARBOHYDRATE UTILIZATION OR CHROMOGENIC SUBSTRATES

Principles of Identification

Identification of bacteria and yeast may be facilitated by the use of automated or packaged kit systems by which organisms are identified with computer-assisted or computer-derived books of **numeric codes.** These numeric codes are generated based on the metabolic profiles of each organism. Each metabolic reaction, or phenotype, is translated into one of two responses: plus (+) for positive reactions and minus (−) for negative reactions. These plus/minus, or "on-off" sequences, are catalogued as binary numbers and stored in a

TABLE 5-8

Rapid Biochemical Tests Performed on Isolated Colonies

Test	Bacterial Enzyme	Mode of Action	Applications
Indole	Trytophanase	Hydrolysis of substrate tryptophane in indole develops a red color upon addition of paradimethyl aminobenzaldehyde	Positive reaction (red color) identifies *Escherichia coli, Proteus vulgaris* Aids in the identification of anaerobes
Spot indole (DMAC)	Tryptophanase	Organism from blood agar or any tryptophane-containing medium is placed on a swab, and reagent is added Hydrolysis of tryptophane to indole is indicated by the production of blue color upon addition of paradimethyl amino-cinnamaldehyde	Aids in the identification of anaerobes
ONPG	β-Galactosidase	An ester linkage of ortho-nitrophenyl moieties to various carbohydrates Hydrolysis results in release of yellow ortho-nitrophenol	Determines lactose fermentation (yellow color) in slow lactose fermenters Differentiates *Neisseria lactamica* from pathogenic *Neisseria*
Oxidase	Cytochrome *c* oxidase	A blue compound is produced when tetramethyl-para-phenylenediamine reacts with cytochrome *c*	Differentiation of nonfermenters Aids in the identification of *Neisseria* sp., *Aeromonas* sp., *Vibrio* sp., and *Campylobacter* sp.
Catalase	Catalase	Breakdown of hydrogen peroxide into oxygen and water, resulting in rapid production of bubbles	Differentiation of staphylococci from streptococci, and of *Listeria* from streptococci
Bile solubility		Autocatalyzes colony in the presence of the surfactant sodium deoxycholate (bile salts)	Presumptive identification of *Streptococcus pneumoniae* in sputum, blood, and CSF cultures
PYR (*L*-pyrrolidonyl-*B*-naphthylamide)	*L*-Pyrroglutamyl-aminopeptidase	Hydrolysis of amide substrate with formation of the free *B*-naphthylamine, which combines with cinnamaldehyde, a reagent, to form a bright red color	Identification of group A streptococci Differentiates *Enterococcus* from group D streptococci
Rapid urease	Urease	Rapid hydrolysis of urea by enzyme urease releases the end product ammonia; the alkalinity causes the phenol red indicator to change from yellow to red	Screening test for *Cryptococcus, Proteus, Klebsiella,* and *Yersinia enterocolitica*
Rapid hippurate		Enzymatic hydrolysis of hippurate visualized by addition of triketohydrindene hydrate	Speciation of *Streptococcus agalactiae, Campylobacter jejuni, Listeria*

computer database. Binary codes are computer converted to an octal code **profile number** that represents the identifying phenotype of specific organisms. Once metabolic profiles have been translated into numbers, a percentage probability of correct identification is assigned based on the comparison of the unknown profile to known profiles within the database. As more organisms are included in the database, the genus and species designations and probabilities become more precise. All commercial suppliers of multi-component biochemical test systems provide users with one or more of the following: a computer, a computer-derived code book, or access to a telephone inquiry center to facilitate matching profile numbers with species.

Manual Rapid Tests

Rapid tests for detection of end products resulting from carbohydrate metabolism or enzymatic tests using **chromogenic substrates** produce reaction end points in minutes to hours. Plastic cupules, reaction chambers, or filter paper strips contain desiccated or dehydrated reagents or substrates. In general, a suspension of bacterial cells or a loopful of an isolated colony is added to the system or rubbed off to a reaction area. The reaction end point is measured by growth/no growth or a color change.

Test kits using conventional carbohydrate metabolism take advantage of one test inoculum distributed to multiple reaction sites to yield more than one result. To obtain more rapid results, con-

TABLE 5-9

Commercially Available Manual and Automated Systems for Microbial Identification

Name	Manufacturer	Principle	Organism(s) Identified
Manual			
API/bioMerieux Vitek	bioMerieux Vitek[1]	Carbohydrate utilization/ chromogenic substrate	Enterobacteriaceae, other GN bacilli, *Staphylococcus, Streptococcus, Enterococcus, Neisseria,* GP bacilli, yeast, anaerobes
Crystal E/NF	Becton Dickinson Microbiology Systems[2]	Carbohydrate utilization/ chromogenic substrate	Enterobacteriaceae, other GN bacilli, *Neisseria, Haemophilus,* GP cocci, GP bacilli
MicroID (RapID)	Remel[3]	Carbohydrate utilization/ chromogenic substrate	Enterobacteriaceae, other GN bacilli, *Neisseria, Haemophilus, Streptococci, Enterococci,* yeast, anaerobes, UTI, GP bacilli
Biolog Microplate	Biolog[4]	Carbohydrate utilization	GP, GN, yeast, anaerobes
Enterotube	Becton Dickinson Microbiology Systems	Carbohydrate utilization/ chromogenic substrate	Enterobacteriaceae, other GN bacilli
MicroScan (TouchScan)	Dade MicroScan Inc.[5]	Carbohydrate utilization/ chromogenic substrate	GP, GN, urinary tract, *Haemophilus, Neisseria*
Oxi-Ferm	Becton Dickinson Microbiology Systems	Carbohydrate utilization	Non-fermenter GN bacteria
Uni-Tek	Remel	Carbohydrate utilization	Non-fermenters, yeast
Bacti-Card	Remel	Chromogenic substrate	*Neisseria*/Moraxella, *Escherichia coli, Streptococcus,* yeast
Gonochek	EY Laboratories[6]	Chromogenic substrate	*Neisseria*/Moraxella
Quad-Ferm	bioMerieux Vitek	Chromogenic substrate	*Neisseria*/Moraxella
Automated			
Vitek (AMS)	bioMerieux Vitek	Carbohydrate utilization/ chromogenic substrate	Enterobacteriaceae, other GN bacilli, *Neisseria, Haemophilus,* Streptococci, Enterococci, Staphylococci, GP bacilli, yeast, anaerobes
MicroScan (Autoscan, Walkaway)	Dade MicroScan Inc.	Carbohydrate utilization/ chromogenic substrate/ fluorogenic substrate	Enterobacteriaceae, other GN bacilli, *Neisseria, Haemophilus,* Streptococci, Enterococci, Staphylococci, GP bacilli, yeast, anaerobes
Sensititre	AccuMed Intl[7]	Carbohydrate utilization/ chromogenic substrate	GN, GP
Pasco	Becton Dickinson Microbiology Systems/Difco[2]	Carbohydrate utilization/ chromogenic substrate	GN, GP

GN, Gram-negative organisms; *GP,* gram-positive organisms.
[1]Hazelwood, Mo.
[2]Sparks, Md.
[3]Lenexa, Kan.
[4]Hayward, Calif.
[5]West Sacramento, Calif.
[6]San Mateo, Calif.
[7]Westlake, Ohio

ventional methods have been modified by decreasing the test substrate medium volume and increasing the concentration of bacteria in the inoculum.

Methods based on enzyme substrates have certain advantages over conventional methods. Because enzymatic methods involve preformed enzymes, they do not require multiplication of the organism (growth independent). Therefore, endpoints are reached in minutes to a few hours. The tests are very sensitive for the presence of the enzyme although not always specific for genus and species identification. However, sensitivity does depend on the concentration and stability of the substrate, the enzyme, and the age of the inoculum. Several of the more rapid modifications of conventional methods for bacterial and yeast identification are listed in Table 5-9. Figure 5-36 displays one of the common manual test kits commercially available in the clinical microbiology laboratory.

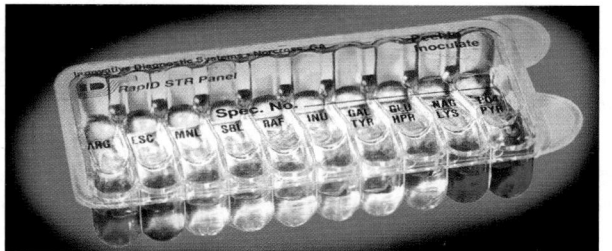

A

REMEL/IDS RapID STR Color Guide   992-144

Test	Cavity	Positive Reactions	Negative Reactions	Comments
ARG	1	● ●	○ ○	*Without the addition of any reagents, read cavities 1-10 and record results:*
ESC	2	●	○ ○ ○	**Cavity 1:** Development of a red or dark orange color is a positive test; a yellow or yellow-orange color is a negative test.
MNL	3	○ ○	● ●	**Cavity 2:** Development of a black color is a positive test; a clear, tan, or a light brown color is a negative test.
SBL	4			**Cavities 3-5:** Development of a yellow or yellow-orange color is a positive test; a red or orange color is a negative test.
RAF	5			
INU	6	○ ○	●	**Cavity 6:** Development of a yellow or orange color is a positive test; a red color is a negative test.
GAL	7	○	○ ○	**Cavities 7-10:** Development of a significant yellow color is a positive test; a very pale or clear color is a negative test.
GLU	8			
NAG	9			
PO4	10			
TYR	7	● ●	○ ○ ○	
HPR	8			**Cavities 7-8:** Development of a purple color, without regard to intensity, is a positive test; a clear, tan, or yellow color is a negative test.
LYS	9	● ●	● ● ○	**Cavities 9-10:** Development of a very dark purple color is a positive test; a light to medium purple color is a negative test.
PYR	10			

Add RapID STR Reagent to cavities 7-10. Allow at least 30 seconds but no longer than 3 minutes for color development.

Note: The RapID Color Guides are intended as an educational aid to be used in conjunction with the Technical Insert for the product. The reaction colors shown in the charts represent the typical shades of positive and negative colors.

800-447-3641   or   **800-225-5443**
(Technical Service)

PRINTED IN U.S.A.   3/98

B

Figure 5-36 _____

RapID Streptococci panel for the identification of *Streptococcus* species. **A,** The commercial test well cartridge containing appropriate substrates. **B,** The interpretive color guide to reactions. (Courtesy Remel, Lenexa, Kan.)

Automated Rapid Tests

In general, most automated systems use turbidity, colorimetry, and fluorescent assay principles. Panels of freeze-dried or lyophilized reagents are provided in microtiter trays or sealed cards. Panels are incubated and read by the system hardware with interpretation of results provided by the software. Advantages of automated systems include the interface to laboratory information systems leading to decreased turnaround times for reporting of results. Other advantages include statistical prediction of correct identification, increased data acquisition and epidemiological analysis, and automated standardization of identification profiles that can reduce analytical errors. If these systems are used in conjunction with automated susceptibility testing, these data may be linked to the pharmacy for patient management applications. Theoretically, early reporting of results can shorten length of hospital stay, augment therapeutic management of appropriate antibiotics, and therefore cut hospital costs.

Vitek

The **Vitek System** (AMS) was first introduced to perform automated antimicrobial susceptibility tests. In 1982, the Enterobacteriaceae-plus Biochemical Card (EBC+) was introduced, providing automatic identification of these organisms within 8 hours of incubation. Today, these 30 microwell cards contain substrates for the identification of numerous gram-positive and gram-negative bacteria and yeast. A suspension of the organism is prepared in saline, and the card is attached to the bacterial suspension by a transfer tube and placed in the filling module of the instrument. The card is inoculated by a vacuum-release method. The card is then placed in the reader-incubator module of the instrument, where it is optically scanned and read on a periodic basis. The computer software collates the readings and matches them to the automated database for final identification. A new release, Vitek 2, was introduced in 1999. This new system includes new hardware, software, and increased automation, resulting in less hands-on time.

MicroScan

The **MicroScan System** consists of plastic, standard-sized 96-well microtiter trays in which up to 32 reagent substrates are included for the identifica-

tion of bacteria and yeast (TouchScan, AutoScan). Some trays, called Combo trays, also include broth microdilutions of various antibiotics in certain of the wells for performing susceptibility tests. MicroScan panels are supplied containing either frozen or dehydrated substrates. For dehydrated antimicrobic panels, shipping is more convenient and allows for room temperature storage and a longer shelf life. The wells are inoculated with a heavy suspension of the organism to be identified and incubated at 35° C for 15 to 18 hours. The panels can be interpreted visually, after which the biochemical results are converted into a seven- or eight-digit biotype number that can be identified with a code book supplied by the manufacturer. Alternatively, an automated tray reader can be used to detect bacterial growth or color changes by differences in light transmission. As with other automated systems, the organism identification is accomplished electronically by collating the readings and matching them to the system's software database for final identification.

The MicroScan Walkaway, the most recent ver-

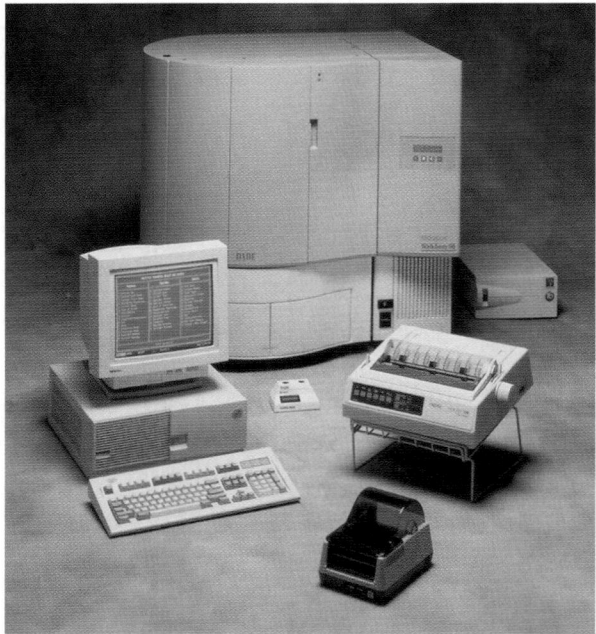

Figure 5-37

MicroScan Walkaway featuring the test platform and automated data management system. (Courtesy Dade MicroScan Inc, West Sacramento, Calif.)

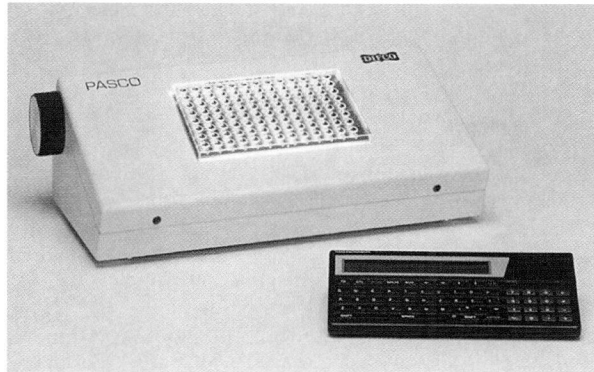

sion of MicroScan automation, is fully automated with capabilities to incubate more than one panel, automatically add reagents to conventional panels when required, read and interpret panel results, and print results, all without operator intervention (Figure 5-37). Rapid fluorescence panels in addition to the conventional MicroScan panels are available for use in the Walkaway instrument. The rapid panels use fluorescent labeled compounds and require only a 2-hour incubation for bacterial identification. Fluorometric reactions detect changes in pH as a result of carbohydrate fermentation. The resultant acid production causes a drop in pH and a decrease in fluorescence.

Sensititre

The **Sensititre System** may be purchased as either a manual enteric identification system or in the form of an automated identification system. The manual plate contains media for performing 23 standard biochemical tests, plus a control, which are dried in the wells of a standard-sized 96-well microtiter tray. Each tray contains four duplicate sets of biochemical wells, permitting simultaneous identification of four organisms per tray. The system contains conventional biochemical tests and is inoculated and read manually.

The Gram-Negative AutoIdentification System uses fluorescent technology to detect bacterial growth and enzyme activity. The system consists of 32 newly formulated biochemical tests, including selected classic biochemical media reformulated to yield a fluorescent signal. Each biochemical test medium, along with an appropriate fluorescent indicator, is dried into the individual wells of the Sen-

sititre plate. Each plate is designed to test three separate organisms. Because these are dried plates, they may be stored at room temperature. All autoidentification tests are read on the Sensititre AutoReader for the presence or absence of fluorescence. The results are transmitted to a computer for analysis and identification.

Pasco

Pasco panels are used for the identification of gram-negative and gram-positive organisms using conventional biochemical tests (Figure 5-38). Panels utilize a microwell plate formatted into 104 microtubes. These microtubes contain appropriate batteries of frozen substrates as well as antimicrobial agents for determining identification and susceptibility of various organisms. Isolated colonies from primary plates are mixed to the appropriate turbidity standard and poured into an inoculum tray. Identification and susceptibility panels are inoculated by placing a standardized template inoculator containing 104 microtips into the inoculum tray and transferring to the appropriate gram-negative or gram-positive panel. Organism identification is achieved by using the Pasco Electracode or the automated Pasco Data Management System. The computer assisted identification system employs the biochemical tests on the panel and off panel reactions such as oxidase and catalase results to generate a biotype code number and subsequent identification.

Evaluation of Rapid Methods

Most rapid and automated procedures are designed to provide results with greater speed and precision than traditional methods. Whether greater efficiency and productivity are achieved depends largely upon the laboratory and the institution(s) that it supports. Therefore both manual and automated systems should be evaluated on site before changing or augmenting current protocols. The best studies are prospective, side-by-side comparisons of the current in-house or reference (often conventional) procedure to the new system for accuracy, cost effectiveness, and effect on work flow. These systems often offer decreased sensitivity and specificity for the identification of the biochemically inert bacteria and some fastidious organisms. Therefore, supplemental and differential media and conventional biochemicals must still be kept on hand to support the identification of these organisms.

Bibliography

Bascomb S, Manafi M: Use of enzyme tests in characterization and identification of aerobic and facultatively anaerobic gram-positive cocci, *Clin Microbiol Rev* 11:318, 1992.

Espinel-Ingroff A et al: Comparison of RapID Yeast Plus System with API 20C System for identification of common, new, and emerging yeast pathogens, *J Clin Microbiol* 36:883, 1998.

Forbes BA et al, editors: Overview of conventional methods for bacterial identification. In *Bailey and Scott's diagnostic microbiology,* ed 10, St Louis, 1998, Mosby, p 167.

Funke G et al: Evaluation of the RapID CB Plus System for identification of coryneform bacteria and *Listeria* spp., *J Clin Microbiol* 36:2439, 1998.

Funke G et al: Evaluation of VITEK 2 System for rapid identification of medically relevant gram-negative rods, *J Clin Microbiol* 36:1948, 1998.

Koneman EW et al, editors: *Color atlas and textbook of diagnostic microbiology,* ed 5, Philadelphia, 1997, Lippincott-Raven.

Miller JM, O'Hara CM: Substrate utilization systems for the identification of bacteria and yeasts. In Murray PR, Baron EJ, et al, editors: *Manual of clinical microbiology,* ed 6, Washington, DC, 1995, American Society for Microbiology, p 103.

O'Hara CM, Tenover FC, Miller JM: Parallel comparison of accuracy and API 20E, Vitek GNI, Microscan Walk/Away Rapid ID, and Becton-Dickinson Cobas Micro ID-E/NF for identification of member of the family Enterobacteriaceae and common gram-negative, non-glucose fermenting bacilli, *J Clin Microbiol* 31:3165, 1993.

Payne WJ et al: Clinical laboratory applications for monoclonal antibodies, *Clin Microbiol Rev* 1:313, 1988.

Stager CE, Davis JR: Automated systems for identification of microorganisms, *Clin Microbiol Rev* 5:302, 1992.

Woods GL, Washington JA: The clinician and the microbiology laboratory. In Mandell GL, Bennett JE, et al, editors: *Principles and practice of infectious disease,* ed 4, New York, 1995, Churchill Livingstone, p 169.

D. MOLECULAR APPLICATIONS IN THE CLINICAL LABORATORY

Gerri S. Hall

HYBRIDIZATION FORMATS
  Probe Labels
  Probe Target

APPLICATIONS OF PROBE TECHNOLOGY
  Probes for Culture Confirmation
    Bacteria
    Probes for *Mycobacterium* sp.
    Fungi

Probes for Rapid Diagnosis of Infectious Diseases
  Respiratory infections
  Sexually transmitted diseases
  Miscellaneous infectious diseases

AMPLIFICATION
  Detection of the Amplicon

CLINICAL APPLICATIONS OF AMPLIFICATION
  Technical Considerations for Implementation
    of Amplification
  Measures to Control Contamination
  Commercially Available Amplification Systems
  Detection of *Mycobacterium tuberculosis*
  Other Available Assays

KEY TERMS

Nucleic acid hybridization	Complementary
RNA	Cycle
DNA	Oligonucleotide
Probe	Primer
Nucleic acid sequence	DNA polymerase
Target	Taq polymerase
Sandwich hybridization	Amplicon
"In-solution" hybridization	Ligase Chain Reaction (LCR)
"In situ" hybridization	Nucleic Acid Based Sequence Amplification (NASBA)
Amplification	
Polymerase Chain Reaction (PCR)	Strand Displacement Amplification (SDA)
Annealing	

The goal of the clinical microbiology laboratory is to provide the clinician with evidence of the presence or absence of an infectious agent that may be causing a particular illness. Traditionally, this diagnosis relied upon methods that detected the pathogen, either directly through culture or antigen detection, or indirectly through serologic methods that would enable the detection of antibodies made in response to the pathogen. The indirect methods could also involve the detection of metabolic by-products of the agent, such as in the detection of toxins.

For some infectious agents reliable culture or serologic methods are not available or these methods may require long periods of turnaround time. Examples of these include *Mycobacterium leprae,* human papilloma virus (HPV) or *Mycobacterium tuberculosis. M. leprae* and HPV are not easily nor routinely cultured in the lab. With *M. tuberculosis,* at least 10 to 12 days are required before cultural isolation is completed and more time is then needed for conventional identification. Because the laboratory is unable to provide definitive evidence of such infections, diagnosis depends primarily upon the clinical picture. The introduction of nucleic acid hybridization and amplification techniques has allowed the clinical lab to decrease the time to detection in many situations and thereby enhance the laboratory's role in the diagnosis of these infectious diseases.

Nucleic acid hybridization is key to the molecular techniques discussed in this chapter. This process provides for the formation of stable double-stranded nucleic acid molecules from complementary single-stranded molecules. The single-stranded molecules can be **RNA or DNA,** and the resultant hybrids formed can be DNA-DNA, RNA-RNA, or DNA-RNA. A **probe** is a labeled single-strand sequence of nucleic acid that is complementary to the **nucleic acid sequence** to be detected and can be either DNA or RNA. The targeted nucleic acid sequence is referred to as the **target,** and it too can be RNA or DNA. This target can be located within the specimen, or in a colony, either from an agar plate or broth culture.

The nucleic acid probe is traditionally constructed from specific nucleic acid fragments (sequence) of the organism (target), or the probe may be a synthetically produced oligonucleotide of spe-

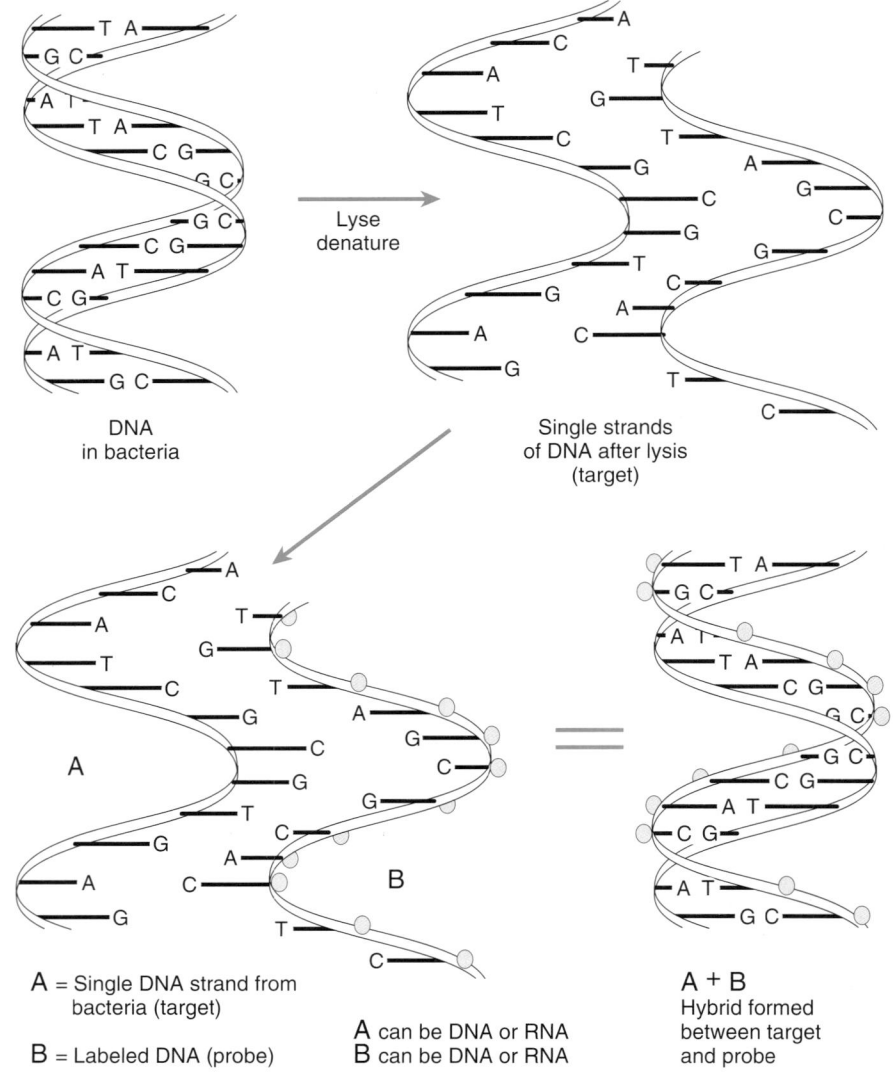

A = Single DNA strand from bacteria (target)

B = Labeled DNA (probe)

A can be DNA or RNA
B can be DNA or RNA

A + B
Hybrid formed between target and probe

Figure 5-39 _____

Hybridization format.

Box 5-1

Hybridization Formats for DNA Probes

Solid-support hybridization
- Filter
- Modified filter: microtiter tray or test tube
- Sandwich hybridization

In-solution hybridization
In situ hybridization
Southern hybridization

cific sequences. In a probe assay, the target and probe must be allowed to come together and hybridize, and the conditions whereby this may occur are referred to as the hybridization format or method (Figure 5-39).

HYBRIDIZATION FORMATS

Box 5-1 lists various hybridization formats that are available for probe testing. Solid support is the

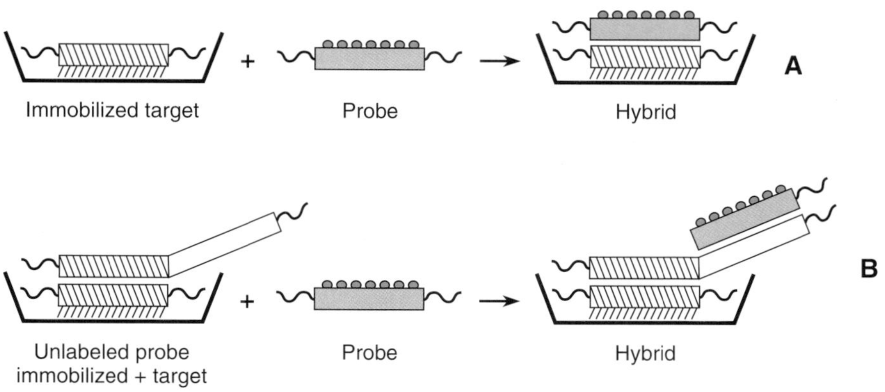

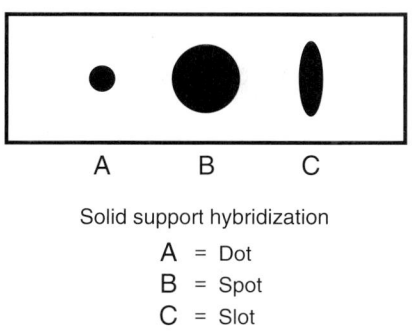

Figure 5-40

A, Solid-state hybridization. **B,** Sandwich hybridization.

conventional approach in which the target nucleic acid is secured to a membrane (nitrocellulose or nylon fiber filter paper) (Figure 5-40, *A*). The probe is then overlaid to attach to target, if present, and after a series of washes, detected as a dot, spot, or blot, depending upon the manner in which the nucleic acid is added to membrane (Figure 5-41). Modifications of this method include use of a microtiter tray well or inside of a test tube as the solid support. **Sandwich hybridization** (Figure 5-40, *B*) is a type of solid support that utilizes two probes, one unlabeled and attached to the solid support and the other labeled and added after the target, if present, has been allowed to hybridize to the first probe. This "sandwich" may help to reduce background nonspecific binding, at the expense of some reduced sensitivity.

"In-solution" hybridization (Figure 5-42) involves movement of both target and probe in a liquid environment, providing for kinetics of interaction that may be 5 to 10 times faster than solid-support hybridization. The required differential separation and removal of the unbound probe has been facilitated by the use of hydroxyapatite, magnetic beads, or differential chemical hydrolysis, depending upon the commercial application of the probe technology.

"In-situ" hybridization occurs in formalin-fixed or paraffin-embedded tissue, which may contain the suspected target. A positive reaction provides a localization of the target nucleic acid within the cellular and subcellular detail of the tissue and as such is ideal for probing of viruses such as HPV, herpes simplex virus (HSV), or Epstein Barr virus (EBV), for example. Although southern hybridization is mentioned in the table, it remains a research tool for detection of very specific nucleic acid fragments and it will not be further discussed.

Probe Labels

To detect the hybridization reaction that may have occurred between probe and target, a label or marker is needed. In most cases, this involves labeling of the probe with any of the markers listed in Box 5-2. Conventional and research methods have utilized radioactive probes to maximize sensitivity of the reaction. These have included radioactive phosphorus (^{32}P), iodine (^{125}I), and sulfur (^{35}S). Clinical labs have been less comfortable

Figure 5-41

Resultant reactions of solid support hybridization.

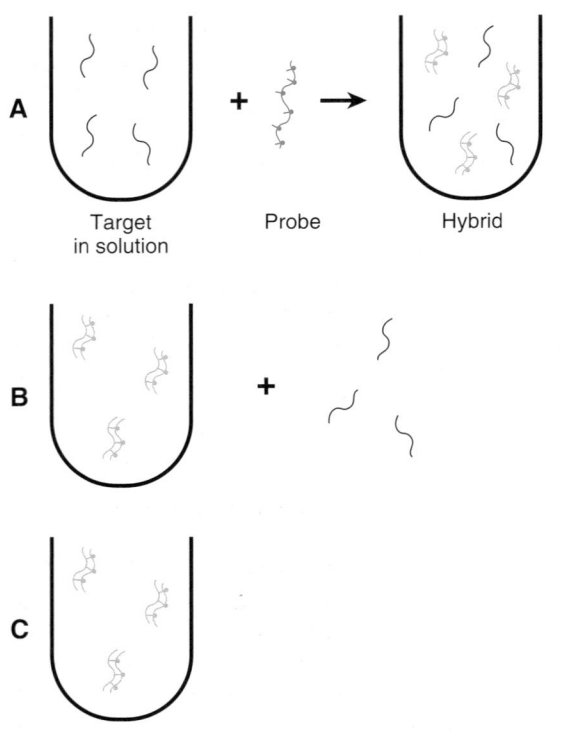

Figure 5-42
In-solution hybridization. **A,** Hybridization. **B,** Separation.
C, Detection of hybrids.

with these labels because they have short half-lives, require elaborate equipment or lengthy incubations, in addition to the need for proper disposal and handling of radioactive substances.

Biotinylated nucleotide probes incorporate biotin into the DNA, with addition of a biotin-binding protein, usually avidin, after hybridization; the

---

avidin is linked to an enzyme such as alkaline phosphatase or horseradish peroxidase, allowing for a colored product (the hybridized probe target). Haptens, such as sulfone or digoxigenin, act as labels with some probe products, with resultant visualization of the hybrid being made by colorimetric, chemiluminescent, or microscopic means. The sensitivities of these probe labels have increased over the years and approach or even exceed that of radioactivity. Chemiluminescense labeling may be the most sensitive method for probe detection. This type of label is utilized by many of the commercial companies that produce probes.

Probe Target
Target material for probe technology can be DNA or RNA. Most commercial probes utilize DNA as a target with DNA or RNA as the probe. Gen-Probe Inc. (San Diego, CA) utilizes ribosomal RNA (rRNA) as the target for chemiluminescent DNA probes. The advantage of RNA as the target is that it increases the sensitivity, because of the higher number of copies of rRNA as compared with DNA per cell.

APPLICATIONS OF PROBE TECHNOLOGY

Probes for Culture Confirmation
Bacteria
Several acridinium ester-labeled probes (e.g., Accuprobe, Gen-Probe, San Diego, CA) can be purchased for culture confirmation of a variety of microbes. A list of gram-positive and gram-negative bacteria that can be identified by Accuprobe products is given in Table 5-10. Daly and colleagues (1991) reviewed the performance of these probes. The procedure used to perform the probe assays for bacteria is shown in Figure 5-43, *A* with modification as noted for use with *Mycobacterium* sp. (see Figure 5-43, *B*). Culture confirmation can be completed in 1.5 to 2 hours or less. Application of the culture confirmation probes to positive blood culture bottle isolates has been reported by Davis and Fuller (1991). A Leader Luminometer (Genprobe, San Diego Inc., San Diego, CA) is required to obtain results, which are recorded as relative light units (RLU). The RLU values needed for a positive result may vary according to the test kit but

---

Box 5-2

Labels for DNA/RNA Probes

Radioactive labels
 ^{32}P
 ^{125}I
 ^{35}S
Biotinylated nucleotides (biotin-avidin probes)
Enzyme-conjugated probes
 Alkaline phosphatase
 Horseradish peroxidase
Probes directly labeled with antibody
Chemiluminescense
Chemical (e.g., digoxigenin)
Fluorescein labels

TABLE 5-10

Organisms for Which Accuprobe DNA Probe Products Are Available to Confirm Culture Results

Bacteria	
Gram-negative	*Neisseria gonorrhoeae*
	Campylobacter jejuni
	Campylobacter coli
	Campylobacter lari
	Haemophilus influenzae
Gram-positive	Group A *Streptococcus*
	Group B *Streptococcus*
	Streptococcus pneumoniae
	Enterococcus spp.
	Staphylococcus aureus
	Listeria monocytogenes
Mycobacteria	*Mycobacterium tuberculosis* complex
	Mycobacterium avium complex
	Mycobacterium avium
	Mycobacterium intracellulare
	Mycobacterium gordonae
Fungi	*Histoplasma capsulatum*
	Blastomyces dermatitidis
	Cryptococcus neoformans
	Coccidioides immitis

are included in the package inserts sold with the tests.

Some research probes, not commercially available, detect gastrointestinal pathogens, such as *E. coli.* Biotinylated DNA probes have been used to hybridize with colonies of *E. coli* to detect enterotoxigenic (ETEC), enteroinvasive (EIEC), enteropathogenic (EPEC), enterohaemorrhagic (EHEC), and diffuse adherence (DAEC) *E. coli* strains causing diarrhea. Dix and associates in 1990 and Moncla and colleagues in 1991 have reported on a DNA probe that can detect anaerobes and other bacteria associated with periodontal disease.

Probes for *Mycobacterium* sp.

Four commercial probes are available for the culture confirmation of *Mycobacterium* sp. Accuprobe (Gen-Probe Inc., San Diego, CA) utilizes the same format as previously described for other bacteria to detect *Mycobacterium tuberculosis* complex (*Mycobacterium tuberculosis, Mycobacterium bovis, Mycobacterium africanum,* and *Mycobacterium microti*) and *Mycobacterium avium* complex (*M. avium* and *Mycobacterium intracellulare*); *Mycobacterium gordonae;* and *Mycobacterium kansasii.* For all, isolates from solid medium or broth (BACTEC, MGIT, or from one of the automated mycobacterial detection systems) can be probed in 1.5 to 2 hours.

Many reports in the literature have verified the specificity of the probe. Sensitivity is not in question with solid media, and testing from broth has a good sensitivity provided the amount of growth in the broth is sufficient. Figures 5-44 and 5-45 suggest how such probes can be used for identification in the routine laboratory. This can be accomplished by obtaining a growth index (GI) in the BACTEC greater than or equal to 100, for example, or by holding a MGIT tube at least 1 day past its positive fluorescence. Table 15-10 also lists the *Mycobacterium* sp. that can be confirmed by Accuprobe.

Fungi

Accuprobes (Gen-Probe Inc., San Diego, CA) for fungal identification are available for *Histoplasma capsulatum, Blastomyces dermatitidis, Cryptococcus neoformans,* and *Coccidioides immitis* (see Table 5-10). The same format for hybridization (e.g., in-solution hybridization using an acridinium ester label and chemiluminescent detection) is employed. A DNA probe for *Candida albicans* was reported by Cheung and Hudson (1988), but it was found to be genus specific but not species specific, and it is not commercially available.

Probes for Rapid Diagnosis of Infectious Diseases

Respiratory infections

Probes have been available from Gen-Probe Inc. (San Diego, CA) for detection of *Legionella* sp. and *Mycoplasma pneumoniae.* However, use of a radioactive label on the probe and lack of much interest among clinicians and labs for their use have made them somewhat obsolete. Direct specimen probes for viral respiratory pathogens are available from a variety of manufacturers, including ENZO Diagnostics, Inc. (Syosset, NY) and Digene (Silver Springs, MD). In situ probes for EBV, cytomegalovirus (CMV), and adenovirus are available, but in general, for research use only.

Sexually transmitted diseases

Commercial probes are available for the diagnosis of *Neisseria gonorrhoeae* and *Chlamydia trachomatis.* The PACE system (Gen-Probe Inc., San Diego, CA) utilizes a chemiluminescent detection method, described earlier for bacteria. The same specimen collection tube can be used to collect one speci-

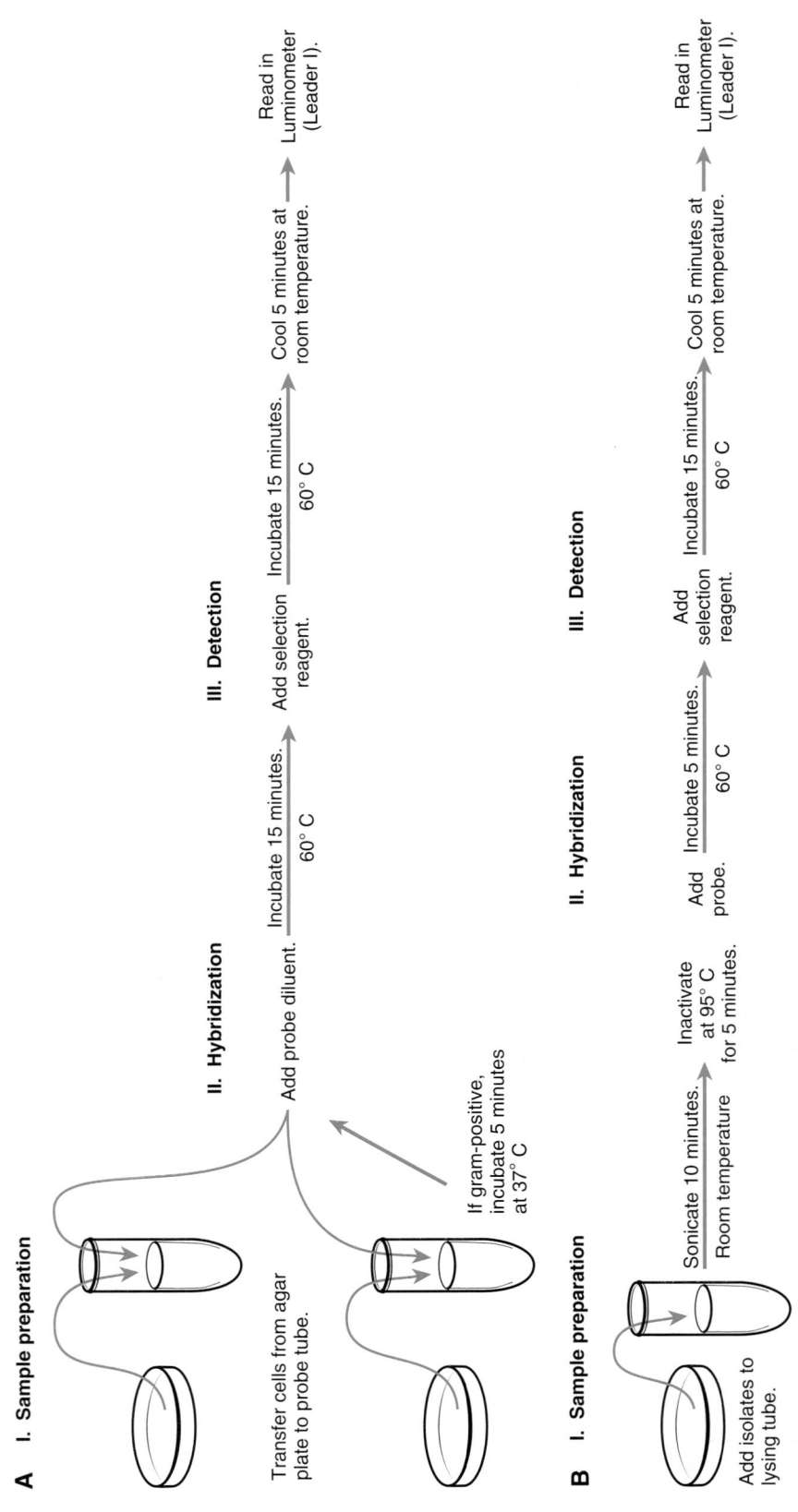

Figure 5-43

Culture identification by Accuprobe. **A,** Gram-positive and gram-negative organisms. **B,** Mycobacteria and fungi.

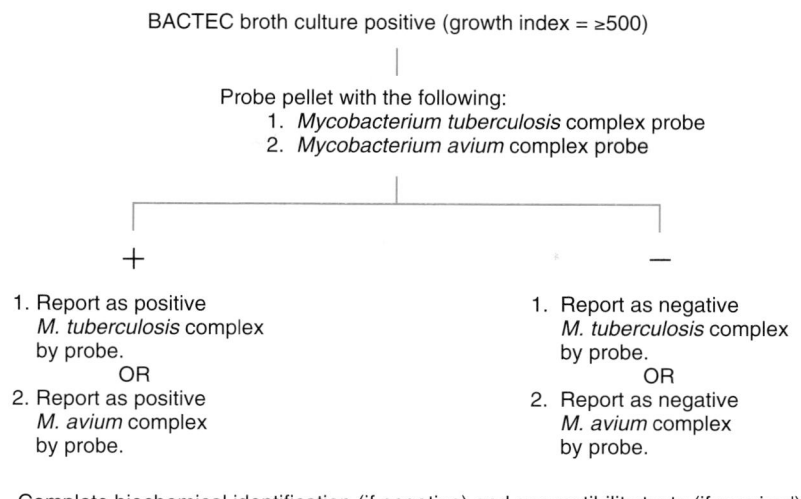

BACTEC broth culture positive (growth index = ≥500)

Probe pellet with the following:
1. *Mycobacterium tuberculosis* complex probe
2. *Mycobacterium avium* complex probe

+

1. Report as positive
   M. tuberculosis complex
   by probe.
   OR
2. Report as positive
   M. avium complex
   by probe.

−

1. Report as negative
   M. tuberculosis complex
   by probe.
   OR
2. Report as negative
   M. avium complex
   by probe.

Complete biochemical identification (if negative) and susceptibility tests (if required).

Figure 5-44

Accuprobe analysis of BACTEC positive mycobacterial cultures.

men for both procedures. After collection of the cervical or urethral specimen, cells are lysed, releasing the target nucleic acid, if present. At this point, all organisms are killed, and thus, if culture is desired in conjunction with the probe assay, separate specimens would have to be collected.

The PACE system for direct detection of pathogens differs from the cultural confirmation application from Gen-Probe. In the PACE procedure, after hybridization with specific probe, the unbound probe is removed via a magnetic bead separation step. The added magnetic beads will attract the bound probe (probe-target complex, if present), and when tubes are placed on a magnetic separation rack and then decanted, the unbound probe is eliminated in the supernatant. The remaining

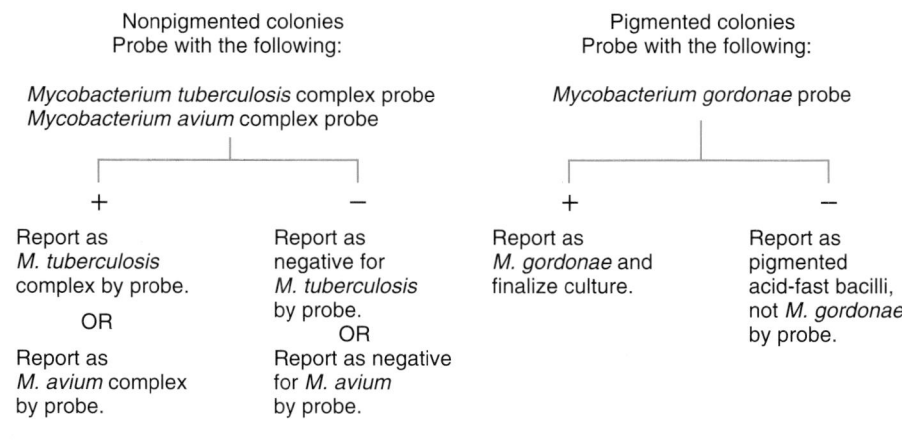

Nonpigmented colonies
Probe with the following:

Mycobacterium tuberculosis complex probe
Mycobacterium avium complex probe

+

Report as
M. tuberculosis
complex by probe.

OR

Report as
M. avium complex
by probe.

−

Report as
negative for
M. tuberculosis
by probe.
OR
Report as negative
for *M. avium*
by probe.

Pigmented colonies
Probe with the following:

Mycobacterium gordonae probe

+

Report as
M. gordonae and
finalize culture.

−

Report as
pigmented
acid-fast bacilli,
not *M. gordonae*
by probe.

Complete identification (if negative alone) and perform susceptibility testing as required

Figure 5-45

Gen-Probe identification of mycobacterial culture positive on solid media by DNA probe.

Definitions

Amplicon: The final product of PCR containing the target sequence of interest; this short, discrete DNA molecule is defined at each of its four ends by the primer sequences used in the amplification.

Anneal: The process by which oligonucleotides "attach" to targeted DNA sequence

Autoradiograph: The image formed on x-ray film resulting from the radioactive emissions of ^{32}P

Complementary: Certain nucleotidases that align opposite each other in the two strands of DNA: G pairs with C and A pairs with T

Cycle: A set of three different temperature settings, performed sequentially, for DNA denaturation, primer annealing, and primer extension

Denaturation: The use of high temperatures (94° C) to separate the double-stranded DNA into single-stranded DNA

DNA: Deoxyribose nucleic acid, composed of a double helix consisting of pair nucleotides and a ribose backbone

DNA amplification: The process by which a single molecule of DNA is manipulated to increase its concentration exponentially

DNA polymerase: A specific enzyme that catalyzes the formation of additional strands of double-stranded DNA for the DNA template

DNA template: The starting ds DNA

End labeling: The addition of a radioactively labeled phosphate group to the 5' end of a oligonucleotide probe

Extension: The process by which primed DNA is synthesized by the action of *Taq* polymerase

Genomic DNA: DNA contained in a cell's chromosome

Nucleotides: Building blocks of the nucleic acids of which DNA is composed; four bases make up DNA: A, adenine; T, thymine; C, cytosine, and G, guanine.

Oligonucleotides: Short strands of single-stranded DNA of defined sequence, less than 50 bases in length; examples are the primers and probes used in PCR.

PCR: Polymerase chain reaction—a primer-mediated, temperature-dependent technique for the enzymatic amplification of a specific DNA sequence.

Primer: A short DNA sequence that anneals to a specific area of the target DNA; DNA polymerase initiates synthesis from this point

Primer-dimer: PCR product that is composed mainly of the primers used in the amplification; these products are formed independently of the DNA template and accumulate exponentially.

Probe: In PCR, a radioactively labeled, single-stranded DNA oligonucleotide, usually 40 to 45 bases long, which is used to specifically identify complementary regions of the amplified PCR product

Taq Polymerase: A heat-stable DNA polymerase isolated from the bacterium *Thermus aquaticus*

Target DNA: A sequence of known nucleotides specifically chosen for amplification

material is resuspended and read in the luminometer as with the Accuprobe products.

For the identification of *Trichomonas vaginalis, Gardnerella vaginalis* (as a marker for bacterial vaginosis), and *Candida albicans,* a probe called AFFIRM (Becton Dickinson, Sparks, MD) is marketed. All three agents are detected in about 45 minutes; the assay requires a small piece of equipment.

For the diagnosis of HSV and HIV, probes are available commercially from a variety of manufacturers, including PathoGene (ENZO, Syosset, NY) and HSV Disk (Diagnostic Hybrids, Inc., Athens, OH). HPV can be detected by probes manufactured by Digene (Silver Springs, MD), BioPap (ENZO Diagnostics, Inc., Syosset, NY) and DAKO Biotinylated HPV Probes (DAKO Corporation, Carpentera, CA).

Miscellaneous infectious diseases

Probes have been reported in the literature for the direct detection of *Plasmodium* sp., *Borrelia burgdorferi,* hepatitis B virus, hepatitis C virus, and a variety of other infectious diseases. Other applications of probe technology are listed in Box 5-3.

AMPLIFICATION

Clinical microbiology and molecular pathology laboratories have more recently adapted amplification methodologies for detection of pathogens and/or their products in infectious material. The methods potentially can approach the sensitivities of culture and are in general higher than those of probes. **Amplification** is a molecular procedure that increases the number of nucleic acid copies in a specimen to millions in a very short period of time (often less than 5 hours). With its inception, it first appeared that amplification would take over all conventional methods in the clinical lab. However, it has become obvious that the technique, although excellent in some areas, may not always be the method of choice. Its successes include identification of organisms for which culture methods are long and tedious, for which there are no culture methods available, or for diseases in which the need to know the answer very rapidly overrides the costs.

The first method of amplification was **Polymerase Chain Reaction (PCR).** It remains a major mode of this molecular technique and leads the way in many

---

Box 5-3

Applications of Probe Technology

Outside clinical microbiology
　Genetic defect detection
　Food microbiology
　Plant pathology
Within clinical microbiology
　▪ Direct detection of microbes in clinical
　　specimens
　▪ Organisms not able to be cultivated
　▪ Organisms with long incubation times
　▪ Diseases with unknown etiologies
　Identification of cultural isolates
　Stain identification
　Identification of toxins, virulence factors
　Identification of resistance markers
　Identification of microbes in environmental
　　specimens
　Identification of resistance factors

---

applications. Originally described by Mullis in 1990, it involves a repeating three-step process in which DNA target material is denatured, **annealing** primers (oligonucleotides) are applied to the single stranded DNA and then enzymatically extended to synthesize **complementary** strands of the DNA. A typical reaction involves a total of 25 to 40 cycles. Each **cycle** is a sequential series of three different temperature settings. Table 5-11 identifies the action of each step in the amplification process. The methodology is

---

TABLE 5-11

Reaction Steps Required for Amplification of DNA by PCR

Step	Temperature (° C)	Action
Denaturation	94	Double-stranded DNA broken into single strands (dsDNA → ssDNA)
Primer annealing	55	Attachment of oligonucleotide primers to complimentary regions on ssDNA
Extension	72	Synthesis of dsDNA (5' → 3'); catalyzed by *Taq* DNA polymerase

similar to the in vivo mode of DNA replication. The following components are required:

1. A short single-stranded DNA (ssDNA) molecule, known as an **oligonucleotide** primer that initiates the DNA for replication
2. A DNA polymerase enzyme that catalyzes the formation of additional molecules of double-stranded DNA (dsDNA)
3. The individual building blocks of DNA, the deoxynucleotide bases (dATP, dCTP, dGTP, and dTTP or dUTP)

Table 5-12 lists the role of each component of the reaction.

Nucleic acid sequence information is available for most organisms of clinical importance. Careful evaluation of this information determines the target for amplification. Microorganisms typically contain unique regions in their genetic material that is characteristic of a particular strain. **Primers** designed to recognize these unique regions permit highly specific identification of a single strain or species. Conversely, the amplification may be intentionally nonspecific. If primers are chosen that flank a region shared by a diverse group of organisms, the resulting amplification would yield the detection of more than one type of organism.

Proper selection of a pair of oligonucleotide primers is essential to the ultimate success of the amplification. Primers are short pieces (18 to 28 nucleotides in length) of single-stranded DNA. They flank the two sides of the target sequence and serve to define the ends of the DNA that has been targeted for amplification. The length of the primers, the temperature used for the reaction, as well as other requirements need to be adhered to eliminate artifacts that might lower amplification efficiency.

DNA polymerase is the enzyme that catalyzes the formation of a new strand of dsDNA identical in content to the original DNA template. Today, **Taq polymerase** is the enzyme most often utilized. It is heat stable and retains full activity after repeat denaturing steps. It is not necessary to add more enzyme during the procedure.

Detection of the Amplicon

As was discussed for probe technology, a variety of formats are available for detection of the product amplicon. These include for amplification: an EIA-type colored format for detection as is used in PCR or chemiluminescense used by some other manufacturers. Radioactivity is often used for detection of PCR amplicons in research and/or homebrew applications (methods developed in house).

A number of biotech companies have commercialized amplification techniques for use in the clinical microbiology lab. PCR is commercially produced by Roche Molecular Systems (Branchburg, NJ). In addition, Table 5-13 lists other commercial companies and the types of amplification that they provide for use in a clinical lab. The principle of Transcription Mediated Amplification (TMA) is the method of Gen-Probe Inc. (San Diego, CA). In this procedure, rRNA is the target material and a transcriptase enzyme is used to produce **amplicons** in a thermal-stable environment.

TABLE 5-12

Component Required for Amplification of DNA by PCR

Reagent	Usual Concentration	Action
KCl	50 mmol	Provides proper salt concentration
Tris-HCl, pH 8.3	10 mmol	Maintains proper pH for efficient action of enzyme
Gelatin	0.01%	Stabilizes enzyme
$MgCl_2 \cdot 6H_2O$	1.5-2.5 mmol	Provides cation required for proper functioning of enzyme
Deoxynucleotides (dATP, dCTP, dTTP or dUTP, dGTP)	200 μmol	Building blocks of DNA required for synthesis of new DNA strands
Sense strand primer	50-100 pmol	Anneals to (+) ssDNA; provides starting point for DNA replication
Anti-sense strand primer	50-100 pmol	Anneals to (−) ssDNA; provides starting point for DNA replication
Template DNA	1 μg	Contains target DNA to be amplified
Enzyme (*Taq* or other thermostable DNA polymerase)	2.5 U	Catalyzes formation of dsDNA
UNG (uracil-*n*-glycosylase)	5 U	Cleaves PCR products that contain UTP

TABLE 5-13

Commercially Available Amplification Products/Manufacturers

PCR	Polymerase chain reaction	Roche Molecular Systems
TMA	Transcription mediated amplification	Gen-Probe, Inc.
LCx	Ligase chain reaction	Abbott Labs
SDA	Strand displacement amplification	Becton Dickinson Microbiology Systems
NASBA (NucliSense)	Nucleic acid sequence based amplification	Organon Teknika
bDNA	Branched chain Hybrid capture	Chiron Digene, Inc.
CPT	Cycling probe technology	ID Biomedical

Because ssRNA is the target, no denaturation of the nucleic acid is needed. The principle of the procedure is shown in Figure 5-46. **Ligase Chain Reaction (LCR),** a product of Abbott Laboratories (Chicago, IL), consists of three steps, as in PCR: denaturation of the target nucleic acid, annealing of primers, an enzymatic ligation of the primers by a thermostable DNA ligase. Two pairs of primers are used in the LCx process and these are designed to hybridize to adjacent target sequences. After annealing, these primers are linked by the ligase enzyme. What results are two chimeric single-stranded oligonucleotides, each containing one member of both primer pairs. As the cycle proceeds, the ligated oligonucleotides act as synthetic target molecules for further rounds of primer annealing and ligation. The amplicon is a short sequence of dsDNA, 40 to 50 nucleotides long, containing one molecule each of the original four primers. The LCR procedure is very similar to PCR; however, in addition it can be used to detect single nucleotide changes, that is, point mutations. Its applicability extends to use in genetic screening, for example, for detection of a mutation that may be responsible for a specific disease or for detection of a mutation that might confer resistance to antibiotics.

Another type of target amplification that is thermally stable is that of **Nucleic Acid Based Sequence Amplification (NASBA),** a system developed by Organon Teknika (Raleigh-Durham, NC). The acronym *NucliSense* has recently been introduced in place of *NASBA*. This amplification procedure utilizes two enzymes: reverse transcriptase, a RNase, and RNA polymerase. An RNA target is first reverse transcribed to produce a cDNA copy; these cDNA copies are transcribed into ssRNA molecules by the RNA polymerase. The recognition site for the polymerase is specified so that only correctly primed DNA sequences are transcribed. The amplicon is RNA.

Strand Displacement Amplification (SDA) is the amplification product of Becton Dickinson Microbiology Systems (Sparks, MD). A PCR process occurs first, in which dsDNA target material is denatured, primers are annealed, and complementary DNA is synthesized by a DNA polymerase. The newly formed strands are phosphorothiolated because of the incorporation of an alpha-thio-modified nucleotide triphosphate. The specific primers that anneal to specific target sites also contain a specific restriction endonuclease recognition site (HincIII). When HincIII is added to the reaction mixture, the second phase of SDA, different from PCR, is initiated. HincIII-produced nicks in the non-phosphorothiolated DNA strands give rise to priming sites for DNA polymerase and as the polymerase proceeds along the template, it "displaces" the nicked strand as an intact molecule that is then capable of performing as a template for further reactions. The polymerase simultaneously, to replace the nicked strand, synthesizes an exact replica of it. The thermal stable process of nicking, cDNA synthesis and strand displacement results in millions of copies of amplicons.

Signal amplification has been utilized by the Chiron Corp. (Emeryville, CA) in a method referred to as branched chain cDNA amplification. By using a series of probes, one of which is a capture probe and another a detector probe, the specific RNA target is captured and attached to a substrate—a microtiter plate. The signal or detector probe is specific for the captured target. This latter probe has attached to it many "branches" that can themselves attach to enzyme molecules, which can then be detected with a chemiluminescent substrate. The number of branches per detector molecule is specific and consistent, and hence the number of these molecules that are attached to the appropriate target are quantifiable. This method of amplification is often referred to as the "Christmas tree method," because the branches are said to light up with the detector when positive for correct

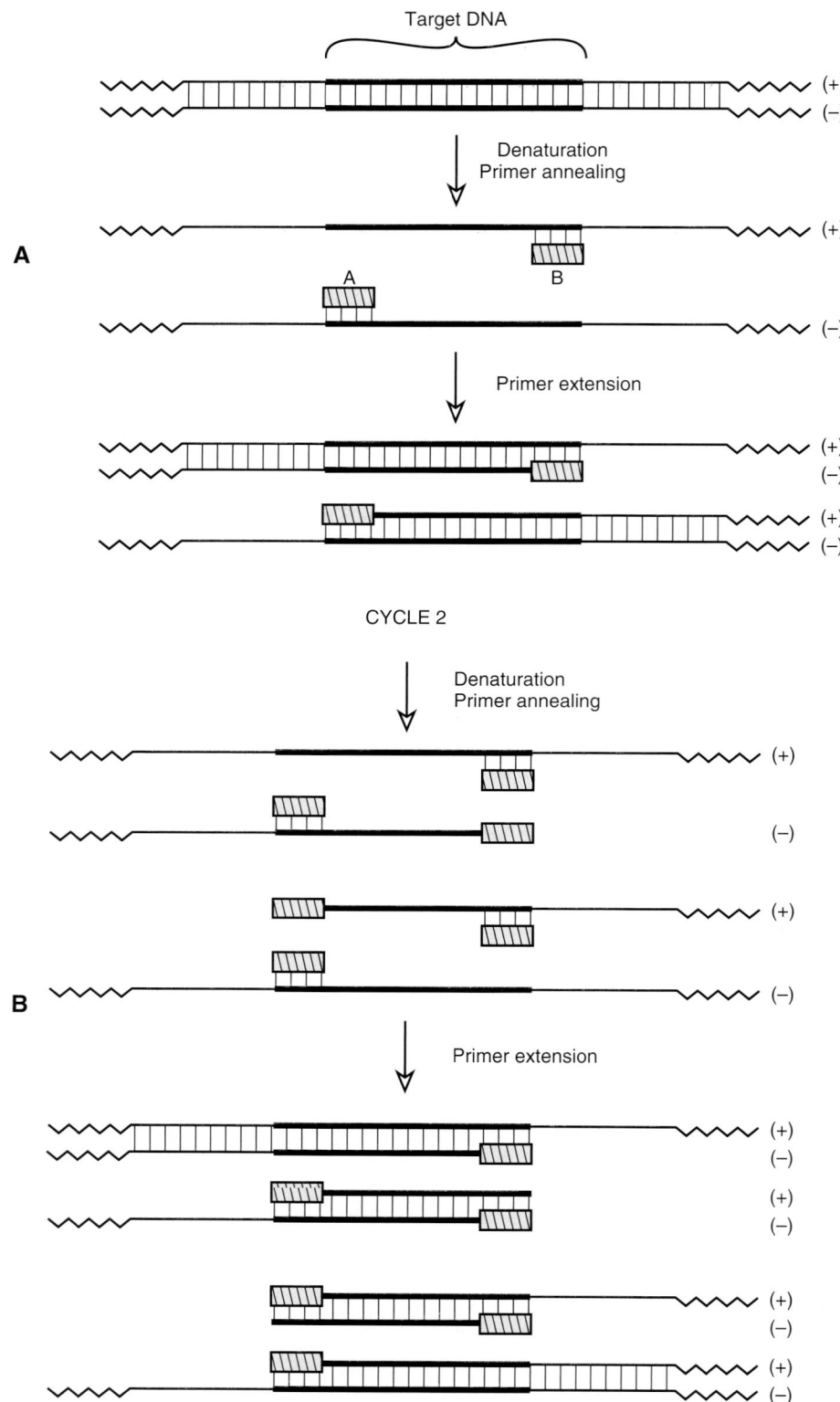

CYCLE 1

Target DNA

Denaturation
Primer annealing

A

Primer extension

CYCLE 2

Denaturation
Primer annealing

B

Primer extension

Figure 5-46 _____

Schematic of the mechanism of amplification of genomic DNA by polymerase chain reaction. **A,** The first cycle results in the generation of two long products, defined at one end by a primer sequence. **B,** The second cycle results in the generation of two long products and two intermediate products (defined at three ends by primer sequences).

CYCLE 3

Denaturation
Primer annealing

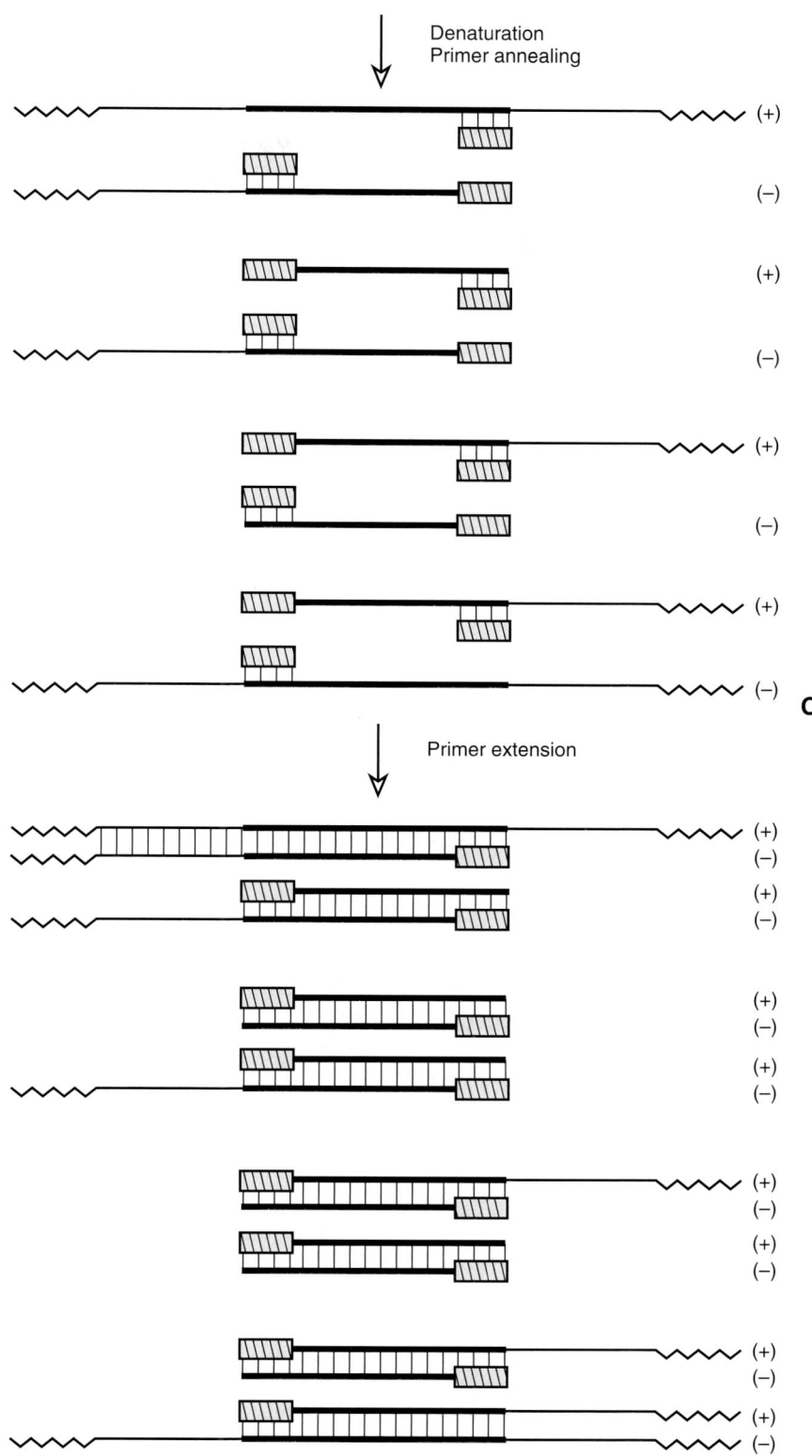

Primer extension

C

Figure 5-46, cont'd

C, The third cycle results in the generation of two short products defined at all four ends by primer sequences. (Adapted from *New England Journal of Medicine* 322:179, 1990.)

target and look like a Christmas tree. Because the signal and not the target is amplified, the potential exists for much less contamination of subsequent reactions, as compared with amplification systems in which the target itself is amplified.

Digene Diagnostics (Silver Springs, Md.) has formulated a method of probe hybridization, which does not require any amplification, but which can provide a very sensitive method for the detection of target material in clinical specimens. The method is referred to as hybrid capture. The target material (specimen) is applied in solution, to a probe-labeled tube and if complementary, the probe and target will hybridize on the inside wall of the tube. A capture probe, specific for the hybrid only, is added and captures any hybrids that have been formed. The capture probe is then detected.

A final method of amplification that has been investigated most recently is that of cycling probe technology, being employed by ID Biomedical Labs (Burnaby, Canada). The method is a gene-based method for detection of specific target sequences. CPT utilizes a chimeric DNA-RNA-DNA probe containing an RNase H-sensitive scissile link that is cleaved by RNase H when hybridized to a complementary DNA sequence. The cleaved probe fragments dissociate from the target, thereby releasing the target for hybridization with another probe molecule. The cycle of hybridization, RNase H–mediated probe cleavage, and probe dissociation repeats multiple times, resulting in an accumulation of cleaved probe fragments, which are then used for detection. No products are available with this technology; however, its use is reported for the detection of the mecA gene of *S. aureus* and the resistance genes of vancomycin-resistant enterococcal strains.

CLINICAL APPLICATIONS OF AMPLIFICATION

The detection of many pathogens is possible through the use of PCR (Table 5-14). In addition, any of the other amplification methods may be employed for specific detections. In clinical microbiology laboratories, often a combination of "home-brew" is used, that is, PCR procedures that are developed by the lab itself, and use of commercially available purchased kits in which

TABLE 5-14

Clinically Important Pathogens That Have Been Identified Through the Use of PCR

Viruses	Parvovirus
	Herpes simplex virus
	Rotavirus
	Papillomavirus
	Human herpesvirus 6
	Dengue virus
	Varicella-zoster virus
	Rubella virus
	Adenovirus
	Rhinovirus
	Hepatitis B virus
Bacteria	*Borrelia burgdorferi*
	Vibrio cholerae
	Helicobacter pylori
	Rickettsia tsutsugamushi
	Staphylococcus aureus
	Chlamydia trachomatis
	Shigella dysenteriae
	Chlamydia psittaci
	Treponema pallidum
	Enterotoxigenic *Escherichia coli*
	Mycobacterium tuberculosis
	Legionella pneumophila
Parasites	*Plasmodium falciparum*
	Toxoplasma gondii
	Entamoeba histolytica
	Pneumocystis carinii
	Trypanosoma cruzi

amplification can be performed. Some labs perform only in-house assays and others employ only the use of "kits" manufactured by commercial companies. What system a lab uses depends upon the availability of the lab to develop molecular procedures and/or the availability of manufactured kits. For some labs, when a request for amplification is made, the specimen is sent out to a reference lab that can perform the appropriate assay.

The choice of which application a clinical laboratory adapts for use must be carefully considered. One of the following criteria must be met:

1. Amplification should supplement existing technology: In many cases, current culture techniques are sufficient to identify a bacterial pathogen. Amplification may be used to enhance the diagnosis. An example is its use in the detection of enterotoxigenic strains of *E. coli,* which contain a characteristic heat-

labile toxin. PCR primers that flank this gene permit a specific detection of the organism. Related organisms that lack this gene are not detected, although all *E. coli* strains can be cultured.

2. Amplification could replace existing technology: An example might be in the detection of *Chlamydia trachomatis* in genital specimens. Culture requires at least 48 hours and studies have shown that the sensitivity of the amplification methods is up to 30% more sensitive than culture.

3. Amplification represents new diagnostic technology: PCR, for example, is of most benefit in the diagnosis of fastidious organisms that cannot be detected by conventional culture techniques, such as human papillomavirus (HPV).

Technical Considerations for Implementation of Amplification

- Determination of the appropriate specimen: Usually the same source as for culture
- Construction of primers and probes, if developed in house: Usually primers are designed to detect the most conserved regions of the target material
- Optimization of amplification conditions: As determined through in-house evaluations or by following the manufacturers' instructions contained in protocols and package inserts
- Choice of a detection format: Usually non-isotopic; often dictated by the manufacturer
- Interpretation of test results: Reporting of results as positive or negative often not sufficient; the lab needs to give the limits of the assay and the problems that may occur and interpretations of the results
- Quality assurance and quality control: Strictly adhere to manufacturers' instructions; or in the case of development of in-house assays, a strict set of QA and QC guidelines to follow for maximum efficiency and accuracy must be employed

Measures to Control Contamination

For any of the amplification methods, adherence to policies that minimize the chance of contamination from one specimen to the next is mandatory. Required cleaning policies should be followed as completely as possible. The use of different areas for reagent preparation, specimen preparation, amplification and detection may be necessary; for some commercial "kit" methods, separate rooms are not suggested, although proper precautions are still necessary. Things to consider to ensure contamination-free procedures include the following: dedicated supplies and reagents, including color coding of reagents that belong to certain procedures; specific protected pipettors; unidirectional work flow (Figure 5-47) from clean (pre-amplification) to "dirty" (post-amplification) activities; dedicated labcoats and gloves; careful and cautious attention to performance. Prevention of carryover of amplicon, particularly in target-based systems, is perhaps that which needs the most controls and care. In some amplification systems, inherent methods are incorporated within the system so that the amplicons are prevented from contaminating the future reactions. One of these is the use of deoxyuridine triphosphate (dUTP) in the amplicon instead of deoxythymidine triphosphate (dTTP). Before the start of the subsequent amplifications, uracil-N-glycosylase (UNG) is added to the reaction material. UNG specifically digests any DNA sequences that contain uracil, thus eliminating any prior amplicon material from contaminating future amplifications. This method is employed by Roche Molecular Systems in the manufacturing of products for PCR. Other systems employ ultraviolet light or attempt to reduce carryover by performing all applications in one tube, hence reducing the number of transfers; or by using RNA as target, which is a more labile amplicon. In the case of Chiron's branched chain reaction, amplifying signal rather than target theoretically provides a system much less prone to contamination. Regardless of any of these additional methods, strict adherence to proper lab techniques is essential.

Commercially Available Amplification Systems

Many amplification methods exist for sexually transmitted diseases. The detection of *Chlamydia trachomatis* is done by means of one of three methods: Ligase Chain Reaction (LCx, Abbott Labs), Polymerase Chain Reaction (Amplicor PCR, Roche Molecular Systems) or Transcription Mediated Amplification (TMA, Gen-Probe, Inc.). In addition,

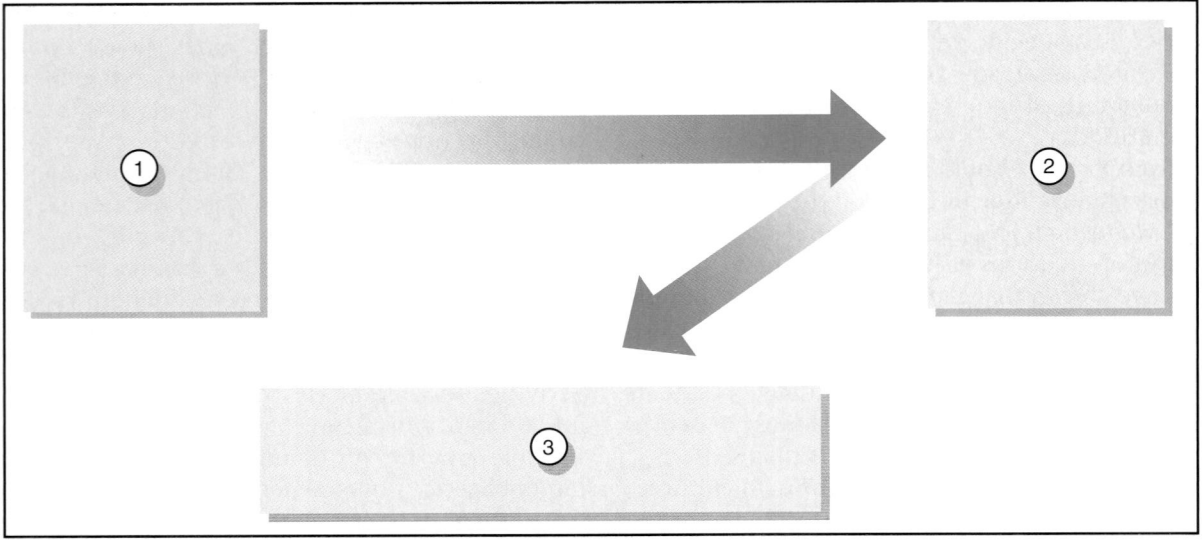

Dedicated equipment and reagent requirements in a PCR laboratory are as follows:

Area 1: Sample preparation
- Positive-displacement pipettes or pipettors with aerosol-resistant tips
- Gloves and laboratory coat
- Refrigerator, freezer, water bath or dry-heat block, laminar flow biosafety cabinet
- Cell lysis reagents

Area 2: Reagent preparation and PCR set-up
- Amplification reagents and supplies
- Positive-displacement pipettes or pipettors with aerosol-resistant tips
- Laminar-flow biosafety cabinet or dead air box
- Gloves and laboratory coat
- Refrigerator and freezer
- Water bath or dry-heat block

Area 3: Amplification and detection
- Thermal cycler
- Pipettors with aerosol-resistant tips
- Detection equipment (electrophoresis unit, incubator, plate washer, plate reader, water bath)
- Refrigerator and freezer
- Reagents and supplies for detection

Figure 5-47

Unidirectional workflow in a polymerase chain reaction (PCR) laboratory.

LCx is approved for the simultaneous detection of *Neisseria gonorrhoeae,* and the other two amplification methods are pending approval by the FDA. Urine can be the sample for detection of both sexually transmitted diseases by LCx with sensitivities that approach or equal that of detection in genital samples. TMA and PCR will have this application available soon as well. Other companies (Becton Dickinson's ProbeTec SDA and Digene's Hybrid Capture Assay) will also have their versions of *Chlamydia* and *Neisseria* amplification in the future. With LCx, automation became a possibility for amplification, thus reducing the hands-on time for amplification. Roche PCR will soon be available

for *C. trachomatis* and hopefully, *N. gonorrhoeae* in their automated equipment, the COBAS. TMA products will be available in the future in the automated Tigris, a very large high-volume instrument as well as use of the VIDAS (bioMerieux Vitek, St. Louis, MO) for the smaller lab. The Probe Tec amplification system, when FDA approved, will be released in an automated format, with everything post–specimen preparation, performed in an instrument (see Table 5-13).

HIV quantitative viral loads can be detected by means of PCR, Chiron branched chain DNA, and NASBA. Qualitative detection of HIV can be accomplished as well; however, outside of neonatal requirements, antibody tests remain the screen assay employed for initial primary HIV diagnosis. Human papilloma virus (HPV) can be detected by in situ methods but more recently a method of hybrid capture (Digene) has allowed for the detection of the virus in solution from PAP smears or thin prep specimens. Both high- and low-risk genotypes can be detected by this format in a relatively rapidly and easily performed assay.

Detection of *Mycobacterium tuberculosis*

For the detection of *M. tuberculosis* directly in clinical respiratory specimens, two amplification methods are presently commercially available and FDA approved: TMA and PCR. Both can be performed on respiratory specimens that are acid-fast smear positive from patients who have never been previously diagnosed with tuberculosis. The FDA has placed these restrictions on the use of the products. The assays each require about 5 hours, are presently in hands-on formulations only, but do provide a rapid and very specific answer to help clinicians more appropriately treat suspected cases of tuberculosis and help to prevent its spread by isolation of patients and appropriate chemotherapy. These assays are expensive to perform, so they cannot be applied to every specimen request for mycobacterial detection.

Other Available Assays

HCV and HBV can be detected by PCR and Chiron's cDNA amplification. CMV can be detected with a high degree of sensitivity in blood buffy coats by means of PCR or the Digene Hybrid capture assay. Quantitation is also available, although not FDA approved as yet.

Amplification methods are available for a wide variety of agents without benefit of commercial availability. Most are in a PCR format. These are most often performed in research labs or commercial companies. For example, some of these methods detect *Bordetella pertussis, Chlamydia pneumoniae, Mycoplasma pneumoniae, Bartonella henselae,* and *Borrelia burgdorferi.* Amplification methods are also available for detection and determination of the viral load for diseases such as HIV, HCV, CMV, and HSV (specifically in cerebrospinal fluid).

Because there are many research labs willing to perform amplification assays for almost any or-

ganism, it is important for the lab to remember that it plays an integral role in helping clinicians to use this powerful tool effectively. For organisms in which detection by culture or serology is still adequate, amplification may not be necessary. For diseases in which the etiology is unknown, amplification may become the gold standard. In most cases, the request is being made because the method is there and felt to be the best. It is important to keep abreast of what is available and how good the methods are: how sensitive and specific the test is; what are the potential chances of false positives or false negatives; what is the expense; and how important it is for a definitive and rapid identification to be made.

In almost all cases, amplification will remain an adjunct test and therefore an added cost to the microbiological examination of the specimen. Cultures are usually still needed for subsequent susceptibility testing, epidemiology, or in specimens in which mixed infections may be possible and only one of the pathogens is detectable by amplification. When amplification is being researched for its potential introduction in the lab, cost savings may not be noted in the microbiology lab; actually, increased costs may be incurred. However, the cost saving to the patient and to the hospital overall may be very great and need to be considered in the outcome analysis of any new test.

Bibliography

Allard U et al: Polymerase chain reaction for detection of adenoviruses in stool samples, *J Clin Microbiol* 28:2659, 1990.

Baselski VS: The role of molecular diagnostics in the clinical microbiology laboratory, *Clin Lab Med* 16:49, 1996.

Bjorkholm B et al: Rapid PCR detection of *Helicobacter pylori*–associated virulence and resistance genes directly from gastric biopsy material, *J Clin Microbiol* 36:3689, 1998.

Cartwright CP: Techniques and diagnostic applications of in vitro nucleic-acid amplification, *Clin Microbiol Newsl* 16:33, 1994.

Cherian T et al: PCR-enzyme immunoassay for detection of *Streptococcus pneumoniae* DNA in cerebrospinal fluid samples from patients with culture-negative meningitis, *J Clin Microbiol* 36:3605, 1998.

Chernesky MA et al: Ability of commercial LCr and PCR assays to diagnose *C. trachomatis* in men by testing first-void urine, *J Clin Microbiol* 35:982, 1997.

Cheung LL, Hudson JB: Development of DNA probes for *Candida albicans, Diagn Microbiol Infect Dis* 10:171, 1988.

Clewley JP: Polymerase chain reaction assay of Parvovirus B19 DNA in clinical specimens, *J Clin Microbiol* 27:2647, 1989.

Daly JA et al: Use of nonradioactive DNA probes in culture confirmation tests to detect *Streptococcus agalactiae, Haemophilus influenzae* and *Enterococcus* spp. from pediatric patients with significant infections, *J Clin Microbiol* 29:80, 1991.

Davis TE, Fuller DD: Direct identification of bacterial isolates in blood cultures by using a DNA probe, *J Clin Microbiol* 29:2193, 1991.

Della-Latta P, Whittier SD: Comprehensive evaluation of performance, laboratory application, and clinical usefulness of two direct amplification technologies for the detection of *Mycobacterium tuberculosis* complex, *Am J Clin Pathol* 110:201, 1998.

Dix K et al: Species specific oligonucleotide probes for the identification of periodontal bacteria, *J Clin Microbiol* 28:319, 1990.

Echeverria P et al: Comparative study of synthetic oligonucleotide and cloned polynucleotide enterotoxin gene probe to identify enterotoxigenic *Escherichia coli, J Clin Microbiol* 25:106, 1987.

Ellner PD, Kiehn TE: Rapid detection and identification of pathogenic mycobacteria by combining radiometric and nucleic acid probe methods, *J Clin Microbiol* 26:1349, 1988.

Gelfand DH, White TJ: Thermostable DNA polymerases. In Innis MA et al: *PCR protocols: a guide to methods and applications,* San Diego, 1990, Academic Press.

Gicquelais KG et al: Practical and economical method for using biotinylated DNA probes with bacterial colony blots to identify diarrhea-causing *Escherichia coli, J Clin Microbiol* 28:2485, 1990.

Goessens WHF et al: Comparison of three commercially available amplification assays, AMP CT, LCx and COBAS AMPLICOR for detection of CT in first void urine, *J Clin Microbiol* 35:2628, 1997.

Gomes TAT et al: DNA probes for identification of enteroinvasive *Escherichia coli, J Clin Microbiol* 25:2025, 1987.

Hillier SL, Briselden AM: Evaluation of a rapid oligonucleotide test for direct detection of *Gardnerella vaginalis* and *Trichomonas vaginalis* from vaginal specimens, abstract presented at ASM meeting, New Orleans, May 1992.

Ho S et al: Direct polymerase chain reaction test for detection of *Helicobacter pylori* in humans and animals, *J Clin Microbiol* 29:2543, 1991.

Iwen PC, Blair TMH, Woods GL: Comparison of the Gen-Probe PACE 2 system, direct fluorescent antibody and cell culture for detecting *Chlamydia trachomatis* in cervical specimens, *Am J Clin Pathol* 95:578, 1991.

Kain K, Lanar DE: Determination of genetic variation with *Plasmodium falciparum* by using enzymatically amplified DNA from filter paper disks impregnated with whole blood, *J Clin Microbiol* 29:1171, 1991.

Kehl SC et al: Evaluation of the Abbott LCx assay for detection of *Neisseria gonorrhoeae* in endocervical swab specimens from females, *J Clin Microbiol* 36:3549, 1998.

Kejian G, Bowden DS: Digoxigenin-labeled probes for the detection of hepatitis B virus DNA in serum, *J Clin Microbiol* 29:506, 1991.

Kesslet HH et al: Rapid diagnosis of enterovirus infection by a new one-step reverse transcription-PCR assay, *J Clin Microbiol* 35:976, 1997.

Kiehn TE, Edwards FF: Rapid identification using a specific DNA probe of *Mycobacterium avium* complex from patients with acquired immunodeficiency syndrome, *J Clin Microbiol* 25:1551, 1987.

Kuritza AP et al: DNA probes for identification of clinically important *Bacteroides* species, *J Clin Microbiol* 23:343, 1986.

Kwok S, Higuchi R: Avoiding false positives with PCR, *Nature* 339:237, 1989.

Lees MI, Newnan DM, Garland SM: Comparison of a DNA Probe assay with culture for the detection of *Chlamydia trachomatis, J Med Microbiol* 35:159, 1991.

Lim SD et al: Genotypic identification of pathogenic *Mycobacterium* species by using a nonradioactive oligonucleotide probe, *J Clin Microbiol* 29:1276, 1991.

Lyles CM et al: Comparison of two measures of human immunodeficiency virus (HIV) type 1 Load in HIV risk groups, *J Clin Microbiol* 36:2647, 1998.

McCreedy BJ et al: Laboratory design and workflow. In Persing DH et al, editor: Diagnostic molecular principles and applications, Washington, DC, American Society for Microbiology, p 149.

McLaughlin GL et al: Optimization of a rapid non-isotopic DNA probe assay for *Plasmodium falciparum* in the Gambia, *J Clin Microbiol* 29:1517, 1991.

Moncla BJ et al: Use of synthetic oligonucleotide DNA probes for identification and direct detection of *Bacteroides forsythus* in plaque samples, *J Clin Microbiol* 29:2158, 1991.

Mullis K et al: Specific amplification of DNA in vitro: the polymerase chain reaction, *Cold Spring Harbor Symp Quantit Biol* 51:263, 1986.

Panke ES et al: Comparison of Gen-Probe DNA probe test and culture for the detection of *Neisseria gonorrhoeae* in endocervical specimens, *J Clin Microbiol* 29:883, 1991.

Pasculle AW, Veto GE et al: Laboratory and clinical evaluation of a commercial DNA probe for the detection of *Legionella* sp., *J Clin Microbiol* 27:2350, 1989.

Pasternack R et al: Comparison of manual Amplicor PCR, Cobas Amplicor PCR, and LCx assays for detection of *C. trachomatis* infection in women using urine specimens, *J Clin Microbiol* 35:402, 1996.

Persing DH: Polymerase chain reaction: trenches to benches, *J Clin Microbiol* 29:1281, 1991.

Piersimoni C et al: Comparative evaluation of the new Gen-Probe *Mycobacterium tuberculosis* amplified direct test and the semiautomated Abbott LCx *Mycobacterium tuberculosis* assay for direct detection of *Mycobacterium tuberculosis* complex in respiratory and extrapulmonary specimens, *J Clin Microbiol* 36:3601, 1998.

Popovic-Uroic T et al: Evaluation of an oligonucleotide probe for identification of *Campylobacter* species, *Lab Med* 22:533, 1991.

Poulakkainen M et al: Comparison of performances of two commercially available tests, a PCR and an LCr test, in detection of urogenital *C. trachomatis* infection, *J Clin Microbiol* 36:1489, 1998.

Reagan DR et al: Characterization of the sequence of colonization and nosocomial candidemia using DNA fingerprinting and a DNA probe, *J Clin Microbiol* 28:2733, 1990.

Rotbart HA: Nucleic acid detection systems for enteroviruses, *Clin Microbiol Rev* 4:156, 1991.

Scholl DR et al: Clinical application of a novel sample processing technology for the identification of salmonellae by using DNA probes, *J Clin Microbiol* 28:237, 1990.

Sommerfelt H et al: Cloned polynucleotide and synthetic oligonucleotide probes used in colony hybridization are equally efficient in the identification of enterotoxigenic *Escherichia coli, J Clin Microbiol* 26:2275, 1988.

Stary A et al: Comparison of LCr and culture for detection of *N. gonorrhoeae* in genital and extragenital specimens, *J Clin Microbiol* 35:239, 1997.

Stary A et al: Performance of transcription mediated amplification and LCr assays for detection of *Chlamydia* infection in urogenital samples obtained by invasive and noninvasive methods, *J Clin Microbiol* 36:2666, 1998.

Tenover FC et al: DNA probe culture confirmation assay for identification of thermophilic *Campylobacter* species, *J Clin Microbiol* 28:1284, 1990.

Wise DJ, Weaver TL: Detection of Lyme disease bacterium, *Borrelia burgdorferi,* by using the polymerase chain reaction and a non-radioisotopic gene probe, *J Clin Microbiol* 29:1523, 1991.

Wolcott M: Advances in nucleic acid based detection methods, *Clin Microbiol Rev* 5:370, 1992.

Wylie JL et al: Comparative evaluation of Chlamydiazyme, PACE 2, and AMP-CT assays for detection of *Chlamydia trachomatis* in endocervical specimens, *J Clin Microbiol* 36:3488, 1998.

Yamakami Y et al: Evaluation of PCR for detection of DNA specific for *Aspergillus* species in sera of patients with various forms of pulmonary aspergillosis, *J Clin Microbiol* 36:3619, 1998.

Zhang G, Weintraub A: Rapid and sensitive assay for detection of enterotoxigenic *Bacteroides fragilis, J Clin Microbiol* 36:3545, 1998.

LEARNING ASSESSMENTS

1. In what situations would molecular applications be most beneficial?

2. What is nucleic acid hybridization? What are the different hybridization formats?

3. Which bacterial cultures can be confirmed by probes?

4. What probes are available for rapid diagnosis of infectious diseases at different body sites?

5. How do amplification techniques provide higher sensitivity in detecting infectious materials?

CHAPTER 6

Host-Parasite Interaction

A. INDIGENOUS MICROBIAL FLORA

Hal S. Larsen

FLORA
Origin of Microbial Flora
Characteristics of Indigenous Microbial Flora

USUAL FLORA AT DIFFERENT BODY SITES
Usual Flora of the Skin
Usual Flora of the Mouth
Usual Flora of the Respiratory Tract
Usual Flora of the Gastrointestinal Tract
Usual Flora of the Genitourinary Tract

OBJECTIVES

1. Define the following terms: *parasitism, usual* or *indigenous flora, commensal, symbiont, opportunist, resident flora, transient flora,* and *carrier.*
2. Describe some factors that determine the nature of the usual flora at various body sites.
3. List the predominant flora of various body sites in a healthy individual.
4. Describe the role of the usual microbial flora in the pathogenesis of infectious disease.
5. Describe the role of the indigenous flora in host defense against infectious diseases.
6. Describe how the human host protects itself from microbial invasion by the following:
   - Epithelial linings in the different organ systems
   - Secretion of fluids that contain antibacterial substances
   - Phagocytes

KEY TERMS

Usual or indigenous flora
Resident flora
Transient flora
Parasite
Symbiont
Commensal
Carrier
Carrier state

CASE STUDY

A 48-year-old woman had a complete hysterectomy. After 3 days of uneventful hospitalization, the patient was discharged from the hospital with a 10-day regimen of prophylactic antimicrobial. On the fifth day after her discharge, she noticed the presence of creamy-white, cheesy material on her tongue and buccal cavity. Wet mount preparations of the material showed budding yeast cells and hyphal elements.

FLORA

Origin of Microbial Flora

The fetus is in a sterile environment until birth. During the first few days of life, the newborn is introduced to the many and varied microorganisms present in the environment. Each organism has the opportunity to find an area on or in the infant that it is adapted to. Those that find their niche colonize various anatomic sites and become the predominant organisms. Others are transient or fail to establish themselves at all. Within a short time following birth, the infant's microbial flora is similar to that of other individuals.

Characteristics of Indigenous Microbial Flora

Microorganisms that are commonly found on or in body sites of healthy persons are termed **usual or indigenous flora.** The different body sites may have the same or different flora, depending on local conditions. Local conditions select for those organisms that are suited for growth in a particular area. For example, the environment found on the skin surface is different from that found in the mouth.

The microorganisms that colonize an area for months or years are termed ***resident flora.*** In contrast, ***transient flora*** are present at a site temporarily. Transient flora come to visit but do not usually live or stay. Organisms that constitute the indigenous flora can be classified as ***parasites*** (live at the expense of the host), ***symbionts*** (benefit the host), or ***commensals*** have neutral effect on the host).

Some pathogenic organisms may establish themselves in a host without manifesting symptoms. These hosts are capable of transmitting the infection. They are termed ***carriers,*** and the condition is called the ***carrier state.*** The carrier state may be acute (short-lived) or chronic (lasting for months, years, or permanently). An example of a chronic carrier state is found in *Salmonella typhi* infection. This organism may establish itself in the bile duct and be excreted in the stool over years. In contrast, *Neisseria meningitidis* may be found in the throat of asymptomatic individuals during an outbreak of meningitis. After a few days or weeks at most, these individuals no longer harbor the organism, so the carrier state was acute. The most transient of carrier states is inoculation of a person's hands or fingers with an organism (e.g., *Staphylococcus aureus* from a wound) that is carried only until the hands are washed.

A number of factors determine which microorganisms are able to colonize the various body sites: the nutritional status of the site, oxidation-reduction potentials, antibody and other anti-bacterial substances, pH, and interference by already established organisms. These conditions may change with age, nutritional status, disease states, and drug or antibiotic effects. The changes may predispose an individual to infection by the usual flora (i.e., opportunistic infection). For example, two groups at increased risk for gram-negative rod pneumonia are diabetics and alcoholics. As described in the previous case study, antibiotics may reduce a particular population of bacteria (e.g., gram-positive), allowing the proliferation of other organisms such as *Candida albicans*. An increase in age brings with it a decrease in the effectiveness of the immune response. As a result, the incidence of infection by opportunistic organisms increases.

USUAL FLORA AT DIFFERENT BODY SITES

The human host is colonized by approximately 100 different species of microorganisms. The effectiveness of the various host defenses is evidenced by the relatively low incidence of infection in uncompromised individuals by members of the usual or indigenous flora. However, infections caused by microbial flora are commonly seen in the clinical microbiology laboratory. The clinical microbiologist must know the types of microorganisms found at the various body sites.

Usual Flora of the Skin
The skin contains a wide variety of microorganisms, most of which are found on the most superficial layers of cells and the upper parts of hair follicles. Microorganisms such as *Propionibacterium*

acnes colonize the deep sebaceous glands. Superficial antisepsis of the skin does not eliminate this organism, which may be found as a contaminant in those culture specimens that require invasive procedures (e.g., blood, cerebrospinal fluid), as a result of contamination of the needle. More organisms are found in moist areas of the skin than in dry areas.

Normal skin has a number of mechanisms to prevent infection. These include the mechanical separation of microorganisms from the tissues, fatty acids that inhibit many microorganisms, excretion of lysozyme by sweat glands, and the desquamation of the epithelium. Washing may decrease the number of skin bacteria by 90%, but the numbers return to normal within a few hours. Washing removes transient pathogens that may cause infection through a variety of mechanisms. Box 6-1 lists the microorganisms most commonly found on the skin. Other organisms have been isolated from the skin but are found only occasionally or rarely and are therefore not listed.

Usual Flora of the Mouth
The mouth contains large numbers of bacteria, with *Streptococcus* being the predominant genus. Many organisms bind to the buccal mucosa and tooth surfaces. Bacterial plaques that develop on teeth may contain as many as 10^{11} streptococci per gram. Plaque also results in a low oxidation-reduction potential at the tooth surface; this sup-

---

Box 6-1

Microorganisms Found on the Skin

Common

Candida spp.
Micrococcus spp.
Staphylococcus spp.
Clostridium spp.
Diphtheroids

Less common

Streptococcus spp.
Acinetobacter spp.
Bacteroides spp.
Gram-negative rods (fermenters and nonfermenters)
Moraxella spp.

Box 6-2

Microorganisms Found in the Mouth

Common

Staphylococcus epidermidis
Streptococcus mitis
Streptococcus sanguis
Streptococcus salivarius
Streptococcus mutans
Peptostreptococcus spp.
Veillonella spp.
Lactobacilus spp.
Actinomyces israelii
Bacteroides spp.

Prevotella/Porphyromonas
Bacteroides oralis
Treponema denticola
Treponema refringens

Less common

Staphylococcus aureus
Enterococcus spp.
Eikenella corrodens
Fusobacterium nucleatum
Candida albicans

---

ports the growth of strict anaerobes, particularly in crevices and in the areas between the teeth. A partial list of microorganisms found in the mouth appears in Box 6-2.

Usual Flora of the Respiratory Tract

The respiratory tract consists of the mouth (previously discussed), nasopharynx, oropharynx, nose, trachea, bronchi, and lungs. The trachea, bronchi, and lungs are protected by the action of ciliary epithelial cells and by the movement of mucus. The tissues of these structures are normally sterile as a result of this protective action. The organisms found in the mouth, nasopharynx, oropharynx, and nose are similar but show some differences. The most common microorganisms found in the *nose* are *S. aureus* and *Staphylococcus epidermidis*. The population of the nasopharynx mirrors that of the nose, although the environment is different enough from that of the nose to select

for several additional organisms. Those organisms found as usual flora of the nose and nasopharynx are outlined in Box 6-3.

The oropharynx contains a mixture of streptococci. A number of species of the viridans group can be isolated, including *Streptococcus mitis, Streptococcus mutans, Streptococcus milleri, Streptococcus sanguis,* and *Streptococcus salivarius.* In addition, diphtheroids and *Moraxella catarrhalis* can be readily isolated. Hospitalized patients often show colonization with gram-negative rods. The usual flora of the oropharynx is listed in Box 6-4.

Usual Flora of the Gastrointestinal Tract

The gastrointestinal tract comprises the esophagus, stomach, small intestine, and colon. Microorganisms usually do not multiply in the esophagus and stomach but are present in ingested food and as transient flora. Most microorganisms are destroyed in the stomach and those that survive

---

Box 6-3

Microorganisms Found in the Nose and Nasopharynx

Common

Staphylococcus aureus
Staphylococcus epidermidis
Diphtheroids
Haemophilus parainfluenzae
Streptococcus spp.

Less common

Streptococcus pneumoniae
Moraxella catarrhalis
Haemophilus influenzae
Neisseria meningitidis
Moraxella spp.

Box 6-4

Microorganisms Found in the Oropharynx

Common

α-Hemolytic and nonhemolytic streptococci
Diphtheroids
Staphylococcus aureus
Staphylococcus epidermidis
Streptococcus pneumoniae
Streptococcus mutans
Streptococcus milleri
Streptococcus mitis
Steptococcus sanguis
Streptococcus salivarius
Moraxella catarrhalis

Haemophilus parainfluenzae
Anaerobic streptococci
Bacteroides spp.
Prevotella/Porphyromonas
Bacteroides oralis
Fusobacterium necrophorum

Less common

Streptococcus pyogenes
Neisseria meningitidis
Haemophilus influenzae
Gram-negative rods

---

generally are protected by being enmeshed in food and move to the small intestine. The small intestine contains few microorganisms. However, microorganisms are prevalent in the colon, where a count between 10^8 and 10^{11} bacteria per gram of solid material is normal. Although we usually think of the facultative anaerobes as being the predominant organisms, anaerobes far outnumber the facultative gram-negative rods, making up over 90% of the microbial flora of the large intestine. The population may be altered by antibiotics. In some cases, certain populations or organisms are eradicated or suppressed and other members of the indigenous flora are able to proliferate. This can be the cause of a severe necrotizing enterocolitis *(Clostridium difficile)*, diarrhea *(C. albicans, S. aureus)*, or other superinfection. The bacteria constituting the usual intestinal flora also carry out a variety of metabolic degradations and syntheses that appear to play a role in the health of the host.

A summary of the organisms found in the gastrointestinal tract is shown in Box 6-5.

Usual Flora of the Genitourinary Tract

The kidneys, bladder, and fallopian tubes are normally free of microorganisms. The urethra is colonized in its outermost segment by those organisms found on the skin. During childbearing years, the vagina is colonized with lactobacilli and anaerobic gram-negative rods and gram-positive cocci. Many organisms are inhibited by the low pH (4 to 5) of the vagina. Microorganisms expected to be isolated from the genitourinary tract are listed in Box 6-6.

The microbial flora have beneficial effects. The development of immunologic competence depends on this flora. The immune system is constantly primed by contact with the microorganisms. Animals born and raised in a germ-free environment have a poorly functioning immune

Box 6-5

Common Microorganisms Found in the Gastrointestinal Tract

Bacteroides spp.
Clostridium spp.
Enterobacteriaceae
Eubacterium spp.
Fusobacterium spp.

Peptostreptococcus spp.
Peptococcus spp.
Staphylococcus aureus
Enterococcus spp.

Box 6-6

Microorganisms Found in the Genitourinary Tract

Common

Lactobacillus spp.
Bacteroides spp.
Clostridium spp.
Peptostreptococcus spp.
Staphylococcus aureus
Staphylococcus epidermidis
Enterococcus spp.
Diphtheroids

Less common

Group B streptococci
Enterobacteriaceae
Acinetobacter spp.
Candida albicans

system. Exposure to otherwise innocuous organisms can be fatal to such animals. The microbial flora produces conditions at the microenvironmental level that block colonization by extraneous pathogens. When the composition of the indigenous flora is altered (e.g., by antibiotic therapy with broad-spectrum antibiotics), other organisms capable of causing disease may fill the void. *C. albicans* may greatly multiply and cause diarrhea or infections in the mouth or vagina, as in the case presented earlier. *C. difficile* produces a colitis as a result of its proliferation following antibiotic therapy.

The microbial flora play an important role in both health and disease. Eradication of the usual flora may have profound negative effects, and yet, many common infections are caused by members of the usual flora. Knowledge of these organisms helps in the collection and processing of specimens and the identification of isolates.

LEARNING ASSESSMENT

1. How did the patient in the case study develop the yeast infection in her mouth?

2. What is the difference between resident and transient flora?

3. What is a carrier?

4. What is the significance of the carrier in the pathogenesis of disease?

5. What determines the composition of the indigenous flora at the different body sites?

B. PATHOGENESIS OF INFECTION

Hal S. Larsen

PATHOGENICITY
  Pathogens
  Opportunistic Pathogens

VIRULENCE

HOST RESISTANCE FACTORS
  Physical Barriers
  Cleansing Mechanisms
  Antimicrobial Substances
  Indigenous Microbial Flora
  Phagocytosis
    Chemotaxis
    Attachment
    Ingestion
    Killing
  Inflammation
  Immune Responses

INFECTIOUS AGENT FACTORS
  Adherence
  Proliferation
  Tissue Damage
    Exotoxins
    Endotoxins
  Invasion
  Dissemination

ROUTES OF TRANSMISSION
  Airborne Transmission
  Transmission by Food and Water
  Close Contact
  Cuts and Bites
  Arthropods
  Zoonoses

EPIDEMIOLOGY
  Definitions
  Surveillance and Reporting

OBJECTIVES

1. Define the following terms: *pathogen, opportunistic pathogen,* and *virulence.*
2. Differentiate the mechanisms of infections caused by true pathogens from those caused by opportunistic pathogens.
3. Describe the various factors and mechanisms by which the human host protects itself from microbial invasion.
4. Discuss the sequence of events in the phagocytosis and killing of an infectious agent.
5. Discuss the conditions that must be present or events that must occur for a microorganism to cause disease.
6. Name the different characteristics of infectious agents that enable them to cause disease in the host.
7. Name the routes of transmission that microorganisms use to infect a host and give examples of each.
8. Define the following terms: *carrier, endemic, epidemic, incidence rate, incubation period, index case, morbidity, mortality, nosocomial infection, reservoir,* and *surveillance.*
9. Explain how public health agencies monitor, investigate, and report infectious diseases.

KEY TERMS

Pathogen	Degranulation
Opportunistic pathogen	Respiratory burst
Opportunistic infection	Inflammation
Iatrogenic infection	Adherence
Virulence	Adhesins
Virulence factors	Exotoxins
Lysozyme	Endotoxins
Antibodies	Invasion
β–Lysins	Dissemination
Interferon	Zoonosis
Bacteriocins	Droplet nuclei
Phagocytosis	Close contact
Lysosomes	Epidemiology
Diapedesis	Endemic
Chemotaxis	Epidemic
Chemotactic agents	Incubation period
Opsonization	Morbidity rate
Opsonins	Surveillance

CASE STUDY

A 52-year-old man was taken to the emergency room in a disoriented and unresponsive state, experiencing shortness of breath. The patient had previous history of poorly controlled diabetes, chronic obstructive pulmonary disease, and Kaposi's sarcoma of the right leg. He had a history of homosexual activities and for several years had received steroid therapy.

On admission, physical examination showed that the patient was slightly febrile and in respiratory failure. A few days later he became progressively anemic, his mental status deteriorated, and a diagnosis of meningitis was made. India ink preparation of his CSF showed encapsulated budding yeasts, which were later identified as *Cryptococcus neoformans*.

PATHOGENICITY

The relationship that exists between the human host and the microbial world is exceedingly complex. Each is in constant interaction with the other and with numerous additional influences, all of which affect the host-microbe relationship. Factors such as nutrition, stress, genetic background, and other diseases present all have an effect on the outcome of the meeting of human and microbe. The relationship is an equilibrium that is in constant motion and subject to change. This part of Chapter 6 discusses the role of each of these factors in host-parasite relationships and how each interacts with the others to prevent or initiate a disease process.

Pathogens

A *pathogen* is a microbe that can cause disease in a susceptible host. Years ago, this definition applied to relatively few organisms. Obviously, certain bacteria such as *Yersinia pestis* and *Bacillus anthracis* were pathogenic in nearly all situations. Others such as *Serratia marcescens* and *Leuconostoc* spp. were considered to be nonpathogenic. Our understanding of host-parasite interactions and our ability to isolate, grow, and identify organisms have improved steadily over the years. In addition, patient populations have changed, which means they have a longer life span and are more susceptible to highly invasive medical procedures, transplants, and so on. As a result, organisms that are found as normal flora and in the environment are being seen with increasing frequency in clinical settings. Therefore our definition of *pathogen* must be expanded to apply to virtually any microorganism when conditions for infection are met. We must also broaden our view of the human host. The potential pathogen list for a 20-year-old healthy college student is much smaller than for a 90-year-old person, a transplant recipient, or a 20-year-old college student with acquired immune deficiency syndrome.

Opportunistic Pathogens

The majority of microorganisms that humans encounter cause disease only if a significant change occurs in host resistance or within the organism itself. These innocuous organisms are called *opportunistic pathogens.* They are usually part of the indigenous flora, but the classic pathogens may also be found among the opportunistic organisms when host defenses weaken. The infections caused by these organisms are *opportunistic infections.* Infections caused by these organisms seldom occur in healthy individuals. In fact, some assume that the infected individual is not "normal" (in terms of body defenses) when infection by an oppor-

TABLE 6-1

An Abbreviated List of Opportunistic Microorganisms

Conditioning Compromising Host Defenses	Organism(s)
Foreign bodies (catheters, shunts, prosthetic heart valves)	*Staphylococcus epidermidis*
	Propionibacterium acnes
	Aspergillus spp.
	Candida albicans
	Viridans streptococci
	Serratia marcescens
	Pseudomonas aeruginosa
Alcoholism	*Streptococcus pneumoniae*
	Klebsiella pneumoniae
Burns	*Pseudomonas aeruginosa*
Hematoproliferative disorders	*Cryptococcus neoformans*
	Varicella-zoster virus
Cystic fibrosis	*Pseudomonas* spp.
Immunosuppression (drugs, congenital disease)	*Candida albicans*
	Pneumocystis carinii
	Herpes simplex virus
	Aspergillus spp.
	Diphtheroids
	Cytomegalovirus
	Staphylococcus spp.
	Pseudomonas spp.

tunistic pathogen occurs. Table 6-1 lists some of the common opportunistic microorganisms.

An **iatrogenic infection** occurs when an infection is the result of medical treatment or procedures. For example, many patients who have indwelling urinary catheters develop a urinary tract infection. The catheter was a necessary procedure in the medical treatment of the individual, but its use has resulted in an infection. Patients who are given immunosuppressive drugs because they have received a transplant are more susceptible to infection. Because any infection in such a patient would probably be because of the physician-ordered drug therapy, it would be an iatrogenic infection.

VIRULENCE

Virulence is the relative ability of a microorganism to cause disease, or the degree of pathogenicity. It is usually measured by the numbers of microorganisms necessary to cause infection in the host. Those organisms that can establish infection with a relatively low infective dose are considered more

virulent than those that require high numbers for infection. This generalization is somewhat misleading because the severity of disease between different organisms varies. If a microorganism requires a relatively high infective dose but the disease it causes is often fatal, we tend to think of the microorganism as *highly virulent.* On the other hand, a different organism may require a low infective dose but produces a relatively mild disease. A number of organism characteristics or factors contribute to virulence: capsules, toxins, enzymes, cell wall receptors, pili, and others. These **virulence factors** allow the pathogen to evade or overcome host defenses and cause disease. Many virulence factors are well defined, such as diphtheria and cholera toxins, the capsule of *Streptococcus pneumoniae,* and the pili of *Neisseria gonorrhoeae.* The exact role, if any, of other factors in disease production (e.g., coagulase, streptokinase, lipase, and IgA protease) is unclear.

HOST RESISTANCE FACTORS

Physical Barriers

Healthy skin is an effective barrier against infection. The stratified and cornified epithelium presents a mechanical barrier to penetration by most microorganisms. Organisms that can cause infection by penetrating the mucous membrane epithelium usually cannot penetrate unbroken skin. Only a few microorganisms are capable of entering the body by way of intact skin. Some of these microorganisms, and others that normally enter when the skin barrier is compromised, are listed in Table 6-2.

Most of the organisms listed in Table 6-2 require help in breaking the skin barrier (e.g., animal or arthropod bite). Those capable of penetrating normal, healthy skin are few and include *Leptospira* spp., *Francisella tularensis, Treponema* spp., and some fungi. Even these organisms probably require microscopic breaks in the skin surface. Healthy, intact skin is clearly the primary mechanical barrier to infection. The skin also has substantial numbers of microbial flora. These organisms are usually not pathogens. Some, however, such as *Staphylococcus aureus,* commonly cause infections. This flora contributes to a low pH, competition for nutrients, and production of bacteri-

TABLE 6-2

MIcroorganisms That Infect Skin or Enter the Body Via Skin

Microorganisms	Disease	Comments
Arthropod-borne viruses	Various fevers, encephalitides	150 distinct viruses, transmitted by infected arthropod bites
Rabies virus	Rabies	Bites from infected animals
Vaccinia virus	Skin lesion	Vaccination against smallpox
Rickettsieae	Typhus, spotted fevers	Infestation with infected arthropods
Leptospira	Leptospirosis	Contact with water containing infected animal urine
Staphylococci	Boils, impetigo	Most common skin invaders
Streptococci	Impetigo, erysipelas	
Bacillus anthracis	Cutaneous anthrax	Systemic disease following local lesion at inoculation site
Treponema pallidum and *pertenue*	Syphilis, yaws	Warm, moist skin is more susceptible
Yersinia pestis	Plague	Bite from infected rat flea
Plasmodium spp.	Malaria	Bite from infected mosquito
Dermatophytes	Ringworm, athlete's foot	Infection restricted to skin, nails, and hair

With permission from Mims CA: *The pathogenesis of infectious disease,* New York, 1977, Academic Press.

cidal substances by the resident organisms. These conditions serve to prevent colonization by transient organisms. Additionally, the low pH resulting from long-chain fatty acids secreted by sebaceous glands ensures that relatively few organisms can survive and prosper in the acid environment of the skin.

Cleansing Mechanisms

Normally the term *cleansing* brings to mind a liquid. One of the most effective cleansing mechanisms humans have, however, is the desquamation of the skin surface. The keratinized squamous epithelium or outer layer of skin is being continuously shed. Many of the microorganisms colonizing the skin are disposed of with the sloughing of the epithelium.

More obvious is the cleansing action of the fluids of the eye and the respiratory, digestive, urinary, and genital tracts. The eye is continually exposed to microorganisms, which means this organ has some highly developed antimicrobial mechanisms. Tears bathe the cornea and sclera. This not only lubricates the eye but also washes foreign matter and infectious agents away from the surface. Additionally, tears contain IgA and lysozyme.

The respiratory tract is also continuously exposed to microorganisms and is protected by nasal hairs, ciliary epithelium, and mucous membranes. A continuous flow of mucus occurs from the membranes lining the nasopharynx, which traps particles and microbes and sweeps them to the oro-

pharynx, where they are either expectorated or swallowed. The trachea is lined with ciliary epithelium. These cells have hair-like extensions (cilia) that sweep particles and organisms upward toward the oropharynx. This material is then expectorated or swallowed. Heavy smokers have a significant reduction in ciliated epithelial cells and therefore are more prone to respiratory infections. The purpose of these mechanisms is to prevent infectious agents and other particles from reaching the bronchioles and lungs. Under normal conditions, they are very effective, and the air moving into and out of the lungs is sterile.

Bacteria are swallowed either as part of the mouth flora and upper respiratory tract or in liquids and food. Most bacteria are easily destroyed by the low pH found in the stomach. Some bacteria, however, are able to survive and pass into the small intestine. The number of bacteria in the intestine increases as the distance from the stomach increases. The number of bacteria in the distal portion of the colon is extremely high. The organisms do not normally gain entrance to the body from the intestine. The mucous secretions and peristalsis serve to prevent the organisms from attaching to the intestinal epithelium. Additionally, secretory antibody and phagocytic cells lining the mucosa defend against infection.

The genitourinary tract is cleansed by the voiding of urine. Consequently, only the outermost portions of the urethra have a microbial population. The vagina contains a large population of organisms as part of the indigenous flora. The acidity of the vagina, resulting from the breakdown of glycogen by the resident flora, tends to inhibit transient organisms from colonizing.

Antimicrobial Substances

A variety of substances produced in the human host have antimicrobial activity. Some are produced as part of phagocytic defense and are discussed later. Others, such as fatty acids, HCl in the stomach, and secretory IgA have already been mentioned. A substance that plays a major role in resistance to infection is **lysozyme,** a low–molecular-weight (approximately 20,000 daltons) enzyme that hydrolyzes the peptidoglycan layer of bacterial cell walls. In some bacteria, the peptidoglycan layer is directly accessible to lysozyme. These bacteria are killed by the enzyme alone. In other bacteria, the peptidoglycan layer is exposed after other agents have damaged the cell wall (e.g., antibody and complement, hydrogen peroxide). In these cases, lysozyme acts with the other agents to cause death of the infecting bacteria. Lysozyme is found in serum and tissue fluids and tears, breast milk, saliva, and sweat.

Antibodies, especially secretory IgA, are found in mucous secretions of the respiratory, genital, and digestive tracts. They may serve as opsonins, thereby enhancing phagocytosis, or they may fix complement and neutralize the infecting organism.

Serum also contains low–molecular-weight cationic proteins termed **β-lysins.** These proteins are lethal against gram-positive bacteria and are released from platelets during coagulation. The site of action is the cytoplasmic membrane.

These antimicrobial substances and systems work best together. A combination of antibody, complement, lysozyme, and β-lysin is significantly more effective in killing bacteria than each alone or than any combination in which one or more are missing.

Proliferation of viruses is inhibited by **interferon.** The interferons are a group of cellular proteins induced in eukaryotic cells in response to virus infection or other inducers. Uninfected cells that have been exposed to interferon are refractory to virus infection. A number of bacteria, viruses, and their products induce interferon production. The interferon produced binds to the surface receptors on noninfected cells. This binding stimulates the cell to synthesize enzymes that inhibit viral replication over several days. The antiviral effect of interferon is only one action it exhibits. One type of interferon plays an important role in the immune response. It inhibits cell proliferation and tumor growth and enhances phagocytosis by macrophages, activity of natural killer cells, and generation of cytotoxic T cells.

Indigenous Microbial Flora

Nonpathogenic microorganisms compete with pathogens for nutrients and space. This competition lessens the chance that the pathogen will colonize the host. Some normal flora species produce **bacteriocins,** substances that inhibit the growth of closely related bacteria. These proteins are produced by a variety of gram-positive and gram-negative bacteria and appear to give the secreting bacterium an advantage, because they can eliminate other bacteria that would compete for nutrients and space. Some species of bacteria produce metabolic byproducts that result in a microenvironment hostile to potential pathogens. Vitamins and other essential nutrients are synthesized by certain bacteria in the intestine and appear to contribute to the overall health of the host.

Phagocytosis

Phagocytosis is an essential component in the resistance of the host to infectious agents. It is the primary mechanism in the host defense against extracellular bacteria and a number of viruses and fungi. The polymorphonuclear neutrophils (PMNs) and macrophages (monocytes in the peripheral blood) are the body's first line of defense.

The stem cells for neutrophils arise in the bone marrow, where they differentiate to form mature neutrophils. During this maturation, the cells synthesize myeloperoxidase, proteases, cathepsin, lactoferrin, lysozyme, and elastase. These products are incorporated into membrane-bound vesicles called **lysosomes.** The lysosomes contain the enzymes and other substances necessary for the killing and digestion of the engulfed particles. They show up as azurophilic granules on a Wright's stain. The PMN also has receptors on the cell membrane for some complement components that stimulate cell motion, the metabolic burst, and secretion of the lysosome contents into a phagosome. The PMN is an end-stage cell and has a circulating

TABLE 6-3

Tissue Distribution of Monocytes/Macrophages

Cell Name	Tissue Distribution
Monocyte	Blood
Kupffer cell	Liver
Alveolar macrophage	Lung
Histiocyte	Connective tissue
Peritoneal macrophage	Peritoneum
Microglial cell	Central nervous system
Mesangial cell	Kidney
Macrophage	Spleen, lymph nodes

half-life of 6 to 7 hours. It may migrate to the tissues, where its half-life is less than a week.

Macrophages also originate in the bone marrow. They circulate as monocytes for 1 to 2 days and then migrate through the blood vessel walls into the tissues and reside in specific tissues as part of the reticuloendothelial system. These cells are widely distributed in the body and play a central role in specific immunity and in nonspecific phagocytosis (Table 6-3).

Four activities must occur for phagocytosis to take place and be effective in host defense: (1) migration to the area of infection (chemotaxis), (2) attachment of the particle to the phagocyte, (3) ingestion, and (4) killing.

Chemotaxis

The PMNs circulate through the body, followed by movement into the tissues by an action called *diapedesis,* which is movement of the neutrophils between the endothelial cells of the blood vessels into the tissues. The body is under constant surveillance by these and other phagocytic cells. When an infection occurs, massive numbers of PMNs accumulate at the site. This accumulation is not a random event but rather is a directed migration of PMNs into the area needing their services. This migration is called *chemotaxis* (a chemical "taxi" or chemically caused movement). Several substances serve as **chemotactic agents.** These are certain components of complement, a number of bacterial products, and products from damaged tissue cells and products from responding immune cells. The initial contact of the PMN with an invading organism may be random. As the organism causes the body's defense mechanisms to respond via inflammation, however, directed

migration of phagocytes occurs (chemotaxis, Figure 6-1). The speed and magnitude of this response are easily visualized by recalling how quickly a splinter or similar injury becomes infected and how much pus is produced.

Attachment

One of the most effective defenses bacteria have against phagocytosis is the capsule. This structure prevents attachment of the organism to the neutrophil's membrane, which must occur before ingestion can take place. Attachment is facilitated by specific antibodies to the microorganism. The neutrophil membrane has a variety of receptors; these include the Fc portion of IgG1, IgG3, and the C3b component of complement. In addition, these three factors can and do bind to the invading microorganism. The result is that the invading microorganisms are coated with one or more of these factors. The receptor on the PMN for the particular factor coating the bacterium binds to the factor and forms a bridge that brings the particle into close physical contact with the leukocyte membrane. The coating of the bacterium with antibody or complement components results in enhanced phagocytosis by the PMN. This process or phenomenon is called *opsonization* (Figure 6-2).

The antibody and complement components are termed *opsonins.* Opsonization can be accomplished by three different types of responses: (1) IgG1 or IgG3 binds to the organism; (2) the antibody response is insufficient for opsonization

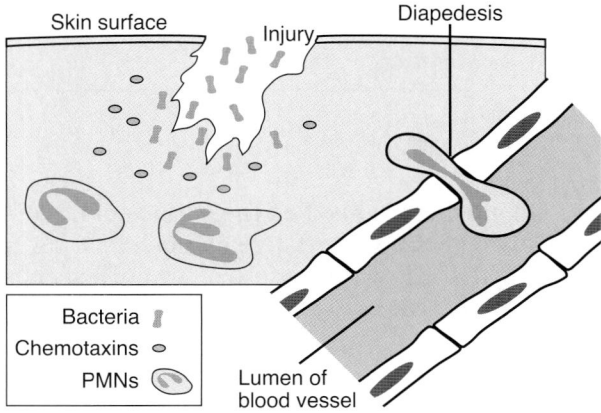

Figure 6-1

Phagocytosis: chemotaxis. *PMNs,* Polymorphonuclear neutrophils.

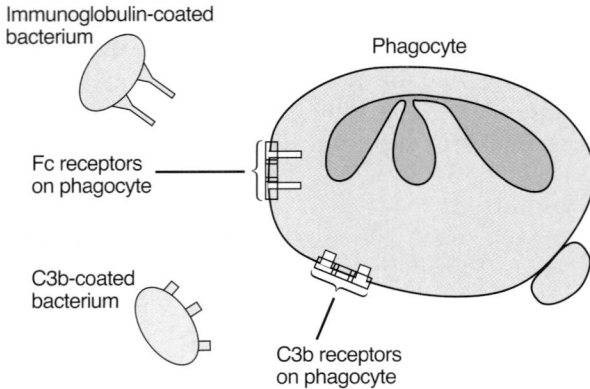

Figure 6-2 _____

Phagocytosis: attachment.

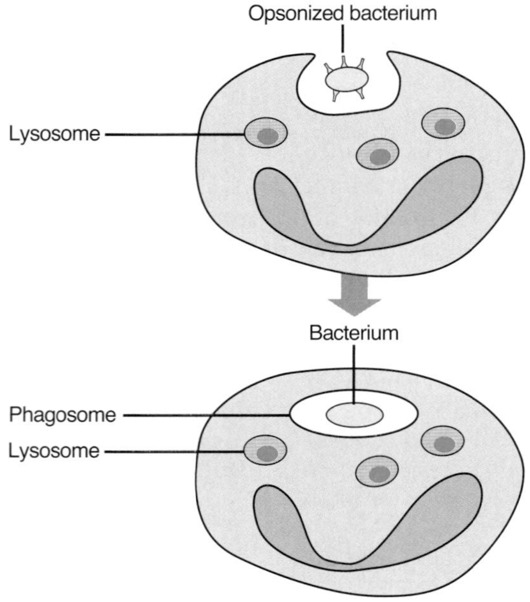

Opsonized bacterium

Lysosome

Bacterium

Phagosome
Lysosome

Figure 6-3 _____

Phagocytosis: ingestion.

but complement is fixed on the surface of the organism; or (3) the alternative complement pathway is activated by the endotoxin or polysaccharides of the organism.

Ingestion

The next step of phagocytosis is ingestion. This process occurs rapidly following attachment (Figure 6-3). The cell membrane of the phagocytic cell invaginates and surrounds the attached particle.

The particle is taken into the cytoplasm and enclosed within a vacuole called a *phagosome.* The phagosome fuses with lysosomes, which are vacuoles containing hydrolytic enzymes. The lysosomes release their contents into the phagosome, a process called **degranulation.** The list of enzymes found within the lysosomes is long—more than 60 enzymes, including proteases, lipases, RNase, DNase, peroxidase, and acid phosphatase. Several of these are important in the killing and digestion of the engulfed bacterial cell.

Killing

The phagocytosis of a particle triggers a significant increase in the metabolic activity of the neutrophil or macrophage. This increase is termed a *metabolic* or **respiratory burst.** The cell demonstrates increases in glycolysis, the hexose monophosphate shunt pathway, oxygen use, and production of lactic acid and hydrogen peroxide. The hydrogen peroxide produced at this time diffuses from the cytoplasm into the phagosome. It acts in conjunction with other compounds to exert a bactericidal effect. In addition, other enzymes from the lysosome have antimicrobial action. They include lactoferrin, which chelates iron and prevents bacterial growth, lysozyme, and several basic proteins. The usual result is that a phagocytosed organism is quickly engulfed, killed, and digested (Figure 6-4). Organisms that are "intracellular" (e.g., *Mycobacterium tuberculosis, Listeria monocytogenes, Brucella* spp.) are able to survive phagocytosis and, in fact, may actually multiply within the phagocyte. Obviously, other defense mechanisms must play a major role in immunity to these intracellular organisms.

The importance of phagocytosis is seen in patients with defects in the numbers or function of phagocytic cells. Such patients have frequent infections in spite of possessing high levels of serum antibody.

Microorganisms have developed a number of ways of countering phagocytosis (Table 6-4). Many of the organisms listed in Table 6-4 are common isolates, which is not surprising, because they have developed a means to interfere with phagocytosis, thereby increasing their pathogenicity.

Inflammation

Inflammation is the body's response to injury or foreign body. A hallmark of inflammation is the ac-

TABLE 6-4

Types of Interference with Phagocytic Activities

Microorganisms*	Type of Interference†	Mechanism (or Responsible Factor)
Streptococci	Kill phagocyte	Streptolysin induces lysosomal discharge into cell cytoplasm
	Inhibit chemotaxis	Streptolysin
	Resist phagocytosis	M substance
	Resist digestion	
Staphylococci	Kill phagocyte	Leucocidin induces lysosomal discharge into cell cytoplasm
	Inhibit opsonized phagocytosis	Protein A blocks Fc portion of Ab
	Resist killing	Cell wall mucopeptide
Bacillus anthracis	Kill phagocyte	Toxic complex
	Resist killing	Capsular polyglutamic acid
Haemophilus influenzae	Resist phagocytosis (unless Ab present)	Polysaccharide capsule
Streptococcus pneumoniae		
Klebsiella pneumoniae	Resist digestion	
Pseudomonas aeruginosa	Resist phagocytosis (unless Ab present)	"Surface slime" (polysaccharide)
	Resist digestion	
Escherichia coli	Resist phagocytosis (unless Ab present)	$\begin{cases} \text{O antigen (smooth strains)} \\ \text{K antigen (acid polysaccharide)} \end{cases}$
	Resist killing	K antigen
Salmonella typhi	Resist phagocytosis (unless Ab present)	Vi antigen
	Resist killing	
Cryptococcus neoformans	Resist phagocytosis	Polysaccharide capsule
Treponema pallidum	Resist phagocytosis	Cell wall
Yersinia pestis	Resist killing	Protein-carbohydrate cell wall
Mycobacteria	Resist killing and digestion	Cell wall structure
	Inhibit lysosomal fusion	?
Brucella abortus	Resist killing	Cell wall substance
Toxoplasma gondii	Inhibit attachment to PMN	?
	Inhibit lysosomal fusion	?

From Mims CA: *The pathogenesis of infectious disease,* New York, 1977, Academic Press.
*Often only the virulent strains show the type of interference listed.
†Sometimes the type of interference listed has been described only in a particular type of phagocyte (polymorph or macrophage) from a particular host, but it generally bears a relationship to pathogenicity in that host.

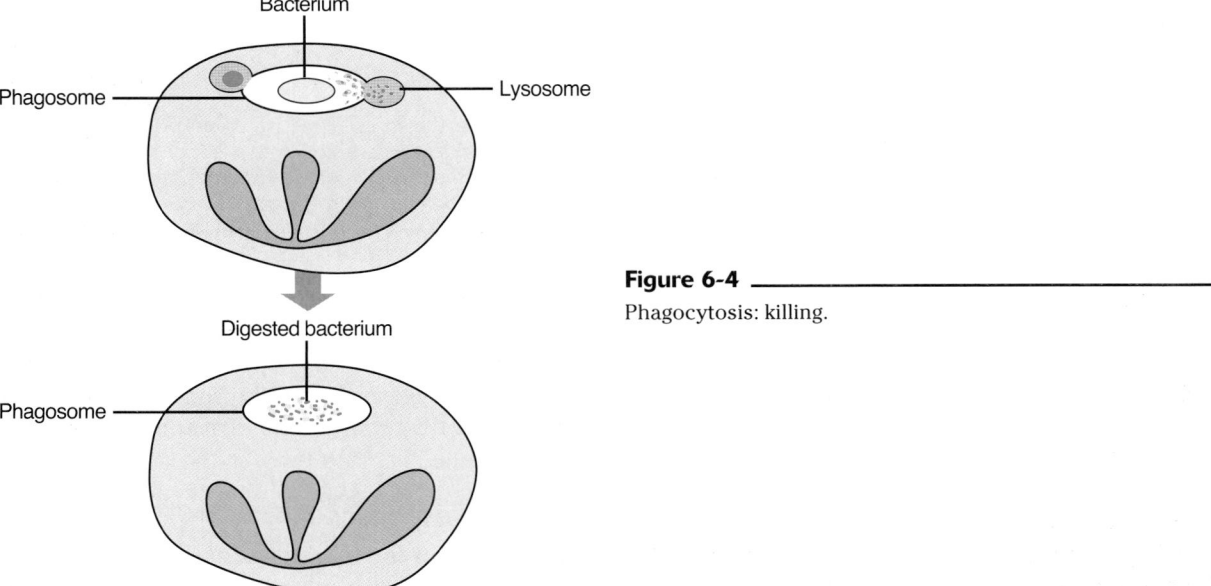

Figure 6-4
Phagocytosis: killing.

TABLE 6-5

Summary of Defenses of the Human or Animal Host to Infection and Evasionary Mechanisms Attributed to Various Microorganisms

Host Defense	Mechanism of Evasion by Microorganism	Example
Hydrodynamic flow	Attachment	Pili, surface proteins, lipoteichoic acid
		Pseudomembrane of diphtheria
Mucus barrier	Attachment	Mannose-sensitive pili
	Penetration	
Deprivation of essential nutrients	Systems of high-affinity uptake	Iron metabolism
Lysozyme in secretions	Resistance to lysis	Substitution of peptidoglycan
Surface immunoglobulins	Absent or low immunogenicity	Hyaluronic acid, capsules
	Antigenic heterogeneity	Pili, capsules, lipopolysaccharide (LPS), M protein, etc.
	Masking of antigens	Capsules, IgA-binding proteins
	Destruction	IgA protease
Unbroken surface (epithelial cell surface)	Penetration	*Neisseria gonorrhoeae, Shigella* spp.
Unknown defenses in lymphatics (intercellular space)		*N. gonorrhoeae, Shigella* spp.
Serum defenses		
Recognition by antibody	Antigenic heterogeneity	Pili, capsules, LPS, M protein, etc.
	Masking of antigen	Capsules, Ig-binding proteins
	Destruction of antibody	
	Antigenic variation	Borreliae
Complement system	Failure to activate alternative pathway	Sialic acid capsules
	Inactivation of complement components	Cleavage of C3b in empyema fluids
	Resistance to bacteriolysis	ColV plasmid, etc.
	Formation of abscess	*Bacteroides fragilis* capsule
Localization		
Fibrin trapping	Fibrinolysis	*Streptococcus*
Abscess formation	Collagenase, elastase	*Pseudomonas, Clostridium*
Secondary immune response	Nonspecific B-cell activation	LPS, lipoprotein, etc.
	Inhibition of delayed hypersensitivity	Anergy of miliary tuberculosis
	Rapidly fatal (toxin)	Anthrax, plaque, *Clostridium*
Phagocytosis	Inhibition of chemotaxis	*Brucella, Salmonella, Neisseria, Staphylococcus, Pseudomonas*
	Inhibition of attachment and ingestion	Capsules, M protein, Ig-binding proteins, gonococcal pili
	Inhibition of metabolic burst	*Salmonella typhi*
	Inhibition of degranulation	Mycobacteriaceae
	Resistance to permeability inducing cationic protein	Gram-positive cell wall, smooth LPS, polyanionic capsules
	Resistance to oxidative attack	Catalase, superoxide dismutase, carotenoid pigments
	Escape from phagosome	*Mycobacterium bovis, Legionella pneumophila*
	Destruction of phagocyte	*Streptococcus pneumoniae, Streptococcus pyogenes, Staphylococcus aureus, Pseudomonas aeruginosa*

Adapted from Gotschlich EC: Thoughts on the evolution of strategies used by bacteria for evasion of host defenses, *Rev Infect Dis* 5:S779, 1983.

cumulation of large numbers of phagocytic cells. These leukocytes release mediators or cause other cell types to release mediators. The mediators cause erythema as a result of greater blood flow, edema from an increase in vascular permeability, and continued phagocyte accumulation, resulting in pus. The enzymes released by the phagocytes digest the foreign particles, injured cells, and cell debris. After the removal of the invading object, the injured tissue is repaired.

Immune Responses

A discussion of the responses of the immune system to infection is beyond the scope of this chapter. A brief discussion, however, in an attempt to furnish an appreciation of its role and complexity, is in order.

The wide variety and complexity of infectious agents necessitate flexibility in the immune mechanisms of the host. Microorganisms with polysaccharide antigens induce predominantly humoral responses (B lymphocyte). These antigens tend to be T-cell independent. Protein antigens cause a response by both T and B cells. Although a number of the parasite's antigens are virulence factors, an antibody response to a particular factor seldom results in immunity. An exception to this is antibody to M protein (anti–M protein) of *Streptococcus pyogenes.* Anti–M protein confers immunity to the host. Viral and fungal infections are dealt with primarily via cellular immune responses (T lymphocytes, natural killer cells). The route of infection may also determine the type of immune response elicited. Antibody is important in immunity to influenza virus but seems to have a smaller role in herpes simplex virus infections. Infections caused by mycobacteria invariably result in a cellular (T-cell and macrophage) response. The same is true of infections due to *L. monocytogenes* and other intracellular organisms. Complement and other substances are activated by bacterial cellular products (endotoxin).

The balance between health and infectious disease is complex and mediated by humoral and cellular factors. The relative importance of each factor depends on the parasite, route of infection, condition and genetic makeup of the host, and other factors yet to be clearly characterized.

Table 6-5 summarizes the defenses used by the human host against infection.

INFECTIOUS AGENT FACTORS

Adherence

Most infectious agents must attach to host cells before infection occurs. In some diseases caused by exotoxins (e.g., botulism, staphylococcal food poisoning), adherence is not important. In virtually all other cases, however, the bacterium, virus, or fungus require **adherence** to the host cell before infection and disease progress. The cell surface structures that mediate attachment are called ***adhesins.*** The host cells must possess the necessary receptors for the adhesins. If the host or the infectious agent undergoes a mutation that changes the structure of the adhesin or the receptor, adherence likely will not take place and the virulence of the infectious agent is affected.

Virus infections depend on the cell's maintaining an appropriate receptor for the virus particle. Infection of the cell occurs only if attachment is the initial event. The main adhesins in bacteria are the pili (fimbriae) and surface polysaccharides. Pili enable bacteria to adhere to host cell surfaces. For example, the strains of *Escherichia coli* that cause traveler's diarrhea use their pili to adhere to cells of the small intestine, where they secrete a toxin that causes the disease symptoms. Similarly, pili are essential for gonococci to infect the epithelial cells of the genitourinary tract. Antibodies to the pili of *N. gonorrhoeae* are protective by preventing the organism from attaching to the epithelial cells.

Proliferation

To establish itself and cause disease, a pathogen must be able to replicate after attachment to host cells. Numerous host factors work to prevent proliferation. Secretory antibody, lactoferrin, and lysozyme have been mentioned previously. To be successful in establishing infection, infectious agents must be able to avoid or overcome these local factors. For example, lactoferrin competes with bacteria for free iron; meningococci can use lactoferrin as a source of iron. They are not inhibited by the presence of lactoferrin and, in fact, are able to use it for growth. On the other hand, the nonpathogenic *Neisseria* spp. are usually unable to use the iron in lactoferrin and are inhibited by its presence.

Several pathogens *(Haemophilus influenzae, N. gonorrhoeae, Neisseria meningitidis)* produce an IgA protease that degrades the IgA found at mucosal surfaces. Other pathogens (influenza virus, *Borrelia* spp.) circumvent host antibodies by shifting key cell-surface antigens. The host produces antibodies against the "old" antigens, which are no longer effective.

An extremely important event in the life of an invading pathogen is phagocytosis. Evasion of phagocytosis is essential for most pathogens to be able to survive and multiply. The most common characteristic of bacteria that allows for such evasion is a polysaccharide capsule. Many of those possessing a capsule are highly virulent (as in the case study) until its removal, at which point their virulence becomes extremely low. Some pathogens are able to survive phagocytosis. Those that do have developed several methods to prevent being killed. Some prevent fusion of phagosomes and lysosomes, others have a resistance to the effects of the lysosomal contents, and still others escape into the cytoplasm.

Tissue Damage

Generally, disease from infection is noticeable only if tissue damage occurs. This damage may be from toxins, either **exotoxins** or **endotoxins,** or from inflammatory substances that cause host-driven, immunologically mediated damage.

Exotoxins

Many of the bacterial exotoxins are highly characterized. Most are composed of two subunits: the first is nontoxic and serves to bind the toxin to the host cells; the second is toxic. The toxin gene is commonly encoded by phage, plasmids, or transposons. Therefore only those carry the extra-chromosomal DNA coding for the toxin gene produce toxin. Isolates of *Corynebacterium diphtheriae* therefore have to be tested for toxin production and identified as to genus and species. Other pathogenic bacteria show similarities. Table 6-6 lists many of the bacterial exotoxins that are important in disease production.

Endotoxins

Gram-negative bacteria have endotoxins. Endotoxins are composed of the lipopolysaccharide portion of the cell wall. The toxicity is caused by the lipid A portion of the lipopolysaccharide. The effects of endotoxin consist of dramatic changes in blood pressure, clotting, body temperature, circulating blood cells, metabolism, humoral immunity, cellular immunity, and resistance to infection.

Endotoxin stimulates the fever centers in the hypothalamus. An increase in body temperature occurs within an hour after exposure. Exposure to endotoxin also causes hypotension. Severe hypotension occurs within 30 minutes after exposure. Septic or endotoxic shock is a serious and potentially life-threatening problem. Unlike shock caused by fluid loss, such as that seen in severe bleeding, septic shock is unaffected by fluid administration. The endotoxin also initiates coagulation, which can result in intravascular coagulation. This process depletes clotting factors and activates fibrinolysis so that fibrin split products accumulate in the blood. These fragments are anticoagulants and can cause serious bleeding. Another feature of patients with endotoxic shock is severe neutropenia, which can occur within minutes following exposure. It results from sequestration of neutrophils in capillaries of the lung and other organs. Leukocytosis follows neutropenia because neutrophils are released from the bone marrow.

Endotoxin has a wide variety of effects on the immune system. It stimulates proliferation of B lymphocytes in some animal species, activates macrophages, activates complement, and has an adjuvant effect with protein antigens. It also stimulates interferon production and causes changes in carbohydrates, lipids, iron, and sensitivity to epinephrine. A severe infection with gram-negative bacteria can lead to serious and often life-threatening problems.

A comparison of bacterial exotoxins and endotoxins is given in Table 6-7.

Invasion

Pathogens exhibit invasion to some degree or another. *Invasion* is the process of penetrating and growing in tissues. With some organisms, the invasion is localized and involves only a few layers of cells. With others, it involves deep tissues; for example, the gonococcus organism is invasive and may infect the fallopian tubes.

Dissemination

Dissemination is the spread of organisms to distant sites (i.e., organs and tissues). With some organisms, such as *Salmonella* spp., dissemination is an important aspect of the disease. Other organisms such as *C. diphtheriae* do not spread beyond their initial site of infection, yet the disease they produce is serious and often fatal. Certain organisms that survive phagocytosis may be disseminated rapidly to many body sites, but the organisms themselves are not invasive. The phagocyte simply carries the organism, but the bacterium itself is incapable of penetrating tissues. *C. perfringens* is an example

TABLE 6-6

Exotoxins of Pathogenic Bacteria

Bacterium	Disease Caused in Humans	Toxins
Bacillus anthracis	Anthrax	Complex lethal edema-producing toxin
Bordetella pertussis	Whooping cough	Lethal, dermonecrotizing toxin
Clostridium botulinum	Botulism	**6 type-specific lethal neurotoxins**
Clostridium oedematiens	Gas gangrene	1. Alpha, lethal, dermonecrotizing
		2. Beta, lethal, dermonecrotizing, hemolytic
		3. Gamma, lethal, dermonecrotizing, hemolytic
		4. Delta, hemolytic
		5. Epsilon, lethal, hemolytic
		6. Zeta, hemolytic
Clostridium perfringens	Gas gangrene and enteritis necroticans	1. **Alpha, lethal, dermonecrotizing, hemolytic**
		2. Beta, lethal
		3. Gamma, lethal
		4. Delta, lethal
		5. Epsilon, lethal, dermonecrotizing
		6. Eta, lethal (?)
		7. Iota, lethal, dermonecrotizing
		8. Theta, lethal, cardiotoxic, hemolytic
		9. Kappa, lethal, proteolytic
		10. **Enterotoxin**
Clostridium septicum	Gas gangrene	Alpha, lethal, hemolytic
Clostridium sordellii	Gas gangrene	1. Edema-producing toxin
		2. Hemorrhagic toxin
Clostridium tetani	Tetanus	1. **Tetanospasmin, lethal, neurotoxic**
		2. Neurotoxin, nonspasmogenic
		3. Tetanolysin, lethal, cardiotoxic, hemolytic
Corynebacterium diphtheriae	Diphtheria	**Diphtheria toxin, lethal, dermonecrotizing**
Escherichia coli	Diarrhea	1. **Heat-labile enterotoxin**
		(2. Heat-stable enterotoxin)
Pseudomonas aeruginosa	Pyogenic infections	**Exotoxin A**
Staphylococcus aureus	Pyogenic infections, enterotoxemia	1. Alpha, lethal, dermonecrotizing, hemolytic
		2. Beta, lethal, hemolytic
		3. Gamma, lethal, hemolytic
		4. Delta, hemolytic
		5. **Exfoliating toxin**
		6. **Enterotoxin**
Streptococcus pyogenes	Pyogenic infections, scarlet fever, rheumatic fever	1. Dick toxin, erythrogenic, nonlethal
		2. Streptolysin O, lethal, hemolytic, cardiotoxic
		3. Streptolysin S, lethal, hemolytic
Vibrio cholerae	Cholera	**Cholera toxin, lethal, enterotoxic**
Salmonella typhimurium	Enteritis	**Enterotoxin?**
Shigella sp.	Dysentery	**Enterotoxin**
Yersinia pestis	Plague	Murine toxin

From Braude AI, Davis CE, Fierer J, editors: *Infectious diseases and medical microbiology,* Philadelphia, 1986, WB Saunders.
Boldface indicates toxins that produce harmful effects of infectious disease.

of a highly invasive organism that may not necessarily disseminate.

Infectious agents have a wide variety of mechanisms that allow them to cause disease. Some, such as capsules and toxins, are common to more than one organism. Others tend to be specialized, such as the tissue tropism of the gonococcus.

Some simple explanations of how infectious diseases occur may be tempting. Microorganisms produce many extracellular factors that appear to aid in infection; however, the exact role of most of these is unknown. Also, although our knowledge of pathogenesis has grown dramatically over the past few years, only six or so organisms whose

TABLE 6-7

Differences Between Bacterial Exotoxins and Endotoxins

	Exotoxins	Endotoxins
Parent organisms	Gram-positive and gram-negative	Gram-negative
Within or without parent organism	Within and without	Within
Chemical nature	Simple protein	Protein-lipid-polysaccharide
Stability to heating (100° C)	Labile	Stable
Detoxification by formaldehyde	Detoxified	Not detoxified
Neutralization by homologous antibody	Complete	Partial
Biologic activity	Individual to toxin	Same for all toxins
Toxicity compared with strychnine as 1	100 to 1,000,000	0.1

Modified from Braude AI, Davis CE, Fierer J, editors: *Infectious diseases and medical microbiology*, Philadelphia, 1986, WB Saunders.

precise mode and method of infection are known. More knowledge and understanding are needed.

ROUTES OF TRANSMISSION

The route by which a pathogen may be transmitted to a susceptible host is often explained by the characteristics of that pathogen. Although some organisms may be naturally transmitted by more than one route, most have a limited number of routes. These routes can be characterized as in the air, via food and water (ingestion), through close contact (includes sexual transmission), through cuts and bites, and via arthropods; animal diseases that can infect humans are transmitted through animal contact **(zoonoses).** A summary of the routes of transmission is given in Table 6-8.

Airborne Transmission

Respiratory spread of infectious disease is common. Often, the respiratory secretions are aerosolized by coughing, sneezing, and talking. Very small particles, referred to as ***droplet nuclei,*** are the residue from the evaporation of fluid from larger droplets and are light enough to remain airborne for long periods. Pathogens that are spread through the air generally must be resistant to drying and inactivation by ultraviolet light. Some infectious agents may be transmitted by dust particles that have become airborne. As discussed earlier in this chapter, the body has a number of defenses against airborne infectious agents. The nasal turbinates, oropharynx, and larynx provide a twisting, mucous-lined passageway that makes direct access to the lower respiratory tract mechanically difficult. In addition, the lower portions of the respiratory tract contain ciliary epithelium that sweeps organisms upward. For a microorganism to cause disease, it must circumvent these defenses, penetrate the mucous layer, and attach to the epithelium. The host also produces secretory IgA, lysozyme, alveolar macrophages, and other humoral factors that act on a pathogen that manages to get beyond the physical defenses.

Respiratory tract infections are the most common reason that patients of all ages seek medical attention. Although most upper respiratory tract infections are self-limiting and can be treated by the patient with over-the-counter medications, some are more serious. Streptococcal sore throat, sinusitis, otitis media, acute epiglottitis, and diphtheria can be serious and even life-threatening. Viral diseases causing the common cold and infectious mononucleosis are usually not life-threatening but can result in much discomfort and absenteeism from work or school.

Although all the diseases just mentioned can be spread via aerosols, some may also be transmitted via the fingers and hands, especially true for the common cold–causing rhinovirus. The fingers and hands are contaminated with infectious nasal secretions because of hand-to-nose contact. The infectious virus particles are passed from the infected individual to a susceptible recipient via hand-to-hand or hand-to-face contact. The recipient transmits the virus picked up from the hands of the infected individual by touching the face and nose. In this case, the disease is transmitted via the respiratory route, but not in the normal, classic manner of respiratory transmission.

Transmission may also result from contact with inanimate objects contaminated with the infectious agent. For example, a door knob is contami-

TABLE 6-8

Common Routes of Transmission*

Route of Exit	Route of Transmission	Example
Respiratory	Aerosol droplet inhalation	Influenza virus; tuberculosis
	Nose or mouth → hand or object → nose	Common cold (rhinovirus)
Salivary	Direct salivary transfer (e.g., kissing)	Oral-labial herpes; infectious mononucleosis
	Animal bite	Rabies
Gastrointestinal	Stool → hand → mouth and/or stool → object → mouth	Enterovirus infection; hepatitis A
	Stool → water or food → mouth	Salmonellosis; shigellosis
Skin	Skin discharge → air → respiratory tract	Varicella; poxvirus infection
	Skin to skin	Human papillomavirus (warts); syphilis
Blood	Transfusion or needle prick	Hepatitis B; cytomegalovirus infection; malaria; human immunodeficiency virus (AIDS)
	Insect bite	Malaria; relapsing fever
Genital secretions	Urethral or cervical secretions	Gonorrhea; herpes simplex; *Chlamydia* infection
	Semen	Cytomegalovirus infection
Urine	Urine → hand → catheter	Hospital-acquired urinary tract infection
	Urine → aerosol (rare)	Tuberculosis
Eye	Conjunctival	Adenovirus
Zoonotic	Animal bite	Rabies
	Contact with carcasses	Tularemia
	Arthropod	Plague; Rocky Mountain spotted fever; Lyme disease

From Sherris JC, editor: *Medical microbiology: an introduction to infectious diseases,* ed 2, New York, 1990, Elsevier.
*The examples cited are incomplete, and in some cases more than one route of transmission exists.

nated by the hand and fingers of an infected individual, and the virus is transmitted to a susceptible person's hand and fingers when that person opens the door. Control of such transmission is often as simple as frequent handwashing.

Infections of the lower respiratory tract are less common but more serious than those of the upper respiratory tract. The organisms causing these infections have managed to bypass host defenses, or the host defenses have been compromised (e.g., by alcoholism, heavy smoking), allowing the pathogen access to the deeper portions of the respiratory tract.

The most common microorganism causing lower respiratory tract infection of individuals over age 30 is *S. pneumoniae.* The pneumococcus is often seen in aspiration pneumonia, a common type of hospital-acquired pneumonia. Pneumococcal pneumonia begins suddenly and is a serious, life-threatening disease, particularly in elderly patients. Among younger people, the common causes of pneumonia are *Mycoplasma* organisms and viruses. The onset of these pneumonias is more gradual than with pneumococcal pneumonia, and the outcome is far more favorable.

In chronic lower respiratory tract infections, the survival of the infecting agent within phagocytes plays a role in the pathogenic mechanism. *M. tuberculosis,* the agent of tuberculosis, a chronic debilitating infection, is the classic example of an intracellular pathogen. This organism is highly virulent, is invasive, and survives well and multiplies within phagocytes.

Transmission by Food and Water

Transmission of gastrointestinal infections is usually a result of ingestion of contaminated food or water. In some situations, infection occurs via the fecal-oral route.

The digestive tract is colonized with vast numbers of different microorganisms. Under usual conditions, the gut flora maintains a harmless relationship with the host. Gastric enzymes and juices in the stomach act to prevent survival of most organisms, but many survive and colonize the small intestine and colon.

Gastrointestinal infections result from organisms that are able to survive the harsh conditions of the stomach and competition with the microbial flora and to produce damage to the tissues of the gastrointestinal tract. This damage is a result of either a preformed toxin or disruption of the normal functioning of the intestinal cells by invasion of the pathogen or production of a toxin within the intestine.

Organisms that can cause disease by means of a preformed toxin include *Clostridium botulinum, Bacillus cereus,* and *S. aureus.* The severity of disease ranges from a mild diarrhea to a rapidly fatal intoxication. Food poisoning by *B. cereus* and *S. aureus* is relatively common and is self-limiting. Botulism, caused by *C. botulinum,* although rare, can be life-threatening.

Other bacteria produce a toxin after infection of the intestinal tract. Generally, to be effective as a disease producer, an organism must survive, adhere to, and colonize the intestinal mucosa and either produce a toxin or invade deeper tissues. A commonly seen cause of diarrhea and intestinal infection is *E. coli.* This organism is a member of the intestinal flora; however, some strains of *E. coli* produce cytotoxins that cause alterations in the biochemical activity of the intestinal epithelial cells, resulting in problems with fluid and electrolyte control by the intestinal cells. These strains of *E. coli,* referred to as *enterotoxigenic,* are a common cause of "traveler's diarrhea" and other intestinal problems.

Probably the classic intestinal pathogen is *Vibrio cholerae,* the cause of cholera. This organism produces an enterotoxin that causes the outpouring of fluid from the cells into the lumen of the intestine. Massive amounts (up to 20 L per day) can be lost. Other intestinal pathogens are *Clostridium difficile, Shigella* spp., *Aeromonas hydrophila, Campylobacter jejuni,* and *Salmonella* spp. The infective dose, severity, and incidence of disease vary with the agent.

A number of viruses also cause diarrheal disease. They multiply within the cells of the intestinal mucosa and affect the normal functioning of the cells. Viral agents in this category include hepatitis, rotavirus, adenovirus, coxsackievirus, and Norwalk-like agents. The incidence of diarrhea caused by these agents is high, especially in situations in which people are in close contact (daycare centers, nurseries, military camps). Numerous parasites, such as *Fasciolopsis buski, Giardia lamblia, Entamoeba histolytica,* and *Balantidium coli,* also infect the gastrointestinal tract.

Close Contact

All of the routes of transmission of infectious diseases require **close contact.** Obviously, for a respiratory pathogen to be transmitted via aerosols, the susceptible host must be relatively close. For this discussion, however, close contact refers to passage of organisms by salivary, skin, and genital contact. Two prominent infections passed by direct transfer of saliva (e.g., kissing) are herpes simplex and infectious mononucleosis. Skin-to-skin transfer of infectious disease is not as common as some of the other routes, but diseases such as warts (human papillomavirus), syphilis, and impetigo result when material from infectious lesions inoculates a susceptible host's skin. The list of sexually transmitted diseases is a long one. In North America, the most commonly transmitted venereal diseases or agents are gonorrhea, herpes simplex, hepatitis, *Chlamydia* spp., syphilis, *Trichomonas* spp., and AIDS.

Cuts and Bites

The classic example of a bite-wound infection is rabies. In fact, human rabies is relatively rare. Of more concern with animal, and especially human bites, is infection by the mouth flora. Dog- and cat-bite infections often yield *Pasteurella multocida,* but the possibilities are extensive. Human bites are extremely dangerous because they are difficult to treat and because the human oral flora comprises many different organisms in extremely high numbers.

Arthropods

Infection as a result of a tick, flea, or mite bite is a common occurrence in many parts of the world. The diseases spread by arthropods include malaria, relapsing fever, plague, Rocky Mountain spotted fever, Lyme disease, typhus, and untold numbers of regional hemorrhagic fevers. In most cases, the infectious agent multiplies in the arthropod, which then feeds off a human host and transmits the microorganism.

Zoonoses

The route of transmission known as *zoonosis* depends on contact with animals or animal products. Certain diseases of animals may also infect humans who have contact with then. These diseases may be passed by animal bites (rabies), arthro-

TABLE 6-9
Zoonoses

Disease	Organism
Anthrax	*Bacillus anthracis*
Brucellosis	*Brucella* spp.
Erysipeloid	*Erysipelothrix rhusiopathiae*
Leptospirosis	*Leptospira interrogans*
Tularemia	*Francisella tularensis*
Ringworm	*Trichophyton* spp., *Microsporum* spp.
Lyme disease	*Borrelia burgdorferi*
Plague	*Yersinia pestis*
Rocky Mountain spotted fever	*Rickettsia rickettsii*
Yellow fever	Flavivirus
Encephalitis	Alphavirus
Colorado tick fever	Orbivirus
Leishmaniasis	*Leishmania* spp.
Rabies	Rhabdovirus
Blastomycosis	*Blastomyces dermatitidis*
Tuberculosis	*Mycobacterium bovis*
Q fever	*Coxiella burnetii*
Ornithosis	*Chlamydia psittaci*
Gastroenteritis	*Campylobacter* spp., *Salmonella* spp.
Listeriosis	*Listeria monocytogenes*
Giardiasis	*Giardia lamblia*
Toxoplasmosis	*Toxoplasma gondii*
Tapeworms	*Taenia saginata*
	Taenia solium
	Diphyllobothrium latum
	Echinococcus spp.
Trichinosis	*Trichinella spiralis*

pod vectors (plague), contact with secretions (brucellosis), and contact with animal carcasses and products (tularemia, listeriosis). The diseases are transmitted by routes already discussed. The common factor is that, regardless of the route, the disease is a disease of animals that is transmitted to humans. A partial list of zoonotic diseases and infecting organisms is shown in Table 6-9.

EPIDEMIOLOGY

Epidemiology is the study of the occurrence, distribution, and causes of disease and injury. This definition includes not only infectious diseases but also problems as diverse as gunshot injuries and heart attacks. The emphasis in this section is on infectious diseases, but the principles of epidemiologic study are the same regardless of the disease or problem studied.

Definitions

Several terms are helpful in describing the incidence and effect of disease in a population and include the following:

▪ Carrier: A **carrier** is a person or animal who harbors and spreads a microorganism that causes disease but does not become ill. The two types of carriers are a casual carrier and a chronic carrier. A casual carrier harbors the microorganism temporarily for a few days or weeks; examples of microorganisms maintained in this fashion are *C. diphtheriae, N. meningitidis,* and *S. pyogenes.* A chronic carrier remains infected for a relatively long time, sometimes throughout life; the typhoid bacillus may be carried chronically.

▪ Endemic: When an organism or disease is constantly present in a population, that disease or organism is termed *endemic.* It is indigenous to a geographic area or population. Some microorganisms or diseases are endemic for one geographical area but not for another. Schistosomiasis is endemic to parts of the Middle East but not for many other parts of the world. Cholera is endemic for large portions of the globe. In the United States, we have a more-or-less constant incidence of common colds, streptococcal pharyngitis, and gonorrhea.

▪ Epidemic: When a disease affects a significantly large number of people at the same time in a geographic area, an **epidemic** occurs. The number of cases per given time is not the only measure. Ten cases of diphtheria in a short time could be considered an epidemic because diphtheria is not often seen. Ten cases of streptococcal pharyngitis during that same period are probably normal, however, because it is an endemic disease. A classic example of an epidemic is influenza. Epidemics of varying degrees happen every year. Periodically (in intervals of 10 to 20 years), worldwide epidemics of influenza affect tens of millions of people; they are termed *pandemics.* Currently, cholera is in its seventh pandemic; it has spread throughout world regions and even continents.

▪ Incidence rate: The number of times a new event occurs in a given period is called the *incidence rate.* It is usually given as cases or infections per 1000 or 100,000 population. It allows a prevalence comparison between diseases or infections.

- Incubation period: The time between exposure to a pathogen and the onset of symptoms is the ***incubation period.*** The incubation period is often difficult to determine because individuals have difficulty pinpointing the date or time of exposure. An individual may be infectious during the incubation period; this situation presents a difficult public health problem because no symptoms are present to identify the infectious person when transmission of the organism is taking place.
- Index case: The first case of a disease, which serves as a source of infection, is the *index case.*
- Morbidity rate: The rate at which an illness occurs, the **morbidity rate,** is the number of cases of a disease in a specified population during a defined time interval. The morbidity rate can be a measure of the infectiousness of an organism.
- Mortality rate: The mortality rate is the number of deaths caused by a disease in a population. Organisms that are highly virulent often have a high mortality rate.
- Nosocomial infections: An infection acquired during hospitalization is termed a *nosocomial infection.*
- Reservoir: The reservoir is the source of an infection. It may be a person, an animal, or something in the environment.
- Surveillance: ***Surveillance*** is the collection of data pertaining to disease occurrence. It is carried out at various levels (physician, city, county, state, federal, international) with a system for reporting to public health agencies.

Surveillance and Reporting

Certain infectious diseases are required by law to be reported to public health authorities. Generally, these are diseases that have a significant effect on the population (venereal diseases) or have the potential for grave consequences (anthrax, plague). A reporting system exists in place in the United States, by which local public health authorities report to a state health agency, which in turn reports to the Centers for Disease Control and Prevention (CDC) at the national level. The CDC works closely with worldwide health agencies such as the World Health Organization (WHO) and the national health agencies of other countries. These organizations monitor the incidence of disease to determine the current health status of the world's population.

At the local level, surveillance and reporting may consist of investigating an outbreak of food poisoning at a church picnic. The state might become involved if the origin of the food poisoning was determined to be a vendor who distributes to other areas of the state. If the vendor is a multistate distributor, the national authorities might be included. Legionellosis, AIDS, Lyme disease, and many others provide examples of full case studies in the methods and procedures used to investigate and monitor an epidemic and the organization of the public health system. These methods and procedures can be complex and cannot be discussed here, but they involve statistical analysis of minute details of a disease outbreak. The clinical laboratory plays a significant role in providing support for these investigations.

Bibliography

Braude AI, Davis CE, Fierer J, editors: *Infectious diseases and medical microbiology,* Philadelphia, 1986, WB Saunders.

Gotschlich EC: Thoughts on the evolution of strategies used by bacteria for evasion of host defenses, *Rev Infect Dis* 5:S778, 1983.

Mims CA: *The pathogenesis of infectious disease,* New York, 1977, Academic Press.

Sherris JC, editor: *Medical microbiology: an introduction to infectious diseases,* New York, 1990, Elsevier.

Spitznagel JK: Microbial interactions with neutrophils, *Rev Infect Dis* 5:S806, 1983.

LEARNING ASSESSMENT

1. What host resistance factor is compromised in the patient described in the case study?

2. What microbial factor contributes to the virulence of the infecting organism?

3. What is the difference between true pathogens and opportunistic pathogens?

4. How does inflammation play a role as a host immune defense?

5. What is the difference between exotoxins and endotoxins?

CHAPTER 7

General Concepts in Specimen Collection and Handling

Merrily Rausch, Joy G. Remley

BASIC PRINCIPLES OF SPECIMEN COLLECTION
  Appropriate Collection Techniques
    Aspirates and tissues
    Swabs
    Need for repeat cultures

PATIENT EDUCATION AND PREPARATION
  Patient Education: Patient-Collected Samples
    Urine
    Sputum
    Stools
  Patient or Site Preparation

PRESERVATION, STORAGE, AND TRANSPORT
  OF SPECIMENS
  Use of Preservatives
  Use of Anticoagulants
  Use of Holding and Transport Media
  Unprotected Specimens
  Storage of Specimens
  Mailing Etiologic Agents

SAFETY
  Protection of the Specimen Transporter
  Protection of the Specimen Processor

LABELING AND REJECTION OF SPECIMENS
  Requisitions
    Source
    Diagnosis/history
    Test requested
  Unacceptable Specimens

PROCESSING OF CLINICAL SAMPLES
  FOR OPTIMAL ORGANISM RECOVERY
  Prioritization During Processing
  Gross Examination of Specimens
  Direct Examination Techniques
    Smear preparation
    When direct smear is not useful
  Primary Inoculation of Routine Specimens
    Selection of primary culture media for routine
      specimens
    Selection of temperature and environmental
      conditions
    Primary isolation media for unusual and
      fastidious bacteria
    Initial processing techniques for primary
      inoculation
  Processing Nonroutine Specimens
    Types of nonroutine specimens

OBJECTIVES

1. Describe the basic principles of specimen collection for materials received in the form of aspirates, tissues, and swabs.
2. Describe patient education for the following patient-collected specimens: urine (clean-catch), sputum, and stool.
3. Discuss patient preparation before specimen collection for procedures such as blood, cervical, and wound cultures.
4. Demonstrate a knowledge of mechanisms for maintaining organism viability relating to preservation, storage, and transport of specimens.
5. Demonstrate an awareness of safe practices related to specimen transport, processing, and labeling.
6. Explain prioritization guidelines used during processing to prevent degradation of the specimen.
7. Discuss multiple techniques for smear preparation and primary media inoculation.
8. Use charts for selection of routine primary culture media and media for unusual and fastidious bacteria.
9. Utilize a standardized thought process to determine methods for processing nonroutine specimens.

KEY TERMS

Polymicrobic
Holding medium
Midstream urine
    collection
Etiologic agents
Universal or standard
    precautions
Noninvasive specimen
Invasive specimen
Direct examination

Cytocentrifugation
Nonselective media
Selective media
Differential media
Enriched media
Indigenous flora
Inoculum counter-
    streak technique
Nonroutine specimen
Nosocomial infection

CASE STUDY

A 67-year-old female exhibited the following presenting symptoms: fever, shortness of breath, chest pain, and a productive cough. An x-ray examination of the chest showed infiltration on her right lower lobe. A transtracheal aspirate was sent to the laboratory for examination and culture. Direct smear examination showed numerous polymorphonuclear cells (PMNs), a moderate amount of gram-positive cocci, and numerous gram-negative rods. The routine aerobic culture showed usual respiratory flora. Anaerobic culture produced no growth after 48 hours of incubation. The microbiology technologist determined whether a delay had occurred during the transport to the laboratory.

Adequate collection, transport, and processing of clinical specimens for microbiologic evaluation are important requirements in the diagnosis of infectious disease. The medical support team meets these requirements through cooperative efforts. This team may consist of individuals with varied knowledge and backgrounds. Nevertheless, all team members—clinical practitioners, nurses, and laboratory practitioners—must be instructed in the basic principles of specimen collection and the requirements of rapid transport, proper storage, and preservation of different specimen types. It is the responsibility of the laboratory practitioner to recognize and reject suboptimal specimens and to inform and educate the other team members. For proper team functioning and the rapid diagnosis and treatment of infectious disease, all members of the team should participate in ongoing communication and education.

This chapter discusses the following topics:

- The basic principles of specimen collection
- Methods for processing clinical specimens for optimal recovery of common bacterial pathogens as well as unusual organisms
- Methods of preservation and proper use of transport media
- Selection of culture media
- Methods for processing nonroutine samples

BASIC PRINCIPLES OF SPECIMEN COLLECTION

The laboratory can make accurate and useful determinations only if a specimen has been collected properly. The following basic principles of specimen collection may serve as guidelines to ensure appropriate collection processes:

- If at all possible, a culture specimen should be taken in the acute phase of the infection and before antibiotics are administered.
- The collection process is initiated by a written order followed by selection of a site to culture. Failure to select an appropriate site to culture leads to misleading culture results and may adversely affect patient management.
- It is important to culture the infecting agents while avoiding the usual flora and colonizing organisms.
- Test results must always be carefully compared with the suspected diagnosis. For example, if gas is observed in the tissues of an amputation site and the suspected diagnosis is gas gangrene caused by *Clostridium perfringens,* the laboratory practitioner should be suspicious of inadequate site selection when the organism is not seen on direct examination or recovered in culture. Failure to recover the organism could be the result of a true absence of the organism or inadequate sampling of the site.

Appropriate Collection Techniques

Aspirates and tissues

Aspirates of sterile body fluids are collected using sterile technique and generally present the laboratory with few problems relating to quality and quantity of specimen. A piece of tissue is another excellent specimen provided that the sample is taken from along the active line of infection. Tissue samples must be protected from drying during transport. Several drops of sterile saline may be used to prevent the tissue from drying.

Lesions, wounds, and abscesses seem to present the most problems related to quantity and quality. Because infection typically elicits a white cell response in the host, an aspirate of pus is the ideal specimen. In deep wounds or abscesses a sample collected from the wall of the abscess, in addition to a sample of pus, provides an enhanced opportunity for thorough assessment. When multiple sites appear infected, an aspirate of a fluctuant, unopen wound is far superior to a swab from an open, draining wound.

Swabs

Swabs are used only as a last resort and are considered inferior to other collection methods. The volume of specimen collected by swabbing a wound tends to be inadequate, and the attempt to extract the material from the swab is often ineffective. If a swab must be used instead of an aspirate or piece of tissue, four basic rules must be followed: (1) clean the wound, (2) explore the wound, (3) obtain fresh culture material, and (4) obtain adequate quantity of material.

CLEAN THE WOUND

All organisms like to feed on pus. These organisms may consist of endogenous flora from the skin and mucous membranes, contaminants from the air, and organisms from the patient's or caregiver's hands. The goal should be to grow only those organisms responsible for the production of the pus. Cleaning the wound kills organisms and also clears any nonviable anaerobic organisms from the wound surface. A 3% solution of hydrogen peroxide can be used to clean the wound. One advantage of hydrogen peroxide is that it kills organisms only for as long as it bubbles. In contrast, povidone-iodine is advantageous as a wound packing because it releases iodine molecules hour after hour, decreasing the numbers of organisms in the wound. A swab contaminated with povidone-iodine may adversely affect the laboratory's ability to grow organisms associated with infection.

EXPLORE THE WOUND

Exploration of the wound, with emphasis on finding any existing sinus tracts, will better define its extent. Organisms found deep in sinus tracts may be very different from those found on the surface and may require special antibiotic therapy for their eradication. Nasopharyngeal swabs, which contain a very small head on a flexible wire, are ideal for probing sinus tracts.

OBTAIN FRESH CULTURE MATERIAL

Material submitted for culture must always be fresh. Pus should never be obtained from slow-draining lines, bags, or bottles, where material may have been sitting for a prolonged period. Many specimens are **polymicrobic** (i.e., they contain more than one organism). If pus sits in a container, detection of slow-growing organisms in a specimen taken from it may be difficult or impossible owing to overgrowth of more rapidly growing organisms. This result may affect subsequent decisions about therapy. For the same reason, a swab collection system should contain a **holding medium** to protect organisms without permitting rapid multiplication during transport.

OBTAIN ADEQUATE QUANTITY OF MATERIAL

Quantity of material is equally as important as freshness. Wounds with a small opening may need to be sampled with a smaller swab, such as the nasopharyngeal swab, to obtain material from inside them. When smaller swabs are substituted, more of them will be necessary to gather adequate amounts of material. Allowing the swab to remain in the wound for a time while the wound is pressed may also be necessary to obtain adequate specimen. The common practice of dabbing at a wound does not permit the necessary saturation of the swab.

Thorough evaluation of a wound *always* includes both smear and culture. A minimum of two swabs per culture is required. The value of the smear is to determine the adequacy of the specimen, identify classic pathogens, and determine the need for the use of special media, special incubation atmospheres, and length of incubation. Organisms such as *Actinomyces* species and *Nocardia* species would probably not be grown unless they were first seen on a smear because cultures would not routinely be held long enough. When a single swab is received, the smear must be eliminated. Culture is still a more sensitive and definitive test. Additionally, quantity of culture material or numbers of swabs must be determined on the basis of the number of tests requested. A request for acid-fast, fungal, viral, and routine bacterial cultures cannot be fulfilled using just two swabs.

Need for repeat cultures

It is important to remember that even with therapy, wounds do not generally change overnight. Repetitious culturing of wounds is a waste of time and money. Most wounds can be easily accessed and sampled thoroughly and should not require repeat culture for 4 to 5 days. Monitoring the situation with a Gram stain is far more economically efficient than repeat culturing.

PATIENT EDUCATION AND PREPARATION

Patient Education: Patient-Collected Samples

Not all specimens are collected by hospital personnel. Specimens such as urine, sputum, and stool are commonly obtained by the patient and most often require extensive patient education. Patients should never be asked whether they know how to collect a particular type of specimen. An affirmative response does not always mean that the patient has learned correct techniques. Attaching printed instructions in multiple languages to a collection device does not ensure that patients will read them. The most effective educational tool is to give the patient a preprinted sheet of instructions using simple language and pictures to help the patient follow along and understand as the procedure is verbally described. Box 7-1 contains more extensive patient teaching tips.

Urine

Explanation of urine collection must include instructions for skin preparation and an explanation of **midstream urine collection.** Patients must be asked to void without collecting the first portion of the specimen but instead to collect the middle portion (midstream). This technique helps eliminate contaminating organisms. The technique should also be used by personnel collecting catheterized specimens to eliminate organisms carried up the urethra during catheterization. Having separate urine collection instructions for male and female patients helps clarify the task. The collection of the first morning specimen provides a more concentrated sample with the potential for optimal results.

Sputum

Lower respiratory tract specimens are among the most difficult specimens to collect adequately and may require the help of a respiratory therapist. The patient should be instructed to remove dentures,

Box 7-1

Patient Teaching Tips

Deal with patient's immediate concerns first.

Assess current understanding, and build on it.

Create learning environment—patients should know they are being taught.

Establish mutual learning outcomes with patient. Keep sessions short; separate long and complex material into short segments.

Avoid too much detail; use examples patient can relate to; teach skills in logical progression.

Have patient use as many senses as possible. This includes hearing, seeing, touching, writing, speaking, and doing. Patients remember 90% of what they say and do, but only 10% of what they hear. Learning requires active participation.

Have patient practice new skills; expect a demonstration by the patient of skill taught.

Document what patient said or did to demonstrate learning.

Think teaching; incorporate it into your cares.

Modified from Abbott Northwestern Hospital: Patient Education Department handout, Minneapolis, 1986, Abbot Northwestern Hospital.

rinse the mouth, gargle with water, and then expectorate with the aid of a deep cough. First morning specimens may be more successful owing to the volume of secretions that collect in the lungs overnight.

If the specimen is being collected for the purpose of diagnosing disease but appears normal, it should not be sent to the laboratory; another specimen should be collected. Infectious secretions exhibit such abnormalities as pus, blood, and dark flecks.

If patients are unable to expectorate a respiratory specimen, the specimen may be aspirated with the aid of a Leuken's trap (Figure 7-1). If secretions are too thick to aspirate, saline nebulization may be used to loosen them, as long as care is taken to prevent excessive dilution of the specimen.

Stools

Kits should be provided for the collection of stool specimens. Three-vial kits are recommended. Each such kit contains a vial with a preservative for parasites, a vial with a preservative for enteric pathogens, and a clean vial for examination of the raw specimen and any additional testing. To maintain a 1:3 ratio of stool to preservative, the recommended amount of stool specimen per vial should not be exceeded. Thoroughly mixing formed specimens with the preservative is also important to protect the organisms or parasites. Specimens should not be collected within 4 days of the patient's receiving barium. Barium will appear as a white chalky substance in the specimen. Patients should also be instructed to avoid contamination of the stool with urine. Multiple specimens may be necessary, particularly for diagnosing parasitic infections. Each specimen must be collected on a different day to take into account the life cycles of parasites.

Patient or Site Preparation

Preparation of the patient or the specimen site before specimen collection contributes to optimal recovery of infecting agents. Removal of an eschar before culture or biopsy of certain wounds or burns allows for more accurate wound assessment. Removing the mucous plug before obtaining a specimen for cervical culture increases the chances for recovery of cervical pathogens. Table 7-1 lists ways in which patients or sites may be prepared before specimen collection for each body site.

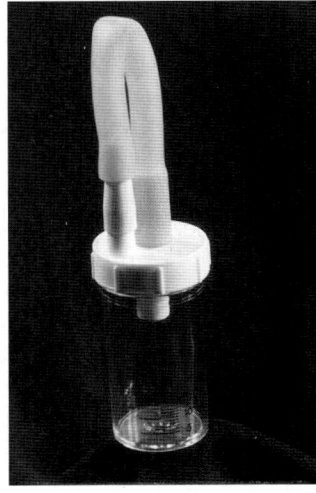

Figure 7-1

Leuken's trap.

TABLE 7-1

Patient or Site Preparation

Site	Preparation
Blood cultures	Skin preparation: alcohol, 2% tincture of iodine, alcohol
Body fluids (sterile)	Skin preparation as for blood cultures
Catheter tips	Iodine preparation before insertion
	Ointment or blood removed with alcohol
Drainage sites	Aspirate or tissue preferable
	Must get to source of drainage
Eye	Skin cleansed around eye
	Purulent material collected on swab or corneal scrapings placed on media at bedside
	Topical anesthetic used only for corneal scraping
Fungal scrapings	70% alcohol or gauze soaked in sterile water or saline used for cleaning, then periphery scraped with scalpel
Genitalia	
Cervix/vagina	Speculum
	Mucous plug removed before culturing
	Vesicles unroofed before bases are scraped
Urethra	Patient instructed not to urinate for 1 hr before collection
	Dacron swab
	Swab inserted 2-4 cm for 2-3 seconds and rotated gently while swab is withdrawn
Lesion/wound/abscess	
Lesion/abscess	Unopen abscess: skin preparation as for blood cultures
	Open wounds: packing removed, wound cleaned with 3% H_2O_2
Burn wounds	Eschar removed before culturing or taking biopsy specimen
Biopsy	Skin preparation as for blood cultures
Sputum	Patient instructed to remove dentures, rinse mouth, and gargle with water
	May enlist aid of respiratory therapy
Stool	Contamination with urine and barium to be avoided
Urine	Perineal area cleansed with antiseptic towelette before collection according to instructions on collection kit

PRESERVATION, STORAGE, AND TRANSPORT OF SPECIMENS

Unfortunately, patients rarely come to the laboratory for a culture, allowing specimens to be processed immediately without transport delay. Transportation and preservation of the specimen is a problem whether the specimen comes from a nursing station three floors above the laboratory or from an outpatient facility, nursing home, or doctor's office across town. The following are major concerns:

- Overgrowth of rapidly growing organisms
- Death of organisms resulting from changes in temperature and pH
- Inaccurate quantitation of organisms in urine and quantitative tissue
- Loss of organisms resulting from drying
- Protection from oxygen
- Protection from clotting
- Safety of the transporter

Maintenance or protection of the primary specimen can be aided by the use of preservatives, anticoagulants, holding media, and even culture media.

Use of Preservatives

Two major specimen types protected by preservatives are urine and stool. Boric acid is used in commercial products to maintain accurate urine colony counts. Phosphate-buffered saline (PBS) helps preserve feces so that fragile organisms, such as *Shigella* species, will not die because of temperature and pH changes. Formalin, polyvinyl alcohol (PVA), and Schaudinn's solution all help preserve parasite trophozoites and cysts so they will remain in recognizable form.

Use of Anticoagulants

The use of anticoagulants is important for any specimen that might clot because organisms bound up in clotted material are difficult to grow. Sodium polyanethol sulfonate (SPS) is the most common anticoagulant used for microbiology specimens. The concentration of SPS must not exceed 0.025% (w/v); some *Neisseria* species and anaerobic streptococci are inhibited by concentrations of 0.025% to 0.05%. Vacutainer tubes (Becton Dickinson) containing SPS are convenient for bone marrow aspirates or synovial fluids that tend to clot.

Heparin is another anticoagulant that can be used selectively in microbiology, but it is routinely used for viral culture as opposed to bacterial cultures. Heparin may inhibit the growth of gram-positive organisms and yeast. Citrate and ethylenediaminetetraacidic acid (EDTA) should not be used for microbiology specimens.

Use of Holding and Transport Media

Swab collection systems contain a holding medium that maintains viability of the organisms but does not permit an increase or decrease in numbers of organisms. Modified Stuart transport medium and Cary-Blair transport medium are commonly used. Studies have shown that many transport media perform equally well at refrigerator temperature, but they should be tested against one another at room temperature when one is attempting to select a superior product.

Unlike other specimens, blood is usually placed in a broth culture medium immediately after collection instead of in a preservative or a holding medium. The major reason is the need to quickly grow and identify the organism present in a potentially life-threatening condition, such as bacteremia. The numbers of organisms present in bacteremia are usually low, and efforts must be made to enhance these numbers quickly. Organisms generally multiply quickly in broth culture.

Unprotected Specimens

Many specimen types are transported without special protection. These include sputums, body fluids, tissues, catheters, medical devices, and specimens for sterility culture. The need to process such specimens without delay as soon as they arrive in the laboratory should be reinforced.

Storage of Specimens

Processing all specimens without delay is probably impossible. The laboratory must make decisions regarding the storage of specimens that cannot be processed immediately. Decisions should be based on knowledge of organisms found in each type of specimen and the stability of those organisms. Box 7-2 separates organisms that are fragile (suspectible to temperature, environmental, and pH changes) from those that are hardy (not readily affected by these changes).

Should specimens be stored at refrigerator temperature, room temperature, or incubator temperature? Urine, viral blood specimens, catheters, and swabs should be refrigerated, but bacterial blood specimens, cerebrospinal fluid (CSF), and cultures processed onto agar plates at the bedside should be placed in an incubator. Room temperature is most appropriate for specimens such as hair and nails for isolation of fungus.

Storage of respiratory and stool cultures presents special problems. Respiratory specimens are likely to contain *Streptococcus pneumoniae.* Although this organism is fragile and may not tolerate the cold well, a respiratory specimen is also likely to be polymicrobic. Overgrowth becomes a problem without refrigeration. Stool specimens may contain *Shigella,* an extremely fragile,

---

Box 7-2

Stability of Organisms

Fragile organisms

Streptococcus pneumoniae
Neisseria gonorrhoeae
Neisseria meningitidis
Salmonella
Shigella
Haemophilus influenzae
Anaerobes
Mycoplasma
Viruses
Chlamydia
Unpreserved parasites

Hardy organisms

Enterics
Pseudomonads
Enterococcus
Other *Streptococcus*
Staphylococcus
Yeast
Fungi
Mycobacteria
Legionella
Clostridium difficile toxin

temperature-sensitive organism, but also contain many other species of gram-negative rods, making overgrowth an even bigger problem than with respiratory specimens. Most laboratories choose to refrigerate both specimen types if processing will be delayed, even though organism viability is not guaranteed. Although the Gram stain is often helpful in diagnosing *S. pneumoniae* even when it is unconfirmed by culture, the Gram stain does not differentiate *Salmonella* and *Shigella* from other gram-negative rods in a stool specimen. The best solution is to process stool specimens without delay.

Mailing Etiologic Agents

Mailing or shipping **etiologic agents** or biohazardous materials is governed by federal regulations devised by the U.S. Department of Health and Human Services. An etiologic agent is a viable microorganism or its toxin that causes, or may cause, human disease. Such material must be placed in a securely closed, watertight container such as a vial or test tube, known as the *primary container* (Figure 7-2). The primary container is placed in a secondary container with sufficient absorbent material (e.g., paper towels) between them to absorb the contents in case of breakage. The secondary

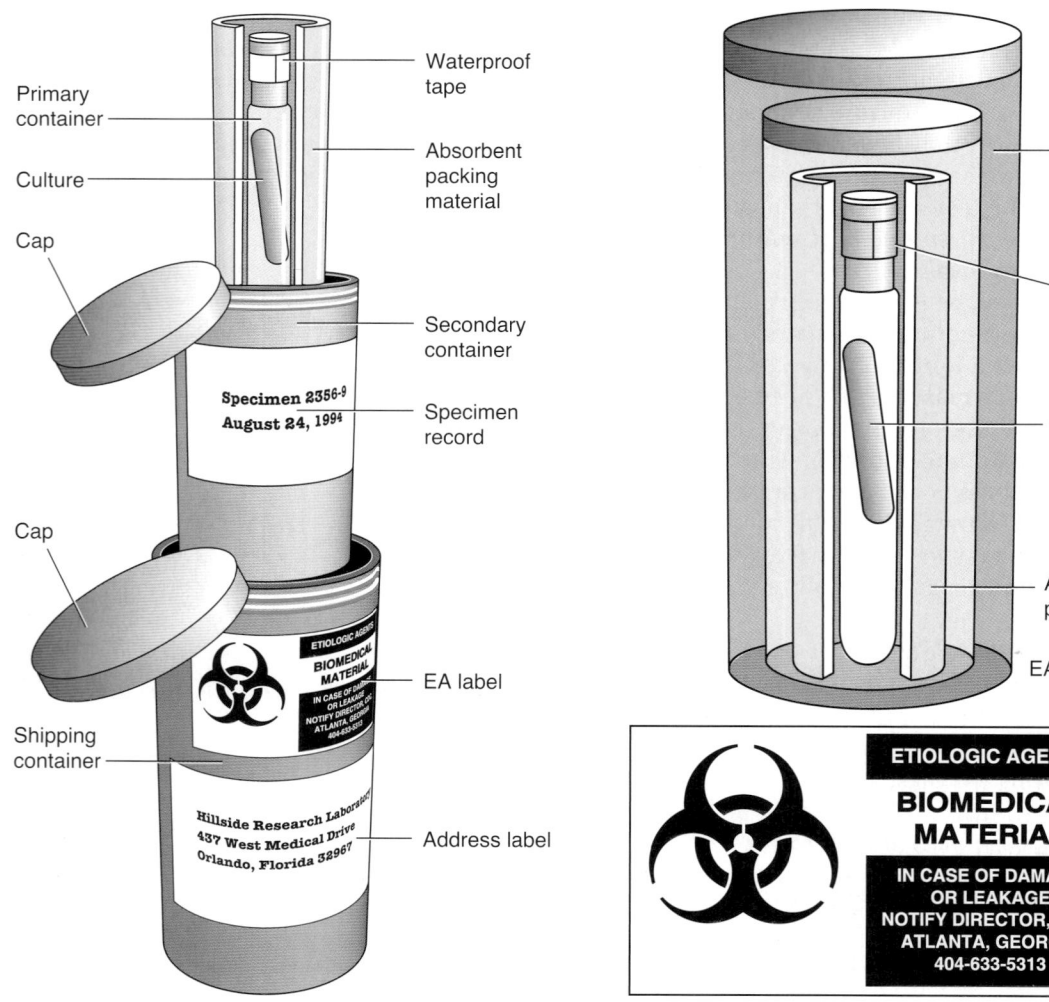

Figure 7-2

Packaging and labeling of etiologic agents. *EA,* Etiologic agent.

container is then placed in an approved mailing container. An etiologic agent label must be placed on the mailing container. This label contains a biohazard symbol and a phone number for The Centers for Disease Control, Atlanta, Georgia (CDC), allowing for notification in the event of leakage.

The regulations also address such topics as mailing of serum samples, maximum volumes of samples to be mailed, and lists of dangerous pathogens that must be sent by registered mail or an equivalent system. The regulations are subject to change. Regulations are published in the *Federal Register.**

SAFETY

Protection of the Specimen Transporter

Protection of the transporter and laboratory personnel from infectious agents in the specimen is as important as protection of the specimen. Leaking specimens and specimens with needles attached present the greatest hazards. In compliance with the rules of **Universal or Standard Precautions** instituted by CDC, all specimens must be transported in leakproof secondary containers. Plastic bags with permanent seals and separate pouches on the outside for requisitions are recommended. After arrival in the laboratory, the bag is opened by tearing along a semiperforated line. Zip-lock bags are not recommended because they are difficult to close and may leak during transport.

Transporting personnel should refuse to transport routine specimens without the protection of a secondary container. Refusing to accept syringes with needles attached is also appropriate. Needle sticks are among the most common and most hazardous laboratory accidents. They are probably also the most easily prevented. A needle must be replaced with a tight-fitting rubber stopper or a stopcock to put resistance on the plunger. Another option is to transfer the aspirated material to another type of container or sterile screw-capped tube, provided enough material exists to fill the tube (to eliminate air that could mix with the specimen and harm any anaerobes present).

---

*Refer to NCCLS Document H5-A3, Vol. 14, No. 7: *Procedures for the handling and transport of diagnostic specimens and etiologic agents,* ed 3, (Approved Standard), Villanova, Pa, May 1994, NCCLS.

As with everything else, there is an exception to the rule. In some cases, a valuable aspirate is so small that most of it is in the needle instead of the syringe. When this happens, the specimen can be transported "individually" (with needle attached) to the microbiology laboratory and placed in the hands of a laboratory employee to process immediately. Under no circumstances should such a specimen be sent by routine transportation mechanisms.

Protection of the Specimen Processor

All health care workers must adhere to strict safety guidelines in daily practice. Laboratory personnel are at risk for accidental infection if they do not use common sense and take appropriate precautions. All individuals handling patient specimens must wear protective clothing and open specimens only in a biohazard hood. It is the responsibility of all medical staff to alert the laboratory and other health care workers when extremely dangerous pathogens are to be considered. Pathogens such as *Brucella, Francisella tularensis,* hepatitis B virus, and *Mycobacterium tuberculosis* are extremely hazardous and must be handled only in laboratories with sufficient safety procedures. Microbiology personnel must routinely participate in safety education.

LABELING AND REJECTION OF SPECIMENS

Requisitions

The laboratory requisition must include enough information to enable the laboratory to do the best job. All that the laboratory knows about the patient is learned from the requisition. All microbiology requisitions should include information about the source, the diagnosis or history, and the test requested.

Source

The source should be specific. Listing only "wound" or "drainage" is insufficient. The source should include the anatomic location and the type of wound. Is it from the head or the leg? Is it a bite, a puncture wound, a surgical incision, or a skin abrasion?

Diagnosis/history

The diagnosis sometimes leads the technologist to suspect growth of a specific organism that may re-

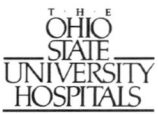

LABORATORY RELEASE

UNACCEPTABLE SPECIMEN: TRANSFER OF RESPONSIBILITY

PATIENT IDENTIFICATION

SPECIMEN	REQUISITION
NAME _____	NAME _____
MEDICAL RECORD NO. ⬚⬚⬚⬚⬚⬚⬚⬚⬚	MEDICAL RECORD NO. ⬚⬚⬚⬚⬚⬚⬚⬚⬚
HOSPITAL NO. (4 DIGIT) ⬚⬚⬚⬚	HOSPITAL NO. (4 DIGIT) ⬚⬚⬚⬚
NURSING STATION _____	NURSING STATION _____
ATTENDING DR. _____	ATTENDING DR. _____
SPECIMEN TYPE_____	SPECIMEN TYPE_____

TEST(S) REQUESTED: _____

PROBLEM

DATE _____ TIME _____ REPORTED BY _____ SUPERVISOR REVIEW _____

☐ INVASIVE ☐ NONINVASIVE (STATE EXCEPTION IN COMMENT AREA.)

☐ NO LABEL ☐ LABEL AND REQUISITION NOT MATCHED

☐ INCOMPLETE INFORMATION ☐ (SUSPECTED) MISDRAW OR MISIDENTIFICATION

COMMENTS: _____
_____
_____
_____
_____
_____

(Continue on separate sheet.)

UNRESOLVED (NOT PROCESSED)

UNIT NOTIFIED:_____ NAME: _____
_____
STAFF DECLINED RESPONSIBILITY (NAME) _____

RELEASE

THIS SPECIMEN WAS OBTAINED FROM:

NAME: _____

MEDICAL RECORD NO. ⬚⬚⬚⬚⬚⬚⬚⬚⬚⬚

LAB USE ONLY	I AM ASSUMING FULL RESPONSIBILITY FOR PROPER IDENTIFICATION OF THIS SPECIMEN
	DATE _____ TIME _____
	_____
	PRINT FULL NAME/TITLE
	_____
	(SIGNATURE)

WHITE—QA COMMITTEE   YELLOW—LABORATORY   PINK—STAFF

Figure 7-3 _____

Laboratory release form. (Courtesy Ohio State University Hospitals.)

quire special media, a different incubation environment, or a longer incubation time. Additionally, knowing that the patient has osteomyelitis or pyelonephritis may affect the extent to which an organism is characterized and may suggest a need for susceptibility testing. Knowledge of a patient's antibiotic therapy is useful for correlation of test results.

Test requested

Every test requested should have a written order on the patient's chart. Most laboratories require a separate requisition for each test requested. Test requisitioning may also be electronically ordered from terminals at remote sites, such as nursing stations. Computer screens are usually formatted to require all information necessary to complete the ordering of a specific test or tests. A properly completed requisition is an important part of specimen collection.

Unacceptable Specimens

The information on the requisition must match the information on the specimen label. If names or sources do not match, the specimen should be collected again. The laboratory should not assume responsibility or liability for questionable information.

Perhaps the best approach to this issue is to divide specimens into two groups, invasive and noninvasive. A **noninvasive specimen,** such as urine, sputum, stool, and wounds, must always be recollected if it is received unlabeled or misidentified in any way. An **invasive specimen,** such as blood culture, sterile body fluid, amniotic fluid, or operating room specimen, may be processed if the person responsible for the error comes to the laboratory and signs a laboratory release form (Figure 7-3). This assigns all responsibility and liability to the person signing the form. The responsibility of the individual may be emphasized by giving him or her a copy of the signed release form.

All rejected specimens require a documented phone call to the collection site to expedite recollection of a specimen. This should be followed by written documentation to verify receipt of the specimen in the laboratory and the reason for its rejection.

Other suboptimal specimens that must be rejected are as follows:

- Leaking specimens
- Syringes with needles attached
- Stools contaminated with urine or barium
- Anaerobes on inappropriate sources
- Unpreserved specimens more than 2 hours old
- Refrigerated blood cultures
- Dried-up specimens
- Specimens in formalin

Processing a suboptimal specimen always yields suboptimal results.

PROCESSING OF CLINICAL SAMPLES FOR OPTIMAL ORGANISM RECOVERY

Prioritization During Processing

All specimens require prompt processing after arrival in the laboratory. Processing every specimen as soon as it is received is often impossible. Laboratory staffing and specimen load may have a significant impact on timely processing. The laboratory must set guidelines for prioritizing specimens on the basis of a number of variables. A four-level scheme of prioritization may be used. The first level requires immediate attention, whereas processing of fourth-level specimens may be delayed. Table 7-2 lists clinical samples and the ways each can be prioritized in a four-level system.

TABLE 7-2
Levels of Specimen Prioritization

Level	Description	Specimens
1	Critical/invasive	Cerebrospinal fluid Brain Blood Heart valves Pericardial fluid Amniotic fluid Bronchoalveolar lavage Vitreous/aqueous fluids
2	Unpreserved May degrade or overgrow	Sputum Tissue Stool Body fluids not listed for level 1 Drainage from wounds Pus Bone
3	Accuracy of quantitation affected	Urine Quantitative tissue Catheter tip
4	Protected/preserved	Swabs in holding medium (aerobic and anaerobic)

Level 1 specimens should be classified as "critical" because of their invasive nature or the severity of disease. They require immediate processing.

Level 2 specimens are unprotected and may quickly degrade or have rapid overgrowth of contaminating flora, changing the nature of such a specimen. Laboratory personnel must quickly provide an optimal growth environment for the fastidious organisms that may be found in these specimens.

Level 3 specimens require quantitation. Urine, catheter tips, and quantitative tissue biopsy specimens are level 3. Delay in processing level 3 specimens may adversely affect the accuracy of quantitation.

If processing of level 2 and level 3 specimens is postponed, some type of protection or preservation must be initiated. This may mean refrigerating urine specimens or placing blood culture bottles in the incubator until a spinal fluid specimen is processed. Placing a small undercounter refrigerator at the site of specimen processing is convenient for the laboratory worker and makes it more likely that urine specimens will be refrigerated during peak workload times.

Level 4 specimens are all other protected specimens arriving in the laboratory in holding media. Processing of level 4 specimens may be delayed to process higher-level specimens.

All specimens must be processed in a timely manner. Batch processing should be avoided when possible.

Gross Examination of Specimens

Observing and documenting the gross appearance of a specimen may provide useful information to both the microbiologist and the physician. The physical characteristics of the specimen must be documented in the written report. Relevant questions to answer include the following:

- Was it a swab or an aspirate?
- Was the stool formed or liquid?
- Was the specimen bloody?
- What was the volume?
- Was the fluid clear or cloudy?

Observations should also be made to determine the adequacy of the specimen:

- Is there evidence of improper collection or transport?

- Is the container leakproof and sterile?
- Does the transport medium cover the swab or is the swab dry?
- Is there enough specimen to perform all tests requested?
- Is the fluid clotted?
- Is there evidence of barium in the stool?

Gross appearance may determine the need for special processing.

- Should anaerobe cultures be performed owing to purulence, foul smell, gas, or sulfur granules in the specimen?
- Are worms or proglottids present in the specimen?

Direct Examination Techniques

Direct examination, regardless of the stain used, may be utilized to (1) determine the quality of the specimen, (2) aid in diagnosis of infectious disease, (3) guide routine culture interpretation, and (4) dictate the need for nonroutine processing.

Lack of material for direct examination makes all these goals impossible or extremely difficult to achieve. Because the direct smear should be used as a guide to routine culture evaluation and interpretation whenever possible, the culture plates should not be viewed until the direct smear has been evaluated. Direct microscopic examination is a requirement in critical situations, such as meningitis, to guide therapy choices when therapy must be initiated before culture results are available.

Smear preparation

Specimens may be received in many forms. Preparation of the direct smear depends on the type of material received. Techniques vary according to whether the specimen is a tissue, swab, or fluid.

TISSUES
See Chapter 8 for a detailed explanation of the preparation of tissue specimens.

SWABS
If swabs are submitted, the swab must be carefully rolled back and forth across a dry, clean slide.

ASPIRATES AND BODY FLUIDS
When the specimen is an aspirate or a body fluid, at least four techniques are available for smear

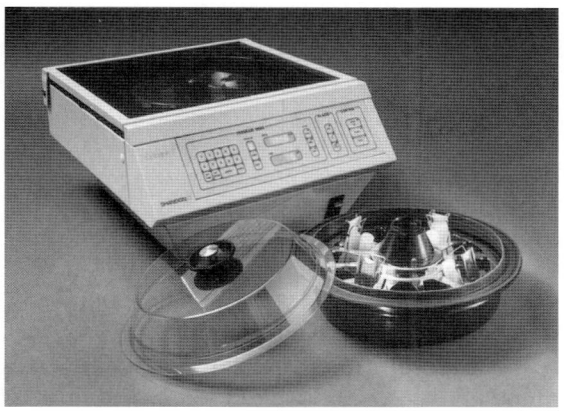

Figure 7-4

Cytospin 2. (Courtesy Shandon, Inc., Pittsburgh, Pa.)

preparation: single drop, centrifuged sediment, layered, and cytocentrifuged (alone or with additives).
Single-drop smear A sterile pipette may be used to place a single drop of fluid on a slide. This technique is useful if high numbers of organisms are likely or the specimen is thick. Care must be taken to keep the smear thin enough to read.
Centrifuged sediment smear Fluids in which small numbers of organisms may be present may be centrifuged at 1500 g for 15 minutes, and the sediment used to prepare the slide.
Layered smear Low-volume fluids such as CSF may not provide a sediment. An alternative technique is to use the majority of the fluid by layering it onto a slide. A drop of fluid may be placed on a slide and allowed to dry and another drop added on top of it, producing a layered smear. Care should be taken not to spread the drops too diffusely. This technique is advantageous for CSF smears for mycobacteria.
Cytocentrifuged smear An alternative to spinning the entire specimen is **cytocentrifugation.** Cytocentrifugation—with devices such as the Cytospin 2 (Shandon Inc, Pittsburgh, Pa; Figure 7-4) or the Aerospray Gram Slide Stainer/Cytocentrifuge (Wescor, Inc, Logan, Utah)—is a technique used to concentrate a small amount of body fluid (0.1-0.5 mL) directly onto a circular area of a microscopic slide. This technique concentrates both cellular material and organisms in a monolayer and provides a small area to scan. The blotter used with the device absorbs the excess fluid not centrifuged onto the slide. This technique may be used for many types of body fluids, including bron-

choalveolar lavage. Up to 12 slides may be spun at once, and different stains may be applied and examined. Some researchers have noted that the cytocentrifuge slide preparation may increase sensitivity of the CSF Gram stain up to 2 logs over conventional concentrated smears. This significant increase in sensitivity enhances visualization of the small numbers of organisms sometimes found in CSF.

Bacterial and cellular morphology is superior in cytocentrifuge preparations. In our experience, the cytocentrifuge preparation has been useful for all body fluids and has proved to be more sensitive than smears made from concentrated fluids. Given the superiority of cytocentrifuge smears, a cytocentrifuge is a worthwhile piece of equipment for all microbiology laboratories. Figure 7-5 shows a direct smear of a CSF prepared by cytocentrifugation and by the single drop method. The cytocentrifuge smear shows a concentration of both cells and organisms with clearing of the background material.

Additives Other substances may be added to the body fluid. Sterile albumin may be added to clear CSF to help minimal cellular material adhere to the slide. When the cytocentrifuge procedure is utilized for extremely mucoid bronchoalveolar lavage specimens, dithiothreitol solution (Sputolysin Test, Behring Diagnostics Inc, Somerville, N.J.) may be

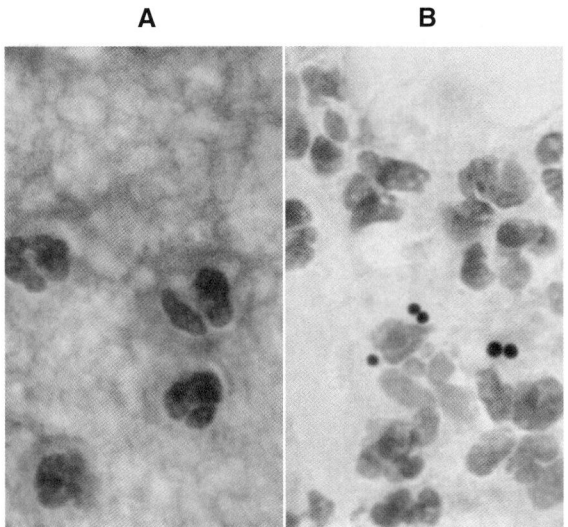

Figure 7-5

Comparison of single-drop smear and cytocentrifuged smear. **A,** Single-drop smear. **B,** Cytocentrifuged smear.

added as a mucolytic agent before the specimen is placed in the cytocentrifuge funnel.

When direct smear is not useful

Direct examination is not appropriate or useful for some types of specimens. A Gram-stained smear from a throat swab or nasopharyngeal swab cannot differentiate pathogenic from nonpathogenic streptococci. Many laboratories do not perform direct smears from urine specimens because culture results are available within 24 hours. Unless the urine smear is specified as a "stat" procedure, its results may not be available before the culture results. A direct urine smear may provide useful information only if it is made and read immediately after collection. Its ability to detect organisms is in the range of 10^5 organisms per mL. If one organism is seen on smear, it represents 100,000 organisms per mL. Urine smears should be made using a loopful of unspun urine. Direct examination techniques are included in Table 7-3.

Primary Inoculation of Routine Specimens

Selection of primary culture media for routine specimens

Selection of aerobic primary media is somewhat standardized for the routine bacterial culture. Individual laboratories may favor one medium over another, however, on the basis of past experience,

patient population considerations, or other special circumstances. Several basic goals must be met in selecting routine media regardless of the specific choice.

TYPES OF CULTURE MEDIA

To meet these goals, an understanding of medium types is needed. Culture media may be divided into categories defined by ability to support bacterial growth. These categories are as follows:

Nonselective media This type, **nonselective media,** support the growth of most nonfastidious microbes, usually in agar plate form. Sheep blood agar is the standard nonselective medium used in the United States.

Selective media This type, **selective media,** support the growth of one type of microbe over another. A selective medium may contain inhibitory substances to prevent the growth of some microbes. Such media may be created by adding antibiotics or other inhibitory chemicals to nonselective media. MacConkey agar is selective for enteric gram-negative bacilli, and CNA (Columbia agar with colistin and nalidixic acid) is selective for gram-positive organisms.

Differential media This type, **differential media,** allow grouping of microbes on the basis of different characteristics displayed on the medium. Media may be differential and nonselective; for ex-

---

TABLE 7-3

Initial Processing Techniques for Bacterial Specimens

Specimen Type	Cytocentrifuge Smear	Routine Smear	Liquefaction	Filtration	Inoculum Counter-Streak
Amniotic fluid	✓				
CSF	✓				✓
Synovial fluid	✓				
Other body fluids	✓			If >10 ml	If <10 ml
Bronchial lavage	✓				
Bile		✓			
Bone marrow		✓			
CAPD	✓			If >10 ml	If <10 ml
Peritoneal/ascitic	✓				
Pericardial fluid	✓				If <10 ml
Lesion/wound/abscess on swabs		✓	Vortex		
Organ/tissue/biopsy		Touch prep/imprint	"Stomach"		
Aspirate/drainage		✓			
Bone		✓	Grind		
Urine					
Organ perfusate	✓			If >10 ml	If <10 ml
Medical device soak solution				If >10 ml	If <10 ml

CSF, Cerebrospinal fluid; *CAPD,* continuous ambulatory peritoneal dialysis.

ample, sheep blood agar can differentiate organisms on the basis of hemolysis. Media may be differential and selective; for example, MacConkey agar differentiates gram-negative bacilli on the basis of lactose fermentation.

Enriched media In **enriched media,** growth enhancers have been added to nonselective agar to allow fastidious organisms to flourish. Chocolate agar is an enriched medium.

Enrichment broth Enrichment broth is designed to encourage the growth of small numbers of a particular organism while suppressing other flora present. LIM broth is an enrichment broth used to enhance the growth of group B streptococci.

Broth media Broth media may enhance small numbers of most aerobes, anaerobes, and microaerophils and some fastidious organisms. Thioglycolate (THIO) broth is an example of a primary broth medium.

REQUIREMENTS FOR ROUTINE PRIMARY PLATING MEDIA
The routine primary plating media chosen for use in a laboratory should include the following items:

- A nonselective agar plate
- An enriched medium for fastidious organisms, if the source is a normally sterile body fluid or a site in which fastidious organisms are expected
- A selective and differential medium for enteric gram-negative bacilli for most routine bacterial cultures
- A selective plate for gram-positive organisms for specimens from anatomic sites in which mixed gram-positive and gram-negative organisms are suspected
- Additional selective media for specific pathogens as needed (body site specimens from which pathogenic *Neisseria* may be isolated require a selective *Neisseria* plate).
- A broth medium (Some laboratories have chosen to eliminate broth media in routine processing. Other laboratories include a thioglycolate broth when plating specimens of body fluids, tissues, lesions, wounds, and abscesses. A broth should be considered at least for plating normally sterile body fluids or specimens from blood- or brain-related sites.)
- A potato dextrose agar plate for yeast isolation

Table 7-4 lists selection of primary media for specific anatomic sites. Equivalent media may be substituted.

Selection of temperature and environmental conditions

Once the medium is selected, temperature and environmental conditions must also be considered.

- Environmental conditions are chosen according to the growth requirements of the **indigenous flora** or pathogen(s) suspected for the body site from which the specimen is taken.
- Fastidious organisms may require increased CO_2 or an anaerobic environment for growth.
- Most routine bacterial culture plates are incubated at 35° to 37° C for 48 hours.
- Broth cultures, when included, are routinely held 5 to 7 days.

Primary isolation media for unusual and fastidious bacteria

Temperature requirements and length of incubation vary for individual organisms. Unusual organisms may require special processing and selection of a medium beyond the routine. It is helpful if the clinician indicates to the laboratory that an unusual organism is suspected. Table 7-5 lists a variety of unusual or fastidious organisms, recommended media, and incubation requirements.

Initial processing techniques for primary inoculation

LIQUEFACTION OF SPECIMENS
As previously stated, most specimens arrive in the laboratory in one of three forms: swab, tissue, or liquid (fluid). The objective of the laboratory should be to convert all specimens for culture to a liquid form (liquefy) without significant dilution of the organisms. Liquefaction permits equal distribution of organisms onto each medium inoculated. To accomplish this task, swabs are placed in 0.5 to 1.0 mL of broth, then vortexed to produce an even suspension of organisms. A sterile pipette is used to dispense inoculum onto plates and into broth. A separate swab is used to make the smear. Tissues are ground in tissue grinders or "stomached" in a Stomacher Lab Blender (Seward Medical, Ltd, Tekmar, Cincinnati, Ohio) in small amounts of broth.

TABLE 7-4

Selection of Primary Culture Media for Routine Specimens

Specimen Type	Gram Stain	BAP	Choc CO$_2$	MAC	PD	CNA	THIO Broth	TM (CO$_2$)	Special Medium Comments
Body fluids	✓	✓	✓	✓	✓		✓		
Amniotic fluid	✓	✓	✓	✓	✓		✓	✓	
CSF	✓	✓	✓		✓		✓		
Synovial fluid	✓	✓	✓	✓	✓		✓	✓	
Bile	✓	✓	✓	✓	✓				
Bone marrow	✓	✓	✓	✓	✓		✓		
CAPD									
<10 ml	✓	✓	✓	✓	✓		✓		
>10 ml	✓		Filter				✓		
Peritoneal/ascitic	✓	✓	✓	✓	✓		✓		
Pericardial	✓	✓	✓	✓	✓		✓		
General sources									
Bone	✓	✓	✓	✓	✓		✓		
Lesion/wound/abscess	✓	✓	✓	✓	✓	✓	✓		
Wound aspirate	✓	✓	✓	✓	✓	✓	✓		
Tissue/biopsy	✓	✓	✓	✓	✓		✓		
Eye/ocular	✓	✓	✓		✓		✓		Bedside inoculation Infants: add TM (CO$_2$)
Aqueous/vitreous	✓	✓	✓		✓		✓		
Urogenital									
Urine									
Catheter/void		✓		✓		✓			Clear: BAP only Cloudy: CNA MAC
Upper tract	✓	✓	✓	✓	✓	✓	✓		
Genital: male or female	✓	✓	✓	✓	✓	✓		✓	
Placenta	✓	✓	✓	✓	✓		✓	✓	
IUD	✓								
Urogenital screens									
Neisseria			✓					✓	
Group B beta hemolytic streptococci		✓							LIM
Yeast					✓				
Gardnerella						✓			HBT
Gastrointestinal									
Feces	✓							CT 4° Optional	CIN (25° C), HE, SMAC CBA or 0.45-μm filter on BAP (42° C, 10% CO$_2$)
Duodenal aspirate	✓	✓	✓	✓	✓	✓			
Gastric aspirate (infant)	✓	✓	✓	✓	✓		✓		
Respiratory sources									
Throat		✓	✓						
Nasopharyngeal/nasal		✓	✓						
Sputum	✓	✓	✓	✓					
Bronchial lavage	✓	✓	✓	✓	✓				
Bronchial brush	✓	✓	✓	✓	✓		✓		
Sinus aspirate	✓	✓	✓	✓	✓	✓	✓		
Pleural fluid	✓	✓	✓	✓	✓		✓		
Lung tissue	✓	✓	✓	✓	✓		✓		
Respiratory screens									
Group A beta hemolytic streptococci		✓							
Staphylococcus aureus		✓							MS or MS + oxac
Neisseria			✓					✓	
Yeast				✓					

BAP, Sheep blood agar; *CBA, Campylobacter* blood agar; *Choc,* chocolate agar; *CIN,* cefsulodin-irgasor-novobiocin agar; *CNA,* Columbia colistin–nalidixic acid agar; *CT, Campylobacter* THIO broth; *HBT,* human blood bilayer medium; *HE,* Hektoen-enteric medium; *IUD,* intrauterine device; *MS,* mannitol salt agar; *MS + oxac,* mannitol salt agar with oxacillin; *PD,* potato dextrose agar with antibiotics; *LIM,* Todd Hewitt (Broth) C̄ CNA special broth medium; *SMAC,* sorbitol-MacConkey agar; *THIO,* thioglycolate; *TM,* Thayer-Martin or other *Neisseria*-selective agar; *MAC,* MacConkey; *CSF,* cerebrospinal fluid; *CAPD,* continuous ambulatory peritoneal dialysis.

TABLE 7-5

Unusual and Fastidious Bacteria: Primary Isolation Media

Organism	Recommended Isolation Media*	Special Considerations	Specimen Selection
Anaerobes	Anaerobic blood agar supplemented with vitamin K and hemin (Schaedler, CDC anaerobic blood agar)	Prereduce all anaerobic media and hold 6-7 days Nonselective	Aspirate Tissues Sterile body fluids
	Kanamycin/vancomycin laked blood agar (KV laked blood)	Selective for *Bacteroides*	
	Phenylethyl alcohol sheep blood agar (PEA), anaerobic	Inhibits facultative gram-negative rods and inhibits *Proteus* swarming	
	Bacteroides bile esculin agar (BBE)	Optional; presumptive identification of *Bacteroides fragilis* group	
	Thioglycolate broth with vitamin K and hemin	Recommended for body fluids and tissues only	
Actinomyces	See Anaerobic media selection (above)	Hold broth 3 weeks	Direct smear diagnosis for IUDs
Bordetella pertussis	Bordet-Gengou Charcoal–horse blood agar (Regan-Lowe)	Bedside inoculation; incubate at high humidity and 35° C in air for 6-7 days; CO_2 not recommended Direct fluorescent antibody test—supplement to culture	Use calcium alginate swabs; collect 2 nasopharyngeal swabs Bronchial washing Throat, PCR-Option to culture
Brucella	Vented biphasic or broth blood culture bottles for blood and body fluids (Castenada)	Potentially dangerous pathogen; process all cultures in biohazard hood with gloves and protective clothing Hold blood bottles 30 days at 35°-37° C in CO_2 and subculture every 4-5 days Hold 10 days at 35°-37° C in 10% CO_2	Bone marrow Blood
	Modified Thayer-Martin or 5% sheep blood agar, *Brucella* agar with 5% serum	Use in potentially contaminated specimens	Abscesses/tissues
Clostridium botulinum	Anaerobic media (see above)	Reference lab test Toxin assay for diagnosis	Feces Serum, feces
Corynebacterium diphtheriae	Nonselective 5% sheep blood agar	Not fastidious 35° C in air	Throat Nasopharyngeal Skin
	Loeffler serum slant Potassium tellurite medium	Rabbit serum enhances growth Need toxigenicity testing to confirm a diagnosis	
	Tinsdale or cysteine-tellurite blood agar	Supports growth of only some strains	
Francisella	Commercial chocolate agar Modified yeast extract agar	Potentially dangerous pathogen; highly infectious by aerosol or penetration of unbroken skin; process all cultures in biohazard hood with gloves and protective clothing Increased CO_2 required; 3-5 days required for visible growth	Lymph node aspirate Sputum Throat Bronchial washing Ulcer biopsy (advancing edge of lesion)
Haemophilus ducreyi (chancroid)	Fresh commercial chocolate agar Addition of vancomycin in contaminated cultures	35° C, 3%-5% CO_2 with high humidity; hold for 5 days	Genital lesion
Helicobacter pylori	Skirrow Chocolate agar	Hold 5 days Increased CO_2 and humidity Geimsa/Gram stain Direct smear may be used diagnostically	Gastric aspirate/biopsy

*Representative media listed—equivalent media may be substituted. *BCYE*, Buffered charcoal yeast extract agar; *BHI*, brain-heart infusion agar; *SPS*, sodium polyanethol sulfonate.

Continued

TABLE 7-5

Unusual and Fastidious Bacteria: Primary Isolation Media—cont'd

Organism	Recommended Isolation Media*	Special Considerations	Specimen Selection
Nocardia	Grows well on routine media 5% sheep blood agar, BHI Grows well on BCYE	Hold for 5-7 days in 3%-5% CO_2	Blood—specimen of choice
Streptobacillus moniliformis (rat bite fever)	Serum-supplemented media (rabbit, calf, or horse serum)	Fastidious microaerophilic Practical laboratory tests not available Reference lab test inhibited by SPS High humidity at 35°-37° C in 10% CO_2 Citrate used as anticoagulant	Joint fluid Abscess fluid Lymph node
Vibrio	TCBS (thiosulfate-citrate-bile-sucrose agar) Grows well on routine stool media	Selective and differential; not cost-effective to use as routine medium in many parts of the country	Stool Lesion

*Representative media listed—equivalent media may be substituted.

The broth-tissue suspension is then processed (Figure 7-6). It is important to remember, however, that the direct smear must be made from the original material before liquefaction.

Other specimens, such as normally sterile body fluids, pus, urine, and even sputum, are inoculated directly onto selected media. Extremely tenacious or mucoid specimens may be digested with substances such as Sputolysin before media inoculation. Methods used to increase the recovery of organisms from body fluids include inoculum counter-streak technique and filtration.

INOCULUM COUNTER-STREAK TECHNIQUE

The **inoculum counter-streak technique** is used when the numbers of organisms are expected to be low but the volume of specimen received is not adequate for filtration (Figure 7-7). The technique uses a larger volume of inoculum than conventional processing, thereby increasing the sensitivity of

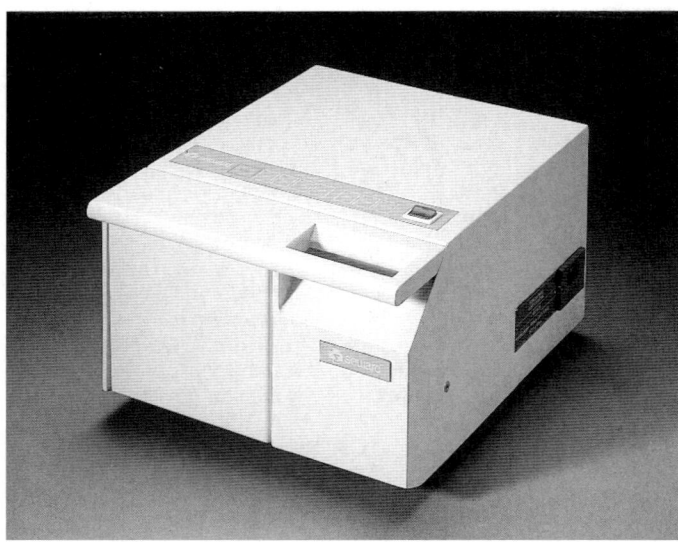

Figure 7-6

Stomacher lab blender. (Courtesy Seward Medical, Ltd., Tekmar, Cincinnati.)

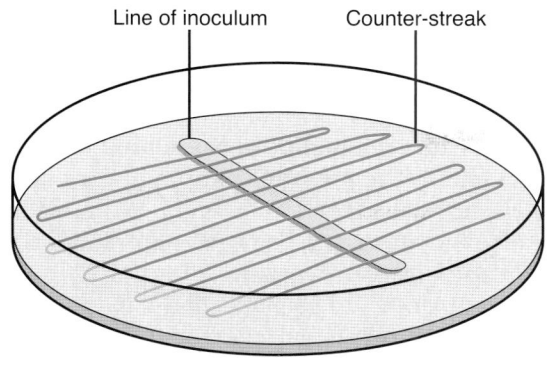

Figure 7-7

Inoculum counter-streak technique.

isolation. If the entire specimen is used, any existing organisms should be recovered. A sterile pipette is used to inoculate the plate from edge to edge across its center. A loop is then used to counter-streak the plate perpendicular to the inoculum line.

The number and type of plate media inoculated may be modified, depending on the volume of fluid received. The objective is to use a large volume of specimen. This technique is a good choice for processing spinal fluids because a CSF specimen could be plated to one plate or to three plates depending on the volume received. If there is only enough specimen for one plate, chocolate agar should be inoculated. Media priority should be established ahead of time.

FILTRATION

Some body fluids and sterility cultures require concentration by filtration when large quantities are received. When the specimen consistency is thin enough to avoid filter clogging, filtration with a Nalgene filter unit is recommended (Procedure 7-1).

Filtration is an excellent technique for processing continuous ambulatory peritoneal dialysis (CAPD) fluids because of the ability to easily obtain a large volume of specimen and the likelihood that the specimen will have low numbers of organisms.

For attempting to recover *Campylobacter* from stool specimens, a filtration technique is both cost-effective and efficient. Liquefied stool is passed through a 0.45-μm membrane filter (HT-450 filter; Gelman Sciences, Ann Arbor, Mich.). The filter is placed on a blood agar plate at 42° C in 10% CO_2. After 30 minutes the filter is removed, and the blood agar plate is returned to the microaerophilic environment, permitting *Campylobacter* to grow luxuriantly.

Processing Nonroutine Specimens

Routine specimens have standardized processing procedures already established in the microbiology laboratory. Examples are urine, stool, sputum, and wound specimens.

In contrast, **nonroutine specimens** may be processed often by the laboratory but have no standardized, established processing procedure. They include vein grafts (both real and artificial),

---

PROCEDURE 7-1. Nalgene Filtering Procedure

Processing should take place in a biohazard hood.

1. Attach a Nalgene filter unit to the Nalgene hand vacuum pump. Attach one end of the tubing to the vacuum pump and the other end to the container to be evacuated.

2. Remove the lid and fill the container with the fluid to be filtered.

3. Manually pump the hand vacuum until all fluid has passed through the filter. Air is exhausted at the rate of 15 mL per stroke for the smaller pump and 36 mL per stroke for the larger pump.

4. Remove the filter according to the manufacturer's instructions, and place it on the surface of an agar plate. Chocolate agar is recommended.

If a fluid is extremely cloudy, filter clogging may be a problem. If the filter does clog, a set of agar plates should be inoculated using the inoculum counter-streak technique.

multiple-lumen catheters, heart valves, implant soak solutions, perfusates, water samples, and equipment suspected of playing a role in **nosocomial infection.** As technology advances, laboratories are receiving many more requests to culture new specimen types that have no established culture procedure. Hospitals with transplant programs may find it necessary to culture food before consumption by immunosuppressed patients. Even when standardized procedures do not exist, a standardized thought process can be implemented to ensure that even the strangest specimen is appropriately cultured. This process begins by asking the series of questions listed below.

- **Is the specimen likely to contain low numbers or high numbers of organisms?** If there are low numbers of organisms, concentration of the specimen is advantageous. When few organisms are anticipated, large amounts of specimen yield better results.
- **If the number of organisms is extremely low, is it important to enhance them?** Some specimens, such as perfusates, are being checked for sterility. In this case, the presence of even one organism is significant. Other specimens, such as foods, may have a tolerance limit of a given number or kinds of bacteria; they must be processed using a quantitative or semiquantitative procedure so that colony counts may be determined. Use of a broth is important when growth must be enhanced, but it can confuse results for specimens requiring colony counts.
- **Does the specimen contain any preservatives or growth inhibitors that must be counteracted?** Sometimes, the effects of a preservative can be eliminated or reduced by dilution or use of a specific medium, such as standard method agar or D/E neutralizing broth.
- **What is a reasonable amount to culture? Are all areas of the specimen homogeneous, or will the portion chosen for culture affect the results?** A 12-cm piece of vein received for culture may contain plaque on only a relatively small portion. Sampling one spot may not be representative of the whole. In that case, sampling and grinding small pieces from multiple sites along the 12-cm piece is necessary.
- **Are the organisms to be found in a specific specimen likely to be fastidious or nonfastidious?** The choice of medium, temperature(s), environment, and length of incubation depends on whether the organisms are fastidious or nonfastidious.
- **Is there any normal flora associated with the specimen?** The presence of normal flora might make special collection techniques important. It also dictates rapid or protected transportation and timely processing.
- **Is the objective to select a single agent from a mixed culture?** An enriched or selective medium is helpful for this type of isolation. If an outbreak of methicillin-resistant staphylococci occurs, for example, wherein equipment or personnel specimens are being cultured, an appropriate amount of methicillin may be placed in the screening medium to eliminate methicillin-sensitive staphylococci.
- **Is there a need to culture both external and internal surfaces?** The surface to be cultured becomes important in devising beneficial methods of culturing catheters and other inanimate objects.

Types of nonroutine specimens

IMPLANT SOAK SOLUTION AND PERFUSATES
Before implantation, valves, corneas, organs, and other medical devices are maintained in soak solutions. At present, no standardized procedure for culturing a soak solution exists. If contamination is present, it is probably at an extremely low level. A large volume of soak solution and some form of concentration of the soak is required because even one organism in this setting may be important. A broth with heavy inoculation, a cytocentrifuge smear, and a large volume of filtered specimen placed on a chocolate agar plate should provide adequate opportunity for low numbers of organisms to grow. The Nalgene filtering procedure previously described works well for this type of specimen. Perfusates are processed in the same manner as implant soak solutions.

WATER STERILITY SPECIMENS
A specimen of water from sources such as whirlpools, stills, and reagent water also requires concentration to provide adequate opportunity to detect microbes. The Millipore Sampler is one product designed for this purpose. The sampler is designed to use 18 mL of water to fill the sam-

ple case, but only 1 mL of water is actually absorbed (Procedure 7-2).

The National Committee for Clinical Laboratory Standards (NCCLS) Document C3-A2, Vol. 11, No. 13, entitled *Preparation and Testing of Reagent Water in the Clinical Laboratory* and approved in August 1991, outlines other options for water testing.

EQUIPMENT

Because of the lack of access to the contaminated site, contaminated equipment may be extremely difficult to culture. An attempt should be made to culture any reservoir where moisture might collect or proper cleaning might be difficult. If culturing dry surfaces is necessary, the use of a moistened swab may be beneficial. Cleansing and assembling techniques should be reviewed at the time of culturing. Single-use, disposable equipment is preferred when possible.

INTRAUTERINE DEVICES (IUDS)

Intrauterine devices are usually cultured for the purpose of identifying *Actinomyces.* A Gram stain of the material should adequately identify the presence of this organism. Cultures require lengthy incubation and manipulation when the information obtained from them is no more helpful in guiding patient management than the smear results.

VASCULAR CATHETER TIPS

Vascular catheter tips are submitted to the laboratory for culture to aid in diagnosis of catheter-related infections. Standardization of the procedure is important.

In 1977 Maki and colleagues determined that diagnosis of catheter site infection and catheter-related septicemia could be made on the basis of organism colony counts after rolling a 5- to 7-cm segment of the catheter across a blood agar plate. More than 15 colonies indicated site infection, whereas catheter-related septicemia correlated with more than 1000 colonies. Many laboratories elect to use this method because of its ease of use. It is far more valuable in predicting catheter-related infection than use of a broth culture. If a catheter containing even one colony is placed in a broth, it will yield a "positive" culture. Even the Maki method demonstrated that only 1.6% of positive catheter cultures accurately predicted septicemia, giving this method a very low positive predictive value.

In the 1980s and 1990s, newer methods were developed that increase the positive predictive value. They involve techniques that culture both the internal and external surfaces of the catheter. Sheretz and colleagues used a 3-minute sonication procedure to remove organisms from both the internal and external walls of the catheter. The catheter is placed in 10 mL of broth and sonicated in a water bath for 1 minute, centrifuged 15 seconds, and plated in two dilutions. For central venous and arterial catheters, sonication has been shown to be superior to the roll plate method of Maki and associates. However, many laboratories may hesitate to change to this technique because of the time, equipment, and manipulation involved.

Results of catheter tip culture can be adversely affected by delay in transport and processing, because the tip is an unprotected specimen. As the surface area dries, organisms may die, yielding inaccurate results. If the catheter tip is extremely long or transported with an excessive amount of

---

PROCEDURE 7-2. Procedure for Using a Millipore Sampler

1. Pour water into the sample case to the upper line (18 mL).

2. Insert paddle, close case tightly, and place case on a flat surface with grid side facing down.

3. Do not agitate, and do not exceed 30 seconds or medium might be lost through the membrane.

4. Remove paddle from case. Empty water.

5. Insert paddle back into case and incubate with grid side down.

blood on it, the colony count and its interpretation may be significantly affected. If care is not taken during their removal, catheters may become contaminated with multiple skin organisms, again adding to the interpretive confusion and the cost of processing a specimen. With these issues in mind, it may not be appropriate to identify and perform susceptibility testing on all organisms found in quantities greater than 15 colonies on a culture. Laboratories should set rules based on clinical relevance and cost-effectiveness for highly mixed cultures. Some laboratories no longer accept catheter tips for culture, whereas other laboratories set strict standards for submission of catheter tips.

Bibliography

Bobadilla M, Sifuentes J, Garcia-Tsao G: Improved method for bacteriological diagnosis of spontaneous bacterial peritonitis, *J Clin Microbiol* 27:2145, 1989.

Chapin-Robertson K, Dahlberg SE, Edberg SC: Clinical and laboratory analysis of cytospin-prepared Gram stains for recovery and diagnosis of bacteria from sterile body fluids, *J Clin Microbiol* 30:377, 1992.

Costello MJ et al: Guidelines for specimen collection, transportation, and test selection, *Lab Med* 24:19, 1993.

Department of Labor, Occupational Safety and Health Administration: Occupational exposure to bloodborne pathogens; proposed rule and notice of hearing, *Federal Register,* p 23041, May 30, 1989.

Doyle PW et al: Clinical and microbiological evaluation of four culture methods for the diagnosis of peritonitis in patients on continuous ambulatory peritoneal dialysis, *J Clin Microbiol* 27:1206, 1989.

Fody ED: *Clinical laboratory handbook for patient preparation and specimen handling,* Fascicle III, Northfield, Ill, 1985, College of American Pathologists.

Fuller D et al: Comparison of BACTEC Plus 26 and 27 media with and without fastidious organism supplement with conventional methods for culture of sterile body fluids, *J Clin Microbiol* 32:1488, 1994.

Gill VJ et al: Optimal use of the cytocentrifuge for recovery and diagnosis of *Pneumocystis carinii* in bronchoalveolar lavage and sputum specimen, *J Clin Microbiol* 26:1641, 1988.

Isenberg HD et al: *Cumitech 9: Collection and processing of bacteriological specimens,* Washington, DC, 1979, American Society for Microbiology.

Isenberg HD et al: *Manual of clinical microbiology,* ed 5, Washington, DC, 1991, American Society for Microbiology.

Maki DG, Weise CE, Sarafin HW: A semiquantitative culture method for identifying intravenous catheter–related infection, *N Engl J Med* 296:1305, 1977.

Males et al: Addi-Check filtration, Bactec, and 10-ml culture methods for recovery of microorganisms from dialysis effluent during episodes of peritonitis, *J Clin Microbiol* 23:350, 1986.

National Committee for Clinical Laboratory Standards: *Protection of laboratory workers from infectious disease transmitted by blood, body fluids, and tissue: tentative guideline* (NCCLS Document M29-T), Villanova, Penn, 1989, NCCLS.

Pezzlo M: *Clinical microbiology procedures handbook,* Washington, DC, 1992, American Society for Microbiology.

Rosett W, Hodges GR: Antimicrobial activity of heparin, *J Clin Microbiol* 11:30, 1980.

Shanholtzer CJ, Schaper PJ, Peterson LR: Concentrated Gram stain smears prepared with a cytospin centrifuge, *J Clin Microbiol* 16:1052, 1982.

Sheretz RJ et al: Three-year experience with sonicated vascular catheter cultures in a clinical microbiology laboratory, *J Clin Microbiol* 28:76, 1990.

Weinstein MP: Clinical evaluation of a urine transport kit with lyophilized preservative for culture, urinalysis, and sediment microscopy, *Diagn Microbiol Infect Dis* 3:501, 1985.

Yeung C, May J, Hughes R: Infection rate for single-lumen versus triple-lumen subclavian catheters, *Infect Control Hosp Epidemiol* 9:154, 1988.

LEARNING ASSESSMENTS

1. Which sample is the least desirable for culture?
   a. Aspirate
   b. Tissue
   c. Swab

2. Which specimen is most difficult to protect or preserve?
   a. Blood culture
   b. Sputum culture
   c. Urine culture

3. Which of the following methods should be used to protect a blood culture?
   a. Refrigeration
   b. Incubation
   c. Storage at room temperature

4. Which of the following methods should be used to protect a urine culture?
   a. Refrigeration
   b. Incubation
   c. Storage at room temperature

5. Which of the following items are reasons to reject a specimen for culture?
   a. Specimen preserved in formalin
   b. Specimen collected after the administration of antibiotics
   c. Specimen dried up
   d. Duplicate culture within the same week
   e. Syringe with needle attached
   f. All of the above

Continued

LEARNING ASSESSMENTS—cont'd

6. Which of the following items apply to the technique of cytocentrifugation?
   a. Is the most inexpensive way to prepare a smear
   b. Requires a very large sample size
   c. Provides a small but concentrated area to scan
   d. Offers increased sensitivity over conventional smears
   e. Can detect only 10^5 organisms or more
   f. All of the above

7. MacConkey's agar is an example of which of the following?
   a. Nonselective media
   b. Selective media
   c. Differential media
   d. Enriched media

8. Sheep blood agar is an example of which of the following?
   a. Nonselective media
   b. Selective media
   c. Differential media
   d. Enriched media

9. In which of the following instances would the inoculum counter-streak method be most advantageous?
   a. The specimen is cloudy and of high volume
   b. The specimen is of a low volume and likely to have few organisms
   c. The objective is to select a single agent from a mixed culture

CHAPTER 8

Microscopic Examination of Infected Materials

Leona W. Ayers

PREPARATION OF SAMPLES
  Smears from Swabs
  Smears from Thick Liquids or Semisolids
  Smears from Thick, Granular, or Mucoid Materials
  Smears from Thin Fluids
  Cytocentrifuge Preparations
    Cytocentrifuge technique

STAINS

MICROSCOPES

TERMINOLOGY FOR DIRECT EXAMINATIONS

EXAMINATION OF PREPARED MATERIAL
  Characterization of Background Materials
  Search for Microorganisms
  Evaluation of Choice of Antibiotic
  Direct Examination Summary
  Initiation of Special Handling for Unsuspected
    or Special Pathogens

GRADING OR CLASSIFYING MATERIALS
  Contaminating Materials
    Criteria
    Gram smear report
    Culture identification guidelines
    Antibiotic susceptibility testing
  Local Materials
    Criteria
    Gram smear report
    Culture identification guidelines
    Antibiotic susceptibilty testing
  Purulence
    Criteria
    Gram smear report
    Culture identification guidelines
    Antibiotic susceptibilty testing

Mixed Materials
  Criteria
  Gram smear report
  Culture identification guidelines
  Antibiotic susceptibility testing

REPORTS OF DIRECT EXAMINATIONS

EXAMPLES OF SAMPLE OBSERVATIONS
  AND REPORTS

QUALITY CONTROL IN DIRECT MICROSCOPIC
  INTERPRETATIONS

DIRECT EXAMINATION SHOWING LOCAL
  AND CONTAMINATING MATERIALS

DIRECT EXAMINATION IN COMMON BACTERIAL
  INFECTIONS

DIRECTION EXAMINATION IN GRAM-POSITIVE
  BACILLARY INFECTIONS

DIRECT EXAMINATION IN UNCOMMON
  GRAM-POSITIVE BACILLI

DIRECT EXAMINATION IN GRAM-POSITIVE
  BACILLI WITH FILAMENTS AND BRANCHES

DIRECT EXAMINATION IN SELECTED GRAM-
  NEGATIVE BACTERIAL INFECTIONS

DIRECT EXAMINATION IN SELECTED GRAM-
  NEGATIVE BACILLARY INFECTIONS

DIRECT EXAMINATION IN POLYMICROBIAL
  INFECTIONS

DIRECT EXAMINATION IN FUNGAL INFECTIONS

DIRECT EXAMINATION IN PARASITIC
  INFECTIONS

DIRECT EXAMINATION IN VIRAL INFECTIONS

OBJECTIVES

1. List the modifications in compound light microscopes that expand their use for direct examination of infected material.

2. Given a list of stains commonly used in the medical diagnostic laboratory, select the stain type for determining whether a microbe is a bacillus, fungus, mycobacterium, or viral inclusion.

3. Given a gram-stained direct smear of infected material, describe the local material, contaminating material, purulence, and associated microorganisms using the descriptive terminology presented.

4. List the common species associated with the following morphology:
   - Gram-negative bacilli, small, pleomorphic
   - Gram-positive cocci, groups
   - Gram-positive yeast and pseudohyphae
   - Hyphae, septate, branched 45-degree angle
   - Enlarged cell with intranuclear and cytoplasmic inclusions

5. Explain the application of quality control and quality improvement activities in the laboratory to the results of the direct microscopic examination and culture.

KEY TERMS

Purulence
Gram stain
Cytocentrifugation
Simple stains
Differential stains
Probe-mediated stains
Gram-positive bacteria
Gram-negative bacteria

Acid-fast bacilli
Colony-forming units (CFUs)
Monomicrobial
Polymicrobial
Amorphous debris
Curschmann's spiral
Microbial morphotypes

CASE STUDY

A 75-year-old male patient with history of COPD, heavy smoking, and alcohol abuse came to his physician with a fever, chills, and a productive cough. Sputum samples were collected and sent to the laboratory for direct smear and culture. Blood cultures also were drawn three times within 24 hours of admission to the hospital. The direct smear was gram stained, which is shown on Plate 9. The sputum culture produced a heavy growth of alpha-hemolytic colonies. Blood cultures yielded similar results after 24 hours of incubation.

Direct microscopy for visualization of microorganisms has been possible for just more than 200 years but was not a practical reality until Koch established the germ theory of disease in the 1880s. By 1880 a Scottish surgeon had published his direct observations of cluster-forming cocci in **purulence** from human disease. He named these cocci *Staphylococcus*. In 1884 Christian Gram developed the **Gram stain,** which today allows us to directly examine a pus specimen for the gram-positive cocci *Staphylococcus*. Differential staining and microscopy underpin the laboratory diagnosis of infectious diseases.

This underpinning in the diagnostic microbiology laboratory, as in the case study, is the ability to combine the rapid response of direct specimen examination with culture isolation and antibiotic susceptibility testing to achieve the following:

- Confirm that the material submitted for study is representative
- Identify the cellular components and debris of inflammation and thereby establish the probability of infection
- Identify specific infectious agents using direct visual detection supported by appropriate culture isolations and immune antibody techniques

TABLE 8-1
Preparing Infected Materials for Visual Examination

Preparation	Specimen or Organism Type
For gross examination	
Wet preparation	Parasites
	Materials >1 mm in size
For microscopic examination	
Wet preparation (direct or sedimented)	Fluids or semisolids
Cytocentrifuged (direct or presedimented)	Clear or slightly turbid fluids
Smear	Clear or slightly turbid fluids
1. Drop	Pus or fluid
	Tissue homogenate
	Swab rinse
2. Pellet	Blood culture
	Dilute specimen
3. Rolled	Swabbed material
4. Imprint (touch preparation)	Tissue

- Provide antibiotic susceptibilities of isolated pathogens to guide treatment
- Develop epidemiologic data

In more than 88% of instances, the physician has a correct idea about the diagnosis after taking a patient history and performing a physical examination. In the remaining instances, in which the diagnosis is not evident, assistance comes from laboratory or radiologic studies. With infectious diseases the physician has an idea of the likely etiology from the rate of symptom progression and is able to evaluate the extent of the infectious process. The physician is greatly pressured to begin immediate treatment of symptomatic patients. Specimens are collected and sent to the laboratory to confirm the physician's idea about the patient's illness. The ability of the laboratory to respond to the physician in a timely manner with useful results is key to keeping the treatment moving in the correct direction or changing treatment direction if the physician's presumptive diagnosis proves incorrect. The diagnostic microbiology laboratory has the opportunity to respond to the physician during the treatment decision-making or early in presumptive therapy. Direct visualization of pathogens becomes primary or direct evidence to confirm or refute the physician's initial clinical impression. If this impression is incorrect, reconsideration is facilitated, and additional studies can be undertaken as needed. Culture results usually are too late to alter presumptive therapy. At best, they confirm the correctness of the therapeutic choices already made and implemented.

PREPARATION OF SAMPLES

The preparation of samples for routine, brightfield microscopy has the objective to prepare material in a manner that facilitates adequate examination within a reasonable time. For smears, specimens should be examined grossly to determine the best approach (Table 8-1). Both thick, but not opaque, and thin (monolayer) smear areas should be produced by the smear process chosen.

Smears from Swabs

Smears should not be prepared from a swab after it has been used to inoculate culture media. Ideally, if the sample can be collected only on swabs, two swabs are submitted. Smears from swabs are prepared by rolling the swab back and forth over contiguous areas of the glass slide to deposit a thin layer of sample material (Figure 8-1). This preserves the morphology and relationships of the microorganisms and cellular elements. The swab should *never* be rubbed back and forth across the slide, because important material on the opposite side of the swab might not be deposited and smear elements could be broken up.

Smears from Thick Liquids or Semisolids

Swabs also can be used as the tool for preparation of smears from thick liquid or semisolid specimens such as feces (Figure 8-2). The swab is immersed in the specimen for several seconds and then used to prepare a thin spread of material on the glass slide for staining and viewing. This swab method

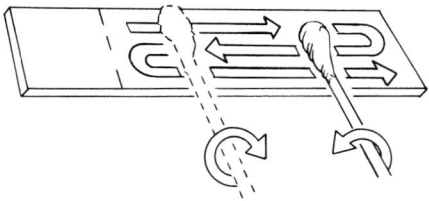

Figure 8-1
Smear preparation of a sample collected on a swab. The swab should be rolled back and forth across the slide to completely deposit the sample.

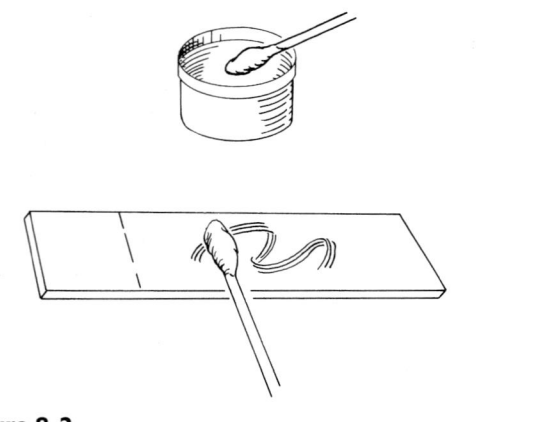

Figure 8-2

Smears from opaque thick liquids or semisolids, such as stool, can be made using a swab to sample and smear the material.

of preparation is adequate but may produce less desirable results than other methods.

Smears from Thick, Granular, or Mucoid Materials

Opaque material must be thinly spread so that a monolayer of material is deposited in some areas. It is most desirable to have both thick and thin areas. Granules within the material must be crushed so that their makeup can be assessed. A better presentation of granules is possible if granules or grains are "fished" from the surrounding materials and crushed on a separate slide using the technique shown in Figure 8-3. Granules that are too hard to crush between two glass slides probably do not represent infectious materials. More likely,

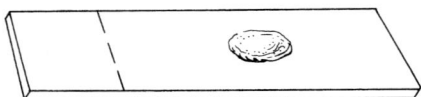

Drop or place the sample onto the surface of a labeled glass slide.

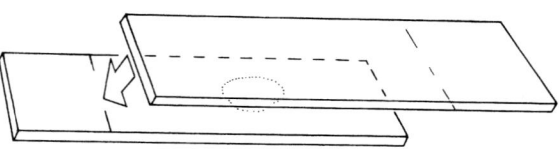

Place the second slide face down over the material.

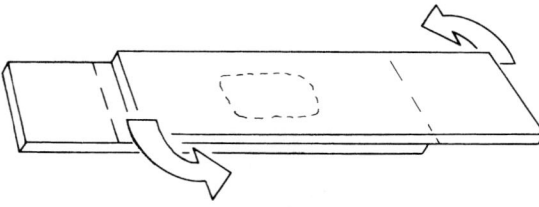

Press to flatten or crush the material, and rotate the two glass surfaces against each other.

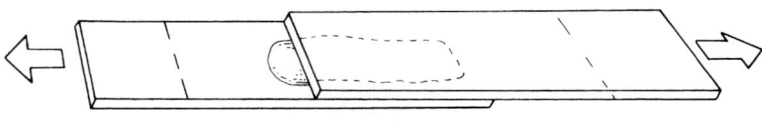

Pull to spread.

Figure 8-3

Preparation of smears from thick, granular, or mucoid samples.

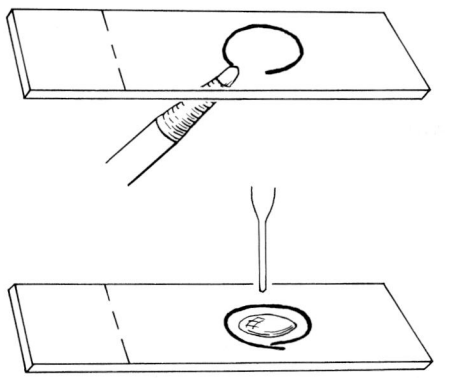

Figure 8-4

Smears from thin fluids can be prepared by placing a single drop of fluid or resuspended fluid sediment on a well-marked area of the slide.

they are small stones or foreign bodies. Examination using a dissecting microscope may help to characterize the nature of hard granules.

The following steps should be used to prepare a smear from thick, granular, or mucoid materials:

1. Place a portion of the sample on the labeled slide and press a second slide, with the label down, onto the sample to flatten or crush the components.
2. Rotate the two glass surfaces against each other so the shear forces break up the material.
3. Once the material is flattened and sufficiently thinned, pull the glass slides smoothly away from each other to produce two smears.
4. If the material is still too thick, repeat the first three steps with another (third) glass slide. The best smear or both smears can be retained for staining.

Slides of material from difficult sample sites, scant samples, or patients with critical illnesses should not be discarded until the culture evaluation is complete.

Smears from Thin Fluids

"Thin" specimens of fluids such as urine, cerebrospinal fluid (CSF), and transudates should be dropped but not spread on the slide. The area of sample drop should be marked on the reverse side of the slide using a wax pencil or placed within the circle or well of a premarked slide. **Cytocentrifu-**

gation is preferred for this type of specimen, if available.

Thin fluid can be prepared by drawing up a small quantity of the fluid or a resuspended sediment of the fluid into a pipette and depositing it as a drop of fluid onto a clearly marked area on the slide (Figure 8-4). The material may not be grossly visible after staining because of a low protein or cell count. The fluid should not be spread over a larger area of the slide unless it is turbid. Turbid or thick fluids can be more efficiently prepared by the previously described method.

Cytocentrifuge Preparations

Cytocentrifugation is an excellent method for preparing nonviscous fluids such as CSF and bronchoalveolar lavage fluids. The cytocentrifugation process deposits cellular elements and microorganisms from the specimen onto the surface of a glass slide as a monolayer. The cellular elements are deposited within a discrete area for easy viewing (Figure 8-5). The protein is dissipated into a filter pad, leaving the background clearer for viewing gram-negative morphotypes. Cell morphology is good, and the concentrating effect shortens viewing time and increases the volume of cellular material reviewed.

Cytocentrifuge technique

A cytocentrifuge with a closed bowl is preferred for microbiology. The bowl can be loaded and un-

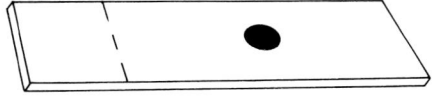

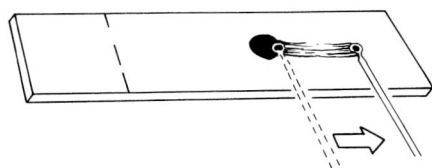

Figure 8-5

Cytocentrifuge preparations deposit the concentrated sample within a limited area for viewing. If the deposit is too heavy, a portion of the material may be smeared to produce a thin area.

loaded within a biohazard chamber to avoid possible infectious aerosols. The steps of the technique are as follows:

1. Small aliquots of fluid (0.1 to 0.2 mL) are placed in the cytocentrifuge holders.
2. The material is spun for 10 minutes.
3. The slide is removed. If the deposit of cells is too heavy, a portion of the cellular deposition can be smeared (see Figure 8-5).
4. The sediment is fixed and decontaminated in 70% alcohol for 5 minutes.

STAINS

Staining imparts an artificial coloration to the smear materials that allows them to be visualized using the magnification provided by a microscope. There are many types of stains, each with specific applications. Stains can be categorized as **simple stains, differential stains,** and **probe-mediated stains.** Simple stains are directed toward coloring the forms and shapes present, differential stains are directed toward coloring specific components of those elements present, and diagnostic antibody or DNA probe—mediated stains are directed specifically at an organism identification. Stains most commonly used in the diagnostic laboratory are listed in Table 8-2. Four of the stains—Gram, acid-fast, calcofluor white, and rapid modified Wright-Giemsa—should be available in all diagnostic microbiology laboratories (Procedures 8-1 to 8-4). Most other stains are directed toward specific organism groups and should be available where needed.

MICROSCOPES

Examination of specimens should begin with gross visual inspection and proceed to the level of magnification needed to visualize the pathogen or determine that no pathogen is present. The ordered tests provide a guide to the examination, but a routine approach to specimen management should include an examination procedure that will discover unexpected pathogens. In most diagnostic microbiology laboratories, this procedure consists of visual inspection at the time of smear and culture preparation, and microscopic examination of a gram-stained preparation for structures too small to be seen with the unaided eye.

Microscopes vary both in their ability to resolve small structures and their modifications. Microscopes are divided into two basic types: compound light microscopes, with common re-

TABLE 8-2

Stains for Infected Materials

Stains	Applications
General morphology	
Wright-Giemsa	Bronchoalveolar lavages
	Tzanck preparations
	Samples with complex cellular backgrounds (visualizes bacteria, yeast, parasites, and viral inclusions)
Selected morphology	
Leifson	Flagella
Methylene blue	Metachromatic granules of *Corynebacterium diphtheriae*
Acid-fast stains	
Ziehl-Neelsen	Sediments for mycobacteria (concentrated smears)
	Partial acid-fastness of *Nocardia* spp.
Fluorochrome	Sediments for mycobacteria (concentrated smears) (auramine and rhodamine)
	Preferred acid-fast stain
Kinyoun	Acid-fast stain modification of Ziehl-Neelsen method for cryptosporidia and cyclospora parasites in stool specimens
Calcofluor white stain	Bronchoalveolar fungi and some parasitic cysts
	Differentiates them from background materials of similar morphology
Gram stain	
Traditional	Routine stain for diagnostic area
	Yeast differentiated from all other organisms
Enhanced	Provides the same differential staining but enhances red-negative organisms by staining the background material a green to gray-green
Genus (species)-specific stains	
Antibody or DNA probe stains	Used for the specific identification of selected pathogens, such as *Chlamydia trachomatis, Bordetella pertussis, Legionella pneumophila;* herpes simplex virus, varicella-zoster virus, cytomegalovirus, adenovirus, and respiratory viruses

PROCEDURE 8-1.   Gram Stain

Principles

This Gram staining method was developed empirically by the Danish bacteriologist Christian Gram in 1884. The sequential steps provide for crystal violet (hexamethyl-*p*-rosanaline chloride) to color all cells and background material a deep blue, and for Gram's iodine to provide the larger iodine element to replace the smaller chloride in the stain molecule. Bacteria with thick cell walls containing teichoic acid retain the crystal violet–iodine complex dye after decolorization and appear deep blue; they are **gram-positive bacteria.** Other bacteria with thinner walls containing lipopolysaccharides do not retain the dye complex; they are **gram-negative bacteria.** The alcohol-acetone decolorizer damages these thin lipid walls and allows the stain complex to wash out. All unstained elements are subsequently counterstained red by safranin dye. The differential ability of the Gram stain makes it useful in microbial taxonomy. The quickness and ease with which the method can be performed makes it an ideal choice for the clinical laboratory setting.

Application

The Gram stain is used routinely and as requested in the clinical microbiology laboratory for the primary microscopic examination of specimens submitted for smear and culture. It is ideally suited for those specimen types in which bacterial infections are strongly suspected, but it may be used to characterize any specimen. Cerebrospinal fluid, sterile fluids, expectorated sputum or bronchoalveolar lavages, and wounds and exudates are routinely stained directly. Urine and stool may not be routinely stained directly. Samples sent for focused screening cultures usually are not stained. The Gram stain is regularly used to characterize bacteria growing on culture media.

Procedure

1. Dry the material on the slide so it does not wash off during the staining procedure. Adherence can be improved by fixation in 70% to 95% alcohol or gently warming the slide to remove all water from the material.

2. Place the smear on a staining rack, and overlay the surface of the material to be stained with the stains in sequence as shown in the figures.

3. Place the smear in an upright position in a staining rack, allowing the excess water to drain off and the smear to dry. Never blot a critical smear. Never put immersion oil on a smear until it is completely dry.

4. Examine the stained smear using the low-power objective, then select an area to examine more closely using a 40¥ to 60¥ oil objective. Suspicious areas are evaluated using the 100¥ oil objective of the microscope.

Results

Gram-positive bacteria stain dark blue to blue-black. All other elements stain safranin red. Individual structures absorb a different amount of safranin, so some will have prominent staining (strong avidity) and others will be weakly stained (low avidity). Among the gram-negative bacteria the enterics have strong avidity and stain a bright red; pseudomonads are less avid and stain moderately well. Anaerobic bacilli and other thin-walled gram-negative organisms, such as *Borrelia, Legionella,* and *Spirillum,* stain weakly. Always check the quality of the stain before moving to interpretation.

Precautions

The Gram stain reaction may vary from the expected in a number of well-recognized circumstances. If the crystal violet is rinsed too vigorously before it is complexed with the iodine, it will wash away and leave poor or no staining of gram-negative organisms. If the decolorization is too vigorous or prolonged, the gram-positive complex will be removed, and the normally gram-positive organisms will not stain. If the decolorization is insufficient, organisms may be falsely gram-positive, and organisms in the thicker areas of the sample may be ob-

Continued

PROCEDURE 8-1. Gram Stain—cont'd

scured. If the safranin is left on the slide for a prolonged period (minutes), the gram-positive complex will be leached from the positive cells; however, failure to leave the safranin in place for sufficient time will result in failure to stain gram-negative bacteria and background mate-rials. Gram stain characteristics may be atypical in antibiotic-treated and dead or degenerating organisms. Typical morphotypes should be sought. Any sample that raises questions about quality of stain or method should be restained.

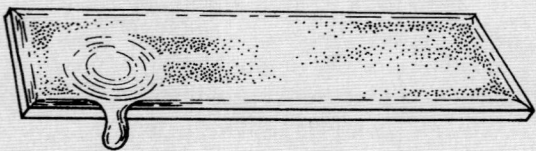

Flood the slide with crystal violet and allow to stand for 30 seconds.

The crystal violet stain is not tied into the organism until the iodine is added. Any rinsing between the crystal violet and the iodine steps must be very brief.

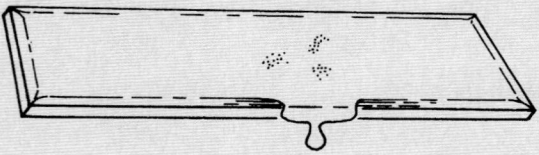

Flood with Gram's iodine and allow to stand for 30 to 60 seconds.

The dilute iodine solution can be used to wash away the crystal violet, and no water rinse is employed.

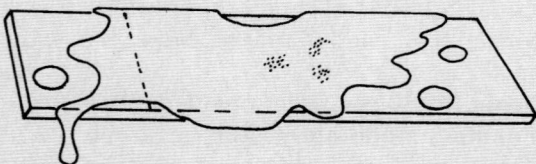

Decolorize the slide with acetone or absolute alcohol or a mixture of the two decolorizers and wash immediately with water.

Acetone is a more rapid decolorizer and may give better results, but the reaction must be stopped with water as soon as the purple color disappears.

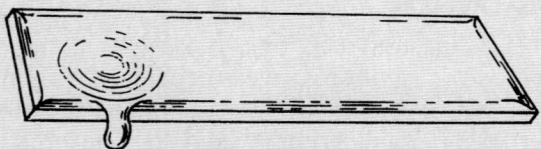

Flood with safranin or dilute carbolfuchsin or neutral red for 30 seconds to 1 minute (anaerobes). Rinse very lightly with water.

The counterstain must not be left in place too long. Anaerobes may stain better at 1 minute or with dilute carbolfuchsin.

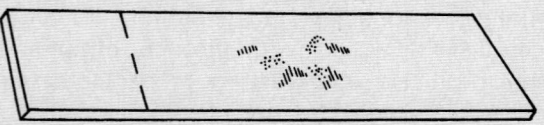

Check the staining reactions before proceeding with smear interpretation.

PROCEDURE 8-2. Acid-Fast Staining of Mycobacteria

Principles

The primary stain binds to mycolic acid in the cell walls of the mycobacteria and is retained after the decolorizing step with acid alcohol. The counterstain does not penetrate the mycobacteria to affect the color of the primary stain.

Application

The direct smear examination is a valuable diagnostic procedure for the detection of mycobacteria in clinical specimens.

Materials

    Difco TB auramine-rhodamine T stain
    Carbolfuchsin stain (prepared by laboratory)
    0.5% acid alcohol (0.5% HCl in 70% ethanol)
    2% acid alcohol (prepared by laboratory)
    1% sulfuric acid (partial acid-fast)
    0.5% aqueous potassium permanganate solution.
    0.3% aqueous methylene blue solution (prepared by laboratory)
    Microscope slides 1 × 3 inches
    Sterile water

Procedure

Fluorescent Stain

1. Cover smears with Difco TB auramine-rhodamine T stain, and stain for 25 minutes.
2. Wash in running tap water.
3. Move slides to slide rack on acid alcohol collection container.
4. Flood smears with 0.5% acid alcohol and decolorize for 2 minutes.
5. Wash smears in running tap water.
6. Move slides to original staining rack.
7. Flood smears with potassium permanganate counterstain for 4 minutes.
8. Wash smears in running tap water.
9. Air dry.

10. Examine smears with the 16× and 40× objectives of the fluorescent microscope equipped with a filter system comparable to a BG-12 exciter filter and an OG-1 barrier filter. Examine each smear for 3 to 5 minutes.

Kinyoun Stain

1. Cover smears with carbolfuchsin and stain for 5 minutes.
2. Wash slides with running tap water.
3. Move slides to staining rack on acid alcohol collection container.
4. Decolorize with acid alcohol until no more color appears in the washings.
5. Wash slides with running tap water, and move them to original staining rack.
6. Flood slides with methylene blue counterstain for 1 minute.
7. Wash with running tap water, drain, and air dry.
8. Examine smears with 100¥ oil immersion lens.

Modified Kinyoun Stain (Partial Acid-Fast)

1. Flood the slides with carbolfuchsin stain for 5 minutes.
2. Rinse with running tap water.
3. Flood slides with 70% ethanol, and rinse with tap water. Repeat until excess red dye is removed.
4. Move slides to rack on acid collection container.
5. Continuously drop 1% sulfuric acid on the smear until the washing becomes colorless.
6. Rinse with running tap water.
7. Move slides to original staining rack.
8. Counterstain with methylene blue for 30 seconds.

Continued

PROCEDURE 8-2. Acid-Fast Staining of Mycobacteria—cont'd

Modified Kinyoun Stain (Partial Acid-Fast)—cont'd

9. Rinse with running tap water and air dry.
10. Examine smears with 100× oil immersion objective.

Ziehl-Neelsen Stain

1. Cover smear with a piece of filter paper cut slightly smaller than the slide.
2. Layer filter paper with carbolfuchsin stain. With Bunsen burner, heat the smears gently until steaming occurs. Stain for 5 minutes without additional heating.
3. Proceed as for Kinyoun method, beginning with step 2.

Results

Fluorescent Stain

Mycobacteria stain bright orange. Count the number of **acid-fast bacilli** seen on the smear and report as follows:

Number of Acid-Fast Bacilli	Report
1 to 20	Number seen
21 to 80	Few
81 to 300	Moderate
300+	Numerous

Kinyoun and Ziehl-Neelsen Stains

Mycobacteria stain red, whereas the background material and nonacid–fast bacteria stain blue.

PROCEDURE 8-3. Calcofluor White Stain/Fungi-Fluor Kit*

Principle

Calcofluor white is a colorless dye that binds to cellulose and chitin. It fluoresces when exposed to long-wavelength ultraviolet and short-wavelength visible light. Special filters are required for optimal use.

Application

Calcofluor white may be used as a specific stain for rapid screening of clinical specimens for fungal elements. This stain may be useful when morphology is ambiguous and the nonspecific staining of other techniques such as Grocott's methenamine silver (GMS) gives confusing results.

Materials

Stock Solution

A 1% (w/v) aqueous solution of calcofluor white is prepared by dissolving the powder in distilled water with gentle heating. The stock solution is stable for 1 year at room temperature.

Working Solution

0.1% calcofluor white containing 0.01% to 0.08% Evans blue as a counterstain.

Procedure

1. Add 1 to 2 drops of working calcofluor white solution or solution A (Fungi-Fluor) to fixed smear or imprint for 1 to 2 minutes.
2. Coverslip or rinse and dry.
3. Examine specimen on fluorescent microscope using the following set of filters: G 365, LP 450, and FT 395.
4. Add Fungi-Fluor solution B if quenching of nonspecific staining is desired. (The quenching with solution B may be excessive [1:4 dilution preferred].)

Results

Yeast cells, pseudohyphae, and hyphae display a bright apple-green or blue-white fluorescence. The central body of the *Pneumocystis* cyst also fluoresces; with quenching (Fungi-Fluor solution B), the cysts of *Pneumocystis* are visible.

*Polysciences, Arrington, Pa.

PROCEDURE 8-4. Rapid Modified Wright-Giemsa Stain

Principle

The Wright-Giemsa stain is available in a modification that requires only 1 to 3 minutes. This neutral dye is a combination of basic thiazine dyes and acid eosin that attach to oppositely charged sites on proteins. The results are metachromatic.

Application

Wright-Giemsa (modified) is a rapid stain for smears and imprints to fully stain background materials and cells and a wide variety of microorganisms.

Precautions

Avoid getting reagents in eyes or on skin or clothing; if this does occur, flush with copious quantities of water. Use with adequate ventilation. If stain is discarded into sink, flush with large volumes of water to prevent azide build-up, which may react with lead and copper plumbing to form highly explosive metal azides.

Procedure

1. Prepare smear or imprint. Fix with alcohol.
2. Dip slide in fixative solution five times for 1 second each time. Allow excess to drain.
3. Dip slide in solution I five times for 1 second each time. Allow excess to drain.
4. Dip slide in solution II five times for 1 second each time. Allow excess to drain.
5. Rinse slide with tap water.
6. Allow to dry. Examine.

Note: The intensity of each stain may be altered by increasing or decreasing dips in solutions I and II. Never use fewer than three dips of 1 full second each.

Results

Blood cells stain as with Wright stain. The cytoplasm is basophilic. The chromatin of white cells is purple. Bacteria are blue. Parasitic protozoan nuclei are red.

---

solving limits of 1 to 10 μm and enlargements up to 2000×; and electron microscopes with enlargements greater than 1,000,000× (Table 8-3). The microbiology laboratory uses several modifications of the compound light microscope, but the workhorse of the laboratory is the brightfield microscope.

TERMINOLOGY FOR DIRECT EXAMINATIONS

The microscopist must have a consistent vocabulary for the description of materials seen in viewed samples. This vocabulary must be shared by the microbiology and medical communities, so

TABLE 8-3

Observing Microbial Pathogens

Tools	Magnification (×)	Application
Eyes	0	Gross examination
Magnifying glass	5	Gross examination
Dissecting microscope	2.5 to 30	Gross detailed examination and manipulation
Compound light microscope		
Brightfield	10 to 2,000	Cells stained
Darkfield	10 to 400	Cells not readily stained for brightfield microscopy
Phase-contrast	10 to 400	Living or unstained cells
Fluorescence	10 to 400	Preparations using fluorochrome stains, which can directly stain cells or be connected to antibodies that attach to cells
Electron microscopes		
Transmission electron	150 to 10 million	Determine ultrastructure of cell organelles
Scanning electron	20 to 10,000	Determine surface shapes and structures

TABLE 8-4

Gram Stain Morphology and Associated Organisms

Morphotype Description	Most Common Organisms
Bacteria	
Cocci	
Gram-positive cocci	*Aerococcus, Enterococcus, Leuconostoc, Pediococcus, Planococcus, Staphylococcus, Stomatococcus, Streptococcus*
Gram-positive cocci	
Pairs	*Staphylococcus, Streptococcus, Enterococcus*
Tetrads	*Micrococcus, Staphylococcus, Peptostreptococcus*
Groups	*Staphylococcus, Peptostreptococcus, Stomatococcus*
Chains	*Streptococcus, Peptostreptococcus*
Clusters, intracellular	Microaerophilic *Streptococcus*, viridans streptococci, *Staphylococcus*
Encapsulated	*Streptococcus pneumoniae, Streptococcus pyogenes* (rarely), *Stomatococcus mucilaginosus*
Gram-positive diplococci (lancet-shaped)	*Streptotoccus pneumoniae*
Gram-negative diplococci	Pathogenic *Neisseria, Moraxella catarrhalis*
Bacilli	
Gram-positive bacilli	
Small	*Listeria monocytogenes, Corynebacterium*
Medium	*Lactobacillus*, anaerobic bacilli
Large	*Clostridium, Bacillus*
Diphtheroid	*Corynebacterium, Propionibacterium, Rothia*
Pleomorphic, gram-variable	*Gardnerella vaginalis*
Beaded	Mycobacteria, antibiotic-affected lactobacilli, and corynebacteria
Filamentous	Anaerobic morphotypes, antibiotic-affected cells
Filamentous, beaded, branched	*Actinomycetes, Nocardia, Nocardiopsis, Streptomyces, Rothia*
Bifid or V forms	*Bifidobacterium*, brevibacteria
Gram-negative coccobacilli	*Bordetella, Haemophilus* (pleomorphic)
Masses	*Veillonella*
Chains	*Prevotella, Veillonella*
Gram-negative bacilli	
Small	*Haemophilus, Legionella* (thin with filaments), *Actinobacillus, Bordetella, Brucella, Francisella, Pasteurella, Capnocytophaga, Prevotella, Eikenella*
Bipolar	*Klebsiella pneumoniae, Pasteurella, Bacteroides*
Medium	Enterics, pseudomonads
Large	Devitalized clostridia or bacilli
Curved	*Vibrio, Campylobacter*
Spiral	*Campylobacter, Helicobacter, Gastrobacillum, Borrelia, Leptospira, Treponema*
Fusiform	*Fusobacterium nucleatum*
Filaments	*Fusobacterium necrophorum* (pleomorphic)
Yeast, fungi, and algae	
Yeast	
Small	*Histoplasma, Torulopsis*
Medium	*Candida*
With capsules	*Cryptococcus neoformans*
Thick-walled, broad-based bud	*Blastomyces*
Hyphae	
Septate	Fungi
Aseptate	Zygomycetes
With arthroconidia	*Coccidioides*
With branches 45-degree angle	*Aspergillus*
Pseudohyphae	*Candida*
Spherule (endospores)	*Coccidioides*
Sporangia with endospores	*Protothecae*
Viruses	
Single or multinuclear cells with intranuclear inclusions	Herpes virus, measles virus
Enlarged cells with intranuclear inclusions or cytoplasmic inclusions	Cytomegalovirus
Cells with dark "smudged" nuclei	Adenovirus

that when observations are reported, everyone will be able to understand the implications of the descriptions. Common observations can be coded so they are consistent among observers. The use of computers for recording coded observations and generating reports of the findings further extends the need for uniform terminology. Only unusual findings should be individually described in a report.

The background of the sample being evaluated should be described in sufficient detail to convey the composition of the material. The presence of cells representing a response to injury supports the probability of infection and directs attention toward specific types of pathogens. Common morphotype descriptions and the most prevalent associated species are shown in Table 8-4. Examples of useful descriptive phrases with quantitation are listed in Table 8-5.

Microorganisms can be described in such a way that, based on prevalence, the description implies the identification of the organism. For example, the observation of a gram-negative bacillus, small and pleomorphic, from the spinal fluid of an infant implies that *Haemophilus influenzae* is the infecting agent.

EXAMINATION OF PREPARED MATERIAL

A limited number of microbial pathogens from commonly sampled infected sites are regularly encountered by the technologist or microbiologist. The simple Gram stain or acid-fast stain is the fastest and least expensive method for presumptive diagnosis in these common clinical settings. Organisms are readily seen, because more than 10^5 **colony-forming units (CFUs)** of infecting organisms per mL are commonly present in clinically evident infections.

Two types of infection are important to distinguish, those caused by a *single* species, or **monomicrobial,** and those caused by *multiple* species, or **polymicrobial.** The single agents of infection or those causing classic infections are easily recognized by microscopy and require limited interpretations. Infections caused by common single species, or by classic infectious agents, include *Streptococcus pneumoniae* pneumonia, *Staphylococcus aureus* abscesses or pyodermas, *H. influenzae* tracheobronchitis or meningitis in infants, *Clostridium perfringens* gas gangrene, *Nocardia* sp. lung abscesses, and gonococcal urethritis.

Polymicrobial presentations in smears require more interpretation and must take into account smear background, the morphology of the organisms, and the anatomic location of the suspected infection as well as accompanying clinical symptoms. Polymicrobial infections usually arise from displaced normal or altered flora, and culture will yield the same species that can be isolated in culture from uninfected but contaminated specimens. These infections usually represent displacement of environmental, skin, oropharyngeal, gastrointestinal, or vaginal flora into tissues, with subsequent infection. Commonly encountered infections of this type are surgical wound (skin flora) infection, aspiration (oropharyngeal flora) pneumonia, perirectal (fecal flora) abscesses, and tuboovarian (vaginal flora) abscess.

Characterization of Background Materials

The laboratory professional always should look at the slide material with the unaided eye before beginning the microscopic examination. The distribution and consistency of the material should be noted. The microscope's low-power objective

TABLE 8-5

Descriptions of Background Material

Cells and Structures	Associations
Amorphous debris (light, moderate, or heavy)	Necrosis, heavy protein fluid
Black particulate debris	Smoke inhalation, crack cocaine
Charcot-Leyden crystals	Eosinophils
Epithelials with contaminating bacteria	Passage of specimen through contaminated area during collection
Curschmann's spirals present (sputum)	Bronchospasm, obstruction, asthma
Epithelial cells (light, moderate, or heavy)	Epithelial surface involved or adjacent to collection site
Intracellular organisms	Inferred association in infection
Local material (light, moderate, or heavy)	Reflection of collection site
Mononuclear cells present	Chronic inflammation
Mucus (light, moderate, or heavy)	Irritation of glandular surface
Purulence (none, light, moderate, or heavy)	Acute inflammation, exudation
Red blood cells	Trauma, hemorrhage

(2.5× to 10×) should be used first to evaluate the general content of the material on the slide. Specimens can be homogeneous or heterogeneous and may contain pathogens evenly distributed throughout the specimen or limited to one visual field. A mental inquiry checklist should be followed until the habit of searching a slide systematically is developed. Items that should be included in such a checklist appear here and on following pages in **bold type** preceded by a bullet (▪).

▪ **Is *there evidence of contamination by normal (resident) microbial flora?*** The laboratory professional should look for squamous epithelial cells, bacteria without the cells of inflammation, food, or other debris. Does this material constitute the entire sample, or is a representative sample also available in a manner that can be recognized? Contamination of specimens not collected from sterile sites diminishes the value of culture studies.

▪ **Is *necrotic (amorphous) debris in the background?*** Infection with organisms such as *C. perfringens* and *Nocardia* spp. may elicit few polymorphonuclear neutrophils (PMNs). The inflammatory cells that do migrate into the area of infection can be lysed. Patients with leukopenia also may have few inflammatory cells within their inflammatory debris. **Amorphous debris** usually is the remains of tissue mixed with the breakdown products or fluids of acute inflammation and always should be searched for organisms. *Mycobacterium tuberculosis* organisms stain poorly as beaded gram-positive bacilli or not at all with Gram stain; they can appear within necrotic debris as negative images.

▪ **Are *unexpected structures present?*** The characteristic coiled structure of a **Curschmann's spiral** is more easily recognized on low power. This structure must not be confused with parasitic larvae, which also can be found in sputum using low-power magnification. Large granules, grains, or fungal forms such as spherules or fungal mats can best be recognized at low power.

Search for Microorganisms

After the full extent of the material has been examined on low power, a representative area should be selected for viewing with the oil-immersion lens.

A 40× or 60× lens is preferred for scanning, and a 100× lens is used for final evaluation. In infection, the organism will be intimate with the purulence of necrotic debris. All grains or granules and the background should be examined carefully. The delicate gram-positive filaments of *Nocardia* spp. may blend into the background. *H. influenzae* may be present in large numbers, hidden within the mucus, in acute exacerbations of chronic bronchitis. Intracellular and extracellular forms should be noted. Strict criteria for **microbial morphotypes** should be maintained. The examiner must not be distracted by precipitated gram-positive stain, keratohyaline granules, or other artifacts. Organisms should be evaluated for shape, size, and Gram reaction. Because cell wall–damaged bacteria, antibiotic-treated bacteria, or dead bacteria may appear falsely gram-negative, their shapes and sizes are critical "co-characteristics." The classic misleading smear example is the observation of gram-negative, lancet-shaped diplococci mixed with the predominant gram-positive forms. The inexperienced observer may misinterpret this as mixed infection rather than the simple presence of dead pneumococci in a classic infection.

▪ ***Examine more than one area of the smear.*** More than one organism should be found if possible. It is rare not to be able to find more than one, because in infection, organisms are usually distributed throughout the specimen. Care should be taken in the interpretation of very low numbers of bacteria, especially in the absence of inflammation or necrosis and in specimens from nonsterile sites. Small numbers of organisms in samples from sterile sites must be seriously considered. However, additional smears can be made and examined if the likelihood of contamination is high.

▪ ***Do not overinterpret the findings.*** Specific diagnosis should be limited to a small number of instances in which the smear is classic in its presentation and extent of infection is not an issue. If acid-fast bacteria are suspected, the acid-fast stain should be performed before an opinion is rendered. If a fungal element is not clearly gram-positive, a calcofluor stain should be performed. Both of these follow-up stains can be performed on the decolorized, Gram-stained preparation.

Evaluation of Choice of Antibiotic

The symptomatic patient with suspected infection most likely will be treated with antibiotics. The physician expects the laboratory to affirm or reject the antibiotic choice made after the presumptive diagnosis. Antibiotic choice should be kept in mind as the smear is viewed. There are a number of important observations.

- *Is there evidence of purulence?* Remember that purulence with red blood cells, neutrophils, protein background, and necrosis reflects acute inflammation. Mononuclear cells, including lymphocytes, monocytes, and macrophages, reflect chronic inflammation. Patients who are cytopenic do not have the cellular response seen in normal individuals. Purulence, blood, and necrosis can be present if traumatic tissue damage occurs in the absence of infection.
- *Is there a single most probable etiologic microorganism?* If so, is the morphology sufficiently characteristic to presume identification? Is there a specified antibiotic for treatment of infections with this agent? Will antibiotic susceptibility testing be necessary, or will identification of the suspected pathogen be sufficient?
- *Is the infection monomicrobial or polymicrobial?* Are morphotypes present that characterize the source of the organisms? Can the mixture of organisms be characterized?
- *If antibiotics are to be used, will the suspected pathogens be susceptible?* Specific considerations should be made about the likelihood of the following:
  1. Penicillinase or β-lactamase producers such as *S. aureus, Haemophilus* sp., and the gonococci
  2. Enterococci, which have limited susceptibility to antibiotics and therefore may require synergistic antibiotic action for killing
  3. Species resistant to aminoglycosides, penems, and cephems, such as the *Bacteroides fragilis* group and *Pseudomonas aeruginosa*
  4. Fungal organisms, which will be unresponsive to antibacterial antibiotics

Direct Examination Summary

Once this stepwise evaluation of the smear has been completed, the information yielded, along with the clinical setting, allows for reasonable management of infected patients until the subsequent steps of culture isolation, susceptibility testing, or antibody or antigen detection can take place.

Initiation of Special Handling for Unsuspected or Special Pathogens

The direct microscopic examination of infected materials, along with specimen site and historical information, may suggest modifications in routine culture techniques to allow the isolation of a suspected pathogen. Modifications might involve ordering other culture tests, adding special media, increasing incubation time, or changing incubation temperature or atmosphere. If recognition or suspicion of such pathogens does not occur from smear or history, the isolation of certain pathogens will not be made, and diagnosis will be delayed or missed.

Some pathogens will not grow in culture and are usually unsuspected. A common one is the nematode parasite *Strongyloides stercoralis,* which can be seen in the sputum and bronchoalveolar fluid of patients with a hyperinfestation syndrome. Visual recognition can lead to a request for stool examination for parasite load and prompt treatment. Untreated hyperinfestations are associated with death of the patient.

Other pathogens that will grow in culture but not in routine bacterial culture can be recognized on smear and redirected for appropriate culture. Organisms such as *Legionella* sp., *Mycobacterium* sp., viruses, and *Bartonella* sp. must be placed on appropriate media for culture confirmation of infection.

GRADING OR CLASSIFYING MATERIALS

Microscopic examination also immediately discloses that a specimen is unlikely to be helpful in diagnosis or culture management. The specimen may be just blood rather than infected material, or it may be oropharyngeal surface debris or some other normal surface material. Processing and culture interpretation of such nonrepresentative specimens may lead to delayed treatment because of a falsely negative culture or to inappropriate antibiotic treatment owing to a falsely positive culture from growth of normal flora or antibiotic-altered flora.

Several grading or classification systems have been derived to aid the technologist in arriving at decisions relating to culturing the specimen or interpretation of growth from culture of a specimen. Most evaluations are aimed at specimens such as sputum, for which collection is complicated by contamination with throat and mouth flora because culture alone may be misleading. The objective is to separate the representative sample from the contaminated sample before culture or culture evaluation. Barlett's method for scoring sputum and the Murray-Washington method for contamination assessment document the association of 10 to 20 squamous epithelial cells (SECs) per 10× microscopic field with unacceptable specimens and 10 to 25 PMNs per 10× field with significant specimens. Heineman's method emphasizes the ratio between the SECs and PMNs.

Many diagnostic microbiology laboratories use the documented observations related to SECs and PMNs but attempt to coordinate observations related to background materials, which consist of local materials, contaminating materials, and purulence, and to describe the relationship of microorganisms to these background materials. The body site of the sample and the classification of the smear together determine the extent of culture evaluation.

Contaminating Materials

Contaminating materials (Plate 1) are recognized as those not coming from the collection site, not contributed by the inflammatory response from the tissues, or not likely to contain the infecting organism. They usually have been added to the specimen in the course of collection from or through a nonsterile area. The most bothersome contaminating materials are those containing microorganisms that will grow in culture and may confuse the culture evaluation. Expectorated sputum, which collects in the lower lung airways and is expelled through the mouth, is the most common contaminated specimen managed by the clinical laboratory.

Criteria

< 25 polymorphonuclear cells per low-power field (LPF) and > 10 epithelial cells and/or mixed bacteria per LPF.

Gram smear report

Quantitate the contaminating materials as 1+ (light), 2+ (moderate), 3+ (moderately heavy), or 4+ (heavy).

Culture identification guidelines

"New culture" using careful collection technique should be requested. If culture is requested, organism identification should be limited to brief evaluation for *S. aureus,* streptococci or viridans streptococci, *Lactobacillus,* diphtheroids, and β-hemolytic streptococci. Gram-negative rods are reported as enterics (coliforms, nonlactose fermenters, or *Proteus* spp. [spreading colonies]), pseudomonads (oxidase-positive). Pathogenic *Neisseria* (identified), *Haemophilus* spp. (smear only), yeast (note only), and any primary pathogen.

Antibiotic susceptibility testing

None appropriate except on primary pathogens.

Local Materials
Criteria

< 25 polymorphonuclear leukocytes (WBCs) per LPF and < 10 contaminating epithelial cells per LPF along with cellular and fluid elements *local* to the area sampled.

The local constituents may vary as follows:

- Respiratory secretions (Plate 3) mucus, alveolar pneumocytes (macrophages), ciliated columnar cells, goblet cells, and occasionally metaplastic epithelial cells (smaller than normal squamous epithelial cells)
- Cerebrospinal fluid (Plate 5) cellular elements
- Cavity fluid (Plate 8) macrophages, few mixed WBCs, mesothelial cells, and proteinaceous fluid
- Wounds—blood and proteinaceous fluids
- Amniotic fluid (Plate 2) anucleate squamous cells and heavy proteinaceous fluid
- Cervix—mucus, columnar epithelial cells, goblet cells, metaplastic squamous epithelial cells, and leukocytes (vary with menstrual cycle)
- Prostatic secretions or semen—spermatozoa and mucus

Gram smear report

Quantitate local microbial flora as 1+ to 4+ (see "Contaminating Materials").

Culture identification guidelines

The designation "usual flora" or a brief presumptive description of colony-type growth may be used (see "Contaminating Materials").

Antibiotic susceptibility testing

None appropriate.

Purulence

Criteria

> 25 polymorphonuclear leukocytes (WBCs) per LPF and no or few (< 10) epithelial cells with mixed bacteria per LPF. Mucus and/or heavy proteinaceous material may be present.

Gram smear report

Quantitate only organisms intimately associated with the WBCs, mucus, or proteinaceous exudate. Use the following system: 1+ (≤ 1 organism per oil immersion field [OIF]), 2+ (few organisms per OIF), 3+ (moderate number per OIF), and 4+ (many per OIF). Quantitate contaminating materials separately—should be ≤ 1 + (none or few).

Culture identification guidelines

Correlate colony growth with Gram-stained smear. Identify: *S. pneumoniae* from viridans streptococci, β-hemolytic streptococci (Lancefield groups A, B, and D; C, F, and G if indicated clinically), *S. aureus* (inventory for epidemiology), *H. influenzae, Haemophilus parainfluenzae* (test for β-lactamase production), *Haemophilus aphrophilus,* pathogenic *Neisseria,* gram-negative bacillic yeast (*Cryptococcus neoformans* only; note presence of other genera), filamentous fungi (transparent tape preparation in biosafety hood), and other organisms as indicated by smear findings.

Antibiotic susceptibility testing

S. aureus, gram-negative nonfastidious bacilli, and other organisms as appropriate or specifically requested.

Mixed Materials

Mixed materials consist of purulent exudate, contaminating materials, and local materials in a single smear.

Criteria

> 25 polymorphonuclear leukocytes (WBCs) per LPF and > 10 epithelial cells and/or contaminating bacteria per LPF. Local secretions may also be present.

Gram smear report

For mixed materials, quantitate only those organisms intimately associated with purulent exudate. Also quantitate the amounts of other elements, contaminating materials, and local materials.

Culture identification guidelines

A "new culture" *may* be requested for mixed specimens. A new specimen *must* be requested if the specimen shows the presence of purulence and uninterpretable culture results. If a new culture specimen cannot be obtained, evaluation should proceed as for contaminating materials.

Antibiotic susceptibility testing

Use purulence guidelines for testing organisms that appear significant.

REPORTS OF DIRECT EXAMINATIONS

Reports of the results of direct specimen examination should be made available as soon as they are completed. The availability of computer-managed reporting using direct physician access through computer terminals in patient care areas, as well as paper reporting, facilitates immediate reporting of results. Reports of direct examinations should be simple and include all information elements needed by the physician to understand the report. The report lists the type of material submitted and clearly states whether the observed microbes are of significance. The format for computer-managed microscopic reports from direct specimen examinations at The Ohio State University is shown in the samples given in Box 8-1.

Only those elements useful in characterizing the specimen should be included in the report. Interpretative comments also may be included when, on the basis of specimen type, background materials, and organism morphology, there is little doubt about the nature of the process or the offending infectious agent. All telephone reports of direct examinations should be recorded in the report.

Box 8-1

Sample Reports of Direct Microscopic Examinations

Respiratory culture **Acc. no. XXXX**

Source: Sputum: expectorated
Microscopic Purulence heavy
Contaminating bacteria, yeast and epithelials heavy
Gram-positive diplococci: consistent with pneumococci

Called to Dr. Doe at 8:00 PM 4/13/99

Respiratory culture **Acc. no. XXXXX**

Source: Sinus: ethmoid contents
Microscopic Purulence moderate
Local materials light
Red blood cells present
Gram-negative bacilli: consistent with pseudomonas

Called to Dr. Doe at 11:35 AM 4/5/99

EXAMPLES OF SAMPLE OBSERVATIONS AND REPORTS

Study the examples of direct observations and the associated reports and comments given in Plates 1 to 108. Practice to determine whether you can make a similar report using only the observation provided. Then read each report to see whether you obtain similar impressions of the specimen and pathogen from the observation and written report.

QUALITY CONTROL IN DIRECT MICROSCOPIC INTERPRETATIONS

Quality control issues, such as quality of specimens submitted and adequacy of culture interpretation, can be monitored using the results of direct examination. Quality control practice that monitors both the smear and culture interpretation should be an ongoing work activity. Correlation between the two results should be made for each patient. Explanations for discrepant results should be sought within the work material. This repeated inspection

of results enables each observer to practice self-education and improve observation skills. Review of these quality control activities allows corrections to be made in specimen collection, specimen management, and culture management.

Quality improvement activities often are suggested by results of quality control monitoring of direct specimen examination. For example, it may be documented that sputum specimens of poor quality are consistently submitted from certain doctors' offices, clinics, or nursing stations in the hospital. This observation becomes the basis for planning corrections that move outside the laboratory to involve the community of patients served.

Historically, the process of infectious disease diagnosis began with observations from direct specimen examination. We should continue the process of direct specimen examination for all of those instances in which this activity provides the opportunity to support or refute clinical diagnoses or discover unsuspected diagnoses.

Bibliography

Balows A et al, editors: *Manual of clinical microbiology,* ed 5, Washington, DC, 1991, American Society for Microbiology.

Bartlett RE: *Medical microbiology: quality, cost, and clinical relevance,* New York, 1974, John Wiley & Sons.

Broaddus C et al: Bronchoalveolar lavage and transbronchial biopsy for the diagnosis of pulmonary infections in the acquired immunodeficiency syndrome, *Ann Intern Med* 102:747, 1985.

Chapin-Robertson K, Dahlver SE, Edberg SC: Clinical and laboratory analysis of Cytopsin-prepared Gram stains for recovery and diagnosis of bacteria from sterile body fluids, *J Clin Microbiol* 30:377, 1992.

Cordonnier C et al: Diagnostic yield of bronchoalveolar lavage in pneumonitis occurring after allogeneic bone marrow transplantation, *Am Rev Respir Dis* 132:1118, 1985.

Golden JA et al: Bronchoalveolar lavage as the exclusive diagnostic modality for *Pneumocystis carinii* pneumonia, *Chest* 90:18, 1986.

Goswitz JJ et al: Utility of slide centrifuge Gram's stain versus quantitative culture for diagnosis of urinary tract infection, *Am J Clin Pathol* 99:132, 1993.

Heineman HS, Chawla JK, Lofton WM: Misinformation from sputum cultures without microscopic examination, *J Clin Microbiol* 6:518, 1977.

Kokoskin E et al: Modified technique for efficient detection of microsporidia, *J Clin Microbiol* 32:1074, 1994.

La Scolea LJ Jr, Dryja D: Quantitation of bacteria in cerebrospinal fluid and blood of children with meningitis and its diagnostic significance, *J Clin Microbiol* 19:187, 1984.

Lewis JF, Alexander J: Microscopy of stained urine smears to determine the need for quantitative culture, *J Clin Microbiol* 4:372, 1976.

Magee CM et al: A more reliable Gram staining technique for diagnosis of surgical infections, *Am J Surg* 130:341, 1975.

Mengel M: The use of the cytocentrifuge in the diagnosis of meningitis, *Am J Clin Pathol* 84:212, 1985.

Murray PR, Washington JA: Microscopic and bacteriologic analysis of expectorated sputum, *Mayo Clin Proc* 50:339, 1975.

Ognibene FP et al: The diagnosis of *Pneumocystis carinii* pneumonia in patients with the acquired immunodeficiency syndrome using subsegmental bronchoalveolar lavage, *Am Rev Respir Dis* 129:929, 1984.

Olson ML et al: The slide centrifuge Gram stain as a urine screening method, *Am J Clin Pathol* 96:454, 1991.

Ryan NJ et al: A new trichrome-blue stain for detection of microsporidial species in urine, stool, and nasopharyngeal specimens, *J Clin Microbiol* 31:3264, 1993.

Shanholtzer CJ, Schaper PJ, Peterson LR: Concentrated Gram stain smears prepared with a Cytospin centrifuge, *J Clin Microbiol* 16:1052, 1982.

Smith JW, Barlett MS: Laboratory diagnosis of *Pneumocystis carinii* infection, *Clin Lab Med* 2:383, 1982.

Spengler M et al: The Gram stain—the most important diagnostic test of infection, *JACEP* 7(12):434, 1978.

Stover DE et al: Bronchoalveolar lavage in the diagnosis of diffuse pulmonary infiltrates in immunosuppressed host, *Ann Intern Med* 101:1, 1984.

Van Scoy RE: Bacterial sputum cultures, a clinician's viewpoint, *Mayo Clin Proc* 52:39, 1977.

Vestal AL: *Procedures for the isolation and identification of mycobacteria.* Pub. no. CDC75-8230, Atlanta, 1975, US Dept of Health, Education, and Welfare.

LEARNING ASSESSMENT

1. Direct smear examination of clinical samples is a rapid means to presumptively identify etiologic agents of infectious disease: true or false?

2. The presence of an infectious disease process can be assessed on a direct smear based on which of the following?
   a. The presence of numerous inflammatory cells
   b. Morphology of the bacteria present
   c. Types of bacteria present
   d. The presence of numerous epithelial cells

3. Which of the following stains may be used for direct smear examination?
   a. Gram stain
   b. Acid-fast stain
   c. Wright or Giemsa stain
   d. Calcofluor-white stain
   e. All of the above

4. Which of the following stains is best used to detect mycobacterial organisms in clinical samples?
   a. Gram stain
   b. Giemsa stain
   c. Acid-fast stain
   d. Lacto-phenol-cotton blue stain

5. Calcofluor white is a colorless dye that binds with which of the following structures?
   a. Cell wall containing mycolic acid
   b. Chitin
   c. Peptidoglycan layer
   d. Metachromatic granules

Continued

LEARNING ASSESSMENT—cont'd

6. Cytocentrifugation is an excellent method for which of the following types of samples?
   a. Heavily contaminated
   b. Nonviscous fluids
   c. Thick purulent material
   d. Filled with mucous

7. A monobacterial type of infection can be immediately suspected based on the direct microscopic examination of the clinical sample: true or false?

8. In a Wright-Giemsa stained smear, bacteria would appear as which of the following colors?
   a. Red
   b. Blue
   c. Purple
   d. Orange

DIRECT EXAMINATION SHOWING LOCAL AND CONTAMINATING MATERIALS

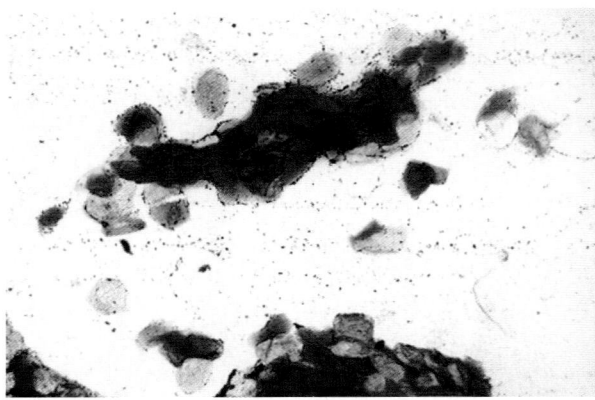

Plate 1

Expectorated sputum, smear, Gram stain, light microscopy, low-power view (LPV). Purulence none. Contaminating bacteria and epithelial cells heavy. No pathogens seen. Please submit carefully collected sample of lower respiratory tree material. The sample is saliva, not sputum. There could be several reasons for submission of this sample to the laboratory. The patient could have been poorly directed and simply "spit" into the collection container, or the patient's cough may not be productive of sputum.

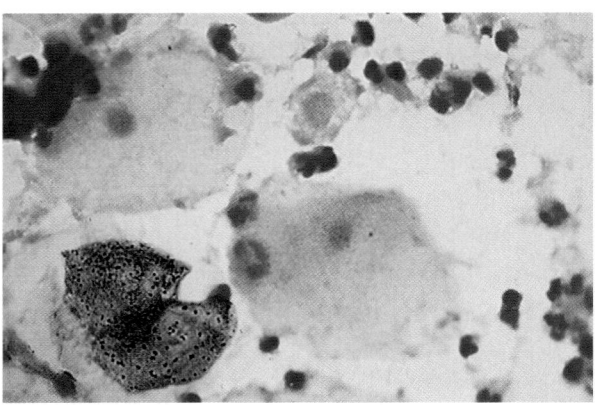

Plate 2

Amniotic fluid, cytocentrifuge preparation, Gram stain, light microscopy, medium-power view (MPV). Purulence moderate. Local materials moderate. No organisms seen. The presence of purulence (neutrophils or "polys") indicates a process suspicious for infection. The absence of organisms in this normally sterile fluid is a critical observation. Squamous epithelial cells are local to this specimen type and confirm that the sample is amniotic fluid. The blue keratohyalin granules must never be mistaken for bacteria.

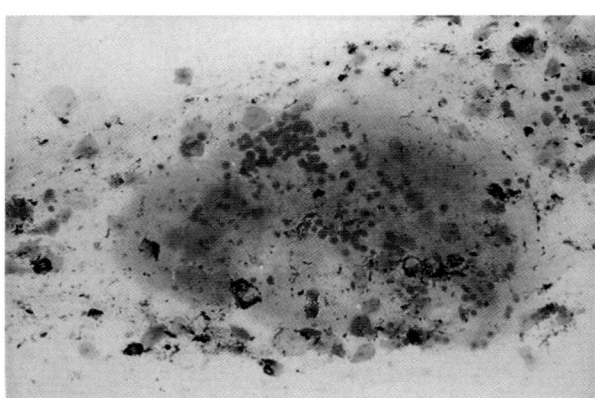

Plate 3

Expectorated sputum, smear, Gram stain, light microscopy, LPV. Purulence none. Local materials moderate. Contaminating bacteria and epithelials heavy. No pathogens seen. The bolus of sputum, consisting of mucus with entrapped alveolar macrophages, confirms that lower respiratory tree material is present. There is no evidence of an infectious process. The sputum is heavily coated by contaminating materials from the oropharynx or mouth. Contaminating organisms will grow in a routine sputum culture.

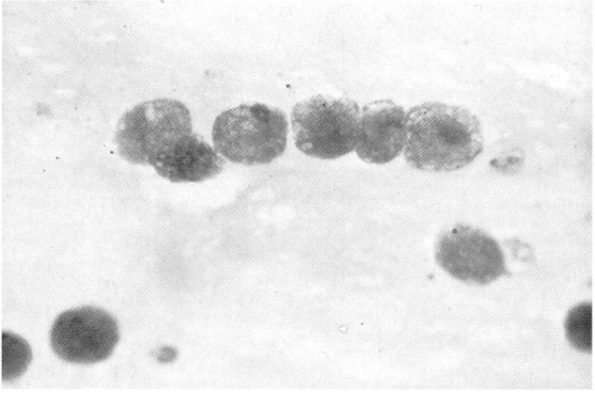

Plate 4

Aspirated sputum, smear, Gram stain, light microscopy, high-power view (HPV). Purulence none. Local materials moderate. No organism seen. The alveolar macrophages and mucus (pink-stained background) are the local materials from the surface of the tracheobronchial tree. This smear confirms that sputum was sampled and there is no suspicion for infection and no evidence of significant contamination. Routine culture of this specimen still will grow insignificant oral flora because culture is more sensitive than direct examination.

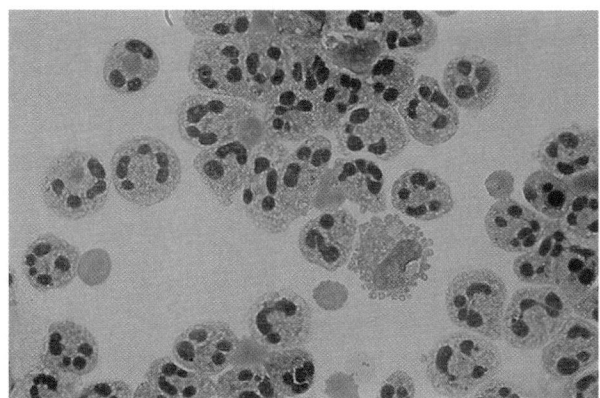

Plate 5 _____

Cerebrospinal fluid (CSF), cytocentrifuge preparation, Gram stain, light microscopy, HPV. Purulence moderate. No organisms seen. CSF is a sterile fluid and normally does not have purulence. The presence of neutrophils is critical. Careful observation for bacteria is mandatory. Acridine orange stain may be helpful in clinical settings in which bacteria are low in number and gram-negative. Cytocentrifuged sediments commonly have a concentration of organisms sufficient for routine microscopy ($\geq 10^5$/mL).

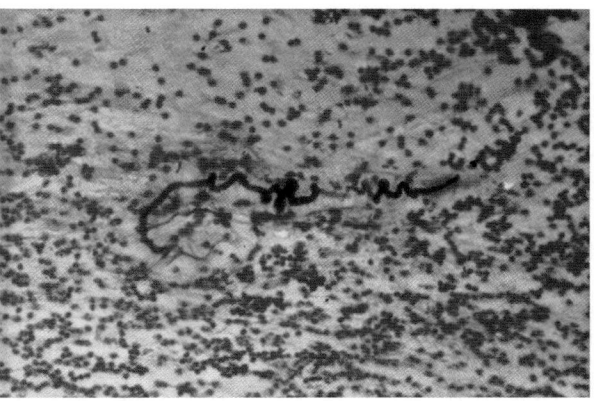

Plate 6 _____

Expectorated sputum, smear, Gram stain, lgiht microscopy, MPV. Purulence heavy. Local materials—Curschmann's spiral light. No organisms seen. The Curschmann's spiral is material local to the tracheobronchial tree but is not normal, so it is specifically reported. This spiral may present in a variety of sizes depending on the size of bronchus involved.

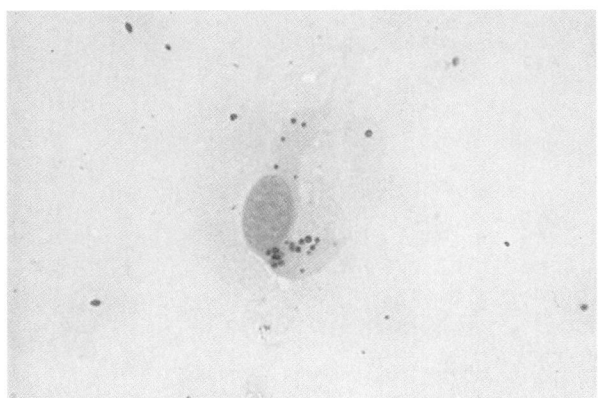

Plate 7 _____

Trauma eye, vitreous aspirate, smear, Gram stain, light microscopy, HPV. Purulence none. No organisms seen. Local materials light. The light protein background and the pigment-containing cell are normal material local to the vitreous of the eye. This local material confirms that the sample is representative. The ability to see this brown pigment cell in smear material is related to the eye trauma. The important emphasis is the absence of purulence.

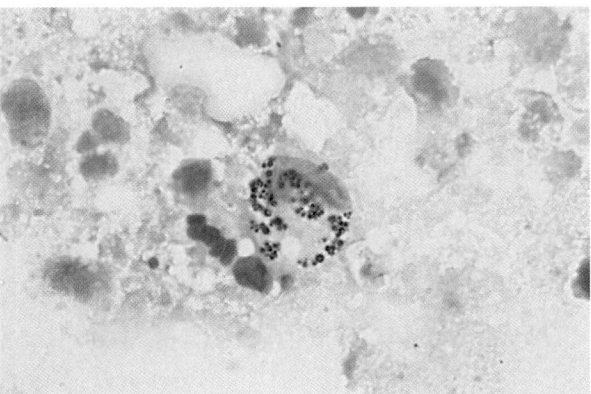

Plate 8 _____

Eye, vitreous aspirate, smear, Gram stain, light microscopy, HPV. Purulence light. Amorphous debris moderate. Local materials light. No organisms seen. This smear suggests that there has been ongoing injury. The pigment has been phagocytized and is seen within a large macrophage. Pigment must never be mistaken for bacteria, and bacteria must never be overlooked if mixed with local materials.

DIRECT EXAMINATION IN COMMON BACTERIAL INFECTIONS

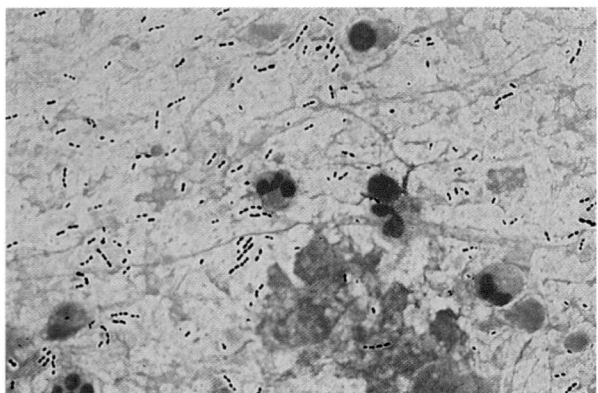

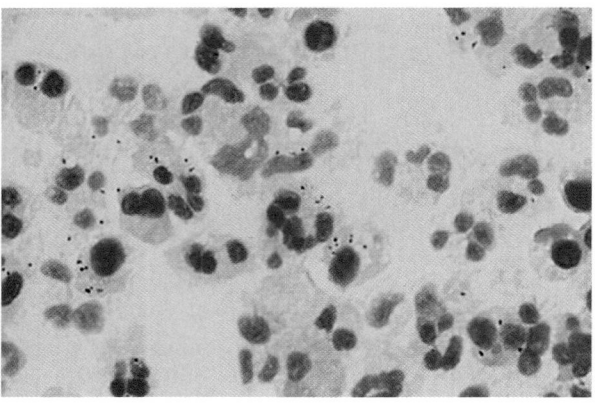

Plate 9

Expectorated sputum, smear, Gram, stain, light microscopy, medium-power view (MPV). Purulence light. Amorphous debris moderate. Gram-positive diplococci, encapsulated, extracellular. *Impression*: Pneumococcal disease.

    This is a typical smear presentation for early pneumococcal pneumonia. The pneumococci have proliferated to high numbers, and the lung is responding with increased mucus and fluid release. There is early migration of the neutrophils, but phagocytosis of the diplococci is limited. Routine bacterial culture of this sample should yield a heavy growth of *Streptococcus pneumoniae.*

Plate 10

Expectorated sputum, smear, Gram stain, light microscopy, high-power view (HPV). Purulence heavy. The presence of gram-positive diplococci, intracellular morphology suggest antibiotic effect. *Impression*: Pneumococcal disease.

    This is a typical smear presentation of a treated but unresolved pneumococcal pneumonia. Neutrophils cover the field, the diplococci are largely intracellular and partially digested, and the background amorphous material is gone. Routine bacterial culture of this sample may be negative for typical colonies of *S. pneumoniae.* A few colonies may be found by a careful search among the contaminating normal flora colonies.

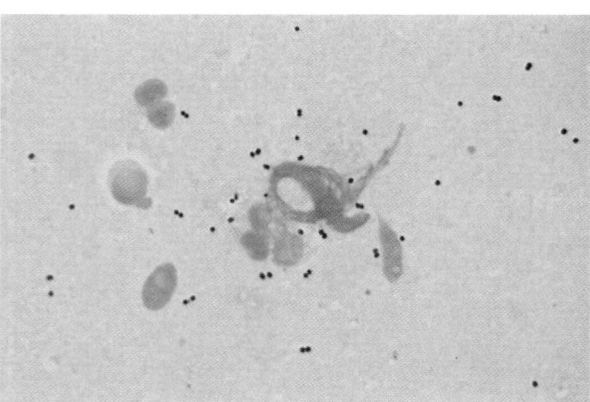

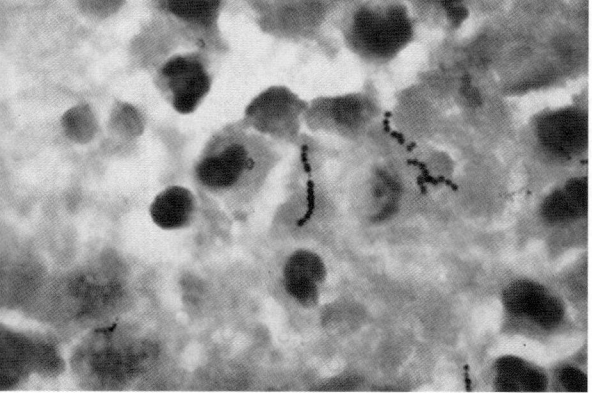

Plate 11

Aspirated sputum, smear, Gram stain, light microscopy, MPV. Purulence light. Amorphous debris heavy. Gram-positive cocci, pairs, encapsulated, extracellular. Initial antibiotic therapy can be directed toward streptococci and staphylococci *(Stomatococcus)*. Routine bacterial culture isolated a pure growth of an encapsulated strain of *Streptococcus pyogenes.* The heavy amorphous background is protein-rich edema fluid from the capillary bed damaged by *S. pyogenes* toxins. The patient subsequently died from the infection despite correct antibiotic therapy and a correct diagnosis.

Plate 12

Wound, smear, Gram stain, light microscopy, MPV. Purulence moderate. Amorphous debris moderate. Gram-positive cocci, chains, extracellular. *Impression*: Streptococcal disease.

    The presence of typical chains of *Streptococcus* on a background showing purulence with poorly preserved "polys" and amorphous debris is suggestive of hemolytic streptococci with tissue cytotoxicity. Routine bacterial culture yielded a pure growth of *S. pyogenes.*

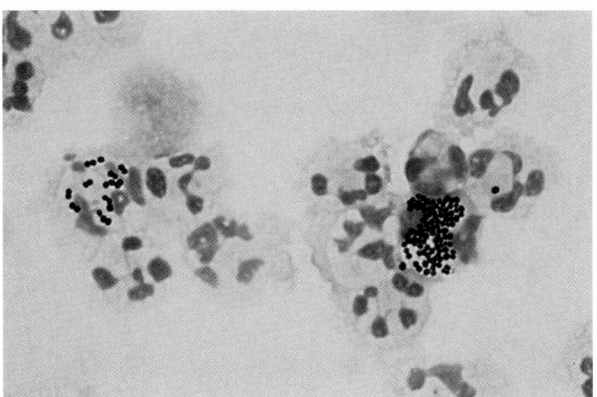

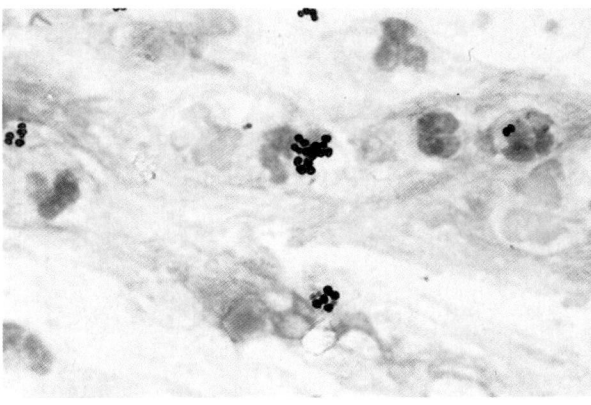

Plate 13

Bronchoalveolar lavage, cytocentrifuge preparation, Gram stain, light microscopy, HPV. Purulence moderate. Gram-positive cocci, pairs, short chains, groups, intracellular. *Impression*: Staphylococcal disease.

The background supports infection, the specimen is directly from the alveolar spaces of the lung, and the organism morphology is typical for staphylococci. Routine bacterial culture yielded a pure growth of methicillin-resistant *Staphylococcus aureus* (MRSA).

Plate 14

Expectorated sputum, smear, Gram stain, light microscopy, MPV. Purulence light. Local materials moderate. Gram-positive cocci, pairs, groups, intracellular and extracellular. *Impression*: Staphylococcal disease.

Smear morphology is typical for staphylococci, but no staphylococcal colonies were present on the culture plates. *Stomatococcus mucilaginosus* colonies were present in high numbers. Careful correlation between direct and culture examinations demonstrated this organism to be the probable cause of infection. The presumptive report implying or suggesting staphylococci followed by a *negative* culture report without explanation raises doubts about competence of the laboratory.

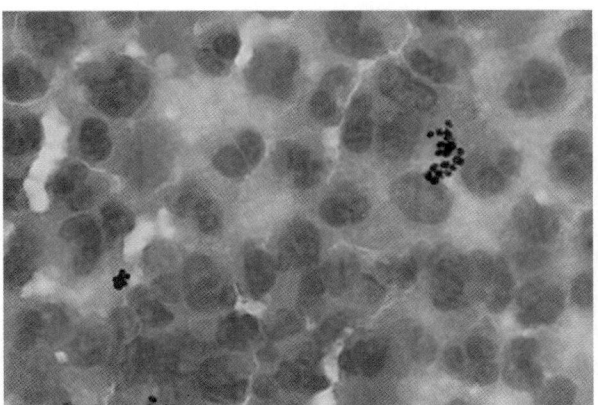

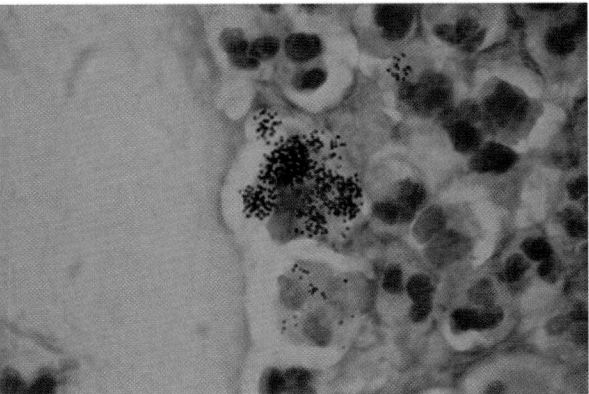

Plate 15

Abscess aspirate, smear, Gram stain, light microscopy, MPV. Purulence heavy. Gram-positive cocci, groups, extracellular. *Impression*: Staphylococcal disease.

Aerobic and anaerobic culture plates were negative at 24 hours. There was culture isolation of *Staphylococcus aureus* from this same abscess 5 days previously. The patient was being treated with clindamycin. Because the cocci in the smear did not appear antibiotic damaged, another species of gram-positive coccus was sought. The anaerobic culture grew *Peptostreptococcus* organisms, which are clindamycin resistant.

Plate 16

Bone aspirate, smear, Gram stain, light microscopy, MPV. Purulence heavy. Amorphous debris moderate. Gram-positive cocci, remnants, intracellular. Morphology suggests prominent antibiotic effect. Culture records confirmed a *S. aureus* osteomyelitis currently under antibiotic treatment. Bacterial culture was negative.

DIRECT EXAMINATION IN GRAM-POSITIVE BACILLARY INFECTIONS

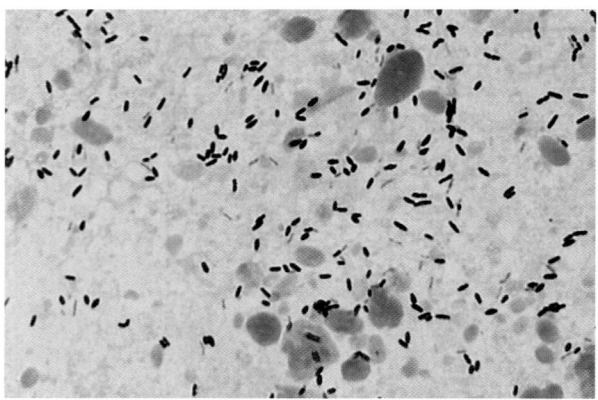

Plate 17

Amniotic fluid, cytocentrifuge, Gram stain, light microscopy, medium-power view (MPV). Purulence light. Local materials moderate. Gram-positive bacilli, small. Morphology consistent with *Listeria monocytogenes*. *Impression*: Congenital listeriosis.

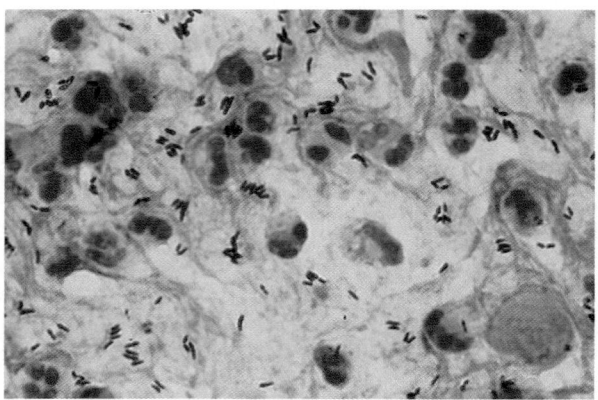

Plate 18

Expectorated sputum, smear, Gram stain, light microscopy, MPV. Purulence moderate. Local materials moderate. Gram-positive bacilli, diphtheroid. Morphology suggests coryneform infection. Routine bacterial culture grew *Corynebacterium pseudodiphtheriticum*.

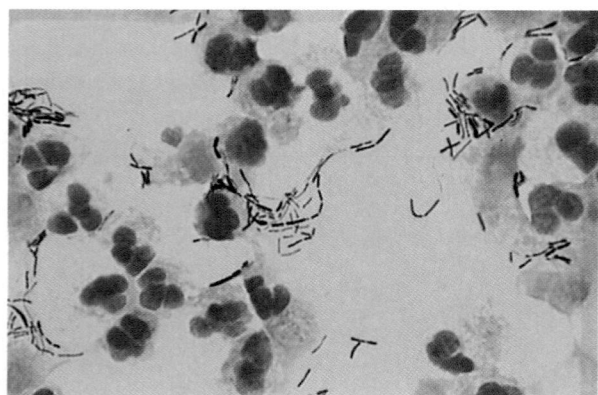

Plate 19

Urine, cytocentrifugation, Gram stain, light microscopy, MPV. Purulence moderate. Gram-positive bacilli, medium, long, chaining. Morphology consistent with *Lactobacillus* spp. *Impression*: Cystitis.

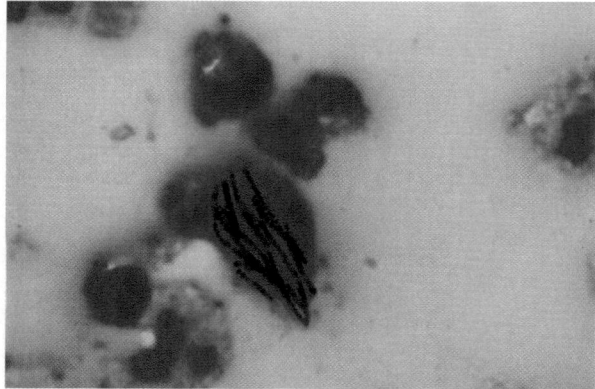

Plate 20

Amniotic fluid, cytocentrifuge preparation. Gram stain, light microscopy, high-power view (HPV). Purulence light. Local materials moderate. Gram-positive bacilli, medium, long, intracellular. Morphotype consistent with *Lactobacillus* spp. *Impression*: Amnionitis.

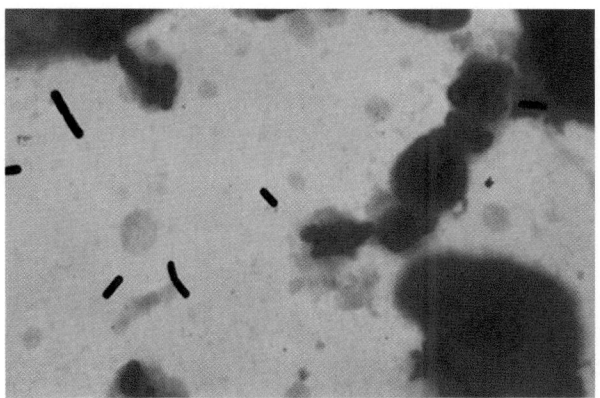

Plate 21

Amniotic fluid, smear, Gram stain, light microscopy, MPV. Purulence light. Local materials moderate. Gram-positive bacilli, large. Morphology consistent with *Clostridium perfringens*. *Impression*: Amnionitis.

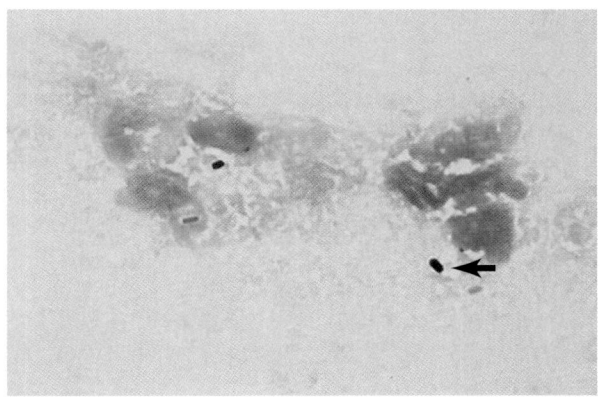

Plate 22

Wound cellulitis, smear, Gram stain, light microscopy, MPV. Purulence none. Amorphous debris moderate. Gram-positive bacilli, large. Gram-negative bacilli, large. Morphology consistent with *Clostridium sp. Impression*: Gas gangrene. Note that the growth rate of this organism is rapid and that both viable (gram-positive) and nonviable (gram-negative) bacilli can be present in the smear material.

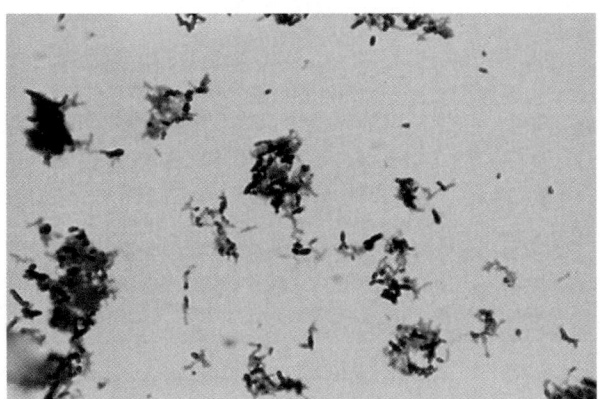

Plate 23

Colony from blood agar, smear, Gram stain, light microscopy, HPV. Gram-positive bacilli, diphtheroid, variably Gram-staining. Morphotype consistent with *Gardnerella vaginalis* (see Plate 24).

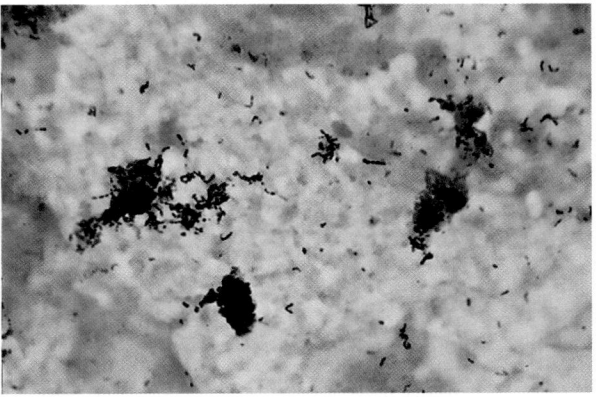

Plate 24

Amniotic fluid, smear, Gram stain, light microscopy, HPV. Local material heavy. Gram-positive bacilli, diphtheroid, variably Gram-staining. Morphotype consistent with *G. vaginalis. Impression*: Amnionitis.

| DIRECT EXAMINATION IN UNCOMMON GRAM-POSITIVE BACILLI

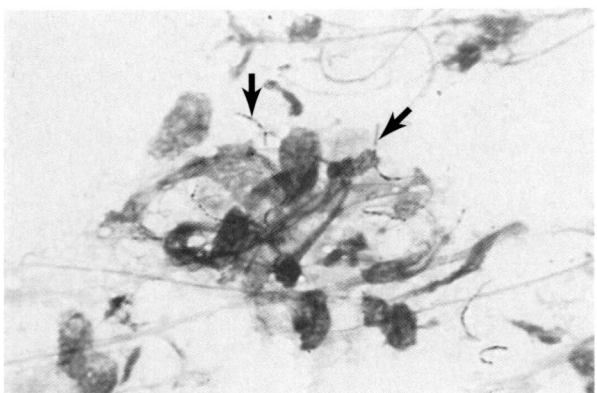

Plate 25

Abscess aspirate, smear, Gram stain, light microscopy, high-power view (HPV). Purulence moderate. Amorphous debris light. Gram-positive bacilli, beaded. Suspect mycobacteria: initiate additional testing (see Plate 26).

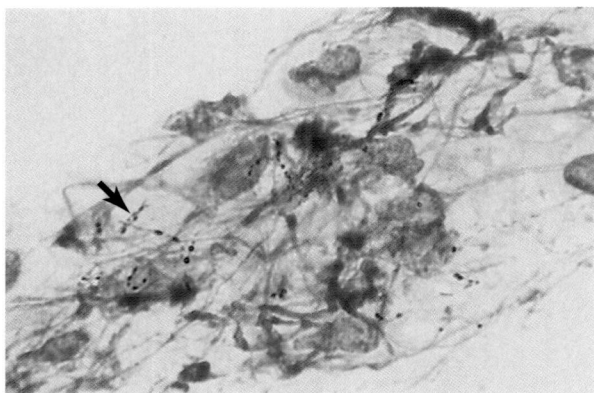

Plate 26

Abscess aspirate, smear, acid-fast stain (Ziehl-Neelsen), light microscopy, medium-power view (MPV). Purulence moderate. Acid-fast bacilli, numerous. Mycobacterial cultures grew *Mycobacterium kansasii.*

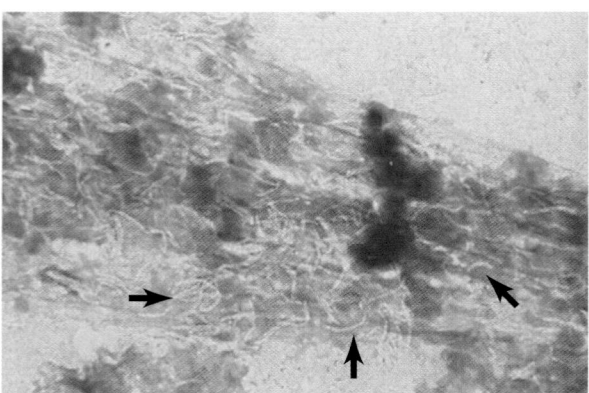

Plate 27

Expectorated sputum, smear, Gram stain, light microscopy, MPV. Amorphous debris heavy. Bacillary shapes, negative image. Oil removed from smear, decolorized with acid alcohol, and immediately restained with Ziehl-Neelsen acid-fast stain. Acid-fast bacilli numerous. Specimen recovered; acid-fast culture requested by laboratory. Suspicious for tuberculosis.

Plate 28

Expectorated sputum, concentrated smear, fluorochrome acid-fast stain, fluorescent microscopy, MPV. Typical acid-fast bacteria, numerous. *Impression*: Tuberculosis. The patient had been placed in respiratory isolation following physical examination and history and was immediately begun on antituberculosis therapy following receipt of the direct examination report. *Mycobacterium tuberculosis* was identified from culture.

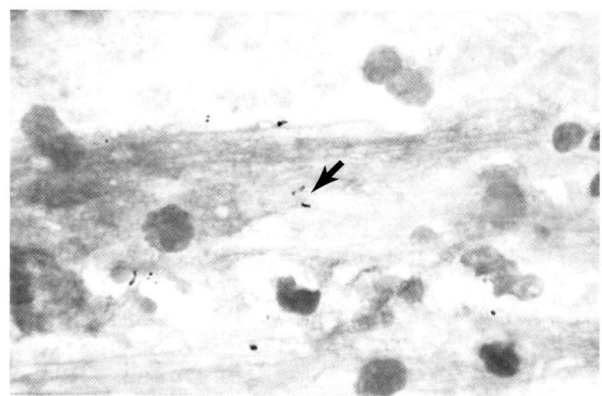

Plate 29 ─────────────

Expectorated sputum, smear, Gram stain, light microscopy, MPV. Purulence light. Local materials light. Amorphous debris moderate. Gram-positive bacilli, medium, beaded. Follow-up acid-fast stain positive. Chest radiograph with right upper lobe mass. Culture isolation of *Rhodococcus equi.*

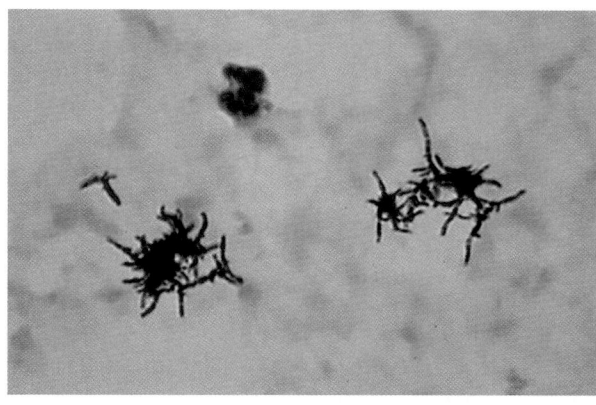

Plate 30 ─────────────

Blood culture, sediment smear, Gram stain, light microscopy, MPV. Blood. Gram-positive bacilli, branched, beaded. Morphology consistent with *Actinomyces* or *Propionibacterium* spp. Culture isolation of *Actinomyces israelii.*

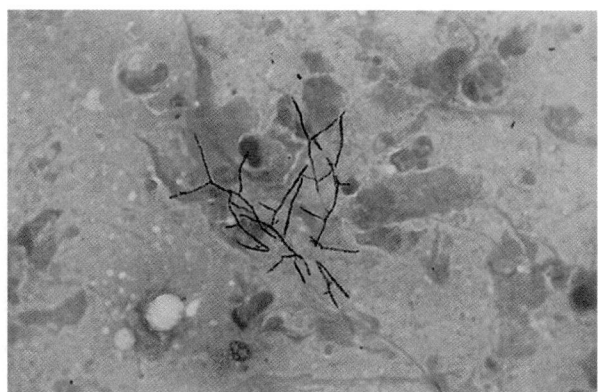

Plate 31 ─────────────

Expectorated sputum, smear, Gram stain, light microscopy, MPV. Purulence light. Local materials light. Amorphous debris moderate. Gram-positive bacilli, branched, beaded. Morphotype consistent with *Nocardia* or *Actinomyces.*

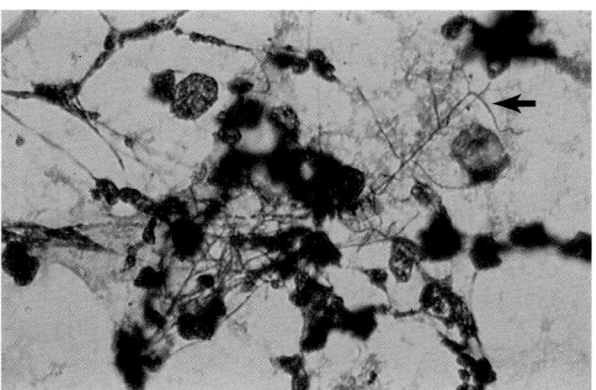

Plate 32 ─────────────

Expectorated sputum, smear, partial acid-fast stain, light microscopy, MPV. Partially acid-fast bacilli, branched, beaded. Morphology consistent with *Nocardia* spp. *Impression*: Nocardiosis.

DIRECT EXAMINATION IN GRAM-POSITIVE BACILLI WITH FILAMENTS AND BRANCHES

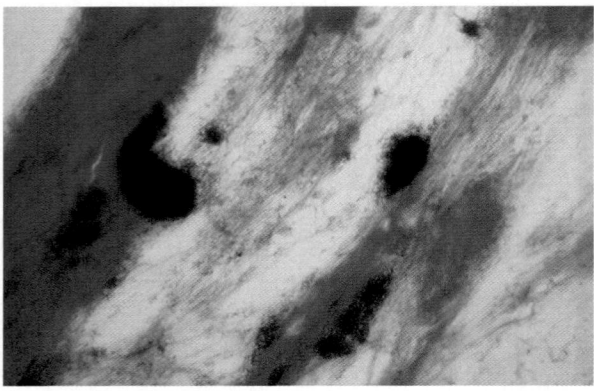

Plate 33

Jaw abscess aspirate, smear, Gram stain, light microscopy, low-power view (LPV). Purulence heavy. Granules present. Suspicious for *Actinomyces* (see Plate 34).

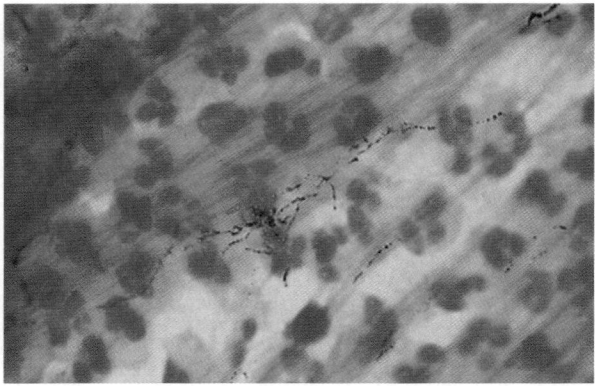

Plate 34

Jaw abscess aspirate, smear, Gram stain, light microscopy, high-power view (HPV). Purulence heavy. Gram-positive bacilli, filamentous, beaded, branched, partial acid-fast stain negative. Morphology consistent with *Actinomyces* spp. *Impression*: Actinomycosis (lumpy jaw).

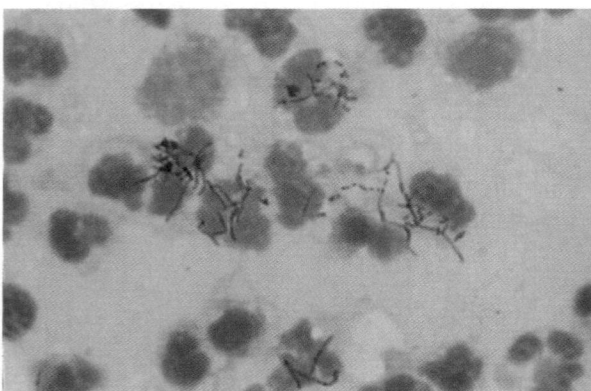

Plate 35

Cutaneous sinus tract aspirate, smear, Gram stain, light microscopy, HPV. Purulence heavy. Gram-positive bacilli, filamentous, beaded, branched, partial acid-fast stain negative. Morphology consistent with *Actinomyces* spp. (see Plate 36). *Impression*: Actinomycosis.

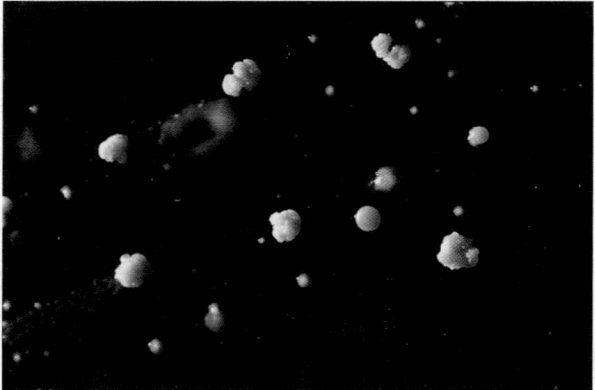

Plate 36

Cutaneous sinus tract aspirate, colonies on anaerobic blood agar plate. Mixed colony morphotypes. Molar tooth colonies. Morphology consistent with *Actinomyces israelii. Impression*: Mixed anaerobic infection–actinomycosis.

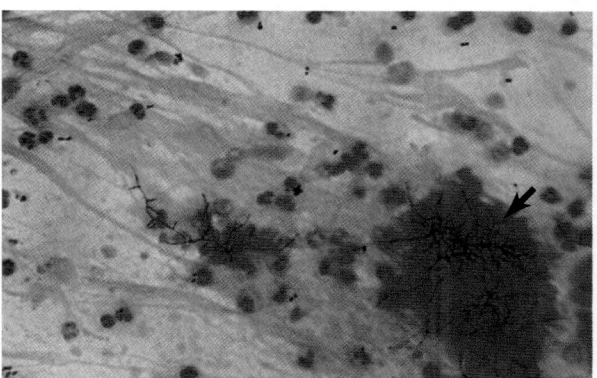

Plate 37

Expectorated sputum, smear, Gram stain, light microscopy, HPV. Purulence heavy. Local materials moderate. Grain present. Gram-positive bacilli, filamentous, beaded, branched. Suspicious for *Nocardia* or *Actinomyces* (see Plate 38).

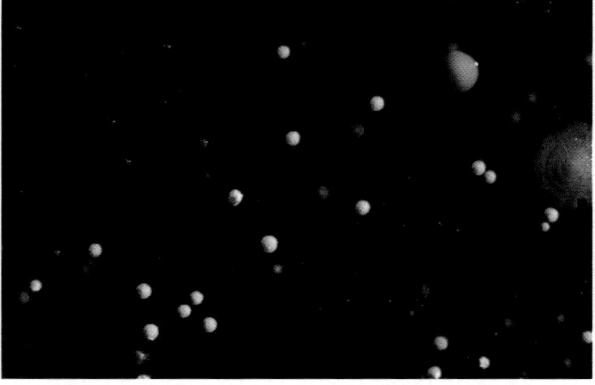

Plate 38

Expectorated sputum, chalky white colonies on plate with 5% sheep's blood agar at 5 days' incubation. Routine sputum culture. Morphology consistent with *Nocardia, Nocardiopsis,* or *Streptomyces* spp.

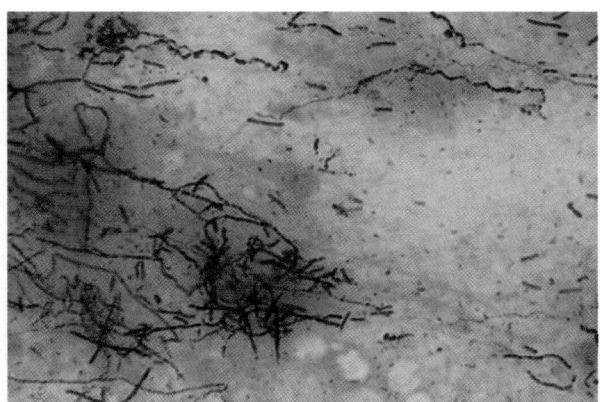

Plate 39

Sinus tract granule, crush-pull smear, Gram stain, light microscopy, HPV. Amorphous debris moderate. Gram-positive bacilli, filamentous, beaded, branched, partial acid-fast negative. Gram-positive bacilli, regular. Gram-negative bacilli, small. Gram-positive cocci. Morphology suggests mixed anaerobic infection with actinomycetes. *Impression*: Actinomycosis. Culture isolation of *Actinomyces naeslundii.*

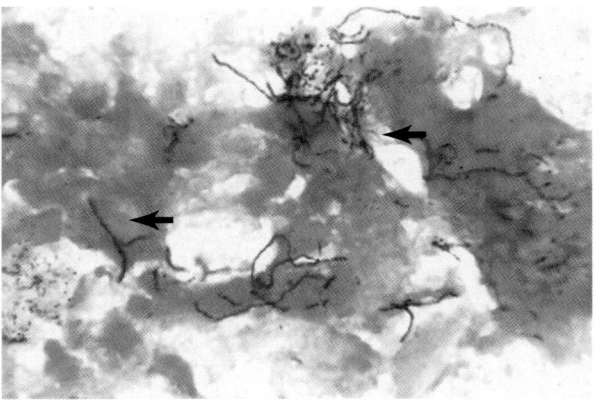

Plate 40

Surgical biopsy of abnormal area in jawbone, smear, Gram stain, light microscopy, HPV. Amorphous debris heavy. Gram-positive bacilli, filamentous, beaded, branched, partial acid-fast stain negative. Morphology suggests actinomycete. Aerobic and anaerobic cultures negative.

| DIRECT EXAMINATION IN SELECTED GRAM-NEGATIVE BACTERIAL INFECTIONS

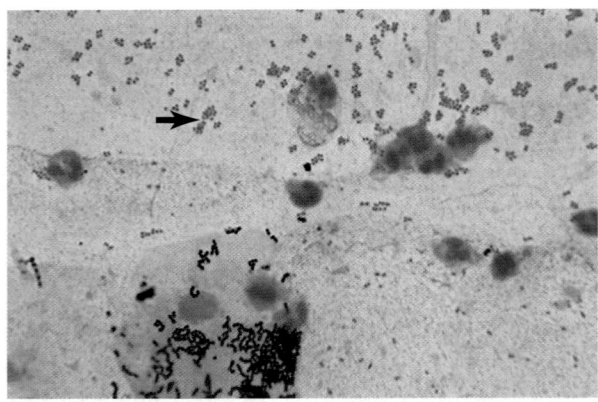

Plate 41 _____

Expectorated sputum, smear, Gram stain, light microscopy, medium-power view (MPV). Mixed materials, type I, layered. Contaminating bacteria and epithelial cells moderate. Purulence light. Gram-negative diplococci. Morphology suggests pathogenic *Neisseria* or *Moraxella* spp. Routine bacterial culture isolated *Moraxella catarrhalis.*

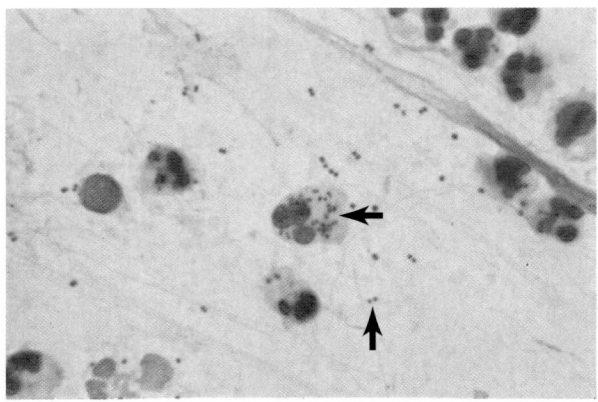

Plate 42 _____

Expectorated sputum, smear, Gram stain, light microscopy, MPV. Purulence moderate. Local materials moderate. Gram-negative diplococci, intracellular, extracellular. Morphology suggests pathogenic *Neisseria* or *Moraxella* spp. Routine bacterial culture isolated *Neisseria meningitidis.*

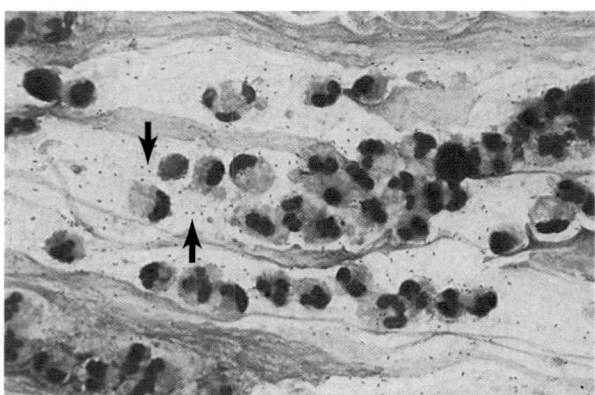

Plate 43 _____

Expectorated sputum, smear, Gram stain, light microscopy, high-power view (HPV). Purulence moderate. Local materials heavy. Mucus present. Gram-negative coccobacilli, intracellular, extracellular. Morphology consistent with *Haemophilus influenzae.*

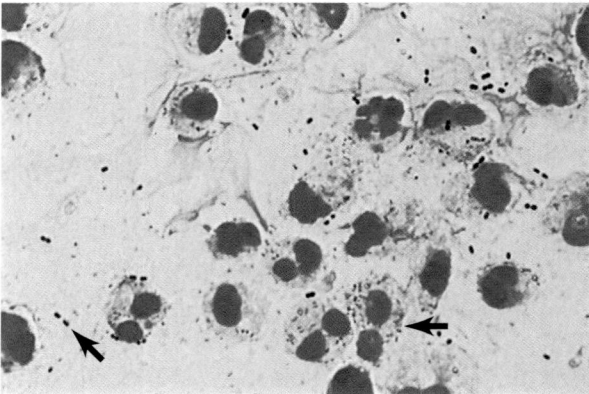

Plate 44 _____

Expectorated sputum, smear, Gram stain, light microscopy, HPV. Purulence heavy. Local materials moderate. Gram-negative bacilli, small, pleomorphic, intracellular, extracellular. Gram-positive diplococci, encapsulated, intracellular, extracellular. Morphology consistent with *H. influenzae* and *Streptococcus pneumoniae. Impression*: Polymicrobial infection.

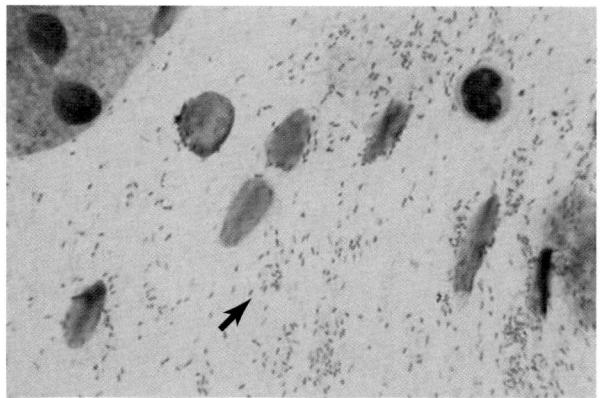

Plate 45 _____

Bronchoalveolar lavage, cytocentrifuge preparation. Wright-Giemsa stain, light microscopy, HPV. Purulence none. Lymphocytes present. Local materials moderate. Small bacilli, numerous (see Plate 46).

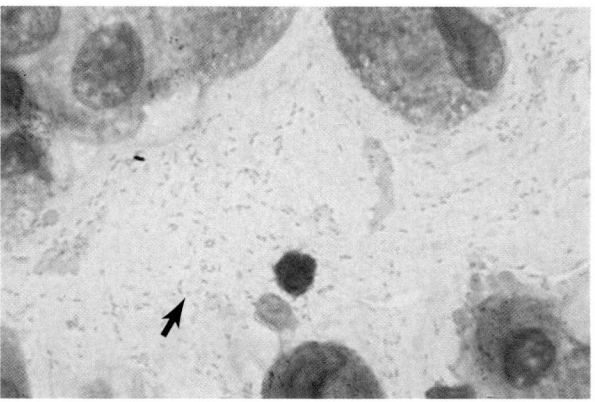

Plate 46 _____

Bronchoalveolar lavage, cytocentrifuge preparation, Gram stain, light microscopy, HPV. Purulence none. Lymphocytes present. Local materials moderate. Gram-negative bacilli, small (see Plate 47).

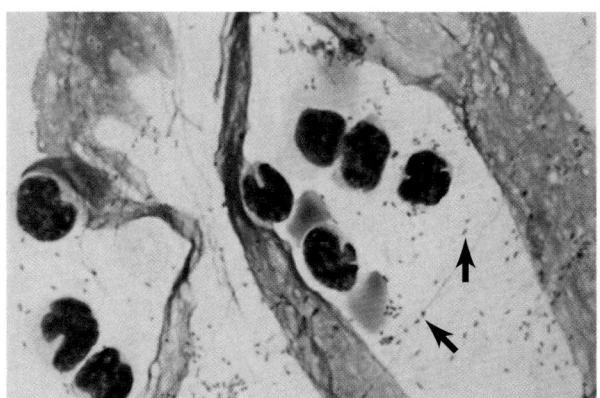

Plate 47 _____

Bronchoalveolar lavage, cytocentrifuge preparation, Wright-Giemsa stain, light microscopy, HPV. Purulence none. Lymphocytes present. Local materials moderate. Gram-negative bacilli, small (see plate 48).

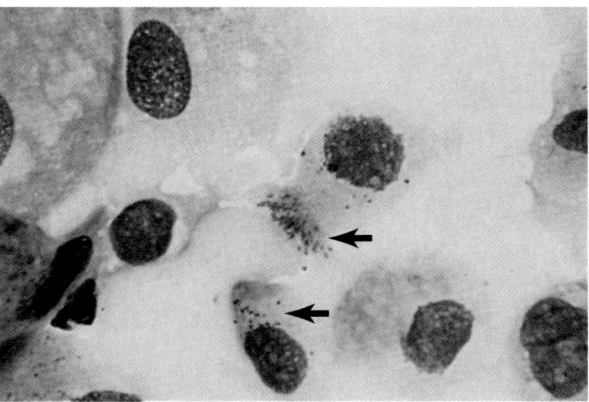

Plate 48 _____

Bronchoalveolar lavage, cytocentrifuge preparation. Wright-Giemsa stain, light microscopy, HPV. Purulence none. Lymphocytes present. Local materials moderate. Ciliated columnar epithelial cells with numerous small bacilli adherent to cilia. Morphology consistent with _Bordetella pertussis._ _Impression_: Whooping cough.

DIRECT EXAMINATION IN SELECTED GRAM-NEGATIVE BACILLARY INFECTIONS

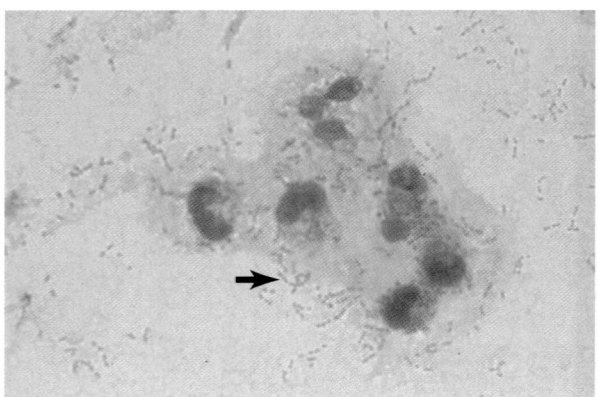

Plate 49

Cerebrospinal fluid (CSF), drop smear, Gram stain, light microscopy, high-power view (HPV). Purulence moderate. Gram-negative coccobacilli, chains. Morphotype suggests *Bacteroides* spp. *Impression*: Gram-negative bacillary meningitis.

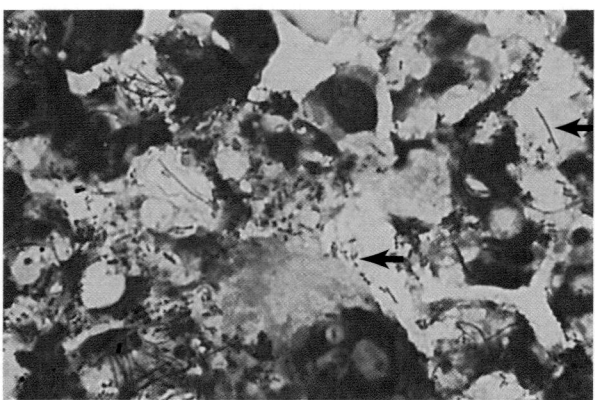

Plate 50

Amniotic fluid, cytocentrifuge preparation, Gram stain, light microscopy, HPV. Purulence moderate. Local materials moderate. Gram-negative coccobacilli. Gram-negative bacilli, filamentous, medium, fusiform. Morphology suggests gram-negative bacillary anaerobic infection. *Impression*: Amnionitis, mixed anaerobic bacteria.

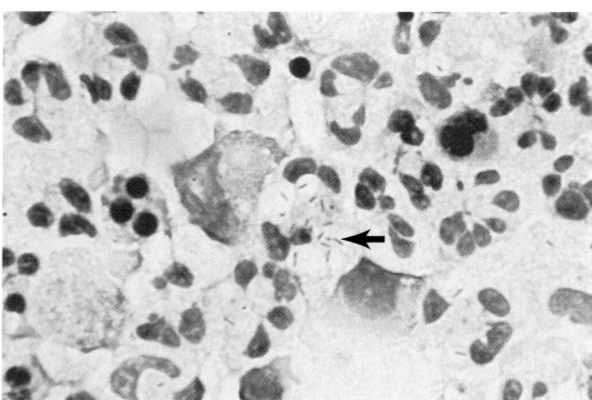

Plate 51

Bronchoalveolar lavage, cytocentrifuge preparation, Gram stain, light microscopy, HPV. Purulence moderate. Local materials light. Gram-negative bacilli, small, intracellular within phagocytic vacuoles (see Plate 52).

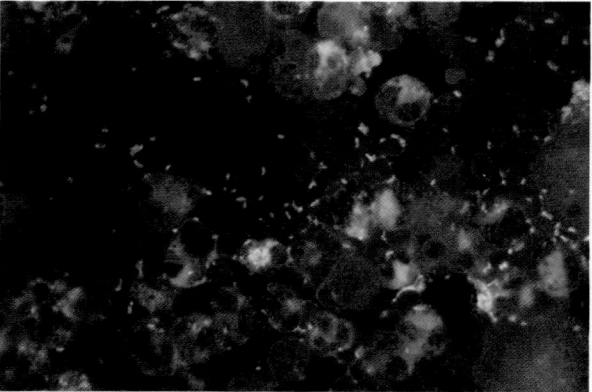

Plate 52

Bronchoalveolar lavage, cytocentrifuge preparation, direct fluorescent antibody (DFA). *Legionella pneumophila,* polyvalent antisera, fluorescent microscopy, HPV. Immunofluorescence positive. *Impression*: Legionnaires' disease.

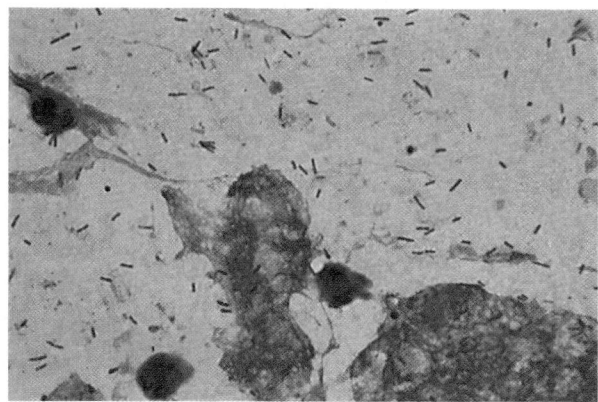

Plate 53

Expectorated sputum, smear, Gram stain, light microscopy, medium-power view (MPV). Purulence light. Local materials light. Mucus moderate. Gram-negative bacilli, medium. *Impression*: Enteric bacillary infection.

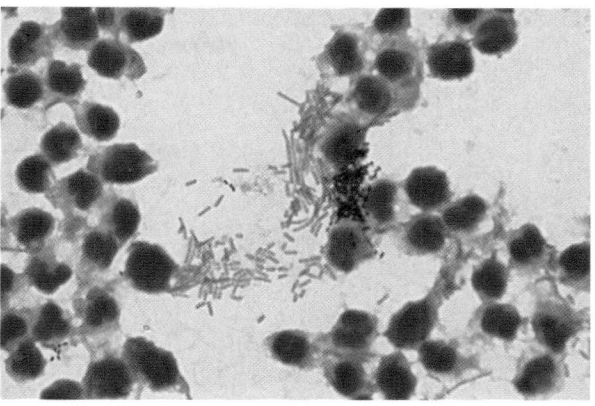

Plate 54

Urine, direct drop smear, Gram stain, light microscopy, MPV. Purulence heavy. Gram-negative bacilli, medium. Gram-positive cocci. Urine culture grew *Escherichia coli* and *Enterococcus faecalis*. The smear is consistent with a bacterial density of 10^5 colony forming units per mL of urine.

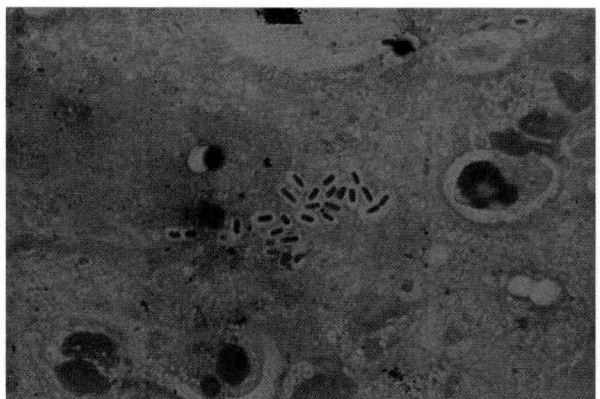

Plate 55

Decubitus skin ulcer, smear, Gram stain, light microscopy, HPV. Purulence moderate. Amorphous debris heavy. Gram-negative bacilli, medium, encapsulated. Yeast. Morphology suggests *Klebsiella pneumoniae*. *Impression*: Enteric bacillary disease.

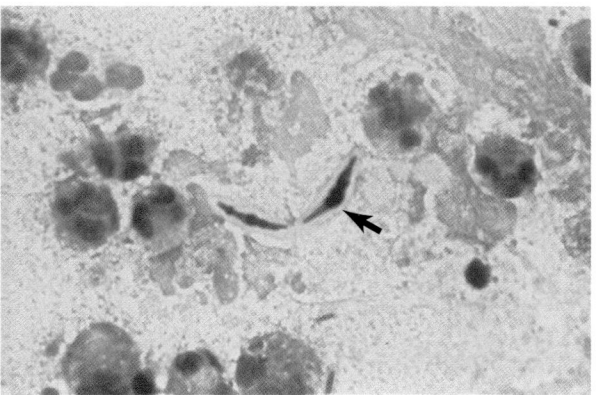

Plate 56

Expectorated sputum, smear, Gram stain, light microscopy, HPV. Purulence moderate. Mucus moderate. Gram-negative bacilli, aberrant, encapsulated. Morphology suggests antibiotic-affected *K. pneumoniae*. *Impression*: Enteric bacillary disease, partially treated.

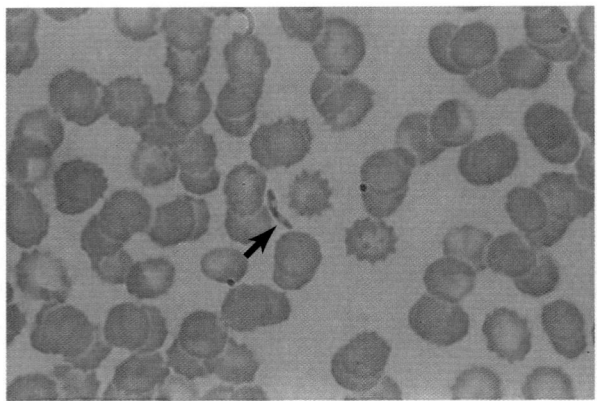

Plate 57 _____

Peripheral blood, smear, Wright/Giemsa stain, light microscopy medium-power view (MPV). Bacilli, medium, bipolar staining (see Plate 58).

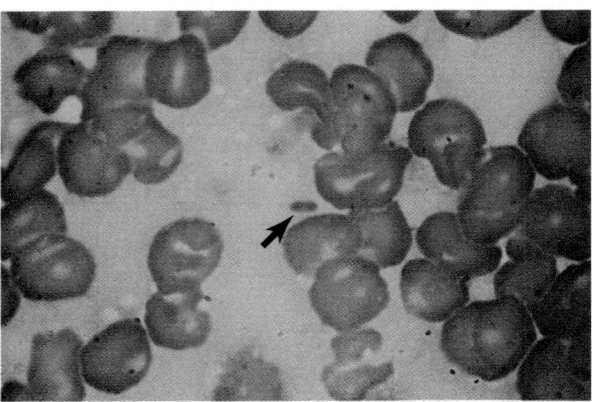

Plate 58 _____

Peripheral blood, smear, Gram stain, light microscopy, high-power view (HPV). Local materials moderate. Gram-negative bacillus, medium, with prominent bipolar staining. Suspicious for *Yersinia pestis*. *Impression*: Bubonic plague.

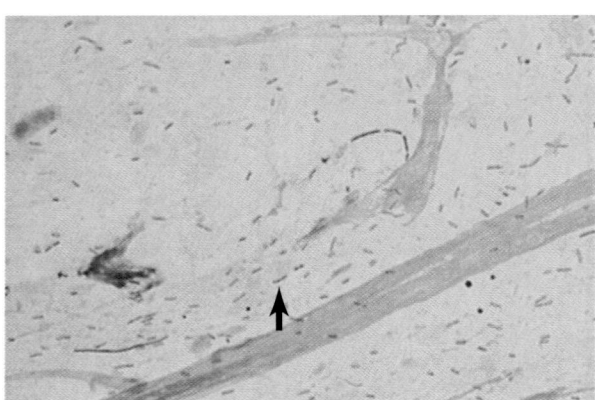

Plate 59 _____

Expectorated sputum, smear, Gram stain, light microscopy, HPV. Purulence none. Local materials none. Mucus present. Gram-negative bacilli, regular, chains. Morphotype suggests *Pseudomonas aeruginosa*. *Impression*: *Pseudomonas* infectious disease.

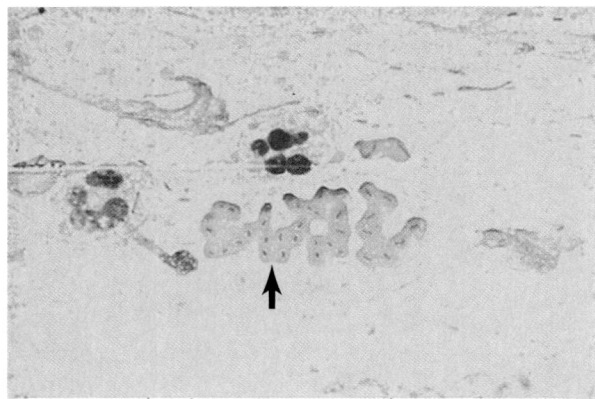

Plate 60 _____

Expectorated sputum, smear, Gram stain, light microscopy, HPV. Purulence light. Local materials none. Mucus present. Gram-negative bacilli, regular, enveloped in prominent slime layer. Morphotype suggests mucoid *P. aeruginosa*. *Impression*: Pseudomonas infectious disease.

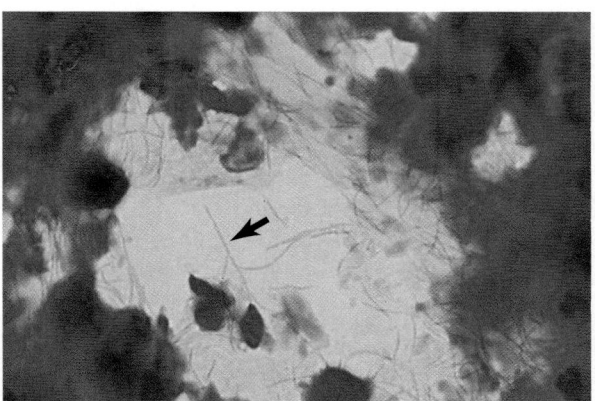

Plate 61

Amniotic fluid, cytocentrifuge preparation, Gram stain, light microscopy, HPV. Purulence light. Local material moderate. Gram-negative bacilli, fusiform. Morphology suggests *Fusobacterium nucleatum*. *Impression*: Amnionitis anaerobic bacteria.

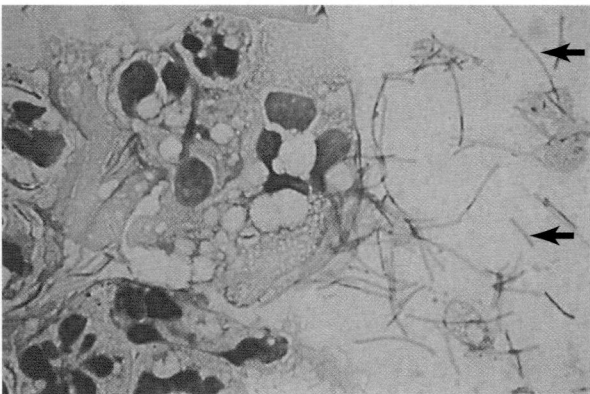

Plate 62

Amniotic fluid, cytocentrifuge preparation, Gram stain, light microscopy, HPV. Purulence moderate. Local material moderate. Gram-negative bacilli, medium and long forms. Morphology suggests *Fusobacterium* spp. *Impression*: Amnionitis, anaerobic bacteria.

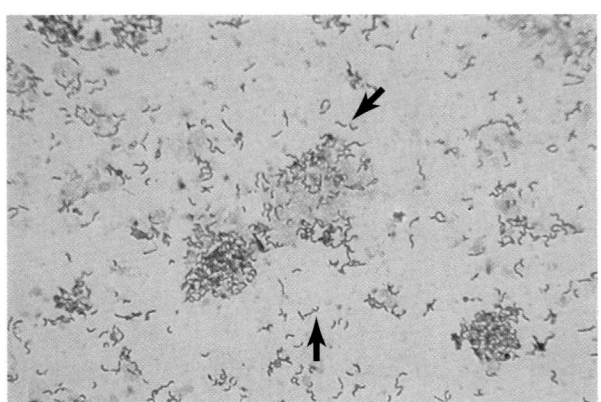

Plate 63

Colonies on blood agar medium, subculture from blood culture, smear, Gram stain, light microscopy, HPV. Local material light. Gram-negative bacilli with spirals, gull-wings. Morphology suggests *Campylobacter* spp.

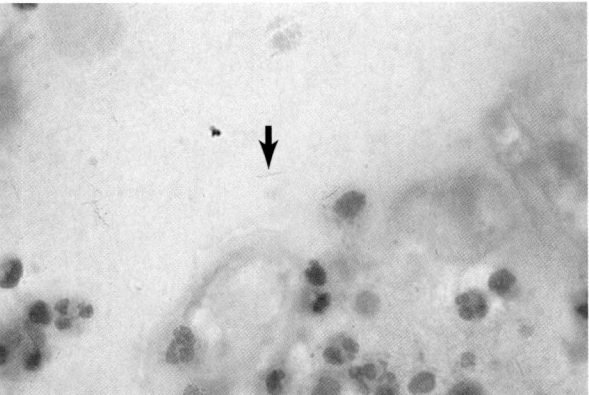

Plate 64

Amniotic fluid, drop smear, Gram stain, light microscopy, HPV. Purulence moderate. Local materials moderate. Gram-negative bacilli, spiral. *Impression*: Amnionitis.

DIRECT EXAMINATION IN POLYMICROBIAL INFECTIONS

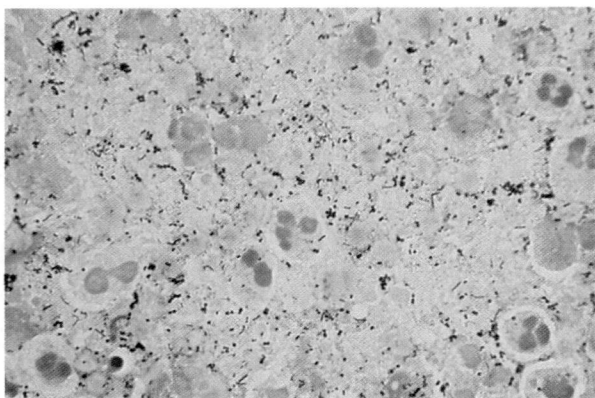

Plate 65

Buccal space abscess, smear, Gram stain, light microscopy, high-power view (HPV). Purulence heavy. Gram-positive cocci, pairs, chains. Gram-positive bacilli, small, diphtheroid, medium, branched. Gram-negative coccobacilli. Morphology suggests polymicrobial infection from mouth flora. *Impression*: Polymicrobial infection, oropharyngeal flora.

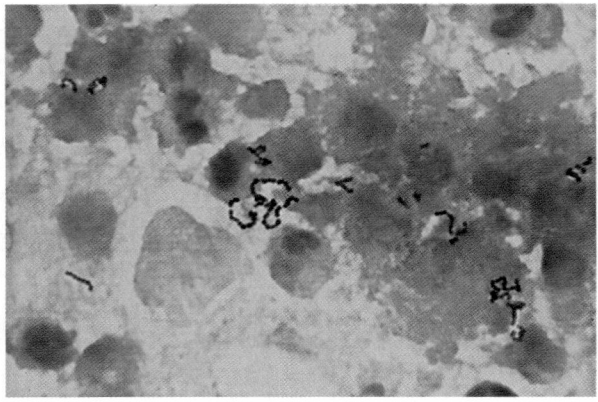

Plate 66

Maxillary sinus aspirate, smear, Gram stain, light microscopy, HPV. Purulence heavy. Gram-positive cocci, chains. Gram-negative coccobacilli, large masses. Morphotype suggests mixed infection with streptococci and anaerobic Gram-negative coccobacilli. *Impression*: Polymicrobial infection, aerobic and anaerobic species.

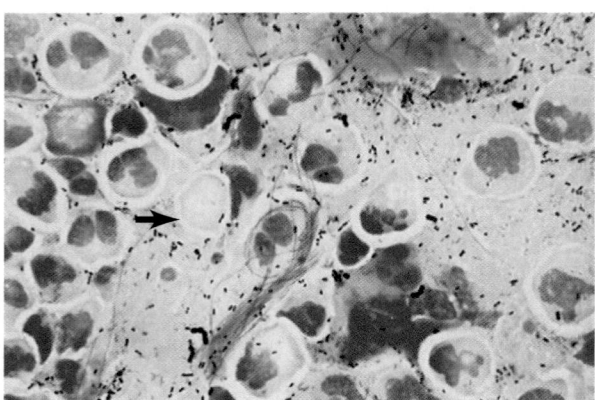

Plate 67

Cervix, smear, conventional Gram stain, light microscopy, medium-power view (MPV). Purulence heavy. Gram-positive cocci, pairs. Gram-negative coccobacilli. Gram-negative filaments. Trichomonads *(arrow) (Trichomonas vaginalis)* (compare with Plate 68). *Impression*: Trichomoniasis with mixed aerobic and anaerobic bacterial flora.

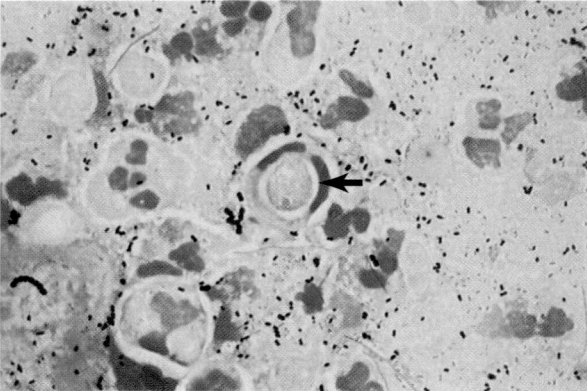

Plate 68

Cervix, smear, *enhanced* Gram stain, light microscopy, MPV. Purulence heavy. Gram-positive cocci, pairs. Gram-negative coccobacilli. Gram-negative filaments. Trichomonads *(arrow) (Trichomonas vaginalis)*. *Impression*: Trichomoniasis with mixed aerobic and anaerobic bacterial flora.

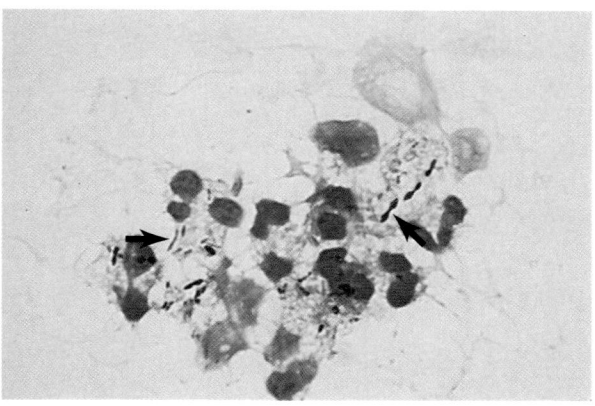

Plate 69

Eye, vitreous aspirate, smear, Gram stain, light microscopy, MPV. Purulence moderate. Gram-positive diplococci, encapsulated, lancet-shaped. Gram-negative bacilli, small, pleomorphic. Morphotype suggests mixed infection with *Streptococcus pneumoniae* and *Haemophilus influenzae*. *Impression*: Vitritis, mixed infection.

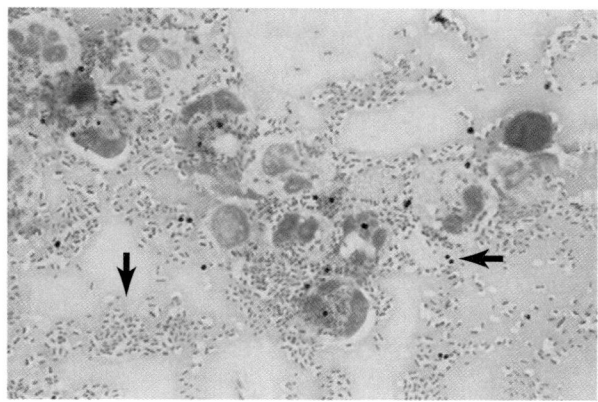

Plate 70

Wound, smear, Gram stain, light microscopy, MPV. Purulence heavy. Gram-negative bacilli, medium. Gram-positive cocci, pairs. *Impression*: Enteric bacillary infectious disease.

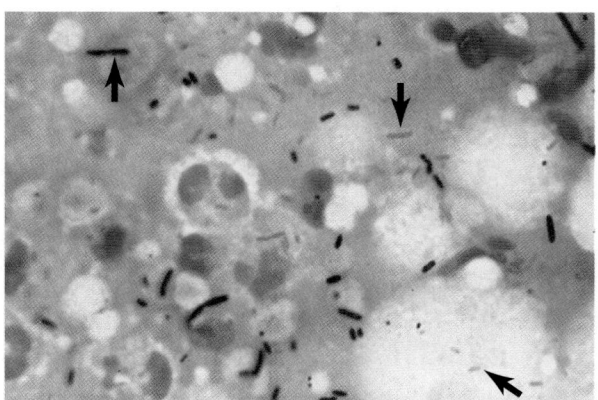

Plate 71

Drainage, ruptured appendix, smear, light microscopy, HPV. Purulence heavy. Gram-positive bacilli, large and medium forms. Gram-negative bacilli, small, bipolar. Gram-positive cocci. Morphology suggest polymicrobial infection with fecal flora. *Impression*: Polymicrobial infection, fecal flora.

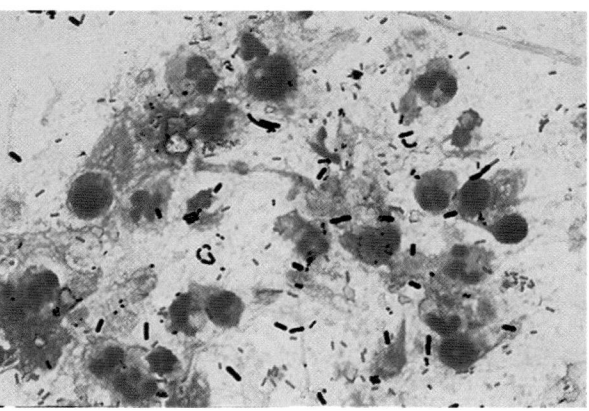

Plate 72

Aspirated sputum, smear, Gram stain, light microscopy, MPV. Purulence light. Local material light. Gram-positive bacilli, large. Gram-negative bacilli, medium, intracellular. Gram-positive cocci, pairs, chains. Morphology suggests polymicrobial infection with fecal flora. *Impression*: Polymicrobial infection, fecal flora.

DIRECT EXAMINATION IN FUNGAL INFECTIONS

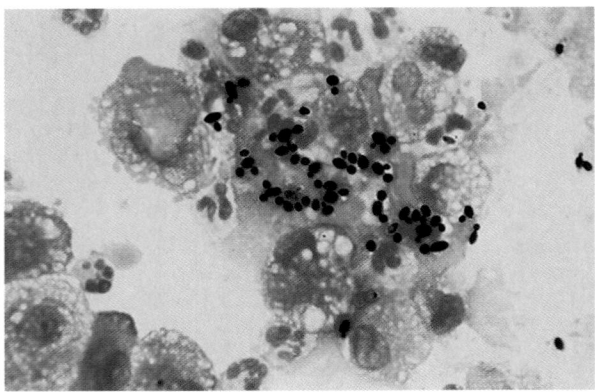

Plate 73

Bronchoalveolar lavage, cytocentrifuge preparation, Gram stain, microscopy, high-power view (HPV). Purulence light. Local materials moderate. Gram-positive yeast with buds. Morphotype consistent with *Candida* spp. *Impression*: Candidiasis.

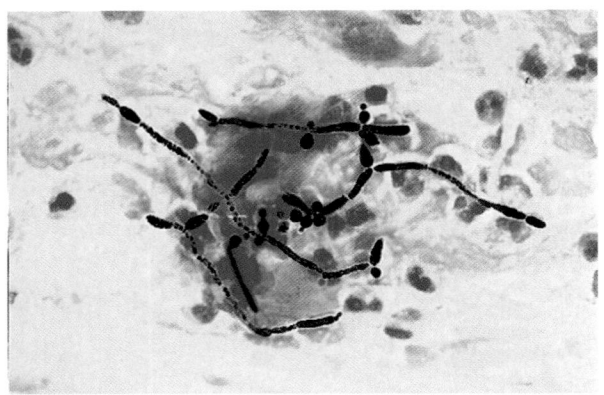

Plate 74

Expectorated sputum smear, Gram stain, light microscopy, HPV. Purulence light. Local materials moderate. Gram-positive pseudohyphae. Morphotype consistent with *Candida* spp. *Impression*: Candidiasis.

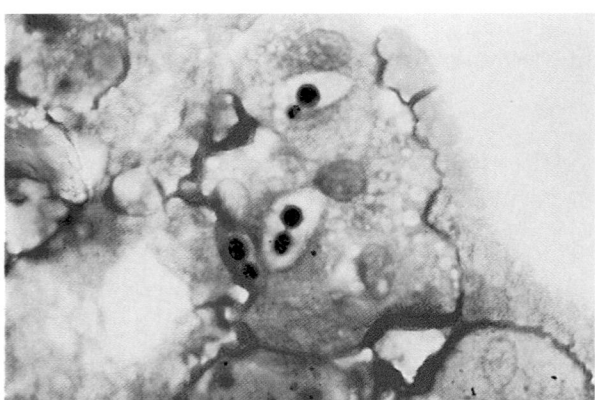

Plate 75

Bronchoalveolar lavage, cytocentrifuge preparation, Gram stain, light microscopy, HPV. Local materials moderate. Red blood cells present. Gram-variable yeast with capsules. Morphology suggests *Cryptococcus* (see Plate 76).

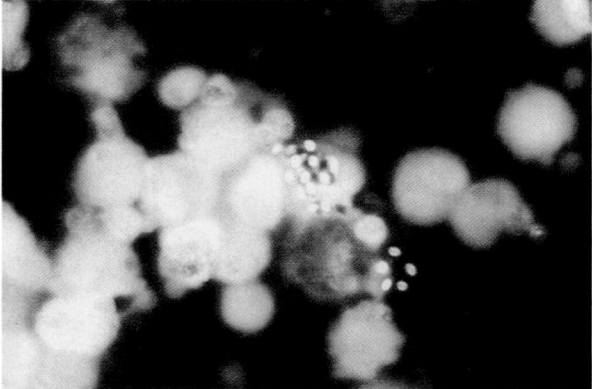

Plate 76

Bronchoalveolar lavage, cytocentrifuge preparation, calcofluor white stain, fluorescence microscopy, HPV. Fluorescent yeast, small, with capsules. Morphology suggests *Cryptococcus neoformans*. *Impression*: Cryptococcosis.

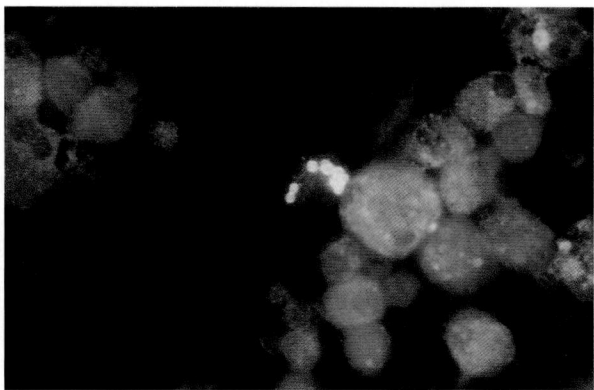

Plate 77

Bronchoalveolar lavage, cytocentrifuge preparation, calco-fluor white stain, light microscopy, HPV. Fluorescent yeast (2 to 4 μm), small, budding. Morphology suggests *Histo-plasma capsulatum. Impression*: Histoplasmosis.

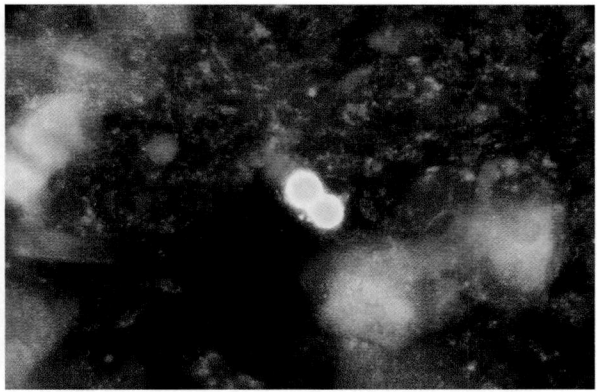

Plate 78

Expectorated sputum, smear, calcofluor white stain, fluorescence microscopy, medium-power view (MPV). Yeast (8 to 20 μm), round, thick-walled, broad-based bud. Morphology suggests *Blastomyces dermatitidis. Impression*: Blastomycosis.

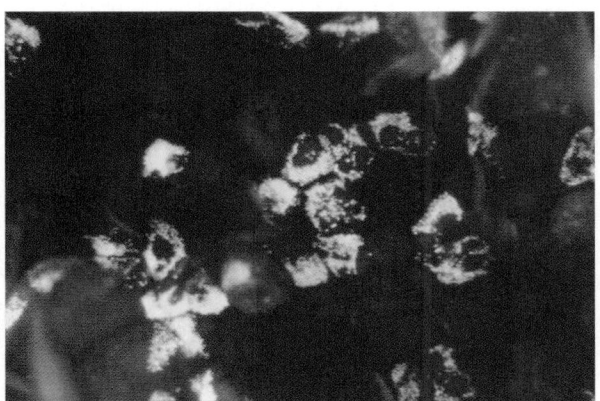

Plate 79

Expectorated sputum, smear, calcofluor white stain, fluores-cence microscopy, MPV. Eosinophils. These cells are another component that stains with calcofluor white. The granules from ruptured eosinophils stain brightly and should not be interpreted as remnants of fungi or parasites.

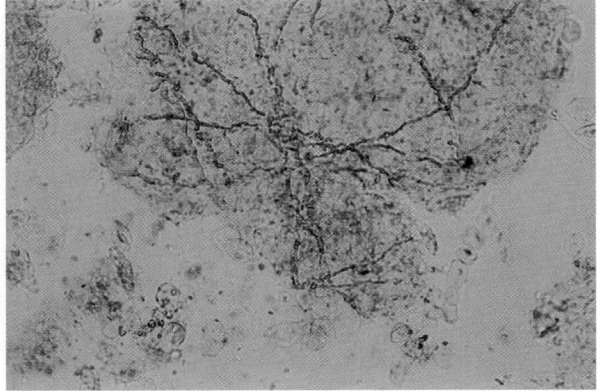

Plate 80

Skin scales, scrapings, KOH wet preparation, light mi-croscopy, high-power view (HPV). Hyphae present, septate, thin. Morphology suggests dermatophyte.

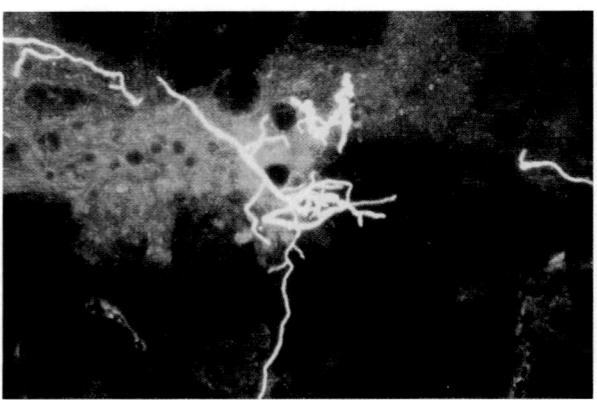

Plate 81 _____

Skin scales from scrapings, calcofluor white stain, fluorescence microscopy, HPV. Hyphae, thin. Morphology suggests dermatophyte. *Impression*: Dermatophytosis.

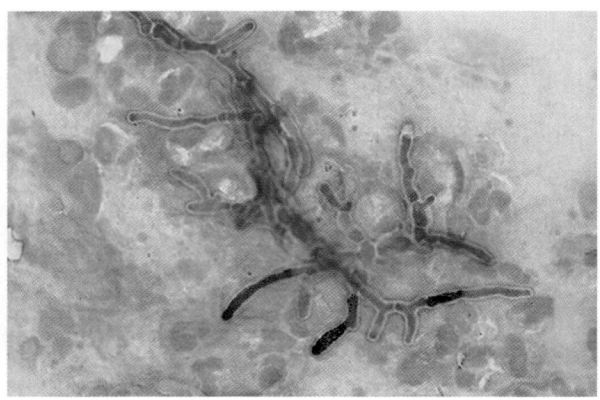

Plate 82 _____

Expectorated sputum, smear, Gram stain, light microscopy, HPV. Purulence light, Local materials heavy. Gram-variable hyphae present (3 to 10 μm), septate, branched 45-degree angle. Morphology suggests *Aspergillus* spp. (see Plate 83).

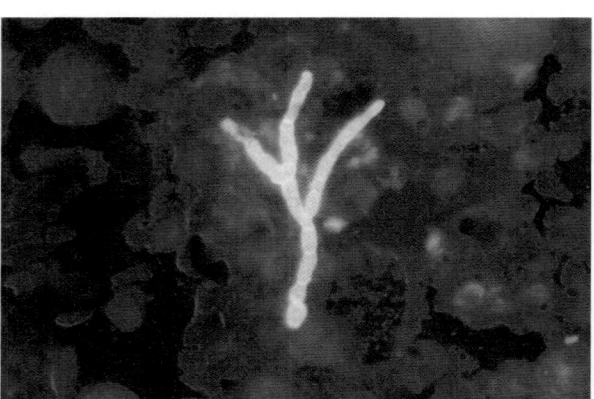

Plate 83 _____

Expectorated sputum, smear, calcofluor white stain, fluorescence microscopy, medium-power view (MPV). Fungal hyphae present (3 to 10 μm), septate, branched 45-degree angle. Morphology suggests *Aspergilus* spp. *Impression*: Aspergillosis.

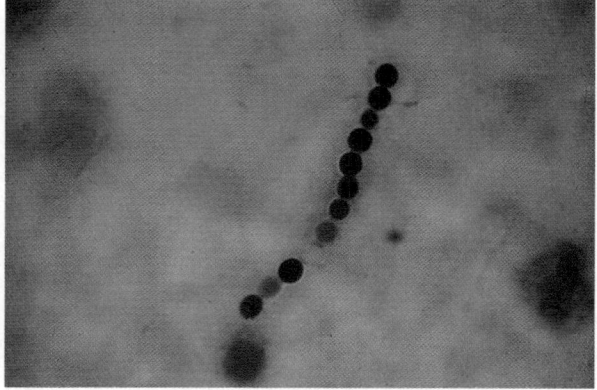

Plate 84 _____

Expectorated sputum, smear, Gram stain, light microscopy, HPV. Purulence none. Local materials moderate. Gram-positive conidia (2 to 4 μm), in chain. Morphotype suggests *Aspergillus* spp. in cavity with air interface. *Impression*: Cavitary aspergillosis. Care must be taken not to mistake these conidia for streptococci or for yeast (see Plate 85).

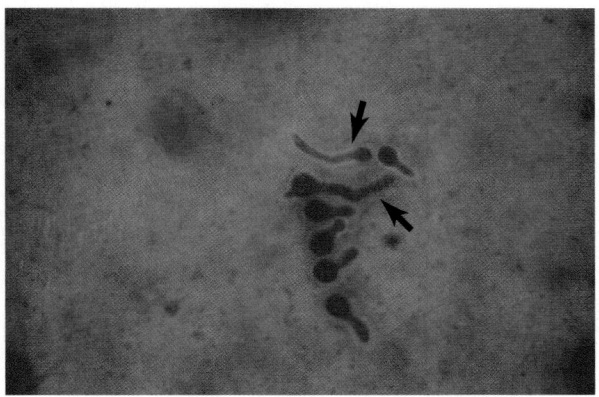

Plate 85 _____

Expectorated sputum, smear, Gram stain, light microscopy, HPV. Purulence none. Local materials moderate. Gram-negative conidia (2 to 4 μm), sporulating. Care must be taken not to confuse these conidia with yeast germ tubes.

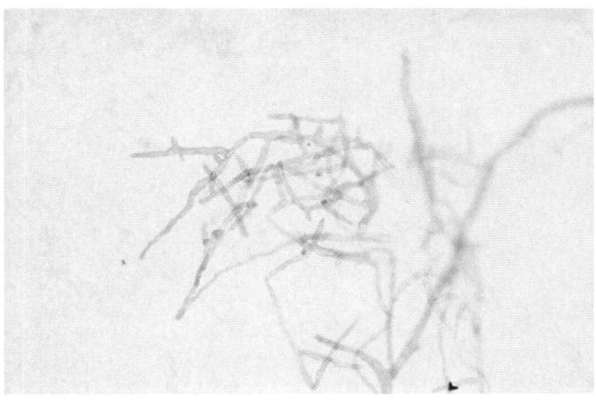

Plate 86 _____

Brain abscess, smear, toluidine blue stain, light microscopy, MPV. Fungal hyphae present (3 to 10 μm), septate, branched 45-degree angle. Morphology suggests *Aspergillus* spp. *Impression*: Cerebral aspergillosis.

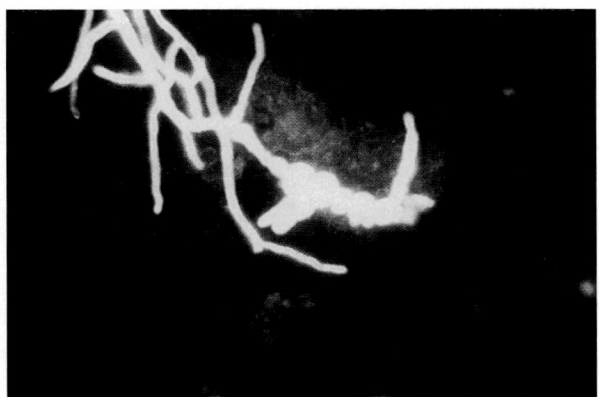

Plate 87 _____

Soft tissue abscess, smear, calcofluor white stain, fluorescence microscopy, HPV. Fungal hyphae, septate, branched chlamydospores. *Impression*: Mycosis.

These hyphae were not clearly visible on the Gram stain smear but stain brightly here. A dermatophyte was isolated in culture.

DIRECT EXAMINATION IN PARASITIC INFECTIONS

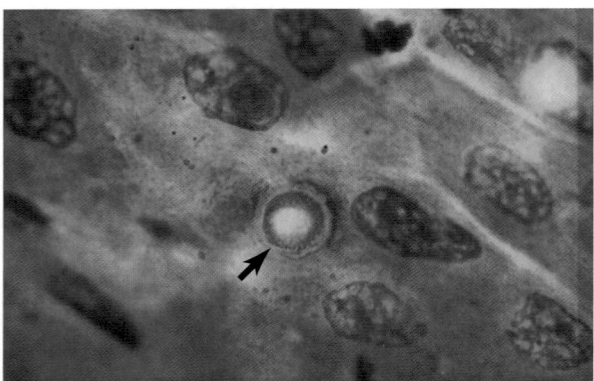

Plate 88

Cornea, scraping, Wright-Giemsa stain, light microscopy, high-power view (HPV). Purulence none. Local materials moderate. Parasitic precyst (13 μm). Morphology consistent with *Acanthamoeba* spp.

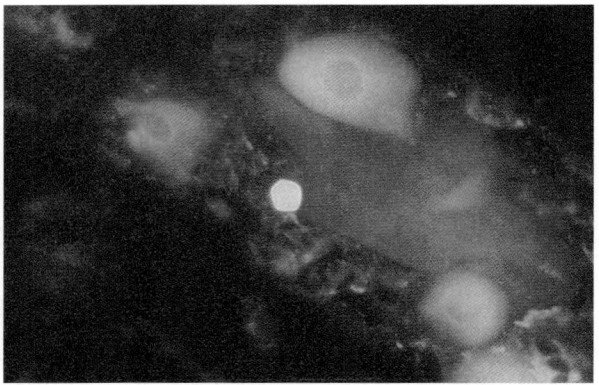

Plate 89

Cornea, scraping from Plate 88, calcofluor white stain, fluorescence microscopy, medium-power view (MPV). Polyhedral parasitic cyst (13 μm). Morphology consistent with *Acanthamoeba* cyst. *Impression*: *Acanthamoeba* keratitis.

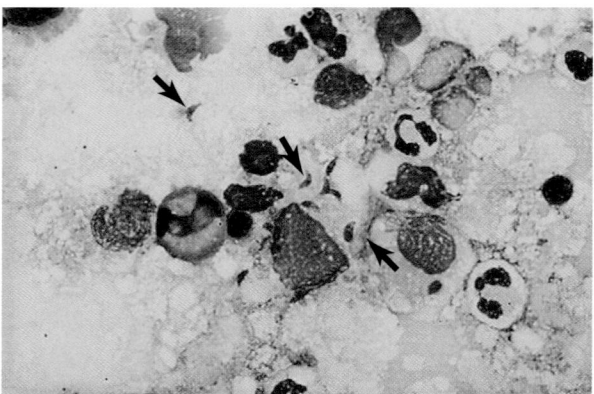

Plate 90

Bronchoalveolar lavage, cytocentrifuge preparation, Wright-Giemsa stain, light microscopy, HPV. Purulence light. Local materials light. Amorphous debris light. Crescent-shaped cells with central nucleus (see Plate 91).

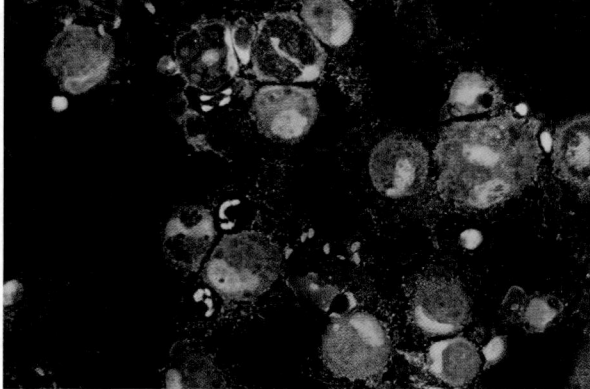

Plate 91

Bronchoalveolar lavage, cytocentrifuge preparation, acridine orange stain, fluorescence microscopy, HPV. Crescent-shaped cells composed of RNA. Morphology consistent with trophozoites (tachyzoites) of *Toxoplasma gondii. Impression*: Toxoplasmosis.

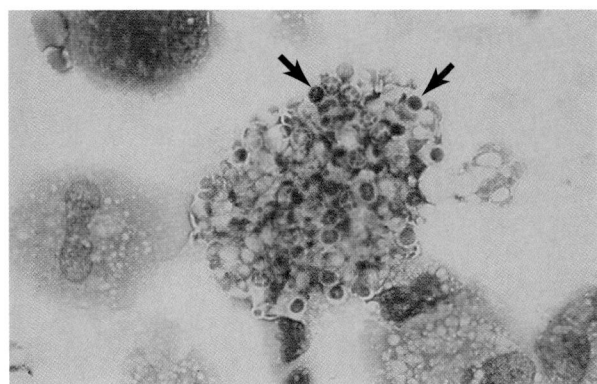

Plate 92

Bronchoalveolar lavage, cytocentrifuge preparation, Gram stain, light microscopy, HPV. Purulence none. Local materials moderate. Alveolar cast composed of gram-negative matrix and intracystic bodies. Morphology consistent with *Pneumocystis carinii* (see Plate 93).

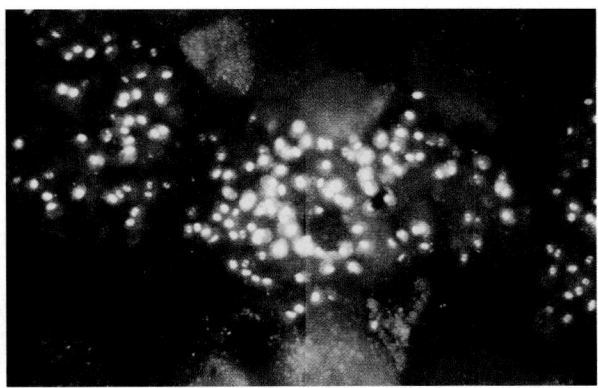

Plate 93

Bronchoalveolar lavage, cytocentrifuge preparation, calcofluor white stain, fluorescence microscopy, HPV. Fluorescent cysts with coccoid bodies. Morphology consistent with *P. carinii*. *Impression*: Pneumocystosis.

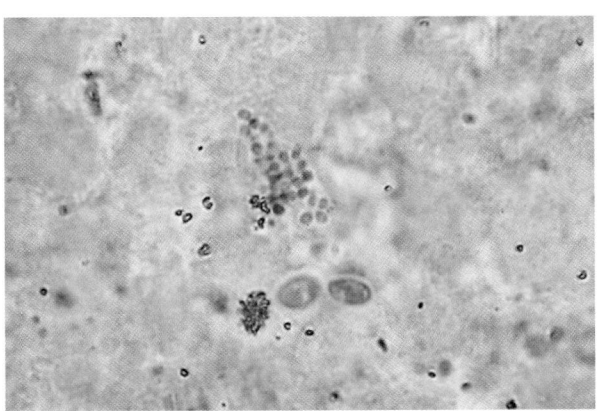

Plate 94

Diarrheic stool, smear, modified Weber stain, light microscopy, 2000× oil. Purulence none. Parasite spores small (1.5 × 0.9 μm). Morphology consistent with enterocytozoon (see Plate 95).

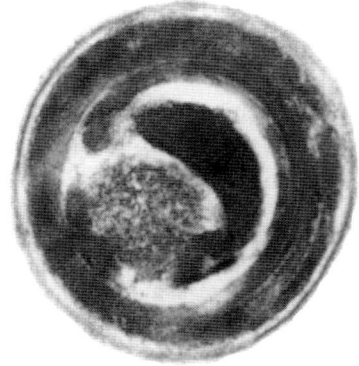

Plate 95

Diarrheic stool from concentration, transmission electron microscopy, 57,000×. Endospore layer and polar tubes present. Morphology consistent with *Enterocytozoon bieneusi*. *Impression*: Intestinal microsporidiosis.

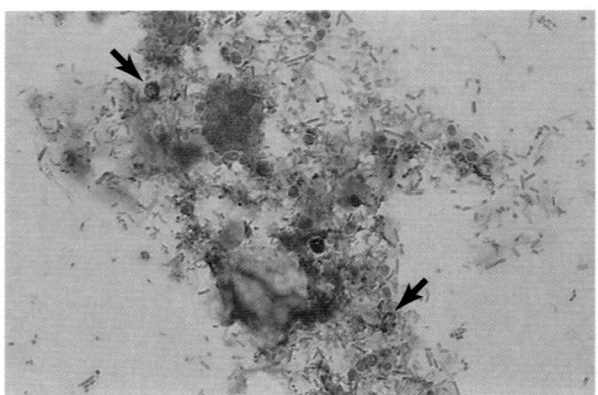

Plate 96 _____

Watery, frothy diarrheic stool, smear, acid-fast stain, medium-power view (MPV). Purulence none. Local materials heavy. Acid-fast oocysts (4 to 6 μm) (see Plate 97). The measurement is taken to clearly separate this oocyst from the 8 to 10 μm oocysts of *Cyclospora* spp.

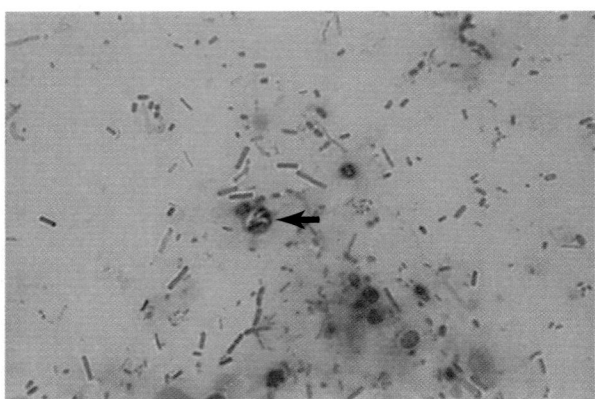

Plate 97 _____

Watery, frothy diarrheic stool from Plate 96, smear, acid-fast stain, high-power view (HPV). Acid-fast oocysts (4 to 6 μm). Sporulated oocysts containing four sporozoites. Morphology consistent with *Cryptosporidium parvum. Impression*: Cryptosporidiosis.

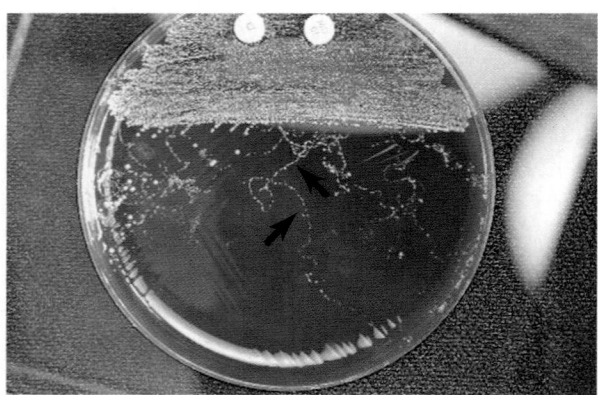

Plate 98 _____

5% Sheep's blood agar plate inoculated with expectorated sputum, 24-hour incubation with 5% CO_2 in air. Note the heavy bacterial growth in the area of primary inoculation with thin trails of colonies lacing the surface of the agar (see Plate 99).

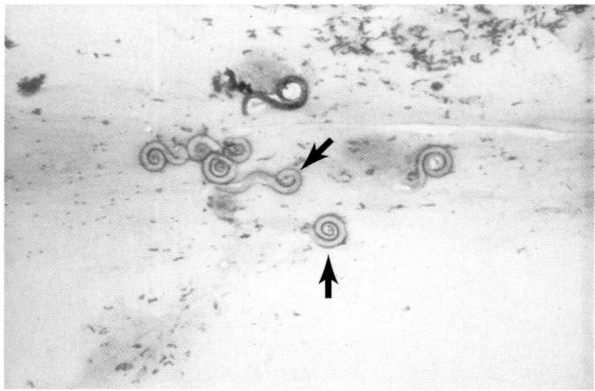

Plate 99 _____

Aspirated sputum, Gram stain, light microscopy, low-power view (LPV). Purulence none. Local materials moderate. Mucus present. Coiled nematode larvae. Morphology consistent with *Strongyloides stercoralis. Impression*: *Strongyloides* hyperinfestation syndrome.

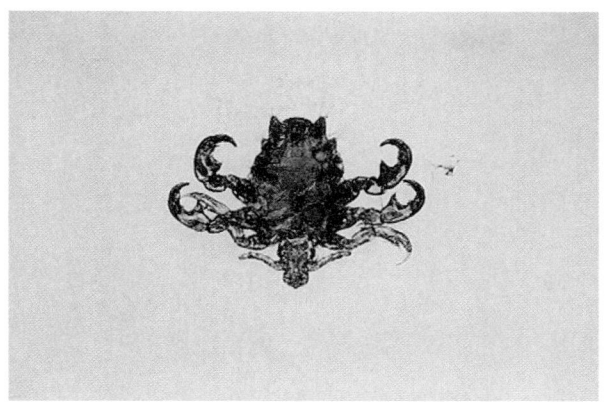

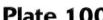

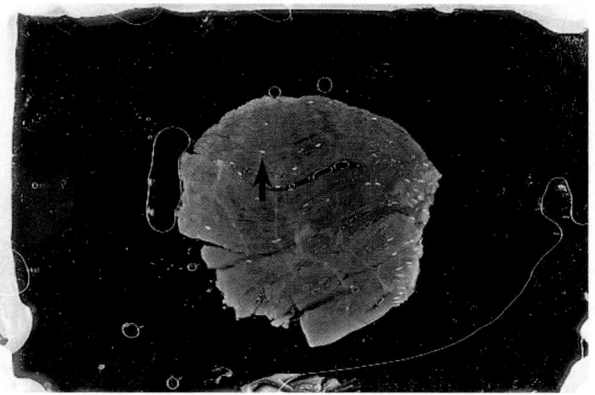

Plate 100

Parasite, pubic hair from surgical patient, unstained mount, light microscopy, LPV. Three pair of legs are identified with characteristic claws at tips. Morphology consistent with *Phthirus pubis* (crab louse). *Impression*: Louse infestation.

Plate 101

Muscle tissue, directly viewed. Encysted calcified larvae. Morphology consistent with *Trichinella spiralis. Impression*: Trichinosis.

DIRECT EXAMINATION IN VIRAL INFECTIONS

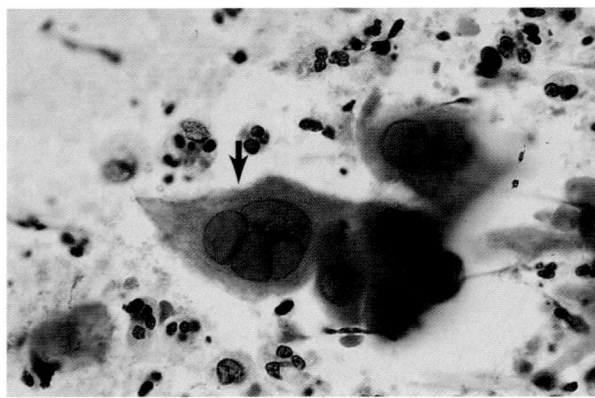

Plate 102

Skin, vesicle fluid, Tzanck preparation, hematoxylin and eosin (H&E) stain, light microscopy, medium-power view (MPV). Purulence moderate. Local materials light. Multinucleated epithelial cells present. Intranuclear inclusions present. Morphology consistent with herpes viral inclusions. *Impression*: Herpes simplex infection.

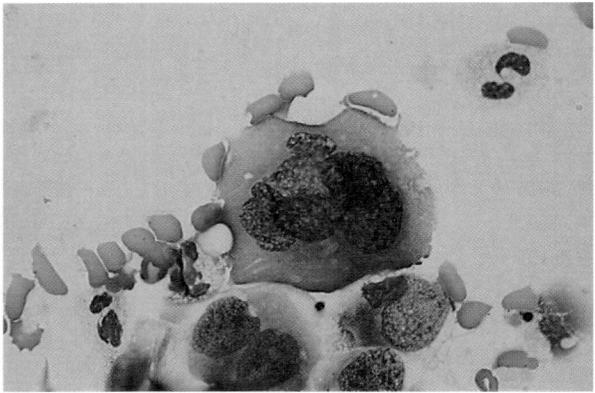

Plate 103

Bronchoalveolar lavage, cytocentrifuge preparation, rapid Wright-Giemsa stain, light microscopy, MPV. Purulence light. Local materials light. Red blood cells present. Multinucleated epithelial cells present. Intranuclear inclusions present. Morphology consistent with herpes viral inclusions. *Impression*: Herpes simplex infection. Compare with Plate 102. Note the change in appearance of the herpes-infected cells with the change in the type of fixation and stain. The H&E stain more clearly shows the "ground-glass" appearance of the nuclear inclusion rimmed by the cell nuclear chromatin. The rapid Wright's stain provides an adequate visual presentation and is more time efficient.

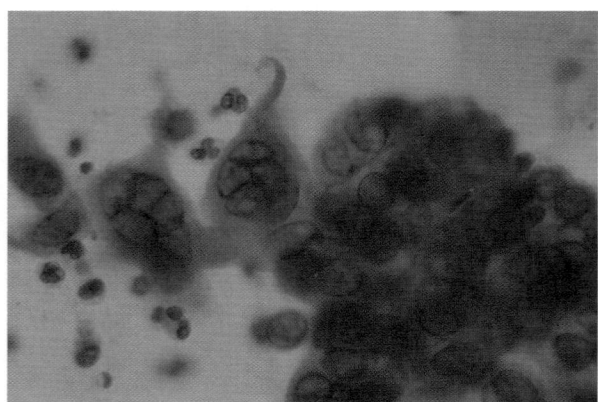

Plate 104

Skin, vesicle fluid, Tzanck preparation, Wright-Giemsa stain, light microscopy, high-power view (HPV). Purulence light. Multinucleated epithelial cells present. Intranuclear inclusions present. Morphology consistent with herpes viral inclusions. *Impression*: Varicella-zoster infection.

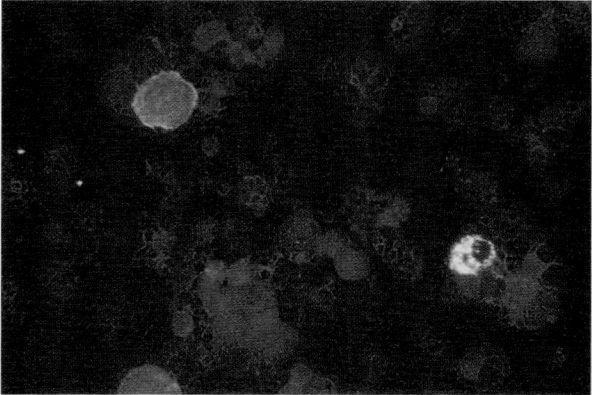

Plate 105

Skin, vesicle fluid, Tzanck preparation, antibody stain for herpes simplex virus, fluorescent microscopy, MPV. Immunostaining positive. Herpes simplex infection, confirmed.

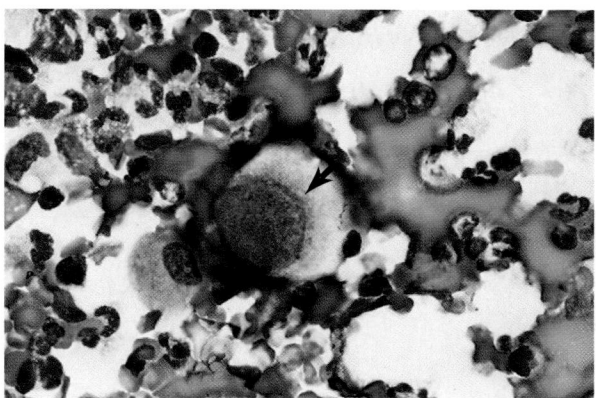

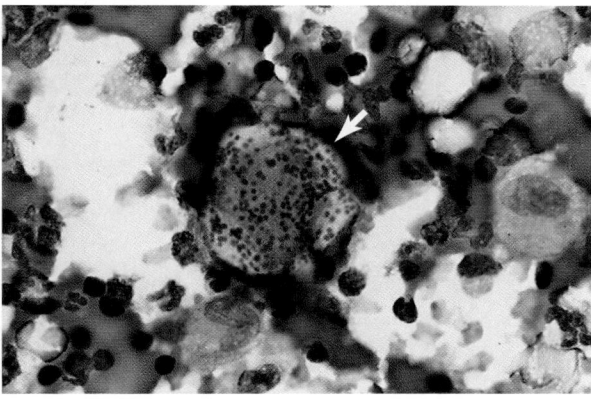

Plate 106

Bronchoalveolar lavage, cytocentrifuge preparation, Wright-Giemsa stain, light microscopy, MPV. Purulence light. Blood moderate. Local materials light. Enlarged pneumocyte with intranuclear inclusion. Morphology consistent with cytomegalovirus. Observe the characteristic nuclear changes for cytomegalovirus. The cell and the nucleus are enlarged, the nucleus is granular, and the nuclear membrane is indistinct. Blood is an indication of capillary damage. *Impression*: Cytomegalovirus disease.

Plate 107

Bronchoalveolar lavage, cytocentrifuge preparation, Wright/Giemsa stain, light microscopy, MPV. Purulence light. Blood moderate. Local materials light. Enlarged pneumocyte with intracytoplasmic inclusions. Morphology consistent with cytomegalovirus. The large, regular-sized, magenta cytoplasmic viral inclusions, when present, are characteristic of this virus. *Impression*: Cytomegalovirus disease.

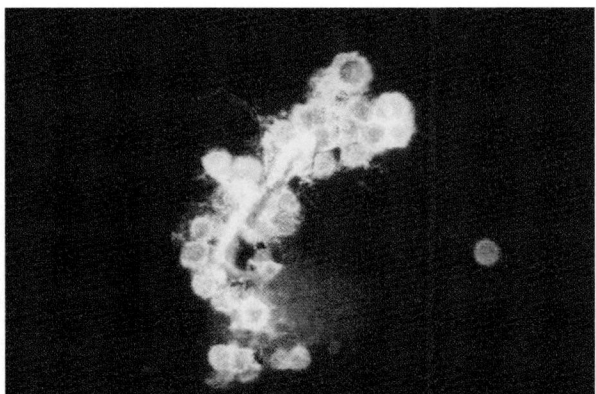

Plate 108

Bronchoalveolar lavage, cytocentrifuge preparation, IFA adenovirus stain, fluorescence microscopy, HPV. Prominent specific fluorescent staining of infected cells. *Impression*: Adenovirus infection. The necrosis and cellular debris associated with adenovirus within the bronchi can be easily overlooked, because the necrotic, virus-infected "smudge" cells may not be recognized. Specific immunostaining should be performed on the basis of clinical suspicion and compatible background material.

CHAPTER 9

Use of Colonial Morphology for the Presumptive Identification of Microorganisms

George Manuselis

IMPORTANCE OF COLONIAL MORPHOLOGY
AS A DIAGNOSTIC TOOL

INITIAL OBSERVATION AND INTERPRETATION
OF CULTURES

GROSS COLONY CHARACTERISTICS USED
TO DIFFERENTIATE AND PRESUMPTIVELY
IDENTIFY MICROORGANISMS
Hemolysis
    α Hemolysis
    β Hemolysis

Size
Form or Margin
Elevation
Density
Color
Consistency
Pigment
Odor

COLONIES WITH MULTIPLE CHARACTERISTICS

GROWTH OF ORGANISMS IN LIQUID MEDIA

OBJECTIVES

1. Describe how growth on blood, chocolate, and MacConkey agars is used in the preliminary identification of isolates.
2. Differentiate α hemolysis from β hemolysis.
3. Describe how gross colony characteristics are used in the presumptive identification of microorganisms.
4. Using colonial morphology, differentiate among the following microorganisms:
   - Staphylococci and streptococci
   - *Streptococcus agalactiae* and *Streptococcus pyogenes*
   - α-Hemolytic *Streptococcus* and *Streptococcus pneumoniae*
   - *Neisseria* species and Staphylococci
   - Yeast and Staphylococci
   - "Diphtheroids" and Staphylococci
   - Lactose fermenters from lactose nonfermenters
   - *Proteus* species from other Enterobacteriaceae

KEY TERMS

Colonial morphology	Hemolysis	Filamentous	Consistency
Lactose fermenter	Transillumination	Rhizoid	Brittle
Nonfermenter	α Hemolysis	Swarming	Creamy
Escherichia/Citrobacter- like organisms	β Hemolysis	Elevation	Butyrous
Klebsiella/Enterobacter- like organisms	Form	Umbilicate	Pigment
	Margin	Umbonate	Streamers
	Smooth	Density	Turbidity

CASE STUDY

An exudate from an infected leg wound on a 25-year-old man was cultured on blood agar plate (BAP) and MacConkey agars. Direct smear examination showed numerous WBCs and a moderate number of gram-positive cocci in pairs and clusters and few gram-negative bacilli. After overnight incubation, two colony morphotyes were visible on the BAP. The first was a medium β-hemolytic, which was yellowish-white and creamy-buttery looking. The second was also β-hemolytic but larger and gray. The MacConkey agar showed dark pink dry-looking colonies. Based on the Gram stain results and colonial characteristics of the isolates, appropriate biochemical tests were set up to identify the causative agent of the leg-wound infection.

The mastery of **colonial morphology** (colony characteristics and form) and interpretation of gram-stained smears from clinical specimens and microbial colonies cannot be overemphasized. Although gram-stained smears provide initial identification of microorganisms by microscopic characterization, growth characteristics of microorganisms on certain types of laboratory media facilitate description of colonial morphology for their identification processes.

Close your eyes and imagine the physical characteristics of a parent, relative, or friend. The height, weight, shape, color or style of hair, eyes, freckles, color of skin, even the voice or laugh may make people distinctive even in a crowd or when their back is facing you. In the same manner, many specific microorganisms have characteristics that distinguish them in a crowd of other genera or species.

This chapter explains how characterization of colonies on culture media facilitates presumptive identification of commonly isolated organisms. It discusses the characteristics that are used to describe morphology of certain groups of organisms and how these characteristics are used to differentiate one species from a closely related species and one genera from another.

IMPORTANCE OF COLONIAL MORPHOLOGY AS A DIAGNOSTIC TOOL

In many ways, the usefulness of colonial morphology extends the capabilities of the microbiologist and, ultimately, the clinical laboratory. The ability to provide a presumptive identification by colonial morphology may include the following:

- **Provide a presumptive diagnosis to the physician in times of critical need.** Even in this age of rapid identification systems, incubation times and procedures can be protracted. In a critical situation, the microbiologist makes an educated judgment about the presumptive identity before performing diagnostic procedures.
- **Enhance the quality of patient care through rapid reporting of results and by increasing this cost-effectiveness of laboratory testing.** This may best be illustrated by using sputum cultures as an example. Because the upper respiratory tract contains many indigenous organisms, to identify every organism in culture would be a time-consuming, cost-prohibitive, and insurmountable task. You should be able to differentiate potential pathogens from the "usual" inhabitants of the upper respiratory tract and direct the diagnostic workup only to potential pathogens. Moreover, potential pathogens are presumptively identified by colonial characteristics, and preliminary reporting initiates immediate therapy.
- **Play a significant role in quality control, especially of automated procedures and other commercially available identification systems.** When commercial and automated systems are used, a mixed inoculum will produce biochemical test results or erroneous interpretation of

reactions that significantly alters the identification. The ability of the microbiologist to determine whether the inoculum is mixed and to ascertain whether the results generated by a commercial or automated system correlate with the suspected identification of the organism is an important component of quality control, accomplished by being able to recognize organisms by their colonial characteristics.

INITIAL OBSERVATION AND INTERPRETATION OF CULTURES

Generally, microbiologists observe the colonial morphology of organisms isolated on primary culture after 18 to 24 hours of incubation. Incubation time may certainly vary according to when the specimen is received and processed in the laboratory, which may affect the "typical" morphology of a certain isolate. For example, young cultures of *Staphylococcus aureus* may appear smaller and may not show the distinct β hemolysis older cultures produce. In addition, the microbiologist must be aware of factors that may significantly alter the colonial morphology of growing microorganisms. These factors include the medium's ingredients, its inhibitory nature, and antibiotics present in the medium.

The interpretation of primary cultures, commonly referred to as *plate reading,* is actually a comparative examination of microorganisms growing on a variety of culture media. Many specimens, such as sputum and wounds, that arrive in the clinical laboratory are plated on blood agar (BAP), chocolate agar (CHOC), and MacConkey (MAC). Therefore as a culture set from a specimen, growth on these three culture media illustrates the comparative colonial examination of plate reading.

First, the ability to determine which organisms grow on selective and nonselective media aids the microbiologist in making an initial distinction between gram-positive and gram-negative isolates. BAP and CHOC support the growth of a variety of fastidious and nonfastidious organisms, gram-positive and gram-negative bacteria. As illustrated in the previous case study, two colony morphotypes were observed on BAP. Because the gram-stained smear showed both gram-positive and gram-negative bacteria, two types of organisms

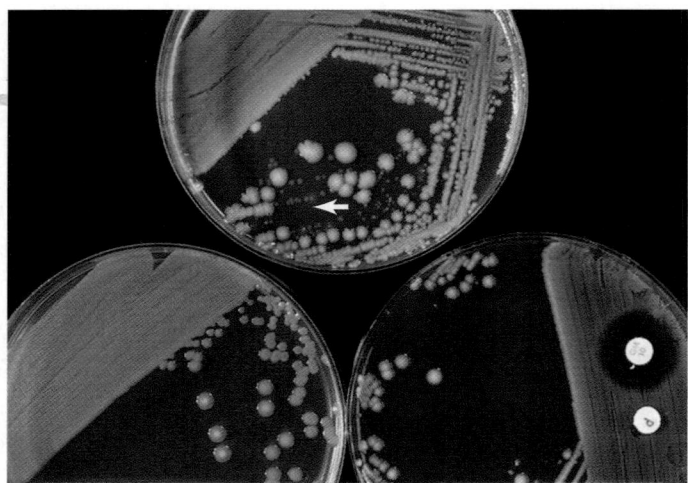

Figure 9-1

Clockwise from the top: chocolate agar (CHOC), blood agar (BAP), MacConkey agar (MAC). The large colonies growing on all three plates are gram-negative rods (enterics). These gram-negative rods grow larger, gray, and mucoid on BAP and CHOC. Notice the smaller grayish brown fastidious colonies of *Haemophilus* organisms growing on CHOC *(arrow)*, which are not growing on BAP or MAC.

must be observed on a nonselective medium such as BAP.

Although BAP supports fastidious organisms, highly fastidious species such as *Haemophilus* species and *Neisseria gonorrhoeae* do not grow on it. Chocolate agar provides nutritional growth requirements to support highly fastidious organisms such as *Haemophilus* species and *N. gonorrhoeae*. Therefore a gram-negative bacillus that grows on CHOC but not on BAP or MAC will be suspected to be *Haemophilus* species, whereas gram-negative diplococci with the same growth pattern will be suspected to be *N. gonorrhoeae* (Figure 9-1). The microbiologist then is able to provide a presumptive identification and determine how to proceed in identifying the isolated organisms.

Second, MacConkey agar, which inhibits gram-positive organisms and some fastidious gram-negative organisms, such as *Haemophilus* and *Neisseria* species, supports most gram-negative rods, especially the Enterobacteriaeceae. Growth on BAP and CHOC but not on MAC, therefore, is indicative of a gram-positive isolate or of a fastidious gram-negative bacillus or coccus.

Gram-negative rods are better described on MacConkey agar because these organisms produce similar-looking colonies on BAP and CHOC media: large, gray, and mucoid. MAC is best used, however, to differentiate **lactose fermenters** from lactose **nonfermenters.** Lactose fermenters are easily detected by the color change they produce on the media; as the pH changes when lactose is fermented, the organisms produce dark pink to red colonies (Figure 9-2, *A*). Again, in the case study presented, dry, dark-pink colonies were observed on MacConkey agar, indicating the presence of a lactose-fermenting, gram-negative rod. Colonies of nonfermenters remain clear and colorless (Figure 9-2, *B*). This differentiation is particularly important in screening for enteric pathogens from stool cultures. Most enteric pathogens do not ferment lactose.

Certain enteric pathogens produce a characteristic colony on MAC that is helpful in presumptive identification. ***Escherichia/Citrobacter*–like organisms** produce a dry, pink colony with a surrounding "halo" of pink, precipitated bile salts (Figure 9-3). ***Klebsiella/Enterobacter*–like organisms** produce large, mucoid pink colonies that occasionally have cream-colored centers (Figure 9-4).

Microorganisms grow on culture media in the same proportion or concentration in which they are present in the clinical specimen. Because many specimens are polymicrobic, this trait can be beneficial in identifying different colony types. The reader should remember that this is a comparative analysis of the growth on the three types of culture media.

A 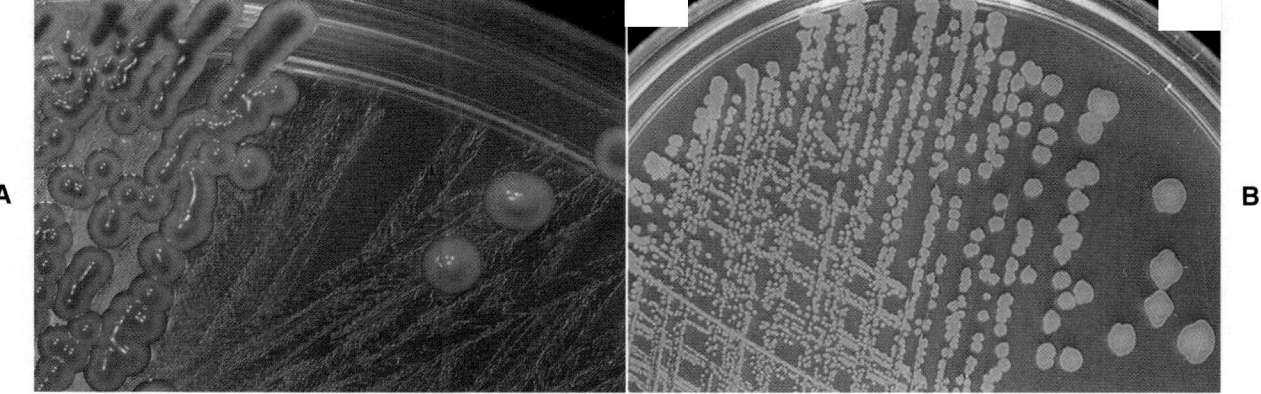 B

Figure 9-2

A, Example of lactose-fermenting gram-negative rods producing pink colonies on MAC. **B,** Example of non–lactose-fermenting gram-negative rods producing colorless colonies on MAC.

A 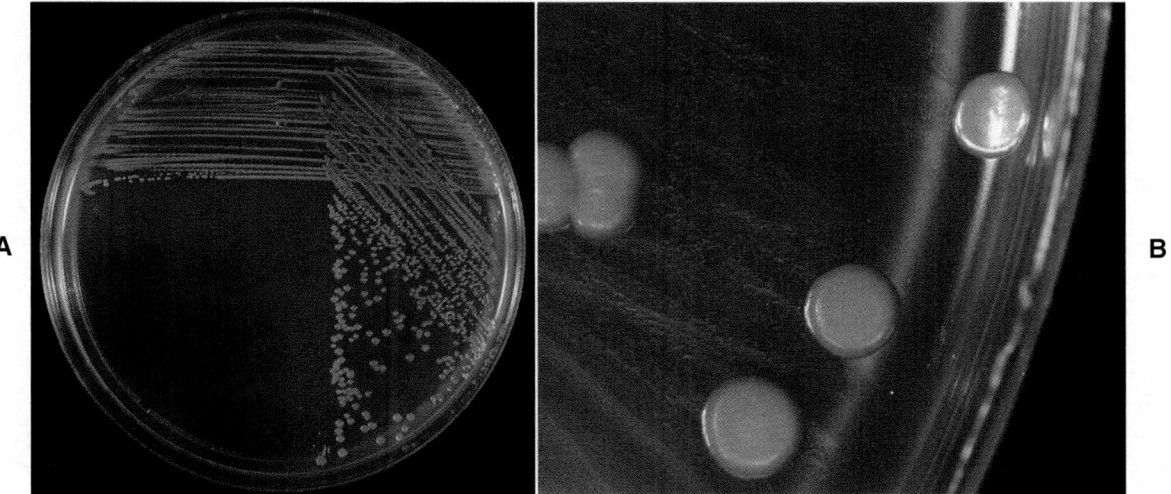 B

Figure 9-3

A, Lactose-fermenting *Escherichia/Citrobacter*–like organisms growing on MacConkey agar (MAC). Notice the dry appearance of the colony and the pink precipitate of bile salts extending beyond the periphery of the colonies. **B,** Close-up of dry, flat *Escherichia/Citrobacter*–like lactose fermenters growing on MAC. Compare with Figure 9-4, *B.*

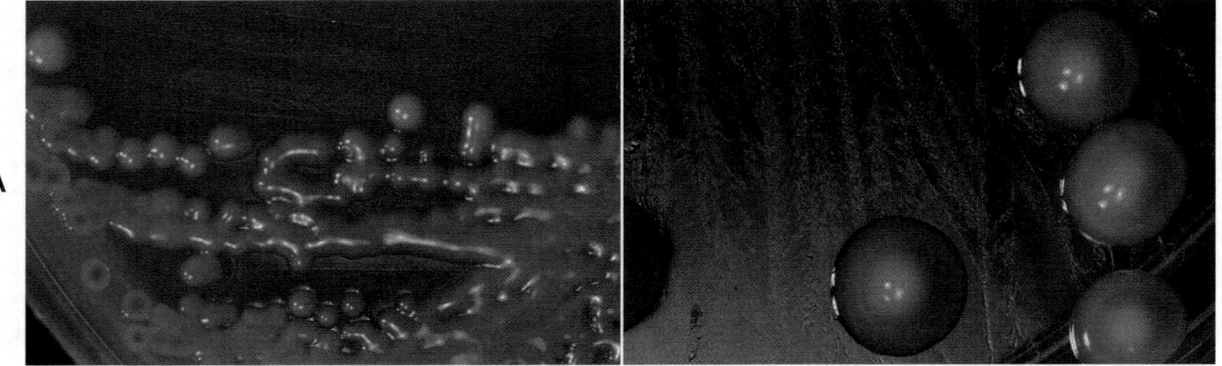

Figure 9-4

A, *Klebsiella/Enterobacter*–like lactose fermenters growing on MacConkey agar (MAC). Notice the pink, heaped, mucoid appearance. **B,** Close-up of *Klebsiella/Enterobacter*–like colonies on MAC. Notice the mucoid, heaped appearance and the slightly cream-colored center after 48 hours' growth.

GROSS COLONY CHARACTERISTICS USED TO DIFFERENTIATE AND PRESUMPTIVELY IDENTIFY MICROORGANISMS

By observing the colonial characteristics of the organisms that have been isolated, the microbiologist is able to make an educated guess about the identification of the isolate. The following descriptions are routinely used to examine colony characteristics.

Hemolysis

On blood agar, **hemolysis** is a reaction observed in the media immediately surrounding or underneath the colony. Often, the colony has to be removed with a loop to visualize the hemolytic pattern. Hemolysis on blood agar is helpful in the presumptive identification, particularly of streptococci. It is important to determine whether true hemolysis is present or whether discoloration of the media is because of growth of the organism on the plate. Proper technique requires the passing of bright light through the bottom of the plate **(transillumination)** to determine whether the organism is hemolytic (Figure 9-5).

Although there are many types of hemolysis, only **α hemolysis** and **β hemolysis** are illustrated in this chapter.

α Hemolysis

α Hemolysis is partial clearing of blood around the colony that results in a green discoloration of the

medium. Examples of organisms that produce α hemolysis include *Streptococcus pneumoniae* and certain viridans streptococci. (For a comparison of the colonial morphology of these two organisms, see Figure 9-23.)

β Hemolysis

β Hemolysis is complete clearing of blood around the colonies because of the complete lysis of red

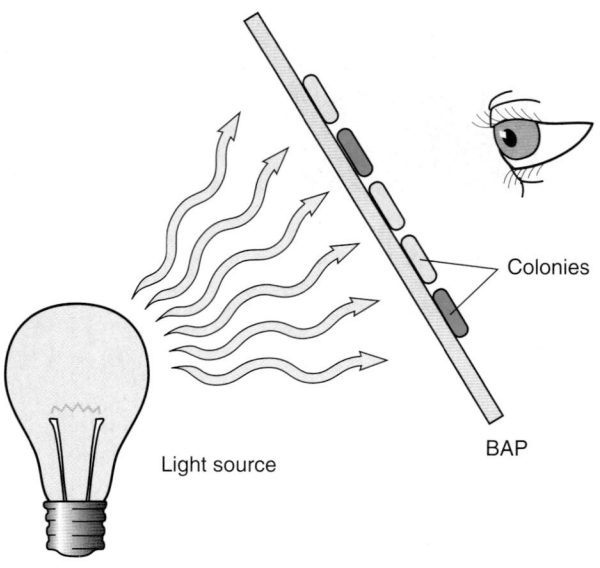

Figure 9-5

The use of transillumination to determine whether the colonies are hemolytic.

blood cells. Certain organisms such as group A β-hemolytic streptococci *(Streptococcus pyogenes),* produce a wide clear zone of hemolysis, whereas others, such as group B β-hemolytic streptococci *(Streptococcus agalactiae)* and *Listeria monocytogenes,* produce a narrow, diffuse zone of hemolysis. These features are helpful hints in the identification of certain species of bacteria. (For a comparison of the colonial characteristics of group A and group B streptococci, see Figure 9-24.) Chocolate agar does not display true hemolysis, because the red cells in the medium have already been lysed. Organisms that are α-hemolytic or β-hemolytic on blood agar usually show a green coloration around the colony on chocolate agar (Figure 9-6). This coloration, therefore, should not be mistaken for a hemolytic characteristic.

Size

Colonies may be described as large, medium, small, or pinpoint. Rarely, however, does a microbiologist take a ruler and actually measure a colony. Size is generally a visual comparison between genera or species. For example, gram-positive bacteria, in general, produce smaller colonies than gram-negative bacteria. *Staphylococcus* species are usually larger than *Streptococcus* species. Figure 9-7 shows colonies of gram-negative rods in comparison with gram-positive cocci.

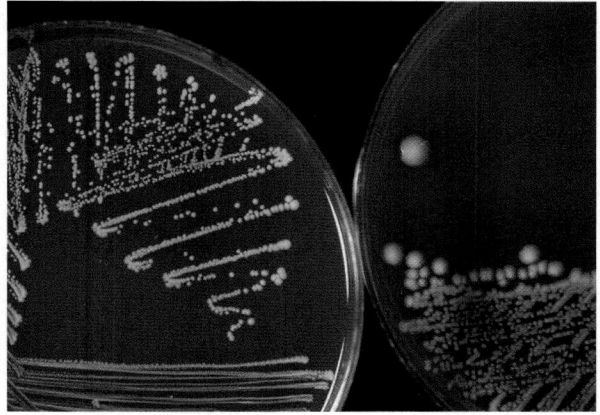

Figure 9-7 _____

Left, Blood agar (BAP): Small white colonies are gram-positive cocci; *right,* BAP: Large gray, mucoid colonies are enteric gram-negative rods.

Form or Margin

The edge of the colonies should be observed and the **form,** or **margin,** described as ***smooth, filamentous***, *rough* or ***rhizoid,*** or *irregular* (Figure 9-8). Colonies of *Bacillus anthracis* on visual examination are described as "Medusa heads" because of the filamentous appearance. Certain genera such as *Proteus* species (especially the species *Proteus mirabilis* and *Proteus vulgaris*), may swarm on nonselective agar such as blood or chocolate. ***Swarming*** is a hazy blanket of growth on the surface that extends way beyond the streak lines. Figure 9-9 shows swarming colonies of *Proteus* sp. Diphtheroids produce colonies that have rough edges (Figure 9-10), whereas yeasts produce colonies that are described as *stars* or colonies *with feet or pedicles.* (For a comparison of the colonial morphology of yeast and staphylococci, see Figure 9-25.)

Elevation

The **elevation** should be determined by tilting the culture plate and looking at the side of the colony (Figure 9-11). Elevation may be *raised, convex, flat,* **umbilicate** (depressed center, an "inny"), or **umbonate** (raised or bulging center, an "outy"). *S. pneumoniae* typically produces umbilicate colonies unless the colonies are mucoid because of the presence of polysaccharide capsule. *S. aureus* typically produces convex colonies. In comparison,

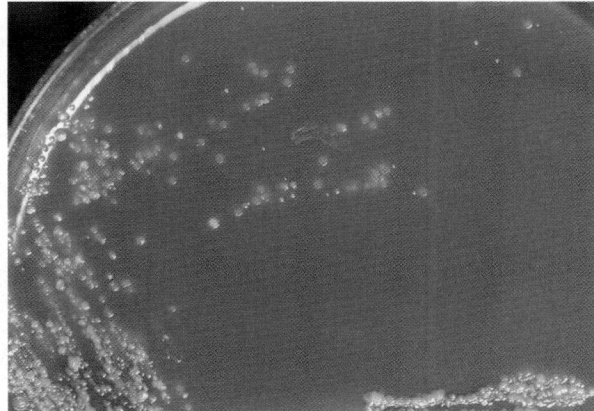

Figure 9-6 _____

Chocolate agar (CHOC) does not display true hemolysis, because the red cells in the medium have already been lysed. Bacteria that are hemolytic on blood agar (BAP) usually are green around the colony on CHOC.

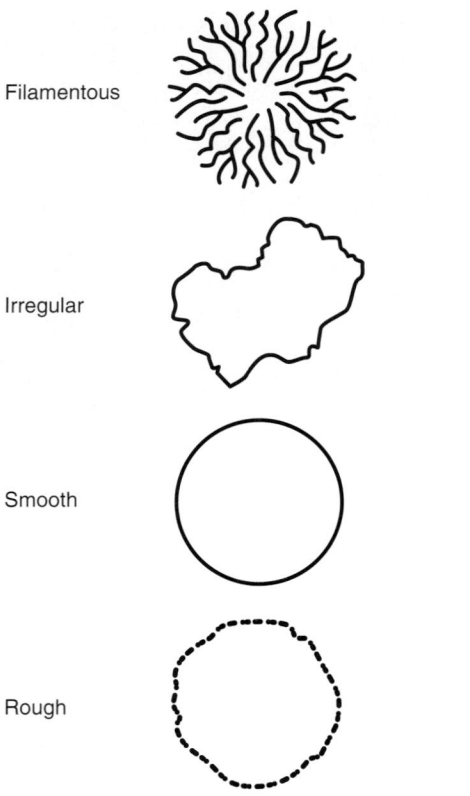

Filamentous

Irregular

Smooth

Rough

Figure 9-8 _____

Illustration of form or margin to describe colonial morphology.

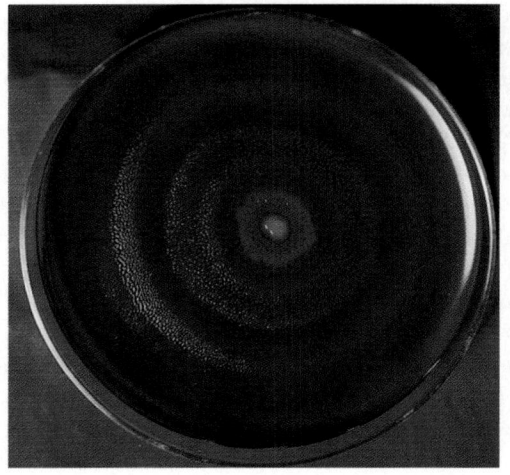

Figure 9-9 _____

Swarming colonies of *Proteus* sp.

Flat

Raised

Convex, or dome

Umbilicate

Umbonate

Figure 9-11 _____

Illustration of elevations to describe colonial morphology.

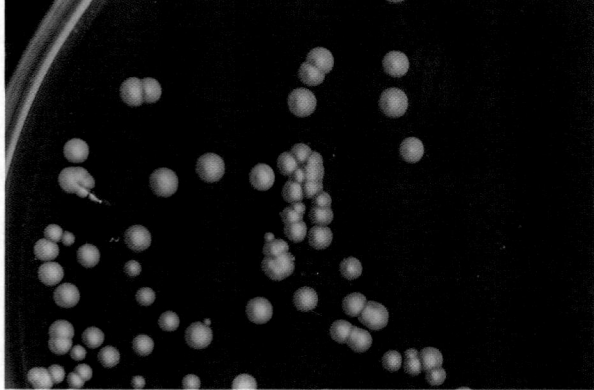

Figure 9-10 _____

"Diphtheroid" colonies with rough edges, dry appearance, and umbonate center growing on blood agar.

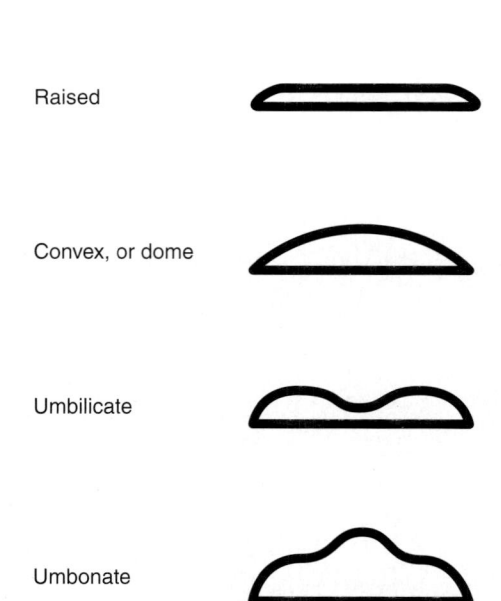

β-hemolytic streptococci generally produce flat colonies.

Density

The **density of** the colony can be *transparent, translucent,* or *opaque.* β-Hemolytic streptococci, except for group B *(S. agalactiae),* are described as translucent. *S. agalactiae* produces colonies that are semiopaque, with the organisms concentrated at the center of the colony, sometimes described as a *bull's-eye* colony. Staphylococci and other gram-positive bacteria are usually opaque. Most gram-negative rods are also opaque. *Bordetella pertussis* is described as shiny, like a *half-pearl,* on blood-containing media.

Color

Color, in contrast with pigmentation, is a term used to describe in general a particular genus. Colonies may be *white, gray, yellow,* or *buff.* Coagulase-negative staphylococci are white (Figure 9-12), whereas *Enterococcus* species may be gray. Certain *Micrococcus* species and *Neisseria* (nonpathogenic) species are yellow or off-white (Figure 9-13). Diphtheroids are buff. Most gram-negative rods are gray.

Consistency

Consistency is determined by touching the colony with a sterile loop. Colony consistency may be **brittle** (splinters), **creamy (butyrous),** *dry,* or

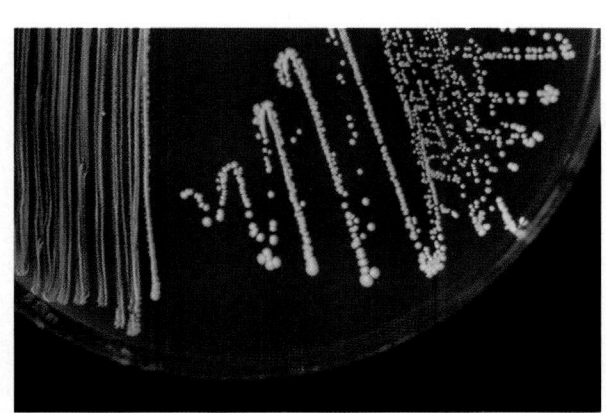

Figure 9-12 ⎯⎯⎯⎯⎯⎯⎯⎯⎯⎯⎯⎯⎯⎯⎯⎯

Example of white colonies of coagulase-negative staphylococci on blood agar.

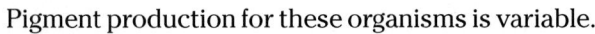

Figure 9-13 ⎯⎯⎯⎯⎯⎯⎯⎯⎯⎯⎯⎯⎯⎯⎯⎯

Example of the yellow colonies characteristic of certain nonpathogenic species of *Neisseria* organisms on blood agar.

waxy; occasionally, the entire colony adheres *(sticky)* to the loop. *S. aureus* is creamy, whereas certain *Neisseria* species are sticky. *Nocardia* sp. produces colonies that are brittle, crumbly, and wrinkled, resembling bread crumbs on a plate. Diphtheroid colonies are usually dry and waxy. Most β-hemolytic streptococci are dry (except for mucoid types), and when pushed by a loop, the whole colony remains intact.

Pigment

Pigment production is an inherent characteristic of a specific organism confined generally to the colony. Examples of organisms that produce pigment include the following:

- *Pseudomonas aeruginosa*—green, sometimes a metallic sheen (Figure 9-14)
- *Serratia marcescens*—brick-red (Figure 9-15)
- *Kluyvera* species—blue
- *Chromobacterium violaceum*—purple
- *Prevotella melaninogenica*—brown-black (anaerobic)

Pigment production for these organisms is variable.

Odor

For safety reasons, inhaling at the surface of the plate to check for odor is not a good idea. Odor should be determined when the lid of the culture plate is removed and its odor dissipates into the surrounding environment. Examples of microor-

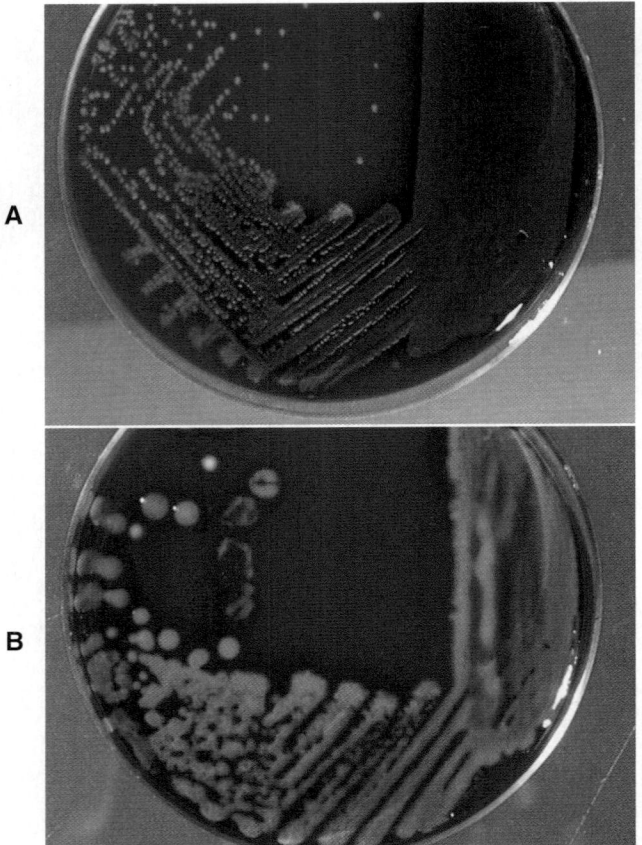

A

B

Figure 9-14 _____

A, *Pseudomonas aeruginosa* illustrating the metallic sheen and green pigmentation of colonies on blood agar plate (BAP).
B, Not all strains of the same organism have the same colonial appearance. This is a mucoid strain of *P. aeruginosa* on BAP.

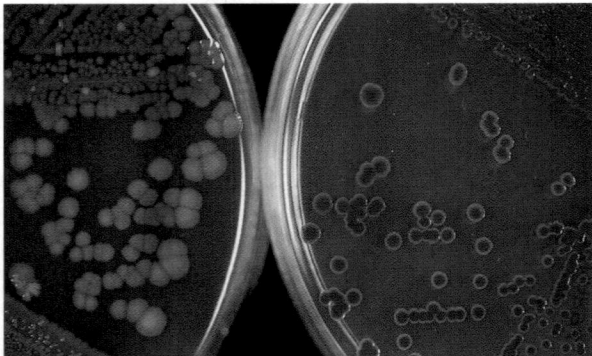

Figure 9-15 _____

Brick-red pigment of *Serratia marcescens,* which is evident on the MacConkey agar on the right. This brick-red pigment should *not* be confused with lactose fermentation. The pigment is slightly visible on chocolate agar *(left).*

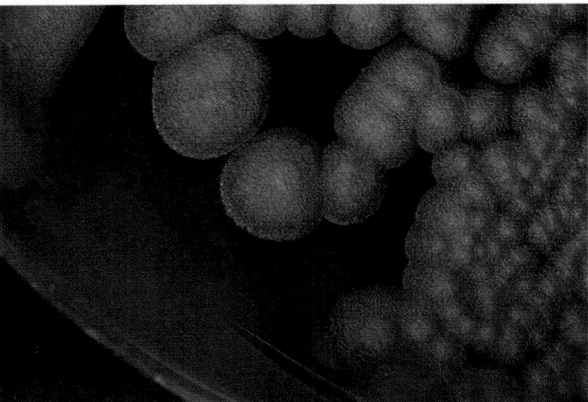

Figure 9-16 _____

Large, rough, greenish-appearing, hemolytic colonies of *Bacillus cereus* on blood agar.

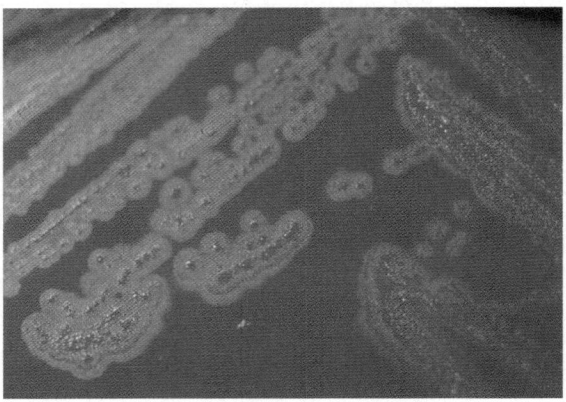

Figure 9-17 _____

Small, "fuzzy-edged," umbonate center–appearing colony of *Eikenella corrodens* on chocolate agar. This organism has the tendency to "pit" the agar.

ganisms that produce distinctive odors include the following:

- *S. aureus*—old sock (stocking that has been worn continuously for a few days without washing)
- *P. aeruginosa*—fruity or grape-like
- *Proteus mirabilis*—putrid
- *Haemophilus* species—musty basement
- *Nocardia* species—freshly plowed field

COLONIES WITH MULTIPLE CHARACTERISTICS

In addition to the organisms already mentioned, other bacteria fit in multiple descriptive categories of colonial morphology. *Bacillus cereus* forms large, rough, greenish, hemolytic colonies on blood agar (Figure 9-16). *Eikenella corrodens* forms a small, "fuzzy-edged" colony with an umbonate center on blood or chocolate agar (Figure 9-17).

GROWTH OF ORGANISMS IN LIQUID MEDIA

Important clues to an organism's identification can also be detected by observing the growth of the organism in liquid media such as thioglycolate. **Streamers** or vines and *puff balls* are associated with certain species of streptococci (Figure 9-18). **Turbidity** (and usually gas if the media contains glucose) is produced by enterics (Figure 9-19). Yeast and *Pseudomonas* species produce scum at the sides of the tube (Figures 9-20 and 9-21). In addition, yeast occasionally grows below the surface, in the microaerophilic area of the media (Figure 9-22).

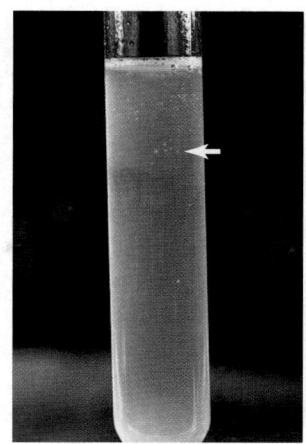

Figure 9-19

Turbidity produced by enterics when growing in thioglycolate. Notice the gas bubbles at the surface of and in the middle of the medium.

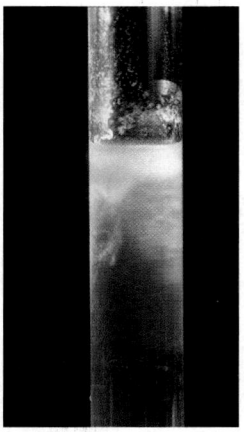

Figure 9-20

Production of "scum" by yeast at the surface of the thioglycolate.

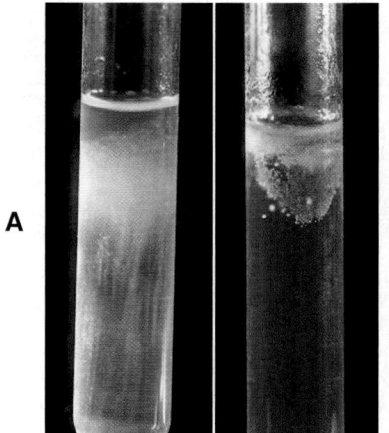

A **B**

Figure 9-18

A, "Vine" or "streamer" effect exhibited by certain species of streptococci when growing in thioglycolate. Notice the effect is more prevalent toward the bottom of the tube. **B,** Example of the "puffed balls" effect exhibited by certain streptococcal species when growing in thioglycolate.

Figures 9-23 (*S. pneumoniae* and α-hemolytic streptococci), 9-24 (*S. pyogenes* and *S. agalactiae*), and 9-25 (staphylococci and yeast) show the difference between various organisms by colonial morphology.

The colonial morphology described in this chapter is not infallible. Variations do occur quite frequently. Therefore the morphologies described

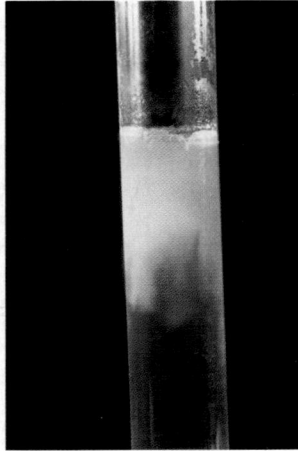

Figure 9-21 —————————————

Illustration of *Pseudomonas* organisms producing surface "scum" at the sides of the thioglycolate. Occasionally, *Pseudomonas aeruginosa* produces a diffusible green pigment and a metallic sheen at the surface.

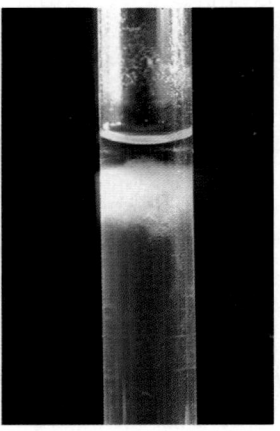

Figure 9-22 —————————————

Yeast growing in the microaerophilic area of thioglycolate.

Streptococcus pneumoniae	α-Hemolytic *Streptococcus (viridans)*
Translucent, may resemble a water droplet; umbilicate, or flat with "penny" edge; entire margin, wide and strong zone of α hemolysis	Translucent, grayer, rough margin, umbonate center

A

Umbilicate

"Penny" edge

Umbonate center

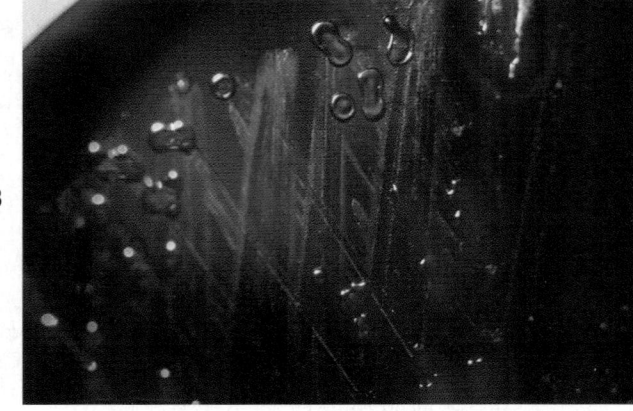

B

Figure 9-23 —————————————

A, Differentiation of *Streptococcus pneumoniae* and α-hemolytic streptococci by colonial morphology. **B,** *Streptococcus pneumoniae* growing on BAP. Notice the strong zone of α hemolysis, umbilicate center, and wet (mucoid) appearance of the colonies.

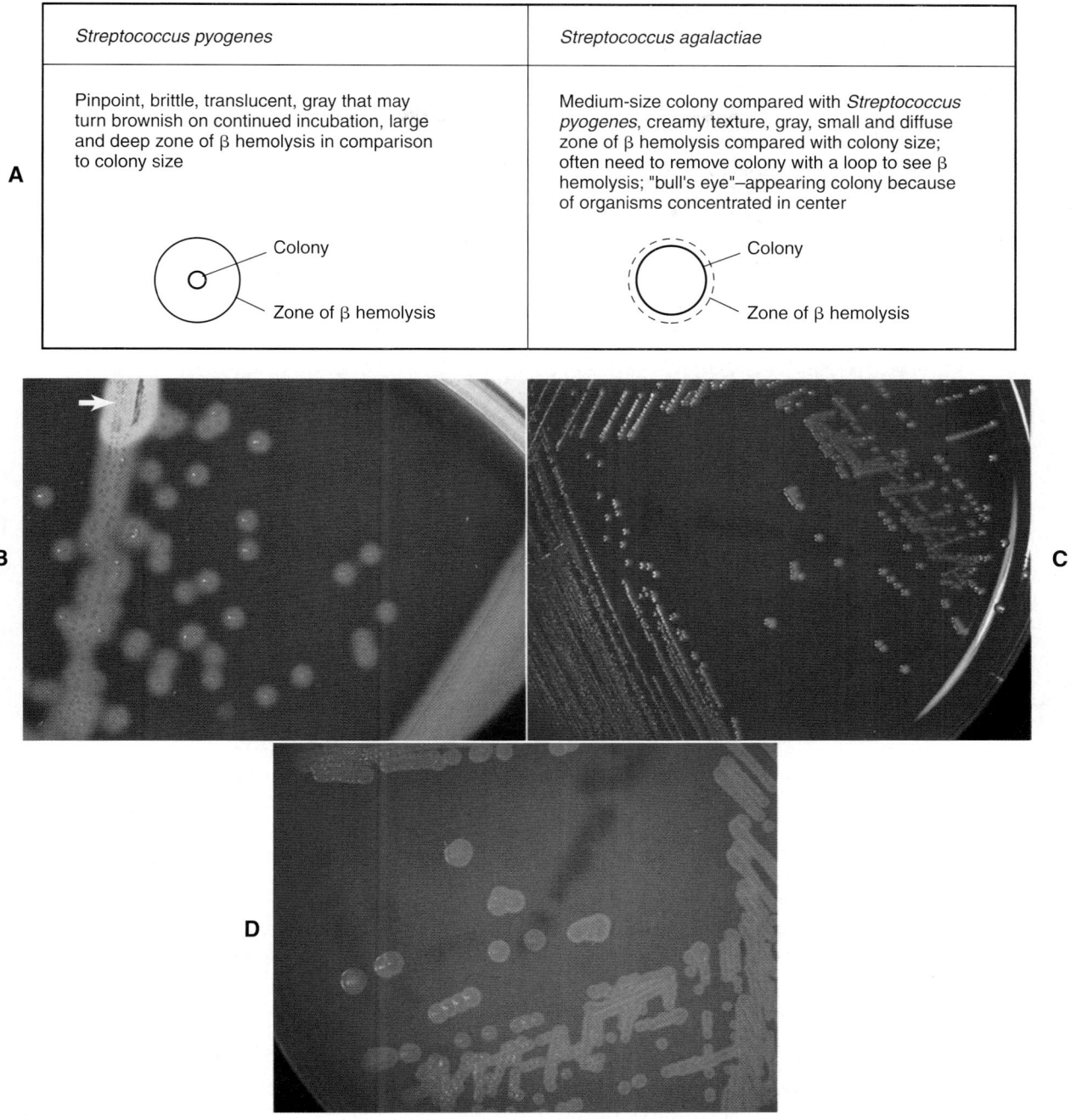

Streptococcus pyogenes	*Streptococcus agalactiae*
Pinpoint, brittle, translucent, gray that may turn brownish on continued incubation, large and deep zone of β hemolysis in comparison to colony size	Medium-size colony compared with *Streptococcus pyogenes*, creamy texture, gray, small and diffuse zone of β hemolysis compared with colony size; often need to remove colony with a loop to see β hemolysis; "bull's eye"–appearing colony because of organisms concentrated in center

A

B

C

D

Figure 9-24

A, Differentiation of *Streptococcus pyogenes* and *Streptococcus agalactiae* by colonial morphology. **B,** Pinpoint colony of *S. pyogenes* exhibiting large, deep zone of β hemolysis on BAP. **C,** Colonies of *S. agalactiae* growing on BAP. This organism produces a larger colony and a smaller, more diffuse zone of hemolysis than *S. pyogenes*. Notice that the hemolysis is not evident in this photograph. Compare with **B. D,** Colonies of *S. agalactiae* growing on BAP. Through the use of transillumination, the hemolytic pattern is now evident; hemolysis is diffuse and remains close to the periphery of the colony. The same colonial morphology is produced by *Listeria monocytogenes,* a gram-positive rod. Compare with **B.** Arrow: *S. pyogenes* produces two hemolysins; one is oxygen stable (S) and the other is oxygen labile (O). Stabbing the medium with an inoculating loop carries the organism into areas where anaerobic conditions are more prevalent, allowing the enhanced hemolysin (O) to be visualized.

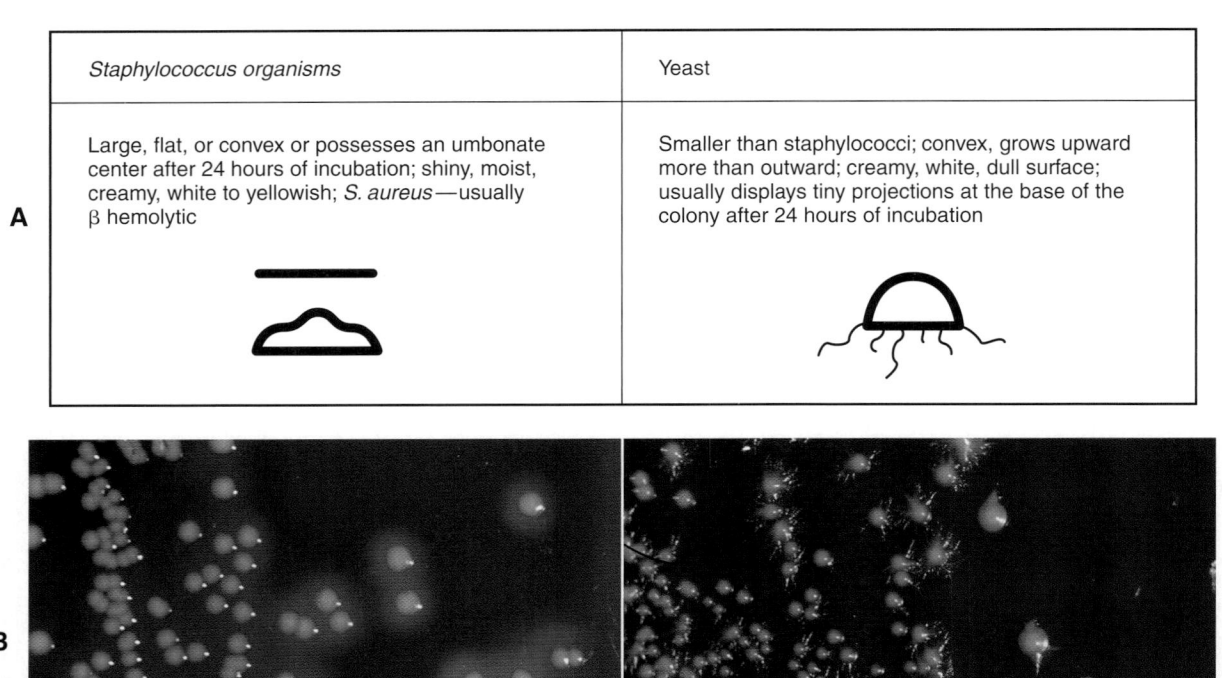

Staphylococcus organisms	Yeast
Large, flat, or convex or possesses an umbonate center after 24 hours of incubation; shiny, moist, creamy, white to yellowish; *S. aureus*—usually β hemolytic	Smaller than staphylococci; convex, grows upward more than outward; creamy, white, dull surface; usually displays tiny projections at the base of the colony after 24 hours of incubation

Figure 9-25

A, Differentiation between staphylococci and yeast by colonial morphology. **B,** Large, white, convex, shiny, moist, β-hemolytic colonies of *Staphylococcus aureus* growing on blood agar plate (BAP). **C,** "Heaped" or convex, white, dull appearance and butyrous texture of *Candida albicans* on BAP. Notice the tiny projections or "feet" at the edge of the colonies.

are general characteristics for any given organism. The identification process must include Gram stain and biochemical reactions in addition to colonial morphology.

Microbiologists become frustrated when changes in colony morphology, Gram staining, and biochemical reactions occur in microorganisms that produce characteristic features. Many times, organisms exhibit characteristics far different from those previously described for them. The ability to recognize these differences and changes in characteristics make this discipline a challenge.

Bibliography

Koneman EW et al: *Color atlas and textbook of diagnostic microbiology,* ed 4, Philadelphia, 1992, JB Lippincott.

Le Beau LJ: Effective lighting systems for photography of microbial colonies *J Biol Photographic Assoc* 44:4, 1976.

LEARNING ASSESSMENT

1. What do the dark pink colonies on MacConkey agar indicate?

2. Why were there two colony types that grew on the SBA but only one on the MacConkey agar?

3. What bacterial species would you suspect when you find α-hemolytic colonies from a respiratory sample?

4. How would you describe the colonies produced on MacConkey by nonfermenting gram-negative bacilli?

5. How would you differentiate β hemolysis from α hemolysis?

6. What would you suspect if you notice "puff balls" growing on the broth medium?

7. Swarming colonies is a characteristic of which bacterial species?

PART II

Laboratory Identification of Significant Isolates

CHAPTER 10

Staphylococci

Hal S. Larsen, Connie R. Mahon

GENERAL CHARACTERISTICS

CLINICALLY SIGNIFICANT SPECIES
Staphylococcus aureus
Virulence factors
Epidemiology
Infections caused by *S. aureus*
Staphylococcus epidermidis
Staphylococcus saprophyticus
Other Coagulase-Negative Staphylococci

LABORATORY DIAGNOSIS
Specimen Collection and Handling
Microscopic Examination
Isolation and Identification
Cultural characteristics
Identification methods
Rapid methods of identification

ANTIMICROBIAL SUSCEPTIBILITY

METHICILLIN-RESISTANT STAPHYLOCOCCI

OBJECTIVES

1. Give the general characteristics of the genus *Staphylococcus.*
2. Differentiate between staphylococci and other gram-positive cocci.
3. Describe the virulence factors associated with staphylococci.
4. Describe the clinical infections associated with staphylococci.
5. Name the differential tests that may be used to identify the clinically relevant *Staphylococcus* species.
6. State which characteristics should be utilized to identify a *Staphylococcus*-like organism isolated from a clinical sample.
7. Explain the reason methicillin resistance is a serious clinical problem.

KEY TERMS

Catalase
"Bunches of grapes"
"Buttery-looking"
Coagulase
Coagulase-negative
  staphylococci
Enterotoxin F
S. aureus phage group I
Toxic shock syndrome
Toxic shock syndrome
  toxin-1 (TSST-1)
Exfoliative toxin
Cytolytic toxins
α Hemolysin
β Hemolysin
Panton-Valentine
  leukocidin
Protein A

Bullous impetigo
Furuncles
Carbuncles
Scalded skin syndrome
Ritter's disease
Phage group II
  staphylococci
Toxic epidermal
  necrolysis (TEN)
Osteomyelitis
Slime
Clumping factor
Free coagulase
Novobiocin
  susceptibility
β-Lactamase
Methicillin-resistant
  staphylococci

CASE STUDY

A 19-year-old woman complained of fever and flank pain. Dysuria, urgency to urinate, and blood-tinged urine were also noted. A urinalysis revealed many white blood cells and white blood cell casts. A urine culture grew white, nonhemolytic colonies on blood agar. The colony count was 45,000 CFU/ml. No growth appeared on MacConkey's agar. The organism was catalase positive and slide- and tube-coagulase negative and produced a 21-mm zone of inhibition in the presence of a novobiocin disc.

Gram-positive cocci are common isolates in the clinical microbiology laboratory. Although most are members of the indigenous microbial flora, some species are definite agents of serious infectious disease. This chapter discusses the most commonly encountered staphylococci and their characteristics, the infections they produce, and their laboratory identification. Infections caused by *Staphylococcus aureus, Staphylococcus epidermidis,* and *Staphylococcus saprophyticus* are emphasized.

GENERAL CHARACTERISTICS

The staphylococci are **catalase**-producing, gram-positive cocci that belong to the family Micrococcaceae. On stained smears, they are spherical cells (0.5 to 1.5 μm) that appear singly, in pairs, and in clusters that have been described as looking like **"bunches of grapes."** These organisms are non-motile and non–spore-forming, and most are facultatively anaerobic, except for *Staphylococcus saccharolyticus* which is an obligate anaerobe. Colonies produced after 18 to 24 hours of incubation appear creamy, white or light gold, and **"buttery-looking."** Some species produce β-hemolytic zones around the colonies. Staphylococci are common isolates in the clinical laboratory and are responsible for several suppurative types of infections. These organisms are normal inhabitants of the skin and mucous membranes of humans and other animals.

Species of staphylococci are initially differentiated by the **coagulase** test. Coagulase-producing (coagulase-positive) staphylococci are *S. aureus, Staphylococcus intermedius, Staphylococcus delphini,* and some strains of *Staphylococcus hyicus* and *Staphylococcus schleiferi.* With the exception of *S. aureus,* these are animal-associated species and thus are rarely isolated from human samples. Consequently, for the vast majority of clinical laboratory situations, coagulase-positive isolates from human sources are considered to be *S. aureus. S. aureus* causes cutaneous infections such as boils, carbuncles, and purulent abscesses. Toxin-induced diseases, such as food poisoning, scalded skin syndrome, and toxic shock syndrome, are also associated with this organism.

Staphylococci that do not produce coagulase are **coagulase-negative staphylococci.** The most clinically significant species in this group are *S. epidermidis* and *S. saprophyticus. S. epidermidis* has been known to cause various hospital-acquired infections, whereas *S. saprophyticus* is mainly associated with urinary tract infections in young females who are sexually active.

Currently, 33 recognized species of coagulase-negative staphylococci exist. The groups listed in Table 10-1, consisting of species of coagulase-negative staphylococci, are established. Most of these species have been isolated from humans usually found inhabiting the skin and mucous membranes. Certain species are found in very specific sites. Others have been isolated from animals and animal products.

In addition to the genus *Staphylococcus,* the family Micrococcaceae includes the nonpathogenic genera *Planococcus* and *Micrococcus.* However, some investigators, have written that the three genera are not as closely related as previously thought. Micrococci are catalase-producing, coagulase-negative, gram-positive cocci found in the environment and as residents of the indigenous skin flora. Micrococci, especially *Micrococcus luteus,* have a tendency to produce a yellow pigmented colony. It is not unusual to isolate them from clinical samples. Because they are considered nonpathogens, they are differentiated from the potentially pathogenic coagulase-negative staphylococci. Differentiating characteristics of micrococci and staphylococci are shown in Table 10-2.

TABLE 10-1
Groups of Coagulase-Negative Staphylococci and Their Clinical Source and Significance

Species	Source*	Species	Source*
S. epidermidis group		S. simulans species group	
S. epidermidis	**Human**, animal	S. simulans	Animal, human
S. haemolyticus	**Human**	S. carnosus	Animal
S. hominis	Human	S. intermedius group	
S. capitis ssp. capitis	Human	S. schleiferi ssp. schleiferi	**Animal**, human
S. capitis ureolyticus	Human	S. sciuri group	
S. caprae	Human, animal	S. sciuri	Animal, human
S. auricularis	Human	S. lentus	Animal, human
S. saccharolyticus	Human	S. vitulinus	Animal
S. warneri	Human, animal	S. hyicus group	
S. pasteuri	Animal, human	S. chromogenes	**Animal**
S. saprophyticus group		Unspecified species group	
S. saprophyticus	**Human**	S. caseolyticus	Animal
S. cohnii ssp. cohnii	Animal, human	S. felis	Animal
S. cohnii ssp. urealyticum	Animal, human	S. hyicus	Animal
S. xylosus	Animal, human	S. lugdunensis	**Human**, animal
S. arlettae	Animal	S. muscae	Animal
S. equorum	Animal, human	S. piscifermentans	Animal
S. gallinarum	Animal		
S. kloosii	Animal		
S. lentus	Animal		

Courtesy Leona W. Ayers, M.D.
***Boldface** indicates common in human or veterinary disease.

TABLE 10-2

Differentiation Between Staphylococci and Micrococci in the Routine Laboratory

Test	Staphylococci	Micrococci
Anaerobic acid production from glucose	+	−*
Growth of furoxone–Tween 80–oil red 0 agar	−	+
Aerobic acid production from glycerol in the presence of erythromycin	+	−
Resistance to bacitracin (0.04 UI)	R(+)†	S
Lysozyme (50-μg disk)	R	S
Lysostaphin test	S(−)†	R

From Schumacher-Perdreau F: Clinical significance and laboratory diagnosis of coagulase-negative staphylococci, *Clin Microbiol Newsl* 13:97, 1991.
*Micrococcus kristinae, Micrococcus varians are positive.
†Some strains show opposite reaction.

CLINICALLY SIGNIFICANT SPECIES

Staphylococcus aureus

Virulence factors

Enterotoxins, cytolytic toxins, and cellular components such as protein A have been described as being responsible for the pathogenicity and virulence of *S. aureus*.

ENTEROTOXINS

Staphylococcal enterotoxins are heat-stable exotoxins that cause diarrhea and vomiting in humans. Enterotoxins A and D are resistant to gastric and digestive juices and have been associated with food poisoning. **Enterotoxin F,** previously described as "pyrogenic exotoxin C," is produced by **S. aureus phage group I** and causes toxic shock syndrome. This enterotoxin is now referred to as *toxic-shock syndrome toxin-1 (TSST-1)*.

EXFOLIATIVE TOXIN

Produced by phage group II, **exfoliative toxin** is also known as *epidermolytic toxin.* It causes the epidermal layer of the skin to slough off and is known to cause scalded skin syndrome, or Ritter's disease.

CYTOLYTIC TOXINS

S. aureus produces other extracellular proteins that affect red blood cells and leukocytes. These hemolysins and leukocidins are **cytolytic toxins**

with properties different from those of previously described toxins. *S. aureus* produces α, β, and δ hemolysins. In addition to hemolyzing red blood cells, α toxin **(α Hemolysin)** is capable of destroying platelets and causing severe tissue damage. **β Hemolysin,** also referred to as *hot-cold lysin,* acts on the sphingomyelin of red blood cell membranes. The "hot-cold" feature associated with this toxin is seen as an enhanced hemolytic activity on incubation at 37° C and subsequent exposure to cold (4° C). δ Hemolysin, although it has been described to cause injury in most cells in culture and to leukocytes, is considerably less lethal than α or β hemolysin.

Staphylococcal leukocidin **(Panton-Valentine leukocidin),** is an exotoxin lethal to polymorphonuclear leukocytes. Although its exact role in staphylococcal infections is unclear, it has been implicated as contributing to the invasiveness of the organism by suppressing phagocytosis.

ENZYMES

Several enzymes are produced by both coagulase-positive and coagulase-negative staphylococci. Examples are coagulase, hyaluronidase, and lipase. Coagulase is mainly produced by *S. aureus*. Although the exact role of coagulase in pathogenicity remains uncertain, it is considered a virulence marker. Many strains of *S. aureus* produce hyaluronidase. This enzyme hydrolyzes hyaluronic acid present in the intracellular ground substance that makes up connective tissues, permitting the easy spread of infection. Lipases are produced by both coagulase-positive and coagulase-negative staphylococci. Lipases act on substances present on the surface of the skin, particularly fats and oil secreted by the sebaceous glands. This activity allows colonization of the organisms in the area.

PROTEIN A

Protein A is one of several cellular components that have been identified in the cell wall of *S. aureus*. Probably the most significant role of protein A in infections caused by *S. aureus* is its ability to bind the Fc portion of the immunoglobulin, thereby avoiding phagocytosis.

Epidemiology

S. aureus inhabits the anterior nares of human carriers. Nasal carriage in patients admitted to the hospital is common. Because close contact among patients and hospital personnel is not unusual, transfer of organisms often takes place. Consequently, increased colonization in patients and hospital workers frequently occurs. In addition to nasal carriage, colonization in the perineum is also common among carriers.

Hospital outbreaks may occur in infant nurseries, in burn units, and among patients who have undergone surgery or other invasive procedures. Transmission of *S. aureus* may occur by direct contact with unwashed contaminated hands and by fomites. Community-acquired infections caused by *S. aureus* are usually associated with poor hygiene and fomite transmission and develop from individuals who are carriers themselves.

Infections caused by *S. aureus*

As with most infections the development of staphylococcal infection is determined by the virulence of the strain, size of the inoculum, and status of the host's immune system. Any event that compromises the host's ability to resist infection encourages colonization and infection. Individuals with normal defense mechanisms are able to combat the infection more easily than those with impaired immune systems. Once the organism has transgressed the initial barriers, it activates the host's immune system for an acute inflammatory response, which leads to the proliferation of polymorphonuclear and phagocytic cells. However, the organisms are able to resist the action of inflammatory cells, by eliciting the help of toxins and enzymes, thereby establishing a focal lesion.

SKIN AND WOUND INFECTIONS

Infections caused by *S. aureus* are suppurative and pyogenic. Typically the abscess is filled with pus and surrounded by necrotic tissues and damaged leukocytes. Some of the common skin infections caused by *S. aureus* are boils, carbuncles, furuncles, folicullitis, and bullous impetigo. These opportunistic infections occur usually as a result of previous skin injuries such as cuts, burns, and surgical wounds. **Bullous impetigo** caused by *S. aureus* is different from streptococcal impetigo, in that staphylococcal pustules are larger and surrounded by a small zone of erythema. Bullous impetigo is a highly contagious infection easily spread by direct contact, fomites, or autoinocu-

lation. Boils and **furuncles** are superficial abscesses, although furuncles may progress into deeper tissues. Multiple lesions may develop from a furuncle, resulting in colonies of lesions described as **carbuncles.**

Staphylococcal infections may also occur secondary to skin diseases of different etiologies. Dry, irritated skin combined with poor personal hygiene encourages the development of infection. Some of these infections manifest because of increased colonization of the organisms in blocked hair follicles, sebaceous glands, and sweat glands. Immunocompromised individuals, particularly those who are receiving chemotherapy, are debilitated by chronic illnesses, or have undergone instrumention procedures, are predisposed to developing staphylococcal infections.

FOOD POISONING

S. aureus produces enterotoxins that have been identified and associated with gastrointestinal upset, most commonly enterotoxins A and D. The source of contamination is usually an infected food handler. Staphylococcal food poisoning occurs when an individual ingests food contaminated with enterotoxin-producing strains. The heat-stable toxins are preformed in inadequately refrigerated rich foods such as creamy sauces and mayonnaise. The enterotoxins do not cause any detectable odor or change in the appearance or taste of the food. Symptoms appear rapidly, approximately 2 to 8 hours after ingestion of the food, and resolve within 6 to 8 hours. Although no fever is associated with this condition, nausea, vomiting, abdominal pain, and severe cramping are common. Headaches may also occur.

SCALDED SKIN SYNDROME

Scalded skin syndrome, or **Ritter's disease,** is an extensive exfoliative dermatitis that occurs primarily in newborns and previously healthy young children. This syndrome is caused by staphylococcal exfoliative or epidermolytic toxin produced by **phage group II staphylococci,** probably present at a lesion distant from the site of exfoliation. The disease has also been recognized in adults. Cases of staphylococcal scalded skin syndrome (SSSS) in adults occur most commonly among patients with chronic renal failure and those with compromised immune systems. Although the mortality rate is low (0% to 7%) in cases seen among children, the rate in adults is as high as 50%.

The severity of the disease varies from being a localized skin lesion in the form of bullous impetigo to a more extensive generalized condition. Bullous impetigo manifests as a localized lesion that contains seropurulent material. This lesion may progress to the generalized form, which is cutaneous erythema followed by profuse peeling of the epidermal layer of the skin. The typical pattern in which the erythema occurs is origination from the face, neck, axillae, and groin and then extension to the trunk and extremities. The duration of the disease is brief, about 2 to 4 days. Incidence of spontaneous recovery among children is high.

The toxin is metabolized and excreted by the kidneys. Investigators believe that this may be the reason why the incidence of SSSS is higher among children less than 5 years and among adults with chronic renal failure and impaired immune systems.

Toxic epidermal necrolysis (TEN), a clinical manifestation with multiple etiologies, has a very similar initial presentation to that of SSSS. Differential diagnosis between SSSS and TEN must be made, because therapies of these two forms of exfoliative disease differ. Whereas TEN is resolved by the administration of steroid therapy, steroids aggravate SSSS. Prompt antimicrobial therapy should be initiated, particularly in adult cases of SSSS, in which the mortality rate is high.

TOXIC SHOCK SYNDROME

Toxic shock syndrome (TSS) is a multisystem disease characterized by high fever, hypotension, and shock. It was first described by Todd in 1978. The syndrome has since been attributed to a toxin released by certain strains of *S. aureus,* known as *TSST-1.* Although the first cases of TSS occurred in seven children of both sexes, an increased incidence of the infection affecting predominantly young menstruating women was observed 2 years later. The association of TSS with tampon use was then established. The syndrome was also seen in males as well as in nonmenstruating females. It was later found that any wound caused by a strain of *S. aureus* that produces TSST-1 may cause TSS.

The initial clinical presentation of TSS consists of high fever, rash, and signs of dehydration, particularly if the patient has had watery diarrhea and vomiting for several days. In extreme cases, patients may be severely hypotensive and in shock. The rash is found predominantly on the trunk but also spreads all over the body.

Laboratory findings include an elevated leukocyte count with the differential blood count showing an increase in band forms and metamyelocytes. The number of platelets is decreased and although there is no evidence of bleeding, disseminated intravascular coagulation is likely. The effects of dehydration on the kidneys are manifested by elevations in creatinine and blood urea nitrogen. Cultures of focal lesions may yield *S. aureus,* but blood cultures are usually negative.

Supportive therapy to replace vascular volume loss is given, along with an appropriate β-lactamase–resistant antimicrobial. *S. aureus* does not need to be isolated to confirm the diagnosis of TSS.

Most patients with TSS recover, although 2% to 5% of cases may be fatal. Recurrence of TSS in menstruating women is as high as 60%. Multiple recurrences that become less severe and shorter in duration have led investigators to hypothesize that immunity to the organism or effect of the toxin eventually develops. Preventive measures such as avoidance of tampon use, use of low absorbency tampons, and more frequent tampon changes have greatly decreased the risk of TSS.

OTHER INFECTIONS

Staphylococcal pneumonia has been known to occur as a bacterial infection secondary to influenza A. Although rare, the infection has a high mortality rate. Staphylococcal pneumonia, which develops as either a contiguous lower respiratory tract infection or a complication of bacteremia, is characterized by multiple abscesses and focal lesions in the pulmonary parenchyma. Infants and immunocompromised patients, such as the elderly and patients receiving chemotherapy or immunosuppressants, are most affected.

Staphylococcal bacteremia leading to secondary pneumonia and endocarditis has been observed among intravenous drug addicts. Fever is the most striking symptom of endocarditis, which must be suspected in an intravenous drug abuser with fever. The organisms gain entrance into the blood, originating from a focal lesion that could be present on the skin or in the respiratory or genitourinary tract.

Staphylococcal **osteomyelitis** occurs as a manifestation secondary to bacteremia. The infection develops when the organism is present in a wound or other focus of infections and gains entrance into the blood. It may lodge in the diaphysis of the long bones and establish an infection. Symptoms include fever, chills, swelling, and pain around the affected area.

Septic arthritis, seen in children and patients with a history of rheumatoid arthritis and intravenous drug abuse, has also been attributed to *S. aureus*. The organisms may be recovered from aspirated joint fluid.

Staphylococcus epidermidis

The role of *S. epidermidis* as an etiologic agent of disease has become increasingly evident. Infections caused by *S. epidermidis* are predominantly hospital acquired. Some of the predisposing factors are instrumentation procedures such as catheterization, prosthetic heart valve implantation, and immunosuppressive therapy. *S. epidermidis* is probably the most common cause of hospital acquired urinary tract infections. Prosthetic valve endocarditis caused by *S. epidermidis* has also increased from 25% of cases in the 1970s to approximately 50% in the 1980s, with about 70% mortality. Other infections caused by *S. epidermidis* occur in intravascular catheters, CSF shunts, and other prosthetic devices. Septicemia has been reported in patients who are immunocompromised.

Infections associated with the use of instruments, such as the use of indwelling catheters and prosthetic devices, are often caused by isolates shown to produce an adherence factor described as **slime.** Slime-producing strains of *S. epidermidis* are able to adhere to and form colonies on the surface of these devices. Slime-producing strains also utilize this adherence factor to inhibit the action of lymphocytes and neutrophils. A laboratory test to detect slime production has been described, but its value in the treatment of the clinical infection is questionable.

Staphylococcus saprophyticus

S. saprophyticus has been associated with urinary tract infections in young, sexually active females. This species is found to adhere more effectively to the epithelial cells lining the urogenital tract than other coagulase-negative staphylococci. It is rarely found in other skin areas or mucous membranes. When present in urine cultures, *S. saprophyticus* may be found in low numbers and yet considered significant.

Other Coagulase-Negative Staphylococci

Other species of coagulase-negative staphylococci (CNS) are found as normal flora in humans and animals. They are not commonly seen as pathogens, although their role in some infections is well established. Therefore they cannot be automatically discarded as contaminants in all cases.

S. haemolyticus is the second most commonly isolated of the CNS, with *S. epidermidis* being the first. It has been reported in wounds, bacteremia, endocarditis, and urinary tract infections. Of notable interest is the emergence of vancomycin resistance in some *S. haemolyticus* isolates.

Two species that are not commonly seen but have established themselves as opportunistic pathogens are *Staphylococcus lugdunensis* and *Staphylococcus schleiferi.* A wide range of infections have been associated with these organisms (e.g., endocarditis, septicemia, prosthesis infections).

| LABORATORY DIAGNOSIS

Specimen Collection and Handling

Proper specimen collection, transport, and processing are essential elements in the correct diagnosis and interpretation of any bacterial culture result. Clinical materials collected from infected sites should be transported to the laboratory without delay to prevent drying, maintain the proper environment, and minimize the growth of contaminating organisms. Although the recovery of staphylococci requires no special procedures, specimens should be taken from the actual site of infection after appropriate cleansing of the surrounding area to avoid contamination by the skin flora.

Microscopic Examination

Microscopic examination of stained smears prepared directly from clinical samples (Figure 10-1) provides information that is helpful in the early diagnosis and treatment of the infection and must always be performed. Numerous gram-positive cocci, along with polymorphonuclear cells in purulent exudates, joint fluids, aspirated secretions,

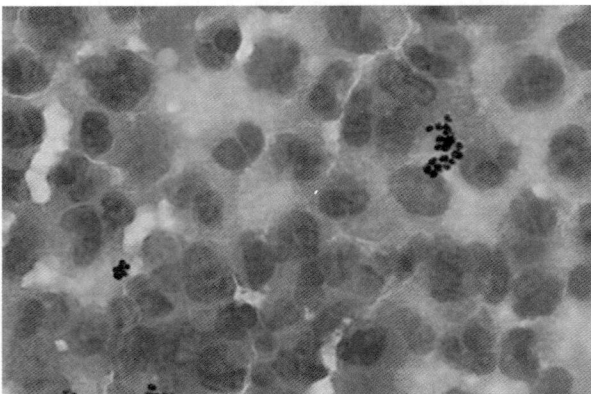

Figure 10-1 _____

Numerous gram-positive cocci in clusters, with many PMNs from an aspirated abcess in staphylococcal disease. *PMNs,* Polymorphonuclear cells.

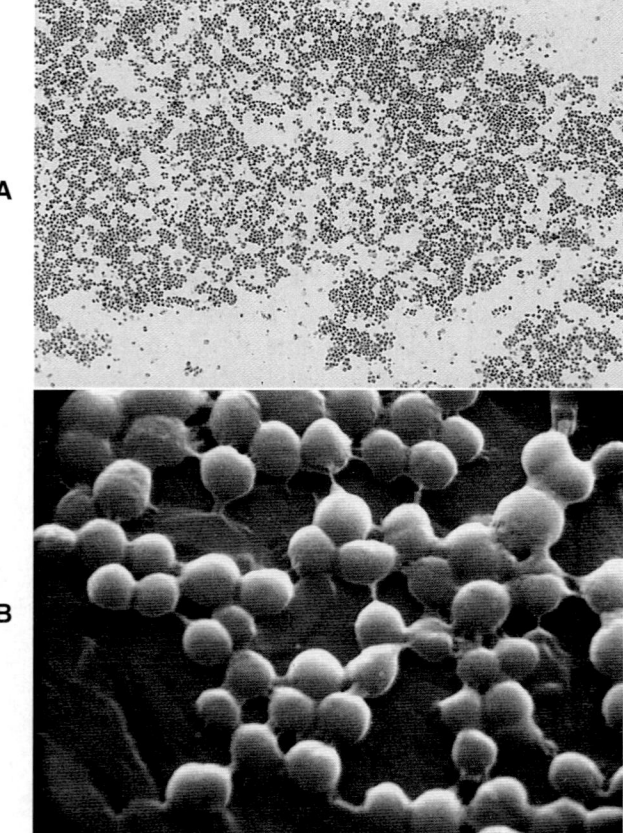

Figure 10-2 _____

A, Microscopic morphology of *Staphylococcus* sp. on Gram stain. Gram-negative–looking cells show how older cells become easily decolorized. **B,** Scanning electron micrograph showing the typical "clusters" of staphylococci.

and other body fluids, are easily seen. A culture should be done regardless of the results of the microscopic examination, because the genus or species cannot be appropriately identified by microscopic morphology alone (Figure 10-2).

Isolation and Identification

Staphylococci grow easily on routine laboratory culture media, particularly sheep's blood agar. A fluid medium such as thioglycolate is usually included in the primary isolation scheme. A selective medium such as mannitol salt agar, Columbia colistin–nalidixic acid agar (CNA), or phenylethyl alcohol (PEA) agar can be used for heavily contaminated specimens.

Cultural characteristics

Staphylococci produce round, smooth, white, creamy colonies on blood agar after 18 to 24 hours of incubation at 35° to 37° C. *S. aureus* may produce hemolytic zones around the colonies (Figure 10-3), which may produce pigment (e.g., yellow, tan, orange). *S. epidermidis* colonies are usually small to medium-sized, nonhemolytic, white colonies. *S. saprophyticus* forms slightly larger colonies, with approximately 50% of the strains producing a yellow pigment. Identification of staphylococci on the basis of colony morphology alone is not recommended.

Identification methods

Staphylococci have been traditionally differentiated from micrococci on the basis of oxidation-

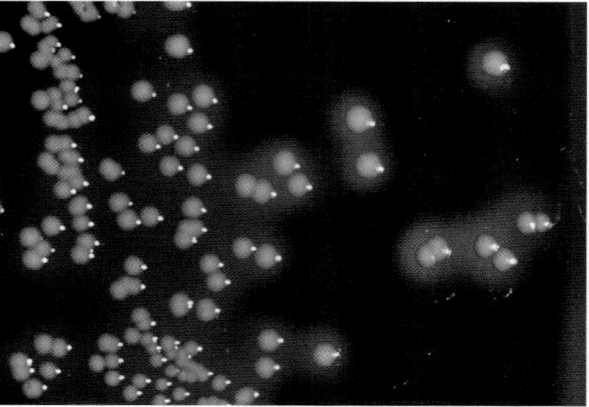

Figure 10-3 _____

Staphylococcus aureus growing on sheep's blood agar showing hemolytic, creamy, buttery-looking colonies.

TABLE 10-3

Differentiation Among Staphylococci from Other Gram-Positive Cocci

Characteristic	Staphylococci	Enterococci	Streptococci	Aerococci	Planococci	Stomatococci	Micrococci
Strict aerobe	−	−	−	−	+	−	+
Facultative anaerobe	d	+	+	+	−	+	−
Motility	−	d	−	−	+	−	−
Growth on NaCl agar							
5% NaCl	+	+	d	+	+	−	+
6.5% NaCl	+	+	d	+	+	−	+
12% NaCl	d	(±)	−	+	+	−	d
Catalase	+	−	−	−	+	±	+
Benzidine test	+	−	−	−	+	+	+
Anaerobic acid from glucose	d	+	+	(+)	−	+	−
Lysostaphin (200 µg/mL)	−	+	+	+	+	+	+*
Erythromycin (9.04 µg/mL)	+	+	−	ND	ND	ND	−†
Bacitracin (0.04-U disk)	+	+	d	−	ND	−	−
Furazolidone (100-µg disk)	−	−	−	−	−	−	+

Modified from Kloos WE, Lambe DE: Staphylococcus. In Balows A et al, editors: *Manual of clinical microbiology,* ed 5, Washington, DC, 1991, American Society for Microbiology.
+, 90% or more species or strains positive; ±, 90% or more species or strains weakly positive; −, 90% or more species or strains negative; *d,* 11%-89% of species or strains positive; ( ), delayed reaction; *ND,* not determined.
*Some strains of *M. luteus, M. roseus,* and *M. sedentarius* demonstrate susceptibility to lysostaphin, presumably because of contaminating levels of endo-β-*N*-acetylglucosaminidase activity.
†A few *Micrococcus* strains demonstrate high-level (MIC >µg/mL) erythromycin resistance.

fermentation (O/F) reactions produced on O/F glucose medium. Staphylococci ferment glucose, whereas micrococci fail to produce acid under anaerobic conditions. However, the O/F tests do not sufficiently discern certain weak acid producers, such as *Micrococcus kristinae,* and those staphylococci that fail to grow or produce acid anaerobically (*Staphylococcus saprophyticus, Staphylococcus auricularis, Staphylococcus hominis, Staphylococcus xylosus,* and *Staphylococcus cohnii*). Tests to differentiate micrococci from staphylococci are shown in Table 10-2. Table 10-3 outlines the key characteristics for differentiating staphylococci from other gram-positive cocci.

S. aureus is identified by the coagulase test (Figure 10-4). The cell-bound coagulase, also referred to as ***clumping factor,*** clots human, rabbit, or pig plasma and is considered a major marker for *S. aureus.* Pig plasma forms a stronger clot and is less susceptible to autolysis than rabbit plasma. The enzyme is easily detected by the slide method and is used to screen colonies that morphologically resemble *S. aureus.* A suspension of the suspected organism is prepared on a glass slide and mixed with a drop of rabbit plasma. If clumping occurs, the isolate is identified as *S. aureus.* Isolates that do not produce cell-bound coagulase should be tested for extracellular free coagulase by the tube

method. **Free coagulase** is an extracellular enzyme that causes a clot to form when bacterial cells are incubated with plasma (Figure 10-5). The clot formed in the tube may have a tendency to undergo autolysis, giving the appearance of a negative result. The laboratory professional should look for clot formation after 4 hours of incubation at 37° C. If no clot appears, the tube should be left at room temperature to incubate overnight, and

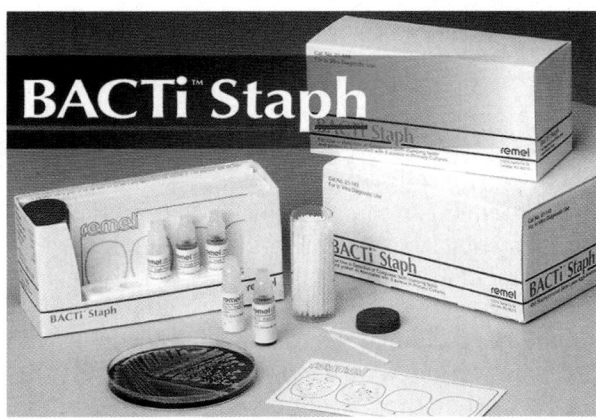

Figure 10-4

(Bacti Staph) cell-wall–bound "clumping factor" and "protein A." Latex agglutination method is available commercially. (Courtesy Remel Lenexa, Kan.)

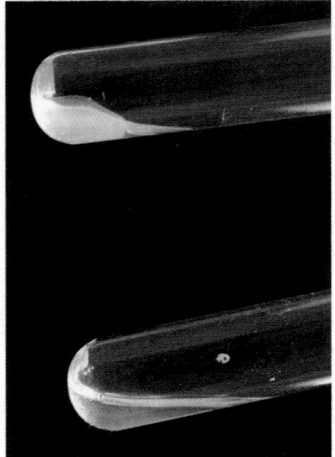

Figure 10-5 _____
Tube coagulase test detects extracellular enzyme "free coagulase." Top tube is coagulase positive.

TABLE 10-4 _____
Groups of Coagulase-Positive Staphylococci and Their Clinical Source and Significance

Species	Source*
S. aureus group	
S. aureus	**Human**, animal
S. aureus ssp. *anaerobius*	Animal
S. hyicus group	
S. hyicus	**Animal**
S. intermedius group	
S. intermedius	**Animal**
S. schleiferi ssp. *coagulans*	**Animal**
S. delphini	Animal

Courtesy Leona W. Ayers, M.D.
***Boldface** indicates common in human or veterinary disease.

checked the following day. Because 5% of *S. aureus* organisms do not produce cell-bound coagulase, any negative slide coagulase test result must be confirmed with the tube method. Table 10-4 groups the coagulase-positive staphylococci, identifying their clinical source and significance. The laboratory professional must be aware that staphylococci other than *S. aureus* organisms produce bound or free coagulase (Table 10-5).

Isolates that do not produce either bound or free coagulase are reported as coagulase-negative staphylococci (Figure 10-6). Urine isolates that are coagulase negative are further tested to presumptively identify *S. saprophyticus*. Presumptive identification of *S. saprophyticus* is accomplished by testing for **novobiocin susceptibility** using a 5-μg novobiocin disk (Figure 10-7). *S. saprophyticus* is resistant to novobiocin, but most other coagulase-negative staphylococci are susceptible.

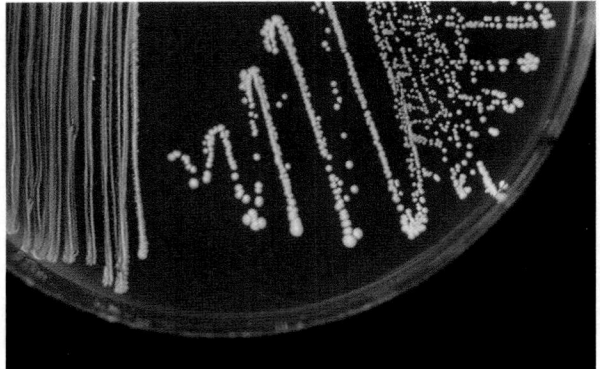

Figure 10-6 _____
Coagulase-negative staphylococci growing on sheep's blood agar in nonhemolytic, white, creamy colonies.

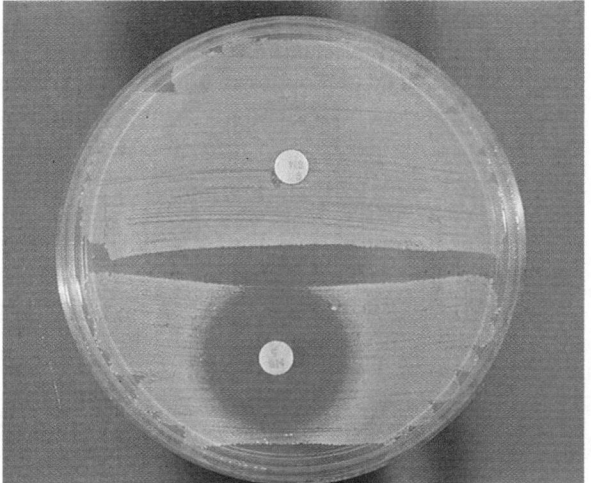

Figure 10-7 _____
Novobiocin susceptibility test to differentiate coagulase-negative staphylococci isolate from urine samples. *Staphylococcus saprophyticus (top)* is resistant to novobiocin, indicated by the *lack* of a zone of inhibition around the disk.

TABLE 10-5

Key Tests for Identification of the Most Clinically Significant Staphylococcus Species

Test	S. aureus	S. epidermidis	S. haemolyticus	S. lugdunensis	S. schleiferi	S. saprophyticus	S. intermedius	S. hyicus
Colony pigment*	+	−	d	d	−	d	−	−
Staphylocoagulase	+	−	−	−	−	−	+	d
Clumping factor*	+	−	−	(+)	+	−	d	−
Heat-stable nuclease	+	−	−	−	+	−	+	+
Alkaline phosphatase	+	+	+	−	+	−	+	+
Pyrrolidonyl arylamidase*	−	−	+	+	−	−	+	−
Ornithine decarboxylase	−	(d)	−	+	−	−	−	−
Urease*	d	+	−	d	(+)	+	+	d
β-Galactosidase*	−	−	−	−	+	+	+	−
Acetoin production	+	+	+	+	+	+	−	−
Novobiocin resistance*	S	S	S	S	S	R	S	S
Polymyxin B resistance*	S	R	S	S/R	S	S	S	R
Acid (aerobically from)								
D-Trehalose	+	−	+	+	d	+	+	+
D-Mannitol	+	−	d	−	−	d	(d)	−
D-Mannose	+	(+)	−	+	+	−	+	+
D-Turanose	+	(d)	(d)	(d)	−	+	d	−
D-Xylose	−	−	−	−	−	−	−	−
D-Cellubiose	−	−	−	−	−	−	−	−
Maltose	+	+	+	+	−	+	(±)	−
Sucrose	+	+	+	+	−	+	+	+

Modified from Kloos WE, Lambe DE: Staphylococcus. In Balows A et al, editors: *Manual of clinical microbiology*, ed 5, Washington, DC, 1991, American Society for Microbiology.

+, 90% or more strains positive; −, 90% or more strains negative; d, 11%-89% of strains positive; ( ), delayed reaction R, resistant; S, sensitive.

*Descriptions are the same as for Table 10-3.

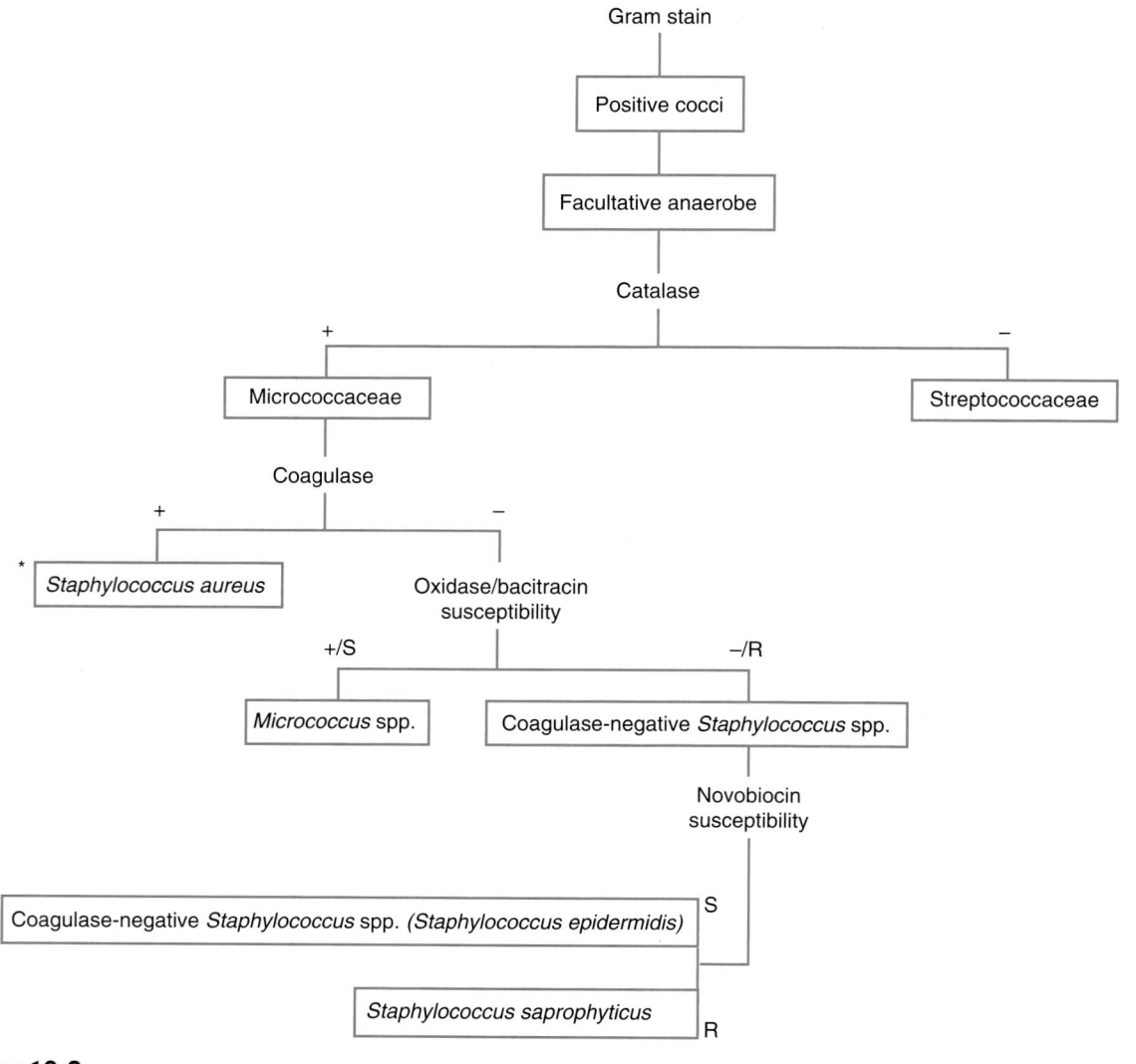

Figure 10-8 _____

Schema for the identification of staphylococcal species. NOTE: Other *Staphylococcus* spp. that are coagulase positive besides *S. aureus* include *S. lugdunensis* (which is often latex test positive), *S. intermedius* (tube positive and latex positive), and *S. delphini* (tube positive and latex positive). (Modified from Kloos WE, Jorgensen JH: Staphylococci. In Lennette EH et al, editors: *Manual of clinical microbiology,* ed 4, Washington, DC, 1985, American Society for Microbiology.)

Figure 10-8 shows the schema for the identification of clinically significant staphylococci.

Although *S. epidermidis* and *S. saprophyticus* are the most clinically significant species of coagulase-negative staphylococci, other species are becoming more important clinically. Table 10-5 outlines some key tests for identification of the clinically significant species of *Staphylococci,* including coagulase-negative isolates.

Rapid methods of identification

There are a number of rapid test kits on the market for differentiating *S. aureus* from the coagulase-negative staphylococci. Among these are the Bacto Staph latex test (Difco), color slide staph test (Seradyn), and Bacti Staph (Remel) (see Figure 10-4). These kits utilize plasma-coated latex particles. The plasma detects both clumping factor (with fibrinogen) and protein A in the cell wall of *S. aureus* (immunoglobulin G). Another test kit available is the Staphyloslide test (Becton Dickinson Microbiology System), which detects clumping factor using sensitized sheep's red blood cells with fibrinogen.

Rapid identification of staphylococci may be performed using the API-Staph Ident. Identification is made on the basis of positive reactions observed in microcupules that contain substrates for carbohydrate utilization. A four-digit profile code is produced from the reactions. Species identification is derived from a computer-based profile book.

ANTIMICROBIAL SUSCEPTIBILITY

Infections by staphylococcal strains that do not produce **β-lactamase** can be treated with penicillin. However, the incidence of penicillin resistance, especially in *S. aureus,* is so high (85% to 90%) that other antibiotics must often be used. There is considerable variability in the susceptibility patterns of staphylococcal isolates. Therefore it is extremely important to perform antimicrobial susceptibility tests on all isolates, especially those from serious infections. Various β-lactamase–resistant penicillins have been developed to treat infections caused by penicillin-resistant staphylococcal species, especially *S. aureus.* The most notable of these is methicillin. As with the initial success of penicillin in the treatment of staphylococcal infections, methicillin treatment appeared to solve the problem of β-lactamase production by clinical isolates. Unfortunately, the solution was temporary.

METHICILLIN-RESISTANT STAPHYLOCOCCI

One of the major problems that has concerned clinicians since the mid-1980s is the evolution of **methicillin-resistant staphylococci,** specifically methicillin-resistant strains of *S. aureus* (MRSA) and *S. epidermidis* (MRSE). The increased number of resistant strains being isolated has been seen worldwide. Some isolates of MRSA are also resistant to multiple agents, including aminoglycosides. Previously limited to large institutions, outbreaks of MRSA are now quite common in all hospital settings in the

United States. Transmission of these strains has been attributed to cross-contamination among infected patients and carriers. Hospital personnel have been implicated as possible human vectors. Similarly, MRSE has also emerged in hospitalized patients and patients who have undergone prosthetic heart valve surgery.

Vancomycin remains the antimicrobial of choice for endocarditis caused by MRSA and MRSE. Because of adverse effects related to this drug, its use is reserved for patients with systemic infections such as bacteremia, endocarditis, and pneumonia. It has been reported that administration of vancomycin in combination with rifampin or gentamicin enhances the therapeutic effects of vancomycin against MRSE. However, similar to the experience encountered with methicillin, the possible emergence of vancomycin-resistant *S. aureus* has been a major concern. Intermediate resistance to vancomycin by *S. aureus* has already been reported. Resistance to vancomycin by *S. aureus* has also been demonstrated in vitro, when the enterococcal plasmid gene encoded for resistance was transferred by conjugation in *S. aureus.* Emergence of highly resistant *S. aureus* strains is likely to present a great therapeutic challenge in the near future.

Prevention and control of nosocomial infections caused by MRSA, MRSE, and vancomycin-resistant *S. aureus* depend on proper hand-washing techniques and adherence to established infection control measures by health care providers.

Bibliography

Baddour LM, Christensen GD: Prosthetic valve endocarditis due to small-colony staphylococcal variants, *Rev Infect Dis* 9:1168, 1987.

Bergdoll MS: Enterotoxins. In Easmon CSF, Adlam C, editors: *Staphylococci and staphylococcal infections,* New York, 1983, Academic Press.

Berkley SF et al: The relationship of tampon characteristics to menstrual toxic shock syndrome, *JAMA* 258:917, 1987.

Bonventr PF et al: Production of staphylococcal enterotoxin F and pyrogenic exotoxin C by *Staphylococcus aureus* isolates from toxic shock syndrome–associated sources, *Infect Immun* 40:1023, 1983.

Christensen GD et al: Adherence of slime-producing strains of *Staphylococcus epidermidis* to smooth surfaces, *Infect Immun* 37:318, 1982.

Davis P et al: Toxic-shock syndrome: epidemiologic features, recurrence, risk factors, and prevention, *N Engl J Med* 303:1429, 1980.

Dunne WM, Franson TR: Coagulase-negative staphylococci: the Rodney Dangerfield of pathogens, *Clin Microbiol Newsl* 8:37, 1986.

Elias PM, Fritsch P, Epstein E: Staphylococcal scalded skin syndrome, *Arch Dermatol* 113:207, 1977.

Eng RHK et al: Species identification of coagulase-negative staphylococcal isolates from blood cultures, *J Clin Microbiol* 15:439, 1982.

Fleurette J et al: Clinical isolates of *Staphylococcus lugdunensis* and *S. schleiferi:* bacteriological characteristics and susceptibility to antimicrobial agents, *Res Microbiol* 140:107, 1989.

Friedman et al: *Staphylococcus epidermidis* septicemia in children with leukemia and lymphoma, *Am J Dis Child* 138:715, 1984.

Fritsch P, Elias P, Varga J: The fate of staphylococcal exfoliation in newborn and adult mice, *Br J Dermatol* 95:275, 1976.

Garbe P et al: *Staphylococcus aureus* isolates from patients with nonmenstrual toxic shock syndrome, *JAMA* 253:2538, 1985.

Gill VJ, Selepak AT, Williams ED: Species identification and antibiotic susceptibilities of coagulase-negative staphylococci isolated from clinical specimens, *J Clin Microbiol* 18:1314, 1984.

Goldberg N: Staphylococcal scalded skin syndrome mimicking acute graft-vs-host disease in a bone marrow transplant recipient, *Arch Dermatol* 125:85, 1989.

Haller PR: Infections in intravenous drug abusers, *Postgrad Med* 83:95, 1988.

Hebert GA et al: Characteristics of coagulase-negative staphylococci that help differentiate these species and other members of the family Micrococcaceae, *J Clin Microbiol* 26:1939, 1988.

Helgerson S. Mallery B, Foster L: Toxic shock syndrome in Oregon, *JAMA* 252:3402, 1984.

Holt JG et al, editors: Gram-positive cocci. In Bergey: *Bergey's manual of determinative bacteriology,* ed 9, Baltimore, 1994, Williams & Wilkins.

Humphreys H, Keane C: Methicillin-resistant *Staphylococcus aureus* and vancomycin-resistant enterococci, *Lancet,* 350 (9079):737, 1997.

Jeljaszewicz J, Ciborowski P, editors: *The staphylococci.* Proceedings of the VIth International Symposium on Staphylococci and Staphylococcal Infections, New York, 1991, Gustav Fischer Verlag.

Jorgensen JH: Laboratory and epidemiologic experience with methicillin-resistant *Staphylococcus aureus* in the USA. *Eur J Clin Microbiol* 5:693, 1986.

Karchmer AW, Archer GL, Dismukes WE: *Staphylococcus epidermidis* causing prosthetic valve endocarditis: microbiologic and clinical observations as guides to therapy, *Ann Intern Med* 98:44, 1983.

Kloos WE, Bannerman TL: Update on clinical significance of coagulase-negative staphylococci, *Clin Microbiol Rev* 7:11, 1994.

Kloos WE, Musselwhite MS: Distribution and persistence of *Staphylococcus* and *Micrococcus* species and other aerobic bacteria on human skin, *Appl Microbiol* 30:381, 1975.

Kloos WE, Wolfshoh JF: Identification of *Staphylococcus* species with the APISTAPH-IDENT system, *J Clin Microbiol* 16:509, 1982.

Koontz F, Pfaller M: Coagulase-negative staphylococci: why and when to do what, *Clin Microbiol Newsl* 11:125, 1989.

Levine G, Norden CW: Staphylococcal scalded-skin syndrome in an adult, *N Engl J Med* 287:1339, 1972.

Lowy FD: Medical progress: *S. aureus* infections, *N Engl J Med* 339(8):520, 1998.

Macdonald A, Smith G, editors: *The staphylococci.* Proceedings of the Alexander Ogston Centennial Conference, Aberdeen, Scotland, 1981, Aberdeen University Press.

Maple PA, Hamilton-Miller JM, Brumfitt W: World-wide antibiotic resistance in the methicillin-resistant *Staphylococcus aureus, Lancet* 1(8637):537, 1989.

Marrie TJ et al: *Staphylococcus* as a cause of urinary tract infection, *J Clin Microbiol* 16:427, 1982.

Marsik FJ, Brake S: Species identification and susceptibility to 17 antibiotics of coagulase-negative staphylococci isolated from clinical specimens, *J Clin Microbiol* 15:640, 1982.

Melish M, Glasgow L: Staphylococcal scalded skin syndrome: the expanded clinical syndrome, *J Pediatr* 78:958, 1971.

Molinari JA: Microbial disease trends and acquired antibiotic resistance: part 2: evolving microbial pathogens antibiotic-resistant *Staphylococcus aureus, Compendium of Continuing Education in Dentistry,* 18(4):320, 1997.

Morrison V, Oldfield E: Postoperative toxic shock syndrome, *Arch Surg* 118:791, 1983.

Petitti D, Reingold A, Chin J: The incidence of toxic shock syndrome in northern California, *JAMA* 255:368, 1986.

Pfaller M, Herwaldt LA: Laboratory, clinical, and epidemiological aspects of coagulase-negative staphylococci, *Clin Microbiol Rev* 1:281, 1988.

Reingold AL et al: Non-menstrual toxic shock syndrome, *Ann Intern Med* 96(2):871, 1982.

Roberson JR et al: Evaluation of methods for differentiation of coagulase-positive staphylococci, *J Clin Microbiol* 30:3217, 1992.

Schleivert PM et al: Identification and characterization of an exotoxin from *Staphylococcus aureus* associated with toxic shock syndrome, *J Infect Dis* 143:509, 1981.

Schumacher-Perdreau F: Clinical significance and laboratory diagnosis of coagulase-negative staphylococci, *Clin Microbiol Newsl* 13:97, 1991.

Schwalbe RS, Stapleton JT, Gilligan PH: Emergence of vancomycin resistance in coagulase-negative staphylococci, *N Engl J Med* 316:927, 1987.

Sheagren JN: *Staphylococcus aureus:* the persistent pathogen, part 1, *N Engl J Med* 310:1368, 1984.

Sheagren JN: *Staphylococcus aureus:* the persistent pathogen, part 2, *N Engl J Med* 310:1437, 1984.

Sorrell TC et al: Vancomycin therapy for methicillin-resistant *Staphylococcus aureus, Ann Intern Med* 97:344, 1982.

Todd J: Toxins, test tubes, and tampons, *Am J Med* 84:579, 1988.

Wiseman G: The hemolysins of *Staphylococcus aureus, Bacteriol Rev* 39:317, 1987.

LEARNING ASSESSMENT

1. What is the identity of the isolate described in the case study at the beginning of the chapter?

2. In what patient population does this organism normally cause infection?

3. In what way is the organism differentiated from other similar isolates?

4. What types of infections does *S. aureus* produce?

5. What is responsible for the staphylococcal infection, scalded skin syndrome?

6. How does protein A contribute to the virulence of *S. aureus?*

7. What are the two types of coagulase produced by *S. aureus?* How is each type detected in the laboratory?

8. In what clinical condition would coagulase-negative staphylococci be significant?

9. What is the role of slime in infections caused by *S. epidermidis?*

CHAPTER 11

Streptococcaceae

Hal S. Larsen

STREPTOCOCCUS AND *ENTEROCOCCUS:*
  GENERAL CHARACTERISTICS
  Cell Wall Structure
  Classification
    Hemolytic patterns
    Physiologic characteristics
    The Lancefield classification scheme
    Biochemical identification
  Noncultural Identification

CLINICALLY SIGNIFICANT STREPTOCOCCI
  AND THEIR ASSOCIATED DISEASES
  Streptococcus pyogenes (Group A Streptococci)
    Antigenic structure
    Virulence factors
    Clinical infections
    Laboratory diagnosis
  Streptococcus agalactiae (Group B Streptococci)
    Antigenic structure
    Virulence factors
    Clinical infections
    Laboratory diagnosis

  Other Groups
    Groups C and G
    Group D
  Enterococcus
  Streptococcus pneumoniae
    Antigenic structure
    Virulence factors
    Clinical infections
    Laboratory diagnosis
  Viridans Streptococci
    Clinical infections
    Laboratory diagnosis
  Nutritionally Variant Streptococci

STREPTOCOCCUS-LIKE ORGANISMS
  Aerococcus
  Leuconostoc
  Pediococcus
  Gemella

OBJECTIVES

1. Describe the general characteristics of *Streptococcus* and related organisms.
2. Explain the Lancefield classification of the streptococci.
3. Discuss the importance of hemolysis patterns on blood agar in the identification of streptococcal isolates.
4. Contrast the significance of the streptococci commonly isolated in the clinical laboratory, both those that occur as normal flora and those that are potential pathogens.
5. Describe the virulence factors associated with the Streptococcaceae.
6. Explain how infection caused by the Streptococcaceae is established.
7. Give the characteristic features of streptococci in direct smears and from culture.
8. Given the microscopic and colonial morphology of an organism isolated from a clinical sample, describe the appropriate biochemical tests for presumptively identifying the organism.
9. State the principle and purpose of each differential test used in the identification of the Streptococcaceae.
10. Discuss the major serologic tests used to detect antibodies that are produced after recent streptococcal infections.

KEY TERMS

Streptococcus
Enterococcus
Hemolytic pattern
Beta (β) hemolysis
Alpha (α) hemolysis
Nonhemolytic
α-Prime hemolysis
Lancefield classification
C carbohydrate
Group A streptococci
  (*Streptococcus pyogenes*)

Group B streptococci
  (*Streptococcus agalactiae*)
Bacitracin
Sulfamethoxazole and trimethoprim (SXT)
Optochin
Bile solubility
S. pneumoniae
Hippurate hydrolysis
PYR hydrolysis test
CAMP test
Bile esculin hydrolysis test

NaCl test
M protein
Hyaluronidase (spreading factor)
Streptolysin O
Pharyngitis
Scarlet fever
Impetigo
Erysipelas
Cellulitis
Rheumatic fever
Acute glomerulonephritis
Streptococcal toxic shock syndrome

Toxic shock syndrome
Group D streptococci
C-reactive protein
Pneumonia
Viridans streptococci
Nutritionally variant streptococci (NVS)
Aerococcus
Leuconostoc
Pediococcus
Gemella

CASE STUDY

A 9-year-old boy complained of fever and sore throat over a 3-day period. On examination by his physician, his pharynx was red and both tonsils were swollen. There was a pronounced cervical adenopathy. A swab of the tonsillar area was taken and inoculated to sheep's blood agar plate (BAP). After 24 hours of incubation, small, shiny, translucent colonies showing β-hemolysis were noted.

The organisms included in the Streptococcaceae are gram-positive cocci that are usually arranged in pairs or chains. Most are facultative anaerobes. The growth requirements can be complex, with the use of blood or enriched medium necessary for their isolation. Their role in human disease ranges from well-established and common to rare but increasing. Clinical microbiologists have ample opportunity to become well acquainted with the members of the Streptococcaceae.

STREPTOCOCCUS AND ENTEROCOCCUS: GENERAL CHARACTERISTICS

Members of **Streptococcus** and **Enterococcus** are gram-positive spherical cells arranged in chains or pairs (Figure 11-1). Compared with cells of other gram-positive cocci, however, the cells of *Streptococcus* and *Enterococcus* appear somewhat more elongated than spherical. They are more likely to appear in chains when grown in broth culture (Figure 11-1 *B*).

The metabolism is fermentative, with lactic acid the primary product. A key characteristic of both genera is that they are catalase negative. Growth is poor on nutrient media such as trypticase soy agar. On media enriched with blood, serum, or glucose, however, growth is more pronounced. The colonies are usually small and somewhat transparent. In addition, some species require increased carbon dioxide for good growth.

Other gram-positive cocci resemble streptococci. These genera, including *Aerococcus, Lactobacillus, Leuconostoc,* and *Pediococcus,* are considered later in this chapter. This chapter discusses characteristics, clinical infections, and laboratory diagnosis associated with each species.

The role of the Streptococcaceae in disease has been known for over 100 years. The range of infections caused by these organisms is wide and well-studied. As we have also seen with other organisms, however, the roles in disease of the usual microbial flora, the previously unknown or poorly characterized species, and the saprophytes are becoming more prominent.

Cell Wall Structure

As a group, the Streptococcaceae possess a typical gram-positive cell wall consisting of mucopeptide (peptidoglycan) and teichoic acid as well as a capsule in young cultures. All streptococci except the viridans group have a layer of C carbohydrate, which can be utilized to serologically classify an isolate. A schematic diagram of the streptococcal cell wall is shown in Figure 11-2. Other cell-wall antigens are present in specific C carbohydrate groups and are explained in the discussions of the individual groups.

Classification

Several different approaches to classification have been used. Of these, four remain useful to the laboratory professional. These four classification schemes are (1) hemolytic pattern on sheep's

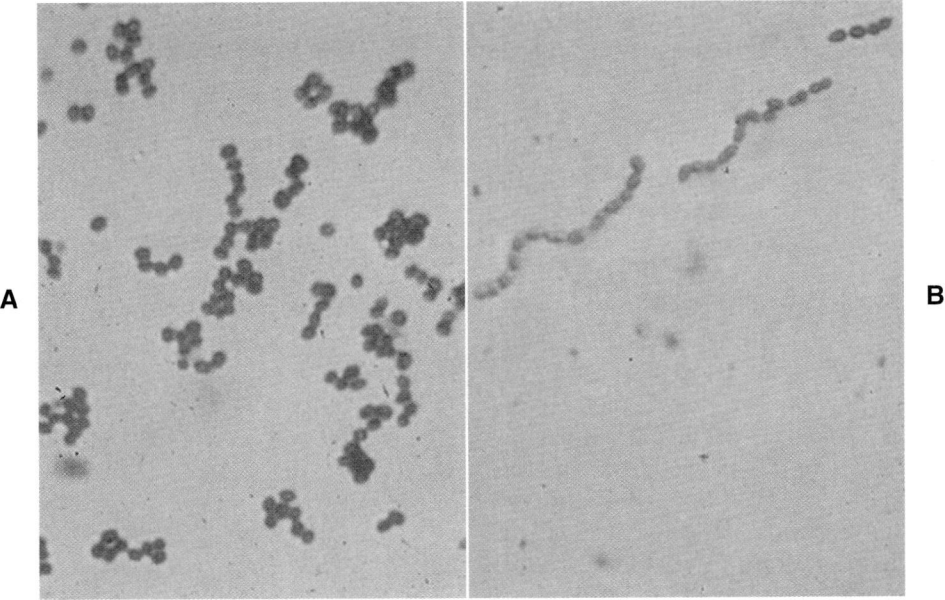

Figure 11-1

Gram stain of *Streptococcus.* **A,** Solid medium. **B,** Liquid medium.

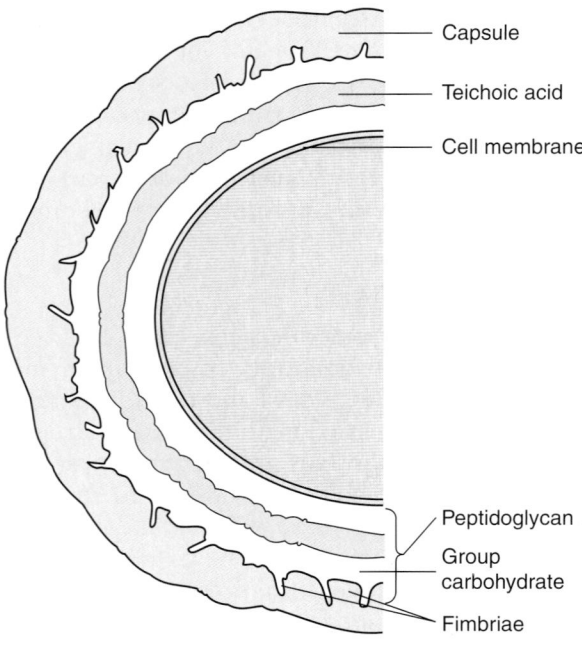

Figure 11-2

Schematic representation of streptococcal cell wall.

the color of the agar; such a colony is termed **non-hemolytic.** Some references term this result as gamma (γ) hemolysis. Because no lysis of the red cells occur, however, γ *hemolysis* is confusing and is not used in this chapter. Some isolates belong-

TABLE 11-1
Types of Hemolysis

Hemolysis	Description
Alpha (α)	Partial lysis of red blood cells around colony
	Greenish discoloration of area around colony
Beta (β)	Complete lysis of red blood cells around colony
	Clear area around colony
Nonhemolytic	No lysis of red blood cells around colony
	No change in agar
Alpha-prime (α′) or wide zone	Small area of intact red blood cells around colony surrounded by a wider zone of complete hemolysis

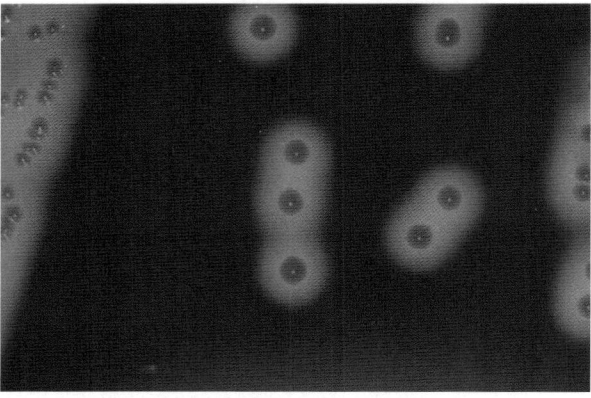

Figure 11-3

A β-hemolytic streptococcal colony on blood agar.

blood agar, (2) physiologic characteristics (type of infection, site of origin, etc.), (3) serologic group or type of C carbohydrate present (Lancefield classification), and (4) biochemical characteristics. Each scheme is used to some degree, and the identification process for a streptococcal isolate in the clinical laboratory may utilize features from each scheme.

Hemolytic patterns

The laboratory professional often makes an initial classification on the basis of the **hemolytic pattern** of the isolate on sheep's blood agar. Although hemolysis patterns can be helpful during the initial work-up of an isolate, it must be kept in mind that many species of streptococci may show more than one type of hemolytic pattern. The types of hemolysis possible are outlined in Table 11-1.

When the red blood cells in the agar surrounding the colony are completely lysed, the resulting area is clear. It is referred to as **beta (β) hemolysis** (Figure 11-3). A partial lysis of the red cells results in a greenish discoloration of the area surrounding the colony. It is termed **alpha (α) hemolysis** (Figure 11-4).

When the red cells immediately surrounding the colony are unaffected, there is no change in

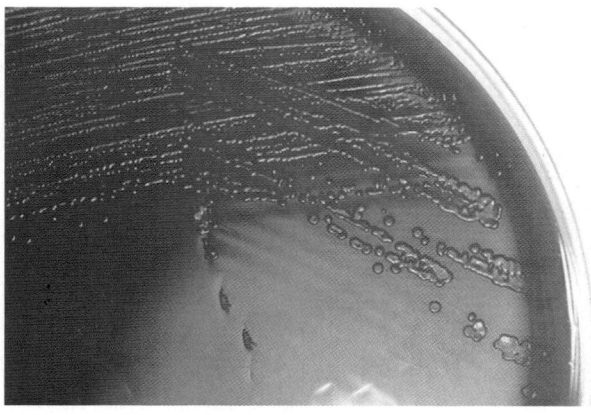

Figure 11-4

An α-hemolytic streptococcal colony on blood agar.

ing to the viridans group produce what is called *wide-zone* or **α-prime hemolysis.** The colonies are surrounded by a very small zone of no hemolysis and then a wider zone of β hemolysis. This reaction may be mistaken for β hemolysis at first glance. The use of a dissecting microscope or the scanning objective shows the narrow zone of intact red cells and the wider zone of complete hemolysis.

Physiologic characteristics

Streptococci have also been classified according to physiologic characteristics. This classification divides the species into four groups: pyogenic streptococci, lactic acid streptococci, enterococci, and viridans streptococci. The *pyogenic streptococci* are those that produce pus; these organisms are mostly β-hemolytic and constitute the majority of the Lancefield groups. The *lactic acid streptococci* are nonhemolytic organisms often found in dairy products; they are part of Lancefield group N. The *enterococci* comprise those species found as part of the flora of the human intestine; this group of organisms is now part of the genus *Enterococcus.* The *viridans streptococci* are not part of Lancefield's classification because they do not have a C carbohydrate; they are widely found as normal flora in the upper respiratory tract of humans. The viridans streptococci are α-hemolytic or nonhemolytic and are often seen as opportunistic pathogens. For the most part, this physiologic classification is historical. Nevertheless, the terms *enterococci* and *viridans streptococci* remain and are still used to describe clinical isolates.

The Lancefield classification scheme

The most commonly used classification scheme was developed in the 1930s by Rebecca Lancefield. The **Lancefield classification** is based upon extraction of **C carbohydrate** from the streptococcal cell wall by placing the organisms in dilute acid and heating for 10 minutes. The soluble antigen was used to immunize rabbits to obtain antisera to the various C carbohydrate groups. After first recognizing the antigen in β-hemolytic streptococci, Lancefield was able to divide the streptococci into serologic groups (designated by letters). Organisms in group A possess the same antigenic C carbohydrate, those in group B have the same C carbohydrate, and so on.

Some of the groups contain several different streptococcal species, whereas others have only one species. For example, ***Streptococcus pyogenes*** is the only member of group A. Therefore the terms *S. pyogenes* and **group A streptococci** describe the same organism, because practically, no other organisms are in this Lancefield group. The same is true of group B, the only member of which is ***Streptococcus agalactiae.*** The terms ***group B streptococci*** and *S. agalactiae* are therefore interchangeable. The other Lancefield groups contain varying numbers of species. Group D streptococci contain several species, including *Streptococcus bovis* and *Streptococcus equinus.*

In addition, streptococcal species other than those that produce β hemolysis are found to possess C carbohydrate. Some are found as usual flora in animals or as animal pathogens, and others may be found in both humans and animals. The Lancefield groups most commonly seen in human infections are A, B, C, D, F, and G, although not all Lancefield groups commonly cause human infection.

Classification of *Streptococcus* and *Enterococcus* is shown in Table 11-2.

Biochemical identification

Biochemical identification can be performed even by small laboratories. Although definitive identification requires a large number of characteristics or perhaps serologic methods, presumptive identification can be accomplished relatively easily with a few key tests and characteristics. Presumptive identification, in the great majority of cases, possesses a high enough rate of accuracy to be useful to the clinician and does not require the exhaustive additional tests that are needed to meet the criteria for definitive identification, especially for those species in groups A, B, and D as well as *Streptococcus pneumoniae* and *Enterococcus.* Speciation of the viridans streptococci, however, does require a considerable increase in the number of tests. The laboratory professional must evaluate the needs of the clinicians and patient population served, the cost of an expanded identification scheme, the resources and abilities of the laboratory, and the usefulness of the data produced.

Table 11-3 outlines the biochemical characteristics used to presumptively identify selected members of the Streptococcaceae.

SUSCEPTIBILITY TESTING

Susceptibility to various antimicrobials can be useful in the early differentiation of gram-positive cocci.

TABLE 11-2

Classification of Streptococcus *and* Enterococcus

Species	Lancefield Group Antigen	Hemolysis Type(s)	Common Terms	Disease Association(s)
S. pyogenes	A	β*	Group A strep	Rheumatic fever; scarlet fever; pharyngitis; glomerulonephritis; pyogenic infections
S. agalactiae	B	β*	Group B strep	Neonatal sepsis; meningitis; puerperal fever; pyogenic infections
S. equisimilis *S. equi* sp. *zooepidemicus* *S. equi*	C	β	Group C strep	Pharyngitis (?); impetigo; pyogenic infections
S. bovis *S. equinus*	D	α, none	*Nonenterococcus*	Endocarditis; urinary tract infections; pyogenic infections
E. faecalis *E. faecium* *E. durans*	D	α, β, none	*Enterococcus*	Urinary tract infections; pyogenic infections
Other species	F, G	β, (α, none)		Pyogenic infections
S. pneumoniae	—	α	*Pneumococcus*	Pneumonia; meningitis; pyogenic infections
S. mutans group *S. sanguis* group *S. mitis* group *S. salivarius* group	—	α, none	Viridans strep (all four groups referred to as *viridans strep*)	Endocarditis; dental caries; abscesses in various tissues

*Occasionally, isolates are found that are nonhemolytic.

Bacitracin has been used for many years to differentiate group A streptococci from other groups of β-hemolytic streptococci. A low concentration of bacitracin (0.04 U) selectively inhibits the growth of group A streptococci. Procedure 11-1 shows the presumptive identification of *S. pyogenes* using bacitracin susceptibility. The PYR test has replaced the bacitracin susceptibility test for group A streptococci because its reaction is more definitive.

Susceptibility to **sulfamethoxazole and trimethoprim (SXT)** can be used in conjunction with that to bacitracin to improve the accuracy of group A identification (Figure 11-5). Groups A and B are resistant to SXT, whereas groups other than A and B are sensitive. Figure 11-6 shows resistance of group A β-hemolytic streptococci to SXT. The pattern shown by *S. pyogenes* when both bacitracin and SXT disks are used is susceptibility to bacitracin and resistance to SXT. The pattern shown by *S. agalactiae* (group B) is resistance to both bacitracin and SXT. If the blood agar contains SXT, a bacitracin disk may be placed directly on the primary inoculum, because growth of the majority of interfering respiratory flora will be inhibited but *S. pyogenes* and *S. agalactiae* will grow. This method is helpful to screen for group A streptococci from throat cultures. The sheep's blood agar containing SXT is inoculated with the throat swab, and a bacitracin disk is placed onto the agar. Those β-hemolytic colonies that grow and are susceptible to bacitracin are presumptively identified as *S. pyogenes*.

Vancomycin is an effective antimicrobial for treating infections caused by gram-positive organisms. Until the mid-1980s, resistance to vancomycin was rarely seen in clinical isolates. Vancomycin resistance is now being seen more commonly, although it is still not widespread. Gram-positive isolates should be tested routinely for vancomycin susceptibility. Table 11-3 lists the usual patterns of vancomycin susceptibility for a number of gram-positive cocci. In particular, *Pediococcus* and *Leuconostoc* are resistant to vancomycin. Some *Streptococcus* isolates and a significant number of *Enterococcus* isolates demonstrate resistance to this antimicrobial.

The differentiation of *S. pneumoniae* from other α-hemolytic streptococcal isolates can be accomplished by the use of **optochin** susceptibility. This is done in the same fashion as the bacitracin disk method. The suspected isolate is inoculated onto a blood agar plate. A disk saturated with a solu-

TABLE 11-3

Biochemical Identification of Streptococcus and Related Organisms

Characteristic	S. pyogenes	S. agalactiae	Other β-hemolytics*	Enterococcus	Group D streptococci	S. pneumoniae	Viridans streptococci	Aerococcus	Pediococcus	Leuconostoc
Hemolysis type	β	β	β	α, β, none	α, none	α	α, none	α, none	α, none	α, none
Susceptibility to										
Vancomycin	S	S	S	S(R)	S	S	S	S	R	R
Bacitracin	S	R†	R†	R	R	S	R†	S	R	R
SXT	R	R	S	R	V	S	S	S		
Optochin	R	R	R	R	R	S	R			
Hydrolysis of										
Hippurate	−	+	−	−†	−	−	−†	+	+	−
PYR	+	−	−	+	−	−	−	+	−	−
CAMP	−	+	−	−	−	−	−	−	−	−
Leucine aminopeptidase	+	+	+	+	+	+	+	−	+	−
Bile esculin	−	−	−	+	+	−	−†	V	+	V
Growth in 6.5% NaCl	−	−	−	+	−	−	−	+	V	V

R, Resistant; *S*, susceptible; *S(R)*, greater percentage susceptible; *V*, variable; +, present; −, absent.
*β-Hemolytic groups other than A, B, and D.
†Exceptions may occur.

PROCEDURE 11-1. Bacitracin Susceptibility

Purpose:	To differentiate *S. pyogenes* from other β-hemolytic groups
Principle:	Group A streptococci are susceptible to low levels (0.04 U) of bacitracin, whereas other groups are resistant. Rare strains of group A streptococci are resistant (approximately 1%), whereas some strains of groups B, C, and G streptococci are sensitive (5% to 10%). Sensitivity to bacitracin *presumptively* identifies an isolate as *S. pyogenes.* This procedure was designed for use only with pure cultures.
Specimen:	Isolated colonies on sheep's blood agar
Media:	5% sheep's blood agar plate
Reagent:	Bacitracin disk (0.04 U)
Procedure:	1. Streak surface of agar plate to obtain confluent growth. 2. Aseptically place bacitracin disk onto inoculated surface. Press down gently on the disk to ensure complete contact with the agar surface. 3. Invert and incubate plates at 35° C for 18 to 24 hours.
Interpretation:	Positive result (susceptible) = Any zone of inhibition around the bacitracin Negative result (resistant) = Uniform lawn of growth up to the edge of the disk (Figure 11-5)
Controls:	Positive: Group A *Streptococcus* (bacitracin susceptible) Negative: Group B *Streptococcus* (bacitracin resistant)

---

tion of optochin (ethylhydrocuprein hydrochloride) is placed onto the inoculated area. A zone of inhibition around the disk is presumptive evidence of *S. pneumoniae.* Other α-hemolytic species of streptococci are resistant to optochin.

BILE SOLUBILITY

Another characteristic that correlates well with optochin susceptibility is **bile solubility.** The test for bile solubility takes advantage of the very active autocatalytic enzymes that **S. pneumoniae**

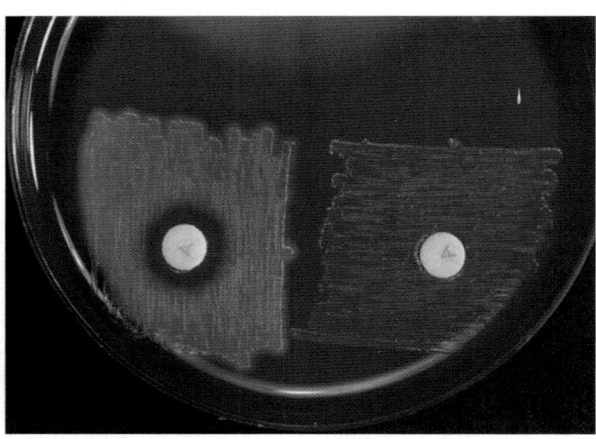

Figure 11-5

Group A streptococcus on blood agar showing susceptibility to bacitracin. *Left*, positive (susceptible); *right*, negative (resistant).

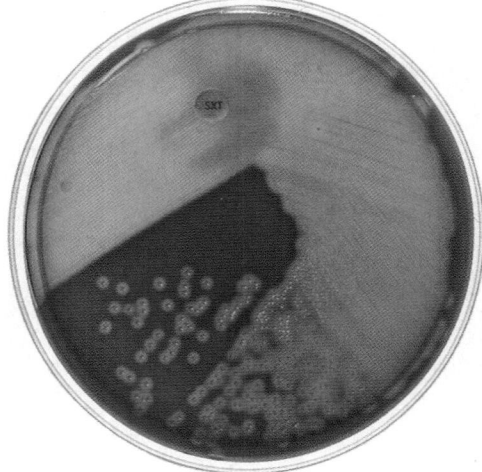

Figure 11-6

Group A streptococcus on blood agar showing resistance to SXT disk.

PROCEDURE 11-2. Hippurate Hydrolysis

Purpose: To differentiate *S. agalactiae* from other β-hemolytic streptococci

Principle: The enzyme, hippuricase, hydrolyzes hippuric acid to form sodium benzoate and glycine. Subsequent addition of Ninhydrin results in the release of ammonia from the oxidative deamination of the α-amino group in glycine as well as the reduced form of Ninhydrin, hydrindantin. The ammonia reacts with residual Ninhydrin and hydrindantin to give a purple-colored complex. Some isolates of group D streptococci also hydrolyze hippurate; however, these isolates are less likely to be β-hemolytic, and their colony morphology is different from that of group B streptococci. An isolate that is hippurate positive and bile esculin negative has a very high probability of being *S. agalactiae.*

Specimen: Isolated colonies on sheep's blood agar

Reagents: *Sodium hippurate (1%):*

Sodium hippurate	1 g
Distilled water	100 mL

Dispense 0.5-mL aliquots in small capped vials. Store at $-10°$ C. Storage life is 6 months.

Ninhydrin reagent:

Ninhydrin	3.5 g
Acetone-butanol mixture (1:1)	100 mL

Store at room temperature. Storage life is 12 months.

Procedure: 1. Inoculate the solution of sodium hippurate heavily with colonies 18 to 24 hours old until a milky suspension is obtained.
2. Incubate tube for 2 hours at 35° C.
3. Add 0.2 mL of Ninhydrin reagent.
4. Mix and incubate for 10 to 15 minutes.

Interpretation: Positive result = Deep purple color (indicates hippurate hydrolysis)
Negative result = No color change (or very slight purple color)

Controls: Positive: *S. agalactiae*
Negative: *S. pyogenes*

possesses. Under the influence of a bile salt, the organism's cell wall lyses during cell division. A suspension of *S. pneumoniae* in a solution of sodium deoxycholate lyses and the solution becomes clear. Other α-hemolytic organisms do not lyse, and the solution remains cloudy.

HYDROLYSIS
A useful test to differentiate group B streptococci from other β-hemolytic streptococci is **hippurate hydrolysis.** *Streptococcus agalactiae* possess the enzyme hippuricase, which hydrolyzes sodium

hippurate to form sodium benzoate and glycine. This hydrolysis can be detected by adding Ninhydrin, which reacts with the α-amino groups to form a purple color. Procedure 11-2 describes the test.

A test that provides a high probability for presumptive separation of group A enterococci and enterococci from the other streptococcal species is the **PYR hydrolysis test** (Figure 11-7). It is more specific than bacitracin susceptibility. A number of commercial systems are on the market, and the reader is referred to the specific package insert. The PYR test takes advantage of the fact that

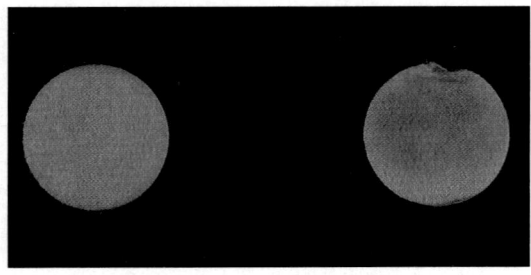

Figure 11-7 _____

The PYR test for *Streptococcus pyogenes* and *Enterococcus*. A positive test gives a bright red color change. *Left,* negative; *right,* positive.

S. pyogenes and *Enterococcus* spp. are able to hydrolyze the substrate PYR. (Substrates utilized in the PYR test are L-pyrrolidonyl-β naphthylamide, and L-pyroglutamic acid-β naphthylamide.) It is as specific as bile esculin and NaCl broth (see later) for *Enterococcus* and more specific than bacitracin for *S. pyogenes.*

Following hydrolysis of the substrate by the peptidase, the resulting β-naphthylamide produces a red color upon the addition of 0.01% cinnamaldehyde reagent (0.01%, *p*-dimethylaminocinnamaldehyde). The substrate is usually impregnated into paper disks, which are moistened and inoculated with the suspected isolate. After 2 minutes to allow for hydrolysis, the cinnamaldehyde reagent is dropped onto the disk. A pink or cherry red color appears within 1 minute if the reaction is positive. A negative reaction is indicated by no color change. The genera that are PYR positive include *Enterococcus, Aerococcus,* and *Gemella.* The only member of *Streptococcus* that is PYR positive is *S. pyogenes.* The PYR test (Procedure 11-3) is an excellent addition to the test menu for the presumptive identification of the gram-positive cocci.

CAMP TEST

Another test that is used to presumptively identify group B streptococci is the **CAMP test.** *CAMP* is an acronym based on the first letters of the surnames of the individuals who first described the reaction: Christie, Atkins, and Munch-Petersen. The CAMP test can be performed three ways. The first is with the use of a β-lysin–producing strain of *S. aureus,* and the second is with the use of a disk impregnated with the β-lysin. Both methods take advantage of the enhanced hemolysis that takes place when the β-lysin and the hemolysins

---

PROCEDURE 11-3. **PYR Hydrolysis Test**

Purpose:	To differentiate those gram-positive cocci that will hydrolyze the substrate L-pyrrolidonyl-beta-naphthylamide (PYR) from those that are PYR negative
Principle:	PYR-impregnated disks serve as the substrate to produce beta-naphthylamine, which is detected in the presence of N,N-methyl-aminocinnamaldehyde by the production of a red color
Specimen:	Isolated colonies on sheep's blood agar
Procedure:	1. Lightly moisten a PYR-impregnated disk with sterile water.
	2. Using a sterile loop or applicator, rub one or more isolated colonies on the surface of the disk.
	3. NOTE: Incubation time and temperature varies slightly by manufacturer. Incubate as indicated in the manufacturer's instructions (2 to 15 minutes).
	4. Add a drop of color developer and observe for a red color on the disk within 5 minutes.
Interpretation:	Positive result = Red color Negative result = Colorless
Controls:	Positive: *Enterococcus faecalis* Negative: *Streptococcus agalactiae*

PROCEDURE 11-4. CAMP Test

Purpose:	To differentiate *S. agalactiae* from other β-hemolytic streptococci
Principle:	Group B streptococci produce a CAMP factor that enhances the lysis of sheep red cells by staphylococcal β-lysin. A positive reaction can be observed in 5 to 6 hours with incubation in carbon dioxide (18 hours with incubation in ambient air).
Specimen:	1. Isolated colonies on sheep's blood agar 2. β-Lysin–producing *S. aureus* on blood agar
Medium:	Sheep's blood agar plate
Procedure:	1. Inoculate *S. aureus* along a line down the center of the agar plate. 2. Inoculate the streptococcal isolate along a thin line 2 cm long and perpendicular to, but not touching, the *S. aureus* streak. 3. Incubate plate at 35° C for 18 hours.
Interpretation:	Positive result = Arrowhead-shaped area of enhanced hemolysis where the two streaks (staphylococcal and streptococcal) approach each other Negative result = No enhanced hemolysis
Controls:	Positive: *S. agalactiae* Negative: *S. pyogenes*

produced by group B streptococci are in contact. The result is a characteristic arrow-shaped hemolysis pattern (Figure 11-8). Procedure 11-4 describes how to perform the CAMP test.

In addition, a rapid CAMP test utilizing the extracted β-lysin from the strain of *S. aureus* that produces it is currently in use. It involves placing a drop of the extracted β-lysin on the area of confluent growth of the suspected group B streptococci. After incubation at 37° C for at least 20 minutes, enhanced hemolysis is observed (Figure 11-9).

BILE ESCULIN AND NaCl TESTS

Two tests that have been mainstays in identification schemes for group D streptococci and *Entero-*

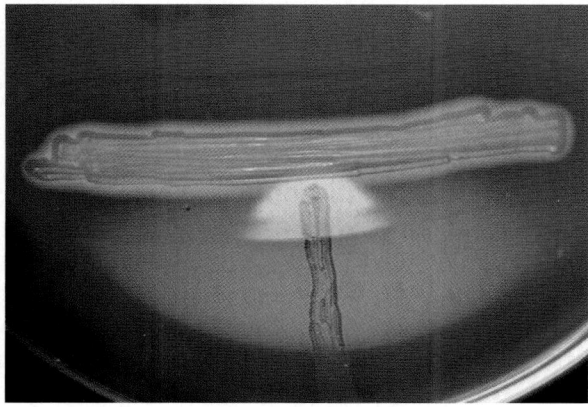

Figure 11-8
The CAMP test for presumptive identification of group B streptococci. *Streptococcus agalactiae* shows the classic arrow shape near the staphylococcus streak.

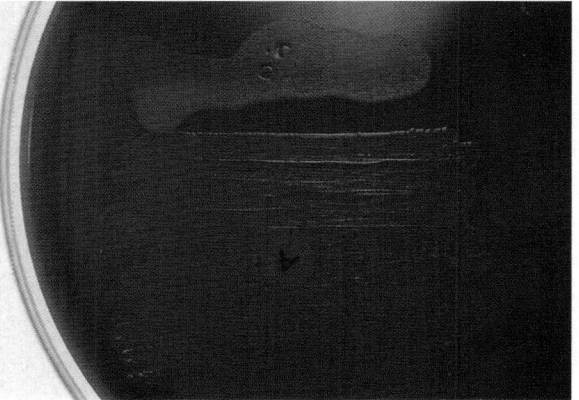

Figure 11-9
A modification of the CAMP test showing the enhanced hemolysis produced by *Streptococcus agalactiae* when a drop of extracted hemolysin is placed on the colony.

PROCEDURE 11-5.   Bile Esculin Hydrolysis

Purpose:	To differentiate group D streptococci and *Enterococcus* from other gram-positive cocci
Principle:	Group D streptococci and *Enterococcus* grow in the presence of bile and also hydrolyze esculin to esculetin and glucose. Esculetin diffuses into the agar and combines with ferric citrate in the medium to give a black complex.
Specimen:	Isolated colonies on blood agar
Media:	Bile esculin agar
Procedure:	1. Pick one or two isolated colonies from the blood agar plate and inoculate to a bile esculin agar slant. 2. Incubate at 35° C for 18 to 24 hours. NOTE: A positive result is often seen within 4 hours. A negative result should be incubated for an additional 24-hour period.
Interpretation:	Positive result = Blackening of the agar slant Negative result = No blackening of the agar slant (NOTE: Growth alone—does not constitute a positive result)
Controls:	Positive: Group D *Streptococcus* Negative: Viridans *Streptococcus*

coccus are the **bile esculin hydrolysis test** (Procedure 11-5 and Figure 11-10) and the **NaCl test,** growth in 6.5% NaCl (Procedure 11-6).

Group D streptococci and *Enterococcus* can grow in the presence of 40% bile and hydrolyze esculin. The resulting product is a black complex in the agar, indicating a positive reaction.

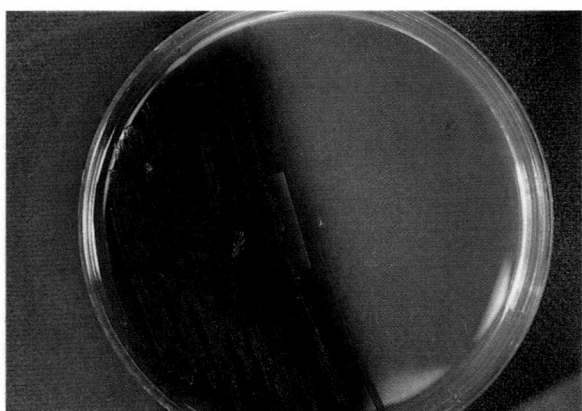

Figure 11-10

The bile esculin test. A positive test *(left)* shows blackening of the agar. Right side is negative.

Growth in 6.5% sodium chloride broth is used to identify the non–β-hemolytic, catalase-negative, gram-positive cocci (Figure 11-11). *Enterococcus, Aerococcus,* and some species of *Pediococcus* and *Leuconostoc* grow in a 6.5% NaCl broth when incubated for 24 hours. Group D streptococci, however, do not grow in a 6.5% NaCl broth.

LEUCINE AMINOPEPTIDASE TEST
Leucine aminopeptidase (LAP) is helpful in differentiating *Aerococcus* and *Leuconostoc* from other gram-positive cocci. As Table 11-3 outlines, *Streptococcus, Enterococcus,* and *Pediococcus* are LAP positive. *Aerococcus* and *Leuconostoc* are LAP negative.

Noncultural Identification

Identification of streptococci, particularly group A, can be made by the direct detection of the group-specific antigen, from either isolated colonies or, in some cases, a direct clinical specimen such as a throat swab.

Identification from isolated colonies can be accomplished by extracting the C carbohydrate by means of acid or heat. The extract containing the specific group carbohydrate is then utilized in a

PROCEDURE 11-6. NaCl Test

Purpose:	To differentiate those gram-positive cocci that will grow in 6.5% NaCl from those that are inhibited by this salt concentration
Principle:	*Enterococcus, Aerococcus,* and some species of *Pediococcus* and *Leuconostoc* can withstand a higher salt concentration than other gram-positive cocci.
Specimen:	Isolated colonies on sheep's blood agar
Medium:	6.5% NaCl broth (nutrient broth base)
Procedure:	1. Pick one or two isolated colonies from the blood agar plate and inoculate into 5 mL of NaCl broth.
	2. Incubate tube at 35° C for 3 days. Check for growth daily.
Interpretation:	Positive result = Turbidity
	Negative result = No turbidity
Controls:	Positive: *Enterococcus faecalis*
	Negative: Viridans *Streptococcus*

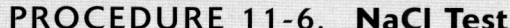

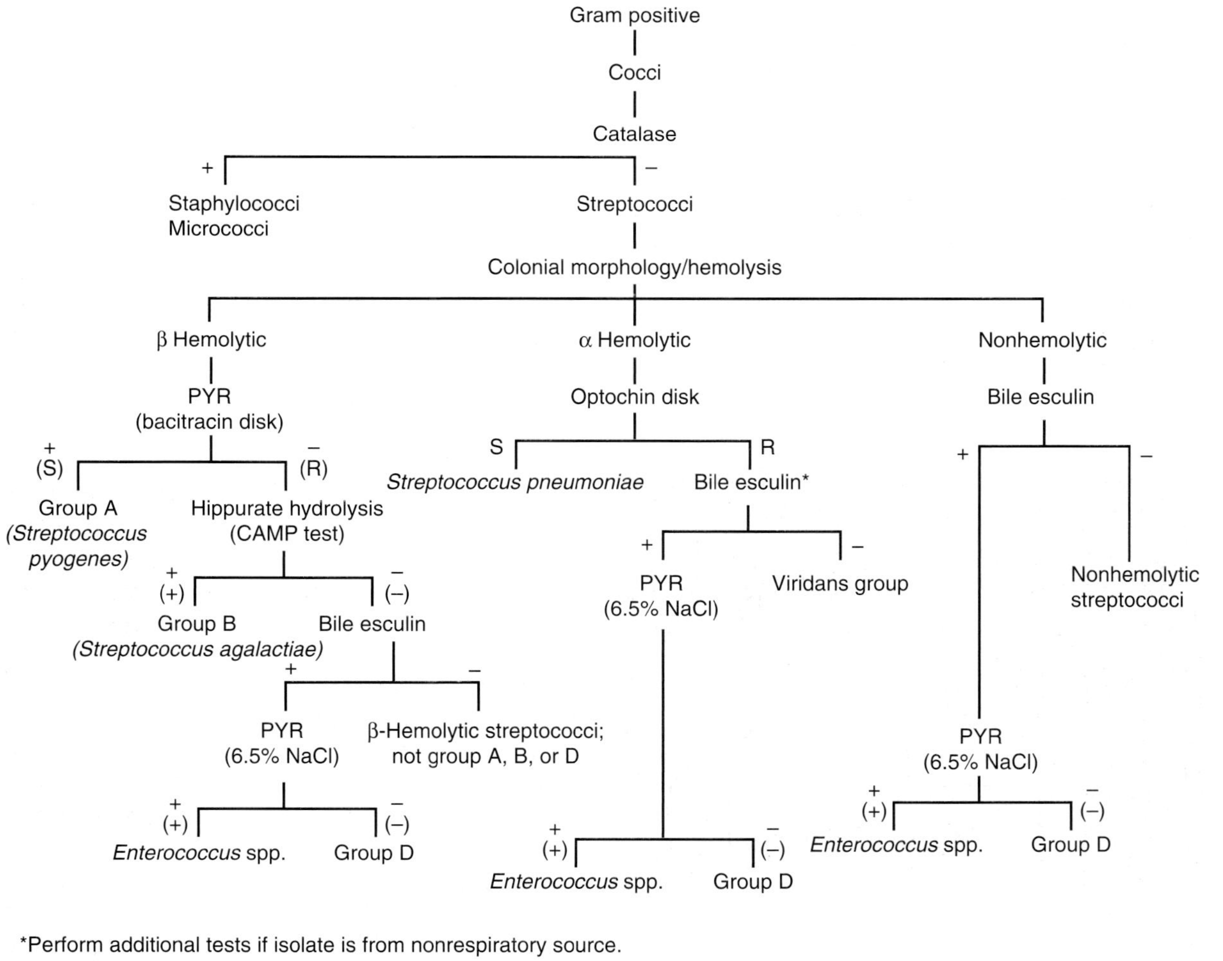

*Perform additional tests if isolate is from nonrespiratory source.

Figure 11-11

Schematic diagram for the presumptive identification of gram-positive cocci.

capillary precipitin test or a slide agglutination test. In the capillary precipitin test, antiserum to the specific group carbohydrate is overlaid by the solution containing the streptococcal extract. After 5 to 10 minutes, the interface between the extraction solution and the antiserum is examined carefully for a white precipitate, which indicates a positive reaction. Each extract can be tested with a number of antisera specific to the various group antigens.

The slide agglutination test utilizes a carrier particle for the group-specific antiserum. In the coagglutination test, the specific antiserum is conjugated to kill *S. aureus* cells containing high amounts of protein A. Another carrier particle often used is latex. Both types of particles serve as holders for the antiserum. When an antibody (carrier particle + specific group carbohydrate antiserum)-antigen (group carbohydrate extraction solution) reaction occurs, it is visualized macroscopically as agglutination of the particles (Figure 11-12).

These methods give a definitive identification as to the Lancefield group the isolate belongs to, but, when the group comprises several species, the methods do not give a species identification. Of course, if the results indicate that the isolate belongs to group A or B, then it can be identified as *S. pyogenes* or *S. agalactiae,* respectively. The cost of these methods is much higher than that of the standard cultural approaches. Consequently, few clinical laboratories routinely utilize them to identify all streptococcal isolates.

Also more than two dozen different products are available, many of which utilize an ELISA system, to detect group A streptococci from throat swabs. These are designed primarily for use in the clinic and the physician's office. Although a positive finding allows the physician to treat for *S. pyogenes* without waiting for culture results, a negative result necessitates a follow-up throat culture. This is because the sensitivity of direct detection methods for group A streptococci has not been high enough to ensure confidence that the negative result is not a false-negative. Additionally, the cost of using direct detection methods can be significantly higher than that of culture only. If the direct test is negative and a subsequent culture is performed to confirm the result, the total cost is almost twice as much as a culture only. The direct detection method for group A streptococci can be a valuable diagnostic tool in the right context; however, the cost and sensitivity must be weighed carefully against desired and actual results.

CLINICALLY SIGNIFICANT STREPTOCOCCI AND THEIR ASSOCIATED DISEASES

Streptococcus pyogenes (Group A Streptococci)
Antigenic structure
The structure of group A streptococci is illustrated in Figure 11-13. *S. pyogenes* shows a cell wall structure similar to that of other streptococci and gram-positive bacteria. The group antigen is unique, placing the organism in Lancefield group A. An antigen that is not found in the other Lancefield groups is referred to as the **M protein.** This is a molecule that is attached to the peptidoglycan of the cell wall and extends to the surface of the cell wall. The M protein is essential to virulence.

Virulence factors
In addition to M protein, a number of extracellular products are produced by *S. pyogenes,* including hemolysins, toxins, and enzymes.

The best-defined virulence factor is M protein. More than 80 different serotypes of M protein exist, which are labeled M5, M10, M23, and so on. Re-

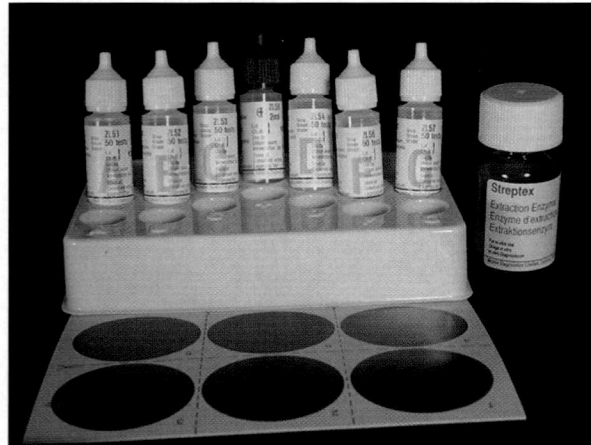

Figure 11-12 ⎯⎯⎯⎯⎯⎯⎯⎯⎯⎯⎯⎯⎯⎯⎯
Slide agglutination test for grouping streptococci.

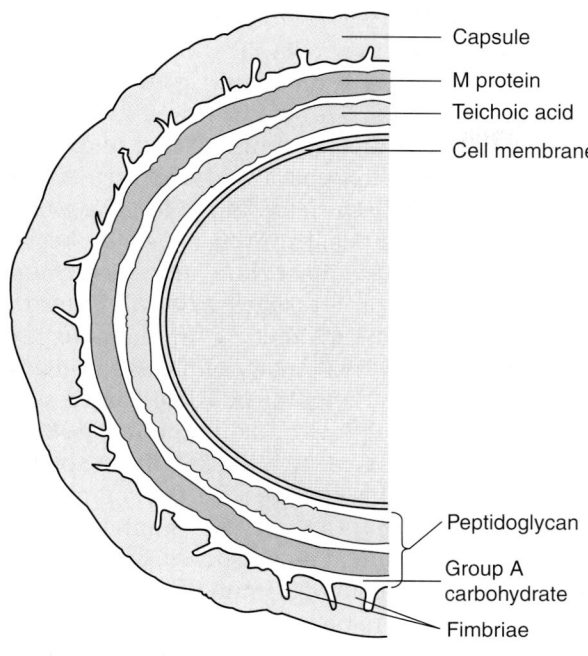

Capsule
M protein
Teichoic acid
Cell membrane

Peptidoglycan

Group A
carbohydrate

Fimbriae

Figure 11-13

A schematic representation of the group A streptococcal cell wall.

sistance to infection with *S. pyogenes* appears to be related to the presence of type-specific antibodies to the M protein. This means that an individual with antibodies against M5 is protected from infection by *S. pyogenes* with the M5 protein but remains unprotected against infection with the roughly 80 remaining M protein serotypes. The M protein molecule causes the streptococcal cell to resist phagocytosis. It also plays a role in adherence of the bacterial cell to mucosal cells.

Other products produced by *S. pyogenes* are streptolysin O, streptolysin S, deoxyribonuclease, streptokinase, **hyaluronidase,** and erythrogenic toxin. Although all of these products have been postulated to play a role in virulence, the exact role each has in infection is not clear.

A hemolysin that is responsible for hemolysis on blood agar plates is **streptolysin O.** The *O* refers to the fact that this hemolysin is *oxygen labile.* It is active only in the reduced form, which is achieved in an anaerobic environment. This hemolysin lyses leukocytes, platelets, and other tissue cells as well as red blood cells. Streptolysin O is highly antigenic, and the infected host readily forms anti-

bodies to the hemolysin. These can be measured in the antistreptolysin-O test to determine whether an individual has had a recent infection with *S. pyogenes.* A second hemolysin is produced that is oxygen stable and so is referred to as *streptolysin S.* The hemolysis seen around colonies that have been incubated aerobically is due to streptolysin S. It is nonantigenic. Streptolysin S also lyses leukocytes.

Streptococcus pyogenes secretes four different deoxyribonucleases (DNases), A, B, C, and D. All strains form at least one deoxyribonuclease. The most common is DNase B. These enzymes are antigenic, and antibodies to DNase can be detected following infection.

Filtrates of group A streptococci cause the lysis of fibrin clots, through the action of streptokinase on plasminogen. The plasminogen is converted into a protease (plasmin), which lyses the fibrin. Antibodies to streptokinase can be detected following infection but are not specific indicators of group A infection, because groups C and G also form streptokinase.

Another name for hyaluronidase is **spreading factor.** This enzyme was so named because it acts to solubilize the ground substance of mammalian connective tissues (hyaluronic acid). It was postulated that the bacteria utilize this enzyme to separate the tissue and then spread the infection. No real evidence exists, however, that hyaluronidase favors the spread of *S. pyogenes* through the tissues.

Some strains of *S. pyogenes* cause a red spreading rash referred to as *scarlet fever* (see section on pyodermal infections). This condition is caused by erythrogenic toxin. It is a protein exotoxin, and three types (A, B, and C) are known. The role, if any, in pathogenesis is unknown.

Clinical infections

Infections resulting from *S. pyogenes* are common and include **pharyngitis, scarlet fever,** skin infections, and other septic infections. In addition, rheumatic fever and glomerulonephritis may occur as a result of infection with group A streptococci.

BACTERIAL PHARYNGITIS

The most common clinical expressions of group A streptococcal infection are pharyngitis and tonsillitis. The majority of cases of bacterial pharyngitis are due to infection with *S. pyogenes.* Other groups, particularly C and G, have the capability to produce significant acute pharyngitis but are much less commonly seen.

"Strep throat" is most commonly seen in children between 5 and 15 years of age. After an incubation period of 1 to 4 days, an abrupt onset of illness ensues, with sore throat, malaise, fever, and headache. It is not unusual to see nausea, vomiting, and abdominal pain as well. The tonsils and pharynx are inflamed. The cervical lymph nodes are swollen and tender. The disease ranges in intensity, however, and all of these symptoms may not be seen. In fact, it is not unusual to isolate a nearly pure culture of *S. pyogenes* from the throat of a child who complains only of a mild sore throat and fever. The symptoms subside within 3 to 5 days unless complications, such as peritonsillar abscesses, occur. The disease is spread by droplets and close contact. Although clinical criteria have been proposed, the diagnosis of streptococcal sore throat relies on a throat culture. Approximately one third of those complaining of sore throat have a throat culture positive for *S. pyogenes*.

PYODERMAL INFECTIONS

Skin infections with group A streptococci result in the syndrome of impetigo, cellulitis, erysipelas, wound infection, or gangrene. **Impetigo,** a localized skin disease, begins as small vesicles that progress to weeping lesions. The lesions crust over after several days. Impetigo is usually seen on very young children (2 to 5 years) and affects exposed areas of the skin. Inoculation of the organism occurs through minor abrasions or insect bites. **Erysipelas** is an infection of the skin and subcutaneous tissues. It is an acute spreading skin lesion that is uncommonly seen. The lesion is intensely erythematous with a plainly demarcated, but irregular edge. It is most often seen in elderly patients. **Cellulitis** may develop following deeper invasion by streptococci. The infection can be serious, even life threatening, with bacteremia or sepsis present. In patients with peripheral vascular disease or diabetes, cellulitis may lead to gangrene.

As mentioned earlier, infection with strains of *S. pyogenes* that produce the erythrogenic toxin may result in *scarlet fever*. This condition, which appears within 1 to 2 days following infection, is characterized by a diffuse red rash that appears on the upper chest and spreads to the trunk and extremities. The rash disappears over the next 5 to 7 days and is followed by desquamation.

POSTSTREPTOCOCCAL INFECTION

There are two serious complications of group A streptococcal disease, rheumatic fever and acute glomerulonephritis.

Rheumatic fever is a complication of *S. pyogenes* pharyngitis. It is characterized by fever and inflammation of the heart, joints, blood vessels, and subcutaneous tissues. Attacks usually begin within a month after infection. The most serious result is a chronic, progressive damage to the heart valves. Repeated infections may produce further valve damage. By 1980, many clinicians considered rheumatic fever eradicated. There was a resurgence of rheumatic fever during the late 1980s, however, and it is once again a significant problem. The cause of this resurgence is not completely clear. It appears to be a result of a number of factors, including clinical management of bacterial pharyngitis, epidemiologic changes, and bacteriologic factors. The pathogenesis of rheumatic fever is poorly understood. Several theories have been proposed, including antigenic cross-reactivity between streptococcal antigens and heart tissue, direct toxicity resulting from bacterial exotoxins, and actual invasion of the heart tissues by the organism. Most evidence favors cross-reactivity as being responsible for the effects.

Another potential result of infection with group A streptococci is **acute glomerulonephritis** (AGN). In contrast to rheumatic fever, AGN may occur after a cutaneous or pharyngeal infection. It is more common in children than adults. The pathogenesis appears to be a result of immunologic mechanisms. Circulating immune complexes are found in the serum of patients with AGN, and it is postulated that these antigen-antibody complexes deposit in the glomerulus. Complement is subsequently fixed, and an inflammatory response causes damage to the glomerulus, resulting in impairment of kidney function.

INVASIVE STREPTOCOCCAL INFECTIONS

Streptococcal toxic shock syndrome A number of reports in recent years associated group A streptococcal infections with toxic shock. The initial streptococcal infection was severe (pharyngitis, peritonitis, cellulitis, wound infections), and symptoms developed that were very similar to those of staphylococcal **toxic shock syndrome.** All isolates were group A streptococcus, and all produced the toxin associated with scarlet fever. It has been proposed that this toxin plays a major role in the pathogenesis of this disease.

ANTIMICROBIAL THERAPY

The group A streptococci are susceptible to penicillin, which remains the drug of choice. For patients allergic to penicillin, erythromycin can be used. For patients who have a history of rheumatic fever, prophylactic doses of penicillin are given to prevent any recurrent infections that may cause additional damage to the heart valves.

Laboratory diagnosis

Colonies of *S. pyogenes* on blood agar are small, transparent, and smooth with a well-defined area of β hemolysis. A Gram stain will reveal gram-positive cocci with some short chains. Examination of Gram stains of upper respiratory specimens or skin swabs is of little value, because these areas have considerable amounts of normal gram-positive cocci.

An essential step in the diagnosis of streptococcal pharyngitis is proper sampling. The tongue should be depressed, and the swab rubbed over the posterior pharynx and each tonsillar area. If exudate is present, it should also be touched with the swab. Care should be taken to avoid the tongue and uvula.

Transport media are not required for normal conditions. The organism is resistant to drying and can be recovered from swabs after several hours of holding. A blood agar plate is inoculated and streaked for isolation. Incubation should be at 35° C to 37° C either in ambient air or under anaerobic conditions. Studies have shown that the normal respiratory flora tend to overgrow the β-hemolytic streptococci when incubated in increased CO_2. Several selective media, such as sheep's blood agar containing trimethoprim-sulfamethoxazole, have been recommended for better recovery of β-hemolytic streptococci from throat cultures. The plate is observed after 24 hours for the presence of β-hemolytic colonies. If none are found, incubation should continue for 24 hours longer before the culture is read as negative. Suspect colonies can be Lancefield-typed using serologic methods, which will give a definitive identification, or biochemical tests can be performed. The correlation between the presumptive identification using biochemical methods and the definitive serologic method is high. Therefore many laboratories utilize the less-expensive biochemical methods. A key test that should be done is bacitracin susceptibility or PYR hydrolysis. *S. pyogenes* is susceptible to bacitracin and hydrolyzes PYR, whereas the other β-hemolytic groups are resistant to bacitracin and are PYR negative.

When the isolate's origin is not from the throat (i.e., blood, sputum), additional tests should be part of the early identification scheme. In this case, hippurate hydrolysis or the CAMP test, bile esculin test, and NaCl broth growth should also be included. The reactions shown by some of the catalase-negative, gram-positive cocci to various biochemical tests are outlined in Table 11-3.

Some immunologic tests used to detect past infection with *S. pyogenes* include antistreptolysin-O, anti-DNase, antistreptokinase, and antihyaluronidase titers.

Streptococcus agalactiae (Group B Streptococci)

Antigenic structure

All strains of *S. agalactiae* have the group B–specific antigen, an acid-stable polysaccharide located in the cell wall. Additionally are three major serotypes, labeled I, II, and III. These type-specific antigens are capsular polysaccharides and can be detected by precipitin tests. The terminal position in the repeating unit is composed of sialic acid, which is an important virulence factor.

Virulence factors

The capsule is another important virulence factor in group B streptococcal infections. Antibodies against the type-specific antigens protect mice against strains of *S. agalactiae* with the homologous polysaccharide in the capsule. The capsule prevents phagocytosis but is ineffective after opsonization. Sialic acid appears to be the most significant component of the capsule. Studies with mutant strains of *S. agalactiae* that lacked the sialic acid component of the capsule showed that loss of capsular sialic acid was associated with loss of virulence. The capsular sialic acid appears to be a critical virulence determinant. It is postulated that the sialic acid in the surface of the bacterial cell inhibits activation of the alternative pathway of complement.

Other products produced by *S. agalactiae* include a hemolysin, the CAMP factor, neuraminidase, deoxyribonuclease, hyaluronidase, and protease.

No evidence exists that any of these products plays a role in the virulence of this organism.

Clinical infections

Group B streptococci (GBS) have been known for many years as the cause of mastitis in cattle. It was not until Lancefield defined streptococcal classification that their role in human disease was recognized.

Streptococcus agalactiae is a significant cause of invasive disease in the newborn. Two clinical syndromes are used to describe neonatal group B streptococcal disease: early-onset infection (less than 7 days old) and late-onset infection (at least 7 days old). Early-onset disease accounts for approximately 80% of the clinical cases in newborns and is caused by vertical transmission of the organism from the mother. Colonization of the vagina and rectal area with GBS is found in 10% to 30% of pregnant women. Most infections of infants occur in the first 3 days after birth, usually within 24 hours. This infection is commonly associated with obstetric complications, prolonged rupture of membranes, and premature birth. It is often a pneumonia or meningitis with bacteremia. The mortality rate is high, and death usually occurs if treatment is not started quickly. The most important determining factor seems to be the presence of group B streptococci in the vagina of the mother. It is recommended that all pregnant women should be screened for GBS at 35 to 37 weeks' gestation.

Late-onset infection occurs between 1 week and 3 months after birth and usually is seen as meningitis. This infection is uncommonly associated with obstetric complications. Also, the organism is rarely found in the mother's vagina prior to birth. The mortality rate is considerably less than that of early-onset disease, but it is high enough to be of serious concern.

The incidence of group B streptococcal infections drops dramatically after the neonatal period. In adults, infection affects two types of patients. The first is the young, previously healthy woman who becomes ill after childbirth or abortion; endometritis and wound infections are most common. The second type of patient is the elderly person with a serious underlying disease or immunodeficiency.

The drug of choice for treating group B infections is penicillin, although this group is less susceptible to penicillin than group A streptococci. The clinical response to antibiotic therapy is often poor in spite of the heavy doses given. Some clinicians recommend a combination of ampicillin and an aminoglycoside for treating group B streptococcal infections.

Laboratory diagnosis

Group B streptococci grow on blood agar as grayish white mucoid colonies surrounded by a small zone of β hemolysis (Figure 11-14). Group B streptococci are gram-positive cocci that form short chains in clinical specimens and longer chains in culture. Presumptive identification is based on biochemical reactions. The most useful test is hippurate, hydrolysis or the CAMP test. Table 11-3 lists the reactions of *S. agalactiae* in various tests. These tests enable the organism to be readily differentiated from other β-hemolytic streptococcal isolates. Figure 11-15 demonstrates how bacitracin and the CAMP test can be used to differentiate *Streptococcus*. The definitive identification can be made by extracting the group antigen and reacting it with specific anti–group B antisera in a precipitin or agglutination procedure.

Other Groups

Groups C and G

In spite of their different Lancefield antigens, groups C and G are now believed to belong to the same species. The name *Streptococcus dysgalactiae* has been proposed for strains isolated from human infections. Isolates from animal sources in-

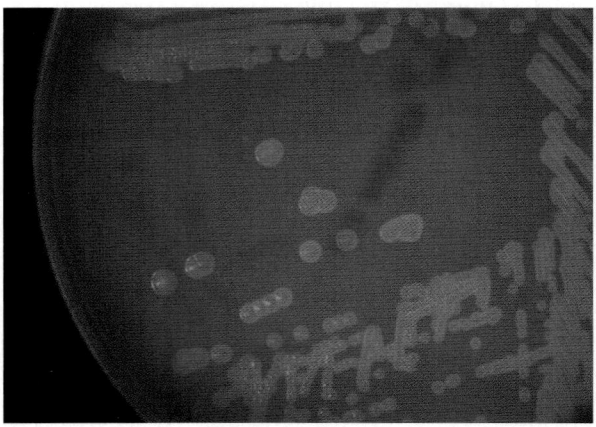

Figure 11-14

Streptococcus agalactiae colony growing on blood agar.

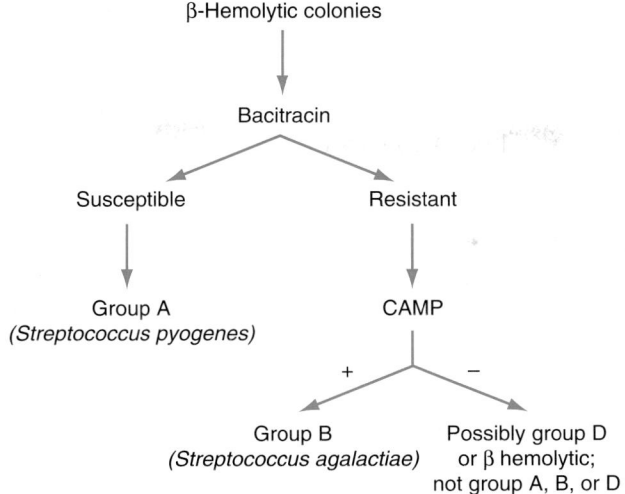

Figure 11-15 ———————————————————————
Schematic diagram for differentiation of group A from group B streptococci.

clude *Streptococcus equi* and *S. equi* ssp. *zooepi-demicus* (group C), and *Streptococcus canis* (group G). Group C and G are β hemolytic on sheep BAP.

Group D

The **group D streptococci** include *Streptococcus bovis* and *Streptococcus equinus*. Until the mid-1980s, the group D streptococci were subdivided into the enterococcal and nonenterococcal groups, with the understanding that those found in the intestinal tract were part of the enterococcal group. Both groups were bile esculin positive, but the nonenterococcal organisms would not grow in a nutrient broth with 6.5%, NaCl. As more became known about the molecular characteristics of each of these subgroups, however, the enterococcal group was placed in a new genus, *Enterococcus,* but the nonenterococcal group remained part of the group D streptococci. Although *S. bovis* is considered a nonenterococcal isolate, it can be found in the intestinal tract.

The group D streptococci may produce bacterial endocarditis, urinary tract infections, and other diseases, such as abscesses and wound infections. An association has been made between bacteremia resulting from *S. bovis* and the presence of gastrointestinal tumors. Isolation of *S. bovis* from a blood culture may be the first indication that the patient has an occult tumor. It is important to dis-

tinguish the group D streptococci from *Enterococcus,* because group D is susceptible to penicillin, whereas *Enterococcus* is usually resistant.

The group D streptococci can be presumptively identified as indicated in Table 11-3. The differentiation of nonhemolytic streptococci is outlined in Figure 11-16. Normally, hemolysis is absent (Figure 11-17) or α hemolysis is seen, although isolates can be β hemolytic on occasion. A key reaction of this group is that it is positive for bile esculin but fails to grow in 6.5% NaCl broth. In addition, it can be separated from *Enterococcus* with the PYR test, because group D is negative but *Enterococcus*

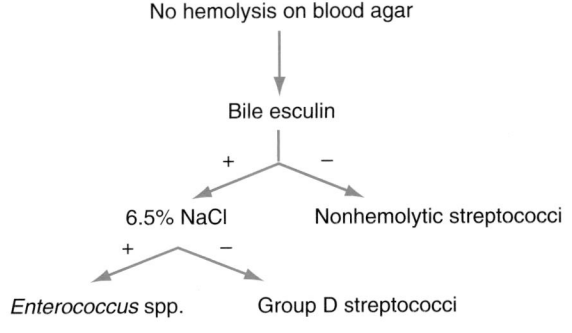

Figure 11-16 ———————————————————————
Schematic diagram for identification of nonhemolytic streptococci.

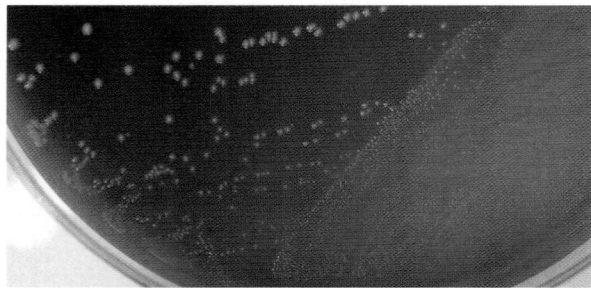

Figure 11-17

Enterococcus sp. growing on blood agar.

is positive. Serotyping should be done to identify an isolate as *S. bovis* because it cannot be positively distinguished from some of the viridans group on the basis of biochemical tests alone (see Table 11-3).

Enterococcus

As already mentioned, *Enterococcus* was previously referred to as group D *Streptococcus* enterococcus. This genus is found in the intestinal tract. The species found in this genus include *Enterococcus faecalis,* which is the most common isolate, *Enterococcus faecium, Enterococcus avium,* and *Enterococcus durans.* They share a number of characteristics with the group D streptococci, including the group D antigen. They show resistance to several of the commonly used antibiotics, so differentiation with *Streptococcus* and susceptibility testing is important. The diseases caused by *Enterococcus* are similar to those seen with group D streptococcal infection.

It is not difficult to differentiate between *Enterococcus* and group D isolates. In addition to being positive for bile esculin, *Enterococcus* grows in 6.5% NaCl broth and is PYR positive. The use of bile esculin, PYR, and 6.5% NaCl to differentiate *Enterococcus* from group D streptococcus is shown in Figure 11-18. It may be worth mentioning that the catalase test result may be confusing when one is trying to differentiate *Enterococcus* species from catalase-producing *Staphylococcus* species. *Enterococcus* species can give a weakly positive (slight bubbling) catalase test reaction on a culture 24 to 48 hours old.

Streptococcus pneumoniae

Also known as the pneumococcus, *S. pneumoniae* is often isolated from a variety of infections.

Antigenic structure

The cell wall of *S. pneumoniae* contains an antigen, referred to as *C substance,* that is similar to the C carbohydrate of the various Lancefield groups. A β-globulin in human serum, called the **C-reactive protein** reacts with this C substance to form a precipitate. This is a chemical reaction and not an antigen-antibody combination. The amount of C-reactive protein increases during inflammation and infection. The key antigen of the pneumococcus is the capsular antigen. There are some 82 different capsular types based on chemical variations of the capsular polysaccharide. Isolates from certain sources, for example, cases of lobar pneumonia, show a predominance of a particular capsular type or types. The capsule is antigenic and can be identified with appropriate antiserum. In the presence of specific anticapsular serum, the capsule swells (quellung reaction). This reaction not only allows for identification of *S. pneumoniae* but serves to specifically serotype the isolate as well.

Virulence factors

The characteristic of *S. pneumoniae* that is clearly associated with virulence is the capsular polysaccharide. Laboratory strains that have lost the ability to produce a capsule are nonpathogenic. In addition, opsonization of the capsule renders the organism nonvirulent. Several toxins are produced, including a hemolysin, an immunoglobulin A protease, neuraminidase, and hyaluronidase. None of these has been shown to have a role in disease production.

Clinical infections

Streptococcus pneumoniae is an important human pathogen, causing **pneumonia,** sinusitis, otitis me-

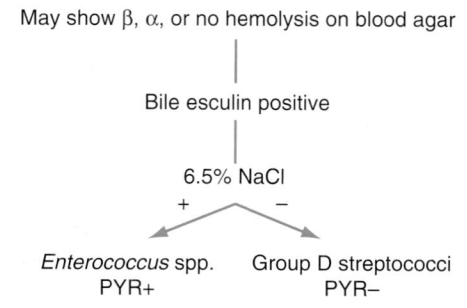

Figure 11-18

Schematic diagram for differentiation of group D streptococci from *Enterococcus.*

dia, bacteremia, and meningitis. It is a common isolate in the clinical microbiology laboratory, both as a pathogen and as a member of the normal respiratory flora.

The most common cause of bacterial pneumonia, it is especially prevalent in the elderly as well as in patients with underlying disease. Of the more than 80 capsular serotypes, about a dozen account for the majority of pneumococcal pneumonia cases. Pneumonia resulting from *S. pneumoniae* is not usually a primary infection but rather is a result of disturbance of the normal defense barriers. Such predisposing conditions as alcoholism, anesthesia, malnutrition, and viral infections of the upper respiratory tract may lead to pneumococcal disease. The most common type of pneumococcal pneumonia is lobar pneumonia. This form is characterized by a very sudden onset with chills, dyspnea, and cough. The infection begins with aspiration of respiratory secretions, which often contain pneumococci. The infecting organisms in the alveoli stimulate an outpouring of edema fluid, which serves to facilitate the spread of the organism to adjacent alveoli. The process stops when the fluid reaches fibrous septa that separate the major lung lobes. This accounts for the "lobar" distribution of the infection, and hence the name. The majority of isolates from pneumococcal lobar pneumonia are types 1, 2, and 3.

For an individual to contract pneumococcal pneumonia, the organism must be present in the nasopharynx, the individual must be deficient in specific circulating antibody against the capsular type of the colonizing strain of *S. pneumoniae,* and there must be some predisposing factor such as a viral infection. The disease may be complicated by a pleural effusion that is usually sterile (empyema). The laboratory may receive fluid from a pleural aspirate for culture. An infected effusion contains many white cells and pneumococci, which are visible on Gram stain. Even with antibiotics, the mortality is relatively high (5% to 10%); without therapy, however, the mortality rate approaches 50%.

Other upper respiratory tract infections caused by *S. pneumoniae* include sinusitis and otitis media. *S. pneumoniae* is the most common isolate in children under the age of 3 years with recurrent otitis media.

The pneumococcus is the most common cause of bacterial meningitis in adults but also affects all age groups. Meningitis usually follows other infections with *S. pneumoniae,* such as otitis media and pneumonia. The course of the disease is rapid, and the mortality rate is near 40%. Direct smears of the spinal fluid often reveal leukocytes and numerous gram-positive cocci in pairs.

Pneumococci may also be involved in other infections, such as endocarditis, peritonitis, and bacteremia. Bacteremia often occurs during the course of a serious infection. Consequently, samples for blood culture are often taken simultaneously with sputum or a fluid aspirate.

Pneumococcal infections are usually treated with penicillin, because the majority of isolates are susceptible. Some strains have shown resistance, and these are treated with erythromycin or chloramphenicol.

A vaccine containing the polysaccharide capsular material of the most commonly encountered types is available. It is recommended for those at risk of developing pneumococcal disease (e.g., asplenic individuals, elderly, patients with cardiac or pulmonary disease). The vaccine has been successful in reducing the incidence and severity of pneumococcal disease.

Laboratory diagnosis
MICROSCOPY
The cells are characteristically seen on Gram stain as gram-positive cocci in pairs (diplococci). The ends of the cells are slightly pointed, giving them an oval or lancet shape (Figure 11-19). The cocci

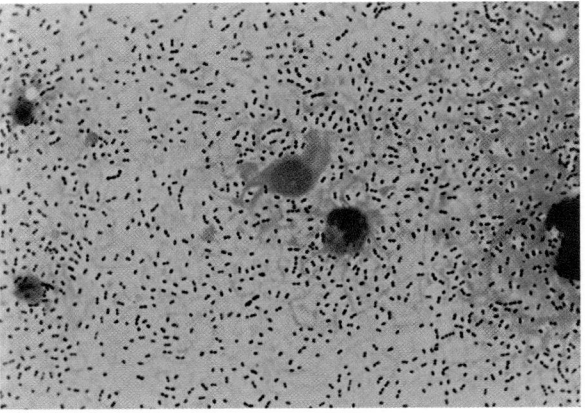

Figure 11-19

Gram stain of *Streptococcus pneumoniae.* Direct smear of sputum from a patient with pneumonia caused by *S. pneumoniae.* Note the clear, nonstained area around the organism that represents the capsule.

may occur singly, in pairs, or in short chains but are most often seen as pairs. As the culture ages, the Gram reaction becomes variable, with gram-negative cells seen. The capsule can be demonstrated by using a capsule stain.

CULTURAL CHARACTERISTICS

The nutritional requirements of *S. pneumoniae* are complex. Media such as brain-heart infusion agar, trypticase soy agar with 5% sheep's blood, or chocolate agar are necessary for good growth. Some isolates require increased CO_2 for growth during primary isolation. The organism can utilize a wide range of carbohydrates and is a facultative anaerobe. Isolates produce a significant zone of α hemolysis surrounding the colonies. Young cultures have a round, glistening, wet, mucoid, dome-shaped appearance (Figure 11-20). As the colonies become older, autolytic changes result in a collapse of each colony's center, giving it the appearance of a coin with a raised rim. The tendency of *S. pneumoniae* to undergo autolysis can make it difficult to keep isolates alive. Clinical isolates and stock cultures require frequent subculturing (every 2 to 3 days) to ensure viability. The colonies may closely resemble those of the viridans streptococci, but a presumptive differentiation is not difficult to make.

IDENTIFICATION

The greatest problem in laboratory diagnosis is distinguishing *S. pneumoniae* from the viridans streptococci. The procedures used most com-

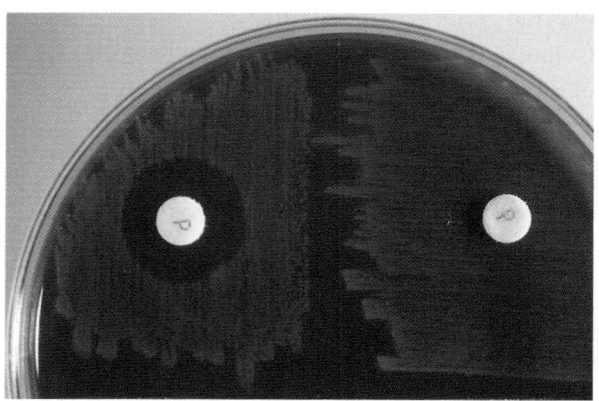

Figure 11-21 ⎯⎯⎯⎯⎯⎯⎯⎯⎯⎯⎯⎯⎯⎯⎯⎯

S. pneumoniae on blood agar showing susceptibility to optochin. *Left,* Susceptible *S. pneumoniae; right,* resistant viridans streptococci.

monly to accomplish this are optochin susceptibility, bile solubility, and the quellung reaction.

Optochin susceptibility is the most commonly used procedure of the three just listed. It takes advantage of the fact that *S. pneumoniae* is susceptible to optochin (ethylhydrocuprein hydrochloride), whereas other α-hemolytic species are resistant. A filter paper disk impregnated with optochin is placed on a blood agar plate that has been inoculated with the suspected *S. pneumoniae*. The plate is incubated at 35° C for 18 to 24 hours. If growth is inhibited around the disk, the isolate is susceptible to optochin and is presumed to be *S. pneumoniae*. The viridans streptococci are resistant to optochin and will grow up to the edge of the optochin disk (Figure 11-21). The differentiation of α-hemolytic streptococci is outlined in Figure 11-22.

The bile solubility test evaluates the ability of *S. pneumoniae* to lyse in the presence of bile salts. It correlates with optochin susceptibility; that is, an isolate that is *S. pneumoniae* will be optochin susceptible and bile soluble. This test also differentiates pneumococcus from the viridans streptococci. *S. pneumoniae* has an autolytic amidase that hydrolyzes the peptidoglycan cell wall layer. This enzyme is activated by surface-active agents, such as bile or bile salts (and detergents such as Dreft), resulting in lysis of the organisms. When a heavy suspension of *S. pneumoniae* is added to a solution of sodium desoxycholate, the cloudiness of the broth clears after incubation at 35° C for 3 hours. A suspension of viridans streptococci remains cloudy.

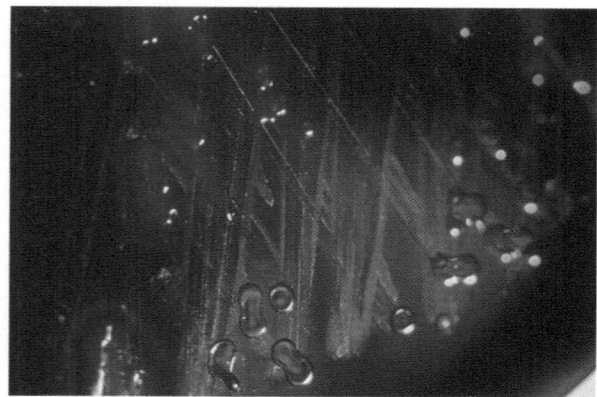

Figure 11-20 ⎯⎯⎯⎯⎯⎯⎯⎯⎯⎯⎯⎯⎯⎯⎯⎯⎯⎯⎯⎯⎯⎯⎯⎯⎯⎯⎯

Streptococcus pneumoniae colonies on blood agar. The colonies demonstrate a characteristic mucoid appearance and a concave center.

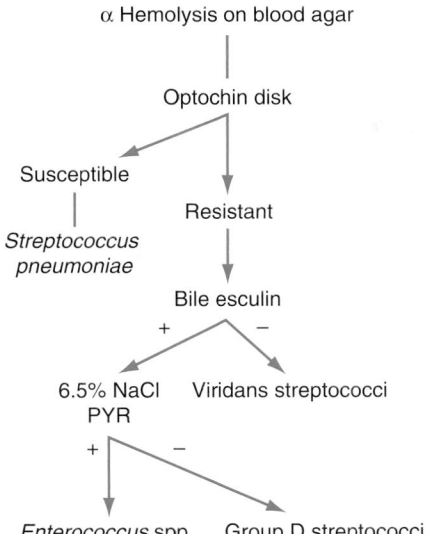

Figure 11-22

Schematic diagram for the differentiation of α-hemolytic streptococci from *Streptococcus pneumoniae.*

Although currently seldom used, the quellung reaction identifies an isolate as *S. pneumoniae* as well as determines its capsular type. This reaction can be used to identify the organism directly from sputum, spinal fluid, and other sources. The antipneumococcal serum is mixed with the material (clinical specimen or isolated colony) along with methylene blue and then examined using the oil-immersion objective. A positive reaction occurs when the pneumococci are mixed with homologous capsular antiserum: the capsule becomes more refractile and swollen.

Viridans Streptococci

Traditionally, the viridans group includes those α-hemolytic streptococci that lack Lancefield group antigens and do not meet the criteria for *S. pneumoniae.* The term *viridans* (green) is not entirely

correct, because the group also includes non-hemolytic species. Identification of the **viridans streptococci** to the species level is a difficult task, partly because there is not widespread agreement on a classification scheme. This lack of agreement among taxonomists results in confusion for the student and the laboratory professional at the bench. Those species commonly isolated from human infections are listed in Table 11-4.

Clinical infections

The viridans streptococci are oropharyngeal commensals. The fact that they are normal upper respiratory flora and are relatively susceptible to most antibiotics has kept them from being identified down to the species level. Although their virulence is low, they cause disease if host defenses are compromised. Viridans streptococci are the most common cause of subacute bacterial endocarditis. They have also been implicated in meningitis, dental caries, abscesses, osteomyelitis, and empyema. Those that cause endocarditis produce dextran, which may allow the organism to adhere to the damaged vascular endothelium. Generally, the course of endocarditis is very slow; symptoms may be present for weeks or months. Individuals whose heart valves have been damaged by rheumatic fever are especially susceptible to endocarditis resulting from viridans streptococci.

Treatment of viridans streptococci infections is with penicillin. Although some resistant strains have been reported, most remain susceptible.

Laboratory diagnosis

Viridans streptococci show typical *Streptococcus* characteristics on Gram stain. The colonies produced are small and are surrounded by a zone of α hemolysis. Some isolates are non-hemolytic. They are bile insoluble and optochin resistant, characteristics that distinguish them from *S. pneu-*

TABLE 11-4

Commonly Isolated Groups of Viridans Streptococci

	Mannitol	Sorbitol	Voges-Proskauer	Arginine	Esculin	Urease
S. mutans group	+	+	+	−	+	−
S. salivarius group	−	−	+	−	+	+/−
S. sanguis group	−	−	−	+	+	−
S. mitis group	−	−	−	−	−	−

Modified from Facklam RR, Washington JA: *Streptococcus* and related catalase-negative gram-positive cocci. In Balows A et al, editors: *Manual of clinical microbiology,* ed 5, Washington, DC, 1991, American Society for Microbiology.

moniae. The lack of β hemolysis separates the viridans streptococci from groups A, B, C, and G. Perhaps the two groups that might be confused with the viridans streptococci are *Enterococcus* and group D *Streptococcus.* Growth in 6.5% NaCl broth differentiates the viridans group from *Enterococcus,* because the viridans streptococci fail to grow (see Figure 11-22). Some strains of *Streptococcus salivarius* can be misidentified as *S. bovis,* however, because a significant number of *S. salivarius* isolates are bile esculin positive. The *Streptococcus milleri* group is composed of strains that may have A, C, F, G, or no Lancefield antigen. These are minute colony types showing α, β, or no hemolysis. When β hemolytic, the zone size is several times the size of the colony. When growing in pure culture or in high concentration, a characteristic sweet odor ("honeysuckle or butterscotch") may be present. A positive Voges-Proskauer test result and a negative PYR test result identify a β-hemolytic isolate as *S. milleri. Streptococcus milleri* has been isolated from abscesses and other pyogenic infections but is rarely involved in endocarditis. A single name, *Streptococcus anginosus,* has been proposed for those organisms belonging to the *S. milleri* group.

The speciation of members of the viridans streptococci group involves performing a considerable number of biochemical tests. This makes it difficult for identifying isolates to the species level without the use of a commercial system developed specifically for that purpose. Several commercial systems identify the viridans streptococci, but no one system can identify all possible species. Also, such systems are relatively expensive.

Nutritionally Variant Streptococci

A subgroup of the viridans streptococci that are nutritionally deficient have been isolated from patients with endocarditis and otitis media. These bacteria are also known as *pyridoxal-dependent* or *vitamin B₆–dependent, thiol-dependent,* and *symbiotic* streptococci. Pyridoxal is not present in most liquid and solid bacteriologic media. This group of organisms were found as satellites around an organism that produces pyridoxal. **Nutritionally variant streptococci (NVS)** may be seen as satellites around colonies of staphylococci, *Escherichia coli, Klebsiella* spp., *Enterobacter* spp., and yeasts.

The NVS colonies are small, measuring 0.2 to 0.5 mm in diameter. On Gram staining, the morphology can vary from that of classic gram-positive streptococci to gram-negative or gram-variable pleomorphic forms. The nutritional state of the organisms determines the state of morphology, with those in close proximity to pyridoxal-producing helper bacteria showing typical *Streptococcus* morphology. As the optimal concentrations or required nutrients decrease, the cells become pleomorphic, even showing globular and filamentous forms.

Many manufacturers of bacteriologic media now include pyridoxal (vitamin B₆) in their media used to grow *Streptococcus* to detect NVS. Isolates of NVS have been reported to resemble existing species of viridans streptococci rather than to form a separate species. Most isolates are susceptible to penicillin, but resistant strains have appeared. Susceptibility to other antibiotics (i.e., erythromycin, penicillin in combination with an aminoglycoside) is the norm.

Nutritionally variant streptococci are part of the normal oral flora and may cause endocarditis. Cases of otitis media and wound infections have also been found that were caused by NVS.

When a laboratory finds positive Gram reactions but negative cultures, NVS should be considered, especially if the Gram stain showed variable morphology and staining characteristics. The specimen should be cultured on a pyridoxal-supplemented medium or plated with a staphylococcal streak, and great care should be taken with inspection of the plates. The NVS are identified by their requirement for pyridoxal or by demonstrating satellitism. In addition, the NVS are bile esculin negative, do not grow in 6.5% NaCl, and are PYR positive. The viridans streptococci are PYR negative.

STREPTOCOCCUS-LIKE ORGANISMS

Streptococcus-like organisms are genera that resemble *Streptococcus* and *Enterococcus* in microscopic and colonial morphology. They particularly resemble the viridans streptococci on blood agar. They may be recognized when antibiotic susceptibility testing of a "streptococcal" isolate shows it to be vancomycin resistant. Because the streptococci show universal sensitivity to vancomycin, further investigation is done, which shows the isolate to be a nonstreptococcal organism. The vancomycin-

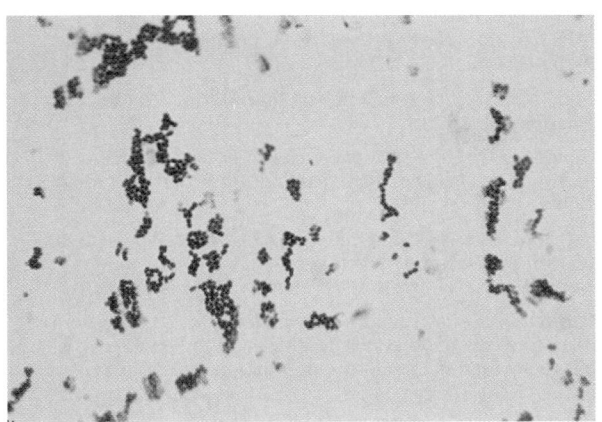

Figure 11-23 _____
Gram stain of *Leuconostoc* sp.

resistant, gram-positive coccus isolate is likely a member of *Leuconostoc* or *Pediococcus*. *Aerococcus* is normally susceptible to vancomycin.

Aerococcus

The only recognized species is *Aerococcus viridans*. It is a gram-positive, nonmotile, spherical cell that tends to form tetrads when grown in broth media. On blood agar the colonies are α-hemolytic and resemble viridans streptococci. ***Aerococcus*** has been isolated from dust, meat, raw vegetables, and various environmental sources, including hospital rooms. It has also been found in the upper respiratory tract and on the skin. It had been considered an airborne contaminant but in later years has been shown to cause endocarditis, urinary tract infections, and other infections. Aerococcal infection is rare and is normally found in immunocompromised patients. As with so many former "nonpathogens," the incidence can be expected to increase as more is known of the organism.

Aerococcus differs from streptococci in microscopic appearance. Unlike *Streptococcus,* it does not form chains but rather tends to form tetrads. Detection usually depends on whether microscopy is performed and the tetrad arrangement of the cells is observed. Table 11-3 lists some of the biochemical characteristics of *Aerococcus* in comparison with the other gram-positive cocci. It is PYR positive and bile esculin variable, and it grows in 6.5% NaCl broth. Because of these characteristics, it may easily be confused with *Enterococcus;* however, *Enterococcus* is LAP positive.

Leuconostoc

Leuconostoc resembles *Streptococcus* and appears as coccobacilli in pairs and occasional short chains (Figure 11-23). It also resembles the viridans streptococci (Figure 11-24) or *Enterococcus* on blood agar. Isolates are usually resistant to vancomycin. Three species of *Leuconostoc* have been isolated from human infections; they are *Leuconostoc lactis, Leuconostoc mesenteroides,* and *Leuconostoc paramesenteroides.* The organisms are found on plants, vegetables, dairy products, wine, and sugar solutions. They have been isolated from cases of meningitis, endocarditis, and septicemia. Like *Enterococcus,* they may grow in 6.5% NaCl and they hydrolyze esculin, but they are PYR and LAP negative. The formation of gas from glucose metabolism distinguishes *Leuconostoc* from *Streptococcus.*

Pediococcus

Members of ***Pediococcus*** form round cells arranged in pairs, tetrads, and clusters. There are eight species, of which *Pediococcus acidilactici* and *Pediococcus pentosaceus* have been isolated from human infections. Pediococci have been isolated from saliva, stool, urine, and wounds. They are found on plants and in alcoholic beverages. Pediococci are also used in the bioprocessing and biopreservation of cheese, meats, vegetables, and soy products. In addition, they have importance as silage additives. They are very rarely seen as causing human disease, but a number of cases of sep-

Figure 11-24 _____
Leuconostoc sp. colonies growing on blood agar. *Leuconostoc* spp. may produce α hemolysis and may resemble viridans streptococci.

ticemia and bacteremia have been documented. *Pediococcus* appears to be universally resistant to vancomycin. To confirm an organism as *Pediococcus,* a Gram stain is very helpful. Cocci found in clusters and tetrads are consistently seen. The bile esculin and LAP reactions are positive, the PYR reaction is negative, and growth is variable in 6.5% NaCl broth. In addition, the organism grows at 45° C.

Gemella

Gemella isolates are similar in colonial morphology and habitat to the viridans streptococci. Strains have been isolated from cases of endocarditis and from wounds and abscesses.

Bibliography

Barreau C, Wagener G: Characterization of *Leuconostoc lactis* strains from human sources. *J Clin Microbiol* 28:1728, 1990.

Bartter T et al: Toxic strep syndrome: a manifestation of group A streptococcal infection, *Arch Intern Med* 148:1421, 1988.

Bosley GS et al: Phenotypic characterization, cellular fatty acid composition, and DNA relatedness of aerococci and comparison to related genera, *J Clin Microbiol* 28:416, 1990.

Campos JM: Noncultural diagnosis of group A streptococcal pharyngitis, *Clin Microbiol Newsl* 9:152:1987.

Chenoweth C, Schaberg D: The epidemiology of enterococci, *Eur J Clin Microbiol Infect Dis* 9:80, 1990.

Christensen JJ et al: *Aerococcus*-like organism, a newly recognized potential urinary tract pathogen, *J Clin Microbiol* 29:1049, 1991.

Christensen JJ, Korner B, Kjaergaard H: *Aerococcus*-like organism—an unnoticed urinary tract pathogen, *Acta Pathol Microbiol Immunol Scand* 97:539, 1989.

Colman G: *Streptococcus* and *Lactobacillus.* In Parker MT, Duerden BI, editors: *Topley & Wilson's principles of bacteriology, virology and immunity,* vol 2, ed 8, Philadelphia, 1990, BC Decker.

Dascal AS et al: PYR-positive *Aerococcus* spp., *Clin Microbiol Newsl* 12:38, 1990.

Facklam RR, Washington JA II: *Streptococcus* and related catalase-negative gram-positive cocci. In Balows A, et al, editors: *Manual of clinical microbiology,* ed 5, Washington, DC, 1991, American Society for Microbiology.

Facklam RR, Collins MD: Identification of *Enterococcus* species isolated from human infections by a conventional test scheme, *J Clin Microbiol* 27:731, 1989.

Fischetti VA: Streptococcal M protein: molecular design and biological behavior, *Clin Microbiol Rev* 2:285, 1989.

Friedland IR, Snipelisky M, Khoosal M: Meningitis in a neonate caused by *Leuconostoc* sp., *J Clin Microbiol* 28:2125, 1990.

Gerber MA: Comparison of throat cultures and rapid strep tests for diagnosis of streptococcal pharyngitis, *Pediatr Infect Dis J* 8:820, 1989.

Ginsburg I: *Streptococcus.* In Braude AI, Davis CE, Fierer J, editors: *Infectious diseases and medical microbiology,* ed 2, Philadelphia, 1986, WB Saunders.

Golledge CL: Bacteremia due to *Leuconostoc* species, *Clin Microbiol Newsl* 11:29, 1989.

Golledge CL et al: Septicemia caused by vancomycin-resistant *Pediococcus acidilactici, J Clin Microbiol* 28:1678, 1990.

Gray BM: Streptococcal infections. In Evans AS, Brachman PS, editors: *Bacterial infections of humans, epidemiology and control,* ed 2, New York, 1991, Plenum Medical Book Co.

Hamoudi AC et al: Clinical relevance of viridans and non-hemolytic streptococci isolated from blood and cerebrospinal fluid in a pediatric population, *Am J Clin Pathol* 93:270, 1989.

Hayden GF, Murphy TF, Hendley JO: Non-group A streptococci in the pharynx, *Am J Dis Child* 143:794, 1989.

Kellogg JA: Suitability of throat culture procedures for detection of group A streptococci and as reference standards for evaluation of streptococcal antigen detection kits, *J Clin Microbiol* 28:165, 1990.

Kiska DL: Staphylococcal and streptococcal toxic shock syndrome, *Clin Microbiol Newsl* 19:33, 1997.

Klein JO: Diagnosis of streptococcal pharyngitis: an introduction, *Pediatr Infect Dis J* 8:813, 1989.

Mastro TD et al: Vancomycin-resistant *Pediococcus acidilactici:* nine cases of bacteremia, *J Infect Dis* 161:956, 1990.

Meier FA et al: Clinical and microbiological evidence for endemic pharyngitis among adults due to group C streptococci, *Arch Intern Med* 150:825, 1990.

Murray BE: The life and times of the enterococcus, *Clin Microbiol Rev* 3:46, 1990.

Park JW, Grossman O: *Aerococcus viridans* infection, *Clin Pediatr* 29:525, 1990.

Roddey OF et al: Comparison of immediate and delayed culture for isolation of group A streptococci, *Pediatr Infect Dis J* 8:710, 1989.

Ross PW: Streptococcal diseases. In Parker MT, Duerden BI, editors: *Topley & Wilson's principles of bacteriology, virology and immunity,* vol 3, *Bacterial diseases,* ed 8, Philadelphia, 1990, BC Decker.

Ruoff KL: Gram-positive vancomycin-resistant clinical isolates, *Clin Microbiol Newsl* 11:1, 1989.

Ruoff KL: Nutritionally variant streptococci, *Clin Microbiol Rev* 4:184, 1991.

Ruoff KL: Recent taxonomic changes in the genus *Enterococcus, Eur J Clin Microbiol Infect Dis* 9:75, 1990.

Ruoff KL: An update on streptococcal taxonomy, *Clin Microbiol Newsl* 10:1, 1988.

Ruoff KL et al: Species identities of enterococci isolated from clinical specimens, *J Clin Microbiol* 28:435, 1990.

Shulman ST: Streptococcal pharyngitis: clinical and epidemiologic factors, *Pediatr Infect Dis J* 8:816, 1989.

Swenson JM, Facklam RR, Thornsberry C: Antimicrobial susceptibility of vancomycin-resistant *Leuconostoc, Pediococcus,* and *Lactobacillus* species, *Antimicrob Agents Chemother* 34:543, 1990.

Technical Information, Todd Hewitt wCNA (LIM BROTH) TI # 64810-A, Remel, Lenexa Kan. 97.

Tenover FC: Laboratory methods for surveillance of vancomycin-resistant enterococci, *Clin Microbiol Newsl* 20:1, 1998.

Turner JC et al: Association of group C β-hemolytic streptococci with endemic pharyngitis among college students, *JAMA* 264:2644, 1990.

Wasilauskas BL: Viridans streptococci: methods and rationale for species identification, *Clin Microbiol Newsl* 9:125, 1987.

Wessels MR et al: Definition of a bacterial virulence factor: Sialylation of the group B streptococcal capsule, *Proc Natl Acad Sci USA* 86:8983, 1989.

LEARNING ASSESSMENTS

1. Name three tests that could be performed on an isolate or initial swab to give the presumptive identity of the isolate described in the case presented.

2. What is the most likely identity of the isolate?

3. What serious sequelae may develop if the infection described in the case is untreated?

4. What other types of infection does this organism cause?

5. What antimicrobial is most commonly used to treat this infection?

6. With what invasive infections has this organism recently been associated?

7. Which streptococcal species causes the most common community-acquired bacterial pneumonia?

8. Differentiate the clinical significance of group B streptococci infection in a pregnant woman from a newborn.

9. Why is enterococci an important nosocomial pathogen?

10. How would you recover nutritionally deficient streptococci from clinical samples such as blood?

CHAPTER 12

Corynebacterium and Other Non–Spore-Forming Gram-Positive Rods

Hal S. Larsen

CORYNEBACTERIUM
General Characteristics
Corynebacterium diphtheriae
  Physiology
  Virulence factors
  Clinical infections
  Laboratory diagnosis
Other *Corynebacteria*
  Corynebacterium jeikeium
  Corynebacterium urealyticum
  Corynebacterium ulcerans
  Corynebacterium pseudotuberculosis
  Corynebacterium xerosis
  Corynebacterium pseudodiphtheriticum
  Corynebacterium striatum
  Corynebacterium kutscheri
Arcanobacterium
Rhodococcus
Undesignated CDC Coryneform Groups
Rothia dentocariosa

LISTERIA MONOCYTOGENES
General Characteristics
Physiology
Virulence Factors
Clinical Infections
  Disease in pregnant women
  Disease in the newborn
  Disease in the immunosuppressed host
Laboratory Diagnosis
  Microscopy
  Cultural characteristics
  Identification

ERYSIPELOTHRIX RHUSIOPATHIAE
General Characteristics
Clinical Infections
Laboratory Diagnosis
  Microscopy
  Cultural characteristics
  Identification

OBJECTIVES

1. List the general characteristics of *Corynebacterium* spp., *Listeria monocytogenes,* and *Erysipelothrix rhusiopathiae.*
2. Explain the clinical significance of these organisms. Describe how the infections they cause are acquired.
3. Describe the distinctive features of the microscopic morphology in direct smears from clinical specimens and/or primary media of these organisms.
4. Name the media required for the isolation of the major pathogens discussed.
5. Describe the colonial morphology of each of the pathogens discussed.
6. List the differential procedures used to diagnose infections caused by *Corynebacterium* spp.
7. Differentiate *Listeria monocytogenes* from other non–spore-forming gram-positive rods and streptococci.
8. Describe the motility patterns of *Listeria monocytogenes* in hanging drop and semisolid medium.
9. Differentiate *Erysipelothrix rhusiopathiae* from other non–spore-forming gram-positive rods.

KEY TERMS

Corynebacterium
Corynebacterium diphtheriae
Pleomorphic
Diphtheria toxin
Diphtheria
Babès-Ernst granules
Loeffler medium
Tinsdale agar
Elek test
Corynebacterium jeikeium
Corynebacterium urealyticum
Corynebacterium ulcerans
Corynebacterium pseudotuberculosis

Corynebacterium xerosis
Corynebacterium pseudodiphtheriticum
Corynebacterium striatum
Corynebacterium kutscheri
Arcanobacterium haemolyticum
Rhodococcus equi
Rothia
Listeria monocytogenes
Tumbling motility
Umbrella pattern motility
Erysipelothrix rhusiopathiae

The gram-positive non–spore-forming rods comprise a heterogeneous group of organisms that include *Corynebacterium, Arcanobacterium, Rhodococcus, Listeria,* and *Erysipelothrix.* Many of these are poorly characterized, hence classification often changes. A wide range of clinical conditions results from infection with these organisms. Although their frequency of isolation in the clinical laboratory is not as great as that of many other organisms (i.e., *Escherichia coli, Staphylococcus au-*

CASE STUDY

A 76-year-old woman receiving corticosteroid therapy for a malignant tumor complained to her physician of fever and headache of 7 days' duration. Her headache had become progressively worse and her temperature was elevated. A complete blood count was performed and showed a slightly elevated white count with normal distribution. A lumbar puncture was performed with the following laboratory results:

- 250 WBC/cu mm
- Glucose 30 mg/DL (Serum glucose was 105 mg/DL)
- Protein 180 mg/DL

The Gram-stained smear of the cerebrospinal fluid (CSF) did not show any microbial forms.

The CSF was inoculated onto blood and chocolate agars. Two days later, beta hemolytic colonies grew on the blood agar. Similar colonial growth was present on the chocolate agar. Gram stain morphology revealed a pleomorphic Gram-positive bacillus. The isolate showed the following biochemical characteristics:

- Christie, Atkins, and Munch-Peterson (CAMP) (positive)
- Catalase (positive)
- Esculin hydrolysis (positive)
- Hippurate hydrolysis (positive)
- Motile at room temperature

reus, Streptococcus), members of this group are often seen. The frequency of isolation is increasing, and some of the lesser-known members (i.e., *Rhodococcus, Arcanobacterium*) are becoming more prominent.

CORYNEBACTERIUM

General Characteristics

The genus **Corynebacterium** consists of a large group of bacteria, animal and human pathogens as well as free-living saprophytes and plant pathogens. They are found worldwide in fresh and salt water, soil, and air. The *corynebacteria* are closely related to mycobacteria and nocardiae; these three groups collectively may be referred to as the CMN group. They have common cell wall structures. The classification of the diphtheroids (or coryneforms) is not well characterized. Consequently, there is a low rate of identification for clinical isolates. Even when sent to a reference laboratory, 30% to 50% of the coryneform-like isolates are unable to be identified to the species level.

The premier pathogen of the group is **Corynebacterium diphtheriae,** which has been extensively studied and is well characterized. Other species that produce disease in humans are *Corynebacterium bovis* (not recognized as a species in the genus *Corynebacterium* by *Bergey's Manual of Systematic Bacteriology*), *Corynebacterium ulcerans* (not recognized as a species in the genus *Corynebacterium* by *Bergey's Manual of Systematic Bacteriology*), *Corynebacterium equi (Rhodococcus equi), Corynebacterium haemolyticum (Arcanobacterium haemolyticum), Corynebacterium xerosis, Corynebacterium jeikeium, Corynebacterium pseudodiphtheriticum,* and *C. pseudotuberculosis.*

The nondiphtheria *corynebacteria* are commonly isolated from clinical specimens. They usually are dismissed as contaminants. As with many previously "nonpathogenic" organisms, however, the coryneforms are being isolated from a variety of body sites, especially in immunocompromised patients.

Corynebacterium diphtheriae
Physiology

The diphtheria bacillus, like other *corynebacteria,* is a facultative anaerobe. It grows best under aerobic conditions, with the optimal growth temperature of 37° C, although multiplication occurs within the range of 15° to 40° C. Growth requirements are complex, with eight essential amino acids. The organism ferments glucose and maltose, producing acid but not gas. It does not produce urease but reduces nitrate to nitrite.

The growth medium markedly affects morphology and toxin production. In stained smears, diphtheria bacilli characteristically appear in palisades or as individual cells lying at sharp angles to one another in V and L formations. When grown on suboptimal media, such as Loeffler coagulated serum, the cells are **pleomorphic** and stain irregularly with methylene blue. Club-shaped swellings and beaded forms are common. The amount of toxin produced is influenced by the growth conditions. The iron content of the medium must be growth rate–limiting for full toxin production. The addition of iron to iron-starved cultures inhibits toxin production very quickly.

C. diphtheriae is readily killed by heat and most of the usual disinfectants. It is, however, resistant to drying and remains viable in the environment for weeks.

Virulence factors

The major virulence factor associated with *C. diphtheriae* is the **diphtheria toxin.** This toxin is produced by those strains of *C. diphtheriae* that are infected with a temperate bacteriophage, which carries the structural gene *(tox)* for diphtheria toxin. Nontoxigenic strains can be converted to tox^+ by infection with the appropriate bacteriophage. Only toxin-producing, *C. diphtheriae* causes the infection **diphtheria;** however, *C. ulcerans* and *C. pseudotuberculosis,* which belong to what is called the "*C. diphtheriae* group," may also produce the toxin when they become infected with the *tox*-carrying bacteriophage.

Diphtheria toxin is a simple protein of 62,000 daltons. It is exceedingly potent and is lethal for humans in amounts of 130 ng per kg of body weight. The toxicity of the toxin is because of its ability to block protein synthesis in eukaryotic cells. The toxin is secreted by the bacterial cell and is nontoxic until exposure to trypsin. The trypsinization results in two polypeptide fragments, A and B, which are linked together by a disulfide bridge. Both fragments are necessary for cytotoxicity. Fragment A is responsible for the toxicity; fragment B binds to receptors on the eukaryotic cells and mediates the entry of fragment A into the cytoplasm following cleavage by cellular enzymes. On reaching the cytoplasm, fragment A disrupts protein synthesis. Fragment A splits nicotinamide adenosine dinucleotide (NAD) to form nicotinamide and adenosine diphosphoribose (ADPR). ADPR binds to and inactivates elongation factor 2 (EF-2), an enzyme required for elongation of polypeptide chains on ribosomes. The reaction can be summarized as follows:

$$NAD^+ + \underset{\text{active}}{EF\text{-}2} \rightleftharpoons ADPR\text{-}\underset{\text{inactive}}{EF\text{-}2} + nicotinamde + H^+$$

Toxin production depends on a lysogenic state in which the bacterium is infected with a bacteriophage that carries the *tox⁺* gene, which codes for the production of diphtheria toxin.

Production of the toxin in vitro depends on a number of environmental conditions: an alkaline pH (7.8 to 8.0), oxygen, and, most importantly, iron concentration in the medium. The amount of iron needed for optimal toxin production is less than the amount needed for optimal growth. Strangely, the toxin is released in significant amounts only when the available iron in the culture medium is exhausted.

Clinical infections

Diphtheria, which occurs in two forms, respiratory and cutaneous, is found worldwide but is uncommon in North America and Western Europe. Those cases that occur are invariably in unimmunized populations. Humans are the only natural hosts for *C. diphtheriae.*

The organism is carried in the upper respiratory tract and spread by droplet infection or hand-to-mouth contact. The incubation period averages 2 to 5 days. The illness begins gradually and is characterized by low-grade fever, malaise, and a mild sore throat. The most common site of infection is the tonsils or pharynx. The organisms rapidly multiply on the epithelial cells and trigger an inflammatory reaction. The infecting toxigenic strain of *C. diphtheriae* produces toxin locally, causing tissue necrosis and exudate formation. This combination of cell necrosis and exudate forms a very tough gray to white pseudomembrane, which attaches to the tissues. It may appear on the tonsils and then spread downward into the larynx and trachea. There is the potential for suffocation if the membrane spreads

and blocks the air passage or if it is dislodged, perhaps as the result of sampling for a throat culture.

The toxin also is absorbed and produces a variety of systemic effects. The systemic manifestations of the disease involve the kidneys, heart, and nervous system, although all tissues possess the receptor for the toxin and may be affected. Death often is a result of cardiac failure. Another effect of the toxin is a demyelinating peripheral neuritis, which may result in paralysis following the acute illness.

Other nonrespiratory sites may be infected, although much less often than the upper respiratory tract. In the cutaneous form of diphtheria, which is prevalent in the tropics, the toxin also is absorbed systemically, but systemic complications are less common than from upper respiratory infections with *C. diphtheriae.*

Diphtheria is treated by prompt administration of antitoxin. Commercial diphtheria antitoxin is produced in horses. Consequently, hypersensitivity to horse serum precludes its administration. Approximately 10% of patients who receive the antitoxin develop an allergic reaction to the horse serum. Antibiotics have no effect on toxin that is already circulating, but they do serve to eliminate the focus of infection as well as prevent the spread of the organism. The drug of choice is penicillin. Erythromycin is the drug used for penicillin-sensitive individuals.

Laboratory diagnosis

MICROSCOPY

C. diphtheriae is a gram-positive, nonsporulating, nonmotile bacillus. The organism is highly pleomorphic and appears in palisades or as individual cells lying at sharp angles to another in V and L formations. This particular arrangement associated with *C. diphtheriae* has been described by westerners as "Chinese characters" (Figure 12-1), although it may be demonstrated by other *Corynebacterium* species.

The organisms often stain irregularly, especially when stained with methylene blue, giving them a beaded appearance. The metachromatic areas of the cell, which stain more intensely than other parts, are called **Babès-Ernst granules.** They represent accumulation of polymerized polyphosphates. The presence of the Babès-Ernst granules indicates the accumulation of food reserves and varies with

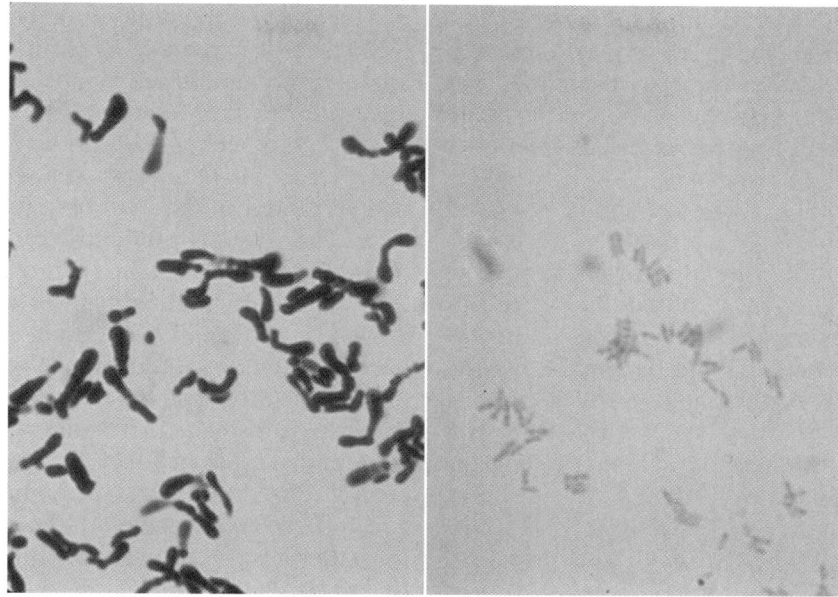

Figure 12-1

Left, Microscopic Gram stain of diphtheroid. *Right,* Microscopic Loeffler methylene blue stain of *Corynebacterium* spp. (Courtesy Cathy Bissonette.)

the type of medium and the metabolic state of the individual cells.

CULTURAL CHARACTERISTICS

Although *C. diphtheriae* will grow on nutrient agar, better growth is usually obtained on a medium containing blood or serum, such as Loeffler serum agar or Pai slant. Characteristic microscopic morphology is demonstrated well when organisms are grown on **Loeffler medium.** On blood agar (Figure 12-2), the organism may have a very small zone of hemolysis.

Tinsdale agar, which contains sheep's blood, bovine serum, cystine, and potassium tellurite, is used as both a selective and differential medium. When grown on Tinsdale agar, corynebacteria form black or brownish colonies.

This appearance is not unique for *C. diphtheriae,* however, so care must be taken not to presumptively identify other genera that produce black colonies *(Staphylococcus* and *Streptococcus)* as *Corynebacterium.* A brown halo surrounding the colony is a useful differentiating feature, because only *C. diphtheriae, C. ulcerans,* and *C. pseudotuberculosis* produce a brown halo on Tinsdale agar. Media containing tellurite (e.g., cystine-tellurite

agar) can be used to isolate *C. diphtheriae.* Tellurite salts present in the medium inhibit the growth of most respiratory flora but *C. diphtheriae* is able to grow. Colonies of *C. diphtheriae* and *C. ulcerans* are gray or gray-black. *Listeria* may develop gray colonies.

Three biotypes of *C. diphtheriae* can be distinguished by their growth characteristics on Tins-

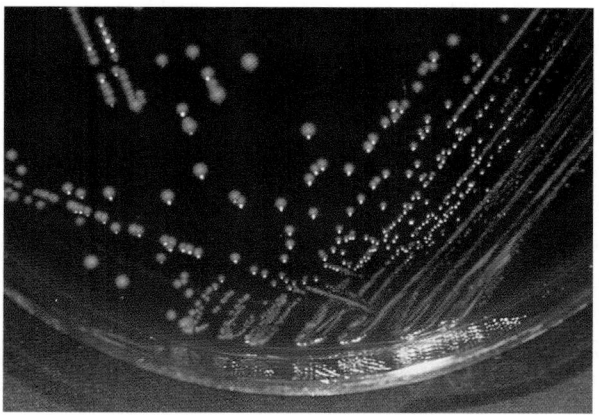

Figure 12-2

Corynebacterium diphtheria growing on blood agar plate. (Courtesy Cathy Bissonette.)

dale agar: *mitis, intermedius,* and *gravis.* The colonies of each differ in size and color. Practically, however, there is little reason to classify an isolate by biotype, because there appears to be little, if any, correlation between disease severity and biotype.

IDENTIFICATION

The biochemical identification of medically important corynebacteria is outlined in Table 12-1. Tinsdale medium is useful for differentiations because only *C. diphtheriae, C. ulcerans,* and *C. pseudotuberculosis* form a brown halo. *C. diphtheriae* is distinguished from the other two species by its lack of urease production. A schematic diagram to presumptively identify *C. diphtheriae* is shown in Figure 12-3.

TEST FOR TOXIGENICITY

The identification of an isolate as *C. diphtheriae* does not mean that the patient has diphtheria. Diagnosis of diphtheria depends on showing that the isolate produces diphtheria toxin. This can be done by either in vivo or in vitro testing. In vivo testing is rarely done because the in vitro methods are reliable, less expensive, and free from the need to use animals. The procedure used for in vivo testing is discussed only to provide a historical perspective.

The in vivo test to determine toxin production by an isolate is carried out in guinea pigs. Approximately 24 hours before the test, one guinea pig is injected with diphtheria antitoxin. The next day, the protected guinea pig and an untreated guinea pig each are injected with a suspension of the suspected organism that has prepared from Loeffler slants. If the isolate produces diphtheria toxin, the untreated animal will die within 3 to 5 days, and the antitoxin-treated animal will survive.

The in vitro diphtheria toxin detection procedure is an immunodiffusion test first described by Elek. In the **Elek test,** organisms (controls and unknowns) are streaked on media of low iron content to optimize toxin production. The organisms are each streaked in a single straight line parallel to each other and 10 mm apart on an Elek plate. A filter paper strip impregnated with diphtheria antitoxin is laid along the center of the plate on a line at right angles to the lines of control and unknown organisms (Figure 12-4). The plate is then incubated at 35° C and examined after 18, 24, and 48 hours. Lines of precipitation are best seen by transmitted light against a dark background. The white precipitin lines start about 4 to 5 mm from the filter paper strip and are at an angle of about 45 degrees to the line of growth. If an isolate is positive for toxin production, and it is placed next to the positive control, the toxin line of the positive control should

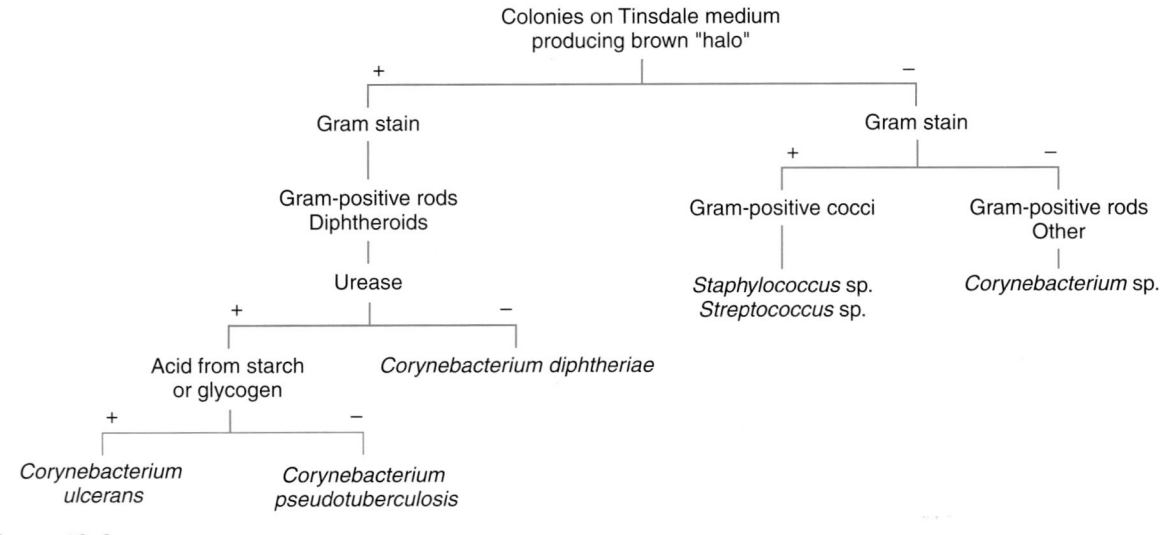

Figure 12-3

A schematic diagram of the presumptive identification of *Corynebacterium diphtheriae.*

TABLE 12-1

Identification of Corynebacteria

Characteristic	Corynebacteria diphtheriae	Corynebacteria ulcerans	Corynebacteria pseudotuberculosis	Corynebacteria xerosis	Corynebacteria jeikeium	Corynebacteria urealyticum	Corynebacteria pseudodiphtheriticum	Corynebacteria striatum	Corynebacteria kutscheri
Tinsdale halo	+	+	+	–	–	–	–	–	–
Catalase	+	+	+	+	+	+	+	+	+
β Hemolysis	V	V	+	–	–	–	–	–	–
Nitrate reduction	+	–	V	+	–	–	+	+	+
Urease	–	+	+	–	–	+	+	–	+
Hydrolysis									
Gelatin	–	+*	–	–	–	–	–	–	–
Esculin	–	–	–	–	–	–	–	–	+
Carbohydrate fermentation									
Glucose	+	+	+	+	+	–	–	+	+
Maltose	+	+	+	+	V	–	–	–	+
Sucrose	–	–	–	+	–	–	–	+	+

+, Present or positive; –, absent or negative; *V*, variable.
*25° C.

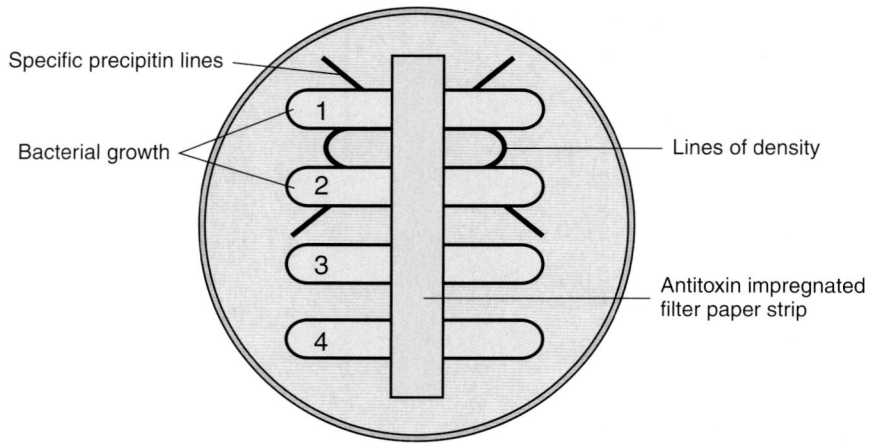

Figure 12-4

Colonial Elek test for toxin-producing strains of *Corynebacterium diphtheriae*. *1,* Positive control; *2,* unknown (toxigenic); *3,* negative control; *4,* unknown (nontoxigenic).

join the toxin line of the positive unknown to form an *arch of identity* (see Figure 12-4). The Elek test requires that reagents and antisera be carefully controlled and titrated. For this reason, and because of the difficulty of the test, it is performed only in certain reference laboratories.

Other Corynebacteria

Corynebacterium jeikeium

Named after Johnson and Kaye, who first reported human infections caused by it, **Corynebacterium jeikeium** shows a high degree of antimicrobial resistance. These organisms appear to be part of the usual skin flora. Infections have been limited to those patients who are immunocompromised or have undergone invasive procedures.

The presence of catheters or prosthetic devices also contributes to infection with *C. jeikeium,* and in fact, it is the most common cause of diphtheroid prosthetic valve endocarditis in adults. *C. jeikeium* has been reported to be typically resistant to a wide range of antimicrobials. Most strains are susceptible to vancomycin but show variable susceptibility to tetracycline and erythromycin.

Corynebacterium urealyticum

Corynebacterium urealyticum has now been described as a urinary pathogen. The species is a slow-growing organism, so cultures must incubate at least 48 hours before growth is detected. Urine isolates with very small, nonhemolytic, white colonies that have characteristic diphtheroid morphology are likely *C. urealyticum* suspects. The isolate should be catalase positive and should rapidly produce urease (within minutes following inoculation on a Christensen urea slant) to be presumptively called *C. urealyticum.* In addition, *C. urealyticum* does not ferment glucose. It also has shown resistance to a wide variety of antimicrobials, such as β-lactam, aminoglycoside, and macrolide.

Corynebacterium ulcerans

A veterinary pathogen causing mastitis in cattle and other domestic and wild animals, **Corynebacterium ulcerans** has been isolated from patients with diphtheria-like illness. A significant number of isolates produce the diphtheria toxin, although the amount of toxin elaborated is much less than by *C. diphtheriae.*

Human infections usually are acquired through contact with animals or by ingestion of unpasteurized dairy products. The organism has been isolated from skin ulcers and exudative pharyngitis. It grows well on Loeffler and Tinsdale media, giving a brown halo around the colonies on Tinsdale medium. The organisms grow well on blood agar and show a narrow zone of hemolysis. Unlike *C. diphtheriae, C. ulcerans* does not reduce nitrate. It gives a positive gelatin reaction at room temperature. It may be that this organism, which has not been fully accepted as a species, has been classified as a subgroup of *C. diphtheriae.*

Corynebacterium pseudotuberculosis

Closely resembling *C. diphtheriae* on blood agar and Gram morphology, **Corynebacterium pseudotuberculosis** also gives a brown halo on Tinsdale medium. It is urease positive and gelatin negative. It produces a dermonecrotic toxin that causes death of a variety of cell types. Like *C. ulcerans*, *C. pseudotuberculosis* is a veterinary pathogen. Human infections usually have been associated with contact with sheep. The organism is susceptible to penicillin and erythromycin.

Corynebacterium xerosis

Corynebacterium xerosis is commonly found on skin and mucocutaneous sites. Opportunistic infections associated with this organism include prosthetic valve endocarditis, bacteremia associated with intravenous catheters, postsurgical wound infections, and pneumonia. Human infection with *C. xerosis* is rare, and affected patients are invariably immunosuppressed. This organism grows well on blood agar and forms pigmented (yellow to tan) colonies.

Corynebacterium pseudodiphtheriticum

Part of the normal flora of the human nasopharynx, **Corynebacterium pseudodiphtheriticum** very rarely causes infection, but when infection occurs, it takes the form of endocarditis. Respiratory and urinary tract infections as well as cutaneous wound infections resulting from this organism have been seen in immunosuppressed patients, including those with acquired immune deficiency syndrome (AIDS). *C. pseudodiphtheriticum,* unlike other *corynebacteria*, does not show the characteristic pleomorphic morphology. The cells stain evenly and often lie in parallel rows (palisades). The species grows well on standard laboratory media, reduces nitrate, and hydrolyzes urea.

Corynebacterium striatum

Corynebacterium striatum is a slow-growing, pleomorphic species that often produces a yellowish green soluble pigment. It is found in the nasopharynx and is a rare cause of infection.

Corynebacterium kutscheri

Primarily an animal pathogen, **Corynebacterium kutscheri** microscopically resembles *C. diphtheriae*, but the colonies are yellow to gray on blood agar.

Arcanobacterium

Arcanobacterium haemolyticum was formerly known as *Corynebacterium haemolyticum*. This organism produces small colonies on sheep's blood agar that demonstrate a narrow zone of hemolysis after 24 hours of incubation that is similar in appearance to the β-hemolytic streptococci. It has been recovered from patients with pharyngitis and so must be distinguished from *C. diphtheriae* and *C. ulcerans* as well as group A streptococcus. *A. haemolyticum* is catalase negative, whereas *C. diphtheriae* and *C. ulcerans* are catalase positive. A Gram stain of the isolated colony in question quickly eliminates the possibility of group A streptococci, because *A. haemolyticum* is a gram-positive rod.

Rhodococcus

Rhodococcus equi (formerly known as *Corynebacterium equi*) may demonstrate filaments, some with branching. The colonies resemble *Klebsiella* on blood agar and form a salmon-pink pigment upon prolonged incubation, especially at room temperature. The species may be partially acid fast. Biochemical identification is difficult because it does not ferment carbohydrates and shows a variable reaction to a number of characteristics (i.e., nitrate reduction, urease). A major clue to identification of *Rhodococcus* is the salmon-pink pigment, followed by a Gram stain showing characteristic diphtheroid gram-positive rods with traces of branching.

R. equi is found in soil. It is the cause of respiratory infection in animals. Human infection is rare, although an increased incidence in immunosuppressed patients, particularly AIDS patients, is being reported.

Undesignated CDC Coryneform Groups

Several coryneform bacilli remain characterized by Centers for Disease Control and Prevention (CDC) group numbers and letters while awaiting proper species designation. All of these organisms have been isolated from a wide range of clinical samples, and they should be regarded as potential nosocomial pathogens or opportunistic pathogens in the immunocompromised patient.

Rothia dentocariosa

A member of the normal human oropharyngeal flora, *R. dentocariosa* may be found in saliva and supragingival plaque. It has been isolated from patients with endocarditis. Microscopically, this organism resembles coryneform bacilli, producing gram-positive short rods but also branching filaments that resemble those of facultative actinomycetes. When placed in broth, however, the species produces coccoid cells, a characteristic differentiating it from the *Actinomyces*. **Rothia** is catalase and nitrate positive, nonmotile, and urease negative.

LISTERIA MONOCYTOGENES

General Characteristics

The genus *Listeria* comprises seven species, of which **Listeria monocytogenes** is the only human and animal pathogen. It is a coccobacillus that often appears coccoid in culture. It is gram-positive, aerobic, and nonsporulating. *L, monocytogenes* grows well on routine laboratory media, producing β hemolysis on sheep's blood agar. Colonies are small, smooth, and translucent, and they show a very narrow ring of hemolysis. They may be confused with group B streptococci because the resemblance is striking. *L. monocytogenes* is widespread in the environment. It has been recovered from soil, water, vegetation, and animal products. It also has been isolated from crustaceans, flies, and ticks. It has long been known to cause illness in many species of wild and domestic animals, including sheep, cattle, swine, horses, dogs, cats, rodents, birds, and fish.

The first human infection was described relatively recently (1926). Since then, the incidence has increased somewhat, and listeriosis is now recognized as an uncommon but serious infection primarily of neonates, pregnant women, and immunocompromised hosts. Infection also may occur in healthy individuals.

Physiology

The optimal growth temperature for *L. monocytogenes* is 30° to 35° C, but growth occurs over a wide range (0.5° to 45° C). It can grow in a high salt concentration (up to 10% NaCl). A source of carbohydrate is essential for growth. The organism prefers a slightly increased CO_2 tension for isolation. It is catalase positive, which differentiates it from *Streptococcus,* and motile at room temperature, which, along with β hemolysis, excludes the corynebac-

teria. In wet mount preparations, *L. monocytogenes* exhibits "tumbling motility" when viewed microscopically. The use of motility medium demonstrates the characteristic "umbrella" pattern when the organism is incubated at room temperature (25° C) but not at 35° C (Figure 12-5).

L. monocytogenes gives a positive CAMP reaction when *Staphylococcus aureus* is used to augment the enhanced hemolysis. A more pronounced CAMP reaction is seen with *L. monocytogenes* when *R. equi* is used in place of *S. aureus*.

Virulence Factors

L. monocytogenes produces a number of products that have been proposed as virulence factors. These include hemolysin (listeriolysin O), catalase, superoxide dismutase, phospholipase C, and a surface protein, p60. Protein p60 induces phagocytosis through increased adhesion and penetration into mammalian cells. Listeriolysin O damages the phagosome membrane, effectively preventing killing of the organism by the phagocyte. The correlation between listeriolysin O production and virulence is strong. Nonhemolytic isolates are found to be avirulent and demonstrate no intracellular spread of the organism.

Clinical Infections

The infectious dose and portal of entry of listeriosis have not been determined, but animal studies as well as analysis of human outbreaks seem to

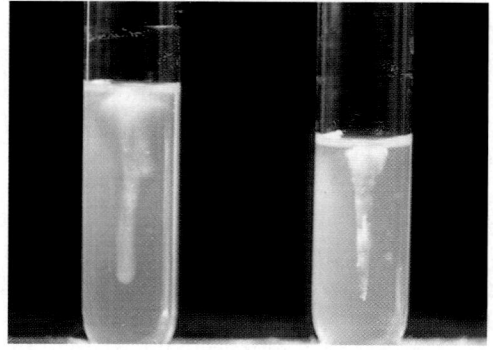

Figure 12-5 _____

Umbrella motility: *Listeria.* Motility test for *Listeria monocytogenes* showing the typical "umbrella" pattern, which occurs towards the surface of the medium, when this organism is incubated at room temperature. Tube on the left is positive. Tube on right is negative control.

indicate that the ingestion of contaminated food with subsequent systemic spread through the intestine is likely. The clinical manifestations of listeriosis differ among patient groups. Infections of newborns and immunocompromised adults are the most common, but disease in healthy individuals, particularly in pregnant women, also occurs.

Disease in pregnant women

During pregnancy, listeriosis is most commonly seen during the third trimester. It has been postulated that *L. monocytogenes* is responsible for spontaneous abortion and stillborn neonates. A pregnant woman with listeriosis may experience a flu-like illness, with fever, headache, and myalgia. At this point, the organism is in the blood stream and has seeded the uterus and fetus. It may progress and result in premature labor or septic abortion within 3 to 7 days. It appears that the infection often is self-limited, because the source of the infection is eliminated when birth occurs.

Disease in the newborn

Infection of the neonate with *L. monocytogenes* is extremely serious. Fatality rates are high, approaching 50% if the fetus is born alive. There are two forms of neonatal listeriosis: early-onset and late-onset. Early-onset listeriosis results from an intrauterine infection that can cause illness at or shortly after birth. The result is most often sepsis. Early-onset disease may be associated with aspiration of infected amniotic fluid.

Late-onset disease occurs several days to weeks after birth. Affected infants generally are full term and healthy at birth. The disease is most likely to manifest as meningitis. The fatality rate is lower than in early-onset infection, although it also is a very serious, often fatal infection.

Disease in the immunosuppressed host

Invasive listeriosis occurs most commonly in persons who are immunosuppressed or older adults, and particularly in patients receiving chemotherapy, as demonstrated in the opening case study. The most common manifestations are central nervous system infection and endocarditis. Affected patients usually have the presenting symptoms of meningitis, meningoencephalitis, or sepsis. Diagnosis is made by culturing *L. monocytogenes* from the blood or spinal fluid.

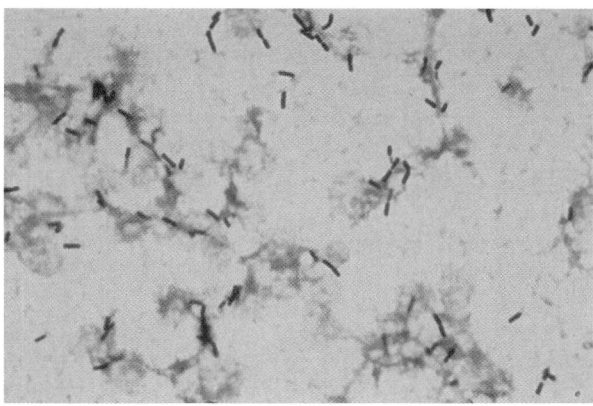

Figure 12-6
Microscopic Gram stain of *Listeria monocytogenes* in the blood. (Courtesy Cathy Bissonette.)

Infection of apparently healthy individuals may occur through the intestinal tract when they eat food contaminated with *L. monocytogenes*. Outbreaks have occurred as a result of eating contaminated cheese, coleslaw, and chicken. Recently, contaminated ice cream, hot dogs, and luncheon meats have served as vehicles for this food-borne disease. The young, the immunocompromised, and older adults are the most vulnerable. The manifestation in these cases is nearly always meningitis, and the fatality rate is high. The antibiotics that have been effectively used to get at listeriosis are penicillins, aminoglycosides, and macrolides. Resistance is not common, although some strains are resistant to one or more antibiotics.

Laboratory Diagnosis

Microscopy

In direct smears (Figure 12-6), *L. monocytogenes* appears as a gram-positive coccobacillus. With subculturing, it tends to appear as coccoid forms. Older cultures often appear gram variable. They may be found singly, in short chains, or in palisades. Depending upon the culture conditions, *L. monocytogenes* may resemble *Streptococcus* when found in the coccoid form and *Corynebacterium* when the bacillus forms prevail. Organisms are not usually seen on the spinal fluid smear.

Cultural characteristics

L. monocytogenes grows well on blood agar and chocolate agar, as well as nutrient agars and broths

TABLE 12-2

Differentiation of Listeria Monocytogenes *and Other Gram-Positive Bacteria*

Organism	Catalase	Esculin Hydrolysis	Motility	β Hemolysis	Growth in 6.5% NaCl
Listeria monocytogenes	+	+	+	+	+
Corynebacterium spp.	+	−	V	V	V
Streptococcus agalactiae	−	−	−	+	V
Enterococcus spp.	−*	+	−	V	+

+, Present or positive; −, absent or negative; *V,* variable.
*May be weak.

such as brain-heart infusion and thioglycolate. The colonies are small, round, smooth, and translucent. They are surrounded by a narrow zone of β hemolysis, which may be visualized only if the colony is removed. The colonies and hemolysis are similar to those seen with *Streptococcus agalactiae* or group B streptococci (Figure 12-7, *A*). Growth is normally complete in 1 or 2 days.

Because *L. monocytogenes* grows at 4° C, an unusual characteristic, a technique called *cold enrichment* may be used to isolate the organism from clinical specimens. This technique calls for inoculation of the specimen into broth and incubation at 4° C for several weeks. Subcultures are made at weekly intervals and examined for *L. monocytogenes.* The length of time required for isolation using this technique lessens its importance in the clinical setting, because treatment must begin early in the infectious process.

Identification

The diagnosis of listeriosis depends on isolating *L. monocytogenes* from blood, cerebrospinal fluid, or swabs of lesions. Table 12-2 lists the characteristics of *L. monocytogenes* and other gram-positive bacteria.

L. monocytogenes is differentiated from group B streptococci by a positive catalase test, **tumbling motility,** and a negative hippurate hydrolysis test. It gives a positive CAMP reaction. However, *Listeria monocytogenes* produces a "block" type hemolysis. This type of hemolysis is in contrast to the "arrowhead" type produced by group B streptococci (see Figure 12-7, *B*). The positive CAMP reaction distinguishes *L. monocytogenes* from the other *Listeria* species, which are CAMP negative. Motility at room temperature is a characteristic **umbrella pattern motility** (see Figure 12-5).

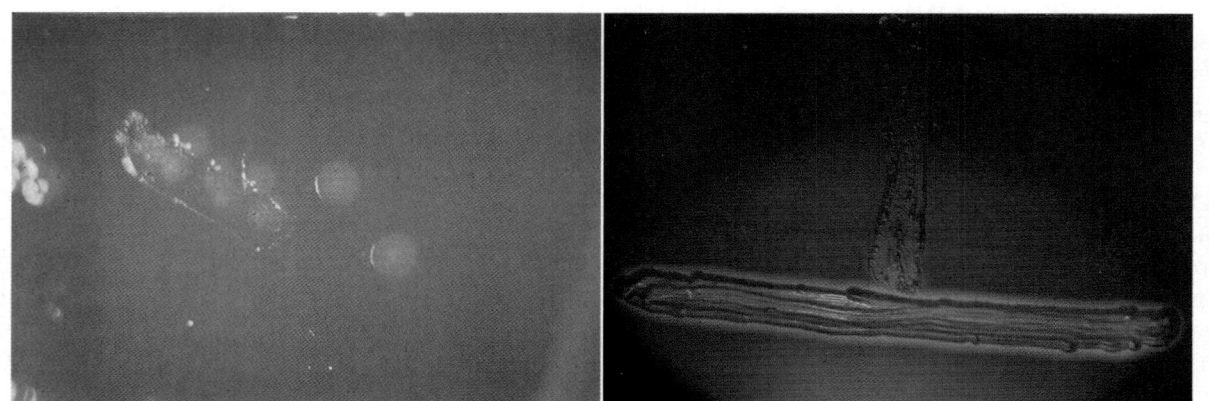

A   **B**

Figure 12-7

A, β Hemolysis: *Listeria* on blood agar plate. Colonial *Listeria monocytogenes* growing on blood agar with colonial morphology similar to that of group B β-hemolytic streptococci. **B,** Conventional CAMP test with *Listeria monocytogenes* showing "block" hemolysis at the junction with the *Staphylococcus.* (Courtesy Cathy Bissonette.)

ERYSIPELOTHRIX RHUSIOPATHIAE

General Characteristics

Erysipelothrix rhusiopathiae is the only species in the genus. It is a gram-positive, nonsporulating, pleomorphic rod that has a tendency to form long filaments. It is found worldwide and is a commensal or a pathogen in a very wide variety of vertebrates and invertebrates. Domestic swine are the major reservoir. Human cases are relatively rare, with infections resulting from occupational exposure. Those individuals whose work involves handling fish and animal products are most at risk. The usual route of infection is through cuts or scratches on the skin. The organism is resistant to salting, pickling, and smoking and survives well in environmental sources such as water, soil, and plant material.

Clinical Infections

E. rhusiopathiae produces three types of disease in humans: septicemia, endocarditis, and erysipeloid. Systemic infection is very uncommon and rarely develops from localized infection. Endocarditis has been seen in patients who have had valve replacements but also in individuals with apparently normal heart valves.

Erysipeloid is a localized skin infection that resembles streptococcal erysipelas. The lesions usually are seen on the hands or fingers because the organisms usually are inoculated through work activities. The incubation period is 1 to 4 days. The infected area is painful and swollen and gives rise to a characteristic lesion: a sharply defined, slightly elevated, purplish red zone that spreads peripherally as discoloration of the central area fades. Low-grade fever, arthralgia, lymphangiitis, and lymphadenopathy may occur. A mild form of the disease lasts 2 to 4 weeks, but it may continue for months. Erysipeloid is a self-limiting infection that normally heals within 3 to 4 weeks. A problem is that second attacks can occur and relapses are common.

Antibiotic therapy is effective, with penicillins, cephalosporins, erythromycin, and clindamycin being useful. The incidence of *E. rhusiopathiae* infections is low.

Laboratory Diagnosis

Microscopy

E. rhusiopathiae is a thin, rod-shaped, gram-positive organism that may form long filaments (Figure 12-8). It is arranged singly, in short chains, or in a V shape. The last arrangement is similar to that seen with the corynebacteria.

Cultural characteristics

The specimen received by the clinical laboratory is from a tissue biopsy or aspirates from skin lesions. These should be inoculated to a nutrient

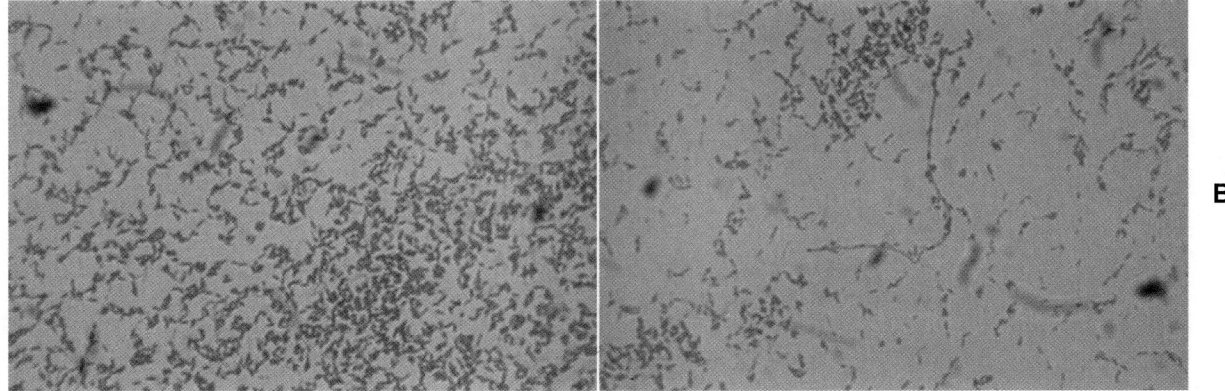

A   B

Figure 12-8

A, Gram stain of *Erysipelothrix rhusiopathiae* at 24 hours. **B,** Gram stain of *E. rhusiopathiae* at 72 hours showing the tendency to form long filaments, which are easily decolorized. (Courtesy Cathy Bissonette.)

TABLE 12-3

Characteristics of Listeria, Corynebacterium, Erysipelothrix, *and Other Related Gram-Positive Bacilli*

Organism	Catalase	Motility	Esculin Hydrolysis	Acid from Glucose	H_2S from TSI Agar	Hemolysis Type	Nitrate Reduction	Urease Production
Corynebacterium spp.	+	−	V	V	−	V	V	V
Listeria monocytogenes	+	+*	+	+	−	β	−	−
Erysipelothrix rhusiopathiae	−	−	−	+	+	None, α	−	−
Kurthia spp.	+	+	−	−	−	None	−	−
Lactobacillus spp.	−	−	−	−	−	None	−	−
Arcanobacterium haemolyticum	−	−	−	+	−	β	−	−
Rhodococcus spp.	+	−	−	−	−	None	V	+
Rothia dentocariosa	+	−	+	+	−	None	+	−
Oerskovia	+	+	+	+	−	None	V	V

+, Positive; −, negative; *V,* variable.
*Motile at 25° C.

broth with 1% glucose and incubated in 5% CO_2 at 35° C. Subcultures should be made daily to blood agar plates.

On blood agar, the colonies are nonhemolytic or α hemolytic and are pinpoint after 24 hours of incubation. After 48 hours of incubation, two distinct colony types are seen. A smaller, smooth form is transparent, glistening, and convex with entire edges. The larger, rough colonies are flatter with a matte surface, curled structure, and irregular edges.

Identification

A comparison of *Erysipelothrix* with *Listeria* is shown in Figure 12-9. Table 12-3 lists the characteristics of *Erysipelothrix* and other related gram-positive bacilli. Identification is based on the Gram stain, hydrogen sulfide production, lack of motility, indole and catalase activities, and a negative Voges-Proskauer reaction. An additional test that can be used to differentiate *Erysipelothrix* from *L. monocytogenes* is susceptibility to neomycin; *Erysipelothrix* is resistant and *L. monocytogenes* is susceptible.

A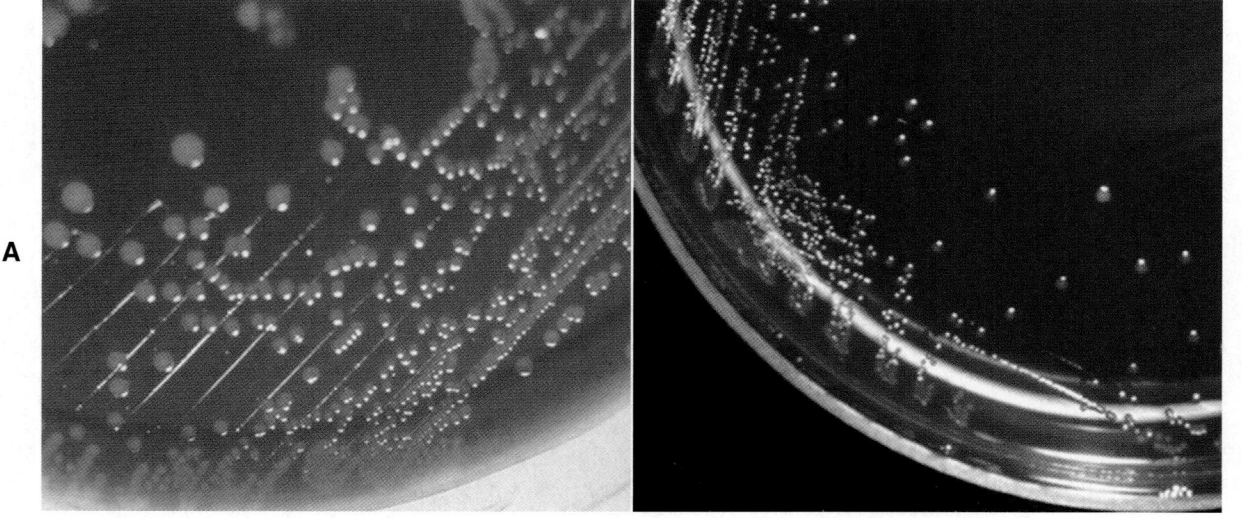B

Figure 12-9

Comparison of colony morphology of *Listeria* **(A)** and *Erysipelothrix* **(B)** growing on blood agar. (Courtesy Cathy Bissonette.)

Bibliography

Brooks R, Joynson DHM: Bacteriological diagnosis of diphtheria, *Assoc Clin Pathologists Broadsheet* 125:576, 1990.

Camilli A, Goldfine H, Portnoy DA: *Listeria monocytogenes* mutants lacking phosphatidylinositol-specific phospholipase C are avirulent, *J Exp Med* 173:751, 1991.

Clarridge JE: When, why, and how far should coryneforms be identified? *Clin Microbiol Newsl* 8:32, 1986.

Cossart P et al: Listeriolysin O is essential for virulence of *Listeria monocytogenes:* direct evidence obtained by gene complementation, *Infect Immun* 57:3629, 1989.

Courtieu AL: Latest news on listeriosis, *Comp Immun Microbiol Infect Dis* 14:1, 1991.

Dietrich MC, Watson DC, Kumar ML: *Corynebacterium* group JK infections in children, *Pediatr Infect Dis J* 8:233, 1989.

Janda WM: *Corynebacterium* species and the coryneform bacteria. Part I: new and emerging species in the genus *Corynebacterium, Clin Microbiol Newsl* 20:41, 1998.

Janda WM: *Corynebacterium* species and the coryneform bacteria. Part II: new and emerging species in the genus *Corynebacterium, Clin Microbiol Newsl* 20:53, 1998.

Lachica RV: Same-day identification scheme for colonies of *Listeria monocytogenes, Appl Environ Microbiol* 56:1166, 1990.

Lipsky BA et al: Infections caused by nondiphtheria *corynebacteria, Rev Infect Dis* 4:1220, 1982.

Mounier J et al: Intracellular and cell to cell spread of *Listeria monocytogenes* involves interaction with F-actin in the enterocyte cell line Caco-2, *Infect Immun* 58:1048, 1990.

Reboli A, Farrar WE: *Erysipelothrix rhusiopathiae:* an occupational pathogen, *Clin Microbiol Rev* 2:354, 1989.

Ronci-Koenig TJ et al: Infections due to *Corynebacterium* Group D2, *Arch Intern Med* 150:1965, 1990.

Schuchat A, Swaminathan B, Broome CV: Epidemiology of human listeriosis, *Clin Microbiol Rev* 4:169, 1991.

Weinheimer LA, Sass E: Clinically significant *Rhodococcus equi* isolates from AIDS patients at Parkland Memorial Hospital, *Clin Lab Sci* 5:140, 1992.

LEARNING ASSESSMENT

1. What is the most likely identity of the isolate described in "Case Study"?

2. What factors may predispose patients to an infection with this organism?

3. What other organism may give similar clinical and laboratory findings? How is this organism differentiated from *Listeria* sp.?

4. How is *Erysipelothrix rhusiopathiae* infection acquired?

5. What are the clinical manifestations caused by *E. rhusiopathiae?*

6. What are the biochemical features of *E. rhusiopathiae?*

7. In what special patient population is *Rhodococcus equi* particularly significant.

8. What is the clinical significance of *Corynebacterium* sp. other than *C. diphtheriae?*

CHAPTER 13

Aerobic Gram-Positive Bacilli

Hal S. Larsen

BACILLUS
  General Characteristics
  Bacillus anthracis
    Physiology
    Virulence factors
    Clinical infections
    Complications and treatment
    Laboratory diagnosis
  Other *Bacillus* Species
    Bacillus cereus
    Bacillus subtilis

AEROBIC ACTINOMYCETES
  Nocardia Species
    General characteristics
    Physiology
    Virulence factors
    Clinical infections
    Laboratory diagnosis
  Other Actinomycetes
    Actinomadura species
    Streptomyces species

KEY TERMS

Edema factor
Lethal factor
Protective antigen
Anthrax
Woolsorter's disease
Cutaneous anthrax
Black eschar
Pulmonary anthrax
Gastrointestinal anthrax
Bamboo rods
Medusa head
String of pearls
Bacillus cereus food poisoning
Mycetoma
Sulfur granules
Eumycotic mycetoma
Actinomycotic mycetoma
Paraffin bait technique
Aerobic actinomycetes

CASE STUDY

A cattle rancher in the Southwestern part of the United States sought medical treatment after suffering for several days with malaise, myalgia, headache, and nausea. He showed his physician several partially healed sores on his arms that he noticed 2 weeks before. Blood was drawn for culture and one of three blood culture bottles showed growth after 24 hours. Gram stain showed a large, gram-positive rod. No growth appeared on MacConkey agar. The colonies on sheep blood agar were β-hemolytic, frosted-glass appearing, and motile.

This chapter discusses a large group of bacteria that are commonly encountered in the microbiology laboratory. Most are found in the environment and can be easily isolated from water and soil. The majority are not highly pathogenic but are being isolated from clinical infections with increasing frequency. Bacteria that belong to the gram-positive aerobic bacilli include the spore-forming *Bacillus* species and the filamentous *Nocardia* species, *Actinomadura* species, and *Streptomyces* species. Figure 13-1 shows a schematic diagram for the presumptive identification of aerobic gram-positive bacteria, including spore-formers, non–spore-formers, and gram-positive cocci.

BACILLUS

General Characteristics

Members of the genus *Bacillus* are aerobic, gram-positive, rod-shaped organisms that form endospores (Figure 13-2). On Gram stain, however, spores do not stain and appear only as "empty spaces." Spore stain is used to demonstrate the presence of spores (Figure 13-3). More than 50 species of *Bacillus* are widely found in the environment. Members of the genus can be isolated from soil from all climates—the subarctic and desert regions, ther-

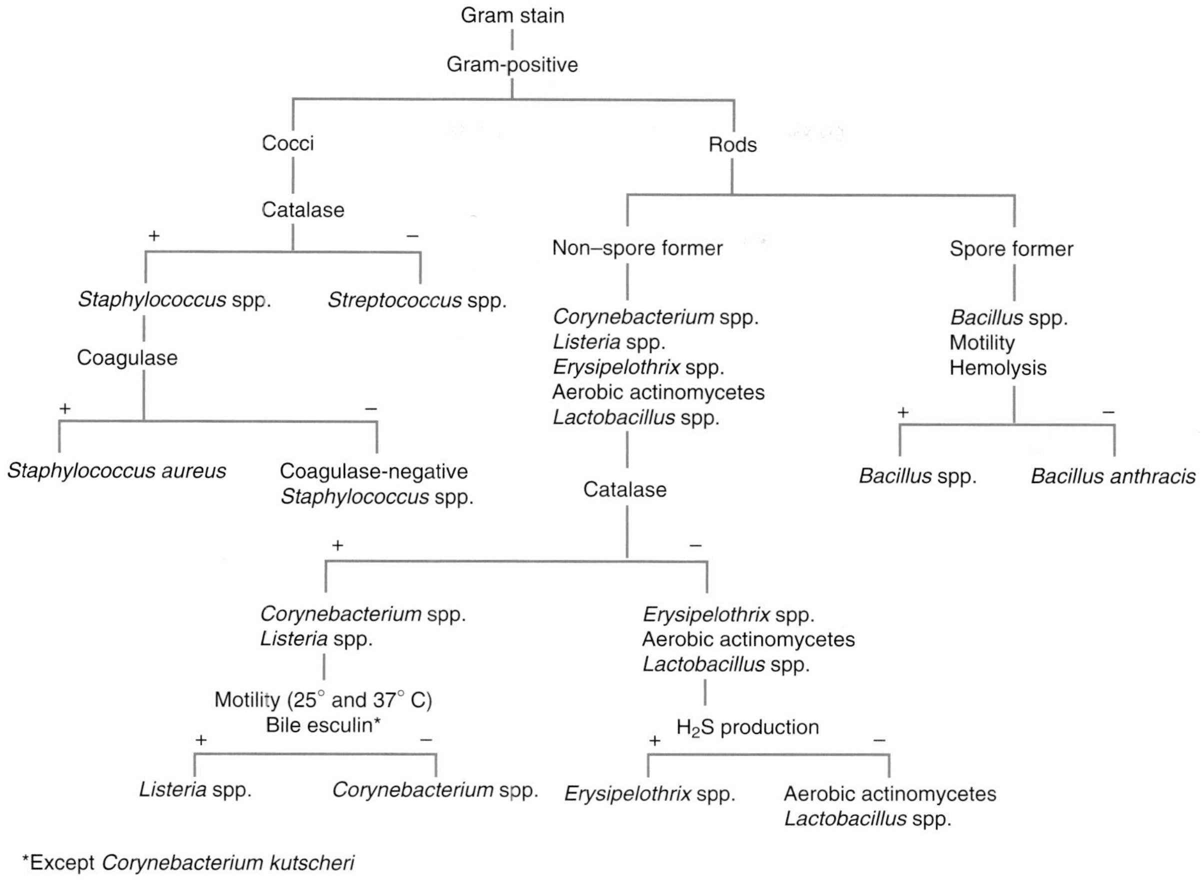

Gram stain
|
Gram-positive

Cocci　　　　　　　　　　　　　　　　　Rods

Catalase

＋　　　　　　　　　－　　　　　　　Non–spore former　　　　　　Spore former

Staphylococcus spp.　　*Streptococcus* spp.　　*Corynebacterium* spp.　　　*Bacillus* spp.
　　　　　　　　　　　　　　　　　　　Listeria spp.　　　　　　　　Motility
Coagulase　　　　　　　　　　　　　　*Erysipelothrix* spp.　　　　　Hemolysis
　　　　　　　　　　　　　　　　　　　Aerobic actinomycetes
＋　　　　　　　　－　　　　　　　　*Lactobacillus* spp.　　　　　　　＋　　　　　　　　－

Staphylococcus aureus　　Coagulase-negative　　　　　　　　　　　　*Bacillus* spp.　　*Bacillus anthracis*
　　　　　　　　　Staphylococcus spp.　　　　　Catalase

　　　　　　　　　　＋　　　　　　　　　　　　　　　　－

Corynebacterium spp.　　　　　　　*Erysipelothrix* spp.
Listeria spp.　　　　　　　　　　　Aerobic actinomycetes
　　　　　　　　　　　　　　　　　　Lactobacillus spp.

Motility (25° and 37° C)
Bile esculin*　　　　　　　　　H₂S production
＋　　　　　　　　－　　　　＋　　　　　　　－

Listeria spp.　　*Corynebacterium* spp.　　*Erysipelothrix* spp.　　Aerobic actinomycetes
　　　　　　　　　　　　　　　　　　　　　　　　　　　　　Lactobacillus spp.

*Except *Corynebacterium kutscheri*

Figure 13-1 _____

Schematic diagram for the identification of gram-positive bacteria.

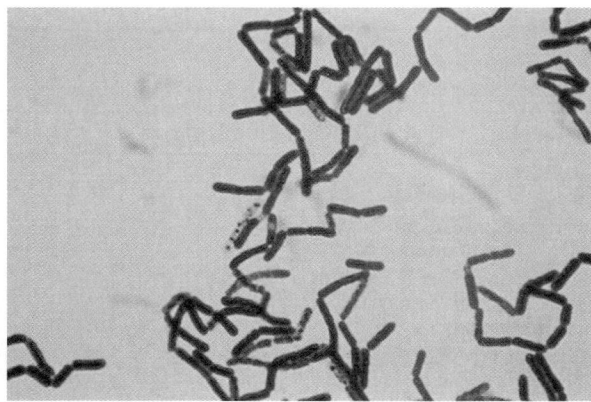

Figure 13-2 _____

Gram stain of *Bacillus* sp. (Courtesy Cathy Bissonette.)

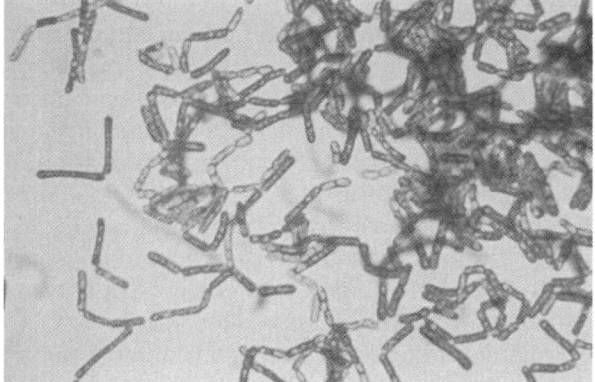

Figure 13-3 _____

Spore stain of *Bacillus* sp. (Courtesy Cathy Bissonette.)

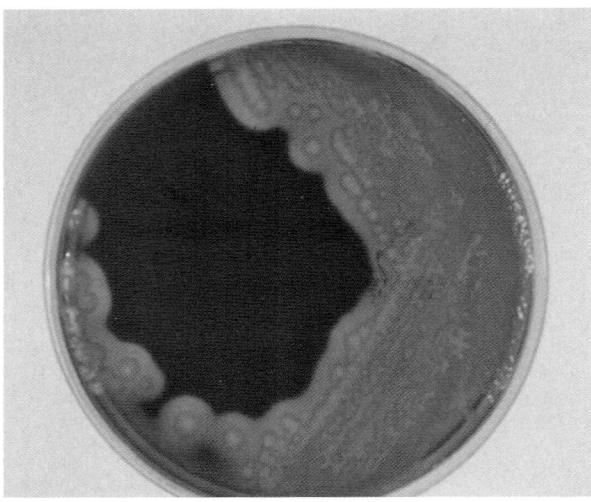

Figure 13-4

Bacillus cereus colony on blood agar. (Courtesy Cathy Bissonette.)

mal springs, fresh and salt water, and plant materials. The temperature range for growth depends on the species but includes temperatures as low as $-5°$ C and as high as $75°$ C. The survival of *Bacillus* sp. in nature is because of the formation of the endospores, which are resistant to conditions to which vegetative cells are intolerant.

Most species grow well on blood agar and other common enriched media. As a result, *Bacillus* sp. are found as contaminants in specimens from a number of sources. The different species show a wide variety of metabolic characteristics. They are catalase positive and form endospores under aerobic conditions. They can be divided into three morphologic groups on the basis of the location and size of the endospore. In group 1, the spores are oval or cylindrical and are located centrally or terminally. The key characteristic placing a species in group I is the spore. Regardless of location, it does not distend the vegetative cell. Organisms belonging to group II have oval spores that are central or terminal and cause the vegetative cell to swell. Morphologic group III consists of species showing round, terminal, swollen spore.

Colony characteristics vary considerably among the species and are often influenced by the type of medium used. Pigment formation is seen in a number of species. Pigment colors range from pink to blue-black and may vary according to growth conditions and substrates. Most species, however, are

unpigmented. Historically, *Bacillus anthracis,* the causative agent of anthrax, has been the most important member of this genus; however, anthrax is now rarely seen in the United States. Other species, most notably *Bacillus cereus* (Figure 13-4), are seen in the clinical laboratory as pathogens and contaminants. Several species are pathogenic for insects.

Bacillus anthracis
Physiology
B. anthracis is a gram-positive or gram-variable rod. It is catalase positive and aerobic or facultative. Spore formation takes place aerobically; this feature, along with a positive catalase test, differentiates *Bacillus* sp. from clostridia. It is nonmotile, distinguishing it from other members of the genus *Bacillus.* Although *B. anthracis* ferments glucose, it fails to ferment mannitol, arabinose, and zylose. It produces lecithinase, therefore, an opaque zone can be seen around colonies growing on egg-yolk agar. This species grows in high salt (7% NaCl) and low pH (<6). Unlike *B. cereus, B. anthracis* is susceptible to penicillin (10 U/mL). It is nonhemolytic on sheep's blood agar. Characteristics especially important to differentiate *B. anthracis* from the closely related *B. cereus* are found in Table 13-1.

Virulence factors
The virulence of *B. anthracis* depends on a glutamic acid capsule and a complex toxin. The capsule, which protects the organism from phagocytosis, is a polypeptide of D-glutamic acid. This

TABLE 13-1

Differentiation of Bacillus anthracis *and* Bacillus cereus

Characteristic	B. anthracis	B. cereus
Hemolysis on sheep blood agar	−	+
Motility	−	+
Lecithinase production	+	+
Fermentation of salicin	−	+/−
Growth in penicillin (10 U/mL) agar	−	+
String of pearls reaction	+	−
Gelatin hydrolysis	−	+
Growth on phenylethyl alcohol agar (PEA)	−	+
Pathogenicity for mice by injection	+	−

Modified with permission from Braude AI, Davis CE, Fierer J, editors: *Infectious diseases and medical microbiology,* Philadelphia, 1986, WB Saunders.
All cultures incubated at 36° to 37° C.

particular isomer of glutamic acid is resistant to hydrolysis by host proteolytic enzymes because it is the "unnatural" form. Although the capsule is necessary for virulence, antibodies against the capsule do not confer immunity.

The anthrax toxin consists of three factors:

- **Edema factor** (EF)
- Protective antigen (PA)
- **Lethal factor** (LF)

The effect of edema factor and lethal factor is seen when either is combined with protective antigen. Edema results from the combination of **protective antigen** with edema factor, whereas death occurs when protective antigen and lethal factor combine. The toxin increases vascular permeability and interferes with phagocytosis. The genes for the synthesis of the toxin are located on a plasmid. If a virulent isolate is repeatedly cultured in vitro, the plasmid is eventually lost, and the organism is no longer virulent.

Clinical infections

Anthrax is a common disease in livestock worldwide. The disease is not spread from animal to animal, but rather from animals feeding on plants contaminated with the spores. Humans are infected primarily as a result of contact with the animals or animal products. The incidence of human anthrax in the United States is very low; less than 5 cases per year are reported. Worldwide, however, cases number several thousand. The disease is enzootic in many parts of the world, including Central and South America. A number of names have been given to infections with *B. anthracis*. The majority refer to occupational associations. Terms such as **"woolsorter's disease"** and "ragpicker's disease" were used to describe infection with the spores of *B. anthracis* as a result of handling contaminated animal fibers, hides, and other animal products.

In humans, three forms of anthrax include the following:

- Cutaneous
- Inhalation or pulmonary
- Gastrointestinal

All three forms of infection result from wound contamination, inhalation, or ingestion of spores, which germinate within the host tissue.

CUTANEOUS ANTHRAX

Wounds contaminated with anthrax spores acquired through skin cuts, abrasions, or insect bites may become **cutaneous anthrax.** The overwhelming majority of anthrax cases in the world are cutaneous. In this form of anthrax, a small pimple or papule appears at the site of inoculation 2 to 3 days after exposure. A ring of vesicles develops; the vesicles coalesce to form an erythematous ring. A small dark area appears in the center of the ring and eventually ulcerates and dries, forming a depressed black necrotic central area known as an *eschar* (**"black eschar,"** "malignant pustule"). The lesion is painless and does not produce pus unless it becomes secondarily infected with a pyogenic organism. The eschar is normally 1 to 3 cm in diameter, although it may be more extensive. The eschar begins to heal after 1 to 2 weeks. The lesion dries, separates from the underlying base, and falls off, leaving a scar. Usually the infection remains localized, but regional lymphangitis and lymphadenopathy appear. If septicemia occurs, symptoms of fever, malaise, and headache are seen. Normally, in uncomplicated cases, no systemic symptoms are present.

INHALATION OR PULMONARY ANTHRAX

Pulmonary anthrax, or "woolsorter's disease" as it is sometimes known, is acquired when spores are inhaled into the pulmonary parenchyma. The infection begins as a nonspecific illness consisting of mild fever, fatigue, and malaise 2 to 5 days after exposure to the spores. It resembles an upper respiratory tract infection such as that seen with colds and "flu." This initial, mild form of the disease lasts 2 to 3 days. It is followed by a sudden severe phase in which respiratory distress is common. The severe phase of the disease is extremely serious. The respiratory problems (dyspnea, cyanosis, pleural effusion) are followed by disorientation, then coma, and death. The course of the severe phase (onset of respiratory symptoms to death) may last for only 24 hours.

GASTROINTESTINAL ANTHRAX

Gastrointestinal anthrax occurs when the spores are inoculated into a lesion on the intestinal mucosa following ingestion of the spores. The symptoms of gastrointestinal anthrax include abdominal pain, nausea, anorexia, and vomiting. Bloody diarrhea may also occur. Because this form of the disease is difficult to diagnose, the fatality rate is higher than in the cutaneous form. Fortunately, gastrointestinal anthrax accounts for less than 1% of the total cases worldwide; it has never been reported in the United States.

Complications and treatment

Approximately 5% of patients with anthrax (cutaneous, pulmonary, gastrointestinal) develop meningitis. The symptoms are typical of any bacterial meningitis and occur very rapidly. Unconsciousness and death, if they occur, follow 1 to 6 days after initial exposure.

Recovery from infection appears to confer immunity. An effective vaccine is available for those who are at risk for occupational exposure. In addition, vaccines are available for veterinary use.

Most isolates of *B. anthracis* are sensitive to penicillin, which is the drug of choice for treatment of anthrax. The organism is also sensitive to many of the broad-spectrum antibiotics, including gentamicin, erythromycin, tetracycline, and chloramphenicol.

Laboratory diagnosis

MICROSCOPY

B. anthracis is a large, square-ended, gram-positive rod found singly or in chains. The spores are seen as unstained spots within the cells. When they are in chains, the ends of the single cells fit snugly together. This, together with the unstained central spore, gives the appearance of **bamboo rods.** Only young cultures are gram-positive. As the cells become older, or if they are under nutritional stress, they become gram-variable.

CULTURAL CHARACTERISTICS

On blood agar, colonies of *B. anthracis* are nonhemolytic, large (3 to 5 mm), gray, and flat with an irregular margin because of outgrowths of long filamentous projections of bacteria that can be seen with a dissecting microscope. The term ***Medusa head*** has been used to describe the colony of *B. anthracis.* Colonies hold tightly to the agar surface and when the edges are lifted with a loop, they stand upright without support. This has been described as having the appearance or characteristics of beaten egg whites.

IDENTIFICATION

Caution should always be used in working with an isolate suspected of being *B. anthracis.* Work should be done in a bacteriologic biologic safety hood, and the area should be disinfected when the work is completed.

An isolate with the appropriate colonial and microscopic morphology may be suspected of being *B. anthracis* if it (1) is nonhemolytic on blood agar, (2) is nonmotile, and (3) produces lecithinase. A presumptive identification can be made by inoculating the suspected isolate onto agar containing penicillin (0.05 to 0.5 U/mL). After incubation for 3 to 6 hours at 37° C, the areas of inoculation are examined microscopically for the presence of large spherical bacilli in chains; this phenomenon is referred to as a ***string of pearls.*** The isolate should be forwarded to the state health laboratory for confirmatory identification. Species identification of bacilli can be accomplished by the use of the API 20E and 50CH systems (bioMerieux Vitek, Hazelwood, Mo.).

Other *Bacillus* Species

Bacillus cereus

B. cereus is a relatively common cause of food poisoning and opportunistic infections in the susceptible host. Food poisoning because of *B. cereus* takes two forms: diarrheal and emetic.

The diarrheal syndrome, usually associated with ingestion of meat or poultry, is characterized by an incubation period of 8 to 16 hours. Afflicted individuals suffer abdominal pain and diarrhea. About 25% of individuals experience vomiting. Fever is uncommon. The average duration of the illness is 24 hours. The diarrheal form is clinically indistinguishable from the diarrhea caused by *Clostridium perfringens*.

The emetic form has the predominant symptoms of abdominal cramps and vomiting. Diarrhea is present in about one third of those affected. This form has been associated with ingestion of fried rice, particularly when prepared in Oriental restaurants. The average duration of the illness is 9 hours. For both the diarrheal and emetic forms of ***Bacillus cereus* food poisoning,** the illness is usually mild and self-limiting. The two forms of illness are caused by two distinct enterotoxins produced by *B. cereus.* A comparison of the enterotoxins is shown in Table 13-2.

TABLE 13-2

Comparison of Enterotoxins Produced by Bacillus cereus

Characteristic	Type of Enterotoxin	
	Diarrheal	Emetic
Clinical syndrome		
Incubation period	8 to 16 hr	1 to 5 hr
Diarrhea	Very common	Fairly common
Vomiting	Occasional	Very common
Duration of illness	12 to 24 hr	6 to 24 hr
Foods implicated	Meat products, soups, vegetables, puddings, sauces	Fried or boiled rice
Enterotoxin		
Molecular weight	ca. 50,000	<5,000
Stability to heat	−	+
Fluid accumulation in ligated rabbit ileal segment	+	−
Increased vascular permeability in guinea pig or rabbit skin	+	−
Lethal for mice after intravenous injection	+	−
Stimulation of adenylate cyclase–cAMP system in intestinal epithelial cells	+	−
Response when fed to rhesus monkeys	Diarrhea	Vomiting

Modified from Braude AI, Davis CE, Fierer J, editors: *Infectious diseases and medical microbiology,* Philadelphia, 1986, WB Saunders.

B. cereus is similar to *B. anthracis* in many ways, morphologically and metabolically. Differentiation between *B. cereus* and *B. anthracis* is outlined in Table 13-1. The organism can be grown aerobically at 37° C on blood agar. A β-hemolytic frosted–glass-appearing colony that is aerobic, spore forming, gram-positive, and motile, ferments salicin, and is lecithinase positive is likely *B. cereus.* It also differs from *B. anthracis* in being resistant to penicillin and nonpathogenic for mice.

Culture of the suspected food may be done to quantitate and isolate *B. cereus.* If more than 10^5 *B. cereus* per gram of food are present and other pathogens are absent, then food poisoning by this organism is confirmed. The stool of patients with food poisoning may also be examined for *B. cereus,* although the organism is part of the normal fecal flora. To confirm the organism as the cause of the disease, the viable counts from the stool should also be at least 10^5 per gram. Quantitative cultures must be done because *B. cereus* may be found in small numbers in a significant proportion of healthy people.

Opportunistic infections caused by *B. cereus,* particularly of the eye, are becoming more common. *Bacillus* species are contaminants of illicit drug paraphernalia and have been documented as causes of meningitis, septicemia, osteomyelitis, and a number of other types of infections.

Unlike *B. anthracis, B. cereus* is resistant to penicillin and many of the other cell-wall antibiotics (e.g., ampicillin, cephalothin, methicillin). Treatment with a clindamycin and gentamicin combination has been successful.

Bacillus subtilis

Infections by other members of the genus are rare. They occasionally cause gastrointestinal illness. They are seen, however, as contaminants. One of the more commonly seen species is *Bacillus subtilis.* The colonies of *B. subtilis* are large and may be pigmented. Pigment colors range from pink and yellow to orange or brown. Identification can be made using the API 20E and 50CH systems.

AEROBIC ACTINOMYCETES

Nocardia and *Actinomyces* organisms are similar morphologically to fungi. These organisms demonstrate filamentous hyphae in culture that are similar microscopically to those seen with fungi. On close inspection, however, differences are observed. These genera are true bacteria and can be differentiated from fungi and from each other. Although they are not commonly seen in most laboratories, they are responsible for significant human diseases.

Nocardia Species

General characteristics

The organisms in this genus are aerobic, gram-positive bacilli that often form branched hyphae. The hyphae are easily disrupted into rods and cocci. Even though *Nocardia* species is, strictly speaking, gram-positive, organisms will often stain gram variable and may be weakly acid fast. The colonial and microscopic morphology, and the types of infections caused, resemble those of the fungi, but these organisms are true bacteria. *Nocardia* species grow well on standard nonselective media. Growth may take a week or more. The organisms in this genus are commonly found in soil. Generally, infections caused by *Nocardia* organisms are seen in immunocompromised patients. Reports of infection in patients with no apparent illness or immunosuppressive therapy are increasing, however. The species of medical importance are *Nocardia asteroides, Nocardia brasiliensis,* and *Nocardia caviae.* Of

the total aerobic actinomycetes received by the Centers For Disease Control and Prevention (CDC) from October 1985 through February 1988, 27% were *N. asteroides* and 6% were *N. brasiliensis* (McNeil et al, 1990). The majority of isolates received for identification were from sputum and wounds.

Physiology

The growth requirements of *Nocardia* organisms are not as well defined as those of many other medically important bacteria. These organisms show an oxidative-type metabolism and as a genus, they use a wide variety of sugars. They do not require specific growth factors as do *Haemophilus* and *Francisella* organisms. *Nocardia* species grow well on most common nonselective laboratory media at temperatures between 25° and 37° C, although 3 to 6 days or longer may pass before growth occurs. Some characteristics of the aerobic actinomycetes are listed in Table 13-3.

Virulence factors

The role of such factors as toxins and extracellular proteins in nocardiosis is unclear. No virulence factors have been identified, although virulence

TABLE 13-3

Characteristics of Selected Aerobic Actinomycetes of Medical Importance

Characteristic	Nocardia asteroides	Nocardia caviae	Nocardia brasiliensis	Actinomadura madurae	Streptomyces griseus
Aerial hyphae	+	+	+	V	+
Acid fastness	V	V	V	−	−
Rifampin resistance	+	+	+	V	V
Hydrolysis of					
Esculin	+	+	+	+	V
Casein	−	−	+	+	+
Hippurate	V	V	−	−	−
Xanthine	−	+	−	−	V
Starch	V	V	V	+	+
Tyrosine	−	V	+	+	+
Acid from					
Arabinose	−	V	−	+	V
Cellobiose	−	−	−	+	+
Glucose	+	+	+	+	+
Inositol	−	+	+	V	V
Mannitol	−	V	+	+	+
Xylose	−	−	−	+	+
Growth at 10° C	−	V	V	−	+

+, 90% or more of the strains tested were positive.
−, 90% or more of the strains tested were negative.
V, Variable.
Modified from Mishra SK, Gordon RE, Barnett DA: Identification of nocardiae and streptomycetes of medical importance, *J Clin Microbiol* 11:730, 1980.

has been correlated with alterations in the components in the cell envelope. The precise role of the various cell-wall molecules in virulence is unknown. *Nocardia* organisms produce a superoxide dismutase and catalase that may give it resistance to oxidative killing by phagocytes. It also produces an iron-chelating compound called *nocobactin*. A correlation has been reported between the amount of nocobactin produced by the organism and its virulence.

Clinical infections

Nocardia species are found worldwide in soil and on plant material. Infection occurs by two routes: pulmonary and cutaneous. Pulmonary infection by *Nocardia* organisms occurs from the inhalation of the organism, which is present in dust or soil. The disease appears to be associated with impaired host defenses, because most persons seen with nocardiosis have an underlying disease or compromised immune defenses. Even so, a significant number of seemingly normal patients show an infection with *Nocardia* organisms and no obvious immune impairment.

Infection with *Nocardia* organisms is serious. Approximately 40% of the diagnoses are made at autopsy. The mortality rate is high, and those who survive often suffer significant tissue damage.

PULMONARY FORM

The majority of the pulmonary form are caused by *N. asteroides*. The most common manifestation of infection is a confluent bronchopneumonia that is usually chronic but may be acute or relapsing. The disease generally progresses more rapidly than tuberculosis but is measured in months rather than years. In the acute form, which is often seen in patients with underlying immune defects, the time course is a matter of weeks.

The initial lesion in the lung is a focus of pneumonitis that advances to necrosis. The abscesses that form may extend into the tissue and coalesce with each other. Extensive tissue involvement and damage result. Unlike some pneumonias, little inflammatory response or scarring, no encapsulation of the abscesses, and no granuloma formation occurs. Dissemination to other organs, especially the brain, may occur, with reports in the literature of involvement of virtually every organ. The sputum is thick, sticky, and purulent. Unlike

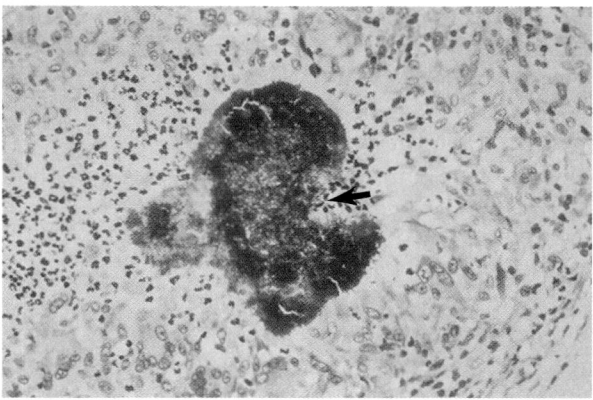

Figure 13-5

Gross appearance of sulfur granules collected from draining sinus tracts. These granules contain masses of filamentous organisms with pus materials.

with infection by the anaerobic actinomycetes, no sulfur granules or sinus tract formation exist.

CUTANEOUS FORM

The second route of infection is cutaneous, or inoculation of the organism into the skin or subcutaneous tissues. *N. brasiliensis* is the most frequent cause of this form of nocardiosis, which is usually seen in the hands and feet as a result of outdoor activity. The trauma most likely is minor, such as from a thorn or wood sliver.

The infection begins as a localized subcutaneous abscess that is invasive and quite destructive of the tissues and underlying bone. These lesions are termed **mycetomas** (certain species of fungi also form mycetomas). Mycetomas are characterized by swelling, draining sinuses, and granules. About half of the mycetomas seen clinically are caused by the actinomycetes, and the remaining half are caused by fungi. As the infection progresses, burrowing sinuses open to the skin surface and drain pus. The pus may be pigmented and contain **sulfur granules** (Figure 13-5), which are masses of filamentous organisms bound together by calcium phosphate. They often appear yellow or orange and have a distinct granular appearance.

Treatment of *Nocardia* infection often involves drainage and surgery and antimicrobials. The organisms are resistant to penicillin but susceptible to sulfonamides. Antifungal agents, of course, have no activity against *Nocardia* organisms; this fact underscores the importance of laboratory diagnosis, because many of the clinical manifestations of pulmonary and cutaneous infection are shared with other organisms, including fungi. This organism represents a classic example of a situation in which laboratory results are absolutely essential to proper antimicrobial treatment.

Laboratory diagnosis

MICROSCOPY

The gram-positive branching filaments characteristic of *Nocardia* organisms are often seen in sputum and exudates or aspirates from skin or abscesses. The specimen often contains coccobacillary bodies as well. The Gram reaction may be weak or irregular, causing a "beading" appearance similar to the appearance of chains of gram-positive cocci. This morphology may easily confuse the microscopist. If the isolate is also acid fast, the possibility of its being a *Norcardia* organism is high.

Wet mounts should also be performed. Granules may be seen in specimens from cutaneous infection. Sampled tissue and pus from the draining sinuses are the specimens of choice for direct examination. The granules may be visualized by separating them from the pus with an inoculating needle and then washing in sterile saline. The granules of *N. asteroides, N. brasiliensis,* and *N. caviae* are soft, white-to-cream colored, and 0.5 to 1 mm in size. They may be crushed between two glass slides to visualize the branching and cellular morphology, comprised of gram-positive, interwoven, thin (0.5 to 1.0 mm in diameter) filaments. The granules may also be used to inoculate the appropriate growth media. The granules of a fungal mycetoma **(eumycotic mycetoma)** are composed of broad, interwoven, septate hyphae that are wider (2 to 5 mm) than those of the actinomycetes **(actinomycotic mycetoma).**

CULTURAL CHARACTERISTICS

Colonies of *Nocardia* organisms may have a chalky, matte, or velvety appearance and may be pigmented.

TABLE 13-4

Colonial and Microscopic Appearance of Aerobic Actinomycetes*

Genus and Species	Macroscopic Appearance†	Microscopic Appearance‡
Actinomadura species		Fine, intertwining, branched filaments with delicate aerial hyphae; nonfragmenting and may form short chains of spores
Actinomadura madurae	Waxy, heaped, folded, membranous, and tough; white, tan, pale orange, pink, or red	
Actinomadura pelletieri	Heaped, irregular, waxy, and granular; areas of bright and dark red; sparse aerial hyphae	
Mycobacterium species		Do not show aerial filaments
Nocardia species (*Nocardia asteroides, Nocardia brasiliensis, Nocardia caviae*)	Orange colonies, glabrous, heaped, and folded; may also be white to pink with aerial hyphae; dry, crumbly, and adherent	Fine, intertwining, branched filaments with delicate aerial hyphae; may have hyphal fragmentation to produce spores from aerial hyphae
Nocardiopsis dassonvillei	Orange colonies, glabrous, heaped, and folded; may also be white to pink with aerial hyphae; dry, crumbly, and adherent	
Rhodococcus species		Do not show aerial filaments
Streptomyces somaliensis	Leathery, heaped, and folded; wide range of pigmentation from cream to brown-black; white aerial hyphae	Fine, intertwining, branched filaments with delicate aerial hyphae; nonfragmenting and often form chains of spores

From Howard BJ et al, editors: *Clinical and pathogenic microbiology,* St Louis, 1987, Mosby.
*On Sabouraud dextrose agar at 25° C.
†A dissecting microscope is best for macroscopic observation.
‡Slide cultures must be set up if the original culture shows no aerial hyphae.

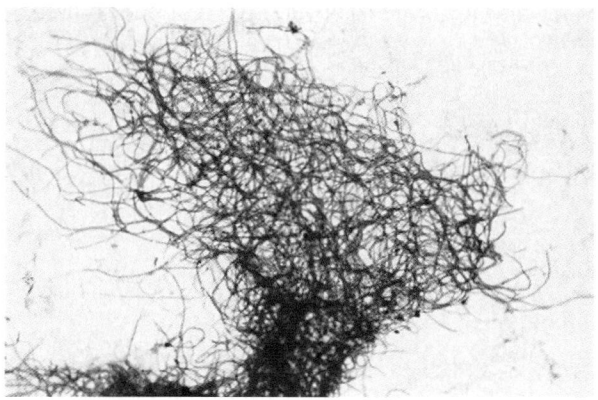

Figure 13-6

Acid-fast stain of *Nocardia* species, showing partially acid-fast appearance.

They have a dry, crumbly appearance that is likened to that of bread crumbs. Table 13-4 outlines the colonial appearance of the aerobic actinomycetes.

IDENTIFICATION

Nocardia organisms grows well on standard non-selective laboratory media, including those used for fungal cultures. Media containing antibiotics used for isolating fungi should not be used, however, because *Nocardia* organisms are sensitive to many of the antimicrobial agents used in these media. The possibility of isolating *Nocardia* organisms is increased by the **paraffin bait technique,** which takes advantage of the fact that *Nocardia* organisms use paraffin as an energy source and other aerobic bacteria do not.

An isolate showing branching filaments that are gram-positive and partially acid fast should be suspected of belonging to the *Nocardia* species (Figure 13-6). Tentative identification of the aerobic actinomycetes is outlined in Table 13-3. Confirmation is normally performed by a reference laboratory experienced in identification of the actinomycetes.

Other Actinomycetes

Actinomadura species

The **aerobic actinomycetes** of clinical importance belonging to *Actinomadura* species include *Actinomadura madurae, Actinomadura pelletieri.* They were formerly classified as members of the *Nocardia* species. They are etiologic agents of mycetomas, which is identical to that caused by *No-cardia.* The colonial appearance is outlined in Table 13-4.

The microscopic and colonial morphology of *Actinomadura* species is very similar to that of *Nocardia* species, and it would be difficult, if not impossible, for an inexperienced technologist to detect a difference. Differentiation can be made using metabolic variations, as shown in Table 13-3. *A. madurae* is cellobiose and xylose positive, whereas the *Nocardia* organisms do not produce acid from these two carbohydrates. Treatment parallels that for infections with *Nocardia* organisms.

Streptomyces species

Streptomyces species comprises approximately 23 species. According to Mishra and colleagues (1980), *Streptomyces griseus* is the third most common aerobic actinomycete, after *N. asteroides* and *N. brasiliensis. Streptomyces* species are also soil microorganisms and resemble the other aerobic actinomycetes, previously discussed, with regard to morphology and the diseases they cause. Tables 13-3 and 13-4 compare the colonial morphology and metabolic characteristics of *Streptomyces* organisms with those of other members of the aerobic actinomycetes. Isolates from this genus may also need to be identified by reference laboratories.

Bibliography

Beaman BL: *Nocardia:* pathogenesis and host resistance. In Ortiz-Ortiz L, Bojalil LF, Yakoleff V, editors: *Biological, biochemical, and biomedical aspects of actinomycetes,* London, 1984, Academic Press.

Bowden GH, Goodfellow M: The actinomycetes: *Actinomyces, Nocardia* and related genera. In Parker MT, Duerden BI, editors: *Topley & Wilson's principles of bacteriology, virology and immunity,* vol 2, *Systematic bacteriology,* ed 8, Philadelphia, 1990, BC Decker.

Braude AI, Davis CE, Fierer J, editors: *Infectious diseases and medical microbiology,* Philadelphia, 1986, WB Saunders.

Knudson GB: Treatment of anthrax in man: history and current concepts, *Mil Med* 151:71, 1986.

Land G, McGinnis MR et al: Aerobic pathogenic *Actinomycetales.* In Balows A, Hausler WJ, Jr et al, editors: *Manual of clinical microbiology,* ed 5, Washington, DC, 1991, American Society for Microbiology.

McNeil MM, Brown JM et al: Comparison of species distribution and antimicrobial susceptibility of aerobic actinomycetes from clinical specimens, *Rev Infect Dis* 12:778, 1990.

Mishra SK, Gordon RE, Barnett, DA: Identification of nocardiae and streptomycetes of medical importance, *J Clin Microbiol* 11:728, 1980.

Shawar RM, More DG, LaRocco MT: Cultivation of *Nocardia* spp. on chemically defined media for selective recovery of isolates from clinical specimens, *J Clin Microbiol* 28:508, 1990.

Turnbull P: Anthrax. In Parker MT, Duerden BI, editors: *Topley & Wilson's principles of bacteriology, virology and immunity*, vol 3, *Bacterial diseases,* ed 8, Philadelphia, 1990, BC Decker.

Turnbull P, Kramer J, Melling J: *Bacillus.* In Parker MT, Duerden BI, editors: *Topley & Wilson's principles of bacteriology, virology and immunity,* vol 2, *Systematic bacteriology,* ed 8, Philadelphia, 1990, BC Decker.

Turnbull PCB, Kramer JM: *Bacillus.* In Balows A et al editors: *Manual of clinical microbiology,* ed 5, Washington, DC, 1991, American Society for Microbiology.

Williams RP: *Bacillus anthracis* and other aerobic spore-forming bacilli. In Braude AI, Davis CE, Fierer J, editors: *Infectious diseases and medical microbiology,* ed 2, Philadelphia, 1986, WB Saunders.

LEARNING ASSESSMENT

1. Based on the clinical symptoms presented in the case study, what organism or organisms could have caused the patient's infection?

2. What is the most likely presumptive identity of the blood culture isolate?

3. What characteristics eliminate the suspicion of a virulent pathogen?

4. What precautions should be taken in the clinical setting if this organism is suspected?

5. What is the most likely source of the isolate?

6. What causes mycetoma?

7. How are the etiologic agents of mycetoma differentiated?

8. How are *Nocardia* species differentiated from other aerobic actinomycetes?

CHAPTER 14

Neisseria Species and Moraxella Catarrhalis

Karen S. Long, John G. Thomas, Jean Barnishan

GENERAL CHARACTERISTICS

PATHOGENIC *NEISSERIA* SPECIES
Neisseria gonorrhoeae
    Virulence factors
    Epidemiology
    Clinical infections
    Laboratory diagnosis
    Presumptive identification
    Antimicrobial resistance
    Treatment
Neisseria meningitidis
    Virulence factors
    Clinical infections
    Treatment
    Vaccine
    Laboratory diagnosis

Moraxella catarrhalis
    Clinical infections
    Laboratory diagnosis

NONPATHOGENIC *NEISSERIA* SPECIES
    Identification
    Neisseria polysaccharea
    Neisseria cinerea
    Kingella denitrificans
    Neisseria lactamica
    Neisseria mucosa
    Neisseria sicca
    Neisseria subflava
    Neisseria flavescens
    Neisseria elongata
    Neisseria weaveri

OBJECTIVES

1. List some general characteristics of the *Neisseria* genus.
2. Discuss the function of pili as virulence factors.
3. Define *AHU strains* of *Neisseria gonorrhoeae* and discuss their role in gonococcal infections.
4. Discuss potential complications of asymptomatic gonococcal infections in women.
5. Define *ophthalmia neonatorum*.
6. List some risk groups for epidemic meningococcal meningitis.
7. Discuss clinical findings in meningococcemia.
8. Discuss the importance and need for correct collection and transportation of specimens for *Neisseria gonorrhoeae*.
9. Compare and contrast the usefulness of the direct Gram stain in the diagnosis of gonorrhea in men and women.
10. List two selective media for *Neisseria gonorrhoeae* and *Neisseria meningitidis*.
11. State the reference method for carbohydrate utilization in the *Neisseria* species.
12. Discuss some drawbacks of nonculture detection methods for *Neisseria gonorrhoeae*.
13. Indicate the reason for β-lactamase testing of all *Neisseria gonorrhoeae* isolates.
14. Disucss the pathogenic significance of *Moraxella catarrhalis*.
15. Differentiate the "pathogenic" and "nonpathogenic" *Neisseria* species.

KEY TERMS

Gonorrhea
Asymptomatic
  gonococcal infection
AHU strains
Pelvic inflammatory
  disease (PID)
Fitz-Hugh–Curtis
  syndrome
Ophthalmia
  neonatorum

JEMBEC
Plasmid-mediated
  penicillinase-
  producing *Neisseria
  gonorrhoeae* (PPNG)
Waterhouse-
  Friderichsen
  syndrome

CASE STUDY

A 20-year-old sexually active woman in college was admitted to the emergency room with complaints of low-grade fever and pain, redness, and swelling of multiple joints. Aspirates from both ankles and an elbow were sent to the laboratory for culture and Gram stain. Direct smear preparations showed "many PMNs and several intracellular and extracellular gram-negative diplococci." However, cultures on blood agar, chocolate agar, MacConkey agar, and Thayer Martin failed to produce any growth after several days of incubation. The culture was reported as "No growth in 5 days." Further history revealed that the patient had been recently treated at a local community hospital for culture-confirmed bacterial meningitis.

The family Neisseriaceae currently contains the true *Neisseria* species, *Kingella kingae,* and *Kingella denitrificans;* the *Eikenella, Simonsiella,* and *Alysiella* species; and Centers for Disease Control and Prevention groups EF 4-a and EF 4-b. These organisms, along with *Acinetobacter* and *Moraxella* species, belong to the class *Proteobacteria.* The taxonomic status of *Moraxella catarrhalis* remains unresolved.

Characteristics of the family and differential characteristics of these genera are shown in Figure 14-1. At present, the genus *Neisseria* contains 12 species and biovars that can be isolated from hu-

mans; the genus *Moraxella* subgenus *Branhamella* contains one such species.

This chapter discusses only the morphologically and biochemically similar species of *Neisseria* and *Moraxella catarrhalis.*

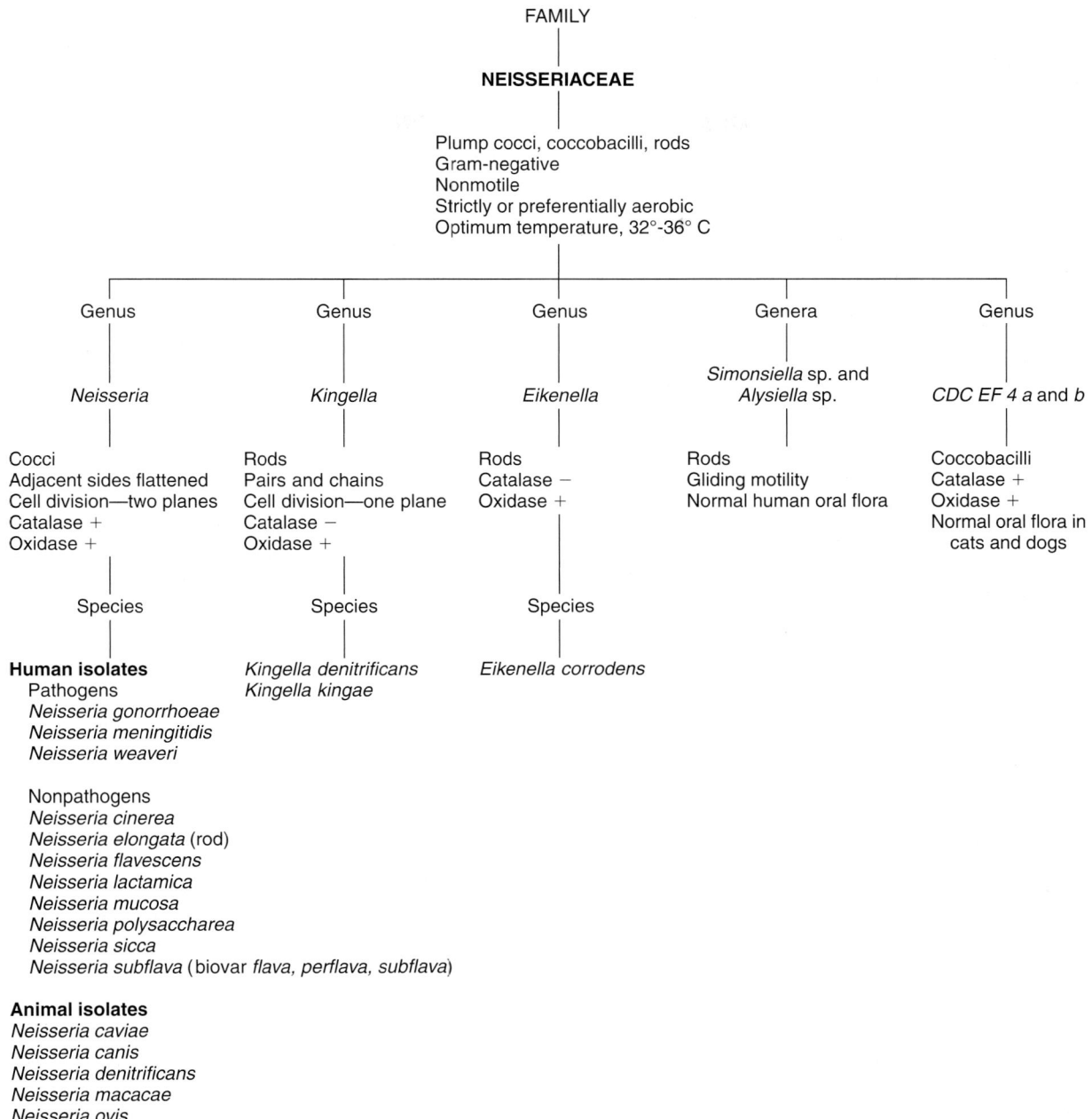

FAMILY

NEISSERIACEAE

Plump cocci, coccobacilli, rods
Gram-negative
Nonmotile
Strictly or preferentially aerobic
Optimum temperature, 32°-36° C

Genus	Genus	Genus	Genera	Genus
Neisseria	*Kingella*	*Eikenella*	*Simonsiella* sp. and *Alysiella* sp.	*CDC EF 4 a* and *b*
Cocci Adjacent sides flattened Cell division—two planes Catalase + Oxidase +	Rods Pairs and chains Cell division—one plane Catalase − Oxidase +	Rods Catalase − Oxidase +	Rods Gliding motility Normal human oral flora	Coccobacilli Catalase + Oxidase + Normal oral flora in cats and dogs

Species (Neisseria)

Species (Kingella)

Species (Eikenella)

Human isolates
Pathogens
Neisseria gonorrhoeae
Neisseria meningitidis
Neisseria weaveri

Kingella denitrificans
Kingella kingae

Eikenella corrodens

Nonpathogens
Neisseria cinerea
Neisseria elongata (rod)
Neisseria flavescens
Neisseria lactamica
Neisseria mucosa
Neisseria polysaccharea
Neisseria sicca
Neisseria subflava (biovar *flava, perflava, subflava*)

Animal isolates
Neisseria caviae
Neisseria canis
Neisseria denitrificans
Neisseria macacae
Neisseria ovis
Neisseria parelongata (rod)

Figure 14-1

Characteristics of the family and the six genera. *Moraxella catarrhalis,* although morphologically and biochemically similar to the *Neisseria* spp., is no longer a member of the *Neisseriaceae* family, so is not included here.

TABLE 14-1

Pathogenicity and Host Range for Species of
Neisseria *Organisms and* Moraxella (Branhamella)

Species	Pathogenicity	Infected Host
N. gonorrhoeae	Primary pathogen	Humans only
N. meningitidis	Primary pathogen	Humans only
N. lactamica	Opportunistic pathogen	Warm-blooded animals
N. sicca	Opportunistic pathogen	Warm-blooded animals
N. subflava	Opportunistic pathogen	Warm-blooded animals
N. mucosa	Opportunistic pathogen	Warm-blooded animals
N. flavescens	Opportunistic pathogen	Warm-blooded animals
N. cinerea	Opportunistic pathogen	Warm-blooded animals
N. polysaccharea	Opportunistic pathogen	Warm-blooded animals
N. elongata	Opportunistic pathogen	Warm-blooded animals
M. catarrhalis	Opportunistic pathogen	Humans only

GENERAL CHARACTERISTICS

Essentially all species of *Neisseria* are aerobic gram-negative diplococci, cytochrome oxidase, and catalase positive; *Neisseria elongata,* which is catalase negative and rod shaped, is the only known exception. *Neisseria* species are capnophilic and have optimal growth in a moist atmosphere. The natural habitat of *Neisseria* species are the mucous membranes of the respiratory and urogenital tracts. Table 14-1 shows the pathogenicity and host range of *Neisseria* and *Moraxella* species.

Neisseria gonorrhoeae and *Neisseria meningitidis* are the primary human pathogens of the genus. *N. gonorrhoeae* is always pathogenic, but *N. meningitidis* may be found as a commensal inhabitant of the upper respiratory tract of carriers. All other *Neisseria* species are considered opportunistic pathogens. You should recognize and differentiate these species from *N. gonorrhoeae* and *N. meningitidis* in isolates from clinical specimens. Pathogenic *Neisseria* species are fastidious organisms, requiring enriched media for optimal recovery.

PATHOGENIC *NEISSERIA* SPECIES

Neisseria gonorrhoeae

Humans are the only natural host for *N. gonorrhoeae,* the agent of gonorrhea. **Gonorrhea** is an acute pyogenic infection of columnar and transitional epithelium; infection may be established at any site where these cells are found. Gonococcal infections occur primarily in the urethra, endocervix, anal canal, pharynx, and conjunctiva. Disseminated infections from the primary site may also occur.

Virulence factors

The pathogenic *Neisseria* species have several characteristics that contribute to their virulence. These virulence factors include the presence of the following:

- Capsule
- Pili
- Cell-wall proteins
- Lipopolysaccharide (endotoxin)
- IgA protease that cleaves IgA on mucosal surfaces

A schematic diagram of the cellular structure of *N. gonorrhoeae* is shown in Figure 14-2.

N. gonorrhoeae is divided into five morphologically distinct colony types, T1 through T5, based on the presence or absence of pili, the fine hair-like projections that are important in the initial attachment of the organism to host tissues. Pili also inhibit phagocytosis of the organism by neutrophils and aid in the exchange of genetic material from cell to cell. Types T1 and T2, which possess pili, are virulent forms, whereas T3 through T5, devoid of pili, are avirulent strains. Piliated organisms usually predominate when first isolated from uncomplicated genitourinary infections, but on subculture, pili are lost and colony types T3 through T5 appear. Antigenic variation allows the gonococcus to regain its pili, contributing to the organism's ability to evade the defenses of the immune system.

The capsule, cell wall proteins (proteins I to III), and the lipopolysaccharides act to prevent phagocytosis of the organism. Moreover, the lipopolysaccharide endotoxin is a major in vivo virulence factor of gram-negative bacteria that mediates damage to body tissues.

Protein I (PI), representing about 60% of the total weight of the outer membrane, demonstrates antigenic variability and has been used for enzyme-linked immunosorbent assay (ELISA) and coagglutination tests for gonococcal serotyping. Several distinct PII proteins are detectable; the gonococcus can rapidly change the expression of this protein, which may account for recurrent infections. Strains with high-molecular-weight (HMW) PI and expressing PII are usually found in symptomatic genital infections; whereas low-molecular-weight PI strains that lack PIIs are found in disseminated infections. Protein III is believed to be the major binding site on the outer membrane for IgG-blocking antibody.

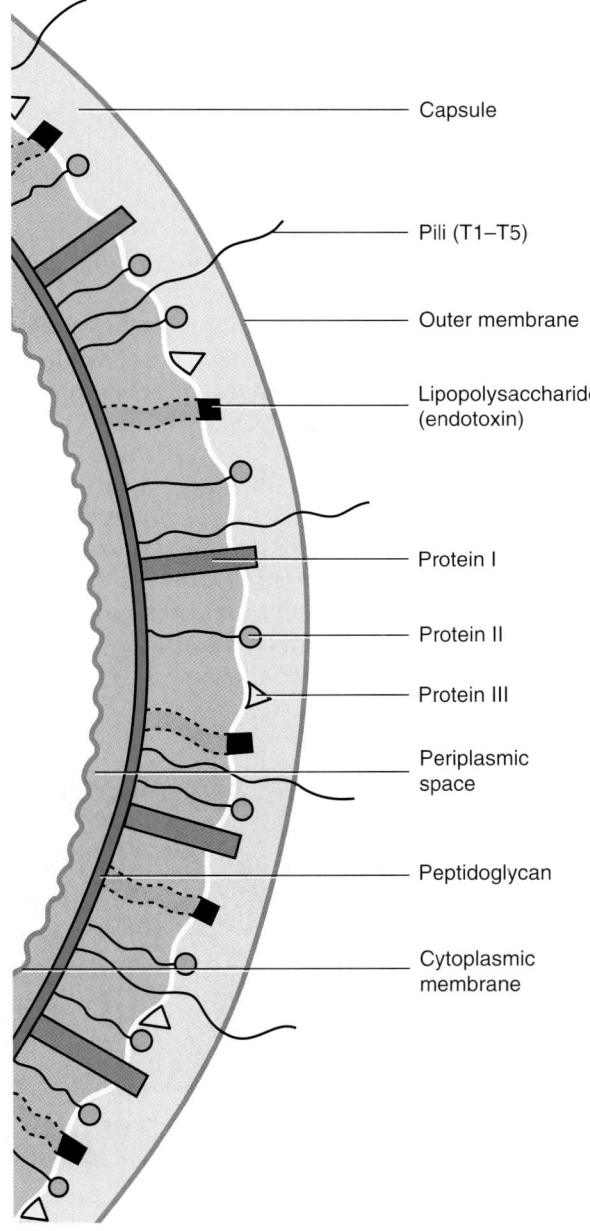

Figure 14-2 ────────────────
Cellular structure of *Neisseria gonorrhoeae.*

Capsule

Pili (T1–T5)

Outer membrane

Lipopolysaccharide (endotoxin)

Protein I

Protein II

Protein III

Periplasmic space

Peptidoglycan

Cytoplasmic membrane

Epidemiology

Infections are transmitted most commonly by sexual contact. The primary reservoir is the asymptomatic carrier. Since 1965, gonorrhea has been the most commonly reported sexually transmitted bacterial infection in the United States. Reported cases increased steadily through the 1960s and 1970s but declined somewhat through the 1980s. The fear of acquired immune deficiency syndrome (AIDS) and a subsequent reduction in high-risk sexual behavior are thought to contribute to this decline. Actual numbers of infected individuals are probably much higher than reported, owing to a large reservoir of asymptomatic carriers and other unreported cases.

Clinical infections

DISEASE IN THE MALE

Gonorrhea has a short incubation period, approximately 2 to 7 days after acquiring the organism. In men, acute urethritis, usually resulting in purulent discharge and dysuria, is the common manifestation. **Asymptomatic gonococcal infection** in men is uncommon; only 3% to 5% of cases may be asymptomatic, whereas 95% show acute infections. *N. gonorrhoeae* strains with a nutritional requirement for arginine, hypoxanthine, and uracil **(AHU strains)** are often isolated from asymptomatic men. Complications in males include ascending infections such as prostatitis and epididymitis.

DISEASE IN THE FEMALE

The endocervix is the most common site of infection in women, resulting in vaginal discharge and dysuria. However, up to 50% of cases in women may be asymptomatic. Symptoms of infection, when present, include dysuria, lower abdominal pain, and vaginal bleeding. Untreated gonococcal cervicitis is a major cause of **pelvic inflammatory disease (PID)** in women, which may cause sterility, ectopic pregnancy, or perihepatitis **(Fitz-Hugh–Curtis syndrome).**

DISSEMINATED INFECTIONS

Blood-borne dissemination of *N. gonorrhoeae* occurs in less than 1% of all infections, resulting in purulent arthritis as seen in the case study and rarely septicemia. Fever and a rash on the extremities may also be present. The majority of disseminated gonococcal infections are attributed to

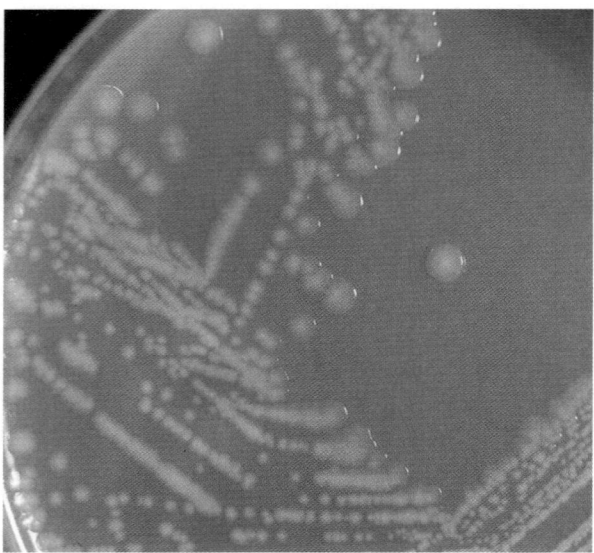

Figure 14-3 _____

Virulent *Neisseria gonorrhoeae* after 24 hours of growth on modified Thayer-Martin (MTM) agar.

the AHU strains and occur in women, having been acquired from infected but asymptomatic males.

INFECTIONS IN OTHER SITES

Other conditions associated with *N. gonorrhoeae* include anorectal and oropharyngeal infections. Infections in these sites are more common in homosexual males but can also occur in women. Most infections are asymptomatic or have nonspecific symptoms. Pharyngitis is the chief complaint in symptomatic oropharyngeal infections, whereas discharge, rectal pain, or bloody stools may be seen in rectal gonorrhea. Approximately 30% to 60% of females with genital gonorrhea have concurrent rectal infection.

Newborns can acquire **ophthalmia neonatorum,** a gonococcal eye infection, during vaginal delivery through an infected birth canal. This condition, which can result in blindness if not immediately treated, is rare in the United States because application of antimicrobial eye drops or silver nitrate is legally required at the birth of every infant. Ocular infections can occur in adults owing to inoculation of the eye with infected genital secretions or, rarely, as a result of a laboratory accident.

Laboratory diagnosis

SPECIMEN COLLECTION, TRANSPORT, AND PROCESSING

Specimens collected for the recovery of *N. gonorrhoeae,* as noted previously, may come from typical sources or from other sites, such as the rectum, blood, pharynx, and joint fluid. The laboratory should be notified when cultures from sites such as the rectum or throat are requested, because normal laboratory protocols for such specimens would not recover the organism.

The specimen of choice for genital infections in males is the urethra, and in females, the endocervix. In males, purulent discharge can be collected directly onto a swab for culture. When no apparent discharge is present, the swab is inserted 2 to 3 cm into the anterior urethra and slowly rotated to collect the specimen. Swabs for rectal culture should be inserted 4 to 5 cm into the anal canal. Disinfectants should be avoided in preparing the patient for collection of the specimen. Because *N. gonorrhoeae* is extremely susceptible to drying and temperature changes, direct plating of the specimen to gonococcal-selective media gives optimal results (Figure 14-3).

Calcium alginate and some cotton swabs have been shown to be inhibitory to *N. gonorrhoeae,* so Dacron or rayon swabs are preferred. Inoculated swabs should be placed in a transport system such as Amies medium with charcoal, transported to the laboratory immediately, and plated within 6 hours. Several commercial transport systems,

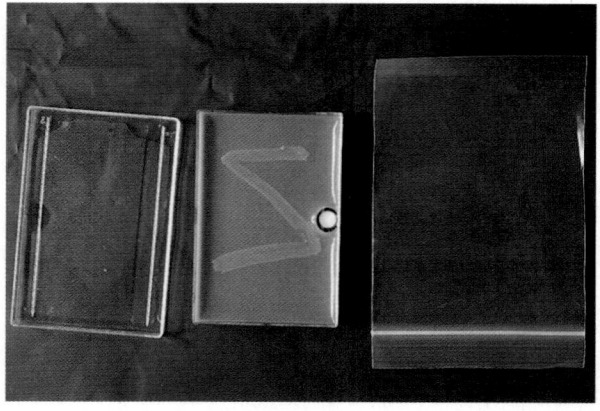

Figure 14-4 _____

Twenty-four hour growth of *Neisseria gonorrhoeae* on a JEMBEC plate streaked in a characteristic Z pattern.

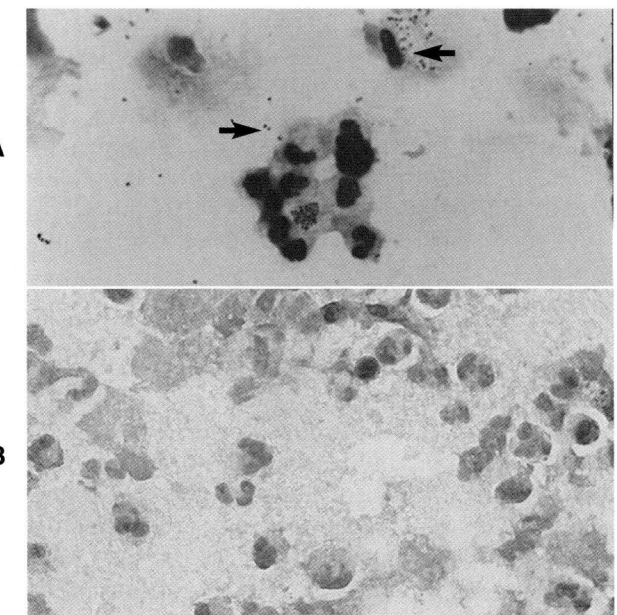

Figure 14-5

A, Direct Gram-stained smear of male urethral discharge showing intracellular and extracellular gram-negative diplococci, which is diagnostic of *Neisseria gonorrhoeae.* **B,** A direct smear with more than five PMNs per field, but no bacteria may suggest nongonococcal urethritis (NGU).

such as **JEMBEC** plates (*James E. Martin Biological Environmental Chamber*) (Figure 14-4), Bio-Bag, Gono-Pak, and Transgrow, contain selective media and a carbon dioxide atmosphere to provide optimal conditions until the specimen reaches the laboratory. These systems are especially useful when the clinic or physician's office is some distance from the laboratory.

DIRECT MICROSCOPIC EXAMINATION

Direct Gram stains should be prepared from urogenital specimens when the culture is collected. Gram stain is not recommended for pharyngeal specimens, in which saprophytic *Neisseria* species are often present. Demonstration of gram-negative intracellular diplococci from a symptomatic male with discharge correlates at a rate of 95% with culture and is presumptive evidence of gonococcal infection (Figure 14-5, *A*). Because women have vaginal and cervical saprophytic flora that resemble gonococci, direct Gram stain correlates in only 50% to 70% of cases with culture. The direct

Gram stain may be helpful in a symptomatic woman with discharge, but culture is necessary for confirmation.

A Gram stain with more than five polymorphonuclear neutrophils (PMNs) per field but no bacteria (Figure 14-5, *B*) may suggest nongonococcal urethritis with organisms such as *Chlamydia trachomatis* or *Ureaplasma urealyticum*.

CULTURE

Cultivation of *N. gonorrhoeae* requires the use of chocolate agar, but this enriched medium also supports the growth of many other organisms found as saprophytes in specimens collected for recovery of gonococci. To prevent overgrowth of the normal flora and to enhance the recovery of the pathogenic species, a selective medium containing inhibitors for gram-negative and gram-positive organisms and yeast is used. Commonly used selective media are described in Table 14-2.

TABLE 14-2

Selective Media for the Isolation of Neisseria Gonorrhoeae *and* Neisseria Meningitidis

Selective Medium	Inhibitory Agents	Suppressed Organisms
Thayer-Martin (TM)	Vancomycin	Gram-positive
	Colistin	Gram-negative
	Nystatin	Yeast
Modified Thayer-Martin (MTM)	Vancomycin	Gram-positive
	Colistin	Gram-negative
	Nystatin	Yeast
	Trimethoprim	Swarming *Proteus* species
Martin-Lewis (ML)	Vancomycin	Gram-positive
	Colistin	Gram-negative
	Anisomycin	Yeast
	Trimethoprim	Swarming *Proteus* species
New York City (NYC)	Vancomycin	Gram-positive
	Colistin	Gram-negative
	Amphotericin B	Yeast
	Trimethoprim	Swarming *Proteus* species
GC-LECT	Vancomycin	Gram-positive
	Lincomycin	Gram-positive
	Colistin	Gram-negative
	Amphotericin B	Yeast
	Trimethoprim	Swarming *Proteus* species
		Capnocytophaga spp.

New York City, a transparent agar, has the added advantage of supporting the growth of the possible urogenital pathogens *Mycoplasma hominis* and *U. urealyticum.* Over the past several years, up to 10% of *N. gonorrhoeae* strains have been reported as sensitive to vancomycin. To recover these sensitive strains, including a nonselective chocolate agar as a primary plating medium is good practice.

Several other genera will grow on selective gonococcal media. Some of these are *Acinetobacter* sp., *Capnocytophaga* sp., and *K. denitrificans.* These are differentiated from *N. gonorrhoeae* by the oxidase and catalase tests.

All specimens received in the laboratory for recovery of *Neisseria* species should be held at room temperature and plated as soon as possible. Media should be warmed to room temperature before inoculation, because *Neisseria* species are susceptible to cold. Specimens on swabs should be rolled in a Z pattern on the media and cross-streaked with a loop to facilitate growth of isolated colonies.

INCUBATION

Inoculated plates should be incubated at 35° C in a 3% to 5% carbon dioxide atmosphere. This is easily accomplished by use of a candle extinction jar

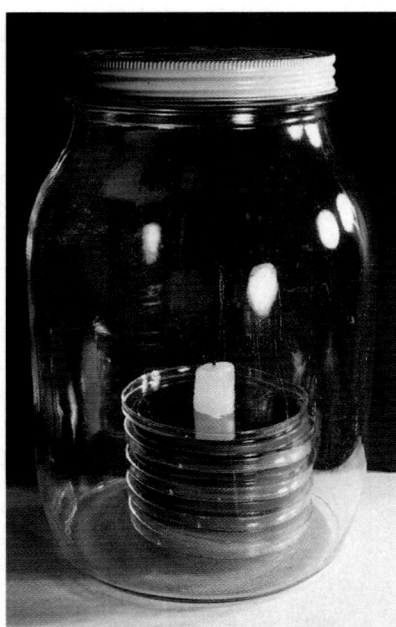

Figure 14-6 _____

Candle extinction jar with inoculated modified Thayer-Martin agar plates.

(Figure 14-6) or a commercially available CO_2 incubator. Sufficient humidity is provided by the moisture evaporating from the media in a closed jar; most commercially available CO_2 incubators are automatically humidified, or a pan of water can be placed in the bottom. Scented or colored candles may be inhibitory to the gonococci, so only white wax candles are used in the candle extinction jar.

Presumptive identification

IDENTIFICATION

Microscopic morphology The Gram stain must be performed on all suspected *Neisseria* species isolates to verify the appearance of gram-negative kidney bean–shaped diplococci. Some gram-negative rods, such as *Kingella* and *Acinetobacter* species, are occasionally able to grow on gonococcal-selective media. To differentiate these from the gram-negative diplococci, the organism can be streaked to a plate with a 10-U penicillin disk added (Figure 14-7). After growth, the edge of the zone of inhibition is stained to visualize the morphology.

Colonial morphology Cultures are examined daily for growth and held for 72 hours. Colonies of *N. gonorrhoeae* on chocolate or selective agar are small, gray, translucent, and raised after 24 to 48 hours of incubation. As noted previously, five colony types of *N. gonorrhoeae* have been described: T1 and T2 have pili and are considered virulent types; these colonies are smaller and raised and they appear bright in reflected light. Types T3 through T5 do not have pili and usually grow as larger, flatter colonies. The AHU (atypical) strains produce smaller colonies that grow more slowly; they are often more difficult to identify with biochemical methods.

The gonococci can produce autolytic enzymes that may make the isolate nonviable, so primary plates should not be incubated in the candle jar once sufficient growth is obtained. A fresh subculture should be used for identification tests.

Oxidase test The filter paper or direct plate oxidase test must be done on all isolates. In the filter paper method, oxidase reagent (1% dimethyl-*p*-phenylene-diaminedihydrochloride or tetramethyl-*p*-phenylene-diamine-dihydrochloride) is placed on filter paper, and a colony from the plate is rubbed onto the reagent with an applicator stick or a nonnichrome needle. A purple color should develop in 10 seconds in a positive reaction on a fresh isolate

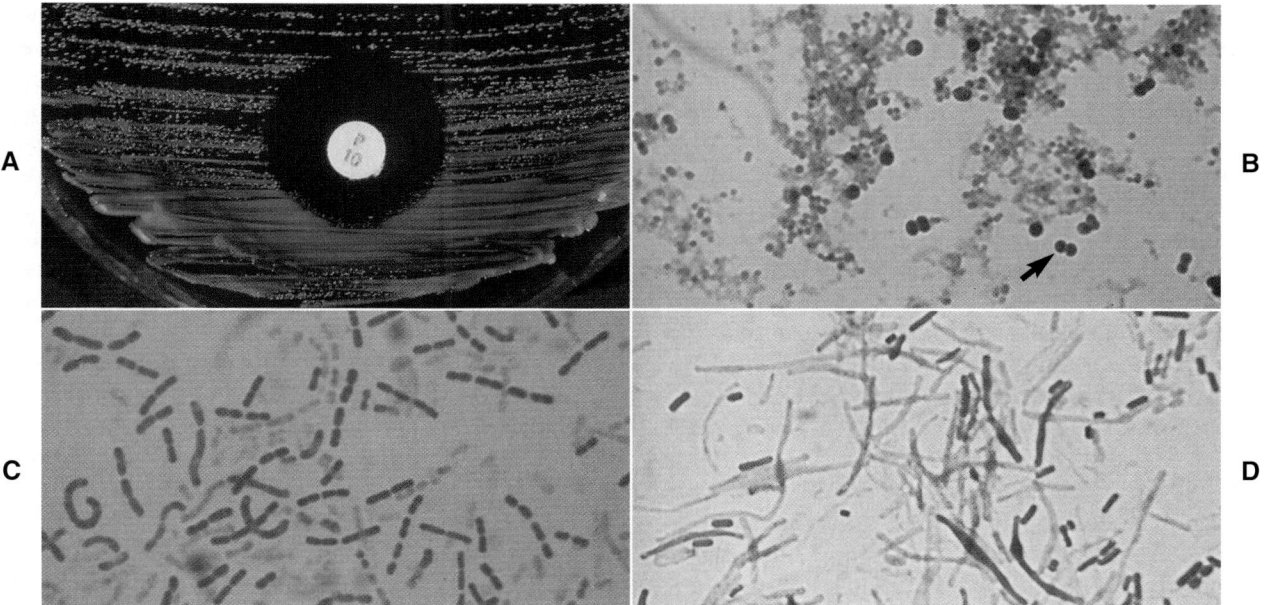

Figure 14-7

A, To differentiate some gram-negative rods from the gram-negative diplococci, the organism can be streaked to a plate and a 10-U penicillin disk added. After growth, the edge of the zone of inhibition is stained to visualize microscopic morphology. **B,** The microscopic morphology of *Neisseria gonorrhoeae* remains a gram-negative diplococci using the 10-U penicillin disk. **C,** The gram-negative rod microscopic morphology of *Kingella* species after the penicillin disk test. **D,** The elongated gram-negative rod microscopic morphology of *Acinetobacter* species after the penicillin disk test.

(Figure 14-8, *A*). Alternatively, the oxidase reagent may be dropped directly on a colony. The colony turns pink then black in a positive reaction (Figure 14-8, *B*). If subculture of the positive colony is needed, it must be done while the colony is still pink; when black, the organism is no longer viable.

Definitive identification To make a presumptive diagnosis of gonorrhea if an oxidase-positive, gram-negative diplococcus was recovered from gono-coccal-selective media was once acceptable, but this procedure is no longer recommended. Oxidase-positive, gram-negative diplococci, such as *Neisseria cinerea* and *N. meningitidis,* and *M. catarrhalis* can grow on selective media from sites where gonorrhea is expected. These organisms would be incorrectly reported as *N. gonorrhoeae*

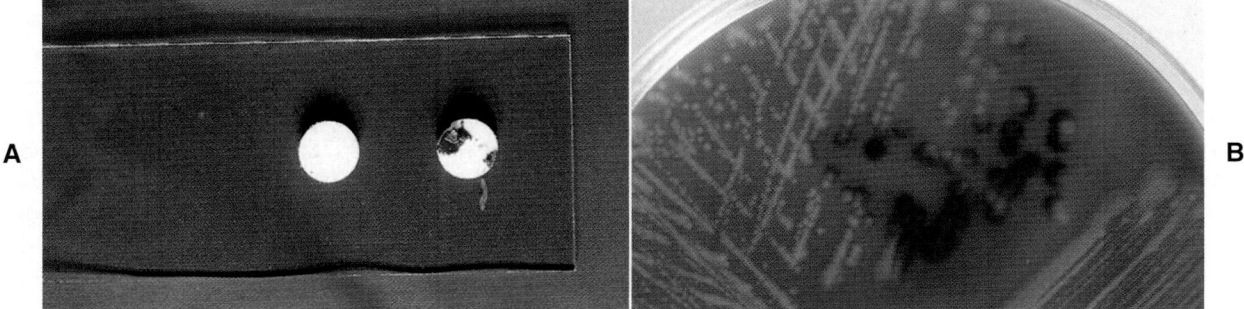

Figure 14-8

A, The oxidase disk test. Negative control is on the left and the positive reaction (purple) is on the right. **B,** Example of a positive oxidase reaction when the reagent is dropped directly on the colony.

if no further identification were done. Many different methods are currently used for the speciation of *Neisseria* and *Moraxella* species or for confirmation only of *N. gonorrhoeae* isolates. Both culture and nonculture tests are available for the detection of *N. gonorrhoeae* and are listed by type in Table 14-3. All have advantages and disadvantages. The selection of a particular method depends on the demographic profile of the patients, sensitivity and specifity of the method with low- or high-prevalence groups, cost of materials and technical time, and number of tests performed.

Carbohydrate utilization methods The traditional method for the identification of *Neisseria* species has been by carbohydrate utilization in cystine trypticase agar (CTA), containing 1% of the individual carbohydrate with phenol red as an indicator. Yellow is produced in 24 to 72 hours if the organism uses the particular carbohydrate, as shown in Figure 14-9 and described in Procedure 14-1. Many problems are associated with this method, however, and it has largely been replaced by newer, faster, and more accurate methods.

The rapid carbohydrate degradation tests require pure cultures but can be read in 2 to 4 hours rather than the 24 to 72 hours needed for the CTA carbohydrate test. These rapid tests also detect acid production from various carbohydrates but they are based on the presence of preformed enzymes for carbohydrate utilization rather than on bacterial growth. Problems noted with these methods, however, include the following:

▪ Weak acid production from glucose by certain strains of *N. gonorrhoeae*
▪ Misidentification of sucrose-negative strains of *Neisseria subflava* as *N. meningitidis*
▪ Species of *N. cinerea* that give positive glucose reactions

Additional tests such as superoxol or colistin susceptibility are needed when acid production is equivocal. The superoxyl test uses 30% H_2O_2 and is performed in the same way as the catalase test. Colonies of *Neisseria gonorrhoeae* produce immediate, vigorous bubbling. *Neisseria meningitidis* and *Neisseria lactamica* produce weak delayed bubbling in this reagent. Other *Neisseria* spp. produce weak delayed bubbling or none at all.

Chromogenic substrate tests detect enzymes that hydrolyze the substrates and produce colored end products. Only strains that are isolated on se-

lective media should be tested, but the advantage of these tests is the identification of *Neisseria* species strains with aberrant carbohydrate utilizations. Problems noted with these tests include misidentification of nonpathogenic species, such as *N. cinerea*, *Neisseria sicca*, *N. subflava*, and *Neisseria mucosa*, as *N. gonorrhoeae* or *N. meningitidis*.

The multitest conventional-chromogenic enzyme methods combine enzyme substrate tests with other biochemical tests and allow identification of strains isolated on selective or nonselective media. These tests can also speciate other genera, such as *Haemophilus*.

Characteristics of significant species of *Neisseria*, *Moraxella*, and *Kingella* are shown in Table 14-4. Key differentiating reactions of the major pathogens include use of glucose only by *N. gonorrhoeae*, whereas *N. meningitidis* uses glucose and maltose. *M. catarrhalis* is asaccharolytic but, unlike the *Neisseria* species, is DNase and butyrate esterase positive.

Immunologic methods Immunologic methods employ monoclonal antibodies for the identification of *N. gonorrhoeae*. These methods do not require pure or viable organisms and can be done from the primary plates. Immunologic methods include coagglutination and fluorescent antibody testing.

The coagglutination tests use monoclonal antibodies attached to a carrier particle; agglutination occurs with *N. gonorrhoeae*. No reported cross-reaction with *N. cinerea* exists, but rare isolates of *N. lactamica* have been reported as *N. gonorrhoeae*.

The fluorescent antibody (FA) method uses monoclonal antibodies that recognize epitopes on the principal outer membrane protein (PI) of *N. gonorrhoeae*. The method is extremely sensitive and specific; no demonstrated cross-reactivity with *N. cinerea* or other *Neisseria* species has occurred. The FA method also microscopically confirms the diplococci's morphologic appearance.

Nonculture methods Alternatives to culture for *N. gonorrhoeae* are available. These methods detect gonococcal antigen or nucleic acid directly in cervical urine and/or urethral exudates. Enzyme-linked immunosorbent assays (ELISAs) and nucleic acid probe technology are currently available, including nonculture, nonamplified, and nonculture amplified (see Table 14-3).

The nucleic acid probe test is a nonisotopic chemiluminescent DNA probe that hybridizes specifically with ribosomal RNA (rRNA) of *N. gon-*

TABLE 14-3

Selected Test Methods for Identification of Neisseria *and Related Species*

Method Type and Name	Manufacturer(s)	Principle	Notes
Conventional			
Cystine Trypticase Agar (CTA) with carbohydrates (1%)	Various	Acid production from carbohydrate utilization	Requires pure culture Must be incubated 24-48 hr
Rapid carbohydrate degredation		Acid production from carbohydrate utilization; detected by preformed enzymes	Requires pure culture Read in 2-4 hr
BBL-MINITEK	BD Microbiology Systems (Cockeysville, Md)		
QuadFERM+	bioMerieux, Inc. (Hazelwood, Mo)		Includes acidometric β-lactamase
Neisseria-Kwik	MicroBioLogics (St. Cloud, Minn)		
Gonobio-Test	IAF Production, Inc (Laval, Quebec, Canada)		
Chromogenic substrate			
Gonochek II	EY Laboratories (San Mateo, Calif)	Detects enzyme production	Confirms isolates only from selective media
Modified conventional/ chromogenic enzyme		Combines enzyme substrate with other biochemical tests Speciates *Neisseria* and *Haemophilus* species	Isolates from selective or nonselective media
BBL Crystal Neisseria/ Haemophilus ID kit	BD Microbiology Systems (Cockeysville, Md)		
Neisseria-Haemophilus Identification (NHI)	bioMerieux, Inc. (Hazelwood, Mo)		
RapID NH System	Remel, Inc. (Lenexa, Kan)		
Microscan HNID Panel	Baxter Healthcare Corp. Microscan Division (W Sacramento, Calif)		
Immunologic coagglutination		Monoclonal antibodies used to detect *N. gonorrhoeae* Slide agglutination	Does not require pure or viable culture
Phadebact Monoclonal GC	Boule Daignostics (Sweden)		
GonoGen II	BD Microbiology Systems (Cockeysville, Md)		
FA monoclonal antibody			
Syva Microtrak *Neisseria gonorrhoeae* culture confirmation test	Syva Co. (Palo Alto, Calif)	Fluorescent-labeled monoclonal antibodies to detect *N. gonorrhoeae*	Does not require pure culture Requires UV microscope
Nonculture Tests			Not recommended for rectal or pharyngeal sites Cannot identify β-lactamase-producing strains
Nonculture nonamplified: *Neisseria gonorrhoeae* PACE 2	Gen-Probe (San Diego, Calif)	DNA probe for direct detection of gonococcal rRNA from specimen	Uses a chemiluminescent labeled, single-stranded DNA probe
AccuProbe *Neisseria* Culture Confirmation Test	Gen-Probe (San Diego, Calif)	Nucleic acid hybridization for confirmation of *N. gonorrhoeae* culture	Uses a chemiluminescent labeled, single-stranded DNA probe
Nonculture amplified: Ligase Chain Reaction Assay (LCx)	Abbott Diagnostics (Chicago, Ill)	Thermophilic amplification of target gene. For *N. gonorrhoeae* and *Chlamydia trachomatis*	Specimens include urogenital and male and female urine

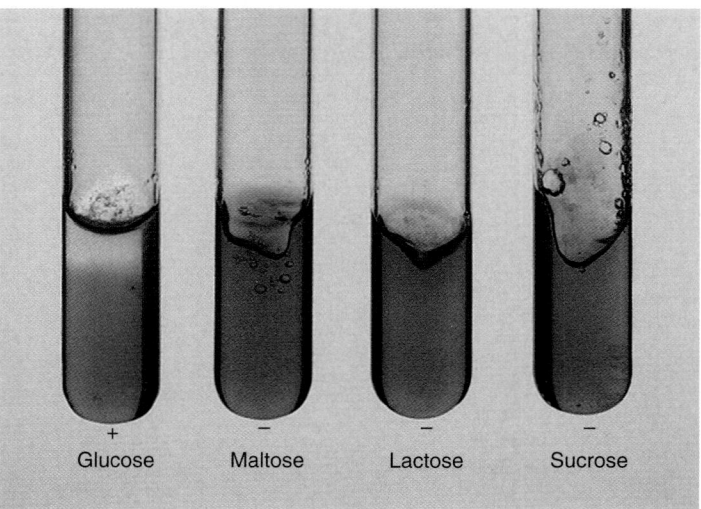

Figure 14-9

Conventional CTA sugars. Yellow color at the top of the media is considered positive. Acid is produced in the glucose tube only, identifying this organism as *Neisseria gonorrhoeae.*

orrhoeae. These methods are rapid and sensitive but they do have some drawbacks. Some disadvantages of the nucleic acid probes include the following:

- Lesser sensitivity than cervical culture in females, so should be used in high-risk populations only
- Not approved for pharyngeal or rectal specimens and should not be used in children or sexual abuse cases

- Cannot identify a *N. gonorrhoeae* infection produced by a β-lactamase–producing strain
- Do not allow for recovery of an organism to be used for susceptibility testing
- False-positive results reported with some strains of *N. lactamica* and *N. cinerea*

Probe technology can be expensive. This method is probably not cost-effective if it is the only probe test used in the laboratory or if low volumes of *N. gonorrhoeae* tests are requested.

PROCEDURE 14-1. CTA Carbohydrate Method

1. Prepare a heavy inoculum in saline of a pure isolate from a fresh subculture of the organism. The subculture must *not* be from a selective agar.

2. Inoculate the top portions only of the following CTA media: glucose, maltose, lactose, and sucrose, plus a carbohydrate-free CTA control.

3. Incubate tightly capped tubes at 35° to 37° C in a non–carbon dioxide atmosphere.

Incubation in an acid CO_2 atmosphere can produce the appearance of carbohydrate degradation in all tubes and, hence, false-positive reactions.

4. Yellow at the top of the media in 24 to 48 hours is considered positive. Bright yellow throughout the media usually indicates contamination with other organisms.

TABLE 14-4

Characteristics of Significant Species of Neisseria, Moraxella *and* Kingella

Characteristic	N. gonorrhoeae	N. meningitidis	N. lactamica	N. cinerea	N. sicca	N. flavescens	Moraxella	Kingella
Pigment on nutrient agar	−	−	−	−	+	+	−	−
Catalase on 3% H_2O_2	+	+	+	+	+	+	+	−
Superoxol (30% H_2O_2)	+	−	−	−	−	−	−	−
Growth on								
MTM, ML, NYC	+	+	+	d	−	−	d	+
Nutrient medium @35° C	−	−	+	+	+	+	+	−
Acid production from								
Glucose	+	+	+	+*	+	−	−	+
Maltose	−	+	+	−	+	−	−	−
Sucrose	−	−	−	−	+	−	−	−
Lactose	−	−	+	−	−	−	−	−
Fructose	−	−	−	−	+	−	−	−
DNase	−	−	−	−	−	−	+	−
Reduction of								
NO_3†	−	d	d	+	+	+	+	−
NO_2	−	−	−	−	−	−	+	+
Tributyrin hydrolysis	−	−	−	−	−	−	+	NT
Enzymes produced								
β-*D*-Galactosidase	−	−	+	−	−	NT	−	−
γ-Glutamylamino-peptidase	−	+	−	−	−	NT	−	−
Hydroxyprolylamino-peptidase	+	−	−	+	NT	+	−	+

+, Most strains (>90%) positive; −, most strains (>90%) negative; d, some strains positive, some negative; *MTM,* modified Thayer-Martin agar; *ML,* Martin-Lewis agar; *NT,* not tested; *NYC,* New York City medium.
*Occasional strains may give weak glucose reactions in some rapid carbohydrate tests.
†0.1% (W/V) nitrate.

Added to the expense is the need to repeat the probe test after the equivocal results are obtained.

As noted previously, in low-prevalence populations, such as children, or in cases of suspected sexual abuse direct specimen detection methods are highly recommended to *not* be used. The specimens should be cultured onto selective gonococcal media, and isolates must be identified to species level by the use of two procedures with different principles. The organism should also be frozen in case further testing is needed. With various methods, isolates such as *N. cinerea, M. catarrhalis,* and *K. denitrificans,* all of which closely resemble *N. gonorrhoeae* biochemically, have been incorrectly reported as *N. gonorrhoeae.* Potentially serious medical, social, and legal ramifications could obviously result.

Additional and future methods As mentioned previously, some strains of *N. gonorrhoeae* have a specific need for one or more nutritional factors to be included in artificial media for growth to occur. These strains are called *auxotypes;* of the approximately 30 known auxotypes, the most common is AHU, which requires arginine, hypoxanthine, and uracil. The AHU strains are usually highly susceptible to penicillin, commonly recovered from patients with disseminated gonococcal infection, and can cause asymptomatic urethritis in males.

The auxotyping procedure is labor intensive. For this reason the procedure is not recommended for the routine clinical microbiology laboratory.

Detection of *N. gonorrhoeae* antigens in clinical specimens has also been accomplished using a polymerase chain reaction (PCR) amplification and hybridization technique. The method is highly sensitive and specific and is now available commercially. A PCR method will be available shortly to allow detection of both *N. gonorrhoeae* and *C. trachomatis* from the same specimen.

Antimicrobial resistance

Until 1976, almost all strains of *N. gonorrhoeae* in the United States were susceptible to penicillin. The first **plasmid-mediated penicillinase-producing *Neisseria gonorrhoeae* (PPNG)** strains were isolated in that year, largely imported from Southeast Asia or Africa. By 1980, more than half of the reported PPNG cases were of domestic origin. Penicillinase-producing gonococcal strains are now endemic in New York City, Los Angeles, and Florida, with as many as 30% of isolates in some places exhibiting this type of resistance. It is, therefore, important that all *N. gonorrhoeae* isolates recovered be tested for β-lactamase (penicillinase) production. The β-lactamase test should be performed from isolates on the primary culture plate, because the plasmid may be lost on subculture.

The CDC has developed a scheme to define PPNG prevalence in various locations. If less than 1% of gonorrhea cases reported are PPNG, the area is defined as *nonendemic*. An endemic area is characterized as 1% to 3% of cases being PPNG, whereas hyperendemic areas are defined as having a greater than 3% incidence of PPNG. This method of surveillance reporting is still evolving.

MECHANISMS OF RESISTANCE

Antimicrobial resistance may develop in several ways. In addition to plasmid-mediated penicillin resistance, in which the organism acquires a new plasmid with genes for β-lactamase production, chromosome-mediated resistance was initially

noted in the United States in 1983. These isolates are β-lactamase negative; the resistance mutants are randomly selected from the gonococcal population. Resistance of these strains is because of a combination of mutations at several chromosomal loci. Chromosomal resistance to penicillin or tetracycline is usually low level. High-level tetracycline resistance is plasmid mediated and was first observed in the United States in 1985.

Spectinomycin resistance, first reported in 1981 in the United States, is not yet prevalent in this country. Resistance to spectinomycin is because of a chromosomal mutation resulting in high-level resistance to the antibiotic. The mechanisms of resistance of *N. gonorrhoeae* are summarized in Table 14-5.

Treatment

Several single-dose antimicrobials are currently recommended for uncomplicated gonococcal therapy by the U.S. Public Health Service. These agents are generally active against organisms with plasmid or chromosomal resistance to other antimicrobials and cure uncomplicated gonorrhea of the pharynx and rectum and urogenital sites. As chromosomal resistance to penicillin increases, however, resistance to multiple antimicrobials may occur.

In 1997 the National Committee for Clinical Laboratory Standards (NCCLS) issued revised guidelines for dilution antimicrobial susceptibility tests (Document M7-A4). A disk susceptibility revision (Document M100-S8) was released in 1998. These documents have considerably expanded the number of reportable antimicrobials. The NCCLS guidelines should be followed in the performance of susceptibility testing, because criteria have been

---

TABLE 14-5

Resistance of Neisseria Gonorrhoeae *in the United States*

Type	Acronym	First Observed	Mechanism
Plasmid-mediated penicillin resistance	PPNG	1976	Plasmid codes for β-lactamase production
Chromosome-mediated resistance	CMRNG	1983	Selection of mutants for low-level penicillin and tetracycline resistance
Plasmid-mediated, high-level tetracycline resistance	TRNG	1985	Plasmid codes for tetracycline resistance
Chromosome-mediated spectinomycin resistance	—	1981	Mutation causes high-level resistance

PPNG, Penicillinase-producing *N. gonorrhoeae; CMRNG,* chromosomally mediated resistant *N. gonorrhoeae; TRNG,* tetracycline-resistant *N. gonorrhoeae.*

developed specifically for testing of *N. gonorrhoeae* isolates, including appropriate control strains.

Neisseria meningitidis

Although the meningococcus *N. meningitidis* can be found in the nasopharynx and oropharynx of 3% to 30% of asymptomatic individuals, it is an etiologic agent of endemic and epidemic meningitis, meningococcemia, and rarely pneumonia, purulent arthritis, or endophthalmitis. *N. meningitidis* has also been recovered from urogenital and rectal sites as a result of oral-genital contact.

Virulence factors

The virulence factors associated with *N. meningitidis* include pili, the polysaccharide capsule, and endotoxin production. Many virulent strains produce IgA$_1$ protease, an enzyme that aids invasiveness. Of the 13 meningococcal serogroups, the encapsulated strains A, B, C, Y, and W-135 are most often associated with epidemics. Group A strains are often incriminated in worldwide epidemics. Serogroups B and C are most common in the United States, with Group B frequently involved in community-acquired disease. Serogroup Y primarily causes meningococcal pneumonia, whereas W-135 is often responsible for invasive disease.

Clinical infections

The primary source of epidemic meningitis are oral secretions or respiratory droplets from asymptomatic carriers, especially among close contacts in closed populations such as college dormitories and military barracks. Epidemic meningitis most often occurs in young adults. It is characterized by abrupt onset of frontal headache, stiff neck, and, sometimes, fever. Meningococcemia, or sepsis, may occur with or without meningitis and carries a 25% mortality rate, even if treated. Petechial skin lesions may develop during bacteremic spread, and thrombosis is common. In some cases, the disease is fulminant and spreads rapidly, causing disseminated intravascular coagulation (DIC), septic shock, or hemorrhage in the adrenal glands (**Waterhouse-Friderichsen syndrome;** Figure 14-10). Death may occur in 12 to 48 hours from onset. Individuals with a deficiency in complement components C5 to C8 are at increased risk of meningococcemia. Meningococcal pneumonia usu-

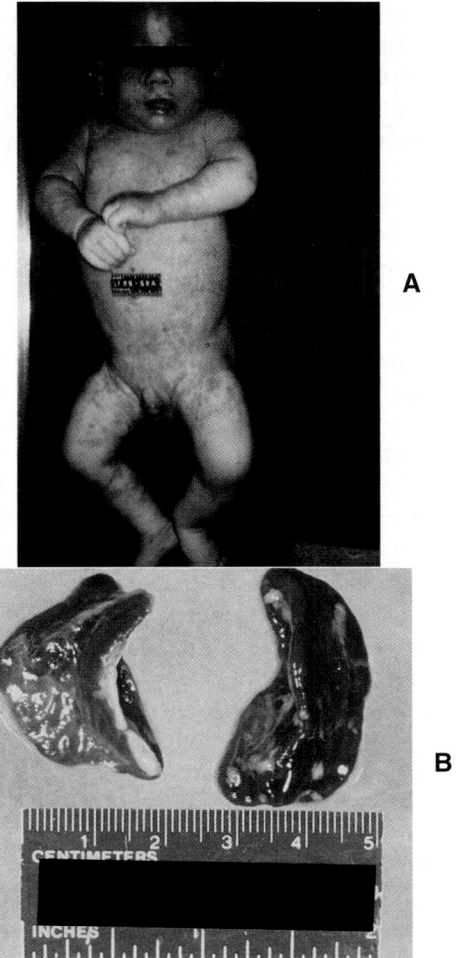

Figure 14-10 _____

A, Petechial skin rash associated with meningococcemia in a baby. **B,** Waterhouse-Friderichsen syndrome illustrating hemorrhage (dark red areas) in the adrenal glands.

ally affects older individuals with underlying pulmonary problems.

Treatment

The drug of choice for treatment of meningitis is penicillin, but rifampin or a sulfonamide is recommended as prophylaxis for close contacts.

Vaccine

Univalent Group A and Group C vaccines and a quadrivalent vaccine containing A, C, Y, and W-135 have been developed. These vaccines are recommended for managing epidemics not sporadic cases. These vaccines are poorly immunogenic, however, in children less than 2 years of age. No vaccine for serogroup B exists because humans do not develop antibody to this group. The quadrivalent vaccine is recommended for the following groups:

- Military recruits
- Asplenic patients more than 2 years of age
- Travelers to areas with epidemic A or C disease

Laboratory diagnosis

SPECIMEN COLLECTION AND TRANSPORT

Culture specimens for *N. meningitidis* may come from a wide variety of sterile and nonsterile sites. These include cerebrospinal fluid (CSF), blood, nasopharyngeal swabs and aspirates, and, less commonly, sputum and urogenital sites. Collection and transport should be performed as specified by the laboratory for the various specimen types.

When commercial blood culture systems are used, data from the manufacturer should be consulted to see whether *N. meningitidis* can be routinely recovered or if techniques such as blind subculture (subculture to chocolate agar of bottle with no apparent visual growth) are required.

DIRECT MICROSCOPIC EXAMINATION

On Gram-stained smears from specimens such as CSF, the meningococci appear as intracellular and

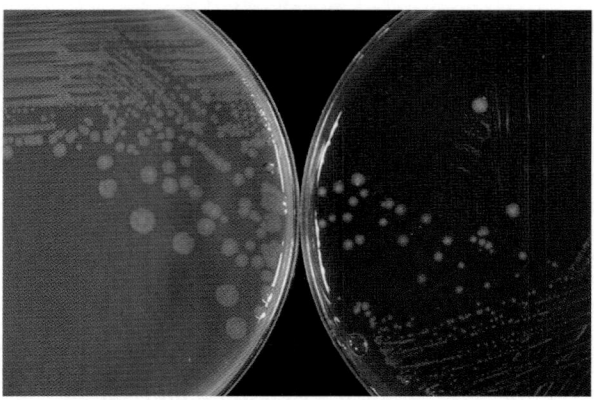

Figure 14-12 _____

Growth of *Neisseria meningitidis* after 48 hours on chocolate agar (CHOC) on the left and blood agar (BAP) on the right. Of the classic pathogens, only the meningococcus grows on BAP and CHOC.

extracellular gram-negative diplococci (Figure 14-11). Encapsulated strains may have a halo around the organisms. The highest yield of positive CSF Gram stains is obtained when specimens are concentrated. A number of investigators have reported that concentration by cytocentrifugation is superior to that by traditional centrifugation and has the potential to increase Gram stain detection by 10 to 100 fold.

In a patient with disseminated meningococcemia who has petechiae from hemorrhage of surface blood vessels, an impression Gram stain smear is often positive for gram-negative diplococci.

CULTURE

Culture using selective and nonselective media for the isolation of *N. meningitidis* and *M. catarrhalis* should, like cultures for *N. gonorrhoeae,* be incubated under carbon dioxide. Both these species and the saprophytic *Neisseria* species will grow on sheep's blood agar and chocolate agar. *N. meningitidis* will grow on gonococcal-selective agars and produce small gray, sometimes mucoid, convex colonies on sheep's blood or chocolate agar (Figure 14-12). *M. catarrhalis* is usually inhibited by the colistin in the medium, but some species resistant to colistin may grow. *N. lactamica,* a generally nonpathogenic species that may mimic *N. meningitidis,* can also grow on selective media. The lactose-positive characteristic may be delayed or nonexis-

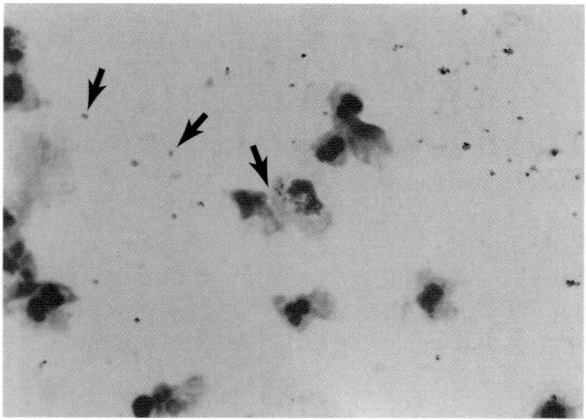

Figure 14-11 _____

Direct Gram-stained smear of CSF illustrating intracellular and extracellular gram-negative diplococci of *Neisseria meningitidis.*

tent. A rapid *o*-nitrophenyl-β-D-galactopyranoside (ONPG) test (which detects lactose utilization) is usually positive in 30 minutes for *N. lactamica.*

Some species of the saprophytic *Neisseria* may be yellow and often produce dry colonies on sheep's blood and chocolate agar.

IDENTIFICATION

The oxidase and catalase tests should be performed on all isolates. Any of the carbohydrate utilization tests described earlier can be used to speciate *N. meningitidis.* Optimal results in these tests are obtained when a fresh subculture of the organism is used. Serogrouping the meningococci is most commonly done by slide agglutination.

Immunologic methods Immunologic methods such as latex agglutination and counterimmunoelectrophoresis are commercially available in kit form and are used to detect the group-specific surface antigens of *N. meningitidis.* These bacterial antigen tests, when performed on CSF, blood, or urine, often allow more rapid detection of a causative organism, but they should not replace culture and Gram stain.

Moraxella catarrhalis

M. catarrhalis, formerly known as *Neisseria catarrhalis,* was transferred to the genus *Branhamella* in 1974. The species was reassigned as a subgenus of *Moraxella* in 1984 and is currently called *Moraxella catarrhalis.* As noted previously, the taxonomic status of this organism is unresolved.

Growth on chocolate agar is seen in Figure 14-13, *A.*

Clinical infections

Isolated only from humans, *M. catarrhalis* is a normal commensal of the respiratory tract. This organism has become an opportunistic pathogen and has been associated with a number of infections, such as pneumonia, sinusitis, otitis media, and systemic disease. Predisposing factors in the pathogenesis include advanced age, immunodeficiency, neutropenia, and chronic debilitating diseases such as chronic obstructive pulmonary disease. *M. catarrhalis* has been reported as the third most common cause of acute otitis media and sinusitis in children (Figure 14-13, *B*). The presence of intracellular gram-negative diplococci in these specimens may alert the microbiologist to possi-

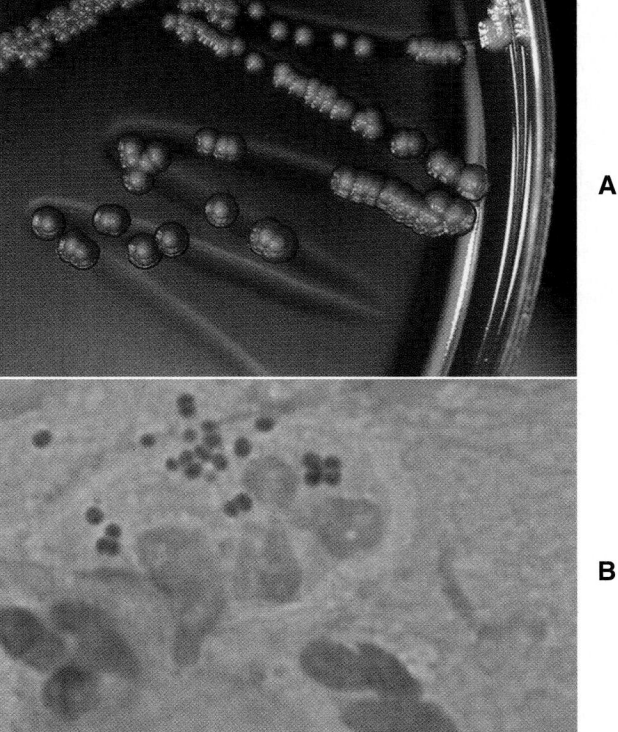

Figure 14-13 _____

A, Growth of *Moraxella catarrhalis* after 48 hours, illustrating the wagon-wheel appearance on chocolate agar. **B,** Direct smear of an otitis media specimen illustrating intracellular gram-negative diplococci. The organism was identified biochemically as *M. catarrhalis* from cultures.

ble infection with *M. catarrhalis.* Most isolates produce β-lactamase, making them resistant to ampicillin and amoxacillin, which are commonly used for otitis media.

Laboratory diagnosis

SPECIMEN COLLECTION AND IDENTIFICATION

Specimen collection for *M. catarrhalis* should be determined by the laboratory according to the various specimen types. The organism will grow on both sheep's blood and chocolate agars, producing smooth, opaque, gray to white colonies. *M. catarrhalis* is usually inhibited on gonococcal selective agars by the colistin in the media, but some species resistant to this antimicrobial may grow. Like *Neisseria* species, *M. catarrhalis* is oxidase and catalase positive. The organism is asaccharolytic in carbohydrate degradation tests, and it may be differentiated from *Neisseria* species by positive DNase and butyrate esterase reactions (see Table 14-4).

NONPATHOGENIC *NEISSERIA* SPECIES

Other *Neisseria* species exist as normal inhabitants of the upper respiratory tract. Referred to as *commensals, saprophytes,* or *nonpathogens,* these species are occasionally isolated from the genital tract. The commensal *Neisseria* species rarely cause disease but have sporadically been implicated in meningitis, endocarditis, prosthetic valve infections, bacteremia, pneumonia, empyema, bacteriuria, osteomyelitis, and ocular infections (Table 14-6). One must keep in mind that the incidence of infections caused by the commensal *Neisseria* spp. is extremely low and that the main reason for the microbiologist to be familiar with these organisms is to accurately separate them from the pathogenic species.

Identification

In the clinical laboratory, when isolated from respiratory specimens, the commensal *Neisseria* species are usually identified only by Gram stain

TABLE 14-6

Infections Reported to be Caused by Neisseria *Species other than* N. Gonorrhoeae *and* N. Meningitidis

Infection	*Neisseria* species
Meningitis	N. lactamica
	N. sicca
	N. subflava
	N. mucosa
	N. flavescens
Endocarditis	N. sicca
	N. subflava
	N. mucosa
Prosthetic valve infection	N. sicca
Bacteremia	N. lactamica
	N. flavescens
	N. cinerea
Pneumonia	N. sicca
Empyema	N. mucosa
Bacteriuria	N. subflava
Osteomyelitis	N. sicca
Ocular infection	N. mucosa
Dog bite	N. weaveri

and gross colony morphology and called *Neisseria species* or *usual oral flora.* Further identification by biochemical tests is not done. When they are isolated from selective agar medium or sterile body sites, differentiation from the pathogenic *Neisseria* may be required. Identification of the *Neisseria* species is traditionally based on the following:

- Gram stain
- Colony morphology
- Catalase
- Oxidase
- Growth on selective agar media for pathogenic *Neisseria*
- Acid production from carbohydrates

These tests and observations do not always adequately differentiate all the commensal species from one another or from the pathogens. In addition, insufficient test parameters and equivocal carbohydrate reactions have led to confusion between the pathogenic and commensal *Neisseria* spp. Additional tests used to help further differentiate these organisms include the following:

- Growth on nutrient agar at 35° C
- Growth on blood or chocolate agar at 22° C
- Reduction of nitrate and nitrite
- DNase activity

Table 14-7 lists the colonial morphology and primary isolation sites of the *Neisseria* species and related organisms. Table 14-8 lists the traditional and additional tests used to identify the *Neisseria* species and some related genera. The organisms are divided into 3 groups and include the following:

- Group 1: Traditional pathogens
- Group 2: Commensal *Neisseria* species that may grow on selective medium
- Group 3: Commensal *Neisseria* species that do not usually grow on selective medium

Groups 2 and 3 are further divided on the basis of their activities in carbohydrates. Saccharolytic organisms are able to split carbohydrates, whereas asaccharolytic organisms are unable to do so.

Neisseria polysaccharea

N. polysaccharea was first described by a group of French investigators in 1974, who isolated the organism from throats of healthy children while conducting meningococcal carriage rate surveys.

TABLE 14-7

Colonial Morphology and Primary Isolation Sites of Neisseria *and Related Organisms*

Organism	Colonial Morphology*	Primary Isolation Sites
N. gonorrhoeae	Small (0.5-1.0 mm), grayish white, translucent, raised with entire edge Usually easily emulsified Smaller than *N. meningitidis* Up to 5 different colonial morphologies from primary culture	Male: urethra Female: endocervix Laboratory should be notified about looking for this organism from other sites so appropriate media can be used
N. meningitidis	1-2 mm, bluish gray (serogroup B may be yellowish) Serogroup A & C may be mucoid. translucent, convex with smooth glistening surface, and may be greenish cast in agar around colonies Usually easily emulsified	Nasopharynx and oropharynx (carriers) Spinal fluid: meningitis Blood: meningococcemia Lower respiratory tract: meningococcal pneumonia
N. polysaccharea	Small, gray (sometimes yellowish) translucent, raised Resembles *N. gonorrhoeae* colony	Nasopharynx of infants and children
N. lactamica	Small, grayish white (often with a yellow ring), translucent slightly butyrous Resembles *N. meningitidis* but smaller	Nasopharynx of infants and children Rarely found in adults
N. cinerea	Small (1.0-1.5 mm), grayish white, translucent, raised with entire edge and slightly granular Resembles *N. gonorrhoeae*	Nasopharynx
K. denitrificans	Small (≤0.5 mm), gray, semitransparent, convex, may pit the agar Colonial morphology of those that do not pit the agar similar to *N. gonorrhoeae*	Upper respiratory tract
M. catarrhalis	3-5 mm, grayish white, opaque 48-hr colony may have elevated center, thinner wave-like periphery (wagon wheel) Often granular, difficult to emulsify Colony can be swept across plate intact (hockey puck)	Upper respiratory tract
N. mucosa	Large (up to 4 mm), grayish to buff yellow, translucent and mucoid, smooth surface, entire edge Viscous (sticky) consistency	Nasopharynx
N. sicca	Large (up to 3 mm), grayish white, opaque, deeply wrinkled, dry, irregular (bread crumb) colony Firmly adherent, difficult to impossible to emulsify	Nasopharynx, saliva, sputum
N. subflava biovars	0.5-2 mm, pale greenish yellow to yellow, smooth surface with entire edge Often adherent	Nasooropharynx
N. flavescens	Colonies similar to *N. meningitidis* but with golden yellow pigment	Pharynx (not often isolated from clinical specimens)
N. elongata	Large (up to 3 mm), grayish white with yellowish tinge, low convex to almost flat Corroding of agar may occur Clay-like colony, difficult to emulsify	Nasopharynx
N. weaveri	Small, semiopaque with a smooth appearance	Wounds from dog bites

*On chocolate agar at 24 to 48 hours.

The organism produces large amounts of extracellular polysaccharide when grown in media containing 1% or 5% sucrose; thus the species name, polysaccharea. *N. polysaccharea's* colonial morphology and carbohydrate utilization (glucose and maltose; but rarely sucrose positive) have led to its misidentification as the pathogenic *N. meningitidis*. Differential tests to separate *N. polysaccharea* from *N. meningitidis* are ability to grow on nutrient agar at 35° C and production of polysaccharide from 1% or 5% sucrose (see Table 14-8). Additional differential tests to separate *N. polysaccharea* from *N. subflava* biovar *subflava* (refer to Table 14-8) are growth on blood or chocolate agar

TABLE 14-8
Differential Tests for Commensal Neisseria and Related Genera

Organism	Growth on ML, MTM or NYC	Traditional Tests		Acid Produced From					Additional Tests		Reduction of		
		Catalase	Oxidase	Glucose	Maltose	Lactose (ONPG)	Sucrose	Fructose	Growth on Blood or Chocolate Agar at 22°C	Growth on Nutrient Agar at 35°C	Nitrate	Nitrite	DNase
Group 1: Traditional pathogens													
N. gonorrhoeae	+	+	+	+	−	−	−	−	−	−	−	−	−
N. meningitidis	+	+	+	+	+	−	−	−	−	−	−	V	−
Group 2: Commensal species—possible growth on selective agar media													
Saccharolytic													
K. denitrificans	V	−	+	(+)	−	−	−	−	+	+	+	V	−
N. lactamica	+	+	+	+	+	+	−	−	V	+	−	V	−
N. polysaccharea	+	+	+	+	+	−	V	−	−	+	−	V	−
Asaccharolytic													
N. cinerea	V	+	+	−	−	−	−	−	−	+	−	+	−
M. catarrhalis	V	+	+	−	−	−	−	−	V	+	+	+	+
Group 3: Commensal species—no growth on selective agar media													
Saccharolytic													
N. mucosa	−	+	+	+	+	−	+	+	+	+	+	+	−
N. sicca	−	+	+	+	+	−	+	+	+	+	−	+	−
N. subflava biovars:													
subflava	−	+	+	+	+	−	−	−	+	+	−	V	−
flava	−	+	+	+	+	+	−	+	+	+	−	V	−
perflava	−	+	+	+	+	−	+	+	+	+	−	V	−
Asaccharolytic													
N. flavescens	−	+	+	−	−	−	−	−	+	+	−	+	−
N. elongata	−	−	+	−	−	−	−	−	+	+	−	+	−
N. weaveri	−	+	+	−	−	−	−	−	+	+	−	+	−

+, Positive; −, negative; (+), positive (delayed); *V*, variable; *ML*, Martin-Lewis agar; *MTM*, modified Thayer-Martin agar; *NYC*, New York City medium.

at 22° C and lack of yellow pigment production (see Table 14-7).

Neisseria cinerea

N. cinerea was first described in 1906 but subsequently misclassified as a subtype of *M. catarrhalis* *(Neisseria pseudocatarrhalis)*. It was called *N. cinerea* in 1939. The organism has received considerable attention in the past 10 years because of its misidentification as *N. gonorrhoeae* in some commercial identification systems. Although *N. cinerea* is glucose negative in CTA sugars, in some commercial kits the glucose was read as positive, making it biochemically identical to *N. gonorrhoeae*. The colonial morphology of this organism is also similar to the T3 colonies of *N. gonorrhoeae* (Figure 14-14). Useful tests for differentiation of *N. cinerea* from *M. catarrhalis* are reduction of nitrate and negative DNase reaction (see Table 14-8). Useful observation for differentiation from *N. flavescens* is lack of yellow pigment production (see Table 14-7).

Kingella denitrificans

CDC first described *K. denitrificans* in 1972 and gave it the designation TM-1 because of its isolation from throat cultures plated on Thayer-Martin medium in carrier surveys of *N. meningitidis* and *N. lactamica*. In 1976, it was placed in the genus *Kingella* and given the species name *denitrificans* because of its ability to reduce nitrate. This organism is normal flora in the upper respiratory tract and rarely causes disease, although endocarditis due to it have been reported. *Kingella* species colonial mor-

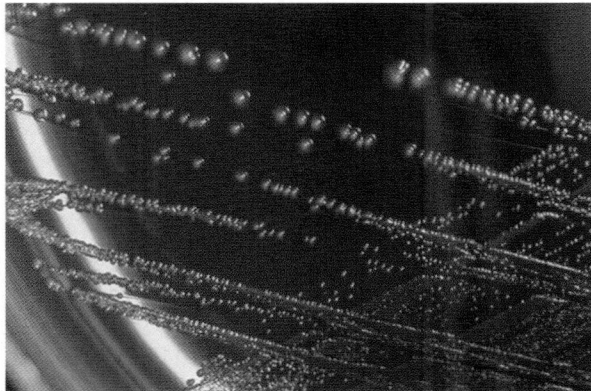

Figure 14-14 ─────────────────────

Colonial morphology of *Neisseria cinerea* on blood agar (48-hour culture).

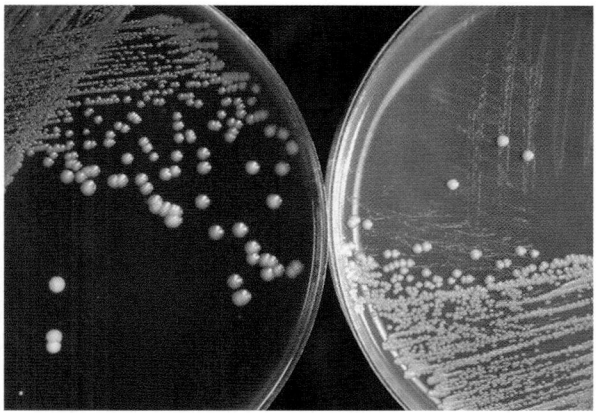

Figure 14-15 ─────────────────────

Culture of *Neisseria lactamica* after 48 hours on blood agar *(left)* and chocolate agar *(right)*. This organism resembles *Neisseria meningitidis.*

phology (if it does not pit the agar) and carbohydrate utilization (only glucose positive) have led to its misidentification as a pathogenic *Neisseria* *(N. gonorrhoeae)*. The Gram stain is the most definitive differential test to separate these organisms. Although *Kingella* species is a gram-negative rod, at times coccoidal forms may predominate, and the penicillin disk test discussed earlier will reveal its true rod form. Additional differential tests include negative catalase reaction, ability to grow on agar medium at various temperatures, and reduction of nitrate (see Table 14-8).

Neisseria lactamica

N. lactamica was reported as early as 1934 but did not become widely recognized as being separate from *N. meningitidis* until 1968. It is commonly found in the nasopharynx of infants and children and, like *N. polysaccharea,* is commonly encountered in meningococcal carrier surveys. The carriage rate of this species in children appears to peak at about 2 years of age and to steadily decline from there. It is rarely isolated from adults. It is the only *Neisseria* species that uses lactose; thus its species designation, *lactamica.*

N. lactamica can be misidentified as *N. meningitidis* because of its similar colony morphology (a little smaller), its carbohydrate reactions (glucose, maltose, but rarely sucrose positive), and some cross-reaction with meningococcal typing sera (Figure 14-15). The definitive test for differentiation from

N. meningitidis and all other *Neisseria* species is use of lactose or positive ONPG reaction.

Neisseria mucosa

The colonies of *N. mucosa* are large, often adherent to the agar, and very mucoid, giving the species its name. It is usually isolated from the nasopharynx of children or young adults. It has also been isolated from the airways of dolphins. This organism has been documented to cause pneumonia in children. It has the same carbohydrate pattern as *Neisseria sicca* and *N. subflava* biovar *perflava,* but differs from these species in its ability to reduce nitrite to nitrogen gas, its colonial morphology, and its lack of pigment production (see Tables 14-7 and 14-8).

Neisseria sicca

The colonies of *N. sicca* are usually dry, wrinkled, adherent, and "breadcrumb like" (see Table 14-7 and Figure 14-16). The word *sicca* in Latin means "dry." *N. sicca* and *N. subflava* biovar *perflava* are usually the two most common *Neisseria* species found in the respiratory tract of adults. Differentiation of this organism from *N. mucosa* and *N. subflava* biovar *perflava* has been discussed (see "*N. mucosa*").

Neisseria subflava

N. subflava's species name means "less yellow" (Figure 14-17). It consists of three biovars that dif-

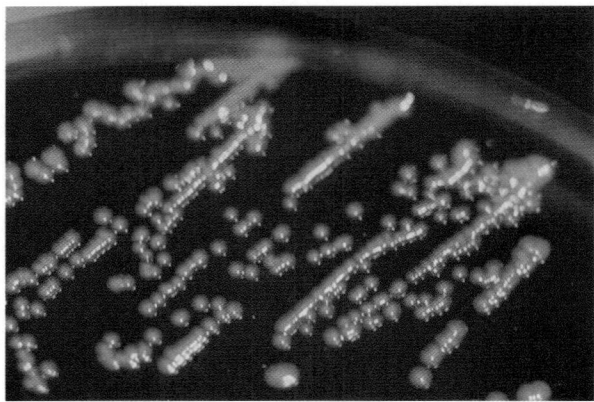

Figure 14-17

Yellow pigmentation of *Neisseria subflava* on blood agar (48-hour culture).

fer from one another by their carbohydrate utilization patterns. Differentiation of this species from *N. polysaccharea* is through its ability to grow on blood or chocolate agar at 22° C.

Neisseria flavescens

N. flavescens (*flavescens* means "yellow") is a yellow-pigmented *Neisseria* species that is asaccharolytic (does not use carbohydrates). It can be differentiated from *N. cinerea* by its ability to grow on blood or chocolate agar at 22° C.

Neisseria elongata

N. elongata is unique among the members of the *Neisseria* species, in that it is a rod and is catalase negative (sometimes weakly positive). It can be differentiated from *K. denitrificans* by its inability to reduce nitrate.

Neisseria weaveri

N. weaveri is also unique among the *Neisseria* species because it is a rod. It is normal oral flora in dogs and can be found in humans in infections caused by dog bites. It is named after Dr. Weaver from CDC because of his extensive research of this organism. It was previously known as CDC group M5 and is catalase positive; it does not produce acid from any of the carbohydrates traditionally used to identify the *Neisseria* species. *N. weaveri* does not reduce nitrate but does reduce nitrite to gas. This organism is usually sensitive to penicillin.

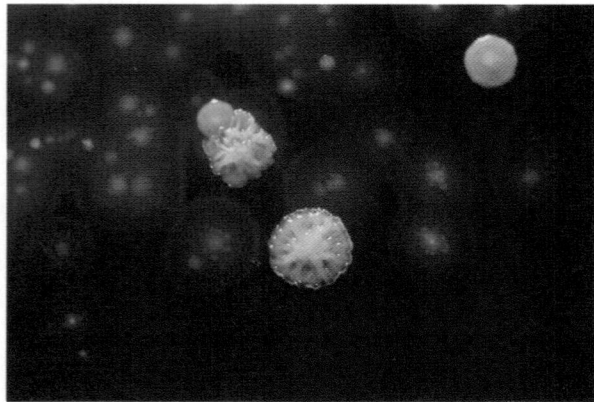

Figure 14-16

Dry, wrinkled breadcrumb-like colonial morphology of *Neisseria sicca* on blood agar (48-hour culture).

Bibliography

Neisseria species and *Moraxella catarrhalis.* In Koneman EW et al editors: *Color atlas and textbook of diagnostic microbiology,* ed 5, Philadelphia 1997, Lippincott.

Carroll KC, Aldeen WE et al: Evaluation of the Abbott LCx ligase chain reaction assay for detection of *Chlamydia trachomatis* and *Neisseria gonorrhoeae* in urine and genital swab specimens from a sexually transmitted disease clinic population, *J Clin Microbiol* 36(6):1630, 1998.

Chapin-Robertson K, Reece ES, Edberg SC: Evaluation of the Gen-Probe Pace II assay for the direct detection of *Neisseria gonorrhoeae* in endocervical specimens, *Diagn Microbiol Infect Dis* 15:645, 1992.

Dillon JR, Carballo M, Pauze M: Evaluation of eight methods for identification of pathogenic *Neisseria* species: Neisseria-Kwik, RIM-N, Gonobio-Test, Minitek, Gonochek II, Gonogen, Phadebact Monoclonal GC OMNI Test, and Syva MicroTrak Test, *J Clin Microbiol* 26:493, 1988.

Dolter J, Bryant L, Janda JM: Evaluation of five rapid systems for the identification of *Neisseria gonorrhoeae* in urogenital samples, *Diagn Microbiol Infect Dis* 13:217, 1990.

Granato PA, Franz MR: Use of the Gen-Probe PACE system for the detection of *Neisseria gonorrhoeae* in urogenital samples, *Diagn Microbiol Infect Dis* 13:217, 1990.

Holmes B, Costas M, On SLW et al: *Neisseria weaveri* sp. nov. (formerly CDC group M-5 from dog bite wounds of humans), *Int J Syst Bacteriol* 43:687-693, 1993.

Judson FN: Gonorrhea, *Med Clin North Am* 74:1353, 1990.

Judson FN: Management of antibiotic resistant *Neisseria gonorrhoeae,* *Ann Intern Med* 110:5, 1989.

Knapp JS: Historical perspectives and identification of *Neisseria* and related species, *Clin Microbiol Rev* 1:415, 1988.

Knapp JS, Rice RJ: *Neisseria* and *Branhamella.* In Murray PR et al: *Manual of clinical microbiology,* ed 6, Washington, DC, 1995, American Society for Microbiology.

National Committee for Clinical Laboratory Standards: *Performance standards for antimicrobial susceptibility,* ed 6, Villanova, Pa, 1997, National Committee for Clinical Laboratory Standards.

National Committee for Clinical Laboratory Standards: *Performance standards for antimicrobial susceptibility testing,* Villanova, Pa, 1998, National Committee for Clinical Laboratory Standards (supplement).

Panke ES, Yang LI et al: Comparison of Gen-Probe DNA probe test and culture for the detection of *Neisseria gonorrhoeae* in endocervical specimens, *J Clin Microbiol* 29:883, 1991.

St. Louis ME et al: HIV prevention through early detection and treatment of other sexually transmitted diseases—United States, *Morbid Mortal Weekly Rep* 47:1-24, 1998.

Welch WD, Cartwright G: Fluorescent monoclonal antibody compared with carbohydrate utilization for rapid identification of *Neisseria gonorrhoeae,* *J Clin Microbiol* 26:293, 1988.

Whittington WL, Knapp JS: Trends in resistance of *Neisseria gonorrhoeae* to antimicrobial agents in the United States, *Sex Transm Dis* 15:202, 1988.

Whittington WL, Rice RJ et al: Incorrect identification of *Neisseria gonorrhoeae* from infants and children, *Pediatr Infect Dis J* 7:3, 1988.

LEARNING ASSESSMENT

1. Why did the cultures from the patient in the case study fail to produce growth?

2. What organism or organisms should be considered as a possible cause of the arthritis in this patient?

3. What serogroup of *N. meningitidis* is most prevalent in the United States?

4. Why is vaccine against *N. meningitidis* not routinely used in the United States?

5. What complications may likely result from *N. gonorrhoeae* infection if it remains untreated?

6. Is *M. catarrhalis* a significant isolate? Explain.

CHAPTER 15

Haemophilus and Other Fastidious Gram-Negative Rods

A. *HAEMOPHILUS* SPECIES, HACEK GROUP, *PASTEURELLA*, *BRUCELLA*, AND *FRANCISELLA* SPECIES

George Manuselis, Jean Barnishan

HAEMOPHILUS SPECIES
  General Characteristics
  Haemophilus influenzae
    Historical perspective
    Virulence factors
    Clinical manifestations of *Haemophilus influenzae* infections
  Infections Associated with Other *Haemophilus* Species
  Laboratory Diagnosis
    Specimen processing and isolation
    Microscopic morphology
    Colony morphology
    Laboratory identification
  Treatment

HACEK GROUP AND *CAPNOCYTOPHAGA* SPECIES
  Haemophilus aphrophilus
  Actinobacillus actinomycetemcomitans
  Cardiobacterium hominis
  Eikenella corrodens
  Kingella Species
  Capnocytophaga Species

PASTEURELLA SPECIES
  General Characteristics
  Pasteurella multocida

BRUCELLA SPECIES
  General Characteristics

FRANCISELLA SPECIES
  Francisella tularensis

OBJECTIVES

1. Characterize each of the bacterial species mentioned in this chapter by morphology, habitat, and nutritional requirements.
2. Describe the modes of transmission of each of the organisms characterized.
3. Explain the clinical significance of these organisms when isolated in the clinical laboratory.
4. Name the appropriate specimens for the recovery of these organisms.
5. Determine the appropriate culture media required to isolate each of the organisms.
6. Describe the microscopic and colonial morphology.
7. Describe the methods of identification currently used to diagnose infections caused by these organisms.

KEY TERMS

X factor (hemin)
V factor (NAD)
Satellitism
Encapsulated
Nonencapsulated
"Pinkeye"
Chancroid

Buboes
"School of fish"
Porphyrin
δ-Aminolevulinic acid
  (ALA)
HACEK

CASE STUDY

A 2-year-old unvaccinated child was seen in the emergency room with headache and fever. The spinal fluid was sent to the lab for culture and sensitivity. The Gram stain showed many white blood cells and many gram-negative rods (small).

This chapter describes miscellaneous gram-negative bacilli that are fastidious. Most of these organisms require special nutrients and environmental growth factors for isolation and identification.

The organisms to be covered in this chapter include the following genera:

- *Haemophilus*
- HACEK
- *Legionella*
- *Bordetella*
- *Pasteurella*
- *Brucella*
- *Francisella*

Two of the genera, *Haemophilus* and *Pasteurella,* belong to the family Pasteurellaceae. Characteris-

tically, members of Pasteurellaceae are gram-negative, pleomorphic, coccoid to rod-shaped cells that are nonmotile and aerobic or facultatively anaerobic, form nitrites from nitrates, and are oxidase and catalase positive.

The genera *Pasteurella, Brucella,* and *Francisella* are etiologic agents of true zoonotic infections.

Legionella species are facultative intracellular parasites that have a wide range of pathogenic potential in humans. *Legionella pneumophila,* the most common isolated species, gained immediate notoriety as the causative agent of a relatively fatal respiratory infection at the 1976 American Legion Convention in Philadelphia. The new family, Legionellaceae, and the new genus, *Legionella,* were named after this famous outbreak.

Three of the four recognized species of the genus *Bordetella* are associated with human disease. *Bordetella pertussis* and *Bordetella parapertussis* are primary human respiratory pathogens that cause whooping cough or pertussis, and *Bordetella bronchiseptica,* an opportunistic human pathogen, causes pneumonia and wound infections. These three species are implicated mostly in diseases of childhood.

Figure 15-1 depicts the prevalence of some of these fastidious organisms in relation to other gram-negative bacilli found in clinical specimens.

HAEMOPHILUS SPECIES

General Characteristics

The genus *Haemophilus* consists of gram-negative, pleomorphic coccobacilli or rods that may vary microscopically from small coccobacilli in direct

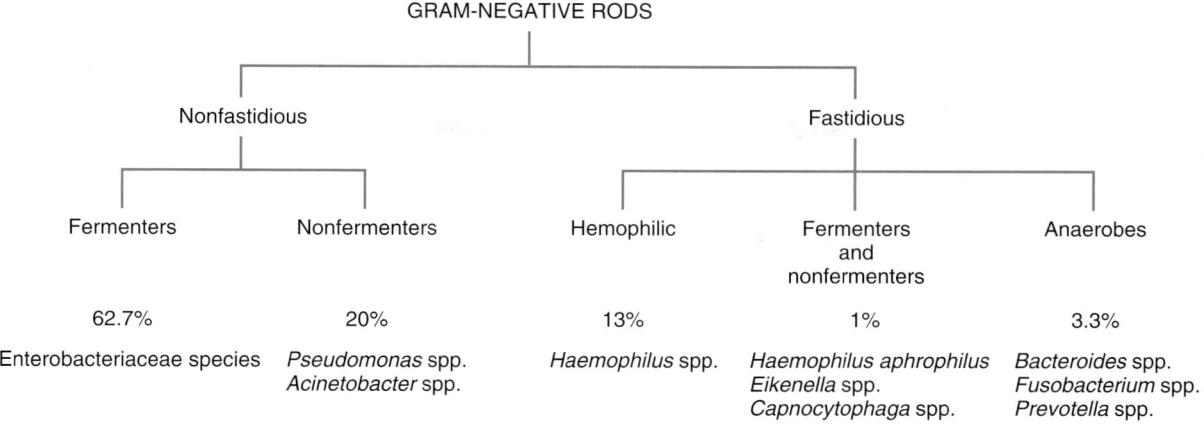

GRAM-NEGATIVE RODS

Nonfastidious		Fastidious		
Fermenters	Nonfermenters	Hemophilic	Fermenters and nonfermenters	Anaerobes
62.7%	20%	13%	1%	3.3%
Enterobacteriaceae species	*Pseudomonas* spp. *Acinetobacter* spp.	*Haemophilus* spp.	*Haemophilus aphrophilus* *Eikenella* spp. *Capnocytophaga* spp.	*Bacteroides* spp. *Fusobacterium* spp. *Prevotella* spp.

Figure 15-1

Prevalence of gram-negative rods isolated from cultures in a large tertiary hospital. Data on *Pasteurella, Brucella, Legionella,* and *Bordetella* are not included. (Data from Clinical Microbiology Laboratory, OSU Medical Center, 1992-1994.)

smears of clinical material to long filaments occasionally seen in smears of colony growth. They are nonmotile and aerobic or facultatively anaerobic, ferment carbohydrates, are generally oxidase and catalase positive, reduce nitrates to nitrites, and are obligate parasites on the mucous membranes of humans and animals.

In accordance with *Bergey's Manual of Systematic Bacteriology,* 10 species of *Haemophilus* are associated with humans: *Haemophilus influenzae, Haemophilus parainfluenzae, Haemophilus haemolyticus, Haemophilus parahaemolyticus, Haemophilus aphrophilus, Haemophilus paraphrophilus, Haemophilus paraphrohaemolyticus, Haemophilus aegyptius, Haemophilus segnis,* and *Haemophilus ducreyi.* In addition, six species are associated with animals and three species of uncertain status. Most members of the genus are nonpathogenic or produce opportunistic infections. Therefore the emphasis of this section is on the major pathogenic species, *H. influenzae, H. aegyptius,* and *H. ducreyi.*

The genus name *Haemophilus* is derived from the Greek words meaning "blood-lover." As the name implies, *Haemophilus* organisms require preformed growth factors present in blood: **X factor** (hemin, hematin) and/or **V factor** (nicotinamide-adenine dinucleotide [NAD]). Traditionally, a small, gram-negative bacillus (coccobacillus) is assigned to this genus, based on its requirements for the X and/or V factor. Species with the prefix *para-* require V factor only for growth. In addition, the pro-duction of hemolysis on 5% horse's or rabbit's blood agar is an important differential characteristic. Although certain species are also hemolytic on a sheep's blood agar plate, the organisms will not grow in pure culture on this medium.

Both X and V factors are found within red blood cells and are important for in vitro growth. Most laboratories use blood agar containing sheep erythrocytes prepared by commercial sources. Only X factor is directly available in this medium. *Haemophilus* species that are V factor dependent do not grow because the red cells are still intact and the sheep blood contains enzymes (NADases) that hydrolyze V factor. To alleviate this problem most clinical laboratories use chocolate agar to facilitate the recovery of *Haemophilus* species from clinical specimens. The lysing of the red cells by heat in the preparation of chocolate agar releases both X and the V growth factors and inactivates the enzymes that hydrolyze V factor.

A phenomenon that helps in the recognition of *Haemophilus* species that require V factor is satellitism. **Satellitism** occurs when an organism such as *Staphylococcus aureus, Streptococcus pneumoniae,* or *Neisseria* species produces V factor (NAD) as a byproduct of its metabolism. The *Haemophilus* organisms isolate obtains X factor from the sheep's blood agar and V factor from one of these organisms. On sheep's blood agar plate, tiny colonies of *Haemophilus* organisms may be seen growing or engaging in "satellitism" around the V factor—producing organism. Figure 15-2 illustrates *H. in-*

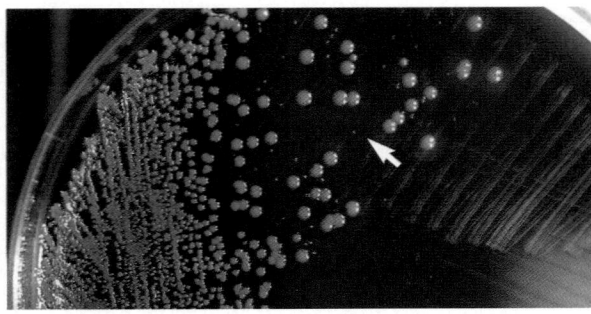

Figure 15-2

Haemophilus influenzae satellitism around and between the large, white, hemolytic staphylococci. The small, gray, glistening colony is *H. influenzae.*

fluenzae satellitism around colonies of *S. aureus.* Except for *H. aphrophilus* and *H. ducreyi,* all clinically significant *Haemophilus* species require V factor for growth and display this unusual growth pattern.

The indigenous flora of the healthy upper respiratory tract consists of many different genera and species of organisms (see Chapter 26). Approximately 10% of this normal bacterial flora in adults consists of *Haemophilus* spp., with the majority of the organisms being *H. parainfluenzae* and nonencapsulated *H. influenzae.* Of the two, *H. parainfluenzae* is the predominant species.

Colonization trends begin in infancy with **encapsulated** strains and average 2% to 6% throughout childhood. In selected populations, such as children who attend day care centers, colonization may reach as high as 60%. **Nonencapsulated** strains of *H. influenzae* in healthy children average 2% of the normal bacterial flora.

Haemophilus influenzae
Historical perspective
Influenza, commonly referred to as the "flu," is a viral infectious disease characterized by acute inflammation of the upper airways. Symptoms often progress to intense inflammation of the mucous membranes lining the nose (coryza), headache, bronchitis, and severe generalized muscle pain (myalgias).

Haemophilus influenzae was named erroneously from the influenza pandemic that ravaged the world between 1889 and 1890. The basis for this assumption was the frequent isolation of this bacillus from the nasopharynx of influenza patients and from postmortem lung cultures. After viral culture

techniques became available, it became apparent that the disease influenza was caused by a virus and that the actual role of *H. influenzae* was that of a secondary invader.

Virulence factors
H. influenzae, the major clinical pathogen of the species, has a wide range of pathogenic potential. The following virulence factors may play a role in the invasiveness of this organism and in the initiation of infection:

- Capsule
- IgA proteases
- Outer membrane proteins and lipo-oligosaccharide (LOS)
- Adherence

Capsule Of all the potential virulence factors, the capsule, if present, plays the most significant role. The serologic grouping of *H. influenzae* into six serotypes, a, b, c, d, e, and f, is based on the capsular polysaccharide. Most invasive infections caused by encapsulated strains of *H. influenzae* belong to capsular serotype b (Hib) and occur primarily in young children. In contrast with the other serotypes, a, c, d, e, and f, the serotype b capsule is a unique polymer composed of ribose, ribitol, and phosphate. The capsule plays a significant role in the pathogenesis of invasive disease. Scientific evidence suggests that the antiphagocytic property and anticomplementary activity of the type b capsule are important factors in virulence.

Not all strains of *H. influenzae* are encapsulated. Therefore two patterns of disease attributed to *H. influenzae* emerge. The first is invasive disease caused by encapsulated (typable) strains predominantly of serotype b in which bacteremia (hematogenous spread) plays a significant role. The second pattern of disease is a more localized infection caused by the contiguous spread of nonencapsulated (nontypable) strains and occurs within or in close proximity to the respiratory tract. Examples of invasive disease include meningitis, cellulitis, arthritis, and epiglottitis, which are found in the pediatric population. Examples of localized infection include pneumonia and sinusitis, which occur primarily in the adult population.

Exceptions to the encapsulated and nonencapsulated categorizations and to whether these organisms appear in the adult or pediatric population do occur. Nonencapsulated strains can cause meningitis in the adult population, especially in the immunocompromised or debilitated person, and can cause neonatal sepsis and invasive lower respiratory tract infections in children.

The other serotypes, a, c, d, e, and f, rarely cause disease in humans. Reports of infections with these serotypes have included pneumonia and bacteremia caused by serotypes a, d, and f in immunocompromised adults, and neonatal sepsis caused by serotype c.

IgA proteases Secretory IgA is present on human mucosal surfaces in organ system areas for which *H. influenzae* has a predilection. Of all the species of *Haemophilus, H. influenzae* is the only one that produces this enzyme. Because this enzyme has the ability to cleave secretory IgA, its production may contribute to the organism's virulence potential.

Adherence The role of adherence as a virulence factor is not well defined. Studies indicate that most nonencapsulated strains are adherent to human epithelial cells, whereas most serotype b strains are not. The lack of this adherent capability in type b organisms may explain the tendency for type b strains to cause systemic infections. The presence of this adherent capability by nonencapsulated strains may explain the tendency for these strains to cause more localized infections.

Outer membrane components and LOS Although the role of these antigens is not well defined, antibody directed against these antigens may play a significant role in human immunity. Each one of these components may be responsible for a specific capability, such as invasiveness, attachment, and antiphagocytic function. LOS has been shown to have a paralyzing effect on the sweeping motion of ciliated respiratory epithelium.

Clinical manifestations of *Haemophilus influenzae* infections

INFECTIONS CAUSED BY ENCAPSULATED (TYPABLE) STRAINS

Meningitis Until recently serotype b has been a common cause of pediatric meningitis in children between the ages of 3 months and 6 years. Blood stream invasion and bacteremic spread follow colonization, invasion, and replication of this organism in the respiratory mucous membranes. Headache, stiff neck, and other meningeal signs are usually preceded by mild respiratory disease.

Epiglottitis Serotype b is the most common cause of this syndrome. The manifestations include rapid onset, acute inflammation, and intense edema that may cause complete airway obstruction, requiring an emergency tracheostomy. The peak incidence in children occurs between the ages of 2 and 4 years.

Arthritis The bacteremic spread of serotype b is the most common cause of arthritis seen in children younger than 2 years of age.

Cellulitis Serotype b is the usual culprit in cases of cellulitis in children younger than 2 years of age. The most common infected site is the cheek, although infection may occur in other areas of the upper extremities. Cellulitis of the cheek is characterized by rapid onset, pain, edema, and a reddish-blue color on the inflamed area. Pediatricians usually diagnose the disease based on the age of the child, symptoms, appearance, and proximity of the cellulitis to the oral mucosa.

Other infections caused by typable strains include acute pharyngitis and pneumonia. Pneumonia in children is usually caused by Hib. The mean age at infection is approximately 14 months.

With the advent of the Hib vaccine, pediatric hospital laboratories are reporting a significant decrease in invasive disease among children. It still remains a problem in the elderly and debilitated population who have not been vaccinated.

INFECTIONS CAUSED BY NONENCAPSULATED (NONTYPABLE) STRAINS

Infections usually caused by nontypable strains of *H. influenzae* include otitis media, bronchitis, sinusitis, pneumonia in elderly patients, and genital tract infections. Table 15-1 summarizes infections caused by *H. influenzae* in different population groups.

Infections Associated with Other *Haemophilus* Species

Haemophilus aegyptius is a species that is genetically similar to *H. influenzae*. Because of their similar identifying characteristics, it is difficult to differentiate *H. influenzae* from *H. aegyptius* in the clinical laboratory. Formerly a separate species of the genus, *H. aegyptius* is now known as *H. influenzae* biogroup *aegyptius*. Both organisms can cause conjunctivitis in primarily the pediatric population. *H. influenzae* biogroup *aegyptius* causes

TABLE 15-1

Infections Caused by Haemophilus influenzae *in Different Population Groups*

Invasive Type b* Pediatric Population	Nonencapsulated in Pediatric Population	Nonencapsulated in Adult Population
Meningitis 　CSF 50%-95% culture positive 　Blood 50%-95% culture positive Cellulitis 　Skin 75%-90% culture positive 　Blood 50%-75% culture positive Epiglottitis 　Blood 90%-95% culture positive Conjunctivitis 　Eye 50%-75% culture positive 　Blood <10% culture positive	Otitis media 　Tympanocentesis 50%-70% culture positive	Pneumonia, bronchitis 　Sputum 25%-75% culture positive 　Blood 10%-30% culture positive Sinusitis 　Sinus aspirate 50%-75% culture positive

Modified from Murray PR: Pasteurellaceae. In Murray PR, Drew LW, Kobayashi GS, Thompson JH, editors: *Medical microbiology,* St Louis, 1990, Mosby.
*May cause invasive disease in immunocompromised and debilitated adults.

both a more acute, contagious, purulent conjunctivitis, commonly referred to as **"pinkeye,"** and a severe systemic disease known as Brazilian purpuric fever (BPF) in hot climates. BPF is characterized by recurrent or concurrent conjunctivitis, high fever, vomiting, petechiae, purpura, septicemia, and shock. The mortality rate for BPF may reach as high as 70%.

Haemophilus ducreyi is the etiologic agent of **chancroid,** a highly communicable sexually transmitted disease. After an incubation period of approximately 4 to 14 days, a nonindurated, painful lesion with an irregular edge develops, generally on the genitalia or perianal areas. The most common sites of infection are on the penis of males or on the labia or within the vagina of females. Suppurative (forming or discharging pus), enlarged, draining, inguinal lymph nodes **(buboes)** are common in the majority of infected patients (Figure 15-3).

Haemophilus parainfluenzae, H. aphrophilus, and *H. paraphropilus* have a very low incidence of pathogenicity and have been implicated most often as causative agents of endocarditis.

Laboratory Diagnosis
Specimen processing and isolation
Haemophilus species have been associated with many diseases in humans. Almost any specimen submitted for routine bacteriology examination may harbor this organism. Common sources include blood, cerebrospinal fluid, middle-ear exudate, joint fluids, upper and lower respiratory tract specimens, swabs from conjunctivae, vaginal swabs, and abscess drainage. *Haemophilus* species die rapidly in clinical specimens; therefore prompt transportation and processing is vital for the isolation of this organism. This is especially true of genital specimens submitted for *H. ducreyi. H. ducreyi* is extremely fastidious. Specimens from genital sites submitted for the isolation of this organism should first be cleaned with sterile gauze moistened with sterile saline. A cotton swab, premoistened with sterile phosphate-buffered saline (PBS), should then be used to collect material from the base of the ulcer. Processing in the laboratory must take place within 10 minutes of collection for maximum recovery.

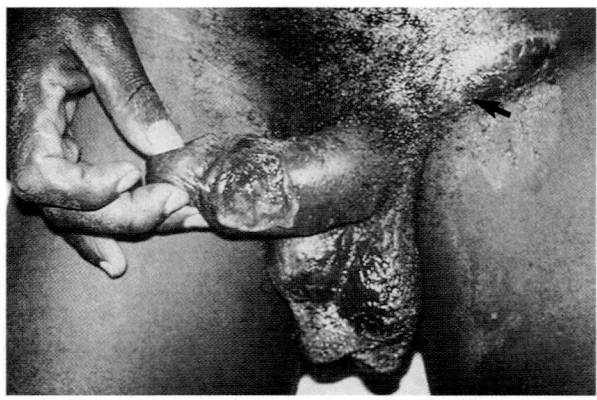

Figure 15-3

Lesions of chancroid on the penis, showing draining buboe *(arrow)* in the adjacent groin area. Chancroid is caused by *Haemophilus ducreyi.*

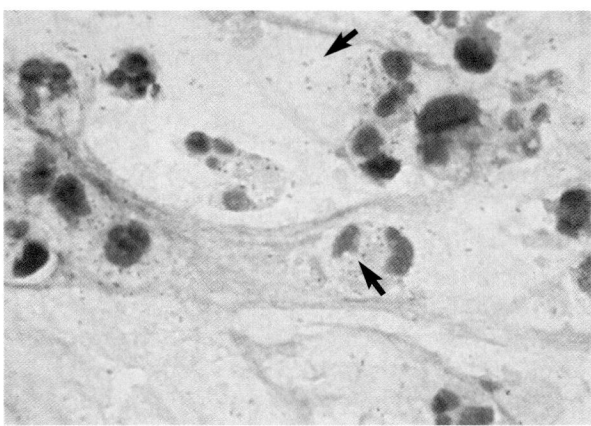

Figure 15-4

Direct smear of *Haemophilus influenzae* in cerebrospinal fluid in a case of meningitis. Note the intracellular and extracellular gram-negative coccobacilli.

It is important to remember that most conventional media do not support the growth of *Haemophilus* species because of the lack of one or more growth factors. When attempting to isolate *H. influenzae,* a common medium to use is chocolate agar incubated between 33° C and 37° C with 5% to 10% carbon dioxide added. Chocolate agar contains both X factor (hemin) and V factor (NAD), which are required growth factors for *H. influenzae.* It has been shown that chocolate agar supplemented with bacitracin (300 mg/L) is an excellent medium for the isolation of *Haemophilus* species from respiratory specimens. The bacitracin is added to reduce overgrowth of normal respiratory flora. Growth on chocolate agar is usually seen after 18 to 24 hours of incubation. However, specimens submitted for *H. ducreyi* should be held for at least 9 days, and specimens for *H. aegyptius* should be held for at least 4 days before reporting a negative result.

Because of their fastidious nature, specimens submitted for *H. ducreyi* and *H. aegyptius* must be plated using special media. For *H. aegyptius,* chocolate agar supplemented with 1% IsoVitaleX (BBL Microbiology Systems, Cockeysville, MD) is required. For *H. ducreyi,* the use of GC agar (GIBCO Laboratories, Grand Island, NY) containing 1% to 2% hemoglobin, 5% fetal calf serum, 10% CVA enrichment, and 3 μg of vancomycin has been proved to be reliable. The use of vancomycin in this media helps reduce commensal flora from genital specimens and allows the visualization of *H. ducreyi.* The culture plates for the recovery of this organism should be incubated in a carbon dioxide atmosphere containing high humidity. High humidity is provided by placing the plates, along with sterile gauze moistened with sterile water, in an open plastic bag ("baggy") in the incubator. Sterile gauze is recommended in lieu of regular nonsterile paper towels to decrease fungal contamination of the plates.

Microscopic morphology

As is common with most of the species of *Haemophilus,* the microscopic morphology varies from a small gram-negative coccobacilli to long filaments. The coccobacillary or small, regular rod microscopic morphology is the more predominant form found in clinical specimens. Encapsulated forms of *H. influenzae* may be observed in Gram-stained direct smears as clear, nonstaining areas ("halos") surrounding the organisms in purulent secretions. Figure 15-4 illustrates the microscopic morphology of *H. influenzae* in a direct smear of cerebrospinal fluid from a patient with meningitis. Figure 15-5 is an example of a Gram stain of an isolated colony of *H. influenzae.*

Gram stains of genital lesions caused by *H. ducreyi* may show gram-negative coccobacilli arranged in groups commonly referred to as the **"school of fish"** formation.

Colony morphology

As mentioned previously (see Chapter 9), most clinical specimens are plated on a variety of culture media and read as a culture set after 24 hours of incubation. Usually blood agar plate, chocolate agar, and MacConkey agar are inoculated simultaneously

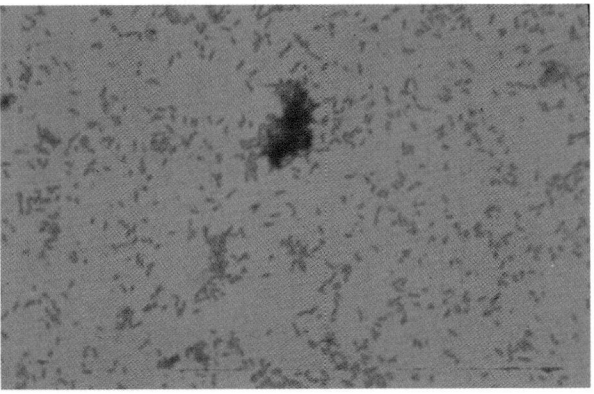

Figure 15-5

Gram stain of a *Haemophilus influenzae* colony. Note the slightly more elongated rods.

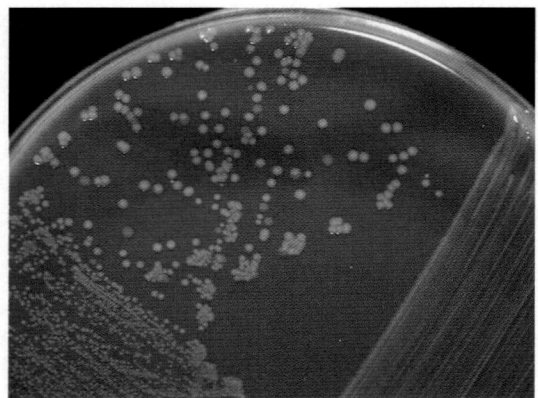

Figure 15-6 —————————————————

Example of *Haemophilus influenzae* growing on CHOC agar. Notice the gray mucoid colonies characteristic of encapsulated strains.

from clinical specimens from areas of the human body where *Haemophilus* organisms may be isolated. Colonies of *Haemophilus* organisms on chocolate agar appear translucent, moist, smooth, and convex, with a distinct "mousy" or "bleach-like" odor. *Haemophilus influenzae* produces a more grayish-appearing colony. Figure 15-6 shows the typical colony morphology of *H. influenzae*. The encapsulated strains grow larger and more mucoid than the nonencapsulated strains.

The first clue that the isolate may belong to the *Haemophilus* group is the growth of gram-negative pleomorphic coccobacilli on chocolate agar, with no growth on sheep's blood agar in pure culture.

Because of their fastidious nature, *Haemophilus* species do not grow on MacConkey agar or other enteric isolation media.

Laboratory identification

Several tests can be used in the clinical laboratory for the identification of *Haemophilus* isolates. These include testing for growth factors (X and V), traditional biochemicals, hemolysis on rabbit's or horse's blood agar, oxidase, and catalase. The porphyrin test is an alternative method for the determination of X factor requirements. In place of traditional biochemicals, several commercial systems can be used to identify and biotype *Haemophilus* species. They include the Minitek System (BBL Microbiology Systems, Cockeysville, MD), the RapID-NH (Innovative Diagnostics, Norcross, GA), HNID (MicroScan, West Sacramento, CA), and NHI (BioMerieux Vitek, Hazelwood, MO). Latex agglutination (Murex Diagnostics, Inc., Norcross, GA; Wampole Laboratories, Cranbury, NJ; BBL Microbiology Systems, Cockeysville, MD) and coagglutination tests (Boule Diagnostics, Huddings, Sweden) have proved to be specific and sensitive in the detection of Hib in cerebrospinal fluid and, to a slightly lesser extent, in other body fluids. Of all the species that require V factor, *H. segnis* is the only organism that is oxidase negative.

Testing for X and V factor requirements using impregnated strips is the traditional approach. This method entails making a suspension of the isolate in trypticase soy broth. Care must be taken not to transfer any X factor–containing media to the broth

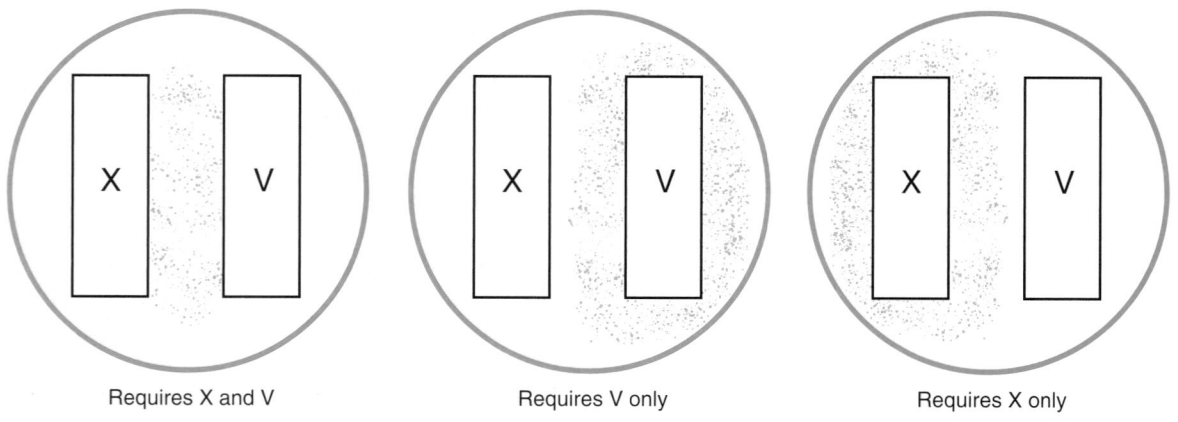

Requires X and V   Requires V only   Requires X only

Figure 15-7 ———

Illustrations of reactions obtained when testing for X and V factor requirements using impregnated strips.

(carryover may produce erroneous or less than definitive results). The organism suspension is then inoculated onto media devoid of X and V factors. Mueller-Hinton agar or trypticase soy agar are acceptable. Allow the plate to dry. Using sterile forceps, place a strip containing X factor on the plate. Press the strip onto the agar using the forceps. Place the V factor strip parallel to the X factor strip approximately 15 mm away. Again, using the forceps, press the V factor strip onto the agar surface. Incubate at 35° C to 37° C in 5% to 10% carbon dioxide for 18 to 24 hours. Observe plates for growth around the strips. Figure 15-7 illustrates the reactions obtained when testing for X and V factor requirements using impregnated strips. Figures 15-8 through 15-10 illustrate the actual identification of unknowns using the impregnated strips. When using this traditional approach it is important to know under what culture conditions the organisms were isolated. *Haemophilus* organisms are facultative anaerobes. When they are grown anaerobically they do not require heme but still require NAD. If a *H. influenzae* organism was incubated anaerobically, it could be misidentified as *H. parainfluenzae*.

The **porphyrin** test is an alternative method for differentiating the heme-producing strains of *Haemophilus* species. The principle of the test is based on the ability of the organism to produce enzymes that convert **δ-aminolevulinic acid (ALA)** into porphyrins or protoporphyrins. Porphobilinogen can be detected by the addition of

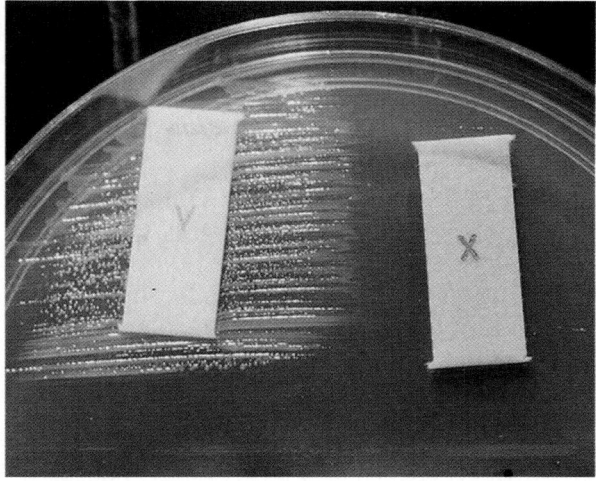

Figure 15-9 _____
This organism is utilizing V factor only. It would be identified as *Haemophilus parainfluenzae*.

p-dimethylaminobenzaldehyde (Kovacs reagent). After the addition of Kovacs reagent, a red color forms in the lower aqueous phase if porphobilinogen is present. Porphyrins can be detected using an ultraviolet light (Wood lamp). Porphyrins fluoresce reddish orange under ultraviolet light. The main advantage of this test is that X factor (heme) is not required; therefore the problem of carryover is eliminated. The disadvantage is that

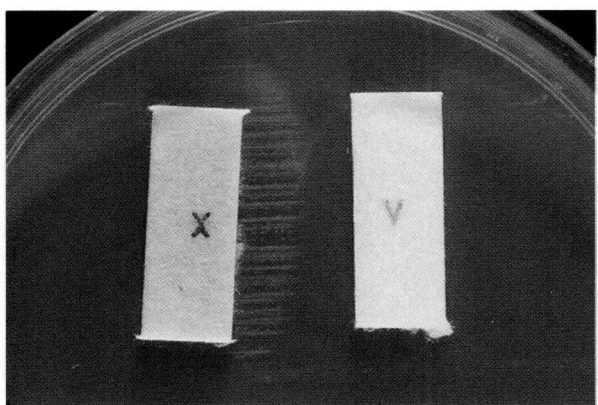

Figure 15-8 _____
This organism would be identified as *Haemophilus influenzae* because it is utilizing both X and V factors.

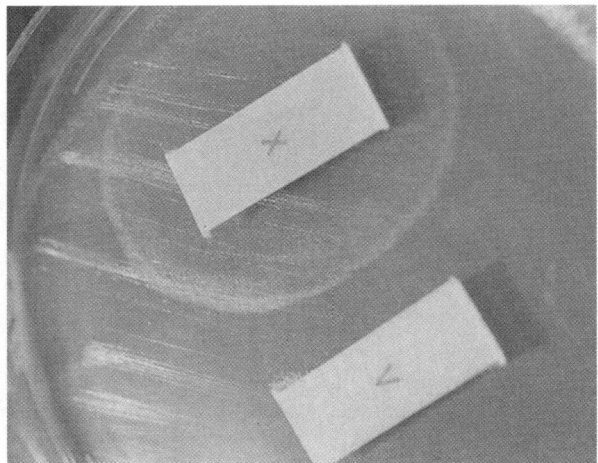

Figure 15-10 _____
This organism is positive for X factor only. The probable species is *Haemophilus aphrophilus* because this species may appear to be hemin dependent on initial isolation.

primary identification is based on a "negative" test result. In the case of *H. influenzae,* the ultraviolet light test is negative (no fluorescence), and after the addition of Kovacs reagent no color change occurs. *Haemophilus* species that can biosynthesize their own heme are porphyrin positive (X strip negative); species that are porphyrin negative cannot synthesize their own heme and therefore are found to be X factor positive when the impregnated strip is used. Figure 15-11 illustrates a positive porphyrin test.

H. aprophilus is not a "true" *Haemophilus* organism because it does not have a strict requirement for X or V factor. It appears at times to be X factor–dependent by impregnated strips (Figure 15-10); but the porphyrin test is positive, meaning *H. aprophilus* can synthesize its own heme. Figure 15-12 is an example of *H. aprophilus* that is not X and/or V factor dependent and is growing all over the trypticase soy agar plate.

Reagents for the porphyrin test can be purchased commercially from Remel Microbiology Products (Lenexa, KS). The ALA Disk is a 1- to 6-hour test that uses ALA reagent impregnated on a filter paper disk. Alternatively, Remel offers a *Haemophilus* Quad Plate, which can be used to identify *Haemophilus* isolates. The Quad Plate contains four zones: X factor only, V factor only, X and V factors, and X and V factors with horse's blood. The *Haemophilus* isolate may be identified based

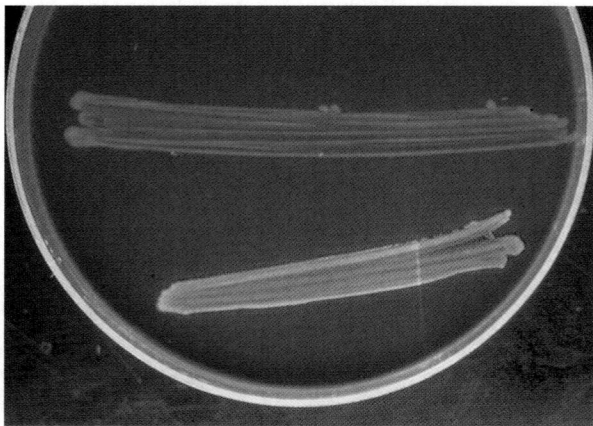

Figure 15-11 _____

Under ultraviolet light, the organism on the bottom is exhibiting a positive porphyrin reaction. The organism on the top is porphyrin negative.

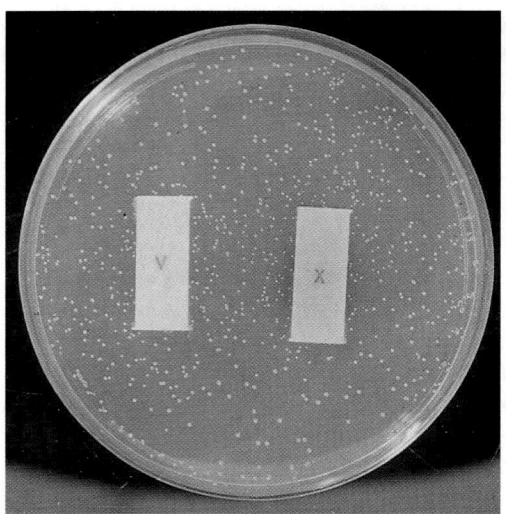

Figure 15-12 _____

A *Haemophilus aprophilus* organism that is not X factor—dependent and is growing all over the trypticase soy agar plate.

on the factor(s) required for growth and the presence of hemolysis.

Table 15-2 lists the differential tests for *Haemophilus* species. Table 15-3 lists the differential tests for *Haemophilus* biogroups.

Treatment

The current recommended treatment of life-threatening illness caused by *H. influenzae* is cefotaxime, ceftriaxone, or cefuroxime. Alternative drugs include trimethoprim-sulfamethoxazole, imipenem, and ciprofloxacin. Also effective is chloramphenicol. Because of the increased resistance to ampicillin, and the possibility of resistance to chloramphenicol, combination therapy with ampicillin and chloramphenicol may also be used for initial therapy. Non–life-threatening *H. influenzae* infection may be treated with amoxicillin-clavulanate, an oral second- or third-generation cephalosporin, trimethoprim-sulfamethoxazole, or ampicillin-sulbactam. For the treatment of *H. ducreyi,* erythromycin, ceftriaxone, or a fluoro-quinolone is recommended. Infections with *H. aprophilus* can be treated with penicillin and gentamicin, or cephalothin and gentamicin.

Because of increased resistance to ampicillin by *Haemophilus* species due to enzyme production (β-lactamase) or, to a lesser extent, altered

TABLE 15-2

Differential Tests for Haemophilus *Species*

	Oxidase	Catalase	Hemolysis (Horse, Rabbit Blood)	Carbon Dioxide Enhances Growth	TSI	Glucose	Pyruvate	Sucrose	Mannose	Fructose	Mannitol	Maltose	Xylose	Lactose	Nitrate	Esculin	Ornithine	Indole	Urea
Factor X+, V+, Porphyrin−																			
H. influenzae	+	+	−	−	NG	+	+	−	−	V	−	−	+	−	+	−	See biotype chart		
H. influenzae ssp.	+	+	−	−	NG	V	+	−	−	V	−	−	+	−	+	−	−	−	+
H. haemolyticus	+	+	+	−	NG	+	−	−	−	V	−	−	V	−	+	−	−	V	+
Factor X−, V+, Porphyrin+																			
H. parainfluenzae	+	V	−	V	NG	+	−	+	V	+	−	+	−	−	+	−	+		
H. segnis	−	V	−	−	NG	W	−	W	−	W	−	W	−	−	+	−	See biotype chart		
H. paraphrophilus	+	−	−	+	A/A	+	−	+	+	+	−	+	V	+	+	−	−	−	−
H. parahaemolyticus	+	V	+	−	NG	+	−	+	−	+	−	+	−	−	+	−	V	−	+
H. paraphrohaemolyticus	+	+	+	+	A/A	+	−	+	−	+	−	+	−	−	+	−	−	−	+
Factor X+, V−, Porphyrin−																			
H. ducreyi	−	−	+/−	+/−	NG	−	−	−	−	−	−	−	−	−	+	−	+		
Factor X−, V−, Porphyrin+																			
H. aphrophilus*	+/−	−	−	+	A/A	+	V	+	V	+	−	+	−	+	+	−	−	−	−

V, Variable; W, weak reaction; A, acid; −, + = 90% or greater; NG, no growth +/−, more positive than negative.
*On initial isolation, may appear to be hemin dependent.

TABLE 15-3

Differential Tests for Haemophilus *Biogroups*

Haemophilus Biogroups	Ornithine	Indole	Urea	Distribution of Biotypes			
				Meningitis and Epiglottitis	Ear Infection	Conjunctivitis	Upper Respiratory Tract
H. influenzae							
Biotype I	+	+	+	••••	••	•	•
Biotype II	−	+	+	•	••	••	•
Biotype III	−	−	+	•	•	••	•
Biotype IV	+	−	+	•	•	•	•
Biotype V	+	+	−	•	•	•	•
Biotype VI	+	−	−	•	•	•	•
Biotype VII	−	+	−	•	•	•	•
Biotype VIII	−	−	−	•	•	•	•
H. parainfluenzae							
Biotype I	+	−	−				
Biotype II	+	−	+				
Biotype III	−	−	+				

−, + = 90% or greater; • = 0%-25%; •• = 26%-50%; ••• = 51%-75%; •••• = 76%-100%.

penicillin binding proteins, several rapid tests to detect β-lactamase production are available, including the chromogenic cephalosporin and acidometric tests.

Either the chromogenic cephalosporin test (Cefinase, Becton-Dickinson, Cockeysville, MD) or the acidometric (Beta-Test, Medical Wire and Equipment Co., Wiltshire, England) can be used. A positive β-lactamase test means that the *Haemophilus* species is resistant to ampicillin and amoxicillin.

In the chromogenic cephalosporin test, a disk impregnated with Cefinase is moistened with one drop of water. Using a sterile loop, smear several colonies onto the disk surface, or use forceps to wipe the moistened disk across the colonies. If the β-lactam ring of the Cefinase is broken by the enzyme, a color reaction occurs. A positive result is a red color on the area where the culture was applied. The reaction occurs usually within 5 minutes.

In the acidometric test, a strip impregnated with benzylpenicillin, and a pH indicator, bromcresol purple, is moistened with one or two drops of sterile distilled water. Using a sterile loop, several colonies are smeared onto the test strip. If the β-lactamase ring of the benzylpenicillin is broken by the enzyme, penicilloic acid is formed, causing a drop in pH. This drop in pH is demonstrated by a color change from purple (negative) to yellow (positive) on the strip within 5 to 10 minutes.

HACEK GROUP AND *CAPNOCYTOPHAGA* SPECIES

HACEK is an acronym consisting of the first initial of each genus represented in the group:

- *Haemophilus aphrophilus*
- *Actinobacillus actinomycetemcomitans*
- *Cardiobacterium hominis*
- *Eikenella corrodens*
- *Kingella* sp.

This group of gram-negative bacilli have in common the need for an environment with increased CO_2 (a candle extinction jar or incubator with 5% to 10% CO_2). Their predilection for attachment to heart valves (usually damaged or prosthetic) makes them an important cause of endocarditis. Members of this group include both fermentative and nonfermentative gram-negative bacilli. All of the members are usual flora of the oral cavity, allowing for their introduction in the blood stream and resultant infections. All are opportunists and require an immunocompromised host or host tissue.

Although not a strict member of the HACEK group, another gram-negative bacillus, *Capnocytophaga* sp., is included in this series of discussions because it is similar in its requirement for CO_2 to enhance growth and its isolation from blood cultures. Unlike the other members of the group, it is not as commonly involved in endocarditis as it is in septicemia in the granulocytopenic patient. Table 15-4 summarizes the key reactions and characteristics of HACEK and *Capnocytophaga* species.

Haemophilus aphrophilus

Haemophilus aphrophilus is described in the beginning of this chapter and is not further reviewed here. Figures 15-13 and 15-14 illustrate the colonial and microscopic morphology of *H. aphrophilus*.

Actinobacillus actinomycetemcomitans

Actinobacillus actinomycetemcomitans is a member of a genus that includes animal pathogens or animal endogenous flora that in general do not routinely cause infections in humans. All are small rods to coccoid gram-negative bacilli that are nonmotile. *A. actinomycetemcomitans* is found as mouth flora in humans. Clinically it has been isolated from blood, lung tissue, abscesses of the mouth, and sinuses. However, it has been isolated from the blood as the causative agent of subacute bacterial endocarditis with an insidious and protracted presentation.

A. actinomycetemcomitans is fastidious, as all members of the HACEK group are, requiring increased CO_2 at least for initial isolation from clinical specimens. It is a fermenter, although the addition of serum to the carbohydrate containing tubes is often necessary to demonstrate this. The isolates may require more than 24 hours for isolation; distinctive star formation in the center of the colonies is often seen at 48 hours. Figures 15-15 and 15-16 depict the colonial and microscopic morphology. In broth, the organism is granular and may adhere to the sides of the tube. Isolates are catalase positive, variable in the oxidase reaction,

TABLE 15-4

Summary of Key Reactions and Characteristics of HACEK *and* Capnocytophaga *Species*

	Catalase	Oxidase	Glucose	Maltose	Sucrose	Lactose	Comments
Haemophilus aphrophilus Gram stain: small coccobacillus Colony morphology: high, convex, granular, yellowish	−	v	+	+	+	+	
Actinobacillus actinomycetemcomitans Gram stain: very small coccobacillus Colony morphology: small colonies that adhere to agar	+	v	+	+	−	−	
Cardiobacterium hominis Gram stain: straight rods, spindles, rosettes Colonial morphology: smooth, opaque, adherent to agar	−	+	+	+	+	−	Indole+
Eikenella corrodens Gram stain: straight rods Colonial morphology: usually pits the agar	−	+	−	−	−	−	Smells like bleach Ornithine +
Kingella kingae Gram stain: coccoid to straight rods, chains and pairs, square ends Colonial morphology: 2 types—spreading, corroding or smooth, convex β-hemolysis under colony	−	+	+	+	−	−	Nitrate −
Capnocytophaga spp. Gram stain: long, thin rod; tapered ends Colonial morphology: flat colonies, irregular in shape, may appear purple	−	−	+	+	−	v	Esculin v

+, Positive; −, negative; v, variable.

do not grow on MacConkey agar, and are negative for urease, indole, esculin, and citrate. Fermentations are positive for glucose (with or without gas), and are somewhat variable for xylose, mannitol, and maltose. The isolates do not ferment lactose or sucrose. They demonstrate sensitivity to penicillin in vitro, although this agent is not always successful clinically. In addition, isolates are susceptible to aminoglycosides, third-generation cephalosporins, quinolones, SXT, rifampin, chloramphenicol, and

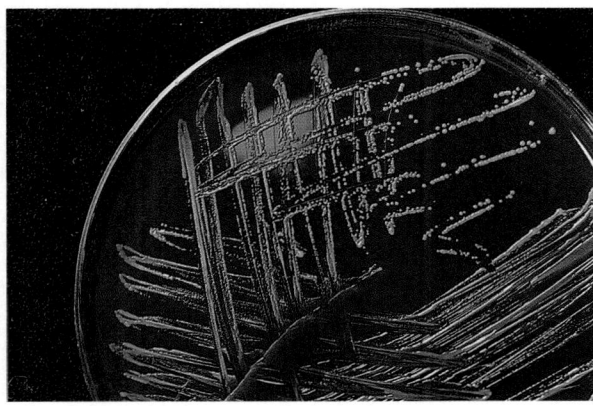

Figure 15-13

Haemophilus aphrophilus growing on BAP.

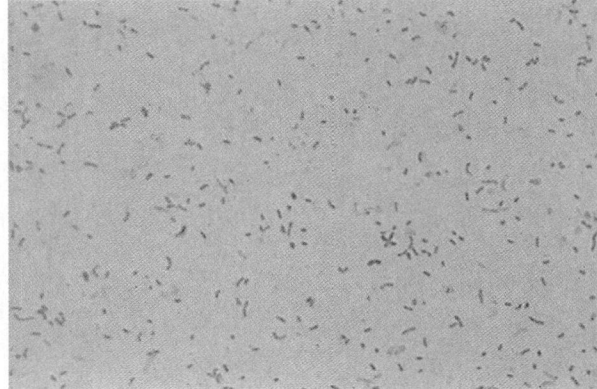

Figure 15-14

Gram-stain, microscopic morphology of *Haemophilus aphrophilus* (1000×).

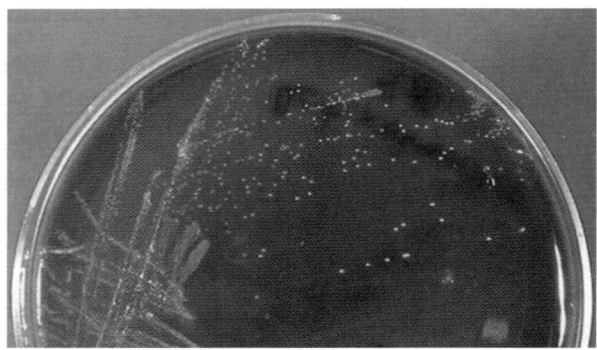

Figure 15-15

Actinobacillus actinomycetemcomitans on blood agar. Notice the star-shaped centers of the colonies.

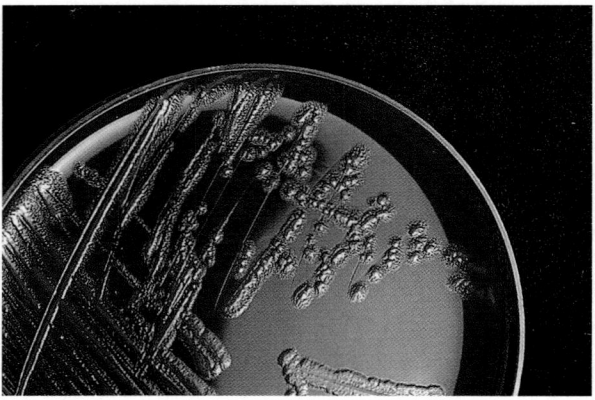

Figure 15-17

The 48-hour growth of colonies of *Cardiobacterium hominis* on BAP.

tetracycline. Resistance is common to vancomycin and erythromycin. Usual treatment for endocarditis is with a penicillin and an aminoglycoside.

Cardiobacterium hominis

Cardiobacterium hominis (IID, *Pasteurella*-like), a pleomorphic, nonmotile, fastidious, gram-negative bacillus, is another member of the HACEK group. *C. hominis* is normal flora of the nose, mouth, and throat, and may be present in the gastrointestinal tract. The usual clinical manifestation is that of endocarditis, often presenting with very large vegetations and no demonstrable fever. Rarely, isolates cause meningitis.

Gram stains of the bacilli often show false-positive reaction. The organisms tend to form rosettes,

swellings, and, in yeast extract, stick-like structures. They grow on blood and chocolate agar, but do not grow on MacConkey agar. Figures 15-17 and 15-18 illustrate the colonial and microscopic morphology. On agar, pitting may be produced. *C. hominis* is a fermenter, but as with *A. actinomycetemcomitans,* reactions may be weak and serum may be needed to enhance them. This organism ferments glucose, mannitol, sucrose (unlike *A. actinomycetemcomitans*), and maltose. Isolates are oxidase positive, catalase negative, and indole positive, the latter two traits helping to further differentiate them from *Actinobacillus* sp. They are negative for urease, nitrate, gelatin, and esculin. Sensitivity can be seen to

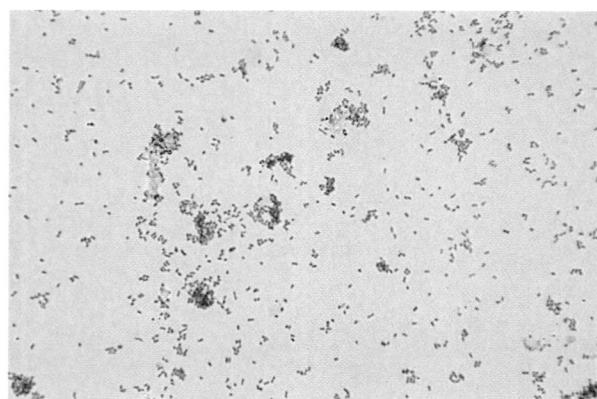

Figure 15-16

Gram-stain, microscopic morphology of *Actinobacillus actinomycetemcomitans* (1000×).

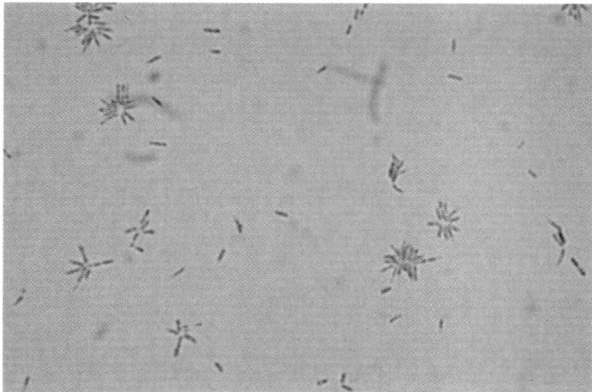

Figure 15-18

Gram stain of *Cardiobacterium hominis* showing typical "rosettes" (1000×).

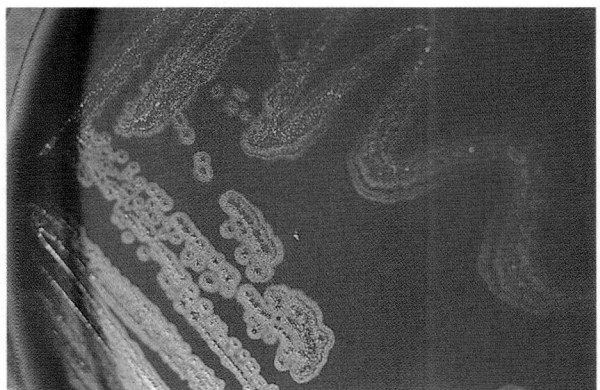

Figure 15-19 _____
Growth of *Eikenella corrodens* on CHOC.

Figure 15-20 _____
Gram stain morphology of *Eikenella corrodens* (1000×).

β-lactams, chloramphenicol, and tetracycline with variable response to aminoglycosides, erythromycin, clindamycin, and vancomycin. Usual modes of therapy include penicillin and an aminoglycoside.

Eikenella corrodens

Eikenella corrodens is a member of the usual flora of the oral and bowel cavities. Most infections that are associated with these organisms have been mixed and occur often as a result of trauma, especially after human fights or bites (i.e., "clenched fist wounds," or after the skin has been broken by human teeth). They have been reported as the cause of meningitis, empyema, pneumonia, osteomyelitis, arthritis, and postoperative tissue infections. In drug addicts, they have been implicated in cellulitis as a result of direct inoculation of the organisms into the skin after oral contamination of needle paraphernalia (because of licking the needle clean instead of sterilizing). They show a predilection for attachment to heart valves and thus cause endocarditis.

Eikenella corrodens (HB-1) are fastidious gram-negative coccobacilli that grow best under conditions of increased CO_2 and hemin with or without added cholesterol. They are nonmotile, oxidase positive, and nonsaccharolytic, and therefore are very similar to the *Moraxella* sp. Unlike the latter, however, they are catalase negative and often produce a yellow pigment. About 45% of the isolates of *E. corrodens* pit or corrode the surface of the agar. Figures 15-19 and 15-20 illustrate the colonial and microscopic morphology. In broth medium, they may adhere to the sides of the tube and produce granules. A bleachlike odor from the agar surface may be obvious. They do not usually grow on MacConkey or eosin-methylene blue agar, and they are LDC and ODC positive, and ADH negative. Characteristically, they are resistant to clindamycin and the aminoglycosides. In vitro, isolates demonstrate sensitivity to penicillin, ampicillin, cefoxitin, chloramphenicol, carbenicillin, and imipenem.

Kingella Species

Members of the genus *Kingella* are coccobacillary to short rods that exist in pairs or short chains (Figure 15-21). They are nonmotile but may demonstrate a "twitching" motility. They are nutrition-

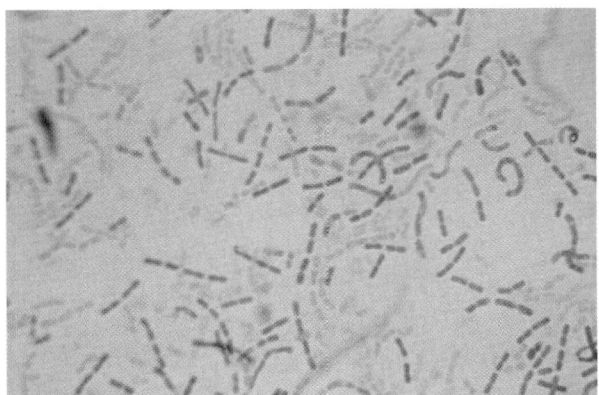

Figure 15-21 _____
Gram stain of *Kingella kingae* illustrating the plump rods in chains. Compare with the other members of the HACEK group (1000×).

ally fastidious, oxidase positive, catalase negative, fermenters of glucose and other sugars.

Kingella denitrificans may grow on Thayer Martin medium and, if it does not pit the agar as many strains do, may resemble *Neisseria gonorrhoeae.* Gram stain morphology as a rod with square ends and in chains should aid in distinguishing *Kingella* sp. It is positive for glucose fermentation and nitrate reduction and may grow at 42° C. It is negative for urease, indole, esculin, gelatin, and citrate and does not grow on MacConkey agar. This species is rarely isolated as a pathogen but has been associated with bacteremia and abscesses.

Kingella indologenes differs from *K. denitrificans* in being positive for indole and fermentation of maltose and sucrose. The rods are more plump than those of *K. denitrificans.* Eye infections with this species have been reported.

Kingella kingae is a weakly fermenting member of the genus. It is negative for sucrose but positive for glucose and maltose; it may produce a yellow-brown pigment, unlike other *Kingella* sp. This organism has two types of colony morphology, a spreading, corroding colony or a smooth, convex, and β-hemolytic colony. It is biochemically inactive otherwise. Isolates have been obtained clinically from blood, bone, joint fluid, urine, and wounds. Most isolates are from children less than 5 years old. Isolates of *Kingella* are usually susceptible to most agents, including penicillin.

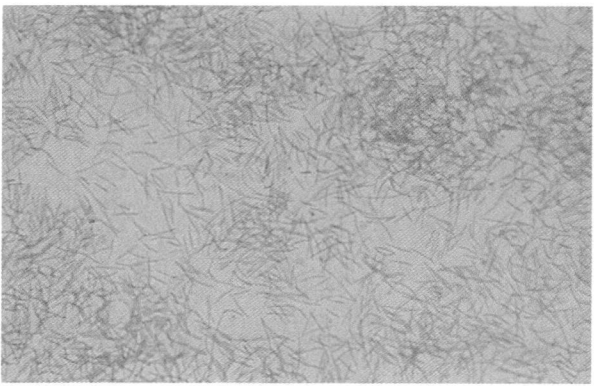

Figure 15-23 _____
Gram stain of *Capnocytophaga* organisms (1000×).

Capnocytophaga Species

Capnocytophaga species, including *Capnocytophaga ochracea (Bacteroides ochraceus), Capnocytophaga gingivalis,* and *Capnocytophaga sputigena,* are fastidious, pitting fermentative gram-negative bacilli that are normal flora of the mouth and oral cavities. They are thin and often fusiform on Gram stain, resembling *Fusobacterium* sp., and may produce a gliding motility on agar surfaces, although flagella are usually absent. Like HACEK organisms, they may require an increased CO_2 atmosphere for isolation and an extra day of incubation for culture. On agar surfaces, they often produce a yellow-orange pigment and are nonhemolytic. Figures 15-22 and 15-23 depict the colonial and microscopic morphology. They ferment (although TSI tubes may be negative without enrichment) sucrose, glucose, maltose, and lactose. They are negative for most biochemical reactions, although they may reduce nitrates and hydrolyze esculin.

Common sites of clinical isolation include blood cultures from the granulocytopenic who has oral ulcers (source of the *Capnocytophaga*), juvenile periodontal disease, and endocarditis. *C. ochracea,* the most common isolate clinically, is susceptible to ampicillin, penicillin, imipenem, erythromycin, clindamycin, ureidopenicillins, piperacillin, tetracycline, chloramphenicol, third-generation cephalosporins, quinolones, and metronidazole. It is resistant to trimethoprim and aminoglycosides and shows variable response to aztreonam and first- and second-generation cephalosporins.

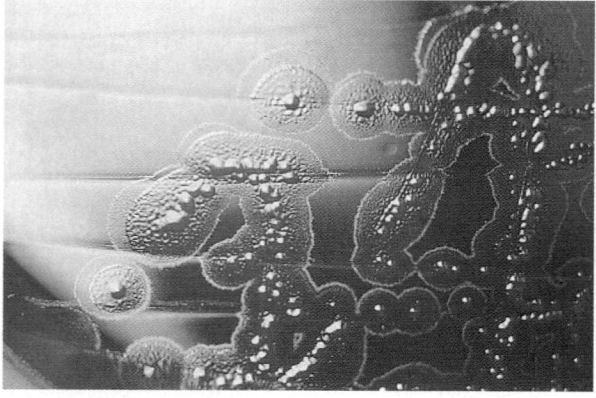

Figure 15-22 _____
Growth of *Capnocytophaga* organisms on CHOC. Notice the movement away from the center of the colony. Compare this growth to *Eikenella.*

PASTEURELLA SPECIES

General Characteristics

The genus *Pasteurella* consists of gram-negative, pleomorphic coccobacilli that vary microscopically from ovoid to short rods to filamentous forms; bipolar staining is common. They are nonmotile and catalase positive. Most isolates are oxidase positive and facultatively anaerobic; they ferment glucose with weak to moderate acid production. *Pasteurella* organisms may exhibit weak acid production from glucose without gas. In triple sugar iron (TSI) agar it gives the appearance of what is referred to as a "sick" TSI reaction. Figure 15-24 compares the TSI reactions of other gram-negative rods with the "sick" acid production of *Pasteurella multocida.*

The various species form grayish colonies that are similar in appearance. All species grow on blood agar plate and chocolate agar; species vary in their ability to grow on MacConkey agar, although most cannot. The ability to grow on blood agar plate without "feeder" organisms or in pure culture and the characteristic bipolar staining of the organism may help differentiate these species from *Haemophilus* species on first observation. Figure 15-25 presents an example of the colony morphology of *Pasteurella.*

Pasteurella species parasitize primarily the mucous membranes of the upper respiratory and gastrointestinal tracts of mammals and birds. They are rare inhabitants of the upper respiratory tract of humans. These organisms can be primary pathogens or secondary invaders and are pathogenic for a wide range of hosts. Humans acquire infections primarily through animal exposure. Table 15-5 lists several *Pasteurella* species associated with infections in humans.

Pasteurella multocida

Currently more than 17 species of *Pasteurella* are known. The most commonly isolated species is *Pasteurella multocida.* This species now includes three subspecies: *multocida, septica,* and *gallicida.* *P. multocida* consists of five serogroups: A, B, D, E, and F, which are based on capsular antigens.

P. multocida produces nonhemolytic colonies that may be mucoid in appearance on blood agar plate after 24 hours of incubation. After 48 hours,

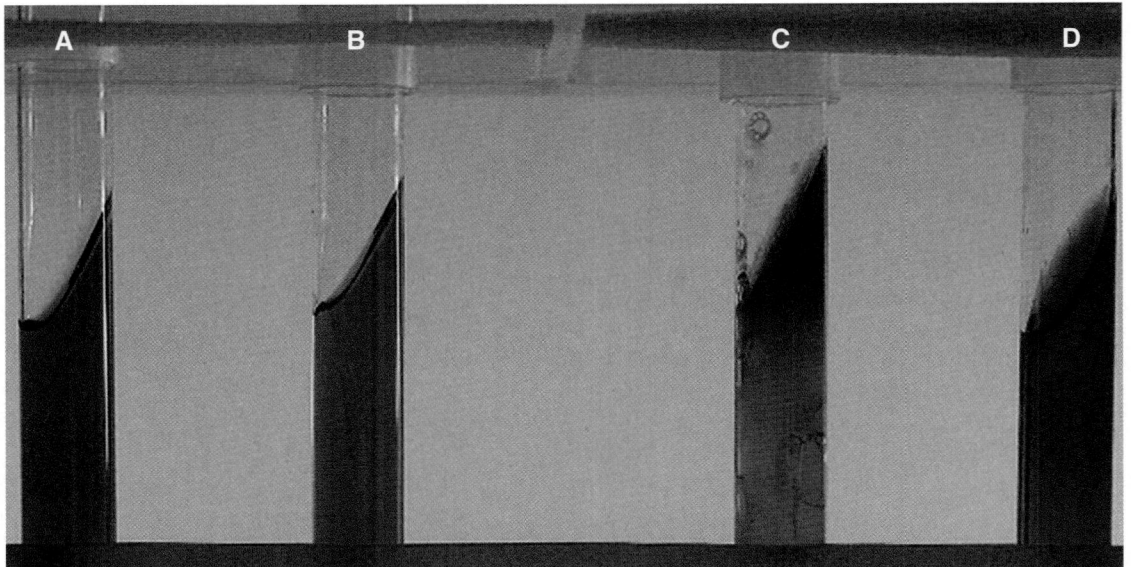

Figure 15-24

The triple sugar iron (TSI) reactions of other gram-negative rods are compared with the weak ("sick") acid production of *Pasteurella multocida.* **A,** Uninoculated. **B,** *Pasteurella multocida.* **C,** *Citrobacter* (a member of Enterobacteriaceae). **D,** Nonfermenter.

TABLE 15-5
Differential Characteristics of Pasteurella Species Associated with Human Infections

Species/Subspecies	Normal Habitat	Hemolysis	Oxidase	Catalase	ODC	Indole	Growth on MacConkey	Urease	Comments
P. multocida ssp. multocida ssp. septica ssp. gallicida	Oral cavities of healthy domestic dogs, cats, and other animals (swine, horses, cattle)	−	+	+	+	+	−	+	Most common isolate from human specimens. Most infections are associated with dog bites, cat bites, and scratches. May cause respiratory tract infections, including lung abscesses, pneumonia, empyema, and tonsillitis. Usually underlying disease present or immune complications Differentiated by acid production from dulcitol and sorbitol. Rare clinical isolates, primarily of veterinary interest. Subsp multocida is SORB +, DULC−, septica is SORB and DULC−, gallicida is SORB and DULC+
P. pneumotropica (Actinobacter pneumotropica)	Respiratory tract of dogs, cats, and some rodents	−	+	+	+	+	V	+	Human infections acquired by mostly dog and cat bites
P. haemolytica	Severe infections in cattle, sheep, swine, and poultry	+	+	+	V	+	V	+	72% are β-hemolytic on initial isolation but may lose this characteristic on subculture. Rare human infections caused by occupational or recreational exposure to animals.
P. aerogenes	Oropharyngeal and intestinal flora in swine	−	+	+	V	−	+	+	Human infections caused by bites or occupational exposure
P. dogmatis	Respiratory tracts of dogs and cats	−	+	+	−	+	−	+	Human infections caused by bites and scratches of dogs and cats
Pasteurella new species 1	Oropharyngeal of dogs and cats	−	+	−	−	+	+	V	Also known as Pasteurella "gas." Caused by bites. Xylose negative, may produce gas from glucose
P. canis	Biotype 1 is found in the oral cavity of dogs	−	+	+	+	V	−	−	Wound infections caused by dog bites
P. bettyae	Isolated from genitourinary tract including vagina, cervix, Bartholin glands, and amniotic fluid	−	V	V	−	+	V	−	Pathogen may be sexually transmitted. Formally known as CDC group HB-5
P. caballi	Upper respiratory tract of horses	−	+	−	V	−	−	−	One reported case of a finger lesion in a veterinarian

V, 20%-80% Positive; +, >90% positive; −, >90% negative.

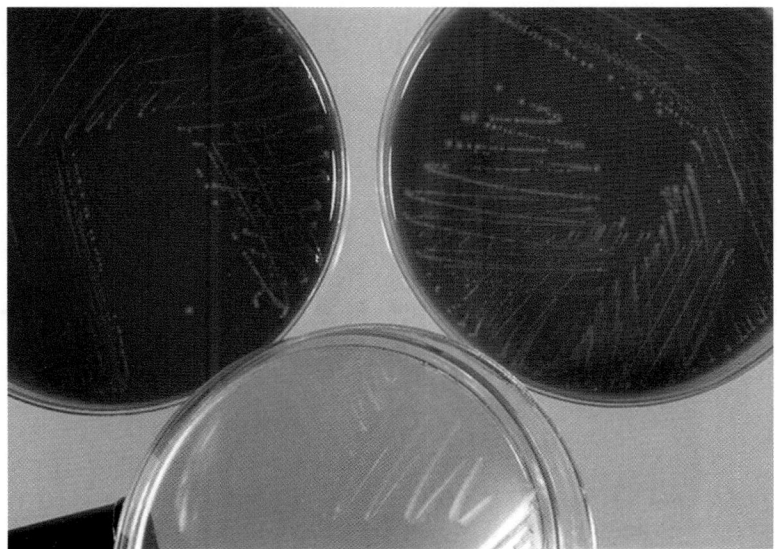

Figure 15-25

Pasteurella multocida growing on blood agar plate and *CHOC.* The MacConkey agar plate is negative for growth.

a narrow green to brown halo can surround the colony.

The most common form of infection caused by *P. multocida* seen in humans is cellulitis. This infection occurs primarily from bites or scratches inflicted by dogs and cats. The organisms are usually transmitted from the animal to the bite site or by the animals' licking preexisting abrasions.

BRUCELLA SPECIES

General Characteristics

Infection with *Brucella* species (Brucellosis) is commonly referred to as "undulant fever." The fever is characterized by remittent fevers, which fluctuate regularly at consistent intervals and can persist for days, months, or years when the disease becomes chronic. Brucellosis is considered a zoonosis that humans acquire from animals or animal products.

The genus *Brucella* consists of six species: *Brucella melitensis, Brucella abortus, Brucella canis, Brucella suis, Brucella neotomae,* and *Brucella ovis.* Four species that originate in animal reservoirs are pathogenic to humans (although the remaining two have caused rare infections): *B. melitensis, B. abor-*

tus, B. canis, and *B. suis. B. melitensis* is the most common cause of brucellosis.

In the animal hosts, *Brucella* species can induce spontaneous abortion secondary to bacteremia in pregnant females. Urine and milk contain the infective organisms. The brucellae primarily infect humans through contact with infected animals and animal products; occupational exposure and ingestion of contaminated milk are the major means of infection.

The brucellae are strict aerobes, have a gram-negative coccobacillary microscopic morphology, and are non–spore-forming, nonmotile, nonencapsulated, intracellular parasites. Traditional biochemical tests demonstrate they are oxidase positive and catalase positive, require carbon dioxide for growth (some species), are hydrogen sulfide positive using the more sensitive lead acetate method (most species), and are urease positive within 2 hours. Blood and bone marrow cultures and acute and convalescent sera for serologic testing are usually submitted for examination. Serologic tests are the primary means of diagnosis of brucellosis. See Table 15-6 for the characteristics of *Brucella* spp. Because *Brucella* organisms are considered to be a type 3 biohazard, isolates should be sent to appropriately equipped reference laboratories.

TABLE 15-6

Differential Characteristics of Brucella *Species Associated with Human Infections*

Species	Natural Host	Serum Agglutination (Patient Antibodies)	H₂S (Lead Acetate)	Urease	CO₂ (Enhanced Growth)	Growth in Dyes	
						Thionine	Fuchsin
B. melitensis	Goat or sheep	+	−	V	−	−	−
B abortus	Cattle	+	+	+<2 hr	+/−	+	−
B. suis	Swine	+	+	+<0.5 hr	−	−	+
B. canis	Dogs	−	−	+<0.5 hr	−	−	−

+, >90% positive; −, >90% negative; +/−, more positive than negative; *V,* variable.

FRANCISELLA SPECIES

Francisella tularensis

Francisella tularensis is a highly infectious, strictly aerobic, nonmotile, small, gram-negative coccobacillus. In addition, it is a facultatively intracellular parasite. *F. tularensis* causes tularemia, an acute, febrile, granulomatous disease characterized by rapid onset and flulike symptoms. Like *Pasteurella* and *Brucella* organisms, *F. tularensis* is considered a zoonotic infection. For a detailed description of their respective disease processes, see Chapter 34.

Two biovars cause disease in North America, *F. tularensis* biovar *tularensis* (type A) and *F. tularensis* biovar *palearctica* (type B). Type A is the more virulent strain, and humans are usually infected by rabbits, sheep, and ticks. Type B is more often transmitted by rodents and mosquitoes.

Because *Francisella* species are a type 3 biohazard, isolates should be sent to reference laboratories for processing and identification. Serologic testing is most frequently used for confirmation.

Bibliography

Balows A et al: *Manual of clinical microbiology,* ed 5, Washington, DC, 1991, American Society for Microbiology.

Baron EJ, Finegold S: *Diagnostic microbiology,* ed 8, St Louis, 1990, Mosby.

Isenberg HD: *Clinical microbiology procedures handbook,* Washington, DC, 1992, American Society for Microbiology.

Joklik WK et al, editors: *Zinsser microbiology,* ed 20, East Norwalk, Conn, 1992, Appleton & Lange.

Koneman EW et al: *Color atlas and textbook of diagnostic microbiology,* ed 5, Philadelphia, 1997, JB Lippincott.

Mandell GL, Douglas RG, Bennett JE, editors: *Principles and practices of infectious diseases,* ed 3, New York, 1990, Churchill Livingstone.

Murray PR et al: *Medical microbiology,* St Louis, 1990, Mosby.

Sanford JP: *Guide to antimicrobial therapy,* Dallas, 1993, Antimicrobial Therapy, Inc.

LEARNING ASSESSMENTS

1. The spinal fluid collected from the patient described in the case study at the beginning of the chapter should be inoculated on which of the following primary media? Circle all that apply.
   a. Blood agar
   b. Chocolate agar
   c. Brain heart infusion agar
   d. MacConkey agar

2. The organism was later identified as *Haemophilus influenzae*. Draw the results of the "X" and "V" strip testing.

3. What would be the appearance of this organism on MacConkey agar?

4. The porphyrin test for this organism would be _____, because the organism _____ biosynthesize heme. The end result of the test would show _____ fluorescence.
   a. Negative; cannot; negative
   b. Positive; cannot; positive
   c. Negative; can; positive
   d. Positive; can; negative

5. The most common biotype and serotype of this organism would be:
   a. Biotype III; serotype a
   b. Biotype I; serotype b
   c. Biotype II; serotype c
   d. Biotype I; serotype d

Continued

LEARNING ASSESSMENTS—cont'd

6. The β-lactamase test was positive. The patient should be treated with which of the following?
   a. Ampicillin
   b. Penicillin
   c. All of the above
   d. None of the above

7. What other organisms are most likely to be causative agents of spinal meningitis but are not necessarily in this age group?

8. What is HACEK?

B. *LEGIONELLA* SPECIES

A. Christian Whelan

EPIDEMIOLOGY

CLINICAL INFECTIONS
  Legionnaires' Disease
  Pontiac Fever

LABORATORY DIAGNOSIS
  Specimen Collection and Handling
  Direct Microscopic Examination
    Nonspecific stains
    Direct fluorescent antibody test
  DNA Probe
  Culture and Identification
  Urine Antigen Test
  Serology
  Antimicrobial Susceptibility

KEY TERMS

Legionnaires' disease
Legionella micdadei
Pontiac fever
Fluorescein
  isothiocyanate (FITC)
L-cysteine

Buffered charcoal yeast
  extract (BCYE)
"Ground glass"
  appearance
Urine antigen test

In 1976, during an American Legion convention in Philadelphia, 221 persons became ill with pneumonia, and 34 of them died of a mysterious disease. *Legionella pneumophila,* the agent of this outbreak, became the first named member of the family Legionellaceae. Currently, the genus includes more than 30 species and 50 serogroups. *Legionella pneumophila* contains 14 serogroups.

The isolation of *Legionella* species from patient specimens and environmental sources has been recently made possible for most microbiology laboratories with the advent of commercial media and other diagnostic methods currently available. An understanding of the microscopic and colonial morphology of the *Legionella* species, their nutritional requirements, the pathogenesis of infection, and the advantages and disadvantages of the various laboratory tests available to diagnose infections enables the technologist and clinical microbiologist to arrive at a reliable laboratory diagnosis.

Legionella species are ubiquitous gram-negative rods acquired by humans primarily through the inhalation of aerosols. Clinically, infected patients may present with a wide variety of conditions, rang-

CASE STUDY

A group of two dozen retirees from the tobacco industry arranged to go on a 2-week cruise of the Caribbean Islands. Typical accommodations included small cabins for couples, three meals a day with a late night buffet, full bar, recreation such as casino and floorshows that lasted well into the evening.

The group got a block of rooms together and spent time socializing over drinks and cigarettes in the cabins, saunas, and poolside. In the fifth day of the cruise, several members of the party asked to see the ship's doctor because of worsening cough. Within the next few days, 10 members of the retiree party and several other passengers were acutely ill with pneumonia, and required medical evacuation to a hospital. Chest x-rays revealed progressive patchy lobar pneumonia that improved after erythromycin was administered.

ing from asymptomatic infection to life-threatening disease. The laboratory diagnosis of *Legionella* infection depends on the results of procedures such as the following:

- Isolation using special media
- Urine antigen detection
- Direct fluorescent antibody (DFA)
- Serology

The isolation and presumptive identification of the most common *Legionella* species can be accomplished by the microbiology laboratory using commercially available media, reagents, and kits.

EPIDEMIOLOGY

Most members of Legionellaceae are found worldwide, occurring naturally in aquatic sources, such as lakes, rivers, hot springs, and mud. Because *Legionella* species can tolerate chlorine concentrations below 2 to 3 mg per L, they resist water treatment and subsequently gain entry into and colonize human-made water supplies. Hot water systems, cooling towers, and evaporative condensers are major artificial reservoirs. Other sources include cold water systems, ornamental fountains, whirlpools, humidifiers, and industrial process waters. The factors that contribute to the ability of *Legionella* species to colonize these sources include the following:

- The ability to multiply over the temperature range of 20° C to 43° C and survive for varying periods at 40° C to 60° C
- The capacity to adhere to pipes, rubber, plastics, and sediment and persist in piped water systems even when flushed
- The ability to survive and multiply within free-living protozoa and in the presence of commensal bacteria and algae

Legionella species are transmitted to human hosts from these environmental sources primarily via aerosolized particles, like those produced by normal tap water pressure. Most outbreaks of disease originate from potable water distribution contamination. Other means of transmission include aspiration of contaminated water or secretions, direct inoculation by respiratory therapy equipment, and immersion of wounds in contaminated water. Transmission between humans has not been demonstrated.

CLINICAL INFECTIONS

Pathogenic *Legionella* species cause intracellular infections in humans but also survive in an extracellular environment. Some species have been recovered only from environmental sources. Clinical manifestations of *Legionella* infections include febrile disease with pneumonia (legionnaires' disease) or without pulmonary involvement (Pontiac fever) and asymptomatic infection. These differing presentations may be influenced by several factors,

including the organism's ability to enter and survive and multiply within the host cells, especially bronchoalveolar macrophages, and the ability to produce proteolytic enzymes. In addition, host factors, such as a suppressed immune system, chronic lung disease, alcoholism, and heavy smoking, predispose individuals to Legionnaires' disease. The mode of transmission and the number of infecting organisms in the inoculum also probably play a role in the clinical features of the infection. When *Legionella* infections are diagnosed early, they can usually be treated successfully with erythromycin or a combination of erythromycin and rifampin. Alternative drugs include doxycycline, minocycline, trimethoprim-sulfa-methoxazole, azithromycin, and clarithromycin. Ciprofloxacin is the drug of choice in transplant recipients.

Legionnaires' Disease

Legionnaires' disease can present in three major patterns:

- Sporadic cases, usually in the community—the most common presentation
- Epidemic outbreaks characterized by short duration and low attack rates
- Nosocomial clusters occurring in compromised patient populations

Pneumonia is the predominant manifestation of *Legionella* disease and places the organism among the top four causes of community-acquired bacterial pneumonia (along with *Streptococcus pneumoniae, Mycoplasma pneumoniae,* and *Chlamydia pneumoniae*). The mortality rate is reported at 15% to 30% and may approach 50% in patients with nosocomial pneumonia if the correct diagnosis is not made early. *Legionella pneumophila* serogroup 1 accounts for most cases (approximately 85%). Other *L. pneumophila* serogroups, commonly 4 and 6, and ***Legionella micdadei*** are more frequently implicated in clinical infections than the other *Legionella* species.

The incubation period for Legionnaires' disease is 2 to 10 days. Patients typically present with a nonproductive cough, fever, headache, and myalgia. Later, as pulmonary infiltrates develop, sputum may be bloody or purulent. Rales, dyspnea, and shaking chills are clinical manifestations of progressing disease.

Dissemination via the circulatory system may lead to extrapulmonary infections with or without pneumonia. Infections of the kidneys, liver, heart, central nervous system, lymph nodes, spleen, and bone marrow as well as cutaneous abscesses have been described. Bacteremia, renal failure, liver function abnormalities, watery diarrhea, nausea, vomiting, headache, confusion, lethargy, and other central nervous system abnormalities have been associated with these infections.

Pontiac Fever

The nonpneumonic form of *Legionella* infection, **Pontiac fever,** usually has an incubation period of about 2 days. Patients are previously healthy individuals who complain of flulike symptoms of fever, headache, and myalgia that last 2 to 5 days and then spontaneously subside. The incidence of Pontiac fever in the general population is unknown. *L. pneumophila* is responsible for most cases of this illness.

LABORATORY DIAGNOSIS

Several methods such as direct examination, culture, and antigen and antibody detection are available for the laboratory diagnosis of infections caused by *Legionella* species. Most laboratories utilize more than one method to maximize their diagnostic capabilities.

Specimen Collection and Handling

Specimens for culture and direct examination commonly include sputum, bronchoalveolar lavage (BAL), and bronchial washings. Ingram and Plouffe recommend that sputum purulence screens not be used and that all sputum specimens be accepted for culture. Transtracheal aspiration, lung tissue, blood, wound and abscess material, and pleural, peritoneal, and pericardial fluids may also be submitted. Water from environmental sources may be cultured for epidemiologic investigation. Urine is collected for antigen detection.

Respiratory secretions and body fluids (except blood) are submitted in sterile, leakproof containers. Small pieces of tissue may be overlaid with sterile water. Saline or buffer should not be used in processing or transporting specimens because of the inhibitory effects of sodium on *Legionella* species. Refrigerate these specimens if more than 2 hours pass between collection and processing,

because overgrowth of contaminating flora may inhibit growth of *Legionella* species when transport of the specimens is prolonged. When samples are to be transported to a reference laboratory, place the samples on wet ice. Freeze the specimens at $-70°$ C if processing will be delayed for several days.

For blood cultures, the Isolator (Wampole Laboratories, Cranbury, NJ) system, which utilizes the lysis centrifugation method, is preferred. Approximately 10 mL of blood is collected in a special lysis centrifugation tube and transported to the laboratory for processing. *Legionella* species can also be isolated from typical Bactec blood culture bottles.

Collect at least 50 to 100 mL of water for culture in a sterile, leakproof container.

Urine specimens for antigen testing are collected in sterile, leakproof containers and assayed within 24 hours of collection. If testing is delayed, specimens should be stored at $2°$ C to $8°$ C or frozen at $-20°$ C.

Direct Microscopic Examination

The rapid and accurate diagnosis of *Legionella* infections is challenging to the clinician because clinical symptoms, radiologic presentations, and standard laboratory tests infrequently implicate the causative agent. Direct examination of stained specimens offers a rapid method for detecting *Legionella* species.

Nonspecific stains

When visualized microscopically in clinical specimens, *Legionella* species are pleomorphic, weakly staining gram-negative rods approximately 1 to 2 μm by 0.5 μm in size. The organisms may be found within macrophages and segmented neutrophils and extracellularly (Figure 15-26). The staining intensity of the organisms can be enhanced by extending the safranin counterstaining time to at least 10 minutes. *L. micdadei* is weakly acid fast in tissue or in other clinical samples, and stains best with the modified Kinyoun procedure (see Chapter 8). Other stains including Diff-Quik (Baxter Scientific, Kansas City, MO) and Giemsa may be used to facilitate detection of the organisms. However, all of these nonspecific staining methods are most useful for examination of specimens from normally sterile sites.

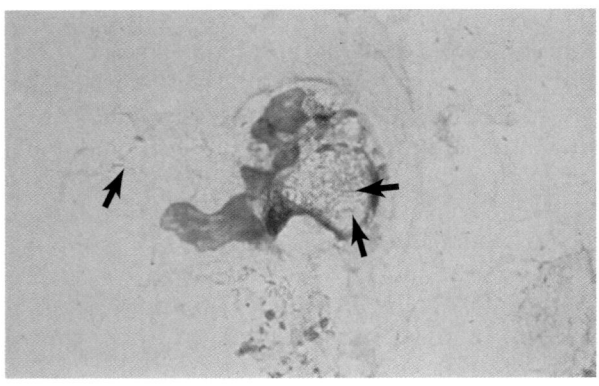

Figure 15-26

Gram stain of specimen demonstrating intracellular and extracellular *Legionella pneumophila* (1000×).

Direct fluorescent antibody test

The direct fluorescent antibody (DFA) test is a rapid laboratory procedure available for detection of the more common species of *Legionella* in clinical samples from the lower respiratory tract. It is described in Chapter 8. The test is especially useful if the result is positive; however, a negative result does not rule out *Legionella* infection. Available are **fluorescein isothiocyanate (FITC)** labeled conjugates that detect all known serogroups of *L. pneumophila* (Genetic Systems, Seattle, WA) and *L. pneumophila* groups 1 to 7, *Legionella bozemanii,* *Legionella dumoffii, Legionella gormanii, Legionella longbeachae* groups 1 and 2, *L. micdadei,* and *Le-*

gionella jordanis (SciMedx, Denville, NJ). The conjugate binds to the antigen in the cell membrane of the organisms, and these antigen-antibody complexes are detected using a fluorescence microscope when the ultraviolet blue light excites the FITC. The organisms thus appear as bright yellow to green, short or coccobacillary rods with intense peripheral staining (Figure 15-27).

Although the specificity of the DFA test has been reported to be 94% to 99%, some species of *Pseudomonas, Bacteroides, Corynebacterium,* and other bacteria may cross-react with the polyvalent conjugates. The microscopist must have experience with the morphologic and staining features of *Legionella* species, so atypical organisms will not be misidentified. Some laboratories prefer not to use polyvalent reagents for direct specimen examination because of these cross-reactions.

The sensitivity of DFA testing for direct specimen examination is approximately 25% to 80% when compared with that of culture. Therefore DFA should not be the only test used. To visualize organisms, approximately 10,000 to 100,000 organisms per mL of specimen must be present. Other factors such as excessively thick smears, which tend to obscure organisms, and the technical skill of the observer may influence the sensitivity of the test.

It is recommended that the DFA is performed when requested by the clinician or when (1) suspicious organisms are seen, or (2) many neutrophils and no organisms are seen on Gram stained or spe-

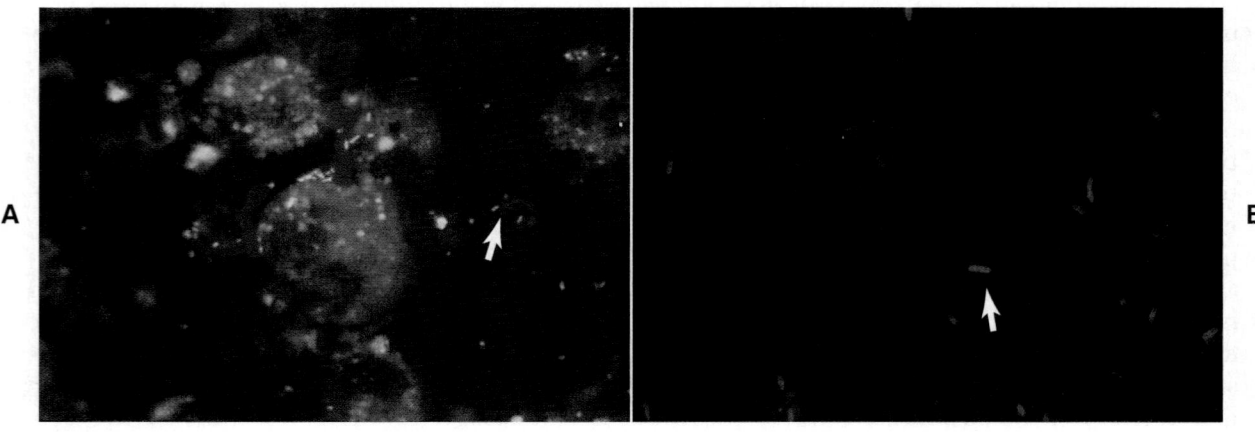

A **B**

Figure 15-27

A, *Legionella pneumophila* in specimen smear stained by direct fluorescent antibody (DFA) technique (450×). **B,** *Legionella pneumophila* in specimen smear stained by DFA technique (1000×). Note intense peripheral staining of the organisms.

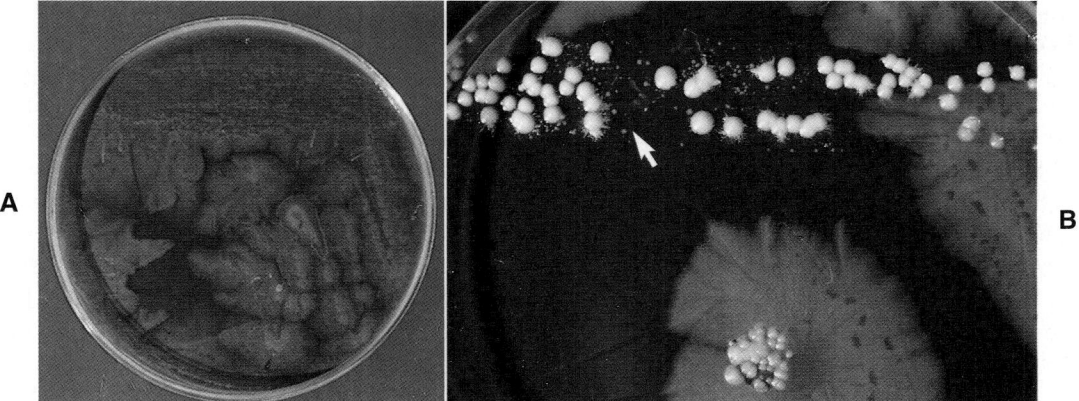

Figure 15-28

A, Nonselective buffered charcoal yeast extract (BCYE) agar plate inoculated with sputum specimen. Note overgrowth of respiratory flora. **B,** Selective BCYE agar plate inoculated with same sputum specimen, which has been acid-washed prior to inoculation. Much of the respiratory flora has been eliminated. *Legionella* colonies are the smallest ones in the first quadrant. (Courtesy Richard Brust.)

cially stained smears. Because the sensitivity of the DFA test is less than that of culture, specimens should not be submitted for DFA testing only.

The DFA test also provides a useful method of confirming that an isolate is a *Legionella* species and of identifying the more common species and serogroups of the genus.

DNA Probe

A DNA probe is commercially available in kit form to detect the presence of all known species and serogroups of *Legionella* in clinical specimens (Gen-Probe, San Diego, CA). The I^{125}-labeled, single-stranded DNA probe combines with the target organism's ribosomal RNA, and the labeled DNA-RNA hybrids are detected in a gamma scintillation counter.

With a specificity of 99% to 100% and a sensitivity of 70% to 75% compared with culture, the test can be used as a substitute for DFA. Finkelstein and colleagues reported that the diagnostic performance of the DNA probe assay was superior to that of DFA testing, even though the probe test sensitivity was 31% to 67%, depending on the diagnostic criteria.

The polymerase chain reaction (PCR) technique increases the sensitivity of the probe; however, the technique is not currently available for clinical use. Advantages of the probe are that the procedure is less tedious and time-consuming than that of the DFA and is free from subjective interpretation. Also, the probe can reliably identify all *Legionella* colonies to the genus level. However, inherent disadvantages of the radioactive probe (short shelf life, expensive equipment, disposal restrictions) limit its use to high-volume laboratories.

Culture and Identification

The single most important test for Legionnaires' disease is culture of the organism. *Legionella* species are fastidious, aerobic bacteria that are unable to grow on sheep's blood agar and require the amino acid L-**cysteine** for growth. The organisms may appear as tiny colonies on chocolate agar that contains L-cysteine. However, **buffered charcoal yeast extract (BCYE)** is the recommended medium for *Legionella* isolation and is available commercially as nonselective and semiselective media. Semiselective BCYE contains polymyxin B, anisomysin, and either vancomycin (PAV) or cefamandole (PAC) and improves recovery of *Legionella* species from highly contaminated specimens. However, growth of some *Legionella* species is inhibited by semiselective media; therefore BCYE with and without antibiotics should be used for culture. Tzielan et al reported maximum recovery using a combination of BCYE without the antimicrobials PAC and PAV.

Acid treatment of specimens contaminated with bacteria before inoculation also enhances isolation of *Legionella* species (Figure 15-28). In this procedure, an aliquot of the specimen is first diluted 1:10 with a 0.2 N KCl-HCl solution and allowed to stand for 5 minutes. Then the medium is inoculated with a portion of the acid-treated specimen (Procedure 15-1).

Inoculated medium is incubated at 35° C to 37° C in air for at least 7 days. Usually within 3 to 5 days *Legionella* species are visible as grayish-white or blue-green, convex, glistening colonies measuring approximately 2 to 4 mm in diameter. When these colonies are viewed with a dissecting microscope illuminated from above, they show a characteristic appearance (Figure 15-29). The central portion of young colonies have a **"ground-glass" appearance,** light gray and granular, whereas the periphery of the colony has pink and/or light blue or bottle-green bands with a furrowed appearance. Plates should be examined daily, because older colonies lose these characteristic features and may be mistaken for other bacteria. Plates with suspicious colonies can also be illuminated with a longwave ultraviolet light (366 nm) and examined for differences in colonial autofluorescence to detect possible mixed *Legionella* infections (Box 15-1).

The physical and biochemical properties of *Legionella* species are listed in Box 15-2. However, biochemical testing has limited value in the presumptive identification of isolates to the species level. The confirmation of the suspected colonies and their presumptive identification as *Legionella*

PROCEDURE 15-1. *Legionella* Species Isolation

Materials:

1. Buffered charcoal yeast extract (BCYE) non-selective and selective plates
2. KCl/HCl buffer, pH 2.2
   Add 5.3 mL of 0.2 N HCl and 25 mL of 0.2 N KCl to 100 mL of distilled water. Adjust pH to 2.2 with HCl or KCl.
   Dispense 4.5 mL into small screw-capped tubes, and autoclave for 10 minutes at 121° C.
   Store under refrigeration. Expiration 6 months.

Method:

1. Prior to medium inoculation, perform the following techniques to obtain the proper inoculum:
   Centrifuge liquid specimens in excess of 2 mL at 3,000 rpm for 10 minutes and 50-mL water samples at 3,000 rpm for 30 minutes. Use the sediment as inoculum.
   Homogenize pieces of tissue in 1 mL of sterile distilled water using a sterile tissue grinder.
   Prepare concentrates from Isolator or other blood culture bottles.

2. Inoculate one BCYE plate and one selective BCYE plate with an aliquot of the sample, and streak for isolation. Note that for water samples this step should be omitted. Proceed to step 3.

3. Additionally, specimens likely to be contaminated with bacterial flora are processed as follows:
   Add 0.5 mL of specimen to 4.5 mL of sterile HCl-KCl buffer pH 2.2 in a sterile screw-capped tube. Place three to four sterile glass beads in the tube if the specimen is excessively mucoid. Recap the tube, mix the specimen with the buffer, and break up the mucus using a vortex mixer.
   Let the suspension stand for 5 minutes.
   Pipet 0.1 mL of the suspension to a nonselective BCYE plate and 0.1 mL to a selective BCYE plate.
   Spread the inoculum over the surface of each plate.

4. Incubate the plates aerobically at 35° C to 37° C for 7 days.

5. Examine cultures daily using a dissecting microscope illuminated from above.

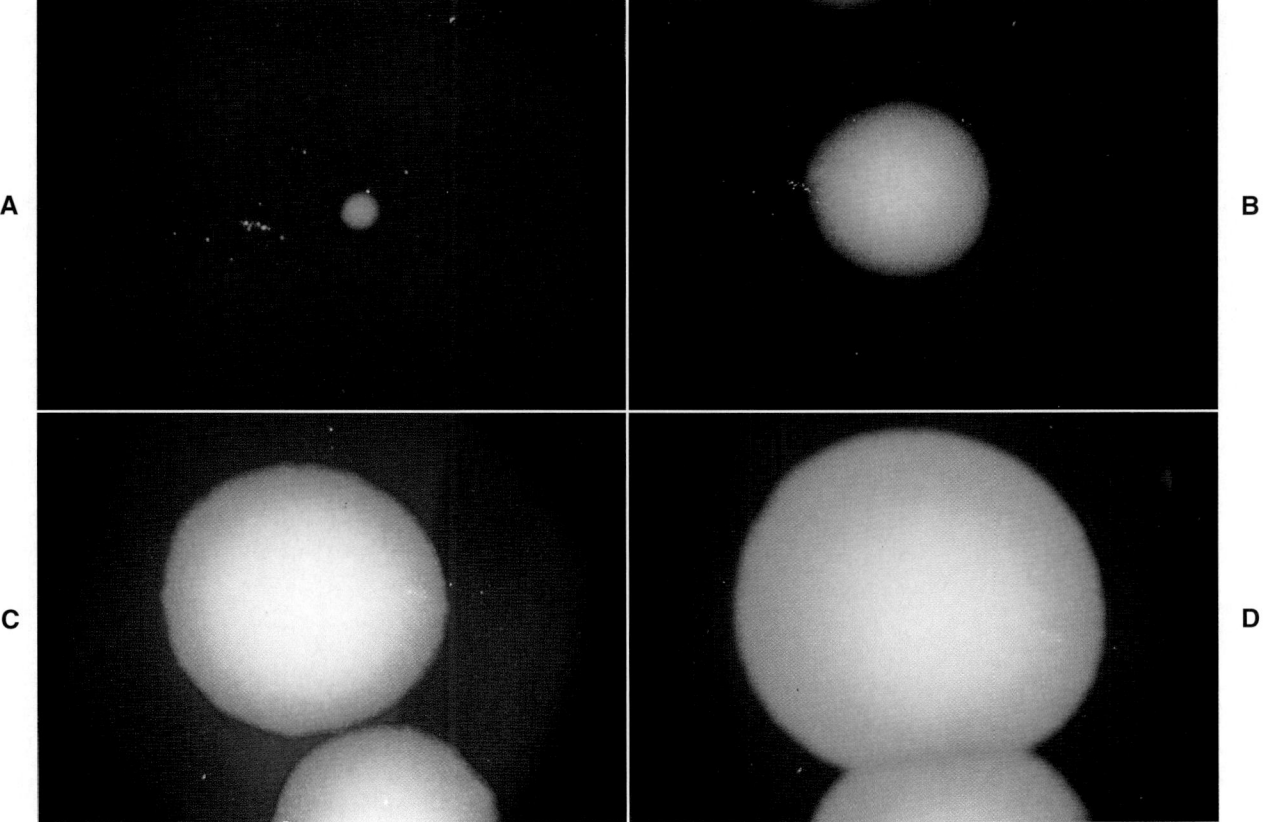

Figure 15-29

A, *Legionella pneumophila* colony on buffered charcoal yeast extract (BYCE) agar after 3 days of incubation, viewed with a dissecting microscope (20×). **B,** Same colony after 4 days of incubation. **C,** Same colony after 5 days of incubation. **D,** Same colony after 7 days of incubation.

species can be achieved in the microbiology laboratory using growth requirement for L-cysteine testing, Gram stain, direct fluorescent antibody tests, and nucleic acid probe (Figure 15-30). The confirmation of the suspected colonies and their presumptive identification as *Legionella* species can be achieved in the microbiology laboratory using the following protocol:

- Prepare a smear from the suspicious colony growing on BCYE medium, and perform the Gram stain. *Legionella* species are thin, gram-negative rods that may show size variation from 2 to 20 μm in length.
- Subculture the isolate to BCYE with L-cysteine and to either sheep's blood agar or BCYE

without L-cysteine. *Legionella* species grow only on BCYE medium supplemented with L-cysteine.
- Prepare smears from colonies that require L-cysteine for growth, and test with polyvalent and monovalent conjugates to determine specific species and serogroup.

Definitive identification is usually performed at reference, public health, or state laboratories.

Urine Antigen Test

Several FDA-approved platforms such as radioimmunoassay, microplate enzyme immunoassay, and a rapid immunochromographic assay, have been developed by Binax, Inc. (Portland, ME) to detect

Box 15-1

Grouping of *Legionella* Species Based on Colonial Autofluorescence*

Negative

L. pneumophila
L. micdadei
L. longbeachae
L. jordanis
L. oakridgensis
L. fairfieldensis
L. feeleii
L. maceachernii
L. hackeliae
L. cincinnatiensis
L. jamestowniensis
L. spiritensis
L. waltersii
L. shakespearei
L. santicrucis
L. israelensis
L. moravica
L. brunensis
L. quinlivanii
L. lansingensis
L. adelaidensis
L. sainthelensi

L. geestiana
L. quarteirensis
L. nautarum
L. worsleiensis
L. londiniensis

Blue-White

L. dumoffii
L. bozemanii
L. gormanii
L. anisa (variable)
L. parisiensis
L. cherrii
L. steigerwaltii
L. tucsonensis

Yellow-Green

L. birminghamensis
L. wadsworthii

Red

L. rubrilucens
L. erythra

Modified from Winn WC Jr: *Legionella.* In Murray PR et al, editors: *Manual of clinical microbiology,* ed 7, Washington, DC, 1999, American Society for Microbiology. *Colonies are exposed to long-wave ultraviolet light (366 nm). (Mineralight Lamp, UVP Inc., San Gabriel, Calif.)

L. pneumophila serogroup 1 soluble antigen from urine, in the **urine antigen test.** It is estimated that this serotype is responsible for up to 85% of legionellosis cases, and urine is a convenient specimen to obtain. The antigen can be detected as early as day 3 of the infection and can persist up to a year (consequently the test is of limited value in persons with a recent history of *Legionella* infection). Prolonged antigenuria has been associated with immunosuppression, renal failure, and chronic alcoholism. Furthermore, early antimicrobic intervention with macrolides may decrease antigen excretion in some patients.

The enzyme immunoassays have gained the most acceptance in clinical laboratories because of speed and ease. Compared with culture, the plate assay reports sensitivities of 90% to 94% and the specificity ranges from 97% to 100%. The 15-minute NOW *Legionella* Test is a visually read immunochromographic assay that has a sensitivity and specificity of 95%. One word of caution: sensitivity and specificity do not always tell the whole story (see Chapter 4). With a sensitivity of 95% and a specificity of 95%, the positive predictive value drops to 90.5, which means 1 out of every 10 positive test results is a false positive. Furthermore, as the prevalence of *Legionella* species declines, the false positive rate increases. Therefore it is important to confirm results with culture, especially when determining the dynamics of this organism in a given patient population. Despite some limitations, these rapid tests represent an important step forward in timely diagnosis of *Legionella* infections.

Serology

The indirect fluorescent antibody (IFA) assay is the most common method employed for the serologic diagnosis of Legionnaires' disease, although other platforms such as EIA are available. For IFA, heat- or formalin-killed bacteria are fixed to a microscope slide. Higher titers can be seen with heat treated organisms; however, less cross-reactivity occurs with formalin preparations. Cross-reacting immunoglobulins have been reported in patients with an infection caused by gram-negative bacilli, *Mycoplasma,* and *Chlamydia.*

The sensitivity of serological tests are reported as 75% to 80%, with a specificity of 90% to 100%. The specificity of the test is enhanced when paired

Box 15-2

Common Phenotypic Characteristics of *Legionella*

Slow growth (3 to 5 days)
Characteristic "ground glass" colony morphology
Lightly staining gram-negative bacillus
Requires L-cysteine for primary isolation
No growth on unsupplemented blood agar
Asaccharolytic
Catalase or oxidase: weakly positive

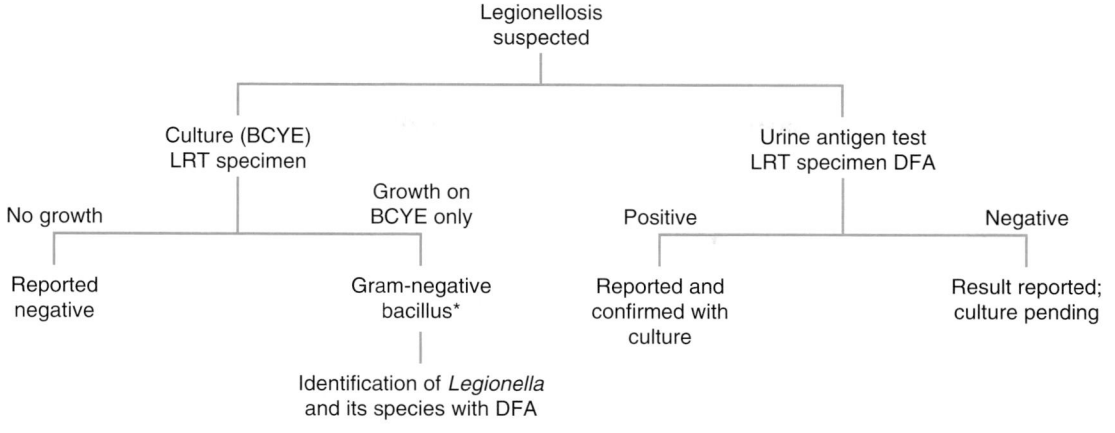

Figure 15-30

Schema for identification of *Legionella* organisms. *LRT,* Lower respiratory tract; *DFA,* direct fluorescent antibody.
*Biohazard precautions; consider organisms such as *Francisella* sp.

sera from patients with symptoms of legionellosis are tested. A fourfold rise in IFA titer to at least 1:128 from the acute serum phase, obtained within 1 week of onset of symptoms, to the convalescent serum phase, 3 to 6 weeks later, is evidence of recent infection. However, patients with disease may not demonstrate a rise in titer for 8 weeks or longer after symptoms commence.

A single antibody IFA titer of at least 1:256 in conjunction with compatible illness indicates a probable case of *Legionella* infection according to the definition of the Centers for Disease Control and Prevention (CDC). However, antibody titers may remain elevated months to years after acute infection; thus a single titer of 1:256 or greater is more suggestive of infection during an outbreak than in sporadic cases.

Antimicrobial Susceptibility

Susceptibility testing of *Legionella* species is not standardized or performed routinely. When infections are diagnosed early, they can usually be treated successfully with erythromycin or a combination of erythromycin and rifampin. This is particularly important in nosocomial infections, because they usually involve compromised patients and the disease often takes an aggressive course. Alternative drugs include newer macrolides (azithromycin, clarithromycin), fluoroquinolones such as ciprofloxacin, doxycycline, and trimethoprim-sulfamethoxazole.

Bibliography

Bangsborg JM et al: Legionellosis in patients with HIV infection, *Infection* 18:342, 1990.

Birtles RJ et al: Evaluation of urinary antigen ELISA for diagnosing *Legionella pneumophila* serogroup 1, *Infection* 43:685, 1990.

Buesching WJ et al: Enhanced primary isolation of *Legionella pneumophila* from clinical specimens by low-pH treatment, *J Clin Microbiol* 17:1153, 1983.

Dominguez JA et al: Comparison of Binax *Legionella* urinary antigen enzyme immunoassay (EIA) with the Biotest *Legionella* urine antigen EIA for detection of *Legionella* antigen in both concentrated and unconcentrated urine samples, *J Clin Microbiol* 34:1579, 1998.

File TM et al: The role of atypical pathogens: *Mycoplasma pneumoniae, Chlamydia pneumoniae,* and *Legionella pneumophila* in respiratory infection, *Infect Dis Clin N Amer* 12:569, 1998.

Finkelstein R et al: Diagnostic efficacy of a DNA probe in pneumonia caused by *Legionella* species, *J Med Microbiol* 38(3):183-6, 1993.

Goetz A, Yu VL: Screening for nosocomial legionellosis by culture of the water supply and targeting of high-risk patients for specialized laboratory testing, *Am J Infect Control* 19:63, 1991.

Gray JJ et al: Serological cross-reaction between *Legionella pneumophila* and Citrobacter freundii in indirect immunofluorescence and rapid microagglutination tests, *J Clin Microbiol* 29:200, 1991.

Hackman BA et al: Comparison of Binax *Legionella* urinary antigen EIA kit with Binax RIA urinary antigen kit for detection of *Legionella pneumophila* serogroup 1 antigen, *J Clin Microbiol* 34:1579, 1996.

Hart CA, Makin T: *Legionella* in hospitals: a review, *J Hosp Infect* 18 (suppl A):481, 1991.

Ingram JG, Plouffe JF: Danger of sputum purulence screens in culture of *Legionella* species, *J Clin Microbiol* 32:209, 1994.

Kazandjian D et al: Rapid diagnosis of *Legionella pneumophila* serogroup 1 infection with the Binax enzyme immunoassay urinary antigen test, *J Clin Microbiol* 35:954, 1997.

Muder RR et al: Other *Legionella* species. In Mandell GL et al, editors: *Principles and practice of infectious diseases,* ed 4, New York, 1995, Churchill Livingstone.

Tzielan CL et al: Growth of 28 *Legionella* species on selective culture media: a comparative study, *J Clin Microbiol* 31:2764, 1993.

Winn WC Jr: *Legionella.* In Murray PR et al, editors: *Manual of clinical microbiology,* ed 7, Washington, DC, 1999, ASM Press.

Yu VL: Personal communication, *Legionella* update, 1993.

LEARNING ASSESSMENTS

1. What three bacterial agents are the main causes of community-acquired primary atypical pneumonia?

2. What risk factors contributed to more severe form of the disease in patients presented in the *Legionella* case?

3. What factors contributed to the above infection?

4. What are the advantages and disadvantages of DFA testing for *Legionella* species?

5. What is the culture medium of choice for the recovery of *Legionella* species?

C. BORDETELLA

A. Christian Whelen

GENERAL CHARACTERISTICS

EPIDEMIOLOGY

VIRULENCE FACTORS

CLINICAL INFECTIONS

LABORATORY DIAGNOSIS
  Specimen Collection and Transport
  Direct Fluorescent Antibody Test
  Nucleic Acid Detection
  Culture and Identification
  Serology

ANTIMICROBIAL SUSCEPTIBILITY

KEY TERMS

Pertussis
Filamentous
  hemagglutinin (FHA)
Pertussis toxin (PT)
Tracheal cytotoxin (TC)
Adenylate cyclase
Whooping cough

Catarrhal phase
Paroxysmal phase
Convalescent phase
Regan-Lowe transport
  medium
Bordet-Gengou potato
  infusion agar

CASE STUDY

An 8-month-old boy was taken to the pediatric clinic after a 3½ week history of cough with progressive severity. He was recently adopted from a poor family who lived in a country that until 1991 was controlled by the former Soviet Union. Originally, he had a coldlike illness with runny nose, but recently had coughed so long and hard that he had vomited. Episodes left him exhausted and gasping for air.

GENERAL CHARACTERISTICS

Members of the genus *Bordetella* are small gram-negative bacilli or coccobacilli. At least seven species are recognized: *Bordetella pertussis, Bordetella parapertussis, Bordetella bronchiseptica, Bordetella avium, Bordetella hinzii, Bordetella holmesii,* and *Bordetella trematum.* All are obligately aerobic bacteria, grow best at 35° C to 37° C, do not ferment carbohydrates, and are relatively inactive in biochemical test systems. Both *B. pertussis* and *B. parapertussis* are primary human pathogens of the respiratory tract, caus-

ing whooping cough or pertussis; the latter organism is usually associated with a milder form of the disease. Both of these organisms are fastidious to primary isolation, requiring special collection and transport systems as well as culture media. *B. bronchiseptica* and *B. avium* are respiratory tract pathogens of wild and domestic birds and mammals and are generally nonfastidious and recoverable on routine microbiologic culture media. *B. bronchiseptica* is also an opportunistic human pathogen, causing pneumonia and wound infections. *B. holmesii* and *B. trematum* have only recently been described as respective agents of immunocompromised bacteremia and wound or ear infection. *B. hinzii* appears to be an avian commensal.

EPIDEMIOLOGY

Infections resulting from *Bordetella* species are acquired through the respiratory tract via the aerosol route. The bordetellae are uniquely adapted to adhere to and replicate on ciliated respiratory epithelial cells. The organisms remain localized to the respiratory tract, but toxins and other virulence factors are produced and have systemic effects.

Pertussis is one of the most highly communicable diseases of childhood, infecting more than 90% of susceptible household contacts. Even in well-immunized populations such as the United States, periodic outbreaks occur every few years and isolated cases occur at all times. Major epidemics have emerged after well-documented decreases in immunization rates. Immunity is short-lived, and *B. pertussis* appears to be maintained in the human population by adults who become transiently colonized with the organism when exposed to it. Adults may or may not experience respiratory symptoms, typically persistent cough, and provide the reservoir for transmitting the organism to susceptible individuals.

Concern over complications with the whole-cell, inactivated vaccine that has been used for almost 5 decades in the United States has led to the development of multivalent, acellular formulations. These vaccines target some of the virulence factors listed below, and clinical trials have demonstrated immunity equivalent to the whole cell preparations with fewer side effects.

VIRULENCE FACTORS

B. pertussis produces a variety of virulence factors that play a role in pathogenesis of disease. The first is believed to be the attachment to ciliated epithelial cells, which appears to be facilitated primarily by **filamentous hemagglutinin (FHA)** and pertactin (69 kDa outer membrane protein). **Pertussis toxin (PT)** is a protein exotoxin that produces a wide variety of responses in vivo. The main activity of PT is modification of host proteins by ADP-ribosyl transferase, which interferes with signal transduction. *B. parapertussis* and *B. bronchiseptica* contain the structural gene for PT, but do not express the complete operon. **Adenylate cyclase** toxin (ACT) inhibits host epithelial and immune effector cells by inducing supraphysiologic concentrations of cyclic AMP. **Tracheal cytotoxin (TC)** contributes to pathogenesis by causing ciliostasis, inhibiting DNA synthesis, and promoting cell death. Other virulence factors have been proposed, but their current roles in disease remain unclear.

CLINICAL INFECTIONS

Classic pertussis or **whooping cough** resulting from *B. pertussis* occurs following exposure to the organism through the respiratory tract and a 1- to 2-week incubation period. The initial symptoms are generally nonspecific and resemble the "common cold" or "flu." These include sneezing, mild cough, runny nose, and perhaps conjunctivitis. At this stage, known as the *catarrhal phase* of the

disease, the infection is highly communicable because of the large number of organisms in the respiratory tract. However, cultures are not often performed at this stage because the symptoms are nonspecific. The catarrhal phase may last for 1 to 2 weeks and is followed by the **paroxysmal phase** of the disease. The hallmark of this phase is the sudden attack of severe, repetitive coughing followed by the characteristic "whoop" at the end of the coughing spell. The whooping sound is caused by the rapid gasp for air following the prolonged bout of coughing. Coughing spells may occur many times a day and are sometimes followed by vomiting. Young children may experience apnea, become cyanotic, and require aid in maintaining a patent airway. Many of these symptoms may be either absent or altered in very young infants, partially immunized children, or adolescents and adults; in addition *B. parapertussis* generally causes disease with milder symptoms. The **convalescent phase** of disease generally begins within 4 weeks of onset with a decrease in frequency and severity of the coughing spells. Complete recovery may require weeks or months.

LABORATORY DIAGNOSIS

Current laboratory diagnosis of pertussis generally employs culture isolation with or without DFA testing. Organisms do not survive well outside the host, so culture lacks sensitivity. Detection with DFA is about 60% to 70% sensitive when compared with culture and can lack specificity. Although serologic diagnosis identifies more cases, it is not generally utilized because it has not been standardized and is not widely available. Some newer tests, such as PCR amplification and detection of *B. pertussis* DNA, show significant promise for accurate and rapid diagnosis.

Specimen Collection and Transport

The specimen of choice for culture and DFA testing of *Bordetella* species is secretions collected from the posterior nasopharynx; throat cultures yield lower sensitivity and should be discouraged. Nasopharyngeal specimens may be collected either by aspiration through a small catheter, which is preferred, or pernasal swab. The swabs should be of either calcium alginate or Dacron (polyester) with a flexible wire shaft. Generally, two swabs are collected, one through each external nares; the swabs should be inserted as far back as possible into the nasopharynx, rotated, held a few seconds, and then gently withdrawn. In practice, swabs are used more commonly than aspiration methods.

Nasopharyngeal swab specimens should be plated directly onto culture media at the bedside, or transferred to an appropriate transport system. Bedside plating is often dependent upon close proximity to the processing laboratory, because fresh media must be provided to medical personnel on short notice. Alternatively, a transport system should be selected based on anticipated transport time. If the transit time is to be 2 hours or less, the swab can be expressed into a solution of 1% casein hydrolysate (casamino acids) broth. For up to 24 hours, Amies transport media with charcoal is appropriate. Specimens should be transported at room temperature and transferred to culture media as soon as they arrive at the laboratory. In situations requiring overnight or several-day transport, half-strength charcoal agar containing 10% horse blood and 40 mg/L cephalexin **(Regan-Lowe transport medium)** should be used. This medium is prepared in screw-capped containers and is inoculated by streaking the surface and then submerging the swab in the agar and leaving it in place. The inoculated Regan-Lowe medium may be sent to the processing laboratory immediately or following incubation for 1 or 2 days at 35° C (preferred method). The processing laboratory may test any growth on the transport medium directly for *Bordetella* spp. and use the swab to inoculate an isolation medium.

Direct Fluorescent Antibody Test

Although the DFA test can be used along with culture, the lack of sensitivity diminishes the clinical utility of a negative result. The test is generally helpful if the result is positive, but false-positive test results can occur, even in experienced hands. Thus, the DFA test should always be used in conjunction with, not as a replacement for, culture. Slides for DFA testing may be prepared directly from swab specimens or following expression of the material from the swab to a solution of 1% casein hydrolysate. At least two slides should be prepared; these are dried, heat-fixed, and stained on the same day of collection or stored at −70° C and heat-fixed

immediately before staining. Polyclonal fluorescent labeled conjugates for both *B. pertussis* and *B. parapertussis* are normally used so that each reagent can serve as a negative control for the other. On microscopic examination, the organisms appear as small, fat rods or coccobacilli with intense peripheral yellow-green fluorescence and darker centers. Recently a monoclonal antibody directed against *B. pertussis* lipopolysaccharide (LPS) has shown promise. This reagent, named BL-5, and one specific for *B. parapertussis* is produced and packaged in Canada (Biotex Laboratories Inc., Edmonton, Alberta).

Nucleic Acid Detection

Detection of *Bordetella* spp. nucleic acid from nasopharyngeal, with or without amplification, may provide considerable improvement in diagnostics. This methodology could circumvent many of the problems associated with specimen transport and bacterial cultivation, although it too has limitations. Furthermore, routine susceptibility testing is not required because of predictable response to erythromycin. A growing number of studies have shown the clinical utility of PCR in the laboratory diagnosis of pertussis. Several bordetellae nucleic acid targets have been exploited, and primers have been designed to amplify single or multiple species. Unique, conserved sequences such as PT promoters, ACT gene, or insertion sequences appear to hold the most promise; however, commercial development will be required prior to widespread application.

Culture and Identification

Since the original development of **Bordet-Gengou potato infusion agar** with glycerol and sheep's blood, few alternative formulations have been successful. The most successful of these is charcoal agar supplemented with 10% horse blood and 40 mg/L cephalexin. This medium is identical in composition to the transport medium of Regan and Lowe except that it contains agar at full strength. The medium has a shelf life of up to 8 weeks and is commercially available. Care should be taken to ensure the appropriate concentration of cephalexin in the medium. Some strains of *B. pertussis* have been reported to be inhibited at 40 mg/L or above. For this reason, it may be advisable to also plate a medium without cephalexin.

Plates for the recovery of *Bordetella* spp. should be incubated at 35° C in air for a minimum of 7 days. It is important to ensure adequate moisture during this period to prevent plates from drying out. Most isolates of *B. pertussis* are detected in 3 to 5 days, whereas *B. parapertussis* is detected a day or so sooner. A stereomicroscope should be used to detect the colonies before they become visible to the unaided eye. On charcoal–horse blood (CHB), young colonies are smooth, glistening, and silver, resembling mercury droplets (Figure 15-31). Older colonies turn whitish-gray as they age.

Suspicious colonies should be Gram stained; small gram-negative rods or coccobacilli should be further screened for *B. pertussis* and *B. parapertussis* using agglutinating antisera or fluorescein-labeled antisera. For the fluorescent antibody test from a plate isolate, slides should be carefully prepared so that organisms are well dispersed on the slide. This ensures that individual cells show characteristic peripheral staining. The agglutination test requires a larger quantity of bacteria, so subculture from the primary isolation plate is sometimes necessary.

When the results of fluorescent staining or agglutination are clear, confirmatory testing is not required. *B. pertussis* and *B. parapertussis* can be adequately identified and separated with these serologic reagents alone. If these tests yield equivocal results, suspicious organisms should be sub-

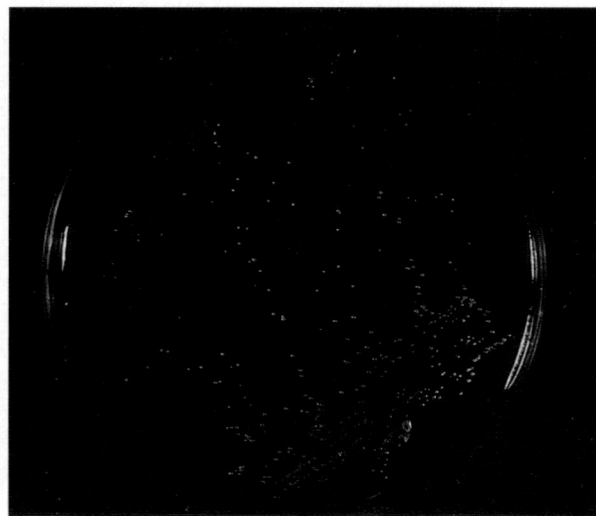

Figure 15-31 ——————————————————

Five-day-old colonies of *Bordetella pertussis* on charcoal–horse blood agar *(incident light from lower right corner)*.

TABLE 15-7 ——————————————————

Differential Characteristics of Bordetella *Species Infecting Humans*

	Species		
Characteristics	*B. pertussis*	*B. parapertussis*	*B. bronchiseptica*
Growth on Charcoal– horse blood	+ (3-5 days)	+ (2-3 days)	+ (1-2 days)
Blood agar	−	+	+
MacConkey agar	−	−	+
Catalase	+	+	+
Oxidase	+	−	+
Urease production	−	+ (24 hr)	+ (4 hr)
Nitrate reduction	−	−	+
Motility	−	−	+

cultured to CHB agar, routine blood agar, and chocolate agar (the latter to assess for *Haemophilus* sp. that may have broken through on selective CHB). Growth patterns should be observed, serologic tests repeated, and additional biochemical tests performed (Table 15-7) to confirm the identification. Box 15-3 summarizes the laboratory diagnosis of pertussis by culture.

Serology

Serologic diagnosis of pertussis can be used to study outbreaks and to document seroconversion following immunization or infection. Unfortunately, the tests have not been sufficiently standardized for routine diagnostic purposes. If serologies are to be performed, reference sera available from the Laboratory of Pertussis (Food and Drug Administration, Bethesda, MD) should be used for quality control. Optimal diagnostic sensitivity requires paired sera and testing for multiple immunoglobulin class-antigen combinations (e.g., IgG to FHA and PT, along with IgA to FHA). Testing for IgM as an acute phase antibody has been disappointing and currently is of little assistance. Serology also tends to be retrospective; several weeks are often required to demonstrate a diagnostic response. Enzyme immunoassay (EIA) for IgG or IgA antibody to FHA from a single serum specimen or from nasopharyngeal aspirates have been developed but have not gained widespread acceptance.

Box 15-3

Summary of Laboratory Diagnosis of Pertussis by Culture

1. Using calcium alginate or Dacron, flexible wire swabs, collect two pernasal specimens from the posterior pharynx.
2. Transfer to transport system a, b, or c:
   a. 1% casein hydrolysate (1 to 2 hr holding time)
   b. Amies transport medium with charcoal (24 hr holding time)
   c. Half-strength charcoal agar with horse blood and cephalexin (incubate 1 to 2 days at 35° C before transport to laboratory)
3. Prepare and read 2 smears for DFA test for *B. pertussis.*
4. Inoculate charcoal–horse blood agar (with cephalexin). Incubate in moist chamber (without carbon dioxide) at 35° C for 7 days.
5. Examine plates at 2 days, and daily thereafter, for typical colonies; use stereomicroscope.
6. Screen *B. pertussis/parapertussis*-like colonies with Gram stain and fluorescent antibody test or agglutinating antisera.
7. Confirm identification of equivocal results by subculture, repeat antisera tests, and biochemical tests.

ANTIMICROBIAL SUSCEPTIBILITY

Erythromycin is the drug of choice for treatment of pertussis as well as for prophylaxis of individuals exposed to patients with disease. Although erythromycin is important for eradication of the organism and prevention of secondary cases, it has clinical efficacy only if treatment is started during the catarrhal phase of disease. Trimethoprim-sulfamethoxazole is used as an alternative treatment. A number of newer antimicrobials including fluoroquinolones (ciprofloxacin) and macrolides (azithromycin, clarithromycin) are active in vitro, but clinical trials are lacking. Routine antimicrobic susceptibility testing of *B. pertussis* or *B. parapertussis* is not necessary because of predictable sensitivity to macrolides. The susceptibility of *B. bronchiseptica* is not predictable, although the organism is usually susceptible to the aminoglycosides. Laboratory susceptibility tests should be done to support the clinical management of patients with opportunistic *B. bronchiseptica* infection.

Bibliography

Cherry JD: Epidemiological, clinical, and laboratory aspects of pertussis in adults, *Clin Infect Dis* 28(suppl 2):112, 1999.

Ewanowich CA et al: Major outbreak of pertussis in northern Alberta, Canada: analysis of discrepant direct-fluorescent antibody and culture results by using polymerase chain reaction methodology, *J Clin Microbiol* 31:1715, 1993.

Friedman RL: Pertussis: the disease and new diagnostic methods, *Clin Microbiol Rev* 1:365, 1988.

Gilchrist MJR: Pertussis: pathophysiology and prevention, *Clin Microbiol Newsl* 12:17, 1990.

Hallander HO et al: Comparison of nasopharyngeal aspirates with swabs for culture of *Bordetella pertussis*, *J Clin Microbiol* 31:50, 1993.

Hewlett EL: A commentary on the pathogenesis of pertussis, *Clin Infect Dis* 28(suppl 2):S94, 1999.

Hoppe J: Update on epidemiology, diagnosis, and treatment of pertussis, *Euro J Clin Microbiol Infect Dis* 15:189, 1996.

Hoppe JE: *Bordetella.* In Murray PR et al, editors: *Manual of clinical microbiology,* ed 7, Washington, DC, 1999, American Society for Microbiology.

Koneman EW et al, editors: *Color atlas and textbook of diagnostic microbiology,* ed 5, Philadelphia, 1997, Lippincott.

Kurzynski TA et al: Comparison of modified Bordet-Gengou and modified Regan-Lowe media for the isolation of *Bordetella pertussis* and *Bordetella parapertussis*, *J Clin Microbiol* 26:2661, 1988.

Lind-Brandberg L et al: Evaluation of PCR for diagnosis of *Bordetella pertussis* and *Bordetella parapertussis* infections, *J Clin Microbiol* 36:679, 1998.

McNicol P et al: Evaluation and validation of a monoclonal immunofluorescent reagent for direct detection of *Bordetella pertussis*, *J Clin Microbiol* 33:2868, 1995.

Muller FMC, Hoppe JE, Wirsing von Konig CH: Laboratory diagnosis of pertussis: state of the art in 1997, *J Clin Microbiol* 35:2435, 1997.

Thomas MG: Epidemiology of pertussis, *Rev Infect Dis* 11:255, 1989.

Wirsing von Konig CH et al: Evaluation of a single-sample serological technique for diagnosing pertussis in unvaccinated children, *Eur J Clin Microbiol Infect Dis* 18:341, 1999.

Woolfrey BF, Moody JA: Human infections associated with *Bordetella bronchiseptica*, *Clin Microbiol Rev* 4:243, 1991.

LEARNING ASSESSMENTS

1. Public health infrastructure has declined in former Soviet-block countries since the collapse of communism. Why is this important in the spread and transmission of pertussis?

2. Immunization is not recommended after age 7. Are adults immune to this infection?

3. What are the clinical samples of choice?

4. What transport media are appropriate for maximum recovery?

GENERAL CHARACTERISTICS
  Microscopic and Colonial Morphology
  Classification
  Virulence and Antigenic Factors
  Clinical Significance

OPPORTUNISTIC MEMBERS OF THE FAMILY
ENTEROBACTERIACEAE AND ASSOCIATED
INFECTIONS
  Escherichia coli
    Clinical infections
  Other *Escherichia* Species
  Klebsiella, Enterobacter, Serratia, and *Hafnia*
    Species
    Klebsiella species
    Enterobacter species
    Serratia species
    Hafnia species
  Proteus, Morganella, and *Providencia* Species
    Proteus species
    Morganella species
    Providencia species
  Edwardsiella Species
  Erwinia and *Pectobacterium* Species
  Citrobacter Species

PRIMARY INTESTINAL PATHOGENS
AND RELATED HUMAN INFECTIONS
  Salmonella Species
    Classification
    Virulence factors
    Antigenic structures
    Clinical infections
  Shigella Species
    Clinical infections
  Yersinia Species
    Yersinia pestis
    Yersinia enterocolitica
    Yersinia pseudotuberculosis

NEW GENERA AND BIOTYPES
  Budivicia species
  Buttiauxella species
  Cedecea species
  Ewingella species
  Kluyvera species
  Koserella species
  Leminorella species
  Moellerella species
  Obesumbacterium species
  Rahnella species
  Tatumella species
  Xenorhabdus species

LABORATORY DIAGNOSIS
  Specimen Collection and Transport
  Isolation and Identification
    Direct microscopic examination
    Culture
    Identification

BIOCHEMICAL PRINCIPLES AND REACTIONS
ON CONVENTIONAL MEDIA
  Lactose Fermentation and Utilization
    of Carbohydrates
    Triple sugar iron (TSI) agar
    o-Nitrophenyl-p-D-galactopyranocide
  Glucose Metabolism and Its Metabolic Products
    Methyl red test
    Voges-Proskauer test
    Miscellaneous reactions

SCREENING STOOL CULTURES FOR PATHOGENS

SEROLOGIC GROUPING
  Salmonella Species
  Shigella Species

OBJECTIVES

1. Give the general characteristics of organisms that belong to the family Enterobacteriaceae.
2. Describe the antigenic structures of this group of organisms, and explain how these structures are used for identification.
3. Given the organism's characteristic growth on nonselective and selective differential media, presumptively identify the isolate.
4. Explain the different reactions that may be observed in the triple sugar iron (TSI) agar.
5. Describe the reactions involved and the products of metabolism tested in the following miscellaneous reactions:
   ▪ Indole test
   ▪ Methyl red and Voges-Proskauer tests
   ▪ Nitrate reduction test
   ▪ Citrate utilization
   ▪ Urease production
   ▪ Phenylalanine deaminase
   ▪ Decarboxylase test
   ▪ Nitrate reduction test
   ▪ Lysine iron agar
6. Given the key reactions for identification, place an unknown organism in its proper tribe or genus.

KEY TERMS

Enterics
Fermentation
O antigen
H antigen
K antigen
Vi antigen
K antigen
Enteropathogenic
  E. coli (EPEC)
Enterotoxigenic E. coli
  (ETEC)
Enteroinvasive E. coli
  (EIEC)
Enterohemorrhagic
  E. coli (EHEC)
Enteroaggregative
  E. coli (EaggEC)
Traveler's diarrhea

Shiga toxin (Stx)
SMAC plate
Triple sugar iron (TSI)
  agar
Kligler iron agar (KIA)
Sulfide, indole, motility
  (SIM)
Motility, indole, and
  ornithine (MIO)
β-galactosidase
β-galactoside permease
Methyl red–Voges-
  Proskauer (MRVP) test
Indole
Deaminase
Decarboxylase
Nitrate reduction

CASE STUDY

A 65-year-old hospitalized male patient complained of draining abscess on his right hip. Drainage was aspirated from the infected site and sent to the laboratory for direct smear, culture, and susceptibility testing. The direct smear showed moderate polymorphonuclear cells (PMNs), few gram-negative rods, some intracellular. After 24 hours of incubation, blood agar plate and chocolate agar plate showed moderate growth of medium-size mucoid colonies, whereas the MacConkey agar showed moderate growth of oxidase negative, nonlactose-fermenting organisms. Biochemical tests to identify the isolate and susceptibility tests were performed.

The family Enterobacteriaceae includes several genera and species; clinical isolates in general acute care facilities consist primarily of *Escherichia coli, Klebsiella pneumoniae,* or *Proteus mirabilis.* It is important, however, to be aware of the other species, because they also cause infectious diseases.

This chapter is divided into three major areas. The first discusses clinically significant enteric species that cause opportunistic infections, the second covers primary intestinal pathogens and their related human infections, and the third describes methods of identification of these organisms.

GENERAL CHARACTERISTICS

The family Enterobacteriaceae, often referred to as **"enterics,"** consists of a large number of diverse organisms. Described in this section are the general characteristics of the members in this family: their morphology, classification, virulence and antigenic factors, and clinical significance. Members of this family have four major features:

- All ferment glucose
- All reduce nitrates to nitrites
- None produce cytochrome oxidase
- All except *Klebsiella, Shigella,* and *Yersinia* organisms are motile; with a rare exception, the flagellar arrangement is peritrichous if the organism is motile

Microscopic and Colonial Morphology

Members of the family Enterobacteriaceae are gram-negative, non–spore-forming, facultatively anaerobic bacilli. On gram-stained smears, they may appear as coccobacilli or straight rods. Colonial morphology on nonselective media, such as sheep's blood agar or chocolate agar, is of little value in their initial identification. With the exception of certain members (e.g., *Klebsiella*) that produce characteristically large and very mucoid colonies, all members of this family produce large, moist, gray colonies on nonselective media and are therefore indistinguishable.

A wide variety of differential and selective media, such as MacConkey agar, and highly selective media, such as Hektoen enteric (HE) agar and XLD (xylose-lysine deoxycholate) agar, are available for the presumptive identification of enteric pathogens. These media contain one or more carbohydrates, such as lactose and sucrose, which show the ability of the species to ferment any carbohydrate. **Fermentation** is indicated by a color change on the medium, which results from a drop in pH detected by a pH indicator incorporated into the medium. Nonfermenting species are differentiated by lack of color change, and colonies retain the original color of the medium. Species that produce hydrogen sulfide (H_2S) may be readily distinguished when placed on HE or XLD agar. HE and XLD agars contain sodium thiosulfate and ferric ammonium citrate, which produce blackening of H_2S–producing colonies. These features have been used to initially differentiate and characterize certain genera. Definitive characterization and identification depend on the biochemical reactions and serologic antigenic structures demonstrated by the particular species.

Classification

The use of tribes in classifying the members in this family was proposed by Ewing in 1963 and has since been continued and extended in subsequent editions of *Edwards and Ewing's Identification of Enterobacteriaceae.* In classifying species into tribes, Ewing grouped bacterial species with similar biochemical characteristics. Within the tribes, species are further classified into their respective genera. Differentiation of each genus and definitive identification of species are based on biochemical characteristics. Table 16-1 lists the bacterial species in the family Enterobacteriaceae and their respective tribes. Table 16-2 shows the biochemical features that differentiate the tribes. Although the concept of using tribes in the classification of bacteria has not been used in *Bergey's Manual of Systematic Bacteriology,* this classification has been an effective way of placing species in groups based on similar biochemical features.

Virulence and Antigenic Factors

The virulence of the members of Enterobacteriaceae is controlled by a number of factors, such as the ability to colonize, adhere, produce various toxins, and invade tissues. Some species also possess plasmids that may mediate resistance to antimicrobials. Many members of this family possess antigens that can be used for identifying different serologic groups. These antigens include the following:

- **O antigen,** or somatic antigen, a heat-stable antigen located in the cell wall
- **H antigen,** or flagellar antigen, a heat-labile antigen found in the flagellum
- **K antigen,** or capsular antigen, a heat-labile polysaccharide found in certain species, such as the K1 antigen of *E. coli* and **Vi antigen** of *Salmonella typhi*

Clinical Significance

Members of the family Enterobacteriaceae are ubiquitous in nature. With the exception of a few

TABLE 16-1

Classification of the Family Enterobacteriaceae

Tribe	Genus	Species	Tribe	Genus	Species
I. Escherichieae	*Escherichia*	coli	V. Klebsielleae, cont'd	*Enterobacter*	aerogenes
		blattae			cloacae
		vulneris			agglomerans
		fergusonii			complex
		hermannii			amnigenus
	Shigella	dysenteriae			sakazakii
		flexneri			gergoviae
		boydii			dissolvens
		sonnei			nimipressuralis
II. Edwardsielleae	*Edwardsiella*	tarda			asburiae
		hoshinae			cancerogenus
		ictaluri			(taylorae)
III. Salmonelleae	*Salmonella*				hormaechei
	Subgroup I	(Most serotypes)		*Hafnia*	alvei
		typhi		*Serratia*	marcescens
		choleraesuis			liquefaciens
		paratyphi A			rubidaea
		gallinarum			fonticola
		pullorum			odorifera
	Subgroup II				plymuthica
	Subgroup III				ficaria
	(Arizona)			*Pantoea*	agglomerans
	Subgroup IV		VI. Proteeae	*Proteus*	mirabilis
	Subgroup V				vulgaris
IV. Citrobacteriaceae	*Citrobacter*	freundii			penneri
		koseri *(diversus)*			myxofaciens
		amalonaticus		*Morganella*	morganii
V. Klebsielleae	*Klebsiella*	pneumoniae ssp.		*Providencia*	alcalifaciens
		pneumoniae			stuartii
		pneumoniae ssp.			rettgeri
		ozaenae			rustigianii
		oxytoca	VII. Yersinieae	*Yersinia*	pseudotuberculosis
		rhinoscleromatis			pestis
		planticola			enterocolitica
		terrigena			frederiksenii
		ornithinolytica			kristensenii
					intermedia
					ruckeri
					aldovae

Modified from Ewing WH: *Edwards and Ewing's identification of Enterobacteriaceae,* ed 4, East Norwalk, Conn, 1986, Appleton & Lange.

species, most are present in the intestinal tract of animals and humans as commensal flora. Some species exist as free-living organisms in soil, water, and sewage, while others are known to be plant pathogens.

Based on the clinical infections they produce, members of the family Enterobacteriaceae may be divided into two categories: (1) opportunistic pathogens and (2) primary intestinal pathogens.

The opportunistic pathogens are often a part of the usual intestinal flora of both humans and animals. Outside their habitat, these organisms may produce serious extraintestinal opportunistic infections as previously described in the case presented. For example, *E. coli,* a member of the bowel flora, may cause fatal meningitis in the newborn, and septicemia or wound and urinary tract infections in persons of any age group. Other organisms found in the environment can be equally devastating if infections develop in a compro-

TABLE 16-2

Biochemical Characteristics of Tribes of Enterobacteriaceae

Tests or Substrate	Escherichieae	Edwardsielleae	Citrobacteriaceae	Salmonelleae*	Klebsielleae	Proteeae†	Yersinieae
Hydrogen sulfide (TSI agar)	−	+	+ or −	+	−	+ or −	−
Urease	−	−	(+ᵂ) or −	−	− or (+)	+ or −	+
Indole	+ or −	+	− or +	−	−	+ or −	+ or −
Methyl red	+	+	+	+	−	+	+
Voges-Proskauer	−	−	−	−	+	−	−
Citrate (Simmons)	−	−	+	+	+	d	−
KCN	−	−	+ or −	−	+	+	−
Phenylalanine deaminase	−	−	−	−	−	+	−
Mucate	d	−		d	+ or −	−	
Mannitol	+ or −	−	+	+	+	− or +	+

Modified from Ewing WH: *Edwards and Ewing's identification of Enterobacteriaceae,* ed 4, East Norwalk, Conn, 1986, Appleton & Lange, p 43.
+, 90% or more positive within 1 or 2 days; (+), positive reaction after 3 or more days (decarboxylase tests: 3 or 4 days); −, no reaction (90% or more) in 30 days; + *or* −, most cultures positive; some strains negative; − *or* +, most strains negative; some cultures positive; *d,* different reactions, +, (+), −; *w,* weakly positive reaction.
*Salmonella biosers *typhi* and *paratyphi* A and some rare bioserotypes fail to utilize citrate in Simmons medium. Cultures of bioser *paratyphi* A and some rare bioserotypes may fail to produce hydrogen sulfide; an occasional strain of almost any serotype of *Salmonella* genus may be hydrogen sulfide negative.
†Some cultures of *Proteus mirabilis* may yield positive Voges-Proskauer tests.

mised host or in wounds contaminated with soil or water.

The primary intestinal pathogens, *Salmonella* organisms, *Shigella* organisms, and *Yersinia enterocolitica,* are considered true pathogens; they are not commensal flora in the gastrointestinal tract of humans. These organisms produce infections that result from the ingestion of contaminated food and water. Table 16-3 describes the diseases commonly associated with members of Enterobacteriaceae.

TABLE 16-3

Bacterial Species and the Infections They Commonly Produce

Bacterial Species	Diseases
Escherichia coli	Bacteriuria, septicemia, neonatal sepsis, meningitis, and diarrheal syndrome
Shigella spp.	Diarrhea, dysentery
Edwardsiella spp.	Diarrhea, wound infection, septicemia, meningitis, enteric fever
Salmonella spp.	Septicemia, enteric fever, diarrhea
Citrobacter spp.	Opportunistic and nosocomial infections (wound, urinary)
Klebsiella spp.	Bacteriuria, pneumonia, septicemia
Enterobacter spp.	Opportunistic and nosocomial infection, wound infection, septicemia, bacteriuria
Serratia spp.	Opportunistic and nosocomial infection, wound infection, septicemia, bacteriuria
Proteus spp.	Wound infection, septicemia, bacteriuria
Providencia spp.	Opportunistic and nosocomial infections, wound infection, septicemia, bacteriuria
Morganella spp.	Opportunistic and nosocomial infections
Yersinia	
pestis	Plague
pseudotuberculosis	Mesenteric adenitis, diarrhea
enterocolitica	Mesenteric adenitis, diarrhea
Erwinia spp.	Wounds contaminated with soil or vegetation
Pectobacterium spp.	Wounds contaminated with soil or vegetation

Modified from Washington J: *Laboratory procedures in clinical microbiology,* ed 2, New York, 1981, Springer-Verlag.

OPPORTUNISTIC MEMBERS OF THE FAMILY ENTEROBACTERIACEAE AND ASSOCIATED INFECTIONS

Escherichia coli

E. coli, the most significant species in the genus *Escherichia,* is recognized as an important potential pathogen in humans. A gram-negative bacillus, it is a common isolate from the colon flora. *E. coli* has a distinctive colony morphology on certain laboratory media, such as MacConkey agar. Although it may appear as a non–lactose-fermenter or as a mucoid colony, *E. coli* usually produces a dry, pink (lactose positive) colony with a surrounding pink area of precipitated bile salts on MacConkey agar. Figure 16-1 illustrates the different colonial morphologies of *E. coli* growing on MacConkey agar. In addition, *E. coli* may appear as a β-hemolytic colony on blood agar plate (BAP).

Most strains of *E. coli* are motile and generally possess both sex pilli and adhesive fimbriae. The organism also possesses O, H, and K antigens. *E. coli* O groups have shown cross-reactivity with similar antigens in other members of Enterobacteriaceae, notably with shigellae. Typing for H antigens is useful in completing the serogrouping of a particular strain. The capsular K antigen, located on the bacterial surface, often masks the O antigen during bacterial agglutination by specific antiserum. Some *E. coli* K antigens are identical to capsular antigens of other species. The K1 antigen has been found to

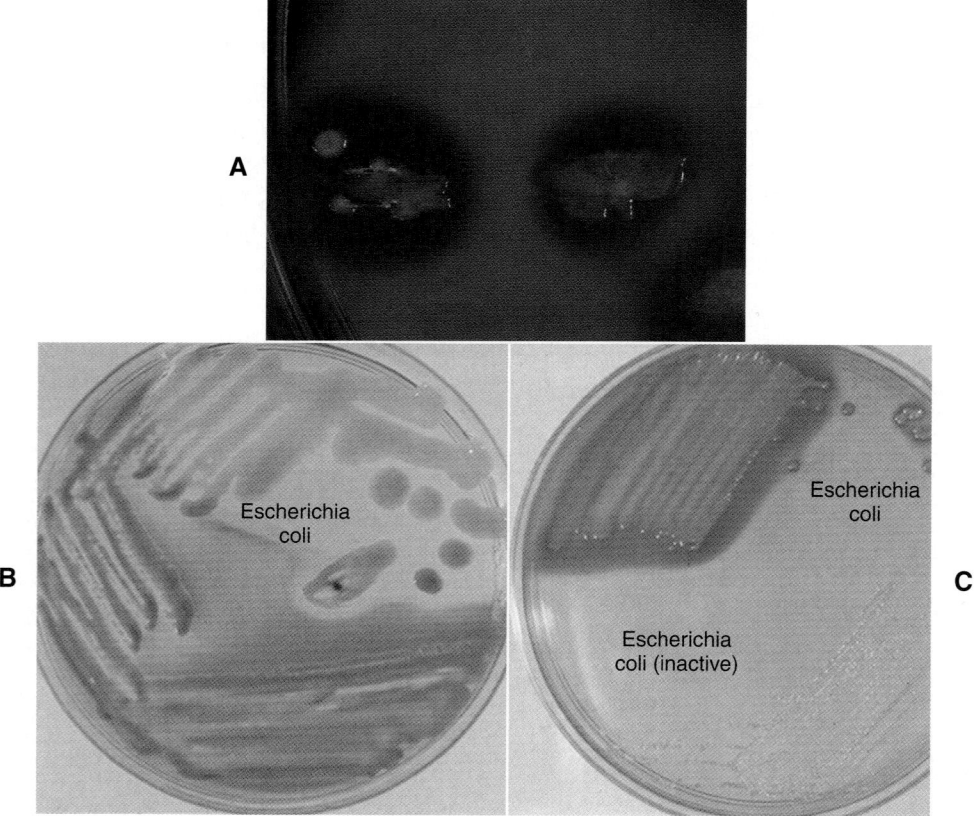

Figure 16-1

A, The typical dry, lactose-positive *Escherichia coli* growing on MacConkey agar. Note the pink precipitate surrounding the individual colonies. **B,** Mucoid colonies of *E. coli* growing on MacConkey agar. **C,** Non–lactose-fermenting (inactive) *E. coli* compared with typical *E. coli* on MacConkey agar. (**B** and **C,** Courtesy Jean Barnishan.)

be identical to the capsular antigen in group B *Neisseria meningitidis,* suggesting a virulence property of K antigens.

Characteristically, *E. coli* does the following:

- Ferments glucose, lactose, trehalose, and xylose
- Has positive indole and methyl red tests
- Does not produce H_2S, DNase, urease, or phenylalanine deaminase
- Does not grow in the presence of potassium cyanide
- Cannot utilize citrate as a sole source of carbon
- May be motile or nonmotile
- Produces a negative result with Voges-Proskauer test

Clinical infections

First described by Theodore Escherich in 1885, *E. coli* was considered a nonharmful member of the colon flora. Since then, *E. coli* has been associated with a wide range of diseases and infections, including meningeal (particularly in the newborn), gastrointestinal, urinary tract, wound, and bacteremic infections in all age groups.

GASTROINTESTINAL INFECTIONS

E. coli may cause several types of diarrheal illnesses. There are five major categories of diarrheogenic *E. coli,* based on definite virulence factors, clinical manifestations produced, epidemiology, and different O:H serotypes. These include the following:

- **Enteropathogenic (EPEC)**
- **Enterotoxigenic (ETEC)**
- **Enteroinvasive (EIEC)**
- **Enterohemorrhagic (EHEC)** serotype O157:H7
- **Enteroaggregative (EaggEC)**

The serotypes associated with these categories and the features associated with the intestinal infections produced by these strains are summarized in Chapter 28.

Enteropathogenic *E. coli* Whereas the enteropathogenic *E. coli* (EPEC) strain has been known to cause infantile diarrhea since the 1940s, its pathogenic role has remained controversial over the last two decades. Certain O serogroups of EPEC were identified in the late 1960s and 1970s as a cause of diarrhea, but only certain H types within each O serogroup were connected to the intestinal infections. O serogrouping could not, however, differentiate these *E. coli* strains from strains of normal flora. In 1978, Levine and colleagues attempted to settle the dispute concerning the pathogenic role of EPEC by challenging volunteers with EPEC strains that lacked the toxins of ETEC and the invasiveness of EIEC. This study showed that these EPEC strains caused distinct diarrhea. Subsequent studies further showed the adhesive property of EPEC strains, a characteristic not seen in ETEC or EIEC strains. The pathogenesis of enteroadherent EPEC is fully described in Farthing and Keusch's textbook *Enteric Infections: Mechanisms, Manifestations,* and *Management.*

Diarrheal outbreaks due to EPEC have occurred in hospital nurseries and day care centers. Cases in adults are rarely seen. The illness is characterized by low-grade fever, malaise, vomiting, and diarrhea. The stool contains large amounts of mucus, but gross blood is not usually present.

Detection of diarrheal illness due to EPEC depends primarily on the index of suspicion of the clinician. In cases of severe diarrhea in children younger than 1 year, infection with EPEC should be suspected. Serologic typing with pooled antisera may be performed to identify EPEC serotypes. However, serotyping for EPEC has been used chiefly for epidemiologic studies rather than for diagnostic purposes.

Enterotoxigenic *E. coli* Enterotoxigenic (ETEC) strains are associated with diarrhea of infants and adults in tropical and subtropical climates, especially in developing countries, where it is one of the major causes of infant bacterial diarrhea. In the United States and other developed countries, ETEC diarrhea is the most common cause of a diarrheal disease sometimes referred to as **"traveler's diarrhea."** This diarrheal illness is often acquired by travelers from industrialized countries when they visit developing countries. ETEC infection is commonly acquired by consuming contaminated food or water. Poor hygiene, inadequate sources of drinking water, and lack of proper sanitation are major contributing factors in the spread and transmission of the disease. A high infective dose of the organisms (10^6 to 10^{10} organisms) is necessary to initiate disease in an immunocompetent host. Protective mechanisms such as stomach acidity have been described as inhibiting colonization and initiation of disease; those suffering from achlorhydria seem to be at greater risk than are normal individuals.

Colonization of ETEC on the proximal small intestine has been recognized to be mediated by adhesion fimbriae that permit ETEC to bind to specific receptors on the microvilli. Once enterotoxigenic strains of *E. coli* are established, they may release into the small intestine one or both of the toxins they produce: a heat-labile toxin (LT) and a heat-stable toxin (ST). The action of the LT is similar to that of *Vibrio cholerae* toxin. Two fragments (A and B) make up the LT; the B fragment binds on the receptor site present on the GM_1 ganglioside of the intestinal mucosa. This binding facilitates the entry of the A fragment, which then acts on adenyl cyclase, activating the conversion of adenosine triphosphate (ATP) to cyclic adenosine monophosphate (cAMP). The accumulation of cAMP in the intestinal mucosa initiates the hypersecretion of electrolytes and fluids into the lumen, resulting in a watery diarrhea. The ST, on the other hand, stimulates guanylate cyclase, causing the increased production of cyclic guanosine monophosphate (cGMP) and subsequent hypersecretion.

The usually self-limiting disease caused by ETEC is characterized by nonbloody, watery diarrhea, nausea, abdominal cramps, and low-grade fever. No evidence exists of mucosal penetration or invasion. The illness may last from 1 to 5 days. Diagnosis of ETEC infections is made primarily by the characteristic presenting symptoms and the isolation of solely lactose-fermenting organisms on differential media. Testing for toxins or colonizing factors remains in the research and reference laboratories, and its use is not justified in the clinical laboratory for diagnostic purposes. Enzyme-labeled oligonucleotide probes have been reported to detect ETEC in fecal specimens. This method is undergoing further testing to determine its efficacy. ETEC infections must be differentiated, however, from other diarrheal illnesses which may appear similar (see Chapter 28).

Enteroinvasive *E. coli* Enteroinvasive strains of *E. coli* (EIEC) are strains very different from the strains of EPEC and ETEC. Enteroinvasive strains produce dysentery with direct penetration, invasion, and destruction of the intestinal mucosa. This diarrheal illness is very similar to that produced by shigellae. The EIEC infections seem to occur in adults and children alike. Direct transmission of EIEC from person to person via the fecal-oral route with subsequent occurrence of an outbreak was reported by Harris and colleagues in 1985.

The clinical infection is characterized by fever, severe abdominal cramps, malaise, and watery diarrhea accompanied by toxemia. Scanty stool containing pus, mucus, and blood follows the watery diarrhea. The organisms may be easily misidentified because of their similarity to shigellae.

EIEC strains may be nonmotile and do not ferment lactose; cross-reactions between shigellae and EIEC O antigens have been seen. Isolates may be mistaken for nonpathogenic *E coli;* although EIEC do not decarboxylate lysine, more than 80% of *E. coli* decarboxylate lysine. For these reasons, cases of diarrheal illness resulting from EIEC may be underreported. Although EIEC and *Shigella* have been found to be similar in morphology and in clinical presentation, the infective dose of EIEC necessary to produce disease is much higher than that of shigellae.

The enteroinvasiveness of EIEC has to be demonstrated for definitive identification. The tests currently available to determine the invasive property of EIEC are not widely used in most clinical microbiology laboratories. The Sereny test, which determines the organisms' ability to produce keratoconjunctivitis in the guinea pig, is one of the assays previously used to determine the virulence of both shigellae and EIEC. DNA probes to identify EIEC strains have been studied and compared with the Sereny test, with comparable results. Other more recent developments in detecting invasiveness include monolayer cell cultures with Hep-2 cells.

Recently, DNA probes to screen stool samples for EIEC have been developed, which eliminate the need for various other tests to identify EIEC.

Enterohemorrhagic *E. coli* In 1982, the O157:H7 strain of *E. coli* was first recognized during an outbreak of hemorrhagic diarrhea and colitis. The enterohemorrhagic *E. coli* (EHEC) strain serotype O157:H7 has since been associated with hemorrhagic diarrhea, colitis, and hemolytic-uremic syndrome (HUS). HUS is characterized by low platelet count, hemolytic anemia, and kidney failure.

The classic illness caused by EHEC is characterized by a watery diarrhea that progresses to a bloody diarrhea and crampy abdominal pain, with low-grade fever or no fever at all. The diarrheic stool contains no leukocytes, which differentiates it from dysentery caused by shigellae or EIEC strain infection. The infection is potentially fatal, especially in young children in day care centers and schools and among the elderly in nursing homes. Processed meats, such as undercooked hamburger served at fast food restaurants, unpasteurized milk, and apple cider, have been implicated in the spread of infection.

E. coli O157:H7 produces two cytotoxins: verotoxins I and II. Verotoxin I is a phage-encoded cytotoxin identical to the **Shiga toxin (Stx)** produced by *Shigella dysenteriae* type I. This verotoxin shows damage on vero cells (African green monkey kidney cells), hence the term *vero*toxin. It also reacts with and is neutralized by the antibody against Shiga toxin. In contrast with verotoxin I, the second cytotoxin (verotoxin II) is not neutralized by the antibody to Shiga toxin and is immunologically different from but biologically similar to verotoxin I. These verotoxins have also been called Shiga-like toxins but are more recently referred to as Shiga toxin 1 (Stx 1) and Shiga toxin 2 (Stx 2); *E. coli* strains that produce these toxins are called Shiga toxigenic *E. coli* (STEC). Several different STEC strains and not just O157.H7 have been reported, and these other serotypes can cause clinical syndromes similar to that produced by O157:H7 *E. coli*. Box 16-1 lists non–O157:H7 EHEC isolated from patients with bloody diarrhea, hemorrhagic colitis, or hemolytic uremic syndrome.

In the laboratory, verotoxin-producing *E. coli* may be identified by one of three methods:

- Stool culture on highly differential medium, with subsequent serotyping
- Finding the verotoxin in stool filtrates
- Demonstration of a fourfold or greater increase in verotoxin-neutralizing antibody titer

Stool culture for *E. coli* O157:H7 may be performed using MacConkey agar containing sorbitol instead of lactose. *E. coli* O157:H7 does not ferment sorbitol in 48 hours, a characteristic that differentiates it from most *E. coli*. The use of this differential medium facilitates the primary screening of *E. coli* O157:H7, which ordinarily would not be distinguished from other *E. coli* on lactose-containing MacConkey or other routine enteric agar. *E. coli* O157:H7 appears colorless on sorbitol–MacConkey agar. Although isolation of other non–sorbitol-fermenting organisms may occur in up to 15% of cultures, *E. coli* O157:H7, when present, produces a heavy growth. A latex agglutination test for rapid presumptive detection of *E. coli* O157:H7 has also been reported useful; isolates must be tested with the negative control to detect nonspecific agglutination.

The commercially available MUG assay (4-methylumbelliferyl β-D-glucuronide) is a biochemical test that may be used to screen for O157:H7, in addition to testing for sorbitol fermentation. *E. coli* O157:H7 rarely produces the enzyme β-glucuronidase, whereas 92% of the other strains do. If the enzyme is present, MUG is cleaved, and a fluorescent product is formed that is detectable with ultraviolet light.

Sorbitol-negative colonies are subsequently subcultured for serotyping using *E. coli* O157:H7 antiserum. ELISA or latex agglutination tests may be used to detect the O157 antigen. This somatic antigen, which is usually the specific target of these commercial assays, may present a problem with regards to specificity because other enteric bacteria may produce false positive results. It is therefore important to confirm the identification of MUG-negative or sorbitol-negative colonies as *E. coli* isolates. A latex test to detect H7 is also now available. When testing colonies taken directly from

---

Box 16-1

Non–O157:H7 Enterohemorrhagic *Escherichia coli* Recovered From Patients with Diarrhea, Hemolytic Colitis, or Hemolytic Uremic Sydrome

O6:H31	OX3:H21	O113:H21
O48:H7	O26	O26:H11
O111:H2	O98:NM	O103:H2
O104:H21	O121:H19	O145:NM

From Nauschuetz W: Emerging foodborne pathogens: enterohemorrhagic *Escherichia coli, Clin Lab Sci* 11:298, 1998.

SMAC plate, the test for H7 may first be negative. It is helpful to grow these isolates in motility media first to enhance agglutination of H7 latex particles. Following the serotyping with *E. coli* O157:H7 antiserum, the isolates are tested for Shiga toxin production. Investigative reports have shown that all *E. coli* O157:H7 strains have so far been found to produce high levels of cytotoxins. STEC strains may be detected using cell culture assays using Vero cells. Because other toxins present in diarrheic stools may produce similar cytopathic effect, this test must be verified with specific antitoxins to Stx 1 and 2.

Free verotoxins present in stool samples have been detected in samples that yielded negative culture results. It had been previously reported that patients with hemorrhagic colitis shed the organism for only a brief period of time; nevertheless, verotoxins may still be detected in the stool. A recently approved ELISA (EHEC Premier, Meridian Diagnostics Inc, Cincinnati, OH) to detect Stx directly from stools can be used for bloody stools, although not all patients with this type of infection produce bloody diarrhea. Gene amplification assay that would amplify the genes that code for Shiga toxins and identify these strains may also be useful in detecting STEC infections. A fourfold increase in verotoxin-neutralizing antibody titer has been demonstrated in patients with hemolytic-uremic syndrome and in whom verotoxin or verotoxin-producing *E. coli* had been detected.

Enteroaggregative *E. coli* Enteroaggregative *E. coli* (EaggEC), first referred to as enteroadherent-enteroaggregative *E. coli,* cause diarrhea by adhering to the mucosal surface of the intestine. These strains are found to adhere to Hep2 cells, packed in an aggregative pattern on the cells and in between the cells. These organisms produce symptoms such as watery diarrhea, vomiting, dehydration, and occasionally, abdominal pain. These symptoms may persist for more than 2 weeks.

OTHER *E. COLI* INFECTIONS

Urinary tract infections *E. coli* is known to be the most common cause of urinary tract and kidney infections in humans. The *E. coli* that cause urinary tract infections usually originate in the large intestine as resident or transient members of the colon flora and may exist as a dominating or minority strain. Strains that cause urinary tract infections are believed to be selected from the fecal flora because of their special adaptation to the urinary tract epithelial mucosa. Moreover, strains isolated from urinary tract infections and acute pyelonephritis in immunocompetent hosts differ from those isolated in hosts compromised by instrumentation (e.g., catheterization) or by other defects of the urinary tract.

E. coli strains that cause acute pyelonephritis in immunocompetent hosts have been shown to be dominating and resident members of the colon flora. These isolates from pyelonephritis infections, which belong to certain serotypes, were also shown to be resistant to the bactericidal activity of serum. Isolates from immunocompromised hosts, on the other hand, consist of a wide variety of strains. Similarly, strains isolated from asymptomatic bacteriuria (ABU) cannot be attributed to a particular population of the colon flora isolates. In addition, isolates from ABU are susceptible to the bactericidal activity of the serum. No specific serotype has been identified.

Among the factors that contribute to the virulence of urethrogenic *E. coli* is the capability of the organism to adhere to the epithelial cells lining the urinary tract. This capability is mediated by adhesins. Another factor is the ability to produce hemolysins and aerobactin. Hemolysins kill leukocytes and inhibit phagocytosis and chemotaxis. Aerobactin is an extracellular iron chelator.

Septicemia and meningitis *E. coli* remains one of the most common causes of septicemia and meningitis among neonates, accounting for approximately 40% of the cases of gram-negative meningitis. Similar infections resulting from this organism are uncommon among older children.

The newborn usually acquires the infection in the birth canal just before or during delivery, when the mother's vagina is heavily colonized. Infection may also result if contamination of the amniotic fluid takes place. Although several strains of *E. coli* have been identified, based on serotypes and enterotoxin production, and associated with diarrheic illnesses, these strains have not been associated with neonatal sepsis or meningitis.

The capsular antigen K1 present in certain strains of *E. coli* has been the most documented virulence-associated factor in neonatal meningeal infections. *E. coli* K1 antigen is also immunochemically identical with the capsular antigen of group B *Neisseria meningitidis.* The association of K1 antigen was established when *E. coli* strains possessing capsular K1 antigen were isolated from neonates with septicemia or meningitis. Fatality rates for infants with meningitis caused by *E. coli* K1 strains also were higher than those for infants infected with non–K1 strains.

In addition to the neonatal population, *E. coli* also remains as a clinically significant isolate in blood cultures from adults. *E. coli* bacteremia in adults may result primarily from a genitourinary tract infection or from a gastrointestinal source.

Other *Escherichia* Species

Escherichia hermannii, formerly called *E. coli* atypical or enteric group II, is a yellow-pigmented organism that has been isolated from spinal fluid, wounds, and blood. Reports of isolating *E. hermannii* from foodstuffs such as raw milk and beef, the same sources of *E. coli* O157:H7, have been published. However, its clinical significance is not fully established.

The newest species added to this genus, *Escherichia vulneris,* has been isolated from humans with infected wounds. More than half of the strains of *E. vulneris* may also produce yellow-pigmented colonies. Figure 16-2 compares the colonial morphology of *E. hermannii* with that of *E. vulneris. Escherichia blattae* is an indole-negative species currently found only in the feces of cockroaches.

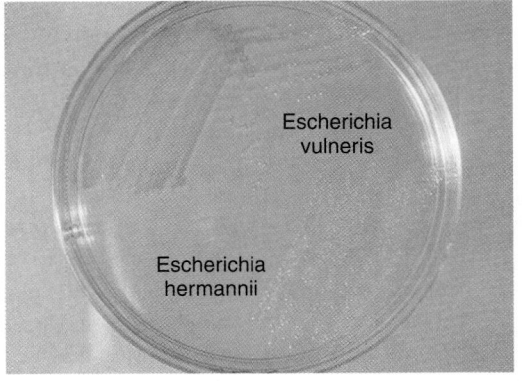

Figure 16-2 _____

Comparison of the colonial morphology of *Escherichia vulneris* and a yellow pigmented *Escherichia hermannii* on MacConkey agar. *Escherichia vulneris* may also produce a yellow-pigmented colony, but the yellow is more prevalent in *E. hermannii.* (Courtesy Jean Barnishan.)

Klebsiella, Enterobacter, Serratia, and *Hafnia* Species

Members of these genera are usually found in the intestinal tract of humans and animals or free-living in soil, water, and plants. These bacterial species have been associated with a wide variety of opportunistic and nosocomial infections, particularly pneumonia and wound and urinary tract infections.

Klebsiella, Enterobacter, Serratia, and *Hafnia* organisms demonstrate variable biochemical reactions. Characteristic of these genera are the following:

- Some species are motile, and some are non-motile
- Most grow on Simmons sodium citrate and in potassium cyanide broth
- None produce hydrogen sulfide
- None (rare) deaminate phenylalanine
- Few hydrolyze urea slowly
- All give a negative reaction with the methyl red test and a positive reaction with the Voges-Proskauer test. With a few exceptions, indole is not produced

Klebsiella species

Usually found in the gastrointestinal tracts of humans and animals, the genus *Klebsiella* consists of several species, namely *Klebsiella pneumoniae, Klebsiella oxytoca, Klebsiella ozaenae* and *Klebsiella rhinoscleromatis.* The absence of motility distinguishes *Klebsiella* species from other members of the family Enterobacteriaceae. Differential features of *Klebsiella* species are shown in Table 16-4.

K. pneumoniae is the most commonly isolated species. *K. pneumoniae* has the distinct feature of possessing a polysaccharide capsule. The capsule offers the organism protection against phagocytosis and antimicrobial absorption, thus contributing to its virulence. This capsule is also responsible for the moist, mucoid colonies characteristic of *K. pneumoniae.* Occasionally evident in direct smears from clinical materials, this capsule is sometimes helpful in providing a presumptive identification. Figure 16-3 illustrates the mucoid appearance of *K. pneumoniae* on MacConkey agar.

Colonization of gram-negative rods in the respiratory tract of hospitalized patients, particularly

TABLE 16-4

Differentiation of Common Species within the Genus Klebsiella

Test or Substrate	*K. pneumoniae*			*K. oxytoca*			*K. ozaenae*			*K. rhinoscleromatis*		
	Sign	% +	(% +)	Sign	% +	(% +)	Sign	% +	(% +)	Sign	% +	(% +)
Urease	+	95.4	(0.1)	+	90		d	14.5^w	(14.8)	−	0	
Indole	−	0		+	100		−	0		−	0	
Methyl red	− or +	11.3		+	100		+	97.7		+	100	
Voges-Proskauer	+	93.7		+	96		−	0		−	0	
Citrate (Simmons)	+	96.8	(0.6)	+	95		d	28.1	(32.4)	−	0	
Gelatin (22° C)	−	0	(0.2)	(+) or −	64		−	0		−	0	
Lysine decarboxylase	+	97.2	(0.1)	+	99		− or +	35.8	(6.3)	−	0	
Malonate	+	92.5		+	100		−	6		+ or −	50	
Mucate	+	92.8		+	95		− or +	25		−	0	
Sodium alginate (utilization)	+ or (+)	88.5	(9.2)	nd			− or (+)	0	(11)	−	0	
Gas from glucose	+	96		+	100		d	55.5	(9.4)	−	0	
Lactose	+	98.7	(1)	+	100		d	26.2	(61.3)	d	6	(70)
Dulcitol	− or +	33		+ or −	53		−	0		−	0	
Organic acid media												
Citrate	+ or −	64.4		nd			− or +	18		−	0	
D-Tartrate	+ or −	67.1		nd			− or +	39		−	0	

Modified from Ewing WH: *Edwards and Ewing's identification of Enterobacteriaceae,* ed 4, East Norwalk, Conn, 1986, Appleton & Lange.

+, 90% or more positive within 1 or 2 days; (+), positive reaction after 3 or more days (decarboxylase tests: 3 or 4 days); −, no reaction (90% or more); + *or* −, most cultures positive; some strains negative; − *or* +, most strains negative; some cultures positive; + *or* (+), most reactions occur within 1 or 2 days; some are delayed; *d,* different reactions, +, (+), −; *nd,* no data; *w,* weakly positive reaction.

of *Klebsiella pneumoniae,* increases with the length of hospital stay. *K. pneumoniae* is a frequent cause of lower respiratory tract infections among hospitalized patients and in other immunocompromised hosts, such as newborns, the aged, and seriously ill patients on respirators. Other infections com-

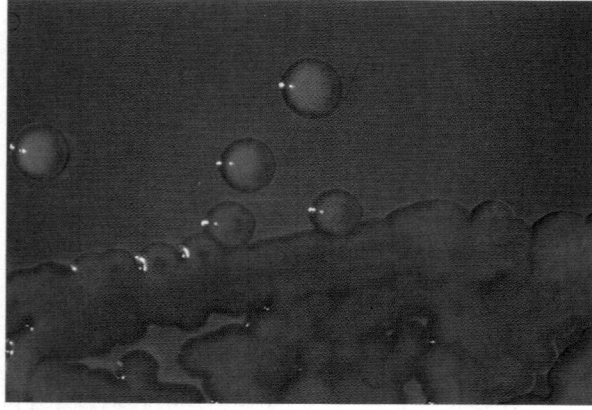

Figure 16-3

Mucoid appearance of *Klebsiella pneumoniae* on MacConkey agar.

monly associated with *K. pneumoniae* involving immunocompromised hosts are wound infections, urinary tract infections, and bacteremia. Reports exist of nosocomial outbreaks of *Klebsiella* infections resistant to multiple antibiotics in newborn nurseries. These outbreaks have been attributed to the plasmid transfer of antimicrobial resistance. Other *Klebsiella* species have been associated with a number of infections. *K. oxytoca* is identical to *K. pneumoniae* except for its production of indole. It produces infections similar to those caused by *K. pneumoniae*. *K. ozaenae* has been isolated from nasal secretions and cerebral abscesses.

K. rhinoscleromatis has been isolated from patients with rhinoscleroma, an infection of the nasal cavity that manifests as an intense swelling and malformation of the entire face and neck. Cases of rhinoscleroma have been reported in Africa and South America. Both *K. ozaenae* and *K. rhinoscleromatis* are not considered true species but are viewed as biochemically inactive strains of *K. pneumoniae*. Organisms of *Klebsiella* group 47, proposed name *Klebsiella ornithinolytica* (indole- and ornithine decarboxylase–positive) and *Klebsiella plan-*

ticola, have been isolated from the urine, respiratory tracts, and blood of humans. *Klebsiella terrigena* has been found in soil and water isolates but has not been implicated in human diseases.

Enterobacter species

The genus *Enterobacter* is composed of 12 species, one of which consists of two biotypes. Clinically significant *Enterobacter* species that have been isolated from clinical samples include *Enterobacter cloacae, Enterobacter aerogenes, Enterobacter agglomerans, Enterobacter gergoviae, Enterobacter sakazakii,* and *Enterobacter hormaechei* (newly proposed name). Members of this genus are characterized as motile. The colony morphology of many of the species resembles that of *Klebsiella* when growing on MacConkey agar. *Enterobacter* species grow on Simmons citrate and in potassium cyanide broth; the methyl red is negative and the Voges-Proskauer test is positive. Unlike *Klebsiella,* however, *Enterobacter* species usually produce ornithine decarboxylase; lysine decarboxylase is produced by most species but not by *E. agglomerans* or *E. cloacae.*

E. cloacae and *E. aerogenes* are the two most common isolates from this genus. Distinguishing characteristics between *E. cloacae, E. aerogenes,* and *K. pneumoniae* are shown in Table 16-5. These two species have been isolated from wounds, urine, blood, and spinal fluid.

E. agglomerans gained notoriety with a nationwide outbreak of septicemia resulting from contaminated intravenous fluids. More recently designated as *E. agglomerans* complex, it includes species that are lysine, ornithine, arginine negative or "triple decarboxylases negative." More than 13 hybridization groups (G) have been described in this complex. *E. agglomerans* HG XIII, which may produce a yellow pigment, has been transferred to a new genus: *Pantoea,* a primarily plant pathogen. *E. agglomerans* is now renamed as *Pantoea agglomerans.*

Figure 16-4 depicts a yellow-pigmented *P. agglomerans. Enterobacter gergoviae* is found in respiratory samples but is rarely isolated from blood cultures. *Enterobacter sakazakii,* a yellow-pigmented *Enterobacter* species, has been documented as a pathogen in neonates causing meningeal and bacteremic infections. It has also been isolated from cultures taken from brain abscesses and respiratory and wound infections. Figure 16-5 illustrates the colonial morphology of *E. sakazakii. E. hormaechei* has been isolated from human sources such as blood, wounds, and sputum.

Enterobacter amnigenus biotypes 1 and 2 and *Enterobacter intermedius* are found naturally in soil and water. *Enterobacter dissolvens* and *Enterobacter*

TABLE 16-5

Diagnostic Features of Enterobacter cloacae, Enterobacter aerogenes, *and* Klebsiella pneumoniae

Test or Substrate	E. cloacae			E. aerogenes			K. pneumoniae		
	Sign	%+	(%+)	Sign	%+	(%+)	Sign	%+	(%+)
Urease	+ᵂ or −	74.6		−	5.0ʷ		+	95.4	(0.1)
Motility	+	92.4		+	91.7		−	0.	
Lysine decarboxylase	−	0		+	97.5		+	97.3	(6.3)
Arginine dihydrolase	+	92.4	(2)	−	0		-	0	
Ornithine decarboxylase	+	93.7	(1.3)	+	95.9	(0.8)	−	0	
Gelatin (22° C)	(+)	0.6	(94.2)	(+) or −	0	(61.2)	−	0	(0.2)
Adonitol, gas	− or +	21.7	(1.3)	+	94.2		d	84.4	(0.3)
Inositol									
Acid	d	13	(8)	+	96.7		+	97.2	(0.9)
Gas	−	4.1	(1.5)	+	93.4		+	92.5	(1.5)
Jordan D-tartrate	− or +	27.4		+ or −	78.3		+	94.4	
Sodium alginate (utilization)	−	0		−	0		+ or (+)	88.9	(8.9)

Modified from Ewing WH: *Edwards and Ewing's identification of Enterobacteriaceae,* ed 4, East Norwalk, Conn., 1986, Appleton & Lange.
+, 90% or more positive within 1 or 2 days; (+), positive reaction after 3 or more days (decarboxylase tests: 3 or 4 days); −, no reaction (90% or more) in 30 days; + or −, most cultures positive, some strains negative; − or +, most strains negative, some cultures positive; + or (+), most reactions occur within 1 or 2 days, some are delayed; *d,* different reactions, +, (+), −; *w,* weakly positive reaction.

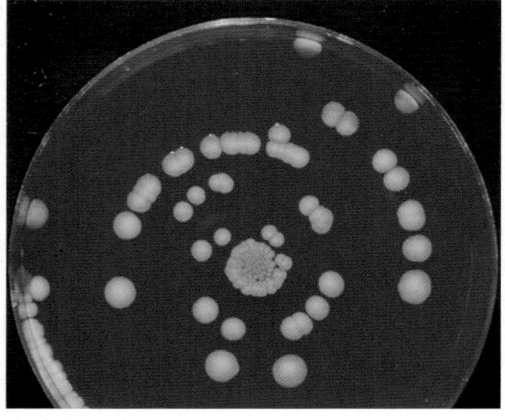

Figure 16-4 _____

Yellow-pigmented *Pantoea agglomerans* (formerly *Enterobacter agglomerans*) blood agar plate. (Courtesy Jean Barnishan.)

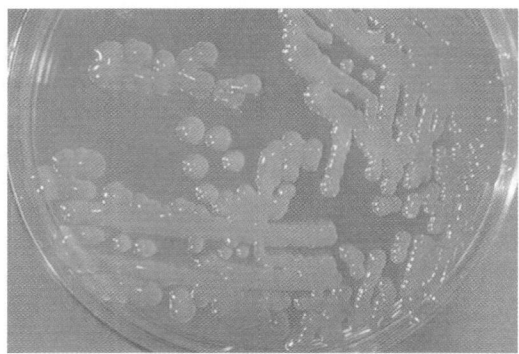

Figure 16-5 _____

Mucoid, yellow-pigmented colonies of *Enterobacter sakazakii* growing on brain-heart infusion agar. (Courtesy Jean Barnishan.)

nimipressuralis are newly recognized species with unknown clinical significance. *Enterobacter asburiae* is similar biochemically to *E. cloacae* and has been isolated from blood, urine, feces, sputum, and wounds.

Serratia species

The genus *Serratia* is composed of *Serratia marcescens, Serratia liquefaciens, Serratia rubidaea, Serratia odorifera, Serratia plymuthica, Serratia ficaria,* and *Serratia fonticola. Serratia* species are opportunistic pathogens associated with nosocomial outbreaks. With the exception of *S. fonticola,*

Serratia species ferment lactose slowly (positive for orthonitrophenyl galactoside [ONPG]) and are differentiated from the tribe by their ability to produce extracellular DNase. *Serratia* species are also known for their resistance to a wide range of antimicrobials. Susceptibility tests must be performed on each isolate to determine appropriate antimicrobial therapy.

S. marcescens and *S rubidaea* produce a characteristic pink to red pigment, especially when the cultures are left at room temperature. Figure 16-6 illustrates the pigmentation of *S. marcescens* and *S. rubidaea.*

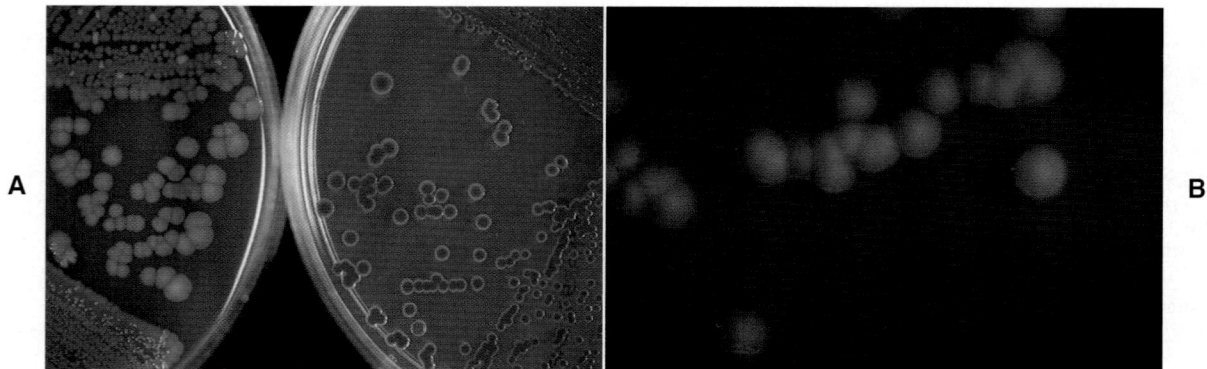

Figure 16-6 _____

A, Example of brick-red pigment of *Serratia marcescens* when growing on MacConkey agar. **B,** Pinkish red pigmentation of *Serratia rubidaea* growing on MacConkey agar.

S. marcescens is the species that is usually considered clinically important. It has frequently been found in hospital-acquired infections of the urinary or respiratory tract and in bacteremic outbreaks in nurseries and cardiac surgery and burn units. Contamination of antiseptic solution used for joint injections has resulted in an epidemic of septic arthritis. *S. plymuthica* osteomyelitis was found following a motorcycle accident. *S. odorifera* contains two biogroups and, as the species name implies, emits a dirty, musty odor resembling that of potatoes. *S. odorifera* biogroup 1 is isolated predominately from the respiratory tract and is positive for sucrose, raffinose, and ornithine. In addition, biogroup 1 may be indole positive (60%). *S. odorifera* biogroup 2 is negative for sucrose, raffinose, and ornithine and has been isolated from blood and cerebrospinal fluid. Biogroup 2 may also be indole positive (50%). *S. liquefaciens* and *S. rubidaea* have also been isolated from human sources.

Hafnia species

The genus *Hafnia* is composed of one species, *Hafnia alvei*. However, there are two distinct biotypes recognized: *H. alvei* and *H. alvei* biotype 1. Biotype 1 grows in the beer wort of breweries and has not been isolated clinically. *Hafnia* has been isolated from a number of anatomic sites in humans and in the environment. *Hafnia* species are not known to cause gastroenteritis but are occasionally isolated from stool cultures. A delayed positive citrate reaction is a major characteristic of *Hafnia* species.

Proteus, Morganella, and Providencia Species

Members of the *Proteus, Morganella,* and *Providencia* genera are normal intestinal flora and are recognized as opportunistic pathogens. Members of the tribe are differentiated from other members of the family Enterobacteriaceae by their ability to deaminate phenylalanine and oxidatively deaminate lysine. All fail to ferment lactose.

Proteus species

The genus *Proteus* consists of four species: *Proteus mirabilis, Proteus vulgaris, Proteus penneri,* and *Proteus myxofaciens*. *P. mirabilis* and *P. vulgaris* are widely recognized human pathogens. Both species have been isolated from urine, wounds, and ear

and bacteremic infections. *P. mirabilis* and *P. vulgaris* are easily identified in the clinical laboratory because of their characteristic colony morphology. Both species produce swarming colonies on nonselective media, such as sheep's blood agar. The colonies also produce a distinct odor, sometimes described as "burned chocolate." Both species also produce hydrogen sulfide and hydrolyze urea. *P. mirabilis* is differentiated from *P. vulgaris* by the indole and ornithine decarboxylase tests; *P. mirabilis* does not produce indole from tryptophan and is ornithine positive, whereas *P. vulgaris* produces indole and is ornithine negative. *P. vulgaris* is sucrose positive and gives an acid/acid reaction in triple sugar iron agar.

Formerly a *P. vulgaris* strain, *P. penneri* is a newly recognized species that also swarms on nonselective media. *P. myxofaciens,* a species that has been isolated only from gypsy moths, is characterized by the large amount of slime it produces.

Morganella species

The genus *Morganella* has only one species, *Morganella morganii,* formerly known as *Proteus morganii*. *M. morganii* has been implicated in diarrheal illness, but its role as an etiologic agent of diarrheal disease remains to be further examined. It is, however, a documented cause of urinary tract infections and has been isolated from other human body sites.

Providencia species

The genus *Providencia* consists of four species: *Providencia alcalifaciens, Providencia stuartii, Providencia rettgeri* (formerly *Proteus rettgeri*), and *Providencia rustigianii*. *Providencia rettgeri* is a documented pathogen of the urinary tract and has caused occasional nosocomial outbreaks. Similarly, *P. stuartii* has been incriminated in nosocomial outbreaks in burn units and has been isolated from urine cultures. Infections caused by *P. stuartii* and *P. rettgeri,* especially in immunocompromised patients, are particularly difficult to treat because of their resistance to antimicrobials.

P. alcalifaciens is usually found in the feces of children with diarrhea; however, its role as a cause of diarrhea has not been proved. The new species *P. rustigianii* is rarely isolated, and its pathogenicity also remains unproven. Table 16-6 shows the differentiating characteristics of *Proteus, Providencia,* and *Morganella.*

Edwardsiella Species

The genus *Edwardsiella* is composed of three species: *Edwardsiella tarda, Edwardsiella hoshinae,* and *Edwardsiella ictaluri. E. tarda* is the only recognized human pathogen. Members of this genus are negative for urea and positive for lysine decarboxylase, hydrogen sulfide, and indole and do not grow on Simmon citrate.

E. tarda is an opportunist, causing bacteremic and wound infections. Its pathogenic role in cases of diarrhea remains a controversy. *E. hoshinae* has been isolated from snakes, birds, and water. *E. ictaluri* causes enteric septicema in fish.

Erwinia and *Pectobacterium* Species

Both species are plant pathogens and are not significant in human infections. *Erwinia* organisms grow poorly at 37° C and fail to grow on selective media, such as eosin–methylene blue agar, MacConkey agar, and other differential media typically used for the isolation of enterics. Identification of these organisms will be more for academic interest than for the evaluation of their significance as causative agents of infection. Most *Erwinia* species have been placed under other genera and are given new designations.

Citrobacter Species

Earlier classifications of the family Enterobacteriaceae included the genus *Citrobacter* under the tribe Salmonelleae, which formerly had consisted of the genera *Salmonella, Citrobacter,* and *Arizona.* However, recent changes in the classification and nomenclature of bacterial species belonging to the tribe Salmonelleae (Ewing, 1986) have caused the reclassification of the genus *Citrobacter* into its own tribe and of *arizona* as a subspecies of *Salmonella.* The genus *Citrobacter* consists of *Citrobacter freundii, C. koseri (diversus),* and *Citrobacter amalonaticus.* Most *Citrobacter* species hydrolyze urea slowly and ferment lactose, producing colonies on MacConkey agar that resemble those of *E. coli* (see Figure 16-1, *A*). All grow on Simmons citrate and give positive reactions in the methyl red test.

C. freundii can be isolated in diarrheal stool cultures, and although it is a known extraintestinal pathogen, its pathogenic role in intestinal disease

---

TABLE 16-6

Differentiating Characteristics of Species of Proteus, Providencia, *and* Morganella

Test	*Proteus penneri*	*Proteus mirabilis*	*Proteus vulgaris*	*Providencia alcalifaciens*	*Providencia stuartii*	*Providencia rettgeri*	*Morganella morganii*
Indole	−	−	+	+	+	+	+
Methyl red	+	+	+	+	+	+	+
Voges-Proskauer	−	− or +	−	−	−	−	−
Simmons citrate	−	+ or (+)	d	+	+	+	−
Christensen urea	+	+ or (+)	+	−	− or +	+	+
H₂S (TSIA)	−(70%)	+	+	−	−	−	−
Ornithine decarboxylase	−	+	−	−	−	−	+
Phenylalanine deaminase	+	+	+	+	+	+	+
Acid produced from							
Sucrose	+	d	+	d	d	d	−
Mannitol	−	−	−	−	d	+	−
Salicin	−	−	d	−	−	d	−
Adonitol	−	−	−	+	−	+	−
Rhamnose	−	−	−	−	−	+ or −	−
Maltose	+	−	+	−	−	−	−
Xylose	+	+	+ or (+)	−	−	− or +	−
Arabitol	−	−	−	−	−	+	−
Swarms	+	+	+	−	−	−	−

Modified from Washington J: *Laboratory procedures in clinical microbiology,* ed 2, New York, 1981, Springer-Verlag.
+, 90% or more positive reaction within 1 or 2 days; −, no reaction (90% or more) in 30 days; − *or* +, most strains negative; some cultures positive; + *or* (+), most reactions occur within 1 or 2 days; some are delayed; *d,* different reactions; + *or* −, most cultures positive; some strains negative.

is not established. *C. freundii* has been associated with infectious diseases acquired in hospital settings; urinary tract infections, pneumonias, and intraabdominal abscesses have been reported. A report involving *C. freundii* in a case of endocarditis in an intravenous drug abuser was published by Plantholt and Trofa in 1987, the third case reported in medical literature and the first to be cured by antimicrobial therapy alone. One of the previously reported cases of *C. freundii* endocarditis required aortic valve replacement when antimicrobial therapy failed; the other case was fatal.

Because most *C. freundii* (80%) produce hydrogen sulfide and some strains (50%) fail to ferment lactose, the colonial morphology of *C. freundii* on primary selective media may be easily mistaken for that of *Salmonella* species when isolated from stool cultures. It is therefore important to be able to differentiate *C. freundii* from *Salmonella*. Differentiation can be done by using a minimal number of biochemical tests, such as urea hydrolysis and lysine decarboxylase. Most *C. freundii* (70%) hydrolyze urea, but all (100%) fail to decarboxylate lysine, whereas *Salmonella* species fail to hydrolyze urea and most decarboxylate lysine.

C. koseri (diversus) is a pathogen documented as the cause of nursery outbreaks of neonatal meningitis and brain abscesses.

C. amalonaticus is frequently found in feces, but no evidence exists that it is a causative agent of diarrhea. It has been isolated from sites of extraintestinal infections, such as blood and wounds.

PRIMARY INTESTINAL PATHOGENS AND RELATED HUMAN INFECTIONS

Salmonella and *Shigella* organisms produce gastrointestinal illnesses in humans. *Salmonella* species inhabit the gastrointestinal tracts of animals. Humans acquire the infection by ingesting the organisms in contaminated animal food products or insufficiently cooked poultry, milk, eggs, and dairy products. Other *Salmonella* species are found only in humans, and infections are transmitted by human carriers.

Infections caused by *Shigella* species are associated with human carriers responsible for spreading the disease; no animal reservoir has been identified. *Shigella* dysentery usually indicates improper sanitary conditions and poor personal hygiene.

Yersinia species infections, on the other hand, are transmitted by a wide variety of wild and domestic animals. *Yersinia* species infections range from gastrointestinal disease, to mediastinal lymphadenitis, to fulminant septicemia and pneumonia.

Salmonella Species

Members of the genus *Salmonella* produce significant infections in humans and in certain animals. *Salmonella* organisms are gram-negative, facultatively anaerobic rods that morphologically resemble other enteric bacteria. On selective and differential media used primarily to isolate enteric pathogens, Salmonellae produce clear, colorless, non–lactose-fermenting colonies; colonies with black centers are seen if the media contain indicators for hydrogen sulfide production. The biochemical features for the genus include the following:

- In almost every case they do not ferment lactose.
- They are negative for indole, the Voges-Proskauer test, phenylalanine, and urease.
- Most produce hydrogen sulfide on triple sugar iron agar.
- They do not grow in potassium cyanide.

Classification

Until recently, the genus *Salmonella,* a large and complex group of organisms, comprised three biochemical discrete species: *Salmonella enteritidis, Salmonella choleraesuis,* and *Salmonella typhi.* Genetic studies have shown, however, that bacterial species in the genus *Salmonella* are very closely related and that only one species, *Salmonella enterica,* must be designated. Additional changes in the *Salmonella* classification include the classification of the genus into seven subgroups with designated subspecies. Subgroup I includes species that cause infections in humans. Members of subgroup I have very similar biochemical characteristics with the exception of *S. typhi, S. choleraesuis,* and *S. paratyphi.* These bacterial species are less active biochemically and are the most serious pathogens for humans, causing enteric fevers. Table 16-7 shows the characteristic features of *S. typhi, S. choleraesuis,* and *S. paratyphi.* Table 16-8 shows the seven *Salmonella* subgroups.

TABLE 16-7

Biochemical Differentiation of Selected Members of the Salmonella *Group*

Test	Reaction of the following:			
	S. choleraesuis	*S. paratyphi A*	*S. typhi*	*Other*†
Arbinose fermentation	−	+	−	+
Citrate utilization	V	−	−	+
Glucose gas production	+	+	−	+
Lysine decarboxylase	+	−	+	+
Ornithine decarboxylase	+	+	−	+
Rhamnose fermentation	+	+	−	+
Trehalose fermentation	−	+	+	+

Data from Farmer JJ et al: *J Clin Microbiol* 21:46, 1985.
−, ≤9% of strains positive; *V,* 10% to 89% of strains positive; +, ≥90% of strains positive.
†Typical strains in serogroups A through E.

TABLE 16-8

Properties of the Seven Salmonella *Subgroups*[a]

Property or Test	Salmonella Subgroup						
	1	*2*	*3a*	*3b*	*4*	*5*	*6*
DNA hybridization group of Crosa et al[b]	1	2	3	4	5	Not studied	Not studied
Genus according to Ewing (1986)	*Salmonella*	*Salmonella*	*Arizona*	*Arizona*	*Salmonella*	*Salmonella*	*Salmonella*
Salmonella subgenus name formerly used	I	II	III	III	IV		
Subspecies according to Le Minor et al[c]	*choleraesuis*	*salamae*	*arizonae*	*diarizonae*	*houtenae*	*bongor*	*indica*
Flagella are usually monophasic (Mono) or diphasic (Di)	Di	Di	Mono	Di	Mono	Mono	Di
Usually isolated from humans and warm-blooded animals	+	−	−	−	−	−	−
Usually isolated from cold-blooded animals and the environment	−	+	+	+	+	+	+
Pathogenic for humans	++++	+	+	+	+	+?	+?
Differential tests[d]							
Dulcitol fermentation	96	90	0	1	0	92	62
Lactose fermentation	1	1	15	85	0	0	25
ONPG[e] test	2	15	100	100	0	92	50
Malonate utilization	1	95	95	95	0	0	0
Growth in KCN medium	1	1	1	1	95	100	0
Mucate fermentation	90	96	90	30	0	85	100
Gelatin hydrolysis[f]	−	+	+	+	+	−	+
D-Gelacturonic acid fermentation	−	+	−	+	+	100	100
Lysis by bacteriophage 01	+	+	−	+	−	46	88
D-Sorbitol fermentation	+	+	+	+	96	100	0

Modified from Balows A et al: *Manual of clinical microbiology,* ed 5, Washington, DC, 1991, American Society for Microbiology.
[a]Data from Le Minor et al (references 93 and 94 in Farmer et al, 1985).
[b]Crosa JH, Brenner DJ, Ewing WH, Falko S: Molecular relationships among the salmonelleae, *J Bacteriol* 115:307, 1973.
[c]Le Minor L, Popoff MY, Laurent B, Hermant D: Individualisation d'une septieme sous-espèce de *Salmonella: S. choleraesuis* subsp. *indica* subsp. nov, *Ann Microbiol* (Paris) 137B:211, 1986.
[d]Numbers indicate percent positive after 2 days of incubation and are based on actual Centers for Disease Control and Prevention data; symbols are based on the data of Le Minor et al.: +, 90% or more positive; −, 10% or fewer positive.
[e]ONPG, *o*-Nitrophenyl-*p*-D-galactopyranoside.
[f]Rapid film method at 37° C (almost all strains are negative by the tube method at 22° C within 2 days).

Species in subgroups II, III, and IV are usually found in cold-blooded animals, as well as in rodents and birds, which serve as their natural hosts. In addition to these changes, *Arizona,* which used to belong to its own genus, has become a member of the genus *Salmonella* and has been reclassified into subgroup III. *Arizona* infection may cause symptoms identical to those of *Salmonella* infections and may be transmitted to humans from pet turtles, snakes, and fish.

Virulence factors

Factors responsible for the virulence of salmonellae have been the subject of speculation and still remain uncertain. The role of fimbriae in adherence in initiating intestinal infection has been cited. It is apparent that fimbriated strains appear more virulent than nonfimbriated strains.

Another factor that contributes to the invasiveness of salmonellae is their ability to traverse intestinal mucosa. Specific factors that mediate this mechanism have not been established. Last, enterotoxin produced by certain salmonellae strains that cause gastroenteritis has been implicated as a significant virulence factor.

Antigenic structures

Salmonellae possess antigens similar to those of other enterobacteria. The somatic O antigens and flagellar H antigens are the primary antigenic structures used in serologic grouping of salmonellae. A few strains may possess capsular K surface antigens, designated as Vi antigen. The serologic identification of the Vi antigen is important in identifying *S. typhi.*

Figure 16-7 shows the antigenic structures used in serologic grouping and their locations.

The heat-stable O antigen of salmonellae, as is the case with other enteric bacteria, is the lipopolysaccharide (LPS) located in the outer membrane of the cell wall. There are many different O antigens present among the subspecies of *Salmonella;* more than one O antigen may also be found in a particular strain. The O antigens are designated by Arabic numbers.

Unlike the O antigens, flagellar antigens are proteins that are heat-labile and are treatable with ethanol or acid. The H antigens of salmonellae may occur in two phases: phase 1, the specific phase,

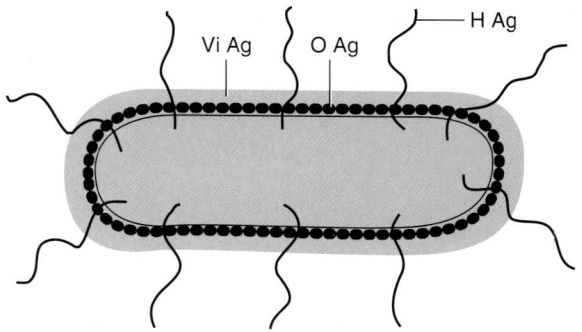

Figure 16-7

The antigenic structures of salmonellae used in serologic typing.

and phase 2, the nonspecific phase. Phase 1 flagellar antigens occur only in a small number of serotypes and determine the immunologic identity of the particular serotype. Phase 1 antigens agglutinate only with homologous antisera. Phase 2 flagellar antigens, on the other hand, occur among several strains. Shared by numerous serotypes, phase 2 antigens react with heterologous antisera.

The heat-labile Vi (coined from the term virulence) antigen is a surface polysaccharide capsular antigen found in *S. typhi* and a few other strains of *Salmonella* subgroup I. The capsular antigen plays a significant role in preventing phagocytosis of the organism. The Vi antigen most often blocks the O antigen during serologic typing but may be removed by heating.

Clinical infections

In humans, salmonellosis may occur in several forms:

- An acute gastroenteritis or food poisoning characerized by vomiting and diarrhea
- Typhoid fever, the most severe form of enteric fever, caused by *S. typhi;* other enteric fevers are caused by other *Salmonella* serotypes (i.e., *S. paratyphi, S. choleraesuis*)
- Nontyphoidal bacteremia
- Carrier state that follows *Salmonella* infection

Humans acquire the infection by ingesting the organisms in food, water, and milk contaminated with human or animal excreta. With the exception of

S. typhi and *S. paratyphi,* salmonellae infect various animals that serve as reservoirs, and sources of human infections. *S. typhi* and *S. paratyphi* have no known animal reservoirs, and infections seem to occur only in humans. Carriers are often the source of infection.

SALMONELLA GASTROENTERITIS

One of the most common forms of "food poisoning," gastrointestinal infection caused by *Salmonella* results from the ingestion of the organisms through contaminated food. The *Salmonella* strains associated with this infection are usually those found in animals; most in the United States belong to the serotypes of *Salmonella enteritidis.* Consequently, the source of the infection has been attributed primarily to poultry, milk, eggs, and egg products as well as to handling pets. Insufficiently cooked eggs and domestic fowl, such as chicken, turkey, and duck, are common sources of infection.

Cooking utensils such as knives, pans, and cutting boards used in preparing the contaminated meat can spread the contamination to other food. Direct transmission from person to person has been reported in institutions. *Salmonella* gastroenteritis, although referred to as *food poisoning,* occurs when a sufficient number of organisms contaminate food that is maintained under inadequate refrigeration, thus allowing growth and multiplication of the organisms. The infective dose necessary to initiate the disease is higher than that required for shigellosis. Approximately 10^6 bacteria may initiate infection, but infections resulting from lower infective doses have been reported.

The symptoms of intestinal salmonellosis, which may appear 8 to 36 hours after ingestion of contaminated food, include nausea, vomiting, fever, and chills, accompanied by watery diarrhea and abdominal pain. The role of enterotoxins in the pathogenesis of *Salmonella* infection remains unclear.

Most cases of *Salmonella* gastroenteritis are self-limiting. Symptoms disappear usually within a few days, with little or no complications. Those who suffer from sickle cell disease and other hemolytic disorders, ulcerative colitis, and malignancy seem to be more susceptible to Salmonellal infection. The infection may be more severe in the very young, the elderly, and those suffering from other underlying disease. Antimicrobial therapy is usu-

ally not indicated in uncomplicated cases. Antimicrobial therapy is believed to prolong the carrier state. Antidiarrheal agents are also restricted in cases of salmonellosis, as these agents may encourage adherence and further invasion. In cases of dehydration, fluid replacement therapy may be indicated.

Dissemination may occasionally occur; in such cases, antimicrobial therapy is required. The antimicrobials of choice include chloramphenicol, ampicillin, and trimethoprim-sulfamethoxazole. Nevertheless, susceptibility testing must be performed.

TYPHOID FEVER AND OTHER ENTERIC FEVERS

The clinical features of enteric fevers include the following:

- Prolonged fever
- Bacteremia
- Involvement of the reticuloendothelial system, particularly the liver, spleen, intestines, and mesentery
- Dissemination to multiple organs

Enteric fever caused by *S. typhi* has been known as typhoid fever, a febrile disease that results from the ingestion of food contaminated with the organisms originating from infected individuals or carriers. *S. typhi* does not have a known animal reservoir; therefore humans are the only source of infection. Other enteric fevers include paratyphoid fevers, which may be due to *S. paratyphi* serovar A, another strict human pathogen; *S. paratyphi* serovar B; and *S. paratyphi* serovar C. Other serovars that have been implicated in cases of septicemia in humans are those of *S. choleraesuis.* The clinical manifestations of paratyphoid fevers are similar to those of typhoid fever but are less severe, and the fatality rate is lower. Therefore, the clinical features of typhoid fever are discussed here in greater detail.

Typhoid fever occurs more often in tropical and subtropical countries, where foreign travelers easily acquire the infection. Improper disposal of sewage, poor sanitation, and lack of a modern water system have caused outbreaks of typhoid fever when the organisms reach a water source. This is uncommon in the United States and other developed countries, where water is purified and treated and handling of wastes is greatly improved. Pasteurization of milk has also diminished the incidence of waterborne typhoid in industrialized countries. Carriers, particularly food handlers, are important sources of infection anywhere in the world. Direct transmission through fomites is also possible. Laboratory workers in the microbiology laboratory have contacted typhoid fever while working with the organisms. Typhoid fever develops approximately 9 to 14 days following ingestion of the organisms. The onset of symptoms depends on the number of organisms ingested; the larger the inoculum, the shorter the incubation period. Characteristically, during the first week of the disease, the patient develops fever, accompanied by malaise, anorexia, lethargy, myalgia, and a continuous dull frontal headache.

When the organisms are ingested, they seem to be resistant to gastric acids and, on reaching the proximal end of the small intestine, subsequently invade and penetrate the intestinal mucosa. At this time, the patient experiences constipation rather than diarrhea. The organisms gain entrance into the lymphatic system and are sustained in the mesenteric lymph nodes. They eventually reach the blood stream and are further spread to the liver, spleen, and bone marrow, where they are immediately engulfed by mononuclear phagocytes. The organisms multiply intracellularly; later, they are released into the blood stream for the second time. The febrile episode becomes more evident during this release of the organisms into the circulatory system. At this time, the organisms may easily be isolated from the blood. Figure 16-8 shows the course of typhoid fever.

During the second and third weeks of the disease, the patient experiences sustained fever with the prolonged bacteremia. The organisms invade the gallbladder and Peyer's patches of the bowel. They also reach the intestinal tract via the biliary tract. "Rose spots" (blanching, rose-colored papules around the periumbilical region) appear during the second week of fever.

Involvement of biliary system sites initiates gastrointestinal symptoms as the organisms reinfect the intestinal tract. The organism now exists in large numbers and may be isolated from the stool. The gallbladder becomes the foci of long-term carriage of the organism, occasionally reseeding the intestinal tract and shedding the organisms in the feces. Necrosis in the gallbladder leading to

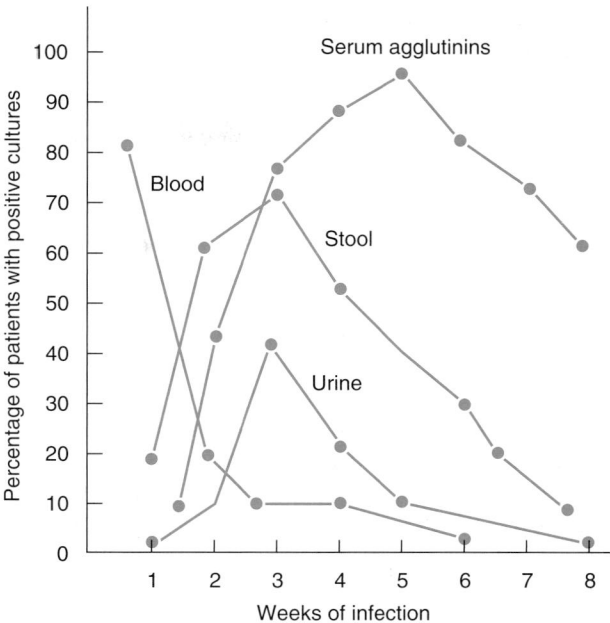

Figure 16-8

Culture and serologic diagnosis of typhoid fever. (Modified from Koneman E et al: *Color atlas in diagnostic microbiology,* ed 3, Philadelphia, 1988, JB Lippincott.)

necrotizing cholecystitis, and necrosis of the Peyer's patches leading to hemorrhage and perforation of the bowel, may occur as serious complications. Pneumonia and thrombophlebitis are other complications that occur in typhoid fever, as well as meningitis, osteomyelitis, endocarditis, and abscesses.

SALMONELLA BACTEREMIA
Salmonella bacteremia, with and without extraintestinal foci of infection caused by nontyphoidal *Salmonella,* is characterized primarily by prolonged fever and intermittent bacteremia. The most commonly associated serotypes of *Salmonella* are *Salmonella typhimurium, S. paratyphi A* and *B,* and *S. choleraesuis.*

Salmonella infection has been observed among two different groups of the population: (1) young children, who experience fever and gastroenteritis with brief episodes of bacteremia; and (2) adults, who experience transient bacteremia during episodes of gastroenteritis or develop symptoms of septicemia without gastroenteritis. The latter manifestations were observed among patients who had underlying illnesses, such as malignancies and liver disease. The risk of metastatic complications could be more severe than the bacteremia itself, even in individuals who do not have underlying diseases. Cases of septic arthritis may also occur in patients who had asymptomatic salmonellosis.

CARRIER STATE

Individuals who recover from the infection may harbor the organisms in the gallbladder, which becomes the site of chronic carriage. Such individuals excrete the organisms in their feces either continuously or intermittently; nevertheless, they become an important source of infection for susceptible persons. The carrier state may be terminated by antimicrobial therapy if gallbladder infection is not evident. Otherwise, cholecystectomy has been the only solution to the chronic state of enteric carriers.

Shigella Species

The genus *Shigella* is very closely related to the genus *Escherichia* and belongs to the tribe Escherichieae. *Shigella* species, however, are not members of the normal gastrointestinal flora, and all *Shigella* species can cause bacillary dysentery. The genus *Shigella* is named after the Japanese microbiologist Kiyoshi Shiga, who first isolated the organism in 1896. The organism, descriptively named *Shigella dysenteriae,* caused the enteric disease bacillary dysentery. Dysentery was characterized by the presence of blood, mucus, and pus in the stool. The disease occurred in an epidemic dimension.

The genus consists of four species that are biochemically similar. *Shigella* species are also divided into four major O antigen groups and must be identified by serologic grouping. The four species and their respective serologic groups are as follows:

- *Shigella dysenteriae* (group A)
- *Shigella flexneri* (group B)
- *Shigella boydii* (group C)
- *Shigella sonnei* (group D)

Several serotypes exist within each species with the exception of *S. sonnei,* which has only one serotype. *S. sonnei* is the most common isolate in the United States.

Characteristics of *Shigella* species are the following:

- They are nonmotile.
- Except for certain types of *S. flexneri,* they do not produce gas from glucose.
- They do not hydrolyze urea.
- When cultured on triple sugar iron agar, they do not produce hydrogen sulfide.
- They do not decarboxylate lysine.

Unlike *Escherichia* species, *Shigella* species do not utilize acetate or mucate as a source of carbon. Table 16-9 shows the biochemical characteristics of *Shigella* species. *S. sonnei* is unique in its ability to decarboxylate ornithine; it slowly ferments lactose, forming pink colonies on MacConkey agar after 48 hours of incubation. *S. sonnei* also yields a positive reaction in ONPG. Figure 16-9 illustrates the growth of *S. sonnei* on MacConkey agar after 24 and 48 hours of incubation. On differential and selective media used primarily to isolate intestinal pathogens, shigellae generally appear as clear, non–lactose-fermenting colonies.

Shigellae are fragile organisms. They are susceptible to the various effects of physical and chemical agents, such as disinfectants and high concentrations of acids and bile. Because they are susceptible to the acid pH of stool, feces suspected of containing *Shigella* organisms should be plated immediately onto laboratory media to increase recovery of the organism.

All *Shigella* species possess O antigens, and certain strains may possess K antigens. *Shigella* K antigens, when present, interfere with the detection

---

TABLE 16-9

Biochemical and Serological Differentiation of Shigella *Species*

	Reaction of the following:			
Test	*S. dysenteriae*	*S. flexneri*	*S. boydii*	*S. sonnei*
Mannitol fermentation	−	+	+	+
ONPG	V	−	V	+
Ornithine decarboxylase	−	−	−	+
Serogroup	A	B	C	D

From Balows A et al, editors: *Manual of clinical microbiology,* ed 4, Washington, DC, 1985, American Society for Microbiology.
−, ≤9% of strains positive; V, 10% to 89% of strains positive; +, ≥90% of strains positive.

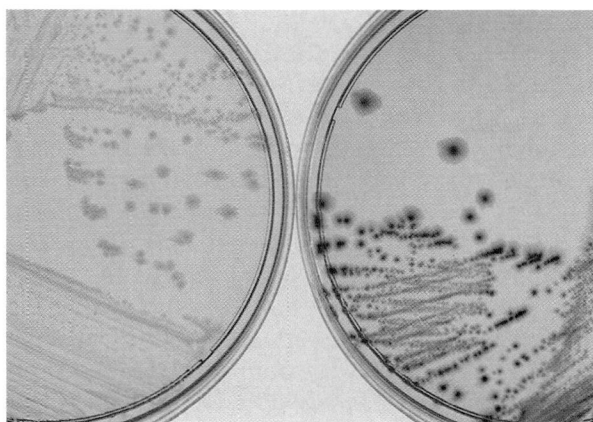

Figure 16-9 _____

Left, Lactose-negative appearance of *Shigella sonnei* growing on MacConkey agar at 18 to 24 hours of incubation. *Right,* Lactose-positive appearance of *S. sonnei* growing on Mac-Conkey agar after 48 hours of incubation.

of the O antigen during serologic grouping. The K antigen is heat-labile and may be removed by boiling the organism in a cell suspension.

Clinical infections

Although all *Shigella* species can cause dysentery, species vary in epidemiology, mortality rate, and severity of disease produced. In the United States, *S. sonnei* is the predominant isolate, followed by *S. flexneri.*

In the United States and other industrialized countries, shigellosis is probably underreported, because most patients are not hospitalized and usually recover from the infection without culture to recover the etiologic agent. *S. sonnei* infection is usually a short, self-limiting disease characterized by fever and watery diarrhea.

The demographics of *S. flexneri* infection have changed during recent years, from the disease's affecting mostly young children to its producing infections in young adults (approximately 25 years old). This observation was made simultaneously with the recognition of the "gay bowel syndrome" in homosexual men, in which *S. flexneri* has been the leading isolate. Conversely, in developing countries, *S. dysenteriae* type 1 and *S. boydii* are the most common isolates. *Shigella dysenteriae* type 1 remains the most virulent species, with significant morbidity and high mortality. Reports exist of mortality rates of 5% to 10%, and perhaps even higher,

resulting from *S. dysenteriae* type 1, particularly among undernourished children during epidemic outbreaks.

Humans are the only known reservoir of *Shigella* organisms. Transmission may occur by direct person-to-person contact, and spread may take place via the fecal-oral route, with carriers as the source. Shigellae may also be transmitted by flies, fingers, and food or water contaminated by infected persons.

Personal hygiene plays a major role in the transmission of *Shigella* organisms. Young children in day care centers, people living in crowded and less-than-adequate housing, and people who participate in anal-oral sex are most likely affected. Children younger than 10 years of age seem to be most affected; those 1 year of age and younger are the most susceptible.

The infection is highly communicable because of the low infective dose required to produce the disease. It has been reported that fewer than 200 bacilli are needed to initiate the disease in some healthy individuals.

Bacillary dysentery caused by *Shigella* species is marked by penetration of intestinal epithelial cells following attachment of the organisms to mucosal surfaces. Local inflammation, shedding of the intestinal lining, and formation of ulcers follow the epithelial penetration. The clinical manifestations of shigellosis vary from asymptomatic to severe forms of the disease. The initial symptoms, marked by high fever, chills, abdominal cramps, and pain accompanied by tenesmus, appear approximately 24 to 48 hours after ingestion of the organisms. The organisms, which originally multiplied in the small intestine, move toward the colon, where they may be isolated 1 to 3 days after the infection develops. Bloody stools containing mucus and numerous leukocytes follow the watery diarrhea, as the organisms invade the colonic tissues and cause an inflammatory reaction.

In dysentery caused by *S. dysenteria* type 1, patients experience more severe symptoms. Bloody diarrhea that progresses to dysentery may appear within a few hours to a few days. Patients suffer from extremely painful bowel movements, which contain predominantly mucus and blood. In young children, abdominal pain is quite intense, and rectal prolapse may result from excessive straining.

Although the effects of shigella toxin have been implicated as the mechanism responsible for the signs of the disease, the connection between the toxin hypothesis and the symptoms remains unclear. However, it has been reported that the detectable toxin levels produced by *S. dysenteriae* type 1 are higher than those produced by other *Shigella* species.

Severe cases of shigellosis may become life-threatening as extraintestinal complications develop. One of the most serious complications is ileus, an obstruction of the intestines, with marked abdominal dilatation, possibly leading to toxic megacolon. Although *Shigella* species infrequently penetrate the intestinal mucosa and disseminate to other body sites, in 1985 Struelens and colleagues reported that as many as 4% of severely ill hospitalized patients in Bangladesh suffered from bacteremia caused by *dysenteriae* type 1. *S. flexneri* bacteremia and bacteremia resulting from other enteric organisms occur, presumably predisposed by ulcers initiated by the shigellae.

Other complications include seizures, which may occur during any *Shigella* species infection, and HUS, a complication exclusively associated with *S. dysenteriae* type 1 shigellosis.

Yersinia Species

The genus *Yersinia* currently consists of 11 named species. *Yersinia* is a relatively new genus added to Enterobacteriaceae. The species *Yersinia pestis* and *Yersinia pseudotuberculosis* were previously classified in the genus *Pasteurella*. *Y. pestis* is the causative agent of plague, a life-threatening disease of rodents transmitted to humans by fleas. *Y. pseudotuberculosis* and *Yersinia enterocolitica* have caused sporadic cases of mesenteric lymphadenitis in humans, especially in children, and generalized septicemic infections in immunocompromised hosts. *Y. enterocolitica* produces an infection that mimics appendicitis. It has also been found to be the cause of diarrhea in a number of community outbreaks. The other members of the genus *Yersinia* species are found in water, soil, and lower animals; occasionally isolates have been found in wounds and the urine of humans. Evidence that other species, in addition to *Y. enterocolitica,* have caused intestinal disease has not been found. *Yersinia ruckeri* is well documented as the causative agent of red mouth disease in fish.

Yersinia pestis

The causative agent of the ancient disease plague still exists in areas where reservoir hosts are found. Plague, caused by *Y. pestis,* is a disease primarily of rodents. It is transmitted to humans by bites of fleas, its most common and effective vector. In humans, plague can occur in two forms: the bubonic, or glandular, form and the pneumonic form. The bubonic form usually results from the bite of an infected insect vector. Characteristic symptoms appear 2 to 5 days after infection. The symptoms include high fever with painful regional lymph nodes as buboes begin to appear.

Pneumonic plague occurs secondary to the bubonic plague when organisms proliferate in the blood stream and respiratory tract. Subsequent epidemic outbreaks may arise from the respiratory transmission of the organisms. The fatality rate in pneumonic plague is high if patients remain untreated.

Y. pestis is a gram-negative, short, plump rod. When stained with methylene blue or Wayson stain, it shows intense staining at each end of the bacillus, referred to as "bipolar staining," which gives it a "safety-pin" appearance. *Y. pestis* may be isolated on routine culture medium. Although it grows at 37° C, it has a preferential growth temperature of 25° C to 30° C. A *Y. pestis*–specific DNA probe for plague surveillance has been studied. If this DNA probe is proved successful, it may be applicable for laboratory diagnostic testing.

Yersinia enterocolitica

Human infections resulting from *Y. enterocolitica* have occurred worldwide, predominantly in Europe, although cases in the northeastern United States and Canada have been reported. It is the most commonly isolated species of *Yersinia.* The organisms have been round in a wide variety of animals, including domestic swine, cats, and dogs. The infection may therefore be acquired from contact with household pets. The role of the pig as a natural reservoir has been greatly emphasized in Europe. Other animal reservoirs, however, have also been identified, and cultures from environmental reservoirs, such as water from streams, have yielded the organism. Human infections have also been reported following the ingestion of contaminated food and possibly water. Other sources of infection include contaminated food, such as market meat and vacuum-packed beef. A major concern regarding the potential risk of transmitting infection with this organism is its ability to survive in cold temperatures; food refrigeration becomes an ineffective preventive measure. In addition, *Y. enterocolitica* sepsis associated with the transfusion of contaminated packed red blood cells has been reported. *Y. enterocolitica* infections manifest in several forms: an acute enteritis, an appendicitis-like syndrome, arthritis, and erythema nodosum. Acute enteritis, the most common form of the infection, is characterized by acute gastroenteritis with fever accompanied by headaches, abdominal pain, nausea, and diarrhea. Stools may contain blood. This form of infection, which often afflicts infants and young children between the ages of 1 and 5 years, is usually mild and self-limiting.

The clinical form that mimics acute appendicitis occurs primarily in older children and adults. It presents with severe abdominal pain and fever; the abdominal pain is concentrated in the right lower quadrant. Enlarged mesenteric lymph nodes and inflamed ileum and appendix are common findings in cases of *Y. enterocolitica* infections.

Arthritis is a common extraintestinal form of *Y. enterocolitica* infection, usually following a gastrointestinal episode or an appendicitis-like syndrome. This form of yersiniosis has been reported more often in adults than in children. The arthritis form exhibits characteristics similar to those of the arthritis seen in other bacterial infections, that is, in infections with *Shigella, Salmonella,* and *Neisseria gonorrhoeae* and in acute rheumatic fever.

Erythema nodosum is an inflammatory reaction characterized by tender, red nodules that may be accompanied by itching and burning. The areas involved include the anterior portion of the legs, whereas some patients have reported nodules on their arms. The reported cases have shown the syndrome to be more common in female patients than in male ones.

The incidence of generalized infection among adults involved those with underlying diseases, such as liver cirrhosis, diabetes, acquired immunodeficiency syndrome (AIDS), leukemia, aplastic anemia, and other hematologic conditions. Cases of liver abscess and acute infective endocarditis caused by *Y. enterocolitica* have also been reported. *Y. enterocolitica* morphologically resembles other *Yersinia* species, which appear as gram-negative coccobacilli with bipolar staining. The organism also grows on routine isolation media, such as blood agar and MacConkey agar. It has an optimal growth temperature of 25° C to 30° C. Cold enrichment has provided better recovery of *Y. enterocolitica.* Appropriate cultures on a specific *Yersinia* media at 25° C should be performed in diarrheal outbreaks of unknown etiology. These organism grow better with cold enrichment, and motility is clearly noted at 25° C but not at 35° C. Fecal samples suspected of containing this organism are inoculated on isotonic saline and kept at 4° C for 1 to 3 weeks.

During recent years, a selective medium to detect the presence of *Y. enterocolitica* was introduced. CIN agar employs cefsulodin, irgasan, novobiocin, bile salts, and crystal violet as the inhibitory agents. This medium, which inhibits normal colon organisms better than MacConkey agar, provides more opportunities to recover *Y. enterocolitica* from feces. This selective medium has since been modified, and media manufacturers such as Difco Bacto (Detroit, MI) have added a differential property to the medium, Yersinia selective agar base, by adding mannitol. Fermentation of mannitol results in a localized drop in pH around the colony. The drop in pH causes the pH indicator neutral red to turn red at the center of the colony, and the bile starts to precipitate. Nonfermentation of mannitol produces a colorless, translucent colony.

Yersinia pseudotuberculosis

Y. pseudotuberculosis, like *Y. pestis,* is a pathogen primarily of rodents, particularly of guinea pigs. In addition to farm and domestic animals, birds are also natural reservoirs; turkey, geese, pigeons, doves, and canaries have yielded positive cultures for this organism.

Y. pseudotuberculosis causes a disease characterized by caseous swellings called pseudotubercles. The disease is often fatal in animals. Human infections, which are rare, are associated with close contact with infected animals or their fecal material or ingestion of contaminated drink and foodstuff. When the organisms are ingested, they spread to the mesenteric lymph nodes, producing a generalized infection. The clinical manifestations include septicemia accompanied by mesenteric lymphadenitis, a presentation similar to appendicitis.

Y. pseudotuberculosis appears as a typical-looking plague bacillus. It may be differentiated from *Y. pestis* by its motility at 18° C to 22° C, production of urease, and ability to ferment rhamnose. Table 16-10 shows differentiating characteristics between *Yersinia* species.

New Genera and Biotypes
Budivicia species
Budivicia aquatica is a group of organisms found by DNA hybridization to be closely related. They are not as closely related to the other members of Enterobacteriaceae but do qualify to belong to the family. These organisms are usually found in water; however, they occasionally occur in clinical specimens.

Buttiauxella species
Buttiauxella agrestis, the only species of *Buttiauxella,* has been isolated from water but not from human specimens. Biochemically, these organisms are similar to both *Citrobacter* species and *Kluyvera* species, but DNA hybridization distinctly differentiates *Buttiauxella* from both genera.

Cedecea species
The genus *Cedecea* is composed of five species: *Cedecea davisae, Cedecea lapagei, Cedecea neteri,* and *Cedecea* species types 3 and 5. Most have been

recovered from sputum, blood, and wounds. Of the five, *C. davisae,* is the most commonly isolated species.

Ewingella species
Ewingella americana is the only species of this genus. *Ewingella* was formerly called "enteric group 40." Most isolates have come from human blood cultures or respiratory specimens. *Ewingella* was first thought to be related to *Cedecea* species; however, DNA hybridization confirmed the finding of a new genus.

Kluyvera species
The genus *Kluyvera* is made up of two closely related species, *Kluyvera ascorbata* and *Kluyvera cryocrescens.* Both have been found in respiratory, urine, and blood cultures and may produce a blue-violet pigment usually but not exclusively on non–blood-containing media. Both species resemble *E. coli* colonies growing on MacConkey agar. Figure 16-10 illustrates the colony characteristics of *Kluyvera* spp. Cephalothin and carbenicillin disk susceptibility tests separate the two species: *K. cryocrescens* shows large zones of inhibition; *K. ascorbata* has small zones. In addition, *K. ascorbata* does not ferment D-glucose at 5° C, whereas *K. cryocrescens* ferments D-glucose at this temperature.

Koserella species
The name *Koserella trabulsii* was proposed in 1985 to replace the designation enteric group 45. These organisms were first thought to be another species of *Hafnia,* but DNA hybridization showed a 15% relatedness, which was not sufficient to include these organisms in that genus. They are biochemically similar to *Hafnia* but differ primarily by yielding negative Voges-Proskauer test results. Koserellae have been isolated from human specimens, but further study will be required to determine their significance in human disease.

Leminorella species
Leminorella is proposed as a genus for the enteric group 57, with two species, *Leminorella grimontii* and *Leminorella richardii.* These organisms produce hydrogen sulfide and have shown weak reactions with *Salmonella* antisera. However, complete biochemical tests will differentiate *Leminorella* species from *Salmonella; Leminorella* species

TABLE 16-10
Differentiation Within the Genus Yersinia

Test	Y. pestis	Y. entero-colitica	Y. pseudo-tuberculosis
Indole	−	d	−
Methyl red	+	+	+
Voges-Proskauer			
25° C	−	d	−
37° C	−	−	−
Motility			
25° C	−	+	+
37° C	−	−	−
β-Galactosidase	+	+	+
Christensen urea	−	+	+
Phenylalanine deaminase	−	−	−
Ornithine decarboxylase	−	+	−
Acid produced from			
Sucrose	−	+	−
Lactose	−	−	−
Rhamnose	−	− or +*	+
Melibiose	−	− or +*	+
Trehalose	−	+ or −	+
Cellobiose	−	+	−

Modified from Washington J: *Laboratory procedures in clinical microbiology,* ed 2, New York, 1985, Springer-Verlag.
*Test results at 25° C.

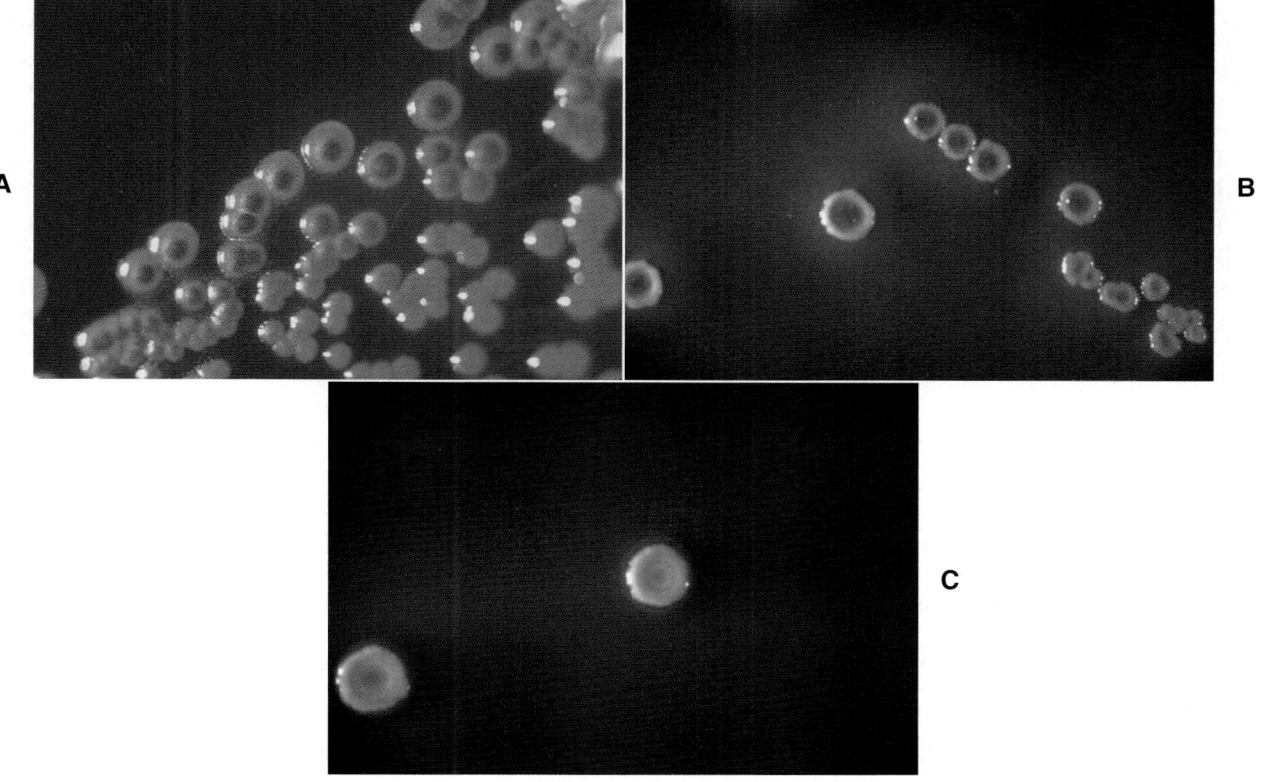

Figure 16-10

A, Blue-violet pigment of *Kluyvera* spp. growing on blood agar plate. The species of this genus resemble the colony morphology of *E. coli* growing on MacConkey agar. **B,** Appearance of *K. cryocrescens* growing on MacConkey agar. **C,** Appearance of *K. ascorbata* growing on MacConkey agar.

are relatively inactive. The clinical significance of these organisms is unknown; however, they have been isolated from urine, feces, and water.

Moellerella species
The new genus *Moellerella,* with one species, *Moellerella wisconsensis,* was formerly called enteric group 46. *Moellerella* is positive for citrate, methyl red, lactose, and sucrose; is negative for lysine, ornithine, arginine decarboxylase, and indole; and resembles *E. coli* growing on enteric media. The clinical significance of this organism has not been established, although it has been isolated from feces in two cases of diarrhea.

Obesumbacterium species
The genus *Obesumbacterium proteus* biogroup 2 are more closely related to *Escherichia blattae* than to other members of Enterobacteriaceae. These

are slow-growing organisms, fastidious at 36° C, and have not been found in human specimens.

Rahnella species
Rahnella aquatilis is the name given to a group of water bacteria. These organisms have no single characteristic that distinguishes them from the other members of Enterobacteriaceae. They resemble *Enterobacter agglomerans;* however, they can be distinguished by a weak phenylalanine reaction; the fact that they are negative for potassium cyanide (KCN), gelatin, lysine, ornithine; motility; and their lack of yellow pigmentation.

Tatumella species
Tatumella ptyseos is the only species of the genus *Tatumella,* the name given to group EF-9. This organism is unusual to Enterobacteriaceae in several ways: stock cultures may be kept frozen in

sheep's blood or may be freeze-dried but will die in a few weeks on agar slants; show more biochemical reactions at 25° C than at 35° C; are motile at 25° C but not at 35° C; and demonstrate large 15- to 36-mm zones of inhibition around penicillin disks. In addition, *Tatumella* organisms are slow-growing, produce tiny colonies, and are relatively nonreactive in laboratory media. These organisms have been isolated from human sources, especially sputum, and may be a rare cause of infection.

Xenorhabdus species

The genus *Xenorhabdus* is composed of *Xenorhabdus nematophilus* and *Xenorhabdus luminescens,* organisms that grow best at 25° C. *X. luminescens DNA* group 5 contains all the human clinical isolates. Colonies are yellow-pigmented, and the organism has been isolated from wounds and blood. *X. nematophilus,* which has been isolated from nematodes, has not been found in human specimens.

| LABORATORY DIAGNOSIS

Specimen Collection and Transport

Members of the family Enterobacteriaceae may be isolated from a wide variety of clinical samples. Most often these bacterial species are isolated with other organisms, including more fastidious pathogens. Therefore, to ensure isolation of both opportunistic and fastidious pathogens, laboratories must provide appropriate collection and transport media, such as Cary-Blair, Amies, or Stuart media. Microbiology personnel must encourage immediate transport of clinical samples to the laboratory for processing, regardless of the source of the clinical sample.

Isolation and Identification

To determine the clinical significance of the isolate, the microbiologist must consider the site of origin. Generally, enteric opportunistic organisms isolated from sites that are normally sterile are highly significant. However, careful examination is critical of organisms recovered from, for example, the respiratory tract, urogenital tract, stool, and wounds in open sites that are inhabited by other indigenous microflora.

Members of the family Enterobacteriaceae are routinely isolated from stool cultures; therefore,

complete identification should be directed only toward true intestinal pathogens. On the other hand, sputum cultures from hospitalized patients may contain enteric organisms that may require complete identification.

Direct microscopic examination

Unlike the case with gram-positive bacteria, in which microscopic morphology may essentially provide a presumptive identification, the microscopic characteristics of enterics are indistinguishable from other gram-negative bacteria. However, smears prepared directly from cerebrospinal fluid, blood, other body fluids, or exudates from an uncontaminated site may be examined microscopically for the presence of gram-negative bacteria. Although this examination is nonspecific for enteric organisms, this presumptive result may aid the clinician in the preliminary diagnosis of the infection, and appropriate therapy can be instituted immediately.

On the other hand, direct smears prepared from samples, such as sputum, that contain indigenous microbial flora do not provide valuable information, because their significance cannot be fully assessed unless the gram-negative bacteria are prevalent and indigenous inhabitants are absent. Direct smear examination of stool samples is not particularly helpful in identifying enteric pathogens but may reveal the inflammatory cells. This information is helpful in determining whether the gastrointestinal disease is toxin-mediated or an invasive process.

Culture

MEDIA

Most laboratories utilize a wide variety of nonselective media, such as blood agar plate and chocolate agar, as well as selective media, such as MacConkey agar, to recover enteric organisms from wounds, respiratory tract secretions, urine, sterile body fluids, and blood. On chocolate agar or on blood agar plate, enteric bacteria produce large, grayish, smooth colonies. On blood agar, plate colonies may be hemolytic or nonhemolytic; if hemolytic, β hemolysis is usually produced. On a selective medium, such as MacConkey agar, lactose-fermenting species produce pink to red colonies as acid is produced from lactose fermentation; crystal violet is precipitated, and neutral red turns red in an acid pH. Non–lactose-fermenting (NLF) species produce clear, colorless colonies on MacConkey agar. Bile and crystal violet are added to the medium to inhibit the growth of gram-positive bacteria.

Stool specimens contain enteric organisms as normal colon flora; therefore in processing stool samples, laboratories may develop their own protocol for the maximum recovery of enteric pathogens. Most microbiologists inoculate stool samples on highly selective media, such as Hektoen enteric (HE) or XLD agar, in addition to MacConkey agar. An enrichment broth has been traditionally inoculated to enhance recovery; this practice is slowly being phased out of the protocol.

On HE agar, lactose-fermenting species produce yellow colonies, whereas NLF species produce green colonies. Certain species of *Proteus* that are NLF and produce hydrogen sulfide appear green with black centers on HE agar. *Citrobacter freundii* usually produces yellow colonies with black centers. On XLD agar, NLF species like *Salmonella* (which produces lysine decarboxylase) produce red colonies with black centers (Figure 16-11).

ENVIRONMENTAL REQUIREMENTS

Members of the family Enterobacteriaceae are facultatively anaerobic and grow at an optimal temperature of 35° C to 37° C, preferably without carbon dioxide. Certain species may grow at low temperatures (1° C to 5° C for *Serratia* and *Yersinia*) or tolerate high temperatures (45° C to 50° C for *E. coli*). Colonies become visible on nonselective and differential media after 18 to 24 hours of incubation.

Identification

Currently, several ways exist to identify members of the family Enterobacteriaceae. Certain laboratories may still prefer to use conventional biochemical tests in tubes, whereas others may prefer miniaturized or automated commercial identification systems. Clinical laboratories that utilize conventional biochemical tests in tubes may find it cumbersome to test an isolate with all of the biochemical tests available. Therefore most of these laboratories develop identification tables and protocol that suit their needs and capabilities. These tables are based on the key features necessary to identify each particular genus and certain species. Figure 16-12 shows an example of a schematic diagram for the identification of commonly isolated enterics using conventional biochemical tests.

Table 16-11 shows the differentiating characteristics of the species, biogroups, and enteric groups of the Enterobacteriaceae.

To identify an isolate, the microbiologist must first determine whether the isolate belongs to the family Enterobacteriaceae. All members of the family (1) are oxidase-negative, (2) utilize glucose fermentatively, and (3) reduce nitrates to nitrites.

Gram-negative isolates, especially non–lactose-fermenters, should be tested for cytochrome oxidase production. This may be accomplished by wetting a tweezer-held disk with oxidase reagent and touching the disk to the colony. A black color change on the disk indicates a positive oxidase test (*non*-Enterobacteriaceae). The oxidase test is best performed off of blood agar plate. Touching an oxidase-impregnated disk to a colony on highly selective media such as CIN may give a false-negative reaction, whereas touching MacConkey agar (differential medium) may give the appearance of a false-positive reaction.

Regardless of the identification system utilized, the microbiologist may presumptively determine utilization of carbohydrates by observing the colo-

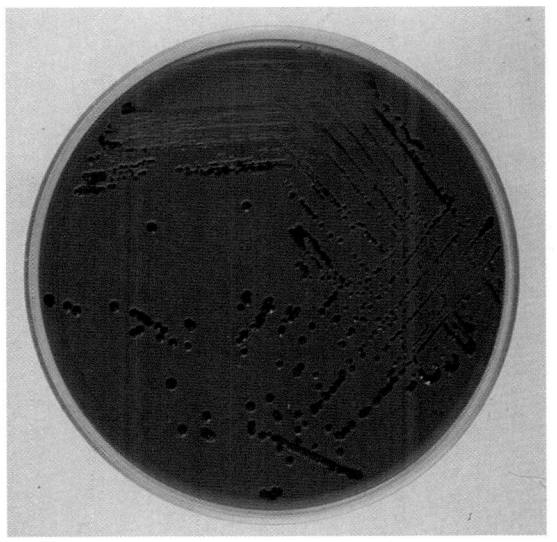

Figure 16-11 ─────────────────────────

Hydrogen sulfide–producing colonies of salmonellae growing on XLD. (Courtesy American Society for Clinical Laboratory Science, Education and Research Fund, Inc., 1982.)

Text continued on p. 496

TABLE 16-11

Biochemical Reactions of the Named Species, Biogroups, and Enteric Groups of the Family Enterobacteriacea*

Species	Indole Production	Methyl Red	Voges-Proskauer	Citrate (Simmons)	Hydrogen Sulfide (TSI)	Urea Hydrolysis	Phenylalanine Deaminase	Lysine Decarboxylase	Arginine Dihydrolase	Ornithine Decarboxylase	Motility (36° C)	Gelatin Hydrolysis (22° C)	Growth in KCN	Malonate Utilization	D-Glucose, Acid	D-Glucose, Gas	Lactose Fermentation	Sucrose Fermentation	D-Mannitol Fermentation	Dulcitol Fermentation
Buttiauxella																				
B. agrestis	0	100	0	100	0	0	0	0	0	100	100	0	80	60	100	100	100	0	100	0
Cedecea																				
C. davisae†	0	100	50	95	0	0	0	0	50	95	95	0	86	91	100	70	19	100	100	0
C. lapagei†	0	40	80	99	0	0	0	0	80	0	80	0	100	99	100	100	60	0	100	0
C. neteri†	0	100	50	100	0	0	0	0	100	0	100	0	65	100	100	100	35	100	100	0
Cedecea sp. 3†	0	100	50	100	0	0	0	0	100	0	100	0	100	0	100	100	0	50	100	0
Cedecea sp. 5†	0	100	50	100	0	0	0	0	50	50	100	0	100	0	100	100	0	100	100	0
Citrobacter																				
C. freundii†	5	100	0	95	80	70	0	0	65	20	95	0	96	15	100	95	50	30	99	55
C. diversus†	99	100	0	99	0	75	0	0	65	99	95	0	0	90	100	98	35	45	100	50
C. amalonaticus†	100	100	0	85	0	80	0	0	85	95	98	0	95	0	100	97	50	15	100	0
C. amalonaticus biogroup 1†	100	100	0	1	0	45	0	0	85	100	99	0	96	0	100	93	19	100	100	4
Edwardsiella																				
E. tarda†	99	100	0	1	100	0	0	100	0	100	98	0	0	0	100	100	0	0	0	0
E. tarda biogroup 1†	100	100	0	0	0	0	0	100	0	100	100	0	0	0	100	50	0	100	100	0
E. hoshinae	13	100	0	0	0	0	0	100	0	95	100	0	0	100	100	35	0	100	100	0
E. ictaluri	0	0	0	0	0	0	0	100	0	65	0	0	0	0	100	50	0	0	0	0
Enterobacter																				
E. aerogenes†	0	5	98	95	0	2	0	98	0	98	97	0	98	95	100	100	95	100	100	5
E. cloacae†	0	5	100	100	0	65	0	0	97	96	95	0	98	75	100	100	93	97	100	15
E. agglomerans† group	20	50	70	50	0	20	20	0	0	0	85	2	35	65	100	20	40	75	100	15
E. gergoviae†	0	5	100	99	0	93	0	90	0	100	90	0	0	96	100	98	55	98	99	0
E. sakazakii†	11	5	100	99	0	1	50	0	99	91	96	0	99	18	100	98	99	100	100	5
E. taylorae†	0	5	100	100	0	1	0	0	94	99	99	0	98	100	100	100	10	0	100	0
E. amnigenus biogroup 1†	0	7	100	70	0	0	0	0	9	55	92	0	100	91	100	100	70	100	100	0
E. amnigenus biogroup 2	0	65	100	100	0	0	0	0	35	100	100	0	100	100	100	100	35	0	100	0
E. intermedius	0	100	100	65	0	0	0	0	0	89	89	0	65	100	100	100	100	65	100	100
Escherichia-Shigella																				
E. coli†	98	99	0	1	1	1	0	90	17	65	95	0	3	0	100	95	95	50	98	60
E. coli, inactive†	80	95	0	1	1	1	0	40	3	20	5	0	1	0	100	5	25	15	93	40
Shigella, serogroups A, B, and C†	50	100	0	0	0	0	0	0	5	1	0	0	0	0	100	2	0	0	93	2
S. sonnei†	0	100	0	0	0	0	0	0	2	98	0	0	0	0	100	0	2	1	99	0
E. fergusonii†	98	100	0	17	0	0	0	95	5	100	93	0	0	35	100	95	0	0	98	60
E. hermannii†	99	100	0	1	0	0	0	6	0	100	99	0	94	0	100	97	45	45	100	19
E. vulneris†	0	100	0	0	0	0	0	85	30	0	100	0	15	85	100	97	15	8	100	0
E. blattae	0	100	0	50	0	0	0	100	0	100	0	0	0	100	100	100	0	0	0	0
Ewingella																				
E. americana†	0	84	95	95	0	0	0	0	0	0	60	0	5	0	100	0	70	0	100	0
Hafnia																				
H. alvei†	0	40	85	10	0	4	0	100	6	98	85	0	95	50	100	98	5	10	99	0
H. alvei biogroup 1	0	85	70	0	0	0	0	100	0	45	0	0	0	45	100	0	0	0	55	0
Klebsiella																				
K. pneumoniae†	0	10	98	98	0	95	0	98	0	0	0	0	98	93	100	97	98	99	99	30
K. oxytoca†	99	20	95	95	0	90	1	99	0	0	0	0	97	98	100	97	100	100	99	55
Klebsiella group 47 indole positive, ornithine positive†	100	96	70	100	0	100	0	100	0	100	0	0	100	100	100	100	100	100	100	10
K. planticola†	20	100	98	100	0	98	0	100	0	0	0	0	100	100	100	100	100	100	100	15
K. ozaenae†	0	98	0	30	0	10	0	40	6	3	0	0	88	3	100	50	30	20	100	2
K. rhinoscleromatis†	0	100	0	0	0	0	0	0	0	0	0	0	80	95	100	0	0	75	100	0
K. terrigena	0	60	100	40	0	0	0	100	0	20	0	0	100	100	100	80	100	100	100	20
Kluyvera																				
K. ascorbata†	92	100	0	96	0	0	0	97	0	100	98	0	92	96	100	93	98	98	100	25
K. cryocrescens†	90	100	0	80	0	0	0	23	0	100	90	0	86	86	100	95	95	81	95	0
Moellerella																				
M. wisconsensis	0	100	0	80	0	0	0	0	0	0	0	0	70	0	100	0	100	100	60	0

From Farmer JJ II et al: Biochemical identification of new species and biogroups of Enterobacteriaceae isolated from clinical specimens, *J Clin Microbiol* 21:46, 1985.
ONPG, *o*-Nitrophenyl-*p*-D-galactopyranoside.
*Each number gives the percentage of positive reactions after 2 days' incubation at 36° C (except *Xenorhabdus*, which was incubated at 25° C). The vast majority of these positive reactions occur within 24 hr. Reactions that become positive after 2 days are not considered.
†Known to occur in clinical specimens.

Salicin Fermentation	Adonitol Fermentation	myo-Inositol Fermentation	D-Sorbitol Fermentation	L-Arabinose Fermentation	Raffinose Fermentation	L-Rhamnose Fermentation	Maltose Fermentation	D-Xylose Fermentation	Trehalose Fermentation	Cellobiose Fermentation	α-Methyl-D-Glucoside Fermentation	Erythritol Fermentation	Esculin Hydrolysis	Melibiose Fermentation	D-Arabitol Fermentation	Glycerol Fermentation	Mucate Fermentation	Tartrate, Jordan	Acetate Utilization	Lipase (Corn Oil)	DNase at 25° C	Nitrate → Nitrite	Oxidase, Kovacs	ONPG	Yellow Pigment	D-Mannose Fermentation
100	0	0	0	100	100	100	100	100	100	100	0	0	100	100	0	60	100	60	0	0	0	100	0	100	0	100
99	0	0	0	0	10	0	100	100	100	100	5	0	45	0	100	0	0	0	0	91	0	100	0	90	0	100
100	0	0	0	0	0	0	100	0	100	100	0	0	100	0	100	0	0	0	60	100	0	100	0	99	0	100
100	0	0	100	0	0	0	100	100	100	100	0	0	100	0	100	0	0	0	0	100	0	100	0	100	0	100
100	0	0	0	0	100	0	100	100	100	100	50	0	100	100	100	0	0	0	50	100	0	100	0	100	0	100
100	0	0	100	0	100	0	100	100	100	100	0	0	100	100	100	0	0	0	50	50	0	100	0	100	0	100
5	0	3	98	100	30	99	99	99	99	55	5	0	0	50	0	98	95	90	80	0	0	99	0	95	0	100
20	98	0	99	0	100	100	100	100	100	99	40	0	2	0	100	98	93	75	75	0	0	100	0	96	0	100
40	0	0	100	100	5	99	99	99	100	100	5	0	10	5	0	70	98	85	75	0	0	99	0	100	0	100
0	0	0	100	100	100	100	100	100	100	100	70	0	0	100	0	55	100	93	82	0	0	100	0	100	0	100
0	0	0	0	9	0	0	100	0	0	0	0	0	0	0	0	30	0	25	0	0	0	100	0	0	0	100
0	0	0	0	100	0	0	100	0	0	0	0	0	0	0	0	0	0	0	0	0	0	100	0	0	0	100
50	0	0	0	13	0	0	100	0	100	0	0	0	0	0	0	65	0	0	0	0	0	100	0	0	0	100
0	0	0	0	0	0	0	100	0	0	0	0	0	0	0	0	0	0	0	0	0	0	100	0	0	0	100
100	98	95	100	100	96	99	99	100	100	100	95	0	98	99	100	98	90	95	50	0	0	100	0	100	0	95
75	25	15	95	100	97	92	100	99	100	99	85	0	30	90	15	40	75	30	75	0	0	99	0	99	0	100
65	7	15	30	95	30	85	89	93	97	55	7	0	60	50	50	30	40	25	30	0	0	85	0	90	75	98
99	0	0	0	99	97	99	100	99	100	99	2	0	97	97	97	100	2	97	93	0	0	99	0	97	0	100
99	0	75	0	100	99	100	100	100	100	100	96	0	100	100	0	15	1	1	96	0	0	99	0	100	98	100
92	0	0	1	100	0	100	99	100	100	100	1	0	90	0	0	1	75	0	35	0	0	100	0	100	0	100
91	0	0	9	100	100	100	100	100	100	100	55	0	91	100	0	0	35	9	0	0	0	100	0	91	0	100
100	0	0	100	100	0	100	100	100	100	100	100	0	100	100	0	100	0	0	0	0	0	100	0	100	0	100
100	0	0	100	100	100	100	100	100	100	100	100	0	100	100	0	100	100	100	0	0	0	100	0	100	0	100
40	5	1	94	99	50	80	95	95	98	2	0	0	35	75	5	75	95	95	90	0	0	100	0	95	0	98
10	3	1	75	85	15	65	80	70	90	2	0	0	5	40	5	65	30	85	40	0	0	98	0	45	0	97
0	0	0	30	60	50	5	30	2	80	0	0	0	0	50	0	10	0	30	2	0	0	100	0	2	0	100
0	0	0	2	95	3	75	90	2	100	5	0	0	0	25	0	15	10	90	0	0	0	100	0	90	0	100
65	98	0	0	98	0	92	96	96	96	96	0	0	46	0	100	20	0	96	96	0	0	100	0	83	0	100
40	0	0	0	100	40	97	100	100	100	97	0	0	40	0	8	3	97	35	78	0	0	100	0	98	98	100
30	0	0	1	100	99	93	100	100	100	100	25	0	20	100	0	25	78	2	30	0	0	100	0	100	50	100
0	0	0	0	100	0	100	100	100	75	0	0	0	0	0	0	100	50	50	0	0	0	100	0	0	0	100
80	0	0	0	0	0	23	16	13	99	10	0	0	50	0	99	24	0	35	10	0	0	97	0	85	0	99
13	0	0	0	95	2	97	100	98	99	15	0	0	7	0	0	95	0	70	15	0	0	100	0	90	0	100
55	0	0	0	0	0	0	0	0	70	0	0	0	0	0	0	0	0	30	0	0	0	100	0	30	0	100
99	90	95	99	99	99	99	98	99	99	98	90	0	99	99	98	97	90	95	75	0	0	99	0	99	0	99
100	99	98	99	98	100	100	100	100	100	100	98	2	100	99	98	99	93	98	90	0	0	100	0	100	1	100
100	100	95	100	100	100	100	100	100	100	100	100	0	100	100	100	100	96	100	95	0	0	100	0	100	0	100
100	100	100	92	100	100	100	100	100	100	100	100	0	100	100	100	100	100	100	62	0	0	100	0	100	1	100
97	97	55	65	98	90	55	95	95	98	92	70	0	80	97	95	65	25	50	2	0	0	80	0	80	0	100
98	100	95	100	100	90	96	100	100	100	100	0	0	30	100	100	50	0	50	0	0	0	100	0	0	0	100
100	100	80	100	100	100	100	100	100	100	100	100	0	100	100	100	100	100	100	20	0	0	100	0	100	0	100
100	0	0	40	100	98	100	100	99	100	100	98	0	99	99	0	40	90	35	50	0	0	100	0	100	0	100
100	0	0	45	100	100	100	100	91	100	100	95	0	100	100	0	5	81	19	86	0	0	100	0	100	0	100
0	100	0	0	0	100	0	30	0	0	0	0	0	0	100	75	10	0	30	10	0	0	90	0	90	0	100

Continued

TABLE 16-11

Biochemical Reactions of the Named Species, Biogroups, and Enteric Groups of the Family Enterobacteriacea—cont'd

Species	Indole Production	Methyl Red	Voges-Proskauer	Citrate (Simmons)	Hydrogen Sulfide (TSI)	Urea Hydrolysis	Phenylalanine Deaminase	Lysine Decarboxylase	Arginine Dihydrolase	Ornithine Decarboxylase	Motility (36°C)	Gelatin Hydrolysis (22°C)	Growth in KCN	Malonate Utilization	D-Glucose, Acid	D-Glucose, Gas	Lactose Fermentation	Sucrose Fermentation	D-Mannitol Fermentation	Dulcitol Fermentation
Morganella																				
M. morganii†	98	97	0	0	5	98	95	0	0	98	95	0	98	1	100	90	1	0	0	0
M. morganii biogroup 1†	100	95	0	0	41	100	100	100	0	95	0	0	91	5	100	91	0	0	0	0
Obseumbacterium																				
O. proteus biogroup 2	0	15	0	0	0	0	0	100	0	100	0	0	0	0	100	0	0	0	0	0
Proteus																				
P. mirabilis†	2	97	50	65	98	98	98	0	0	99	95	90	98	2	100	96	2	15	0	0
P. vulgaris†	98	95	0	15	95	95	99	0	0	0	95	91	99	0	100	85	2	97	0	0
P. penneri†	0	100	0	0	30	100	99	0	0	0	85	50	99	0	100	45	1	100	0	0
P. myxofaciens	0	100	100	50	0	100	100	0	0	0	100	100	100	0	100	100	0	100	0	0
Providencia																				
P. rettgeri†	99	93	0	95	0	98	98	0	0	0	94	0	97	0	100	10	5	15	100	0
P. stuartii†	98	100	0	93	0	30	95	0	0	0	85	0	100	0	100	0	2	50	10	0
P. alcalifaciens†	99	99	0	98	0	0	98	0	0	1	96	0	100	0	100	85	0	15	2	0
P. rustigianii†	98	65	0	15	0	0	100	0	0	0	30	0	100	0	100	35	0	35	0	0
Rahnella																				
R. aquatilis†	0	88	100	94	0	0	95	0	0	0	6	0	0	100	100	98	100	100	100	88
Salmonella																				
Subgroup 1 serotypes†—most	1	100	0	95	95	1	0	98	70	97	95	0	0	0	100	96	1	1	100	96
S. typhi†	0	100	0	0	97	0	0	98	3	0	97	0	0	0	100	0	1	0	100	0
S. choleraesuis†	0	100	0	25	50	0	0	95	55	100	95	0	0	0	100	95	0	0	98	5
S. paratyphi A†	0	100	0	0	10	0	0	0	15	95	95	0	0	0	100	99	0	0	100	90
S. gallinarum†	0	100	0	0	100	0	0	90	10	1	0	0	0	0	100	0	0	0	100	90
S. pullorum†	0	90	0	0	90	0	0	100	10	95	0	0	0	0	100	90	0	0	100	0
Subgroup 2 strains†	2	100	0	100	100	0	0	100	90	100	98	2	0	95	100	100	1	1	100	90
Subgroup 3a strains† *(Arizona)*	1	100	0	99	99	0	0	99	70	99	99	0	1	95	100	99	15	1	100	0
Subgroup 3b strains† *(Arizona)*	2	100	0	98	99	0	0	99	70	99	99	0	1	95	100	99	85	5	100	1
Subgroup 4 strains†	0	100	0	98	100	2	0	100	70	100	98	0	95	0	100	100	0	0	98	0
Subgroup 5 strains†	0	100	0	100	100	0	0	100	100	100	100	0	100	0	100	80	0	0	100	100
Serratia																				
S. marcescens†	1	20	98	98	0	15	0	99	0	99	97	90	95	3	100	55	2	99	99	0
S. marscescens biogroup 1†	0	100	60	30	0	0	0	55	4	65	17	30	70	0	100	0	4	100	96	0
S. liquefaciens group†	1	93	93	90	0	3	0	95	0	95	95	90	90	2	100	75	10	98	100	0
S. rubidaea†	0	20	100	95	0	2	0	55	0	0	85	90	25	94	100	30	100	99	100	0
S. odorifera biogroup 1†	60	100	50	100	0	5	0	100	0	100	100	95	60	0	100	0	70	100	100	0
S. odorifera biogroup 2†	50	60	100	97	0	0	0	94	0	0	100	94	19	0	100	13	97	0	97	0
S. plymuthica†	0	94	80	75	0	0	0	0	0	0	50	60	30	0	100	40	80	100	100	0
S. ficaria†	0	75	75	100	0	0	0	0	0	0	100	100	55	0	100	0	15	100	100	0
"Serratia" fonticola†	0	100	9	91	0	13	0	100	0	97	911	0	70	88	100	79	97	21	100	91
Tatumella																				
T. ptyseos†	0	0	5	2	0	0	90	0	0	0	0	0	0	0	100	0	0	98	0	0
Xenorhabdus																				
X. luminescens (25° C)	50	0	0	50	0	25	0	0	0	0	100	50	0	0	75	0	0	0	0	0
X. nematophilus (25° C)	40	0	0	0	0	0	0	0	0	0	100	80	0	0	80	0	0	0	0	0
Yersinia																				
Y. enterocolitica†	50	97	2	0	0	75	0	0	0	95	2	0	2	0	100	5	5	95	98	0
Y. frederiksenii†	100	100	0	15	0	70	0	0	0	95	5	0	0	0	100	40	40	100	100	0
Y. intermedia†	100	100	5	5	0	80	0	0	0	100	5	0	10	5	100	18	35	100	100	0
Y. kristensenii†	30	92	0	0	0	77	0	0	0	92	5	0	0	0	100	23	8	0	100	0
Y. pestis†	0	80	0	0	0	5	0	0	0	0	0	0	0	0	100	0	0	0	97	0
Y. pseudotuberculosis†	0	100	0	0	0	95	0	0	0	0	0	0	0	0	100	0	0	0	100	0
"Yersinia" ruckeri	0	97	10	0	0	0	0	50	5	100	0	30	15	0	100	5	0	0	100	0
Enteric group 17†	0	100	2	100	0	60	0	0	21	95	0	0	97	3	100	95	75	100	100	0
Enteric group 41†	100	100	0	0	0	50	0	0	0	0	100	0	100	50	100	100	100	100	100	100
Enteric group 45†	0	100	0	100	0	0	0	100	22	100	100	0	78	0	100	89	0	0	100	0
Enteric group 57†	0	70	0	40	100	0	0	0	0	0	0	0	30	0	100	60	0	0	0	50
Enteric group 58†	0	100	0	85	0	70	0	100	0	85	0	100	0	100	85	85	30	0	100	85
Enteric group 59†	10	100	0	100	0	0	0	30	0	60	0	100	0	80	90	100	100	80	0	0
Enteric group 60†	0	100	0	0	50	0	0	0	0	0	100	75	0	100	100	0	0	0	50	0
Enteric group 63	0	100	0	0	0	0	100	0	0	100	65	0	0	0	100	0	0	0	100	0
Enteric group 64	0	100	0	50	0	0	0	0	50	0	100	0	100	100	100	50	100	0	100	0
Enteric group 68†	0	100	50	0	0	0	0	0	0	0	0	0	100	0	100	0	0	100	100	0
Enteric group 69	0	0	100	100	0	0	0	0	100	100	100	0	100	100	100	100	100	25	100	100

†Known to occur in clinical specimens.

Salicin Fermentation	Adonitol Fermentation	myo-Inositol Fermentation	D-Sorbitol Fermentation	L-Arabinose Fermentation	Raffinose Fermentation	L-Rhamnose Fermentation	Maltose Fermentation	D-Xylose Fermentation	Trehalose Fermentation	Cellobiose Fermentation	α-Methyl-D-Glucoside Fermentation	Erythritol Fermentation	Esculin Hydrolysis	Melibiose Fermentation	D-Arabitol Fermentation	Glycerol Fermentation	Mucate Fermentation	Tartrate, Jordan	Acetate Utilization	Lipase (Corn Oil)	DNase at 25° C	Nitrate → Nitrite	Oxidase, Kovacs	ONPG	Yellow Pigment	D-Mannose Fermentation
0	0	0	0	0	0	0	0	0	10	0	0	0	0	0	0	5	0	95	0	0	0	90	0	5	0	98
0	0	0	0	0	0	0	0	0	0	0	0	0	0	0	0	100	0	100	0	0	0	91	0	0	0	95
0	0	0	0	0	0	15	50	15	85	0	0	0	0	0	0	0	0	15	0	0	0	100	0	0	0	85
0	0	0	0	0	1	1	0	98	98	1	0	0	0	0	0	70	0	87	20	92	50	95	0	0	0	0
50	0	0	0	0	1	5	97	95	30	0	60	1	50	0	0	60	0	80	25	80	80	98	0	1	0	0
0	0	0	0	0	1	0	100	100	55	0	80	0	0	0	0	55	0	85	5	45	40	90	0	1	0	0
0	0	0	0	0	0	0	100	0	100	0	100	0	0	0	0	100	0	100	0	100	50	100	0	0	0	0
50	100	90	1	0	5	70	2	10	0	3	2	75	35	5	100	60	0	95	60	0	0	5	0	5	0	100
2	5	95	1	1	7	0	1	7	98	5	0	0	0	0	0	50	0	90	75	0	10	100	0	10	0	100
1	98	1	1	1	1	0	1	1	2	1	0	0	0	0	0	15	0	90	40	0	0	100	0	1	0	100
0	0	0	0	0	0	0	0	0	0	0	0	0	0	0	0	5	0	50	25	0	0	100	0	0	0	100
100	0	0	94	100	94	94	94	94	100	100	0	0	100	100	0	13	30	6	6	0	0	100	0	100	0	100
0	0	35	95	99	2	95	97	97	99	5	2	0	5	95	0	5	90	90	90	0	2	100	0	2	0	100
0	0	0	99	2	0	0	97	82	100	0	0	0	0	100	0	20	0	100	0	0	0	100	0	0	0	100
0	0	0	90	0	1	100	95	98	0	0	0	1	0	45	1	0	0	85	1	0	0	98	0	0	0	95
0	0	0	95	100	0	100	95	0	100	5	0	0	0	95	0	10	0	0	0	0	0	100	0	0	0	100
0	0	0	1	80	10	10	90	70	50	10	0	1	0	0	0	0	50	100	0	0	10	100	0	0	0	100
0	0	0	10	100	1	100	5	90	90	5	0	0	0	0	0	0	0	0	0	0	0	100	0	0	0	100
5	0	5	100	100	0	100	100	100	100	0	8	0	15	8	0	25	96	50	95	0	0	100	0	15	0	95
0	0	0	99	99	1	99	98	100	99	1	1	0	1	95	1	10	90	5	90	0	2	100	0	100	0	100
0	0	0	99	99	1	99	98	100	99	1	1	0	1	95	1	10	30	20	75	0	2	100	0	100	0	100
60	5	0	100	100	0	98	100	100	100	50	0	0	0	100	5	0	0	65	70	0	0	100	0	0	0	100
0	0	0	100	100	0	100	100	100	100	0	0	0	0	75	0	0	100	0	100	0	0	100	0	100	0	100
95	40	75	99	0	2	0	96	7	99	5	0	1	95	0	0	95	0	75	50	98	98	98	0	95	0	99
92	30	30	92	0	0	0	70	0	100	4	0	0	96	0	0	92	0	50	4	75	82	83	0	75	0	100
97	5	60	95	98	85	15	98	100	100	5	5	0	97	75	0	95	0	75	40	85	85	100	0	93	0	100
99	99	20	1	100	99	1	99	99	100	94	1	0	94	99	85	20	0	70	80	99	99	100	0	100	0	100
98	50	100	100	100	100	95	100	100	100	100	0	0	95	100	0	40	5	100	60	35	100	100	0	100	0	100
45	55	100	100	100	7	94	100	100	100	100	0	7	40	96	0	50	0	100	65	65	100	100	0	100	0	100
94	0	50	65	100	94	0	94	94	100	88	70	0	81	93	0	50	0	100	55	70	100	100	0	70	0	100
100	0	55	100	100	70	35	100	100	100	100	0	8	0	40	100	0	0	17	40	77	100	92	8	100	0	100
100	100	30	100	100	100	76	97	85	100	6	91	0	100	98	100	88	0	58	15	0	0	100	0	100	0	100
55	0	0	0	0	11	0	0	9	93	0	0	0	0	25	0	7	0	0	0	0	0	98	0	0	0	100
20	0	30	99	98	5	1	75	70	98	75	0	0	25	1	40	90	0	85	15	55	5	98	0	95	0	100
92	0	20	100	100	30	99	100	100	100	100	0	0	85	0	100	85	5	55	15	55	0	100	0	100	0	100
100	0	15	100	100	45	100	100	100	100	96	77	0	100	80	45	60	6	88	18	12	0	94	0	90	0	100
15	0	15	10	77	0	0	100	85	100	100	0	0	0	0	45	70	0	40	8	0	0	100	0	70	0	100
70	0	0	50	0	0	1	80	90	100	0	0	0	50	20	0	50	0	0	0	0	0	85	0	50	0	100
25	0	0	0	50	15	70	95	100	100	0	0	0	95	70	0	50	0	50	0	0	0	95	0	70	0	100
0	0	0	50	5	5	0	95	0	95	5	0	0	0	0	0	50	0	30	0	30	0	75	0	50	0	100
0	0	0	0	0	0	0	25	0	0	0	0	0	0	0	0	0	0	50	0	0	0	0	0	0	50	100
0	0	0	0	0	0	0	0	0	0	0	0	0	0	0	0	0	0	60	0	0	20	20	0	0	60	80
100	0	0	100	100	70	5	100	97	100	100	95	0	95	0	0	11	21	30	87	0	0	100	0	100	0	100
100	100	0	100	100	100	100	100	100	100	100	0	100	100	100	0	100	0	100	50	0	0	100	0	100	100	100
11	0	0	0	100	22	100	100	100	100	100	0	0	55	80	0	0	0	13	55	0	0	89	0	80	0	100
0	0	0	0	90	0	0	0	90	0	0	0	0	0	0	0	60	100	0	0	0	100	0	0	0	0	0
100	0	0	100	100	0	100	100	100	100	100	55	0	0	0	0	30	0	60	45	0	0	100	0	100	0	100
100	0	0	0	100	0	100	100	100	100	100	10	0	10	60	50	50	0	0	0	100	0	100	0	100	25	100
0	0	0	0	25	0	75	0	0	100	0	0	0	0	0	0	75	0	75	0	0	0	100	0	100	0	100
100	0	0	100	100	0	100	100	100	100	100	65	0	0	0	0	65	0	0	0	0	0	100	0	100	0	100
100	100	0	0	100	0	100	100	100	100	100	0	0	0	0	0	100	50	0	0	0	100	0	100	0	100	100
50	0	0	0	0	0	50	0	100	0	0	0	0	0	0	0	50	0	0	0	0	0	100	100	0	0	100
100	0	0	100	100	100	100	100	100	100	100	100	0	100	100	0	0	100	0	25	0	0	100	0	100	100	100

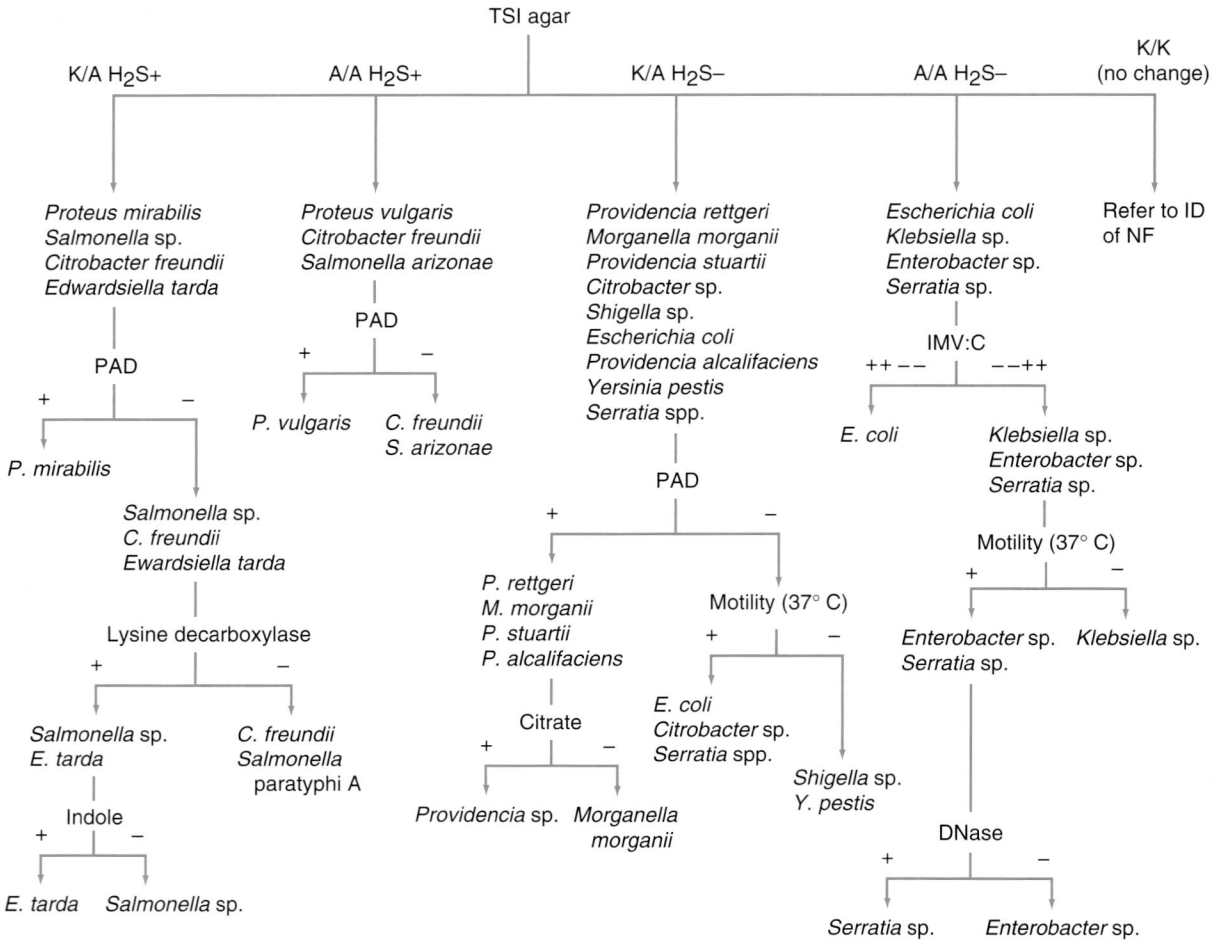

Figure 16-12

Flow chart for the presumptive identification of commonly encountered Enterobacteriaceae on TSI agar. (Data from Koneman E et al: *Color atlas in diagnostic microbiology,* ed 5, Philadelphia, 1997, Lippincott-Raven.) *K,* Alkaline; *A,* acid; *H₂S,* hydrogen sulfide; *TSI,* triple sugar iron; *PAD,* phenylalanine deaminase; *NF,* nonfermenter.

nial morphology of the isolate on a differential or selective medium, such as MacConkey, HE, or XLD.

The traditional biochemical tests to perform include the following:

- **Triple sugar iron (TSI) agar** or **Kligler iron agar (KIA)** to determine glucose and lactose, or sucrose, utilization (sucrose in TSI only) and hydrogen sulfide production
- Lysine-iron agar (LIA) to determine lysine decarboxylase activity
- Urea test to determine hydrolysis of urea
- Simmons citrate as the sole source of carbon
- **Sulfide, indole, motility (SIM)** or **motility, indole, and ornithine (MIO)** test
- Carbohydrate fermentation

BIOCHEMICAL PRINCIPLES AND REACTIONS ON CONVENTIONAL MEDIA

Lactose Fermentation and Utilization of Carbohydrates

Lactose is a disaccharide carbohydrate that consists of glucose and galactose connected by a galactoside bond. Glucose and galactose are released when this bond is cleaved by the enzyme **β-galactosidase.** Lactose degradation has been used to initially differentiate those bacterial species that are capable of fermenting lactose (LF) and those that are NLF species.

Two enzymes are necessary for a bacterium to take up lactose. These are **β-galactoside permease,** which serves as a transport enzyme that facilitates entry of the lactose molecule through the bacterial cell wall, and β-galactosidase, the enzyme that hydrolyzes lactose into glucose and galactose. Glucose becomes available for bacterial metabolism. Needless to say, certain bacterial species may be able to utilize carbohydrates only in their simplest form, glucose, and are not able to attack the disaccharide lactose. Similarly, those bacterial species incapable of fermenting glucose cannot utilize lactose.

Because all members of the family Enterobacteriaceae ferment glucose, this carbohydrate has not been the choice for differential media such as MacConkey or eosin-methylene blue agar. Non–lactose-fermenting species (typical of true enteric pathogens such as *Salmonella* and *Shigella*) are not easily distinguished from lactose-fermenting enterics (common enteric flora). This is the reason that lactose—and not glucose—is incorporated into most gram-negative differential media and highly selective enteric media.

By definition, lactose-fermenters possess both β-galactoside permease and β-galactosidase, and non–lactose-fermenters do not possess β-galactosidase. Some bacterial species lack β-galactoside permease but possess the β-galactosidase. These bacterial species, termed late lactose-fermenters or slow lactose-fermenters, eventually cleave the lactose molecule.

Triple sugar iron (TSI) agar

KIA or TSI agar is very useful in the presumptive identification of enterics, particularly in screening for intestinal pathogens. The formulas for KIA and TSI are identical except that TSI contains sucrose in addition to glucose and lactose. Lactose is present in a concentration 10 times that of glucose (10:1 ratio). In TSI, sucrose is present in concentration 10 times that of glucose. Ferrous sulfate and sodium thiosulfate are added to detect the production of hydrogen sulfide. Phenol red is used as the pH indicator, which is yellow below the pH of 6.8. Uninoculated medium is red, since the pH is buffered at 7.4. Both KIA and TSI are useful in detecting the ability of the microorganism to produce gas from the fermentation of sugars; to detect the fermentation of glucose and lactose in KIA and glucose, lactose, and/or sucrose in TSI; and to detect the production of hydrogen sulfide gas.

Both KIA and TSI agars are poured on a slant (see Figure 16-13). This sets up reaction chambers within the tube; the slant portion is the aerobic chamber being exposed to oxygen; the butt, or deep portion, is the anaerobic chamber, being protected from the air. To inoculate TSI agar, the laboratory professional should pick a well-isolated colony with an inoculating needle and stab the butt (all the way to the bottom) at the base of the slant. Then the laboratory professional streaks the slant by "fish tailing" (moving the needle back and forth) as the needle is being pulled out of the butt.

Based on the reactions shown on the TSI agar, the microbiologist determines whether the isolate ferments glucose only (typical of true enteric pathogens) or whether it ferments glucose, lactose, and/or sucrose (typical of most opportunistic enterics).

The reaction patterns are written with the slant results first, followed by the butt reaction, separated by a backslash (slant reaction/butt reaction), and it is important that the reactions be read within an 18- to 24-hour incubation period. The reaction patterns shown below are an integral part of the identification schema for the family Enterobacteriaceae.

REACTIONS ON KIA OR TSI AGAR
1. **No fermentation**
   Alkaline slant/alkaline butt (ALK/ALK or K/K) or alkaline slant/no change (ALK/no change or K/NC).

   These reactions are typical of organisms that are not members of the Enterobacteriaceae. Although nonenteric bacilli are unable to ferment either lactose or glucose, these organisms can degrade the peptones present in the medium, resulting in the production of alkaline byproducts and changing the indicator to a deep red color.

2. **No lactose (sucrose) fermentation: glucose only**
   Acid slant/acid butt (A/A) (8 to 12 hours).

   KIA and TSI agar contain glucose in a 0.1% concentration. The acid produced from this concentration of glucose is enough to change in indicator to yellow throughout the medium in this time frame. Reading the results after less than 12 hours of incubation gives the false appearance of an organism capable of fermenting glucose and lactose (sucrose). For this reason, KIA or TSI agar must be incubated for 18 to 24 hours.
   Alkaline slant/acid butt (Alk/acid or K/A) (18 to 24 hours).

This reaction is typical of an organism that ferments only glucose. After 18 to 24 hours the glucose concentration is depleted in the slant and the butt. The organism begins oxidative degradation of the peptones in the slant, resulting in alkaline byproducts that change the indicator to a deep red color. Fermentation (anaerobic) of glucose in the butt produces larger amounts of acid, overcoming the alkaline effects of peptone degradation; therefore the butt remains acid (yellow).

3. **Lactose (sucrose) fermentation (18 to 24 hours)**
   Acid/acid (A/A).

   The lactose present in TSI and KIA and the sucrose present in TSI is 10 times the concentration of glucose. The Enterobacteriaceae attack the simple sugar (glucose) first, and then the lactose (sucrose). The acid production from the fermentation of the additional sugar(s) is sufficient to keep both the slant and the butt acid (yellow) when examined at the end of 18 to 24 hours.

4. **Hydrogen sulfide production**
   Alkaline slant/acid butt, H_2S in butt (Alk/Ac H_2S or K/A H_2S) or acid slant/acid butt, H_2S in butt (A/A H_2S).

   Hydrogen sulfide production is another system that is helpful in differentiating the Enterobacteriaceae. Two indicators are present in the medium: sodium thiosulfate and ferrous sulfate. Because the visualization of H_2S production is a two-step process (see below), both indicators must be present. In addition, H_2S is a colorless gas, therefore the second indicator is necessary to visually detect its production.

   1. Bacterium (acid environment) + Sodium thiosulfate = H_2S gas
   2. H_2S + Ferric ions = Ferrous sulfide (black precipitate)

5. **Gas production (aerogenic) or no gas production (nonaerogenic)**
   The production of gas results in the formation of bubbles or splitting of the media in the butt or complete displacement of the media from the bottom of the tube. Figure 16-13 illustrates the reactions on TSI agar.

o-Nitrophenyl-*p*-D-galactopyranoside

Organisms that are slow or late lactose fermenters appear as nonfermenting colonies on primary isolation medium. When placed on TSI or KIA slants, these species produce similar results after 18 to 22 hours of incubation, raising suspicions that the species is an intestinal enteric pathogen. The *o*-nitrophenyl-*p*-D-galactopyranoside (ONPG) test determines whether the organism is a slow or late lactose-fermenter (one that lacks the enzyme permease but possesses β-galactosidase) or a true non–lactose-fermenter. The ONPG is structurally similar to lactose, except that glucose is replaced with ONPG, and ONPG is more easily transported through the bacterial cell wall. β-Galactosidase acts on the ONPG (a colorless compound), cleaves it into galactose and orthonitrophenol, and the compound turns yellow. The compound remains colorless if the organism is a non–lactose-fermenter (Figure 16-14).

Glucose Metabolism and Its Metabolic Products

Lactose degradation results in glucose and galactose available for bacterial consumption. Glucose is metabolized via the Embden-Meyerhof pathway, producing several intermediate byproducts, including pyruvic acid. Further degradation of pyruvic acid produces mixed acids as final end products. However, enterics take two separate pathways: the mixed acid fermentation pathway or the butylene glycol pathway.

The methyl red (MR) and Voges-Proskauer (VP) tests detect the end products of glucose fermentation. Each test detects products from a different pathway.

Methyl red test

If glucose is metabolized by the mixed acid fermentation pathway, acidic end products are produced, which results in a low pH. Red color (indicating a low pH) develops after addition of the indicator methyl red (Figure 16-15):

Glucose → Pyruvic acid → Mixed acid fermentation (pH 4.4)
↓
Red color with methyl red indicator

Voges-Proskauer test

Carbon compounds are degraded to butylene glycol and acetylmethylcarbinol (acetoin), which is further converted to diacetyl. Diacetyl in the presence of potassium hydroxide and α-naphthol forms a red complex. The pH remains at a rela-

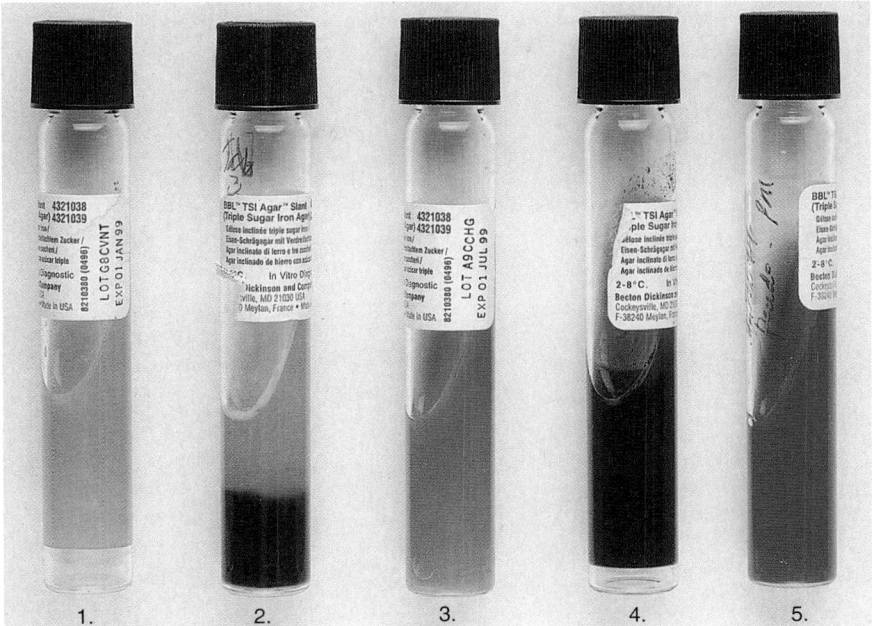

Figure 16-13

Triple sugar iron agar reactions of Enterobacteriaceae. *Left to right:* Tube 1, A/A gas; tube 2, A/A H_2S; tube 3, K/A; tube 4, K/A H_2S; tube 5, K/K.

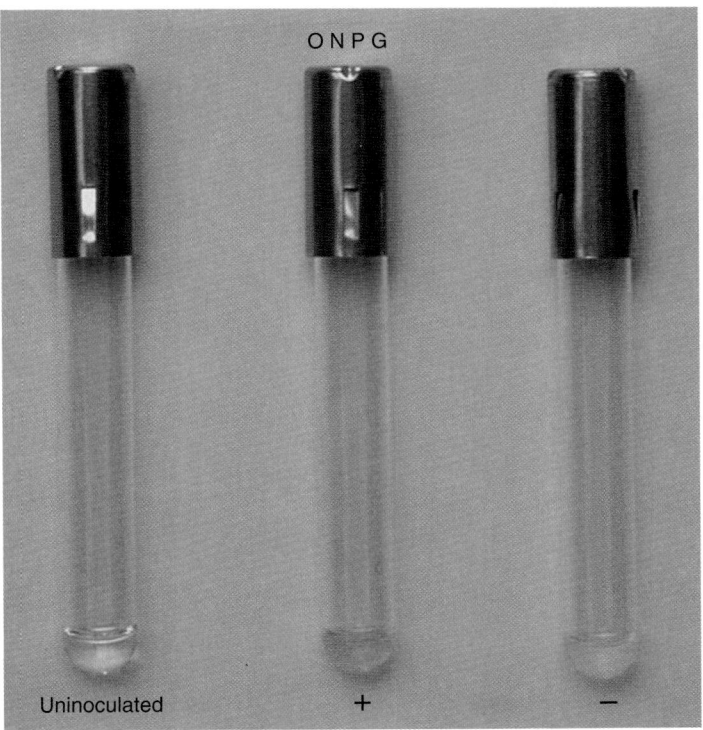

Figure 16-14

Orthonitrophenyl galactopyranoside (ONPG) test. (Courtesy American Society for Clinical Laboratory Science, Education and Research Fund, Inc., 1982.)

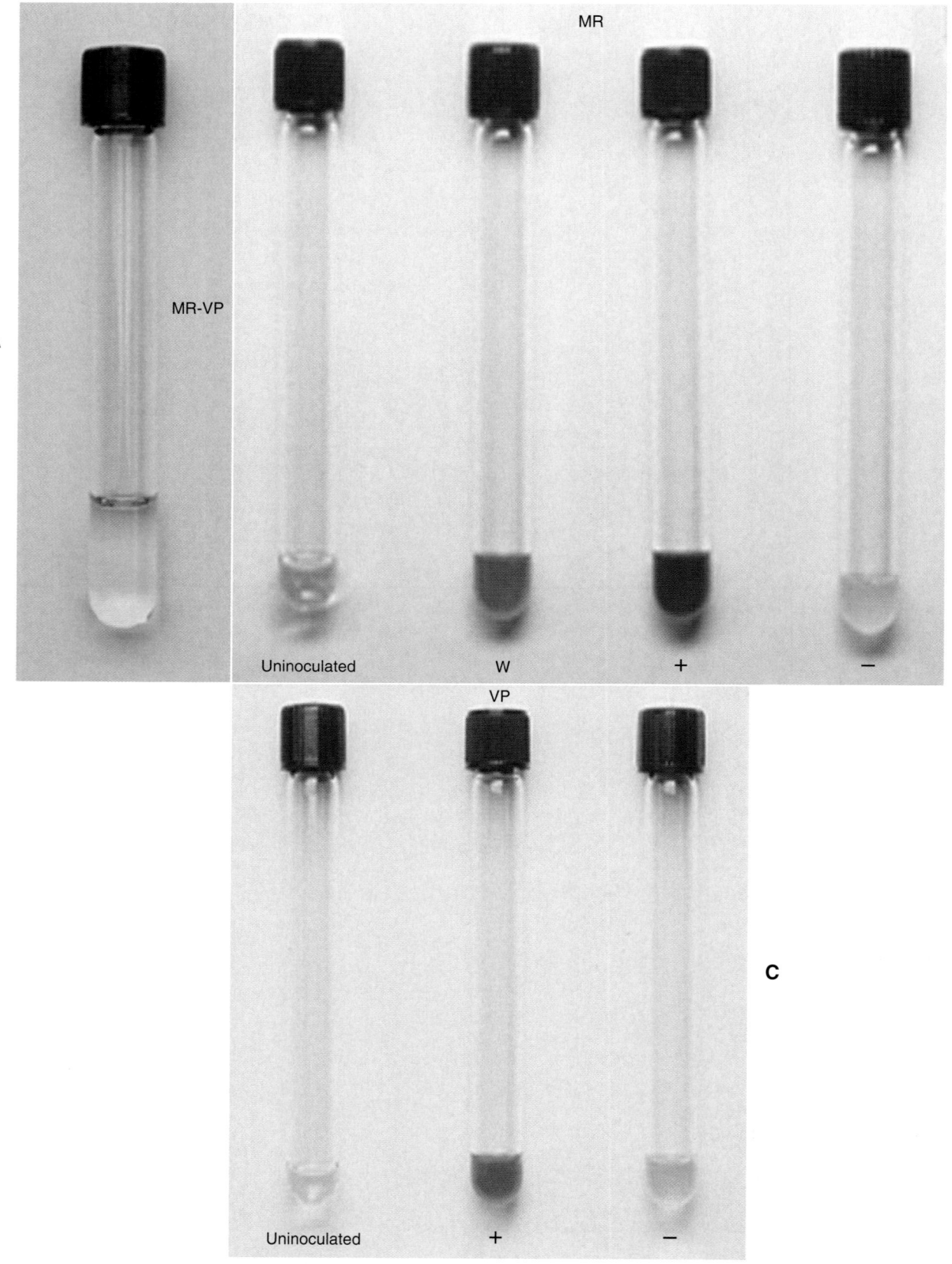

A

MR-VP

B

MR

Uninoculated   W   +   −

C

VP

Uninoculated   +   −

Figure 16-15

A, The methyl red–Voges-Proskauer test is inoculated and incubated overnight. Then it is split equally into two parts, one part for the methyl red test, the other for the Voges-Proskauer test. **B,** Methyl red test. **C,** Voges-Proskauer test. (Courtesy American Society for Clinical Laboratory Science, Education and Research Fund, Inc., 1982.)

tively neutral level. Figure 16-15 illustrates the **methyl red–Voges-Proskauer (MRVP) test:**

VP reaction

Glucose → Pyruvic acid → Acetoin → Diacetyl + KOH +
  └─ α-Naphthol → Red complex
  └─→ Butylene glycol

Miscellaneous reactions

INDOLE PRODUCTION

Indole is one of the degradation products of the amino acid tryptophan. Organisms that possess the enzyme tryptophanase are capable of deaminating tryptophan, with the formation of the intermediate degradation products of indole, pyruvic acid and ammonia. A red color develops after the addition of paradimethylaminobenzaldehyde (PDAB) (Figure 16-16).

CITRATE UTILIZATION TEST

The citrate utilization test determines whether the organism can utilize sodium citrate as the sole source of carbon for metabolism. The alkaline pH that results from use of citrate turns the indicator in the medium from green to blue. It is important to keep the inoculum light, since dead organisms can be a source of carbon, producing a false-positive reaction (Figure 16-17).

UREASE PRODUCTION TEST

The urease test determines whether the organism hydrolyzes urea, releasing a sufficient amount of ammonia to produce a color change. A positive test result is indicated by a bright pink color (Figure 16-18).

MOTILITY TEST

The motility test medium has agar concentrations of 0.4% or less, to allow free spread of organism. A single stab into the medium is made. After overnight incubation, movement away from the stab line or a hazy appearance throughout the medium indicates a motile organism.

MALONATE TEST

The malonate test determines whether the organism is capable of utilizing sodium malonate as its sole source of carbon. A positive test results in increased alkalinity, changing the indicator to blue (Figure 16-19).

CARBOHYDRATE FERMENTATION TESTS

Carbohydrate fermentation tests determine the ability of a microorganism to ferment a specific 1% concentration of carbohydrate incorporated into a basal medium such as purple broth base, producing acid or acid with gas when the test result is positive. Examples of sugars used to differentiate bacteria include maltose, rhamnose, lactose, sucrose, raffinose, and arabinose. The polyhydric alcohols (which end in *ol*) that are collectively called "sugars" include adonitol, dulcitol, mannitol, and sorbitol. A yellow color is considered a positive reaction.

PHENYLALANINE DEAMINASE

Phenylalanine **deaminase** determines whether the organism possesses the enzyme that deaminates phenylalanine to phenylpyruvic acid. Addition of a ferric chloride reagent results in a green color if phenylpyruvic acid is present. This is helpful in initial differentiation of *Proteus, Morganella,* and *Providencia* from the rest of the Enterobacteriaceae (Figure 16-20).

Deamination of phenylalanine

Phenylalanine → Phenylalanine deaminase →
  Phenylpyruvic acid + $(FeCl_3)$ → Green

DECARBOXYLASE TESTS

Decarboxylase tests determine whether the bacterial species possess enzymes capable of decarboxylating (attacking the carboyl group of an amino acid) specific amino acids in the test medium. The three amino acids commonly used to test for Enterobacteriaceae are lysine, ornithine, and arginine. Specific amine products and carbon dioxide are products of decarboxylation. Degradation of the amino acids and their specific end products are shown in the following reaction:

Degradation of amino acids and their specific end products

Lysine (amino acid) → Lysine decarboxylase →
  Cadaverine (amine) + CO_2
Ornithine → Ornithine decarboxylase → Putrescine
Arginine → Arginine dihydrolase → Citrulline →
  Ornithine → Putrescine

Arginine conversion involves a two-step process. First, arginine is converted to citrulline by arginine dihydrolase. Next, citrulline is further con-

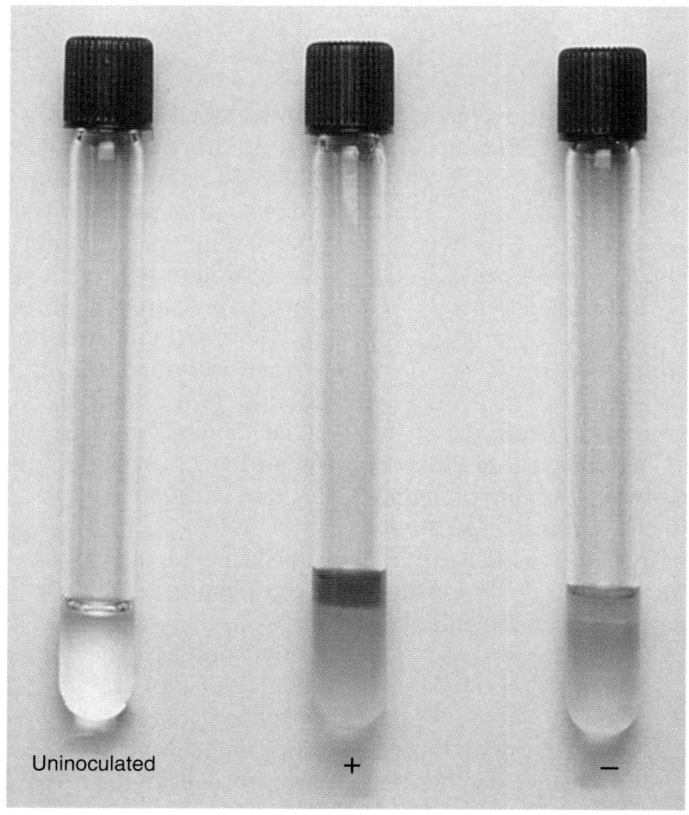

Figure 16-16

Indole broth. (Courtesy American Society for Clinical Laboratory Science, Education and Research Fund, Inc., 1982.)

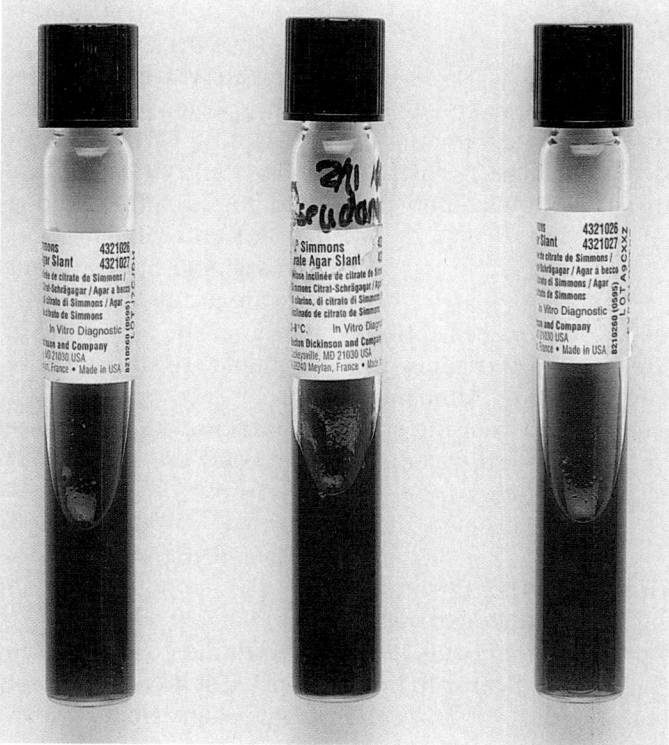

Figure 16-17

Citrate utilization test. *Left,* Uninoculated; *middle,* positive result; *right,* negative result.

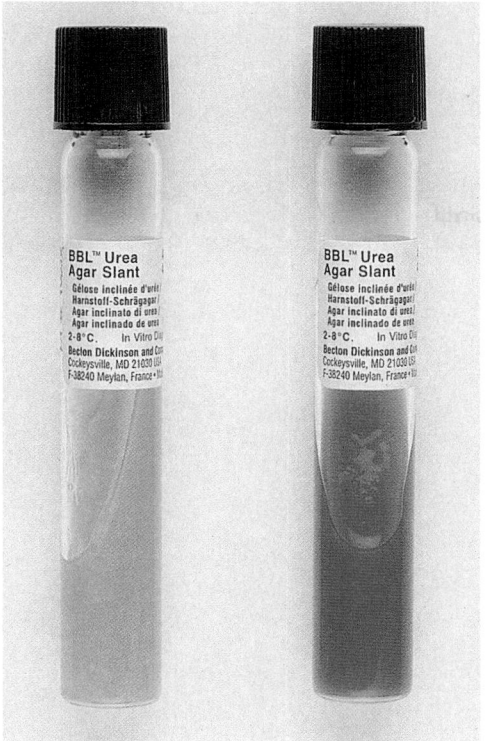

Figure 16-18 _____

Urease test. *Left,* Positive result; *right,* negative result.

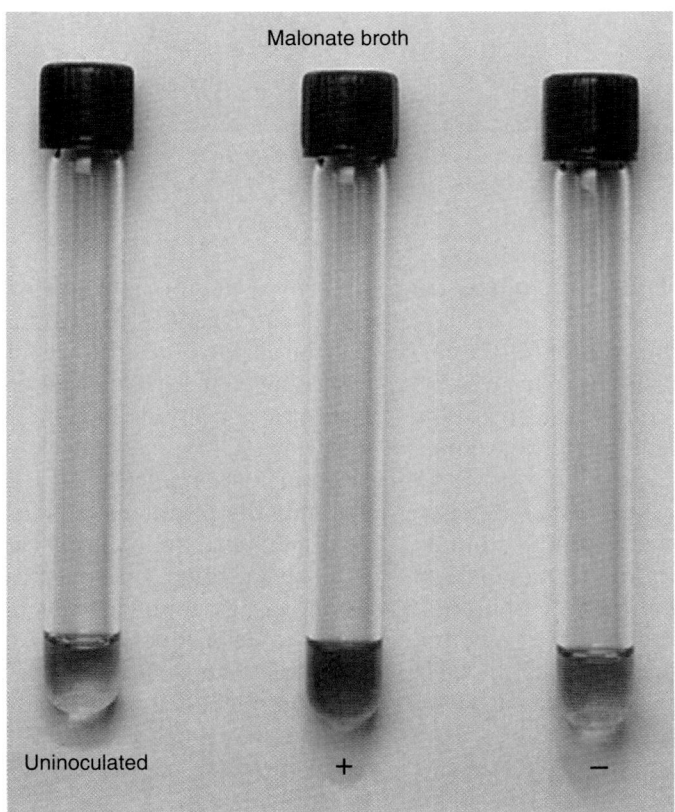

Figure 16-19 _____

Malonate test. (Courtesy American Society for Clinical Laboratory Science, Education and Research Fund, Inc., 1982.)

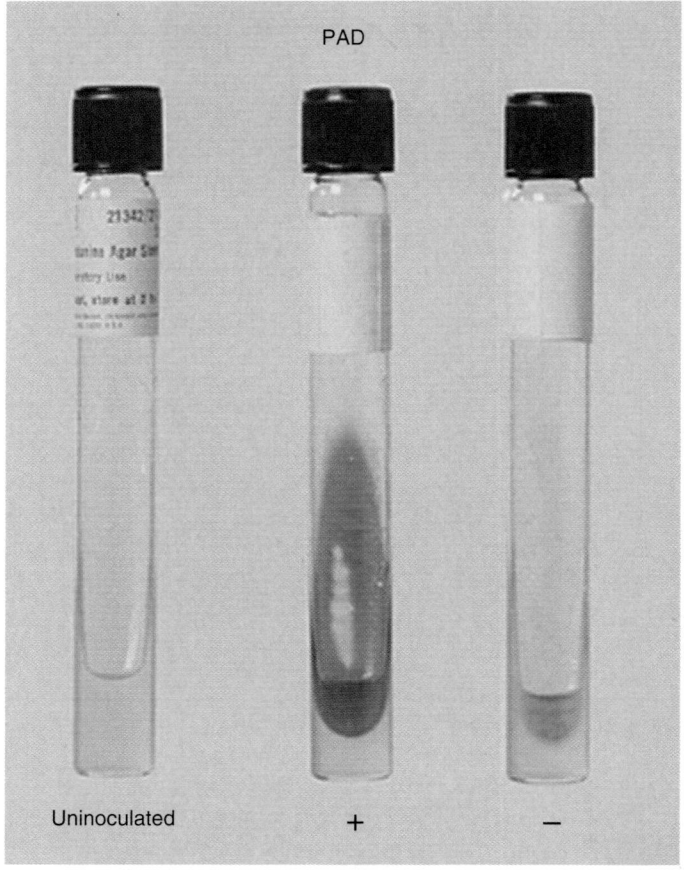

Figure 16-20

Phenylalanine deaminase test. (Courtesy American Society for Clinical Laboratory Science, Education and Research Fund, Inc., 1982.)

verted to ornithine, which is decarboxylated to putrescine.

The test to detect decarboxylation of Enterobacteriaceae contains the Moeller decarboxylase base medium. This base contains glucose, peptone, pH indicator, bromcresol purple and cresol red, and the specific amino acid. The role of glucose in the medium is important because decarboxylases are inducible enzymes produced in an acid pH. In addition, by definition, all members of Enterobacteriaceae are glucose-positive, providing a growth stimulus. The uninoculated medium is purple. A control tube containing only the base medium without the amino acid is tested along with the test organism to determine the viability of the organism. For decarboxylation to take place, two conditions must be met: an acid pH and an anaerobic environment. The control tube determines whether sufficient acid is produced. Both tubes are inoculated with the test organism, are overlayed with a layer of sterile mineral oil, which creates anaerobic conditions, and then are incubated.

During the first few hours of incubation, Enterobacteriaceae organisms attack the glucose first, changing the pH to acid. The change in pH in the medium changes the purple color to yellow. If the organism produces the specific decarboxylase and the amino acid in the medium is attacked, release of the amine products causes an alkaline pH shift. This results in a purple (positive result) color in the broth medium. If the organism does not possess the specific decarboxylase, the medium remains yellow (negative result). The control tube remains the original color.

Modifications of the decarboxylase test to detect other biochemical reactions are also routinely used. Examples of these include MIO (motility, indole, ornithine) test and lysine iron agar (LIA) tests (Figure 16-21).

MOTILITY, INDOLE, ORNITHINE TEST

MIO is a semisolid agar medium used to detect motility and production of indole and ornithine decarboxylase. MIO is useful in differentiating *Klebsiella* species from *Enterobacter* and *Serratia* species. Motility is shown by a clouding of the medium or spreading growth from the line of inoculation. Ornithine decarboxylation is indicated by a purple color throughout the medium. Because MIO is a semisolid medium, it does not have to be overlayed with mineral oil to provide anaerobic conditions. Indole production is detected by the addition of Kovacs reagent; a pink to red color is formed in the reagent area if the test result is positive.

LYSINE IRON AGAR SLANT

The LIA test is a tubed agar slant. It contains lysine as the specific amino acid, glucose, ferric ammonium citrate, and sodium thiosulfate. LIA is used primarily to determine whether the bacterial species decarboxylates or deaminates lysine (see Figure 16-21). Hydrogen sulfide production is also detected in this medium. LIA is inoculated in the same manner as TSI agar slant. LIA is most useful in conjunction with TSI in screening stool specimens for the presence of enteric pathogens. LIA is helpful in differentiating *Salmonella* (lysine-positive) from *Citrobacter* species (lysine-negative).

LIA is also useful in differentiating *Proteus, Morganella,* and *Providencia* species from the rest of the members of Enterobacteriaceae. This group of enterics deaminate (attack the NH_2 group instead of the carboxyl group) amino acids. In the LIA slant, deamination of lysine turns the original purple color slant to a plum or reddish-purple color; the butt remains yellow.

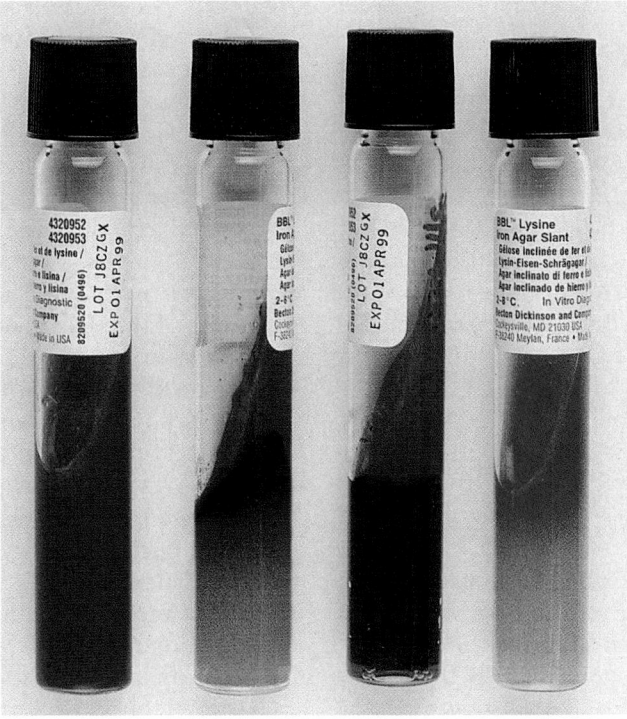

Figure 16-21

Lysine iron agar (LIA) reactions. *Left to right,* K/K (positive decarboxylation without H_2S), K/A H_2S (negative decarboxylation with H_2S), K/K H_2S (positive decarboxylation with H_2S), R/Y (negative decarboxylation, positive deamination without H_2S).

NITRATE REDUCTION TEST

The **nitrate reduction** test determines whether the organism has the ability to reduce nitrate to nitrite and further reduce nitrite to nitrogen.

The organism is inoculated into a nutrient broth containing a nitrogen source. After 24 hours of incubation, sulfanilic acid and *N,N*-dimethyl-1 naphthylamine (NNDN) is added. A red color indicates the presence of nitrite:

Nitrate reduction test reaction

Nutrient broth with 0.1% potassium nitrate →
Nitrate reductase → Nitrite + Sulfanilic acid +
N,N-Dimethyl-1-naphthylamine → Diazo red dye

If no color develops, this may indicate that nitrate has not been reduced or *that nitrate has been further reduced to nitrogen gas (N_2), nitric oxide (NO), or nitrous oxide (N_2O), which the reagents will not be able to detect.* Adding a small amount of zinc dust will help to determine whether the test has produced a true-negative result or whether the lack of color production was due to reduction beyond nitrate. Zinc dust reduces nitrate.

Therefore development of a red color after the addition of zinc confirms a true-negative test result.

POTASSIUM CYANIDE TEST

The KCN test is mentioned briefly here in a historical context. The test is not performed in clinical laboratories because of its potential lethal effects on personnel. The principle of the test is to determine the ability of the organism to live and grow in KCN. The enzymes of certain bacteria, such as *Citrobacter freundii,* are resistant to KCN and therefore grown in the medium; others such as *Salmonella* are sensitive to KCN and do not grow in the medium.

SCREENING STOOL CULTURES FOR PATHOGENS

Because of the mixed microbial flora of fecal specimens, efficient screening methods should be utilized for the recovery and identification of stool pathogens. Enteric pathogens include the following: *Salmonella, Shigella, Aeromonas, Campylobacter, Yersinia, Vibrio,* and *E. coli* O157:H7. All fecal specimens should be screened for *Salmonella, Shigella,* and *Campylobacter* organisms (see Chapter 17). In addition, many laboratories are routinely screening for *E. coli* O157:H7. Screening routinely for the remaining organisms may not be cost-effective; therefore these organisms should be addressed on the basis of patient history (e.g., travel near coastal areas, where certain organisms are endemic) and gross description of the specimen (bloody or watery). It should be noted that any method screening for *Salmonella* and *Shigella* species also screens for *Aeromonas* and *Plesiomonas* species (see Chapter 17), and therefore additional media are not needed.

Fecal pathogens are generally non–lactose-fermenters. These organisms appear as clear or colorless and translucent colonies on MacConkey agar. In addition, many laboratories use selective media, such as HE agar, which detects lactose and sucrose fermentation and H_2S production in conjunction with MacConkey agar. Because media selection varies in many laboratories, only MacConkey agar will be used here as an example.

However, many of the bacteria that compose common fecal flora also appear as non–lactose-fermenters, for example, *Proteus, Providencia, Serratia, Citrobacter,* and *Pseudomonas* as well as the late lactose-fermenting organisms. For this reason, it is necessary to set up screening tests to differentiate these organisms from stool pathogens. An easy approach is to take a well-isolated, NLF colony and perform a screening battery consisting first of an oxidase test and then of inoculation of LIA and TSI agar. The following will serve as an example. After 18 to 24 hours of incubation, the results of the reactions are for the TSI, K/AG, and for the LIA, K/A. Using Table 16-12 and tracing the TSI result to where it intersects the LIA result, you see that this organism could be *Salmonella, Shigella, Aeromonas, E. coli, Enterobacter,* or *Citrobacter.* If the oxidase test performed the previous day yielded a negative result, *Aeromonas* is eliminated as a potential pathogen. Because other potential pathogens are in this category, additional biochemical testing must be performed to identify the organism. When the results of a biochemical identification indicate *Salmonella* or *Shigella,* serotyping must be performed using a commercial typing kit.

If the screening battery pinpoints a group of organisms that are nonpathogens, the process is complete and the culture is discarded (after 48 hours of incubation).

TABLE 16-12

Stool Culture Screening for Enteric Pathogens Utilizing TSI and LIA in Combination

LIA Reactions	TSI Reactions							
	K/A H₂S	K/AG H₂S	K/AG	K/A	A/A H₂S	A/AG	A/A	K/K
R/A		P. vulgaris P. mirabilis *	M. morganii Providencia *	M. morganii Providencia *	P. vulgaris P. mirabilis *		Providencia	Pseudomonas†
K/K H₂S	*	Salmonella Edwardsiella	Salmonella					
K/K	Salmonella Edwardsiella *		Hafnia Klebsiella Serratia	Salmonella Plesiomonas† Hafnia Serratia		Klebsiella Enterobacter E. coli	Serratia	
K/A H₂S	Salmonella	Salmonella Citrobacter		*	Citrobacter			
K/A			Salmonella Shigella Aeromonas† E. coli Enterobacter Citrobacter *	Shigella Yersinia Aeromonas† E. coli Enterobacter *		Aeromonas† E. coli Citrobacter Enterobacter *	Aeromonas† Yersinia Citrobacter Enterobacter *	

Data from the Microbiology Laboratory, OSU Hospitals and Maureta Ott, Columbus, Ohio.

K, Alkaline; A, acid; G, gas; R, deamination (red slant).

*Results of TSI and LIA reactions in this category indicate a potential pathogen; additional tests must be performed.

†Oxidase positive.

SEROLOGIC GROUPING

Once an isolate is biochemically identified as *Salmonella* or *Shigella* sp., serologic grouping of the isolate for the O serogroups (somatic antigen) must be performed for confirmation.

Salmonella Species

Based on the common O antigens, *Salmonella* may be placed into major groups designated by capital letters. Approximately 60 O antigenic groups exist; however, 98% of *Salmonella* isolates from humans belong to serogroups A through G.

Laboratories may report isolates as *Salmonella* groups (A-G) when specific serotyping is not available; isolates may be sent to a reference laboratory for serotyping. If an isolate is suspected of being one of these three serotypes, *S. typhi, S. choleraesuis,* or *S. paratyphi A,* because of its medical implications, it must be biochemically identified and serologically confirmed. Their identification is very important in providing proper therapy for the patient and in limiting any possible complications that may develop. Measures may also be taken to prevent an epidemic outbreak.

It is imperative for any laboratory performing bacteriology to be able to serologically identify *S. typhi,* particularly, and other members of *Salmonella* in O groups A through G. Other isolates can be identified as "biochemically compatible with *Salmonella*" and submitted to a reference laboratory for further testing.

To perform serologic grouping by slide technique, first prepare a saline emulsion from a pure culture of the organism. Serologic typing is best performed on a colony taken from a pure culture growing on nonselective media, such as blood agar plate, although TSI or MacConkey agar can be used for presumptive serologic identification. A slide with wells is easy to use for the agglutination test. A regular microscope slide may be used by marking separate squares with a wax pencil. The laboratory professional places one drop of antisera on the appropriately labeled slide. One drop of bacterial emulsion is added to each drop of antisera. Antisera kits usually consist of a polyvalent A through G, Vi, and serogroups A, B, C_1, C_2, D, E, and G. In the event of a positive agglutination in the Vi antisera with no agglutination in the other groups, the emulsion should be heated to 100° C

for 10 minutes to inactivate the capsular Vi antigen. The emulsion is then cooled and retested with antisera A to G. If the organism agglutinates with group D antisera, it can be reported as *S. typhi.* Larger laboratories usually maintain antisera to serotype salmonellae for all the somatic types. H antigen or flagella typing is usually performed in a reference laboratory that provides epidemiologic information of the common source in outbreaks.

Shigella Species

Similar serogrouping procedures may be used in the serologic testing for *Shigella* species. Serologic grouping of *Shigella* species is based on the O antigen present. *Shigella* species may belong to one of the four serogroups: A, B, C, and D. *S. dysenteriae, S. flexneri, S. boydii,* and *S. sonnei* correspond to these serogroups, respectively. The O antisera used for serogrouping are polyvalent, containing several serotypes within each group (with the exception of group D, which contains only a single serotype).

If agglutination fails, the suspension must be heated to remove the capsular antigen that may be present, and subsequently the agglutination test procedure is repeated.

The members of the family Enterobacteriaceae present a challenge to the microbiologist when isolated from infected sites. The microbiologist must determine the clinical significance of the isolate, particularly those that produce opportunistic infections. Intestinal pathogens, when isolated, must be reported to the clinician as soon as possible. With the development of rapid diagnostic tests to identify these organisms, treatment can be provided when appropriate, and prevention of the spread of disease may be easily accomplished.

Bibliography

Arduino MJ et al: Growth and endotoxin production of *Yersinia enterocolitica* and *Enterobacter agglomerans* in packed erythrocytes, *J Clin Microbiol* 27:1483, 1989.

Azad MA: Colonic perforation in *Shigella dysenteriae 1* infection, *Pediatric Infect Dis* 5:103, 1986.

Bader M et al: Venereal transmission of shigellosis in Seattle—King County, *Sex Trans Dis* 4:89, 1977.

Balows A et al, editors: *Manual of clinical microbiology,* ed 4, Washington, DC, 1985, American Society for Microbiology.

Baron EJ, Finegold S: *Bailey & Scott's diagnostic microbiology,* ed 8, St Louis, 1990, Mosby.

Bean NH et al: Surveillance for foodborne outbreaks—United States, 1988-1992, CDC Surveillance Summaries, October 24, 1996, *MMWR Morb Mortal Wkly Report* 45:737, 1996.

Bitar R, Tarpley J: Intestinal perforation in typhoid fever: a historical and state-of-the-art review, *Rev Infect Dis* 7:257, 1985.

Brenner DJ et al: Atypical biotypes of *E. coli* found in clinical specimens and description of *E. hermanii* sp. nov., *J Clin Microbiol* 15:703, 1982.

Brenner DJ et al: *Escherichia vulneris:* a new species of Enterobacteriaceae associated with human wounds, *J Clin Microbiol* 15:1133, 1982.

Boedexer EC: Enteroadherent (enteropathogenic) *E. coli.* In Farthing MJ, Keusch GT, editors: *Enteric infection: mechanisms, manifestation, and management,* New York, 1988, Raven Press.

Boileau C, D'Hauteville H, Sansonetti P: DNA hybridization technique to detect *Shigella* sp. and enteroinvasive *E. coli, J Clin Microbiol* 20:959, 1984.

Brown JE et al: Purification and biological characterization of Shiga toxin from *Shigella dysenteriae 1, Infect Immun* 36:996, 1982.

Butler T: Plague and other *Yersinia* infections. In Greenough WB, Merigan TC, editors: *Current topics in infectious disease,* New York, 1983, Plenum Med. Book Co.

Candy DCA, Stephen J: *Salmonella.* In Farthing MJ, Keusch GT, editors: *Enteric infection: mechanisms, manifestations, and management,* New York, 1988, Raven Press.

Cherubin CE et al: Septicemia with non-typhoid *Salmonella, Medicine* 53:365, 1974.

Carbonetti NH et al: Aerobactin-mediated iron uptake by *E. coli* isolates from human extraintestinal infections, *Infect Immun* 51:966, 1986.

Chmel H: *Serratia odorifera* biogroup 1 causing an invasive human infection, *J Clin Microbiol* 26:1244, 1988.

Cohen JI, Rodday P: *Yersinia enterocolitica* bacteremia in a patient with the acquired immunodeficiency syndrome, *Am J Med* 86:254, 1989.

Cravioto A et al: An adhesive factor found in strains of *Escherichia coli* belonging to the traditional infantile enteropathogenic serotypes, *Curr Microbiol* 3:95, 1979.

Donahue AR et al: Enzyme-linked immunosorbent assay for *Shigella* toxin, *J Clin Microbiol* 24:65, 1986.

Echeverria P et al: Plasmids coding for colonization factor antigens I and II, heat-labile enterotoxin, and heat-stable enterotoxin A2 in *Esherichia coli, Infect Immun* 51:626, 1986.

Eden CS et al: Host-parasite interaction in the urinary tract, *J Infect Dis* 157:421, 1988.

Eden CS et al: Variable adherence to normal human urinary-tract epithelial cells of *Escherichia coli* strains associated with various forms of urinary tract infection, *Lancet* 2:490, 1976.

Ewing WH: *Edwards & Ewing's identification of enterobacteriaceae,* ed 4, New York, 1986, Elsevier.

Farmer JJ, Howard BJ, Weissfeld AS: Enterobacteriaceae. In Howard BJ et al, editors: *Clinical and pathogenic microbiology,* St Louis, 1987, Mosby.

Farmer JJ et al: Biochemical identification of new species and biogroups of Enterobacteriaceae isolated from clinical specimens, *J Clin Microbiol* 21:46, 1985.

Farmer JJ et al: The *Salmonella-Arizona* group of Enterobacteriaceae: nomenclature, classification and reporting, *Clin Microbiol Newsl* 6:63, 1984.

Farthing MJ, editor: *Enteric infection: mechanisms, manifestations, and management,* New York, 1988, Raven Press.

Forbes BA, Sahm DF, Weissfeld AS: Enterobacteriaceae A. In Forbes BA, Sahm DF, Weissfeld AS: *Bailey & Scott's diagnostic microbiology,* St Louis, 1998, Mosby, p 509.

Freeman BA: *Burrows textbook of microbiology,* ed 22, Philadelphia, 1985, WB Saunders.

Fukushima H et al: *Yersinia pseudotuberculosis* infection contracted through water contaminated by a wild animal, *J Clin Microbiol* 26:584, 1988.

Gavini F et al: Transfer of *Enterobacter agglomerans* (Beijerinck 1988) Ewing and Fife 1972 to *Pantoea* gen. nov. as *Pantoea agglomerans* comb. nov. and description of *Pantoea dispersa* sp. nov., *Int J Syst Bacteriol* 39:337, 1989.

Gomes TA et al: DNA probes for identification of enteroinvasive *Escherichia coli, J Clin Microbiol* 25:2025, 1987.

Griffin PM et al: Illnesses associated with *Escherichia coli* O157:H7 infections: a broad clinical spectrum, *Ann Intern Med* 109:705, 1988.

Griffin PM, Tauxe RV. The epidemiology of infections caused by *Escherichia coli* O157:H7, other enterohemorrhagic *E. coli,* and the associated hemolytic uremic syndrome, *Epidemiol Rev* 13:60, 1991.

Harris JR et al: Person-to-person transmission in an outbreak of enteroinvasive *Escherichia coli, Am J Epidemiol* 122:245, 1985.

Hayes P, Wells JG, Griffin PM: Isolation and identification of *Escherichia coli* O157:H7. BACTinews, published by REMEL, Vol 2, No 2, Lenexa, Kan, April 1994.

Hennessey TW et al: National outbreak of *Salmonella* enteritidis infections from ice cream, *N Eng J Med* 334:1281, 1996.

Horowitz H et al: *Serratia plymuthica* sepsis associated with infection of central venous catheter, *J Clin Microbiol* 25:1562, 1987.

Jacobs J et al: *Yersinia enterocolitica* in donor blood: a case report and review, *J Clin Microbiol* 27:1119, 1989.

Karmali M et al: The association between idiopathic hemolytic-uremic syndrome and infection by verotoxin-producing *E. coli, J Infect Dis* 151:775, 1985.

Kehl KS et al. Evaluation of the premier EHEC assay for detection of Shiga-toxin producing *Escherichia coli, J Clin Microbiol* 35:2051, 1997.

Kelly M, Brenner D, Farmer JJ: Enterobacteriaceae. In Lennette EH, editor: *Manual of clinical microbiology,* ed 4, Washington, DC, 1985, American Society for Microbiology.

Kelly M, Brenner D, Farmer JJ: Enterobacteriaceae. In Balows A et al, editors: *Manual of clinical microbiology,* ed 5, Washington, DC, 1991, American Society for Microbiology.

Keusch GT, Bennish M: *Shigella.* In Farthing MJ, Keusch GT, editors: *Enteric infection: mechanisms, manifestations, and management,* New York, 1988, Raven Press.

Khanna R, Levendoglu H: Liver abscess due to *Yersinia enterocolitica, Dig Dis Sci* 34:636, 1989.

Knutton S, Lloyd D, McNeish A: Identification of a new fimbrial structure in enterotoxigenic *E. coli* (ETEC) serotype O148:H28 which adheres to human intestinal mucosa: a potentially new human ETEC colonization factor, *Infect Immun* 55:86, 1987.

Koneman E et al: *Color atlas in diagnostic microbiology,* ed 5, Philadelphia, 1997, Lippincott-Raven.

Koneman EW et al: The Enterobacteriaceae. In *Color atlas and textbook of diagnostic microbiology,* ed 5, Philadelphia, 1997, Lippincott-Raven, p. 171.

Korhonen TK et al: Serotypes, hemolysin production, and receptor recognition of *Escherichia coli* strains associated with neonatal sepsis and meningitis, *Infect Immun* 48:486, 1985.

Levine MM: *Escherichia coli* that cause diarrhea: enterotoxigenic, enteropathogenic, enteroinvasive, enterohemorrhagic, and enteroadherent, *J Infect Dis* 155:377, 1987.

Levine M et al: *Escherichia coli* strains that cause diarrhea but do not produce heat-labile or heat-stable enterotoxins and are noninvasive, *Lancet* 1:1119, 1978.

Levine M et al: Immunity to enterotoxigenic *Escherichia coli,* *Infect Immun* 17:78, 1979.

Levine M et al: New knowledge on pathogenesis of bacterial enteric infections as applied to vaccine development, *Microbiol Rev* 47:510, 1983.

Lew PD et al: Intra-abdominal *Citrobacter* infections: association with biliary or upper gastrointestinal source, *Surgery* 95:398, 1984.

Lipsky AB et al: *Citrobactor* infections in humans: experience at the Seattle VA Medical Center and review of the literature, *Rev Infect Dis* 2:746, 1980.

March B, Ratnam S: Latex agglutination test for detection of *Escherichia coli* serotype O157, *J Clin Microbiol* 27:1675, 1989.

March SB, Ratnam S: Sorbitol-MacConkey medium for detection of *Escherichia coli* O157-H7 associated with hemorrhagic colitis, *J Clin Microbiol* 23:869, 1986.

McDonough KA et al: Identification of a *Yersinia pestis*–specific DNA probe with potential for use in plague surveillance, *J Clin Microbiol* 26:2515, 1989.

Mathewson JJ, Cravioto A: HEp-2 cell adherence as an assay for virulence among diarrheagenic *E. coli, J Infect Dis* 159:1057, 1989.

Medon PP et al: Identification of enterotoxigenic *Escherichia coli* isolates with enzyme-labeled synthetic oligonucleotide probes, *J Clin Microbiol* 26:2173, 1988.

Nakashima A et al: Epidemic septic arthritis caused by *Serratia marcescens* and associated with benzalkonium chloride antiseptic, *J Clin Microbiol* 25:1014, 1987.

Nauschuetz W: Emerging foodborne pathogens: enterohemorrhagic *Escherichia coli, Clin Lab Sci* 11:298, 1998.

O'Brien AD et al: Purification of *Shigella dysenteriae* 1 (Shiga)-like toxin from *Escherichia coli* O157:H7 strain associated with hemorrhagic colitis, *Lancet* 2:573, 1983.

Pai C et al: Epidemiology of sporadic diarrhea due to verocyto-toxin-producing *E. coli:* a 2-yr prospective study, *J Infect Dis* 157:1054, 1988.

Pai CH, Kelly JK: Shiga-like toxin producing *E. coli.* In Farthing MJ, Keusch GT, editors: *Enteric infection: mechanisms, manifestations, and management,* New York, 1988, Raven Press.

Pai C et al: Sporadic cases of hemorrhagic colitis associated with *E. coli* O157:H7, *Ann Intern Med* 101:738, 1984.

Palmer SR, Rowe B: Investigation of outbreaks of *Salmonella* in hospitals, *BMJ* 287:891, 1983.

Paton AW, Paton JC: Detection and characterization of Shiga toxigenic *Escherichia coli* by using multiplex PCR Assays for stx1, stx2, eaeA, enterohemorrhagic *E. coli* hlyA, Rfb011 and rfbO157, *J Clin Micro* 36:598, 1998.

Pickering, LK, Bartlett AV, Woodward WE: Acute infectious diarrhea among children in day care, *Rev Infect Dis* 8:539, 1986.

Plantholt SJ, Trofa AF: *Citrobacter freundii* endocarditis in an intravenous drug abuser, *S Med J* 80:1439, 1987.

Raj P: Pathogenesis and laboratory diagnosis of *Escherichia coli*–associated enteritis, *Clin Microbiol Newsl* 15:89, 1993.

Ratnam S et al: A nosocomial outbreak of diarrheal disease due to *Yersinia enterocolitica* serotype 0:5 biotype 1, *J Infect Dis* 145:242, 1982.

Riley LW et al: Hemorrhagic colitis associated with a rare *E. coli* serotype, *N Engl J Med* 308:681, 1982.

Robins-Browne RM: *Yersinia enterocolitica.* In Farthing MJ, Keusch GT, editors: *Enteric infection: mechanisms, manifestations, and management,* New York, 1988, Raven Press.

Rothbaum R et al: A clinicopathologic study of enteroadherent *E. coli:* a cause of protracted diarrhea in infants, *Gastroenterology* 83:441, 1982.

Rubin R, Weinstein L: *Salmonellosis: microbiologic, pathologic, and clinical features,* New York, 1977, Stratton International Medical Book Corp.

Sack RB: Enterotoxigenic *E. coli:* identification and characterization, *J Infect Dis* 142:279, 1980.

Sack B et al: Enterotoxigenic *E. coli* isolated from food, *J Infect Dis* 135:313, 1977.

Sansonetti PJ: Enteroinvasive *E. coli.* In Farthing MJ, Keusch GT, editors: *Enteric infection: mechanisms, manifestations, and management,* New York, 1988, Raven Press.

Sarf LD et al: Epidemiology of *E. coli* K1 in healthy and diseased newborns, *Lancet* 1:1099, 1975.

Sowers EG, Wells JG, Strockbine NA: Evaluation of commercial latex reagents for identification of O157 and H7 antigens of *Escherichia coli, J Clin Microbiol* 34:1286, 1996.

Strampfer M, Schoch P, Cunha B: Cerebral abscess caused by *Klebsiella ozaenae, J Clin Microbiol* 25:1553, 1987.

Struelens MJ et al: *Shigella* septicemia: prevalence, presentation, risk factors, and outcome, *J Infect Dis* 152:784, 1985.

Symonds J: Haemorrhagic colitis and *Escherichia coli* O157: a pathogen unmasked, *BMJ* 296:875, 1988.

Taylor D et al: Clinical and microbiologic features of *Shigella* and enteroinvasive *Escherichia coli* infections detected by DNA hybridization, *J Clin Microbiol* 26:1362, 1988.

Wanke CA, Guerrant KL: Enterotoxigenic *E. coli.* In Farthing MJ, Keusch GT, editors: *Enteric infection: mechanisms, manifestations, and management,* New York, 1988, Raven Press.

Washington J: *Laboratory procedures in clinical microbiology,* ed 2, New York, 1985, Springer-Verlag.

Watanakunakorn C: Acute infective endocarditis due to *Yersinia enterocolitica, Am J Med* 86:723, 1989.

Weisfeld A, McNamara A: Enterobacteriaceae. In Howard B, editor: *Clinical and pathogenic microbiology,* ed 2, St Louis, 1994, Mosby.

Wilhelm I et al: Epidemic outbreak of *Serratia marcescens* infection in a cardiac surgery unit, *J Clin Microbiol* 25:1298, 1987.

Wood K et al: Comparison of DNA probes and the Sereny test for identification of invasive *Shigella* and *Escherichia coli* strains, *J Clin Microbiol* 24:498, 1986.

Zbinden R, Blass R: *Serratia plymuthica* osteomyelitis following a motorcycle accident, *J Clin Microbiol* 26:1409, 1988.

LEARNING ASSESSMENT

1. What are the three general characteristics a gram-negative bacilli must possess to belong to the family Enterobacteriaceae?

2. Which of the following tests detect the production of mixed acids as a result of subsequent metabolism of pyruvate?
   a. Methyl red test
   b. Voges-Proskauer test
   c. Citrate test
   d. Indole test
   e. Decarboxylase test

3. The metabolism of glucose to pyruvate by the members of the family Enterobacteriaceae is via Embden-Meyerhof pathway. The subsequent metabolism of pyruvate shows this reaction:

   Glucose → Pyruvate → Acetylmethylcarbinol (acetoin) + Butylene glycol

   This reaction is the basis for:
   a. Oxidase reaction
   b. Methyl red test
   c. Indole test
   d. Voges-Proskauer test
   e. Oxidative/fermentative glucose test

4. An oxidase-negative, gram-negative bacillus that produces an acid slant and acid butt on triple sugar iron agar (TSI) is able to ferment which of the following carbohydrates?
   a. Glucose only
   b. Lactose, glucose, and/or sucrose
   c. Lactose only
   d. Lactose and sucrose, but not glucose
   e. Sucrose only

Continued

LEARNING ASSESSMENT—cont'd

5. A patient who had just returned from Mexico was admitted to the hospital with a 3-day history of vomiting and diarrhea, no fever, and no fecal leukocytes. On admission, a stool culture grew an organism that was identified as an *Escherichia coli.*
   Which of the following strains may be suspected?
   a. Enteropathogenic *E. coli*
   b. Enterotoxigenic *E. coli*
   c. Enterohemorrhagic *E. coli*
   d. Enteroinvasive *E. coli*

6. A gram-negative, oxidase-negative coccobacillus was isolated from the cerebrospinal fluid from an infant in the newborn nursery. The organism produced dark pink colonies on MacConkey's agar and gave the following biochemical results:
   TSI:A/A Gas$^+$H$_2$S$^-$ PAD: negative
   SIM: $=++$ LIA: P/P
   Urease: negative   Citrate: negative
   The most probable identity of this organism is:
   a. *Escherichia coli*
   b. *Enterobacter aerogenes*
   c. *Klebsiella pneumoniae*
   d. *Serratia marcescens*

7. An organism often associated with lobar pneumonia in elderly hospitalized patients
   a. *Klebsiella pneumoniae*
   b. *Escherichia coli*
   c. *Proteus vulgaris*
   d. *Shigella* species
   e. *Citrobacter freundii*

Continued

LEARNING ASSESSMENT—cont'd

8. The most common cause of urinary tract infections in the community
   a. *Klebsiella pneumoniae*
   b. *Escherichia coli*
   c. *Proteus vulgaris*
   d. *Shigella* species
   e. *Citrobacter freundii*

9. An opportunistic pathogen, this organism causes urinary tract and wound infections; may cause the production of kidney stones
   a. *Klebsiella pneumoniae*
   b. *Escherichia coli*
   c. *Proteus vulgaris*
   d. *Shigella* species
   e. *Citrobacter freundii*

10. Acquired by eating improperly cooked or preserved contaminated food, this enteric organism produces dysentery in affected individuals
    a. *Klebsiella pneumoniae*
    b. *Escherichia coli*
    c. *Proteus vulgaris*
    d. *Shigella* species
    e. *Citrobacter freundii*

CHAPTER 17

Vibrio, Aeromonas, Plesiomonas, and Campylobacter Species

Amy M. Carnahan, Gerald Andrews

VIBRIO
  General Characteristics
    Microscopic morphology
    Physiology
    Antigenic structure
    Clinical disease spectrum
  Vibrio cholerae
    Epidemiology
    Clinical infection
  Vibrio parahaemolyticus
    Epidemiology
    Clinical infection
  Vibrio vulnificus
    Epidemiology
    Clinical infection
  Vibrio alginolyticus
  Laboratory Diagnosis
    Specimen collection and transport
    Culture media
    Presumptive identification
    Definitive identification
  Antimicrobial Susceptibility

AEROMONAS
  General Characteristics
    Antigenic structure
  Clinical Infection
    Gastroenteritis
    Wound infection
    Septicemia
    Miscellaneous extraintestinal infections

Laboratory Diagnosis
  Culture media
  Presumptive identification
  Definitive identification
  Antimicrobial Susceptibility

PLESIOMONAS
  Epidemiology
  General Characteristics
    Microscopic morphology
    Antigenic structure
  Clinical Infections
    Gastroenteritis
    Extraintestinal infection
  Laboratory Diagnosis
    Culture media
    Identification
  Antimicrobial Susceptibility

CAMPYLOBACTER AND CAMPYLOBACTER-LIKE
SPECIES
  Epidemiology
    Helicobacter pylori
  General Characteristics
  Clinical Infection
    Helicobacter pylori
  Laboratory Diagnosis
    Specimen collection and transport
    Culture media
    Presumptive identification
    Definitive identification
  Antimicrobial Susceptibility

OBJECTIVES

1. Describe the general characteristics of each of the organisms reviewed in this chapter. Discuss the similarities and differences between each group of organisms.
2. Discuss the various infections associated with each organism and ways the infections are acquired.
3. Describe the microscopic and colonial morphology characteristic of these species.
4. Describe ways to differentiate the bacterial species that cause gastrointestinal illnesses from other diarrheal agents.
5. Describe the appropriate specimen collection, transport, and processing for maximum recovery of each of these organisms.
6. Give the selective media that are appropriate for their recovery.
7. Describe the biochemical tests that will presumptively identify these groups of organisms.
8. Name the confirmatory tests commonly used to identify these isolates.

KEY TERMS

Cholera	Cholera toxin	Kanagawa phenomenon	CAMPY
Vibriostatic	Choleragen	TCBS	Darting motility
O/129 susceptibility	Rice-watery	Microaerophilic	Urea breath test
Halophilic	El Tor	Type B gastritis	

CASE STUDY

A 65-year-old Chinese man, in obvious shock, was examined in the emergency room for a painful swelling of the left hand. His past medical history uncovered bilateral knee joint pain and posthepatic cirrhosis. The day before admission he had pricked his left index finger while selecting shrimp from a fish market. At first he only noticed a local reaction in his finger, but after 12 hours the left hand began to swell accompanied by nausea, vomiting, and diarrhea. The patient was now clammy with a weak pulse, marked swelling, and bullous formation with gangrenous changes apparent on the left hand. A diagnosis of septic shock was made and antibiotic therapy was instituted. Blood and wound cultures subsequently grew an oxidase-positive, gram-negative rod that produced a pink colony on MacConkey agar and green colonies on TCBS agar, and required 3% to 6% NaCl for growth. There was no acceptable identification with any rapid identification system, and final identification was made with conventional biochemicals supplemented with 1% NaCl. The patient suffered a cardiac arrest and died 11 hours after admission.

This chapter covers agents of diarrheal diseases and other infections caused by species of *Vibrio*, *Aeromonas*, *Plesiomonas*, and *Campylobacter*. *Helicobacter pylori*, a newly recognized agent, also is discussed.

VIBRIO

The genus *Vibrio* resides in the family Vibrionaceae and encompasses more than 30 species, although to date only 12 of these species have been implicated in human infections. These microorganisms commonly are found in a wide variety of aquatic environments, including fresh water, brackish or estuarine water, and marine or salt water. Pandemics (worldwide epidemics) of cholera, a devastating diarrheal disease caused by *Vibrio cholerae,* have been documented since 1817, and we are currently in the midst of the seventh such pandemic. An eighth **cholera** epidemic due to a new serogroup, O139, has recently emerged in India and is rapidly spreading. We also have witnessed a general increase in the number of reported cases of *Vibrio* infections caused by other species and originating from both gastrointestinal and extraintestinal sources. The various reasons for this significant rise in the isolation and identification of *Vibrio* clinical isolates include the following:

- Increased travel to either coastal or choleraendemic areas
- Increased consumption of seafood (particularly uncooked)
- Increased use of recreational water facilities, which encourages aquatic exposure
- Larger populations of immunocompromised individuals
- Increased awareness of the existence and significance of these organisms in the clinical microbiology laboratory

General Characteristics

Microscopic morphology

Vibrio species are facultatively anaerobic, asporogenous, gram-negative rods that measure approximately 0.5 µm by 1.5 to 3.0 µm. These organisms possess polar, sheathed flagella when grown in broth, but they can produce peritrichous, unsheathed flagella when grown on solid media. They have been described classically as "curved" gram-negative rods, but this morphology is often seen only in the initial Gram stain of the clinical specimen (Figure 17-1, *A* and *B*). Vibrios usually appear as small, straight gram-negative rods, but they can be highly pleomorphic, especially under suboptimal growth conditions.

Physiology

All 12 clinically significant species are oxidase-positive and able to reduce nitrate to nitrite, except for *Vibrio metschnikovii*. All species generally have the **vibriostatic** compound **O/129 susceptibility** (2, 4-diamino-6, 7-diisopropylpteridine), exhibiting a zone of inhibition to a 150-µg Vibriostat disk (Oxoid, USA) on either a Mueller-Hinton or trypticase soy agar (Figure 17-2). Most vibrios also exhibit a positive string test observed as a mucoid "stringing" reaction after emulsification of colonies in 0.5% sodium desoxycholate.

All species, except for *V. cholerae* and *Vibrio mimicus,* are **halophilic,** or salt-loving, and require the addition of Na^+ for their growth and accurate identification. Vibrios can be differentiated from the closely related genera *Aeromonas* and *Plesiomonas* by means of these key biochemical and growth requirement characteristics, as shown in Table 17-1.

Antigenic structure

Very little is known about the antigenic structure of *Vibrio* species, except for *V. cholerae, Vibrio parahaemolyticus,* and some limited work on *Vibrio fluvialis* and *Vibrio vulnificus*. All strains of *V. cholerae* share a common flagellar (H) antigen. The cholera vibrios are further divided into six serogroups on the basis of their somatic (O) antigen. Strains of *V. cholerae* that agglutinate in O1 antisera are associated with epidemic cholera. Within the *V. cholerae* serogroup are three subtypes: Ogawa (A, B), Inaba (A, C), and Hikojima (A, B, C). Those

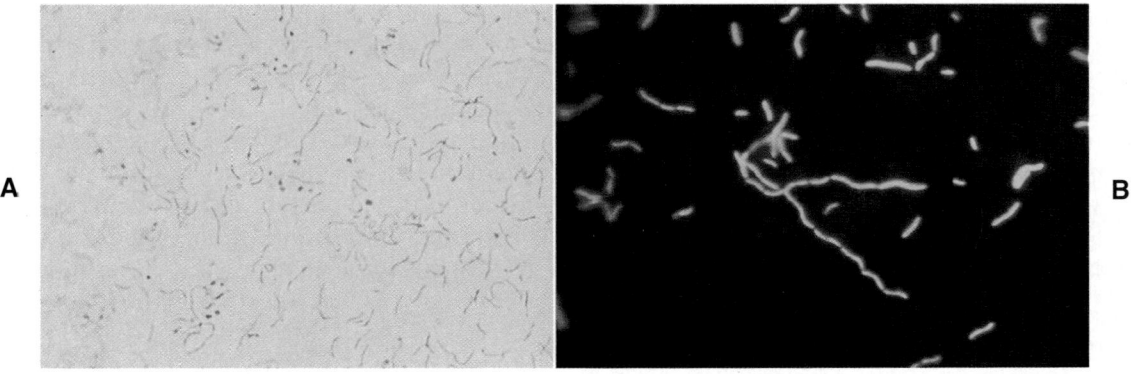

Figure 17-1

A, Microscopic morphology of *Vibrio* sp. on Gram-stained smear. (Courtesy J. Michael Janda.) **B,** Acridine orange stain of *Vibrio cholerae.* (Courtesy Rita R. Colwell.)

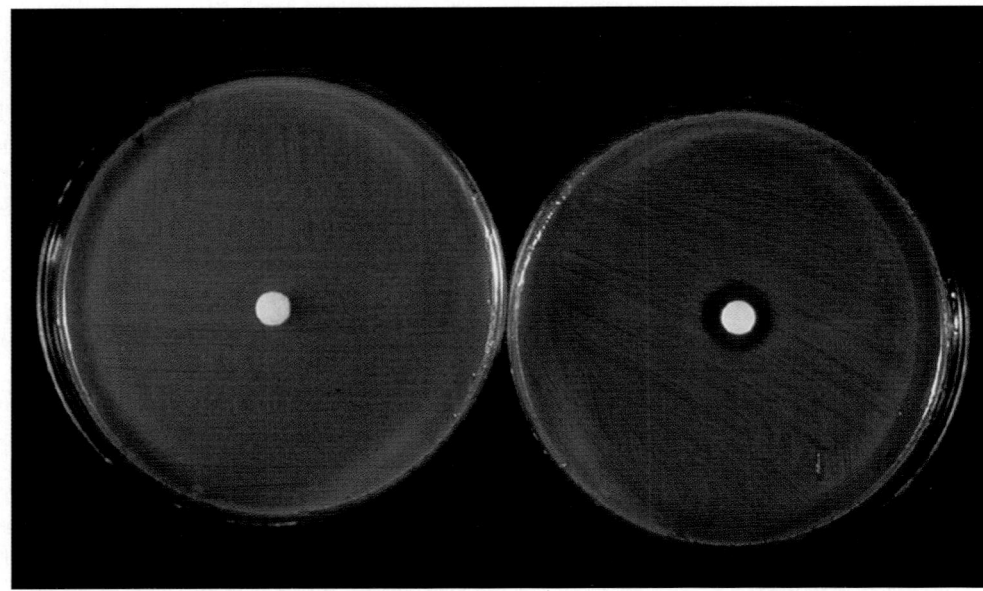

Figure 17-2

O/129 Susceptibility test for *Vibrio* sp. Resistant *(left)*. Susceptible *(right)*.

strains that phenotypically resemble *V. cholerae* but fail to agglutinate in O1 antisera are referred to as non-O1 *V. cholerae* strains.

The species of *V. parahaemolyticus* also can be serotyped by means of its O (somatic) and K (cap-

TABLE 17-1

Salient Features for the Identification of Vibrio, Aeromonas, *and* Plesiomonas

	Vibrio	*Aeromonas*	*Plesiomonas*
Gram reaction	−	−	−
Oxidase activity	+	+	+
Resistance to O/129*			
10 μg	+/−	+	+/−
150 μg	−	+	−
Growth in nutrient			
broth with:			
0% NaCl	−/+	+	+
6.5% NaCl	+	−	−
Acid from:			
Glucose	+	+	+
Inositol	−	−	+
Mannitol	+	+/−	−
Sucrose	+/−	+/−	−
Gelatin liquefaction	+	+	−

Courtesy Carnahan AM: Update on *Aeromonas* identification, *Clin Microbiol Newsl* 13(22):169, 1991.
+, Most strains positive; −, most strains negative; +/− or −/+, predominant reaction first.
*Vibriostatic agent (2, 4-diamino-6, 7-diisopropylpteridine)

sule) antigens, but this generally is used only in outbreaks or large epidemiologic studies conducted by reference laboratories.

Clinical disease spectrum

Vibrio species can originate from a number of clinical sources, and most species have been implicated in more than one disease process, ranging from mild gastroenteritis to cholera and from simple wound infections to fatal septicemia. Table 17-2 shows the various clinical infections associated with *Vibrio* species. The four major *Vibrio* species likely to be encountered in the clinical laboratory are *V. cholerae* (O1 and non-O1), *V. parahaemolyticus*, *V. vulnificus*, and *Vibrio alginolyticus*.

Because most laboratories, except those in coastal areas, have a fairly low frequency of isolation of *Vibrio* species, a good medical history is extremely important. Often the best indication of a possible *Vibrio* infection is the presence of certain recognized factors, such as the following:

- Recent consumption of raw seafood (especially oysters)
- Recent immigration or foreign travel
- Gastroenteritis with cholera-like or rice-water stools

TABLE 17-2

Clinical Infections Associated with Vibrios

Species	Clinical Infection	Frequency
Vibrio cholerae O1	Cholera, gastroenteritis, wound infections, bacteremia	Common
V. cholerae O139	Cholera	Relatively common
V. cholerae non-O1	Gastroenteritis, septicemia, ear infections	Relatively common
Vibrio parahaemolyticus	Gastroenteritis, wound infections	Common
Vibrio vulnificus	Septicemia, wound infections	Common
Vibrio alginolyticus	Wound infections, ear infections, conjunctivitis, respiratory infections, bacteremia	Common
Vibrio mimicus	Gastroenteritis, ear infections	Uncommon
Vibrio damsela	Wound infections	Uncommon
Vibrio fluvialis	Gastroenteritis	Uncommon
Vibrio furnissii	Gastroenteritis	Uncommon
Vibrio hollisae	Gastroenteritis	Uncommon
Vibrio cincinnatiensis	Meningitis	Rare
Vibrio metschnikovii	Septicemia, peritonitis	Rare
Vibrio carchariae	Wound infections	Rare

From Bottone EJ, Janda JM: *Vibrio.* In Howard B et al, editors: *Clinical and pathogenic microbiology,* ed 1, St Louis, 1987, Mosby.

- Accidental trauma incurred during contact with fresh or marine water or associated products (e.g., shellfish, hooks)

Vibrio cholerae

Epidemiology

V. cholerae O1 is the causative agent of cholera, also known as *Asiatic cholera* or *epidemic cholera.* It has been a disease of major public health significance for centuries. Most epidemics occur in developing countries, where it is endemic; in particular, cholera is prevalent in the Bengal region of India and Bangladesh. However, there has been a fairly recent increase in the number of cases of cholera in the United States, particularly off the Gulf Coast, as well as in South America.

Clinical infection

Cholera is an acute diarrheal disease that is spread mainly through contaminated water. However, improperly preserved and handled foods, including fish and seafood, milk, ice cream, and unpreserved meat, have been responsible for outbreaks. The disease manifests in acute cases as a severe gastroenteritis, accompanied by vomiting and followed by diarrhea. The stools produced by cholera patients are described as "rice-water" and the number of stools, which are watery and contain numerous flecks of mucus, may be as many as 10 to 30 per day. If left untreated, cholera can result in such a rapid fluid and electrolyte loss that it leads to dehydration, hypovolemic shock, metabolic acidosis, and death in a matter of hours.

This devastating clinical scenario is the result of a powerful enterotoxin known as **cholera toxin** or **choleragen.** Once ingested, the cholera organisms colonize the small intestine, where they multiply and produce choleragen. The toxin consists of two toxic A subunits and five multiple binding B subunits. There is an initial binding to the GM_1-ganglioside receptor on the cell membrane through the B subunits. Then the A2 subunit facilitates the entrance of the A1 subunit. Once inside the cell, the active A1 subunit stimulates the production of adenylate cyclase through the inactivation of the G protein. This leads to an accumulation of cyclic adenosine monophosphate (cAMP) along the cell membrane, which stimulates a hypersecretion of electrolytes (NA^+, K^+, HCO_3^-) and water out of the cell and into the lumen of the intestine, as shown in Figure 17-3. The net effect is that the gastrointestinal tract's absorptive ability is overwhelmed, resulting in the massive outpouring of **rice-watery** stools.

Treatment and management of cholera are best accomplished by the administration of copious amounts of intravenous or oral fluids to replace those fluids lost. The administration of antibiotics can shorten the duration of diarrhea and thereby reduce fluid losses.

Epidemic *V. cholerae* O1 strains occur in two biogroups: classic and El Tor. El Tor has been the

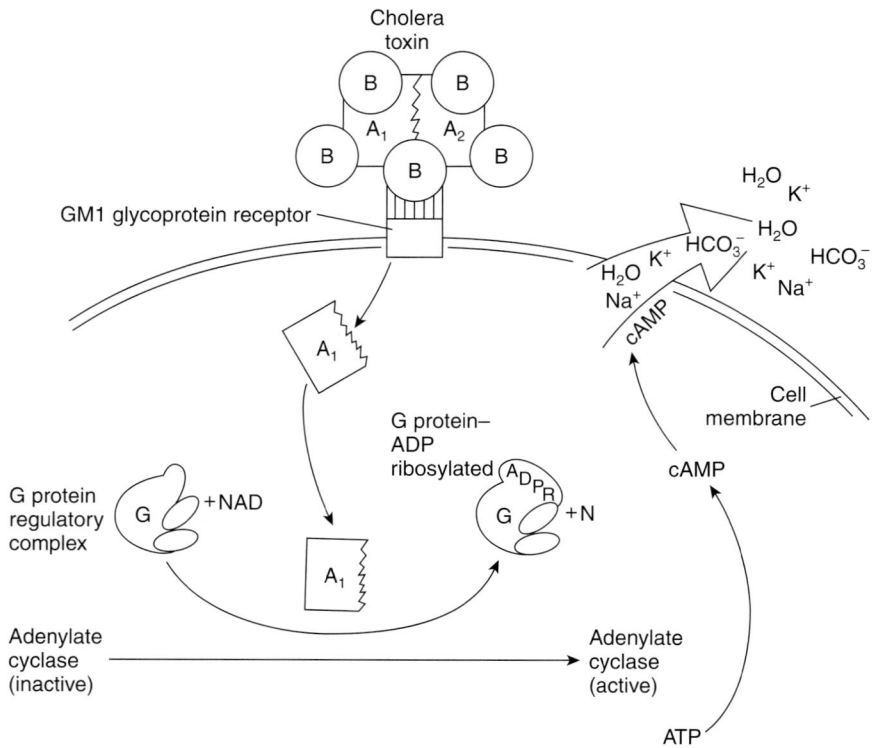

Figure 17-3

The action of cholera toxin. The complete toxin is shown binding to the GM_1-ganglioside receptor on the cell membrane through the binding (B) subunits. The active portion (A_1) of the A subunit enters the cell and inactivates the G protein by ADP-ribosylation. Because the G protein acts to return adenylate cyclase form its active to inactive form, the net effect is persistent activation of adenylate cyclase. The increased adenylate cyclase activity results in accumulation of cyclic adenosine 3' 5'-monophosphate (cAMP) along the cell membrane. The cAMP causes the active secretion of sodium (Na^+), chloride (Cl^-), potassium (K^+), bicarbonate (HCO_3^-), and water out of the cell into the intestinal lumen. (Courtesy Ryan KJ: *Vibrio* and *Campylobacter.* In Sherris J, editor: *Medical microbiology: an introduction to infectious diseases,* ed 2, New York, 1990, Elsevier Science.)

predominant biogroup in the last two pandemics. Recent studies in Bangladesh, however, indicate a rapidly occurring reemergence of the classic biogroup. The **El Tor** biogroup differs from the classic in that El Tor is Voges-Proskauer–positive, hemolyzes erythrocytes, is inhibited by polymyxin B (50 µg), and is able to agglutinate chicken red blood cells. The two biogroups also have different phage susceptibility patterns.

There have been a number of cases of *Vibrio* infections reported involving other serogroups, such as *V. cholerae* non-O1. These strains are phenotypically similar to toxigenic *V. cholerae* O1, but most lack the cholerae toxin gene and appear to cause a milder form of gastroenteritis or cholera-like disease. These non-O1 strains also have been implicated in a variety of extraintestinal infections, including cholecystitis, ear infections, cellulitis, and septicemia.

The emergence of a new *V. cholerae* serogroup O139, originating in Madras, India, in 1992, has led to a widespread occurrence of cholera cases throughout India and Bangladesh. Some of these strains share cross-reacting antigens with *Aeromonas trota.*

Vibrio parahaemolyticus
Epidemiology

V. parahaemolyticus is the second most common *Vibrio* species implicated in gastroenteritis. It was first recognized as a pathogen in Japan in 1950, when it was the culprit in a large food-poisoning outbreak; even today, it is the number-one cause of "summer diarrhea" in Japan. It also has been isolated in Europe, the Baltic area, Australia, Africa, Canada, and nearly every coastal state in the United States. Like other vibrios, *V. parahaemolyticus* is found in aquatic environments, but it appears to be limited to coastal or estuarine areas, despite a halophilic requirement of 1% to 8% NaCl. *V. parahaemolyticus* has a definite association with at least 30 different marine species, including oysters, clams, crabs, lobsters, scallops, sardines, and shrimp. Hence, most cases of gastroenteritis can be traced to recent consumption of raw, improperly cooked, or recontaminated seafood, particularly oysters.

Clinical infection

The gastrointestinal disease caused by *V. parahaemolyticus* is generally self-limited. Patients have watery diarrhea, moderate cramps or vomiting, and little if any fever. Symptoms begin approximately 24 to 48 hours after ingestion of contaminated seafood.

V. parahaemolyticus has occasionally been isolated from extraintestinal sources, such as wounds, and ear and eye infections, and even in a case of pneumonia. Invariably, the patient has a history of recent aquatic exposure or a water-associated traumatic injury to the infected site.

The pathogenesis of *V. parahaemolyticus* is not as clear-cut as in the case of *V. cholerae* and the production of choleragen. However, there is a possible association between hemolysin production and virulence potential, known as the **Kanagawa phenomenon**. It has been observed that most clinical *V. parahaemolyticus* strains produce a heat-stable hemolysin that is able to lyse human erythrocytes in a special high-salt mannitol medium (Wagatsuma agar). These strains are considered to be Kanagawa-positive, whereas most environmental isolates are Kanagawa-negative. There are exceptions to both these observations, however, and the exact role of this hemolysin in pathogenesis of the disease is still not understood. It also is important to note the recent emergence of atypical urease-positive *V. parahaemolyticus* strains from clinical sources along the Pacific coast of North America.

Vibrio vulnificus

After cholera, the second most serious type of *Vibrio*-associated infections are those caused by *V. vulnificus*.

Epidemiology

This vibrio species can be found in marine environments on the Atlantic, Gulf, and Pacific coasts of North America. Until 1976, *V. vulnificus* was commonly referred to as the "lactose-positive" *Vibrio*.

Clinical infection

Infections caused by *V. vulnificus* generally fall into two categories: primary septicemia and wound infections. The former is surmised to occur through a gastrointestinal route following the consumption of shellfish, especially raw oysters. Those patients with liver dysfunction and syndromes that result in increased serum levels of iron (e.g., hemochromatosis, cirrhosis, thalassemia major, hepatitis) are particularly predisposed to this scenario. Within hours, septicemia can develop, with a mortality rate of 40% to 60%. Those patients with wound infections with *V. vulnificus* invariably have a history of some type of traumatic aquatic wound that often presents as a cellulitis. The majority of such patients usually are not immunocompromised, have experienced a mild to severe injury to the infected site, and do not live in a coastal area.

Vibrio alginolyticus

Of the four major *Vibrio* species likely to be encountered in the clinical laboratory, *V. alginolyticus* is the least pathogenic for humans and most infrequently isolated. It is a common inhabitant of marine environments and a strict halophile, requiring at least 3% NaCl and able to tolerate up to 10% NaCl. Nearly all isolates originate from extraintestinal sources, such as eye and ear infections or wound and burn infections, and the organism may be an occupational hazard for people in constant contact with seawater, such as fishermen or sailors.

Laboratory Diagnosis
Specimen collection and transport

Vibrios do not have any fastidious growth requirements, and there are only a few special collection and processing procedures necessary to

TABLE 17-3

Reactions in Eight Key Differential Tests to Divide the 12 Clinically Significant Vibrio *Species into Six Groups*

Test	Group 1		Group 2	Group 3	Group 4
	Vibrio cholerae	*Vibrio mimicus*	*Vibrio metsch-nikovii*	*Vibrio cincin-natiensis*	*Vibrio hollisae*
Growth in nutrient broth:					
With no NaCl added	+	+	−	−	−
With 1% NaCl added	+	+	+	+	+
Oxidase			−	+	+
Nitrate → nitrite			−	+	+
myo-Inositol fermentation	−	−	−	+	−
Arginine dihydrolase					−
Lysine decarboxylase					−
Ornithine decarboxylase					−

Courtesy Kelly MT, Hickman-Brenner FW, Farmer JJ III: *Vibrio.* In Balows A et al, editors: *Manual of clinical microbiology,* ed 5, Washington, DC, 1991, American Society for Clinical Microbiology.Key test results are boxed.
Key test results are boxed.

ensure the recovery of vibrios from clinical material. Whenever possible, body fluids, pus, or tissues should be submitted, but swabs are acceptable if they are transported in an appropriate holding medium, such as Cary-Blair, to prevent desiccation. Buffered glycerol saline is not recommended as a transport or holding medium, because the glycerol is toxic for vibrios. Even strips of blotting paper soaked in liquid stool and placed in airtight plastic bags are considered viable specimens for up to 5 weeks. Stool specimens should be collected as early as possible in the course of the illness, before the administration of any antimicrobial agents, and plated as quickly as possible.

Culture media

The salt concentration (0.5%) in most commonly used laboratory media, such as nutrient agar or blood agar, is sufficient to support the growth of any vibrios present. On blood-containing agars, such as sheep's blood or chocolate agar, vibrios produce medium to large colonies that appear smooth, opaque, and iridescent with a greenish hue. The sheep's blood agar plate should also be examined for the presence of β, α, or γ hemolysis. On MacConkey agar, the pathogenic vibrios usually grow as non–lactose-fermenters. However, lactose-fermenting species such as *V. vulnificus* may be overlooked and incorrectly considered to be members of the Enterobacteriaceae, such as *Escherichia*

coli. It therefore is imperative to determine the oxidase activity of any suspicious *Vibrio*-like colonies. This can be accomplished by either directly testing colonies from sheep's blood or chocolate agar plates with fresh oxidase reagent or subculturing any suspicious lactose-fermenting colonies on MacConkey to a fresh sheep's blood agar plate for next-day testing. This is necessary because lactose-positive colonies from selective-differential media such as MacConkey or CIN (cefsulodin-irgasin-novobiocin) agar may give false-negative oxidase reactions.

If a selective medium is warranted, either because of the clinical history (exposure to seafood or seawater) or for geographic reasons (coastal area resident or recent foreign travel), **TCBS** (thiosulfate citrate bile salts sucrose) agar is the most available and widely used selective medium. It differentiates sucrose-fermenting (yellow) species (Figure 17-4) such as *V. cholerae, V. alginolyticus, V. fluvialis, Vibrio furnissii, Vibrio cincinnatiensis, V. metschnikovii, Vibrio carchariae,* and some *V. vulnificus* from the non–sucrose-fermenting (green) vibrios, that is *V. mimicus, V. parahaemolyticus, Vibrio damsela,* and most *V. vulnificus.* Although TCBS generally inhibits all other organisms, it should be monitored with stringent quality-control measures, as there is great variation in performance from lot to lot, and not all *Vibrio* species grow on TCBS. If an enrichment procedure is desired to enhance isolation

	Group 5			Group 6		
Vibrio damsela	Vibrio fluvialis	Vibrio furnissii	Vibrio alginolyticus	Vibrio parahae-molyticus	Vibrio vulnificus	Vibrio carchariae
−	−	−	−	−	−	−
+	+	+	+	+	+	+
+	+	+	+	+	+	+
+	+	+	+	+	+	+
−	−	−	−	−	−	−
+	+	+	−	−	−	−
			+	+	+	+

of vibrios, alkaline peptone water with 1% NaCl (pH 8.5) can be inoculated (at least 20 mL volume) and incubated for 5 to 8 hours at 35° C before subculturing to TCBS.

Presumptive identification

There are several key tests that can aid in the initial identification of a *Vibrio* isolate. Vibrios can be easily confused with other genera, including *Aeromonas, Plesiomonas,* Enterobacteriaceae, and even *Pseudomonas.* Their general susceptibility to the vibriostatic agent O/129 (150 μg) distinguishes them from *Aeromonas.* Inability to ferment inositol (except for *V. cincinnatiensis*) separates them from *Plesiomonas;* positive oxidase activity sepa-

rates them from the Enterobacteriaceae; and a fermentative metabolism separates them from the oxidative *Pseudomonas* (see Table 17-1).

Definitive identification

After the presumptive identification of *Vibrio,* a number of useful biochemical tests aid in identifying the majority of clinical isolates to the species level. Kelly and colleagues recently outlined eight key differential tests to divide the 12 clinically significant *Vibrio* species into six groups as an initial identification step (Table 17-3). Some of the additional tests necessary to identify the four major clinical *Vibrio* species are summarized in Table 17-4. However, it is important to note that with the halophilic or salt-

TABLE 17-4

Differentiation of the Four Major Clinical Vibrio *Species*

Test or Property	Reaction				
	Vibrio cholerae (Classical)	Vibrio cholerae (El Tor)	Vibrio parahaemolyticus	Vibrio vulnificus	Vibrio alginolyticus
Growth in nutrient broth with:					
0% added NaCl	+	+	−	−	−
3% NaCl	+	+	+	+	+
6% NaCl	−	−	+	+	+
8% NaCl	−	−	+	−	+
10% NaCl	−	−	−	−	+
Sucrose fermentation	+	+	−	−	+
Lactose fermentation	−	−	−	+	−
Voges-Proskauer	−	+	−	−	+

+, Most strains positive; −, most strains negative.

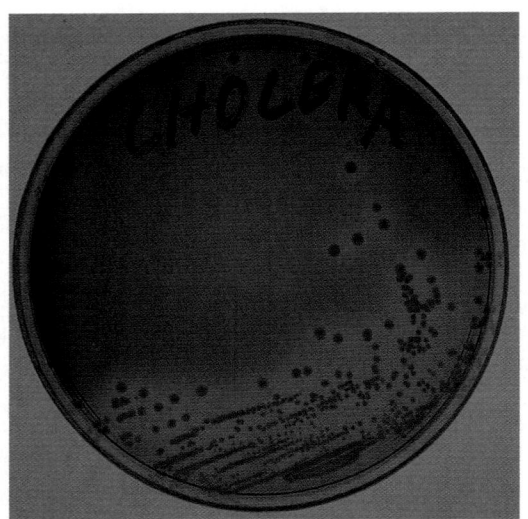

Figure 17-4 ——————————————————————
Vibrio cholerae on TCBS agar.

loving vibrios, it often is necessary to add at least 1% NaCl to most biochemical media to obtain reliable reaction results.

RAPID OR SEMIAUTOMATED IDENTIFICATION SYSTEMS
Although these systems contain databases of the more commonly encountered clinical vibrios, they generally are inadequate for the accurate identification of these species, particularly the less common species. In particular, their inoculating suspensions should contain at least 0.85% NaCl, such as that found with the API-20E identification strips (bioMerieux Vitek, Hazelwood, Mo). Even then, the halophilic vibrios may grow poorly if at all, and they often are confused with other genera, such as *Aeromonas*. Most authors advocate identification with conventional biochemicals, supplemented with additional NaCl where warranted; alternatively, the rapid-system identification should be confirmed at the reference laboratory level.

SEROLOGY
It generally is considered sufficient for most clinical laboratories below the level of reference laboratory to simply screen their presumptive *V. cholerae* isolates with commercially available polyvalent O1 antiserum. However, there have been reports of non-O1 *V. cholerae* misidentified as *V. cholerae* O1 and vice versa. In any case, all isolates with a presumptive identification of *V. cholerae* should be promptly reported to the appropriate public health authorities, and the isolate should be forwarded to the health department and/or a reference laboratory for typing with both O1 and O139 antisera and cholera toxin testing, if warranted.

Antimicrobial Susceptibility

Fortunately, both Mueller-Hinton agar and broth contain sufficient salt to support the growth of the *Vibrio* species most often isolated from clinical specimens. The recommended methods to be employed are standardized disk diffusion (Bauer-Kirby) or dilution susceptibility testing methods.

In general, most strains of *V. cholerae* are susceptible to tetracycline, gentamicin, chloramphenicol, and nalidixic acid, with tetracycline being the drug of choice. Increased resistance from the acquisition of plasmids is relatively uncommon in the United States, but there are reports of multiple resistant strains from both Asia and Africa.

AEROMONAS

The genus *Aeromonas* consists of ubiquitous oxidase-positive, glucose-fermenting, gram-negative rods that are widely distributed in freshwater, estuarine, and marine environments worldwide. They frequently are isolated from retail produce sources and animal meat products. Aeromonads are responsible for a diverse spectrum of disease syndromes among a variety of warm and cold-blooded animals, including fish, reptiles, amphibia, mammals, and humans.

Until recently, they resided in the family Vibrionaceae. However, phylogenetic evidence from molecular studies resulted in the proposal of a separate family Aeromonadaceae. There are currently 13 proposed species of *Aeromonas*, but only seven species or biovars have been isolated with any frequency from clinical specimens.

General Characteristics

Aeromonads are straight, not curved, rods (1.1 to 4.4 μm by 0.4 to 1.0 μm), and most are motile by means of a single polar flagellum. To date, two species, *Aeromonas salmonicida* and *Aeromonas media*, are generally considered nonmotile and not pathogenic for humans. The range of temperature for growth of all aeromonads is from 0° C to 42° C, with a seasonal pattern of increased isolation from

May through October. Most clinical mesophilic strains can be cultured from 4° C to 42° C, and the psychrophilic fish pathogen *A. salmonicida* usually grows only below 37° C.

Antigenic structure

There are currently two serotyping systems developed for mesophilic aeromonads based on the somatic O antigens. The first serotyping schema was developed by Sakasaki and Shimada and established 45 groups among the mesophilic species. A later study by Cheasty et al established 10 additional serogroups, but at present, serotyping is recommended only at the reference laboratory level for epidemiologic purposes.

Clinical Infection
Gastroenteritis

Although aeromonads have been epidemiologically implicated as causative agents of enteric disease since the 1960s, they still are not firmly established as enteric pathogens. Despite numerous case-control studies and case reports, we still are awaiting a successful human volunteer trial. Nevertheless, there are sufficient clinical associations to warrant the screening of stool specimens for the presence of aeromonads, followed by further identification to the level of species. The medical history of patients displaying diarrhea and harboring aeromonads often, but not always, involves aquatic exposure, such as an association with untreated well water or consumption of seafood, particularly raw oysters or clams.

There are currently five diarrheal presentations observed in patients in whom *Aeromonas* has been isolated from their stools, as follows:

1. An acute, secretory diarrhea often accompanied by vomiting
2. An acute, dysenteric form of diarrhea with blood and mucus
3. A chronic diarrhea usually lasting more than 10 days
4. A choleraic type including rice-water stools
5. The nebulous syndrome commonly referred to as "traveler's diarrhea"

Most cases are self-limiting, but in the pediatric and geriatric populations, supportive therapy and antimicrobials are often indicated.

The species *Aeromonas hydrophila*, *Aeromonas veronii* (biovars sobria and veronii), and *A. trota* are most strongly associated with cases of gastroenteritis to date, with a possible pathogenic role for *Aeromonas caviae* among pediatric patients.

Wound infection

This is the second most common type of *Aeromonas* infection. It invariably involves a recent traumatic aquatic exposure and generally occurs on the extremities. The most common presentation is cellulitis, although there are a few instances of myonecrosis with or without gas gangrene, and even a rare case of ecthyma gangrenosum associated with sepsis. Most aeromonad wound isolates are *A. hydrophila*, *A. veronii* biovar veronii, or *Aeromonas schubertii*. The latter species has been isolated almost exclusively from aquatic wound infections and blood.

The most interesting association between aeromonads and wound infections involves the species *A. hydrophila* and the use of leeches for medicinal therapy following plastic surgery. These patients end up with serious aeromonad wound infections following the use of leech therapy to relieve venous congestion. It appears that the leech *Hirudo medicinalis* has a symbiotic relationship with the aeromonads within its gut, where the organisms aid in the enzymatic digestion of the blood ingested by the leech.

Septicemia

Aeromonad sepsis appears to be the most invasive type of *Aeromonas* infection and has a strong association with the species *A. veronii* biovar sobria (formerly identified as *Aeromonas sobria* in clinical isolates). Such patients are most likely to be immunocompromised, with a history of liver disease or dysfunction, hematologic malignancies, hepatobiliary disorders, or traumatic injuries. Also at high risk are individuals diagnosed with leukemia, lymphoma, or myeloma. Although the original source of infection has not been elucidated, it is surmised that it is the gastrointestinal tract, in the biliary tract, or, even more rarely, in the respiratory tract.

Miscellaneous extraintestinal infections

Aeromonads have also been implicated in cases of osteomyelitis, meningitis, pelvic abscesses, otitis, cystitis, endocarditis, peritonitis, cholecystitis, and endophthalmitis in both healthy and immunocompromised individuals.

Laboratory Diagnosis
Culture media
Aeromonads grow quite readily on most media used for both routine cultures and stool cultures. After 24-hour incubation at 35° to 37° C, aeromonads appear as large round, raised, opaque colonies with an entire edge and a smooth, often mucoid surface. Often, an extremely strong odor is present, and pigmentation ranges from translucent and white to buff in color. Hemolysis is variable on blood agar media, with most species displaying β hemolysis. Although aeromonads grow on nearly all enteric media, they often are overlooked on MacConkey agar because a large number of aeromonads ferment lactose. A study by Kelly and colleagues of several media suggests the combined use of ampicillin blood agar and a modified CIN agar may yield the highest recovery of aeromonads. However, the incorporation of ampicillin in the blood agar may inhibit some A. caviae strains as well as the newly proposed species, A. trota, whose hallmark is susceptibility to ampicillin. The use of an enrichment broth generally is not considered necessary. However, if such a medium is warranted for detecting chronic cases or asymptomatic carriers, alkaline peptone water is recommended. This can be inoculated, incubated overnight, and subsequently subcultured to plate media.

Presumptive identification
Because the genera Aeromonas, Plesiomonas, and Vibrio are so closely related, it is necessary to first determine that an isolate is indeed an aeromonad (see Table 17-1). The simplest way of screening for aeromonads is to perform a test for oxidase activity on growth from a blood agar plate. This distinguishes aeromonads from Enterobacteriaceae. Other advantages to the use of a blood agar medium are the simultaneous ability to test for indole production and observe for any hemolysis. The presence and type of hemolysis often are the only clues to an infection involving more than one species of Aeromonas. To distinguish the aeromonads from Vibrio and Plesiomonas, testing for sensitivity to the vibrio-static agent O/129 is recommended in lieu of a salt tolerance, since V. cholerae and V. mimicus grow quite well without additional salt. Finally, the ability to ferment glucose distinguishes Aeromonas from Pseudomonas.

Definitive identification
Definitive identification is accomplished with a small number of biochemical tests and antimicrobial markers using a dichotomous key, Aerokey II (Figure 17-5). When used in conjunction with the additional tests from Table 17-5, the clinical microbiologist should be able to identify nearly all Aeromonas isolates to the level of species. However, it should be noted that the esculin hydrolysis test requires an agar-based medium, not a broth. Any antimicrobial resistance markers and susceptibility studies should be determined by the standard Bauer-Kirby method, because of possible discrepancies in β-lactamase detection by rapid minimal inhibitory concentration (MIC) methods.

RAPID OR SEMIAUTOMATED IDENTIFICATION SYSTEMS
Although these systems can identify an isolate as belonging to the A. hydrophila or A. hydrophila complex, the majority are currently inadequate for identification to the proper species level. This is due to a lack of sufficient discriminatory markers to detect interspecies differences, as well as poor correlation between conventional test results and rapid or miniaturized versions, specifically esculin hydrolysis, decarboxylase reactions, and sugar fermentation.

The presence of species-related disease syndromes (e.g., A hydrophila and A. schubertii from aquatic wounds, A. veronii biovar sobria from septicemia, A. caviae from pediatric diarrhea, and A. hydrophila from medicinal leech therapy cases), coupled with differences in antimicrobial susceptibilities among the species, strongly suggests that conventional identification and antimicrobial susceptibilities should be performed on clinical aeromonad isolates.

Antimicrobial Susceptibility
Although most cases of Aeromonas-associated gastroenteritis are self-limited, antimicrobial therapy often is indicated. It always is warranted in wound infections and septicemia. As a genus, aeromonads are nearly uniformly resistant to penicillin, ampicillin, carbenicillin, and cephalothin. Exceptions are the susceptibility of A. veronii biovar sobria to cephalothin and the susceptibility of A. trota to ampicillin. Otherwise, aeromonads are generally susceptible to third-generation cephalosporins, trimethoprim-sufamethoxazole, aminoglycosides, chloramphenicol, and quinolones.

TABLE 17-5

Differential Characteristics for Mesophilic Clinical Aeromonas Species

Characteristic	Aeromonas hydrophila	Aeromonas veronii biogroup sobria	Aeromonas veronii biogroup veronii	Aeromonas caviae	Aeromonas schubertii	Aeromonas jandaei	Aeromonas trota
Esculin hydrolysis	+	−	+	+	−	−	−
Voges-Proskauer	+	+	+	−	V+	−	−
Pyrazinamidase activity	+	−	−	+	−	−	−
Arginine dihydrolase	+	+	−	V	+	+	+
Fermentation:							
Arabinose	V	−	−	+	−	−	−
Cellobiose	−	−	+	V	−	−	+
Mannitol	+	+	+	+	−	+	+
Sucrose	+	+	+	+	−	−	−
Susceptibility:							
Ampicillin	R	R	R	R	R	R	S
Carbenicillin	R	R	R	R	R	R	S
Cephalothin	R	S	S	R	S	R	R
Colistin*	V	S	S	S	S	R	S
Decarboxylase:							
Lysine	+	+	+	−	+	+	+
Ornithine	−	−	+	−	−	−	−
Indole	+	+	+	+	−	+	+
H₂S†	+	+	+	−	−	+	+
Glucose (gas)	+	+	+	−	−	+	+
Hemolysis (5% sheep erythrocytes)	+	+	+	V	+	+	V

Courtesy Carnahan AM et al: *Aeromonas trota* sp. nov., an ampicillin-susceptible species isolated from clinical specimens, *J Clin Microbiol* 29(6):1209, 1991.
+, Positive; −, negative; V, variable; R, resistant; S, susceptible.
*MIC single dilution 4 μg/mL.
†H₂S from gelatin-cysteine-thiosulphate media.

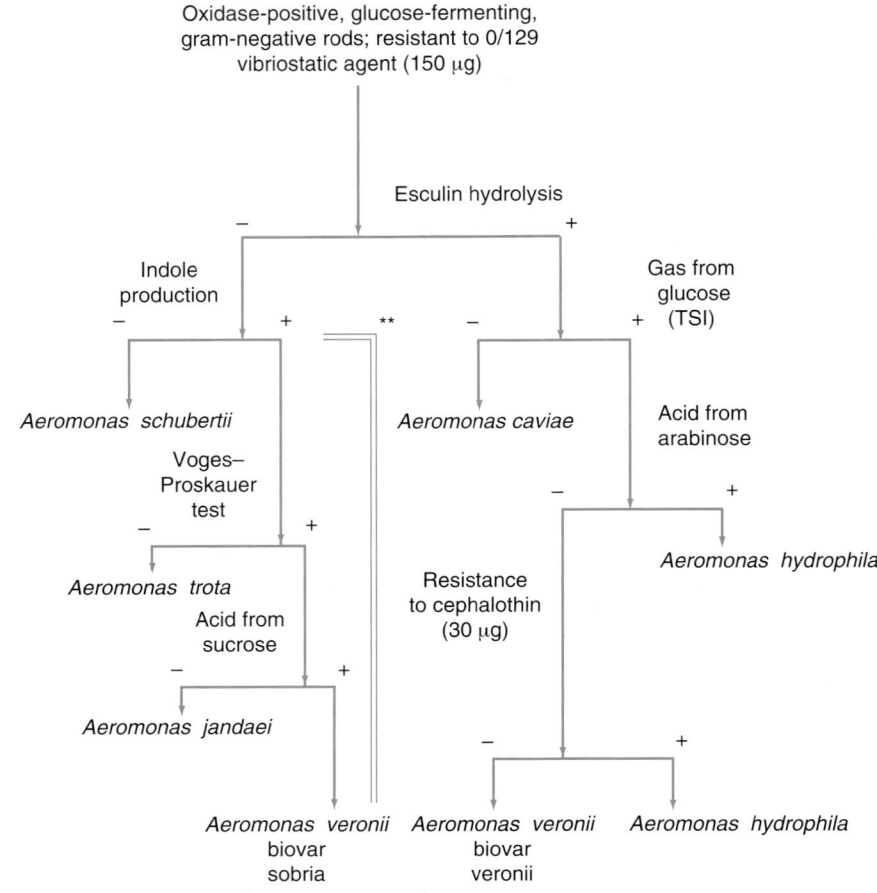

Oxidase-positive, glucose-fermenting,
gram-negative rods; resistant to 0/129
vibriostatic agent (150 μg)

Esculin hydrolysis

Indole
production

Gas from
glucose
(TSI)

Aeromonas schubertii

Aeromonas caviae

Voges–
Proskauer
test

Acid from
arabinose

Aeromonas trota

Aeromonas hydrophila

Acid from
sucrose

Resistance
to cephalothin
(30 μg)

Aeromonas jandaei

Aeromonas veronii
biovar
sobria

Aeromonas veronii
biovar
veronii

Aeromonas hydrophila

** Aerokey II can be modified to end here with an
identification of *A. veronii* biovar sobria

Figure 17-5

Aerokey II—identification key for clinical *Aeronomas* species. (Courtesy Carnahan AM, Behram S, Joseph SW: Aerokey II—a flexible key for identifying clinical *Aeromonas* species, *J Clin Microbiol* 29:2843, 1991.)

PLESIOMONAS

The genus *Plesiomonas* currently resides in the family Vibrionaceae and includes a single species, *Plesiomonas shigelloides*. Like the vibrios and aeromonads, these organisms are oxidase-positive, glucose-fermenting, facultatively anaerobic gram-negative rods that are motile by polar flagella. However, recent phylogenetic studies have presented evidence that the ancestry of *Plesiomonas* is actually closer to the family Enterobacteriaceae, particularly the genus *Proteus,* and it has been proposed that *Plesiomonas* be moved to this genus.

Epidemiology

These microorganisms are found in both soil and aquatic environments, but because of an intolerance to increased NaCl and a minimum growth temperature of 8° C, they are generally found only in the fresh and estuarine waters of tropical and subtropical climates. Like the genus *Aeromonas,* they are widely distributed among both warm- and cold-blooded animals, including dogs, cats, pigs, vultures, snakes, lizards, fish, newts, and shellfish. They have emerged as a potential cause of enteric disease in humans and have also been isolated from a number of extraintestinal infections.

Cases are probably underreported because of the similarity to *E. coli* on most ordinary enteric media. But increased laboratory awareness of the existence of *Plesiomonas,* coupled with the knowledge of previously outlined recreational, immunologic, and gastronomic risk factors, has resulted in a gradual but steady increase in the number of reported cases, mostly in adults.

General Characteristics
Microscopic morphology
Plesiomonads are straight (0.8 to 1 μm by 3 μm) gram-negative rods that occur singly, in pairs, or in short chains or filamentous forms. They do not form spores or capsules and are motile by monotrichous or two to five lophotrichous polar flagella.

Antigenic structure
The genera *Plesiomonas* and *Shigella* share both biochemical and antigenic features, and plesiomonads often cross-agglutinate with *Shigella sonnei, Shigella dysenteriae,* and even *Shigella boydii,* hence the species name *shigelloides.* However, unlike *Shigella, Plesiomonas* appears to possess a much lower virulence potential, with a low symptomatic carriage rate among humans. Plesiomonads can be serotyped by their somatic O antigens (50 groups) and their flagellar H antigens (17 groups), based on a schema by Aldova. Some of the 107 serovars are ubiquitous, and others are confined only to certain regions.

Clinical Infections
Gastroenteritis
Unlike the genus *Aeromonas,* there have been at least two well-documented outbreaks of diarrheal disease in Japan caused by *Plesiomonas.* The most common vehicle of transmission is the ingestion of contaminated water or food, particularly uncooked seafood such as oysters or shrimp. However, only a few possible virulence features have been defined to explain this organism's association with enteric disease. There are at least three major clinical types of gastroenteritis caused by *Plesiomonas,* as follows:

1. The more common watery or secretory diarrhea
2. A second subacute or chronic disease that lasts between 14 days and 2 to 3 months

3. A more invasive, dysenteric form that resembles colitis

On the average, 25% to 40% of all patients present with fever and/or vomiting, and the single most common clinical symptom for all such patients is abdominal pain. Most cases are self-limited, but antimicrobial therapy is indicated in severe and prolonged cases.

Extraintestinal infection
Because of the organism's wide dissemination among the animal population, it is readily apparent that occupational exposure can be a source of such infections for veterinarians, zookeepers, aquaculturists, fish handlers, and athletes participating in water-related sports. Finally, there is the factor of the immune status of the individual patient, with the more serious infections such as bacteremia and meningitis usually occurring only in severely immunocompromised patients or neonates.

Laboratory Diagnosis
Culture media
Plesiomonas grows quite readily on most media routinely used in the clinical laboratory. After 18 to 24 hours incubation at 35° C, shiny, opaque, nonhemolytic colonies appear, with a slightly raised center and a smooth and entire edge. However, since the majority of strains are lactose-fermenters, the easiest screening procedure is an oxidase test performed on colonies from nonselective media, such as sheep's blood agar or chocolate agar. Although a specialized medium is not recommended for the detection of plesiomonads from stool specimens, because certain strains are inhibited on EMB (eosin-methylene blue) or MacConkey agar, IBB (inositol brilliant green bile salts) agar can be employed to enhance the isolation of pleisiomonads. Plesiomonad colonies are white to pink on this medium, and most coliform colonies are either green or pink. In addition, the agar used should not contain ampicillin, because plesiomonads often are susceptible to ampicillin and therefore will be inhibited.

Identification
Plesiomonas can be presumptively differentiated from nearby genera with several key tests (see Table 17-1). Their positive oxidase activity separates them from the Enterobacteriaceae, their sen-

sitivity to the vibriostatic agent O/129 (150 µg) separates them from *Aeromonas,* and their ability to ferment inositol separates them from all *Aeromonas* and nearly all *Vibrio* species.

Most rapid identification systems include *P. shigelloides* in their databases and appear to be able to identify it with a fairly high degree of accuracy. This is in large part because of its unique profile of positive ornithine and lysine decarboxylases and arginine dihydrolase reactions, combined with the fermentation of inositol.

As was previously mentioned, there is a serotyping schema for *Plesiomonas,* although this method is employed when an isolate is referred to the reference laboratory. What is important to reinforce is the possibility of cross-reactivity with *Shigella* antigens, particularly in some rapid serotyping kits, and the absolute necessity of an initial determination of an isolate's oxidase reaction from noninhibitory media.

Antimicrobial Susceptibility

Although most cases of plesiomonad gastroenteritis are self-limited, antimicrobial therapy is indicated in patients with severe or chronic gastroenteritis. Likewise, extraintestinal infections, particularly among neonates, often require antimicrobial therapy. Studies have shown a general resistance to the penicillin class of antibiotics, but penicillins combined with a β-lactamase inhibitor as well as trimethoprim-sulfamethoxazole are active. There are reports of resistance to more than one aminoglycoside (e.g., gentamicin, tobramycin, and amikacin), but the new quinolones appear to be an effective therapy.

CAMPYLOBACTER AND *CAMPYLOBACTER*-LIKE SPECIES

Campylobacter species and *Campylobacter*-like species, which include *Helicobacter* and *Wolinella,* have recently undergone certain changes in taxonomy. Based on RNA (rRNA) sequence studies *Wolinella recta* and *Wolinella curva* have been found to be similar to the campylobacters; although they may appear to be strict anaerobes, they have grown under a **microaerophilic** environment. Hence, *W. recta* and *W. curva* have been transferred to the genus *Campylobacter* as *Campy-*

lobacter rectus and *Campylobacter curvus.* As a result of these hybridization studies, a new genus, *Arcobacter,* and a new family, Campylobacteraceae, have been proposed. A few species have been designated in the new genera *Helicobacter* and *Arcobacter.* These recent changes in taxonomic status are shown in Table 17-6. This table also includes other *Campylobacter* species that have been identified, most of which are rarely isolated from human specimens.

Epidemiology

Campylobacter species have been known to cause abortion in domestic animals, such as cattle, sheep, and swine. Although these organisms were suspected of causing human infections earlier, campylobacters were not established as human pathogens until sensitive isolation procedures and isolation media were developed.

TABLE 17-6

Members of the Family Campylobacteraceae and Other Campylobacter-*Like Organisms*

Current Designation	Previous Designation and Synonyms
Campylobacter jejuni ssp. *jejuni*	*Campylobacter fetus* ssp. *jejuni*
Campylobacter jejuni ssp. *doylei*	*C. fetus* ssp. *jejuni*
Campylobacter coli	*C. fetus* ssp. *jejuni*
Campylobacter lari	*Campylobacter laridis*
Campylobacter fetus ssp. *fetus*	*C. fetus* ssp. *intestinalis*
C. fetus ssp. *venerealis*	*C. fetus* ssp. *fetus*
Campylobacter hyointestinalis	None
Campylobacter sputorum biovar *sputorum*	*C. sputorum* ssp. *sputorum*
C. sputorum biovar *bubulus*	*C. sputorum* ssp. *bubulus*
C. sputorum biovar *fecalis*	*Campylobacter fecalis*
Campylobacter upsaliensis	None
Campylobacter mucosalis	*C. sputorum* ssp. *mucosalis*
Campylobacter concisus	None
Campylobacter curvus	*Wolinella curva*
Campylobacter rectus	*Wolinella recta*
Arcobacter cryaerophilus	*Campylobacter cryaerophila*
Arcobacter nitrofigilis	*Campylobacter nitrofigilis*
Arcobacter butzleri	*Campylobacter butzleri*
Helicobacter pylori	*Campylobacter pylori*
Helicobacter mustelae	*C. pylori* ssp. *mustelae*
Helicobacter felis	None
Helicobacter muridarum	None
Helicobacter fennelliae	*Campylobacter fennelliae*
Helicobacter cinaedi	*Campylobacter cinaedi*

Courtesy Kaplan RL, Weissfeld AS: *Campylobacter, Helicobacter,* and related organisms. In Howard B et al, editors: *Clinical and pathogenic microbiology,* St Louis, 1994, Mosby.

TABLE 17-7

Campylobacter *Species and Their Clinical Significance*

Campylobacter Species	Clinical Significance
Campylobacter fetus ssp. *fetus*	Bacteremia in immunocompromised patients
C. fetus ssp. *venerealis*	Rarely involved in human infections
Campylobacter sputorum biovar *bubulus*	
C. sputorum biovar *fecalis*	
Campylobacter mucosalis	
Aeromonas nitrofigilis	
Helicobacter mustelae	
Helicobacter muridarum	
Helicobacter felis	
Helicobacter pylori	Common cause of duodenal ulcers and type B gastritis; possibly a risk factor in gastric carcinoma
Campylobacter hyointestinalis	Enteric disease in swine; occasionally associated in human enteric illness
Campylobacter lari	Enteritis very similar to that caused by *Campylobacter jejuni*
Campylobacter upsaliensis	Potential pathogen in humans, causing gastrointestinal illness and bacteremia in both immunocompetent and immunocompromised patients
Campylobacter concisus	Involved in periodontal disease; has also been recovered from individuals with gastrointestinal illness
Campylobacter rectus	Associated with periodontal disease; has been recovered from patients with root canal infections and Crohn's disease
Campylobacter jejuni	Most common cause of bacterial diarrhea worldwide
Helicobacter fennelliae	Recovered from homosexual men presenting with proctitis, proctocolitis, and enteritis
Helicobacter cinaedi	Recovered from blood of homosexual patients with AIDS and from blood and feces of children and adult females
A. butzleri	Associated with diarrheal disease in humans and in children with recurring gastrointestinal illness (abdominal cramps)

Today, the most common cause of bacterial gastroenteritis worldwide is *Campylobacter jejuni*. The transmission of campylobacterioses has been attributed to direct contact by exposure to animals and handling infected pets, such as dogs, cats, and birds, and indirectly by the consumption of contaminated water and dairy products and improperly cooked poultry. Person-to-person transmission also has been reported. *Campylobacter* species also are sexually transmitted.

Although the first reported cases of *Campylobacter* gastroenteritis in humans involved primarily children, later investigations showed that the diarrheal disease also occurs in adults. The population that most often manifests the disease includes children younger than 1 year of age and adults between 20 and 29 years of age. Among the other *Campylobacter* species that cause gastrointestinal disease (enteric campylobacters) are *Campylobacter coli* and *Campylobacter lari*.

Campylobacter fetus ssp. *fetus* has been isolated most frequently from blood cultures and is rarely associated with gastrointestinal illness. The majority of infections occur among immunocompromised and elderly patients. Table 17-7 summarizes the clinical significance of *Campylobacter, Arcobacter,* and *Helicobacter* species.

Helicobacter pylori

Until recently, *H. pylori* was unnamed. Within the past few years, it has been strongly associated with gastric and duodenal ulcers. The significance of these organisms had been questioned as early as the beginning of the century, and although the organisms were previously found in human gastric tissue, it was difficult to assess their significance because the samples were taken at autopsy.

Currently, *H. pylori* is recognized as the major cause of chronic superficial gastritis (type B gastritis). *H. pylori* has been identified in more than 75% of gastric ulcer patients.

H. pylori has been reported to colonize 20% to 40% of the adult population in the United States. In developing countries in Africa, Asia, and South America, the incidence is reported to be as high as 80% to 100%. This greater incidence is attributed to poor sanitary conditions. Some data suggests human-to-human transmission and possibility of a human reservoir.

General Characteristics

Campylobacter species are non–spore-forming, curved, gram-negative rods, showing an S-shaped, "seagull-wing" appearance. These organisms are oxidase-positive and motile, using a single polar flagellum. They exhibit a characteristic "darting" motility on hanging drop preparations or when visualized under phase-contrast microscopy. Campylobacters require selective media and a microaerophilic environment for growth and isolation.

Campylobacters were formerly classified with the vibrios because of their characteristic microscopic morphology, but DNA homology studies have shown that *Campylobacter* species do not belong with the vibrios. In addition, unlike the vibrios, which are fermentative, campylobacters are nonfermentative.

Bergey's Manual lists five different species for the genus *Campylobacter: C. fetus, C. jejuni, C. coli, Campylobacter sputorum,* and *Campylobacter concisus. C. fetus* contains two subspecies: *C. fetus* ssp. *fetus* and *C. fetus* ssp. *venerealis.* Formerly designated as subspecies of *C. fetus, C. jejuni* and *C. coli* are now recognized as separate species. In recent years, several other *Campylobacter* species have been described.

Campylobacter pyloridis or *Campylobacter pylori* was first referred to as a *Campylobacter*-like species, but *H. pylori* is now the designated nomenclature for this newly recognized organism. The genus *Helicobacter* includes other renamed *Campylobacter* species as well as newly described organisms (see Table 17-6).

Clinical Infection

Patients infected with *C. jejuni* present with a diarrheal disease that begins with mild abdominal pain within 2 to 10 days after ingestion of the organisms. Cramps and bloody diarrhea may follow the initial signs. Patients may experience fever and chills and, rarely, nausea and vomiting. In most patients, the illness is self-limited and usually resolves in 2 to 6 days. Untreated patients may remain carriers for several months. Other enteric *Campylobacter* infections (i.e., those caused by *C. coli* and *C. lari*) present with similar clinical manifestations.

Helicobacter pylori

Once acquired, *H. pylori* colonizes the stomach for a long time. Unlike other gastrointestinal pathogens, *H. pylori* causes a low-grade inflammatory process, producing a chronic superficial gastritis. Although it does not invade the gastric epithelium, the infection is recognized by the host immune system, which initiates an antibody response. The antibodies produced are not protective, however.

H. pylori is also now recognized as a major cause of **type B gastritis,** a condition formerly associated primarily with stress and chemical irritants. In addition, based on recent data, the strong association between long-term *H. pylori* infection and gastric cancer has raised more questions regarding the clinical significance of this organism. There is speculation that long-term *H. pylori* infection that leads to chronic gastritis is an important risk factor for gastric carcinoma.

Laboratory Diagnosis

Specimen collection and transport

C. fetus ssp. *fetus* may be recovered from several routine blood culture media. *Campylobacter* species that cause enteric illness are isolated from stool samples and rectal swabs (the less-preferred technique). If delay in processing the stool is anticipated, it can be placed in a transport medium such as Cary-Blair to maintain the viability of the organisms. A common stool transport medium, buffered glycerol-saline, is toxic to enteric campylobacters and should therefore be avoided.

H. pylori may be recovered from gastric biopsy materials. Samples must be transported quickly to the laboratory. Stuart medium can be used to maintain the viability of the organisms if delay in processing is anticipated. Tissue samples may also be placed in cysteine Brucella broth with 20% glycerol and frozen at $-70°$ C.

Culture media

An enriched selective agar, **CAMPY** BAP (blood agar plate), is the most commonly used medium in the United States to isolate *C. jejuni* and other enteric campylobacters. This commercially available medium contains Brucella agar base, 10% sheep's blood, and a combination of antimicrobials: vancomycin, trimethoprim, polymyxin B, amphotericin B, and cephalothin. Other selective media that have been successful in recovering

Campylobacter species are Butzler medium and Skirrow medium. Table 17-8 shows the composition of each of these selective media.

Medium V, a modification of the original Butzler medium, contains cefoperazone, rifampin, colistin, and amphotericin B; it seems to inhibit normal colon flora better than the original formulation. CVA medium has been reported to provide better suppression of fecal flora, even when this medium is incubated at 37° C. Incubation at 37° C allows the recovery of *Campylobacter* species that are inhibited at 42° C.

C. fetus ssp. *fetus* and *C. rectus* and *C. curvus* can be isolated using routine culture media.

To recover *H. pylori,* a combination of a nonselective medium, such as chocolate agar, and a selective medium, such as Skirrow, may be used. It is important that the inoculated medium be fresh and moist and that the culture be incubated in an environment with increased humidity.

INCUBATION

There is a double purpose for incubating stool cultures at 42° C to recover *C. jejuni*. First, *C. jejuni* and other enteric campylobacters grow optimally at 42° C. Second, growth of colon organisms is inhibited at this higher temperature. *C. fetus* ssp. *fetus,* on the other hand, is a rare stool isolate, and growth is suppressed at 42° C; therefore to isolate this organism, media should be incubated at 37° C.

Enteric *Campylobacter* species require a microaerophilic and capnophilic environment. The ideal atmospheric environment for these organisms contains a gas mixture of 5% to 10% O_2 and 10% CO_2. Except for *C. rectus* and *C. curvus,* a strict anaerobic environment does not support the growth of most *Campylobacter* species.

Any of the methods described below can be used to obtain the required environment for campylobacters.

With the CAMPY PAK II system (Becton Dickinson Microbiology Systems, Cockeysville, Md), plates are placed in a jar (usually one similar to that used for anaerobic cultures), and a gas-generating envelope is activated when water is added. Once the envelope is activated, it takes approximately an hour to achieve the ideal atmospheric environment. Gas Generating Kit System BR56 (Oxoid, USA) is similar to CAMPY PAK II.

An evacuation replacement system similar to that used to obtain a strict anaerobic condition may also be used. The anaerobic jar is evacuated to a pressure of 15 inches Hg at least twice and refilled each time with one of the following gas mixtures: 10% CO_2, 90% N_2; 5% CO_2, 10% H_2, 85% N_2; or 10% CO_2, 10% H_2, 80% N_2.

The BioBag Type Cfj (Becton Dickinson) consists of a single plate bag and a generator ampule. The inoculated plate is placed in the bag and heat-sealed. Once the generator ampule is crushed, it provides an atmosphere of 5% to 10% O_2 and 8% to 10% CO_2. The plate can be examined at any time without being removed from the bag.

A candle jar may be used if none of the above-mentioned systems can be obtained. However, this method provides the least ideal environmental condition. The incubation time should be extended to 72 hours to more efficiently isolate enteric *Campylobacter* species. This procedure allows facultative organisms present on the medium to reduce the O_2 tension created by the candle to a more suitable concentration for campylobacters.

Another method that relies on the presence of facultative organisms such as *Proteus* and *E. coli* to reduce the oxygen content in the environment is the Fortner principle. In this method, a Campy BAP is inoculated and placed in a bag with a plate inoculated with the facultative organism. It is necessary to incubate the plates for at least 72 hours to allow growth of *Campylobacter* species, which does not take place until the proper environment is achieved.

TABLE 17-8

Selective Media for the Cultivation of Campylobacter *Species*

Medium	Base	Antimicrobial Agent
CAMPY blood agar plate	Brucella agar 10% sheep red blood cells	Vancomycin Trimethoprim Polymyxin B Amphotericin B Cephalothin
Skirrow	Oxoid blood agar base Lysed, defibrinated horse red blood cells	Vancomycin Trimethoprim Polymyxin B
Butzler	Thioglycolate fluid with agar added 10% sheep red blood cells	Bacitracin Novobiocin Actidione Colistin Cefazolin

Other systems such as Kaplan's Poly Bag system and Bacti-Gas Station (Scott Laboratories, Kiskeville, RI) may also be considered as alternatives. The inexpensive Poly Bag system holds up to eight inoculated plates in one bag. The bag is charged with the gas mixture (5% O_2, 10% CO_2, 85% N_2) several times and then tied off with a rubber band. The Bacti-Gas Station comes with reusable environmental bags and a gas cylinder to provide the gas mixture.

Presumptive identification

MICROSCOPIC MORPHOLOGY

Campylobacter species are curved, gram-negative rods that measure approximately 0.2 to 0.5 μm by 0.5 to 5.0 μm. On Gram-stained smears, these organisms stain poorly. For better visualization, carbolfuchsin is recommended as a counterstain; if safranin is used, counterstaining should be extended to 2 to 3 minutes. Enteric campylobacters may appear as long spirals, S shapes, or seagull-wing shapes. These organisms may appear as coccobacilli in smears prepared from older cultures. Phase-contrast or darkfield microscopy of fresh stool samples may show the characteristic **darting motility** typical of enteric campylobacters.

Acrobacter species have a microscopic morphology similar to that of *Campylobacter* species. *H. pylori* also appears similar to campylobacters, but one ultrastructural study has shown that *Helicobacter* has multiple flagella at one pole, unlike the single polar flagellum of campylobacters.

COLONIAL MORPHOLOGY

The typical colonial morphology of *C. jejuni* and other enteric campylobacters is moist, "runny looking," and spreading. Colonies are usually non-hemolytic; some are round and raised, and others may be flat. *Campylobacter fetus* ssp. *fetus* produces smooth, convex, translucent colonies. A tan or slightly pink coloration is observed in some enteric campylobacter colonies. Other *Campylobacter* species produce colonies similar to those of *C. jejuni.* Although most do not produce pigment, *Campylobacter mucosalis* and *Campylobacter hyointestinalis* can produce a dirty yellow pigment.

Definitive identification

Isolates from stool and rectal swabs can be presumptively identified as *Campylobacter* species by observing the characteristic Gram-stained microscopic morphology, the characteristic motility in a hanging-drop preparation using phase-contrast microscopy or darkfield microscopy, and positive oxidase and catalase reactions. The microscopic morphology is very important, as it differentiates *Campylobacter* from other bacterial species (i.e., *Aeromonas* and *Pseudomonas*) that are oxidase-positive and can grow at 42° C in a microaerophilic environment. To observe the typical motility, organisms should be suspended in *Brucella* or tryptic soy broth. Distilled water and saline seem to inhibit motility.

Table 17-9 lists the biochemical tests most useful in definitively identifying the most commonly encountered *Campylobacter, Helicobacter,* and *Arcobacter* species.

H. pylori may be presumptively identified in a gastric biopsy specimen by testing for the presence of a rapidly acting urease reaction. The collected tissue sample may be placed onto a Christensen's urea medium and incubated at 37° C for 2 hours. A rapid color change suggests the presence of *H. pylori.* Urease activity may also be detected by the **urea breath test.** The breath test is reportedly both sensitive and specific and is recommended for monitoring therapy. In this test, the patient is given ^{14}C-labeled urea to drink. Urea degraded by the urease activity of *H. pylori* releases $^{14}CO_2$, which is detected in the exhaled breath by a scintillation counter.

Another detection method, although not specific for *H. pylori,* is to stain the gastric biopsy tissue using Giemsa, Gram, or silver stain to visualize the bacterium.

SEROLOGY

Latex agglutination tests are now available for rapid identification of colonies of enteric campylobacters on primary isolation media. The Meritec-Campy (jcl) test (Meridian Diagnostics, Inc., Cincinnati) and Campyslide (Becton Dickinson) can detect the presence of *C. jejuni, C. coli,* and *C. lari.* Campyslide also identifies *C. fetus* ssp. *fetus.* However, neither system differentiates between the isolated *Campylobacter* species.

Serologic assays for the detection of antibodies to *H. pylori* are also currently available. Specific antibodies in serum may be detected by enzyme-linked immunosorbent assay (ELISA) or by indirect im-

TABLE 17-9
Biochemical Tests to Differentiate Campylobacter, Arcobacter, *and* Helicobacter *Species*

Species	Catalase	Nitrate Reduction	Urease	H₂S Production (TSI)	Hippurate Hydrolysis	Indoxyl Acetate Hydrolysis	Growth at 15° C	Growth at 25° C	Growth at 42° C	Nalidixic Acid (30 µg)	Cephalothin (30 µg)
Campylobacter jejuni ssp. *jejuni*	+	+	−	−	+	+	−	−	+	−	−
Campylobacter jejuni ssp. *doylei*	V	−	−	−	V	+	−	−	−	+	+
Campylobacter coli	+	+	−	−	−	+	−	−	+	+	−
Campylobacter lari	+	+	V	−	−	−	−	−	+	−	−
Campylobacter fetus ssp. *fetus*	+	+	−	−	−	+	−	+	−	+	+
Campylobacter hyointestinalis	+	+	−	+	−	−	−	+	+	+	+
Campylobacter upsaliensis	W	+	−	−	−	+	−	−	+	−	+
Campylobacter concisus	−	+	−	+	−	−	−	−	+	+	−
Campylobacter curvus	−	+	−	+	−	+	−	−	+	+	ND
Campylobacter rectus	−	+	−	+	−	+	−	−	W	+	ND
Arcobacter butzleri	−W	+	−	−	−	+	+	+	V	V	−
Helicobacter pylori	+	V	+	−	−	−	−	−	V	−	+
Helicobacter fennelliae	+	−	−	−	−	+	−	−	−	+	+
Helicobacter cinaedi	+	+	−	−	−	V	−	−	−	+	+

TSI, Triple sugar iron agar slant; +, positive result; −, negative result; *W*, weak; *V*, variable result; *ND*, not determined; −*W*, mostly negative, some weak. All *Campylobacter* species are oxidase positive.

munofluorescent assay (IFA) methods. These methods have been reported to be reasonably sensitive and specific indicators of *H. pylori* infections.

Antimicrobial Susceptibility

Antimicrobial susceptibility testing for *Campylobacter* species is not routinely performed in the clinical microbiology laboratory and is not standardized. The drug of choice for treating intestinal campylobacteriosis is erythromycin, although most patients recover without antimicrobial intervention. Gentamicin is used to treat systemic infections. Tetracycline, erythromycin, and chloramphenicol may be used as substitutes for gentamicin.

Several drug modalities for treating *H. pylori* infections are currently being studied. The most common thought is that triple therapy, which may include amoxicillin, metronidazole or tetracycline, and bismuth, is most effective in eradicating the organism.

Bibliography

Albert MJ et al: Characterization of *Aeromonas trota* strains that crossreact with *Vibrio cholerae* 0139 Bengal, *J Clin Microbiol* 33:3119, 1995.

Aldova E: Experience with serology of *Plesiomonas shigelloides* O-antigenic structure, *J Hyg Epidemiol Microbiol Immunol* 29:201, 1985.

Altwegg M: *Aeromonas caviae.* An enteric pathogen? *Infection* 13:228, 1985.

Baron EG, Peterson LR, Finegold SM: *Bailey and Scott's diagnostic microbiology,* ed 9, St Louis, 1994, Mosby.

Baron S: *Medical microbiology,* ed 3, New York, 1991, Churchill Livingstone.

Blaser MJ et al: *Campylobacter* enteritis: clinical and epidemiologic features, *Ann Intern Med* 91:179, 1979.

Bottone EJ, Janda JM: *Vibrio.* In Howard B et al, editors: *Clinical and pathogenic microbiology,* ed 1, St Louis, 1987, Mosby.

Brenden RA, Miller MA, Janda JM: Clinical disease spectrum and pathogenic factors associated with *Plesiomonas shigelloides* infections in humans, *Rev Infect Dis* 10:303, 1988.

Butzler JP, De Boeck M, Goosens H: New selective medium for isolation of *Campylobacter jejuni* from fecal specimens, *Lancet* 2:818, 1983.

Butzler JP, Skirrow MB: *Campylobacter* enteritis, *Clin Gastroenterol* 8:737, 1979.

Carnahan A: Update on *Aeromonas* identification, *Clin Microbiol Newsl* 13:169, 1991.

Carnahan A, Behram S, Joseph SW: Aerokey II—a flexible key for identifying clinical *Aeromonas* species, *J Clin Microbiol* 29:2843, 1991.

Chan FTH, Mackenzie AMR: Enrichment medium and control system for isolation of *C. festus* ssp. *jejuni* from stools, *J Clin Microbiol* 15:12, 1982.

Clark RB, Janda JM: *Plesiomonas* and human disease, *Clin Microbiol Newsl* 13:49, 1991.

Cover TL, Blaser MJ: *Heliobacter pylori* and gastroduodenal disease, *Annu Rev Med* 43:135, 1992.

Dekeyser P et al: Acute enteritis due to related vibrio: first positive stool cultures, *J Infect Dis* 125:390, 1972.

Edmonds P et al: *Campylobacter hyointestinalis* associated with human gastrointestinal disease in the United States, *J Clin Microbiol* 25:685, 1987.

Famey T et al: An outbreak of *Campylobacter* enteritis associated with failed milk pasteurization, *J Infect* 31:137, 1995.

Fliegelman RM et al: Comparative in vitro activities of twelve antimicrobial agents against *Campylobacter* species, *Antimicrob Agents Chemother* 27:429, 1985.

Fox JG et al: *Campylobacter mustelae,* a new species resulting from the elevation of *Campylobacter pylori* spp. *Mustelae* to species status, *Int J Syst Bacteriol* 39:301, 1989.

Graves TW, Bradley RR, Crutcher JM: Outbreak of *Campylobacter* enteritis associated with cross-contamination of food—Oklahoma, 1996, *MMWR Morb Mort Wiccy Rep* 47:129, 1998.

Haapasalo M: *Bacteroides buccae* and related taxa in necrotic root canal infections, *J Clin Microbiol* 29:940, 1986.

Han YH et al: *Wolinella recta, Wolinella curva, Bacteroides ureolyticus,* and *Bacteroides gracilis* are microaerophiles, not anaerobes, *Int J Syst Bacteriol* 41:219, 1991.

Hoeck FJ et al: Evaluation of the performance of commercial test kits for detection of *Heliobacter pylori* antibodies in serum, *J Clin Microbiol* 30:1525, 1992.

Janda JM: Pathogenic *Vibrio* spp.: an organism group of increasing medical significance, *Clin Microbiol Newsl* 9:49, 1987.

Janda JM: Recent advances in the study of the taxonomy, pathogenicity, and infectious syndromes associated with the genus *Aeromonas, Clin Microbiol Rev* 4:397, 1991.

Janda JM, Duffey PS: Mesophilic aeromonads in human disease: current taxonomy, laboratory identification, and infectious disease spectrum, *Rev Infect Dis* 10:980, 1988.

Janda JM et al: Current perspectives on the epidemiology and pathogenesis of clinically significant *Vibrio* spp., *Clin Microbiol Rev* 1:245, 1988.

Joseph SW, Colwell RR, Kaper JB: *Vibrio parahaemolyticus* and related halophilic vibrios, *Crit Rev Microbiol* 10:77, 1982.

Kaplan RL: *Campylobacter.* In Lennette EH et al, editors: *Manual of clinical microbiology,* ed 3, Washington, DC, 1980, American Society for Microbiology.

Kaplan RL, Barrett JE: *Monograph: Campylobacter,* Kansas City, Mo, 1981, Marion Scientific.

Kaplan RL, Weissfeld AS: *Campylobacter, Helicobacter,* and related organisms. In Howard B et al, editors: *Clinical and pathogenic microbiology,* St Louis, 1994, Mosby.

Karmali MA, Fleming PC: Applicaton of the Fortner principle to isolation of *Campylobacter* from stools, *J Clin Microbiol* 10:245, 1979.

Kelly MT, Hickman-Brenner FW, Farmer JJ III: *Vibrio.* In Balows A et al, editors: *Manual of clinical microbiology,* ed 5, Washington, DC, 1991, American Society for Microbiology.

Kiehlbauch JA et al: *Campylobacter butzleri* sp. nov. isolated from humans and animals with diarrheal illness, *J Clin Microbiol* 29:376, 1991.

Koneman EW et al: *Color atlas of diagnostic microbiology,* ed 4, Philadelphia, 1997, JB Lippincott.

Kreig NR: *Bergey's manual of systemic bacteriology,* vol 1, Baltimore, 1984, Williams & Wilkins.

Mandell Gl, Douglas RG, Bennett JE: *Principles and practice of infectious diseases,* ed 3, New York, 1990, Churchill Livingstone.

Morris JG, Cholera Laboratory Task Force: *Vibrio cholerae* 0139 Bengal. In Wachsmuth I et al, editors: *Vibrio cholera. Molecular and global perspectives,* Washington, DC, 1984, American Society for Microbiology.

Pai CH et al: *Campylobacter* gastroenteritis in children, *J Pediatr* 94:589, 1979.

Paisley JW et al: Darkfield microscopy of human feces for presumptive diagnosis of *Campylobacter fetus* ssp. *jejuni* enteritis, *J Clin Microbiol* 15:61, 1982.

Parsonnet J et al: *Helicobacter pylori* infection and risk of gastric carcinoma, *N Engl J Med* 325:1127, 1991.

Patton CM et al: Human disease associated with *Campylobacter upsaliensis* (catalase-negative or weakly positive *Campylobacter* species) in the United States, *J Clin Microbiol* 27:66, 1989.

Penner JL: The genus *Campylobacter:* a decade of progress, *Clin Microbiol Rev* 1:157, 1988.

Pugina P et al: An outbreak of *Arcobacter (Campylobacter) butzleri* in Italy, *Microbiol Ecol Health Dis* 4:S94, 1991.

Quinn TC et al: Infections with *Campylobacter jejuni* and *Campylobacter*-like organisms in homosexual men, *Ann Intern Med* 101:187, 1984.

Sack RB, Tilton RC, Weissfield AS: *Cumitech* 12. In Rubin SJ, editor: *Laboratory diagnosis of bacterial diarrhea,* Washington, DC, 1980, American Society for Microbiology.

Segreti J et al: High-level quinolone resistance in clinical isolates of *Campylobacter jejuni, J Infect Dis* 165:667, 1992.

Shimada T, Kosako Y: Comparison of two O-serotyping systems for mesophilic *Aeromonas* spp., *J Clin Microbiol* 29:197, 1991.

Skirrow MB: *Campylobacter* enteritis. A "new" disease, *Br Med J* 2:9, 1977.

Smibert RM: Genus *Campylobacter* Sebald and Bernon 1963, 907. In Krieg NR, Holt JG, editors: *Bergey's manual of systemic bacteriology,* vol 1, Baltimore, 1984, Williams & Wilkins.

Soltesz V et al: Optimal survival of *Helicobacter pylori* under various transport conditions, *J Clin Microbiol* 24:562, 1988.

Steele TW, Owen RJ: *Campylobacter jejuni* spp. *doylei* ssp. nov., a subspecies of nitrate-negative campylobacters isolated in central and south Australia, *J Clin Microbiol* 24:562, 1988.

Talley NJ et al: Serodiagnosis of *Heliobacter pylori.* Comparison of enzyme-linked immunosorbent assays, *J Clin Microbiol* 29:1635, 1991.

Tanner ACR et al: *Wolinella* gen. nov., *Wolinella succinogenes (Vibrio succinogenes* Wolin et al) comb. nov., and description of *Bacteroides gracilis* sp. nov., *Wolinella recta* sp. nov., *Campylobacter concisus* sp. nov., and *Eikenella corrodens* from humans with periodontal disease, *Int J Syst Bacteriol* 31:432, 1981.

Tauxe RV et al: Illness associated with *Campylobacter laridis,* a newly recognized *Campylobacter* species, *J Clin Microbiol* 21:222, 1985.

Totten PA et al: *Campylobacter cinaedi* (sp. nov.) and *Campylobacter fennelliae* (sp. nov.): two *Campylobacter* species associated with enteric disease in homosexual men, *J Infect Dis* 151:131, 1985.

Vandamme P, De Ley J: Proposal for a new family Campylobacteracae, *Int J Syst Bacteriol* 41:451, 1991.

Vandamme P et al: Identification of *Campylobacter cinaedi* isolated from blood and feces of children and adult females, *J Clin Microbiol* 28:1016, 1990.

Vandamme P et al: Revision of *Campylobacter, Helicobacter,* and *Wolinella* taxonomy: emendation of generic descriptions and proposal of Arcobacter gen. nov., *Int J Syst Bacteriol* 41:88, 1991.

von Graevenitz A, Altwegg M: *Aeromonas* and *Plesiomonas.* In Balows A, editor: *Manual of clinical microbiology,* ed 5, Washington, DC, 1991, American Society for Microbiology.

Warren JR, Marshall B: Unidentified curved bacilli on gastric epithelium in active chronic gastritis (letter), *Lancet* 1:1273, 1983.

LEARNING ASSESSMENT

1. What genus would you initially suspect in the case described based on the patient's past and present medical history?

2. What additional test(s) would you use to confirm your genus identity?

3. Which species would you suspect this isolate to be based on colonial morphology, media fermentation results, and halophilic requirement?

4. Which biochemical test results would be most helpful in confirming your genus and species identification?

5. What culture medium is best to use when *Vibrio* sp. is suspected from a clinical sample?

6. Which *Campylobacter* species cause gastrointestinal illnesses?

7. What cultural and environmental requirements are needed to recover *Campylobacter jejuni* from stool samples?

8. Why is *Helicobacter pylori* an important pathogen?

9. What invasive procedures are used to determine the presence of *H. pylori?*

10. What noninvasive procedures may be used to detect this organism?

CHAPTER 18

Nonfermenting Gram-Negative Bacilli and Miscellaneous Gram-Negative Rods

Gerri S. Hall

GENERAL CHARACTERISTICS
OF NONFERMENTERS
Clinical Infections
Biochemical Characteristics
Initial Clues to Nonfermenters
Identification Methods

MOST COMMONLY ENCOUNTERED
NONFERMENTATIVE ORGANISMS
The Pseudomonads
Pseudomonas aeruginosa
Pseudomonas fluorescens and Pseudomonas
putida
Stenotrophomonas maltophilia
Acinetobacter Species
Other Pseudomonads
Pseudomonas stutzeri
Pseudomonas mendocina
Pseudomonas pseudoalcaligenes, Pseudomonas
alcaligenes, and CDC Group 1
Pseudomonads and Other Nonfermenters Whose
Names Have Been Changed
Burkholderia cepacia (Pseudomonas cepacia)
Burkholderia gladioli (Pseudomonas gladioli)
Burkholderia pseudomallei (Pseudomonas
pseudomallei)
Sphingomonas paucimobilis (Pseudomonas
paucimobilis)
Brevundimonas diminuta (Pseudomonas
diminuta)

Brevundimonas vesicularis (Pseudomonas
vesicularis)
Ralstonia pickettii (Pseudomonas pickettii)
Shewanella putrefaciens (Pseudomonas
putrefaciens)
Comamonas species
Methylobacterium extorquens

MISCELLANEOUS NONFERMENTING
GRAM-NEGATIVE BACILLI
Nonfermenters with Peritrichous Flagellation
Alcaligenes species
Agrobacterium species
Oligella ureolytica
CDC group IVc-2
Ochrobactrum anthropi
Nonmotile Gram-Negative Bacilli
Flavobacterium species
Sphingobacterium species
Chryseomonas and Flavimonas and Balneatrix
species
Moraxella, Moraxella-like genera,
and Oligella species
Other Gram-Negative Nonfermenters
EO-2 and Psychrobacter species
Dysgonic fermenters (DF)
Eugonic fermenters (EF)
HB-5
Chromobacterium species

OBJECTIVES

1. Describe the general characteristics of nonfermentative gram-negative rods.
2. Differentiate the metabolic pathways utilized by nonfermentative and fermentative organisms.
3. Describe how nonfermentative organisms cause infections.
4. Recognize the initial clues to nonfermentative organisms.
5. Describe the typical reactions and characteristic features of most of the commonly encountered nonfermentative organisms.

KEY TERMS

Asaccharolytic
Fermentative
Nonfermentative
Embden-Meyerhof
  Pathway
Entner-Doudoroff
  Pathway

Oxidizers, or
  saccharolytic
  organisms
Biochemically inert, or
  nonoxidizers
Hugh-Leifson OF
  medium

Oxidase positive
Glucose oxidation
  (OF test)
Pseudomonad
Pyocyanin
Pyoverdin
2-Aminoacetophenone

Nonmotile
Motile
Dysgonic fermenters
  (DF)
Eugonic fermenters (EF)

CASE STUDY

A 25-year-old woman who received a bone marrow transplant as treatment for aplastic anemia had the following presenting symptoms: fever, chills, and malaise of about 2 days duration. Blood cultures were drawn according to standard procedure (i.e., two sets of 20 ml each were sent off to the lab in the blood culture system that was presently being used in the hospital). The patient was admitted, and about 5 hours later, another two sets were sent to the lab because her fever persisted. At this point, the patient was given broad-spectrum antibiotics, with the plan to give her antifungals if the fever persisted. About 12 hours after the first blood culture draw, the clinician was called because 2 of 2 blood cultures tested positive for a gram-negative bacillus. In another 4 hours the other two sets tested positive for what appeared to be the same organism, at least from the gram-stained picture. The next day, the clinician was informed that the gram-negative bacillus had tested negative for lactose fermentation and tested positive for oxidase. The isolate would be further worked up for identification and susceptibility.

This chapter discusses miscellaneous organisms that are becoming more clinically significant because of increasing numbers of immunocompromised patients. The groups of organisms discussed in this chapter are the pseudomonads, *Acinetobacter* species, *Stenotrophomonas maltophilia* and other oxidase-negative ozidizers, HACEK members, *Capnocytophaga* species and **asaccharolytic** species.

Aerobic gram-negative bacilli can be divided into at least two large groups, those that ferment carbohydrates (**fermentative** or fermenters) and those that do not ferment (**nonfermentative** or nonfermenters). Figure 18-1 describes the **Embden-Meyerhof** and **Entner-Doudoroff** pathways that organisms use to break down carbohydrates.

GENERAL CHARACTERISTICS OF NONFERMENTERS

Nonfermentative organisms that can break down carbohydrates oxidatively are also referred to as ***oxidizers or saccharolytic,*** whereas those organisms that are not able to break down carbohydrates either fermentatively or oxidatively are re-

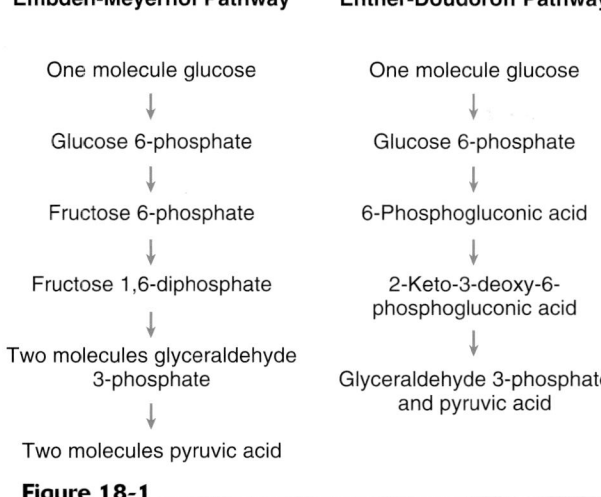

Embden-Meyerhof Pathway

One molecule glucose
↓
Glucose 6-phosphate
↓
Fructose 6-phosphate
↓
Fructose 1,6-diphosphate
↓
Two molecules glyceraldehyde 3-phosphate
↓
Two molecules pyruvic acid

Entner-Doudoroff Pathway

One molecule glucose
↓
Glucose 6-phosphate
↓
6-Phosphogluconic acid
↓
2-Keto-3-deoxy-6-phosphogluconic acid
↓
Glyceraldehyde 3-phosphate and pyruvic acid

Figure 18-1

Two fermentation pathways for glucose degradation.

ferred to as ***biochemically inert or nonoxidizers.*** Nonfermentative gram-negative bacilli and coccobacilli are ubiquitous in the environment. They are found in soil, water, plants, decaying vegetation, and foodstuffs; in hospitals, they are isolated from nebulizers, dialysate fluids, saline, and catheter devices. These organisms are variably resistant to agents such as chlorhexidine and quaternary ammonium compounds.

Clinical Infections

Nonfermenters accounts for approximately 15% of all isolates of gram-negative bacilli found in the clinical microbiology laboratory. Clinically, differences exist among infections caused by each species; however, some common disease manifestations and risk factors are present. Some of the disease manifestations associated with nonfermenting organisms are septicemia, meningitis, osteomyelitis, and wound infections usually following surgery or trauma. Risk factors for development of infection by these organisms are listed in Box 18-1. Immunosuppression, foreign body implantation, and traumatic breaks in a host barrier are the main events preceding infection with one of these organisms.

Biochemical Characteristics

In general, nonfermenters vary in their biochemical and morphologic characteristics. One common feature of this group of organism, however, is their

nonreactivity in triple sugar iron (TSI) agar or Kligler iron agar (KIA) (Table 18-1). A fermenter typically produces an acid (yellow) butt with an acid or alkaline (red) slant on TSI or KIA in 24 hours. A nonfermenter (either an oxidizer or nonoxidizer) produces no change (red) in the butt and slant or may produce an alkaline (red) slant (Figure 18-2). In addition to these types of organisms, some "true" fermenters are fastidious and do not easily acidify the butt or slant of a TSI like other fermenters but do show reactions if more sensitive media are used.

Characteristically, nonfermenters and fastidious fermenters often produce either weak or small amounts of acids from carbohydrates. In media that contain large amounts of peptones (2.0%), such as TSI agar, whatever acids produced are neutralized or "masked" by the alkaline reaction from peptone utilization. To detect small amounts of acids produced, whether fermentatively or oxidatively, Hugh and Leifson developed a medium that contains the same amount of carbohydrates (1%) found in the TSI and KIA media but a lower amount of peptone (0.2%) in the oxidation-fermentation (OF) medium (1%) (Figure 18-3).

Box 18-1

Risk Factors for Diseases Caused by Nonfermentative Gram-Negative Bacilli

Immunosuppression

Diabetes mellitus
Cancer
Steroids
Transplantation

Trauma

Gun shot, knife wounds, punctures
Surgery
Burns

Foreign Body Implantation

Catheters: urinary or blood stream
Prosthetic devices: joints, valves
Corneal implants or contact lenses

Infused Fluids

Dialysate
Saline irrigations

TABLE 18-1

Biochemical Reactions Characteristic of Nonfermenters on TSI, KIA, and of Media

	Triple Sugar Iron (TSI) Agar	Kligler Iron Agar (KIA)	Hugh-Leifson Oxidation-Fermentation (OF) Medium
Carbohydrates (concentration)	Glucose (0.1%)	Glucose (0.l%)	Glucose or other carbohydrate being tested (1%)
	Lactose (1%)	Lactose (1%)	
	Sucrose (1%)		
Peptone	2%	2%	0.2%
Fermenter	Acid butt	Acid butt	Open tube: acid
	Acid or alkaline slant	Acid or alkaline slant	Sealed tube: acid
Nonfermenter			
Oxidizer	Alkaline butt	Alkaline butt	Open tube: acid
Nonoxidizer (asaccharolytic)	Alkaline slant	Alkaline slant	Sealed tube: no acid
	Alkaline butt	Alkaline butt	Open tube: no acid
	Alkaline slant	Alkaline slant	Sealed tube: no acid

Table 18-1 shows the differences in reactions among these groups of organisms. When isolates are tested in **Hugh-Leifson OF medium,** two tubes are inoculated: one is overlayed with sterile mineral oil to create an anerobic environment (closed); the other is left aerobic, without mineral oil overlay (open). When acid is produced in both open and closed tubes, the isolate is determined to be a fermenter; the absence of acid production in the closed tube indicates that the organism is a nonfermenter. The open tube may or may not show acidity. No acid production in the open tube may indicate that the organism is a nonoxidizer.

Initial Clues to Nonfermenters

Initial clues to the presence of a nonfermenter in the clinical laboratory are as follows:

- Long, thin gram-negative bacilli or coccobacilli
- **Oxidase-positive** reaction (although reaction is variable in some and absent in others)
- Nonreactive in 24 hours in commercial kit systems for the identification of Enterobacteriaceae
- TSI: nonreactive (i.e., no acid production in slant or butt)

Figure 18-2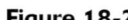

Reactions in triple sugar iron (TSI) agar. *Left to right:* A/A, H₂S, no gas: lactose-fermenter with H₂S; ALK/A, no gas, no H₂S: glucose-fermenter, non–lactose-fermenter; ALK/ALK, no gas, no H₂S: nonfermenter.

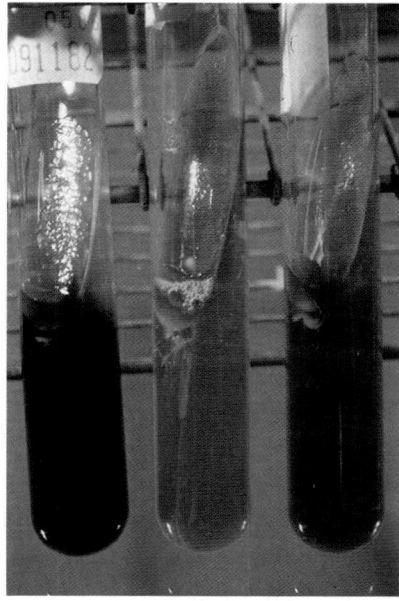

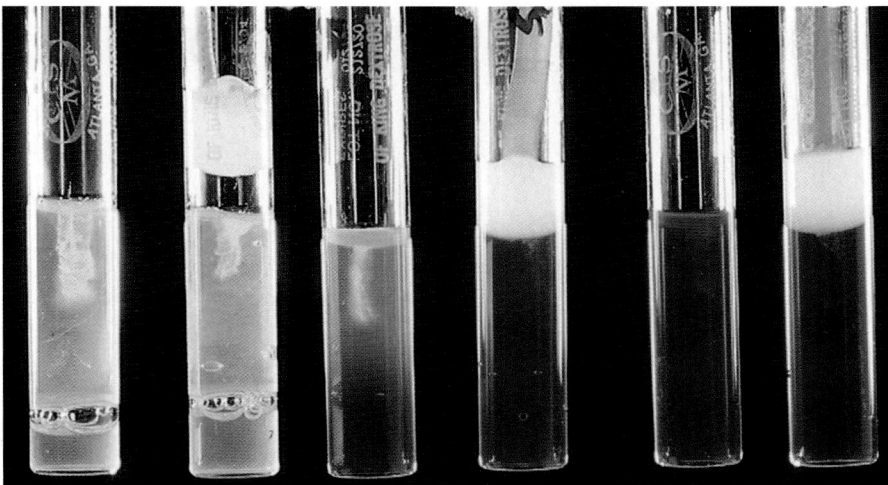

Figure 18-3

Reactions in oxidative fermentation (OF) media. *Left to right:* Fermenter: open and sealed tubes positive for acid production; nonfermenter: open tube positive for acid production, sealed tube negative for acid production; nonfermenter/nonoxidizer: open and sealed tubes negative for acid production.

■ Resistance to antibiotics (i.e., aminoglycosides, cephalosporins, imipenem, penicillins)

The nonfermenters may be organized into smaller groups based on reactions to three tests that are commonly performed to facilitate easy identification: (1) growth on MacConkey agar, (2) oxidase reaction, and (3) **glucose oxidation (OF test).** The eight possible combinations of results are then used to group the nonfermenters as shown in Figure 18-4. Included in this figure are some isolates of nonfermentative gram-negative bacilli not always considered to be with the nonfermenters. They are, however, biochemically quite similar (e.g., *Brucella* sp., *Bordetella* sp.) and are discussed in Chapter 15. Figure 18-4 will be cited in the following detailed discussions of the nonfermenter groups most commonly encountered in the clinical microbiology laboratory, to allow the reader to become familiar with the initial clues for each organism.

Identification Methods

For the identification of nonfermentative gram-negative bacilli, conventional tube biochemical testing, kit systems, or a combination of the two approaches can be used. The majority of clinical isolates are *Pseudomonas aeruginosa, Acinetobacter* sp., or *S. maltophilia.* For these most common isolates, most of the kit systems and automated

identification systems perform adequately, or a limited number of conventional biochemicals can be used to identify these organisms. For the remainder of the nonfermenters, decisions must first be made as to which need to be identified.

The decision to identify organisms depends on the site from which they are isolated; that is, were they isolated from a sterile site in which the nonfermenter is the only isolate or from a nonsterile site in which three or four other bacteria are also present? In the former case, it may be decided that definitive identification and susceptibility testing are required. Use of a kit system with or without a conventional biochemical scheme should be utilized. In the latter case, a genus identification may be appropriate and may be achieved through use of a few biochemical tests (e.g., oxidase, growth on MacConkey agar, glucose utilization, indole, motility). Definitive identification of every nonfermenter can be very time consuming and costly and may not contribute much to the diagnosis of the disease. Figure 18-5 gives an example of results obtained for a large number of nonfermentative gram-negative bacilli using 20 biochemical or morphologic characteristics. If needed, laboratory professionals should consider sending the isolate to a reference laboratory that is better equipped to achieve these identifications in a cost-effective manner.

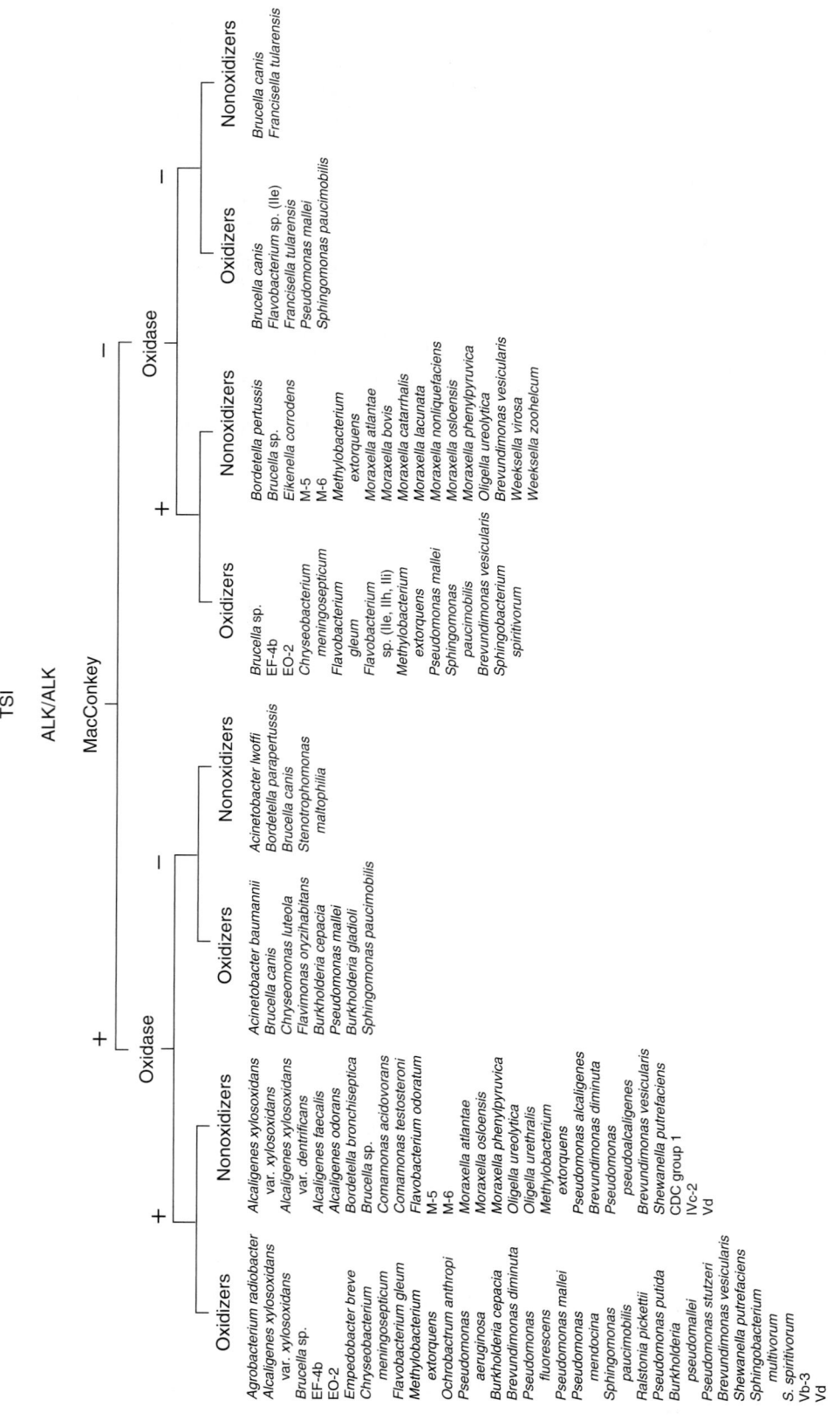

Figure 18-4

Grouping of nonfermenters based on eight possible results.

	MOTILE, STRONGLY SACCHAROLYTIC NONFERMENTERS										MOTILE, WEAK, OR NONSACCHAROLYTIC NONFERMENTERS										
	Pseudomonas aeruginosa	*Pseudomonas fluorescens/putida*	*Burkholderia (Pseudomonas) cepacia*	*Alcaligenes xylosoxidans ssp. xylosoxidans*	*Stenotrophomonas maltophilia*	*Burkholderia (Pseudomonas) pseudomallei*	*Pseudomonas stutzeri*	*Sphingomonas (Pseudomonas) paucimobilis*	*Pseudomonas mendocina*	*Ralstonia (Pseudomonas) pickettii*	*Pseudomonas acidovorans*	*Pseudomonas pseudoalcaligenes*	*Alcaligenes faecalis*	*Alcaligenes xylosoxidans ssp. denitrificans*	*Oligella ureolytica*	*Bordetella bronchiseptica*	*Pseudomonas alcaligenes*	*Brevundimonas (Pseudomonas) diminuta*	*Brevundimonas (Pseudomonas) vesicularis*	*Comamonas sp. (Pseudomonas testosteroni)*	*Shewanella putrefaciens*
Oxidase	+	+	+	+	−	+	+	+	+	+	+	+	+	+	+	+	+	+	+	+	+
Pyocyanin	+/−	−	−	−	−	−	−	−	−	−	−	−	−	−	−	−	−	−	−	−	−
Fluorescein	+	−/+	−	−	−	−	−	−	−	−	−	−	−	−	−	−	−	−	−	−	−
Glucose	+	+	+	+/−	+/−	+	+	+/−	+	+	−	−/+	−	−	−	−	−	−	−	+	−
Xylose	+	+	+/−	+	−	+	−/+	+/−	+	+	−	−	−	−	−	−	−	−	−	−	−
Mannitol	+/−	+/−	+/−	−	−	+	−/+	−	−	−	+/−	−	−	−	−	−	−	−	−	−	−
Lactose	−	−	+/−	−	−	+	−	+/−	−	−	−	−	−	−	−	−	−	−	−	−	−
Maltose	−	−	+/−	−	+	+	+/−	+/−	−	−	−/+	−	−	−	−	−	−	−	−	+	−
42° C	+	−	+/−	+	+/−	+	+	−	+	+/−	−	+	+/−	−/+	−	+	+/−	−/+	+/−	+/−	+/−
Esculin	−	−	−/+	−	+	+/−	−	+	−	−	−	−	−	−	−	−	−	−	−	+	−
Urea	+	−/+	+/−	−	+/−	−/+	−/+	−/+	+/−	+	−	−	−/+	−	+	+	−/+	+/−	−	−	+/−
DNase	−	−	−	−	+	−	−	+	−	−	−	−	−	−	−	−	−	+	+	−	+
ONPG	−	−	+/−	−	+	−	−	+/−	−	−	−	−	−	−	−	−	−	−	−	−	−
Indole	−	−	−	−	−	−	−	−	−	−	−	−	−	−	−	−	−	−	−	−	−
Motility	+	+	+	+	+	+	+	−	+	+	+	+	+	+	+	+	+	+	+	+	+
Flagella	1	>1	>1	P	>1	>1	1	1	1	1	>1	1	P	P	P	P	1	1	1	>1	1
H₂S	−	−	−	−	−	−	−	−	−	−	−	−	−	−	−	−	−	−	−	−	+
N₂ gas	+/−	−	−	−	−	+	+	−	+	−/+	−	−	+	+/−	+	−	−	−	−	−	−
Pigment	B,F,G	F	Y	−	Y	−	B,Y	Y	−	−	−	−	−	−	−	−	−	−	B,Y	−	B
Growth on MAC	+	+	+	+	+	+	+	−	+	+	+	+	+	+	+	+	+	+	−/+	+/−	+

Figure 18-5

Continued

Biochemical and morphologic characteristics of selected nonfermentative gram-negative bacilli. (Data from Ohio State University Hospital.)

| | NONMOTILE, PIGMENTED, INDOLE-POSITIVE NONFERMENTERS | | | | NONMOTILE COCCOBACILLI | | |
| | | | | | | Oxidase negative | |
	Chryseobacterium (Flavobacterium) meningosepticum	*Flavobacterium odoratum*	*Weeksella zoohelcum*	*Weeksella virosa*	*Moraxella sp.*	*Acinetobacter lwoffii*	*Acinetobacter baumannii*
Oxidase	+	+	+	+	+	−	−
Pyocyanin	−	−	−	−	−	−	−
Fluorescein	−	−	−	−	−	−	−
Glucose	+/−	−	−	−	−	−	+
Xylose	−	−	−	−	−	−	+
Mannitol	−/+	−	−	−	−	−	−
Lactose	−	−	−	−	−	−	+
Maltose	−/+	−	−	−	−	+/−	−
42° C	+/−	−	−	−/+	−/+	−	+
Esculin	+	−	−	−	−	−	−
Urea	−/+	+	+	−/+	−	−/+	−/+
DNase	+	+	+	+	−	−	−/+
ONPG	+/−	−	−	−	−	−	−
Indole	+	−	−/+	+	−	−	−
Motility	−	−	−	−	−	−	−
Flagella	−	−	−	−	−	−	−
H₂S	−	−	−	−	−	−	−
N₂ gas	−	−/+	−	−	−	−	−
Pigment	Y	Y	B	B	−	−	−
Growth on MAC	+	+	−	−	+/−	+	+

Flagella

1, Polar monotrichous.

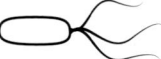

>1, Polar tuft (>1 flagellum).

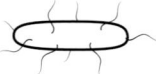

P, Peritrichous.

Figure 18-5, cont'd

For legend see p. 545.

MOST COMMONLY ENCOUNTERED NONFERMENTATIVE ORGANISMS

The Pseudomonads

The genus *Pseudomonas* accounts for a large percentage of nonfermenters isolated in the clinical microbiology laboratory (Table 18-2). Characteristics common to the **pseudomonads** are as follows:

- Gram-negative bacillus or coccobacillus
- Motile with polar or polar tufts of flagella (except *Pseudomonas mallei*)
- Oxidase and catalase positive
- Usually grows on MacConkey agar
- Usually oxidizes carbohydrates

Pseudomonas aeruginosa

Pseudomonas aeruginosa is the most commonly reported isolate of the genus. It is an uncommon part of normal flora; only 4% to 12% of humans carry it as part of normal fecal flora. It may, however, account for 5% to 15% of nosocomial infections.

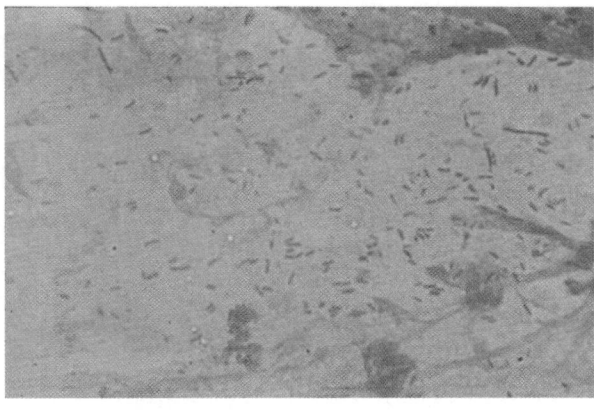

Figure 18-6 _____

Gram stain of bronchial specimen positive for a nonfermentative gram-negative bacillus (e.g., *Pseudomonas aeruginosa*).

CLINICAL INFECTIONS

The clinical diseases documented to be caused by *P. aeruginosa* include bacteremia with ecthyma gangrenosum of the skin; wound infections; pulmonary disease; especially among individuals with cystic fibrosis; nosocomial urinary tract infections; endocarditis; infections after burns; and, in rare cases, central nervous system diseases, including meningitis.

Other conditions associated with *P. aeruginosa* infection are otitis externa, in particular, in swimmers or divers, and a necrotizing skin rash, referred to as *jacuzzi* or *hot tub syndrome,* that develops in users of these recreational facilities. The organisms have a propensity to invade vascular walls of vessels, which further their spread in the body. *P. aeruginosa* accounts for 6.2% of all bacteremias and up to 75% of nosocomial bacteremias. Poor prognostic factors associated with *P. aeruginosa* bacteremia include septic shock granulocytopenia, inappropriate antibiotic therapy, and the presence of septic metastases. In the case described at the beginning of the chapter, *P. aeruginosa* was the identified organism from the blood cultures. Figure 18-6 illustrates the Gram stain of a bronchial specimen containing *P. aeruginosa.*

VIRULENCE FACTORS

P. aeruginosa may produce a variety of factors that lend to its pathogenicity, such as endotoxin, proteases, hemolysin, "slime," lecithinase, elastase, coagulase, DNase, and exotoxin.

TABLE 18-2 _____

Members of Pseudomonas *Genus and Others Whose Names Have Been Changed*

Species	Characteristic(s) of Interest or Distinction
Pseudomonas aeruginosa	Blue-green pigment Grapelike odor
Pseudomonas alcaligenes	
Burkholderia (Pseudomonas) cepacia	Most common isolate
Brevundimonas (Pseudomonas) diminuta	Often in patients with cystic fibrosis
Pseudomonas fluorescens	
Burkholderia (Pseudomonas) gladioli	Fluorescent pigments
Pseudomonas mallei	
Pseudomonas mendocina	Animal pathogen (glanders)
Sphingomonas (Pseudomonas) paucimobilis	
Pseudomonas petucinogena	Yellow pigment
Ralstonia (Pseudomonas) pickettii	
Pseudomonas pseudoalcaligenes	
Burkholderia (Pseudomonas) pseudomallei	Cause of melioidosis
Pseudomonas putida	Fluorescent pigment
Pseudomonas stutzeri	Wrinkled colonies
Brevundimonas (Pseudomonas) vesicularis	
Pseudomonas, CDC Group 1	

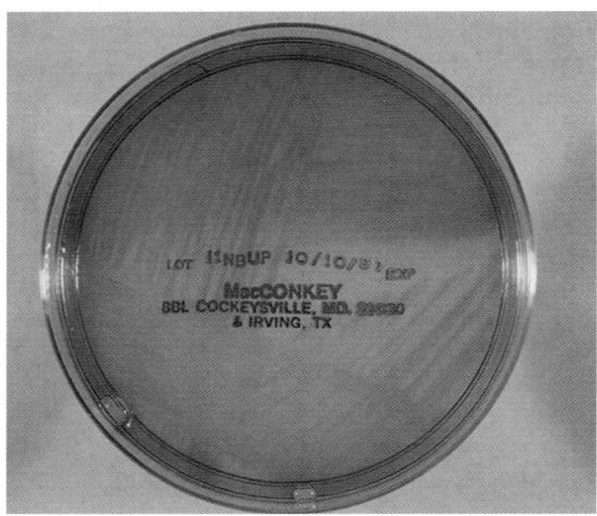

Figure 18-7 _____

Pseudomonas aeruginosa on MacConkey agar. Note blue-green pigment.

IDENTIFYING CHARACTERISTICS

Most isolates are β-hemolytic on sheep's blood agar and produce a characteristic green metallic sheen resulting from the presence of the pigment **pyocyanin.** On MacConkey agar (Figure 18-7), pyocyanin causes colonies of *P. aeruginosa* to appear blue-green. Some strains appear mucoid on blood agar; others may not (Figure 18-8). Pyocyanin is easy to detect on most media, with most strains, but can be specifically determined in media such as Sellers and fluorescent-nitrate (FN) medium. No other strain of a gram-negative nonfermenter produces pyocyanin, so its production is a characteristic used to differentially identify *P. aeruginosa.* Pyocyanin typing can be used to differentiate between strains of *P. aeruginosa* that are of epidemiologic interest. About 4% of clinical strains, however, are apyocyanogenic.

Most *P. aeruginosa* strains also produce **pyoverdin,** a fluorescent pigment that can be detected on Sellers or FN medium. Pyoverdin is produced by other species of *Pseudomonas,* including *Pseudomonas fluorescens,* and *Pseudomonas putida.*

Many strains of *P. aeruginosa* produce a fruity, grapelike odor caused by the presence of **2-aminoacetophenone.** Other key characteristics of *P. aeruginosa* are as follows:

- Gluconate production from glucose via oxidation
- Arginine dihydrolase (ADH) positive
- Growth at 42° C
- Cetrimide positive
- Citrate positive
- Acetamide utilization

TREATMENT

P. aeruginosa is usually resistant to many antibiotics, including penicillin, ampicillin, many cephalo-

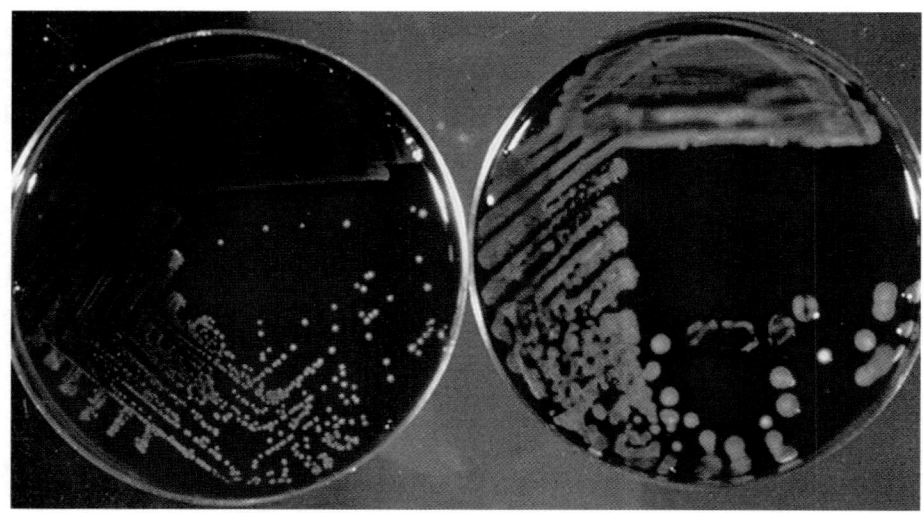

Figure 18-8 _____

Pseudomonas aeruginosa on sheep blood agar. *Left,* Nonmucoid colonies. *Right,* Mucoid colonies. Note discoloration of media, especially on the left.

sporins, and chloramphenicol. It is also usually susceptible to the aminoglycosides, semisynthetic penicillins such as piperacillin, and azlocillin, the third-generation cephalosporins, ceftazidime, and imipenem. Treatment of severe infections with *P. aeruginosa* usually requires double-drug therapy (e.g., ceftazidime with tobramycin or piperacillin with tobramycin).

Pseudomonas fluorescens and *Pseudomonas putida*

Pseudomonas fluorescens and *Pseudomonas putida* are members of the fluorescent group of pseudomonads, along with *P. aeruginosa,* that produce pyoverdin. Neither *P. putida* nor *P. fluorescens* produces pyocyanin or grows at 42° C, differentiating them from *P. aeruginosa.* As to differentiating between the two, *P. putida* is gelatin hydrolysis negative and *P. fluorescens* is positive. They are both of low virulence, rarely causing clinical diseases. Both have been isolated from respiratory cultures, contaminated blood bank products, urine, cosmetics, hospital equipment, and fluids. Both have been documented, although rarely, as causes of urinary tract infections, abscesses (postsurgical), empyema, septic arthritis, and other wound infections. They are, in general, susceptible to aminoglycosides, polymyxin, and piperacillin, but they are resistant to carbenicillin.

Stenotrophomonas maltophilia

S. maltophilia is the third most common nonfermentative gram-negative bacillus isolated in the clinical laboratory. Before 1983, it was believed to be a member of the pseudomonads, it was later reclassified as a member of the plant pathogen genus *Xanthomonas.* Now, because of its genetic sequencing, it is classified as a member of the *Stenotrophomonas* genus. Isolates are fairly ubiquitous in the environment, being common to water, sewage, and plant materials; likewise, the organism is common to the hospital environment, where it is found as a contaminant in blood-drawing equipment, disinfectants, transducers, and the like. *S. maltophilia* is not considered part of the normal human flora, but it may colonize hospitalized patients, especially those who undergo procedures that expose them to contaminated equipment or to antibiotics to which *S. maltophilia* may be resistant. These antimicrobials include cephalosporins, penicillins, imipenem, and aminogly-

cosides. *S. maltophilia* may be susceptible to sulfamethoxazole/trimethoprim (SXT) and possibly ticarcillin-clavulanate or piperacillin/tazobactam.

Clinically, *S. maltophilia* isolated from clinical specimens is initially regarded as a saprophyte or colonizer. With the increased use of agents to which it alone is innately resistant, however, more and more reports of disease production can be attributed to this organism. There are reports of pneumonia; endocarditis (especially in a setting of prior IV drug abuse and/or heart surgery); wound infections, including cellulitis and ecthyma gangrenosum; bacteremia; and, rarely, meningitis and urinary tract infections. Almost all these infections have occurred in a nosocomial setting. Pseudoinfections have also occurred as a result of contaminated collection tubes or cups (e.g., blood collection tubes). The single most important risk factor in the affected individuals was the presence of a venous catheter. Most patients with bacteremia responded well to therapy, unless they had concomitant pneumonia or shock.

IDENTIFYING CHARACTERISTICS

Isolates of *S. maltophilia* can be recognized as nonfermentative gram-negative bacilli with a negative oxidase reaction. In addition, they are positive for catalase, DNase, esculin, and gelatin hydrolysis and for the presence of lysine decarboxylase.

Acinetobacter Species

The genus *Acinetobacter,* in the family Neisseriaceae, consists of 12 DNA hybridization groups (genospecies). Two genospecies are the most common clinical isolates: *Acinetobacter baumannii* (previously referred to as *Acinetobacter calcoaceticus* var. *anitratus*) and *Acinetobacter lwoffii* (previously referred to as *A. calcoaceticus* var. *lwoffii*). The genus has had many synonyms over the years, including *Mima, Herellea,* and even *Diplococcus.*

The *Acinetobacter* species are ubiquitous in the environment (e.g., soil, water, milk, frozen soups) and in the hospital (e.g., ventilators, humidifiers, catheters). About 25% of adults have skin colonization with an *Acinetobacter* spp., and 7% carry the organism in their pharynx. Hospitalized patients may become easily colonized if they were not already harboring the organisms, and thus *Acinetobacter* spp. may be considered insignificant when isolated from urine, feces, vaginal secretions, and many different types of respiratory specimens. As many as 45% of tracheostomy sites may be colonized.

CLINICAL INFECTIONS

These organisms are opportunistic and account for 1% to 3% of all nosocomial infections. *Acinetobacter* species are second only to *P. aeruginosa* in frequency of isolation in the clinical microbiology laboratory. Diseases for which they have been reported responsible include urinary tract infections, pneumonia and/or tracheobronchitis, endocarditis (with up to a 22% associated mortality), septicemia, meningitis (often as a complication of intrathecal chemotherapy for cancer), and cellulitis, most often as a result of contaminated indwelling catheters, trauma, burns, or introduction of a foreign body.

Eye infections caused by *Acinetobacter,* including endophthalmitis, conjunctivitis, and corneal ulcerations, have been reported in the literature. Most of the diseases produced by members of the genus *Acinetobacter* are caused by *A. baumannii* (Figure 18-9). *A. Iwoffii* is less virulent, and its isolation most often indicates contamination or colonization rather than infection.

Isolates of *Acinetobacter* spp., particularly *A. baumannii,* are often resistant to many antimicrobials, including penicillins and first- and second-generation cephalosporins. They demonstrate variable susceptibility to aminoglycosides, imipenem, and aztreonam in vitro.

IDENTIFYING CHARACTERISTICS

Members of the genus *Acinetobacter* have the following cultural and biochemical traits in common. They are all coccobacilli, oxidase negative, catalase positive, and **nonmotile.** *Acinetobacter* organisms possess few growth requirements and thus are capable of growing on most laboratory media, including MacConkey agar. One characteristic feature of this organism is the purplish hue it produces on MacConkey agar. Isolates usually grow better at 30° C than 37° C and at a pH of 5.5 to 6.0. *A. baumannii* species are saccharolytic, and *A. Iwoffii* species are nonsaccharolytic. The purplish hue produced on this medium may cause the species to resemble a lactose-fermenting organism.

Other Pseudomonads
Pseudomonas stutzeri

An initial clue to the identity of *Pseudomonas stutzeri* is its macroscopic appearance—a wrinkled, leathery, adherent colony that may produce a light yellow or brown pigment. Like most members of the family Pseudomonadaceae, it is a saprophyte but has been found to produce a variety of diseases in patients who have septicemia, pneumonia, and endocarditis and surgical patients with wound infections, septic arthritis, conjunctivitis, or urinary tract infections. Isolates in vitro are usually susceptible to aminoglycosides, SXT, ampicillin and polymyxin, tetracyclines, quinolones,

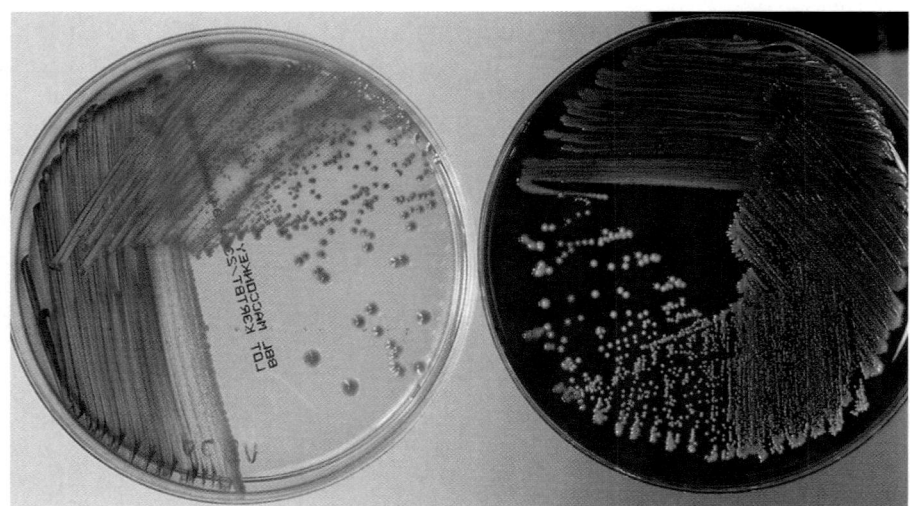

Figure 18-9

Acinetobacer baumannii is saccharolytic, which may cause it to resemble a lactose-fermenting organism on MacConkey agar *(left); A. baumannii* colonies on BAP *(right).*

and third-generation cephalosporins but resistant to chloramphenicol and the first- and second-generation cephalosporins.

Pseudomonas mendocina

Pseudomonas mendocina resembles a nonpigmented *P. aeruginosa* but is acetamide and 2-ketogluconate negative. The organisms are motile by means of a single polar flagellum, oxidize glucose and xylose, grow on MacConkey agar, are positive for oxidase and ADH, and are nonproteolytic. They are found in soil and water and are rarely isolated from humans; if so, they are usually contaminants.

Pseudomonas pseudoalcaligenes, Pseudomonas alcaligenes, and CDC Group 1

One group of pseudomonads, consisting of *Pseudomonas pseudoalcaligenes, Pseudomonas alcaligenes,* and CDC Group 1, are asaccharolytic and oxidase positive. They all grow on MacConkey agar and may or may not reduce nitrates. They differ in their ability to grow at 42° C; *P. pseudoalcaligenes* does, *P. alcaligenes* does not, and CDC Group 1 shows variable growth at this temperature.

Pseudomonads and Other Nonfermenters Whose Names Have Been Changed

Table 18-3 lists the present taxonomy of many nonfermenters to help clarify terminology changes. Box 18-2 summarizes observed characteristics that are common to most nonfermenters.

Burkholderia cepacia (Pseudomonas cepacia)

Burkholderia cepacia has been called *Pseudomonas multivorans, Pseudomonas kingii,* and EO-1. It is a plant pathogen that often attacks onion bulbs.

Clinically, *B. cepacia* is a low-grade, nosocomial pathogen that has most often been associated with pneumonia in patients with cystic fibrosis (CF). It has also been reported to cause endocarditis, specifically in drug addicts, pneumonitis, urinary tract infections, osteomyelitis, dermatitis, and other wound infections resulting from use of contaminated water. It has been isolated from irrigation fluids, anesthetics, nebulizers, detergents, and disinfectants. Research supports the association of *B. cepacia* and increased severity of disease and death in patients with CF. *B. cepacia* is usually susceptible to chloramphenicol, ceftazidime, and SXT

TABLE 18-3

Taxonomic Changes for Some Nonfermenters

New Taxonomy	Old Taxonomy
Alcaligenes faecalis	*Alcaligenes odorans/faecalis*
Alcaligenes xylosoxidans ssp. denitrificans	*Alcaligenes denitrificans,* CDC Group Vc
Alcaligenes xylosoxidans ssp. xylosoxidans	*Achromobacter xylosoxidans,* CDC Group III a,b
Chryseomonas luteola	*Pseudomonas luteola,* CDC Group Ve-1
Chryseobacterium meningosepticum	*Flavobacterium meningosepticum/F. indolgenes*
Comamonas acidovorans	*Pseudomonas acidovorans*
Comamonas testosteroni	*Pseudomonas testosteroni*
Flavimonas oryzihabitans	*Pseudomonas oryzihabitans*
Flavo sp. IIe	CDC Group IIe
Flavo sp. IIh	CDC Group IIh
Flavo sp. IIi	CDC Group IIi
Flavobacterium gleum	CDC Group IIb
Flavobacterium indologenes	CDC Group IIa
Methylobacterium spp.	*Pseudomonas mesophilica*
Ochrobactrum anthropi	*Achromobacter* spp. biovar. 1,2; Vd-1,2
Oligella ureolytica	CDC Group IV-e
Oligella urethralis	*Moraxella urethralis*
Pseudomonas gladioli	*Pseudomonas marginata*
Pseudomonas mendocina	CDC Vb-2
Pseudomonas pickettii	*Pseudomonas thomasii,* Va-1,2 *Pseudomonas pseudoalcaligenes,* biovar 2
Psychrobacter immobilis	*Micrococcus cryophilus*
Shewanella putrefaciens	*Pseudomonas putrefaciens*
Sphingobacterium multivorum	*Flavobacterium multivorum,* IIk-2
Sphingobacterium spiritivorum	*Flavobacterium spiritivorum,* IIk-3
Weeksella virosa	CDC Group IIf (Flavo IIf)
Weeksella zoohelcum	CDC Group IIj (Flavo IIj)
Stenotrophomonas maltophilia	*Pseudomonas (Xanthomonas) maltophilia*
Empedobacter brevis	*Flavobacterium breve*
Myroides odoratus	*Flavobacterium odoratum*

Modified from Gilardi GI: Update on taxonomy of nonfastidious glucose-nonfermenting gram-negative bacilli, *Clin Microbiol Newsl* 12:73, 1990.

but resistant to aminoglycosides, polymyxins, many cephalosporins, and penicillins. Resistance may develop quite rapidly.

The organism grows well on most laboratory media but may lose viability on blood agar in 3 to 4 days without appropriate transfers. Selective media are available that increase recovery of *B. cepacia* from respiratory specimens in patients with CF. Other isolates of *Pseudomonas* sp. may also be recovered, but a selective medium does help to re-

Box 8-2

Characteristics Common to Groups of Nonfermenters

Pigmentation

Yellow

Flavobacterium sp. (fermenter)
Sphingomonas paucimobilis
Chryseomonas luteola
Flavimonas oryzihabitans
Sphingobacterium sp.
Pseudomonas stutzeri (light yellow)

Pink

Methylobacterium sp.

Purple (MacConkey agar)

Acinetobacter sp.

Blue-green

Pseudomonas aeruginosa

Violet

Chromobacterium violaceum (fermenter)

Lavender to lavender-green (blood agar)

Flavobacterium sp.
Stenotrophomonas maltophilia

Tan (occasionally)

P. stutzeri
Shewanella putrefaciens

Wrinkled Colonies

P. stutzeri
Burkholderia pseudomallei

Odors

Sweet

Alcaligenes faecalis
Myroides odoratus
P. aeruginosa (grapes)

Popcorn

EO-4
EF-4ab

Nonmotile

Acinetobacter sp.
Moraxella sp.
Flavobacterium sp. (fermenter)
Sphingobacterium sp. (May "glide")
Oligella sp. (non-*ureolytica*)

Oxidase Negative

Acinetobacter sp.
S. maltophilia
Chryseomonas sp.
Flavimonas sp.
Burkholderia cepacia (+/−)

H₂S Positive

Shewanella putrefaciens

Courtesy Anne Morrissey (Cleveland, OH), George
Manuselis, and Connie Mahon.

duce normal flora overgrowth. The preferred temperature is 30° C. Unlike other members of the genus *Pseudomonas, B. cepacia* may be oxidase negative. It utilizes glucose, maltose, lactose, and mannitol and is lysine decarboxylase (LDC) positive, ornithine decarboxylase (ODC) positive, and arginine dihydrolase (ADH) negative. Isolates are motile by means of polar tufts of flagella. It does not fluoresce like *P. aeruginosa,* but it does produce a nonfluorescing yellow or green pigment that may diffuse into the media. Colonies of *B. cepacia* are nonwrinkled, and this trait may be used to differentiate isolates from *P. stutzeri,* which also produces a yellow pigment.

Burkholderia gladioli (Pseudomonas gladioli)

A plant pathogen, *Burkholderia gladioli* resembles *B. cepacia* and may be mistaken for it. Isolates have been found in cystic fibrosis patients, but these organisms are more susceptible to antimicrobials than *B. cepacia.* A yellow pigment may be produced. These organisms are **motile** by means of one or two polar flagella and are catalase and urease positive. *B. gladioli* organisms oxidize glucose, are mannitol positive and decarboxylase negative, are positive for growth on MacConkey agar, and are 100% resistant to polymyxin. *B. gladioli* produces variable results with oxidase and nitrate reduction, but results are usually negative.

Burkholderia pseudomallei (Pseudomonas pseudomallei)

Clinically, *Burkholderia pseudomallei* is important because it can cause melioidosis, an aggressive granulomatous pulmonary disease caused by ingestion, inhalation, or inoculation of the organisms with further metastatic abscess formation in lungs and other viscera. Overwhelming septicemia may occur. The incubation period in vivo may be prolonged. The organisms are found in water and muddy soils in Southeast Asia (including Vietnam and Thailand), Northern Australia, and Mexico. Local infections, including orbital cellulitis, dacrocystitis, and draining abscesses, may occur. Although isolates may be susceptible in vitro to many antibiotics, including SXT, chloramphenicol, tetracycline, semisynthetic penicillins, and ceftazidime, the clinical response to therapy is usually slow, and relapses are common. Those who have traveled to endemic areas are at risk for infection with *B. pseudomallei*. This organism should be considered especially when a nonfermentative, wrinkled colony is isolated (Figure18-10) that demonstrates bipolar staining on Gram-stained smears. *P. stutzeri,* which may also appear as wrinkled colonies, does not utilize lactose, in contrast to *B. pseudomallei,* which oxidizes lactose.

Sphingomonas paucimobilis (Pseudomonas paucimobilis)

A yellow-pigmented pseudomonad, *Sphingomonas paucimobilis* does not grow on MacConkey agar and requires more than 48 hours for culture on blood agar. Although isolates have been found to produce esterases, endotoxin, lipases, and phosphatases, inherent virulence is limited, and most isolates must be regarded as colonizers or contaminants. This organism can be isolated environmentally from water, including that in swimming pools, as well as from hospital equipment and laboratory supplies.

Documented *S. paucimobilis* infections include peritonitis associated with chronic ambulatory peritoneal dialysis (CAPD), septicemia, meningitis, leg ulcer, empyema, and splenic and brain abscesses. Isolates demonstrate variable resistance to antibiotics, although most are susceptible to aminoglycosides; quinolones; third-generation cephalosporins such as ceftazidime, ceftriaxone, and ceftizoxime; SXT; and ampicillin.

Brevundimonas diminuta (Pseudomonas diminuta)

Brevundimonas diminuta has been found in blood, cerebrospinal fluid (CSF), urine, and wounds; it is usually considered a contaminant. The isolates are motile and possess a short wavelength on their single polar flagellum. *B. diminuta* oxidizes glucose; is indole negative and oxidase positive, and may produce a brown, water-soluble pigment on heart infusion agar with tyrosine added. In vitro the organism demonstrates resistance to ampicillin, cefoxitin, and nalidixic acid.

Brevundimonas vesicularis (Pseudomonas vesicularis)

Like *B. diminuta*, *Brevundimonas vesicularis* is a slender rod, with short-wavelength polar flagella. About 15% of *B. vesicularis* strains may produce a yellow pigment, and some may produce a tan pigment when grown on media with tyrosine. *B. vesicularis* is oxidase positive and oxidizes glucose and maltose. Isolates have been found clinically in CSF, blood, urine, and eye specimens, but like *B. diminuta* and other members of miscellaneous pseudomonads, they usually are colonizers or contaminants.

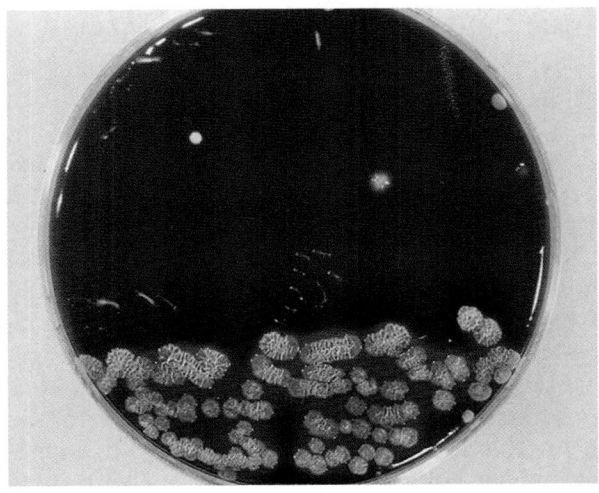

Figure 18-10 ⸻

Burkholderia pseudomallei on sheep blood agar.

Ralstonia pickettii (Pseudomonas picketti)

Isolates of *Ralstonia pickettii* can be found contaminating sterile hospital fluids and, as such, may be isolated from human specimens such as those from urine, nasopharynx, abscesses, wounds, and blood, usually as colonizers or contaminants. These isolates are oxidase, catalase, and urease positive; grow on MacConkey agar; reduce nitrate; oxidize glucose and xylose; and are motile by means of a single polar flagellum. They are susceptible to most agents, except for the aminoglycosides and polymyxin.

Shewanella putrefaciens (Pseudomonas putrefaciens)

Pseudomonas putrefaciens is now *Shewanella putrefaciens* and is a member of "Unknown RNA Homology Group Affiliation." *S. putrefaciens* produces profuse H_2S on TSI agar, possibly resembling H_2S producers of the family Enterobacteriaceae. The oxidase test should differentiate *Shewanella* from the other group. This isolate also produces reddish brown or pink colonies that are often mucoid. Rarely pathogenic, isolates can be obtained from abscesses and traumatic ulcers, but are usually colonizers. Environmental sources such as stagnant water, natural gas, petroleum brine, and spoiled dairy products may contain *S. putrefaciens*. The organisms are usually susceptible to ampicillin, tetracycline, chloramphenicol, erythromycin, and the aminoglycosides.

Comamonas species

Comamonas species was once referred to as *Pseudomonas acidovorans* or *Pseudomonas testosteroni*. These organisms resemble vibrios or spirillum-like bacteria, produce alkalinity in a blue OF media, are usually motile by multitrichous polar flagella, and accumulate hydroxybutyrate. Ubiquitous in soil and water, *Comamonas* species are rarely isolated from clinical specimens but have been found in hospital equipment and fluids. Rarely, isolates reportedly have caused a nosocomial bacteremia, corneal ulcerations, endocarditis in intravenous drug abusers, sepsis, and pyoarthrosis. *Comamonas acidovorans* may be more resistant than other members of the genus, having demonstrated resistance to aminoglycosides. *Acidovorax* is the genus of nonfermenters formerly called *Pseudomonas faecalis* and *Pseudomonas delafieldi,* among other names. These organisms are motile and utilize carbohydrates oxidatively.

Methylobacterium extorquens

Methylobacterium extorquens, formerly *Pseudomonas mesophilica,* produces a characteristic pink to coral pigment, prefers a lower temperature (25°-35° C), produces distinctive vacuoles, and utilizes methanol (hence the newer nomenclature). Isolates are often first seen on fungal media, such as Sabouraud agar, and do not grow as well on blood or chocolate agar. Buffered charcoal yeast extract is also a good medium for their recovery.

Epidemiologically, *M. extorquens* organisms are isolated from soil, sewage, water, and hospital nebulizers and can also be isolated from clinical specimens such as throat swabs and bronchial and even blood specimens. Clinically, these organisms have been reported to cause bacteremia (one case) and skin ulcers. Contaminated tap water has been implicated as a cause of positive blood cultures in a patient receiving irrigations who had recently undergone a bone marrow transplant procedure. The only other pink-pigmented nonfermentative bacilli are a group of coccoid bacteria now classified in the *Roseomonas* genus. These bacteria have been isolated from blood, CSF, sputum, and wounds as well as the environment. Distinguishing them from *Methylobacterium* sp. may be difficult. *Roseomonas* sp. are unable to oxidize methanol or assimilate acetamide. On Sabouraud's agar, they produce pink, mucoid colonies; however, they do not appear black under ultraviolet light as do the *Methylobacterium* sp.

MISCELLANEOUS NONFERMENTING GRAM-NEGATIVE BACILLI

Nonfermenters with Peritrichous Flagellation

Alcaligenes species

The family Alcaliginaceae includes species of *Alcaligenes* and *Bordetella*. The *Alcaligenes* genus includes the following species: *Alcaligenes faecalis (odorans), Alcaligenes piechaudii, Alcaligenes xylosoxidans* ssp. *xylosoxidans,* and ssp. *denitrificans.*

Isolates of *Alcaligenes* are found in water (e.g. swimming pools, tap water, dialysis fluids) and are resistant to disinfectants such as chlorhexidine and quaternary ammonium compounds. They are isolated in specimens from hospitalized patients such as urine, feces, sputum, and wounds. *A. faecalis* has been isolated from blood of patients with and without septicemia. *A. xylosoxidans* ssp. *xylosoxidans* has been associated with otitis media, meningitis, pneumonia, surgical wound infections, urinary tract infections, peritonitis, and bacteremia.

A. piechaudii was reportedly isolated from ear discharge from a patient with diabetes. Gram-stained smears of the exudate were positive for gram-negative bacilli and gram-positive cocci. Both coagulase-negative staphylococci and *A. piechaudii* were repeatedly isolated. The patient recovered once the diabetes was stabilized.

All *Alcaligenes* species possess peritrichous flagella (Figure 18-11), are oxidase positive, usually are nonsaccharolytic, and are obligately aerobic and gram-negative. These organisms usually grow well on most laboratory media, including MacConkey agar. In OF media, most are nonoxidative and produce a deep blue color at the top, except for *A. xylosoxidans* ssp. *xylosoxidans* organisms, which produce an acid reaction in both glucose and xylose (hence the name). All species reduce nitrates to nitrites; both the subspecies of *A. xylosoxidans* and *A. faecalis* can further reduce nitrites to nitrogen gas. Isolates of *Alcaligenes* species are negative for indole production and for esculin and gelatin hydrolysis.

Isolates of members of the genus *Alcaligenes* are usually susceptible to SXT, piperacillin, ticarcillin, carbenicillin, ceftazidime, cefoperazone, and quinolones (although variably). Resistance to the aminoglycosides is common. In addition, *A. piechaudii* may be susceptible to amoxicillin.

Agrobacterium species

The genus *Agrobacterium* is a group of nonfermentative, peritrichously motile plant pathogens that are ubiquitous in soil and water. Three species are known to infect plants: *Agrobacterium tumefaciens,* the cause of crown gall, *Agrobacterium rhizogenes,* the cause of hairy root disease, and *Agrobacterium rubi,* the cause of cane gall. A vari-

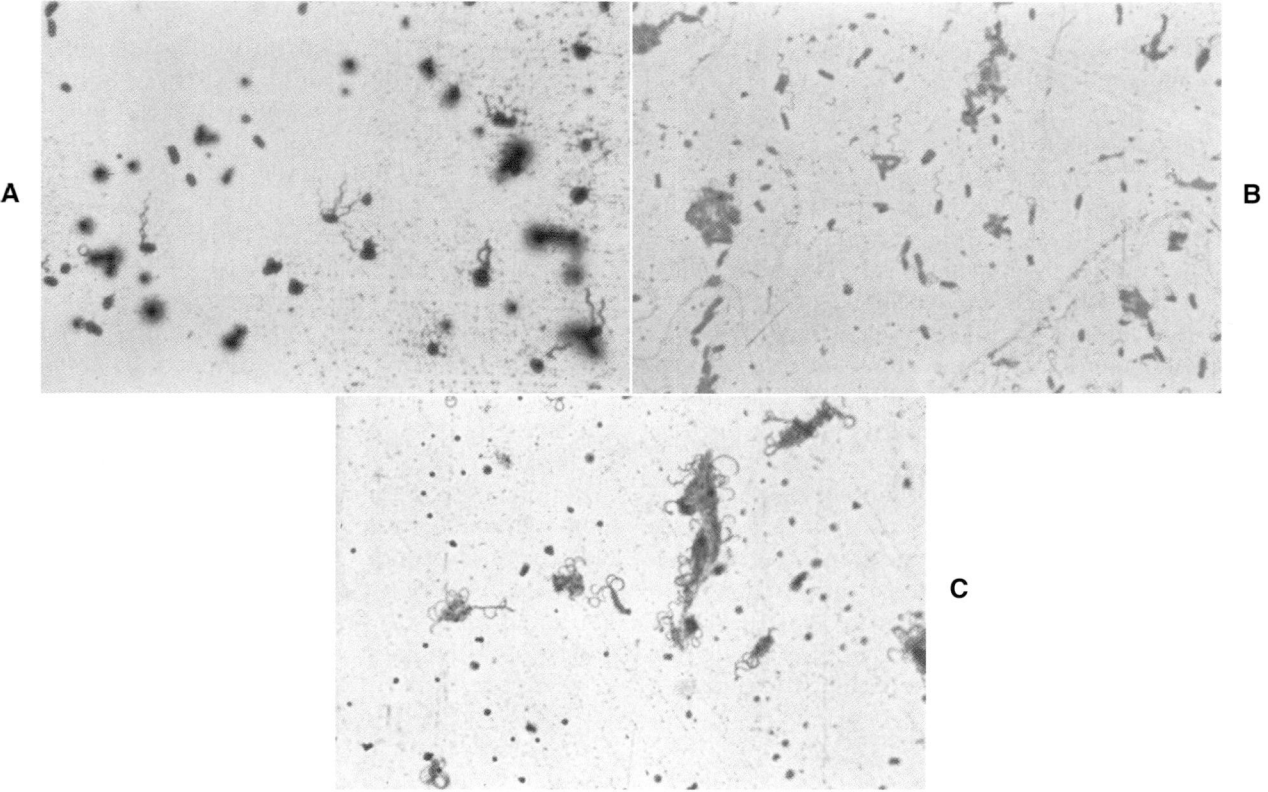

Figure 18-11

Flagella stains of gram-negative bacilli. **A,** Peritrichous flagella (e.g., *Alcaligenes* sp.). **B,** Polar, monotrichous (e.g., *Pseudomonas aeruginosa.* **C,** Polar, multitrichous (e.g., *Comamonas* sp.).

ant of *Agrobacterium tumefaciens, Agrobacterium radiobacter,* is the only member of the genus isolated from human clinical specimens. It has been found in sputum, pleural fluid, synovial fluid, and urine. At one time, this isolate was referred to as *Vd-3.* Infections by the organism have included prosthetic valve endocarditis, septicemia (with pneumonia), and three cases of catheter-related infection.

Isolates of *A. radiobacter* can be recognized by the characteristic production of 3-ketolactone, which is due to the oxidation of lactose at the C-3 glycerol moiety. *A. radiobacter* organisms are oxidase positive, produce H_2S (using lead acetate strips), have peritrichous flagella, and produce positive results when tested for esculin hydrolysis and urease (to differentiate from *Alcaligenes* sp.).

A related group of yellow-pigmented *Agrobacterium*-like, gram-negative bacilli exists; these organisms are also plant pathogens, but they have not yet been adequately characterized or named. Isolates of *Agrobacterium* sp. are usually resistant to penicillins, chloramphenicol, and cefazolin but susceptible to second- and third-generation cephalosporins, polymyxin, SXT, imipenem, and the aminoglycosides.

Oligella ureolytica

Oligella ureolytica (CDC Group IVe) belongs to a genus of bacteria that are nonoxidative, usually nonmotile, small, paired, gram-negative bacilli. They are isolated clinically from the genitourinary tract. *O. ureolytica* is unusual in the genus, because most isolates are motile by means of peritrichous flagella; hence the relationship to *Alcaligenes* sp. as well as to another genus, *Taylorella.* Isolates of *O. ureolytica* are urea positive and reduce nitrates to nitrites. They are also phenylalanine deaminase (PDA) positive, which helps differentiate them from *Alcaligenes* sp. Clinically, urine isolates of this organism have been documented, as well as one report of a blood culture isolate from a patient with obstructive uropathy in which the isolate was believed to be significant. Another species of *Oligella, Oligella urethralis,* is described later in this chapter.

CDC Group IVc-2

CDC Group IVc-2 organisms are morphologically similar to *O. ureolytica* but differ biochemically; they cannot reduce nitrates to nitrites and are PDA negative. They are most like the *Alcaligenes eutrophus* species. CDC IVc-2 is a motile, oxidase-positive, catalase-positive, asaccharolytic, gram-negative bacillus. Isolates are urease positive but negative for gelatin, esculin, and indole. They usually grow on MacConkey agar. Cases of septicemia in two patients undergoing CAPD have been reported. The organisms were isolated in mixed and pure cultures. Isolates are resistant to aminoglycosides, vancomycin, ampicillin, and first- and second-generation cephalosporins. They are usually susceptible to ciprofloxacin, third-generation cephalosporins, piperacillin, and doxycycline, although not many isolates have been tested.

Ochrobactrum anthropi

Ochrobactrum anthropi was at one time referred to as *Achromobacter* biovar 1, 2, or Vd-1, 2. Isolates are positive for oxidase, urease, and H_2S in addition to possessing peritrichous flagella. They are oxidative in OF medium. The organism has been isolated clinically from a case of bacteremia and from urinary tract infections in immunocompromised individuals. One report suggests the significance of *O. anthropi* in osteochondritis of the foot. Resistance has been demonstrated in vitro to chloramphenicol, tetracyclines, aztreonam, cephalosporins, and carbenicillin. Susceptibility has been shown to SXT and the aminoglycosides.

The *Bordetella* genus include the following species: *Bordetella pertussis* (the most common human isolates, usually from the respiratory tract); *Bordetella parapertussis, Bordetella bronchiseptica,* and three newer species, *Bordetella hinzii (A. faecalis), Bordetella trematum,* and *Bordetella holmesii* (CDC group NO-2). The latter is nonmotile and more clearly resembles members of the *Acinetobacter* genus. *B. pertussis* and *B. parapertussis* are also nonmotile. *B. hinzii* has rarely been isolated from blood and sputum; *B. trematum* from ear infections and wounds of humans. *B. holmesii* has been associated with bacteremia. All but *B. trematum* and *B. holmesii* are asaccharolytic and oxidase and urease negative and produce a brown pigment.

Nonmotile, Gram-Negative Bacilli
Flavobacterium species

The genus *Flavobacterium* has basically been renamed. The group consists of isolates of gram-negative, weakly fermentative bacilli that are ubiquitous in soil and water. They are not considered part of the normal human flora. Because isolates often contaminate hospital equipment, patients may become colonized while in the hospital. *Flavobacterium* species are thus responsible for a share of nosocomial nonfermentative, gram-negative infections. Even though the organisms are weak fermenters, the reactions are usually delayed, and the isolates initially appear to be nonfermenters.

Flavobacterium species are long, thin bacilli, often with bulbous ends. They are nonmotile and often possess a yellow intracellular pigment (especially prominent in IIb) (Figure 18-12). On media with blood a lavender-green discoloration of the agar may occur because of the proteolytic activity of the organisms. Some species release a characteristic fruity odor. Most are DNase positive, oxidase positive, and gelatin hydrolysis positive. All except *Flavobacterium odoratum* are indole positive, a distinctive characteristic that separates *Flavobacterium* from other species of nonfermenters. Clinically important species of the genus include *Flavobacterium indologenes*, *Flavobacterium meningosepticum*, *F. odoratum*, *Flavobacterium breve*, and unnamed species IIb, IIe, IIh, and IIi. The species IIb is more common in clinical specimens than all other flavobacteria. *Chryseobacterium* is the new genus name for *F. meningosepticum* and *F. indologenes*. *F. breve* is now called *Empedobacter brevis*, and *F. odoratum* has been renamed *Myroides odoratus*.

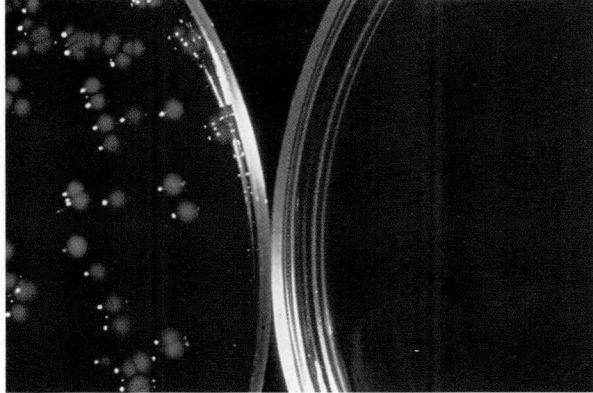

Figure 18-12 _____

Chryseobacterium meningosepticum. Note the growth with yellow pigment on blood agar *(left)* and absence of growth on MacConkey plate *(right).*

Most diseases produced by members of the genus *Flavobacterium* that have been reported are due to *Chryseobacterium meningosepticum.* The disease is typically a meningitis or septicemia in a newborn, especially in conjunction with prematurity. In adults, *C. meningosepticum* may cause pneumonia, endocarditis, bacteremia, and meningitis. Some species in vitro are susceptible to penicillin, which is also an unusual characteristic of gram-negative bacilli, including the nonfermenters. The response to other antibiotics is variable, and an in vitro susceptibility test is needed.

The previously unnamed *Flavobacterium* species, IIf and IIj, have been renamed as members of the genus *Weeksella*. These isolates are nonsaccharolytic and indole positive. *Weeksella virosa* (Flavo IIf) colonies may be mucoid or "slimy" and possess a yellow-green pigment. Isolates have been found from genitourinary specimens and will grow on Thayer-Martin or other *Neisseria gonorrhoeae*–selective media. *Bergeyella* (*Weeksella*) *zoohelicum* is nonmucoid, although its colonies may be sticky; it is urease positive and otherwise similar to *W. virosa*. It has been isolated from many sources, in particular from dog bite wounds.

Sphingobacterium species

Isolates of another genus, *Sphingobacterium*, were at one time regarded as members of the genus *Flavobacterium*. These isolates are aflagellate but do produce a gliding motility characteristic of the genus. They are oxidase, catalase, and esculin positive. Unlike *Flavobacterium* species they are indole negative. What is unique to the group is the presence of sphingophospholipids in the cell wall. They are truly fermenters and oxidize some carbohydrates. Growth on MacConkey agar is sparse to none, but these organisms will grow in the presence of 40% bile. Two species, *Sphingobacterium spiritovorum* and *Sphingobacterium multivorum*, are very similar biochemically, but *S. spiritovorum* produces acid from mannitol, ethanol, and rhamnose, and *S. multivorum* does not. Both produce a yellow pigment similar to that of isolates of *Chryseobacterium*, *Weeksella*, and *Empedobacter* species. Clinically, *S. multivorum* has been isolated from blood of patients with septicemia and from cases of peritonitis. *S. spiritovorum* has also been isolated from clinical specimens and from hospital environments.

There is another species in the genus *Sphingobacterium, Sphingobacterium mizutae,* formerly called *Flavobacterium mizutaii.* They are oxidase positive, indole negative, and esculin positive. *S. mizutae* has been isolated from a case of meningitis in premature birth. Most isolates of *Sphingobacterium* sp. are sensitive to SXT and resistant to penicillins, cephalosporins, aminoglycosides, clindamycin, and polymyxin.

Chryseomonas and *Flavimonas* and *Balneatrix* species

Chryseomonas luteola (formerly CDC Ve-1) and *Flavimonas oryzihabitans* (formerly CDC Ve-2) are gram-negative, nonfermentative, oxidase-negative bacilli. They both are catalase positive and motile, grow on MacConkey agar, and often produce a yellow pigment. *Flavimonas* species specifically may produce wrinkled or rough colonies at 48 hours. *C. luteola,* possessing multitrichous flagella, is positive for esculin, arginine, urease, and nitrate. *Flavimonas* organisms are negative for these biochemicals and possess a single polar flagellum. Both *Flavimonas* spp. and *Chryseomonas* spp. oxidize glucose and other sugars.

The natural habitat of species of *Flavimonas* and *Chryseomonas* is unknown, although *Flavimonas* organisms have been found in Japanese rice paddies and have been isolated from hospital drains and respiratory therapy equipment. These two organisms are rarely isolated from humans, but they have been isolated from wounds, abscesses, and blood cultures, as well as peritoneal fluid, from CAPD and other sources. *Flavimonas* and *Chryseomonas* organisms have been implicated in cases of bacteremia and peritonitis and possibly meningitis, although many times in association with each other or with other bacteria. *C. luteola* has been recovered as the only isolate from a case of prosthetic valve endocarditis and subdiaphragmatic abscess. *Flavimonas* organisms have been isolated from eye cultures and were described as the cause of "sticky eye" in one patient who responded to therapy appropriate for *Flavimonas.* There appears to be higher risk for infection by these organisms in the presence of foreign materials (e.g., catheters), corticosteroid use, and immunocompromised states.

Both *C. luteola* and *F. oryzihabitans* are susceptible to aminoglycosides, third-generation cephalosporins, ureidopenicillins, and quinolones. *Flavimonas* organisms are resistant to first- and second-generation cephalosporins but usually susceptible to penicillin. *C. luteola* is usually sensitive to cephalosporins and penicillin. Both demonstrate variable susceptibilities to tetracycline, chloramphenicol, and SXT. *Balneatrix alpica* is a curved to straight rod and is motile by polar flagella; colonies are pale yellow, becoming brown with age. No growth occurs on MacConkey agar. The isolates are positive for oxidase, indole, nitrate reduction, gelatin, and lecithinase. The organism oxidizes glucose, mannose, fructose, and other sugars. Isolates are usually susceptible to all β-lactams, aminoglycosides, SXT, quinolones, nalidixic acid, and tetracycline.

Moraxella, Moraxella-like genera, and *Oligella* species

Members of the genus *Moraxella* are strongly oxidase positive, nonmotile, and coccobacillary to bacillary gram-negative bacilli. They are, in general, biochemically inert with regard to carbohydrate oxidation and alkalinization. They are strictly aerobic and most often susceptible to penicillin, an unusual characteristic for the nonfermenters. These isolates are opportunists that reside on the mucous membranes of humans and lower animals and can be isolated as such from the respiratory tract, urinary tract, and eyes; however, they rarely cause disease in humans. Members of the genus *Moraxella* commonly encountered include the following:

- *Moraxella nonliquefaciens*
- *Moraxella lacunata*
- *Moraxella osloensis*
- *Moraxella phenylpyruvica*
- *Moraxella atlantae*

M. nonliquefaciens is the most commonly isolated member of the genus. It often resides as normal flora in the respiratory tract and rarely causes disease in humans. Rare cases of bacteremia, keratitis, and endophthalmitis caused by *M. nonliquefaciens* have been reported. The organism is gelatin hydrolysis negative and urease negative and does not usually grow on MacConkey agar. Its phenylalanine deaminase (PD) reaction is negative as well. *M. osloensis* is similar morphologically and biochemically to *M. nonliquefaciens;* unlike the latter, however, it grows and produces an alkaline reaction in acetate medium and acidifies ethanol. *M. osloensis* is found as normal flora in the genitourinary tract.

M. phenylpyruvica has been isolated from urine, blood, CSF, and the genitourinary tract. Unlike the others, it is urease positive and also PD positive. Similar to *M. phenylpyruvica* is *M. atlantae,* a more fastidious member of the genus that will, however, grow on MacConkey agar. It may also spread and pit the agar surfaces of the medium on which it grows. It is gelatin negative, PD negative, and nitrate negative. *M. lacunata,* a common conjunctival isolate, is a small coccobacillus that is usually gelatin positive, urease negative, and unable to grow on MacConkey agar. It may be PD positive.

M-5 and M-6 are two closely related strains of the *Moraxella* genus that are oxidase positive, nonmotile, asaccharolytic coccobacilli. M-5 has been isolated from wounds of animal bites. It is usually PD positive and gelatin positive and often produces a water-soluble yellow-tan pigment. It is nitrate negative but may reduce nitrites. The tentative name of these isolates is *Neisseria parelongata.* M-6 has been isolated from numerous body sites and implicated in cases of endocarditis and osteomyelitis. Unlike the other members of the *Moraxella* and *Moraxella*-like genera, M-6 is catalase negative. It usually does not grow on MacConkey agar. Its tentative name is *Neisseria elongata.* M-6 may be resistant to penicillin but, like most other isolates, is sensitive to the aminoglycosides, ampicillin, chloramphenicol, and many other antimicrobial agents.

Related to the genus *Moraxella* is the genus *Oligella.* Members of this genus include *O. urethralis,* formerly called *Moraxella urethralis.* These are PD, nitrate, and nitrite positive with gas formation, and gelatin negative. They are small coccoid organisms, most often isolated from the gastrointestinal tract. They usually do not grow on MacConkey agar, and unlike members of the genus *Moraxella,* they alkalinize citrate when the test is performed in an aerobic low-glucose peptone (ALP) slant. Unlike other members of the genus *Oligella* (e.g., *O. ureolytica*), *O. urethralis* does not oxidize sugars and is nonmotile (see earlier discussion under *O. ureolytica*).

Other Gram-Negative Nonfermenters

This section discusses a miscellaneous group of nonfermentative bacilli and fastidious gram-negative bacilli that are difficult to place in specific groups.

EO-2 and *Psychrobacter* species

EO-2

Isolates of EO-2 are coccoid, vacuolated, or peripherally staining O-shaped gram-negative bacteria in pairs, short chains, or packets. They are nonmotile, are mucoid on agar plates, and oxidize glucose, xylose, lactose, and mannitol. They do not always grow on MacConkey agar, are oxidase and catalase positive, and reduce nitrates to nitrites. EO-2 isolates are negative biochemically for indole, decarboxylases, esculin, and gelatin but positive for urease. Isolates have been obtained from urine, eye discharge, blood, pleural fluid, CSF, and lung, throat, and genitourinary tract specimens. Their clinical significance is unclear.

PSYCHROBACTER SPECIES

Psychrobacter immobilis organisms are cold-loving (psychrotrophic), nonmotile, oxidase-positive, oxidative diplococci. They resemble *Moraxella* organisms and, like them, are penicillin susceptible. They have been associated with fish, processed meat, and poultry. Clinically, they have been isolated from the eye of a newborn, who had acquired the infection nosocomially via a water source. *P. immobilis* organisms were also reportedly isolated from the blood and CSF of a 2-day-old infant. Isolates grow well at 5° to 25° C but not at 35° to 37° C. They are nitrate positive and can grow on Thayer-Martin medium.

Dysgonic fermenters (DF)

Strains of gram-negative bacilli referred to by the CDC as **dysgonic fermenters (DF)** are a group of slowly growing, fastidious bacilli that do ferment sugars but require the addition of increased CO_2 to the medium or an environment for isolation. (DF-2 and DF-2–like bacilli are two such strains. DF-1 bacilli are now classified under the *Capnocytophaga* genus and are discussed in Chapter 15, along with the HACEK organisms.) DF-2 and DF-2–like bacilli have been named by CDC as members of the genus *Capnocytophaga* as well. DF-2 is now named *Capnocytophaga canimorsus,* and DF-2–like is *Capnocytophaga cynodegmi.* Like other *Capnocytophaga* species, these two species are oxidase and catalase positive with gliding motility. Both are negative for indole and gelatin and are usually nitrite positive. Both ferment glucose and lactose. *C. canimorsus* organisms ferment galactose and glycogen most of the time, whereas *C. cynodegmi* does so less often; *C. cynodegmi* ferments melibiose, raffinose, and sucrose, and *C. canimorsus* does not.

C. canimorsus can cause sepsis, with or without endocarditis, cellulitis, and meningitis. Affected patients are most likely to have asplenia or alcoholism or to be receiving corticosteroids. A previous dog or cat bite is often associated in the majority of clinical cases. Endophthalmitis after corneal transplantation has also been reported.

Capnocytophaga spp. are susceptible to β-lactams, except for the first- and second-generation cephalosporins, which have intermediate to poor activity (except for cefoxitin). There have been reports of β-lactamase–producing strains, but the addition of a β-lactamase inhibitor can restore good activity. DF isolates are also susceptible to quinolones, metronidazole, clindamycin, tetracycline, and imipenem but demonstrate resistance to aminoglycosides, vancomycin, and semisynthetic penicillins.

DF-3

DF-3 is a short rod to a coccobacillary, nonmotile, fastidious, gram-negative fermentative bacillus. It requires increased CO_2 like members of *Capnocytophaga* and addition of serum to enhance the fermentations. It can have a sweet to bitter odor on solid medium and will not grow on MacConkey agar. Indole reaction may be weakly positive, esculin reaction is positive, and the isolates are negative for nitrate and the decarboxylases. Fermentation occurs with glucose, lactose, maltose, and raffinose. Isolates have reportedly been taken from blood, urine, wounds, peritoneal abscesses, and stool specimens. In the last, isolation is often associated with patients who have hypogammaglobulinemia with chronic diarrhea, but the role of DF-3 in disease is unclear. Isolates are susceptible to carbenicillin, chloramphenicol, tetracycline, clindamycin, and SXT but resistant to β-lactams, quinolones, metronidazole, vancomycin, and erythromycin.

Eugonic fermenters (EF)

Eugonic fermenters (EF) are a group of nonfastidious fermenters, as distinguished from unnamed dysgonic fermenters, which are fastidious fermenters. The abbreviation for this group of gram-negative bacilli is EF, and EF-4a and EF-4b are discussed here. Both have been isolated from infected areas following dog and cat bites, respectively. Isolates are nonmotile, short rods to coccobacilli, oxidase and catalase positive. EF-4a is a glucose fermenter, closely resembling *Pasteurella* organisms, but it ferments only glucose. It may produce a yellow to tan pigment, reduces nitrate to gas, may grow on MacConkey agar, and may liquefy gelatin or grow at 42° C. It is negative for indole and urea. EF-4a colonies give off a characteristic popcorn-like odor, a trait shared with EF-4b.

EF-4b is an oxidizer of glucose, not a fermenter, and is usually associated with cat bites or scratches. In addition, EF-4b is gelatin negative and does not reduce nitrates to gas. Both are susceptible to β-lactams, chloramphenicol, tetracycline, and aminoglycosides.

HB-5

HB-5 organisms, still unnamed, are capnophilic (CO_2- requiring) coccobacilli and rods that are facultatively anaerobic, fastidious fermenters. They ferment glucose and fructose and are catalase positive, oxidase positive or negative, and indole positive. They may grow on MacConkey agar and are nonmotile. Isolates have been obtained from placenta, amniotic fluid, blood, rectal sites, abscesses, and urogenital specimens.

Chromobacterium species

Chromobacterium violaceum is a fermentative gram-negative bacillus that may be oxidase positive. It is motile with polar flagella and, as its name implies, produces a violet pigment about 91% of the time. The pigment is violacein, an ethanol-soluble, water-insoluble pigment. The presence of the pigment may hamper proper oxidase reactions. Isolates are usually indole negative, but nonpigmented strains may be indole positive. Isolates ferment glucose and, variably, sucrose; grow on MacConkey agar and most enteric media; reduce nitrate; and grow at 42° C. On Gram stain, the organisms may appear as curved bacilli that may resemble vibrios if the oxidase reaction is positive. When the oxidase reaction is negative, it may resemble enterics.

Reservoirs of *C. violaceum* are soil and water. They are found more commonly in tropical and subtropical climates. They are opportunists, attacking the immunocompromised patient with neutrophil deficits, usually as a result of contamination of wounds with water or soil. They have been isolated from cases of osteomyelitis and abscesses as well as from blood, urine, and gastrointestinal infections. *C. violaceum* organisms are sensitive to chloramphenicol, tetracycline, and SXT but resistant to cephalosporins and variably resistant to penicillin and the aminoglycosides. Many patients do not do well, however, even with adequate therapy, because of their underlying disease.

Bibliography

Baron EJ, Finegold SM: *Bailey & Scott's diagnostic microbiology,* ed 9, St Louis, 1994, Mosby.

Bergogne-Berezin E, Joyl-Guillou ML: An underestimated nosocomial pathogen, *Acinetobacter calcoaceticus, J Antibmicrob Chemother* 16:535, 1985.

Bisbe J et al: *Pseudomonas aeruginosa bacteremia:* univariate and multivariage analyses of factors influencing the prognosis in 133 episodes, *Rev Infect Dis* 10:629, 1988.

Bouvet PJM, Grimont PAD: Taxonomy of the genus *Acinetobacter* with the recognition of *Acinetobacter baumannsii* sp. nov., *Acinetobacter haemolyticus* sp. nov., *Acinetobacter johnsonii* sp. nov., and *Acinetobacter junii* sp. nov., and emended descriptions of *Acinetobacter calcoaceticus* and *Acinetobacter Iwoffii, Int J System Bacteriol* 36:228, 1986.

Carson LA et al: Comparative evaluation of selective media for isolation of *Pseudomonas cepacia* from cystic fibrosis patients and environmental sources, *J Clin Microbiol* 26:2096, 1988.

Centers for Disease Control: *Ochrobactrum anthropi* meningitis associated with cadaveric pericardial tissue processed with a contaminated solution—Utah, 1994, *MMWR* 45:671, 1996.

Cieslak TJ et al: Catheter-associated sepsis caused by *Ochrobactrum anthropi:* report of a case and review of related nonfermentative bacteria, *Clin Infect Dis* 14:902, 1992.

Clark WA et al: *Identification of unusually pathogenic gram-negative aerobic and facultatively anaerobic bacteria,* Atlanta, 1984, Centers for Disease Control.

Dauga C et al: *Balneatrix alpica* gen. nov., sp. nov., a bacterium associated with pneumonia and meningitis in a spa therapy centre, *Res Microbiol* 144:35, 1993.

Dunne WM Jr., Tillman J, Murray JC: Recovery of a *Agrobacterium radiobacter* with a mucoid phenotype from an immunocompromised child with bacteremia, *J Clin Microbiol* 31:2541, 1993.

Edmond MB et al: *Agrobacterium radiobacter:* a recently recognized opportunistic pathogen, *Clin Infect Dis* 16:388, 1993.

Elting LS, Bodey GP: Septicemia due to *Xanthomonas* sp. and non-*aeruginosa Pseudomonas* sp.: incidence of catheter-related infections, *Medicine* 69:296, 1990.

Forlenza SW: *Capnocytophaga:* an update, *Clin Microbol Newsl* 13:89, 1991.

Freney J et al: Septicemia caused by *Sphingobacterium multivorum, J Clin Microbiol* 25:1126, 1987.

Funke G et al: Characteristics of *Bordetella hinzii* strains isolated from a cystic fibrosis patient over a 3-year period, *J Clin Microbiol* 34:966, 1996.

Fyfe JAM, Harris G, Govan GRW: Revised pyocin typing method for *Pseudomonas aeruginosa, J Clin Microbiol* 29:47, 1984.

Gilardi GL: Update on taxonomy of nonfastidous glucose-nonfermenting gram-negative bacilli, *Clin Microbiol Newsl* 12:73, 1990.

Glupczynski Y et al: *Pseudomonas paucimobilis* peritonitis in patients treated with peritoneal dialysis, *J Clin Microbiol* 20:1255, 1984.

Goldman DA, Klinger JD: *Pseudomonas cepacia:* biology, mechanisms of virulence, epidemiology, *J Pediatr* 108:806, 1986.

Gransden WR, Eykyn SJ: Seven cases of bacteremia due to *Ochrobactrum anthropi, Clin Infect Dis* 15:1068, 1992.

Hammerberg O, Bialkowska-Hobrzanska O, Gopaul D: Isolation of *Agrobacterium radiobacter* from a central venous catheter, *Eur J Clin Microbiol Infect Dis* 10:450, 1992.

Hearn YR, Gardner RM: *Achromobacter xylosoxidans:* an unusual neonatal pathogen, *Am J Clin Pathol* 96:211, 1991.

Hollis DG et al: Characterization of centers for disease control group NO-1, a fastidious nonoxidative, gram-negative associated with dog and cat bites, *J Clin Microbiol* 31:746, 1993.

Holmes B, Lewis R, Trevett A: Septicemia due to *Achromobacter* group B: a report of two cases, *Med Microbiol Let* 1:177, 1992.

Hsueh P-R et al: Bacteremic necrotizing fasciitis due to *Flavobacterium odoratum, Clin Infect Dis* 21:1337, 1995.

Hudson MJ et al: Relationship of CDC group EO-2 and *Psychrobacter immobilis, J Clin Microbiol* 25:1907, 1987.

Kaye KM, Macone A, Kazanjian PH: Catheter infection caused by *Methylobacterium* in immunocompromised hosts: report of three cases and review of the literature, *Clin Infect Dis,* 14:1010, 1992.

Kerr KG, Corps CM, Hawkey PM: Infections due to *Xanthomonas maltophilia* in patients with hematologic malignancy, *Rev Infect Dis* 13:762, 1991.

Khardori N: Nosocomial infections due to *Xanthomonas maltophilia (Pseudomonas maltophilia)* in patients with cancer, *Rev Infect Dis* 12:997, 1990.

Kitch T, Jacobs MR, Applebaum PC: *Evaluation of the 4H NF plus method for identification of 86 gram-negative nonfermentative rods,* Abstract #149, ASM General Meeting, 1991, Dallas, Texas, Washington DC, 1991, American Society for Microbiology.

Koneman EW et al: *Color atlas and textbook of diagnostic microbiology,* ed 5, Philadelphia, 1997, JB Lippincott.

Kostman JR, Solomon F, Fekete T: Infections with *Chryseomonas luteola* (CDC Group Ve-1) and *Flavimonas oryzihabitans* (CDC Group Ve-2) in neurosurgical patients, *Rev Infect Dis* 13:223, 1991.

Lampe AS, van Reijden TKJ: Evaluation of commercial test systems for the identification of nonfermenters, *Eur J Clin Microbiol* 3:301, 1984.

Levett PN, Garrett DA, Wickramasuriya T: *Flavimonas oryzi-habitans* as a cause of ocular infection, *Eur J Clin Microbiol Infect Dis* 10:594, 1991.

Lloyd-Puryear M, Wallace D, Baldwin T, Hollis DG: Meningitis caused by *Psychrobacter immobilis* in an infant, *J Clin Microbiol* 29:2041, 1991.

Lorian V, editor: *Antibiotics in laboratory medicine*, ed 4, Baltimore, 1996, Williams & Wilkins.

Marshall WF et al: *Xanthomonas maltophilia*: an emerging nosocomial pathogen, *Mayo Clinic Proceedings* 64:1097, 1989.

Moss CW et al: Cultural and chemical characterization of CDC group EO-2, M-5, and M-6 *(Moraxella)* sp., *Oligella urethralis, Acinetobacter* sp. and *Psychrobacter immobilis, J Clin Microbiol* 26:484, 1988.

Murray PR, Baron EJ, Pfaller MA, editors: *Manual of clinical microbiology,* ed 6, Washington, DC, 1995, American Society for Microbiology.

Oberhofer TR: Use of the API 20E, Oxi/Ferm, and Minitek systems to identify nonfermentative and oxidase positive fermentative bacteria: seven years of experience, *Diagn Microbiol Infect Dis* 1:241, 1983.

Palleroni NJ, Bradbury JF: *Stenotrophomonas,* a new bacterial genus for *Xanthomonas maltophilia* (Hugh 1980) Swings et al 1983, *Int J Syst Bacteriol* 43:606, 1993.

Peel MM et al: *Alcaligenes piechaudi* from chronic ear discharge, *J Clin Microbiol* 26:1580, 1988.

Ramos JM et al: Infection caused by the nonfermentative gram-negative bacillus CDC Group IV c-2: case report and literature review, *Eur J Clin Microbiol Infect Dis* 12:456, 1993.

Rihs JD et al: *Roseomonas,* a new genus associated with bacteremia and other human infections, *J Clin Microbiol* 31:3275, 1993.

Robin T, Janda MJ: *Pseudo-, Santho-, Stenotrophomonas maltophilia:* an emerging pathogen in search of a genus, *Clin Microbiol Newsl* 18:9, 1996.

Ross JP et al: Severe *Burkholderia (Pseudomonas) gladioli* infection in chronic granulomatous disease: report of two successfully treated cases, *Clin Infect Dis* 21:1291, 1995.

Rossau R et al: *Oligella,* a new genus including *Oligella urethralis* comb. nov. (formerly *Moraxella urethralis*) and *Oligella ureolytica* sp. nov. (formerly CDC Group Ive); relationship to *Taylorella equigenitalis* and related taxa, *Int J Syst Bacteriol* 37:198, 1987.

Segers P et al: Classification of *Pseudomonas diminuta* Leifson and Hugh 1954 and *Pseudomonas vesicularis* Busing, Doll, and Fretag 1953 in *Brevundimonas* gen. nov. as *Brevundimonas diminuta* comb. nov. and *Brevundimonas vesicularis* comb. nov., respectively, *Int J Syst Bacteriol* 44:499, 1994.

Tablan OC et al: *Pseudomonas cepacia* colonization in patients with cystic fibrosis: risk factors and clinical outcome, *J Pediatr* 107:382, 1985.

Tenover FC, Mizuki TS, Carlson LG: Evaluation of AutoSCAN-W/A automated microbiology system for the identification of non–glucose-fermenting gram-negative bacilli, *J Clin Microbiol* 28:1628, 1990.

Truant AL et al: Comparison of AMS Vitek, MicroScan and Autobac Series II for the Identification of gram-negative bacilli, *Diagn Microbiol Infect Dis* 12:211, 1989.

Urakami T et al: Further studies of the genus *Methylobacterium* and description of *Methylobacterium aminovorans* sp. nov., *Int J Syst Bacteriol* 43:504, 1993.

Vancanneyt M et al: Reclassification of *Flavobacterium odoratum* (Strutzer 1929) strains to a new genus, *Myoides*, as *Myoides odoratus* comb. nov. and *Myoides odoratimimus* sp. nov., *Int J Syst Bacteriol* 46:926, 1996.

Vandamme P et al: New perspectives in the classification of the flavobacteria: description of *Chrysseobacterium* gen. nov., *Bergeyella* gen. nov., and *Empedobacter* nom. rev., *Int J Syst Bacteriol* 44:827, 1994.

Vandamme P et al: *Moraxella lincolnii* sp. nov., isolated from the human respiratory tract, and reevaluation of the taxonomic position of *Moraxella osloensis, Int J Syst Bacteriol* 43:474, 1993.

Vandamme P et al: *Bordetella trematum* sp. nov., isolated from wounds and ear infections in humans, and reassessment of *Alcaligenes denitrificans* Ruger and Tan 1983, *Int J Syst Bacteriol* 46:849, 1996.

Veys A et al: Application of gas-liquid chromatography to the routine identification of nonfermenting gram-negative bacteria in clinical specimens, *J Clin Microbiol* 27:1538, 1989.

Welch DF et al: Selective and differential medium for recovery of *Pseudomonas cepacia* from the respiratory tracts of patients with cystic fibrosis, *J Clin Microbiol* 25:730, 1987.

Weyant RS et al: *Bordetella holmesii* sp. nov., a new gram-negative sp. associated with septicemia, *J Clin Microbiol* 33:1, 1995.

Willems A et al: *Acidovorax,* a new genus for *Pseudomonas facilis, Pseudomonas delafielddii,* E. Falsen (EF) Group 13, EF Group 16, and several clinical isolates with the sp. *Acidovorax facilis* comb. nov., *Acidovorax delafieldii* comb. nov., and *Acidovorax temperans* sp. nov, *Int J Sys Bacteriol* 40:384, 1990.

Yabuuchi E et al: *Sphingobacterium* gen nov., *Sphingobacterium apiritivorum* comb. nov., *Sphingobacterium multivorum* comb. nov., *Sphingobacterium mizutae* sp. nov., and *Flavobacterium indologenes* sp. nov.: glucose nonfermenting gram-negative rods in CDC groups Ilk-2 and IIb, *Int J Syst Bacteriol* 33:580, 1983.

Yabuuchi et al: Proposal of *Burkholderia* een. nov. and transfer of seven sp. of the genus *Pseudomonas* homology group II to the new genus, with the type sp. *Burkholderia cepacia* (Palleroni and Holmes 1981) comb. nov., *Microbiol Immunol* 36:1251, 1992.

Yabuuchi et al: Transfer of two *Burkholderia* and an *Alcaligenes* sp. to *Ralstonia* gen. nov.: proposal of *Ralstonia pickettii* (Ralston, Palleroni and Doudoroff 1973) comb. nov., *Ralstonia solanacearum* (Smith 1896) comb. nov. and *Ralstonia eutropha* (Davis 1969) comb. nov. 1995, *Microbiol Immunol* 39:897.

Yu PKW et al: Application of QuadFERM + for the identification of fastidious gram-positive and gram-negative bacilli, *Diagn Microbiol Infect Dis* 14:185, 1991.

Zapardiel J et al: Peritonitis with CDC Group IVc-2 bacteria in a patient on continuous ambulatory peritoneal dialysis, *Eur J Clin Microbiol Infect Dis* 10:509, 1991.

LEARNING ASSESSMENTS

1. What is the difference between nonfermentative and fermentative organisms?

2. Where do nonfermenters usually exist?

3. What types of infections do nonfermenters produce?

4. What risk factors are associated with nonfermentative gram-negative bacilli?

5. What are the most common nonfermentative gram-negative bacilli?

6. What are the susceptibility patterns of the most common nonfermenters?

7. What initial clues indicate that an isolate is a nonfermenter?

8. Which of the nonfermenters are commonly isolated form clinical infections?

9. How would you differentiate *Pseudomonas aeruginosa* organisms from other fluorescent pseudomonads?

10. What are the identifying characteristics of *Acinetobacter* species?

11. How would you differentiate *Pseudomonas pseudomallei* from *Pseudomonas stutzeri?*

CHAPTER 19

Anaerobes of Clinical Importance

Paul G. Engelkirk, Janet Duben-Engelkirk

IMPORTANT CONCEPTS IN ANAEROBIC
  BACTERIOLOGY
  Anaerobes Defined
  Why Are They Anaerobes?
    Oxygen toxicity
    Absence of protective enzymes
  Where Anaerobes Are Found
  Anaerobes at Specific Anatomic Sites
    Respiratory tract
    Skin
    Genitourinary tract
    Gastrointestinal tract
  Factors that Predispose Patients to Anaerobic
    Infections
  Indications of Anaerobe Involvement in Human
    Disease

SPECIMEN SELECTION, COLLECTION,
  TRANSPORT, AND PROCESSING
  Specimen Quality
  Specimen Transport and Processing
    Aspirates
    Swabs
    Tissue
    Blood
  Processing Clinical Samples for Maximum
    Recovery of Anaerobic Pathogens
    Macroscopic examination of specimen
    Direct microscopic examination of specimen
    Inoculation of appropriate plated and tubed
      media
    Anaerobic incubation of inoculated media

PROCEDURES FOR IDENTIFYING ANAEROBIC
  ISOLATES
  Preliminary Procedures
    When to examine primary plates
    Indications of the presence of anaerobes
      in culture
    Processing colonies suspected of being
      anaerobes

  Identification of Anaerobic Isolates
    Presumptive identification
    Definitive identifications

FREQUENTLY ENCOUNTERED ANAEROBES
  AND THEIR ASSOCIATED DISEASES
  Gram-Positive Spore-Forming Anaerobic Bacilli
    Clinical infection
    Laboratory diagnosis
    Identification
  Gram-Positive Non–Spore-Forming Anaerobic
    Bacilli
    Clinical infection
    Laboratory diagnosis
    Identification
  Anaerobic Gram-Negative Bacilli
    Clinical infection
    Laboratory diagnosis
    Identification
  Anaerobic Cocci
    Clinical infection
    Gram-positive cocci
    Gram-negative cocci
    Identification

SUSCEPTIBILITY AND β-LACTAMASE TESTING
  Anaerobe Resistance to Antimicrobial Agents
  Susceptibility Testing of Anaerobes
    When to test
    Antimicrobial agents to be tested
  Problems in Susceptibility Testing of Anaerobic
    Isolates
  Susceptibility Testing Options
  Quality-Assurance Considerations Pertaining
    to Susceptibility Testing
  β-Lactamase Testing

TREATING ANAEROBE-ASSOCIATED DISEASES

OBJECTIVES

1. Differentiate obligate anaerobes from facultative organisms.
2. Describe how anaerobes, as part of normal flora, initiate and establish infection.
3. Given the clues to an anaerobic infection (signs and manifestations), name the most probable etiologic agent of the following:
   - Wound botulism
   - Tetanus
   - Gas gangrene
   - Actinomycosis
   - Lung abscess
   - Peritonitis
4. Give the bacteriologic indicators used to recognize anaerobes as the possible causative agent.
5. Describe the clinical infections associated with the following organisms and how they are acquired and manifested:
   - *Clostridium* species
   - Anaerobic, non–spore-forming, gram-positive bacilli
   - *Actinomyces*
   - *Bacteroides* spp.
   - *Fusobacterium* spp.
   - Gram-positive cocci
   - *Veillonella* spp.
6. Describe the laboratory methods of performing cultures and identifying anaerobes:
   - Acceptable and unacceptable specimens
   - Culture environments
   - Isolation media
   - Identification systems
7. Describe the acceptable methods for performing anaerobic antimicrobic susceptibility tests.
8. Given the microscopic, colony morphology, and key reactions in the differentiating tests used to identify anaerobic isolates, identify the most notable species of the following:
   - *Clostridium*
   - Anaerobic, gram-positive, non–spore-forming bacilli
   - Gram-negative, non–spore-forming bacilli
   - Anaerobic cocci

KEY TERMS

Obligate anaerobe
Bacteriostatic
Bactericidal
Exogenous anaerobe
Endogenous anaerobe
Facultative anaerobe

Anaerobic chamber
Aerotolerance test
Capnophilic
Aerotolerant anaerobe
Sodium polyethanol
 sulfate (SPS)

"Roll tubes"
Tetanus
Tetanospasmin
Myonecrosis
Botulism

Pseudomembranous
 colitis
Nagler test
Actinomycosis
Microaerophiles

A 45-year-old male farmer was admitted to the hospital for complications resulting from a tractor accident that caused traumatic injury to his left leg. The patient's leg was painful, bluish, and edematous. A radiograph revealed pockets of gas in the tissue. A complete blood count revealed a marked increase in neutrophils and a total white blood cell count of 33,000/mm^3. A Gram stain of the wound specimen revealed numerous, rectangularly-shaped, gram-positive bacilli, moderate gram-positive cocci in clusters, no spores, and very few leukocytes. The attending physician concluded that the Gram stain results were indicative of contamination rather than infection. Fortunately for the patient, the infectious disease specialist thought differently.

Anaerobic bacteria are significant for a variety of reasons. They are important in human and veterinary medicine because they play a role in serious, often fatal, infections and intoxications. They can be involved in infectious processes in virtually any organ or tissue of the body and consequently can be recovered from most clinical specimens.

This chapter describes the following:

- Anaerobes of clinical importance and their role in disease
- Proper techniques for selecting, collecting, transporting, and processing clinical specimens for anaerobic bacteriology
- Procedures for identifying and testing the susceptibility of anaerobic isolates

IMPORTANT CONCEPTS IN ANAEROBIC BACTERIOLOGY

Anaerobes Defined

In addition to Gram reaction and cellular morphology, bacteria are commonly classified in the clinical microbiology laboratory on the basis of their relationship to oxygen (O_2) and carbon dioxide (CO_2) (Table 19-1).

This classification is easily accomplished by comparing an organism's ability to multiply on a solid medium, usually blood agar, in four different environments:

1. Air (about 21% O_2 and 0.03% CO_2)
2. CO_2 incubator (about 15% O_2 and 5%-10% CO_2)
3. Microaerophilic system (5% O_2)
4. Anaerobic system (0% O_2)

In general, anaerobes are organisms that do not require oxygen for life and reproduction. In addition, oxygen's direct toxic effect may prohibit the growth of these organisms in environments in which oxygen is present. Although the term *anaerobe* is used throughout this chapter as a synonym

TABLE 19-1

Classification of Bacteria on the Basis of Their Relationship to Oxygen and Carbon Dioxide

Category	Requirement	Examples
Obligate aerobe	15%-21% O_2 (as found in a CO_2 incubator or air)	Mycobacteria, fungi
Microaerophile	5% O_2	*Neisseria, Campylobacter* spp.
Facultative anaerobe	Multiplies equally well in the presence or absence of O_2	Enterobacteriaceae, most staphylococci, streptococci
Aerotolerant anaerobe	Reduced concentrations of O_2 (anaerobic system and a microaerophilic environment)	Most strains of *Propionibacterium, Clostridium* spp.
Obligate anaerobe	Strict anaerobic environment (0% O_2)	Most *Bacteroides* spp., many *Clostridium, Eubacterium, Fusobacterium* spp., *Peptostreptococcus* spp., *Porphyromonas* spp., most strains of *Veillonella parvula*
Capnophile	5%-10% CO_2	Some anaerobes, *Neisseria, Haemophilus* spp.

Modified from Engelkirk PG, Duben-Engelkirk J, Dowell VR Jr: *Principles and practice of anaerobic bacteriology*, Belmont, Calif, 1992, Star.

for anaerobic bacteria, the laboratory professional must understand that other types of anaerobic microorganisms, such as certain fungi and protozoa, also exist.

Obligate anaerobes, which grow only in the absence of molecular oxygen, vary in their sensitivity to oxygen and can be classified as *moderate anaerobes* and *strict anaerobes.* A moderate anaerobe, such as *Bacteroides fragilis, Fusobacterium nucleatum,* or *Prevotella melaninogenica,* is unable to multiply in an atmosphere containing more than 2% to 8% O_2. Moderate anaerobes can tolerate exposure to air for several hours on the surface of blood agar but require an anaerobic environment for multiplication. Strict anaerobes, such as *Clostridium haemolyticum, Clostridium novyi* type B, and certain treponemes, cannot multiply in the presence of more than 0.5% O_2 and are killed by only a few minutes' exposure to air. Fortunately, strict anaerobes are seldom associated with human infections. Aerotolerant anaerobes are capable of growing in atmospheres containing molecular oxygen but grow best in an anaerobic environment.

Why Are They Anaerobes?

Several theories have been advanced to explain the anaerobic requirement of certain microorganisms. Common concepts that have been well-studied include oxygen toxicity, absence of protective enzymes, and bacteriostatic and bactericidal effects as oxygen.

Oxygen toxicity

As stated by Margulis and Sagan, "Oxygen is toxic because it reacts with organic matter. It grabs electrons and produces so-called free radicals: highly reactive, short-lived chemicals that wreak havoc with the carbon, hydrogen, sulfur, and nitrogen compounds at the basis of life. Oxygen breaks down or renders useless the small metabolites—food—that otherwise become components in cellular systems. Oxygen combines with the enzymes, proteins, nucleic acids, vitamins, and lipids that are vital to cell reproduction."

Molecular oxygen itself can be toxic to some anaerobes, but substances produced when oxygen becomes reduced are even more toxic. During oxidation-reduction reactions, molecular oxygen is reduced in a stepwise manner by the addition of electrons, as shown in the following equations:

$$O_2 + e^- \rightarrow O_2^- \text{ (superoxide anion)}$$
$$O_2^- + e^- + 2H^+ \rightarrow H_2O_2 \text{ (hydrogen peroxide)}$$
$$H_2O_2 + e^- + H^+ \rightarrow H_2O + OH^\bullet \text{ (hydroxyl radical)}$$
$$OH^\bullet + e^- + H^+ \rightarrow H_2O$$

Absence of protective enzymes

Organisms that use oxygen have one or more enzymes to protect them from superoxide anions and their toxic derivatives (e.g., superoxide dismutase and catalase). Anaerobes are particularly susceptible to these toxic derivatives of oxygen because they lack one or more of the protective enzymes. In phase 1, when anaerobes are exposed to oxygen, electrons that usually would be available for metabolic functions are diverted to the reduction of molecular oxygen, with a consequent decrease in the amount of energy available for growth and synthesis of new cell material. This results in a slowing down or complete cessation of growth—a **bacteriostatic** effect. If the period of exposure to oxygen is brief, the effect may be reversible. If the anaerobes are placed back into an anaerobic environment at this point, electrons would again be available for normal metabolic processes, energy production, and cell growth. However, should the anaerobes remain in the presence of oxygen, phase 2 would occur. Phase 2 is the lethal, irreversible effect of oxygen toxicity due to the previously mentioned superoxide anions, hydroxyl radicals, and hydrogen peroxide. Phase 2 therefore has a **bactericidal** effect.

Strict anaerobes also may require an environment that has a low oxidation-reduction (redox) potential. This may be in part because certain enzymes that are essential for bacterial growth require fully reduced sulfhydryl ($-SH$) groups to be active. Reducing agents such as thioglycollate, cysteine, and dithiothreitol often are added to microbiologic media to obtain a low redox potential.

In vivo, bacteria have a tendency to lower the redox potential at their site of growth. Consequently, anatomic sites colonized with mixtures of organisms frequently provide conditions favorable to the growth of obligate anaerobes.

Where Anaerobes Are Found

Based on scientific evidence, many scientists believe that anaerobes originated about 3 to 4 billion years ago in warm, shallow waters, where they were protected from the sun's deadly ultraviolet rays. It is thought that life on this planet remained anaerobic for hundreds of millions of years.

Today, anaerobes are found only in specific ecologic niches. They can be found in soil, in freshwater and saltwater sediments and as components of the microbial flora of humans and other animals. Anaerobes that exist outside of the bodies of animals are referred to as **exogenous anaerobes** and cause exogenous types of infections. Anaerobes that exist inside the bodies of animals *(indigenous microflora)* are referred to as **endogenous anaerobes** and are the source of endogenous infections.

Anaerobic infections of exogenous origin are usually caused by gram-positive spore-forming bacilli such as *Clostridium.* Clostridia or their toxins initiate infection when spores are ingested through contaminated food or gain access through open wounds contaminated with soil. Although less frequently encountered in human diseases, *Sarcina ventriculi* (an endospore-forming, gram-positive coccus), *Fusobacterium ulcerans, Desulfovibrio desulfuricans,* and *Desulfomonas* spp. gain access to the body through soil-contaminated wounds and may cause exogenous infections.

By far, the anaerobes most frequently isolated from infectious processes in humans are those of endogenous origin. Table 19-2 shows endogenous anaerobes commonly encountered in human infections. Although many different species of anaerobes can be potentially isolated from human clinical specimens, the number of species routinely isolated is relatively small. Approximately two-thirds of clinically significant anaerobe-associated infectious processes involve the anaerobes or groups of anaerobes shown in Figure 19-1.

Anaerobes of endogenous origin can contribute to an infectious disease in any anatomic site of the body if suitable conditions exist for colonization and penetration of the bacteria.

Anaerobes at Specific Anatomic Sites

Anaerobes outnumber aerobes at mucosal surfaces, such as the linings of the oral cavity, gastrointestinal (GI) tract, and genitourinary (GU) tract. These heavily colonized surfaces are the usual portals of entry into the tissues and blood stream for endogenous anaerobes. Under ordinary circumstances, microorganisms that are members of the microbial flora do not cause disease. Indeed, many actually can be beneficial. However, when

TABLE 19-2

Endogenous Anaerobes Commonly Involved in Human Infections

Infection	Anaerobe
Actinomycosis	*Actinomyces israelii,* other *Actinomyces* spp., *Propionibacterium acnes*
Antibiotic-associated diarrhea and pseudomembranous colitis	*Clostridium difficile, Clostridium perfringens* less often
Bacteremia	*Bacteroides* spp., *Fusobacterium* spp., *Peptostreptococcus* spp.
Brain abscess	*Bacteroides* spp., *Fusobacterium* spp., *Clostridium* spp. (infrequently) (These infections are often polymicrobial)
Complication of Vincent's angina (necrotizing ulcerative gingivitis)	*Fusobacterium necrophorum*
Endocarditis	*Bacteroides* spp., gram-positive cocci, non–spore-forming, gram-positive bacilli (Anaerobes are uncommon isolates)
Eye infections	*Peptostreptococcus* spp., *Clostridium* spp., *Bacteroides* spp., *Actinomyces* spp.
Infections of the female urogenital tract	Gram-positive cocci, *Bacteroides* spp., *Clostridium* spp.
Intraabdominal infections, liver abscess peritonitis	*Bacteroides fragilis* group, other *Bacteroides* spp., *Fusobacterium* spp., *C. perfringens,* other *Clostridium* spp., *Peptostreptococcus* spp., *Actinomyces* spp. (frequently polymicrobial)
Myonecrosis (gas gangrene)	*C. perfringens, Clostridium novyi, Clostridium septicum* (80% to 95% of the cases)
Oral, sinus, and dental infections	*Peptostreptococcus* spp., *Porphyromonas* spp., *Wolinella* spp., *Fusobacterium* spp. (often polymicrobial)
Perineal and perirectal infections	*B. fragilis* group, other *Bacteroides* spp., *Fusobacterium* spp., *Clostridium* spp., *Peptostreptococus* spp., *Eubacterium* spp., *Actinomyces* spp.
Pleuropulmonary infections, aspiration pneumonia	*Porphyromonas* spp., *F. nucleatum, Peptostreptococcus* spp., *B. fragilis* group, *Actinomyces* spp., *Eubacterium* spp.

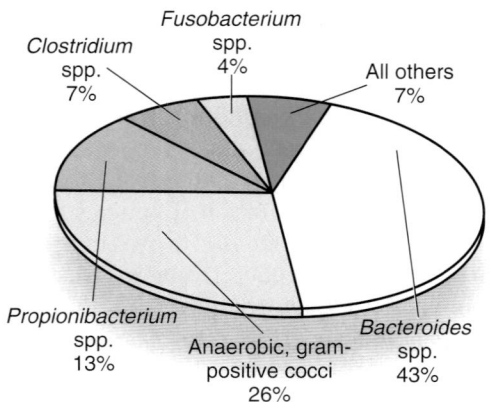

Figure 19-1

Frequency of isolation of anaerobes from clinical specimens. (From Engelkirk PG, Duben-Engelkirk J, Dowell VR Jr: *Principles and Practice of Clinical Anaerobic Bacteriology,* Belmont, Calif, 1992, Star.)

some of these organisms gain access to usually sterile body sites (e.g., blood stream, brain, lungs), they can cause serious or even fatal infections. Knowledge of the composition of the microflora at specific anatomic sites is useful for predicting the particular organisms most likely to be involved in infectious processes that arise at or adjacent to those sites. Finding site-specific organisms at a distant and/or unusual site can serve as a clue to the underlying origin of an infectious process. For example, the isolation of oral anaerobes from a brain abscess may suggest the presence of an oral lesion. Because some anaerobes have fairly predictable susceptibility patterns, such knowledge also may be of value to physicians considering empiric antimicrobial therapy. Table 19-3 summarizes the variety of endogenous anaerobes that may be found at specific body sites.

Repiratory tract

Ninety percent of the bacteria present in saliva, nasal washings, and gingival and tooth scrapings are anaerobes. Gram-negative bacilli and anaerobic cocci are the anaerobes occurring in the highest numbers. These particular anaerobes should be suspected as participants in any infectious process occurring in the oral cavity and in cases of aspiration pneumonia. An oral nidus (origin) should be suspected whenever certain oral anaerobes such as *F. nucleatum* and *Porphyromonas* spp.

are recovered from the blood stream or from abscesses located far from the oral cavity. Certain oral anaerobes produce volatile and foul-smelling metabolic byproducts that undoubtedly contribute significantly to the odor of "bad breath" and exudates from oral lesions and aspiration pneumonia.

Expectorated sputum and oral specimens collected by swab are unacceptable for anaerobic bacteriology. Because they would contain indigenous anaerobes of the oral cavity, it would be difficult to differentiate organisms causing the disease from contaminants present in the specimen.

Skin

The indigenous members of the skin flora include anaerobes. *Propionibacterium acnes,* a common skin colonizer, is frequently isolated from blood cultures. Its presence in blood culture bottles often represents "contamination" from the patient's

TABLE 19-3

Endogenous Anaerobes at Various Anatomical Sites

Site	Anaerobe
Oral cavity	*Bacteroides* spp.
	Fusobacterium spp.
	Peptostreptococcus spp.
	Veillonella spp.
	Gram-positive non–spore-forming bacilli
Upper respiratory tract	*Actinomyces* spp.
	Bacteroides spp.
	Fusobacterium spp. (esp. *Fusobacterium necrophorum*)
	Peptostreptococcus spp.
	Veillonella spp.
	Propionibacterium spp.
	Eubacterium spp.
Skin	*Propionibacterium* spp.
	Peptostreptococcus spp.
	Eubacterium spp.
Urethra	*Bacteroides* spp.
	Fusobacterium spp.
	Peptostreptococcus spp.
Vagina	*Lactobacillus* spp.
	Peptostreptococcus spp.
	Bacteroides spp.
	Propionibacterium spp.
Colon	*Bacteroides* spp.
	Bifidobacterium spp.
	Clostridium spp.
	Eubacterium spp.
	Lactobacillus spp.
	Peptostreptococcus spp.

skin, although its presence also can signify a true bacteremia. *P. acnes,* like coagulase-negative staphylococci, may cause endocarditis. Other anaerobes found on the skin include *Peptostreptococcus* and *Eubacterium* spp. Superficial wound or abscess specimens aspirated by needle and syringe are much better specimens for anaerobic bacteriology than material collected by swabs; the latter often are contaminated with anaerobes of the skin microflora.

Genitourinary tract

Anaerobic bacteria that colonize the distal urethra would be recovered if specimens of voided or catheterized urine were cultured for anaerobes. Although anaerobes can be a rare cause of infectious diseases of the urinary tract, their presence in such specimens generally indicates contamination of the urine with organisms flushed from the distal urethra. Similarly, 50% of the bacteria in cervical and vaginal secretions are anaerobes. Whenever anaerobes are recovered from vaginal and cervical swabs, neither the microbiologist nor the physician can distinguish the indigenous microflora contaminants from the organisms actually contributing to the patient's infectious process. For this reason, GU tract swabs and voided or catheterized urine specimens are unacceptable for anaerobic bacteriology.

Gastrointestinal tract

Of the estimated 500 species of bacteria that inhabit the human body, approximately 300 to 400 live in the colon. Microflora studies have found that anaerobes outnumber **facultative anaerobes** by a factor of 1000:1. Although *B. fragilis* is the most common species of anaerobic bacteria isolated from human soft-tissue infection and anaerobic bacteremia, this species accounts for less than 1% of the human intestinal microflora. *Bacteroides vulgatus, Bacteroides thetaiotaomicron,* and *Bacteroides distasonis* are among the most common species of bacteria isolated from human feces. Other species commonly inhabiting the GI tract include *Bifidobacterium, Clostridium, Eubacterium,* and *Peptostreptococcus* spp.

Stool specimens are not routinely cultured for anaerobes. However, if a patient is suspected of having pseudomembranous colitis and/or antibiotic-associated diarrhea caused by *Clostridium difficile,* diarrheal specimens from that patient should be examined.

Factors that Predispose Patients to Anaerobic Infections

Factors that commonly predispose the human body to anaerobic infections include trauma of mucous membranes or skin, vascular stasis, tissue necrosis, and decrease in the redox potential of tissue.

The precise mechanisms by which anaerobic bacteria cause disease are not known. However, anaerobes produce or possess a variety of enzymes, capsules, and adherence factors thought to play a role in pathogenicity. These are collectively referred to as *virulence factors* (Table 19-4). In addition to those listed in Table 19-4, β-lactamases, chondroitin sulfatase, fibrinolysin, heparinase, leukocidins, and endotoxin all have been suggested as possible virulence factors of anaerobes.

Generally, infectious diseases involving anaerobic bacteria follow some type of trauma to protective barriers such as the skin and mucous membranes. Trauma at these sites allows anaerobes of the indigenous microflora (or soil anaerobes, in some cases) to gain access to deeper tissues. Vascular stasis (blockage of blood flow) prevents oxygen from entering a particular site. This results in an environment conducive to growth and multiplication of any anaerobes that might be present at that site. Similar results may occur in the presence of tissue necrosis and when redox potential in tissue is decreased. Table 19-5 lists examples of conditions that predispose a patient to anaerobic infections.

Indications of Anaerobe Involvement in Human Disease

Infectious processes involving anaerobes are usually purulent, but the absence of leukocytes does not rule out the possibility that anaerobes are contributing to the process. Some of the more serious infectious processes in humans are caused by anaerobes producing cytotoxins and other histotoxic virulence factors that contribute to the necrotizing process by destroying neutrophils, macrophages, and other cells.

Table 19-6 contains a list of indications of anaerobe involvement in infectious processes. Although any of these indicators should alert the physician

TABLE 19-4

Potential Virulence Factors of Anaerobic Bacteria

Potential Virulence Factor	Possible Role of the Virulence Factor	Anaerobes Known or Thought to Possess the Virulence Factor
Polysaccharide capsules	Promote abscess formation; serve an antiphagocytic function	*Bacteroides fragilis, Porphyromonas gingivalis,* and some other anaerobic gram-negative bacilli
Adherence factors	Certain pili, fimbriae, fibrils enable organisms to adhere to cell surfaces	*B. fragilis* and *P. gingivalis* in humans; *Bacteroides nodosus* in sheep
Clostridial toxins/exoenzymes		
Collagenases	Catalyze the degradation of collagen	
Cytotoxins	Toxic to specific types of host cells	
DNAses	Destroy DNA	
Enterotoxins	Toxic to cells of the intestinal mucosa	
Hemolysins	Liberate hemoglobin from red blood cells by lysing the cells	
Hyaluronidase	Catalyze the hydrolysis of hyaluronic acid, the cement substance of tissues	
Lipases	Catalyze the hydrolysis of ester linkages between the fatty acids and glycerol of triglycerides and phospholipids	Certain *Clostridium* spp.
Necrotizing toxins	Cause necrosis (death) of cells	
Neuraminidases	Destroy neuraminic acid, a sialic acid found on cell surfaces	
Neurotoxins	Destroy or disrupt nerve tissue	
Permeases (e.g., ADP-ribosyl-transferases)	Alter the physiology of cells in such a way as to cause severe fluid loss and ionic imbalance	
Phospholipases	Catalyze the splitting of phospholipids, lecithinases	
Proteases	Split proteins by hydrolysis of peptide bonds	
Proteinases	Split the interior peptide bonds of proteins (endopeptidases)	

Modified from Engelkirk PG, Duben-Engelkirk J, Dowell VR Jr: *Principles and practice of anaerobic bacteriology,* Belmont, Calif, 1992, Star.

TABLE 19-5

Examples of Conditions That Predispose a Patient to Anaerobe-Associated Infections or Diseases

Predisposing Condition	Explanation
Human or animal bite wounds	Endogenous anaerobes of the oral cavity enter the wound
Aspiration of oral contents into the lungs after vomiting	Endogenous anaerobes of the oral cavity and other materials (mucus, stomach contents, etc.) enter the lungs
Tooth extraction, oral surgery, or traumatic puncture of the oral cavity	Endogenous anaerobes of the oral cavity gain entrance to traumatized tissue and the blood stream
Gastrointestinal tract surgery or traumatic puncture of the bowel	Endogenous anaerobes of the gastrointestinal tract gain access to traumatized tissue and the blood stream
Genital tract surgery or traumatic puncture of the genital tract	Endogenous anaerobes of the genital tract gain access to traumatized tissue and the blood stream
Introduction of soil into a wound	Clostridial spores in the soil enter the tissues via a traumatic wound, resulting in colonization and multiplication of the bacteria

Modified from Engelkirk PG, Duben-Engelkirk J, Dowell VR Jr: *Principles and practice of anaerobic bacteriology,* Belmont, Calif, 1992, Star.

TABLE 19-6

Indications of Involvement of Anaerobes in Infectious Processes

Indication	Rationale
Infection is in close proximity to a mucosal surface	Anaerobes are the predominant microflora at mucosal surfaces
Infection persists despite aminoglycoside therapy	Aminoglycosides are ineffective against most anaerobes
Presence of foul odor	*Porphyromonas* and *Fusobacterium* spp. produce foul-smelling metabolic end products
Presence of large quantity of gas	*Clostridium* spp. produce large quantities of gas during metabolism
Presence of black color or brick-red fluorescence	Pigmented species of *Porphyromonas* and *Prevotella* produce a pigment that fluoresces brick-red under long-wave ultraviolet light; turns dark brown to black
Presence of sulfur granules	Sulfur granules are often present in patients with actinomycosis
Distinct morphologic characteristics in Gram-stained preparations	The morphology of certain anaerobes is somewhat (but not completely) distinctive: Certain anaerobes such as *Bacteroides* and *Fusobacterium* are quite pleomorphic; *Fusobacterium nucleatum* is fusiform; *Clostridium* spp. are often large, gram-positive rods that may or may not contain spores

Modified from Engelkirk PG, Duben-Engelkirk J, Dowell VR Jr: *Principles and practice of anaerobic bacteriology*, Belmont, Calif, 1992, Star.

to the possible involvement of anaerobes, most are not specific for anaerobes. For example, large quantities of gas in the specimen might be due to organisms such as *Escherichia coli* or a mixture of enteric bacteria other than anaerobes. Similarly, the foul odor usually associated with specimens containing anaerobes could be absent.

Many of the infectious processes involving anaerobes are polymicrobial, consisting of mixtures of obligate anaerobes or mixtures of obligate or microaerotolerant anaerobes and facultative organisms. Symbiotic relationships frequently exist between some of the bacteria involved in polymicrobial infections, which can act synergistically in the production of disease.

SPECIMEN SELECTION, COLLECTION, TRANSPORT, AND PROCESSING

Specimen Quality

When physicians suspect an infection involving anaerobes, they must properly select a clinical specimen and arrange for its proper collection and rapid transport to the laboratory. Although the selection, collection, and transport of clinical specimens are procedures routinely performed outside the laboratory by nonlaboratory professionals, laboratory practitioners can play a major role in accomplishing these steps, which are vital to the successful outcome of an anaerobic culture. The laboratory must provide physicians and other health care workers with proper education, written guidelines, and appropriate devices for collection and transport.

When clinical laboratory professionals provide in-service education to those who select, collect, and transport specimens for anaerobic bacteriology, a rationale must be given for proper specimen selection. The consequences of working up improper or incorrectly collected or transported specimens should be outlined. The laboratory also must develop criteria for the rejection of inappropriate specimens, with the cooperation of hospital medical staff. For example, when a specimen is not acceptable, particularly when collected at surgery, the physician must be notified before the sample is discarded. The reason for rejection should always be stated.

Many types of specimens are acceptable for anaerobic culture; these are listed in Table 19-7. Box 19-1 contains a list of specimens not recommended for anaerobic culture, most of which are collected by swab and are therefore likely to be contaminated by indigenous anaerobic flora at the particular body site.

Specimen Transport and Processing

Regardless of the type of specimen submitted for anaerobic bacteriology, it must be transported and

TABLE 19-7
Acceptable Specimens for Anaerobic Bacteriology

Anatomic Source	Specimens and Recommended Methods of Collection
Central nervous system	Cerebrospinal fluid, aspirated abscess material, tissue from biopsy or autopsy
Dental/ENT specimens	Aspirated abscess material, biopsied tissue
Localized abscesses	Needle and syringe aspiration of closed abscesses
Decubitus ulcers	Aspirated pus
Sinus tracts or draining wounds	Aspirated material
Deep tissue or bone	Specimens obtained during surgery from depths of wound or underlying bone lesion
Pulmonary	Percutaneous transtracheal aspiration: aspirate obtained by direct lung puncture; pleural fluid obtained by thoracentesis
	Biopsied tissue: "sulfur granules" from draining fistula
Intraabdominal	Aspirate from abscess, ascitic fluid, biopsied tissue
Urinary tract	Suprapubic bladder aspiration
Female genital tract	Aspirate from loculated abscess; culdocentesis specimen
Other	Blood, bone marrow, aspirated synovial fluid, biopsied tissue from any normally sterile site

Modified from Engelkirk PG, Duben-Engelkirk J, Dowell VR Jr: *Principles and practice of anaerobic bacteriology,* Belmont, Calif, 1992, Star.

processed as rapidly as possible and with minimum exposure to oxygen. Specimens usually are collected from a warm, moist environment that is low in oxygen. Thus, it is important to avoid "shocking" the anaerobes by exposing them to oxygen or permitting them to dry out. In addition, the amount of time they remain at room temperature should be minimized.

Aspirates

Specimens collected by needle and syringe are better for anaerobic bacteriology than those collected by swab. They are less likely to be contaminated by indigenous microflora, including endogenous anaerobes. Following aspiration of the specimen, any air present in the syringe and needle should be rapidly expelled. To prevent production of a potentially infectious aerosol, place an alcohol-soaked gauze pad over the needle while cautiously expelling the air.

Transporting specimens within a needle and syringe assembly is no longer acceptable because of the hazard of accidental skin puncture. The aspirate should be injected into some type of oxygen-free transport tube or vial, preferably one containing a prereduced, anaerobically sterilized (PRAS) transport medium. PRAS media are prepared by boiling (to remove dissolved oxygen), autoclaving (to sterilize the mixture), and replacing any air with an oxygen-free gas mixture.

Once in the laboratory, aspirates in transport containers should be vortexed to ensure even distribution of the material, especially when the sample is grossly purulent. Using a sterile Pasteur pipette, add one drop of purulent material or two to three drops of nonpurulent material to each plate and streak it in such a manner as to obtain well-isolated colonies. Also inoculate 0.5 to 1 mL of the specimen into the bottom of a tube of enriched thioglycollate broth. Spread one drop evenly over an alcohol-cleaned glass slide for Gram staining.

Swabs

In those rare instances in which swabs are deemed necessary, use commercially available, oxygen-free swabs. Such containers are available from a number of commercial sources. The Accu-CulShure collection instrument (Technology for Medicine, Pleasantville, N.Y.) is a uniquely designed swab that exposes the swab only at the collection site (e.g., the cervix) and protects it from indigenous

Box 19-1

Unacceptable Specimens for Anaerobic Bacteriology

Clinical specimen

Exudates and other material collected by swabs from superficial wounds, abscesses, burns, cysts, or ulcers

Vaginal, cervical, or urethral swabs

Respiratory tract specimens collected by swab, nasotracheal or orotracheal suction, or bronchoscope; expectorated sputum

Stool specimens, rectal swabs

Voided or catheterized urine

Modified from Engelkirk PG, Duben-Engelkirk J, Dowell VR Jr: *Principles and practice of anaerobic bacteriology,* Belmont, Calif, 1992, Star.

microflora contamination both before and after collecting the specimen. Swabs submitted for anaerobic bacteriology always should be transported in oxygen-free transport containers.

On its arrival in the laboratory, place the swab in a tube containing about 1 mL of sterile thioglycollate broth. Vortex the swab vigorously to remove the clinical material and then press it firmly against the inner wall of the tube to remove as much liquid as possible. Inoculate the remaining liquid suspension as previously described for an aspirate.

Tissue

Tissue specimens collected by biopsy or at autopsy from usually sterile sites are acceptable specimens for anaerobic culture. Small pieces of tissue can be placed in oxygen-free transport tubes or vials containing PRAS medium to keep the tissue moist. When inserting either swabs or small pieces of tissue into an anaerobic transport container, care must be taken not to tip the container. This would cause the heavier-than-air, oxygen-free gas mixture to be displaced by room air, thus defeating the primary purpose of using such a transport medium.

Larger tissues present greater transport problems. To resolve this, large tissues may be transported in pouches containing an oxygen-free atmosphere to prevent exposure to oxygen en route to the laboratory. Such bags or pouches are available commercially from Becton Dickinson (Bio-Bags and GasPak Pouches; Cockeysville, Md.) and Remel (Anaerobe Pouches; Lenexa, Kan.) and described in more detail in a later section of this chapter.

To process the tissue or bone fragments in the laboratory, add 1 mL of sterile thioglycollate broth to a sterile tissue grinder. Homogenize the piece of tissue or bone fragment until a thick suspension is obtained. Ideally, this procedure can be performed within an anaerobic chamber. If a chamber is not available, the grinding must be accomplished as quickly as possible at the workbench. Inoculate the suspension as described previously for an aspirate.

Blood

A discussion of the variety of commercially available blood culture systems is beyond the scope of this chapter. Blood must be cultured in such a manner as to recover any and all bacteria or yeasts that may be present. This usually requires aseptic inoculation of both an anaerobic (unvented) and aerobic (vented) bottle. Investigations have shown that single-bottle systems are less efficient in isolating certain organisms (including anaerobes) than two-bottle systems. Once inoculated, blood culture bottles should be rapidly transported to the laboratory, where they are incubated at 35° to 37° C. It is important to note that blood for culture must be carefully collected so as to minimize contamination with skin flora. This usually is accomplished by meticulous preparation of the venipuncture site with a bactericidal agent, such as tincture of iodine or an iodophor.

Quality-assurance considerations relating to specimens are summarized in Table 19-8.

Processing Clinical Samples for Maximum Recovery of Anaerobic Pathogens

To ensure that results are clinically significant, only properly selected, collected, and transported specimens should be processed in the anaerobic bacteriology laboratory. In processing a specimen for anaerobic bacteriology, primary emphasis should be placed on safety, adherence to prescribed procedures, and speed.

Ideally, once a specimen arrives in the laboratory, it is placed immediately in an anaerobic chamber to prevent further exposure of clinical materials to oxygen. Anaerobic chambers allow all steps in the processing of a specimen to be performed in an oxygen-free environment. In those laboratories not equipped with anaerobic chambers, holding systems may be used (described later in this chapter). To comply with mandatory infectious disease safety policies, follow the appropriate safety precautions. Wear disposable latex gloves when handling clinical specimens containing potentially infectious agents and use a laminar flow safety cabinet whenever it is appropriate to do so.

In addition to the initial processing steps previously described, the following procedures also should be performed:

- Macroscopic examination of the specimen
- Preparation of Gram-stained smears for microscopic examination
- Inoculation of appropriate plated and tubed media, including media specifically designed for culturing anaerobes
- Anaerobic incubation of inoculated media

TABLE 19-8

Specimen Quality Assurance

Component	Comments
Specimen selection	Persons responsible for selecting specimens must be familiar with the types of specimens that are suitable for anaerobic bacteriology.
Request slips	Request slips must include patient demographics, specimen type and source, date and time of collection, the requesting physician, and antimicrobial agents the patient may have already taken.
	The time of collection is especially important, because it will determine how quickly the specimen is transported to the laboratory.
	The type of specimen alerts the microbiologists as to the anaerobes to expect, which serves as a guide to media selection.
Specimen collection	Collect with an attempt to minimize contamination of the specimen with organisms of the indigenous microflora.
	Minimize exposure of the specimens to oxygen.
Specimen handling	Label specimen containers with the patient's name, identification number, source of specimen, and date and time of collection.
	In the laboratory, check the name on the specimen container against the name on the request slip to ensure that specimens have not been inadvertently switched.
Specimen transport	Transport specimens rapidly to minimize exposure to oxygen and time spent at room temperature.
	Use appropriate transport devices whenever a delay is anticipated between collection and processing.
	Clinical laboratory personnel must provide the appropriate containers and must instruct health care practitioners in their proper use.
Written laboratory directives or guidelines	Written guidelines to clinicians should include the following: appropriate and inappropriate specimens, specimen collection and transport procedures, and policy regarding specimen duplication.
	Criteria for rejection should include unlabeled specimen container, inappropriate specimen for patient's condition, incorrectly collected and/or transported specimen, too much delay between collection and arrival in the lab, and dried out samples.
Education of clinicians	Clinical laboratory professionals should participate in educating health care practitioners who are involved in patient assessment, test ordering, and specimen collection regarding anaerobic bacteriology.

Modified from Engelkirk PG, Duben-Engelkirk J, Dowell VR Jr: *Principles and practice of anaerobic bacteriology,* Belmont, Calif, 1992, Star.

Macroscopic examination of specimen

Examine each specimen received in the anaerobic bacteriology section macroscopically, and record pertinent observations on some type of a worksheet. Some of the characteristics to note during the macroscopic examination are listed in Table 19-9.

Direct microscopic examination of specimen

Direct smears for Gram stain must be prepared on all specimens received in the laboratory. Examination of a thin Gram-stained smear is one of the most important diagnostic procedures performed in anaerobic bacteriology laboratories. In some laboratories, smears are stained before inoculation of media; microscopic observations then can serve as a guide to selecting the media to be inoculated. In other laboratories, a routine battery of media is inoculated before staining and examining the smear, thus eliminating any further delay in media inoculation. The latter approach is recommended.

Gram-stained smears must be examined for several reasons, as follows:

- The Gram stain reveals the various types and relative number of microorganisms present. The presence of multiple distinct morphologic forms suggests that a polymicrobic infectious process is present. This should be reported to the requesting physician.

- Certain morphotypes may provide a presumptive identification of organisms and serve as a guide to media selection. For example, if large, gram-positive bacilli are seen, clostridia may be suspected. An egg-yolk agar to detect lecithinase or lipase may be added in the primary set-up. Thin, gram-negative bacilli with tapered ends may be fusobacteria. Extremely pleomorphic, gram-negative bacilli with bizarre shapes are suggestive of *Fusobacterium mortiferum* or *Fusobacterium necrophorum*. Tiny, round to oval, gram-negative cocci with a tendency to stain gram-variable are suggestive of *Veillonella* species, whereas gram-negative coccobacilli may be *Bacteroides, Porphyromonas,* or *Prevotella* spp.

- The Gram stain often reveals the presence of leukocytes. However, certain anaerobes produce necrotizing toxins (leukocidins) that destroy leukocytes. Thus, the absence of leukocytes in a Gram-stained smear does not rule out the involvement of anaerobes and never should be used as a criterion for rejecting a wound specimen.
- Finally, the Gram stain can serve as a quality-control technique. Failure to isolate certain organisms observed in the Gram-stained smear might indicate that problems exist with the anaerobic technique being used. However, failure to recover certain morphotypes also could indicate those particular organisms were dead or the patient was receiving antimicrobial agents that inhibited growth of the organisms on the plated media.

Direct smears for Gram stain should be methanol-fixed rather than heat-fixed. Methanol fixation preserves the morphology of leukocytes and bacteria better than heat fixation. Gram-negative anaerobes frequently stain a very pale pink when safranin is used as the counterstain and thus are easily overlooked in Gram-stained smears of clinical specimens and blood cultures. To enhance the red color of gram-negative anaerobes, use of basic fuchsin as the counterstain or counterstaining with safranin for 3 to 5 minutes is recommended. Some *Clostridium* species routinely stain pink, but studies have shown that this problem can be eliminated by performing all steps of the Gram staining procedure under anaerobic conditions (i.e., within an anaerobic chamber).

In addition to the Gram stain, some laboratories routinely examine wet mounts of clinical materials using regular transmitted light, phase-contrast microscopy, or darkfield illumination. These procedures aid in the detection of motile organisms and refractile spores.

Inoculation of appropriate plated and tubed media

The choice of media for use in the anaerobic bacteriology laboratory is an extremely important aspect of successful anaerobic bacteriology. Anaerobes have special nutritional requirements for

TABLE 19-9

Characteristics to Note During the Macroscopic Examination of a Specimen

Questions to Ask	Comments
Is it an appropriate specimen?	Inappropriate specimens should be rejected.
Was it submitted in an appropriate transport container?	Improperly transported specimens should be rejected.
How old is the specimen? Are the date and time of collection recorded on the accompanying request slip?	Specimens that are too old may be cause for rejection.
Is there evidence that the specimen has dried out during transit?	Specimens that have dried out during transport should be rejected.
Does the specimen have a foul odor?	Many anaerobes, especially *Fusobacterium* and *Porphyromonas* spp., have foul-smelling metabolic end products; however, the lack of a foul odor does not exclude anaerobes.
Does the specimen fluoresce brick-red when exposed to a Wood's lamp? (A Wood's lamp emits long-wave [366 nm] ultraviolet light.)	Pigmented species of *Porphyromonas* and *Prevotella* produce substances that fluoresce under long-wave UV light prior to becoming darkly pigmented. Although a brick-red fluorescence is presumptive evidence of these organisms, some members of this group fluoresce colors other than brick-red.
Is the necrotic tissue or exudate black?	Such discoloration may be due to the pigment produced by pigmented species of *Porphyromonas* and *Prevotella.*
Does the specimen contain sulfur granules?	Such granules are associated with actinomycosis, a condition caused by *Actinomyces* spp., *Propionibacterium propionicus,* and closely related organisms, such as *Propionibacterium acnes.*
Is the specimen bloody?	Such information should be included in a preliminary report to the requesting physician.
Is the specimen purulent?	Such information should be included in a preliminary report to the attending physician.

Modified from Engelkirk PG, Duben-Engelkirk J, Dowell VR Jr: *Principles and practice of anaerobic bacteriology,* Belmont, Calif, 1992, Star.

vitamin K, hemin, and yeast extract, and all primary isolation media for anaerobes should contain these three ingredients. Recommendations of different authorities in the area of anaerobic bacteriology with regard to specific media to be included in the primary isolation set-up of anaerobe cultures vary slightly.

MEDIA FOR USE IN THE PRIMARY ISOLATION SET-UP
Table 19-10 lists the primary media recommended for recovery of anaerobes. Although these media are designed for anaerobes, they also support the growth of most aerobes. No single medium exists that supports all common species of anaerobes while inhibiting all aerobes. In addition to those listed in Table 19-10, other nonselective and selective media may be helpful. Table 19-11 lists media designed for specific anaerobes to be used in conjunction with the primary media.

The ideal media for use in the culture of anaerobes are those that have never been exposed to oxygen or have been exposed only briefly. Such media include freshly prepared media and those stored under anaerobic conditions from the time they were made. Media exposed to air for extended periods may contain toxic substances, produced as a result of the reduction of molecular oxygen. Such media may also have redox potentials above that required for anaerobes to initiate growth. Although it is not practical to prepare fresh media each time they are needed, freshly prepared media can be stored within an anaerobic chamber or holding system until used.

An alternative is to use commercial media that have been prepared, packaged, shipped, and stored under anaerobic conditions (i.e., not exposed to oxygen until they are inoculated or not exposed at all when plates are inoculated within an anaerobic chamber). Such PRAS media (shown in Figure 19-2) are available from Anaerobe Systems (San Jose, Calif.). Growth is initiated quickly on PRAS media, and many anaerobes produce sufficient growth after only 24 hours of incubation. Studies have demonstrated that these media perform better than fresh media or other commercially available media.

Reducing agents, such as palladium chloride, are sometimes added to media before autoclaving in an attempt to "prereduce" them. However, care must be taken in selecting the type of reducing agents, as some are toxic to certain anaerobes. Media containing reducing agents are available from a variety of commercial sources. Storing them in gas-permeable cellophane sleeves and/or at refrigerator temperatures may decrease their shelf life. In all likelihood, there is a limit to the length of time that reducing agents can maintain sufficiently low oxidation-reduction potentials when they are in constant contact with oxygen. An enzyme called Oxytase, available from a company of the same name (Mansfield, Ohio) also can be used to convert ordinary media into media suitable for use in anaerobic bacteriology.

ADDITIONAL MEDIA FOR AEROBIC INCUBATION
In addition to the battery of selective anaerobic media to be incubated anaerobically, a variety of plated media to be incubated aerobically in a CO_2 incubator also is inoculated. The specific media vary somewhat from one laboratory to another and depend on the specimen type; nevertheless, blood, MacConkey, and chocolate agar plates usually are included. Some laboratories also routinely include a phenylethyl alcohol reportedly have (PEA) plate or colistin nalidixic acid (CNA) plate. Figure 19-3 shows a typical plating protocol for a wound sample and the types of results that might be expected.

INOCULATION PROCEDURES
In laboratories not equipped with an anaerobic chamber, inoculation of appropriate plated and tubed media could be performed in an area with a suitable nitrogen gas holding system. Such a holding system, which may employ a jar, a box, or other small chamber, allows uninoculated plates to be held under anaerobic conditions until needed. Inoculated plates should be held under near-anaerobic conditions until placed into an anaerobic jar or bag. Care should be taken to ensure that inoculated plates do not remain in the holding jar at room temperature for extended periods (i.e., not longer than 1 hour). Also, because the holding jar should remain as anaerobic as possible, care should be taken to minimize convection currents whenever freshly inoculated plates are added to the jar.

Some microbiologists believe it is better to batch-process specimens than to process each specimen as it arrives in the laboratory; this relieves their concern that freshly inoculated plates

TABLE 19-10

Primary Set-Up Media Recommended for Recovery of Anaerobes

Medium	Orgnisms	Comments
Anaerobic blood agar plate (Brucella blood agar [BRU/BA] is the most popular choice)	Supports growth of virtually all obligate and facultative anaerobes, when incubated anaerobically	An enriched medium containing sheep's blood for enrichment and detection of hemolysis, vitamin K_1 (required by some *Porphyromonas* spp.), and hemin (which enhances growth of some *Bacteroides* spp., including members of the *Bacteroides fragilis* group); similar excellent media (e.g., CDC anaerobe agar, enriched brain heart infusion blood agar, and Schaedler blood agar) are also available for use; variations have been reported in the ability of these different blood agar media to support growth of certain anaerobes (Sheppard et al, 1990)
Bacteroides bile esculin (BBE) agar plate	Supports growth of bile-tolerant *Bacteroides* spp., when incubated anaerobically; some strains of *Fusobacterium mortiferum, Klebsiella pneumoniae,* enterococci, and yeast may grow to a limited extent	A selective medium containing gentamicin (which inhibits most aerobic organisms), 20% bile (which inhibits most anaerobes), and esculin; used primarily for rapid isolation and presumptive identification of members of the *B. fragilis* group, which grow well on BBE (due to their bile-tolerance) and turn the originally light-yellow medium to brown (due to esculin hydrolysis)
Kanamycin-vancomycin-laked blood (KVLB) agar plate	Supports growth of *Bacteroides* and *Prevotella* spp., when incubated anaerobically; yeasts and kanamycin-resistant, facultative, gram-negative bacilli will also grow	A selective medium containing kanamycin (which inhibits most facultative gram-negative bacilli), vancomycin (which inhibits most gram-positive organisms and vancomycin-sensitive strains of *Porphyromonas* spp.), and laked blood (which accelerates production of brown-black pigmented colonies by certain *Prevotella* spp.; used primarily for rapid isolation and presumptive identification of pigmented species of *Prevotella;* a similar medium that substitutes paromomycin for kanamycin inhibits growth of kanamycin-resistant, facultative, gram-negative bacilli
Phenylethyl alcohol (PEA) agar plate (also called phenylethanol agar or phenethyl alcohol agar)	Supports growth of virtually all obligate anaerobes (both gram-positive and gram-negative) and gram-positive, facultative anaerobes, when incubated anaerobically	A selective medium containing phenylethyl alcohol; used primarily to suppress the growth of any facultative, gram-negative bacilli (e.g., *Entero-bacteriaceae*) that might be present in the clinical specimen, especially swarming *Proteus* spp.
Anaerobic broth (e.g., thioglycollate [THIO], chopped meat)	Supports growth of virtually all types of bacteria grown in THIO: obligate aerobes and microaerophiles near the top, obligate anaerobes at the bottom, and facultative anaerobes throughout	Because obligate anaerobes can be overgrown by more rapidly growing facultative organisms present in the specimen and killed by their toxic metabolic by-products, THIO serves only as a backup source of culture material (e.g., in the event that there is no growth on plated media due to a jar failure or the presence of anti-microbial agents in the specimen); chopped meat carbohydrate broth can be used in place of THIO; broth cultures should never be relied on exclusively for isolating anaerobes from clinical material

Modified from Engelkirk PG, Duben-Engelkirk J, Dowell VR Jr: *Principles and practice of anaerobic bacteriology,* Belmont, Calif, 1992, Star.

TABLE 19-11
Additional Selective and Nonselective Media

Medium	Special Use
Cycloserine cefoxitin fructose agar (CCFA)	*Clostridium difficile*
Bacteroides gingivalis blood agar (BGBA)	Dental cutlures for *Prevotella gingivalis*
Egg-yolk agar (EYA)	*Clostridium* spp.
Cadmium sulfate–fluoride–acridine trypticase agar (CFAT)	Dental cutlures for *Prevotella gingivalis*
Josamycin, vancomycin, norfloxacin (JVN)	*Fusobacterium* and *Leptotrichia*
Lactobacillus selective media (LBS)	*Lactobacillus* spp.
Peptostreptococcaceae selective agar (PS)	*Peptostreptococcus* spp.

will remain at room temperature in a holding system that may contain some oxygen. Batch processing is certainly an acceptable alternative for aspirates and specimens received in proper transport containers (i.e., those kept moist under anaerobic conditions). It would be unacceptable, however, to batch-process improperly submitted specimens (e.g., dry swabs) or clinical materials apt to contain rapidly growing bacteria. The delay would further expose anaerobes to molecular oxygen, increase the likelihood of specimens drying out, and decrease the probability of recovering anaerobes.

Anaerobic incubation of inoculated media

After specimens are rapidly processed and inoculated onto the appropriate media, the inoculated plates must be incubated anaerobically at 35° to 37° C. The most common and practical choices for anaerobic incubation systems for clinical laboratories are anaerobic chambers, anaerobic jars, and anaerobic bags or pouches. The choice of system

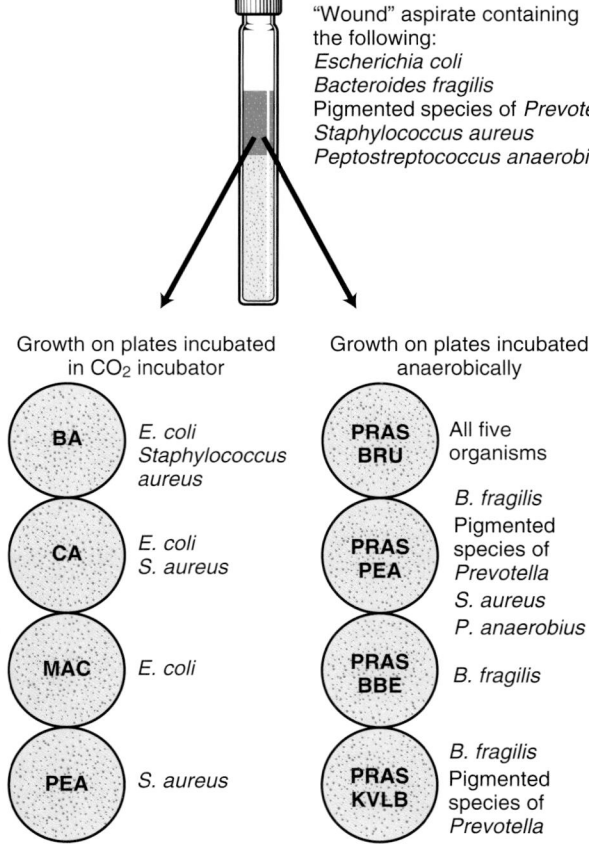

"Wound" aspirate containing the following:
Escherichia coli
Bacteroides fragilis
Pigmented species of *Prevotella*
Staphylococcus aureus
Peptostreptococcus anaerobius

Growth on plates incubated in CO₂ incubator

BA — *E. coli*, *Staphylococcus aureus*
CA — *E. coli*, *S. aureus*
MAC — *E. coli*
PEA — *S. aureus*

Growth on plates incubated anaerobically

PRAS BRU — All five organisms
PRAS PEA — *B. fragilis*, Pigmented species of *Prevotella*, *S. aureus*, *P. anaerobius*
PRAS BBE — *B. fragilis*
PRAS KVLB — *B. fragilis*, Pigmented species of *Prevotella*

Figure 19-3

Culture results that might be obtained from the primary isolation set-up of a hypothetical "wound" specimen. This diagram illustrates the media and atmospheric conditions that would support growth of various organisms contained in the specimen. *BA*, Blood agar; *BBE*, Bacteroides bile-esculin agar; *BRU*, Brucella agar; *CA*, chocolate agar; *KVLB*, kanamycin-vancomycin-laked blood agar; *MAC*, MacConkey agar; *PEA*, phenylethyl alcohol blood agar; *PRAS*, PRAS medium. (From Engelkirk PG, Duben-Engelkirk J, Dowell VR Jr: *Principles and Practice of Clinical Anaerobic Bacteriology*, Belmont, Calif, 1992, Star.)

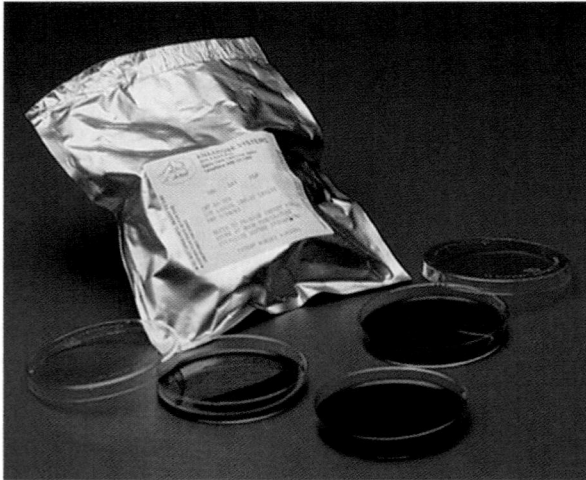

Figure 19-2

Prereduced, anaerobically sterilized (PRAS) plated media. PRAS plated media are manufactured, packaged, shipped, and stored under anaerobic conditions. (Courtesy Anaerobe Systems, San Jose, Calif.)

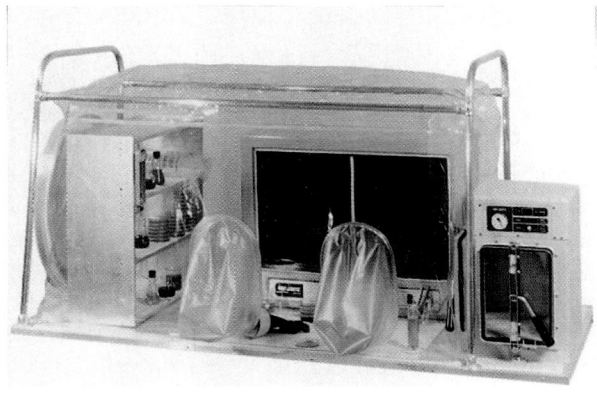

Figure 19-4
"Glove Box" type of anaerobic chamber manufactured by Coy Laboratory Products. The flexible, clear vinyl chambers are available in three lengths (36, 59, and 78 inches), including one fitted with two pairs of gloves so that two microbiologists can use the chamber simultaneously. (From Engelkirk PG, Duben-Engelkirk J, Dowell VR Jr: *Principles and practice of anaerobic bacteriology,* Belmont, Calif, 1992, Star.)

is influenced by a number of factors, including financial considerations, the number of anaerobic cultures performed, and space limitations.

ANAEROBIC CHAMBERS

The ideal anaerobic incubation system is an **anaerobic chamber,** which provides an oxygen-free environment for inoculating media and incubating cultures. Identification and susceptibility tests also can be performed within the chamber, if necessary.

A number of anaerobic chambers are available commercially. Some models, called "glove boxes," are fitted with airtight rubber gloves (Figure 19-4). The microbiologist inserts the hands into the gloves and manipulates specimens, plates, and tubes inside the chamber. Glove boxes traditionally have been constructed of flexible vinyl. They are available from companies such as Coy Corporation (Grass Lake, Mich.), Forma Scientific (Marietta, Ohio), and Lab-Line Instruments (Melrose Park, Ill.).

Gloveless anaerobic chambers are also available commercially (Figure 19-5) (Anaerobe Systems, San Jose, Calif.). Airtight rubber sleeves that fit snugly against the user's bare forearms are used in place of gloves, enabling the microbiologist to work within an anaerobic environment with bare hands. However, to comply with mandatory infectious disease safety precautions, it is recommended that disposable latex gloves be worn if clinical specimens are being processed within gloveless chambers. Subsequent operations may be performed with bare hands. The newer gloveless models have a dissecting microscope mounted on the front of the rigid Plexiglas chamber. This enables the user to observe colony morphology within the chamber, eliminating the need to remove the plates from the chamber and eliminating exposure of the colonies to oxygen.

All anaerobic chambers contain the following:

- Catalyst
- Desiccant
- Hydrogen gas (5% to 10%)
- Carbon dioxide gas (5% to 10%)
- Nitrogen gas (80% to 90%)
- Indicator

Anaerobic chambers contain a catalyst (usually palladium-coated alumina pellets) that removes residual oxygen from the atmosphere within the chamber. With time, the catalyst pellets become inactivated by gaseous metabolic end products produced by the anaerobes. A product called Anatox (Don Whitley Scientific, Shipley, West Yorkshire,

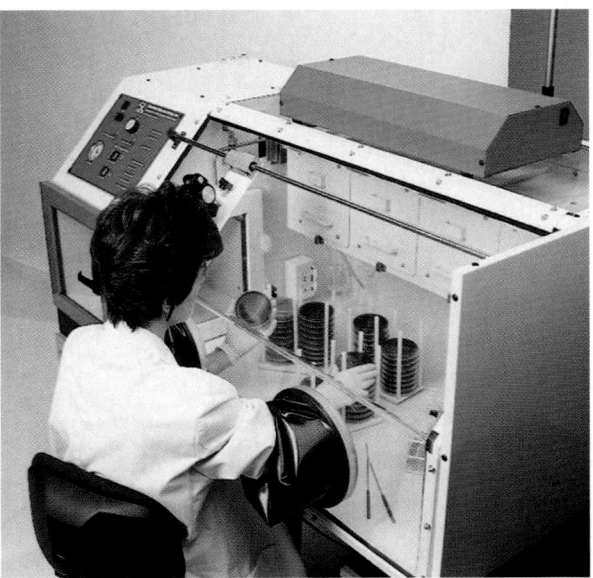

Figure 19-5
"Gloveless" type of anaerobic chamber with dissecting microscope attachment. This stainless steel and Plexiglas chamber was manufactured by Anaerobe Systems. (Courtesy Anaerobe Systems, San Jose, Calif.; Sheldon Manufacturing, Inc., Cornelius, Ore.)

England) has been shown to absorb these metabolites and prolong catalyst life. Silica gel is used as a desiccant to absorb the water formed when hydrogen combines with free oxygen in the presence of the catalyst. The silica gel desiccant turns blue to pink when saturated with water, and it needs to be heated daily to rejuvenate. Carbon dioxide is required for the growth of many anaerobic organisms, and inert nitrogen gas is used as a filler for the remaining percentage of the anaerobic atmosphere. The indicator system can be either methylene blue or resazurin. Methylene blue remains white in the absence of oxygen and turns blue in the presence of oxygen; resazurin goes from colorless in the absence of oxygen to pink in the presence of oxygen.

ANAEROBIC JARS

For small laboratories, where the volume of anaerobic cultures may not justify the purchase of anaerobic chambers, alternative systems are available. One such alternative is the GasPak jar, manufactured by Becton Dickinson (Cockeysville, Md.) (Figure 19-6). The jars have been used in clinical laboratories for many years, enabling even small laboratories to perform satisfactory anaerobic bacteriology. Newer models accommodate a large number of plates as well as microtiter suscepti-

bility trays and anaerobic identification strips or trays. Other systems are available from Adams Scientific (West Warwick, R.I.), Difco Laboratories (Detroit, Mich.), Oxoid (Columbia, Md.), Remel (Lenexa, Kan.), EM Diagnostic Systems (Gibbstown, N.J.), and other companies. None of these systems provide all the features or advantages of anaerobic chambers, and cost analysis may reveal that, over time, a chamber is actually more cost-effective.

Anaerobic jar systems such as the GasPak use an envelope gas generator. When water is added to the GasPak envelope, two gases are generated— carbon dioxide and hydrogen. The two gases have a function similar to that in the anaerobic chamber. Hydrogen is explosive, and if the catalyst is not functioning properly, hydrogen gas will be present in the jar; therefore following incubation, an individual should never open the jar in the vicinity of an open flame. A methylene blue indicator strip is always added to the jar to verify that an anaerobic atmosphere has been achieved. If the catalyst performs properly, water vapor will be present on the inside of the jar and the indicator strip will be colorless. Some of the newer gas-generating packets contain a built-in indicator. Failure to achieve anaerobic conditions could be due to a "poisoned" catalyst or a crack in the jar, lid, or "O" ring.

A "poisoned" catalyst results from the gases (particularly H_2S) produced by anaerobes. The reusable catalyst pellets can be rejuvenated after every use by heating them in a 160° C oven for a minimum of 2 hours. Some of the newer gas-generating packets contain a built-in supply of fresh catalyst, thus eliminating the need to maintain a container of rejuvenated catalyst within the jar.

The major disadvantage of any anaerobic jar system is the plates have to be removed from the jar to be examined. This, of course, exposes the colonies to oxygen, which is especially hazardous to the anaerobes during their first 48 hours of growth. For this reason, a suitable holding system always should be used in conjunction with anaerobic jars. Plates can be removed from the anaerobic jar, placed in an oxygen-free holding system, removed one by one for rapid microscopic examination of colonies, and then quickly returned to the holding system. Plates never should remain in room air on the open bench.

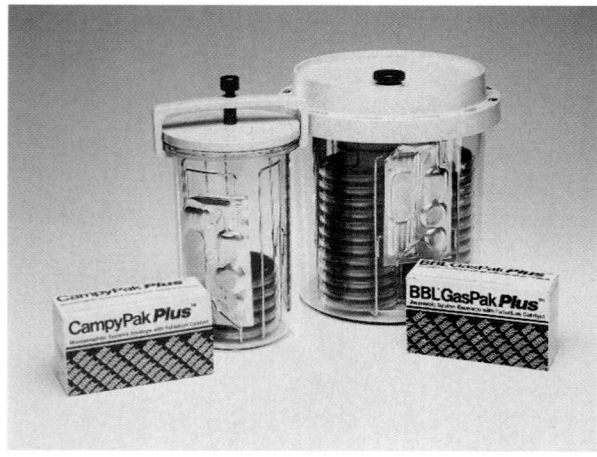

Figure 19-6

Anaerobic jars. This photograph depicts two of the many different types of anaerobic jars that are available commercially. As can be seen in this photograph, the jars can also be used to culture for microaerophilic organisms. (Courtesy Becton Dickinson Microbiology Systems, Cockeysville, Md.)

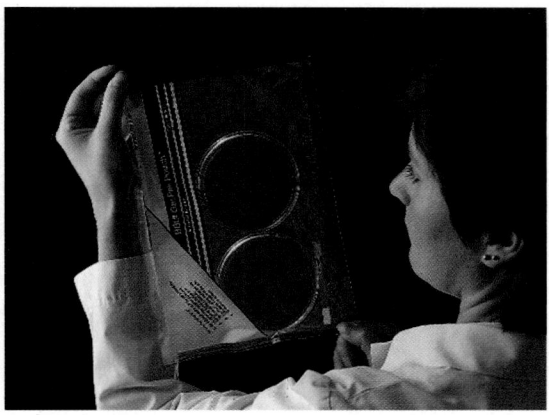

Figure 19-7 _____
Anaerobic pouch. This photograph depicts the GasPak Pouch, one of the commercially available anaerobic bag or pouch systems. Identification and susceptibility testing systems requiring anaerobic incubation can be incubated within some of the bags or pouches. (Courtesy Becton Dickinson Microbiology Systems, Cockeysville, Md.)

ANAEROBIC BAGS OR POUCHES

Other alternatives to an anaerobic chamber are anaerobic bags or pouches (Figure 19-7). Such products are available from Becton Dickinson (Type A BioBag and GasPak Pouch, Cockeysville, Md.) and Remel (Anaerobic Pouch, Lenexa, Kan.). These products will be collectively referred to as bags. One or two inoculated plates are placed into a bag, an oxygen-removal system is activated, and the bag is sealed and incubated. Theoretically, the plates can be examined for growth without removing the plates from the bags—thus without exposing the colonies to oxygen. However, with some of the products, a water-vapor film on the inner surface of the bag or the lid of the plate can sometimes obscure vision. In such cases, the plates must be removed from the bag to observe for growth, and a new bag and oxygen-removal system must be used whenever additional incubation is required. As with the anaerobic jar, plates must be removed from the bags in order to work with the colonies at the bench. Thus, an anaerobic holding system should be used in conjunction with any of the anaerobic bags.

Any of these bags are also useful transport devices. For example, a biopsy specimen can first be placed in a sterile screw-capped tube containing sterile saline, which is then placed in one of these bags. The oxygen-removal system is activated, and the specimen is transported to the laboratory within the bag.

PROCEDURES FOR IDENTIFYING ANAEROBIC ISOLATES

Preliminary Procedures
When to examine primary plates
Plates incubated in an anaerobic chamber can be examined at any time without exposing the colonies to oxygen; however, those in anaerobic jars, bags, or pouches are exposed to the potentially damaging effects of oxygen whenever the containers are opened. Thus, when should anaerobic jars, bags, or pouches be opened? Should they be opened after 24 or 48 hours of incubation? If they are opened at 24 hours, slow-growing anaerobes will be too small to work with. More rapidly growing anaerobes, however, such as some *Clostridium* and *Bacteroides* spp., could be worked up at 24 hours, especially when appropriate PRAS media are used for the primary isolation set-up. Thus, waiting until 48 hours to open jars or bags could delay identification of clinically important anaerobes by a day.

If a holding system is available at the anaerobe workstation and is used in conjunction with jars, bags, or pouches, exposure to oxygen will be minimized, and plates can be removed and examined at 24 hours and then placed immediately into the holding system. As soon as all plates are examined, those requiring additional incubation are returned to an anaerobic system and incubated for an appropriate period before reexamination. Cultures are routinely held 5 to 7 days to allow growth of particularly slow-growing anaerobes and up to 3 weeks whenever *Actinomyces* spp. are suspected.

Indications of the presence of anaerobes in cultures
There are several clues that alert the microbiologist that anaerobes may be present on the primary plates. These include the following:

- A foul odor upon opening an anaerobic jar or bag; some anaerobes, especially *Clostridium difficile, Fusobacterium,* and *Porphyromonas* spp., produce foul-smelling metabolic end products that are readily apparent when the jars, bags, or pouches are opened.

- Colony morphotypes present on the anaerobically incubated blood agar plates but not on the CO_2-incubated blood or chocolate agar plates.
- Good growth (more than 1 mm in diameter) of gray colonies on the BBE (Bacteroides bile-esculin) plate, characteristic of members of the *B. fragilis* group.
- Colonies on either the KVLB (kanamycin-vancomycin-laked blood) agar or anaerobic blood agar plate (e.g., BRU/BA [Brucella/blood agar] plate) that fluoresce brick-red under ultraviolet light or are brown to black in ordinary light, characteristic of pigmented *Porphyromonas* and *Prevotella* spp., although most strains of *Porphyromonas* will not grow on KVLB due to their sensitivity to vancomycin.
- Double zone of hemolysis on blood agar, suggestive of *Clostridium perfringens*.

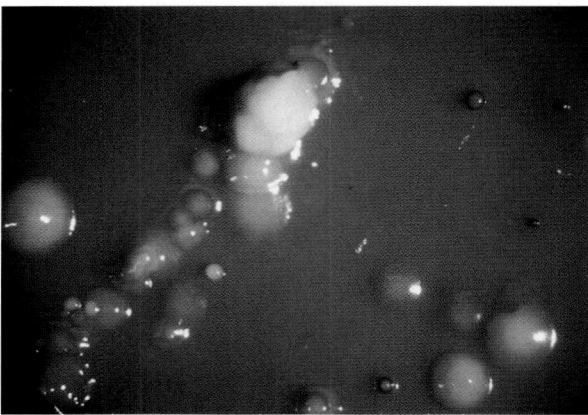

Figure 19-8

Anaerobic blood agar plate from an intrauterine device culture as seen through a dissection microscope. The heavy mixture of sizes and types of colonies makes the task of isolating and identifying colonies very difficult without the enhancement obtained with a dissecting microscope.

Processing colonies suspected of being anaerobes

When anaerobes are suspected, the following steps must be performed and recorded for each colony morphotype present on the anaerobic blood agar plate to initiate presumptive identification of the isolates:

- Describe colony morphology and whether growth occurred on each of the selective (BBE, KVLB) and nonselective anaerobic blood agar plate (BRU/BA) media used.
- Describe Gram-stain reaction and cell morphology.
- Inoculate pure culture/subculture plate; add appropriate disks.
- Set up aerotolerance test.

COLONY MORPHOLOGY

Enumerate, describe, and record each colony morphotype and growth characteristics on a worksheet. The use of a dissecting microscope to observe the fine details of the colonies and pick colonies for isolation is recommended. Figure 19-8 depicts the appearance of colonies as seen through a dissecting microscope. Growth of a particular morphotype can be semiquantitated using terms such as "light," "moderate," and "heavy" or by using some type of coding system (e.g., 1+, 2+). Use Table 19-12 as a guide for characteristic features to note when examining colonies of anaerobic isolates.

GRAM REACTION AND CELL MORPHOLOGY

Prepare a smear for Gram stain. Record the gram reaction and cell morphology on a worksheet. The Gram-stain reaction and morphologic appearance of the organism aid in the presumptive identification of isolates, as shown in a schematic diagram in Figure 19-9.

PURE CULTURE/SUBCULTURE PLATE
AND SPECIAL-POTENCY DISKS

Although the Gram stain is helpful in the initial identification of an anaerobic isolate, certain species of *Clostridium* may stain pink and thus appear to be gram-negative bacilli. To determine the true Gram-stain reaction of the isolate, special-potency disks are used. These disks, in addition to determining the true Gram-stain reaction, may provide a presumptive identification of the suspected anaerobic organism.

Based on the Gram-stain reaction and morphology of the organism, special-potency disks are added to the subculture plate. The disks are placed on the heavily inoculated area of the plate (usually the first quarter or third of the plate, depending on the particular manner of streaking). The specific

TABLE 19-12

Characteristics to Note When Examining Colonies of Anaerobic Bacteria

Characteristic	Suspected Anaerobe
Color/pigment	
Brown-black colonies	If a gram-negative rod, may be a pigmented species of *Porphyromonas* or *Prevotella;* if a gram-positive coccus, may be *Peptococcus niger*
Red, pink, tan, yellow	If a gram-positive rod, may be an *Actinomyces* sp.
Surface (e.g., glistening or dull)	—
Density (e.g., opaque, translucent, transparent)	Members of the *Bacteroides ureolyticus* group (gram-negative bacilli) typically have translucent to transparent colonies
Consistency (e.g., butyrous [butter-like], viscous, membranous, brittle)	—
Form, elevation, margin	—
Fluorescence under ultraviolet light	
Brick-red	If a gram-negative rod, may be a pigmented species of *Porphyromonas* or *Prevotella*
Red	If a gram-negative coccus, may be *Veillonella* spp.
Chartreuse	If a gram-negative rod, may be a subspecies of *Fusobacterium nucleatum;* if a gram-positive rod, may be *Clostridium difficile*
Pitting of the agar	May be *Bacteroides ureolyticus, Bacteroides gracilis,* or *Wolinella* spp. (all gram-negative bacilli)
Double zone of hemolysis	*Clostridium perfringens* (a gram-positive rod)
Extensive swarming	May be *Clostridium tetani* (terminal spores) or *C. septicum* (subterminal spores); both are gram-positive bacilli
Odor	
Like a horse stable	*C. difficile* (a gram-positive rod)
Sweet, unpleasant	If a gram-positive coccus, may be *Peptostreptococcus anaerobius*
Spider-like appearance (having thin, wooly filaments, originating at a single point)	If a gram-positive rod, may be a young colony of *Actinomyces israelii* or *Propionibacterium propionicus*
Molar tooth appearance	If a gram-positive rod, may be an older colony of *A. israelii* or *P. propionicus*
White, bread-crumb appearance	If a gram-negative rod, may be a subspecies of *F. nucleatum*
Ground-glass appearance	If a gram-negative rod, may be a subspecies of *F. nucleatum*
Fried-egg appearance	If a gram-negative rod, may be *Fusobacterium mortiferum* or *Fusobacterium varium,* although other anaerobes also produce such colonies

Modified from Engelkirk PG, Duben-Engelkirk J, Dowell VR Jr: *Principles and practice of anaerobic bacteriology,* Belmont, Calif, 1992, Star.

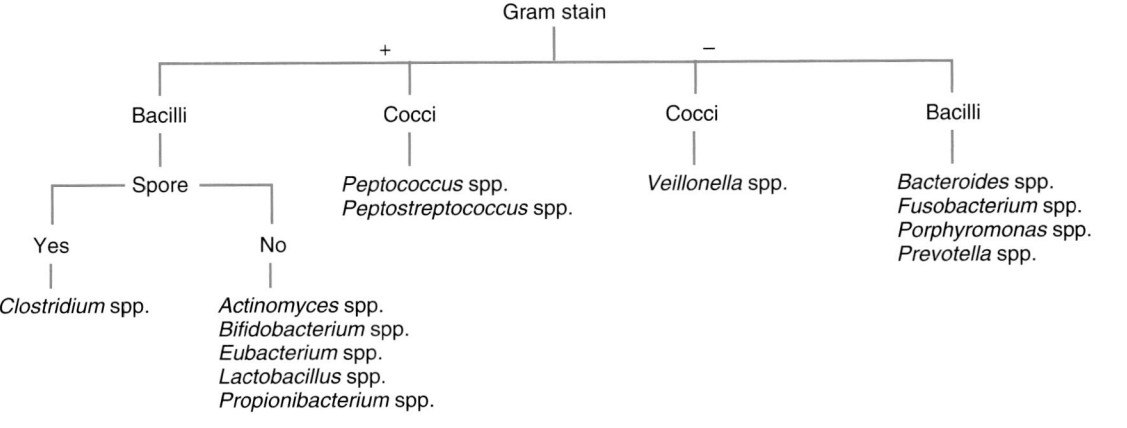

Figure 19-9

Schematic diagram for the initial identification of anaerobic isolates based on Gram stain morphology.

TABLE 19-13

Interpretation of Special-Potency Antimicrobial Disk Results

Vancomycin Result*	Kanamycin Result*	Colistin Result*	Interpretation
Susceptible	Variable	Resistant	Probably a pink-staining, gram-positive bacillus; however, if the kanamycin result is R, it could be a *Porphyromonas* sp.
Sensitive	Resistant	Resistant	*Porphyromonas* spp.
Resistant	Resistant	Resistant	Probably a member of the *Bacteroides fragilis* group, but could be a *Prevotella* sp.
Resistant	Resistant	Variable	*Prevotella* spp.
Resistant	Resistant	Susceptible	Probably a *Prevotella* sp.
Resistant	Susceptible	Susceptible	*Bacteroides ureolyticus, Bilophila wadsworthia,* or a *Fusobacterium* sp.; *Veillonella* spp. (gram-negative cocci) will also produce these results

Courtesy Mangels JI, 1998.
*Vancomycin, 5μg; kanamycin, 1 mg; colistin, 10 μg.

TABLE 19-14

Interpretation of Aerotolerance Test Results

	Aerobe	Capnophilic Aerobe	Facultative Anaerobe	Obligate Anaerobe
Blood agar plate incubated aerobically in a non-CO_2 incubator	+	−	+	−
Chocolate agar plate incubated aerobically in a CO_2 incubator	+	+	+	−
Blood agar plate incubated anaerobically	−	−*	+	+

Haemophilus influenzae will grow on an anaerobically incubated Brucella blood agar plate but can be differentiated from an anaerobe by its growth on the chocolate agar plate incubated in the CO_2 incubator.

TABLE 19-15

Options Available for Identifying Anaerobic Bacteria

Identification Technique	Time to Obtain Results	Extent of Identification Capability
Presumptive identification based on colony morphology, Gram-stain observations, and results of simple tests (e.g., disks, catalase, spot indole)	Same day that the pure culture/subculture (PC/SC) plate is available	Limited capability; many clinically encountered anaerobes cannot be identified
Definitive identification		
Commercially available, preexisting enzyme-based identification systems (e.g., ANIDENT, MicroScan, RapId ANA II, Vitek ANI card)	Same day that the PC/SC plate is available (most systems require 4 hr incubation)	Most of the commonly encountered, clinically significant anaerobes can be identified
Commercially available biochemical-based identification systems (e.g., API 20A, Minitek, Sceptor)	24 to 48 hr after the PC/SC plate is available	Most commonly encountered saccharolytic anaerobes can be identified, but many asaccharolytic anaerobes cannot be
Cellular fatty acid analysis by high-resolution gas-liquid chromatography (GLC) (e.g., the MIDI system)	24 to 48 hr after the PC/SC plate is available	Most clinically encountered anaerobes can be identified
Conventional tubed biochemical tests and fatty acid analysis of GLC	24 to 72 hr after the PC/SC plate is available	Most clinically encountered anaerobes can be identified

Modified from Engelkirk PG, Duben-Engelkirk J, Dowell VR Jr: *Principles and practice of anaerobic bacteriology*, Belmont, Calif, 1992, Star.

disks to be added are shown in Figure 19-10. Interpretation of special-potency antimicrobial disk results is shown in Table 19-13.

AEROTOLERANCE TESTING

The **aerotolerance test** determines whether an isolate is a strict anaerobe or a facultative anaerobe. Incubating the suspected isolate in both aerobic and anaerobic environments determines the true atmospheric requirements of the organism. The subculture plate incubated anaerobically may serve as one of the plates used in the aerotolerance test. Suspected colonies also should be inoculated onto the following additional plates:

- A blood agar plate for incubation in a non-CO_2 incubator. This plate enables differentiation between aerobic and **capnophilic** organisms.
- A chocolate agar plate for incubation in a CO_2 incubator.

With the exception of the subculture plate, several different isolates can be tested on each plate. Incubate all aerotolerance test plates appropriately for 24 to 48 hours. Following incubation, examine the aerotolerance test plates for growth. Theoretically, an anaerobe should grow only on the anaerobically incubated plates. However, some **aerotolerant anaerobes** (e.g., certain *Clostridium, Actinomyces, Propionibacterium, Bifidobacterium,* and *Lactobacillus*) may grow on the CO_2-incubated chocolate agar plate, but they usually grow better on the anaerobically incubated plate. A facultative, noncapnophilic organism will grow on all plates, but a capnophilic aerobe should grow only on the CO_2-incubated chocolate agar plate. *Haemophilus influenzae,* however, will grow on the anaerobic plate and the CO_2-incubated chocolate agar plate but not on the aerobically incubated blood agar plate. Table 19-14 shows how the aerotolerance test is interpreted.

Identification of Anaerobic Isolates

There are various methods available to microbiologists for identifying anaerobic isolates. Table 19-15 lists several options from which the microbiologist may choose. The method and level of identification usually depend on the size and capabilities of the laboratory. There are several reasons why an anaerobic isolate must be identified beyond the microscopic and colonial morphology, as follows:

- Identification of an anaerobic isolate can often indicate to the physician the probable source of the infectious process. For example, *Clostridium septicum* bacteremia suggests colon cancer or other diseases of the colon. Similarly, regardless of the site of isolation, recovery of certain pigmented *Porphyromonas* species suggests an oral origin, whereas isolation of members of the *B. fragilis* group suggests an intestinal origin.
- Empiric therapy is likely to be more effective if the physician's choice of antimicrobial agent(s) is based on knowledge of the infecting organism(s).
- Over time, the identification of anaerobes provides a database of information regarding the role of certain anaerobic bacteria in infectious processes, in much the same way that susceptibility testing results provide a database of information to help physicians select antimicrobial agents for empiric therapy.

Presumptive identification

A presumptive identification of a bacterium is derived from simple colony and Gram-stain observations and the results of several relatively rapid and inexpensive tests. This method of identification has gained popularity in recent years, due primarily to the ever-increasing emphasis on speed and cost reduction. Described below are some rapid, inexpensive tests that are of value in presumptively identifying many of the anaerobes commonly encountered in clinical materials.

AEROTOLERANCE

Results of the aerotolerance test may be used to determine whether the isolate is truly an anaerobic organism.

FLUORESCENCE

Many strains of pigmented *Porphyromonas* and *Prevotella* spp. fluoresce brick-red under long-wave (366 nm) ultraviolet (UV) light. However, some strains fluoresce colors other than brick-red (e.g., brilliant red, yellow, orange, and pink-orange). Certain other anaerobes also fluoresce under UV light

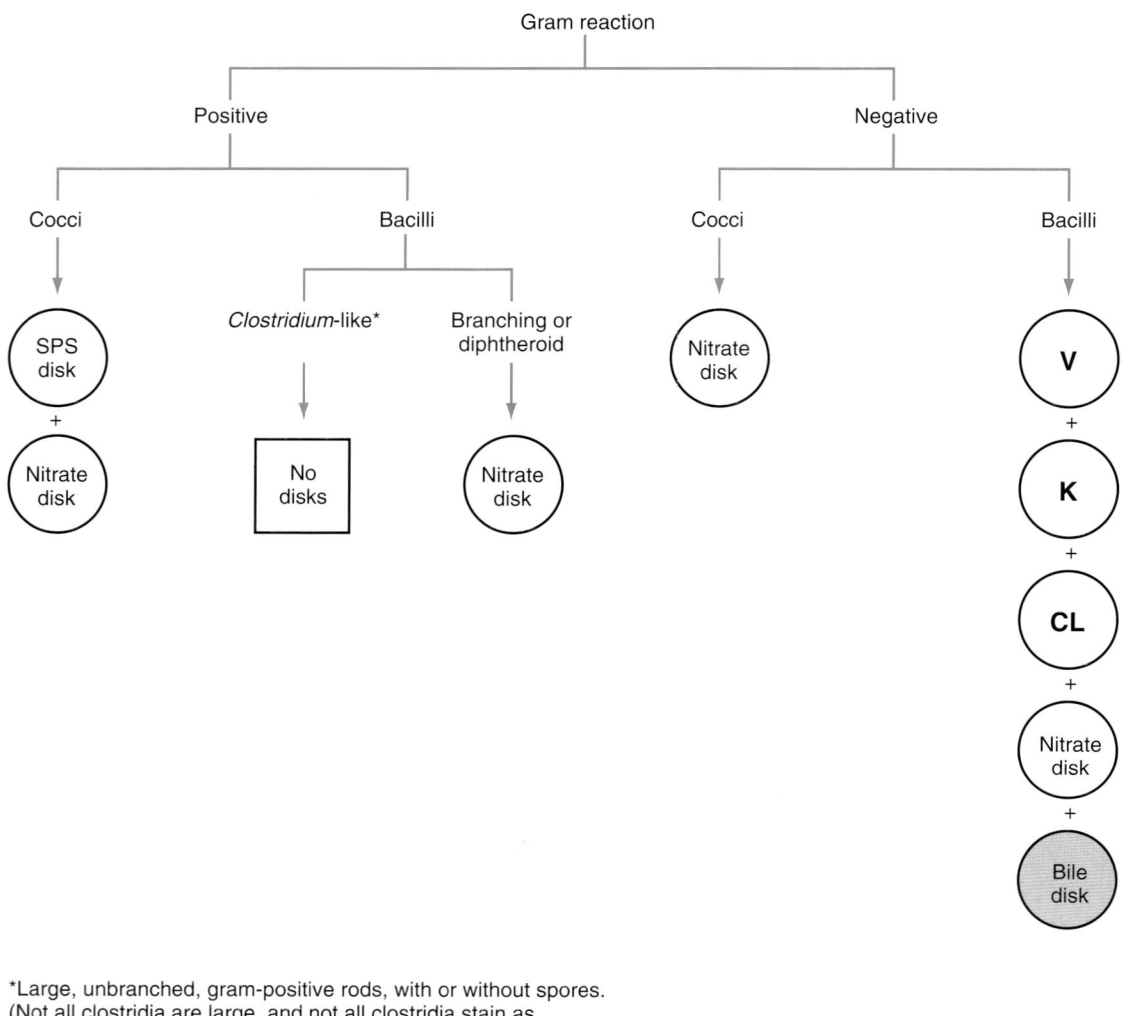

*Large, unbranched, gram-positive rods, with or without spores.
(Not all clostridia are large, and not all clostridia stain as
gram-positive rods.)

Figure 19-10 _____

Disks to add to the pure culture/subculture plate. SPS, Sodium polyanethol sulfonate; V, vancomycin [5 mg]; K, kanamycin [1 mg]; CL, colistin [10 mg]). *Clostridium-like organisms are large, unbranched, gram-positive rods, with or without spores. (Not all clostridia are large, and not all clostridia will stain as gram-positive rods.) (Modified from Engelkirk PG, Duben-Engelkirk J, Dowell VR Jr: *Principles and Practice of Clinical Anaerobic Bacteriology,* Belmont, Calif, 1992, Star.)

(e.g., *F. nucleatum* and *C. difficile* fluoresce chartreuse, and *Veillonella* spp. fluoresce red). The red fluorescence of *Veillonella* is culture medium-dependent; it is weaker than the fluorescence produced by pigmented species of *Porphyromonas* and *Prevotella* and fades completely if the colonies are exposed to air for 5 to 10 minutes. The fluorescence of *Porphyromonas asaccharolytica* is shown in Figure 19-11.

SPECIAL-POTENCY ANTIMICROBIAL DISKS

To verify that the organism is truly a gram-negative bacillus as opposed to a *Mobiluncus* species or a species of *Clostridium* (e.g., *Clostridium ramosum* or *Clostridium clostridioforme*) that may stain gram-negative, add special-potency disks to anaerobic blood agar subcultures. Disks of the proper potency must be pressed firmly to the surface of the plate to ensure uniform diffusion of the agent into

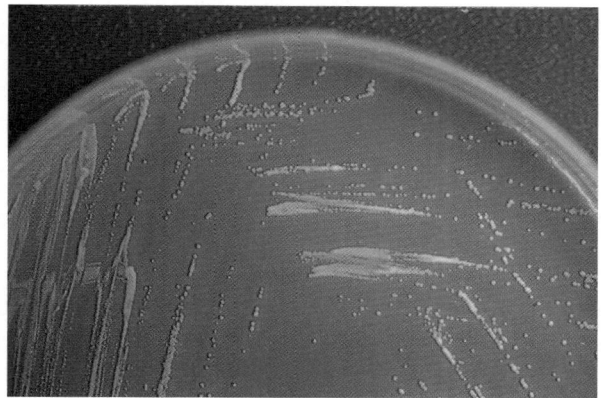

Figure 19-11

Example of the brick-red fluorescence seen when colonies of certain Porphyromonas and Prevotella species are subjected to long-wave ultraviolet light; Porphyromonas asaccharolytica, 72-hour-old culture shown here. (From Engelkirk PG, Duben-Engelkirk J, Dowell VR Jr: *Principles and Practice of Clinical Anaerobic Bacteriology,* Belmont, Calif, 1992, Star.)

the medium. Disk results are analyzed in a stepwise manner (see Table 19-13). The disk results for *C. ramosum* are shown in Figure 19-12.

Sodium polyanethol sulfonate (SPS) disk Add an **SPS** disk to the anaerobic blood agar subculture plate whenever the Gram stain reveals the isolate to be a gram-positive coccus. The SPS disk is used to presumptively identify *Peptostreptococcus anaerobius,* which is susceptible to SPS.

Nitrate disk Perform a nitrate reduction test using a disk that is a miniaturized version of the conventional nitrate reduction test. This determines an organism's ability to reduce nitrate.

Bile disk This disk is used to determine an organism's ability to grow in the presence of relatively high concentrations (20%) of bile. Add a bile disk to the anaerobic blood agar subculture plate whenever the Gram stain reveals the isolate to be a gram-negative bacillus. Good growth on the BBE plate and growth in 20% bile broth also indicate bile resistance. An anaerobic, gram-negative bacillus that is a member of the *B. fragilis* group fits this description.

CATALASE TEST

Using a plastic, disposable inoculating loop or a wooden applicator stick, remove some of the growth from the subculture plate and rub it onto a small area of a glass microscope slide. Perform a catalase test by adding a drop of 15% hydrogen peroxide. Watch for the production of bubbles of oxygen gas. Among other uses, the catalase test is of value in differentiating aerotolerant strains of *Clostridium* (catalase-negative) from *Bacillus* species (catalase-positive).

SPOT INDOLE TEST

Saturate a small piece of filter paper with the spot indole reagent p-dimethylaminocinnamaldehyde (DMCA). Using an inoculating loop, remove some of the growth from the subculture plate and rub it onto the saturated area. Rapid development of a blue or green color indicates a positive test (i.e., production of indole from the amino acid tryptophan), whereas a pink or orange color indicates a negative test. The spot indole test also can be performed directly on a pure culture plate. DMCA was compared to Kovac and Ehrlich reagents for the detection of indole production by anaerobes. It proved to be the most sensitive; the Kovac reagent was the least sensitive of the three.

MOTILITY TEST

Motility may be determined using either very young (4 to 6 hours old) broth cultures or 24- to 48-hour colonies on agar. Motile, gram-negative anaerobes include some *Campylobacter* (e.g., *Campylobacter concisus, Campylobacter curvus,*

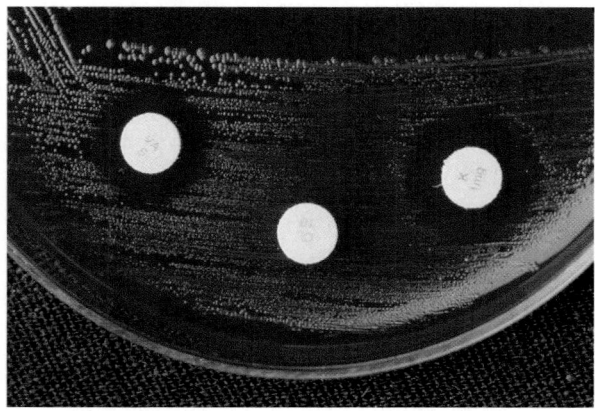

Figure 19-12

Typical special-potency antimicrobial disk results for Clostridium ramosum; susceptible to vancomycin (left) and kanamycin (right), and resistant to colistin (center disk). (Courtesy Anaerobe Systems, San Jose, Calif.)

Campylobacter rectus) and *Mobiluncus* species, among many others.

LECITHINASE AND LIPASE REACTIONS
An egg-yolk agar plate is used to determine the activities of these enzymes. These reactions are of value in identifying many species of clostridia.

PRESUMPTO PLATES
Many of the previously mentioned observations and tests are incorporated into specialized types of plated media, collectively referred to as Presumpto plates or CDC (Centers for Disease Control and Prevention) differential agar media. Three types of quad plates called Presumpto 1, Presumpto 2, and Presumpto 3 are available. These plates contain tests for the determination of growth on 20% bile; lipase and lecithinase production; casein, esculin, gelatin, and starch hydrolysis; hydrogen sulfide and indole production; DNase activity; and glucose, lactose, mannitol, and rhamnose fermentation. Formulations for Presumpto plate media can be found in a 1977 CDC publication by Dowell and colleagues. Presumpto plates are available from several commercial sources, including Remel (Lenexa, Kans.) and Carr-Scarborough Microbiologicals (Stone Mountain, Ga.).

Definitive identifications
Although many laboratories base their identification of anaerobic organisms on presumptive identification criteria, others perform additional procedures to obtain definitive identification. Many anaerobic isolates cannot be identified using presumptive tests. Whenever such anaerobes are encountered, definitive identification is required. A wide variety of techniques exist for making definitive identification, as follows:

- PRAS and non-PRAS tubed biochemical test media
- Biochemical-based and preexisting enzyme-based minisystems
- Gas-liquid chromatographic analysis of metabolic end products
- Cellular fatty acid analysis by gas-liquid chromatography (GLC)

The majority of today's clinical microbiology laboratories use one of the commercially available biochemical-based or preexisting enzyme-based minisystems for making definitive identifications, but it is important to remember that none of them will identify all the anaerobes that could potentially be isolated from clinical specimens. Most are designed to identify those anaerobes discussed earlier that are most frequently encountered in clinical specimens. It is far more important for a system to identify such organisms than to identify obscure anaerobes that are only rarely isolated from clinical specimens or involved in infectious processes.

CONVENTIONAL TUBED BIOCHEMICAL IDENTIFICATION SYSTEMS
The use of tubed biochemical systems originated from studies of rumen contents and sewage sludge by R. E. Hungate in the 1950s and 1960s. Major components of the Hungate technique were oxygen-free, flame-sterilized gassing jets or cannulae, agar-containing media on the inner surfaces of tightly stoppered glass tubes or **"roll tubes,"** and a variety of tightly-stoppered test tubes containing PRAS biochemicals. Roll tubes were inoculated under flowing oxygen-free gas; the tightly-stoppered, inoculated tubes served as their own anaerobic culture chambers.

In general, conventional or traditional systems for the identification of anaerobic isolates employ large test tubes containing a variety of PRAS or non-PRAS biochemical test media. Such media can be either prepared in the laboratory or purchased from commercial sources (e.g., Adams Scientific, West Warwick, R.I.; Carr-Scarborough; and Remel).

Citron and associates described a modified "gold standard" PRAS biochemical method for identifying bile-resistant *Bacteroides* spp. Their abbreviated protocol involves preparing inoculum directly from pure culture plates. PRAS biochemical tubes containing arabinose and trehalose are inoculated using a tuberculin syringe. A catalase test is included for identifying indole-negative species. Rhamnose, salicin, sucrose, trehalose, and xylose are added for identifying indole-positive species. Tests are incubated overnight, and a pH indicator (bromothymol blue) is added after growth occurs. The investigators reported that 98% of 189 clinical isolates were correctly identified using this protocol.

BIOCHEMICAL-BASED MINISYSTEMS

The first commercially available alternatives to conventional tubed media were the biochemical-based identification systems manufactured by Analytab Products (bioMerieux, Hazelwood Mo.) and BBL (Minitek, Cockeysville, Md.), which are still in use in some laboratories. These systems provide many of the same tests as the conventional system but in the form of a small plastic strip or tray; hence the term *minisystem.*

The biochemical-based minisystems are easier and faster to inoculate than a conventional system. Although they can be inoculated aerobically, they require anaerobic incubation. The larger model BBL anaerobic jars and some of the commercially available bags and pouches can be used to incubate biochemical-based minisystem trays and strips if an anaerobic chamber is not available. After 24 to 48 hours of incubation, test results are read, a code number is generated for each isolate, and the numbers are looked up in a compendium codebook. It is important to note the databases from which the codebooks are developed do not contain all the anaerobes that can potentially be isolated from clinical specimens.

PREFORMED ENZYME-BASED MINISYSTEMS

Many of the newer commercial systems are based on the presence of preformed enzymes. Because these minisystems do not depend on enzyme induction, there is virtually no lag time, and results are available in 4 hours. The small plastic panels or cards are easy to inoculate, can be inoculated at the bench, and do not require anaerobic incubation. Most of the systems generate code numbers, which are referenced in a manufacturer-supplied codebook. Like the biochemical-based minisystems, these systems are primarily of value for identifying commonly isolated anaerobes. The databases from which the codebooks are developed do not contain all the anaerobes that can potentially be isolated from clinical specimens. Examples of preexisting enzyme-based minisystems include ANI Card (Vitek Systems, Hazelwood, Mo.), AN-IDENT (Analytab Products, Plainview, N.Y.), RapId Ana II (Innovative Diagnostic Systems, Atlanta, Ga.), and Rapid Anaerobe Identification Panel (Baxter Healthcare, MicroScan Division, West Sacramento, Calif.). In general, the systems use

the same or similar substrates. They contain a number of nitrophenyl and naphthylamide compounds, which are colorless substances that produce yellow or red products, respectively, in the presence of appropriate enzymes.

GAS-LIQUID CHROMATOGRAPHY (GLC)

Laboratories that must routinely definitively identify anaerobic isolates that cannot be identified using one of the previously mentioned commercially available minisystems may wish to incorporate GLC into the identification protocol. Like other types of chromatographic techniques (e.g., gas-solid chromatography, thin-layer chromatography, ion-exchange chromatography), GLC uses the chemical and physical properties of a particular component to separate it from other components in a mixture. All chromatographic techniques have a mobile and stationary phase. In GLC, an inert gas serves as the mobile phase and a liquid serves as the stationary or separating phase. The unknown mixture is usually prepared for separation, volatilized, and carried as a gas through a packed column. Acids are recovered in a specific order, based on their chemical and physical properties. As the column separates the acids, they are identified based on their position on the chromatograph by their relative retention time as compared to a standard. Quantitation of an unknown is based on the area under the peak with respect to a known standard. Figure 19-13 depicts the Capco gas-liquid chromatograph (Dodeca, Fremont, Calif.), specifically manufactured for and commonly used in anaerobic bacteriology laboratories.

Identifying anaerobes through metabolic end product analysis by GLC Identification of anaerobes by GLC analysis of metabolic end products was pioneered by W. E. C. Moore, E. P. Cato, L. V. Holdeman, and others at the Virginia Polytechnic Institute (VPI) in Blacksburg. Their GLC procedure, details of which can be found in the *VPI Anaerobe Laboratory Manual,* is still widely used in laboratories throughout the world. The VPI guidelines for GLC were used for many years at the CDC but were modified by G. L. Lombard, V. R. Dowell, Jr., and their colleagues. The CDC guidelines for GLC can be found in *Gas-Liquid Chromatography Analysis of the Acid Products of Bacteria.* A brief summary of the CDC procedure follows.

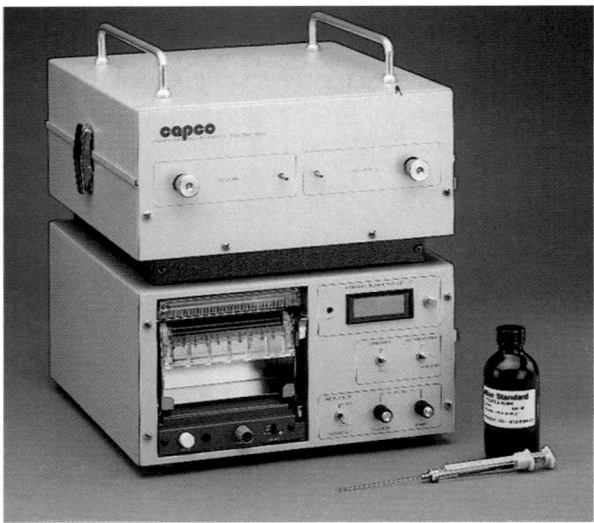

Figure 19-13 _____

The Capco model 700A anaerobe identification system, manufactured by Dodeca. The "turnkey system," which costs approximately $7000, consists of a compact gas-liquid chromatograph with integral recorder and all accessories and supplies (except a tank of helium carrier gas) needed to analyze anaerobic bacteria on the basis of their metabolic products. The dual-column chromatograph is 12.5 inches wide, 13.75 inches deep, and 14 inches high and weighs only 26 lb. (Courtesy Dodeca, Fremont, Calif.)

The anaerobe to be tested is grown in a tube of peptone–yeast extract–glucose medium (PYG), which is available commercially from Adams Scientific (West Warwick, R.I.), Carr-Scarborough, Remel, and other media manufacturers. This medium also contains cysteine hydrochloride, resazurin, and a salt solution. Aliquots of the PYG culture are used to analyze volatile and nonvolatile acids. Short-chain volatile acids produced by anaerobes include formic, acetic, propionic, isobutyric, isovaleric, valeric, isocaproic, butyric, caproic, and heptanoic.

Volatile acids are identified by comparing the elution times of products in the ether extract with those of known acids in a standardized volatile acid mixture that has been chromatographed in the same manner on the same day. Figure 19-14, *A* and *B* shows chromatographs of a volatile acid standard and *Fusobacterium,* respectively.

Nonvolatile, low-molecular-weight aliphatic and aromatic acids produced by anaerobes are identified by comparing the elution times of products

in the chloroform extract with those of known acids in a standardized, nonvolatile acid mixture that has been chromatographed in the same manner on the same day. Nonvolatile, low-molecular-weight aliphatic and aromatic acids produced by anaerobes include pyruvic, lactic, oxalacetic, oxalic, malonic, fumaric, succinic, benzoic, phenylacetic, and hydrocinnamic acids. In Figure 19-14, *C* and *D* chromatographs show the nonvolatile acid standard and *Actinomyces,* respectively.

Identifying anaerobes through cellular fatty acid analysis by high-resolution GLC Cellular fatty acid analysis is another method of identifying anaerobes. The term *cellular fatty acids* refers to fatty acids and related compounds (aldehydes, hydrocarbons, dimethylacetals) that are present within organisms as cellular components. Cellular fatty acids are coded for on bacterial chromosomes, as opposed to plasmids, and are not affected by simple mutations or plasmid loss. Thus, the fatty acid composition of a particular organism is relatively stable when grown under certain growth conditions (medium, incubation temperature, and time). Although fatty acid profiles can be identified manually, computerized, high-resolution gas chromatography and specialized software programs are now available to analyze cellular fatty acids of unknown bacteria and compare the results to patterns of known species.

First grown in pure culture in PYG broth or another standardized medium, the bacterial cells are removed by centrifugation and then saponified to release the fatty acids from the bacterial lipids. After extraction, the methyl esters are analyzed by GLC. A chromatogram depicting the unknown organism's fatty acid composition and a comparison to a database or "library" of fatty acids of known anaerobes are generated as a computer printout or report. The report includes computer-generated statistical values or "similarity indices," which are based on deviations in the unknown organism's fatty acid composition from the known profile in the library. Because no subjective interpretations are required, the identifications are objective and highly reproducible.

Using GLC and related techniques, investigators have been attempting for many years to directly identify anaerobes and other organisms in clinical specimens. Johnson and colleagues, for example, described a method for identifying *C. dif-*

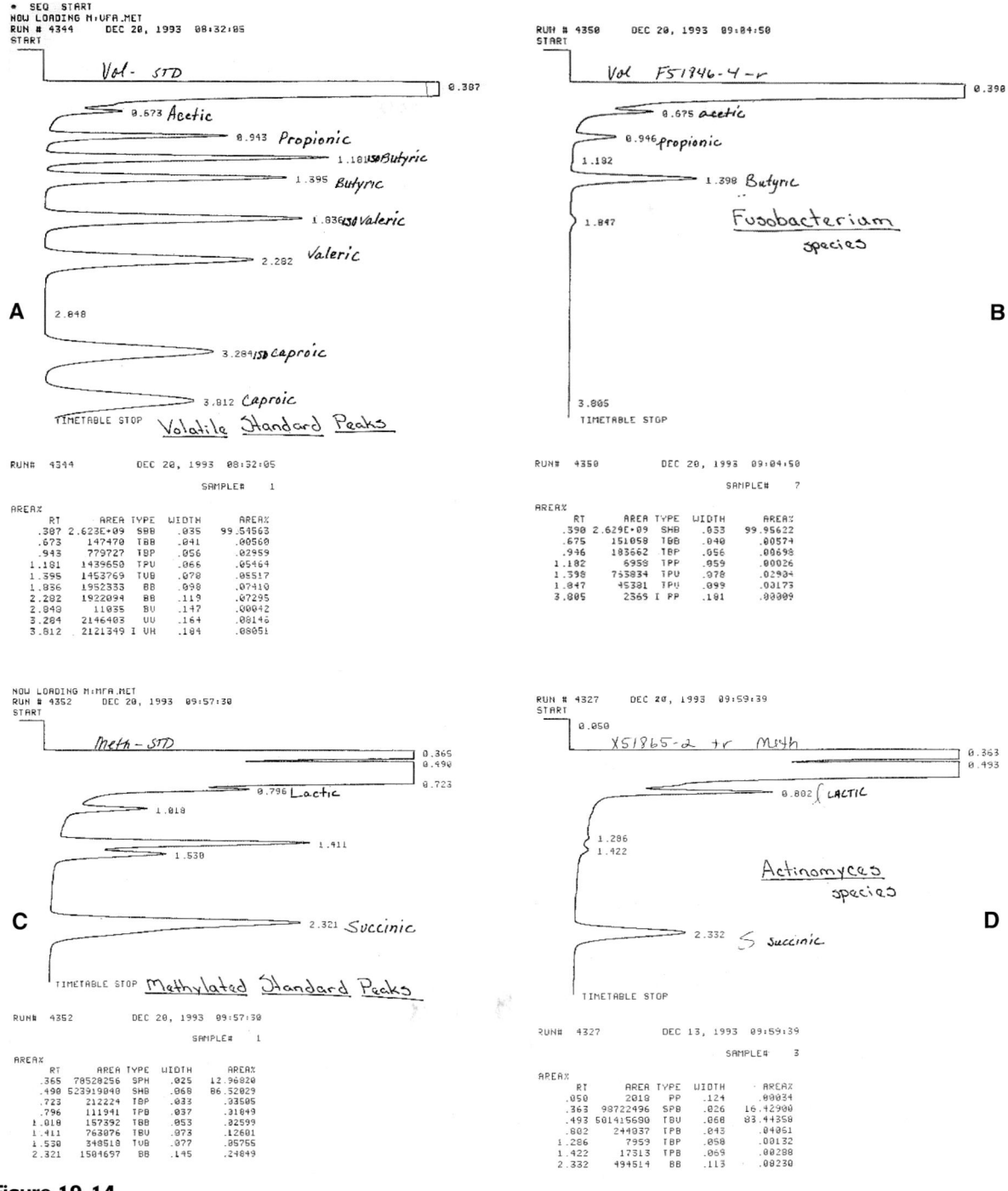

Figure 19-14

A, Volatile acid standard chromatograph. Elution times of known acids and their peaks are depicted in the extract of the standard solution. **B,** Volatile acid chromatograph of unknown identified as *Fusobacterium* species after comparison of the retention times of the acids with those for the standard solution. Numbers located near the acid peaks are retention times. **C,** Methylated acid standard chromatograph. Elution times of known acids and their peaks are depicted in the extract of the standard solution. **D,** Methylated acid chromatograph of an unknown identified as *Actinomyces* species after comparison of the retention times of the acids with those of the standard solution. Numbers located near the acid peaks are retention times in minutes. *RT,* Retention time.

ficile in stool specimens using culture-enhanced GLC. In this technique, GLC is used to detect four distinctive peaks produced by *C. difficile.* In the future, assays of this type (i.e., those performed directly on clinical specimens) will probably be modified to enable use of instrumentation.

FREQUENTLY ENCOUNTERED ANAEROBES AND THEIR ASSOCIATED DISEASES

Taxonomically, anaerobic bacteria encountered in human clinical specimens may be divided into two major groups: those capable of forming endospores (spore-formers) and those incapable of forming endospores (non–spore-formers). The presence or absence of spores, coupled with the Gram-staining reaction and cellular morphology, is often helpful in making the initial or presumptive identification of anaerobic bacteria and determining the appropriate identification tests to be performed.

Gram-Positive Spore-Forming Anaerobic Bacilli

All spore-forming anaerobic bacilli are classified in the genus *Clostridium* and collectively referred to as clostridia. Although all clostridia are capable of producing spores, some species do so readily, whereas others require extremely harsh condi-

tions. Spores may or may not be observed in Gram-stained smears of clinical specimens containing clostridia. With certain species, spores may not be observed in Gram-stained smears of *Clostridium* colonies from an agar plate. It is sometimes necessary to use a heat or alcohol shock method to induce and demonstrate sporulation.

Clostridia may be grouped according to the location of the endospore within the cell. Spores are described as *terminal* when the spore is located at the end of the bacterial cell and *subterminal* when the spore is found at a location other than the end of the cell. Figure 19-15, *A* shows a clostridial species that produces terminal spores, and Figure 19-15, *B* shows a clostridial species that produces subterminal spores.

Certain characteristics may be used to initially identify clostridial isolates. A boxcar-shaped, anaerobic, gram-positive bacillus that produces a characteristic double zone of hemolysis on BRU or BA can be presumptively identified as *C. perfringens.* A heavily swarming, anaerobic, gram-positive bacillus with terminal spores is probably *Clostridium tetani,* whereas one with subterminal spores is most likely *C. septicum.*

Clinical infection
Clostridium species are most frequently encountered in exogenous anaerobic infections or intoxications. Clostridia or their toxins usually gain ac-

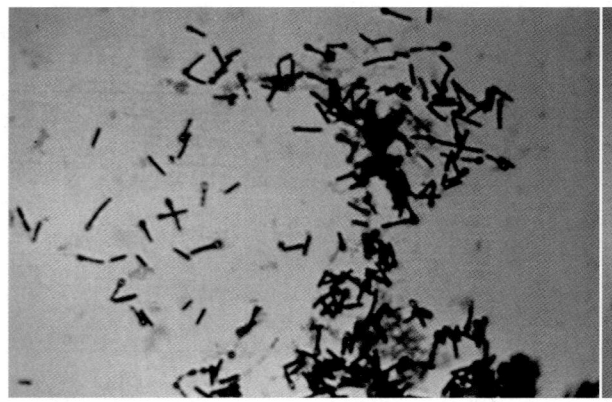
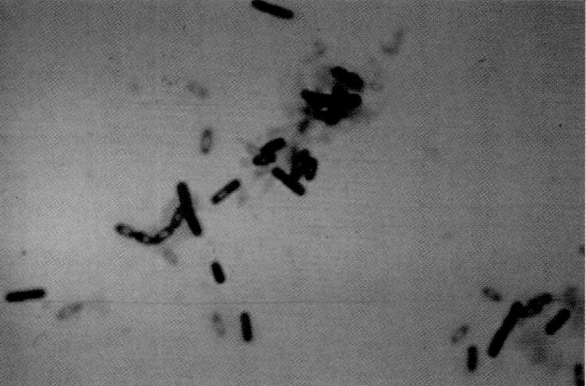

A B

Figure 19-15

A, Classification of some clinically encountered clostridia by endospore location: Gram-stained appearance of terminal spores of *Clostridium tetani.* **B,** Gram-stained appearance of subterminal spores of *Clostridium sordellii. (*Courtesy Bartley SL, Howard JD, Simon R, Centers for Disease Control and Prevention, Atlanta, Ga.)

cess to the body through ingestion or open wounds that have become contaminated with soil.

Clostridia cause classic diseases such as tetanus, gas gangrene (myonecrosis), botulism, and *Clostridium perfringens* food poisoning (foodborne intoxication). In tetanus, gas gangrene, and wound botulism, clostridial spores enter through open wounds and germinate in vivo. The vegetative bacteria then multiply and produce toxins. In foodborne intoxication due to *C. perfringens*, organisms are acquired through consumption of contaminated food. One clostridial infection that is of endogenous origin is antibiotic-associated pseudomembranous colitis caused by *C. difficile*.

TETANUS

The clinical manifestations of **tetanus** are attributed to the neurotoxin (tetanospasmin) produced by the causative agent *C. tetani*. **Tetanospasmin** acts on inhibitory neurons, preventing the release of neurotransmitters. This results in continuous muscular spasms leading to trismus, risus sardonicus (distorted grin), and difficulty in breathing.

Tetanus manifests when spores develop into vegetative cells and multiply at a site of inoculation that provides a low redox potential, giving the organism the opportunity to produce the neurotoxin. The toxin is thereafter transmitted to the central nervous system. Symptoms appear within approximately 7 days after inoculation. The incubation period, however, ranges from 1 to 54 days.

Clinical manifestations include muscular rigidity, usually in the jaws, neck, and lumbar region. Difficulty in swallowing results from muscular spasms in the pharyngeal area. Rigidity of the abdomen, chest, back, and limbs may also occur.

As a result of the widespread use of DPT (diphtheria-pertussis-tetanus) vaccine, tetanus is no longer a common disease in the Untied States. Tetanus in the newborn, or tetanus neonatorum, often results from the use of contaminated instruments, from umbilical infections, or in cases of septic abortions. Therapy for tetanus requires antitoxin injection, muscle relaxants, and constant nursing care, in addition to supportive therapy.

MYONECROSIS OR GAS GANGRENE

Myonecrosis usually occurs when organisms contaminate wounds, through either trauma or surgery. *C. perfringens, Clostridium histolyticum, C. sep-*

ticum, C. novyi, and *Clostridium bifermentans* can cause myonecrosis. Under favorable conditions, the organisms are able to grow, multiply, and release potent exotoxins. In gas gangrene, clostridial exotoxins, such as α toxin produced by *C. perfringens,* cause necrosis of the tissue and allow deeper penetration by the organisms. The onset and spread of myonecrosis are rapid, and the affected extremities often require amputation.

Clinical manifestations of myonecrosis include pain and swelling in the affected area. Bullae, serous discharge, discoloration, and definite tissue necrosis are observed. Treatment of gas gangrene involves extensive surgical débridement of involved tissue, antimicrobial therapy, and sometimes the use of hyperbaric oxygen.

BOTULISM

Occasionally, intoxication (poisoning) may follow ingestion of preformed toxins produced by exogenous anaerobes. Foodborne **botulism** results from the ingestion of preformed botulin, a toxin produced in the food by *Clostridium botulinum*. Botulin is an extremely potent toxin; only a small amount can produce paralysis and death. Botulin attaches to the neuromuscular junction of affected nerves, preventing the release of acetylcholine, which results in a flaccid type of paralysis and death.

Common food sources include home-canned vegetables, homecured meat such as ham, fermented fish, and other preserved foods. Clinical manifestations develop as early as 2 hours or as late as 3 to 8 days following ingestion of food containing the botulin toxin, which is absorbed in the small intestine. Weakness and paralysis are the main features of botulism. Double vision, impaired speech, and difficulty in swallowing are common features. Respiratory paralysis may occur in severe cases. Treatment of foodborne botulism involves the use of antitoxin and supportive care.

Infant botulism, unlike that in adults, follows ingestion of *C. botulinum* spores. The most common associated food source in infant botulism is contaminated honey. The spores germinate, colonize in the colon, and subsequently produce toxins in vivo.

Wound botulism is the result of contamination of wounds with spores of *C. botulinum,* with subsequent germination, multiplication, and production of toxins in vivo. Clinical manifestations that develop in wound botulism are similar to those of foodborne intoxication. Wound botulism is usually treated with penicillin.

***Clostridium perfringens* food poisoning** *C. perfringens* food poisoning, a relatively mild and self-limited GI tract illness, usually follows ingestion of enterotoxin-producing *C. perfringens* in contaminated food. Following an 8- to 12-hour incubation period, the patient experiences diarrhea and crampy abdominal pain for about 24 hours. Other than fluid replacement, therapy is usually unnecessary.

ANTIBIOTIC-ASSOCIATED DIARRHEA
AND PSEUDOMEMBRANOUS COLITIS

C. difficile is the most common but not the sole cause of antibiotic-associated diarrhea and **pseudomembranous colitis.** This organism is found as part of the GI flora of many individuals. Following antimicrobial therapy, many organisms of the GI flora other than *C. difficile* are killed, thus allowing *C. difficile* to multiply and produce abundant quantities of two types of toxins: toxin A, an enterotoxin; and toxin B, a cytotoxin. Bloody diarrhea with associated necrosis of colon mucosa is seen in patients with pseudomembranous colitis.

In addition, *C. difficile* is a common cause of nosocomial (hospital-acquired) infection. The organism is frequently transmitted among hospitalized patients and is often present on the hands of hospital personnel who are caring for such patients.

Table 19-16 shows other clinically encountered *Clostridium* species and associated infections.

TABLE 19-16

Clinically Encountered Clostridium *Species*

Clostridium Species	Associated Infections
C. baratii	War wounds; peritonitis; eye, ear, and prostate infections
C. bifermentans	Wounds, abscesses, bacteremia
C. botulinum	Urinary tract, lower respiratory tract, pleural cavity, and abdominal infections; wounds; abscesses; bacteremia
C. cadaveris	Abscesses, wounds
C. clostridioforme	Abdominal, cervical, scrotal, and pleural infections; septicemia; peritonitis; appendicitis
C. difficile	Antibiotic-associated diarrhea, pseudomembranous colitis, bacteremia (rarely), pyogenic infections; also isolated from the hospital environment
C. hastiforme	War wounds, bacteremia, abdominal abscesses
C. histolyticum	War wounds, gas gangrene; has been isolated from the gingival plaque of institutionalized and primitive populations
C. innocuum	Commonly isolated from infections of the gastrointestinal tract; empyema
C. limosum	Bacteremia, peritonitis, pulmonary infections
C. novyi	Wounds, gas gangrene
C. paraputrificum	Bacteremia, peritonitis, wounds, appendicitis
C. perfringens	Infections derived from colonic contents (e.g., peritonitis, intraabdominal abscesses, and infections of soft tissues below the waist); involved in about 80% of cases of gas gangrene; bacteremia
C. putrefaciens	Bacteriuria (pregnant women with bacteremia)
C. putrificum	Abscesses, wounds, bacteremia
C. ramosum	Infections of the abdominal cavity, genital tract, lung, biliary tract; bacteremia
C. septicum	Bacteremia, suppurative infections, necrotizing enterocolitis, gas gangrene
C. sordellii	Wounds, penile lesions, bacteremia, abscesses, infections of the abdomen and vagina
C. sporogenes	Bacteremia, endocarditis, central nervous system and pleuropulmonary infections, penile lesions, infected war wounds, other pyogenic infections
C. subterminale	Bacteremia (rarely); empyema; infections of the biliary tract, soft tissue, and bone
C. tertium	Appendicitis, brain abscess, infections related to the intestinal tract and soft tissue, infected war wounds, bacteremia; has been isolated from gingival sulcus of patients with periodontitis
C. tetani	Infected gums and teeth, corneal ulcerations, infections of mastoid and middle ear, intraperitoneal infections, tetanus neonatorum, post partum uterine infection, various soft-tissue infections related to trauma (including abrasions and lacerations) and use of contaminated needles; has been isolated from the hospital environment

Modified from Engelkirk PG, Duben-Engelkirk J, Dowell VR Jr: *Principles and practice of anaerobic bacteriology*, Belmont, Calif, 1992, Star.
NOTE: Virtually all *Clostridium* spp. listed here have been isolated from fecal specimens of apparently healthy persons. Such isolates could represent transient rather than permanent residents of the normal colonic flora. Eighteen additional *Clostridium* species isolated from feces but not from clinical specimens or other anatomic sites have been excluded from this list.

TABLE 19-17

Laboratory Confirmation of Selected Clostridial Diseases

Disease	Laboratory Confirmation Procedures
Botulism	
Foodborne	Isolation of *C. botulinum* from the stool specimen or detection of botulin toxin in the serum, stool, or epidemiologically implicated food
	Botulin toxin is initially identified by toxicity to mice; the specific toxin type is determined by neutralization tests using type-specific antitoxins
Infant	Detection of *C. botulinum* and/or botulin toxin in the stool of symptomatic infants
Wound	Isolation of *C. botulinum* from a wound specimen or detection of botulin toxin in the patient's serum or stool
C. perfringens food poisoning	Requires two or more findings
	▪ $>10^5$ colony CFU of *C. perfringens*/gram of implicated food
	▪ Median *C. perfringens* spore count >106/gram of stool from affected patients (such counts have been found in healthy individuals)
	▪ Isolation of the same type of *C. perfringens* from stools of affected patients and from the suspected food (isolates are not always serotypable)
	▪ Presence of *C. perfringens* enterotoxin in stool specimens from ill persons and its absence in stool specimens from well persons
C. difficile–induced diarrhea	Tissue culture cytotoxin assay (CTA); other methods include CIE, ELISA, latex agglutination, and a dot immunobinding assay; positive latex results should be confirmed by CTA, and stools yielding negative dot immunobinding assay results should be further tested using CTA
Tetanus	Laboratory confirmation rarely required; when *C. tetani* is isolated from wounds of patients with tetanus, toxicity and neutralization tests can be performed by intramuscular injection of culture supernatant or whole culture into untreated mice and mice protected with tetanus antitoxin; failure to isolate *C. tetani* from wound cultures does not eliminate the possibility of tetanus

Modified from Engelkirk PG, Duben-Engelkirk J, Dowell VR Jr: *Principles and practice of anaerobic bacteriology,* Belmont, Calif, 1992, Star.

Laboratory diagnosis

Table 19-17 summarizes the laboratory confirmation of major clostridial diseases.

MICROSCOPIC MORPHOLOGY

Clostridial cell wall structure is similar to that of other gram-positive bacteria. However, some species appear gram-variable, and some routinely stain gram-negative. *C. ramosum* and *C. clostridioforme* routinely appear as pink-staining bacilli in Gram-stained preparations. Special-potency antimicrobial disks should always be used to determine the true gram reaction of a pink-staining anaerobic bacillus. Figure 19-12 shows how the special-potency antimicrobial results can be used to determine the true gram reaction of a pink-staining bacillus.

COLONIAL MORPHOLOGY

Whenever clostridia are suspected, either clinically or as a result of Gram-stain observations (i.e., the presence of large gram-positive bacilli, with or without spores), certain media and procedures are added in addition to those routinely used for anaerobic cultures.

Egg-yolk agar (EYA) EYA is useful for detecting enzymes (i.e., lecithinase, lipase, and proteolytic enzymes) produced by some clostridia. Lecithinase-positive organisms produce a colony surrounded by a wide zone of opacity. This opacity is actually in the medium and not a surface phenomenon. The appearance of the lecithinase reaction is shown in Figure 19-16. Lecithinase-positive clostridia include *C. bifermentans, Clostridium sordellii, C. perfringens, C. novyi* type A, and *Clostridium baratii*. It must be noted, however, that a few organisms other than *Clostridium* species also cause this reaction.

Lipase-positive organisms produce a colony covered with an iridescent, multicolored sheen, sometimes described as resembling the appearance of gasoline on water or mother-of-pearl. This multicolored sheen also may appear on the surface of the agar in a narrow zone around the colony. In contrast to the lecithinase reaction, the lipase reaction is essentially a surface phenomenon. The appearance

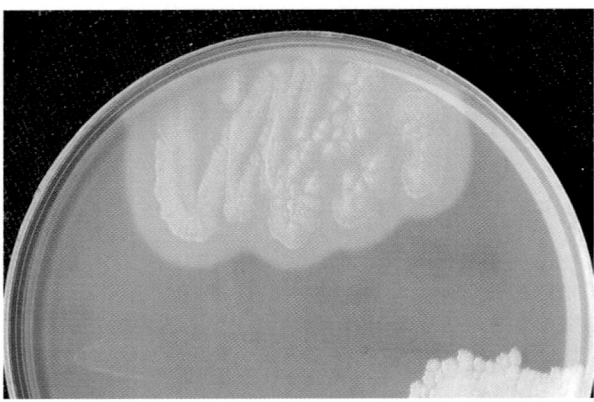

Figure 19-16

Positive lecithinase reaction on egg yolk agar (EYA). The reaction occurs within the agar. Clostridium perfringens is shown here. (Courtesy Anaerobe Systems, San Jose, Calif.)

of the lipase reaction is depicted in Figure 19-17. Examples of lipase-positive clostridia are *C. botulinum*, *C. novyi* type A, and *Clostridium sporogenes*. Other anaerobes that are lipase-positive include *F. necrophorum, Prevotella intermedia,* and some isolates of *Prevotella loescheii.*

Organisms that produce proteolytic enzymes have a completely clear zone (often quite narrow) around their colonies. Proteolysis is best observed by holding the plate up to a strong light source. It is reminiscent of the complete clearing seen with β-hemolytic organisms on BRU/BA plates.

Direct Nagler test If *C. perfringens* is suspected (gram-positive boxcar-shaped bacilli seen on Gram stain), a direct **Nagler test** can be performed as part of the primary isolation set-up. This test employs an EYA plate and a reagent known as *C. perfringens* type A antitoxin. This reagent inhibits the lecithinase reaction produced by *C. perfringens* and three other species of *Clostridium.* Although the test is used to presumptively identify *C. perfringens,* a positive test result is not specific for this organism; *C. baratii, C. bifermentans,* and *C. sordellii* also are Nagler test–positive.

Brucella/blood agar (BRU/BA) Extensive swarming on the BRU/BA plate is characteristic of *C. septicum* and *C. tetani.* A double zone of hemolysis (an inner zone of complete β hemolysis and an outer zone of partial hemolysis) that appears within 24 hours of incubation is characteristic of *C. perfringens,* as shown in Figure 19-18.

Cycloserine-cefoxitin-fructose agar (CCFA) Whenever a patient is suspected of having antibiotic-associated diarrhea or pseudomembranous colitis, a CCFA plate may be inoculated with the patient's fecal specimen. CCFA is a selective and differen-

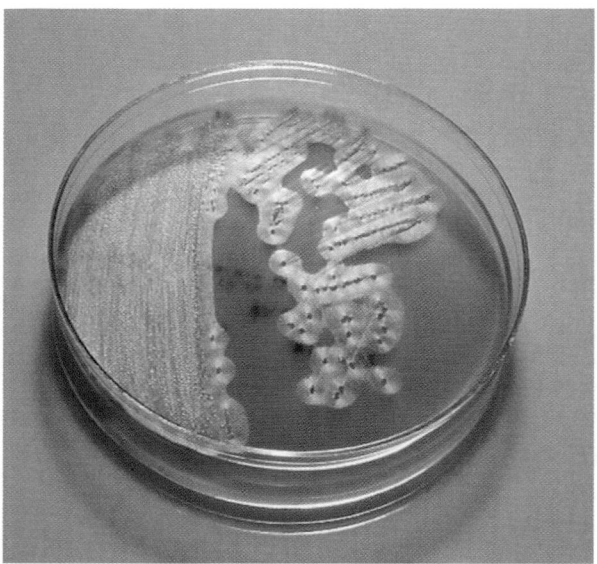

Figure 19-17

Positive lipase reaction on egg yolk agar (EYA). The reaction occurs on the *surface* of colonies and the surrounding medium. *Fusobacterium necrophorum* is shown here. (Courtesy Anaerobe Systems, San Jose, Calif.)

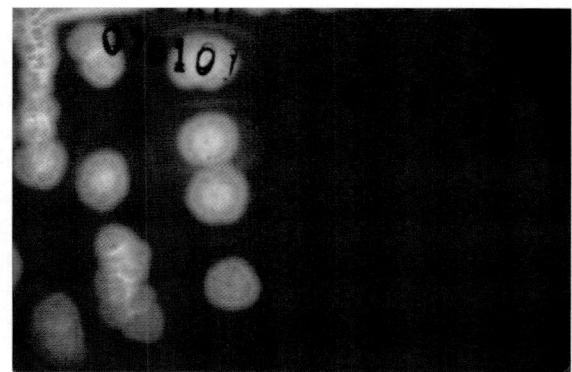

Figure 19-18

Double zone of hemolysis produced by *Clostridium perfringens;* inner zone of *complete* beta-hemolysis; outer zone of *partial* hemolysis. (Courtesy Anaerobe Systems, San Jose, Calif.)

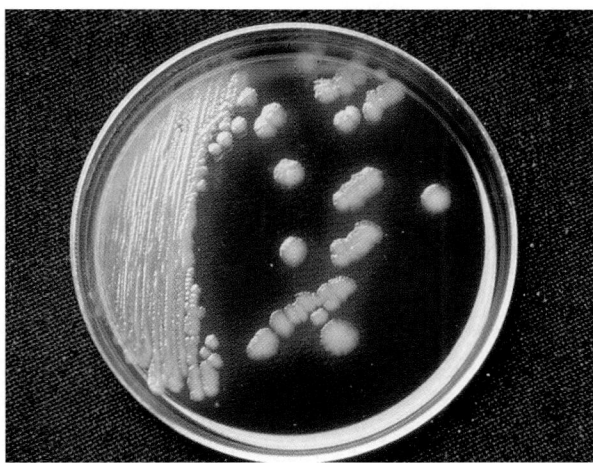

Figure 19-19

The appearance of *Clostridium difficile* on cycloserine-cefoxitin-fructose agar (CCFA); yellow, ground-glass colonies and a yellowing of the medium around the colonies. (Courtesy Anaerobe Systems, San Jose, Calif.)

tial medium for the recovery and presumptive identification of *C. difficile,* the most common cause of those two entities. On CCFA, *C. difficile* produces yellow ground-glass colonies, and the originally pink agar turns yellow in the vicinity of the colonies. The appearance of *C. difficile* on CCFA is shown in Figure 19-19. Although other organisms may grow on CCFA, their colonies are smaller and do not resemble the characteristic colonies of *C. difficile*. *C. difficile* has a characteristic odor resembling a horse stable, and colonies on BRU/BA fluoresce chartreuse under UV light. Organisms that are isolated should then be tested for toxin production on appropriate cell lines.

Bartley and Dowell reported that modified cycloserine mannitol agar (mCMA) and modified cycloserine mannitol blood agar (mCMBA) are superior to modified CCFA (mCCFA) for recovery of *C. difficile* from fecal specimens. In addition, mCCFA fails to inhibit growth of a variety of commonly encountered gram-positive and gram-negative intestinal organisms, whereas mCMBA and mCMA inhibit all such organisms except *Serratia liquefaciens*.

Identification

Presumptive identification of some *Clostridium* spp. is shown in Figure 19-20. Identification of clinically

encountered clostridia using biochemical characteristics is summarized in Table 19-18.

Gram-Positive Non–Spore-Forming Anaerobic Bacilli

Non–spore-forming, anaerobic, gram-positive bacilli include *Actinomyces, Bifidobacterium, Eubacterium, Mobiluncus, Lactobacillus,* and *Propionibacterium* spp. (Table 19-19). Many species are found as part of the indigenous microflora of humans and other animals; therefore infections that result are opportunistic. The microscopic morphology of these organisms varies, raging from very short rods to long, branching filaments. Although certain species of *Lactobacillus* are anaerobic, their role in infectious processes is uncertain, and they will not be described here.

Clinical infection

ACTINOMYCOSIS

Actinomyces spp. and related anaerobic bacteria, such as *Bifidobacterium, Eubacterium,* and *Propionibacterium,* are the usual cause of actinomycosis. This group of organisms has been associated with actinomycosis of the brain, orofacial region, pleuropulmonary region, and genital organs.

Actinomycosis is a chronic, granulomatous, infectious disease characterized by the development of sinus tracts and fistulae, which erupt to the surface and drain pus containing sulfur granules (small colonies of bacteria). Examinations of wet mounts and Gram-stained preparations of pus from draining sinuses are useful diagnostic procedures for demonstrating the non–spore-forming gram-positive bacilli that frequently exhibit branching in clinical materials (Figure 19-21).

BACTERIAL VAGINOSIS

Some investigators believe that bacterial vaginosis (BV) involves endogenous anaerobes of the vagina such as *Mobiluncus* spp. (especially *Mobiluncus curtisii* spp. *curtisii*), which are curved, motile, gram-positive bacteria. In all likelihood, BV is a synergistic infectious process involving a variety of organisms, including *Bacteroides* and *Peptostreptococcus* spp. in addition to *Mobiluncus* spp. and *Gardnerella vaginalis*.

Clinical features of BV include a gray-white, homogenous, malodorous vaginal discharge with small

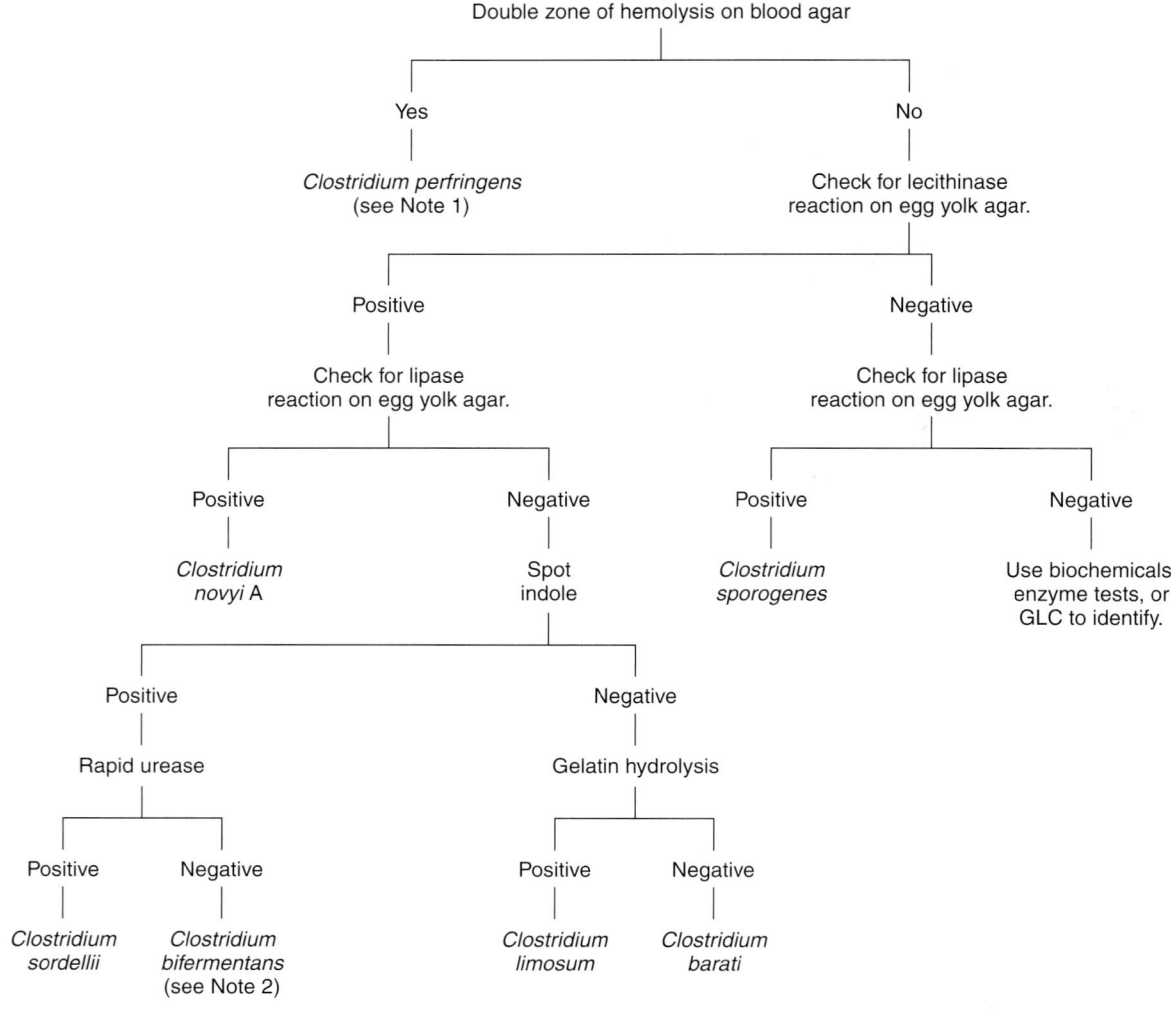

Notes

1. Boxcar-shaped bacilli; lecithinase-positive; reverse CAMP test-positive; subterminal spores, but spores rarely observed
2. Produces chalk-white colonies on egg yolk agar

Figure 19-20 _____

Identification of *Clostridium* species. Use this chart for organisms fulfilling the following three criteria: 1) anaerobic; 2) gram-positive bacilli; and 3) sporeformers. *GLC,* Gas-liquid chromatography. (Data from Mangels, JI, 1998.)

TABLE 19-18

Characteristics of Some Clinically Encountered Clostridia Organisms

Species	Relationship to Oxygen	Swarming on BRU/BA	Double Zone of Hemolysis	Chartreuse Fluorescence	Gram Reaction	Position of Spores	Motility	Flagella	Indole	Indole Derivatives	Esculin Hydrolysis	Lecithinase	Lipase	Proteolysis in Milk	Gelatin Hydrolysis	DNase	Glucose	Lactose	Mannitol	Rhamnose	Urease	Major Acids Produced in PYG
C. bifermentans	MA, AN	−	−	−	+	ST	+	PF	+	−	−	+	−	+	+	−	+	−	−	−	−	A
C. clostridioforme	AN	−	−	−	−+	ST	−+	PF	−	−	+−	−	−	−	−	−	+	+−	−	+−	−	A
C. difficile	AN	−	−	+	+	ST	+	SSF^{PF}	−	−	+−	−	−	−	−+	−+	+	−	+	−	−	A, IB, B, IV, VA, IC
C. novyi type A	AN	−	−	−	+	ST	+−	PF^{NF}	−	−	−	+	+	+	+	NG	+−	−	−	−	−	A, P, B
C. perfringens	MA, AN	−	+	−	+	−ST	−	−	−	−	V	+	−	−	+	+	+	+	−	−	−	A, B
C. ramosum	AN	+	−	−	−	(T)	−	−	−	−	+	−	−	−	−	−	+	+	+−	V	−	A
C. septicum	MA, AN	+	−	−	+	ST	+	PF	−	−	+	−	−	−	+	+	+	+	+	−	−	A, B
C. sordellii	MA, AN	−	−	−	+	ST	+	PF	+	+	−	+	−	+	+	−	+	−	−	−	+	A
C. sphenoides	AN	−	−	−	−	TST	+	PF	+	+	+	−	−	−	−	V	+	+	+	+	−	A, IB, B, IV
C. sporogenes	AN	−	−	−	+	ST	+	PF	−	−	+	−+	+	+	−+	−+	+	−	+	−	−	A, B
C. tertium	FA, AT	+	−	−	+−	T	+	PF	−	−	+	−	−	−	−	+	+	+	+	−	−	A, B
C. tetani	AN	+	−	−	+	T	+	PF	+−	−	−	−	−	+	+	+	+	−	−	−	−	A, P, B

Modified from Engelkirk PG, Duben-Engelkirk J, Dowell VR Jr: *Principles and practice of anaerobic bacteriology*, Belmont, Calif, 1992, Star.

AN, Obligate anaerobe; *MA*, microaerotolerant anaerobe; *AT*, aerotolerant anaerobe; *FA*, facultative anaerobe; *ST*, subterminal; *T*, terminal; *NF*, no flagella; *SSF*, single subpolar flagellum; *PF*, peritrichous flagella; *V*, variable; *NG*, no growth; *A*, acetic acid; *P*, propionic acid; *IB*, isobutyric acid; *B*, butyric acid; *IV*, isovaleric acid; *IC*, isocaproic acid; *(T)*, variable, but usually terminal; *SSF·PF*, most strains SSF, but some PF; *PF·NF*, most strains PF, but some NF; +, most strains positive, but some negative; −+, most strains negative, but some positive; *TST*, mostly terminal, occasionally subterminal; −ST, usually not observed, but subterminal when seen.

bubbles, little or no discomfort, and no inflammation. Although *Mobiluncus* spp. have a typical gram-positive cell wall structure, they frequently stain pink or gram-variable with Gram stain (Figure 19-22).

Other clinically encountered anaerobic, non–spore-forming, gram-positive bacilli and their clinical significance are shown in Table 19-20.

Laboratory diagnosis

ACTINOMYCES SPP.

Actinomyces spp. are straight to slightly curved rods with varying lengths, from short rods to long filaments. Short rods may have clubbed ends and

may be seen in diphtheroid arrangements, short chains, or small clusters. Longer rods and filaments may be straight or wavy and branched. Although the *Actinomyces* are gram-positive, irregular staining may cause a beaded or banded appearance. The typical branching, filamentous, Gram-stained appearance of an *Actinomyces* species depicted in Figure 19-21 is referred to as "*Actinomyces*-like."

Investigators at the Centers for Disease Control and Prevention (CDC) Anaerobic Bacteria Branch found that members of the genus *Actinomyces* are seldom obligate anaerobes. However, some are

TABLE 19-19

Clinically Encountered Gram-Positive Non–Spore-Forming Anaerobic Bacilli

Species	Body Site	Clinical Significance
Actinomyces		
A. israelii	Oral cavity, tonsillar crypts, dental plaque, intestinal and female genital tracts	Principal agent of human cervicofacial, thoracic, and abdominal actinomycosis; lacrimal canaliculitis and conjunctivitis; dacrocystitis; cervicitis and endometritis in women using intrauterine or vaginal contraceptive devices; "sulfur granules" are produced
A. meyeri	Periodontal sulcus	Infrequently isolated from brain abscesses and pleural fluid; less often from abscesses of cervicofacial area, hip, hand, foot, spleen, and bite wounds
A. odontolyticus	Oral cavity	Actinomycosis (rare cause); lacrimal canaliculitis; periodontitis (possibly) and dental caries (possibly)
A. viscosus	Oral cavity, caries, dental plaque, calculus	Periodontal disease; cervicovaginal secretions of women with and without IUDs; uninfected conjunctiva and cornea; cervicofacial and abdominal cases of actinomycosis (occasionally); lacrimal canaliculitis and other infections of the eye; cervicitis and endometritis of women using IUDs (possibly)
Bifidobacterium		
B. bifidum	Colon, vagina	—
B. breve	Colon, vagina	Has been isolated from clinical specimens
B. dentium	Colon, vagina, oral cavity, dental caries, dental plaque	Has been isolated from clinical specimens
B. infantis	Colon (infants), vagina	—
B. longum	Colon	Has been isolated from clinical specimens
B. pseudocatenulatum	Colon (infants)	—
Eubacterium		
E. aerofaciens	Colon	Occasionally isolated from blood cultures and various infections, including subacute bacterial endocarditis, renal abscess fluid, and appendiceal abscess
E. alactolyticum	Oral cavity	Frequently isolated from infected sites; dental calculus and gingival crevice in periodontal disease, root canals, purulent pleurisy, jugal cellulitis, postoperative wounds; abscesses of the brain, lung, intestinal tract, and mouth
E. brachy	Oral cavity	Subgingival samples and supragingival tooth scrapings from persons with periodontal disease, lung abscesses

Modified from Engelkirk PG, Duben-Engelkirk J, Dowell VR Jr: *Principles and practice of anaerobic bacteriology*, Belmont, Calif, 1992, Star.
Note: Ten *Eubacterium* spp. and three *Bifidobacterium* spp. isolated from feces but not from clinical specimens or other anatomic sites have been excluded from this list.
*Although *Mobiluncus* spp. have a typical gram-positive cell wall, they stain pink to gram-variable with Gram-staining procedures.

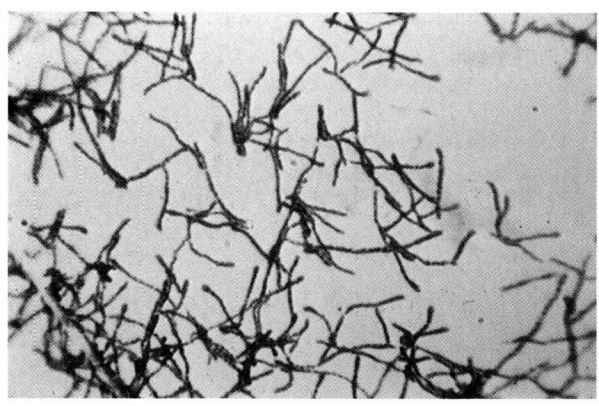

Figure 19-21 _____

Gram-stained appearance of *Actinomyces israelii*, illustrating the term *Actinomyces*-like

TABLE 19-19 ────────────────────────────

Clinically Encountered Gram-Positive Non–Spore-Forming Anaerobic Bacilli—cont'd

Species	Body Site	Clinical Significance
Eubacterium—*cont'd*		
E. combesii	Unknown	Has been isolated from various infections
E. contortum	Colon, vagina	Blood, abdominal aortic aneurysm, wounds
E. lentum	Colon	Blood, postoperative wounds, and various kinds of abscesses (brain, rectal, scrotal, pelvic)
E. limosum	Colon	Rectal and vaginal abscesses, blood, wounds
E. moniliforme	Colon	Blood and various other infections
E. nitritogenes	Colon	Has been isolated from various infections
E. nodatum	Oral cavity	Subgingival samples and supragingival tooth scrapings from persons with periodontal disease
E. rectale	Colon	—
E. saburreum	Dental plaque and gingival crevice	—
E. tenue	Unknown	Abscess following abortion, knee synovial fluid, blood
E. ventriosum	Colon	Mouth abscess, infections of the neck, purulent pleurisy, pulmonary abscesses, bronchiectasis
E. yurii	Unknown	Periodontal pockets, subgingival dental plaque
Mobiluncus*		
M. curtisii subsp. curtisii subsp. holmesii	Vagina	Thought to play a role in bacterial vaginosis
M. mulieris	Vagina	Thought to play a role in bacterial vaginosis
Propionibacterium		
P. acnes	Skin, colon	Acne vulgaris, wounds, blood, pus, and soft-tissue abscesses
P. avidum	Moist areas of the skin (e.g., vestibule of the nose, axilla, perineum, sinuses)	Has been isolated from infected sinuses, chronically infected wounds, and submaxillary abscesses but is probably not the primary cause of these infections
P. granulosum	Oily areas of skin (e.g., forehead or between shoulder blades)	May play some part in the pathogenesis of acne but probably not otherwise pathogenic
P. propionicus	Oral cavity, cervicovaginal secretions of healthy women, secretions from uninfected conjunctiva and cornea	A cause of actinomycosis and lacrimal canaliculitis

*Although *Mobiluncus* spp. have a typical gram-positive cell wall, they stain pink to gram-variable with Gram-staining procedures.

TABLE 19-20

Characteristics of Some Clinically Encountered Gram-Positive Non–Spore-Forming Anaerobic Bacilli

Species	Relationship to Oxygen	48-hr Colony <1 mm Diameter	Red Pigment	β-Hemolysis	Rough Colonies	Branched Rods	Catalase
Actinomyces spp.							
A. israelii	FA, AT, MA, AN	+	−	−	+	+	−
A. meyeri	FA, AT, MA, AN	−+	−	−	−	+	−
A. naeslundii	FA, AT, MA, AN	−+	−	−	−+	+	−
A. odontolyticus	FA, AT, MA, AN	−	+	−	−	+	−
A. pyogenes	FA, AT	−	−	+	−	−	−
A. viscosus	FA, AT, MA, AN	−	−	−	−+	+	+
Bifido-bacterium spp.							
B. dentium	FA, AT, MA, AN	−	−	−	−	−	−
Eubacterium, spp.							
E. alactolyticum	AN	+	−	−	−	−	−
E. lentum	AN	−	−	−	−	−	V
E. limosum	AN	−	−	−	−	−	−
Propioni-bacterium spp.							
P. acnes	FA, AT, MA, AN	−	−	−	−	−	+
P. propionicus	FA, AT, MA, AN	+	−	−	+	+	−

Modified from Engelkirk PG, Duben-Engelkirk J, Dowell VR Jr: *Principles and practice of anaerobic bacteriology,* Belmont, Calif, 1992, Star.
AN, Obligate anaerobe; *MA,* microaerotolerant anaerobe; *AT,* aerotolerant anaerobe; *FA,* facultative anaerobe; *V* or ( ), variable; *A,* acetic acid; *P,* propionic acid; *B,* butyric acid; *C,* caproic acid; *L,* lactic acid; *S,* succinic acid; +⁻, most strains are positive, but some are negative; −⁺, most strains are negative, but some are positive.

quite fastidious, requiring special vitamins, amino acids, and hemin for adequate growth.

Young *Actinomyces* colonies are frequently spider-like or wooly, whereas older colonies may resemble a raspberry or a molar tooth. Depending on the species, colonies may be red, pink, tan, yellow, white, or grayish.

BIFIDOBACTERIUM SPP.

Bifidobacterium spp. are variable in shape, ranging from coccobacilli to long, branching rods. The ends of the cells may be pointed, bent, club-shaped, spatulated, or bifurcated (forked). Cells may appear singly or in chains, as star-like aggregates, "V" arrangements, or "palisade" clusters.

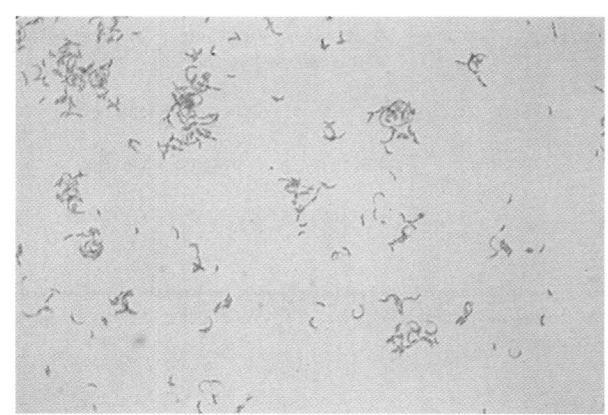

Figure 19-22

Gram-stained appearance of Mobiluncus curtisii ssp. curtisii, illustrating the curved morphology of this organism. (Courtesy Suzette L. Bartley, James D. Howard, and Ray Simon, Centers for Disease Control and Prevention, Atlanta, GA.)

Indole	Gelatin Hydrolysis	Proteolysis in Milk	Glucose	Lactose	Mannitol	Rhamnose	Major Acid Products in PYG
−	−	−	+	+⁻	+⁻	+⁻	A, L, S
−	−	−	+	−⁺	−	−	A, L, S
−	−	−	+	−⁺	−	−	A, L, S
−	−	−	+	−⁺	−	−	A, L, S
−	+	+	+	−	−	−	A, L, S
−	−	−	+	+⁻	−	−	A, L, S
−	−	−	+	+	−	−	A, L
−	−	−	V	−	−	−	A, B, C
−	−	−	−	−	−	−	(A)
−	−	−	+	−	+	−	A, B
+	+	+	+	−	−⁺	−	A, P, (L), (S)
−	−	−	+	+⁻	−	−	A, P, L

Colonies of *Bifidobacterium* spp. are convex, entire, cream to white, smooth, glistening, and soft.

EUBACTERIUM SPP.

Eubacterium spp. may be observed as either uniform or pleomorphic (variable in shape) gram-positive rods. They may be coccoid, diphtheroidal, or filamentous and range in width from thin to plump. *Eubacterium* colonies are usually small, circular, and convex, with an entire margin. An indole-negative, nitrate-positive, anaerobic gram-positive diphtheroid can be presumptively identified as *Eubacterium lentum.*

MOBILUNCUS SPP.

Mobiluncus spp. are found in the healthy vagina but increase dramatically in number in bacterial vaginosis. They are curved, motile bacilli and, although they stain pink or gram-variable with the Gram stain, they are *not* gram-negative organisms. Their cell walls are structurally similar to gram-positive organisms and lack lipopolysaccharide (LPS). Like gram-positive organisms, *Mobiluncus* spp. are susceptible to vancomycin and resistant to colistin. The Gram-stained appearance of *Mobiluncus* is depicted in Figure 19-22.

PROPIONIBACTERIUM SPP.

Propionibacterium spp. are pleomorphic rods that frequently appear as diphtheroids. The Gram-stained appearance of *P. acnes* is shown in Figure 19-23. Because *P. acnes* is a common member of the skin flora, it is frequently isolated from blood culture bottles and often dismissed as a skin

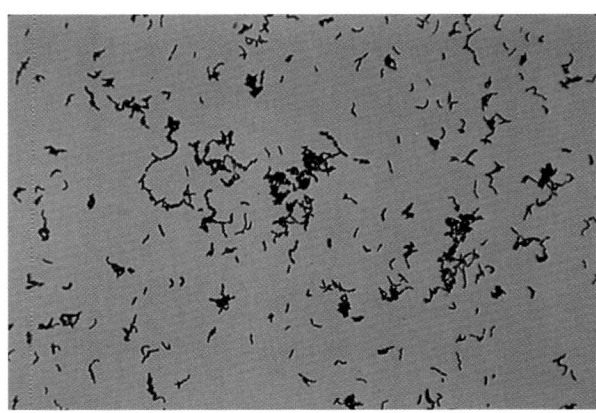

Figure 19-23

Gram-stained appearance of *Propionibacterium acnes,* illustrating the term diphtheroid. (Courtesy Suzette L. Bartley, James D. Howard, and Ray Simon, Centers for Disease Control and Prevention, Atlanta, GA.)

contaminant. However, *P. acnes,* like coagulase-negative staphylococci, can cause subacute bacterial endocarditis and bacteremia and thus is not always a contaminant. A catalase-positive, spot indole–positive, anaerobic gram-positive diphtheroid can be presumptively identified as *P. acnes.*

Like *Actinomyces* spp., *Propionibacterium propionicus* (formerly *Arachnia propionica*) can cause actinomycosis. This organism varies considerably in size and shape, ranging from coccoid and short diphtheroidal rods to long, branched filaments. Individual cells may be of uneven diameter and have distended or clubbed ends.

Identification

Identifying characteristics of clinically encountered non–spore-forming gram-positive bacilli are shown in Table 19-20.

Anaerobic Gram-Negative Bacilli

Many of the non–spore-forming, anaerobic, gram-negative bacilli involved in human infectious processes are found as members of the indigenous microflora. Tables 19-21 and 19-22 list the clinically encountered anaerobic gram-negative non–spore-forming bacilli, their habitat, and clinical significance. At first glance, the variety of such organisms appears overwhelming. Fortunately, only a few of the genera are commonly encountered in clinical specimens, which include the four major groups: *B. fragilis* group, *Porphyromonas* spp., *Prevotella* spp., and *Fusobacterium* spp.

Clinical infection

Anaerobic gram-negative bacilli are frequently found in mixed infections, causing abscesses and sepsis. *B. fragilis* often is isolated from soft-tissue infections. *P. asaccharolytica* is widely distributed in human tissues and fluids, whereas *Porphyromonas gingivalis* and *Porphyromonas endodontalis* are associated primarily with oral infections. *Fusobacterium* spp. are most often found in mixed infections and are associated with gum and other oral lesions.

Laboratory diagnosis

BACTEROIDES SPP.
One of the most clinically important genera of anaerobic gram-negative bacilli is the genus *Bacteroides.* Organisms in this genus have generated

considerable interest due to their frequent involvement in infectious processes and resistance to antimicrobial agents used to treat anaerobe-associated infections. *Bacteroides* spp. are found as part of indigenous microflora of the oral cavity and the gastrointestinal and genitourinary tracts.

The genus *Bacteroides* can be divided into bile-tolerant and bile-sensitive species. In the past, bile-sensitive species were subdivided into pigmented and nonpigmented species. However, in recent years, most pigmented species of bile-sensitive *Bacteroides* have been reclassified into the genera *Porphyromonas* and *Prevotella*. Many nonpigmented species of *Bacteroides* also have been transferred to the genus *Prevotella.*

BILE-TOLERANT *BACTEROIDES* SPP.
As shown in Table 19-21, bile-tolerant *Bacteroides* spp. include members of the *B. fragilis* group and two other species, *Bacteroides eggerthii* and *Bacteroides splanchnicus.* Members of the *B. fragilis* group (which includes *B. fragilis* and eight closely related species) are especially pathogenic. Figure 19-24 illustrates the frequency of isolation of the various members of the *B. fragilis* group. *B. fragilis* is the most common species of anaerobic bacteria isolated from infectious processes of soft tissue and anaerobic bacteremia.

It is important to identify members of the *B. fragilis* group to the species level because of species-to-species variability in both virulence and drug resistance. Penicillin-resistant strains of *B. fragilis* and other members of the *B. fragilis* group have been encountered for a number of years, but there also are reports of resistance to tetracycline, cefotaxime, cefoperazone, moxalactam, clindamycin, and other antimicrobials among isolates of this group. Although members of the *B. fragilis* group were the first anaerobes reported to produce β-lactamases, it is now known that many other anaerobes are also capable of producing them.

Gram-stained smears of *Bacteroides* spp. colonies reveal gram-negative coccobacilli or bacilli, but cells in broth cultures are frequently pleomorphic. The Gram-stained appearance of a typical *Bacteroides* species is shown in Figure 19-25.

Colonies of the *B. fragilis* group on the BBE agar plate are gray and a minimum of 1 mm in diameter. The originally light-yellow medium turns brown in the area around the colonies. Good growth is

TABLE 19-21

Clinically Encountered Bacteroides, Porphyromonas, *and* Prevotella *Species*

Species	Normal Flora Site	Clinical Significance
Bile tolerant		
***Bacteroides fragilis* group**		
B. caccae	Colon	Rarely isolated from clinical specimens
B. distasonis	Colon (common)	Occasionally isolated from clinical specimen
B. fragilis	Colon	The most common anaerobic species isolated from soft-tissue infections
B. merdae	Colon	—
B. ovatus	Colon	Occasionally isolated from clinical specimens
B. stercoris	Colon	—
B. thetaiotaomicron	Colon (common)	Frequently found in clinical specimens
B. uniformis	Colon	Various clinical specimens
B. vulgatus	Colon (common)	Occasionally isolated from infections
Other *Bacteroides* species		
B. eggerthii	Colon	Occasionally isolated from infections
B. splanchnicus	Colon, vagina	Occasionally isolated from infections
Bile sensitive		
Pigmented		
Prevotella		
P. corporis	Unknown	Various clinical specimens
P. denticola	Gingival crevice	Various clinical specimens
P. intermedia	Gingival crevice	Specimens from head, neck, and pleural infections; occasionally isolated from blood, abdominal, and pelvic sites
P. loescheii	Gingival crevice	—
P. melaninogenica	Gingival crevice	Various clinical specimens
Porphyromonas		
P. asaccharolytica	Unknown	Various clinical specimens
P. endodontalis	Unknown	Dental root canals
P. gingivalis	Mouth	—
Nonpigmented *Prevotella*		
P. bivia	Vagina	Infections of the urogenital or abdominal region; occasionally isolated from mouth, blood, chest fluid, breast abscess
P. buccae	Gingival crevice	Chest drainage, blood, sinus aspirate (sinusitis), peritoneal fluid, mandibular cyst
P. buccalis	Oral cavity	—
P. disiens	Vagina, mouth	Abdominal and urogenital infections
P. heparinolytica	Unknown	Periodontitis lesions
P. oralis	Gingival crevice	Infections of the oral cavity and the upper respiratory and genital tracts
P. oris	Gingival crevice	Systemic infections; nonoral isolates from face, neck, and chest abscess and drainage; abdominal wound drainage; peritoneal fluid, blood, spinal fluid
P. oulora	Gingival crevice	—
P. veroralis	Oral cavity	—
P. zoogleoformans	Gingival sulcus	—
Nonpigmented pitting *Bacteroides* species		
B. gracilis	Gingival crevice	—
B. ureolyticus	Buccal cavity, intestinal and urogenital tracts	Infections of the respiratory and intestinal tracts; has been isolated from blood following tooth extractions
Nonpitting *Bacteroides* species		
B. capillosus	Colon, mouth	Cysts and wounds
B. coagulans	Colon, urogenital tract	Occasionally isolated from clinical specimens
B. forsythus	Oral cavity	—
B. galacturonicus	Colon	—
B. pectinophilus	Colon	—

Modified from Engelkirk PG, Duben-Engelkirk J, Dowell VR Jr: *Principles and practice of anaerobic bacteriology,* Belmont, Calif, 1992, Star.

TABLE 19-22

Clinically Encountered Gram-Negative Anaerobic Bacilli (Other Than Bacteroides, Porphyromonas, *and* Prevotella *Species)*

Species	Normal Flora Site	Clinical Significance
Anaerobiospirillum succiniciproducens	Unknown	Blood, feces from diarrhetic patients
Anaerorhabdus furcosus	Colon (infrequent)	Infected appendix, lung, and abdominal abscess
Bilophila wadsworthia	Colon	Intraabdominal specimens from patients with gangrenous and perforated appendicitis
Butyrivibrio		
B. crossotus	Colon	—
B. fibrisolvens	Colon	Eye infection
Campylobacter concisus	Oral cavity	Periodontal disease, wounds
Centipeda periodontii	Oral cavity	Periodontal disease
Desulfomonas pigra	Colon	Peritoneal fluid, pylonidal cyst abscess, ruptured sigmoid colon
Desulfovibrio vulgaris	Colon	Pleural fluid
Fusobacterium		
F. alocis	Gingival sulcus	Submandibular abscess, mouth ulcer
F. gonidiaformans	Intestinal, urogenital tracts	Various types of infections
F. mortiferum	Colon	Blood and various clinical specimens
F. necrogenes	Colon	—
F. nechrophorum	Body cavities	Necrotic lesions, abscess, blood
ssp. *funduliforme*		—
ssp. *nechrophorum*		—
F. nucleatum	Gingival margin and sulcus	Infections of the upper respiratory tract and pleural cavity; occasionally from wounds and other types of infections
F. periodonticum	Oral cavity	—
F. prausnitzii	Colon (very common)	—
F. pseudonecrophorum	Unknown	—
F. russii	Colon	—
F. sulci	Gingival sulcus	—
F. ulcerans	None	Cutaneous tropical ulcers
F. varium	Colon	Purulent infections of the upper respiratory tract, surgical wounds, and peritonitis
Leptotrichia buccalis	Oral cavity, femal periurethral region	—
Megamonas hypermegas	Colon	—
Mitsuokella		
M. dentalis	Oral cavity	Dental root canals
M. multiacidus	Colon	Occasionally isolated from clinical specimens
Selenomonas		—
S. artemidis	Gingival crevice	
S. dianae	Gingival crevice	—
S. flueggei	Gingival crevice	—
S. noxia	Gingival crevice	—
S. sputigena	Gingival crevice	Transtracheal aspirate and pleural fluid; relationship to periodontal disease unknown
Succinimonas amylolytica	Unknown	Wound drainage
Succinovibrio dextrinosolvens	Oral cavity (rare), colon (rare)	Septicemia
Tissierella praeacuta	Colon	Infrequently from lung abscess, gangrenous lesions, blood
Wolinella		
W. curva (*Campylobacter curvus*)	Oral cavity	Lesions in oral cavity, blood; pathogenicity unknown
W. recta (*Campylobacter rectus*)	Gingival crevice	Periodontal pockets, necrotic dental root canals; pathogenicity unknown

Modified from Engelkirk PG, Duben-Engelkirk J, Dowell VR Jr: *Principles and practice of anaerobic bacteriology*, Belmont, Calif, 1992, Star.

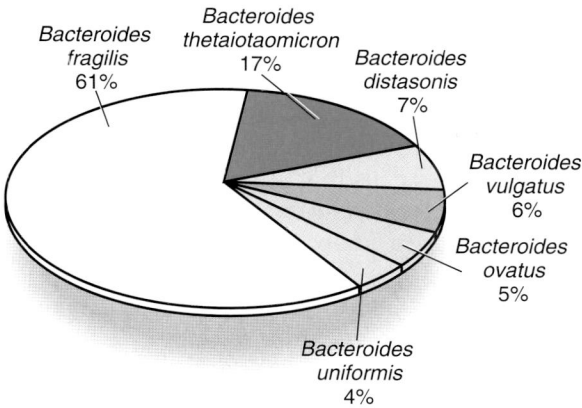

Figure 19-24 _____

Frequency of isolation of members of the Bacteroides fragilis group from clinical specimens. From: Goldstein and Citron (1988). (Redrawn from Engelkirk PG, Duben-Engelkirk J, Dowell VR Jr: *Principles and Practice of Clinical Anaerobic Bacteriology,* Belmont, Calif, 1992, Star.)

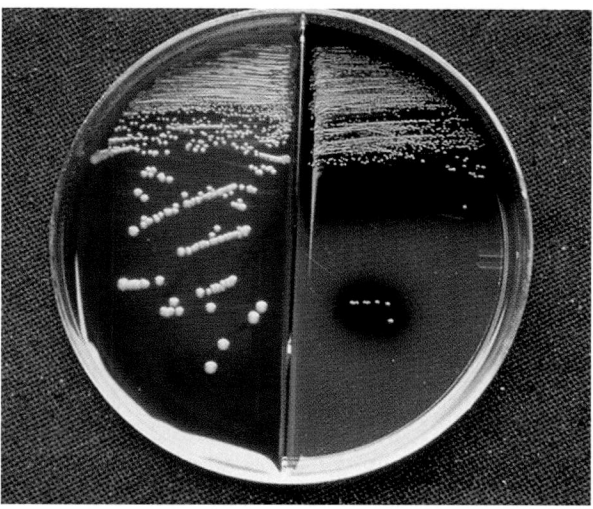

Figure 19-26 _____

Appearance of *Bacteroides fragilis* on a KVLB agar *(left)*/BBE agar biplate *(right);* browning of the BBE medium is the result of esculin hydrolysis. (Courtesy Anaerobe Systems, San Jose, Calif.)

the result of bile tolerance, and browning of the medium is due to esculin hydrolysis. A dark precipitate (stippling) in the medium around the areas of heavy growth is suggestive of the species *B. fragilis,* although some strains of *Bacteroides ovatus* also cause stippling. The appearance of *B. fragilis* group organisms on BBE agar is shown in Figure 19-26.

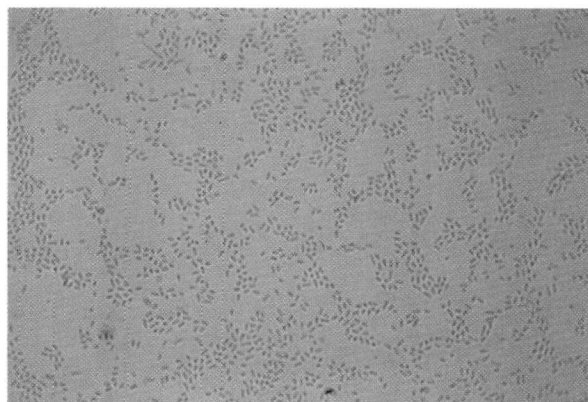

Figure 19-25 _____

Gram-stained appearance of *Bacteroides thetaiotaomicron,* illustrating the typical appearance of *Bacteroides* spp. (Courtesy Suzette L. Bartley, James D. Howard, and Ray Simon, Centers for Disease Control and Prevention, Atlanta, Ga.)

Caution must be taken, however, when interpreting results on BBE agar. *B. vulgatus,* a member of the *B. fragilis* group, does not hydrolyze esculin and therefore does not produce a brown discoloration of the medium. *B. splanchnicus* and *B. eggerthii,* which currently are not members of the *B. fragilis* group, are bile-resistant and esculin hydrolysis–positive; thus, colonies of these organisms have the same appearance on BBE agar as members of the *B. fragilis* group.

Depending on the commercial source, age, and storage conditions of the medium, other organisms such as *F. mortiferum, Klebsiella pneumoniae, Enterococcus* spp., and yeasts may also grow on BBE agar. Their colony size (which tends to be smaller), Gram-stain morphology, and aerotolerance will aid in the recognition of these other organisms.

BILE-SENSITIVE PIGMENTED SPECIES

Certain species of *Prevotella,* namely *Prevotella corporis, P. intermedia, P. loescheii, Prevotella melaninogenica,* and some strains of *Prevotella denticola,* produce protoporphyrin, a dark pigment that causes their colonies to become brown to black with age. *Prevotella* spp. appear as gram-negative coccobacilli or bacilli, very similar to *Bacteroides* spp.

Colony pigmentation (brown to black) may take 2 to 3 weeks of incubation before it becomes evident on routine blood agar plates, but it appears sooner on media containing laked blood (blood that has been frozen and then thawed). For this reason, always subject nonpigmented colonies on KLVB agar (or BRU/BA) to long-wave UV light, such as a Wood's lamp, to detect the typical brick-red fluorescence of pigment-producing *Prevotella* spp. The brick-red fluorescence of such pigmented species under UV light is similar to that shown in Figure 19-11.

Some species of pigmented *Prevotella* fluoresce colors other than brick-red, such as brilliant red, yellow, orange, and pink-orange, and some do not fluoresce at all. Only brick-red fluorescence allows presumptive identification of the pigmented *Prevotella* group.

P. asaccharolytica, Porphyromonas gingivalis, and *Porphyromonas endodontalis* also produce a dark brown to black pigment, protoheme when grown for 6 to 10 days on blood agar plates. Most strains of these fastidious, obligate anaerobes require hemin and menadione, a vitamin K derivative, for growth. *Porphyromonas* also produces brick-red fluorescence and other colors under UV light, similar to *Prevotella,* but certain species do not fluoresce at all. Because most *Porphyromonas* strains are susceptible to vancomycin, they will not grow on media containing 5 mg or more vancomycin per milliliter, such as KVLB agar.

BILE-SENSITIVE NONPIGMENTED SPECIES

Bile-sensitive nonpigmented *Bacteroides* spp. are listed in Table 19-21. This table shows those species that pit the agar and those that are nonpitting. Recent reports have shown that the so-called pitting anaerobes of the *Bacteroides ureolyticus* group (which includes *B. ureolyticus, Bacteroides gracilis, Wolinella curva,* and *Wolinella recta*) are actually **microaerophiles** rather than obligate anaerobes. Moreover, *W. curva* and *W. recta* have recently been reclassified as *C. curvus* and *C. rectus,* respectively.

Not all strains of these pitting organisms actually pit agar, and among those strains that do pit, not all colonies will appear to be pitting. Thus, they may resemble a mixed culture. Nonpigmented *Prevotella* spp. include *Prevotella bivia, Prevotella buccae, Prevotella buccalis, Prevotella disiens, Prevotella oralis, Prevotella oris, Prevotella oulora,* and *Prevotella veroralis.*

FUSOBACTERIUM

Fusobacterium is often described microscopically as long, thin, and tapered rods, a morphology characteristically referred to as *fusiform.* It is important to note, however, that only *F. nucleatum* ssp. *nucleatum* has cells that are consistently fusiform in shape, and clinically encountered bacteria that are fusiform in shape are not necessarily *Fusobacterium* spp.

The Gram-stained appearance of *F. nucleatum* ssp. *nucleatum* is depicted in Figure 19-27. Other fusobacteria, such as *F. mortiferum,* appear pleomorphic, exhibiting globular forms, swellings, and other bizarre shapes. The pleomorphism of *F. mortiferum* is depicted in Figure 19-28. Organisms other than fusobacteria may also have fusiform-shaped cells; examples include *B. gracilis, Bacteroides forsythus,* and microaerophilic *Capnocytophaga* spp.

Certain *Vibrio*-like anaerobes, or *anaerobic vibrions* (curved, motile, gram-negative staining bacilli), have been reclassified as *Anaerobiospirillum, Butyrivibrio, Campylobacter, Desulfovibrio, Selenomonas, Succinovibrio,* and *Mobiluncus* spp. Of these, *C. curvus, C. rectus,* and *Mobiluncus* spp. are encountered most frequently in clinical materials—the *Campylobacter* from oral, GI, and vaginal specimens and the *Mobiluncus* spp. from vaginal specimens. Although cells of *C. curvus* are curved, *C. rectus* cells are straight rods.

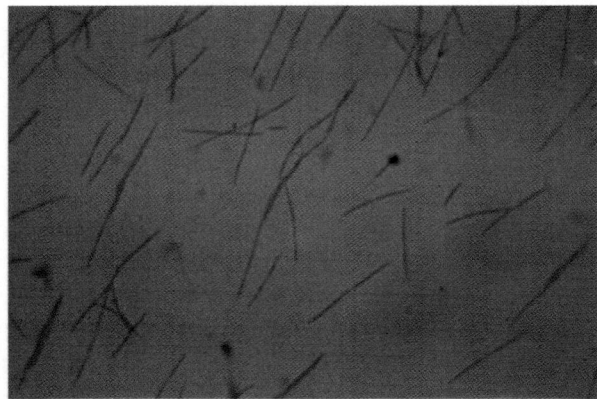

Figure 19-27 _____

Gram-stained appearance of *Fusobacterium nucleatum* ssp. *nucleatum,* illustrating the fusiform morphology of this organism. (Courtesy Suzette L. Bartley, James D. Howard, and Ray Simon, Centers for Disease Control and Prevention, Atlanta, Ga.)

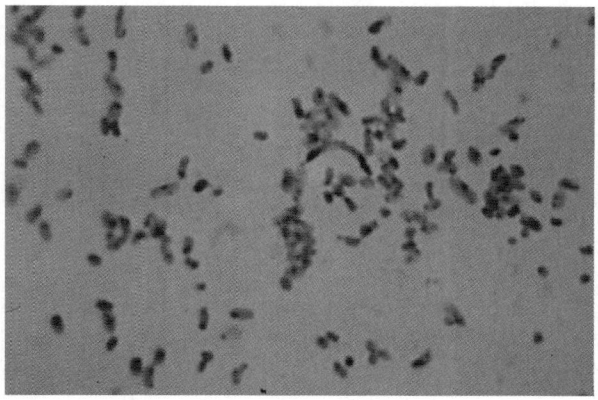

Figure 19-28

Gram-stained appearance of *Fusobacterium mortiferum,* illustrating pleomorphism. (Courtesy Suzette L. Bartley, James D. Howard, and Ray Simon, Centers for Disease Control and Prevention, Atlanta, Ga.)

Identification

Presumptive identification of anaerobic, gram-negative bacilli is shown in Tables 19-23 through 19-27. Definitive identification information is contained in Tables 19-28 and 19-29.

Anaerobic Cocci

Clinical infection

Anaerobic cocci are isolated from a wide variety of infections, including brain abscess, aspiration pneumonia, lung abscess, gingivitis, and other peri-odontal diseases. Table 19-30 describes the various species of anaerobic cocci, where they are found, and infections they cause.

Gram-positive cocci

Most of the gram-positive anaerobic cocci previously classified as *Peptococcus* spp. have been renamed *Peptostreptococcus* spp., with the exception of *Peptococcus niger.* Most of the anaerobic gram-positive cocci isolated from clinical specimens are in the genus *Peptostreptococcus* (Figure 19-29). Other anaerobic gram-positive cocci encountered in clinical materials are *Coprococcus, Gemella, Sarcina,* and certain *Streptococcus* spp.

An SPS-sensitive, anaerobic, gram-positive coccus can be presumptively identified as *P. anaerobius,* whereas an SPS-resistant, spot indole–positive, anaerobic, gram-positive coccus can be presumptively identified as *Peptostreptococcus asaccharolyticus. P. niger* produces colonies that become light gray when exposed to air, but it is only rarely isolated from clinical specimens.

Media preparation, age, and storage conditions are critical for the isolation of clinically significant anaerobic gram-positive cocci. The size and arrangement (e.g., pairs, tetrads, chains, clusters) of the gram-positive anaerobic cocci vary with growth conditions and therefore are not reliable criteria for identification.

Text continued on p. 617

TABLE 19-23

Presumptive Identification of Porphyromonas *spp.*

Porphyromonas sp.	Arginine	α-Fucosidase	Trypsin	N-acetyl-β-glucosaminidase (NAG)	Fluorescence Under UV Light
P. asaccharolytica	Most strains +	+	−	−	+
P. endodontalis	Most strains −	−	−	−	+
P. gingivalis	+	−	+	+	−

Courtesy Mangels JI, 1998.

NOTES:

1. Use this table for an anaerobic gram-negative bacillus that produces the following special potency antimicrobial disk results: vancomycin susceptible, kanamycin resistant, colistin resistant; such an organism could be a pink-staining gram-positive bacillus or a *Porphyromonas* sp.
2. Try performing the Gram stain under anaerobic conditions (Johnson et al, 1995); if still gram-negative, assume the isolate to be a *Porphyromonas* sp.
3. Confirmation of *Porphyromonas* sp.: brick red fluorescence under long-wave (360-nm) UV light (a Wood's lamp) or dark brown to black pigmented colonies; fluorescence usually disappears as pigment develops; pigment production usually occurs within 3 to 14 days, but may take as long as 21 days

Related articles: Hudspeth et al, 1997; Maiden et al, 1996; Durmaz et al, 1995.

TABLE 19-24

Presumptive Identification of Members of the Bacteroides fragilis *Group*

Bile-Resistant Bacteroides spp.	Indole	Catalase	Notes
B. fragilis	−	+	−
B. vulgatus	−	Most strains +	Can be identified as *B. vulgatus* if indole-negative, catalase-positive, and esculin-negative (no browning of BBE medium)
B. distasonis	−	Most strains +	−
B. merdae (rarely isolated)	−	Most strains −	−
B. caccae	−	−	−
B. thetaiotaomicron	+	+	Can be presumptively identified as *B. thetaiotaomicron* if indole-positive and catalase-positive
B. uniformis	+	Most strains −	−
B. ovatus	+	Most strains −	−
B. stercoris (rarely isolated)	+	−	−
B. eggerthii (rarely isolated)	+	−	−

Courtesy Mangels JI, 1998.

NOTES:
1. Use this table for an anaerobic gram-negative bacillus that produces the following special potency antimicrobial disk results: vancomycin resistant, kanamycin resistant, colistin resistant; such an organism is most likely a member of the *B. fragilis* group, but it could be a *Prevotella* sp.
2. If the isolate is growing on the BBE plate (i.e., it is bile resistant), it is a member of the *B. fragilis* group; if it is not growing on BBE, it is a *Prevotella* sp. (see Table 19-25).
3. Further identification of members of the *B. fragilis* group will require inoculation of a biochemical- or enzyme-based ID system.

TABLE 19-25

Presumptive Identification of Prevotella *spp.*

Pigmented Species of Prevotella	Color of Pigmented Colonies	Indole	Lipase	Esculin	Notes
P. melaninogenica	Tan to buff	−	−	Most strains negative	−
P. denticola	Tan to buff	−	−	+	Can be presumptively identified as *P. denticola*
P. loescheii	Tan to buff	−	Most strains negative; some strains weakly positive	−	Can be presumptively identified as *P. loescheii* if indole-negative and lipase-positive
P. corporis	Black	−	−	−	−
P. intermedia	Black	+	Most strains positive	−	Can be identified as *P. intermedia* if indole-positive and lipase-positive
P. bivia	Variable	−	−	−	−

Courtesy Mangels JI, 1998.

NOTES:
1. Some *Prevotella* spp. produce pigmented colonies, whereas others do not; use this table for a pigmented, bile-resistant, anaerobic gram-negative bacillus that produces the following special potency antimicrobial disk results: vancomycin resistant, kanamycin resistant, colistin susceptible; *or* a pigmented, bile-sensitive organism that is resistant to all three antimicrobial agents; in either case, the organism is probably a *Prevotella* sp.
2. Nonpigmented *Prevotella* spp. include *Prevotella bivia, Prevotella buccae, Prevotella buccalis, Prevotella disiens, Prevotella heparinolytica, Prevotella oralis, Prevotella oris, Prevotella oulorum, Prevotella veroralis,* and *Prevotella zoogleoformans.*
3. If the nonpigmented isolate is indole-positive and esculin-positive, it can be identified as *P. heparinolytica;* inoculation of a biochemical- or enzyme-based ID system will be necessary to identify other nonpigmented *Provotella* spp.

TABLE 19-26

Presumptive Identification of the Bacteroides ureolyticus *Group and* Bilophila wadsworthia

Nitrate-Positive Isolates	Agar Pitting	Motility	Urease	Strong Oxidase	Notes
Bacteroides gracilis	Most strains +	−	−	−	—
Bacteroides ureolyticus	Most strains +	−	+	Variable	Agar-pitting, urease-positive isolates can be identified as *B. ureolyticus.*
Campylobacter curvus & *Campylobacter rectus*	Most strains −	+	−	−	—
Campylobacter concisus	Most strains −	+	−	+	—
Biolophila wadsworthia	−	−	Most strains +	−	Bile-resistant; on BBE, will produce clear colonies with black centers (fish eye appearance); strongly catalase-positive

Courtesy Mangels JI, 1998.

NOTES:
1. Use this table for a nitrate-positive, anaerobic gram-negative bacillus that produces the following special potency antimicrobial disk results: vancomycin resistant, kanamycin susceptible, colistin susceptible; such an organism is probably *Bilophila wadsworthia* or a member of the *Bacteroides ureolyticus* group
2. Nitrate-negative, anaerobic gram-negative bacilli that produce these special potency antimicrobial results are probably *Fusobacterium* spp. (see Table 19-27)

TABLE 19-27

Presumptive Identification of Fusobacterium *spp.*

Nitrate-negative Isolates (*Fusobacterium* spp.)	Cell Morphology	Colony Morphology	Indole	Bile Resistant	Notes
Fusobacterium nucleatum	Tapered ends	Breadcrumb-like, speckled, or smooth	+	−	Can be identified as *F. nucleatum* if cells are "fusiform" and indole-positive
Fusobacterium gonidiaformans	Gonidial forms	Smooth	+	−	—
Fusobacterium necrophorum	Round ends, bizarre shapes	Umbonate with greening of the blood agar	+	Most strains −	Can be identified as *F. necrophorum* if lipase-positive
Fusobacterium naviforme	Boat shaped	Mottled	+	−	—
Fusobacterium varium	Round ends	Smooth, fried egg colonies	Most strains +	+	Can be identified as *F. varium* if indole-negative, bile-sensitive, and esculin-negative
Fusobacterium mortiferum	Bizarre shapes	Fried egg colonies	−	+	Can be identified as *F. mortiferum* if esculin-positive
Fusobacterium russi	Round ends	Smooth	−	−	Can be identified as *F. russi* if indole-negative and bile sensitive

Courtesy Mangels JI, 1998.

NOTES:
1. Use this table for a nitrate-negative, anaerobic gram-negative bacillus that produces the following special potency antimicrobial disk results: vancomycin resistant, kanamycin susceptible, colistin susceptible; such an organism is probably a *Fusobacterium* sp.
2. Inoculation of a biochemical- or enzyme-based ID system will be necessary for further identification of *Fusobacterium* spp.

TABLE 19-28

Characteristics of Some Clinically Encountered Nonmotile Gram-Negative Anaerobic Bacilli

Species	Brown-Black Pigmentation	Red Fluorescence	Pitted Colonies	Colonies ≤1 mm Diameter	Catalase	Oxidase	Indole	Inhibited by Bile	Esculin Hydrolysis	Lipase	DNase	Glucose	Lactose	Gelatin Hydrolysis	Proteolysis in Milk	Urease	Rifampin (15 µg)	Butyric	Succinic	Phenylacetic
Bacteroides spp.																				
B. gracilis	−	−	−+	+	−	−	−	+									S	−	+	−
B. ureolyticus	−	−	+−	+	−	+	−	+								+	S	−	+	−
Fusobacterium spp.																				
F. mortiferum	−	−	−	−	−	−	−	−	+		+	+			−		R	+	−+	−
F. necrophorum	−	−	−	−	−	−	+	+			+	+		−+	V		S	+	−	−
F. nucleatum	−	−	−	−	−	−	+	+			−	−					S	+		
F. varium	−	−	−	−	−	−	+−					+				+	R	+		
Porphyromonas spp.	+	+	−	−	−	−	−	−	−					+			S	+	+	
P. asaccharolytica	+	+−					+	+						+	+	−	S	+	+	−
P. endodontalis	+						+	+						+	+	−	S	+	+	+
P. gingivalis																				
Prevotella spp.	+	+	−	−	−	−	−	+	+	−	+	+	+	+	+	−	S	−	+	−
P. intermedia																				

Modified from Engelkirk PG, Duben-Engelkirk J, Dowell VR Jr: *Principles and practice of anaerobic bacteriology,* Belmont, Calif, 1992, Star.
V, Variable; *R,* resistant; *S,* sensitive; +−, most strains are positive but some are negative; −+, most strains are negative but some are positive.

TABLE 19-29

Characteristics of Some Clinically Encountered Bile-Tolerant, Saccharolytic Bacteroides Species (the Bacteroides fragilis Group)

Species	Catalase	Indole	DNase	Penicillin (2 U Disk)	Rifampin (15 µg Disk)	Kanamycin (1 mg Disk)	Arabinose	Cellobiose	Mannitol	Rhamnose	Salicin	Trehalose	Butyric	Succinic
B. caccae	−	−	+	R	S	R	+	+−	−	V	+	+	−	+
B. distasonis	+−	−	−	R	S	R	−	−	−	+	+	+	−	+
B. fragilis	+−	−	−	R	S	R	−	−	−	−	−	−	−	+
B. merdae	−	−	−	R	S	R	−	+	−	+	+	+	−	+
B. ovatus	+	+	+	R	S	R	+	+	+	+	+	+	−	+
B. stercoris	−	+	+	R	S	R	−+	−	−	+	−	−	−	+
B. thetaiotaomicron	+	+	+	R	S	R	+	+	−+	+	−+	+	−	+
B. uniformis	−	+	+	R	S	R	+	+	−	−+	+−	−	−	+
B. vulgatus	−+	−	−	R	S	R	+	−	−	+	−	−	−	+

Modified from Engelkirk PG, Duben-Engelkirk J, Dowell VR Jr: *Principles ad practice of anaerobic bacteriology,* Belmont, Calif, 1992, Star.
V, Variable; *R,* resistant; *S,* sensitive; +−, most strains positive but some are negative; −+, most strains negative but some are positive.

TABLE 19-30

Clinically Encountered Anaerobic Cocci

Genus	Normal Flora Site	Clinical Significance
Gram-positive cocci		
Streptococcus		
S. hansenii	Colon	—
S. pleomorphus	Colon	—
Coprococcus	Three species have been isolated from feces but not from clinical specimens	—
Gemella	Unknown	—
Peptococcus niger	Umbilicus, vaginal area	Only occasionally isolated from human samples; more common among veterinary specimens
Peptostreptococcus		
P. anaerobius	Vagina, colon	Isolated from a wide variety of clinical specimens, including abscesses of the brain, jaw, pleural cavity, ear, pelvic region, urogenital area, and abdominal region; also from blood, spinal fluid, joint cultures, and specimens from cases of osteomyelitis; gingival crevice of persons with gingivitis or periodontal diseases
P. asaccharolyticus	Vagina	Vaginal discharge, skin abscess, peritoneal abscess
P. hydrogenalis	Unknown	Has been isolated from feces and vaginal discharge
P. magnus	Genital tract; rare in colon or gingival crevice	Wounds; abdominal abscess; peritoneal, appendiceal, and urogenital sites; more frequent in anatomic sites below diaphragm
P. micros	Genital tract; infrequently in healthy gingival crevice and intestinal tract	Frequently isolated from clinical specimens, including brain, lung, jaw, head, and neck; bite abscesses, spinal fluid, blood, and abscesses at other body sites; often a major component of the gingival sulcus in periodontal disease
P. prevotii	Skin, vagina, tonsils	—
P. productus	Colon (one of the more predominant members of the fecal flora)	—
P. tetradius	Vagina	Vaginal discharge and various purulent infections
Gram-negative cocci		
Acidaminococcus fermentans	Colon	Rarely isolated from clinical specimens
Megasphaera elsdenii	Colon	Rarely isolated from clinical specimens
Veillonelia		
V. atypica		
V. dispar	Oral cavity	Head, neck, dental, and pulmonary infections; bite wounds
V. parvula		

Courtesy Engelkirk PG, Duben-Engelkirk J, Dowell VR Jr: *Principles and practice of anaerobic bacteriology*, Belmont, Calif, 1992, Star.

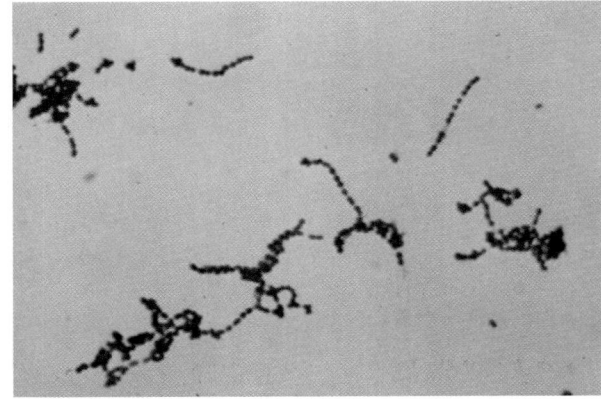

Figure 19-29

Gram-stained appearance of a *Peptostreptococcus* sp. illustrating the chain formation that occurs with some species. (Courtesy Suzette L. Bartley, James D. Howard, and Ray Simon, Centers for Disease Control and Prevention, Atlanta, Ga.)

TABLE 19-31

Characteristics of Some Clinically Encountered Anaerobic Cocci

Species	Relationship to Oxygen	Gram-Stain Reaction	Catalase	Indole	Esculin Hydrolysis	Urease	Nitrate Reduction	Glucose	Lactose	Acids Produced in PYG
Peptostreptococcus spp.										
Peptostreptococcus anaerobius*	AN, MA	+	−	−	−	−	−⁺	+	−	A, IB, IV, IC
Peptostreptococcus asaccharolyticus	AN	+	−⁺	+	−	−	−	−	−	A, B
Peptostreptococcus indolicus†	AN	+	−	+	−	−	+	−	−	A, P, B
Peptostreptococcus magnus	AN	+	−⁺	−	−	−	−	−	−	A
Peptostreptococcus micros	AN	+	−	−	−	−	−	−	−	A
Peptostreptococcus prevotii	AN	+	−⁺	−	−	−	−	−	−	A, P, B
Peptostreptococcus tetradius	AN	+	−	−	−	+	−	+	+	A, B, L
Sarcina spp.										
Sarcina ventriculi‡	AN, MA	+	V	−	+	+	+	+	+	A
Staphylococcus spp.										
Staphylococcus saccharolyticus	AN, MA, AT	+	+	−	−	−	+	+	−	A
Veillonella spp.										
Veillonella parvula	AN, MA	−	+	−	−	−	+⁻	−	−	A, P

Courtesy Engelkirk PG, Duben-Engelkirk J, Dowell VR Jr: *Principles and practice of anaerobic bacteriology*, Belmont, Calif, 1992, Star.

AN, Obligate anaerobe; *MA*, microaerotolerant anaerobe; *AT*, aerotolerant anaerobe; *V*, variable; *A*, acetic acid; *P*, propionic acid; *IB*, isobutyric acid; *B*, butyric acid; *IV*, isovaleric acid; *IC*, isocaproic acid; *L*, lactic acid; +⁻, most strains positive but some are negative; −⁺, most strains negative but some are positive.

*Inhibited by SPS disk.
†Coagulase-positive.
‡Forms endospores.

Gram-negative cocci

Although several genera of anaerobic gram-negative cocci (see Table 19-30) are found in the indigenous microflora, only *Veillonella* spp. are implicated as pathogens. *Veillonella* cocci are very small (0.3 to 0.5 mm in diameter) and inhabit the oral cavity. Other genera of gram-negative cocci (*Acidaminococcus* and *Megasphaera*) live in the gastrointestinal tract but are only rarely isolated from clinical specimens. A nitrate-positive, anaerobic, gram-negative coccus can be presumptively identified as a *Veillonella* spp.

Identification

Schematic diagrams showing the presumptive identification of anaerobic cocci are shown in Figures 19-30 and 19-31. Other characteristics used to identify anaerobic cocci are shown in Table 19-31.

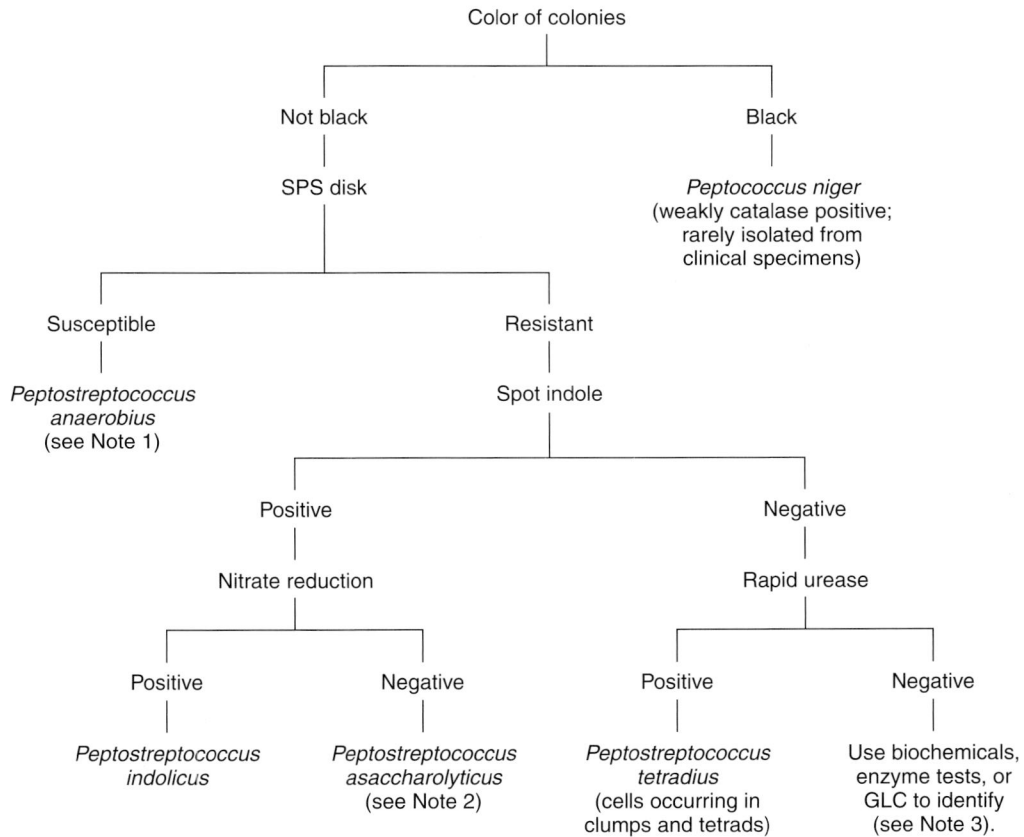

Notes

1. *P. anaerobius* has characteristic cell morphology, colony morphology, and odor. Some strains of *Peptostreptococcus micros* are susceptible to SPS, but they generally produce smaller zones of inhibition and the cells would be less than 0.7 μm in diameter.
2. *P. asaccharolyticus* has characteristic cell morphology, colony morphology, and odor. *Peptostreptococcus hydrogenalis* is also indole-positive but unlike *P. asaccharolyticus* is alkaline phosphatase-positive.
3. *P. micros* can often be identified by its characteristic cell and colony morphology.

Figure 19-30

Identification of anaerobic gram-positive cocci. Anaerobic, gram-positive cocci (AGPC) are susceptible to metronidazole, whereas microaerophilic, gram-positive cocci are not. A 5-mg metronidazole disk can be used to determine metronidazole susceptibility. Although metronidazole-resistant strains of AGPC have been reported, they appear to be rare. *GLC*, Gas-liquid chromatography; *SPS*, sodium polyanethol sulfonate. (Data from Mangels, JI, 1998; Murdoch DA, 1998.)

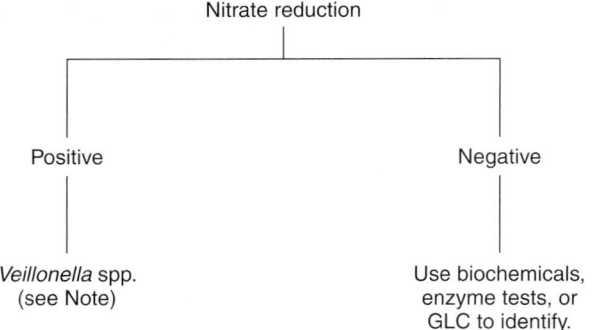

Nitrate reduction

Positive — *Veillonella* spp. (see Note)

Negative — Use biochemicals, enzyme tests, or GLC to identify.

Note

Nitrate-positive, anaerobic, gram-negative cocci can be reported as *Veillonella* species. *Veillonella* spp. are less than 0.5 µg in diameter and are usually in clusters or diplococci. *Veillonella* spp. produce small, convex, translucent to transparent colonies with entire edges. The colonies may fluoresce red under long-wave UV light (a Wood's lamp). Nitrate-negative strains of *Veillonella* do occur.

Figure 19-31

Identification of anaerobic gram-negative cocci. Although they are gram-positive, P. asaccharolyticus and P. indolicus are easily decolorized, and may appear to be gram-negative. A 5-mg vancomycin disk can be used to confirm that anaerobic, gram-negative cocci are truly gram-negative. Gram-negative cocci will be resistant to vancomycin, whereas gram-positive cocci will be susceptible. Although Megasphaera spp. commonly stain gram-positive, they are really gram-negative on the basis of cell wall composition. *GLC*, Gas-liquid chromatography. (Data from Mangels JI, 1992; Murdoch DA, 1998.)

SUSCEPTIBILITY AND β-LACTAMASE TESTING

Antimicrobial susceptibility testing of anaerobes is currently controversial. The information contained in this section should not be considered definitive. Issues that clinicians and microbiologists have not agreed on include the following:

- Clinical significance of the anaerobic isolate
- Predictability of anaerobe susceptibilities
- Cost of susceptibility testing
- Difficulty of performing susceptibility testing on anaerobes

Questions frequently asked are as follows:

- Should susceptibility testing of anaerobes be performed at all in clinical microbiology laboratories?
- Which isolates should be tested?
- Which antimicrobial agents should be tested?
- Which method should be used?

These are all valid questions, and each is addressed in this section.

Traditionally, the isolation, identification, and susceptibility testing of obligate anaerobes have been quite slow when compared to other groups of bacteria. As a result, antimicrobial therapy of anaerobe-associated infectious processes has frequently been initiated on an empiric basis: When physicians suspected the presence of anaerobes, they selected an antimicrobial agent that they thought would be effective. Although not a very scientific approach, empiric therapy undoubtedly has saved many lives.

Anaerobe Resistance to Antimicrobial Agents

Although anaerobe susceptibility patterns were once thought to be quite predictable, the results of numerous studies have shown otherwise. Resistance of anaerobes to antimicrobial agents is no longer limited to the *B. fragilis* group; it occurs among many different anaerobes and involves a variety of antimicrobial agents. In addition to members of the *B. fragilis* group, especially resistant anaerobes include *B. gracilis, C. ramosum,* and *Fusobacterium varium*.

Locally determined patterns of susceptibility and resistance should be used to guide empiric therapy.

Susceptibility Testing of Anaerobes
When to test
The National Committee for Clinical Laboratory Standards (NCCLS) Working Group on Anaerobic Susceptibility Testing of Anaerobic Bacteria cites the following major reasons for susceptibility testing of anaerobic isolates:

- To determine patterns of susceptibility of anaerobes to new antimicrobial agents
- To monitor susceptibility patterns periodically in various medical centers, local communities, and hospitals
- To help manage infections in individual patients

The NCCLS Working Group states that susceptibility testing is not required for many anaerobes isolated from patients. The following specific situations warrant susceptibility testing of anaerobes:

- When the isolate is an organism known to be resistant
- When the usual therapeutic regimens have failed and the infectious process persists
- When the role of antimicrobial agents is pivotal in determining the outcome
- When there exists no precedent for empiric therapy
- When the infection is severe
- When long-term therapy is required

The NCCLS Working Group also suggests that the following specific infectious processes warrant susceptibility testing of anaerobic isolates:

- Brain abscess
- Endocarditis
- Infection of a prosthetic device or vascular graft
- Joint infections
- Osteomyelitis
- Refractory or recurrent bacteremia

Because many anaerobe-associated infectious processes are polymicrobial, deciding which anaerobic isolates warrant susceptibility testing is frequently difficult. The NCCLS Working Group suggests that anaerobes that are recognized as virulent and/or commonly resistant to antimicrobial agents, such as the following, should be considered for testing:

- Members of the *B. fragilis* group
- Other *Bacteroides* species (including *B. gracilis*)
- *Porphyromonas* and *Prevotella* spp.
- *C. perfringens*
- *C. ramosum*
- *C. septicum*
- Certain *Fusobacterium* spp. (including *F. varium*)
- *Bilophila wadsworthia*

Antimicrobial agents to be tested
Initiation of antimicrobial therapy is usually empiric and based on the following knowledge:

- The nature and location of the infectious process. Special characteristics of specific diseases significantly affect the approach to therapy. In bacterial endocarditis, for example, a bactericidal drug must be used. The blood-brain barrier makes certain drugs unsuitable and others less effective for treating brain abscess or meningitis (clindamycin, for example, does not cross the blood-brain barrier).
- The pathogens anticipated in infectious processes of the type being treated. Aspiration pneumonia, for example, would be expected to involve mixed flora of the oral cavity. Intraabdominal infectious processes would be expected to involve mixed gastrointestinal flora. Female genitourinary infectious processes would be expected to involve mixed vaginal flora.
- Factors that might have modified the anticipated flora
- Typical susceptibility patterns of the expected flora
- Gram-stain results
- The severity of the infection

The clinical outcome in any given case will be influenced by a multitude of factors, including the speed with which antimicrobial therapy is initiated; whether the agent crosses the blood-brain barrier; the concentration of agent achieved in serum, tissues, and body cavities or spaces; the degree of protein binding that occurs; and the effect of microbial and other enzymes on the agent.

Recommendations regarding antimicrobial therapy of anaerobe-associated diseases change frequently due to the introduction of new drugs, shifting resistance patterns among anaerobes and other pathogens, and the results of local as well as large-scale, multicenter investigations. The choice of regimen depends on a number of factors, including the type of infection, whether it is community or hospital-acquired, the seriousness of the infection, whether complications exist, the general health of the patient, and last—but certainly not least—the specific organisms that are isolated and their resistance patterns.

The selection of agents to be used in susceptibility testing of anaerobes will certainly be influenced by their availability in the hospital pharmacy, and should include penicillin, clindamycin, metronidazole, imipenem, and ampicillin/sulbactam.

Problems in Susceptibility Testing of Anaerobic Isolates

There is, unfortunately, no general agreement as to a "gold standard" technique, because problems are encountered with all available methods. The problems include a lack of reproducibility, failure of some anaerobes to grow on or in particular media, difficulty in reading endpoints with certain methods, and a lack of comparability between methods. Cost and procedure complexity are other factors that inhibit laboratories from performing susceptibility testing of anaerobes. Of far greater concern, however, are the accuracy of the methods and their correlation with the in vivo or clinical situation.

Susceptibility Testing Options

A variety of methods exist for susceptibility testing of anaerobes. These methods have been described in Chapter 3 of this textbook. The agar dilution method using Brucella agar (with laked blood and vitamin K) is the reference method recommended by the NCCLS. However, the procedure is not practical for use in most clinical microbiology laboratories.

The broth dilution method, whether the macro or micro method is used, uses Brucella broth enriched with hemin, $NaHCO_3$, and vitamin K_1. Macrodilution is reported to be more dependable

than microdilution, but it is less practical due to the commercial availability of frozen or lyophilized microtiter MIC (minimal inhibitory concentration) trays for susceptibility testing of anaerobes.

Two other methods, Spiral Gradient Endpoint (SGE) and PDM Epsilometer (E test), described in Chapter 3, offer alternative methods for anaerobic susceptibility testing. Neither disk diffusion nor broth disk elution procedures are acceptable for susceptibility testing of anaerobes.

To date, none of these susceptibility testing methods has been established as fully reliable for predicting the clinical or bacteriologic outcome of a given anaerobe-associated infectious process.

Quality-Assurance Considerations Pertaining to Susceptibility Testing

An NCCLS-approved method must be used for susceptibility testing of anaerobes. Whichever procedure is selected, it must be performed exactly in accordance with NCCLS guidelines and/or the manufacturer's instructions. Appropriate quality-control (QC) organisms must be used to monitor the accuracy of the method each time it is performed. The QC organisms currently recommended by the NCCLS are as follows:

- *B. fragilis* (ATCC 25285)
- *B. thetaiotaomicron* (ATCC 29741)
- *E. lentum* (ATCC 43055)

This list of organisms is provided solely to illustrate QC standards in effect at present. Readers should use only the most recent edition of any NCCLS standards. These organisms may be obtained directly from the American Type Culture Collection or companies such as Adams Scientific (West Warwick, R.I.), Anaerobe Systems (San Jose, Calif.), and Remel (Lenexa, Kan.).

β-Lactamase Testing

β-lactamases are enzymes that destroy the β-lactam ring of penicillins (penicillinases) and cephalosporins (cephalosporinases), thus rendering these antibiotics ineffective. The first anaerobes shown to produce β-lactamases were members of the *B. fragilis* group. Those produced by *B. fragilis* are primarily cephalosporinases. It is now known that some strains of *Bacteroides, Prevotella, Fusobacterium,* and *Clostridium* produce β-lactamases as well. The ability of an anaerobe to produce β-lactamase enzymes can be determined using simple, commercially available methods (see Chapter 3).

The absence of β-lactamase does not necessarily mean that an organism will be susceptible to β-lactam antibiotics. Anaerobes can be resistant to such agents by mechanisms other than β-lactamase (e.g., by altering the number or type of penicillin-binding proteins or blocking penetration of the drug into the active site through alteration of the bacterial outer membrane pores). Anaerobes known to be resistant to β-lactam drugs by mechanisms other than production of β-lactamase include *B. gracilis, B. wadsworthia,* and some strains of *B. distasonis* and *B. fragilis.* Thus, β-lactamase testing may be used as an adjunct to susceptibility testing but never as a replacement for it. It is not necessary to test all clinically significant anaerobes for β-lactamase production.

TREATING ANAEROBE-ASSOCIATED DISEASES

Finegold states that treatment of anaerobe-associated infectious processes involves a three-pronged attack, as follows:

1. Create an environment in which anaerobes cannot proliferate. Useful measures include removing dead tissue (débridement), draining pus, eliminating obstructions, decompressing tissues, releasing trapped gas, and improving circulation in and oxygenation of tissues. In lesser infections, surgical therapy may be all that is required.
2. Arrest the spread of anaerobes into healthy tissues. Antimicrobial agents play an important role here.
3. Neutralize toxins produced by the anaerobes when such toxins are present. Specific antitoxins can be used.

Bibliography

Allen SD, Siders JA, Marler LM: Current issues and problems in dealing with anaerobes in the clinical laboratory, *Contemp Issues Clin Microbiol* 15:333, 1995.

Appelbaum PC, Spangler SK, Jacobs MR: Evaluation of two methods for rapid testing for beta-lactamase production in *Bacteroides* and *Fusobacterium, Eur J Clin Microbiol Infect Dis* 9:47, 1990.

Bartley SL: Personal communication, 1990.

Brazier JS: Appraisal of Anotox, a new anaerobic atmospheric detoxifying agent for use in anaerobic cabinets, *J Clin Pathol* 35:233, 1982.

Brook I: Recovery of anaerobic bacteria from clinical specimens in 12 years at two military hospitals, *J Clin Microbiol* 26:1181, 1998.

Citron DM et al: Short prereduced anaerobically sterilized (PRAS) biochemical scheme for identification of clinical isolates of bile-resistant *Bacteroides* species, *J Clin Microbiol* 28:2220, 1990.

Citron DM et al: Evaluation of the E test for susceptibility testing of anaerobic bacteria, *J Clin Microbiol* 29:2197, 1991.

Cox ME: Explosive potential of gas mixtures commonly used in anaerobic chambers, *Clin Infect Dis* 25(Suppl 2):S140, 1997.

Cox ME: Testing, reactivating, and cleaning palladium catalysts, *Clin Infect Dis* 25(Suppl 2):S139, 1997.

Dowell VR Jr: Personal communication, 1989.

Dowell VR Jr, Hawkins TM: *Laboratory methods in anaerobic bacteriology: CDC laboratory manual,* Atlanta, 1974, Centers for Disease Control.

Dowell VR Jr, Lombard GL: *Procedures for preliminary identification of bacteria,* Atlanta, 1984, Centers for Disease Control.

Dowell VR Jr et al: *Media for isolation, characterization, and identification of obligately anaerobic bacteria,* Atlanta, 1977, Centers for Disease Control.

Durmaz B et al: Enzymatic profiles of *Prevotella, Porphyromonas,* and *Bacteroides* species obtained with the API ZYM system and Rosco diagnostic tablets, *Clin Infect Dis* 20(Suppl 2):S192, 1995.

Engelkirk PG, Dugen-Engelkirk J, Dowell VR Jr: *Principles and practice of clinical anaerobic bacteriology,* Belmont, Calif, 1992, Star.

Finegold SM: Therapy of anaerobic infections. In Finegold SM, George WL, editors: *Anaerobic infections in humans,* San Diego, 1989, Academic Press.

Finegold SM, George WL, editors: *Anaerobic infections in humans,* San Diego, 1989, Academic Press.

Finegold SM, George WL, Mulligan ME: *Anaerobic infections,* Chicago, 1986, Year Book Medical.

Goldstein EJC, Citron DM: Annual incidence, epidemiology, and comparative in vitro susceptibilities to cefoxitin, cefotetan, cefmetazole, and ceftizoxime of recent community-acquired isolates of the *Bacteroides fragilis* group, *J Clin Microbiol* 26:2361, 1988.

Hentges DJ: Anaerobes as normal flora. In Finegold SM, George WL, editors: *Anaerobic infections in humans,* San Diego, 1989, Academic Press.

Hill G: Spiral gradient endpoint method compared to standard agar dilution for susceptibility testing of anaerobic gram-negative bacilli, *J Clin Microbiol* 29:975, 1991.

Hill GB, Schalkowsky S: Development and evaluation of the spiral gradient endpoint method for susceptibility testing of anaerobic gram-negative bacilli, *Rev Infect Dis* 12(Suppl 2):S200, 1990.

Holdeman LV, Cato EP, Moore WEC, editors: *VPI anaerobe laboratory manual,* ed 4, Blacksburg, 1977, Virginia Polytechnic Institute and State University.

Hudspeth MK et al: Growth characteristics and a novel method for identification (the Wee-Tab system) of *Porphyromonas* species isolated from infected dog and cat bite wounds in humans, *J Clin Microbiol* 35:2450, 1997.

Johnson MJ et al: Techniques for controlling variability in Gram staining of obligate anaerobes, *J Clin Microbiol* 33:755, 1995.

Krieg NR, Holt JG, editors: *Bergey's manual of systematic bacteriology,* vol 1, Baltimore, 1984, Williams & Wilkins.

LaRocco M, Robinson A: Evaluation of three commercial tests for rapid detection of beta-lactamase in anaerobic bacteria, *Eur J Clin Microbiol* 4:593, 1986.

Loesch WJ: Oxygen sensitivity of various anaerobic bacteria, *Appl Microbiol* 18:723, 1969.

Lombard GL, Dowell VR Jr: *Gas-liquid chromatography analysis of the acid products of bacteria,* Atlanta, 1982, Centers for Disease Control.

Maiden MFJ et al: Rapid characterization of periodontal bacterial isolates by using flurogenic substrate tests, *J Clin Microbiol* 34:376, 1996.

Mangels JI: Anaerobic bacteriology. In *Clinical microbiology procedures,* Washington, DC, 1992, American Society for Microbiology.

Mangels JI: Anerobic bacteriology. In *Essential procedures for clinical microbiology,* Washington, DC, 1998, American Society for Microbiology.

Mangels JI, Cox ME, Lindberg LH: Methanol fixation: an alternative to heat fixation of smears before staining, *Diagn Microbiol Infect Dis* 2:129, 1984.

Mangels JI, Douglas BP: Comparison of four commercial Brucella agar media for growth of anaerobic organisms, *J Clin Microbiol* 27:2268, 1989.

Margulis L, Sagan D: *Microcosms: four billion years of microbial evolution,* New York, 1986, Summit Books.

Murdoch DA: Gram-positive anaerobic cocci, *Clin Microbiol Rev* 11:81-120, 1998.

National Committee for Clinical Laboratory Standards: *M11-A. Methods for antimicrobial susceptibility testing of anaerobic bacteria: approved standard,* ed 3, Villanova, Penn, 1997, The Association.

Smith LDS, Williams BL: *The pathogenic anaerobic bacteria,* ed 3, Springfield, Ill, 1984, Charles C Thomas.

Sneath PHA et al, editors: *Bergey's manual of systematic bacteriology,* vol 2, Baltimore, 1986, Williams & Wilkins.

Summauen P et al: *Wadsworth anaerobic bacteriology manual,* ed 5, Belmont, Calif, 1993, Star.

Sutter VL et al: *Wadsworth anaerobic bacteriology manual,* ed 4, Belmont, Calif, 1985, Star.

LEARNING ASSESSMENT

1. What disease did the infectious disease specialist suspect? (Give two names for this disease.)

2. What genus of bacterium do you suspect is causing this disease?

3. What species do you suspect?

4. What is the clinical significance of the gram-positive cocci?

5. If this is an infectious disease, why were so few leukocytes observed on the Gram stain?

CHAPTER 20

The Spirochetes

A. Christian Whelen

LEPTOSPIRES
  General Characteristics
  Virulence Factors and Pathogenicity
  Clinical Infections
  Laboratory Diagnosis
    Cultural characteristics
    Microscopy
    Serologic tests
  Treatment and Prevention

BORRELIAE
  General Characteristics
  Borrelia recurrentis and Other Borreliae
    Clinical infections
    Laboratory diagnosis
    Treatment and prevention

Borrelia burgdorferi
  Clinical infections
  Laboratory diagnosis
  Treatment and prevention

TREPONEMES
  General Characteristics
  Clinical Infections
    Primary stage
    Secondary stage
    Tertiary stage
    Congenital syphilis
    Laboratory diagnosis
    Treatment and prevention
  Other Treponemal Diseases
    Yaws
    Pinta
    Endemic syphilis (bejel)

OBJECTIVES

1. Describe the general characteristics of the *Leptospira*.
2. List the clinical infections caused by *Leptospira* organisms.
3. Describe the diagnostic tests used to identify *Leptospira* organisms in the clinical laboratory.
4. State the general characteristics of the genus *Borrelia*.
5. Describe the etiologic agent and the arthropod vectors of relapsing fever.
6. Describe the etiologic agent and the arthropod vector of Lyme disease.
7. Describe the classic skin lesion—erythema chronicum migrans (ECM)—of Lyme disease.
8. Name the four species of the genus *Treponema* that are pathogenic in humans.
9. Describe the primary, secondary, and tertiary clinical manifestations of syphilis.
10. Describe the diagnostic tests used to identify *Treponema pallidum* in the clinical laboratory.
11. Describe the three nonvenereal treponemal diseases.

KEY TERMS

Zoonotic
Spirochetes
Periplasmic flagella
Fletcher's semisolid medium
Stuart liquid medium
Leptospirosis
Weil's disease
Kelly medium
Antigenic variation
Endemic relapsing fever
Epidemic relapsing fever
Arthropod vectors

Lyme borreliosis
Erythema chronicum migrans (ECM)
Rapid plasma reagin (RPR)
Syphilis
Chancre
Gummas
MHA-TP test
Jarisch-Herxheimer reaction
Yaws
Pinta
Bejel

CASE STUDY

A 16-year-old boy arrived at a local medical clinic in rural California complaining of fever, fatigue, and muscle aches. It was mid-September, and he had been having symptoms for about 2 weeks, except for a 4-day afebrile period. As a candidate for Eagle Scout, he had been active for most of August working with local officials to convert donated land into wildlife management areas. He reported that he had removed numerous ticks; based on some of the ticks' engorgement with blood, he assumed that some of them had escaped detection for several days. He did not notice any rash but revealed that the larger ticks (i.e., the ticks that had been attached the longest) had been discovered on his head hairline. He was concerned that his illness could interfere with one of his favorite fall activities, hunting with his father.

The order Spirochaetales contains two families, Leptospiraceae and Spirochaetaceae. The Leptospiraceae family contains the genus *Leptospira* and the Spirochaetaceae family contains *Borrelia* and *Treponema*. These three genera include the causative agents of important human diseases and **zoonotic** diseases, which are diseases that can be transmitted from animals to humans.

The **spirochetes** are slender, flexuouse, helically shaped, unicellular bacteria ranging from 0.1 to 3 μm wide and from 5 to 20 μm long, with one or more complete turns in the helix. They differ from other bacteria in that they have a flexible cell wall around which several fibrils are wound. These fibrils, termed the ***periplasmic flagella*** (also known as the *axial fibrils, axial filaments, endoflagella,* and *periplasmic fibrils*), are responsible for motility. A multilayered outer sheath similar to the outer membrane of other gram-negative bacteria completely surrounds the protoplasmic cylinder (the cytoplasmic and nuclear regions enclosed by the cytoplasmic membrane–cell wall complex and periplasmic flagella).

The spirochetes exhibit various types of motion in liquid media. They are free living, or survive in association with animal and human hosts as normal flora or pathogens. In addition, they are chemoheterotrophic and can utilize carbohydrates, amino acids, long-chain fatty acids, or long-chain fatty alcohols as carbon and energy sources. Metabolism can be anaerobic, facultatively anaerobic, or aerobic depending on the species. They are gram-negative and reproduce via transverse fission.

LEPTOSPIRES

General Characteristics

Organisms of the genus *Leptospira* are tightly coiled, thin, flexible spirochetes, 0.1 μm wide and 5 to 15 μm long (Figure 20-1). In contrast to both *Treponema* and *Borrelia* organisms, the spirals are very close together, so the organism may be seen as a chain of cocci via microscope. One or both ends of the organism have hooks rather than tapering off. Their motion is rotational. Two species, *Leptospira interrogans* and *Leptospira biflexa,* are recognized as pathogenic and saprophytic leptospiras, respectively. Leptospires are obligately aerobic and can be grown in artificial media such as **Fletcher's semisolid** and **Stuart liquid media.**

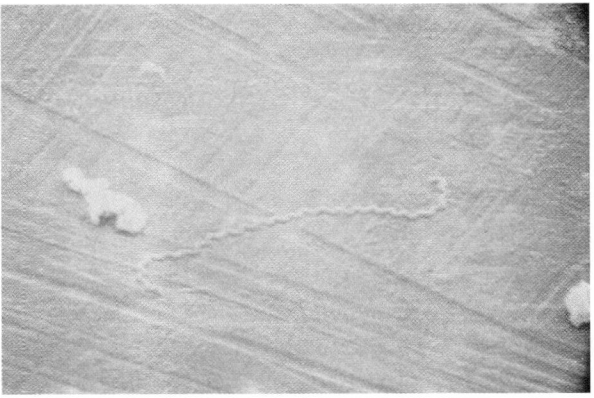

Figure 20-1 _____

Scanning electron micrograph of *Leptospira interrogans* isolated from blood of a patient. The tight coils and bent ends are characteristic of this organism (×2500).

Like the treponemes and borreliae, under electron microscopy leptospires reveal a long axial filament covered by a very fine sheath. All species have two periplasmic flagella. The organisms cannot be stained readily, but they can be impregnated with silver and visualized. Unstained cells are not visible by brightfield microscopy but are visible by darkfield, phase-contrast, and immunofluorescent microscopy.

Virulence Factors and Pathogenicity

Based on the antigenic composition, *L. interrogans* can be divided into multiple serogroups and serovars (serotypes). More than 200 different serovars have been determined; leptospiral disease in the United States is caused by more than 20 different serovars, the most common of which are *Leptospira icterohaemorrhagiae* and *Leptospira canicola.*

The various serogroups of *L. interrogans* are parasitic or pathogenic for a wide range of wild and domestic animals and humans, but the mechanism of pathogenicity is not known. Factors that may play a role in pathogenicity include reduced phagocytosis in the host, a soluble hemolysin produced by some virulent strains, cell-mediated sensitivity to leptospiral antigen by the host, and small amounts of endotoxins produced by some strains. With regard to the endotoxin, the clinical findings in animals with leptospirosis suggest the presence of endotoxemia.

Clinical Infections

Leptospirosis is a zoonotic disease in humans and is primarily associated with occupational exposure. Work with animals or in rat-infested surroundings poses hazards for veterinarians, dairy workers, swineherds, slaughterhouse workers, miners, sewer workers, fish and poultry processors, and so on. In the United States the majority of leptospirosis cases result from recreational exposures and occur most commonly in the summer. In 1992, 54 cases of leptospirosis were reported in the United States; however, many cases may go unrecognized and unreported.

In the natural host, leptospires live in the lumen of renal tubules and are excreted in the urine. Dogs, rats, and other rodents are the principal animal reservoirs of leptospires. Hosts acquire infections directly by contact with the urine of carriers or indirectly by contact with bodies of water contaminated with the urine of carriers. Leptospires can survive in neutral or slightly alkaline waters for months.

Leptospires are most likely to enter the human host through small breaks in the skin or intact mucosa. The initial sites of multiplication are unknown. Nonspecific host defenses do not stop multiplication of leptospires, and leptospiremia occurs during the acute illness. Late manifestations of the disease may be caused by the host's immunologic response to the infection.

The incubation period of leptospirosis is usually 10 to 12 days but ranges from 3 to 30 days after inoculation. The onset of clinical illness is usually abrupt, with nonspecific, influenza-like constitutional symptoms such as fever, chills, headache, severe myalgia, and malaise. The subsequent course is protean, is frequently biphasic, and often results in hepatic, renal, and central nervous system involvement. The major renal lesion is an interstitial nephritis with associated glomerular swelling and hyperplasia that does not affect the glomerulus. The most characteristic physical finding is conjunctival suffusion, but this is seen in less than half of the patients. Severe systemic disease **(Weil's disease)** includes renal failure, hepatic failure, and intravascular disease and may result in death. Duration of the illness varies from less than 1 week to 3 weeks. Late manifestations may be caused by the host immunologic response to the infection.

In patients with a leptospiral bacteremia, immunoglobulin M (IgM) antibodies are detected within a week after onset of disease and may persist in high titers for many months. A month or more after the onset of illness, immunoglobulin G (IgG) antibodies can be detected in some patients. Convalescent serum contains protective antibodies.

Laboratory Diagnosis
Cultural characteristics
Leptospires can be easily cultured from the blood or cerebrospinal fluid (CSF) during the acute phase of the disease. After the first week, the spirochetes may be shed intermittently in the urine, which can also be cultured. Isolation of leptospires is accomplished by direct inoculation of laboratory media.

Microscopy
Although direct demonstration of leptospires in clinical specimens during the first week of the disease by special stains, darkfield, or phase-contrast microscopy is possible, it is not recommended. Direct demonstration is only successful in a small percentage of cases, and false-positive results may be reported because of the presence of artifacts, especially in urine.

Serologic tests
A macroscopic slide agglutination test for rapid screening as well as a more sensitive microscopic agglutination test are available for detection of leptospiral antibodies. These tests are not used frequently because they require the maintenance of appropriate living organisms.

Treatment and Prevention
Leptospires are susceptible to streptomycin, tetracycline, doxycycline, and the macrolide antibiotics in vitro. Although treatment data are too sparse to be definitive, penicillin is considered beneficial and alters the course of the disease if treatment is initiated before the fourth day of illness, after which time penicillin may not alter the course of the disease. Doxycycline appears to shorten the course of the illness in adults and reduce the incidence of convalescent leptospiruria.

Protective clothing (boots and gloves) should be worn in situations involving possible occupational exposure to leptospires; rodent control is also indicated. Drainage of waters known to be contaminated also helps reduce the risk of exposure. Short-term prophylaxis may be accomplished by weekly administration of doxycycline to high-risk groups with short-term occupational exposure.

Vaccination of dogs and livestock prevents the development disease but not the initial infection and leptospiruria. For humans in endemic areas, vaccines have been effectively used in the practice of veterinary medicine.

BORRELIAE

General Characteristics
The genus *Borrelia* comprises several species of spirochetes that are morphologically similar but have different pathogenic properties and host ranges. Most species cause relapsing fever; however, another species, *Borrelia burgdorferi,* is the etiologic agent of Lyme disease. All borreliae are arthropod borne.

The borreliae are gram-negative, highly flexible organisms varying in thickness from 0.2 to 0.5 μm and in length from 3 to 20 μm. The spirals vary in number from three to ten per organism and are much less tightly coiled than those of the leptospires (Figure 20-2). Unlike the leptospires and treponemes, the borreliae stain easily and can be examined under the regular light microscope. Electron-microscopic pictures show the same general patterns as are seen with the treponemes—long periplasmic flagella coated with sheaths of protoplasm and periplasm. From 15 to 20 periplasmic flagella per cell are seen. The borreliae multiply by binary fission.

The borreliae are typically cultivated in the clinical laboratory using **Kelly medium.**

Borrelia recurrentis and Other Borreliae

Borrelia recurrentis causes relapsing fever. As the name suggests, the acute infection causes febrile episodes that subside spontaneously and tend to recur over a period of weeks. The relapses are caused by **antigenic variation;** borreliae systematically change their surface antigens while they are in the host during the course of a single infection.

Borreliae causing relapsing fever can be either tick borne **(endemic relapsing fever)** or louse borne **(epidemic relapsing fever).** The tick-borne borreliae are transmitted by a large variety of soft-shelled ticks of the genus *Ornithodoros.* Species-specific borreliae often bear the same epithet as their vectors (e.g., *Ornithodoros hermsi* transmits *Borrelia hermsi*). These borreliae are widely distributed throughout the eastern and western hemispheres, and transmission to a vertebrate host takes place via infected saliva during tick attachment.

The louse-borne fever, or epidemic relapsing fever, is transmitted via the body louse, *Pediculus humanus humanus,* and humans are the only reservoir. The borreliae infect the hemolymph of the louse. Unlike tick-borne disease, transmission of the louse-borne disease occurs when infected lice are crushed and scratched into the skin rather than through the bite of an infected arthropod.

Clinical infections

After an incubation period of 2 to 15 days, infection by borreliae causes massive spirochetemia, which remains at varying levels of severity during the entire course of borreliosis. The infection is accompanied by sudden high fever, rigors, severe headache, muscle pains, and weakness. The febrile period lasts about 3 to 7 days and ends abruptly with the development of an adequate immune response. The disease recurs several days to weeks later, following a less severe but similar course. The spirochetemia worsens during the febrile periods and wanes between recurrences. Tick-transmitted *B. recurrentis* has a shorter primary febrile attack and afebrile episode than the louse-borne infection, as well as longer, more numerous relapses.

Laboratory diagnosis

MICROSCOPY

During the febrile period, diagnosis of borreliosis is readily made by Giemsa or Wright staining of blood smears. Borreliosis is the only spirochetal disease in which the organisms are visible in blood with brightfield microscopy. The appearance of the spirochete among the red cells is characteristic (see Figure 20-2).

CULTURAL CHARACTERISTICS

Borreliae can be recovered using Kelly medium or animal inoculation (involving suckling Swiss mice or suckling rats). *B. recurrentis, Borrelia hermsi, Borrelia parkeri, Borrelia turicatae,* and *Borrelia hispanica* have been successfully cultivated. Antigenic variation in the spirochetes that cause re-

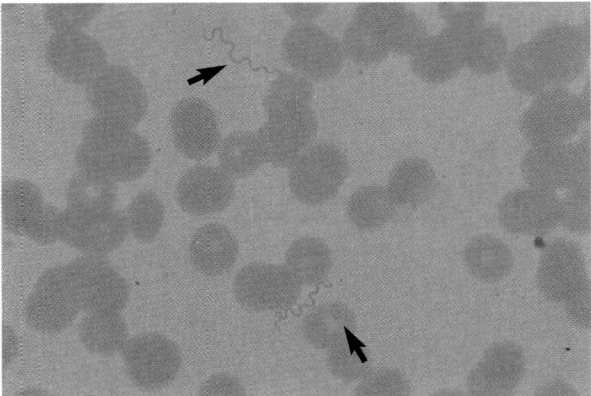

Figure 20-2 _____

Appearance of *Borrelia recurrentis* in blood. Giemsa stain (×850).

lapsing fever makes the serodiagnosis of their diseases difficult and impractical.

Treatment and prevention

Borreliae are susceptible to many antibiotics; however, tetracyclines are the drugs of choice because they reduce the relapse rate and rid the central nervous system of spirochetes.

Relapsing fever is best prevented by control of exposure to the **arthropod vectors.** For tick-borne relapsing fever, exposure control includes wearing protective clothing, rodent control, and the use of repellents. For louse-borne relapsing fever, control is best achieved by the application of good personal and public hygiene, especially improvements in overcrowding and delousing.

Borrelia burgdorferi

B. burgdorferi is the agent of Lyme disease (Lyme borreliosis), which was first described after an outbreak among children in Lyme, Connecticut, in 1975. *B. burgdorferi* is transmitted via *Ixodes* ticks. The majority of cases occur during June through September, when more people are involved in outdoor activities. The disease affects people of all ages and both sexes.

Clinical infections

Lyme borreliosis is characterized in its early stages by symptoms of fever, headache, generalized muscle pain, and perhaps fatigue and weight loss. About 60% of patients exhibit **erythema chronicum migrans (ECM),** the classic skin lesion that is normally found at the site of the tick bite. It begins as a red macule and expands to form a large annular erythema with partial central clearing. Late manifestations of the disease involve the joints and the cardiac and neurologic systems. Arthritis is the most common manifestation, occurring weeks to years later.

Laboratory diagnosis

Early diagnosis and antibiotic treatment are important for preventing neurologic, cardiac, and joint abnormalities that can occur late in the disease. Culture of *B. burgdorferi* from skin biopsies (ECM margin) or joint fluid (in patients with arthritis) permits definitive diagnosis, but it lacks sensitivity. Direct examination of blood or skin specimens are rarely productive.

Diagnosis is typically supported serologically, either by Indirect Fluorescent Antibody (IFA) or Enzyme Immunoassy (EIA). EIA is often used because of its superior sensitivity, specificity, and ease of use. False-positive results are unusual with current kits, especially when initial results are confirmed with a Western blot for specific *B. burgdorferi* antigens; however, a *T. pallidum* infection could produce a false-positive result. Consequently, a nontreponemal test (such as **rapid plasma reagin [RPR]**) for syphilis should be performed on positive sera to exclude the factor of cross reactivity. Serology can also be used to detect antibodies in the CSF, which is indicative of neuroborreliosis.

The IgM antibody response to *B. burgdorferi* begins during the first 10 days after infection but does not peak until 3 to 6 weeks after the onset of the disease. Peak levels of IgG antibodies are not observed until after 4 to 6 months after the illness onset, and they typically persist in untreated patients with late manifestations of Lyme borreliosis. Western blot confirmation of IgM antibody presence includes reactivity for two of the three of the following bands: 24, 39, 41 and kD_2. Confirmation of IgG antibody presence is acceptable when five of the following bands are present: 18, 21, 28, 30, 39, 41, 45, 58, 66, and 93 kD_2.

Treatment and prevention

Doxycycline and amoxicillin are equally effective in treating early stages of Lyme borreliosis without complications. For refractile or late stages, prolonged treatment with ceftriaxone has been effective. Protective clothing and repellents should be worn in areas in which tick exposure is intense. Attached ticks should be removed immediately because pathogen transmission is likely associated with the length of attachment.

TREPONEMES

The genus *Treponema* comprises four species that are pathogenic for humans: *T. pallidum* ssp. *pallidum,* the causative agent for **syphilis;** *T. pallidum* ssp. *pertenue,* the causative agent of yaws; *Treponema carateum,* the causative agent of pinta; and *T. pallidum* ssp. *endemicum,* the causative agent of endemic syphilis. At least six nonpathogenic organisms have been identified in the normal flora, and they are particularly prominent in the oral cavity.

General Characteristics

T. pallidum treponemes are fine, spiral organisms that are about 0.1 to 0.2 μm in thickness and 6 to 20 μm in length. They are difficult to visualize with a light microscope because they are so thin, but they can be seen very easily using darkfield microscopy. The spirals are regular and angular with 4 to 14 spirals per organism (Figure 20-3). Three periplasmic flagella are inserted into each end of the cell. The ends are pointed and covered with a sheath. The cells are motile, with graceful flexuouse movements in liquid.

Clinical Infections

T. pallidum ssp. *pallidum* causes syphilis. This organism is an exclusively human pathogen under natural conditions. Syphilis was first recognized in Europe at the end of the fifteenth century, when it reached epidemic proportions. Two theories have been proposed concerning its introduction to Europe. The first theory suggests that Christopher Columbus's crew brought the disease from the West Indies back to Europe. The second theory suggests that the disease was endemic in Africa and transported to Europe via the migration of armies and civilians. The venereal transmission of

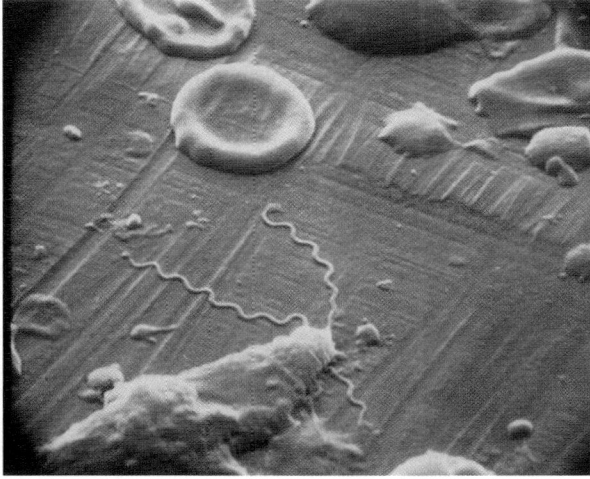

Figure 20-3
Scanning electron micrograph of *Treponema pallidum* (Nichols stain). Two treponemes are shown adjacent to an erythrocyte (×2500).

syphilis was not recognized until the eighteenth century.

The causative agent for syphilis was not discovered until 1905. The word *syphilis* comes from a poem written in 1530 that described a mythical shepherd named Syphilus who was afflicted with the disease as punishment for cursing the gods. The poem represented the compendium of knowledge at the time regarding the disease.

Syphilis is acquired by direct sexual contact with an individual who has an active primary or secondary syphilitic lesion. Consequently, the genital organs—the vagina and cervix in females, and the penis in males—are the usual sites of inoculation. Syphilis can also be acquired by nongenital contact with a lesion (e.g., on the lip) or transplacental transmission to a fetus, resulting in congenital syphilis. After bacterial invasion through a break in the epidermis or penetration through intact mucous membranes, the natural course of syphilis can be broken down into primary, secondary, and tertiary stages based on the clinical manifestations.

Primary stage

After inoculation the spirochetes multiply rapidly and disseminate to local lymph nodes and other organs via the blood stream. The primary lesion develops 10 to 90 days after infection and is a result of an inflammatory response to the infection at the site of the inoculation. The lesion, known as the *chancre,* is typically a single erythematous lesion that is not tender but is firm with a clean surface and raised border. The lesion is teeming with treponemes and is extremely infectious. It may not be apparent in females because it is commonly found on the cervix or vaginal wall. The lesion can also be found in the anal canal of either sex and remain undetected. No systemic signs or symptoms are evident in the primary stages of the disease.

Secondary stage

Approximately 2 to 12 weeks after development of the primary lesion, the patient may experience secondary disease, with clinical symptoms of fever, sore throat, generalized lymphadenopathy, headache, and rash. (The rash is unusual in that it can also occur on the palms and soles.) All secondary lesions of the skin and mucous membranes are highly infectious. The secondary stage may last for several weeks and may relapse. It may also be mild and go unnoticed by the patient.

Tertiary stage

After the secondary stage the disease does not progress in about 25% of cases. Another 25% the disease becomes latent and produces no further clinical symptoms, whereas the remaining 50% of untreated cases develop tertiary symptoms some 2 to 20 years later. These symptoms include the development of granulomatous lesions **(gummas)** in skin, bones, and liver (benign tertiary syphilis); degenerative changes in the central nervous system (neurosyphilis); and syphilitic cardiovascular lesions, particularly aortitis and aortic valve insufficiency. Patients in the tertiary stage are usually not infectious. In the United States the tertiary stage of disease is not often seen because most patients are adequately treated with antibiotics before the tertiary stage is reached.

Congenital syphilis

Treponemes can cross the placenta and be transmitted from an infected mother to her fetus. Congenital syphilis affects many body systems and is therefore very severe and mutilating. All pregnant women should have serologic examinations for syphilis early in pregnancy.

Laboratory diagnosis

DARKFIELD MICROSCOPIC EXAMINATION

Darkfield microscopy is a key aid in the detection of *T. pallidum* in primary and secondary lesions; the treponemes are illuminated against a dark background. In primary syphilis, demonstration of motile treponemes in material from the chancre is diagnostic. However, the darkfield microscopic examination requires considerable skill and experience. The test can be misinterpreted, especially during the examination of specimens from oral lesions, in which nonpathogenic spirochetes are numerous. Furthermore, the lesion material must be examined at the time of collection. If darkfield microscopy is not available, it is best to pursue a serologic-based diagnosis.

SEROLOGIC TESTS

Serology is the dominant tool used for laboratory diagnosis of syphilis. Two major types of serologic tests exist: nontreponemal tests and treponemal

tests. Both have lower sensitivities in the primary stage but have sensitivities of nearly 100% in secondary stages of syphilis. The treponemal tests retain a very high sensitivity in the tertiary stage as well.

Nontreponemal tests The nontreponemal tests detect reaginic antibodies that develop against lipids released from damaged cells. Although they are biologically nonspecific and known to react with organisms of other diseases and conditions (causing false-positive reactions), the nontreponemal tests are excellent screening tests. The antigen employed is a cardiolipin-lecithin complex made from beef hearts.

The two nontreponemal tests widely used today are the Venereal Disease Research Laboratory (VDRL) and RPR tests. These tests are inexpensive to perform, demonstrate rising and falling reagin titers, and correlate with the clinical status of the patient. The VDRL test uses a cardiolipin antigen that is mixed with the patient's serum or CSF. Flocculation occurs in a positive reaction and is observed microscopically. RPR is the most common test used. It is read macroscopically and employs carbon particles as its reaction indicator. The black carbon particles are bound to cardiolipin; when mixed with a positive sera on a disposable card, the particles clump together. Co-agglutination is easily observed without a microscope. Reactive (or weakly reactive) sera should undergo titration and be tested with treponemal tests.

Treponemal tests The treponemal tests detect antibodies specific for treponemal antigens. They are helpful in the detection of late-stage infections and the confirmation of positive nontreponemal test results. Treponemal test titers remain high and usually do not drop in response to therapy as the nontreponemal test results do. Thus they are not useful in following therapy or detecting reinfection. The antigens used are spirochetes derived from rabbit testicular lesions. The two most commonly used treponemal tests are the fluorescent treponemal antibody absorption (FTA-ABS) test and the microhemagglutination test for *T. pallidum* antibody (MHA-TP).

In the FTA-ABS test the patient's serum is absorbed with extracts of a cultivated treponeme that is not *T. pallidum* to remove any nonspecific treponemal antibody. Then the absorbed serum is placed on a slide that has *T. pallidum* organisms affixed to it. After any specific antibody is allowed to react with the organisms, nonbound constituents in the serum are removed by washing. The presence of anti-*T. pallidum* antibody is then detected by application of a fluorescein-labeled anti-human globulin serum and examination of the slide with an ultraviolet (UV) microscope. Positive results are indicated by bright fluorescence of the *T. pallidum* organisms. An FTA-ABS 19S-IgM test has also been developed for evaluation of congenital syphilis, however the test is still considered provisional.

The **MHA-TP test** is an indirect hemagglutination test using *T. pallidum* antigens absorbed to tanned erythrocytes. It is simpler to perform than the FTA-ABS test, does not require an expensive UV microscope, and is slightly less sensitive but slightly more specific than the FTA-ABS test.

Treatment and prevention

Penicillin is the drug of choice for treating patients with syphilis. It is the only proven therapy that has been widely used for patients with neurosyphilis, congenital syphilis, and syphilis during pregnancy. *T. pallidum* is extremely sensitive to penicillin, with a minimal inhibitory concentration of approximately 0.004 U/ml of penicillin. Resistant strains have not developed. Successful therapy requires that penicillin levels (0.03 U/mL) be maintained for 7 to 10 days. Long-acting penicillin such as benzathine penicillin is preferred. Dosages vary according to the stage of disease. Alternative regimens for patients who are allergic to penicillin and not pregnant include doxycycline and tetracycline. A typical **Jarisch-Herxheimer reaction** may occur within hours following treatment and is probably caused by the sudden release of endotoxin from the spirochetes.

For a discussion on interpretation of serologic tests for syphilis and the recommendations for appropriate therapy, please refer to the *Sexually Transmitted Diseases Treatment Guidelines* published by the Centers for Disease Control (see bibliography).

Educating people about sexually transmitted diseases, identifying and treating all sexual contacts of persons infected with syphilis, and reporting each case of syphilis to the health authorities for contact investigation help control the spread of syphilis. In addition, pregnant females should have serologic examinations early and late in the pregnancy. Serologic screening of high-risk populations should also be performed.

Other forms of prevention include the proper use of barrier contraceptives such as condoms.

Other Treponemal Diseases

Three nonvenereal treponemal diseases occur in different geographic locations. These treponematoses are found in developing countries where hygiene is poor, little clothing is worn, and direct skin contact is common because of overcrowding. All three diseases have primary and secondary stages, but tertiary manifestations are uncommon. All diseases respond well to penicillin or tetracycline. These infections are rarely transmitted by sexual contact, and congenital infections do not occur. The three nonvenereal treponemal diseases are the following:

- **Yaws**
- **Pinta**
- Endemic syphilis, or **bejel**

Yaws

Yaws is a spirochetal disease caused by *T. pallidum* ssp. *pertenue*. It is endemic in the humid, tropical belt—the tropical regions of Africa; parts of South America, India, and Indonesia; and many of the Pacific Islands. It is not seen in the United States. The course of yaws resembles that of syphilis but the early-stage lesions are elevated, granulomatous nodules.

Pinta

Pinta, which is caused by *T. carateum,* is found in the tropical regions of Central and South America. It is acquired by person-to-person contact and is rarely transmitted by sexual intercourse. Lesions begin as scaling, painless papules and are followed by an erythematous rash that becomes hypopigmented with time.

Endemic syphilis (bejel)

Bejel is caused by *T. pallidum* ssp. *endemicum* and closely resembles yaws in clinical manifestations. It is found in the Middle East and the arid, hot areas of the world. The primary and secondary lesions are usually papules that often go unnoticed. They can progress to gummas of the skin, bones, and nasopharynx. Darkfield microscopy is not useful because of normal oral spirochetal flora. Poor hygienic conditions are important in perpetuating these infections. Bejel is transmitted by direct contact or sharing contaminated eating utensils.

Bibliography

Brandao AP et al: Macroscopic agglutination test for rapid diagnosis of human leptospirosis, *J Clin Microbiol* 36:3138, 1998.

Centers for Disease Control and Prevention: Recommendations for test performance and interpretation from the Second National Conference on Serologic Diagnosis of Lyme Disease, *MMWR* 44:590, 1995.

Centers for Disease Control and Prevention: 1993 Sexually transmitted diseases treatment guidelines, *MMWR* 42:01, 1993.

Craven RB et al: Improved serodiagnostic testing for Lyme disease: results of a multicenter serologic evaluation, *Emer Infect Dis* 2:136-40, 1996.

Fister RD et al: Comparative evaluation of three products for the detection of *Borrelia burgdorferi* antibody in human serum, *J Clin Microbiol* 27:2843, 1989.

Gussenhoven GC et al: LEPTO dipstick: a dipstick assay for detection of *Leptospira*-specific immunoglobin M antibodies in human sera, *J Clin Microbiol* 35:92, 1997.

Hoffmann H: Lyme Borreliosis—problems of serological diagnosis, *Infection* 24:470, 1996.

Holmes KK, Mårdh P-A, editors: *Sexually transmitted diseases,* ed 2, New York, 1984, McGraw-Hill.

Jaffe HW: The laboratory diagnosis of syphilis, new concepts. *Ann Intern Med* 83:846; 1975.

Joklik WK et al, editors: The spirochetes. In *Zinsser microbiology,* ed 20, Norwalk, Conn, 1992, Appleton & Lange.

Krieg NR, Holt JG, editors: The spirochetes. In *Bergey's manual of systematic bacteriology,* Baltimore, 1984, Williams & Wilkins.

Larsen SA et al, editors: *A manual of tests for syphilis,* Washington, DC, 1990, APHA.

Larsen SA et al: Laboratory diagnosis and interpretation of tests for syphilis, *Clin Microbiol Rev* 8:1, 1995.

Lukehart SA et al: Invasion of the central nervous system by *Treponema pallidum:* implications for diagnosis and treatment, *Ann Intern Med* 109:855, 1988.

Murray PR et al, editors: *Manual of clinical microbiology,* ed 6, Washington, DC, 1995, American Society for Microbiology.

Musher DN: How much penicillin cures syphilis? *Ann Intern Med* 109:849, 1988.

Nadelman RB, Wormser GP: Lyme borreliosis, *Lancet* 352:557, 1998.

Public Health Service: *Syphilis: a synopsis,* PHS publication No. 1660, Washington, DC, 1968, U.S. Government Printing Office.

Rawlings JA: An overview of tick-borne relapsing fever with emphasis on outbreaks in Texas, *Texas Med* 91:56, 1995.

Romanowski B et al: Serologic response to treatment of infectious syphilis, *Ann Intern Med* 114:1005, 1991.

Shapiro ED: Lyme disease, *Ped Rev* 19:147, 1998.

Sigal LH et al: A vaccine consisting of recombinant *Borrelia burgdorgeri* outer-surface protein A to prevent Lyme disease, *New Engl J Med* 339:216, 1998.

Spach D et al: Tick-borne diseases in the United States, *N Engl J Med* 329:936, 1993.

Steer AC: Diagnosis and treatment of Lyme arthritis, *Med Clin North Am* 81:179, 1997.

Steere AC et al: The early clinical manifestations of Lyme disease. *Ann Intern Med* 99:76, 1983.

Steere AC et al: Treatment of the early manifestions of Lyme disease. *Ann Intern Med* 99:22, 1983.

Sung L, MacDonald NE: Syphilis: a pediatric perspective, *Ped Rev* 19:17, 1998.

Winslow WE et al: Evaluation of a commercial enzyme-linked immunosorbent assay for detection of immunoglobin M antibody in diagnosis of human leptospiral infection, *J Clin Microbiol* 35:1938, 1997.

Woods GL: Update on laboratory diagnosis of sexually transmitted diseases, *Gyn Pathol* 15:665, 1995.

LEARNING ASSESSMENT

1. What risk factors are suggestive of *Borrelia* sp. relapsing fever infection?

2. Which tick-borne species of *Borrelia* is associated with a skin rash or lesion?

3. What is the significance of finding partially engorged ticks?

4. What is the test of choice for the laboratory diagnosis of borreliosis?

CHAPTER 21

Chlamydia, Mycoplasma, and Ureaplasma Species

A. *CHLAMYDIA* SPECIES

John G. Thomas, Karen S. Long

GENERAL CHARACTERISTICS

CHLAMYDIA PNEUMONIAE
  Clinical Infections
  Laboratory Diagnosis

CHLAMYDIA TRACHOMATIS
  Clinical Infections
    Trachoma
    Lymphogranuloma venereum
    Other sexually transmitted diseases
    Chlamydia in the newborn

Laboratory Diagnosis
  Direct microscopic examination
Culture
  Cell culture
Nonculture, Nonamplified
  Enzyme immunoassay
Nonculture, Amplified
  Nucleic acid probes/amplification
  Antibody detection
Results Reporting

CHLAMYDIA PSITTACI

OBJECTIVES

1. List the members of the family Chlamydiaceae.
2. Discuss the unique growth cycle of *Chlamydia,* describing elementary (EB) and reticulate (RB) bodies.
3. Describe *Chlamydia* by distinguishing the genus from rickettsiae, viruses, and bacteria.
4. List the major diseases associated with each of the three species of *Chlamydia.*
5. Describe the modes of transmission for each species of the genus.
6. Define the appropriate cultures for detection of the species *Chlamydia trachomatis.*
7. List in descending order (from most important to least important) the appropriate assays for antigen detection, including direct fluorescence, EIA, nucleic acid probe, and PCR for *C. trachomatis.*
8. Discuss the general types of therapy used in the management of chlamydial infections, emphasizing the obligate intracellular parasitic relationship of Chlamydiaceae.
9. Discuss serologic investigations as well as the limitations of complement fixation (CF) and microimmunofluorescence (MIF) and the corresponding rise and fall of these markers in disease.
10. Discuss the problems with serologic cross-reactivity among the three species.

KEY TERMS

TWAR *(Chlamydia pneumoniae)*
Elementary body (EB)
Reticulate body (RB)
Major outer membrane protein (MOMP)

Lymphogranuloma venereum (LGV)
Pelvic inflammatory disease (PID)
Trachoma

CASE STUDY

A 7-day-old newborn was brought by his grandmother to the emergency department of a large city hospital. He had been discharged 3 days after birth, with last nursing note suggesting "fussy." On admission he had a fever of 39° C, loss of appetite, a profuse yellow discharge from the right eye, and general "irritability." Past medical history revealed the mother to be a 17-year-old intravenous drug abuser with no prenatal care, who had a vaginal delivery in the parking lot of a local hospital. The eye discharge was cultured for a variety of organisms and was diagnostic.

Previously unclassified organisms that shared selected characteristics with rickettsieae, bacteria, viruses, and mycoplasma, (Table 21-1) members of the genus *Chlamydia* are recognized today as being unique and therefore are classified into their own order (Chlamydiales) and family (Chlamydiaceae). This section describes the unique growth cycle of *Chlamydia* and the human diseases caused by *Chlamydia.*

There are three species in the genus *Chlamydia: Chlamydia trachomatis, Chlamydia psittaci,* and the newest member, *Chlamydia pneumoniae. C. pneumoniae* was previously referred to as *C. trachomatis,* strain **TWAR.** As shown in Table 21-2, initial differentiation of the *Chlamydia* species was based on selected characteristics of the growth cycle, susceptibility to sulfa drugs, and DNA relatedness. Table 21-2 also shows additional properties of the *Chlamydia* species have helped further differentiate the three species on the basis of natural host, major diseases, and number of antigenic variants, such as serovars.

GENERAL CHARACTERISTICS

Chlamydiae have a unique growth cycle because they are deficient in independent energy metab-

TABLE 21-1

Comparative Properties of Microorganisms

Characteristic	Organisms				
	Chlamydiae	*Viruses*	Bacteria	*Rickettsiae*	*Mycoplasmas*
DNA and RNA	+	−	+	+	+
Obligate intracellular parasites	+	+	−	−	−
Peptidoglycan in cell wall	+	−	+	−	−
Growth on nonliving medium	−	−	+	−	+
Contain ribosomes	+	−	+	+	+
Sensitivity to					
Antibiotics	+	−	+	+	+
Interferon	+	+	−	−	−
Binary fission (replication)	+	−	+	+	+

olism and are therefore obligate intracellular parasites. Replication involves two distinct forms of the organism: an **elementary body (EB),** which is infectious; and a **reticulate body (RB),** also called *initial body,* which is noninfectious. The life cycle (Figure 21-1) begins when the small EB infects the host cell by inducing energy-requiring active phagocytosis. In vivo, host cells are primarily the nonciliated, columnar, or transitional epithelial cells that line the conjunctiva, respiratory tract, urogenital tract, and rectum. During the next 8 hours, they organize into larger, reticulating initial bodies, which then divert the cells' synthesizing functions to their own metabolic needs and begin to multiply by binary fission (Figure 21-2). About 24 hours after infection, the dividing organisms begin reorganizing into infective EBs. At

about 30 hours, multiplication ceases, and by 35 to 40 hours, the disrupted host cell dies, releasing new EBs (Figure 21-3) that can infect other host cells, and the cycle continues.

The EB has an outer membrane similar to that of many gram-negative organisms. The most prominent component of this membrane is the **major outer membrane protein (MOMP).** The MOMP is a transmembrane protein that contains both species-specific and subspecies-specific epitopes that can be defined by monoclonal antibodies.

The chlamydial outer membrane also contains a large lipopolysaccharide (LPS). This extractable LPS (with ketodeoxyoctonate [KDO]) is shared by all members of the genus and is the primary antigen detectable in genus-specific tests and serologic assays for *Chlamydia.*

TABLE 21-2

Initial Differentiation of Chlamydia *species (1988)*

Properties	Species		
	C. trachomatis	*C. psittaci*	*C. pneumoniae*
Inclusion morphology	Round, vacuolar	Variable shape, dense	Round, dense
Glycogen in inclusions	+	−	−
Elementary body morphology	Round	Round	Pear-shaped
Sulfa drug sensitivity	+	−	−
DNA relatedness (against *C. pneumoniae*)	10%	10%	100%
Natural hosts	Humans	Birds	Humans
		Lower animals	
Major human diseases	Sexually transmitted diseases, trachoma	Pneumonia	Pneumonia
	Lymphogranuloma venereum	FUO	Pharyngitis
			Bronchitis
Number of serovars	15	10	1

FUO, Fever of unknown origin.

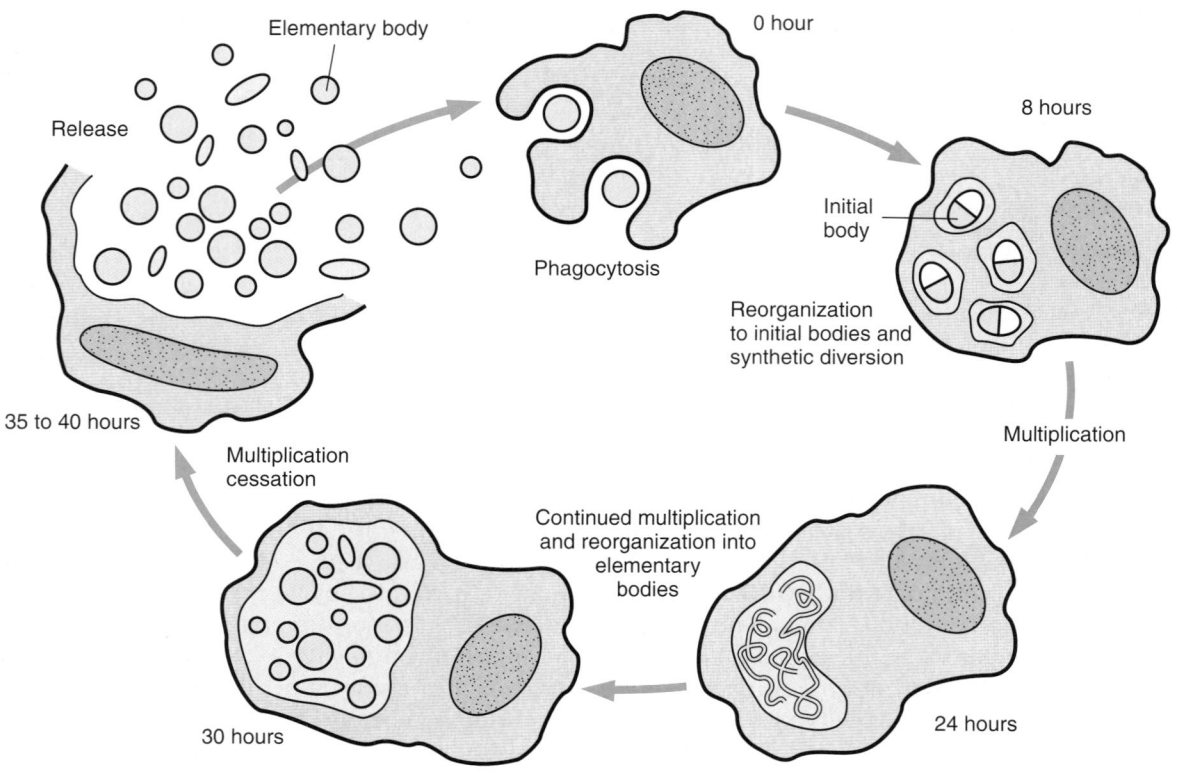

Figure 21-1

Life cycle of *Chlamydia* organisms.

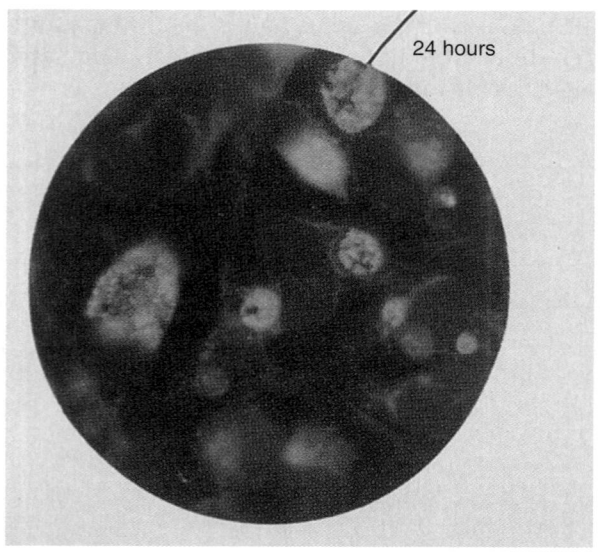

Figure 21-2

Chlamydia spp. growth cycle highlighting reticulate bodies (RBs), sometimes referred to as *initial bodies*. (Courtesy Syva-Microtrak, Palo Alto, Calif.)

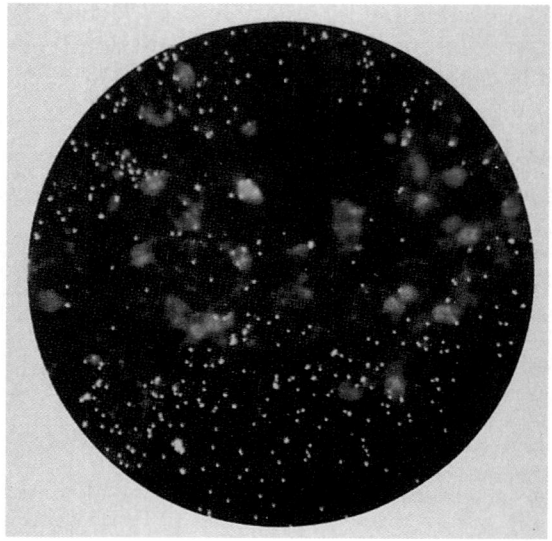

Figure 21-3

Elementary bodies (EBs) and cells in *Chlamydia trachomatis*–positive direct specimen. (Courtesy Syva Microtrak, Palo Alto, Calif.)

CHLAMYDIA PNEUMONIAE

C. pneumoniae is the most recently recognized species of *Chlamydia*. It was formerly known as *Chlamydia* species, strain TWAR. As shown in Table 21-3, TWAR was originally identified in 1965 from a conjunctival culture of a child (TW) enrolled in a Taiwan trachoma vaccine study. In 1983 at the University of Washington, a similar organism was isolated in HeLa cells from a pharyngeal specimen of a college student (AR). Today, *C. pneumoniae* is recognized as an important respiratory pathogen. It is known to be the cause of acute respiratory disease, pneumonia, and pharyngitis (Table 21-4). It also has been isolated from patients with otitis media, effusion, pneumonia with pleural effusion, and aseptic pharyngitis. Most recently, it has been implicated as an important factor in asthma and cardiovascular disease, where *C. pneumoniae* has been isolated from atherosclerotic tissue. Its possible pathogenic role is circumstantial, however. Infection with *C. pneumoniae* has been established as a risk factor for Guillain-Barré syndrome. There also appears to be a relationship between sarcoidosis and *C. pneumoniae*, but considerable work needs to be done to establish the existence and degree of this relationship. A single *C. pneumoniae* serovar has been found to date.

TABLE 21-3

History of Chlamydia pneumoniae *(Strain TWAR)*

Strain	Year	Comments
TW-183	1965	Isolated from a conjunctiva culture of a child in trachoma vaccine study in Taiwan
10L-207	1967	British isolated *Chlamydia* strain from conjunctiva of an Iranian child with trachoma Similar to TW-183
	1978	Retrospective serologic studies of pneumonia epidemic in teenagers and young adults in Finland supports *Chlamydia* agent as etiology
AR-39	1983	University of Washington, first pharyngeal isolate isolated in HeLa cells from college student

Clinical Infections

Infection with *C. pneumoniae* is thought to be fairly common, although probably 90% of infections are asymptomatic or mildly symptomatic. In adults, antibodies have been demonstrated in more than 50% of infections, but there is virtually no antibody detectable in children before the age of 5 years. It is thought that the attack rate is highest between the ages of 6 and 20 years, with a particular emphasis in college-age students. Unlike viral respiratory diseases, there seems to be no seasonal incidence, although some Scandinavian data have indicated the possibility of epidemics every 4 to

TABLE 21-4

Human Diseases Caused by Chlamydia *Species*

Species	Serovars*	Disease	Target
C. trachomatis (15 serovars)	A, B, Ba, C	Hyperendemic blinding trachoma	Human
	D, E, F, G, H, I, J, K	Inclusion conjunctivitis (adult and newborn)	Human
		Nongonococcal urethritis	
		Cervicitis	
		Salpingitis	
		Pelvic inflammatory disease (PID)	
		Endometritis	
		Acute urethral syndrome	
		Proctitis	
		Epididymitis	
		Pneumonia of newborns	
		Perihepatitis (Fitz-Hugh–Curtis syndrome)	
	L_1, L_2, L_3	Lymphogranuloma venereum (LGV)	
C. pneumoniae (strain TWAR)	1	Pneumonia, bronchitis	Human
		Pharyngitis	
		Influenza-like febrile illness	
C. psittaci	10 serotypes	Psittacosis	Bird
		Endocarditis	
		Abortion	

*Predominant serovars associated with disease.

TABLE 21-5

Summary of Key Epidemiologic and Clinical Features of Chlamydia pneumoniae *Infections*

Epidemiologic	Clinical
Virtually no antibody detectable before 5 years of age	Estimated to account for approximately 6% to 10% of outpatient and hospitalized pneumonia
Antibodies present in > 50% of adults	90% of infections are asymptomatic or mildly symptomatic
Attack rate highest between the ages of 6 years and mid-20s, often focusing on college-age students	Biphasic illness: prolonged sore throat and croup-like hoarseness followed by lower respiratory (flu-like) symptoms
No seasonal incidence; epidemics have been reported every 4 to 6 years	Pneumonia and bronchitis, rarely accompanied by sinusitis
Reinfection is common	Fever relatively uncommon
	Chest radiograph shows isolated pneumonitis
	One in 9 infections results in pneumonia
	Sarcoidosis, cardiovascular relationships?

6 years. Reinfection with *C. pneumoniae* appears to be very common and can be either milder or more severe than the initial infection.

The epidemiologic and clinical features of *C. pneumoniae* are shown in Table 21-5.

The clinical picture in college-age students, although it may be varied, is a biphasic clinical course. This infection produces a prolonged sore throat (5 to 7 days) and hoarseness, followed by flu-like lower respiratory symptoms (8 to 15 days). Because of its striking clinical similarity to bacterial pharyngitis, the result of a streptococcal antigen test often is thought to be falsely negative. The second phase of the biphasic illness often results in pneumonia (approximately one of 9 infections) and bronchitis but is rarely accompanied by sinusitis. Fever is relatively uncommon, and radiographs show isolated pneumonitis. *C. pneumo-*

niae is now recognized as the third most common cause of infectious respiratory disease. It accounts for approximately 6% to 10% of outpatient and hospitalized cases of pneumonia.

The mode of transmission, incubation period, and infectiousness of *C. pneumoniae* infections are still largely unknown. It is known, however, that there is no animal reservoir or animal vector. Table 21-6 organizes known data about *C. pneumoniae* and highlights those situations and/or populations at risk that would benefit from detection of *C. pneumoniae,* usually by serologic methods.

Laboratory Diagnosis

C. pneumoniae may be cultured on selected cell lines and visualized with fluorescein-conjugated monoclonal antibodies. Established cell lines H 292 and Hep-2 from the human respiratory tract are more

TABLE 21-6

Who to Evaluate for Chlamydia pneumoniae

Population/Situation	Evaluation Methods	Comments
Surveillance to establish baseline prevalence, both qualitative and quantitative		
Pneumonias requiring hospitalization (age 6 to 20 years)	*C. pneumoniae*–specific IgM and IgG: acute and convalescent, use micro-IF	12% antibody prevalence
Pharyngitis in college students	IgM, single visit	9% antibody prevalence
Retrospective, undiagnosed outbreaks in young adults, college or military	CF or micro-IF, IgG-specific	
Selected patients		
Serious pneumonia, undiagnosed; clinically presents like *Mycoplasma pneumoniae*	*C. pneumoniae*–specific IgM and IgG by micro-IF	Rather than repeat cultures for similar respiratory pathogens (i.e., *Mycoplasma pneumoniae,* establish etiology and impact on diagnosis-related group reimbursement)

Micro-IF, Microimmunofluorescence.

TABLE 21-7

Appropriate Specimens for Detection of Chlamydial Infections

Clinical Manifestation/Site of Infection	Specimen Site/Type	Comments
Inclusion conjunctivitis and trachoma	Conjunctival swab, scraping with spatula or tears	Specimen collection in neonates is difficult
Urethritis	Urethral swab	In males, > 4 cm and do not use discharge
Epidicymitis	Epididymis aspirate	
Cervicitis	Endocervical swab	Remove exudate first
Salpingitis	Fallopian tube (lumen) or biopsy	
Lymphogranuloma venereum	Bubo or cervical lymph node aspirate	
Infant pneumonia	Throat swab, nasopharyngeal aspirate, or lung tissue	
Sexually transmitted disease, male sex partner	Urine	Noninvasive diagnostic procedure EIA antigen detection is 80% accurate; PCR, 98%
Psittacosis	Sputum, lung tissue	
Chlamydia pneumoniae pneumoniae or pharyngitis	Sputum, throat or lung tissue	Tissue culture isolation and direct immuno-fluorescence are relatively new and need further evaluation
Sexually transmitted disease, result clarification	Rectal, vaginal swabs	May be used for supplemental information and in clarifying previous isolates or diagnostic dilemmas

sensitive than human lines (HL), but the traditional HeLa 229 cells are more sensitive than McCoy or L cells. Monoclonal antibodies specific for the *C. pneumoniae* strain are used to identify inclusions in cell culture. It should be noted that a genus-reactive monoclonal antibody can identify *C. pneumoniae* inclusions but cannot differentiate this organism from the other chlamydial species.

Attempts to culture *C. pneumoniae,* if undertaken, should take into account the organism's lability. *C. pneumoniae* seems to be considerably more labile than *C. trachomatis,* although its viability is relatively stable at 4° C. Specimens used for detection of chlamydial infections are listed in Table 21-7.

An indirect fluorescent antibody method has been reported for detecting *C. pneumoniae* in respiratory secretions; the antibody reacts with the MOMP (Figure 21-4). This same antibody can be used to identify infected culture monolayers.

Given the difficulty of and lack of standardization for isolation of *C. pneumoniae,* serologic tests have been the method of choice for detection. A complement fixation (CF) test that uses a genus-specific antigen has been the traditional assay most often employed for *C. pneumoniae* detection. In initial investigations to determine prevalence and reinfection rate, a four-fold rise in CF titer suggested recent chlamydial infection but did not distinguish

among the three known species. The present method of choice is microimmunofluorescence (micro-IF), which is more sensitive and specific than CF. Further, it does not crossreact with *C. trachomatis* and *C. psittaci.* Micro-IF also can distinguish an IgM from an IgG response. Single titer evaluations, although not diagnostic, may be suggestive. An IgM titer greater than 1:32 or an IgG single titer greater than 1:512 may suggest *C. pneumoniae* as a recent

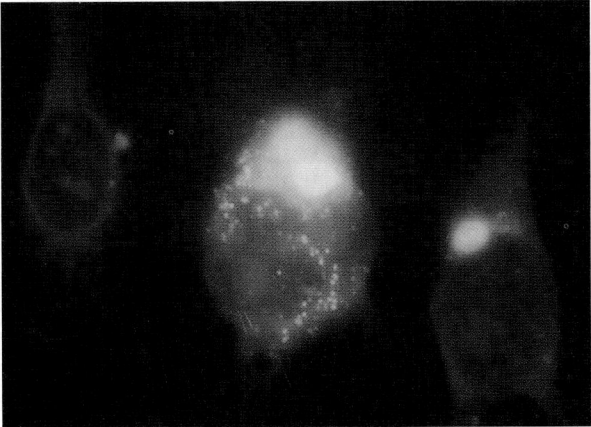

Figure 21-4

Chlamydia pneumoniae detection from direct sputum smear using fluorescent labeled monoclonal antibody, highlighting cytoplasmic inclusions (×700). (Courtesy DAKO Reagents, Carpinteria, Calif.)

TABLE 21-8

Detection of Chlamydia *Species by Various Serologic Methods*

Species of *Chlamydia*	Serologic Findings			
	CF Total	IgM	Micro-IF*	IgG
Chlamydia trachomatis serovars (15 serovars)				
A–C	+	+		+
D–K	(> 1:16)	Newborn		
L1–L3 (LGV)	> 1:64			
Chlamydia pneumoniae (strain TWAR, only known strain)	4-fold rise			4-fold rise
	+	> 1:32		or > 1:512
				(single specimen)
Chlamydia psittaci (10 serovars)	≥ 32			
	+	4-fold rise		> 1:512
	4-fold rise			(single specimen)
	(A/C)	(A/C)		

CF, Complement fixation (using LPS), where > 1:16 is indicative of previous exposure; *A/C,* acute/convalescent sera.
*Detects antibodies (IgM/ and total) against 10 major immunotypes using 4 antigenic pools: C complex: C-V-H-L, B complex: B-E-D, G-F complex: K.

etiologic agent, warranting further evaluation. Table 21-8 summarizes these serologic findings. An IgG titer greater than or equal to 1:16 but less than 1:512 is evidence of past infection or exposure.

Two antibody response patterns have been identified for *C. pneumoniae* infections. In the primary response, most often seen in adolescents, university students, and military trainees, CF antibodies usually appear first. By micro-IF, *C. pneumoniae*–specific IgM does not appear until 3 weeks after onset of symptoms, and often *C. pneumoniae*–specific IgG does not reach diagnostic levels for 6 to 8 weeks. Therefore the traditional convalescent serum obtained approximately 14 to 21 days after onset does not contain micro-IF–detectable *C. pneumoniae* antibody. In contrast, during reinfection, a CF antibody change is not detected, but by micro-IF, and IgG titer of 1:512 or more can appear within 2 weeks. IgM levels may be detectable but are low.

CHLAMYDIA TRACHOMATIS

C. trachomatis is the most common sexually transmitted bacterial pathogen in the United States. There are between 4 million and 10 million new cases each year. Only genital warts caused by human papillomavirus is a more common sexually transmitted disease (STD) in the United States. *Neisseria gonorrhoeae* is a distant third, with approximately 3 million to 4 million new cases per year.

Characterization of LPSs have separated *C. trachomatis* into 15 serovars, further reorganized into 10 immunotypes and grouped into 4 antigenic pools called C complex, D complex, G and F complex, and K complex.

C. trachomatis is unique in that it carries 10 stable cryptic plasmids whose function is currently unknown. This unique characteristic is a major reason for the applications of nucleic acid amplification by polymerase chain reaction (PCR) and identification by hybridization, discussed later.

Clinical Infections

Trachoma

The human diseases caused by *C. trachomatis* and the corresponding associated serotypes are listed in Table 21-4. Initially, *C. trachomatis* was associated with hyperendemic blindness and **trachoma.** This worldwide epidemic was associated with serotypes A, B, Ba, and C. These organisms are shed in feces and spread from person to person, people to fomites, and flies to people. These serotypes are most frequently found near the equator and are seen in climates with high temperature and high humidity, but not in the United States. In India and Egypt, the usual history of the infection ends in blindness in adults. Prevention includes either or both antibiotic treatment and a simple surgical procedure on the eyelid to stop the continual abrasion of the cornea. Figure 21-5 shows a patient with trachoma.

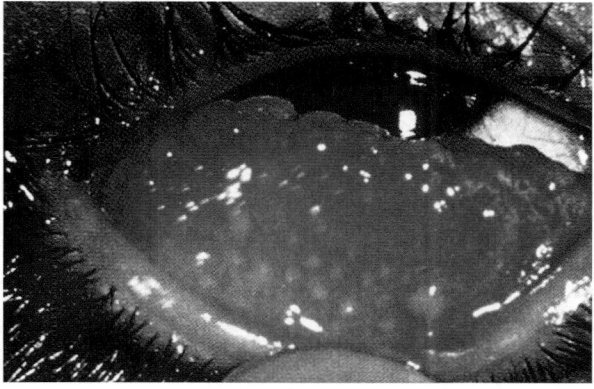

Figure 21-5 _____

Conjunctival scarring and hyperendemic blindness caused by *Chlamydia trachomatis* in ocular infections.

Lymphogranuloma venereum

C. trachomatis serotypes L_1, L_2, and L_3 cause **lymphogranuloma venereum (LGV),** an STD often seen in immigrants from and travelers to endemic parts of the world. In LGV, the patients have inguinal and anorectal symptoms (Figure 21-6). Table 21-4 shows other *C. trachomatis* serovars and the associated human diseases.

Other sexually transmitted diseases

Chlamydial infections in adult men include nongonococcal urethritis (NGU), epididymitis, and prostatitis. Between 45% and 68% of female partners of men with *Chlamydia*-positive NGU yield chlamydial isolates from the cervix. Approximately 50% of current male partners of women with a cervical chlamydial infection are also infected.

Infections in adult women include urethritis, follicular cervicitis (leukorrhea, hypertrophic cervical erosion), endometritis, proctitis, salpingitis, **pelvic inflammatory disease (PID),** and perihepatitis, also called the Fitz-Hugh–Curtis syndrome. Infections can be persistent and subclinical as well as acute and demonstrable. Salpingitis can lead to scarring and dysfunction of the ova ductile transport system, resulting in infertility or ectopic pregnancy. In the United States, this is a major cause of sterility.

Chlamydia in the newborn

Infants can be infected with *Chlamydia* when they travel through an infected birth canal. Chlamydial infection in an infant delivered by cesarean section is a rarity, and infection from seronegative mothers has not been reported. Infants suffering from chlamydial infection experience conjunctivitis, nasopharyngeal infections, and pneumonia (Figure 21-7). The portal of entry is ocular, with colonization of the oropharynx a necessary event before infection. Between 20% and 25% of babies born to *Chlamydia*-culture–positive mothers develop conjunctivitis, 15% to 20% develop nasopharyngeal infection, and 3% to 18% develop pneumonia. Otitis media is a less

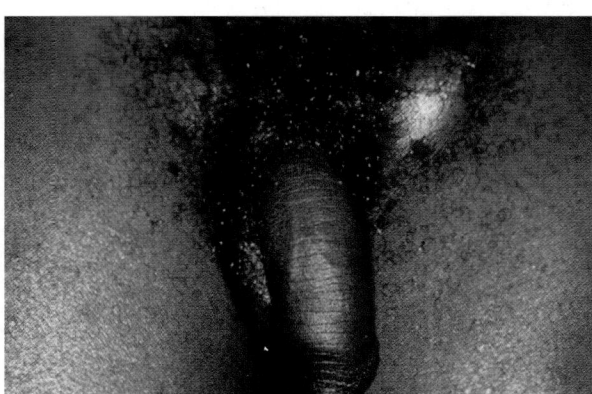

Figure 21-6 _____

Inguinal swelling and lymphatic drainage due to *Chylamydia trachomatis* serovars L_1, L_2, or L_3; that is, lymphogranuloma venereum (LGV).

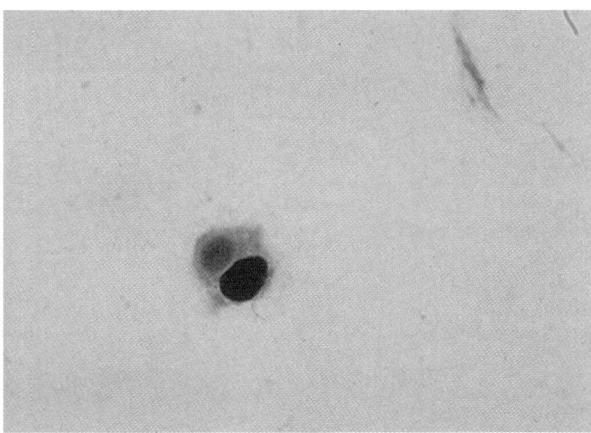

Figure 21-7 _____

Giemsa stain showing inclusion body from ocular swab of 7-day-old newborn who was discharged but then readmitted with fever, weight loss, lack of eating, and "fussiness." At 3 days after delivery, *Neisseria gonorrhoeae* was isolated from ocular discharge, although the patient had been given silver nitrate. Eye cultures confirmed the presence of *Chlamydia trachomatis* and diagnosis of neonatorum ophthalmia.

TABLE 21-9

Inclusion Conjunctivitis in the Neonate Caused by Chlamydia trachomatis

Incubation period	4 to 5 days
Signs	Edematous eyelids
Discharge	Copious, yellow
Course	Untreated, weeks to months
Complications	Corneal panus formation, conjunctival scarring
Giemsa stain of conjunctival scraping	Juxtanuclear inclusion

frequent infection. Babies also may be colonized in the vagina and the rectum. Clinically, it is believed that pneumonia in babies younger than 6 months of age is associated with *C. trachomatis,* unless proven otherwise. This pneumonia also can occur as a mixed infection, often concomitantly with gonococcus, cytomegalovirus, *Pneumocystis,* and other viruses. Table 21-9 shows selected features associated with neonatal inclusion conjunctivitis.

Laboratory Diagnosis

There are numerous methods for laboratory diagnosis of *C. trachomatis.* These methods vary in their sensitivity, specificity, and positive predictive value. Table 21-10 addresses the situations in which the appropriate tests may be most applicable, identifying the population group(s) at greatest risk. Table 21-11 provides the predictive values for these serologic assays as well as isolation, detection, and identification.

The most appropriate tests or combination of assays used depend on the following factors:

- Knowledge of the population at risk
- Capability and facilities available for testing
- Cost of materials
- Ability to batch specimen types
- Experience of technologist

Prevalence in the population to be tested is a very important criterion in determining which method or combination of methods should be used. For any assay, the positive predictive value increases (assuming optimum technical conditions) when the prevalence of the disease in the population is high.

The type of specimen selected for laboratory processing depends on the symptoms of the patient and the clinical presentation. However, re-

TABLE 21-10

Appropriate Chlamydia trachomatis *Assays for Selected Patient Population*

	Patient Population							
	Prenatal		Newborn		Clinics*		Legal Applicablity (Rape or Child Abuse?)	Test of Cure
Assay	Low Risk	High Risk	Eye	Throat	Low Risk	High Risk		
Culture	A/B	A	B	A	A/B	B	Yes	Yes
Nonculture, nonamplified								
DFA	B	A	A	A	B	A	No	No
EIA	A/B	A	A	A	A/B	A	No	No
O/A	—	—	—	—	B	B	No	No
Nonculture, amplified								
Probe	B	B	IUO	IUO	B	A	No	No
PCR	A	A	IUO	IUO	A	A	IUO	IUO
Serology								
CF	B, LGV	B, LGV	NA	NA	B, LGV	B, LGV	No	No
EIA	B	B	A	A	B	B	NA	NA
Micro-IF	NA	B	A	A (IgM)	B	B	No	No

A, Most useful, stands alone; *B,* probable, but needs verification or complementary assay employing conjugate recognizing different *C. trachomatis* macromolecules, i.e., LPS (EIA) vs MOMP (DFA) or competition assay for DNA probes; *C,* least useful; *IUO,* investigational use only; *LGV,* lymphogranuloma venereum; *NA,* not available.
*A *low-risk* population is defined as one with a < 5% incidence, such as in an obstetrics-gynecology or family practice patient group (birth control, annual gynecologic examination, etc.). A *high-risk* population is defined as one with a > 10% incidence, such as those in STD clinics, university or college student health centers, and emergency department patients.

TABLE 21-11

Detection Capabilities of Various Methods for Chlamydia trachomatis

| | SENS* % | SPEC* % | PPV* % | NPV* % | Specimen Site | | | | | Reported Cross-Reactivity | Comments |
					Cervical-Urethral	Rectal	Urine	Eye	False +/−		
Culture	50 to 85	100	73 to 98	90 to 100	+	+	+	+	False −	None	Labor-intensive gold standard for specificity
Nonculture, nonamplified											
DFA	70 to 95	92 to 98	73 to 98	95 to 99	+	+	−	+	False −/+	Staphylococci	Screen only; experience in FA needed
EIA	72 to 95	90 to 99	45 to 92	95 to 99	+	−	LA	LA	False +/−	Streptococci, GC, *Acinetobacter*	Verify with complementary assay
Probe	60 to 90	92 to 98	85 to 99	98 to 99	+	−	−	−	False +/−	Selected bacteria	Screen and verify by repeat culture
Nonculture, amplified											
PCR, LCR, TMA	85 to 95	99 to 100	85 to 95	100	+	−	+	RUO	False −	None reported	No verification necessary
Serology					See Table 21-8					Depends on antigen used	Several methods: CF, MIF

SENS, Sensitivity; *SPEC,* specificity; *PPV,* positive predictive value; *NPV,* negative predictive value; *LA,* limited availability; *RUO,* research use only.
*RANGE: Low to high prevalence as described in the text.

gardless of the source, the specimen should consist of infected epithelial cells and not exudate. Further, it is important to remember that plastic or metal swabs are superior to wooden swabs, which are toxic to cell culture, if swabbing is employed for isolation. Table 21-7 lists the optimum specimens for detection of *Chlamydia* in patients with a variety of clinical manifestations.

Direct microscopic examination

Direct specimen examination by cytologic methods primarily emphasize trachoma and inclusion conjunctivitis. Various investigators have estimated this method as nearly 95% sensitive, but it is technically demanding and influenced by the quality of the specimen from the newborn. Although this method is difficult to use with large batches of endocervical specimens, it does offer rapidity in selected cases, particularly in detecting ocular infection in newborns. When direct fluorescent antibody (DFA) testing is used for endocervical or urethral specimens, the characteristic "green apple" EB is suggestive but needs verification by alternative methods employing a different epitope. Direct specimen examination offers one additional important advantage: It allows for immediate quality control of the specimen, revealing whether the cells present in the field are columnar epithelial. Figure 21-8 shows inclusion bodies demonstrated by direct examination of cytologic stains of endocervical smears.

Culture

Cell culture

Until the development of PCR, chlamydial cell culture was considered the gold standard for detecting infection with *C. trachomatis,* but its utility has been limited because of the inherent technical complexity, time and specimen handling requirements, expense, and labile nature of the organism. Even under the most stringent and optimal conditions, isolation of chlamydiae is only approximately 80% sensitive. Cell lines used for the detection of chlamydiae include McCoy, HeLa 229, BHK-21, and Buffalo Green Monkey kidney. The cell lines are grown on coverslips in 1-dram shell vials or on the surface of multiwell cell culture dishes containing cyclohexamine. The shell vial technique also has been used and found to be more sensitive than the microwell method because multiple blind passes are not necessary to maximize the isolation rate in a 1-dram vial. The specimen is centrifuged onto the cell monolayer and incubated for 72 hours. Fluorescein conjugate and monoclonal antibodies or an iodine or Giemsa stain can be used to detect the chlamydial inclusions (Figure 21-9).

The fluorescent monoclonal antibody stain is considered the most sensitive. There are a number of commercially available fluorescent antibodies. Some researchers use species-specific monoclonal antibodies that bind to the MOMP, whereas others use the genus-specific antibody, which binds

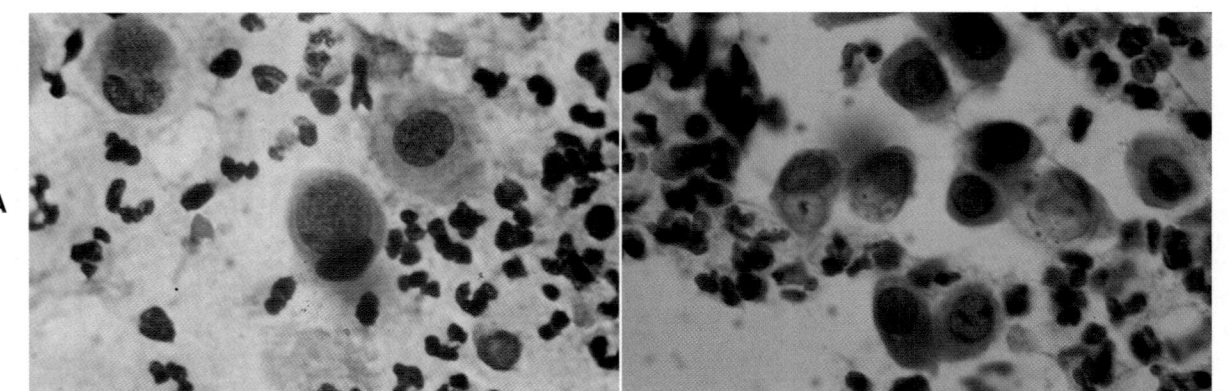

Figure 21-8

A and **B,** Cytologic examination of endocervical specimens demonstrating inclusion bodies consistent with *Chlamydia trachomatis.* Papanicolaou stain. (**B,** ×600).

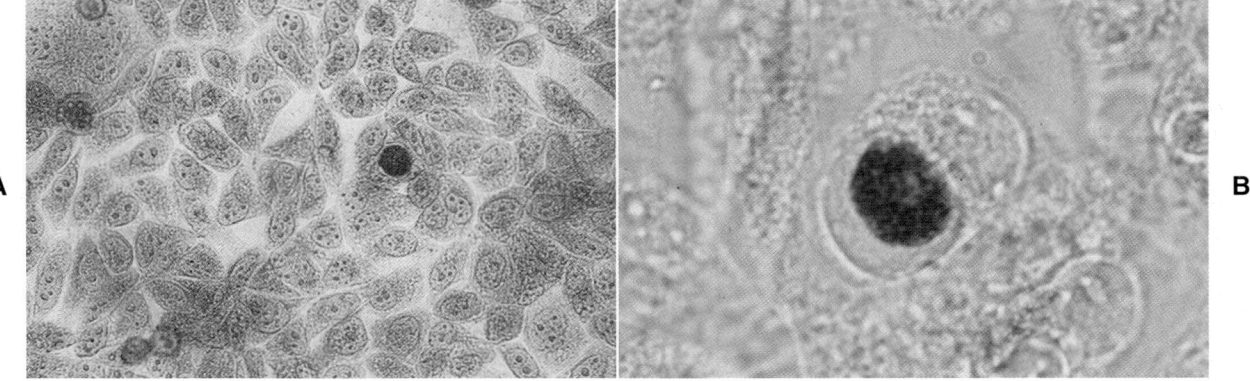

Figure 21-9

Iodine-stained inclusion bodies from *Chlamydia trachomatis*–infected McCoy cells. (**A,** ×40; **B,** ×100.) Note the size and half-moon shape of the inclusion.

to an LPS component. Monoclonal antibodies against the MOMP are reported to offer the brightest fluorescence with consistent body morphology and less nonspecific staining than monoclonal antibodies against the LPS. There have been a great many publications determining the specificity, sensitivity, and positive and negative predictive values of the fluorescent monoclonal antibody method. Published reports show a sensitivity range of 70% to 95% and a specificity range of 92% to 99%.

Nonculture, Nonamplified

Enzyme immunoassay

The most commonly employed rapid antigen assay for the detection of *C. trachomatis* is the EIA. Depending on the manufacturer, the EIA detects either the outer membrane LPS chlamydial antigen or the MOMP. A plethora of commercial kits are available, all having similar advantages. These include the ability to screen large volumes of specimens, obtain objective results, test performance in 3 to 5 hours, and use various specimen types, including urine for males, which may be very important when evaluating partner contact. A summary of the published sensitivity, specificity, and negative and predictive values as well as test specimens is shown in Table 21-11. Basically, however, none of them equals the sensitivity of culture, and most are significantly less sensitive. Discrepancies in sensitivity could be based on differences in sample size, disease prevalence, population charac-

teristics, collection sampling techniques, and laboratory standards.

One additional caution must be observed when EIA is employed for chlamydial antigen detection. A positive result must be considered preliminary and should be verified, because antigen detection methods may give a false-positive result when used in low-prevalence (<5%) populations. Verification of a positive specimen can be made on the same specimen using a monoclonal blocking antibody and a repeated EIA test using DFA or, alternatively, competitive binding for probe assays.

Nonculture, Amplified

Nucleic acid probes/amplification

The newest advances in *Chlamydia* identification have dealt with detection of nucleic acids. Initially, there was only one probe commercially available, a nonisotopically labeled DNA probe that detected urogenital *C. trachomatis* rRNA (Gen-Probe, Pace 2, San Diego, Calif.). Although the sensitivity, specificity, and positive and negative predictive values have been in the same range or higher than those reported for EIA (see Table 21-11), the DNA probe has the added advantage of detecting two sexually transmitted diseases (*N. gonorrhoeae* and *C. trachomatis*) from one sample. A unique "spin off" of EIA is OIA or "optical immunoassay." This membrane capture technology has been available since 1983, and its results are available in less than 30 minutes. Presently it is approved only for physicians' office use and focuses on "near-to-patient" rapid tests approach.

Most recently, target amplification has been reported as both an amplification and a detection method for *C. trachomatis*. Initial reports were very encouraging and suggested an increase in detection from urogenital specimens of greater than 15% to 30% over established EIA and tissue culture methods. Greater recovery was also seen in male urine specimens. Sensitivity, specificity, and predictive values were observed between 85% to 100%. On June 6, 1993, the U.S. Food and Drug Administration (FDA) approved the first commercial PCR assay for *C. trachomatis* detection, Amplicor, marketed by Roche Diagnostic (Roche Diagnostic Systems, Branchburg, N.J.).

Today, the number of commercially-available, FDA-approved systems, has increased to three, including Abbott and Gen-Probe. The specimen selection has expanded to include urine for both men and women, and significant automation for the Roche and Abbott assays (Table 21-12).

Additional observations must be noted, however. The concomitant use of a rapid screen for white cells (leukocyte esterase test) in urogenital specimens may heighten suspicion, demonstrate leukorrhea, and target specimens that would have the highest probability of detecting a true STD infectious agent. Conversely, there are significant, selected clinical limitations for the use of rapid screening methods employing EIA, DFA, or nucleic acid hybridization. As established by the Centers for Disease Control and Prevention (CDC), these assays cannot be used in rape or child abuse cases, nor should they be used in the measurement of treatment success. Because established appropriate antibiotics have a predictable 95% cure rate, the false-positive rate (due to less than 5% potentially uncured) would obscure follow-up results and suggest treatment failure. The nonculture, amplified assays may also be most useful in low-risk patient populations because they have essentially no false-positive result. In fact, these methods will most likely become the "gold standard" often called "expanded gold standard," recognizing the problems with culture.

Antibody detection

Serologic assays can be used in the detection of *C. trachomatis* infections. Historically, these were thought to be limited and problematic. Many individuals have chlamydial antibodies from previous infections, and because chlamydial infections tend to be localized, they do not cause the traditional fourfold rise in antibody titer between acute and convalescent specimens. Today, the interpretation and significance of serologic assays are being reevaluated, and serologic testing is growing as a complementary diagnostic tool in certain selected scenarios such as the following:

- After reorganization of the serologic classification of *C. trachomatis* from 15 serovars to 10 immunotypes, four antigenic pools or complexes of *C. trachomatis* are now recognized.

TABLE 21-12

Summary of Nonculture, Amplified Tests for Chlamydia trachomatis

Test	Manuf. Name	Target	Specimen Source	GC, Simultaneously	Automation	Verification	FDA Approval
PCR	Roche Amplicore	Cryptic Plasmid 6 DNA	Cervical Urethral Male urine Female urine	Yes	All except specimen processing	No manufacturer defined, FDA-approved procedure	Screen
LCR	Abbott LCx	Cryptic Plasmid 6 DNA	Cervical Urethral Male urine Female urine	No	Detection, only	Same	Screen
TMA	GenProbe TM	23s RNA	Cervical Urethral Male urine Female urine	No	None, yet	Same	Screen

PCR, Polymerase chain reaction; *LCR,* ligase chain reaction; *TMA,* transcription mediated amplification.

These are C complex, D complex, G and F complex, and K complex. With micro-IF, when a specific IgM response to a different pool of *C. trachomatis* immunotypes is observed, new infections can be detected in patients who have had previous infections with other immunotypes.

- Ascending infections by *C. trachomatis* involving fallopian tubes and additional organs of the upper female genital tract are almost never detected by endocervical cultures. Hence, patients at risk for chronic infections would be missed with the standard screening methods employing a cervical swab. The best serologic screening of patients at risk, particularly as part of a prenatal work-up, may be for the immunotypes now defined for *C. trachomatis* using the four pools listed previously. Prenatal patient sera are often kept for approximately 1 year following initial serologic evaluations— for example, for hepatitis B virus, human immunodeficiency virus, and the TORCH agents. This is a serum reservoir that needs to be recognized and used more effectively.
- Complement fixation detects genus-reactive antibody, including elevated levels of antibody in systemic infections, such as LGV. Diagnosis of LGV is supported by CF titers of 1:64 or more, as demonstrated in Table 21-8. It must be noted, however, that CF generally is not useful in nonsystemic chlamydial conjunctivitis or routine urogenital tract infections.

Micro-IF detects antibodies to chlamydial EBs; they are serotype-specific antibodies. Hence, high levels of chlamydial IgM by micro-IF are diagnostic of systemic *C. trachomatis* infection in infants. In fact, because same-day diagnosis is possible, IgM micro-IF is the method of choice for diagnosis of *C. trachomatis* pneumonia in infants, preferable even to culture. Further, infants with inclusion conjunctivitis normally do not have detectable IgM antibodies unless they have a systemic infection. Chlamydial IgG is generally not useful in infants, because rising titers are seldom observed, and when they are, they probably reflect maternal antibody.

Results Reporting

With such great latitude in current testing choices, it is very important for each laboratory to clearly report and define results. Some key points in the development of an approach to ordering and reporting results of tests for *C. trachomatis* and related organisms in a patient specimen are as follows:

- Agreeing in advance with the obstetrics/ gynecology and emergency departments on which organisms are associated with which clinical syndrome, then test accordingly, using profiles
- Reporting which tests were and were not performed for each patient profile
- Reporting unusual observations. Pure isolates of *Pseudomonas, Haemophilus, Neisseria meningitidis,* and yeast are not normal, and the physician needs to be aware of their presence.

CHLAMYDIA PSITTACI

C. psittaci is the cause of psittacosis, also known as ornithosis or parrot fever. Diagnosis of psittacosis usually is based on a history of exposure to psittacines and a fourfold rise in CF antibody to the chlamydial group LPS antigen. In adults in the United States, several hundred cases of pneumonia each year are due to *C. pneumoniae,* compared with only a few hundred due to *C. psittaci.* Retrospective serologic testing of sera from patients with acute respiratory disease have shown that many people previously thought to have *C. psittaci* infections due to "transient bird exposure" were, in fact, actually infected with the *C. pneumoniae* organism. Hence, misdiagnosis of *C. psittaci* is a problem, and the physician needs to know the tests that are most appropriate for differentiating these chlamydial isolates (see Table 21-8).

Isolation of *C. psittaci* in culture, although diagnostic, is difficult and is not routinely employed nor recommended in the United States. Therefore almost all diagnoses of *C. psittaci* are based on serologic evaluation. As shown in Table 21-8, a single CF titer greater than 1:32 is suggestive of acute illness in a symptomatic patient during an outbreak of psittacosis. The rise in CF antibodies usually is not demonstrable until the acute illness is over, however, and it often is weak or absent if appropriate antibiotic therapy is given. This is most often a "rule-out" disease. If *C. pneumoniae* and *C. trachomatis*–specific IgG and IgM are not detected by micro-IF and a fourfold rise in chlamydial antibodies is detected by CF, then *C. psittaci* should be strongly suspected. A good history is paramount in evaluating bird exposure, incubation time, and disease process.

Bibliography

Altaie S et al: Evaluation of two ELISAs for detecting *Chlamydia trachomatis* from endocervical swabs, *Diagn Microbiol Infect Dis* 15:579, 1992.

Bass CA et al: Clinical evaluation of a new polymerase chain reaction assay for detection of *Chlamydia trachomatis* in endocervical specimens, *J Clin Microbiol* 31:2648, 1993.

Burnstein GR et al: Incidents *Chlamydia trachomatis* infections among inner-city adolescent females, *JAMA* 280:521, 1989.

Caliendo A: Diagnosis of CT infections using amplification methods: can we afford it? *Clin Microbiol Newsl* 20(9):75, 1998.

Campbel LA et al: Serological responses to *Chlamydia pneumoniae* infection, *J Clin Microbiol* 28:1261, 1990.

Centers for Disease Control: False-positive results with use of *Chlamydia* test in the evaluation of suspected sexual abuse, *MMWR* 39:932, 1991.

Chapin-Robertson K: Use of molecular diagnostics in sexually transmitted disease: critical assessment, *Diagn Microbiol Dis* 16:173, 1993.

Fonte CE, Carlisle J, Lazerson J: Vaginal discharge in a two-month-old infant, *Hosp Pract* Oct:39, 1987.

Glaser JB, Hammerschlag MR, MacCormick WM: Sexually transmitted diseases in the victims of sexual assault, *N Engl J Med* 315:625, 1986.

Grayston JT et al: A new *Chlamydia psittaci* strain, TWAR, isolated in acute respiratory tract infections, *N Engl J Med* 315(3):161, 1986.

Grayston JT et al: Current knowledge of *Chlamydia pneumoniae,* strain TWAR, an important cause of pneumonia and other acute respiratory diseases, *Eur J Clin Microbiol* 8:191, 1989.

Huovinen P et al: Pharyngitis in adults: the presence and co-existence of viruses and bacterial organisms, *Ann Intern Med* 110:612, 1989.

LaScolea LJ Jr: The value of noncultured chlamydial diagnostic tests [editorial], *Clin Micro Newsl* 13:21, 1991.

Loeffelholz M et al: Detection of *Chlamydia trachomatis* in endocervical specimens by polymerase chain reaction, *J Clin Microbiol* 30:2847, 1992.

Moncada J et al: Evaluation of Syva's enzyme immunoassay for the detection of *Chlamydia trachomatis* in urogenital specimens, *Diagn Microbiol Infect Dis* 15:663, 1992.

Nettleman MD et al: Cost effectiveness of culturing for *Chlamydia trachomatis:* a study in a clinic for sexually transmitted diseases, *Ann Intern Med* 105:189, 1986.

Phillips RS et al: Criteria for selective testing of chlamydia, *Am J Med* 186:515, 1989.

Quinn TC et al: Epidemiologic and microbiologic correlates of *Chlamydia trachomatis* infections in sexual partnerships, *JAMA* 276(21):1737, 1996.

Schacter J: Why we need a program for the control of *Chlamydia trachomatis* [editorial], *N Engl J Med* 320:802, 1989.

Scholes D et al: Prevention of PID by screening for cervical chlamydial infection, *N Engl J Med* 1362, 1996.

Sillus M, White P: Rapid identification of *Chlamydia psittaci* and TWAR *(C. pneumoniae)* in sputum samples using an amplified enzyme immunoassay [letters to the editor], *J Clin Pathol* 43:260, 1990.

Stagano S et al: Infant pneumonitis associated with cytomegalovirus, *Chlamydia, Pneumocystis,* and *Ureaplasma:* a prospective study, *Pediatrics* 68:322, 1981.

Washington AE et al: *Chlamydia trachomatis* infections in the United States, what are they costing us? *JAMA* 257:2070, 1987.

Washington AE et al: Cost of and payment source for pelvic inflammatory disease trend and projections, 1938-2000, *JAMA* 266:2565, 1991.

LEARNING ASSESSMENT

1. What organisms should be considered as possible causes of neonatal conjunctivitis?

2. What stains should be performed on the discharge or conjunctival scraping for microscopy examination?

3. For the infant described in the case study, what other clinical conditions could be due to the causative organisms?

4. What are the most common sites of infection in newborns infected with this organism?

5. What sexually transmitted disease (STD) is caused by *Chlamydia trachomatis* serotypes L_1, L_2, and L_3?

6. What other STDs are caused by serotypes of *C. trachomatis?*

7. How does lymphogranuloma venereum (LGV) differ from other STDs caused by *C. trachomatis?*

8. Which *Chlamydia* species is associated with Guillain-Barré syndrome?

9. What is psittacosis?

10. How is this condition usually diagnosed?

B. *MYCOPLASMA* AND *UREAPLASMA* SPECIES

John G. Thomas, Karen S. Long

GENERAL CHARACTERISTICS

CLINICAL INFECTIONS
  Mycoplasma pneumoniae
  Mycoplasma hominis and *Ureaplasma urealyticum*
  Emerging *Mycoplasma* Pathogens

LABORATORY DIAGNOSIS
  Specimen Collection and Transport
  Culture
  Media
  Identification
  Serologic Diagnosis

ANTIMICROBIAL SUSCEPTIBILITY

INTERPRETATION OF LABORATORY RESULTS

OBJECTIVES

1. Describe the general characteristics of *Mycoplasma* and how they differ from other bacterial species.
2. Describe the clinical diseases caused by *Mycoplasma pneumoniae, Mycoplasma hominis,* and *Ureaplasma urealyticum.*
3. Identify the preferred stains for demonstration of the mycoplasmas.
4. Discuss the possible roles of *Mycoplasma hominis* and *Ureaplasma urealyticum* in infections of low-birth-weight and high-risk neonates.
5. Discuss the potential effect of *Mycoplasma fermentans (incognitus* strain) on the immune system and its possible role as a cofactor in HIV-1 disease.
6. List and discuss the various diagnostic methods for *Mycoplasma pneumoniae* infection.
7. Name two selective media for detection of the mycoplasmas.

KEY TERMS

Cell wall deficients (CWDs)
Pleuropneumonia-like organism (PPLO)
AIDS-related mycoplasma
T-strain mycoplasma

CASE STUDY

A premature infant in the neonatal intensive care unit, who weighed 1.5 pounds at birth (LBW), developed signs of meningitis and a lumbar puncture (LP) is performed. White blood cell count of the CSF was "negative," the Gram stain was reported as "no organisms seen," and routine culture at 3 days was "no growth." The infant was still symptomatic at this time, and the pediatric ID physician, after consultation with the microbiology laboratory, ordered additional cultures of the original CSF, which had been placed in the 37° C incubator. An organism was recovered by the laboratory.

This discussion highlights a group of organisms once thought to be viruses because of their size. Mycoplasmas are the smallest free-living organisms in nature; *Mycoplasma* and *Ureaplasma* are two of the six genera in the family Mycoplasmataceae (Table 21-13). Of the approximately 70 species of *Mycoplasma* and *Ureaplasma* identified in plants

TABLE 21-13

Divergent Ecosystems Inhabited by Genera of the Family Mycoplasmataceae

Ecosystem	Mycoplasma	Ureaplasma	Acholeplasma	Spiroplasma	Thermoplasma	Anaeroplasma
Soil and grasses	−	−	−	+	−	−
Crops and plants	−	−	−	+	−	−
Mown hay	−	−	−	−	+	−
Water	−	−	+	−	−	−
Deciduous trees	−	−	−	+	−	−
Humans	+	+	−	−	−	+
Cattle	+	+	−	−	−	+

and animals, the following three species are known to be human pathogens:

- *Mycoplasma pneumoniae,* which causes respiratory disease
- *Mycoplasma hominis,* associated with urogenital tract disease
- *Ureaplasma urealyticum,* associated with urogenital tract disease

In the laboratory, mycoplasmas are common and hard-to-detect contaminants of cell cultures. They also may be emerging or opportunistic pathogens for selected patient populations.

GENERAL CHARACTERISTICS

Mycoplasmas are pleomorphic organisms that do not possess a cell wall (Figure 21-10), a characteristic that makes them resistant to cell-wall–active antibiotics, such as penicillins and cephalosporins. Because of the absence of cell wall, they were originally grouped under the general term **cell wall deficients (CWDs).** Table 21-14 compares features of three genera known to be pathogenic for humans. Generally, mycoplasmas are slowly growing, highly fastidious, facultative anaerobes requiring complex media containing cholesterol and fatty acids for growth; important

TABLE 21-14

CWD and PPLO: Human Pathogens in the Family Mycoplasmataceae

Feature	Mycoplasma	Ureaplasma	Acholeplasma
Cell-wall deficient	+	+	+
Gram stain	−	−	−
Penicillin susceptible	−	−	−
Urease activity	−	+	−
Induced in hypertonic solution and penicillin, lysozyme, or salts	−	−	−
Derivation: Exists in nature as free-living organism	+	+	+
Contains cell wall components but lacks true cell wall	+	+	+
Reverts to parental form (or re-establishes cell wall) when induction is eliminated	−	−	−
Independent replication in vitro 6a sterol (medium) (i.e., cell-free medium)	+	+	−
Pleomorphic shape	+	+	+
Other shared characteristics	Smaller than bacteria—close in size to myxoviruses Limited metabolic activity (i.e., fastidious) Lower GC (guanidine/cytosine) ratio than most bacteria Many mycoplasma contain DNase Smaller genome than bacteria		

CWD, Cell wall deficient; *PPLO,* pleuropneumonia-like organism.

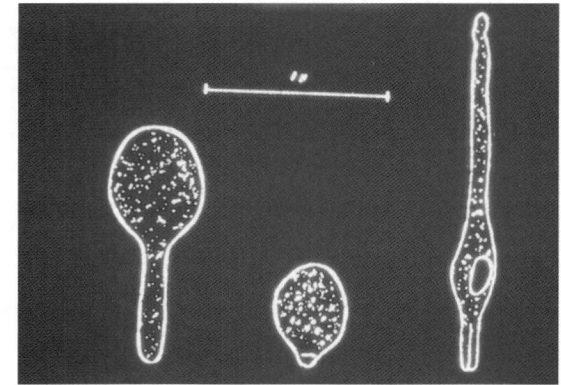

Figure 21-10

Schematic representation of three *Mycoplasma* species demonstrating varied shape and pleomorphism within genera. *Left, Mycoplasma pulmonis; center, Mycoplasma gallisepticum; right, Mycoplasma pneumoniae.*

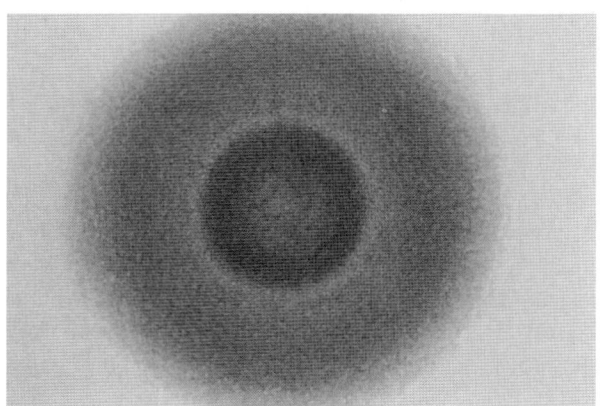

Figure 21-11

Typical large *Mycoplasma* colony showing "fried egg" appearance. (Courtesy Bionique Testing Laboratories, Saranac Lake, N.Y.)

A 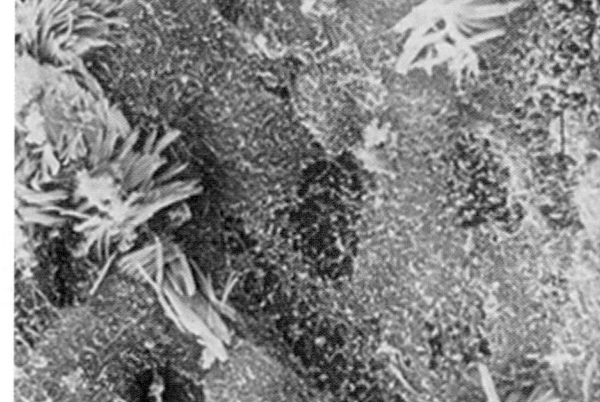 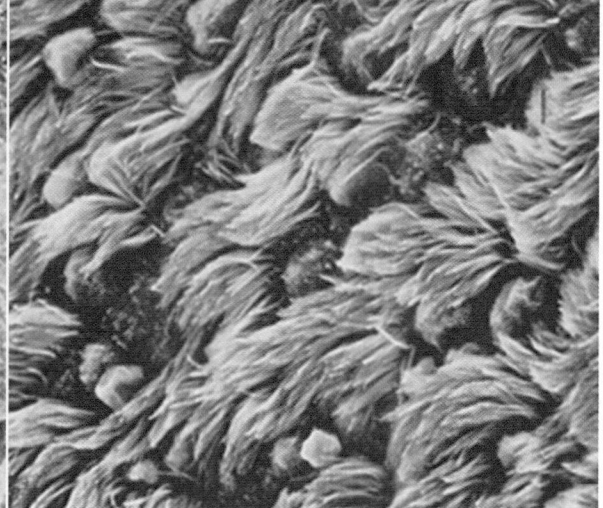 B

Figure 21-12

Electron micrograph of effect of *Mycoplasma pneumoniae* on ciliated tracheal cells. **A,** Infected animal model. **B,** Uninfected animal model.

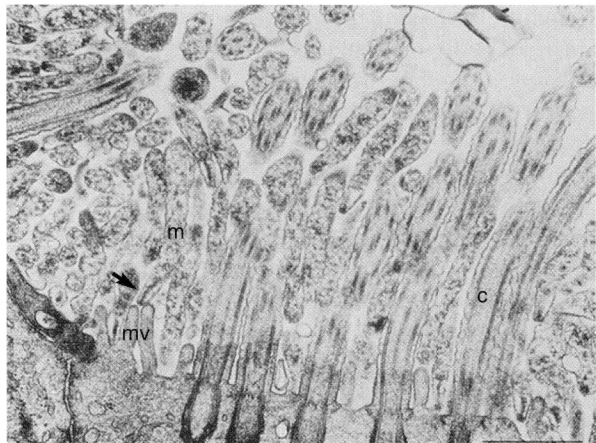

Figure 21-13 _____

Electron micrograph of *Mycoplasma pneumoniae* attaching by specific attachment features to ciliated trachea. *mv,* Microvilli; *m,* mycoplasma, *c,* cilia.

exceptions include aerobic *M. pneumoniae* and the more rapidly growing *M. hominis.* On solid media, mycoplasma form colonies with the center of the colony embedded beneath the surface, giving the classic "fried egg" appearance (Figure 21-11).

The first Mycoplasma was isolated in the late 1800s from a cow with pleuropneumonia. *M. pneumoniae* has been called the Eaton agent, named after the researcher who first isolated it. Until recently, *M. pneumoniae* has been known as a **pleuropneumonia-like organism (PPLO).** The mycoplasmas adhere to the epithelium of mucosal surfaces in the respiratory and urogenital tracts and are not eliminated by mucous secretions or the passage of urine. Figure 21-12 shows electron micrographs depicting ciliated tracheal epithelial cells before and after *M. pneumoniae* infection. Figure 21-13 is an electron micrograph demonstrating the shape of *M. pneumoniae* and its orientation of attachment by a "two-pronged end" structure. Mycoplasma species indigenous to humans are shown in Table 21-15.

CLINICAL INFECTIONS

Mycoplasma pneumoniae

M. pneumoniae may cause bronchitis, pharyngitis, or a relatively common respiratory infection known as primary atypical pneumonia or walking pneumonia. The organism does not occur as a normal commensal; therefore its isolation (when successful) is always significant and pathognomonic. *M. pneumoniae* causes approximately 20% of reported pneumonias in the general population and up to 50% in military settings. School-age children and young adults are especially susceptible to infection. Clinical disease is uncommon in very young children and older adults. Other groups at risk include closed-in populations such as prisoners, college students, and military personnel. Epidemics are known to occur in these populations. Infection is not considered seasonal, but many cases occur in autumn and early winter. Outbreaks

TABLE 21-15 _____

Mycoplasma *Species Indigenous to Humans*

Species	Usual Habitat	Reported Frequency	Colony Morphology*
M. salivarium	Oropharynx	Very common	Large, fried egg
M. orale	Oropharynx	Common	Small, spherical
M. buccale	Oropharynx	Uncommon	Large, fried egg
M. faucium	Oropharynx	Uncommon	Large, fried egg
M. lipophilum	Oropharynx	Rare	Large, fried egg
M. pneumoniae	Oropharynx	Common (with disease)	Small, spherical, granular
M. fementans	Oropharynx	Rare	Small, fried egg, spherical
	Urogenital tract	Uncommon	
M. hominis	Oropharynx	Uncommon	Large, fried egg, vesiculated peripheral zone
	Urogenital tract	Common (9% to 50% women)	
M. genitalium†	Urogenital tract	Common?	
Ureaplasma urealyticum	Urogenital tract	Very common (81% women; 30% to 50% men)	Tiny, spherical, fried egg, granular

*Relative sizes: large = > 100 nm; small = 50 to 100 nm; tiny = < 50 nm.
†Cross-reacted with *M. pneumoniae* DNA probe (when previously available).

also have been noted when adolescents return to school in the fall. Transmission is probably through aerosol droplet spray produced in coughing.

Many infections are completely asymptomatic or very mild; only approximately 3% to 10% of patients demonstrate clinically apparent pneumonia (Figure 21-14). The incubation period is usually 2 to 3 weeks, and early symptoms are nonspecific, consisting of headache, low-grade fever, malaise, and anorexia. Sore throat, dry cough, and earache are accompanying symptoms. Extrapulmonary complications, including cardiovascular, central nervous system, dermatologic, and gastrointestinal problems, are rare but do occur. *M. pneumoniae* is not associated with infections of the urogenital tract. It has, however, been associated with extrapulmonary disease and implicated as a coinfection or cofactor in epidemic group A meningococcal meningitis and infant pneumonitis.

Mycoplasma hominis and Ureaplasma urealyticum

M. hominis and *U. urealyticum* are both associated with infections in the urogenital tract. They are, however, frequently isolated from asymptomatic individuals, making interpretation of a positive culture difficult. Because they are opportunistic pathogens, the immune status of the host is an important factor in the occurrence and severity of disease. In addition, it has been reported that among sexually active individuals, the rate of colonization is directly related to the number of sexual partners. Higher rates of colonization have been noted in African-American men and women and in adults of lower socioeconomic status. The organisms do not persist in infants colonized at birth. Table 21-16 summarizes the known association of genital mycoplasmas with urogenital and newborn diseases.

M. hominis is found in the lower genitourinary tracts of approximately 50% of healthy adults and has not been reported as a cause of nongonococcal urethritis (NGU). The organism may, however, invade the upper genitourinary tract and cause salpingitis, pyelonephritis, pelvic inflammatory disease, or postpartum fevers.

U. urealyticum does not cause disease in the female lower genital tract but has been associated with approximately 10% of cases of nongonococcal urethritis in men, as well as with upper female

TABLE 21-16

Summary of the Association of Genital Mycoplasmas with Urogenital and Newborn Diseases

Disease	Mycoplasma hominis	Ureaplasma urealyticum	Comments
Nongonococcal urethritis	None	Strong	Ureaplasmas cause some cases, but the proportion is unknown
Prostatitis	Weak	None	An association with a few cases of chronic disease has been reported; a causal relation is unproven
Epididymitis	None	None	Mycoplasmas are not an important cause
Reiter disease	None	None	The role of ureaplasmas should be studied
Bartholin gland abscess	Weak	None	*M. hominis* may cause some disease but is not an important cause
Vaginitis and cervicitis	None	None	*M. hominis* often associated with disease, but a causal relation is unproven
Pelvic inflammatory disease	Strong	Weak	*M. hominis* causes some cases, but the proportion is unknown
Postabortal fever	Strong	None	*M. hominis* is responsible for some cases, but the proportion is unknown
Postpartum fever	Strong	None	Recent work indicates *M. hominis* may be a major cause
Urinary calculi	None	Weak	Ureaplasmas cause calculi in male rats, but no convincing evidence exists that they cause natural human disease
Pyelonephritis	Strong	None	*M. hominis* causes some cases
Involuntary infertility	None	Weak	Ureaplasmas are associated with altered motility of sperm
Repeated spontaneous abortion and stillbirth	None	Weak	Maternal and fetal infections have been associated with spontaneous abortion, but a causal relation is unproven
Chorioamnionitis	None	Strong	An association exists, but a causal relation is unproven
Low birth weight	None	Strong	An association exists, but a causal relation is unproven
Neonatal infections, including sepsis, pneumonia, meningitis	Strong	Strong	Further clarification is needed, but importance is growing in a selected prenatal population

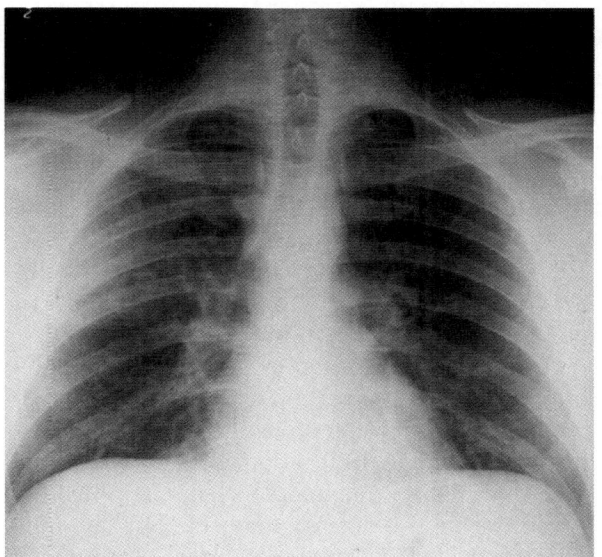

Figure 21-14

Typical chest radiograph of a patient with a 3-week course of atypical pneumonia. Note nonspecific interstitial pneumonia, patchy infiltrate delineated by feathery outline.

genitourinary tract disorders. *U. urealyticum* has been recovered from more than 60% of normal, sexually active females. *Ureaplasma* has been associated with reproduction disorders, chorioamnionitis, congenital pneumonia, and the development of chronic lung disease in premature infants. Although it is not a primary cause of chronic lung disease, Cassell and associates (1988) reported *U. urealyticum* as the most common organism isolated from tracheal aspirates of low-birth-weight infants with respiratory disease. Fourteen percent of infections were in newborns delivered by cesarean section, thus indicating that infection occurred in utero and not during passage through the birth canal.

Both *M. hominis* and *U. urealyticum* can be transmitted to the fetus at delivery and have been reported as the most common organisms recovered from the cerebrospinal fluid of certain high-risk newborns, including preterm and low-birth-weight babies. It has been recommended that culture for these organisms be attempted when the CSF specimen from a newborn with evidence of meningitis is negative for both Gram stain and traditional bacteriology culture (Table 21-17).

M. hominis may be isolated from culture in 24 to 48 hours. This does not include blood cultures, where its growth is inhibited by sodium polyanethole sulfonate (SPS), an additive often found in blood culture media. Identification often is made by typing methods employing immunofluorescence and observation of plate media using a stereoscope. *U. urealyticum* also has been reported to cause chronic inflammatory diseases such as arthritis and cystitis in hypogammaglobulinemic patients.

Lastly, it has been reported that these isolates have been intermittently associated with patients who are immunosuppressed or have endocarditis, sternal wound infections, or arthritis.

Emerging *Mycoplasma* Pathogens

The pathogenicity of *Mycoplasma genitalium,* first isolated in 1980, has not been established, but the organism has been associated with some cases of nongonococcal urethritis and pelvic inflammatory disease. Its prevalence is not known, but it may be primarily a resident of the gastrointestinal tract

TABLE 21-17

Summary of the Recent Association of Genital Mycoplasmas with Neonatal Disease

| Condition/Target Population | Isolates | | Comments |
	Mycoplasma hominis	*Ureaplasma urealyticum*	
Neonatal period, including preterm delivery, very low birth weight. Clinical signs compatible with			These findings need further clarification because most neonatal infections resolve without therapy, but in low socioeconomic groups, "diagnostic work-up" of newborns should now include CSF and blood cultures for detection of *Mycoplasma*. This includes low-birth-weight and preterm newborns, in whom traditional CSF cell counts and cultures would be negative.
Meningitis (CSF)	+	+	
Pneumonia (trachea)	+	+	
Sepsis (blood)	+	+	

that occurs secondarily in the genitourinary or respiratory tract. *M. genitalium* is very difficult to recover from culture and may require 2 to 3 months of incubation. Understanding this organism is important because it crossreacts with *M. pneumoniae* in some direct fluorescent antibody tests, causing a false-positive result.

Mycoplasma fermentans [*incognitus* strain] is a newly described mycoplasma that closely resembles *M. fermentans* and is most likely a new strain rather than a new species. It is more fastidious than *M. fermentans,* growing only on modified SP-4 culture medium, with colonies visible in 10 to 14 days. Recent interest in *M. fermentans* [*incognitus* strain], sometimes called Lo's *Mycoplasma* in recognition of its discoverer, has centered on its relationship to patients infected with the human immunodeficiency virus type 1 (HIV-1). The association of this *Mycoplasma* with the development of acquired immune deficiency syndrome (AIDS) is not clear at present, but *M. fermentans* [*incognitus* strain] may be able to suppress the immune system by reducing the number of T lymphocytes or "turning on" T lymphocytes to produce cytokines. Using polymerase chain reaction (PCR) technology in a serologic study of *Mycoplasma* in AIDS patients, Lo et al (1989) reported co-infection of HIV and *M. fermentans* [*incognitus* strain] in the majority of patients studied. The organism has been identified in thymus, liver, spleen, lymph nodes, brain, and kidney of HIV-1–positive patients. Not surprisingly, it has been referred to as **AIDS-related *mycoplasma.***

| LABORATORY DIAGNOSIS

Specimen Collection and Transport

Owing to the lack of a cell wall, all mycoplasmas are extremely sensitive to drying. Therefore specimens for culture should be delivered immediately to the laboratory. Swabs should be placed in a transport medium such as trypticase soy broth with 0.5% albumin and 400 U/mL of penicillin or SP4 medium (sucrose phosphate buffer, *Mycoplasma* base, horse serum [20%], and neutral red) (see Figure 21-15). On arrival in the laboratory, the specimens should be frozen at −70° C if immediate plating is not possible.

Isolation of *M. pneumoniae* from respiratory sites is attempted infrequently because recovery from culture is difficult (sensitivity is approximately 40%). Growth may take several weeks, and technical expertise is necessary. Diagnosis is usually established serologically, traditionally with acute and convalescent sera collected 2 to 3 weeks apart to demonstrate a four-fold rise in titer. *M. hominis* and *Ureaplasma* are less stringent in their growth requirements but require cholesterol for synthesis of plasma membranes.

Optimally, serum samples for serologic testing should be collected at the onset of symptoms and 2 to 3 weeks later for acute and convalescent measurements; however, this often is not practical. With newer methods, single serum samples collected during the disease may rule out the infection or suggest additional evaluations. A schematic representation of classic clinical and corresponding diagnostic manifestations of *M. pneumoniae* is shown in Table 21-18. As noted previously, many of the early symptoms are nonspecific, and a thorough understanding of the disease process is necessary for interpretation of both serum and culture results.

Culture
Media
Several media have been developed for the recovery of mycoplasmas. They include supplemented PPLO agar, Shephard A-7B agar (for *U. urealyticum*), SP4, Hayflick's biaphasic medium, E agar, and New York City agar, a selective agar for *N. gonorrhoeae* that also supports the growth of *M. hominis* and *U. urealyticum. M. pneumoniae* and *M. genitalium* require glucose (their major source of energy), *M. hominis,* requires arginine, and *U. urealyticum* requires urea. *Ureaplasma* requires liquid medium to have a pH of 6.0 and is difficult to maintain in culture because death occurs rapidly when the urea is depleted. Figure 21-15 presents a schematic representation of media and methods used in the traditional isolation and identification of *Mycoplasma.*

Identification
Mycoplasma-like colonies are stained with Dienes stain because the organisms do not stain well with Gram or acridine orange (AO) stain. It is performed

TABLE 21-18

Major Clinical and Corresponding Diagnostic Manifestation of Mycoplasma pneumoniae

Manifestation	Days After Onset						
	5	10	15	20	25	35	40
Headache and malaise	+1	+3	+3	+2	+1		
Dry cough	+2	+4	+4	+1			
Chest soreness	+3	+3	+1				
Fever							
104° F							
102° F	▮	▮	▪	▪	—		
100° F							
Chest radiograph	+2	+3	+2	+2	+1		
Mycoplasma culture with or without antibiotic treatment	+	+	+	+	+	+	+
Cold agglutinin (titer)	≤1:8	1:32	1:64	1:320	1:320	1:64	1:16
Complement fixation (titer)	≤1:8	≤1:8	1:32	1:64	1:256	1:256	1:128
Mycoplasma-specific Ig							
IgM	−	+	+	+	+	+	+
IgG	−	−	+	+	+	+/−	−

−4, Most severe; +1, least severe; +, present or positive; −, absent or negative; ▮, patient treated without appropriate antibiotic; ▯, patient treated with optimum antibiotic therapy, dose, and duration.

by placing a small block of the agar plate on a glass slide, covering the colony with the stain, adding a coverslip, and examining microscopically under low power. *Mycoplasma* have a typical "fried egg" appearance, the periphery staining a light blue and the center dark blue (Figure 21-16). *Mycoplasma* almost universally show a mixed colony presentation on primary isolation when examined with a stereoscope (Figure 21-17).

A direct plate immunofluorescent (IF) method also can be used. Fluorescent-labeled anti–*M. pneumoniae* antibody is flooded on colonies on the plate; the plate is then washed and examined for immunofluorescence. Another fluorochrome method used to identify *Mycoplasma-* infected eukaryotic tissue culture is the Chen method. It uses a DNA fluorochrome stain (Hoechst 33258), which highlights *Mycoplasma* as small ovoid bodies distributed throughout the glacial acetic acid–fixed cell culture. Figure 21-18 shows Vero cells (a monkey cell line) artificially infected with *Mycoplasma orale* (Figure 21-18, *A*) and *M. salivarium* (Figure 21-18, *C*), respectively. Note the differences in morphotypes and distribution. Vero cell nuclei, which are rich in DNA, fluoresce with Hoechst 33258 stain in the negative control (Figure 21-18, *B*) as well as in the infected cell cultures. This method offers a unique way for diagnostic and clinical virology laborato-

ries to perform quality control on their continuous cell cultures, as required by the College of American Pathologists for laboratory accreditation (personal communication, Bionique Testing Laboratories, Saranac Lake, N.Y., 1993).

M. hominis requires as few as 2 days to form colonies on solid media, whereas *M. pneumoniae* may take approximately 20 days to show typical growth. The characteristic of guinea pig red blood cells (0.4%) adhering to colonies of *M. pneumoniae* and not *M. hominis* is another standard assay that helps distinguish the two species (see Table 21-19). Further, guinea pig cells do not adhere to large-colony mycoplasma, which are common inhabitants of the upper respiratory tract.

Ureaplasma colonies, once called **T-strain mycoplasma** (T for tiny), are extremely small and difficult to see with the naked eye; hence, *Mycoplasma* cultures on solid media should always be examined with a stereoscopic microscope. Figure 21-19 shows both *M. hominis* and *U. urealyticum* grown on New York City agar; the arrow points to the "tiny" ureaplasma. Urease activity of ureaplasma also may be detected on solid agar containing urea and manganese chloride (U9B urease color test medium). Urease-positive colonies are a dark golden-brown color owing to the deposition of manganese dioxide. Both *M. hominis* and *U. urealyticum* require cho-

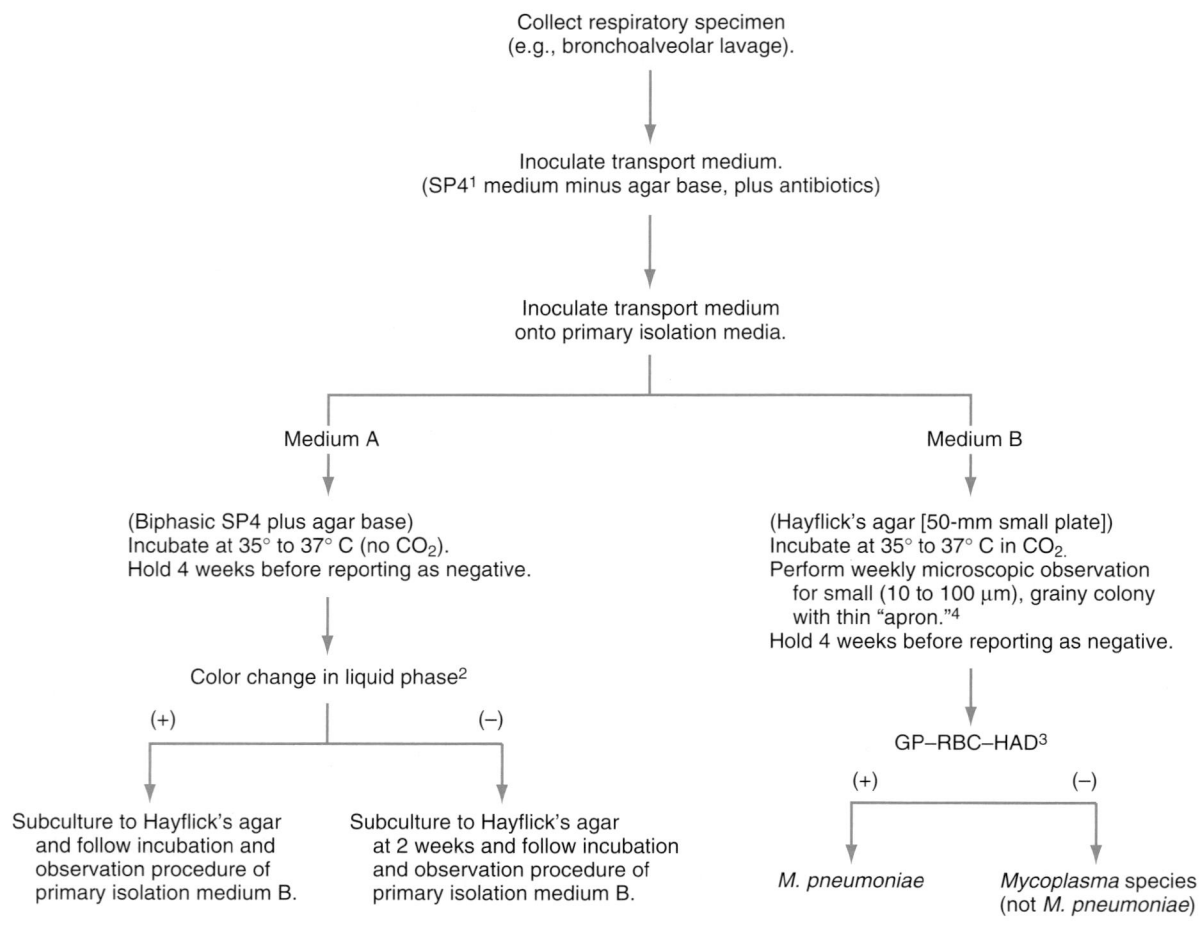

Figure 21-15

Flow diagram for *Mycoplasma* spp. isolation using classic methods.

Within the figure:

Collect respiratory specimen
(e.g., bronchoalveolar lavage).

Inoculate transport medium.
(SP4[1] medium minus agar base, plus antibiotics)

Inoculate transport medium
onto primary isolation media.

Medium A

(Biphasic SP4 plus agar base)
Incubate at 35° to 37° C (no CO_2).
Hold 4 weeks before reporting as negative.

Color change in liquid phase[2]

(+)

Subculture to Hayflick's agar
and follow incubation and
observation procedure of
primary isolation medium B.

(−)

Subculture to Hayflick's agar
at 2 weeks and follow incubation
and observation procedure of
primary isolation medium B.

Medium B

(Hayflick's agar [50-mm small plate])
Incubate at 35° to 37° C in CO_2.
Perform weekly microscopic observation
for small (10 to 100 μm), grainy colony
with thin "apron."[4]
Hold 4 weeks before reporting as negative.

GP–RBC–HAD[3]

(+)

M. pneumoniae

(−)

Mycoplasma species
(not *M. pneumoniae*)

[1]*SP4,* Sucrose phosphate buffer, *Mycoplasma* base, horse serum (20%), neutral red. Medium stabilizes and decontaminates specimen. Storage at −70° C for repeat testing is recommended.

[2]Color change: *positive,* yellow color with no gross turbidity; *negative,* red color.

[3]GP–RBC–HAD = Guinea pig red blood cell hemadsorption. β-Hemolysis test for presumptive identification of *Mycoplasma pneumoniae* may be used in lieu of GP–RBC–HAD.

[4]Thin colony periphery.

Note: Diene's stain can be used for detection of *Mycoplasma* species on Hayflick's agar; plate immunofluorescence using labeled antibody can be used for identification.

lesterol for synthesis of plasma membranes and other undetermined growth factors; horse serum (20% v/v) is the traditional source.

Although uncommon, extragenital *M. hominis* infections are emerging, and this organism should be considered whenever many PMNs are seen on Gram stain but the routine bacterial culture is ster-ile. The isolate grows well anaerobically and will appear as pinpoint (0.05 mm), clear, glistening, raised colonies on Columbia colistin–nalidixic acid (CNA) agar or anaerobic blood agar (CDC formula) in 48 hours. Under these anaerobic conditions, the colonies do not display the typical "fried egg" morphology characteristic of mycoplasma. The anaer-

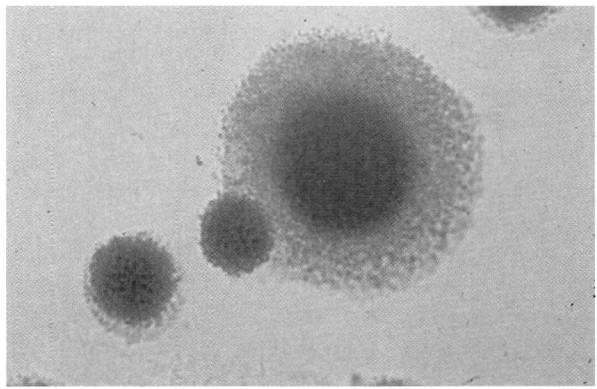

Figure 21-16 _____

Diene's stain of *Mycoplasma* spp. colonies demonstrating typical "fried egg" appearance.

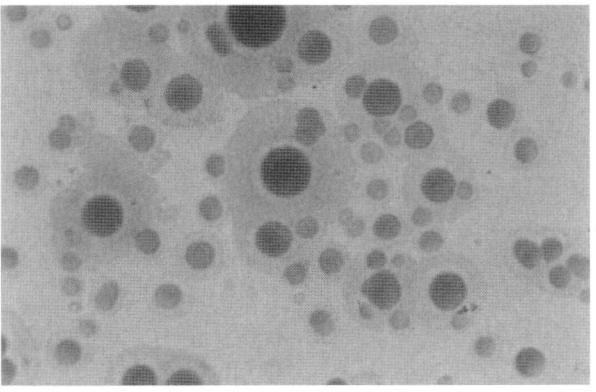

Figure 21-17 _____

Typical mixed sizes of *Mycoplasma* organisms on primary isolation media: *Mycoplasma salivarium.* (Courtesy Bionique Testing Laboratories, Saranac Lake, N.Y.)

A

B

C

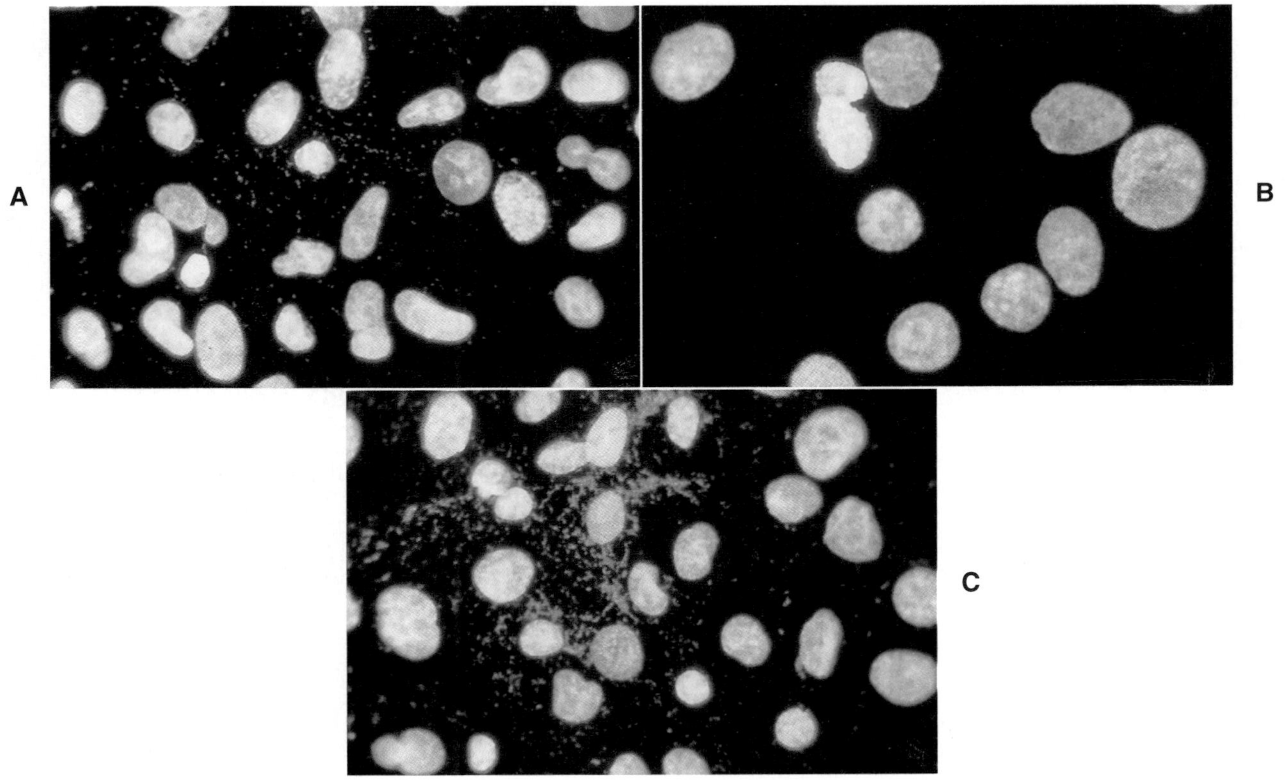

Figure 21-18 _____

Identification of *Mycoplasma*-infected eukaryotic cell culture employing DNA-fluorochrome stain (Hoechst no. 33258 stain). **A,** *Mycoplasma orale.* **B,** Uninfected Vero cell culture highlighting the DNA-rich nucleus. **C,** *Mycoplasma salivarium.* The mycoplasma appear as small pinpoint fluorescent bodies throughout the background. (Courtesy Bionique Testing Laboratories. Saranac Lake, N.Y.)

TABLE 21-19

Comparative Features of Various Laboratory Methods Used in the Detection of Mycoplasma pneumoniae, Mycoplasma hominis, *and* Ureaplasma urealyticum

Detection Method	M. pneumoniae	M. hominis	U. urealyticum
Nonserologic			
Culture	Traditional methods difficult but new "kit" formats simplify protocols	Method of choice, CNA plate, but must differentiate "infection" from "colonization"	Method of choice using urease detection, simultaneously
Indirect immunofluorescence	Respiratory antigen for early-stage infection		
	Research use only, but is promising		
Latex agglutination	Method of choice using polyclonal antibody specific for *M. pneumoniae* in respiratory exudates		
Serologic			
Cold agglutinins	Historical only > 1:16 single titer		
Complement fixation (CF)	Traditional assay *but* < 50% seroconvert; need four-fold rise between acute and convalescent sera > 1:32 single titer may be suggestive		
Indirect hemagglutination		Method of choice but need composite antigen recognizing seven serovars of *M. hominis*	
Latex agglutination	IgM/IgG		
Enzyme immunoassay (EIA)	Method of choice		
	M. pneumoniae reactive IgM, IgG, and IgA, *but* IgM may remain elevated for 1 yr	IgG only	
Immunoblot	IgM, IgG, *M. pneumoniae*-specific		
Polymerase chain reaction	Research only		

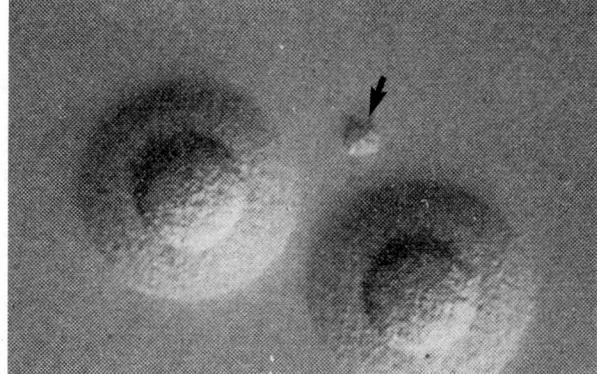

Figure 21-19

Mixed isolation of *Mycoplasma hominis* and *Ureaplasma urealyticum* showing why *U. urealyticum* was originally called "T" for "tiny-strain" *(arrow).*

obic plate should be examined using oblique light. These colonies that do not Gram stain should be subcultured to A7 medium, on which they demonstrate typical "fried egg" growth, stain positive with Dienes stain, and hydrolize arginine if they are *Mycoplasmas* (personal communication, A. William Pasculle, 1992).

Serologic Diagnosis

The cold agglutinin antibody titer has been used for many years as an indicator of primary atypical pneumonia (see Table 21-18), but it is both insensitive and nonspecific for *M. pneumoniae.* Approximately 50% of patients with primary atypical pneumonia produce a detectable cold agglutinin antibody titer.

Until recently, the most commonly used technique for demonstration of *M. pneumoniae* antibodies was micromethod complement fixation (CF), which was time consuming and had inherent technical problems. Enzyme immunoassay (EIA) and indirect hemagglutination methods (IHA) are now available for detection of serum antibodies and in some cases detect either IgM or IgG. Polymerase chain reaction (PCR) methods have been investigated and found to be very specific but are not yet commercially available. Table 21-18 highlights selected features of these immunologic assays and other methods. Detection methods were added for comparative analysis and completeness. It is important to remember that demonstration of a significant rise in antibody titer in conjunction with culture isolation is preferable for definitive diagnosis. The table also highlights another point: Given the number of assays, no one assay is optimum, although methods of choice are indicated in the table.

Serologic methods are available for *M. hominis* or *U. urealyticum,* but they are generally performed by reference laboratories only.

ANTIMICROBIAL SUSCEPTIBILITY

No agent is mycoplasmacidal for *M. pneumoniae,* but erythromycins (particularly the latest generation) and tetracycline can shorten the duration of symptoms in patients with respiratory infections. Because of side effects, tetracycline is used only for treatment of adults. *M. hominis,* which is much more resistant than *M. pneumoniae,* is usually resistant to erythromycin and susceptible to lincomycin, whereas *U. ureaplasma* is generally resistant to lincomycin and sensitive to erythromycin. Both organisms are usually sensitive to tetracycline, but some high-level resistance is emerging. Standard methods have not been developed for susceptibility testing for mycoplasma, and protocols have varied considerably from laboratory to laboratory. With reported antimicrobial resistance, newer broad-spectrum antimicrobials and new strains, such as *M. fermentans* [*incognitus* strain]; however, methods are being reevaluated. Susceptibility testing is usually recommended for clinically significant *M. hominis,* employing broth dilution; although several methods have been reported in the literature, these isolates should be forwarded to a reference laboratory.

INTERPRETATION OF LABORATORY RESULTS

Finally, a word about interpreting and reporting results for *Mycoplasma* generally and *Ureaplasma* specifically. *M. pneumoniae* detected by any method from pulmonary or nonpulmonary specimens should be considered significant and a pathogen. *M. hominis* is not as clear-cut; differentiation from colonization and infection requires detailed clinical analysis and potentially repeat cultures, given its propensity for rapid detection using anaerobic media (CNA) (i.e., within 48 hours). *U. urealyticum* is the most difficult to assess. In urogenital specimens, it has been reported to colonize up to 70% of men and 45% of women with no apparent infection. Its isolation is absolutely not indicative of pathogenicity, and it is incumbent on the laboratory to educate the physician, usually including a statement with culture results suggesting its potential for colonization versus pathogenicity. In nonurogenital specimens, particularly CSF isolates, it is reasonable to evaluate cautiously the clinical significance of ureaplasma.

Table 21-20 is a "reality check." Respiratory specimens received in the laboratory often provide limited clinical information. Specimens are processed and inoculated onto the most appro-

TABLE 21-20

Laboratory Detection of Frequent Respiratory Nonbacterial Pathogens

Epidemiologic Factors						Laboratory Methods		
Age	Age/Organism Frequently Involved	Disease	Season	Specimen Source	Strains	Culture	Noncaulture	
Newborn	1, 3	Pneumonia, aseptic work-up		Tracheal suction	Gram	Traditional, plus mycoplasmal		
Grade school	2, 3	Atypical pneumonia	Fall	Sputum	Gram, acid-fast bacillus	Traditional, plus mycoplasmal	EIA, mycoplasmal, IgM	
College student	1, 2	Biphasic disease with pharyngitis and, later, bronchitis	Spring?	Sputum	Direct FA	Cell culture, mycoplasmal	Cold agglutinin	
Adult	2, 3, 4	Pneumonia or immunocompromised		Sputum Bronchoalveolar lavage specimen	Direct FA, acid-fast bacillus Gomori methenamine silver, toluidine blue, and/or calcofluor white	Cell culture Traditional plus fungal, acid-fast bacillus	IgG, mycoplasmal	

1, Chlamydia pneumoniae (strain TWAR); 2, Mycoplasma pneumoniae (outbreak) and/or M. hominis; 3, viral (outbreak) adenovirus/RSV/influenza (seasonal); 4, other: AFB, fungus, legionnaire bacterium (LDB), or Pneumocystis carinii pneumonia (PCP).

priate media given the most likely candidate for the disease process, clinical presentation, age of patient, and seasonability, recognizing that there is a certain predictability with selected pathogens. Table 21-20 highlights a scheme in which selected stains, cultures, and nonculture techniques may be used for the detection of several pathogens: *Mycoplasma, Chlamydia,* viruses, mycobacteria, fungi, *Legionella,* and *P. carinii.* All respiratory specimens should be stored at $-70°$ C, including an acute serum. The patient would not be charged until the specimen was processed for the most likely pathogen following initial evaluation. This table complements Table 21-19.

Bibliography

Barker CE, Sillis M, Wreghitt TG: Evaluation of Serodia Myco II particle agglutination test for detecting *Mycoplasma pneumoniae* antibody: comparison with u-capture ELISA and indirect immunofluorescence, *J Clin Pathol* 43:163, 1990.

Baseman JB et al: Isolation and characterization of *Mycoplasma genitalium* strains from the human respiratory tract, *J Clin Microbiol* 26:2266, 1988.

Bernet C et al: Detection of *Mycoplasma pneumoniae* by using the polymerase chain reaction, *J Clin Microbiol* 27:2492, 1989.

Cassell GH et al: Association of *Ureaplasma urealyticum* infection of the lower respiratory tract with chronic lung disease and death in very-low-birth-weight infants, *Lancet* 2:240, 1988.

Cassell GH et al: Does *Ureaplasma urealyticum* cause respiratory disease in newborns? *Pediatr Infect Dis J* 7:535, 1988.

Cassell GH et al: *Ureaplasma urealyticum* intrauterine infection: role in prematurity and disease in newborns, *Clin Microbiol Rev* 6:69, 1993.

Cassell GH et al: Protein antigens of genital mycoplasmas, *Rev Infect Dis* 10:S391, 1988.

Chen TR: In situ detection of *Mycoplasma* contamination in cell culture by fluorescent Hoechst 33258 stain, *Exp Cell Res* 104:255, 1977.

Cunningham K: Role of genital mycoplasma in neonatal disease, *Clin Microbiol Newsl* 12:147, 1990.

Dular R, Kajioka R, Kasatiya S: Comparison of Gen-Probe commercial kit and culture technique for the diagnosis of *Mycoplasma pneumoniae* infection, *J Clin Microbiol* 26:1068, 1988.

Huovinen P et al: Pharyngitis in adults: the presence and coexistence of viruses and bacterial organisms, *Ann Intern Med* 110:612, 1989.

Kenny GE: Mycoplasmas. In Balows A, editor: *Manual of clinical microbiology,* ed 5, Washington, DC, 1991, American Society for Microbiology.

Limb DI: Mycoplasmas of the human genital tract, *Med Lab Sci* 46:146, 1989.

Lo SC et al: Virus-like infectious agent (VLIA) is a novel pathogenic mycoplasma: *Mycoplasma incognitus, Am J Trop Med Hyg* 41:586, 1989.

Mansel JK et al: *Mycoplasma pneumoniae* pneumonia, *Chest* 95:639, 1989.

Marjaana Kleemola SR, Karjalainen JE, Raty RKH: Rapid diagnosis of *Mycoplasma pneumoniae* infection: clinical evaluation of a commercial probe test, *J Infect Dis* 162:70, 1990.

Martinez OV et al: *Mycoplasma hominis* septic thrombophlebitis in a patient with multiple trauma: a case report and literature review, *Diagn Microbiol Infect Dis* 12:193, 1989.

McMahon DK et al: Extragenital *Mycoplasma hominis* infections in adults, *Am J Med* 89:275, 1990.

Moore PS et al: Respiratory viruses in *Mycoplasma* as cofactors for epidemic group A meningococcal meningitis, *JAMA* 264:1271, 1990.

Mycoplasma still putative cofactor in AIDS, *ASM News* 57:402, 1991.

Risi GF, Sanders CV: The genital mycoplasmas, *Obstet Gynecol Clin North Am* 16:611, 1989.

Sasaki T et al: Evidence that Lo's Mycoplasma *(Mycoplasma fermentans incognitus)* is not a unique strain among *Mycoplasma fermentans* strains, *J Clin Microbiol* 30:2435, 1992.

Sillis M: The limitations of IgM assays in the serological diagnosis of *Mycoplasma pneumoniae* infections, *J Med Microbiol* 33:253, 1990.

Stagno S et al: Infant pneumonitis associated with cytomegalovirus, *Chlamydia, Pneumocystis,* and *Ureaplasma:* a prospective study, *Pediatrics* 68:322, 1981.

Tilton RC et al: DNA probe versus culture for detection of *Mycoplasma pneumoniae* in clinical specimens, *Diagn Microbiol Infect Dis* 10:109, 1988.

Waites KB et al: Chronic *Ureaplasma urealyticum* and *Mycoplasma hominis* infections of central nervous system in preterm infants, *Lancet* 1:17, 1988.

Waites KB et al: Mycoplasmal infections of cerebrospinal fluid in newborn infants from a community hospital population, *Pediatr Infect Dis* 9:241, 1990.

Yajko DM et al: Evaluation of PPLO, A7B, E, and NYC agar media for the isolation of *Ureaplasma urealyticum* and *Mycoplasma* species from the genital tract, *J Clin Microbiol* 19:73, 1984.

Zahawi MF et al: A study of three blood culture media for isolating genital mycoplasmas from obstetrical and gynecologic patients, *J Infect* 21:143, 1990.

LEARNING ASSESSMENT

1. From what source did the infant described in the case study acquire the infection?

2. Was the infant infected during passage through the birth canal or in utero?

3. Would routine prenatal culture of the mother have yielded this organism?

4. Why was the Gram stain negative?

5. On what gonococcal-selective medium does this organism produce very tiny colonies?

6. What special procedure must be observed on specimens suspected of *Mycoplasma?* Why?

7. What types of culture medium are used to isolate *Mycoplasma* and *Ureaplasma* organisms?

8. Why is "cold agglutinin" titer not a useful diagnostic tool for *Mycoplasma pneumoniae?*

9. What current serologic assays are available to demonstrate *M. pneumoniae* antibodies?

10. How are *Mycoplasma* infections treated?

CHAPTER 22

Mycobacterium tuberculosis and Other Nontuberculous Mycobacteria

James L. Vossler

GENERAL CHARACTERISTICS

SAFETY CONSIDERATIONS
Personnel Safety
Proper Ventilation
Proper Use of Biologic Safety Cabinet
Use of Proper Disinfectant
Other Precautions

SPECIMEN COLLECTION AND PROCESSING
Sputum and Other Respiratory Secretions
Gastric Aspirates and Washings
Urine
Stool
Blood
Tissue and Other Body Fluids

DIGESTION AND DECONTAMINATION
OF SPECIMENS
Decontamination and Digestion Agents
Sodium hydroxide
N-acetyl-L-cysteine
Benzalkonium chloride
Oxalic acid

CONCENTRATION

STAINING FOR ACID-FAST BACILLI
Examination and Interpretation of Smears

CULTURE MEDIA AND ISOLATION METHODS
Egg-Based Media
Serum- or Agar-Based Media
Liquid Media
Other Culture Media for Recovery of Mycobacteria
Isolator Lysis-Centrifugation System

IDENTIFICATION
Laboratory Levels or Extents of Service
Identification of Mycobacteria
Colony morphology
Growth rate and recovery time
Temperature
Photoreactivity
Biochemical Identification
Niacin accumulation
Nitrate reduction
Catalase
Hydrolysis of Tween 80
Iron uptake
Arylsulfatase
Pyrazinamidase
Urease
Inhibitory tests
Slow versus rapid growth
Chromatography
Amplification for Mycobacterium tuberculosis
DNA hybridization
Serology
Susceptibility of Mycobacterium tuberculosis

MYCOBACTERIUM TUBERCULOSIS COMPLEX
Mycobacterium tuberculosis
Clinical disease: primary tuberculosis
Reactivation tuberculosis
Extrapulmonary tuberculosis
Identification of Mycobacterium tuberculosis
Treatment of tuberculosis
Mycobacterium bovis

Continued

NONTUBERCULOUS MYCOBACTERIA: CLINICAL
  SIGNIFICANCE AND DIFFERENTIATION
  Mycobacterium avium Complex
    Epidemiology
    Clinical infections
    Laboratory diagnosis
    Susceptibility testing
  Mycobacterium kansasii
    Epidemiology
    Clinical infections
    Laboratory diagnosis
  Mycobacterium fortuitum-chelonei Complex
    Mycobacterium fortuitum
    Mycobacterium chelonei
  Mycobacterium marinum
  Mycobacterium scrofulaceum
  Mycobacterium xenopi
    Mycobacterium celatum
  Mycobacterium szulgai

  Mycobacterium malmoense
  Mycobacterium simiae
  Mycobacterium ulcerans
  Mycobacterium haemophilum
  Mycobacterium gordonae
  Mycobacterium asiaticum
  Mycobacterium thermoresistibile
  Mycobacterium terrae-triviale Complex
  Mycobacterium nonchromogenicum
  Mycobacterium flavescens
  Mycobacterium smegmatis
  Mycobacterium phlei
  Mycobacterium vaccae
  Mycobacterium gastri
  Mycobacterium paratuberculosis
  Mycobacterium genavense

MYCOBACTERIUM LEPRAE

OBJECTIVES

1. Describe the general characteristics of mycobacteria, and differentiate them from other groups of organisms.
2. Discuss the safety precautions to be followed while working in a mycobacteriology laboratory.
3. Describe the appropriate specimen collection and processing procedures to recover mycobacteria from clinical samples.
4. Explain why clinical samples for mycobacterial isolation require digestion and decontamination procedures.
5. Name the different digestion reagents and their proper uses.
6. Describe the principle and procedures for the stains used to demonstrate mycobacteria in clinical samples and isolates.
7. List the different culture media used for the isolation of mycobacteria.
8. Discuss the different tests used to identify mycobacteria.
9. Describe new methods of detecting mycobacterial species in samples.
10. Discuss the clinical disease caused by *Mycobacterium tuberculosis*.
11. Discuss the clinical significance of nontuberculous mycobacteria.

KEY TERMS

Acid fastness
Nontuberculosis
   mycobacteria (NTM)
Ziehl-Neelson stain
Kinyoun stain
Auramine/auromine-
   rhodamine
   fluorochrome stains
Löwenstein-Jensen (LJ)
Middlebrook 7H10 and
   7H11 agars

Rapid growers
Photochromogens
Scotochromogens
Nonchromogenic
*Mycobacterium
   tuberculosis* complex
Mycolic acids
Pott disease
Nonphotochromogenic

The genus *Mycobacterium* comprises 71 recognized species. The most familiar of the species are *Mycobacterium tuberculosis* and *Mycobacterium leprae*, the causative agents of tuberculosis (TB) and leprosy, respectively. Both diseases have long been associated with chronic illness and social stigma. In addition to tuberculosis and leprosy, *Mycobacterium* organisms produce a spectrum of infections in humans and animals. Until 1985 the incidence of tuberculosis in the United States steadily declined, but the growing number of immunocompromised patients worldwide has led to the resurgence of tuberculosis as well as an explosion of disease caused by nontuberculous mycobacteria (NTMs). Box 22-1 shows the usual clinical significance of *Mycobacterium* species isolates.

These epidemiologic changes have led to certain challenges within the mycobacteriology laboratory, including rapid identification of all clinically significant mycobacteria and antimicrobial susceptibility testing of *Mycobacterium* species. Fortunately, new developments in the field of clinical mycobacteriology are helping to meet these challenges.

These methods may eliminate the need for lengthy culturing for isolation and protracted biochemical methods of identification. Future developments in the application of molecular biology to mycobacteriology may further diminish the time required to increase accuracy, reproducibility, rapidity, and ease of performance and allow cost containment.

This chapter discusses the following subjects:

- The general characteristics of mycobacteria
- Safety precautions that must be observed in the mycobacteriology laboratory

CASE STUDY

The patient is a 56-year-old Caucasian man who came to the emergency department with the complaints of fatigue and mild weight loss (10 lb) over the past 12 months. Upon questioning, the patient also complained of a cough for 3 months that produced white sputum with streaks of red. The patient indicated a history of night fever and chills but denied dyspnea or chest pain. The patient also had a family history of pulmonary tuberculosis from his original home in Mexico. His last PPD approximately 5 years ago was apparently negative by patient report. Vital signs included a temperature of 97.7° F, pulse of 63 beats per minute, respirations 15 per minute, and blood pressure of 96/56.

The patient received an x-ray examination of the chest that revealed infiltrate in the right upper lobe. A computer tomography scan of the chest showed nodular patchy opacity in the right upper lobe. The patient was admitted for further evaluation. A purified protein derivative test showed a 10 × 7 mm induration. Three sputum samples were obtained for acid-fast bacillus (AFB) smears and cultured. The following results were obtained:

Sputum 1: smear negative.
Sputum 2: smear negative.
Sputum 3: induced, smear negative.

Processed samples were inoculated onto Löwenstein-Jensen (LJ) media and into BACTEC 12B bottles. After 12 to 14 days of incubation the BACTEC bottles from all three specimens yielded positive results. Smears of the bottles (GI 40-60) revealed AFB by Kinyoun's CF stain. Direct polymerase chain reaction amplification for *Mycobacterium tuberculosis* of the BACTEC media yielded positive results. A four drug antituberculosis regimen of Isoniazid (INH) 300 mg qd, rifampin 600 mg qd, PZA 1 gram qd, and ethambutol 900 mg qd was recommended.

- Appropriate specimen collection and handling
- Laboratory procedures for isolation and identification of mycobacterial isolates
- Clinically significant *Mycobacterium* species and the infections they produce

Box 22-1

Usual Clinical Significance of *Mycobacterium* Species Isolates

Pathogen

Mycobacterium tuberculosis
Mycobacterium bovis
Mycobacterium ulcerans

Often pathogen, potential pathogen

Mycobacterium kansasii
Mycobacterium marinum

Potential pathogen

Mycobacterium avium complex
Mycobacterium fortuitum
Mycobacterium chelonei
Mycobacterium abscessus
Mycobacterium simiae
Mycobacterium scrofulaceum
Mycobacterium szulgai

Mycobacterium xenopi
Mycobacterium malmoense
Mycobacterium haemophilum
Mycobacterium asiaticum
Mycobacterium genavense

Usual saprophyte, rare pathogen

Mycobacterium gordonae
Mycobacterium flavescens
Mycobacterium gastri
Mycobacterium nonchromogenicum
Mycobacterium terrae
Mycobacterium triviale
Mycobacterium phlei
Mycobacterium smegmatis
Mycobacterium vaccae
Mycobacterium thermoresistibile

| GENERAL CHARACTERISTICS

Mycobacteria are slender, slightly curved or straight rod-shaped organisms 0.2 to 0.4 $\times$ 2 to 10 μm in size. They are nonmotile and do not form spores. The cell wall structure has an extremely high lipid content; thus mycobacterial cells resist staining with commonly used basic aniline dyes at room temperature. Mycobacteria do take up dye with increased staining time or application of heat; however, they resist decolorization with up to 3% hydrochloric acid, and some also resist decolorization with 95% ethanol. These characteristics, referred to as **acid fastness** and *acid-alcohol fastness,* respectively, are basic characteristics distinguishing mycobacteria from other genera and species.

Mycobacteria are strictly aerobic and grow more slowly than most bacteria pathogenic for humans. The most rapidly growing species generally grow on simple media in 2 to 3 days at temperatures of 20° to 40° C. Most mycobacteria associated with disease require 2 to 6 weeks of incubation on complex media at specific optimum temperatures. The growth of *M. tuberculosis* is enhanced by an atmosphere of 5% to 10% carbon dioxide and a growth medium with a pH of 6.5 to 6.8. One of the mycobacteria pathogenic for humans, *M. leprae,* fails to grow in vitro.

Rate of growth, colony morphology, pigmentation, nutritional requirements, optimum incubation temperature, and biochemical test results are traditional characteristics used to differentiate species within the genus *Mycobacterium.* More rapid techniques currently available include a radiometric culture system (BACTEC), which can be used for isolation, susceptibility testing, and distinguishing *M. tuberculosis* from the nontuberculous mycobacteria using a selective growth inhibitor. Additionally, a limited number of species-specific nucleic acid probes offer rapid identification of culture isolates. Researchers have developed polymerase chain reaction (PCR) assays, which increase the sensitivity of nucleic acid probes. Other techniques, such as thin-layer chromatography, gas-liquid chromatography, and, more recently, high-performance liquid chromatography have been used to distinguish mycobacterial species. The application of PCR and chromatography methods has slowly moved out of the research and larger reference mycobacteriology laboratories to routine laboratories and are being increasingly adopted by clinical laboratories.

SAFETY CONSIDERATIONS

The serious nature of tuberculosis disease and the usual airborne route of infection require that special safety precautions be used by anyone handling mycobacterial specimens. The incidence of tuberculosis infection (i.e., skin test positivity) in those who work in the mycobacteriology laboratory is at least three times higher than among other laboratory personnel in a given institution. The hazard of working in a mycobacteriology laboratory is, however, minimal when the laboratory is well designed, appropriate equipment is available, and precautions are followed closely.

Personnel Safety

The administration of the microbiology laboratory must ensure that each employee is (1) provided with adequate safety equipment, (2) trained in safe laboratory procedures, (3) informed of the hazards associated with the procedures, (4) prepared for action following an unexpected accident, and (5) monitored regularly by medical personnel. Laboratory personnel must be responsible for using appropriate safety equipment and following established procedures. The laboratory worker should maintain optimal health. A skin test (Mantoux test) with purified protein derivative (PPD) of tuberculin should be administered the first day of employment and thereafter regularly to persons previously skin test negative (nonreactors). Individuals known to be previously skin test positive (reactors) should be counseled regularly and referred for medical evaluation if their health status changes.

Proper Ventilation

Laboratory design and ventilation play an important role in mycobacteriology laboratory safety. Ideally, the mycobacteriology laboratory should be separate from the remainder of the laboratory and have a nonrecirculating ventilation system. The area in which specimens and cultures are processed should have negative air pressure in relation to other areas; that is, the airflow should be from clean areas, such as corridors, into less clean areas. Six to 12 room air changes per hour effectively remove 99% or more of airborne particles within 30 to 45 minutes. A much higher number of room air changes per hour may cause problems of air turbulence within the biologic safety cabinets.

Proper Use of Biologic Safety Cabinet

Because the route of infection by mycobacteria is primarily through inhalation, it is essential that the dispersal of organisms into the air be minimized and that inhalation of airborne bacilli be avoided. The biologic safety cabinet is the single most important piece of equipment in a mycobacteriology laboratory. Various types of biologic safety cabinets are available, including Class I negative-pressure cabinets and Class II vertical-laminar-flow cabinets. Proper installation, maintenance, and testing are essential to their performance. Each cabinet should be tested and recertified at least yearly by trained personnel with special monitoring equipment. Processing raw specimens or transferring viable cultures outside a safety cabinet should not be permitted.

Ultraviolet (UV) light kills microorganisms. After the safety cabinet work area has been cleaned with disinfectant, the UV light inside the cabinet should be used to further eliminate contamination of surfaces and airborne bacteria. Because of the hazards to skin and eyes associated with excess UV light, the UV light should be turned on only when the cabinet is not in use.

Use of Proper Disinfectant

To prevent the dispersal of infectious aerosols into the laboratory area, all potentially infectious materials should be tightly covered when outside the biologic safety cabinet. Specimens should be centrifuged in aerosol-free safety carriers, and the tubes should be removed from the safety carriers only inside the biologic safety cabinet. Covering the work surface with a towel or absorbent pad soaked in a phenolic disinfectant reduces the accidental creation of infectious aerosols. Specimens taken out of the safety cabinet for transport to a decontamination area must be covered.

In the selection of a disinfectant for the mycobacteriology laboratory, the product brochure should be consulted to make certain that the disinfectant is bactericidal for mycobacteria (tuberculocidal). The following types of disinfectants are suitable for cleaning work areas, but some have limitations on their use.

- **Phenol-soap mixtures** containing orthophenol or other phenolic derivatives are effective with contact periods of 10 to 30 minutes.
- **Sodium hypochlorite** is effective at a concentration of 0.1% to 0.5% (e.g., a 1:50 to 1:10 dilution of most household bleaches). The solution should be made fresh daily, and contact time should be 10 to 30 minutes. Sodium hypochlorite loses effectiveness in the presence of a large amount of protein material.
- **Formaldehyde,** 3% to 8%, or alkaline glutaraldehyde, 2%, is effective. Contact time should be at least 30 minutes.
- **Phenol,** 5%, with a contact time of 10 to 30 minutes is adequate. Phenol is irritating to the skin and hazardous to the eyes.

Other Precautions

For sterilizing a wire inoculating loop, an electric incinerator should be used within the biologic safety cabinet. An alcohol-sand flask can also be used to clean the waxy culture material from the wire before flaming in a Bunsen burner. Disposable sterile applicator sticks or plastic transfer loops are convenient and efficient for making smears and transfers. Splashproof discard containers must be used to prevent aerosol formation and possible cross-contamination of samples.

Protective clothing provides extra safety for the individual working in the mycobacteriology laboratory. Gloves and laboratory coats or gowns are essential. Face masks or respirators are recommended. Some laboratory directors believe that caps and shoe covers should also be worn.

SPECIMEN COLLECTION AND PROCESSING

Mycobacteria may be recovered from a variety of clinical specimens, including respiratory specimens, urine, feces, blood, cerebrospinal fluid (CSF), tissue biopsies, and aspirations of any tissue or organ. Thus successful isolation of mycobacteria from clinical specimens begins with properly collected and handled specimens. Whenever possible, diagnostic specimens should be collected before the initiation of therapy. All specimens should be transported to the laboratory and ideally should be processed as soon as possible after collection. If immediate transport is not possible, the specimen should be refrigerated, but no longer than overnight. Delays in processing lead to false-negative cultures and increased bacterial contamination.

Each specimen should be confined to a single collection in an individual collection container recommended by the laboratory that is to provide the requested diagnostic service. The most commonly recommended containers are a sterile, wide-mouth jar with tightly fitted screw-cap lid and a sterile, disposable (nonpolystyrene), 50-mL centrifuge tube with a leakproof screw-cap lid. Special receptacles containing a 50-mL centrifuge tube for sputum collection are available commercially.

The spectrum of illness caused by *Mycobacterium* spp. is so broad that almost any site may yield an acceptable specimen. Each specimen type, even when properly collected, transported, and processed, may have an intrinsic maximal yield. This can be the result of tubercle burden at the collection site or of environmental effects such as pH that may affect recovery. Emphasis should be placed on collecting the number and types of specimens that, when transported and processed correctly, maximize the diagnostic yield. Box 22-2 lists the types of clinical samples acceptable for mycobacteriologic culture.

Sputum and Other Respiratory Secretions

Although a variety of clinical specimens may be submitted to the laboratory to recover *M. tuberculosis* (MTB) and nontuberculous mycobacteria (NTM), respiratory secretions, such as sputum and bronchial aspirates, are the most common. The number of specimens necessary to obtain culture confirmation and perform susceptibility testing is related to the frequency of smear positivity. According to Bates (1979), "When at least two of the first three sputum smears are positive, then three specimens usually are enough to confirm the diagnosis. If none, or only one of the first three sputum smears is positive, a larger number of specimens is needed for culture confirmation." Smear positivity and culture yield vary with the extent of the disease (i.e., whether there is cavitary or noncavitary pulmonary disease or endobronchial or laryngeal disease).

Box 22-2

Acceptable Specimens for Processing

Respiratory specimens

Spontaneously expectorated sputum
Normal saline–nebulized, induced sputum
Transtracheal aspirate
Bronchoalveolar lavage
Bronchoalveolar brushing
Laryngeal swab
Nasopharyngeal swab

Body fluids

Pleural fluid
Pericardial fluid
Joint aspirate
Gastric aspirate

Peritoneal fluid
Cerebrospinal fluid
Stool
Urine
Pus

Body tissues

Blood
Bone marrow biopsy/aspirate
Solid organ
Lymph node
Bone
Skin

The sputum samples should be 5- to 10-mL samples produced by a deep cough or expectorated sputum induced by inhalation of an aerosol of hypertonic saline. When sputum is not obtainable, bronchoscopy may be performed, at which time samples such as bronchial washing, bronchoalveolar lavage (BAL), or transbronchial biopsy specimens are obtained. Brushings appear to be more commonly diagnostic than washing or biopsy. This may be the result of an inhibitory effect on the mycobacteria of the volumes of lidocaine used in adults during bronchoscopy or of dilution of the specimen with saline. Often, patients are able to produce sputum for several days after bronchoscopy; these samples should be collected and examined.

Gastric Aspirates and Washings

Gastric aspirates are used to recover mycobacteria that may have been swallowed during the night. Use of this type of specimen should only be used for patients who fail to produce sputum by aerosol induction, children under 3 years of age, and nonambulatory individuals. Children with primary pulmonary tuberculosis typically have closed caseous lesions with relatively small numbers of organisms, resulting in a low yield from analysis of sputum. Abadco and colleagues (1992)

have suggested that gastric lavage is better than bronchoalveolar lavage for the detection of mycobacteria in children. They reported that a bacteriologic diagnosis of childhood pulmonary TB could be made in 10% versus 50%, respectively, when BAL was compared with three morning gastric lavage specimens. This has not appeared to be the case in adults. Gastric lavage may offer a diagnostic alternative only in those unable to expectorate sputum and in whom BAL might be contraindicated. Gastric aspirates should be obtained in the morning after an overnight fast. Three specimens should be collected within 3 days. Sterile water, 30 to 60 mL, is instilled either orally or via nasogastric tube aspiration. Prolonged exposure to gastric acid kills mycobacteria and diminishes culture yield. Specimen processing should be done expeditiously, or the specimen should be neutralized with sodium carbonate or another buffer salt to pH 7.0.

Urine

For examination of urine a first morning midstream specimen is preferred. The entire volume of voided urine, or a minimum of 15 mL, is collected in a sterile container. A specimen may be collected through an indwelling catheter with a sterile needle and syringe. Urine specimens should be refrigerated during the interval between collection and processing; specimens should be processed promptly.

As a general rule, pooled specimens collected over 12 to 24 hours are not recommended. Such specimens are more subject to contamination and may contain fewer viable tubercle bacilli.

Stool

Examination of stool specimens for the presence of acid-fast organisms can be useful in identifying patients (such as individuals with AIDS) who may be at risk for developing disseminated mycobacterial disease resulting from *Mycobacterium avium* complex (MAC). Frequently, the number of organisms found in the bowel in these patients is quite high, although it has been reported that 68% of MAC culture-positive stool specimens are acid-fast smear negative. Stool specimens should be collected in clean containers without any preservative and sent directly to the laboratory for processing. If processing within a few hours is not possible, the specimen should be kept frozen at $-20°$ C until processing time. Culture of feces for mycobacteria from patients other than those with or at risk for AIDS is usually not warranted.

Blood

Mycobacteremia, once considered rare, is now often seen in patients with AIDS but less frequently in other immunocompromised hosts. A majority of the infections are caused by MAC. Recovery of the organism from blood is associated with clinical disease. The Isolator lysis-centrifugation system (Wampole Laboratories, Cranbury, N.J.) or direct inoculation of blood into BACTEC 13A Medium (Becton Dickinson Diagnostic Instrument Systems, Towson, Md.) have been shown to be effective for the collection and culture of blood samples. The two collection systems have been considered equivalent, although the isolator system allows for quantitative analysis, which may be used to monitor therapy and evaluate prognosis.

Tissue and Other Body Fluids

At times, tissue and other body fluids may be needed for microscopic examination and culture. Whenever possible, CSF specimens should be from large-volume spinal taps to increase diagnostic yield. Diagnosis of tuberculous meningitis is extremely difficult. Peritoneal (ascitic fluid) smears are also rarely positive for acid-fast bacilli. Culture of large volumes and collection of the specimen into BACTEC bottles or other mycobacterial liquid media may help maximize yield in this and other dilute specimens.

When noninvasive techniques have failed to provide a diagnosis, surgical procedures may need to be considered. Specimens may need to be obtained from the lung, pericardium, lymph nodes, bones, joints, bowel, or liver. The tissue or fluid should be collected aseptically and placed in a sterile container. If the tissue is not processed immediately, a small amount (10 to 15 mL) of sterile saline should be added to prevent dehydration. It may be necessary to collect fluid containing fibrinogen (e.g., pleural, pericardial, peritoneal) into a container with an anticoagulant. The amount of fluids recommended for culture varies—2 mL for cerebrospinal fluid, 3 to 5 mL for exudates and pericardial and synovial fluids, and 10 to 15 mL for abdominal and chest fluids. Immediate processing of these samples is important. When tissue is collected, histologic evaluation may reveal caseating or noncaseating granuloma formation with the presence of multinucleated giant cells. These histologic changes are consistent with but not specific for mycobacterial disease.

DIGESTION AND DECONTAMINATION OF SPECIMENS

To ensure optimal recovery of mycobacteria from clinical specimens, many specimens must be processed before inoculation onto culture media. Each step must be carried out with precision. Specimens from sterile body sites must be simply concentrated (if a large volume) and inoculated. However, specimens that may contain commensalistic bacteria should be decontaminated and concentrated.

Most clinical specimens, such as sputum, contain mucin or organic debris that surround the bacteria within the sample. An abundance of nonmycobacterial organisms, as well as possible mycobacteria, make up the microflora of these specimens. When placed into culture medium, the abundant nonmycobacterial organisms can quickly overgrow the more slowly growing mycobacteria. The purposes of the digestion-decontamination process are (1) to liquefy the sample through digestion of the proteinaceous material and (2) to allow the chemical decontaminating agent to contact and kill the nonmycobacterial organisms. The high lipid content in the cell walls of mycobacteria makes them somewhat less susceptible to the killing action of various chemicals. With liquefaction of the specimen the surviving mycobacteria can be concentrated with centrifugation. Additionally, liquefying the mucin enables the mycobacteria to contact and use the nutrients of the medium to which they are subsequently inoculated.

Specimens that contain mucus and require both digestion and decontamination are sputum, gastric washing, bronchoalveolar lavage, bronchial washing, and transtracheal aspirate. Voided urine, autopsy tissue, abdominal fluid, and any fluid known to be contaminated require decontamination. Specimens from normally sterile sites, such as blood, CSF, synovial fluid, and biopsy tissue from deep organs, do not require decontamination. Sterility should be strictly maintained in collection and transport. Stool decontamination is especially difficult and may require repeated attempts at decontamination.

Decontamination and Digestion Agents

Each laboratory should maintain a proper balance between rate of recovery of mycobacteria and the suppression of contaminating growth. Failure to isolate mycobacteria from patients with signs and symptoms of classic mycobacterial disease may indicate that the decontamination is too harsh. On the other hand, if more than 5% of all specimens cultured are contaminated, the decontamination procedure may be inadequate. The bactericidal action of a decontaminating agent is influenced by the concentration of the chemical agent, exposure time, and temperature; therefore alterations in any of these factors may increase or decrease the bactericidal effect. In general, a range that is considered acceptable in this delicate balance is between 2% and 5% of bacterially contaminated mycobacterial cultures.

The optimal decontamination procedure requires an agent that is mild and yields growth of mycobacteria while controlling contaminants. The use of selective or antibiotic-treated media may diminish the need for harsh decontamination procedures.

Sodium hydroxide

Sodium hydroxide (NaOH), usual concentration 2%, 3%, or 4%, serves as both a digestant and a decontaminating agent. It must be used with caution because it is only slightly less harmful to the mycobacteria than to the contaminating organisms.

N-acetyl-L-cysteine

A combination of a liquefying agent, such as N-acetyl-L-cysteine (NALC) or dithiothreitol, and sodium hydroxide is commonly used. The liquefying agent has no inhibitory effect on bacterial cells; however, liquefaction of the sample allows the decontaminating chemical to come into uniform contact with the contaminating bacteria more readily. When contamination can be controlled with a lower concentration of sodium hydroxide, the recovery of mycobacteria is indirectly improved using the milder procedure, because fewer mycobacteria are lost in the process.

Procedure 22-1 describes NALC-NaOH digestion and decontamination.

Benzalkonium chloride

Another digestant-decontamination procedure uses benzalkonium chloride (Zephiran) combined with trisodium phosphate (Z-TSP). Trisodium phosphate liquefies sputum rapidly but requires long exposure to decontaminate the specimen. Benzalkonium chloride shortens the exposure time and effectively destroys many contaminants, with little bactericidal effect on the tubercle bacilli.

The addition of phosphate buffer to digested specimens results in greater isolation of mycobacteria. Zephiran is bacteriostatic for tubercle bacilli, necessitating either neutralization before planting or use of egg-based media to exploit its inherent neutralizing capacity.

Oxalic acid

Oxalic acid, 5%, is used to decontaminate specimens contaminated with *Pseudomonas aeruginosa,* such as sputum specimens from patients with cystic fibrosis.

PART II · Laboratory Identification of Significant Isolates

PROCEDURE 22-1. NALC-Sodium Hydroxide (NALC-NaOH) Digestion-Decontamination

Principle

Sodium hydroxide (NaOH) acts as both a decontaminating agent and a digestant. Because of the toxicity NaOH has on mycobacteria, the agent should be used at the lowest concentration available. N-acetyl-L-cysteine (NALC) is a mucolytic agent, which allows for a lower concentration of NaOH to be used and thereby optimizes the recovery of mycobacteria from the specimen.

Reagents

NALC-NaOH digestant: Combine equal volumes of 2.94% sodium citrate dihydrate (= 0.1 M) and 4% sodium hydroxide (NaOH). Just before use, add 0.5 g of powdered NALC per 100 mL of mixture. Refrigerate when not in use; discard after 24 hours.

Phosphate buffer, 0.067 M, pH 6.8, or water, sterile, distilled, 30 to 40 mL per specimen.

Bovine albumin fraction V, 0.2% in saline, sterile.

Procedure

1. Working within the biologic safety cabinet, transfer 10 mL (or total specimen if volume is less than 10 mL) to 50-mL screw-cap centrifuge tube. If specimen volume is greater than 10 mL, select most purulent-appearing material. Add an equal volume of NALC-NaOH digestant to each sample.

2. Tighten caps and mix on a test tube mixer until liquefied (5 to 20 seconds per tube), inverting each tube to ensure that NALC-NaOH solution contacts any untreated particles on the upper part of the tube.

3. Let tubes stand at room temperature for 15 minutes. If more decontamination is de-sired, increase the concentration of NaOH rather than the time the specimen is exposed to the digestion-decontamination mixture.

4. Dilute the digested-decontaminated specimens to the 50-mL mark with sterile distilled water or sterile phosphate buffer to minimize the continuing action of the NaOH and lower the specific gravity of the specimen. Tighten caps and invert or swirl to mix.

5. Centrifuge at 3000 g for 15 minutes (or the appropriate combination of relative centrifugal force and time to give 95% sedimentation) using aerosol-free safety cups or in an aerosol-controlled vented centrifuge.

6. Holding the tube so that the sediment is on the upper side of the tube, pour off supernatant into a splashproof discard container of disinfectant.

7. Holding the tube in a horizontal position to keep the sediment as dry as possible, use a sterile applicator stick to remove a small part of the sediment and place it on a marked microscope slide. The smear should be about 1 × 2 cm.

8. Resuspend sediment in 1 to 2 mL of sterile 0.2% bovine albumin solution. If media will be inoculated immediately, the sediment may be resuspended in sterile water or sterile saline.

9. An optional step is to prepare a 1:10 dilution using 0.5 mL of the resuspended sediment in 4.5 mL of sterile water. Dilution decreases the concentration of toxic substances that may inhibit growth of mycobacteria. Inoculate diluted and undiluted specimens to solid media.

CONCENTRATION

The specific gravity of the tubercle bacilli ranges from 1.07 to 0.79. Because of the low specific gravity of the acid-fast bacilli, a low centrifugal force has a buoyant rather than sedimenting effect. Excess mucus will compound this effect. Treatment with mucolytic agents such as NALC splits mucoprotein, allowing greater sedimentation. Kent and Kubica (1985) suggest that a 95% sedimenting efficiency should be the goal for recovery. Therefore concentration centrifugation speeds must be at least 3000 g to maximize recovery.

Lower g force necessitates longer centrifuge time. The consequences of longer centrifuge time are prolonged exposure to the toxic effects of both the digestion-decontamination agents used and the higher temperatures generated by unrefrigerated centrifuges. Alternatives to high-speed centrifugation concentration have been explored. In summary, the digestion-decontamination agent used, its concentration, the length of exposure of the agent to the specimen, and the centrifugation speed and temperature all affect the recovery of *Mycobacterium* species.

STAINING FOR ACID-FAST BACILLI

When Gram stained *Mycobacterium* spp. stain faintly or not at all, giving a beaded appearance because of irregular uptake of the stain and the increased lipid content of the cell wall of *Mycobacterium* organisms. Acid-fast smears are prepared from digested, decontaminated, and concentrated specimens.

The conventional acid-fast staining methods, **Ziehl-Neelsen** and **Kinyoun stain,** use carbolfuchsin solutions for the primary stain, acid-alcohol as a decolorizing agent, and a methylene blue counterstain. The Ziehl-Neelsen staining procedure involves the application of heat with the carbolfuchsin stain, whereas the Kinyoun acid-fast stain is a cold stain. Slides are examined using a 100× oil immersion objective on a light microscope for 15 minutes, viewing a minimum of 300 fields before a slide is called negative.

The **auramine or auramine-rhodamine fluorochrome stains** are more sensitive than the carbolfuchsin stains. Approximately 18% of all culture-positive specimens had smears that were positive on auramine-rhodamine stain but negative on Kinyoun or Ziehl-Neelsen stain. In addition, smears may be screened at a lower magnification (250× to 400×), thus allowing for more fields to be examined in a shorter time frame. A fluorescence microscope equipped with an appropriate filter system is needed for the examination of a fluorochrome-stained smear. The smear is examined under a mercury vapor lamp with a strong blue filtered light. Positive stains reveal bright yellow-orange bacilli against a dark background.

Examination and Interpretation of Smears

Smears being examined for acid-fast organisms should be carefully examined with a minimum of 300 fields (examine three horizontal sweeps of a smear that is 2 cm long and 1 cm wide). Individuals with extensive disease shed large numbers of organisms. However, many individuals have subtle infections wherein less organisms will be shed. Thus the overall sensitivity of the acid-fast smear varies from 20% to 80% depending on the extent of the infection. Even with concentration techniques the number of organisms observed on a smear will be considerably less than organisms seen on an individual with bacterial pneumonia. The U.S. Department of Health and Human Services has made recommendations regarding the interpretation and reporting of acid-fast smears (Box 22-3).

Because of the potential cross contamination of acid-fast bacilli from one smear to another, careful attention should be paid to the staining technique. Staining jars should not be employed. Smears should not come in contact with one another or should be air dried or blotted.

In the interpretation of a smear as positive for acid-fast organisms, laboratory professionals must realize that organisms other than *Mycobacterium* may stain at least partially acid fast. *Nocardia* sp., *Legionella micdadei,* and *Rhodococcus* sp. may all appear acid fast.

CULTURE MEDIA AND ISOLATION METHODS

Mycobacteria are strictly aerobic and grow more slowly than most bacteria pathogenic for humans. The generation time of the mycobacteria is more

Box 22-3

Acid-Fast Smear Interpretation

Carbolfuchsin stain: # acid-fast bacilli seen (1000×)	Fluorochrome stain: # acid-fast bacilli seen (450×)	Quantitative report
0	0	No acid-fast bacilli seen
1-2/300 fields	1-2/70 fields	Doubtful acid-fast bacilli seen; resubmit another specimen for examination
1-9/100 fields	1-2/70 fields	1+
1-9/10 fields	2-18/50 fields	2+
1-9/fields	4-36/fields	3+
>9/fields	>36/fields	4+

Modified from Kent PT, Kubica GP: *Public health myco-bacteriology: a guide for the level III laboratory,* Atlanta, 1985, U.S. Department of Health and Human Service, Public Health Service, Centers for Disease Control.

than 12 hours; *M. tuberculosis* has the longest replication time at 20 to 22 hours. The most rapidly growing species generally grows on simple media in 2 to 3 days at temperatures of 20° to 40° C. Most mycobacteria associated with disease require 2 to 6 weeks of incubation on complex media at specific optimum temperatures. The growth of *M. tuberculosis* is enhanced by an atmosphere of CO_2 between 5% and 10% for the few first weeks of incubation. Mycobacteria require a pH between 6.5 and 6.8 for the growth medium and grow better at higher humidity. One of the mycobacteria pathogenic for humans, *Mycobacterium genavense,* grows in a very limited manner, whereas another, *M. leprae,* fails to grow in vitro.

The many different media available for the recovery of mycobacteria from a clinical specimen are variations of three general types (Table 22-1): egg-based medium, serum albumin agar medium, and liquid medium. Within each general type, there are nonselective formulations and formulations that have been made selective by the addition of antimicrobial agents. Because some isolates do not grow on a particular agar and each type of culture medium offers certain advantages, a combination of culture media is generally recommended for primary isolation. The use of a solid-based medium, such as **Löwenstein-Jensen (LJ),** in combination with a liquid-based medium (such as BACTEC broth, MGIT broth [Becton Dickinson, Cockeysville,

Md.]) is recommended for routine culturing of specimens for the recovery of acid-fast bacilli.

Egg-Based Media

The basic ingredients in an inspissated egg medium, such as LJ, Petragnani, and American Thoracic Society (ATS) media, are fresh whole eggs, potato flour, and glycerol, with slight variations in defined salts, milk, and potato (see Table 22-1). Each contains malachite green to suppress the growth of gram-positive bacteria. LJ medium is most commonly used in clinical laboratories. Selective media that contain antibiotics, such as Gruft modification of LJ and Mycobactosel (Becton Dickinson Microbiology Systems, Cockeysville, Md.), are sometimes used in combination with nonselective media to increase isolation of mycobacteria from contaminated specimens. The nonselective egg-based media have a long shelf-life of 1 year, but distinguishing early growth from debris is sometimes difficult.

Serum- or Agar-Based Media

Serum albumin agar media, such as **Middlebrook 7H10 and 7H11 agars,** are prepared from a basal medium of defined salts, vitamins, cofactors, glycerol, malachite green, and agar combined with an enrichment consisting of oleic acid, bovine albumin, glucose, and beef catalase (Middlebrook OADC enrichment). Middlebrook 7H11 also contains 0.1% casein hydrolysate, which improves recovery of isoniazid-resistant strains of *M. tuberculosis.* The addition of antimicrobial agents to either 7H10 or 7H11 makes the medium more selective by suppressing the growth of contaminating bacteria. Mitchison's selective 7H11 contains polymyxin B, amphotericin B, carbenicillin, and trimethoprim lactate (see Table 22-1).

In contrast to opaque egg-based media, clear agar-based media can be examined using a dissecting microscope for early detection of growth and colony morphology. Drug susceptibility tests may be performed on agar-based media without the alteration of drug concentrations that occurs with egg-based media. When specimens are inoculated to Middlebrook 7H10 and 7H11 media and

incubated in an atmosphere of 10% carbon dioxide and 90% air, 99% of the positive cultures are detected in 3 to 4 weeks, earlier than for those detected on egg-based media.

Certain precautions should be followed in the preparation, storage, and incubation of Middlebrook media. Excess heat and exposure of the prepared media to light can both result in the release of formaldehyde, which is toxic to mycobacterial growth.

Liquid Media

Mycobacterium spp. grow more rapidly in liquid media. Middlebrook 7H9 broth is a nonselective liquid medium used for subculturing stock strains,

TABLE 22-1

Mycobacterial Culture Media

Medium	Composition	Inhibitory Agents
American Thoracic Society (ATS)	Fresh whole eggs, potato flour, glycerol	Malachite green (0.02%)
Löwenstein-Jensen (LJ)	Fresh whole eggs, defined salts, glycerol, potato flour	Malachite green (0.025%)
Petragnani	Fresh whole eggs, egg yolks, whole milk, potato, potato flour, glycerol	Malachite green (0.052%)
Middlebrook 7H10	Defined salts, vitamins, cofactors, oleic acid, albumin, catalase, glycerol, glucose	Malachite green (0.00025%)
Middlebrook 7H11	Defined salts, vitamins, cofactors, oleic acid, albumin, catalase, glycerol, 0.1% casein hydrolysate	Malachite green (0.0001%)
Middlebrook 7H9, 7H12 (BACTEC 12B)	Broth base, casein hydrolysate, bovine serum albumin, catalase, C-14–labeled palmitic acid, deionized water	Polymyxin B Amphotericin B Nalidixic acid Trimethoprim Azlocillin
Middlebrook 7H9, 7H13 (BACTEC 13A)	Broth base, casein hydrolysate, bovine serum albumin, catalase, C-14–labeled palmitic acid, SPS, polysorbate 80	Polymyxin B Amphotericin B Nalidixic acid Deionized water Trimethoprim Azlocillin
Gruft (modification of LJ)	Fresh whole eggs, defined salts, glycerol, potato flour, RNA	Malachite green Penicillin Nalidixic acid
Mycobactosel (BBL) LJ	Fresh whole eggs, defined salts, glycerol, potato flour	Malachite green Cycloheximide Lincomycin Nalidixic acid
Middlebrook 7H10 (selective)	Defined salts, vitamins, cofactors, oleic acid, albumin, catalase, glycerol, glucose	Malachite green Cycloheximide Lincomycin Nalidixic acid
Mitchison's selective 7H11	Defined salts, vitamins, cofactors, oleic acid, albumin, catalase, glycerol, glucose, casein, hydrolysate	Carbenicillin Amphotericin B Polymyxin B Trimethoprim lactate

SPS, Sodium polyanethol sulfonate; *RNA,* ribonucleic acid.

picking single colonies, and preparing inoculum for in vitro testing.

The most sensitive and rapid primary isolation liquid media are Middlebrook 7H12 and 7H13 (BACTEC 12B and 13B Becton Dickinson Diagnostic Instruments Systems, Towson, Md.). The BACTEC system is an automated radiometric culture system for detecting the growth of *Mycobacterium* spp.

The BACTEC broth contains a ^{14}C-labeled substrate (palmitic acid) that is metabolized by mycobacteria, liberating radioactive carbon dioxide ($^{14}CO_2$) into the headspace of the vial. The amount of $^{14}CO_2$ liberated is detected by the BACTEC 460 instrument and interpreted as a "growth index." It is assumed that the release of CO_2 denotes growth of the organism.

The recommended inoculum for the BACTEC 12B 4-mL vial is 0.5 mL of decontaminated concentrated specimen. Antibiotics supplied by the manufacturer—polymyxin B, amphotericin B, nalidixic acid, trimethoprim, and azlocillin (PANTA) reconstituted into polyoxyethylene stearate, a growth-enhancing agent—are added to each vial at the time of inoculation. The Middlebrook 7H13 medium (BACTEC 13B) was introduced for the culturing of larger volumes of blood or bone marrow. Its components are similar to those of the BACTEC 12B vial except that an anticoagulant, sodium polyanethol sulfonate (SPS), and polysorbate 80 have been added. Five milliliters of blood may be added directly to this 30-mL vial.

A number of studies have shown that the radiometric BACTEC isolation method significantly improves the isolation rate of mycobacteria and reduces the recovery time compared with conventional isolation media. The BACTEC vials should be read within 4 days of inoculation. Negative vials should be retested every 3 to 4 days for the first 2 weeks and then once weekly for the remaining 6 weeks. With the BACTEC method, mycobacteria may be detected in clinical specimens in less than 2 weeks.

In general, the time required for isolation and identification of *M. tuberculosis* is reduced from 6 weeks to 3 weeks. The time in which the radiometric system will detect growth reflects the quantity of viable *Mycobacterium* species in the submitted sample, which is indirectly reflected by smear positivity.

In smear-positive samples, *M. tuberculosis* may

be detected as early as 7 to 8 days and *M. avium* as early as 5 to 8 days. In smear-negative samples, MTB and mycobacteria other than *[M.] tuberculosis* (MOTT) are usually detected in 14 to 28 days and 8 to 12 days, respectively, by the BACTEC system. These detection times are an obvious improvement in the recovery time from conventional media. In conventional agar cultures, recovery from smear-positive TB specimens may require 16 days, and from smear-negative specimens, 26 days. By the end of the fourth week, 96.8% of all effectual positives will have been detected, and by the end of the fifth week, 98.8%. The greater sensitivity of the BACTEC system has resulted in a higher yield from smear-negative specimens.

The disadvantage of the BACTEC system is that when the BACTEC vial is positive before a companion agar or egg medium culture, no colony morphology or pigmentation appears to suggest that the growth is of a mycobacterial species other than tuberculosis. The BACTEC system also may not be as good in recovery of all species of *Mycobacterium,* specifically *Mycobacterium fortuitum* and *M. avium* complex. False-positive results from cross-contamination have been reported.

The BACTEC system can also be used for the antimicrobial susceptibility testing of *M. tuberculosis.* Currently, it is not recommended for sensitivity testing of MOTT. Automated, nonradiometric microbial detection systems designed for the recovery of mycobacteria from clinical specimens are also available. These include the Mycobacterial Growth Indicator Tube (MGIT) System (BBL, Becton Dickinson Microbiology Systems, Hunt Valley, Md.), the MB/BACT System (Organon Teknika, Durham, N.C.), and the ESP MYCO Culture System (Difco, Detroit, Mich.).

Other Culture Media for Recovery of Mycobacteria

A chocolate agar plate should be included in the primary isolation media for skin and other body surface specimens for the recovery of *Mycobacterium haemophilum,* which requires hemoglobin or hemin for growth. The plate should be incubated at 30° C, the optimum temperature for recovery of this organism and for *Mycobacterium marinum.*

A biphasic media system for the detection and isolation of mycobacteria, Septi-Chek AFB, is available commercially (BBL Septi-Chek AFB, Becton Dickinson Microbiology Systems, Cockeysville, Md.)

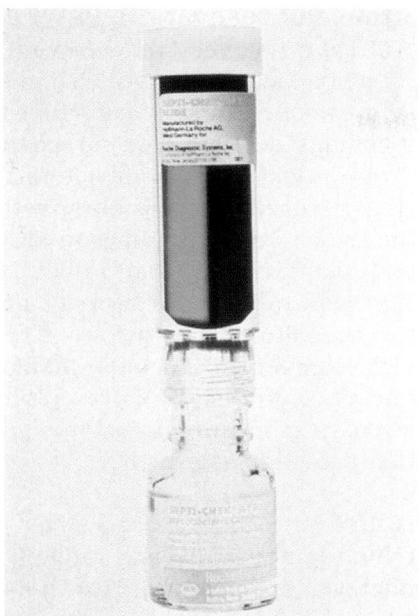

Figure 22-1
Septi-Chek AFB.

(Figure 22-1). The system consists of a bottle containing Middlebrook 7H9 broth with an atmosphere of 5% to 8% CO_2, an enrichment consisting of growth-enhancing factors and antimicrobial agents, and a paddle with agar media. One side of the paddle is covered with nonselective Middlebrook 7H11 agar. One of the two sections on the reverse side of the paddle contains a modified egg-based medium for differentiating *M. tuberculosis* from other mycobacteria, and the other contains chocolate agar for the detection of contaminating bacteria.

The biphasic media system provides for growth for rapid identification and drug susceptibility testing without the need for routine subculturing. The biphasic media system is sensitive and does not require use of radioactivity and a CO_2 incubator. Detection times are shorter than with conventional agar but significantly longer than with the BACTEC system.

Isolator Lysis-Centrifugation System

Isolator (Wampole Laboratories, Cranbury, N.J.) is a collection system that contains saponin to liberate intracellular organisms. After treatment with the saponin, the sample is inoculated into mycobacteria media plates or tubes. The system allows for higher yields and shorter recovery times for mycobacteria. It offers the advantage of yielding isolated colonies and the ability to quantitate mycobacteremia, which may be useful in monitoring the effectiveness of therapy in disseminated *M. avium* complex infection.

For maximal recovery of mycobacteria, many laboratories use a battery of one or more units of an egg-based medium, one agar medium, and the radiometric broth method for primary isolation. A selective medium is often reserved for specimens in which heavy contamination is anticipated.

IDENTIFICATION

Laboratory Levels or Extents of Service

A change in the distribution of mycobacterial laboratory testing led to development of the concepts of levels of service by the American Thoracic Society (ATS) and extents of service by the College of American Pathologists (CAP) to maintain quality of service.

Extents of service, as defined by ATS, are as follows:

1. Specimen collection only. No mycobacteriologic procedures performed, all specimens sent to another laboratory.
2. Acid-fast stain and/or inoculation only. Identification by reference laboratory.
3. Isolation and definitive identification of *M. tuberculosis,* preliminary grouping of nontuberculous *Mycobacterium* spp., with definitive identification at a reference laboratory.
4. Definitive identification of all mycobacterial isolates with assistance in the selection of therapy, with or without drug susceptibility testing.

The CAP's *levels of service* are as follows:

Level I. Specimen collection only. No mycobacteriologic procedures performed. All specimens sent to another laboratory.
Level II. Perform microscopy. Isolate and identify and sometimes perform susceptibility tests for *M. tuberculosis.*
Level III. Perform microscopy. Isolate, identify, and perform susceptibility testing for all species of *Mycobacterium.*

A facility's selection of a level of service depends on the volume of specimens submitted, the ability to perform the requested tests according to comfort and training in performance of each requested test, as well as the time, effort, and funds allocated for the service.

The Centers for Disease Control and Prevention (CDC) has developed separate training courses designed for each level of service as well as manuals for reference.

Procedures available within a particular mycobacteriology laboratory then vary with the level of service of that laboratory. In addition, the methodology within laboratories varies. The CDC, in collaboration with the Association of State and Territorial Public Health Laboratory Directors, surveyed mycobacterial laboratories for their practices in isolation, identification, and susceptibility testing of MTB. Those laboratories that used conventional mycobacteriologic methods for culturing and identification were not able to report results as quickly as those that have already incorporated newer methodologies, amount of time needed being 43 versus 22 days, respectively.

Identification of Mycobacteria

Once an isolate has been recovered in the mycobacteriology laboratory, certain characteristics may be used to classify the isolate before performing biochemical tests. The first step is to confirm that the isolate recovered in broth or solid media culture is an acid-fast organism by performing an acid-fast stain. Then, once the organisms are growing on solid media, phenotypic characteristics such as colony morphology, growth rate, optimum growth temperature, and photoreactivity help speciate mycobacteria. These characteristics do not allow for definitive identification but are presumptive and help in the selection of other, more definitive tests. Table 22-2 summarizes the identification characteristics of clinically important mycobacteria.

Colony morphology

Colonies of mycobacteria are generally distinguished as having either a smooth and soft or a rough and friable appearance. Colonies of *M. tuberculosis* that are rough often also exhibit a prominent patterned texture referred to as *cording* (curved strands of bacilli); this texture is the result of tight cohesion of the bacilli. Colonies of *Mycobacterium intracellulare* may appear to have a dense center, resembling a fried egg.

Growth rate and recovery time

Growth rate and recovery time depend on the species of mycobacteria but are also influenced by media, the temperature of incubation, and the initial inoculum size. The range in recovery time is wide, from 3 to 60 days. Mycobacteria are generally categorized as having visible growth in less than or more than 7 days. **Rapid growers** are able to produce colonies in less than 7 days. Determination of growth rate should be evaluated from the time of subculture, not the time of detection from clinical sample. The inoculum should be sufficiently small to produce isolated colonies. Microscopic agar examination for microcolonies allows earlier detection of growth.

Temperature

The optimum temperature and range at which a mycobacterial species may grow may be extremely narrow, especially at the time of initial incubation. *M. marinum, Mycobacterium ulcerans,* and *M. haemophilum* grow best at 30° to 32° C and poorly, if at all, at 35° to 37° C. At the other extreme, *Mycobacterium xenopi* grow best at 42° C.

Photoreactivity

Mycobacterium spp. have traditionally been categorized into three groups according to their photoreactive characteristics. Species that produce carotene pigment upon exposure to light are **photochromogens.** Species that produce pigment in the light or the dark are **scotochromogens.** Color may range from pale yellow to orange. Growth temperature may influence the photoreactive characteristics of a species. Other species, such as *M. tuberculosis,* are **nonchromogenic** and nonphotoreactive. These colonies are a buff color.

Biochemical Identification

A panel of biochemical tests can identify most mycobacteria isolates, but because growth of *Mycobacterium* spp. is so slow, accomplishing this may take several weeks. Progress in molecular technology has diminished the frequency with which biochemical tests are routinely performed in the identification of mycobacteria. Because mycobacterial species may show only quantitative differences in enzymes used in biochemical identification, no single biochemical test should be relied on for the identification of a species, and for

TABLE 22-2

Identification of Clinically Important Mycobacteria*

Descriptive term	Species (Subspecies)	Colony Morphology	Temp. Growth Range (°C)	Growth Rate (R=Rapid, S=Slow)	Pigment (Photo, Scoto, Nonphoto)	Arylsulfatase 3 Day	Arylsulfatase 2 WK	Carbon Sources: Sodium Citrate	Inositol	Mannitol	Catalase: Semi-Quant >45	Catalase: Heat Stable (68°C)	Catalase: Iron Uptake	Growth on MacConkey	Niacin	Nitrate Reduction	Pyrazinamidase†	Growth on 5% NaCl	Tellurite Reduction	Growth on TCH	Tween Hydrolysis 10 Day	Tween Opacity (1 Week)	Urease‡
Rapid growers	M. fortuitum biovar fortuitum	Smooth (87) Rough (13)	22-40	R	N	+	+	− (99)	− (99)	− (99)	+45	+	+	+	−	+		+	+	+	+/−		+
	M. fortuitum biovar peregrinum	Smooth	22-37	R (97)	N	+ (97)	+ (99)	− (99)	− (99)	+ (99)	+45 (98)	+ (94)	+ (99)	+ (96)	− (99)	+ (99)		+ (75)	+ (97)	+ (99)	+/− (50)	+ (91)	+ (93)
	M. fortuitum‖ third biovariant complex	Smooth	22-37	R	N (99)				+ (99)	+ (99)													
	M. chelonae subsp. chelonae	Smooth/Rough 60/40	22-35	R (97)	N (99)	+ (96)	+ (98)	+ (99)	− (99)	− (99)	+45 (97)	−/+ (53/47)	− (98)	+ (96)	− (92)	− (99)		− (99)	+ (85)	+ (98)	−/+ (93/47)	+ (91)	+ (99)
	M. chelonae subsp. abscessus		22-40					− (99)	− (99)	− (99)								+ (90)					
	M. chelonae (turtlelike)		22-30					+ (99)	− (99)	− (99)			+ (Tank)(99)					− (99)					
	M. fallax§ (looks like M. tb.)	Rough	30-37	R (30°) / S (37°)	N = 99%	− (99)	−	− (99)	− (99)	− (99)	+	(74)	− (99)	− (99)	− (99)	+ (99)		− (99)		+ (99)	+ (99)		− (96)
	Other rapid growers	Smooth or Rough	17-52		P=4% S=38% N=58%	− (72)	+ (75)	− (70)	+ (59)	+ (60)	− (66)	− (63)	+ (56)	− (52)	− (95)	+ (51)		+ (52)	+ (87)	+ (99)	+ (75)	V	+ (66)
	M. ulcerans	Smooth, Rough	25-33	S	N	−						+			−	−	+	−		+	−		−
TB complex	M. tuberculosis	Rough, Cords	33-39	S	N=99%	− (99)	− (93)				− (99)	− (99)		− (99)	+ (98)	+ (99)	+ (98)	− (99)	− (70)	+ (92)	+ (68)	+ (83)	+ (98)
	M. africanum	Rough	35-38	S	N	− (99)	−				−			− (99)	− (95)	− (94)	−	− (99)	− (99)	Var.	−		+ (99)
	M. bovis	7H10=R LJ=S	35-38	S	N=99%	− (99)	− (87)				− (97)	− (99)		− (99)	− (95)	− (94)	− (98)	− (99)	− (55)	− (94)	(84)	(75)	+ (99)

Modified from Kent PT, Kubica GP: *Public health mycobacteriology: a guide for the level III laboratory,* Atlanta, 1985, Centers for Disease Control.

*Test reactions listed as "+" or "−", followed by percentage of strains reacting as indicated. If no percentage is given or space is blank, insufficient data were available or test is of no apparent value.

†Pyrazinamidase data (Wayne Method) from both Wayne and Hawkins. Unless indicated, results are those at 4 days. Strains of *M. tuberculosis* resistant to PZA are often pyrazinamidase negative. Within *M. terrae* complex, *M. nonchromogenicum* usually "+" and *M. terrae* usually "−".

‡Urease data (Murphy-Hawkins Disk Method) primarily from Dr. Jean E. Hawkins.

§Data on *M. fallax* from Levy-Frebault et al (I.J.S.B. 33:336, 1983).

‖Several strains in this complex have varied in carbon sources as follows: "+" sodium citrate, "+" sodium citrate, "+" mannitol, "−" inositol.

Continued

TABLE 22-2
Identification of Clinically Important Mycobacteria—cont'd

Group	Species (Subspecies)	Colony Morphology	Growth Temp. Range (°C)	Growth Rate (R = Rapid, S = Slow)	Pigment (Photo, Scoto, Nonphoto)	Arylsufatase 3 Day	Arylsufatase 2 Wk	Sodium Citrate	Inositol	Mannitol	Catalase Semi-Quant >45	Catalase Heat Stable (68°C)	Iron Uptake	Growth on MacConkey	Niacin	Nitrate Reduction	Pyrazin amidase†	Growth on 5% NaCl	Tellurite Reduction	Growth on TCH	Tween Hydrolysis + 10 Day	Tween Opacity (1 Week)	Urease‡
Nonphotochromogens	M. avium complex	Smooth, Rough, Trans.	22-45	S=99%	N=85% S=12% P=3%	−	+ (51)				− (99)	+ (76)	−	− (68)	− (99)	− (92)	+ (86)4d (99)7d	− (99)	+ (82)	+ (99)	− (98)	− (99)	+ (99)
	M. xenopi	(99) Smooth X	35-45	S	N=80% S=20%	+ (76)	+ (99)				+− (99)	+ (83)	−	− (99)	− (99)	− (94)	+ (51)	− (99)	− (59)	+ (99)	− (99)		− (99)
	M. shimoidei	Rough	30-45	S	N	−	−					+	−		−	−	+		−	+	+		−
	M. gastri	Smooth	25-40	S=80% R=20%	N=99%	− (96)	+ (99)				− (99)	− (99)		− (84)	− (99)	− (99)	+ (99)4d (63)7d	− (99)	− (74)	+ (99)	+ (99)	− (99)	+ (79)
	M. terrae complex	Smooth few Rough	22-37	S=77% R=23%	N=95% S=4% P=1%	− (99)	− (51)				+ (99)	+ (96)	−	− (77)	− (99)	+ (72)	+ (63)4d (88)7d	+ (94)	+ (75)	+ (99)	+ (99)	− (93)	(91)
	M. triviale	Rough	22-37	S	N=99%	− (66)	+ (99)				+ (93)	+ (99)	−	+ (99)	− (97)	+ (99)	+ (60)4d (90)7d	+ (99)	+ (99)	+ (99)	+ (99)		− (86)
	M. malmoense	Smooth	22-37	S	N=90% S=10%	− (99)	− (89)				− (99)	+ (69)		− (99)	− (99)	− (99)	+	− (99)	+ (71)	+ (99)	+ (97)		− (67)
	M. haemophilum (Needs hemin)	Rough	22-35	S	N	−					−	−	−			−	+	−	−	−	−		+
Photochromes	M. simiae	Smooth	22-37	S	P=91% N=9%	− (99)	+ (84)				+ (99)	+ (95)	−		+ (85)	− (85)	+ (99)	− (99)	− (85)	+ (99)	− (85)		+ (64)
	M. kansasii	Smooth Rough	25-40	S=98% R=2%	N=99% S=<1% P=<1%	− (99)	− (55)				+ (99)	+ (95)	−	− (99)	− (99)	+ (99)	− (99)4d (69)7d	− (99)	+ (84)	+ (99)	+ (99)	− (64)	+ (97)
	M. marinum	Smooth	25-35	R=61% S=39%	P=99%	− (66)	+ (99)				− (79)	− (58)	−	− (99)	− (80)	− (96)	+ (99)	− (97)	− (79)	+ (99)	+ (99)		+ (99)
	M. asiaticum	Smooth	33-37	S=99%	P=99%	− (99)	− (67)				+ (91)	+ (91)		− (99)	− (99)	− (99)	+	− (99)	− (70)	+ (99)	+ (91)	− (99)	− (99)
Scotochromogens	M. scrofulaceum	Smooth Rough	22-37	S=95% R=5%	S=97% P=3%	− (99)	− (64)				+ (93)	+ (96)		− (99)	− (99)	− (85)	+ (60)4d (99)7d	− (99)	+ (57)	+ (99)	− (98)	− (99)	+ (99)
	M. szulgai	Smooth Rough	22-37	S	S (99) 37° P 25°	− (99)	+ (62)				+ (99)	+ (81)			− (99)	+ (99)	+	− (99)	− (56)	+ (99)	+− (50)	+ (64)	+ (94)
	M. gordonae	Smooth	22-37	S=99% R=1%	S=99%	− (99)	+ (57)				+ (92)	+ (97)		− (99)	− (99)	− (95)	+ (67)4d (78)7d	− (99)	− (77)	+ (98)	+ (99)	− (99)	− (85)
	M. flavescens	Smooth	25-42	S=59% R=41%	S=99%	− (84)	− (78)				+ (85)	+ (99)		− (99)	− (99)	+ (96)	+ (99)	+ (71)	− (67)	+ (99)	+ (97)	+ (99)	+ (71)

Note: "No 'X' Colony − (99)" indicated for M. gastri / M. terrae complex group and for M. scrofulaceum / M. gordonae group.

†Pyrazinamidase data (Wayne Method) from both Wayne and Hawkins. Unless indicated, results are those at 4 days. Strains of M. tuberculosis resistant to PZA are often pyrazinamidase negative. Within M. terrae complex, M. nonchromogenicum usually "+" and M. terrae usually "−".

‡Urease data (Murphy-Hawkins Disk Method) primarily from Dr. Jean E. Hawkins.

expediency, all necessary biochemical tests should be set up at one time. The biochemical tests are based on the enzymes the organisms possess, the substances that their metabolism produce, and the inhibition of their growth on exposure to selected biochemicals. Appropriate positive and negative controls should be included for each biochemical test.

Niacin accumulation

Most mycobacteria possess the enzyme that converts free niacin to niacin ribonucleotide. However, 95% of *M. tuberculosis* isolates produce free niacin (nicotinic acid) because the species lack the niacin-connecting enzyme. Accumulation of niacin, detected as nicotinic acid, is the most commonly used biochemical test for the identification of MTB. Nicotinic acid reacts with cyanogen bromide in the presence of an aniline to form a yellow pigmented compound (Figure 22-2). Reagent-impregnated strips have eliminated the need to handle and dispose of cyanogen bromide, which is both caustic and toxic. Cyanogen bromide must be alkalinized with sodium hydroxide before disposal.

This test may be negative when performed on young cultures with few colonies. It is recommended that the test be done on egg agar cultures 3 to 4 weeks old and with at least 50 colonies. Tests that yield negative results may need to be repeated in several weeks. The test should not be performed on scotochromogenic or rapidly growing species because *M. simiae,* BCG (bacillus of Calmette-Guérin) strain of *M. bovis, M. africanum, M. marinum, M. chelonei,* and *M. bovis* may be positive, although this occurs rarely. Results are most consistent when the test is performed on egg media.

Nitrate reduction

The production of nitroreductase, which catalyzes the reduction of nitrate to nitrite, is relatively uncommon among other *Mycobacterium* species, but a positive result may be seen in *Mycobacterium kansasii, Mycobacterium szulgai, M. fortuitum,* and *M. tuberculosis.* Sulfanilamide and *N*-naphthylene-diamine added to a solution of bacteria in sodium nitrate turn red in the presence of nitrite (Figure 22-3). When no color change occurs, however, either no reaction has occurred or the reaction has gone beyond nitrite. The addition of zinc detects free nitrate and results in a pink color change in a true-negative reaction. The nitrate reduction test differentiates *M. tuberculosis* from the scotochromogens and *Mycobacterium avium* complex (MAC).

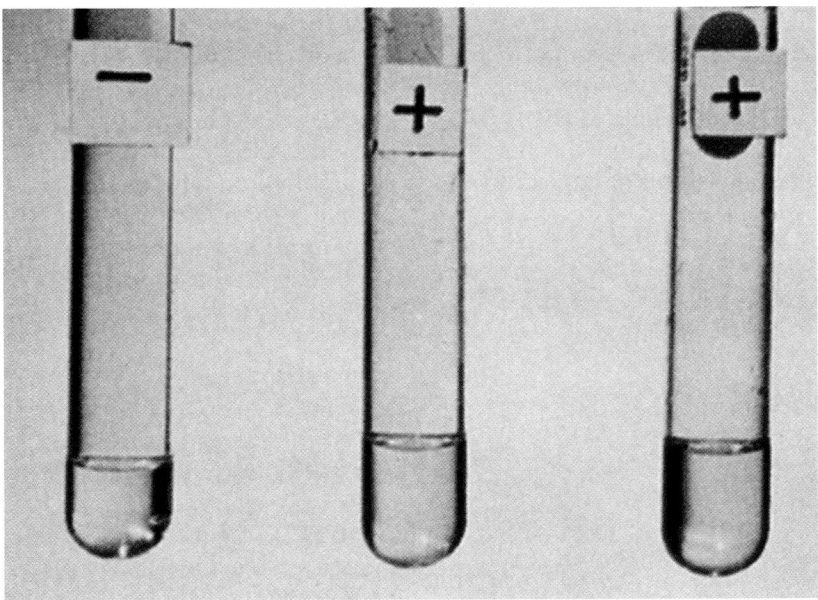

Figure 22-2
Niacin test.

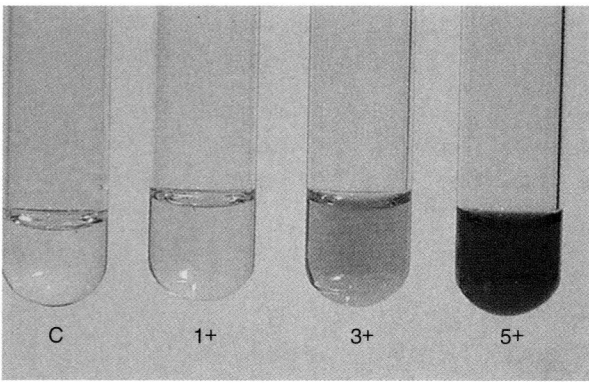

Figure 22-3 —————————————————————

Nitrate reduction test.

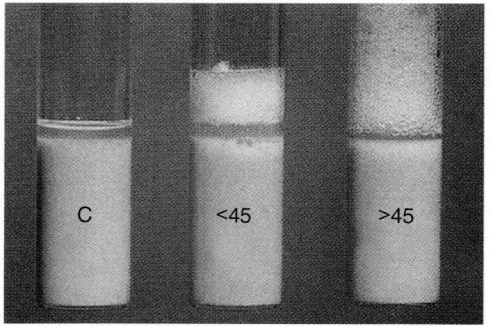

Figure 22-5 —————————————————————

Semiquantitative catalase test.

Catalase

Catalase is an enzyme that can split hydrogen peroxide into water and oxygen. Mycobacteria are catalase positive. However, not all strains produce a positive reaction after the culture is heated to 68° C for 20 minutes. Isolates that are catalase positive have a heat-stable catalase. Most *M. tuberculosis* complex organisms do not produce heat-stable catalase. An exception are certain strains resistant to isoniazid (INH), which may be clinically useful. Other catalase-negative species include *Mycobacterium gastri, M. haemophilum,* and *M. marinum.* Catalase quantity and heat stability are, however, species dependent. Semiquantitation of catalase production uses the addition of Tween 80 (a detergent) and hydrogen peroxide to a 2-week-old culture. The reaction is monitored after 5 minutes, and the resulting column of bubbles is measured (Figures 22-4 and

22-5). The column size is recorded as greater than or less than 45 mm.

Hydrolysis of Tween 80

Some mycobacteria possess a lipase that can split the detergent Tween 80 into oleic acid and polyoxyethylated sorbitol. The time required for the hydrolysis is variable. The products of hydrolysis alter optical rotation of transmitted light, causing a pink color change. This test is helpful in distinguishing scotochromogenic and nonphotochromogenic mycobacteria.

Iron uptake

Some mycobacteria are able to convert ferric ammonium citrate to an iron oxide. After growth of the isolate appears on an egg-based medium slant, rusty-brown colonies appear in a positive reaction upon the addition of 20% aqueous solution of ferric ammonium citrate; this is a result of the iron uptake (Figure 22-6). The test is most useful in distinguishing *Mycobacterium chelonei* which is generally negative, from other rapid growers, which are positive.

Arylsulfatase

Most members of the genus *Mycobacterium* posses the enzyme arylsulfatase. This enzyme hydrolyzes the bond between the sulfate group and the aromatic ring structure in compounds with the formula $R—OSO_3H$. Tripotassium phenolphthalein sulfate is such a molecule, from which phenolphthalein is liberated upon exposure to arylsulfatase. The liberation of phenolphthalein causes a pH change in the presence of sodium bicarbonate, indicated by

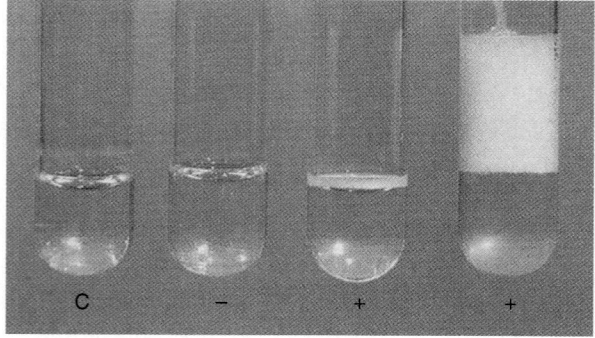

Figure 22-4 —————————————————————

Catalase test.

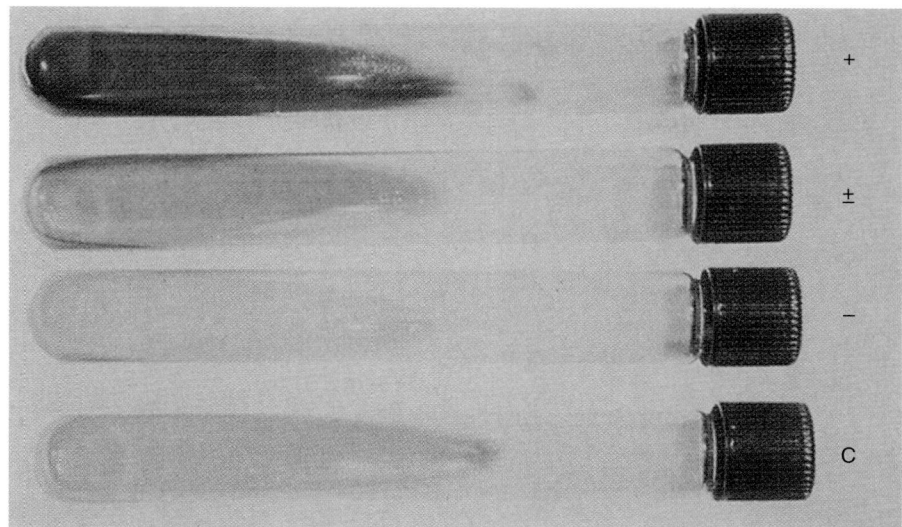

Figure 22-6
Iron uptake.

a pink color change. The *M. fortuitum-chelonei* complex (see later), *M. xenopi,* and *Mycobacterium triviale* have rapid arylsulfatase activity that can be detected in 3 days. *M. marinum* and *M. szulgai* exhibit activity with 14-day incubation.

Pyrazinamidase

The presence of pyrazinamidase allows deamination of pyrazinamide to pyrazinoic acid and ammonia in 4 days, producing a red pigment (Figure 22-7). This test may be useful in distinguishing *M. marinum* from *M. kansasii* and *Mycobacterium bovis* from *M. tuberculosis.*

Urease

Detection of urease activity may be used to distinguish *Mycobacterium scrofulaceum* from *Mycobacterium gordonae* (Figure 22-8).

Inhibitory tests

NAP

NAP (p-nitro-aceytlamino-β-hydroxypropiophenone) is a precursor in the synthesis of chloramphenicol. Since 1960, NAP has been known to selectively inhibit **Mycobacterium tuberculosis complex.** Laszlo and Eidus (1978) later confirmed that 99.5% of more than 5000 strains they tested were inhibited by NAP. The radiometric application of this selective inhibition evolved soon after.

Performance of the test either with isolated MTB colonies or with broth from a BACTEC medium with a growth index of 50 to 100 or more is recommended. An aliquot of the original BACTEC medium is transferred to the BACTEC-NAP vial which contains 5 mg of NAP and no antibiotics. Growth is then closely monitored and compared with the original BACTEC vial, which serves as a growth control. A 20% increase or decrease in growth index is considered significant. About 4 to 6 days more are required for identification if such indirect NAP testing is performed. Testing should be done with positive and negative controls.

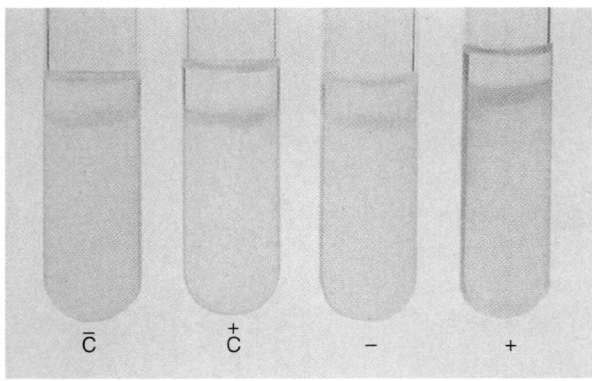

Figure 22-7
Pyrazinamidase test.

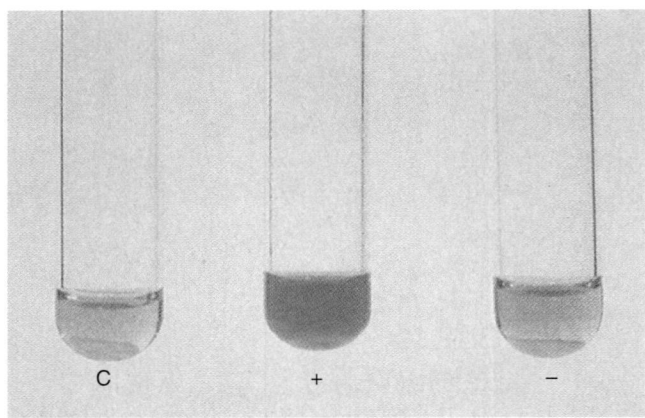

Figure 22-8 _____
Urease test.

Direct specimen BACTEC-NAP testing, eliminating a prior isolation, has been performed and has been reported to identify *M. tuberculosis* in an average of 7.8 days but with diminished sensitivity.

TCH
TCH (thiophene-2-carboxylic acid hydrazide) distinguishes *M. bovis* from *M. tuberculosis*. *M. bovis* is susceptible to lower levels of TCH than MTB. Variability in inhibition exists, depending on the concentration of the inhibitory agent and the temperature of incubation. This selective inhibitory agent has also been applied to radiometric systems.

GROWTH IN 5% NaCl
High salt concentration in egg-based media inhibits the growth of most mycobacterium. *Mycobacterium flavescens, M. triviale,* and most rapidly growing *Mycobacterium* spp. are exceptions that do grow in 5% NaCl.

TELLURITE REDUCTION
Reduction of colorless potassium tellurite to black metallic tellurium in 3 to 4 days is a characteristic of *M. avium* complex (Figure 22-9) and thus is useful in distinguishing *M. avium* complex from other nonchromogenic species. In addition, all rapid growers are able to reduce tellurite in 3 days.

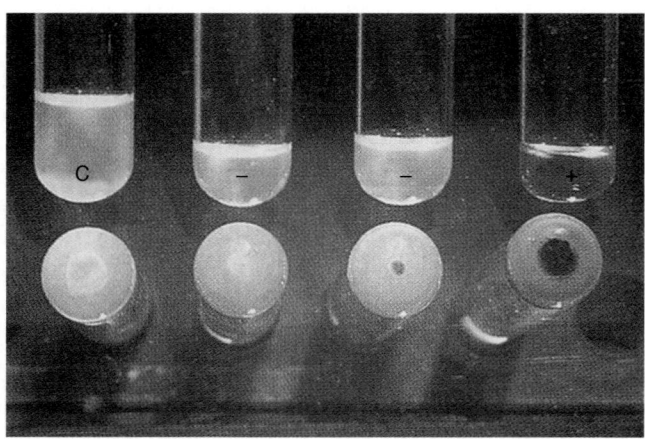

Figure 22-9 _____
Test for tellurite reduction.

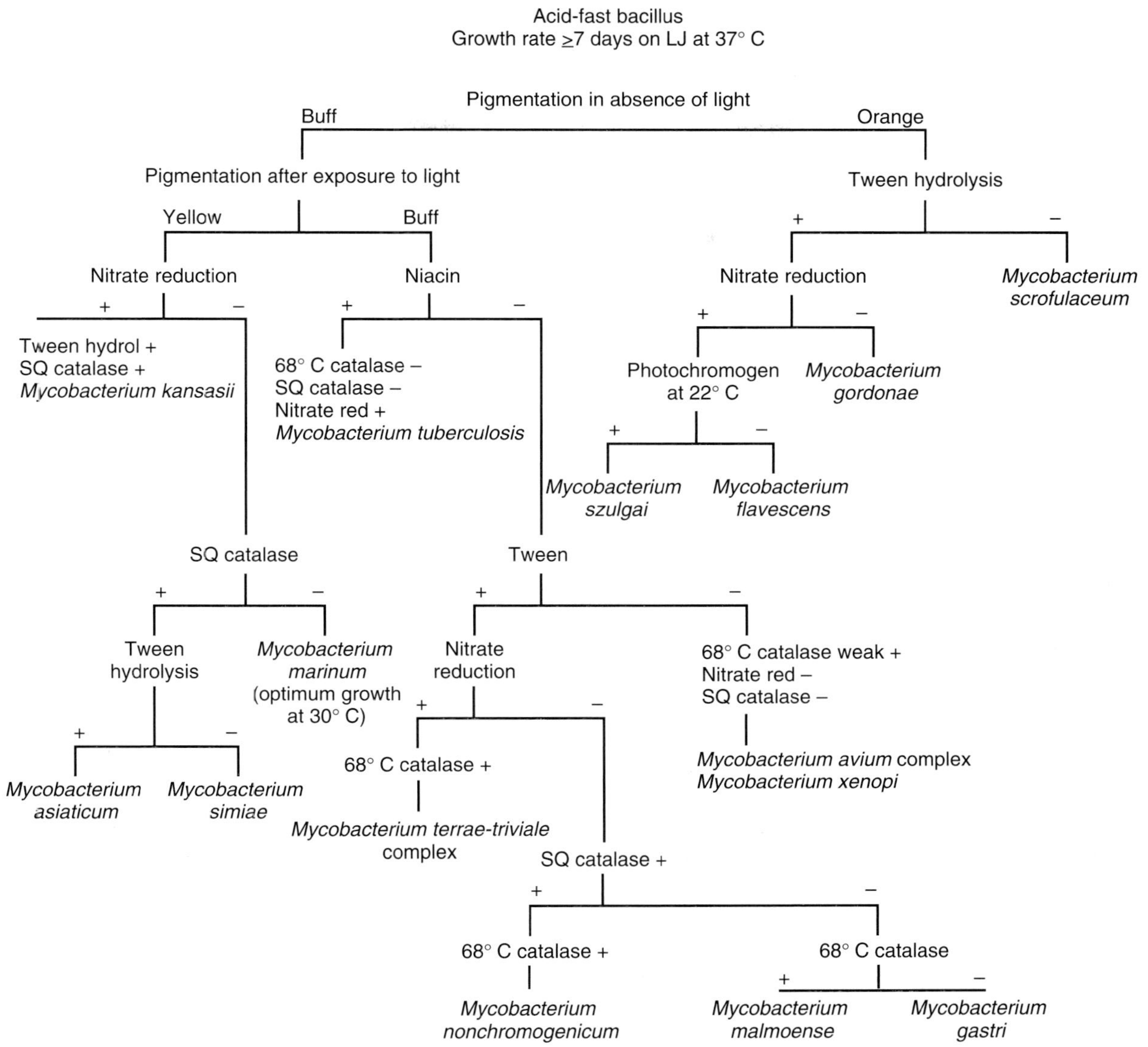

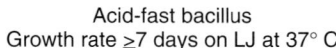

Acid-fast bacillus
Growth rate ≥7 days on LJ at 37° C

Pigmentation in absence of light

Buff   Orange

Pigmentation after exposure to light   Tween hydrolysis

Yellow   Buff   +   −

Nitrate reduction   Niacin   Nitrate reduction   *Mycobacterium scrofulaceum*

+   −   +   −   +   −

Tween hydrol +
SQ catalase +
Mycobacterium kansasii

68° C catalase −
SQ catalase −
Nitrate red +
Mycobacterium tuberculosis

Photochromogen
at 22° C   *Mycobacterium gordonae*

+   −

Mycobacterium szulgai   *Mycobacterium flavescens*

SQ catalase   Tween

+   −   +   −

Tween hydrolysis   *Mycobacterium marinum* (optimum growth at 30° C)

Nitrate reduction

68° C catalase weak +
Nitrate red −
SQ catalase −

Mycobacterium avium complex
Mycobacterium xenopi

+   −   +   −

Mycobacterium asiaticum   *Mycobacterium simiae*

68° C catalase +

Mycobacterium terrae-triviale complex

SQ catalase +

+   −

68° C catalase +   68° C catalase

Mycobacterium nonchromogenicum

+   −

Mycobacterium malmoense   *Mycobacterium gastri*

Figure 22-10 _____

Schematic diagram for the identification of slowly growing *Mycobacterium* species. Exceptional reactions occur. Organisms should be subjected to a battery of morphologic and physiologic tests before final identification is made. *SQ,* Semiquantitative; *LJ,* Löwenstein-Jensen.

GROWTH ON MACCONKEY AGAR

M. fortuitum-chelonei complex can grow on Mac-Conkey agar without crystal violet, whereas most other mycobacteria cannot.

Slow versus rapid growth

Figures 22-10 and 22-11 show schematic diagrams for the identification of slow-growing and rapid-growing *Mycobacterium* species.

Chromatography

The cell walls of *Mycobacterium* organisms contain long-chain fatty acids called **mycolic acids** that may be detected chromographically. The type and quality of mycolic acids are specific to species. Chromatographic species identification of *Mycobacterium* has been of longstanding interest, and methods have changed as technology has evolved. Earlier methods, such as column chromatography

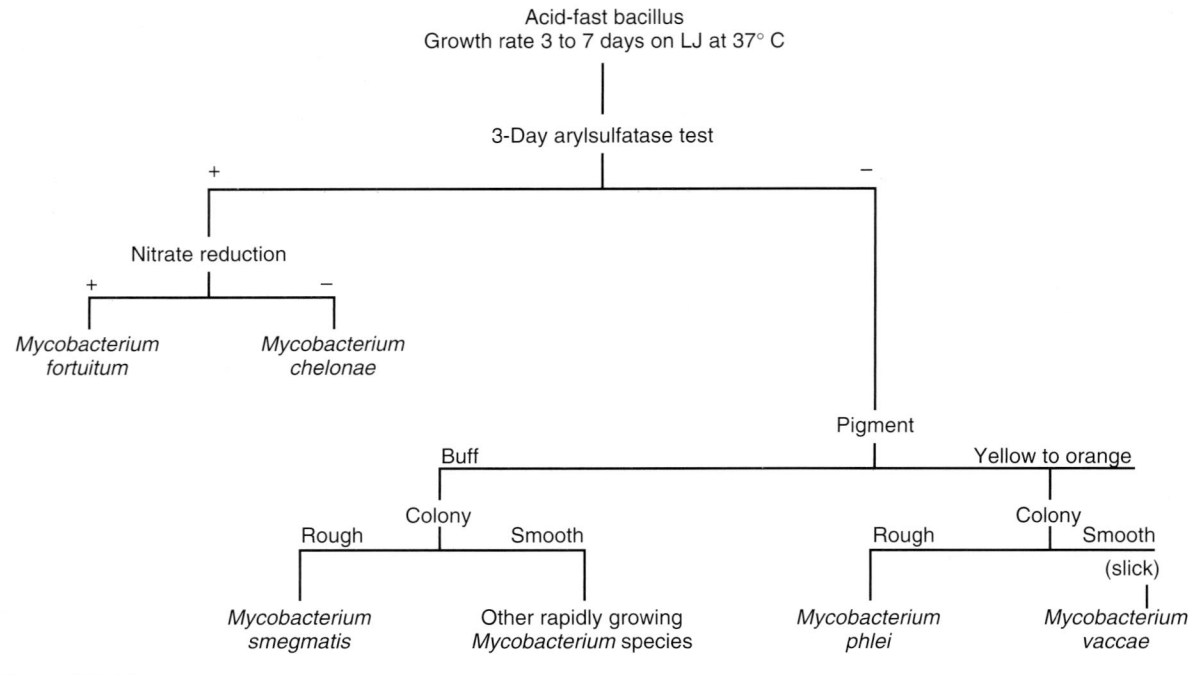

Figure 22-11

Schematic diagram for the identification of rapidly growing *Mycobacterium* species. Exceptional reactions occur. Organisms should be subjected to a battery of morphologic ad physiologic tests before final identification is made. *LJ,* Löwenstein-Jensen.

and thin-layer chromatography, have been replaced by gas-liquid chromatography and, most recently, high-performance liquid chromatography. Current methods allow sufficient amount of mycolic acid to be easily extracted from small quantities of bacterial cultures. Tisdale and associates developed a basic saponification–lipid extraction method that allows correct identification of most mycobacterial species using chromatograms and colony characteristics. Acid methanolysis and higher temperatures have improved mycolic acid separation.

Species identifications made with high-performance liquid chromatography (HPLC) have been shown to agree well with biochemical and probe identifications. Many state health departments and the CDC use this method for identification of mycobacterial isolates. Chromatography is rapid and highly reproducible, but the initial cost of equipment is high.

Amplification for *Mycobacterium tuberculosis*

DNA hybridization

The use of nucleic acid hybridization techniques allows rapid identification of certain common mycobacterial species. Commercially available nu-

cleic acid probes are available for the *M. tuberculosis* complex, the *M. avium* complex, *M. avium, M. intracellulare, M. kansasii,* and *M. gordonae.* These tests are nonisotopically labeled (i.e., an acridine ester–labeled piece of nucleic acid) probes specific to mycobacterial ribosomal RNA (rRNA). The rRNA is released from the cell after lysis and heat. The DNA probe is allowed to react with the test solution. If specific rRNA is present, a stable DNA-RNA complex, or hybrid, is formed. Unbound probe is chemically degraded. The complex is detected by adding an alkaline hydrogen peroxide solution. The hybrid-bound acridine ester is available to cause a chemiluminescent reaction, resulting in the emission of light. The amount of light emitted is related to the amount of hybridized probe. The sensitivity of recognition is about 10^4 organisms per mL. It is estimated that 10^5 to 10^6 (some say as many as 10^7) organisms per mL are required for detection by the Gen-Probe (San Diego, Calif.) procedure. According to the manufacturer, 3 to 6×10^8 organisms per mL are required. In the experience of Gonzalez and colleagues, the amount of organism required for testing "corresponded in the case of MTB to a single colony of at least 1 mm in diameter or in the case of MAC to a barely visible film of growth on the surface of the slant." Most positive results are well above the cut-off value of 10% hybridization. When a probe is used on a contaminated specimen, the obtained percentage hybridization may incorrectly fall below accepted cut-off hybridization levels, leading to falsely negative results.

DNA hybridization identification can be applied to growth on conventional agar as well as to growth in radiometric liquid media such as BACTEC. The combination of radiometric detection and DNA hybridization identification using the probe technology allows rapid recovery and identification. Waiting for the early log phase of growth or an index reading of 500 to 999 increases the sensitivity of probe identification. Ellner and associates (1988), using either BACTEC 12B medium or Middlebrook 7H11 medium and the Gen-Probe, found that 95% of TB cultures could be identified within 4 weeks. With growth on LJ medium, 7 weeks were required for identification.

In addition to hybridization assays, many laboratories have begun using the polymerase chain reaction to identify the *M. tuberculosis* complex. As more molecular methods become commercially available and increasingly automated, identification and detection of mycobacteria will become increasingly faster, less costly, and more specific.

Serology

Serologic diagnostic methods for the detection of mycobacterial antigens has not come into widespread clinical use. Also, because of the lack of antigen specificity and weakness of antibody response in infected individuals, detection of specific antibodies in individuals is not available.

Susceptibility of *Mycobacterium tuberculosis*

Along with increased incidence of mycobacterial disease, the development of multidrug-resistant strains of mycobacteria is being observed. Within any population of *M. tuberculosis,* resistance to a single agent can develop at a fairly well-defined rate. For example, with isoniazid the chance that a resistant isolate will develop is 1 in 10^5; for streptomycin 1 in 10^6, and for both 1 in 10^{11}. In a patient with pulmonary tuberculosis the pulmonary cavity may contain 10^7 to 10^9 bacterial cells. Random drug resistance has a good chance of developing when only one antibiotic is used or if the patient is on multidrug therapy and fails to complete the course of

medication. Therefore the use of three or more drugs to treat mycobacterial infections has become common. So that patients can be placed on appropriate therapy, the CDC currently recommends that, when isolated, *M. tuberculosis* be tested for in vitro susceptibility to isoniazid, rifampin, ethambutol, and streptomycin. Pyrazinamide is to be considered as well. Likewise, testing should be repeated if the patient's cultures for *M. tuberculosis* remain positive after 3 months of therapy.

Susceptibility testing of *M. tuberculosis* requires meticulous technique and experienced personnel in interpreting results. Therefore laboratories who isolate few *M. tuberculosis* isolates should consider sending isolates to a reference laboratory for susceptibility testing. Currently, four methods are used for determining susceptibility of *M. tuberculosis.* They include radiometric, proportional, resistance ratio, and absolute concentration methods.

In clinical correlations with in vitro data, if 1% of a patient's bacilli are resistant to a particular drug, treatment fails. Laboratory tests then must demonstrate the rate of resistant organisms. To do so, the inoculum of bacilli used is adjusted to enable this 1%—usually 100 to 300 colony-forming units (CFU) per mL—to be determined. The test is often referred to as the *proportion method* because it allows one to predict the possibility that the 1% is resistant or not. The methods for determining such resistance include agar dilution, disk elution, and the BACTEC system.

The absolute concentration method involves dispensing of media (usually Middlebrook 7H10) containing appropriate drugs into quadrants of a Petri dish. Acid-fast bacilli are then prepared in an inoculum to yield about 100 to 300 CFU/mL, which entails preparation of a barely turbid broth culture, which is then diluted 10^{-2} and 10^{-4}. The two dilutions provide for a set of plates that should be countable (i.e., 100 to 300 CFU on the control plate). A control plate is set up in each run of drugs so that the numbers of colonies on the test quadrants can be counted and compared with the number on the control quadrant. If the test growth is less than 1% of the control growth, the organism is susceptible; if greater, resistant. By this method, results can be obtained in 2 to 3 weeks, depending on growth of the organism. Plates are kept at 37° C for incubation.

With the radiometric method, laboratories use the BACTEC 460 system. This method uses a liquid containing ^{14}C-labeled growth substrate. Growth is indicated by the amount of ^{14}C-labeled CO_2 released from the liquid. A standardized inoculum is inoculated into a drug free and drug-containing vial. The amounts and rates of CO_2 produced in the absence and presence of the drug are compared to determine susceptibility or resistance.

The BACTEC bottles are read for 4 to 5 days after inoculation. After a growth index (GI) of 30 is achieved in the growth control vial, the readings over the next 2 days are recorded. If the change in GI reading in a drug vial exceeds that in the growth vial, the organism is said to be resistant; if it does not, susceptible.

The resistance ratio method determines the level of resistance in an isolate by comparing growth or inhibition when grown in the presence of an antibiotic to a laboratory reference strain in which the susceptibility pattern is known. The reference strain and the patient strain are run in parallel by inoculating a standard inoculum to media containing twofold serial dilutions of the drug. Resistance is expressed as the ratio of the MIC of the test strain divided by the MIC of the reference strain for each drug.

Table 22-3 lists drugs and their concentrations to be used in susceptibility tests. The susceptibility test is performed on a pure culture, identified as *M. tuberculosis*. A direct susceptibility may be performed, however, using clinical specimens that are positive on smear provided that appropriate dilutions are made on the basis of numbers of acid-fast bacilli seen. The advantage of this direct assay is a quicker susceptibility report—within 2 to 3 weeks of culture, rather than 5 to 7 weeks or more. If, however, cultures are not thoroughly decontaminated, overgrowth is a problem. Likewise, the mycobacteria isolated may be other than *M. tuberculosis*.

Because multidrug-resistant *M. tuberculosis* cases are increasing in the United States, rapidly isolating *M. tuberculosis* and determining its susceptibility in vitro is necessary so that appropriate therapy may be employed. To this end, the laboratory is required to perform the most efficient and rapid tests possible. Researchers are looking for more rapid methods involving amplification, use of luciferase enzymes, and detection of resistance genes. It is hoped that these methods will be available soon for laboratory use.

In vitro susceptibility testing of most NTM is not routinely performed. Correlation between clinical outcome and in vitro test results have not been shown. In addition, no standardized method currently exists for performing these tests. The one exception are the rapidly growing mycobacteria. Broth microdilution, and agar disc diffusion may be employed. The E-test is being used with increasing frequency for performing susceptibility testing on the rapid growers.

TABLE 22-3

Antituberculosis Drugs and Their Recommended Concentrations

Drug	Concentration (µg/mL)*
Primary	
Isoniazid	0.2
Isoniazid	1.0
Streptomycin	2.0
Streptomycin	10.0
Rifampin	1.0
Ethambutol	5.0
Secondary†	
Ethionamide	5.0
Capreomycin	10.0
Cycloserine	20.0
Kanamycin	5.0
Pyrazinamide (at pH 5.5)	25.0

*7H10 Medium.
†Modified from National Committee for Clinical Laboratory Standards: *Antimycobacterial susceptibility testing: Proposed Standard Document M24-P,* vol 10, Villanova, Pa, 1990, NCCLS.

MYCOBACTERIUM TUBERCULOSIS COMPLEX

M. tuberculosis complex consists of *M. tuberculosis, M. bovis* (BCG), *M. africanum,* and *M. microti. M. africanum* has been associated with human cases of tuberculosis in tropical Africa. *M. microti* is not associated with human disease. These two latter species are rarely encountered in the laboratory in the United States and therefore are not included in the following discussion.

Mycobacterium tuberculosis

M. tuberculosis was first described by Robert Koch in 1882; however, the disease tuberculosis is one of the oldest documented communicable diseases. Today there are over 1 billion cases of tuberculosis infection worldwide, with 8 to 10 million new cases of disease and 3 million deaths attributed to tuberculosis per year. A person is "infected" with *M. tuberculosis* when exposed to the organism. Whether or not a person has the disease tuberculosis is determined by that person's cellular immunity, the amount of exposure, and the virulence of the strain.

In the United States before 1985, there was a continual decline in the annual number of tuberculosis cases at a rate of about 5% decrease per year. In 1985 this decline ended, and currently the number of documented tuberculosis cases per year in the United States is increasing (more than 18% cumulative increase since 1985). This increase has been attributed to several factors, including the epidemic of AIDS, increased use of intravenous drugs, and greater spread among inhabitants of closed environments, such as nursing homes, correctional facilities, and shelters for the homeless. In addition, more cases are associated with immigration from endemic areas or higher numbers of migrant workers from such areas in certain states in the United States.

Clinical disease: primary tuberculosis

Clinically, tuberculosis is usually a disease of the respiratory tract. Tubercle bacilli are acquired from persons with active disease and are excreting viable bacilli by means of coughing, sneezing, or talking. Airborne droplet nuclei, 1 to 10 μm, enter the respiratory tract of an exposed individual and are deposited in the lung alveoli. The exposed individual is said to be "infected" with *M. tuberculosis*. After infection in most individuals, *M. tuberculosis* organisms are phagocytized in alveolar macrophages. They are still capable of intracellular multiplication at this time. In a person with adequate cellular immunity, T cells arrive within 4 to 6 weeks with macrophage-activating polypeptides called *lymphokines*. This enables the white blood cells in the area of infection to destroy the intracellular mycobacteria.

There is then a regression and healing of the primary lesion and any disseminated foci of infection by the *M. tuberculosis* organisms. The pathologic features of this infection are the result of the hypersensitivity and local concentration of the antigen (bacterium). If there is little antigen and a great deal of hypersensitivity reaction, a hard tubercle or granuloma may be formed. The *granuloma* is an organization of lymphocytes, macrophages, giant cells, fibroblasts, and capillaries. With this granuloma formation, healing occurs,

along with fibrosis, encapsulation, and scar formation as a reminder of the past infection.

If the antigen load and hypersensitivity reaction are both high, tissue necrosis from enzymes of degenerating macrophages may occur, the tissue response is less organized, and no granuloma is formed. Without granuloma or necrosis, lesions may heal without obvious pathology. With necrosis, a caseous material may be present at the site of the primary lesion as a result of solid or semisolid amorphous material laid down at the site of necrosis.

After this healing of first-degree infection, the bacilli are not totally eradicated, and in the infected individual, there is a potential for reactivation of tuberculosis disease.

Clinical diagnosis of primary tuberculosis is usually limited to detection of a positive tuberculin skin test using purified protein derivative (PPD). Children may demonstrate a nonproductive cough and fever with or without shortness of breath; these symptoms are unusual in adults. Chest radiographs are usually normal, although rarely there may be infiltrates without cavitation in the anterior segment of the upper, middle, or lower lobe with hilar or paratracheal adenopathy. Along with these limited clinical findings there is a paucity of bacteriologic findings. If sputum or bronchial washings are cultured during the primary infection, the yield is only 25% to 30% positive. A small percentage of individuals who are infected with tuberculosis develop progressive pulmonary disease. This is most often due to a failed cellular immune response and hence a failure to stop multiplication of the bacilli. In young children or older adults who are primarily infected and in people with an underlying immunodeficiency, massive lymphohematogeneous dissemination may occur and lead to meningeal or military (disseminated) tuberculosis. In addition, 10% of young adults may progress to active disease from their primary infection. This will look like reactivation tuberculosis in older adults, and the only way to differentiate it is by finding a new PPD positivity.

Reactivation tuberculosis

The risk of reactivation of tuberculosis is about 3.3% during the first year after a positive tuberculin skin test and a total of 5% to 15% thereafter in the person's lifetime. Progression from infection to active disease varies with age and the intensity and duration of exposure. Malnutrition, with or without other factors such as alcoholism, homelessness, incarceration, immunosuppression, and AIDS, can contribute greatly to the progression to active tuberculosis.

Reactivation tuberculosis occurs when there is an alteration or a diminution of the cellular immune system in the infected host that favors replication of the bacilli and progression to disease. The symptoms of disease are slow in developing and consist of fever, shortness of breath, night sweats and chills, fatigue, anorexia, and weight loss. Approximately 20% of individuals may have no symptoms, but the majority of patients eventually have cough, chest pain, and productive sputum. Hemoptysis occurs in 25% of cases. The radiographs of patients with reactivation tuberculosis reveal a patchy or confluent consolidation with increased linear densities extending to the hilum; thick-walled cavities without air-fluid levels usually are found in apical or posterior segments of the upper lobe or superior segment of the middle lobe of the lung. If there is bronchogenic spread of the bacilli, multiple alveolar densities will be seen; rarely is there enlargement of the lymph nodes. If the disease has been chronic, fibrosis, loss of lung volume, and calcifications will be demonstrated.

The PPD test may be negative in up to 25% of these cases; diagnosis is confirmed by smear and culture of sputum, gastric aspirates, or bronchoscopy specimens. Fiberoptic bronchoscopy has been found to yield a 95% recovery; post-bronchoscopic sputa are usually positive as well.

In any case of pulmonary tuberculosis disease, there may be complication if diagnosis and treatment are delayed. These include empyema, pleural fibrosis, massive hemoptysis, adrenal insufficiency (rare), and hypercalcemia (up to 25% of cases). In patients with AIDS and tuberculosis with drug-susceptible bacilli, the risk of progression to disease from infection is quite high, although the clinical findings may vary from those in the non-AIDS patient with reactivation tuberculosis. The diagnosis is usually made by culture and smears, with a rate of sensitivity similar to that in the non-AIDS patient.

Extrapulmonary tuberculosis

Extrapulmonary tuberculosis occurred much less commonly than pulmonary tuberculosis (<15%) before the AIDS epidemic; however, as cases of pulmonary TB in the United States declined, the number of cases of extrapulmonary tuberculosis

remained constant. Cases of extrapulmonary disease have increased since 1988 because it is a common presentation in the HIV-infected individual, although it is most often found in association with pulmonary disease.

Miliary tuberculosis refers to the seeding of many organs outside the pulmonary tree with acid-fast bacilli through hematogenous spread. This usually occurs shortly after primary pulmonary disease but can take place anywhere in the course of acute or chronic tuberculosis. The most common sites of spread of *M. tuberculosis* in its miliary form are spleen, liver, lungs, bone marrow, kidney, adrenal gland, and eyes, usually in that order of preference. Overall, children account for the majority of cases of miliary TB, but it is also a common form of tuberculosis disease in the HIV-infected individual. The mortality is 20% or higher in most literature series; the finding of meningitis is an extremely bad prognostic indicator.

Other forms of extrapulmonary tuberculosis include: pleural, lymphadenitis, gastrointestinal, skeletal, meningeal, peritoneal, genitourinary, and miscellaneous infections. Pleurisy, an unexplained pleural effusion with mononuclear pleurocytosis, manifests as cough, fever, and chest pain, resembling the presentation of bacterial pneumonia; it occurs in about 5% of all cases of tuberculosis. In endemic areas, pleurisy is a presentation in the young individual; in the United States, middle-aged to older persons are most affected. Resolution is common. Acid-fast bacilli are rarely seen in pleural fluid, but cultures may be positive in 20% to 50% of cases; pleural biopsies offer a higher yield of microbiologic diagnosis.

Lymphadenitis is usually a disease of children, appearing as painless head or neck swellings. Lymph node involvement, particularly mediastinal, has been a common extrapulmonary manifestation in AIDS patients.

Genitourinary tuberculosis can involve the kidneys and genital organs. Renal tuberculosis accounts for 2% of all cases of tuberculosis and manifests as typical urinary tract symptoms and sterile pyuria. Cultures may be positive in up to 80% of cases. Male genital tuberculosis usually appears as a scrotal mass and occurs most often along with renal tuberculosis; in women, hematogenous spread is usually the source.

Skeletal tuberculosis of the spine is referred to as **Pott disease.** Back pain is the most common characteristic. Cultures of bone and tissue are needed to confirm the diagnosis. Peripheral skeletal bones and joints also may be involved, with the hip and knee being the most common sites.

Meningitis due to *M. tuberculosis* is usually the result of a rupture of a tubercle into the subarachnoid space and not usually hematogenous spread. In childhood, it occurs rarely after primary pulmonary infection. Most of the infection occurs at the base of the brain, and patients may develop very thick, gelatinous, mass-like lesions there. With more chronic disease, a fibrous mass may surround cranial nerves. Involvement of arteries may cause infarctions. CSF examination usually reveals elevated protein, decreased glucose, and predominance of lymphocytes. Prognosis with this form of extrapulmonary tuberculosis is not good.

Virtually any organ of the body can be infected by *M. tuberculosis,* and other uncommon manifestations include: gastrointestinal infection, peritonitis, cutaneous tuberculosis, laryngitis, otitis, and involvement of urea, adrenal glands, eyes, and breast. Up to 70% of HIV-infected patients may have extrapulmonary tuberculosis alone or, most often, in combination with pulmonary disease. The most common extrapulmonary sites in this population are disseminated (miliary), lymph node involvement (especially mediastinal), genitourinary, and intraabdominal. Bacteremia is not uncommon.

Identification of *Mycobacterium tuberculosis*

Colonies of this slowly growing species are thin, flat, spreading, and friable with a rough appearance. The colonies are classically described as being buff in color (Figure 22-12). Elaboration of cord factor may result in characteristic cord formation. Isoniazid-resistant strains may have somewhat longer recovery times. Optimum growth occurs at 35° to 37° C. Colonies are not photoreactive.

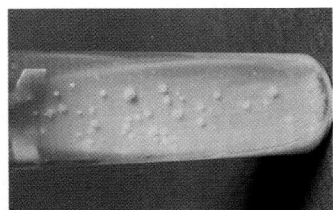

Figure 22-12 _____

Mycobacterium tuberculosis growing on Löwenstein-Jensen (LJ) medium.

Biochemically, *M. tuberculosis* is characteristically positive for niacin accumulation, reduction of nitrate to nitrite, and production of catalase, which is destroyed after heating. Isoniazid-resistant strains may not produce catalase at all. *M. tuberculosis* is inhibited by NAP. This species can be distinguished from *M. bovis* by the inhibition of *M. bovis* by TCH and pyrazinamidase activity.

Treatment of tuberculosis

In a nationwide survey conducted by the CDC in 1991, *M. tuberculosis* isolates resistant to at least one antituberculosis drug was found in 14.9% of cases. Also, resistance to both INH and rifampin was observed in 3.3% of the cases. Thus, treatment of tuberculosis involves the use of more than one antibiotic.

For pulmonary tuberculosis, treatment usually involves a 9-month course of therapy with isoniazid and rifampin, usually once per day the first month and two times a week thereafter. Many regimens also include a 2- to 8-week initial course of streptomycin or ethambutol. Most individuals clear their sputum of acid-fast bacilli within the first 2 months. Pyrazinamide (PZA) may be added to the regimen if there is a suspicion of lowered cellular immunity and a need to obtain bactericidal levels of antituberculous activity intracellularly in macrophages. PZA is usually recommended for a shorter course—initially along with isoniazid and rifampin.

For cases of resistance to isoniazid or rifampin, second-line antituberculosis drugs include capreomycin, cycloserine, kanamycin, amikacin, ciprofloxacin, and ethambutol. With the numbers of cases of multidrug-resistant *M. tuberculosis* increasing, newer agents are being tested in vitro to determine their efficacy.

The two reasons for drug failure are lack of patient compliance with drug therapy and resistance of the isolates. If compliance is an issue, directly observed therapy (DOT) is recommended to ensure proper medication. Otherwise, resistance may be assumed and tested for in vitro.

Mycobacterium bovis

M. bovis produces tuberculosis primarily in cattle but also in other ruminants, as well as dogs, cats, swine, parrots, and humans. The disease in humans closely resembles that caused by *M. tuberculosis* and is treated similarly. In some areas of the world, a significant percentage of cases of tuberculosis are due to *M. bovis,* but in the United States the number of isolates of this organism is very low.

M. bovis is closely related taxonomically to *M. tuberculosis* and belongs to the *M. tuberculosis* complex. It grows very slowly on egg-based medium, producing small, granular, rounded, white colonies with irregular margins after 21 days of incubation at 37° C. Growth is nonpigmented. On Middlebrook 7H10 medium, colonies are similar to those of *M. tuberculosis* but slower to mature. Most strains of *M. bovis* are niacin negative, do not reduce nitrate, and do not grow in the presence of TCH, characteristics that distinguish the species from most strains of *M. tuberculosis.*

NONTUBERCULOUS MYCOBACTERIA: CLINICAL SIGNIFICANCE AND DIFFERENTIATION

There is a large group of mycobacteria, excluding *M. tuberculosis* complex and *M. leprae,* that normally inhabit the environment and can cause disease, often resembling tuberculosis, in humans. These organisms are sometimes referred to as *atypical mycobacteria* or *mycobacteria other than the tubercle bacillus* (MOTT). The term *nontuberculous mycobacteria* (NTM) is used here.

Most NTMs are found in soil and water. They have been commonly implicated as opportunistic pathogens in patients with underlying lung disease, immunosuppression, or percutaneous trauma. AIDS has contributed greatly to the incidence and awareness of nontuberculous mycobacterial disease. Chronic pulmonary disease resembling tuberculosis is the usual clinical presentation associated with these organisms, although a few species are more often associated with cutaneous infections. Infections caused by the nontuberculous mycobacteria are not considered transmissible from person to person. Regional differences in the incidence of nontuberculous mycobacterial disease are quite striking.

Mycobacterium avium Complex
Epidemiology
Organisms within the *M. avium* complex (MAC) are commonly found in the environment and have been recovered from soil, water, house dust, and other environmental sources. Certain areas, such as coastal marshes, have higher concentrations of the organ-

ism. *M. avium* is a cause of disease in poultry and swine, but animal-to-human transmission has not been shown to be an important factor in human disease. Environmental sources, especially natural waters, seem to be the reservoir for human infections. A large increase in *M. avium* complex infections has occurred in the past decade, primarily owing to the number of infections in patients with AIDS.

Clinical infections
Pulmonary disease resulting from MAC infection presents a clinical picture similar to that of tuberculosis: cough, fatigue, weight loss, low-grade fever, and night sweats. Radiologic examination demonstrates cavitary disease in most patients, whereas solitary nodules or diffuse infiltrates may be observed in others. Disseminated disease has become more common, usually occurring in immunocompromised patients or patients with hematologic abnormalities. MAC infections are now the most common systemic bacterial infection in patients with AIDS.

The clinical outcome of *M. avium* complex lung disease is unpredictable; thus the management of affected patients can be difficult. Observation, therapy for underlying pulmonary disease (e.g., bronchodilators, broad-spectrum antibiotics, smoking cessation), and periodic sputum cultures may be all that is required for most patients. For patients with significant symptoms and advanced or progressive radiographic disease, multidrug therapy is indicated. For children with cervical lymphadenitis due to MAC, excisional surgery without chemotherapy is usually successful. A combination of surgical excision and chemotherapy is the usual treatment for adults with localized, nonpulmonary disease.

Most cases of disseminated disease in immunosuppressed patients without AIDS responds to multidrug regimens. Multidrug therapy consisting of ethambutol, rifampin (or rifabutin), clofazimine, and an injectable aminoglycoside has resulted in symptomatic and clinical improvement in most (but not all) patients with AIDS. The treatment of MAC disease may be directed best by physicians experienced in pulmonary or mycobacterial disease.

Laboratory diagnosis
Because the two species within the MAC complex, *M. avium* and *M. intracellulare,* are so similar, most

laboratories do not distinguish between them but report isolates of both species as *M. avium* complex. On primary isolation media, these organisms grow slowly, producing thin, transparent or opaque, homogeneous, smooth colonies. A small proportion of strains may exhibit rough colonies. Usually the colonies are nonpigmented, but they may become yellow with age. Rarely are the colonies pigmented from the onset of detectable growth. Optimum growth temperature is 37° C. On microscopic examination, the cells are short and coccobacillary, uniformly stained without beading or banding. Long, thin, beaded bacilli resembling *Nocardia* species may be seen in stains of very young cultures or under certain other conditions. MAC species are inactive in the majority of physiologic tests used to identify the mycobacteria. Exceptions are the production of a heat-stable catalase and the ability to grow on media containing TCH at 2 μg/mL (see Table 22-2). Nonisotopic nucleic acid probes are available for the identification of MAC as well as the two individual species.

Susceptibility testing

In laboratory tests, members of the *M. avium* complex are generally resistant to the relatively low concentrations of antituberculosis drugs currently used for testing *M. tuberculosis.* Treatment recommendations have been based largely on empiric data rather than in vitro susceptibility testing. For this reason, routine agar dilution susceptibility testing with the antituberculosis agents, as currently performed for testing *M. tuberculosis,* is not recommended for *M. avium* complex isolates. Currently, the usefulness of testing at higher drug concentrations than used for *M. tuberculosis* or determination of minimum inhibitory concentrations is being evaluated. In vitro susceptibility studies using combinations of drugs have shown significant synergism between drugs. The significance of in vitro tests in predicting clinical response and recommendations for testing individual isolates have yet to be determined.

Mycobacterium kansasii
Epidemiology

M. kansasii, along with *M. avium* complex, is one of the two most common causes of nontuberculous mycobacterial pulmonary disease in humans.

In the United States, most cases of *M. kansasii* infections have been reported from the southern states of Texas, Louisiana, and Florida, from Illinois and Missouri in the Midwest, and from California. *M. kansasii* strains have been isolated from water, yet the natural source of human infection is not clear. As with other nontuberculous mycobacteria, infections are not normally considered contagious from person to person.

Clinical infections

The most common manifestation is chronic pulmonary disease involving the upper lobes, usually with evidence of cavitation and scarring. Extrapulmonary infections, including lymphadenitis, skin and soft-tissue infection, and joint infection, have been reported occasionally. Disseminated *M. kansasii* infection rarely occurs in the immunocompetent but has been reported in severely immunocompromised patients, particularly those with AIDS.

For treatment of pulmonary disease caused by *M. kansasii,* a multidrug regimen of isoniazid, rifampin, and ethambutol is currently recommended. Isolates of *M. kansasii* are resistant to pyrazinamide; therefore this drug is not an alternative choice for treatment.

Laboratory diagnosis

Cells of *M. kansasii* are long rods with distinct cross-banding. This slowly growing organism has an optimal growth temperature of 37° C. Colonies are smooth to rough with wavy edges and dark centers when grown on Middlebrook 7H10 agar. Some cording usually can be seen with low-power magnification. Colonies grown in the dark are nonpigmented or buff; when grown in light or exposed to light, colonies become yellow (photochromogenic) (Figure 22-13). With prolonged exposure to light, most strains form dark red crystals of 10 β-carotene on the surface of and inside the colony. Rarely, scotochromogenic and nonchromogenic strains are isolated. Most strains are strongly catalase positive (>45 mm); less commonly isolated are strains that are low catalase producers (<45 mm).

Characteristics that distinguish this species are a growth rate similar to that of *M. tuberculosis* at 37° C, strong photochromogenic properties, ability to hydrolyze Tween 80 in 3 days, strong nitrate

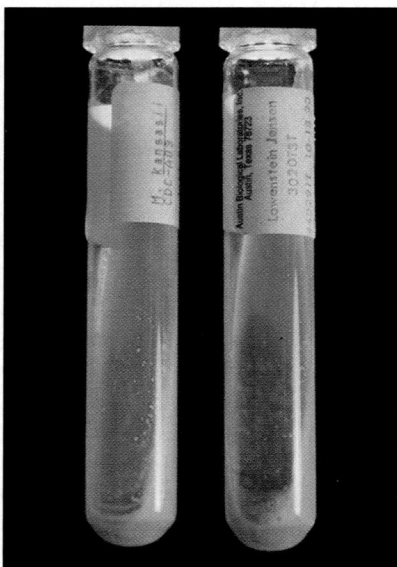

Figure 22-13 _____

Mycobacterium kansasii on Löwenstein-Jensen (LJ) medium showing photoreactivity. *Left,* Before exposure to light; *right,* after exposure to light.

reduction and catalase production, and pyrazinamidase production (see Table 22-2). A nonisotopic nucleic acid probe for the identification of *M. kansasii* isolates is available commercially.

When tested in vitro using the current drug concentrations recommended for *M. tuberculosis,* most strains of *M. kansasii* are susceptible to rifampin and ethambutol, partially resistant to isoniazid and streptomycin, and resistant to pyrazinamide.

Mycobacterium fortuitum-chelonei Complex

The *Mycobacterium fortuitum-chelonei* complex is made up of the species *M. fortuitum* and its biovariants, *M. chelonei* and its subspecies, and *M. abscessus* (formerly *M. chelonei* subsp. *abscessus*). Organisms in this complex are acid-fast and nonpigmented, stain positive, grow in less than 7 days at their optimal temperature, are arylsulfatase positive at 3 days, and grow at 38° C on MacConkey agar without crystal violet. Species within the complex can be differentiated by additional biochemical tests, however. Differentiating features that distinguish *M. fortuitum-chelonei* from other rapidly growing species are shown in Table 22-2.

M. fortuitum and *M. chelonei* are commonly found in the same types of infections, yet the two species vary in their susceptibility to antimicrobial agents, *M. fortuitum* generally being more susceptible. For this reason, determination of species and subspecies of clinically significant isolates may be warranted.

Mycobacterium fortuitum

Common in the environment, *M. fortuitum* has been isolated from water, soil, and dust. The organism has been implicated frequently in infections of the skin and soft tissues, including localized infections and abscesses at the site of puncture wounds. Infections associated with long-term use of intravenous and peritoneal catheters, injection sites, and surgical wounds following mammoplasty and cardiac bypass procedures have been reported. A variety of other infections have been associated with *M. fortuitum.* Differences in susceptibility to antimicrobial agents occur within the three subspecies; thus, in vitro susceptibility testing is often recommended for clinically significant isolates. A test method using a broth microdilution minimum inhibitory concentration determination has been well studied for the rapidly growing mycobacteria.

After 3 to 5 days of incubation at 37° C, colonies of the rapidly growing *M. fortuitum* appear rough or smooth and either nonpigmented, creamy white, or buff. Microscopic examination of growth on cornmeal-glycerol and Middlebrook 7H11 agars after 1 to 2 days of incubation reveals colonies with branching, filamentous extensions, and rough colonies with short aerial hyphae. On microscopic examination, cells are pleomorphic, ranging from long, tapered to short, thick rods. Most cultures, especially older ones, tend to decolorize and appear partially acid-fast on any of the acid-fast staining techniques. Additional characteristics that distinguish *M. fortuitum* from other rapidly growing mycobacteria are the positive 3-day arylsulfatase test and the reduction of nitrate (see Table 22-2). Three biovariants of *M. fortuitum* exist: biovariant *fortuitum,* biovariant *peregrinum* (proposed *M. peregrinum* sp. nov., nom.rev.), and a biovariant referred to as "third group" (*M. fortuitum* ssp. *acetamidolyticum*). Separation of these three biovariants can be made on the ability of the isolate to use mannitol, inositol, or sodium citrate as a sole source of carbon.

Mycobacterium chelonei

M. chelonei is found in the environment and associated with many of the same opportunistic infections as *M. fortuitum*. Both species have been associated with a variety of infections of the skin, lungs, bone, central nervous system, and prosthetic heart valves as well as with disseminated disease. *M. chelonei* exhibits more resistance to antimicrobial agents than *M. fortuitum* but sometimes is susceptible to amikacin and a sulfonamide.

Microscopically, young cultures of *M. chelonei* are strongly acid fast, with pleomorphism ranging from long, tapered to short, thick rods. This rapidly growing mycobacterium produces rough or smooth, nonpigmented to buff colonies within 3 to 5 days of incubation at 37° C. Unlike *M. fortuitum, M. chelonei* does not produce extensive filamentous branching colonies on cornmeal-glycerol agar. A positive 3-day arylsulfatase test, no reduction of nitrate, and growth on MacConkey agar without crystal violet are additional characteristics that differentiate *M. chelonei* from other rapidly growing mycobacteria (see Table 22-2). *M. chelonei* ssp. *chelonae* can be distinguished from *M. abscessus* (formerly designated as *M. chelonei* ssp. *abscessus*) because the former does not grow in the presence of 5% sodium chloride and is able to use citrate as a sole source of carbon. An unnamed mycobacterial species, referred to as *M. chelonei*–like organism (MCLO), does not grow in the presence of 5% sodium chloride, usually uses citrate and mannitol as a sole carbon source, and gives an unusual tan (±) reaction on iron uptake medium.

Mycobacterium marinum

M. marinum has been implicated in diseases of fish and isolated from aquariums. Cutaneous infections in humans have occurred when traumatized skin came in contact with inadequately chlorinated fresh water or with salt water. Outbreaks of cutaneous lesions in lifeguards have been reported. The typical presentation of a tender red or blue-red subcutaneous nodule, or "swimming pool granuloma," usually occurs on the elbow, knee, toe, or finger. In some cases, an abscess develops at the primary site of inoculation, with secondary ascending spread along the lymphatics. Treatment modalities include simple observation of minor lesions, surgical excision, antituberculosis drug therapy, and the use of single antibiotic agents. In the standard in vitro susceptibility testing, as currently used to test *M. tuberculosis, M. marinum* is susceptible to rifampin and ethambutol, resistant to isoniazid and pyrazinamide, and partially resistant or intermediate to streptomycin.

Cells of *M. marinum* are moderately long to long rods with cross-barring. Colonies of this slowly growing organism are smooth to rough (Figure 22-14) and wrinkled on inspissated egg medium but may be smooth when grown on Middlebrook 7H10 or 7H11 agar. *M. marinum* is photochromogenic; young colonies grown in the dark may be nonpigmented or buff, whereas colonies grown in or exposed to light develop a deep yellow color. Growth is optimum at incubation temperatures of 30° to 32° C. This preference for growth at the lower incubation temperatures, along with photochromogenicity, are clues to the identification of *M. marinum.* Some strains of *M. marinum* produce niacin; however, none reduces or produces nitrate heat-stable catalase. The organisms hydrolyze Tween 80 and produce urease and pyrazinamidase (see Table 22-2).

Mycobacterium scrofulaceum

The most common form of disease associated with *M. scrofulaceum* is cervical lymphadenitis in children. The infection manifests in one or more enlarged nodes, often adjacent to the mandible and high in the neck, with little or no pain. Patients are usually treated by surgical incision and drainage; antituberculosis drugs usually are not

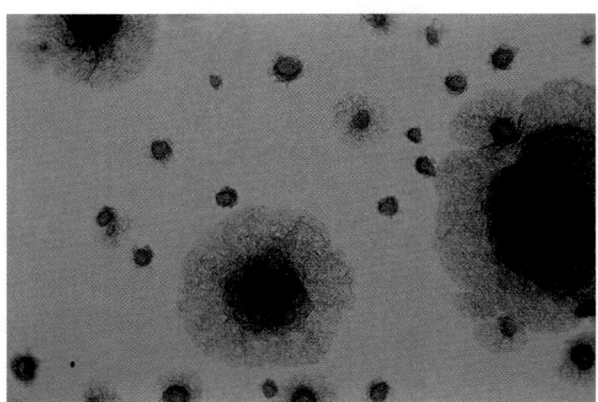

Figure 22-14 _____

Mycobacterium marinum on Middlebrook 7H10 growing rough colonies.

necessary. Pulmonary infections caused by *M. scrofulaceum* have been reported. *M. scrofulaceum* is resistant to isoniazid, streptomycin, ethambutol, and *p*-aminosalicylic acid when tested in vitro using the current procedure for testing *M. tuberculosis.*

On microscopic examination, *M. scrofulaceum* is a uniformly stained, acid-fast, medium to long rod. The organism grows slowly (4 to 6 weeks) at incubation temperatures ranging from 25° to 37° C. Colonies are smooth with dense centers and pigmentation from light yellow to deep orange. The organism is scotochromogenic (Figure 22-15); that is, pigment is produced when cultures are incubated in the absence of light and may darken when exposed to light. Members of this species do not hydrolyze Tween 80 nor reduce nitrate, but they do produce urease and are high (>45 mm) catalase producers (see Table 22-2). These characteristics aid in differentiating this organism from other slowly growing scotochromogens, including certain strains of *M. avium* complex, *M. gordonae,* and *M. szulgai.*

Organisms with characteristics of both *M. scrofulaceum* and *M. avium* complex have been isolated

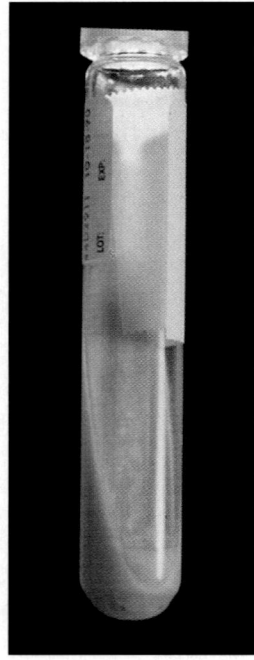

Figure 22-15 ⎯⎯⎯⎯⎯⎯⎯⎯⎯⎯⎯⎯⎯

Mycobacterium scrofulaceum on Löwenstein-Jensen (LJ) medium.

from clinical specimens. These organisms are referred to as *M. avium-intracellulare-scrofulaceum,* or MAIS group. The potential for pathogenicity of these organisms has yet to be determined.

Mycobacterium xenopi

M. xenopi has been recovered from hot and cold water taps (including water storage tanks of hospitals) and birds. The organism was first isolated from an African toad and considered nonpathogenic for humans until recently. Isolation of *M. xenopi* is relatively uncommon in the United States, yet it has been reported as one of the most commonly found nontuberculous mycobacteria in southeast England. The reported human cases of *M. xenopi* infection are mostly slowly progressive pulmonary infections in individuals with predisposing conditions. Preexistent lung disease, alcoholism, malignancy, and diabetes mellitus are some of the conditions associated with reported *M. xenopi* infections. The pulmonary infections presented clinical pictures similar to those seen in patients with *M. tuberculosis, M. kansasii,* or *M. avium* complex infection. Disseminated and extrapulmonary infections have been reported. Strains of *M. xenopi* are susceptible to the quinolones (ciprofloxacin and ofloxacin); some isolates are susceptible to vancomycin, erythromycin, or cefuroxime. In vitro susceptibility to antituberculosis drugs is variable, with resistance to ethambutol only being the most common pattern.

On acid-fast–stained smears, *M. xenopi* are long, filamentous rods. Colonies of this slowly growing mycobacterium on Middlebrook 7H10 agar are small with dense centers and filamentous edges. Microscopic observation (low-power magnification) of colonies growing on cornmeal-glycerol agar reveals distinctive round colonies with branching and filamentous extensions. Aerial hyphae are usually seen in rough colonies. Young colonies on cornmeal agar show a "bird's nest" appearance, with stick-like projections. Optimal growth temperature is 42° C; the organism grows more rapidly at this temperature than at 37° C and fails to grow at 25° C. This organism has been classified with the nonphotochromogenic group; however, colonies frequently are bright yellow on primary isolation when incubated in the absence of light and when exposed to light. Distinctive characteristics, in addition to optimum growth at 42° C and yellow scotochromogenic pigment, are negative reactions for niacin accumulation and nitrate reduction and positive reactions for the production of heat-stable catalase, arylsulfatase, and pyrazinamidase (see Table 22-2).

Mycobacterium celatum

A newly described species, *Mycobacterium celatum* sp. nov. is a slowly growing, nonphotochromogenic organism very similar in biochemical characteristics to *M. xenopi.* Mycolic acid patterns of this new species, as determined by HPLC, are most similar to those of *M. xenopi* but are distinct from other described species. In contrast to *M. xenopi, M. celatum* grows best at 37° C and poorly at 45° C, produces large colonies on Middlebrook 7H10 agar, and is usually resistant to rifabutin.

Mycobacterium szulgai

Of the reported infections with *M. szulgai,* the most common manifestation is pulmonary disease similar to tuberculosis. Extrapulmonary infections, including lymphadenitis and bursitis, also have been reported. This organism is much more susceptible than *M. avium* complex to the conventional antituberculosis drugs.

On microscopic examination of an acid-fast–stained smear, cells of *M. szulgai* are medium to long rods with some cross-barring. When the organism is cultured on egg-based medium at 37° C, smooth and rough colonies are observed. At 37° C, yellow to orange pigment develops in the absence of light and intensifies with exposure to light (scotochromogenic). Colonies grown at 22° C are nonpigmented or buff in the absence of light and develop yellow to orange pigment with light exposure (photochromogenic). Characteristics that differentiate *M. szulgai* from other slowly growing mycobacteria are slow hydrolysis of Tween 80, positive nitrate reduction, and inability to grow in the presence of 5% sodium chloride. The last characteristic, along with photochromogenicity at 22° C, distinguishes *M. szulgai* from *M. flavescens* (see Table 22-2).

Mycobacterium malmoense

Pulmonary disease associated with *M. malmoense* has been reported more commonly outside the United States, such as in Sweden, England, Wales, and Scotland. Reports of cases of chronic pulmonary disease and cervical adenitis in the United States have appeared, however. In laboratory studies using conventional antituberculosis drug resistance

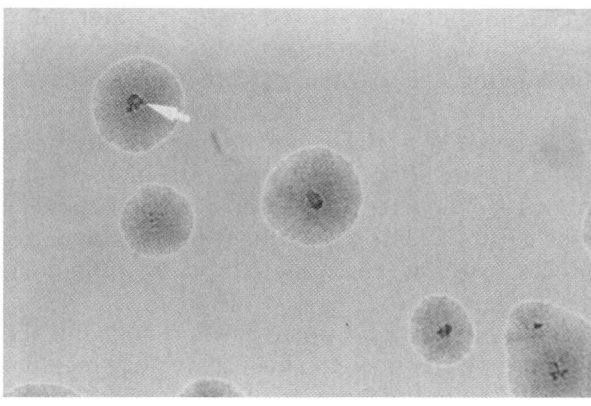

Figure 22-16 _____

Mycobacterium malmoense on Middlebrook 7H10 medium.

testing, *M. malmoense* is resistant to isoniazid, streptomycin, *p*-aminosalicylic acid, and rifampin and is susceptible to ethambutol and cycloserine.

M. malmoense appears as a short coccobacilli without cross-bands on acid-fast–stained smears. Colonies are smooth (Figure 22-16), glistening, and opaque with dense centers. Color is nonpigmented to buff; exposure to light does not produce pigment **(nonphotochromogenic).** Growth rate is slow; optimum growth temperature is 37° C; growth at 22° C may require as much as 7 weeks of incubation. Some strains may require longer incubation (up to 12 weeks) before colonies become visible. For this reason, some investigators suspect that *M. malmoense* may be underreported in the United States, because most laboratories incubate cultures for 6 weeks, 2 to 6 weeks less than the incubation period needed for some strains of this organism. The increase in the isolation of *M. malmoense* may be attributed to the implementation of radiometric culture techniques in larger laboratories.

Differential characteristics of *M. malmoense* are no accumulation of niacin, absence of nitrate reduction, ability to hydrolyze Tween 80, and the usual production of a heat-stable (68° C) catalase. *M. malmoense* can be differentiated from biochemically similar *M. gastri* on the basis of the urease-negative and pyrazinamidase-positive reactions of *M. malmoense* (see Table 22-2).

Mycobacterium simiae

The original strains of *M. simiae* were isolated from the lymph nodes of monkeys. Although the organism has been recovered from tap water, there seems to be significant geographical variation in the incidence. For example, *M. simiae* is rarely isolated in most parts of the United States, but in parts of Texas, it is a relatively common isolate. Infrequent cases of human infection from *M. simiae* have been reported and are most often pulmonary disease in patients with preexisting lung damage. Most isolates are resistant to most antituberculosis drugs in vitro.

Cells of *M. simiae* appear as short coccobacilli. When they are grown on inspissated egg medium at 37° C, smooth colonies appear in 10 to 21 days. Colonies on Middlebrook 7H10 agar are thin, transparent or tiny, and filamentous. The species is usually photochromogenic, being nonpigmented or buff when incubated in the absence of light and yellow when exposed to light. Development of the yellow pigment may require prolonged incubation, whereas some strains may fail to produce pigment on exposure to light. Differential biochemical characteristics are the accumulation of niacin, negative nitrate, reduction, and high level (> 45 mm) of heat-stable catalase (see Table 22-2).

Mycobacterium ulcerans

M. ulcerans is a very rare cause of mycobacteriosis in the United States but has been reported more frequently in other parts of the world. The disease manifests as a painless nodule under the skin after previous trauma. A shallow ulcer develops that may be quite severe. Patients rarely develop fever or systemic symptoms.

The acid-fast cells of *M. ulcerans* are moderately long without beading or cross-banding. Optimal growth temperature is 30° to 33° C with little growth at 25° C and usually none at 37° C. The organism grows slowly, often requiring 6 to 12 weeks of incubation before colonies are evident. Colonies are smooth and rough and nonpigmented or lightly buff, and they do not develop pigment with exposure to light (nonphotochromogenic). *M. ulcerans* produces a heat-stable catalase but is inert to most other conventional biochemical tests.

Mycobacterium haemophilum

The rare infections associated with *M. haemophilum* occur primarily in patients who are immunocompromised. Cases have been reported in patients with Hodgkin's disease and AIDS. Submandibular lymphadenitis, subcutaneous nodules, painful swellings, ulcers progressing to abscesses, and draining fistulas are often the clinical manifestations.

A unique characteristic of this organism is its requirement for hemoglobin or hemin for growth. Isolation of this species is accomplished on media supplying the needed growth supplement, such as chocolate agar, Mueller-Hinton agar with 5% Fildes enrichment, and Löwenstein-Jensen medium containing 2% ferric ammonium citrate. Successful isolation on Middlebrook 7H10 agar with an X-factor disk planted in the inoculated area has been reported (Vadney and Hawkins). Optimum growth temperature is 28° to 32° C; little or no growth occurs at 37° C. Colonies are rough to smooth and nonpigmented. Microscopically, the cells are strongly acid-fast, short, occasionally curved bacilli without banding or beading and arranged in tight clusters or cords.

Mycobacterium gordonae

M. gordonae is commonly found in water taps and soil and is generally referred to as the *tap-water bacillus.* This organism is frequently found in clinical specimens as a causal resident but is rarely implicated in disease. Infections reported in the literature have been isolated cases of meningitis secondary to ventriculoatrial shunts, hepatoperitoneal disease, endocarditis in a prosthetic aortic valve, synovitis, cutaneous lesions of the hand, and possible cases of pulmonary disease. In laboratory in vitro antituberculosis drug resistance tests, *M. gordonae* is resistant to isoniazid, streptomycin, and *p*-aminosalicyclic acid but susceptible to rifampin and ethambutol.

Growth of *M. gordonae* appears on egg-based medium after 10 to 14 days as smooth, yellow-orange colonies pigmented with both absence of and exposure to light (scotochromogenic). Optimum growth temperature range is 22° to 37° C. Differential characteristics are negative nitrate reduction, ability to hydrolyze Tween 80, and the production of heat-stable catalase (see Table 22-2). Isolates of *M. gordonae* can be rapidly identified with the use of a commercially available nucleic acid probe specific to the species.

Mycobacterium asiaticum

Mycobacterium asiaticum is a normally saprophytic *Mycobacterium* species that very rarely causes human infection. The cells are acid-fast coccoid rods. Growth on inspissated egg medium after 15 to 21 days at 37° C is dysgonic and smooth. Members of this species are usually photochromogenic, showing no pigment or buff when cultured in the absence of light and yellow when exposed to light. Occasional strains fail to develop pigment after exposure to light. *M. asiaticum* fails to reduce nitrate and produces a high level (> 45 mm) of heat-stable catalase. No accumulation of niacin and the hydrolysis of Tween 80 are useful characteristics in differentiating this organism from *M. simiae* (see Table 22-2).

Mycobacterium thermoresistibile

Mycobacterium thermoresistibile is uncommonly isolated from clinical specimens. The species is classified as a rapidly growing mycobacterium, yet on primary isolation, it may grow slowly because of its preference for higher incubation temperatures. Thus, it may be mistaken for a slowly growing scotochromogen. On subculture on egg-based medium, the organism produces smooth to rough yellow colonies within 3 to 5 days. Distinctive characteristics of this species are the ability to grow at 52° C and a negative iron uptake test (see Table 22-2).

Mycobacterium terrae-triviale Complex

There have been a few reported cases of human infection associated with the *Mycobacterium terrae-triviale* complex. Rare cases of septic arthritis, synovitis, osteomyelitis, respiratory infection, and tenosynovitis of the fingers, hands, and wrists have been reported. Isolates from the sputum and gastric lavage of humans are not uncommon and often are considered casual residents.

Microscopically, members of the *M. terrae-triviale* complex appear as acid-fast, short to medium coccobacilli. Both species, *M. terrae* and *M. triviale,* grow slowly at an optimum temperature of 37° C and are nonphotochromogenic. The colonies of *M. triviale* on egg-based medium are rough, dry, and heaped, whereas the colonies of *M. terrae* tend to be smoother. Characteristics that differentiate the complex from other mycobacteria are hydrolysis of Tween 80, reduction of nitrate, and the presence of a heat-stable catalase (see Table 22-2).

Mycobacterium nonchromogenicum

Mycobacterium nonchromogenicum is another species that is most commonly saprophytic but on rare occasions pathogenic. Primary lung disease due to *M. nonchromogenicum* has been reported. The cells are acid-fast, moderately long rods. After incubation at 37° C, colonies of this slowly growing, nonphotochromogenic species are smooth to rough, and white to buff. Positive pyrazinamidase and negative nitrate reduction reactions differentiate *M. nonchromogenicum* from the *M. terrae-triviale* complex (see Table 22-2). Because of the similarities among *M. nonchromogenicum, M. terrae,* and *M. triviale,* some observers classify the three species in an *M. terrae* complex.

Mycobacterium flavescens

Isolation of *M. flavescens* from human clinical specimens usually represents contamination or colonization. The cells are coccoid rods that show irregular acid fastness with acid-fast stains. Growth rate is intermediate with soft, yellow-orange, butyrous colonies appearing on egg-based medium after 7 to 10 days at 37° C. Some strains grow well at temperatures up to 45° C. The species is scotochromogenic, pigmentation appearing when isolates are cultivated in the absence and in the presence of light. This organism can grow on routine bacteriologic media, as can other of the more rapidly growing mycobacterial species. Other differential characteristics are the ability to hydrolyze Tween 80, reduction of nitrate, and tolerance to 5% sodium chloride (see Table 22-2).

Mycobacterium smegmatis

Commonly considered saprophytic, *Mycobacterium smegmatis* has been implicated in rare cases of pulmonary, skin, soft-tissue, and bone infections. Microscopically, on acid-fast stain, cells are long and tapered or short rods with irregular acid fastness. Occasionally, rods are curved with branching or Y-shaped forms; swollen with deeper staining, beaded or ovoid forms are sometimes seen. Colonies appearing on egg medium after 2 to 4 days are usually rough, wrinkled, or coarsely folded; smooth, glistening, butyrous colonies may also be seen. Colonies on Middlebrook 7H10 agar are heaped and smooth or rough with dense centers. Pigmentation is rare or late; colonies appear nonpigmented, creamy white, or buff to pink in older cultures. In addition to the rapid growth rate and the nonpigmented, rough colony form, characteristics valuable in the identification of this organism are its negative arylsulfatase reaction, positive iron uptake, ability to reduce nitrate, and growth in the presence of 5% sodium chloride and on MacConkey agar without crystal violet (see Table 22-2).

Mycobacterium phlei

At one time, *M. phlei* was common to the environment, particularly in hay and grass, but it is now only occasionally encountered in human clinical specimens. This organism is classified as a rapidly growing mycobacterium, with growth appearing on egg-based medium after 3 to 5 days at 37° C. Growth also takes place at incubation temperatures of 45° and 52° C. Colonies are usually rough or coarsely wrinkled with a deep yellow to orange pigment. Occasional strains are smooth and butyrous. Typical strains incubated on Middlebrook 7H10 agar show heaped, rough colonies with dense centers. Microscopically, *M. phlei* is short, coccoid rods that stain irregularly with the acid-fast stain (i.e., some cells within the smear do not appear acid fast). Other characteristics, in addition to the rough, orange-pigmented colonies, that differentiate *M. phlei* from other rapidly growing mycobacteria are a negative arylsulfatase reaction, positive iron uptake, and inability to grow on MacConkey agar without crystal violet (see Table 22-2).

Mycobacterium vaccae

Mycobacterium vaccae, a saprophytic organism occasionally isolated from clinical specimens, is a rapidly growing (3 to 5 days) mycobacterium. Colonies on egg-based medium are smooth, moist, and shiny with buff to orange pigment. The organism may be buff at 35° C incubation but turns pigmented at cooler temperatures. Colony morphology on Middlebrook 7H10 agar is varied, often "slick" in appearance; there may be amorphous or poor growth on this medium. Cells are short, coccoid rods staining irregularly acid fast in older cultures. *M. vaccae* is differentiated from other arylsulfatase-negative, rapidly growing mycobacteria primarily on the basis of colony morphology and pigmentation (see Table 22-2).

Mycobacterium gastri

M. gastri has been found in soil and very rarely in human gastric lavage and sputum specimens. When present in clinical specimens, it generally has been regarded as a casual resident not associated with disease. Cells are moderately long to long rods with cross-barring common. Colonies on inspissated egg medium at 37° C are slowly growing, rough, and nonpigmented or buff in both absence and presence of light (nonphotochromogenic). On Middlebrook 7H10 agar, colonies are dense and rough and may have wavy edges. Differentiation of *M. gastri* from other slowly growing, nonphotochromogenic mycobacteria is based on the following characteristics: no niacin accumulation, ability to hydrolyze Tween 80, negative nitrate reduction, and low level of heat-labile catalase (see Table 22-2).

Mycobacterium paratuberculosis

Mycobacterium paratuberculosis is the causative agent of Johne's disease, an intestinal infection occurring as a chronic diarrhea in cattle, sheep, goats, and other ruminants. A *Mycobacterium* species that most closely resembles *M. paratuberculosis* has been reported as being isolated from samples taken from resected terminal ileum of three patients with Crohn's disease. *M. paratuberculosis* is difficult to cultivate because of its very slow growth rate (3 to 4 months) and its need for a mycobactin-supplemented medium for primary isolation. (Mycobactin is an iron-binding hydroxymate compound produced by other mycobacterial species.)

Mycobacterium genavense

A new species, *Mycobacterium genavense,* has been reported as a cause of disseminated infections in patients with AIDS. This slowly growing, fastidious mycobacterium has been recovered in BACTEC cultures but failed to grow on subculture to routine solid media. Dysgonic growth was obtained when subculture medium Middlebrook 7H11 agar was supplemented with mycobactin J. In a reported study (Coyle) of isolates from seven patients with AIDS, the subculture growth from the supplemented medium consistently yielded positive tests for semiquantitative and heat-stable-catalase, pyrazinamidase, and urease.

MYCOBACTERIUM LEPRAE

M. leprae is the causative agent of Hansen disease (leprosy), an infection of the skin, mucous mem-

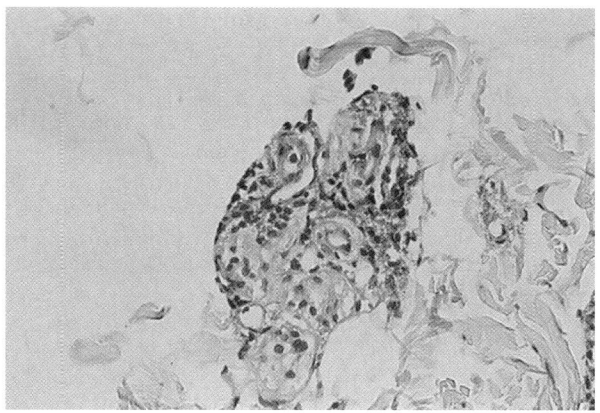

Figure 22-17

Mycobacterium leprae from a skin biopsy from a patient with lepromatous leprosy (acid-fast smear stained with Ziehl-Neelsen stain).

M. leprae is a rod-shaped bacterium usually 1 to 7 μm in length and 0.3 to 0.5 μm wide. After examination of the entire smear, the number of organisms present per oil immersion field (1000×) is reported as the *bacteriologic index* (BI). The number of "solid-staining" cells per 100 total bacilli exmined is reported as the *morphologic index* (MI). "Solid-staining" cells are those with dense, uniform staining of the entire bacillus with even sides and rounded ends in which the length of the bacillus is at least five times the width of the bacillus. The BI and MI aid the clinician in determining the progress of the disease. The definitive laboratory diagnosis is the development of disease in laboratory mice following inoculation of patient biopsy material to the mouse footpad.

branes, and peripheral nerves. The disease is rare in the United States and other Western countries, yet it remains a major problem in other parts of the world. In the United States, the reported cases are generally from areas with a warm climate, including California, Texas, Louisiana, Florida, Hawaii, and Puerto Rico.

There are two major forms of the disease, tuberculoid leprosy and lepromatous leprosy, but there is no distinct separation between these two manifestations. With tuberculoid leprosy, skin lesions and nerve involvement producing areas of anesthesia may occur. Spontaneous recovery often occurs with tuberculoid leprosy. On the other hand, lepromatous leprosy is slowly progressive, malignant, and, if untreated, life threatening. It is characterized by skin lesions and progressive, symmetric nerve damage. Lesions of the mucous membranes of the nose may lead to destruction of the cartilaginous septum, resulting in nasal and facial deformities. Current therapy usually consists of a combination of diaminodiphenylsulfone (dapsone), clofazimine, and rifampin.

Laboratory diagnosis of leprosy depends on the microscopic demonstration of acid-fast bacilli that cannot be cultured from skin biopsy specimens. Organisms are extremely rare and may not be detected in skin scrapings or biopsy specimens from patients with tuberculoid leprosy. However, acid-fast bacilli are usually abundant in samples from patients with lepromatous leprosy (Figure 22-17).

Bibliography

Abadco DL, Steiner P: Gastric lavage is better than bronchoalveolar lavage for isolation of *Mycobacterium tuberculosis* in childhood pulmonary tuberculosis, *Pediatr Infect Dis J* 11:735, 1992.

Abe C et al: Detection of *Mycobacterium tuberculosis* in clinical specimens by polymerase chain reaction and Gen-Probe amplified *Mycobacterium tuberculosis* direct test, *J Clin Microbiol* 31:3270, 1993.

Abe C et al: Comparison of MB-Check, BACTEC, and egg-based media for recovery of Mycobacteria, *J Clin Microbiol* 30:878, 1992.

American Thoracic Society: Diagnosis and treatment of disease caused by nontuberculous mycobacteria, *Am Rev Respir Dis* 142:940, 1990.

American Thoracic Society: Diagnostic standards and classification of tuberculosis, *Am Rev Respir Dis* 142:725, 1990.

American Thoracic Society: Levels of laboratory services for mycobacterial diseases: official statement of the American Thoracic Society, *Am Rev Respir Dis* 128:213, 1983.

Anargyros P, Astill DSJ, Lim FSL: Comparison of impoved BACTEC and Löwenstein-Jensen media for culture of mycobacteria from clinical specimens, *J Clin Microbiol* 28:1288, 1990.

Barnes PF et al: Tuberculosis in patients with human immunodeficiency virus infection, *N Engl J Med* 324:1644, 1991.

Bates JH: Diagnosis of tuberculosis, *Chest* 76:757, 1979.

Beam RE, Kubica GP: Stimulatory effects of carbon dioxide on the primary isolation of tubercle bacilli on agar-containing medium, *Am J Clin Pathol* 50:395, 1968.

Bloch AB et al: Nationwide survey of drug resistant tuberculosis in the United States, *JAMA* 271:665, 1994.

Böttger EC, Hirschel B, Coyle MB: *Mycobacterium genavense* sp. nov, *Int J Syst Bacteriol* 43:841, 1993.

Butler WR et al: *Mycobacterium celatum* sp. nov, *Int J Syst Bacteriol* 43:539, 1993.

Centers for Disease Control: Advisory Council for the Elimination of Tuberculosis: screening for tuberculosis and tuberculosis infection in high-risk populations, *MMWR* 44(RR), 1995.

Chopin-Robertson K et al: Detection and identification of *Mycobacterium* directly from BACTEC bottles by using a DNA-rRNA probe, *Diagn Microbiol Infect Dis* 17:203, 1993.

Clarridge JE et al: Large scale use of polymerase chain reaction for detection of *Mycobacterium tuberculosis* in a routine mycobacteriology laboratory, *J Clin Microbiol* 31:2059, 1993.

Coyle MB, Carlson LDC: Laboratory aspects of *"Mycobacterium genavense,"* a proposed species isolated from AIDS patients, *J Clin Microbiol* 30:3206, 1992.

David HL, Selin MJ: Immune response to mycobacteria. In Rose NR, editor: *Manual of clinical immunology,* ed 2, Washington, DC, 1980, American Society for Microbiology.

Davis TE: *Mycobacterium tuberculosis:* a renewed challenge for the clinical microbiology laboratory, *Clin Microbiol Newsl* 14:97, 1992.

Desmond EP: Clinical features and laboratory identification of *Mycobacterium genavense, Clin Lab Newsl* 16:49, 1994.

DesPrez RM, Heim CR: *Mycobacterium tuberculosis.* In Mandell GL, Douglas RG, Bennett J, editors: *Principles and practice of infectious disease,* ed 3, New York, 1985, Churchill Livingstone.

Driver CR et al: Drug resistance among tuberculosis patients, New York City, 1991 and 1992, *Public Health Rep* 109:632, 1994.

Eisenach KD et al: Detection of *Mycobacterium tuberculosis* in sputum samples using a polymerase chain reaction, *Am Rev Respir Dis* 144:1160, 1991.

Ellner PD et al: Rapid detection and identification of pathogenic mycobacteria by combining radiometric and nuclei acid probe methods, *J Clin Microbiol* 26:1349, 1988.

Fisher JF et al: Utility of Gram's and Geimsa stains in the diagnosis of pulmonary tuberculosis, *Am Rev Respir Dis* 141:511, 1990.

Forbes BA, Hicks KES: Ability of PCR assay to identify *Mycobacterium tuberculosis* in BACTEC 12B vials, *J Clin Microbiol* 32:1725, 1994.

Forbes BA, Hicks KES: Direct detection of *Mycobacterium tuberculosis* in respiratory specimens in a clinical laboratory by polymerase chain reaction, *J Clin Microbiol* 31:1688, 1993.

Gonzalez R, Hanna BA: Evaluation of Gen-Probe DNA hybridization systems for the identification of *Mycobacterium tuberculosis* and *Mycobacterium avium-intracellulare, Diagn Microbiol Infect Dis* 8:69, 1987.

Gordin F, Slutkin G: The validity of acid-fast smears in the diagnosis of pulmonary tuberculosis, *Arch Pathol Lab Med* 114:1025, 1990.

Gross WM, Hawkins JE: Radiometric selective inhibition tests for differentiation of *Mycobacterium tuberculosis, Mycobacterium bovis,* and other Mycobacteria, *J Clin Microbiol* 21:565, 1985.

Guerrant GO, Lambert MA, Moss CW: Gas-chromotographic analysis of mycolic acid cleavage products in mycobacteria, *J Clin Microbiol* 13:899, 1981.

Havlik JA et al: Disseminated *Mycobacterium avium* complex infection: clinical identification and epidemiological trends, *J Infect Dis* 165:577, 1992.

Huebner RE, Good RC, Tokars JI: Current practices in mycobacteriology: results of a survey of state public health laboratories, *J Clin Microbiol* 31:771, 1993.

Inderlied CB, Kemper CA, Bermudez LEM: The *Mycobacterium avium* complex, *Clin Microbiol Rev* 6:266, 1993.

Isenberg HD et al: Collaborative feasibility study of a biphasic system (Roche Septi-Chek AFB) for rapid detection and isolation of Mycobacteria, *J Clin Microbiol* 29:1719, 1991.

Jonas V et al: Detection and identification of *Mycobacterium tuberculosis* directly from sputum sediments by amplification of rRNA, *J Clin Microbiol* 31:2410, 1993.

Kent PT, Kubica GP: *Public health mycobacteriology: a guide for the level III laboratory,* Atlanta, 1985, Centers for Disease Control.

Kiehn TE et al: *Mycobacterium tuberculosis* bacteremia detected by the Isolator lysis-centrifugation blood culture system, *J Clin Microbiol* 21:647, 1985.

Kirihara JM, Hillier SL, Coyle MB: Improved detection times for *Mycobacterium avium* complex and *Mycobacterium tuberculosis* with the BACTEC radiometric system, *J Clin Microbiol* 22:841, 1985.

Kubica GP, Wayne LG: The mycobacteria: a sourcebook, part A and part B, New York, 1984, Marcel Dekker.

Kusunoki S, Takayuki E: Proposal of *Mycobacterium peregrinum* sp. nov., nom.rev., and elevation of *Mycobacterium chelonae* sub. sp. *abscessus* (Kubica et al) to special status: *Mycobacterium abscessus* comb. nov, *Int J Syst Bacteriol* 42:240, 1992.

Laszlo A, Eidus L: Test for differentiation of *M. tuberculosis* and *M. bovis* from other mycobacteria, *Can J Microbiol* 24:754, 1978.

Lipsky BA et al: Factors affecting the clinical value of microscopy for acid-fast bacilli, *Rev Infect Dis* 6:214, 1984.

Morgan MA et al: Comparison of a radiometric method (BACTEC) and conventional culture media for recovery of mycobacteria from smear-negative specimens, *J Clin Microbiol* 18:384, 1983.

Morgan MA et al: Evaluation of the p-nitro-alpha-acetylamino-beta-hydroxypropriophenone differential test for identification of *Mycobacterium tuberculosis* complex, *J Clin Microbiol* 21:634, 1985.

National Committee for Clinical Laboratory Standards: *Antimycobacterial susceptibility testing: Proposed Standard Document M24-P,* vol 10, Villanova, Pa, 1990, NCCLS.

Nolte FS et al: Direct detection of *Mycobacterium tuberculosis* in sputum by polymerase chain reaction and DNA hybridization, *J Clin Microbiol* 31:1777, 1993.

Park CH et al: Rapid recovery of mycobacteria from clinical specimens using automated radiometric technic, *Am J Clin Pathol* 81:341, 1984.

Roberts GD, Koneman EW, Kim YK: *Mycobacterium.* In Balows A et al, editors: *Manual of clinical microbiology,* ed 5, Washington, DC, 1991, American Society for Microbiology.

Roberts GD et al: Evaluation of the BACTEC radiometric method for recovery of mycobacteria and drug susceptibility testing of *Mycobacterium tuberculosis* from smear-positive specimens, *J Clin Microbiol* 18:689, 1983.

Roberts GD, Thompson GP: Bacteriology and bacteriologic diagnosis of tuberculosis. In Schlossberg D, editor: Tuberculosis, ed 3, New York, 1994, Springer-Verlag.

Roberts MC et al: The use of p-nitro-alpha-acetylamino-beta-hydroxypropriophenone in the differentiation of mycobacteria, *Am Rev Respir Dis* 38:759, 1960.

Runyon EH: Identification of mycobacterial pathogens utilizing colony characteristics, *Am J Clin Pathol* 54:578, 1970.

Shafer RW et al: Extrapulmonary tuberculosis in patients with human immunodeficiency virus infection, *Medicine* 70:384, 1991.

Smith MB, Bergman JS, Woods GL: Detection of *Mycobacterium tuberculosis* in BACTEC 12B broth cultures by Roche Amplicor PCR Assay, *J Clin Microbiol* 35:900, 1997.

Sommers HM, McClatchy JK: *CUMITECH 16: laboratory diagnosis of the mycobacterioses,* Washington, DC, 1983, American Society for Microbiology.

Stager CE et al: Role of solid media when using in conjunction with the BACTEC system for mycobacterial isolation and identification, *J Clin Microbiol* 29:154, 1991.

Strong BE, Kubica GP: Isolation and identification of Mycobacterium tuberculosis: *a guide for the level II laboratory,* Atlanta, 1981, Centers for Disease Control.

Telenti A et al: Detection of rifampin-resistant mutations in *Mycobacterium tuberculosis, Lancet* 341:647, 1993.

Telenti A et al: Direct, automated detection of rifampin-resistant *Mycobacterium tuberculosis* by polymerase chain reaction and single-stranded conformation polymorphism analysis, *Antimicrob Agents Chemother* 37:2054, 1993.

Tenover FC et al: The resurgence of tuberculosis: is your laboratory ready? *J Clin Microbiol* 31:767, 1993.

Thibert L, LaPierre S: Routine application of high-performance liquid chromatography for identification of mycobacteria, *J Clin Microbiol* 31:1759, 1993.

Tisdale PA, Roberts GD, Anhalt JP: Identification of clinical isolates of *Mycobacterium* with gas-liquid chromotography alone, *J Clin Microbiol* 10:506, 1979.

Toossi Z, Ellner JJ: Tuberculosis. In Gorbach SL, Bartlett JG, Blacklow NR, editors: *Infectious diseases,* Philadelphia, 1992, WB Saunders.

Vadney FS, Hawkins JE: Evaluation of a simple method for growing *Mycobacterium haemophilum, J Clin Microbiol* 22:884, 1985.

Vannier AM, Tarrand JJ, Murray PR: Mycobacterial cross contamination during radiometric culturing, *J Clin Microbiol* 26:1867-1868, 1988.

Wayne LG, Kubica GP: Family Mycobacteriaceae. Chester 1897, 63, genus *Mycobacterium* (Lehmann and Neuman 1896, 363). In Sneath PHA, Mair NS, Sharpe ME, Holt JG, editors: *Bergey's manual of systematic bacteriology,* vol 2, Baltimore, 1986, Williams & Wilkins.

Welch DF et al: Timely culture for mycobacteria which utilizes a microcolony method, *J Clin Microbiol* 31:2178, 1993.

Whittier PS et al: Evaluation of the Septi-Chek AFB system in the recovery of mycobacteria, *Eur J Clin Microbiol* 11:915, 1992.

Wilson SM et al: Progress toward a simplified polymerase chain reaction and its application to diagnosis of tuberculosis, *J Clin Microbiol* 31:766, 1993.

Woods GL, Washington JA II: Mycobacteria other than *Mycobacterium tuberculosis:* review of microbiologic and clinical aspects, *Rev Infect Dis* 9:275, 1987.

Zhang Y et al: The catalase-peroxidase gene and isoniazid resistance of *Mycobacterium tuberculosis, Nature* 358:591, 1992.

LEARNING ASSESSMENT

1. Describe the current recommendations for the identification of *M. tuberculosis* in the clinical laboratory.

2. Describe why mycobacterial infections have to be treated for 6 months or more, and explain the need to use multiple drugs when treating *M. tuberculosis* infections.

3. Compare and contrast the different levels of mycobacterial laboratory testing, and cite the reasons why smaller-volume laboratories should consider not performing full identification and susceptibility testing on mycobacterial isolates.

4. Discuss the methods used to process clinical specimens for mycobacterial culture and the reasons specimens need to be decontaminated and digested before culture.

5. With respect to laboratory technique, give some problems that may lead to reporting false-negative and false-positive results.

CHAPTER 23

Medically Significant Fungi

Linda A. Smith, Annette W. Fothergill,
Deanna A. Sutton, James L. Harris

GENERAL CHARACTERISTICS
  Yeasts versus Molds
  Septate versus Sparsely Septate
  Hyaline versus Dematiaceous
  Dimorphism
  Reproduction

TAXONOMY
  Zygomycota
  Ascomycota
  Basidiomycota
  Fungi Imperfecti

CLINICAL SITES OF INFECTION
  Superficial Mycoses
  Cutaneous Mycoses
  Subcutaneous Mycoses
  Systemic Mycoses

SPECIMEN COLLECTION, HANDLING,
  AND TRANSPORT
  Hair
  Skin
  Nails
  Blood and Bone Marrow
  Cerebrospinal Fluid
  Abscess Fluid and Wound Exudates
  Respiratory Specimens
  Urogenital and Fecal Specimens

METHODS OF IDENTIFYING FUNGAL AGENTS
  Direct Microscopic Examination of Specimens
    KOH preparation
    KOH with calcofluor white
    India ink
    Tissue stains
  Culture
    Culture media
    Incubation

BEGINNING THE IDENTIFICATION
  Gross Examination of the Culture
  Microscopic Examination for Fungal Structures
    Tease mount
    Cellophane tape preparation
    Slide culture

SAFETY ISSUES

AGENTS OF SUPERFICIAL MYCOSES
  Malassezia furfur
  Piedraia hortae
  Trichosporon beigelii
  Phaeoannellomyces werneckii

AGENTS OF DERMATOPHYTOSES
  Epidemiology
  Clinical Infections
    Infections involving hair and hair follicles
    Infections involving the nail and nail bed
    Athlete's foot
    Systemic infections
  Treatment
  Commonly Encountered Dermatophytes
    Trichophyton mentagrophytes
    Trichophyton rubrum
    Trichophyton tonsurans
    Microsporum canis
    Microsporum gypseum
    Microsporum audouinii
    Epidermophyton floccosum
  Laboratory Diagnosis
    Specimen collection and processing
    Direct microscopic examination
    Culture
    Identification

Continued

AGENTS OF SUBCUTANEOUS MYCOSES
  Sporotrichosis
    Epidemiology
    Clinical infections
    Laboratory diagnosis
  Chromoblastomycosis
    Epidemiology
    Clinical infections
    Laboratory diagnosis
  Eumycotic Mycetoma
    Epidemiology
    Clinical infections
    Laboratory diagnosis
  Subcutaneous Phaeohyphomycosis
    Laboratory diagnosis

AGENTS OF SYSTEMIC MYCOSES
  Blastomyces dermatitidis
    Epidemiology
    Clinical infections
    Laboratory diagnosis
  Histoplasma capsulatum var. *capsulatum*
    Epidemiology
    Clinical infections
    Laboratory diagnosis

  Coccidioides immitis
    Epidemiology
    Clinical infections
    Laboratory diagnosis
  Paracoccidioides brasiliensis
    Epidemiology
    Clinical infections
    Laboratory diagnosis

AGENTS OF OPPORTUNISTIC FUNGAL
  INFECTIONS: THE SAPROBES

AGENTS OF YEAST INFECTIONS
  General Characteristics
  Clinically Significant Yeast Species
    Candida species
    Cryptococcus species
    Rhodotorula species
    Trichosporon beigelii
  Methods of Yeast Identification
    Germ tube production
    Carbohydrate assimilation
    Cornmeal agar morphology
    Potassium nitrate assimilation
    Urease test
    Temperature

OBJECTIVES

1. Describe the general characteristics of fungi.
2. List and describe the growth requirements of fungi.
3. Define the terms associated with fungal structures.
4. Classify fungi into their respective classes.
5. Describe asexual reproduction and sexual reproduction of fungi.
6. Describe the appropriate specimen collection procedures, staining methods, and culture techniques used in the mycology laboratory.
7. Characterize the following different types of mycoses, defining the tissues they affect:
   - Superficial
   - Cutaneous
   - Subcutaneous
   - Systemic
   - Opportunistic saprobic
8. Differentiate the etiologic agents of these mycoses.
9. List the common opportunistic saprobes associated with infections in immunocompromised hosts.

KEY TERMS

Mold
Yeast
Saprobe
Blastoconidia
Mycelium
Hyphae
Rhizoids
Septate hyphae
Hyaline hyphae
Dematiaceous hyphae
Dimorphic fungi
Conidia
Arthroconidia
Zygomycete
Sporangiophore
Sporangiospore
Ascomycota

Ascospore
Basidiomycete
Fungi Imperfecti
Superficial mycoses
Cutaneous mycoses
Subcutaneous mycoses
Systemic mycoses
Dermatophyte
Ectothrix
Endothrix
Macroconidia
Microconidia
Chromoblastomycosis
Eumycotic mycetoma
Pseudohyphae
Germ tube

CASE STUDY

A 45-year-old male presented to his physician with a history of a 3-week nonproductive cough and mild chest pain. He has a history of smoking one to two packs of cigarettes a day and has worked as a farmer in Ohio for the last 20 years. He does not have any disease or condition that would classify him as immunocompromised.

What in the patient history might provide a clue to the organism that is causing the disease?

What specimen and culture requirements would be appropriate to recover the organism?

Fungi constitute an extremely diverse group of organisms and are generally classified as either **molds** or **yeasts.** Some have been recognized as classic pathogens, whereas others are recognized only as environmental **saprobes.** With the advent of chemotherapy, radiation therapy, and diseases such as acquired immunodeficiency syndrome (AIDS) that affect the immune system, the line between pathogen and saprobe has been blurred. The isolation of all organisms, especially in the immunocompromised patient, must initially be considered a significant finding and evaluated in light of the patient history and physical examination results.

This chapter discusses the following:

- General characteristics of fungi, including the basic terminology relating to fungal structures
- Taxonomy and classification of fungi
- Specimen collection and processing appropriate for fungal recovery
- Methods of isolation and identification
- Various types of clinical infections associated with the most commonly encountered fungi, including agents of superficial infections, dermatophytoses, subcutaneous and systemic infections, opportunistic saprobes, and yeasts

GENERAL CHARACTERISTICS

The characteristics of the fungi are different from those of plants or bacteria. Fungi are eukaryotic, that is, they possess a true nucleus with nuclear membrane and mitochondria. Bacteria are prokaryotic, lacking these structures. Unlike plants, fungi lack chlorophyll and must absorb nutrients from the environment. In addition, fungal cell walls are made of chitin, whereas those of plants contain cellulose. Most fungi are aerobes that grow best at a neutral pH, although they tolerate a wide range of pH values. Moisture is necessary for growth, but spores and conidia survive in dry conditions.

Yeasts versus Molds

Yeasts are single vegetative cells that typically form a smooth, creamy bacterial-like colony without aerial hyphae. Identification of yeasts is based primarily on biochemical differences, because their morphologies are similar. Yeasts reproduce by budding, with subsequent production of a **blastoconidium** (daughter cell), as shown in Figure 23-1. This process involves lysis of the yeast cell wall so that a blastoconidium can form. As this structure enlarges, the nucleus of the parent cell undergoes mi-

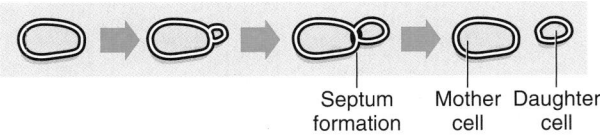

Septum formation   Mother cell   Daughter cell

Figure 23-1
Formation of blastoconidia in yeast.

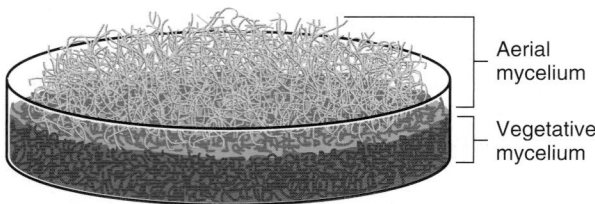

Figure 23-2

Aerial mycelia give mold the "woolly" appearance. Vegetative mycelia are responsible for absorbing nutrients from the medium.

tosis. Once the new nucleus is passed into the daughter cell, a septum forms and the daughter cell breaks free (see Figure 23-1).

Most molds, on the other hand, have a "fuzzy" or woolly appearance that is due to the mycelium (Figure 23-2). The **mycelium** is made up of many long strands of tubelike structures called **hyphae,** which may be aerial or vegetative. Aerial mycelium extends above the surface of the colony and is responsible for the macroscopic appearance. In ad-

dition, it may support the reproductive structures that can be used to identify the different fungal genera. The vegetative mycelium extends downward into the medium to absorb nutrients.

In some species, antler, racquet, or spiral hyphae may aid in identification (Figure 23-3, *A*). Antler hyphae have swollen, branching tips that resemble moose antlers. Racquet hyphae contain enlarged, club-shaped areas. Spiral hyphae are tightly coiled. **Rhizoids** (see Figure 23-3, *B*), rootlike structures, may be seen in some of the Zygomycetes.

Septate versus Sparsely Septate

Hyphae may be *septate* or sparsely septate. **Septate hyphae** (Figure 23-4, *A*) show frequent cross-walls between the cells, whereas sparsely septate hyphae (Figure 23-4, *B*) have few cross-walls at irregular intervals.

Hyaline versus Dematiaceous

Another characteristic useful in identification is pigmentation. **Hyaline hyphae** are lightly pigmented (see Figure 23-4, *A*), whereas **dematiaceous**

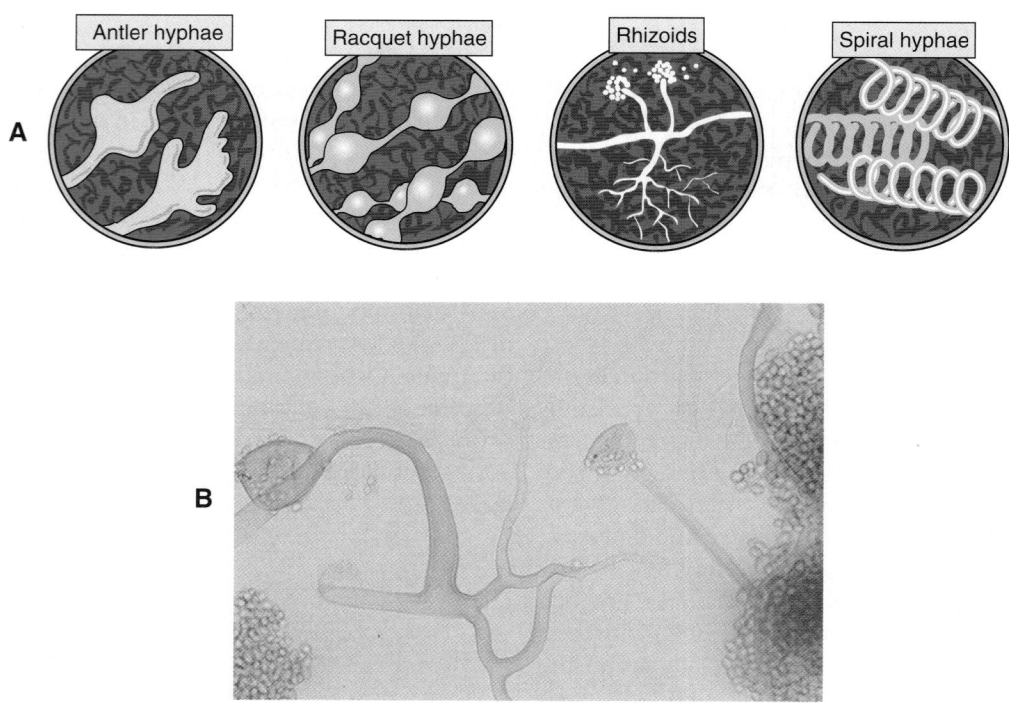

Figure 23-3

A, Specialized structures that are formed in vegetative mycelia by certain fungal species. **B,** *Rhizopus* sp. showing rhizoids.

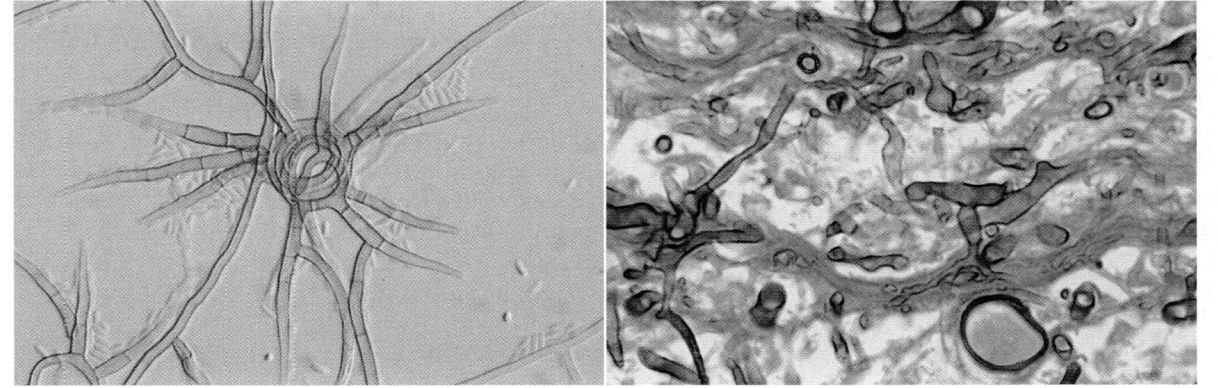

A   B

Figure 23-4

A, *Phaeoacremonium* sp. displaying septate hyphae. Zygomycetous hyphae in tissue **(B)** appears sparsely septate.

hyphae are darkly pigmented (Figure 23-5) because of the presence of melanin in the cell wall.

Dimorphism

Dimorphism refers to the ability of some fungi to exist in two forms. These **dimorphic fungi** include a mold phase and either a yeast or spherule phase. The yeast or tissue state is seen in vivo or when the organism is grown at 37° C with increased CO_2. The mold phase is seen when the organism is grown at room temperature (25° C).

Dimorphic fungal species include *Blastomyces dermatitidis, Coccidioides immitis, Histoplasma capsulatum* var. *capsulatum, Paracoccidioides brasiliensis, Sporothrix schenckii,* and *Penicillium marneffei.*

Reproduction

Fungi may reproduce asexually or sexually. Asexual reproduction results in the formation of **conidia** following mitosis. Asexual reproduction is carried out by specialized fruiting structures known as conidiogenous cells. These structures form conidia, which contain all the genetic material necessary to create a new fungal colony. Two common conidiogenous cells are the *phialide* (vaselike structures that produce phialoconidia) (Figure 23-6) and the *annellide* (ringed structures that produce annelloconidia). Both form their conidia blastically (budding) like many yeasts—the parent cell enlarges and a septum forms to separate the conidial cell. **Arthroconidia** are formed by fragmentation of fertile hyphae (Figure 23-7). In the clinical laboratory, most molds are identified on the basis of the structures formed as a result of asexual reproduction. Sexual

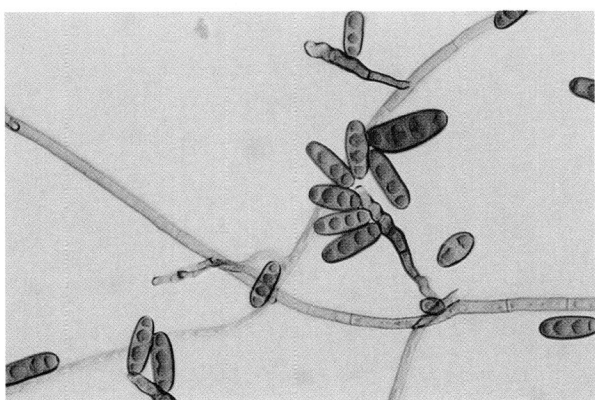

Figure 23-5

Bipolaris sp. is an example of a dematiaceous fungus. Note the dark pigmentation, which is due to the presence of melanin in the cell wall.

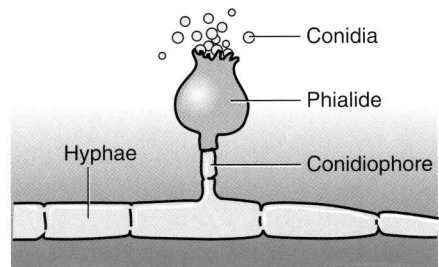

Figure 23-6

An example of asexual reproduction is the production of phialoconidia. Conidia are formed from conidiogenous cells like phialide (a vaselike structure). Phialoconidia are "blown out" of the phialide.

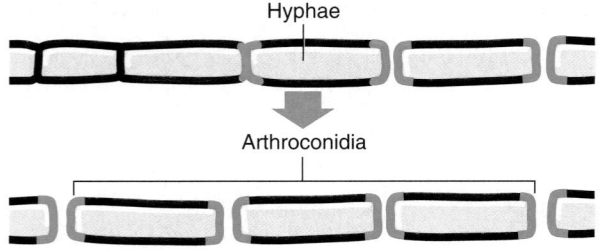

Figure 23-7

Arthroconidia, another form of asexual reproduction, are formed by fragmentation of fertile hyphae.

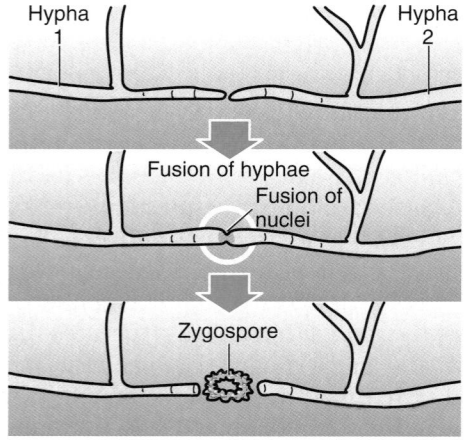

Figure 23-8

Sexual reproduction occurs by the fusion of compatible nuclei with the subsequent production of a zygospore.

reproduction requires the joining of two compatible nuclei, followed by meiosis (Figure 23-8).

| TAXONOMY

Most of the etiologic agents of clinical infections are found in four groups of fungi. They consist of Divisions Zygomycota, Ascomycota, and Basidiomycota, and the Form-Division Fungi Imperfecti.

Zygomycota

Zygomycetes are rapidly growing organisms normally found in the soil. They are often opportunistic pathogens in immunocompromised hosts. Zygomycetes generally produce profuse, gray to white aerial mycelium characterized by the presence of sparsely septate hyphae. Asexual reproduction of Zygomycetes is characterized by the presence of **sporangiophores** and **sporangiospores.** The asexual spores (sporangiospores) are produced in a structure known as a sporangium that develops from a hypha (Figure 23-9). Sexual reproduction occurs with the production of zygospores. Common Zygomycetes include *Mucor, Rhizopus,* and *Absidia* organisms.

Ascomycota

Ascomycota are characterized by the production of sexual spores known as **ascospores** within a saclike structure known as an *ascus.* It is important to note, however, that they are usually identified on the basis of characteristic asexual structures. Representative organisms include *Microsporum* spp., *Trichophyton* spp., and *Pseudallescheria boydii.*

Basidiomycota

Clinically significant **basidiomycetes** are few in number. The only major pathogen is *Filobasidiella neoformans,* the perfect (sexual) form of *Cryptococcus neoformans* var. *neoformans.*

Fungi Imperfecti

The Form-Division **Fungi Imperfecti** contains the largest number of organisms that are etiologic agents of cutaneous, subcutaneous, and systemic mycoses. Organisms are placed within this group when no

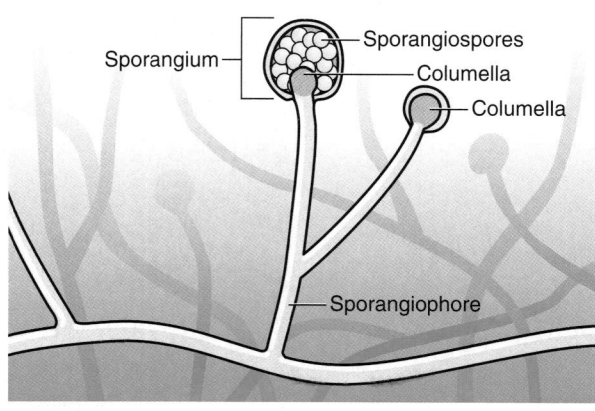

Figure 23-9

Asexual reproduction by *Zygomycetes* is characterized by the production of spores (sporangiospores) from within a sporangium.

mode of sexual reproduction has been identified. Therefore they are identified on the basis of characteristic asexual reproductive structures.

CLINICAL SITES OF INFECTION

Other classifications for mycoses are superficial, cutaneous, subcutaneous, or systemic, according to the tissues affected. Figure 23-10 shows the different layers of tissues where fungal infections may occur.

Superficial Mycoses

Superficial mycoses are infections confined to the outermost layer of skin and/or hair. The clinical infection pityriasis versicolor is characterized by discoloration or depigmentation and scaling of the skin. The agents of tinea nigra cause brown or black macular patches primarily on the palms. Piedra is confined to the hair shaft and characterized by nodules composed of hyphae and a cement-like substance that attaches it to the hair shaft. The fungal species associated with superficial mycoses

include *Malassezia furfur, Piedraia hortae,* and *Trichosporon beigelii.*

Cutaneous Mycoses

Cutaneous mycoses are infections that affect the keratinized layer of skin, hair, or nails. Symptoms include itching, scaling, or ringlike patches of the skin; brittle, broken hairs; and thick, discolored nails. Genera associated with cutaneous infection include *Trichophyton, Epidermophyton,* and *Microsporum* organisms.

Subcutaneous Mycoses

Subcutaneous mycoses involve the deeper skin layers, including muscle and connective tissue. Except in certain patient populations, usually no dissemination occurs through the blood to major organs. Characteristic clinical features include progressive, nonhealing ulcers and the presence of draining sinus tracts. In tropical areas, agents such as *Phialophora* spp. and *Cladosporium* spp. cause chromoblastomycosis, which is characterized by draining sinus tracts and tissue destruction. *Sporothrix schenckii* commonly presents as a lympho-

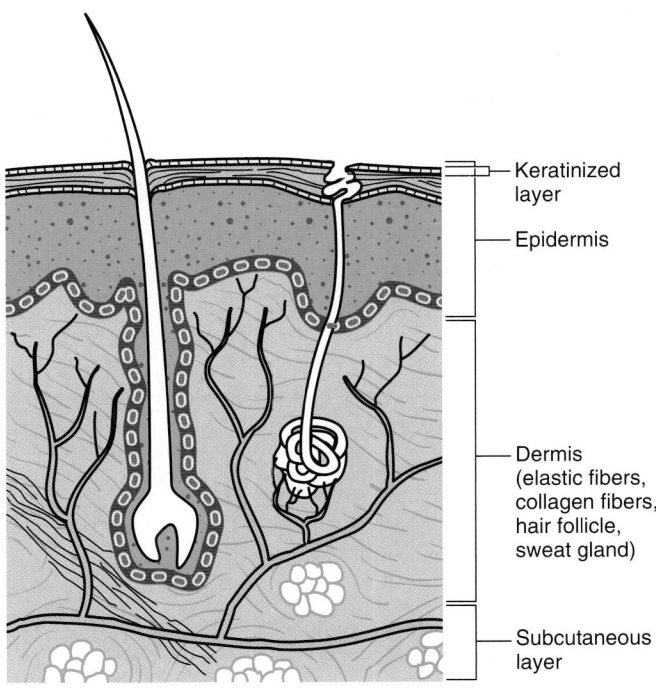

Figure 23-10

Diagram of the layers of skin and tissues in which fungal infections may occur.

cutaneous form, but dissemination into systemic sporotrichosis may occur.

Systemic Mycoses

Systemic mycoses are those infections that affect internal organs or deep tissues of the body. Often the initial site of infection is the lung, from which the organism disseminates hematogenously to other organs. Pulmonary infiltrates may be seen on radiography. Generalized symptoms include fever and fatigue. Chronic cough and chest pain may also accompany these infections. Dimorphic etiologic agents of systemic mycoses include *Histoplasma, Coccidioides,* and *Blastomyces* organisms. Other fungal agents not previously associated with dissemination have been implicated in systemic fungal infections.

SPECIMEN COLLECTION, HANDLING, AND TRANSPORT

Collection of appropriate specimens is the primary criterion for accurate diagnosis of mycotic infections. All specimens for mycology should be transported and processed as soon as possible. Because many pathogenic fungi grow slowly, any delay in processing compromises specimen quality and decreases the probability of isolating the causative agent resulting from overgrowth by contaminants. All work with clinical materials must be carried out under a biologic safety hood. In addition, all laboratories should maintain a protocol for rejection of unsatisfactory or improperly labeled specimens.

Although almost any tissue or body fluid can be submitted for fungal culture, the most common spec-

imens are respiratory secretions, hair, skin, nails, tissue, blood or bone marrow, and cerebrospinal fluid (CSF). Table 23-1 presents the predominant culture sites for recovery of etiologic agents.

Hair, skin, or nails submitted for dermatophyte culture are generally contaminated with bacteria and/or rapidly growing fungi. With these types of specimens, media containing antibiotics should be inoculated. The following procedures are recommended for collecting and processing clinical samples usually submitted for fungal studies.

Hair

Sterile forceps should be used to pull affected hair. A Wood's lamp may be useful in identifying infected hairs. Hairs infected with fungi such as *Microsporum audouinii* fluoresce when a Wood's lamp is shone on the scalp. A less useful method involves cutting the hairs close to the scalp with sterile scissors. Hairs are placed directly into a sterile Petri dish. A few pieces of hair are inoculated onto fungal medium and placed in a 25° C incubator.

Skin

Skin samples are scraped from the outer edge of a surface lesion. Skin must be cleaned with 70% isopropanol before sampling. A potassium hydroxide (KOH) wet mount is prepared with some of the scrapings, and the remainder are inoculated directly on the agar. KOH breaks down tissue and allows fungal hyphae to be seen.

Nails

Nail specimens may be submitted as either scrapings or cuttings and occasionally as a complete nail. Nails are cleaned with 70% isopropyl alcohol

TABLE 23-1

Predominant Culture Sites for Recovery of Etiologic Agents*

Infection	Respiratory	Blood	Bone Marrow	Tissue	Skin	Mucus	Bone
Blastomycosis	+				+	+	+
Histoplasmosis	+	+	+				
Coccidioidomycosis	+				+	+	
Paracoccidioidomycosis	+				+	+	
Sporotrichosis	+			+	+	+	
Chromoblastomycosis				+	+		
Eumycotic mycetoma				+	+		
Phaeohyphomycosis				+	+		

*Organisms may be recovered from multiple sites in disseminated infections.

before scraping the surface. Deeper scrapings are necessary to prepare a KOH preparation and inoculate media. Sterile scissors are used to cut complete nails into small thin strips, which are used to inoculate media.

Blood and Bone Marrow

Blood from septicemic patients can harbor a wide variety of fungal pathogens as well as opportunistic saprobes. Suspicion of fungal agents warrants drawing blood into a lysis centrifugation system such as the Isolator tube (Wampole, Cranbury, N.J.). The lysis of white blood cells and red blood cells releases organisms, which are then concentrated into a sediment during centrifugation. The concentrate obtained is then inoculated onto routine culture media.

Bone marrow may be plated directly onto media.

Cerebrospinal Fluid

Cerebrospinal fluid and other sterile body fluids should be concentrated by centrifugation prior to inoculation. One drop of the concentrate is used for India ink preparations, and the remainder is inoculated to media. If more than 5 mL is submitted, the CSF may be filtered through a membrane filter, and portions of the filter placed on media. Use of media with antibiotics may not be needed, because the body fluids are sterile.

Abscess Fluid and Wound Exudates

Abscess fluid and material from wounds may be plated directly on the media. Tissue should be gently minced before inoculation onto media. Although grinding of tissue has been recommended, this process may destroy fragile fungal elements and prevent recovery of etiologic agents, particularly if a zygomycete is present. Grinding of tissue may be necessary for KOH and calcofluor white preparations. When large sections of tissue are submitted, suspicious areas, such as purulent or discolored sections, are selected for grinding and subsequent culture.

Respiratory Specimens

Respiratory tract secretions (sputum, transtracheal aspirates) and pleural lavage fluids are commonly submitted, because many fungal infections have a primary focus in the lungs. Patients should obtain sputa from a deep cough shortly after the patient arises in the morning. If the patient cannot produce sputum, a nebulizer may be used to induce sputum. All sputum specimens should be collected into a sterile, screw-top container.

The specimens may be inoculated onto media with a sterile pipette if the material is not too viscous. With viscous materials such as a thick tracheal aspirate, either a cotton swab may be used to inoculate the material onto the media, or the specimen may be digested with trypsin and concentrated prior to inoculation. In addition to nonselective media, a medium with antibiotics should be used to prevent bacterial overgrowth. A KOH preparation should also be made. On occasion, mucolytic agents such as N-acetyl-L-cysteine may be used.

Urogenital and Fecal Specimens

Laboratory professionals often receive specimens such as urine, feces, and vaginal secretions for bacteriologic culture; on occasion these specimens grow a yeast that requires identification. Urine submitted specifically for fungal culture should be centrifuged and the sediment used to inoculate media. A first-voided morning urine specimen is preferred.

METHODS OF IDENTIFYING FUNGAL AGENTS

Direct Microscopic Examination of Specimens

The direct examination of clinical material for fungal elements serves several purposes. First, it provides a rapid report to the physician, which may in turn result in the early initiation of treatment. Second, in some cases, specific morphologic characteristics may provide a clue to the genus of the organism. In turn, any special media indicated for species identification can be inoculated immediately. Third, direct examination may provide evidence of infection in spite of negative cultures. Such a situation may occur with specimens from patients who are on antifungal therapy, which may inhibit growth in vitro even though the infection may still be present in the patient.

Although the Gram stain performed in the routine microbiology laboratory often gives the first evidence of infections with yeast, other direct stains give more specific information concerning a mold infection. The types of direct examination used in identification of fungal infections include wet preparations such as KOH, India Ink, and calcofluor white. Histologic stains, such as the periodic acid–Schiff (PAS) stain, Grocott-Gomori methenamine–silver nitrate (GMS) stain, and hematoxylin and eosin (H&E) stain, may be useful.

KOH preparation

A 10% to 20% solution of potassium hydroxide is useful for detecting fungal elements in skin, hair, nails, and tissue. In this procedure, KOH is mixed in equal proportions with the specimen on a slide. The slide is then coverslipped and heated gently. Any fungi present will be visible, because the KOH dissolves keratin and other cellular material in the specimen.

KOH with calcofluor white

If a fluorescent microscope is available, a drop of calcofluor white (fluorescent dye) can be added to the KOH preparation prior to coverslipping. Calcofluor white binds to polysaccharides present in the chitin of the fungus or to cellulose. Fungal elements fluoresce apple green or blue-white, depending on the combination of filters used. Therefore any element with a polysaccharide skeleton fluoresces. The actual fungal structure must be seen before a positive preparation is reported.

India ink

India ink preparations may be used to examine cerebrospinal fluid for the presence of the encapsulated

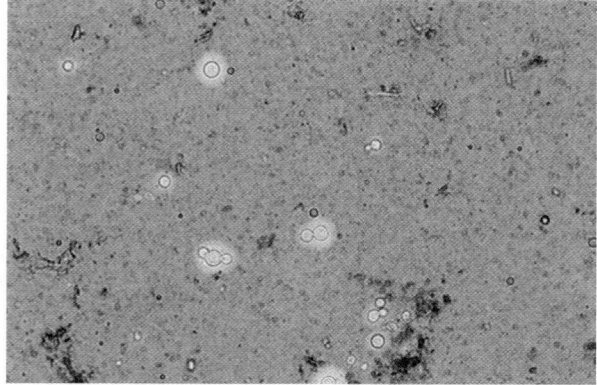

Figure 23-11

India ink preparation is used primarily to examine cerebrospinal fluid for the presence of the encapsulated yeast *Cryptococcus neoformans.* This is an India ink preparation from an exudate containing encapsulated budding yeasts.

TABLE 23-2

Staining Characteristics of Fungi

Stain	Color of Fungal Element	Background Color
Periodic acid–Schiff	Magenta	Pink or green
Grocott-Gomori methenamine–silver nitrate	Black	Green
Giemsa	Purple-blue yeast with clear halo	Pink-purple
India ink	Yeast with clear halo	Black
KOH	Refractile	Clear
KOH-calcofluor	Fluorescent	Dark
Masson-Fontana	Brown	Pink-purple

yeast *Cryptococcus neoformans.* A drop of India ink is mixed with a drop of sediment from a centrifuged spinal fluid specimen, and the preparation is examined on high power. With this negative stain, budding yeast surrounded by a large clear area against a black background (Figure 23-11) is presumptive evidence of *C. neoformans.* White blood cells and other artifacts may resemble encapsulated organisms; therefore careful examination is necessary. Many laboratories, however, now use the latex agglutination test for cryptococcal antigen in place of the India ink examination.

Tissue stains

Common tissue stains used in the histology section for detection of fungal elements are the periodic acid–Schiff (PAS) stain, the Grocott-Gomori methenamine–silver nitrate (GMS) stain, the Giemsa stain, and the Masson-Fontana stain. Giemsa stain is used primarily to detect *Histoplasma capsulatum* in blood or bone marrow (Figure 23-12). PAS attaches to polysaccharides in the fungal wall and stains pink. The Masson-Fontana method stains melanin in the cell wall and identifies the presence of a dematiaceous fungus. Acid-fast stains are used primarily to differentiate *Nocardia* species from other actinomycetes. Table 23-2 lists the characteristic fungal reactions seen with selected stains.

Culture

Culture media

In general, fungi do not share the broad range of nutritional and environmental needs that characterize bacteria; and therefore relatively few types of standard media are needed for primary isolation. These include Sabouraud dextrose agar (SDA), SDA with antibiotics, and brain-heart infusion (BHI) agar enriched with blood and antibiotics. The pH of the Emmons modification of SDA is close to neutral and is a more efficient medium for primary isolation than the original formulation.

The antimicrobials usually included in SDA with antibiotics are chloramphenicol and cyclohexamide. Chloramphenicol inhibits bacterial growth; cyclohexamide inhibits many of the saprobic fungi. Table 23-3 shows the expected growth results with some of the standard fungal media.

Incubation

Most laboratories routinely incubate fungal cultures at room temperature (25° C to 30° C). Fungi grow optimally at this temperature, but bacteria have a slower growth rate. If the etiologic agent suspected is a dimorphic fungus, cultures should also be incubated at 37° C. Cultures are generally maintained for 4 to 6 weeks and should be examined weekly or twice a week for growth. Zygomycetes such as *Mucor* and *Rhizopus* organisms are rapidly growing molds that may fill the tube with aerial mycelium within several days, whereas with slow-growing organisms such as *Fonsecaea* and *Phialophora*, it may be 2 weeks or more before growth is seen.

Data that should be recorded about an isolate include the number of days until first visible growth, whether mold or yeast forms, media on which isolated, temperature at which growth occurred, and morphology of the colonies.

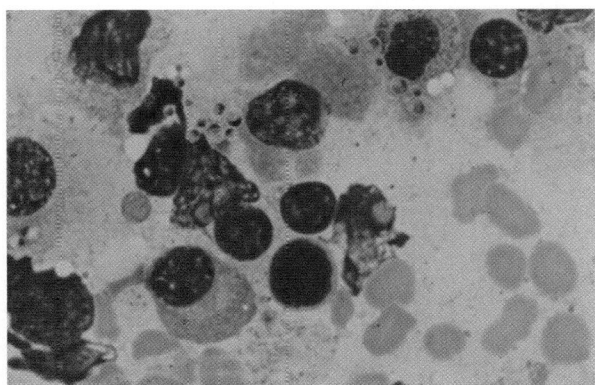

Figure 23-12

Giemsa stain is used primarily to detect organisms in tissue samples. This is a bone marrow stained with Giemsa, showing the yeast phase of *Histoplasma capsulatum* var. *capsulatum*.

TABLE 23-3
Summary of Primary Fungal Culture Media

Medium	Expected Growth Results
At 25° C	
SDA	Initial isolation of pathogens and saprobes
	Dimorphic fungi may exhibit their mycelial phase
SDA with antibiotics	Saprobes are generally inhibited on this medium
	Dermatophytes and most of the fungi considered primary pathogens grow
BHI	Initial isolation of pathogens and saprobes
BHI with antibiotics	Recovery of pathogenic fungi
	Dermatophytes not usually recovered
Inhibitory mold agar	Initial isolation of pathogens except dermatophytes
Cyclohexamide	Primary recovery of dermatophytes
At 37° C	
SDA	The yeast form of dimorphic fungi and other organisms grow
	Dermatophytes grow poorly
BHI with blood	Yeasts such as *Cryptococcus* grow well
	The yeast form of *Histoplasma capsulatum* takes up some of the heme pigment in the medium and becomes light tan with a grainy wrinkled texture

SDA, Sabouraud dextrose agar; *BHI,* brain-heart infusion agar.

BEGINNING THE IDENTIFICATION

Although the number of fungal species known exceeds 100,000, the number typically implicated in human disease is around 100. The number routinely seen is much lower. Therefore identification at least to the genus level is usually possible. The traditional starting place is to decide whether the isolate is a yeast or a mold.

Gross Examination of the Culture

Once an organism has grown, it must be examined for characteristic gross and microscopic morphologic structures, so that identification can be made. Figure 23-13 presents a schematic guideline to how identification may be made. Gross morphologic traits, such as color, texture, and growth rate, are initial observations that should be made. Rapidly growing organisms such as the Zygomycetes usually appear within 1 to 3 days, whereas intermediate growers may take 5 to 9 days, and slow growers up to 2 weeks. Pigment on the reverse side of the colony or in the aerial mycelium

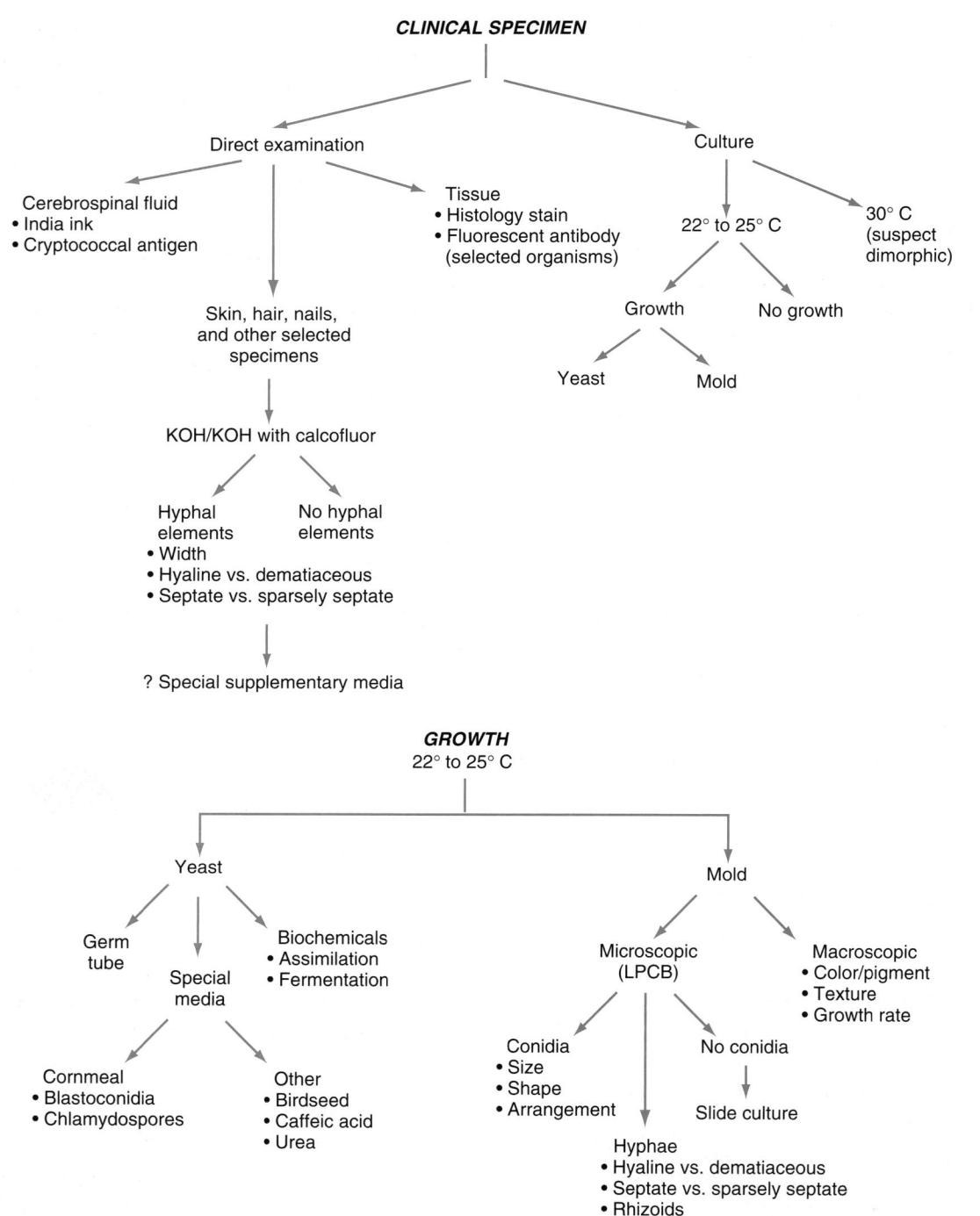

Figure 23-13

Guideline for the identification of fungal isolates. *LPCB,* Lactophenol cotton blue.

can be noted but is not always helpful, especially in the dematiaceous fungi.

Microscopic Examination for Fungal Structures

The most common procedure for microscopic examination is a direct mount of the fungus isolate. A tease mount or cellophane tape preparation may be prepared. On occasion, a slide culture may be prepared, when the initial isolate fails to show conidial production. Characteristics that should be observed are the following:

- Septate versus nonseptate hyphae
- Hyaline or dematiaceous hyphae
- The types, size, shape, and arrangement of conidia

Tease mount

For the tease mount, two teasing needles are used to remove a portion of the mycelium from the middle third of the colony. This is placed into a drop of lactophenol cotton blue (LPCB) on a slide and gently teased apart. The LPCB is used to stain tease mounts or cellophane tape mounts from cultures. The combination of lactic acid, phenol, and the blue dye kills, preserves, and stains the organism.

The preparation is cover-slipped and examined under low (10×) and high (40×) power for characteristic conidial structures. Hyaline hyphae take up the LPCB but dematiaceous fungi retain their dark color. The major disadvantage of the procedure is the disruption of conidia during the teasing process.

Cellophane tape preparation

Cellophane tape preparation involves gently placing a section of transparent tape, sticky side down, on top of the colony and then removing it. The tape is placed onto a drop of LPCB on a slide and examined. An advantage of this procedure is that the conidial arrangement is retained. A major disadvantage is the potential contamination of the colony. A coverslip is not needed if the cellophane tape technique is used, because the tape serves as coverslip.

Slide culture

Slide cultures are useful for demonstrating natural morphology of fungal structures and for encouraging conidiation in some poorly fruiting fungi. Several methods have been devised for constructing these culture chambers, and Procedure 23-1 incorporates the best features of several of these.

PROCEDURE 23-1. Constructing Slide Culture Chambers for Fungi

Prepare and take apart slide cultures within a properly operating biologic safety hood. Fungi suspected of being pathogens are not recommended for observation in slide cultures.

1. Into a 60-mm sterile Petri dish, pour 7 to 8 mL of sterile, 1.5% water agar, and allow to solidify.

2. Lay a sterile coverglass onto the agar. Place on the glass a 5- to 8-mm-square block of nutrient medium (e.g., potato dextrose agar, potato agar, V8 Juice agar, or other sporulation-inducing medium).

3. Inoculate the sides of the block with the desired fungus, and cover the block with a second sterile coverglass and replace the dish lid.

4. Incubate this completed slide culture chamber at room temperature (25° C) for 5 to 10 days. The progress of growth may be monitored by inverting the chamber and examining the fungus on the microscope stage using the low-power objective.

5. When conidia or spores are evident, carefully lift the coverglasses away from the nutrient medium. Mount each coverglass separately in a drop of LPCB on a microscope slide for examination.

SAFETY ISSUES

Universal precautions apply to the mycology laboratory. Because of the additional hazard of airborne conidia, a Class II biologic safety cabinet should be used to reduce personnel exposure to fungal elements. Specimen processing and plating must be done under a properly maintained and operating hood. The use of a hooded electric incinerator is recommended to eliminate the hazards of open gas flames and to contain particles emitted when loops or needles are incinerated. The cabinet should be checked daily to see that none of the airflow inlets or outlets is blocked by supplies, incinerators, or waste disposal jars.

Use of Petri dishes in the mycology laboratory is hazardous, and screw-top tubes are recommended. Screw-capped tubes tend to show less media dehydration than Petri dishes and are more easily handled and stored. The chance for release of airborne conidia is less. On the other hand, Petri dishes have a greater surface area for colony isolation and are easier to manipulate when making preparations for microscopic examination.

AGENTS OF SUPERFICIAL MYCOSES

Four fungal agents are commonly associated with superficial mycoses:

- *Malassezia furfur*
- *Piedraia hortae*
- *Trichosporon beigelii*
- *Phaeoannellomyces werneckii*

Superficial mycoses are fungal diseases that affect only the cornified layers (stratum corneum) of the epidermis. Patients who suffer from superficial fungal infections do not show any overt symptomatology, because the fungal agents do not activate any tissue response or inflammatory reaction. Patients usually seek medical attention for the cosmetic effects caused by these fungi.

Malassezia furfur

Malassezia furfur causes tinea versicolor or pityriasis versicolor, a disease characterized by patchy lesions or scaling of varying pigmentation. Also described as "fawn-colored liver spots," pityriasis may involve the chest, trunk, or abdomen. *M. fur-*

fur has also been implicated in disseminated infections in patients receiving high-dose lipid replacement therapy, particularly in infants.

M. furfur is a common endogenous skin colonizer. Although reasons for overgrowth by *M. furfur* resulting in the clinical manifestations are still unknown, it appears to be related to squamous cell turnover rates. This is evidenced by the higher incidence of tinea versicolor among persons receiving corticosteroid therapy, which decreases the rate of squamous epithelial cell turnover. Some investigators have identified genetic influence, poor nourishment, and excessive sweating as other factors that contribute to the overgrowth of the organism on the skin.

M. furfur is identified in KOH preparations of skin scrapings or by observing yellow fluorescence on a Wood's lamp examination of the infected body site. Microscopic examination of the direct smear in KOH preparations shows budding yeasts, approximately 4 to 8 μm, along with septate, sometimes branched hyphal elements. This microscopic appearance has gained *M. furfur* the term "spaghetti and meatballs" fungi (Figure 23-14). Skin scrapings

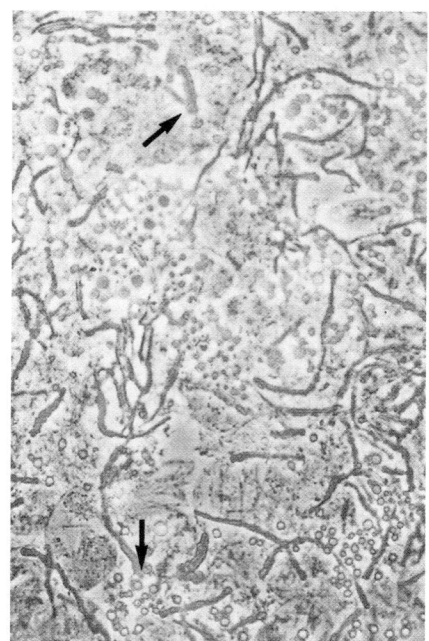

Figure 23-14 ———————————————

Diagram of the typical "spaghetti and meatballs" appearance of *Malassezia furfur* in a potassium hydroxide preparation.

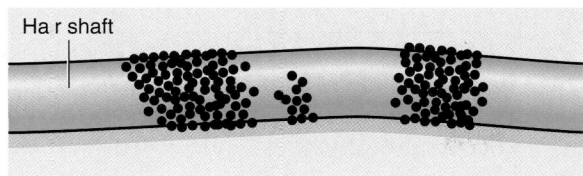

Figure 23-15 _____

Diagram of black piedra on a hair shaft. Black piedra is caused by *Piedraia hortae*.

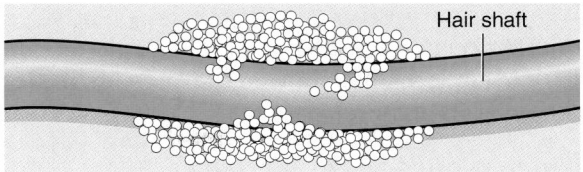

Figure 23-16 _____

Diagram of white piedra caused by *Trichosporon beigelii*.

are seldom cultured. If desired, *M. furfur* can be cultured using a suitable agar medium with fatty acid (oleic acid) overlay.

Recommended treatment using 1% selenium sulfide, found in some medicated shampoo (e.g., Selsun Blue) provides a temporary remedy. The infection usually recurs when treatment is stopped.

Piedraia hortae

Piedraia hortae is the causative agent of black piedra, an infection that occurs on scalp hair. The disease is endemic in tropical areas of Africa, Asia, and Latin America. The organism *P. hortae* produces hard, dark brown to black gritty nodules (Figure 23-15) made of asci containing eight ascospores. When infected hair shafts are removed and placed in 10% to 20% KOH, the nodules may be crushed open to reveal the asci. Thick-walled rhomboid cells containing ascospores are seen.

P. hortae grows slowly on Sabouraud dextrose agar at room temperature. It forms brown colonies that microscopically show dark septate hyphae. Treatment usually consists of removal of infected hair shafts and application of topical fungicides.

Trichosporon beigelii

Trichosporon beigelii causes white piedra, which also occurs on the hair shaft. White piedra is characterized by a soft mycelial mat around facial and genital hair, less commonly scalp hair (Figure 23-16). White piedra is endemic in tropical areas of South America, the Far East, and the Pacific.

Widely distributed in nature, *T. beigelii* is also occasionally found as part of the normal skin flora. It has also been recognized as an opportunistic systemic pathogen. Although rare, systemic disease caused by this fungus is frequently fatal and occurs most often in the immunocompromised host, commonly people who have he-

matologic disorders or malignancies or are undergoing chemotherapy.

Diagnosis is made by finding hyphal elements within the shaft nodule and budding blastoconidia and arthroconidia in culture. *T. beigelii* grows rapidly on primary fungus media. The colonies are cream-colored and yeast-looking. Colonies eventually become wrinkled as they mature. Microscopically, *T. beigelii* produces both arthroconidia and blastoconidia (Figure 23-17). Identification is confirmed by biochemical reactions; *T. beigelii* does not ferment carbohydrates or utilize potassium nitrate but does assimilate glucose, galactose, sucrose, maltose, and lactose, features differentiating it from other *Trichosporon* species.

McManus and Jones (1985) have reported the role of latex agglutination test for cryptococcal antigen in diagnosing disseminated *Trichosporon* infections. They described the presence of a heat-stable antigen produced by *T. beigelii* that shares antigenic sites with the polysaccharide capsule of

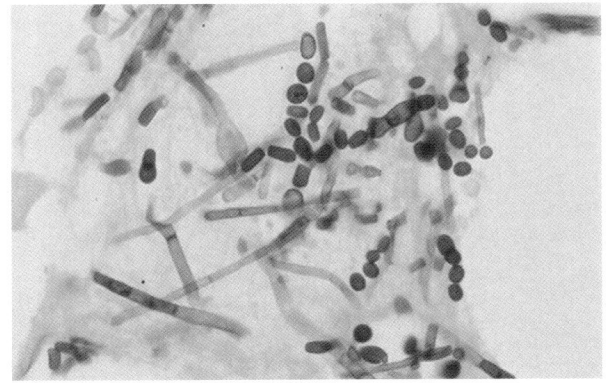

Figure 23-17 _____

Microscopic appearance of *Trichosporon beigelii* on LPCB preparation, showing the presence of both blastoconidia and arthroconidia.

Cryptococcus neoformans. This false-positive result, although misleading the mycologic diagnosis, has nevertheless allowed the early institution of appropriate therapy.

Phaeoannellomyces werneckii

Tinea nigra, characterized by brown to black nonscaly macules that occur most often on the palms of the hands and soles of the feet, is caused by *Phaeoannellomyces werneckii.* The disease is endemic in the tropical areas of Central and South America, Africa, and Asia. It involves no inflammatory or other tissue reaction to the infecting fungus. The clinical presentation is so similar to other conditions, however, especially malignant melanoma, that misdiagnosis could occur, resulting in unnecessary surgical procedures.

Proper diagnosis of tinea nigra can be made by direct examination of skin scrapings placed in 10% to 20% KOH. Microscopic examination shows septate hyphal elements and budding cells (Figure 23-18). When grown in culture medium, *P. werneckii* produces shiny, moist, yeastlike colonies that start with a brownish coloration that eventually turns olive to greenish black. Microscopic examination of the colony shows budding blastoconidia, whereas the older mycelial portion of the colony shows hyphae with blastoconidia in clusters. Annelloconidia are seen in older hyphal colonies. Treatment consists of the application of keratolytic agents.

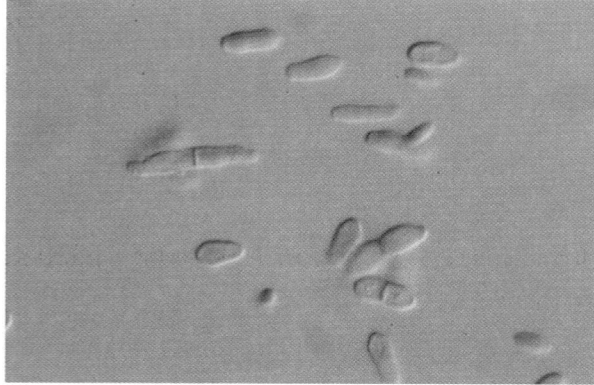

Figure 23-18

Microscopic structures of *Phaeoannellomyces werneckii,* showing characteristic budding annelloconidia. *P. werneckii* causes tinea nigra.

AGENTS OF DERMATOPHYTOSES

Three genera of fungi, *Microsporum, Trichophyton,* and *Epidermophyton* organisms, are etiologic agents of dermatophytoses. Species within these genera are keratinophilic, that is, they are adapted to grow on hair, nails, and cutaneous layers of skin that contain the scleroprotein keratin. Infection of deep tissue by these fungi is rare, but occasionally, extensive inflammation and nail bed involvement may result.

Epidemiology

Most of the agents of dermatophytoses live freely in the environment, but a few have adapted almost exclusively to living on human host tissues, and these are very rarely recovered from any other source. Distribution of many **dermatophyte** species is worldwide, whereas others are found only in restricted geographic regions. Approximately 43 species of dermatophytes and dermatophyte-like fungi have been described, and just over two dozen of these have been documented to cause human infection.

Those dermatophytes that primarily inhabit the soil are termed *geophilic.* Most geophilic fungi produce large numbers of conidia and therefore are among the most readily identified species. *Zoophilic* dermatophytes are typically adapted to live on animals and are not commonly found living freely in soil or on dead organic substrates. They often cause infections in their animal hosts and may be spread as disease agents to humans. Fewer conidia are produced by zoophilic fungi than by geophilic species. A few dermatophytes have become adapted exclusively to human hosts and are termed *anthropophilic.* Although they are encountered almost always as agents of human disease, the infections are seldom inflammatory. Species identification may be quite difficult because most anthropophilic species produce few conidia.

Clinical Infections

Dermatophytoses usually involve a restricted region of the host, and traditionally, these diseases are named with respect to the portion of the body affected. Because the infections were at one time believed to be the result of burrowing worms that formed ring-shaped patterns in the skin, the term *tinea* was applied to each disease, along with a Latin term for the body site. We continue to de-

TABLE 23-4

Various Forms of Dermatophytoses and the Respective Affected Sites

Type of Ringworm	Site Affected
Tinea capitis	Head
Tinea favosa	Head (distinctive pathology)
Tinea barbae	Beard
Tinea corporis	Body—glabrous skin
Tinea manuum	Hand
Tinea unguium	Nails
Tinea cruris	Groin
Tinea pedis	Feet
Tinea imbricata	Body (distinctive lesion)

scribe the various forms of "ringworm" in these terms, as shown in Table 23-4. Each ringworm lesion is the result of a local inoculation on the skin with the etiologic agent; many lesions represent many sites of infection. Lesions enlarge with time, usually with most inflammation occurring at the growing edge. Some cases of ringworm are subclinical, exhibiting only a dry, scaly lesion without inflammation.

Not only are diverse sites on the host involved, but also certain species cause distinctive lesions. The notable example is tinea imbricata, caused by *Trichophyton concentricum*. Over time, involved portions of the trunk develop diagnostically distinctive concentric rings of scaling tissue. In some forms of ringworm, a persistent allergic reaction, the dermatophytid, is manifested in the formation of sterile, itching lesions on body sites distant from the point of infection. Symptoms of dermatophyte infections vary from slight to moderate and occasionally severe.

Infections involving hair and hair follicles
Different body sites manifest different symptoms. Infections in the scalp, where hair follicles are the initiation sites, may be among the most severe and disfiguring forms of the disease. Tinea favosa, or favus, begins as an infection of the hair follicle by *Trichophyton schoenleinii* and progresses to a crusty lesion made up of dead epithelial cells and fungal mycelia. Crusty, cup-shaped flakes called scutula are formed. Hair loss and scar tissue formation commonly follow.

Two distinct forms of tinea capitis, gray-patch ringworm and black dot ringworm, are caused by different species of dermatophyte. Gray-patch ringworm is a common childhood disease easily spread among children. The fungus primarily colonizes the outer portion of hair shafts, the so-called **ectothrix** hair involvement. The lesions are seldom inflamed, but luster and color of the hair shaft may be lost. *Microsporum audouinii* and *Microsporum ferrugineum* are agents of this form of disease. Black-dot ringworm is an **endothrix** hair involvement. The hair follicle is the initial site of infection, and fungal growth continues within the hair shaft, causing it to weaken. The brittle, infected hair shafts break off at the scalp, leaving the "black dot" stubs. *Trichophyton tonsurans* and *Trichophyton violaceum* are the most common fungi implicated in this form of ringworm.

Infections involving the nail and nail bed
Onychomycosis is most often caused by dermatophytes but also may be the result of infection by other fungi. These nail and nail bed infections may be among the most difficult dermatophytoses to treat. Long-term, costly therapy with griseofulvin is considered the best but may still result in unsatisfactory resolution of the disease. Some common agents that infect the nail are the *Trichophyton* species *Trichophyton rubrum, Trichophyton mentagrophytes,* and *T. tonsurans* as well as *Epidermophyton floccosum.*

Athlete's foot
Among the shoe-wearing human population, tinea pedis or ringworm of the foot is a common disease, particularly of men. The gender disparity may be related more to shoe styles than to any physiologic differences between the sexes. Various sites on the foot may be involved, but most often, tinea pedis affects the toe webs or toenails. In more severe cases, the sole of the foot may develop extensive scaling with fissuring and erythema. The disease may progress around the sides of the foot from the sole, giving rise to use of the term "moccasin foot," descriptive of the shape of the lesion. Infections of the glabrous skin range from mild with only minimal scaling and erythema to severely inflamed lesions.

Systemic infections
Immunocompromised persons may suffer systemic dermatophyte infections.

Treatment

Successful treatment of dermatophytic skin infections is usually accomplished with keratinolytic agents, which remove outer layers of skin along with the fungal elements. Systemic treatment with griseofulvin is appropriate for more extensive tinea corporis lesions. Recurring infections are common with most types of ringworm, even with the best therapies. Nail bed infections are often resistant to therapy and may at best remain chronic problems.

Commonly Encountered Dermatophytes

Trichophyton mentagrophytes

In many parts of the world, *Trichophyton mentagrophytes* is the most commonly isolated dermatophyte, and both anthropophilic and zoophilic strains are known. *T. mentagrophytes* infects skin, hair, and nails. Colonial morphology varies with the extent of conidia production. The granular colony form has a powdery appearance owing to abundant microconidia formed, usually in clusters. In the downy form, conidia are less abundant, and the microscopic morphology may resemble that of *T. rubrum.* Compared with other dermatophytes, *T. mentagrophytes* is a relatively rapid-growing fungus. Macroconidia are thin walled, smooth, and cigar shaped with four to five cells separated by parallel cross-walls. These conidia measure about 7 by 20 to 50 μm and are produced singly on undifferentiated hyphae. Microconidia (Figure 23-19) are globose to tear-shaped and measure 2.5 to 4 μm.

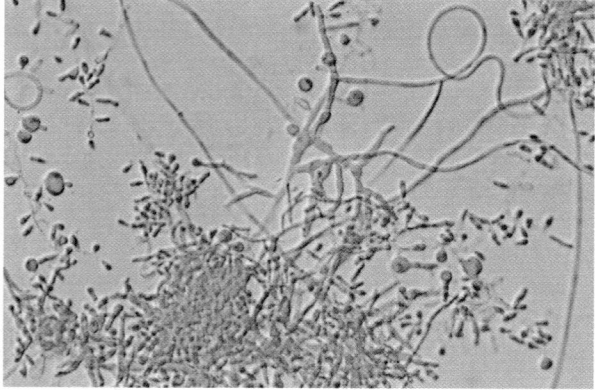

Figure 23-19 _____

Trichophyton mentagrophytes, showing globose, teardrop-shaped microconidia (Nomarski optics, ×1250).

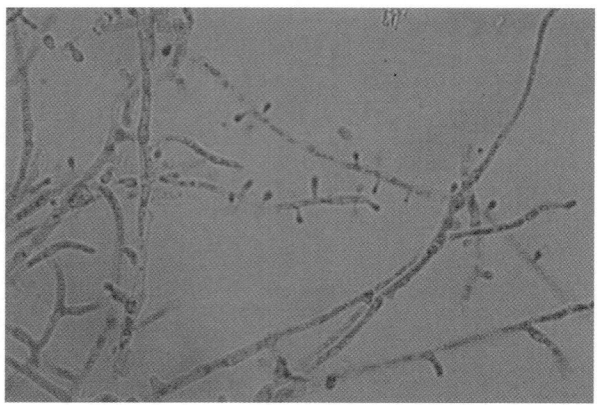

Figure 23-20 _____

Trichophyton rubrum, showing clavate or peg-shaped microconidia.

Trichophyton rubrum

Trichophyton rubrum is recognized as the most common species isolated from many forms of ringworm. It is a relatively slow-growing anthropophilic dermatophyte found wherever human populations live. Skin and nails are common sites infected by *T. rubrum,* but hair is seldom involved. The colonies usually remain hyaline, but with age, they may develop pink to deep burgundy wine–colored pigment on the reverse side. Although *T. rubrum* is known to produce three- to eight-celled cylindrical macroconidia measuring somewhat smaller than those of *T. mentagrophytes,* these are seldom seen in clinical isolates. A typical microscopic picture of *T. rubrum* contains clavate or peg-shaped microconidia (Figure 23-20) formed along undifferentiated hyphae, and even these may be sparse. Pigmentation studies, 5-day urease production, and hair perforation tests are important tools for distinguishing between *T. mentagrophytes* and *T. rubrum.*

Trichophyton tonsurans

Trichophyton tonsurans, which infects skin, hair, and nails, has become the leading cause of tinea capitis in children in many parts of the world, including the United States. When grown on Sabouraud dextrose agar, *T. tonsurans* colonies usually form a rust-colored pigment on the colony's reverse. This dermatophyte is anthropophilic and typically produces only small numbers of peg-shaped microconidia. *T. tonsurans* has an absolute requirement for thiamine, a feature helping to distinguish it from *T. mentagrophytes* and *T. rubrum*.

Microsporum canis

Microsporum canis, a relatively rapid-growing zoophilic dermatophyte found worldwide, is the species of *Microsporum* most commonly isolated from humans. It primarily infects skin and hair. Freshly isolated cultures typically produce many macroconidia and microconidia, and the reverse side of the colony usually develops a lemon-yellow pigment, especially on potato dextrose agar. Macroconidia are spindle shaped with echinulate, thick walls; they measure 12 to 25 μm by 35 to 110 μm and have 3 to 15 cells (Figure 23-21). The tapering, sometimes elongated, spiny distal ends of macroconidia are key features that distinguish this species. Microconidia are abundantly formed by most isolates, and these may be the only conidia present in cultures that have been serially transferred.

Microsporum gypseum

Microsporum gypseum is a rapidly growing geophilic species found in soils all over the world. Infections in humans are not common, but sites involved are primarily skin and hair. Abundant macroconidia and microconidia produced by most isolates of this species result in a powdery, granular appearance on colony surfaces. Colonies that

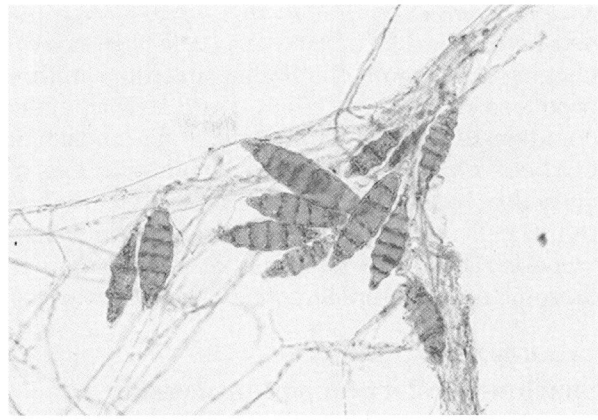

Figure 23-22
Microsporum gypseum, showing fusiform, moderately thick-walled macroconidia containing several cells.

form tan to buff conidial masses are typical of fresh isolates, but this species tends to develop pleomorphic tufts of white, sterile hyphae in aging cultures and after serial transfers. Abundant brown to red pigment may form beneath some strains, but others remain colorless. The fusiform, moderately thick-walled conidia (Figure 23-22) measure 8 to 15 μm by 25 to 60 μm and may have as many as six cells. In some isolates, the distal end of the macroconidium may bear a thin, filamentous tail that is longer than the rest of the conidium. The cell walls are moderately thick.

Microsporum audouinii

A slow-growing anthropomorphic dermatophyte, *Microsporum audouinii* was responsible for most of the gray-patch ringworm of children until a few decades ago, when *T. tonsurans* replaced it. *M. audouinii* commonly infects hair and skin but seldom the nails. Colonies of *M. audouinii* appear cottony-white and generally form little or no pigment on the reverse. Conidia are only rarely produced. Some isolates form chlamydoconidium-like swellings terminally on hyphae.

Epidermophyton floccosum

Epidermophyton floccosum is an anthropomorphic dermatophyte species infecting skin and nails. Colonies of *E. floccosum* are yellow to yellow-green. *Macroconidia* (describing the larger of two sizes of conidia) is used in reference to the conidia of

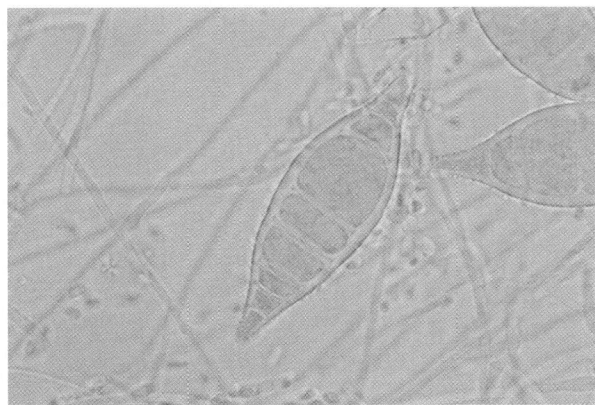

Figure 23-21
Microsporum canis, showing spindle-shaped, echinulate macroconidia with thick walls and tapered ends, which are key features in the identification of this species.

E. floccosum, even though this fungus is unique among the dermatophytes in its lack of microconidia. The smooth, thin-walled macroconidia are produced in clusters or singly. The distal end of the conidium is broad, or spatulate, and reminiscent of a beaver's tail. Occasionally, conidia may be single celled, but usually they are separated into two to five cells by perpendicular cross-walls. *Epidermophyton* isolates are notorious for developing pleomorphic tufts of sterile hyphae in older cultures.

Laboratory Diagnosis
Specimen collection and processing
The affected site should be washed or swabbed briefly with alcohol before collection of the specimen. Properly collected hair, skin scrapings, nail scrapings, or nail clippings are possible sources of the infecting fungi.

Direct microscopic examination
Initial diagnosis of a dermatophyte infection of the skin may be made in a skin scraping mounted in potassium hydroxide. These preparations may be modified by incorporating Parker Quink blue-black ink (Parker Pen USA, LTD, Janesville, WI) or calcofluor white fluorescent brightener into the KOH to enhance detection and observation of fungal elements in the epithelial cells. The KOH acts to dissolve the skin cells, leaving intact the hyaline, septate hyphae, which appear similar among all the various etiologic agents of ringworm.

Culture
Isolation of dermatophytes in pure culture is fundamental in correctly identifying them to genus and species. Short clippings of suspected infected hair, skin scrapings, or nail scrapings are placed on the surface of suitable inhibitory and noninhibitory agar media and incubated at 30° C for up to 4 weeks. Nail clippings should be stuck into the medium or distributed on the agar. It is generally inappropriate to plant whole nails onto the medium surface. Rather, scrapings or clippings of the most suspicious-looking, often deeper, thicker portions of the nail should be removed and placed in culture. Skin scrapings taken from the border of the lesion increase the chance of recovering viable fungal elements. Scalp lesions may be inspected under a Wood's lamp, a source of near ultraviolet wavelength light. Infection of hair by a select few dermatophytes *(M. canis, M. audouinii, M. ferrugineum,* and *T. tonsurans)* cause hair shafts to fluoresce, and the ultraviolet light aids in detection of these infections.

Identification
Differential tests for dermatophytes include nutritional studies, pigment formation on special media, hair perforation tests, and urease production.

HAIR PERFORATION TEST
In the hair perforation test, sterile 5- to 10-mm hair fragments are floated on sterile water supplemented with a few drops of sterile, 10% yeast extract. Conidia or hyphae from the dermatophyte in question are inoculated onto the water surface. Hair shafts are removed and microscopically examined in LPCB at weekly intervals for up to 1 month. *T. rubrum,* which may be morphologically similar to *T. mentagrophytes,* usually causes only surface erosion of hair shafts in this test, whereas *T. mentagrophytes* usually forms perpendicular penetration pegs in the hair shafts (Figure 23-23). Some laboratories also use this test to distinguish penetration-capable *M. canis* from *Microsporum equinum,* which does not penetrate hair.

UREASE TEST
Another test used to help differentiate *T. mentagrophytes* from *T. rubrum* is the 5-day urease test. Tubes of Christensen urea agar are very lightly inoculated

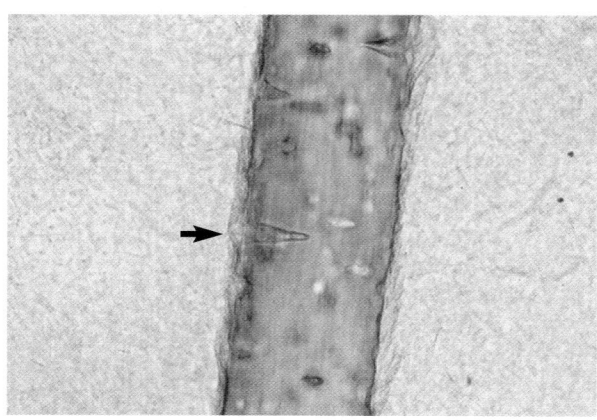

Figure 23-23

A positive hair perforation test shows penetration of the fungal agent in the hair shaft. This is the typical reaction by *Trichophyton mentagrophytes,* whereas *Trichophyton rubrum* causes only surface erosion of hair shaft.

with the dermatophyte and held for 5 days at room temperature. Most isolates of *T. mentagrophytes* demonstrate urease production within that time, whereas most *T. rubrum* isolates require more than 5 days to give a positive reaction.

THIAMINE REQUIREMENT

Some dermatophytes cannot synthesize certain vitamins and therefore do not grow on vitamin-free media. Although several vitamin deficiencies are recognized in fungi, the test for thiamine requirement is perhaps the single most useful nutritional test for dermatophytes. Tubes of media with and without the vitamin are inoculated with a tiny, medium-free portion of hyphae or conidia and observed for growth after 10 to 14 days. Great care must be exercised to avoid transfer of culture media with the inoculum, because even minuscule amounts of vitamin carried over with it can adequately supply the requirement and thereby mask an otherwise negative reaction.

GROWTH ON RICE GRAINS

Poorly sporulating isolates of *M. canis* may be difficult to differentiate from *M. audouinii,* a species that typically forms few spores. Sterile, nonfortified rice is inoculated lightly with hyphae of the isolate under study. After 10 days of incubation at room temperature, the medium is observed for growth. *M. canis* and virtually all other dermatophytes grow well and usually form many conidia, whereas *M. audouinii* does not grow.

OTHER TESTS

By way of a single developmental process, dermatophytes typically form two sizes of reproductive cells, **macroconidia** and **microconidia.** Both of these are anamorphic or asexual conidia and their distinctive size, shape, and surface features make them valuable structures for identification of species. Some dermatophytes are known to also have teleomorphic (sexual) stages, in which ascospores are the reproductive cells. Teleomorphs in this group of organisms are not observed in routine laboratory studies of patient specimens, because dermatophytes are heterothallic, requiring combination of two distinct mating types. Although a few reference laboratories perform mating tests with known "tester strains," this is not a procedure regularly used in clinical laboratories.

AGENTS OF SUBCUTANEOUS MYCOSES

Subcutaneous mycoses are fungal diseases affecting subcutaneous tissues. These mycoses are usually the result of the traumatic implantation of foreign objects into the deep layers of the skin, permitting the fungus to gain entry into the host. The etiologic agents responsible are organisms commonly found in soil or on decaying vegetation. Organisms inciting subcutaneous mycoses belong to a variety of genera in the Form-Class Hyphomycetes. Although some are moniliaceous (hyaline or light colored), many are dematiaceous, producing darkly pigmented colonies and containing melanin in their cell walls. The infections are commonly chronic in nature and usually incite the development of lesions at the site of trauma.

Subcutaneous fungal infections may be grouped together by the disease processes they cause or the etiologic agents involved. This section discusses the following diseases and their respective etiologic agents:

- **Sporotrichosis:** *Sporothrix schenckii*
- **Chromoblastomycosis:** *Fonsecaea compactum, Phialophora verrucosa, Cladophialophora carrioni, Fonsecaea pedrosoi,* and *Rhinocladiella aquaspersa*
- **Eumycotic mycetoma:** *Pseudallescheria boydii, Acremonium falciforme, Madurella mycetomatis, Madurella grisea,* and *Exophiala jeanselmei*
- **Phaeohyphomycosis:** *Exophiala* species and *Wangiella dermatitidis*

Other subcutaneous mycoses rarely seen in the United States are lobomycosis, subcutaneous zygomycosis, and rhinosporidiosis.

Sporotrichosis

Epidemiology

Sporothrix schenckii is commonly recovered from the soil and is associated with decaying vegetation. It is endemic in warm, arid areas such as Mexico and also in moist, humid regions such as Brazil, Uruguay, and South Africa. In temperate countries such as France, Canada, and the United States, most cases of sporotrichosis are associated with gardening, particularly with exposure to rose thorns (rose handler's disease) and sphagnum moss.

Clinical infections

The most commonly seen presentation of *S. schenckii* infection is lymphocutaneous sporotrichosis. This chronic infection is characterized by nodular and ulcerative lesions along the lymph channels that drain the primary site of inoculation. Less commonly seen disease entities include fixed cutaneous sporotrichosis, in which the infection is confined to the site of inoculation and mucocutaneous sporotrichosis, a relatively rare condition. Primary and secondary pulmonary sporotrichosis as well as extracutaneous and disseminated forms of the disease may also occur. Several serologic procedures are available for the diagnosis of sporotrichosis, the most useful being immunodiffusion and latex slide agglutination.

Laboratory diagnosis

SPECIMEN COLLECTION

Clinical samples submitted for examination include aspirates from cutaneous nodules, pus, exudate, and material from curettage or swabbing of open lesions.

DIRECT MICROSCOPIC EXAMINATION

Direct examination of tissue may reveal *S. schenckii* as small, cigar-shaped yeast. Although the organism may occasionally be seen in a gram-stained smear, wet mount of materials are often unrewarding because of the small numbers of organisms present.

CULTURE

Because *S. schenckii* is dimorphic, cultures are examined at 25° C and 37° C. This fungus grows well on most culture media, including those containing cycloheximide (Mycosel [BBL Diagnostics, Cockeysville, MD], Mycobiotic [Difco Laboratories, Detroit, MI]).

Characteristics at 25° C The colonial morphology of *S. schenckii* can be quite variable. At room temperature, colonies are often initially white, glabrous, and yeastlike and turn darker and become more mycelial as they mature. Microscopic examination reveals thin, delicate hyphae bearing conidia developing in a "rosette" pattern at the ends of delicate conidiophores (Figure 23-24, *A*). Dark-walled conidia are also produced along the sides of the hyphae.

Characteristics at 37° C Demonstration of dimorphism is important for specific identification of *S. schenckii*. To induce mycelial to yeast conversion, the fungus in inoculated on blood agar tubes and incubated at 37° C. The formation of yeast colonies may require several subcultures (Figure 23-24, *B*). Complete conversion seldom occurs, but a portion of the colony will develop cigar-shaped yeastlike cells.

Chromoblastomycosis

Epidemiology

Also known as verrucous dermatitidis and chromomycosis, **chromoblastomycosis** occurs worldwide but is most common in tropical and sub-

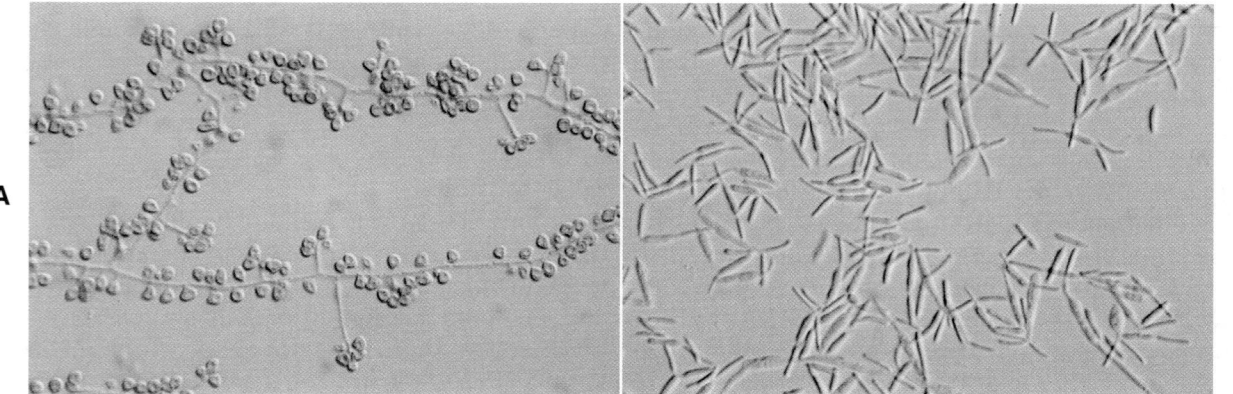

Figure 23-24

A, Mold phase of *Sporothrix schenckii,* indicating hyaline conidia borne at the ends of conidiophore in "rosettes" as well as dematiaceous conidia along the sides of the hyphae (Nomarski optics, ×625). **B,** Yeast phase of *Sporothrix schenckii,* showing cigar-shaped yeast cells typical of the species.

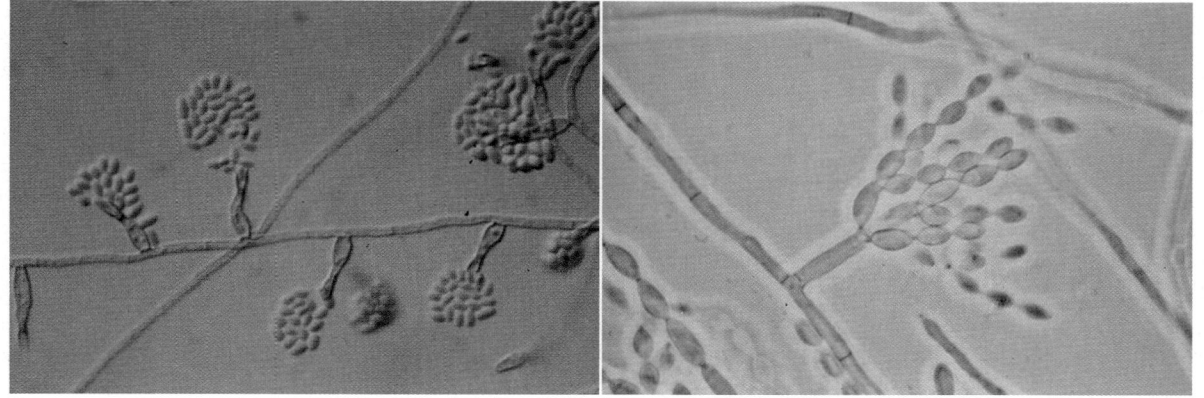

Figure 23-25

A, Conidia of *Phialophora verrucosa* at the tips of phialides with collarettes (Nomarski optics, ×1,250). **B,** Conidial arrangement of *Cladophialophora carrionii.* (Courtesy Dr. Michael McGinnis.)

tropical regions of the Americas and Africa. In the United States, most cases have occurred in Texas and Louisiana. Several organisms are responsible for the disease, and particular organisms appear to reside in specific areas of endemicity throughout the world. Chromoblastomycosis is caused by several etiologic agents, namely *F. compacta, P. verrucosa* (Figure 23-25, *A*), *C. carrionii* (Figure 23-25, *B*), *F. pedrosoi,* and *R. aquaspersa.*

Clinical infections

Chromoblastomycosis is a chronic mycosis of the skin and subcutaneous tissue that develops over a period of months or, more commonly, years. It is mostly asymptomatic in the absence of secondary complications, such as bacterial infections, carcinomatous degeneration, and elephantiasis. Lesions are usually confined to the extremities, often the feet and lower legs, and are a result of trauma to these areas. Lesions of chromoblastomycosis most often appear as verrucous nodules that may become ulcerated and crusted. Longstanding lesions have a cauliflower-like surface. Brown, round sclerotic bodies, which are nonbudding structures occurring singly or in clusters, are seen in tissues. These sclerotic bodies reproduce by dividing in various planes, resulting in multicellular forms. Occasionally, short hyphal elements may also be seen.

Laboratory diagnosis

At present, serologic evaluation of patients for chromoblastomycosis does not provide a practical adjunct to diagnosis.

SPECIMEN COLLECTION
Small punch biopsies of affected skin areas should be submitted for histopathology and culture. The presence of sclerotic bodies in tissue, combined with a compatible clinical picture, is diagnostic. Samples are inoculated onto the usual fungal media.

MICROSCOPIC EXAMINATION
The microscopic morphology of each of the agents is described in Table 23-5. *P. verrucosa* and *C. carionii* are shown in Figure 23-25. Etiologic agents are identified on the basis of characteristic structures, such as arrangement of conidia and how conidia are borne.

CULTURE
Organisms inciting chromoblastomycosis are darkly pigmented or dematiaceous molds. Growth is moderate to slow, and colonies are velvety to woolly, gray-brown to olivaceous black. Species are not differentiated by colonial morphologies, because they all produce similar characteristics.

Eumycotic Mycetoma
Epidemiology
Mycetomas are indolent infections of the subcutaneous tissues that arise at the site of inoculation. Mycetomas may be caused by either fungi or bacteria. Those caused by bacteria are referred to as *actinomycotic mycetomas,* and those caused by fungal agents are referred to as **eumycotic mycetoma.** Although clinical manifestations are similar for the two types of mycetomas, etiology must be deter-

TABLE 23-5

Microscopic Morphology of Fungi Causing Chromoblastomycosis

Organism	Microscopic Morphology
Phialophora verrucosa	Conidiogenous cells dematiaceous, flask-shaped phialides with collarettes Conidia oval, one-celled, occur in balls at tips of phialides
Fonsecaea pedrosoi	Primary one-celled conidia formed on sympodial conidiophores Primary conidia function as conidiogenous cells to form secondary one-celled conidia Some conidia similar to those seen in *Cladosporium* organisms, some like those in *Rhinocladiella* organisms, and others like those in *Phialophora* sp.
Fonsecaea compactum	Similar to *F. pedrosoi* but with more compact conidial heads Conidia are subglobose rather than ovoid
Cladophialophora carrionii	Erect conidiophores bearing branched chains of one-celled, brown blastoconidia Conidium close to tip of conidiophore termed "shield cell" Fragile chains
Rhinocladiella aquaspersa	Conidiophores erect, dark, bearing conidia only on upper portion near the tip Conidia elliptical, one-celled, produced sympodially

mined for appropriate therapy. Mycetomas occur in tropical and subtropical areas but may also be seen in temperate zones. The disease is endemic in India, Africa, and South America.

Although mycetoma is an uncommon mycosis in the United States, the following species are the most commonly incriminated agents: *P. boydii, A. falciforme, M. mycetomatis, M. grisea,* and *E. jeanselmei.*

Clinical infections

Mycetomas are generally confined to the extremities, although they may be observed at other anatomic sites. The lesions are made up of granulomas and abscesses that drain to the outside through sinus tracts. The pus from these lesions contains granules (grains) that are composed of compact mycelial masses. The characteristic granules formed by the different genera of fungi that incite mycetomas are listed in Table 23-6. These

lesions, which are initially confined to the subcutaneous tissue, frequently proliferate to involve the musculature and, in advanced cases, to cause severe destruction of the bone.

Laboratory diagnosis

SPECIMEN COLLECTION

Grains or granules from draining sinus tracts should be examined for color (light or dark), size, and texture (soft or hard) and should be cultured to recover the etiologic agent.

DIRECT MICROSCOPIC EXAMINATION

Direct microscopic examination of the granules immediately differentiates eumycotic from actinomycotic mycetomas. Figure 23-26, *A*, shows the branching filamentous rods of actinomycetes in contrast to the hyphal elements (Figure 23-26, *B*) seen in eumycotic infections. To recover the eumycotic agent, samples are inoculated onto routine fungal media.

CULTURE

P. boydii colonies grow rapidly and produce white to dark gray colonies on potato dextrose agar at 25° C and 35° C. The anamorph (asexual form of the fungus), *Scedosporium apiospermum,* produces oval conidia singly at the tips of conidiogenous cells (cells that make conidia) known as annellides (Figure 23-27). Some strains may produce the teleomorph (sexual form of the fungus) in the laboratory and may form cleistothecia containing ascospores (Figure 23-28). This phenomenon occurs in fungi that are homothallic (i.e., require only one mating strain to produce the sexual form of the fungus).

A. falciforme is a moniliaceous (light-colored) mold. Colonies grow slowly, and are grayish brown, becoming grayish violet. This organism produces mucoid clusters of single or two-celled, slightly

TABLE 23-6

Description of Granules Seen in Eumycotic Mycetomas

Fungus	Color	Size (mm)	Texture
Pseudallescheria boydii	White	0.5–1.0	Soft
Acremonium falciforme	White	0.2–0.5	Soft
Madurella mycetomatis	Black	0.5–5.0	Hard
Madurella grisea	Black	0.3–0.6	Soft
Exophiala jeanselmei	Black	0.2–0.3	Soft

A
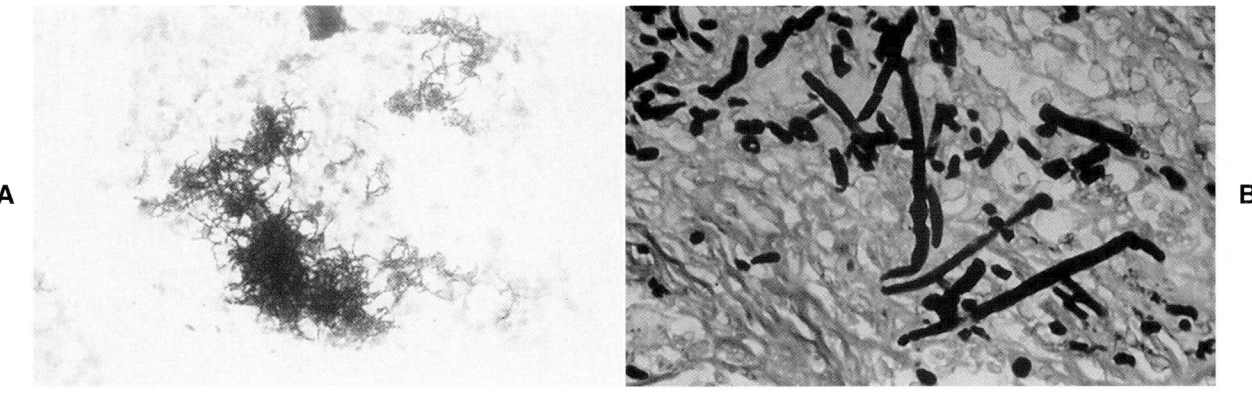
B

Figure 23-26

Actinomycotic mycetoma, showing fine-branching, filamentous rods in tissue sample **(A)**, compared with the hyphal elements **(B)** seen in eumycotic infections (×1250).

curved conidia borne from phialides at the tips of long, unbranched, multiseptate conidiophores, that are held together in mucoid clusters at the apices.

M. mycetomatis grows slowly. It is white initially, then becomes yellow, olivaceous, or brown with a characteristic diffusable brown pigment. Although about half of the isolates produce conidia from the tips of phialides, many remain sterile.

M. grisea grows slowly, produces olive brown to black colonies, and may produce a reddish brown pigment. *M. mycetomatis* grows best at 37° C and may grow at 40° C, but 30° C is the optimum temperature for *M. grisea*.

E. jeanselmei produces olivaceous to black colonies that are initially yeastlike but become velvety at maturity. Their conidia are also borne from annellides, and they aggregate in masses at the tips of the conidiophore, as seen in Figure 23-29.

Subcutaneous Phaeohyphomycosis

Phaeohyphomycosis is a mycotic disease caused by darkly pigmented fungi or fungi that have melanin in their cell walls. This term was coined by Ajello et al in 1974 to separate several clinical infections caused by dematiaceous fungi from those distinct clinical entities known as chromoblastomycosis. In tissue, these fungi may form yeastlike cells that are solitary or in short chains, or hyphae

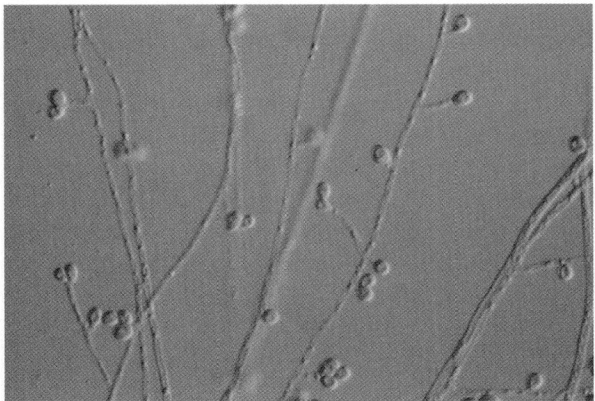

Figure 23-27

The *Scedosporium apiospermum* synanamorph of *Pseudallescheria boydii* (Nomarski optics, ×625).

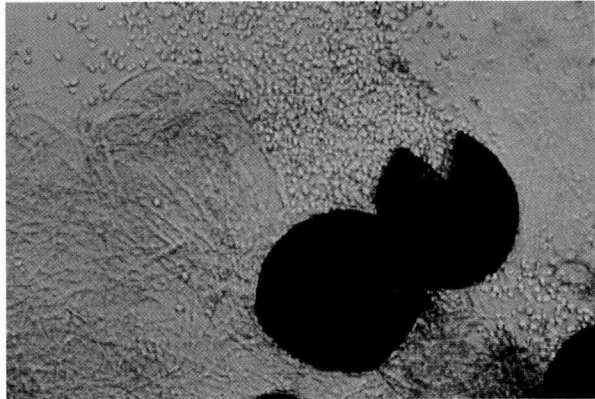

Figure 23-28

Sexual structures (cleistothecia containing ascospores) of *Pseudallescheria boydii* (Nomarski optics, ×325).

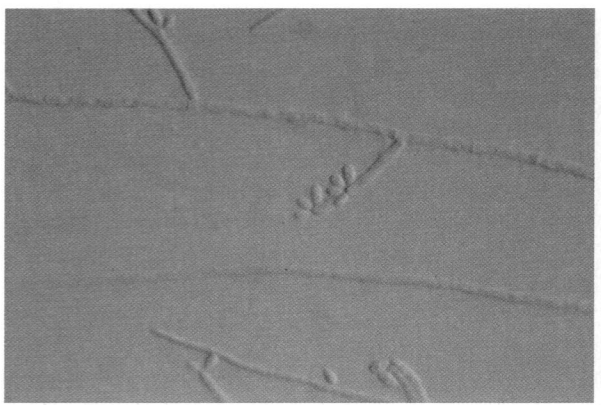

Figure 23-29 _____

Conidia of *Exophiala jeanselmei* borne at the tips of annellides (Nomarski optics, ×1250).

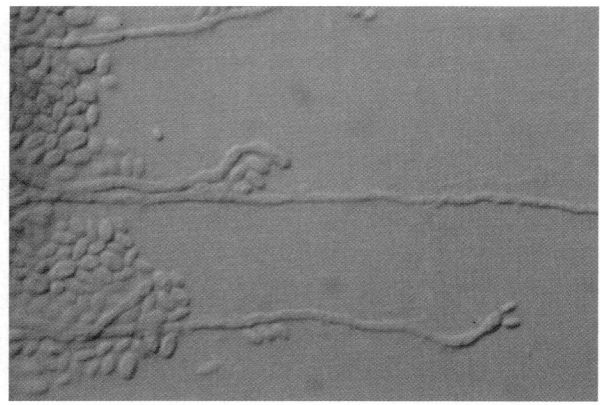

Figure 23-30 _____

Conidia of *Wangiella dermatitidis* borne at the tips of phialides as well as the black yeast synanamorph (Nomarski optics, ×1250).

that are septate, branched, or unbranched, and often swollen to toruloid. Agents responsible for these mycoses are organisms commonly found in nature, encompassing many genera of Hyphomycetes, Coelomycetes, and Ascomycetes.

Fungi that appear to be regularly associated with this condition include *Exophiala* species and *W. dermatitidis*. A more complete list of genera associated with subcutaneous phaeohyphomycosis is found in Box 23-1.

Laboratory diagnosis

SPECIMEN COLLECTION

Biopsy specimens of phaeohyphomycosis lesions should be submitted to the histology laboratory for fungal stains and to the mycology laboratory for culture.

Box 23-1

Dematiaceous Genera Inciting Subcutaneous Phaeohyphomycosis*

Alternaria	*Fonsecaea*
Anthropsis	*Mycocentrospora*
Bipolaris	*Oidiodendron*
Chaetomium	*Phaeosclera*
Cladosporium	*Phialophora*
Curvularia	*Phoma*
Dactylaria (Ochroconis)	*Ulocladium*
Exophiala	*Xylohypha*

_____
*This list is not all inclusive.

MICROSCOPIC EXAMINATION

In addition to the usual stains, such as GMS, H&E, and PAS, laboratory professionals may wish to include the Masson-Fontana stain to detect melanin in the cell walls, thus documenting the dematiaceous nature of the etiologic agent.

CULTURE

E. jeanselmei has been previously described as an agent of mycetoma. Young colonies are black and yeastlike owing to the *Phaeoannellomyces* synanamorph (the black yeast form of the fungus). Older colonies become more filamentous and produce their conidia from conidiogenous cells known as annellides (cells that have annellations or rings at their apices).

W. dermatitidis (Figure 23-30) differs from *E. jeanselmei* (see Figure 23-29) by having conidiogenous cells that are phialides without collarettes and by having its yeast synanamorph in the genus *Phaeococcomyces*. Although both organisms may be yeastlike and mucoid initially, *W. dermatitidis* more frequently retains this morphology as it matures, with only limited mycelium developing. Physiologically, *W. dermatitidis* grows at 40° C and is nitrate negative; *E. jeanselmei* fails to grow at 40° C and is nitrate positive.

AGENTS OF SYSTEMIC MYCOSES

Organisms that cause classic, systemic fungal diseases have historically been categorized together because they share several characteristics such as mode of transmission, dimorphism, and systemic dissemination. Although the term *systemic* generally refers to the organisms described here, it must be understood that any fungus, given an immunocompromised host, has the potential to become invasive and to disseminate to sites far removed from the portal of entry.

The four classic agents of systemic mycoses are the following:

- *Blastomyces dermatitidis*
- *Histoplasma capsulatum* var. *capsulatum*
- *Coccidioides immitis*
- *Paracoccidioides brasiliensis*

These organisms are dimorphic, which refers to their ability to grow in the mold form in their natural environment or in the laboratory at 25° C to 30° C as shown in Table 23-7 or in the yeast or spherule form when incubated at 35° C to 37° C on enriched media. Each agent has a fairly well-defined area of endemicity, and the diseases they all incite are contracted by the inhalation of infectious conidia. Table 23-8 provides a summary of systemic mycoses, their agents, and characteristics. All laboratory procedures to recover and identify these agents must be performed under a certified biologic safety cabinet.

Blastomyces dermatitidis

Epidemiology

Blastomyces dermatitidis causes blastomycosis, also known as Gilchrist's disease, North American blastomycosis, and Chicago disease. It occurs primarily in North America and parts of Africa. In the United States, it is endemic in the Mississippi and Ohio river basins. Sporadic point-source outbreaks have also occurred in the St. Lawrence River basin. The natural reservoir has not been unequivocally established, although the organism has been recovered from the soil and from some natural environments. Apparently, only a very narrow range of conditions supports its growth. In areas where the organism appears endemic, natural disease occurs in dogs and horses, and the disease process mimics that seen in human infections.

Clinical infections

Blastomycosis occurs when the conidia are inhaled. It is most prevalent in middle-aged men, as are other systemic mycoses, presumably owing to men's greater occupational exposure to the soil. Although patients with primary infection may exhibit flulike symptoms, most are asymptomatic and cannot accurately define the time of onset. When the primary disease fails to resolve, pulmonary disease may ensue, with cough, weight loss, chest pain, and fever. Progressive pulmonary

TABLE 23-7

Morphology of Systemic Fungi at 25° C

Fungus	Macroscopic Morphology	Microscopic Morphology
B. dermatitidis	Slow to moderate growth White to dark tan Young colonies tenacious, older colonies glabrous to woolly Spicules in center of colony	Oval, pyriform, to globose smooth conidia borne on short, lateral hypha-like conidiophores
H. capsulatum*	Slow growth White to dark tan with age Woolly, cottony, or granular	Microconidia small, one-celled, round, smooth (2–5 μm) Tuberculated macroconidia large, round (7–12 μm) Hypha-like conidiophores
C. immitis	Rapid growth White to tan to dark gray Young colonies tenacious, older colonies cottony Tend to grow in concentric rings	Alternating one-celled, "barrel-shaped" arthroconidia with disjunctor cells
P. brasiliensis	Slow growth White to beige Colony glabrous, leathery, flat to wrinkled, folded or velvety	Colonies frequently only produce sterile hyphae Fresh isolates may produce conidia similar to those of *B. dermatitidis*

**Histoplasma capsulatum* var. *capsulatum* (teleomorph *Ajellomyces capsulatus*). *Histoplasma capsulatum* var. *duboisii* is endemic in central Africa and is not discussed in this chapter.

TABLE 23-8

Summary of Systemic Mycoses

Fungus	Ecology	Clinical Disease	Tissue Form
B. dermatitidis	Mississippi and Ohio River valleys	Primary lung Chronic skin/bone Systemic, multiorgan	Large yeast (8–12 μm) Broad-based bud
*H. capsulatum**	Ohio, Missouri, and Mississippi River valleys Bird and bat guano Alkaline soil	Primary lung Asymptomatic Immunodeficient hosts prone to disseminated disease	Small, oval yeast (2–5 μm) in histiocytes, phagocytes
C. immitis	Semiarid regions: southwest United States, Mexico, Central and South America In soil	Primary lung Asymptomatic Secondary cavitary Progressive pulmonary Multisystem	Spherules (30–60 μm) containing endospores
P. brasiliensis	Central and South America In soil	Primary lung Granulomatous Ulcerative nasal and buccal lesions Lymph node involvement Adrenals	Thick-walled yeasts (15–30 μm) Multiple buds "Mariner's wheel"

*Histoplasma capsulatum var. *capsulatum* (teleomorph *Ajellomyces capsulatus*). *Histoplasma capsulatum* var. *duboisii* is endemic in central Africa and is not discussed in this chapter.

or invasive disease may follow, resulting in ulcerative lesions of the skin and bone. In the immunodeficient patient, multiple organ systems may be involved, and the course may be rapidly fatal.

Laboratory diagnosis

At present, still no practical, reliable serologic procedures exist for the diagnosis or prognosis of blastomycosis. Diagnosis requires identification of the organism in tissue or isolation and identification in culture.

SPECIMEN COLLECTION

In pulmonary disease, the first morning sputum may be submitted for direct microscopic examination and culture. Specimens must be processed immediately. Bronchial washings and other pulmonary secretions may also be examined for cytology.

Exudative material from cutaneous lesions and tissue must also be examined directly for yeasts.

DIRECT MICROSCOPIC EXAMINATION

Microscopic examination of tissue or purulent material in cutaneous skin lesions may reveal large, spherical, refractile yeast cells, 8 to 15 μm in diameter, with a double-contoured wall and buds connected by a broad base (Figure 23-31). Potas-

sium hydroxide (10%) or calcofluor white may be used to aid examination for the presence of the yeast cells.

CULTURE

Although demonstration of characteristic yeast cells in direct smear examination is usually diagnostic, cultures should also be performed, particularly when smears are negative. Because the yeast

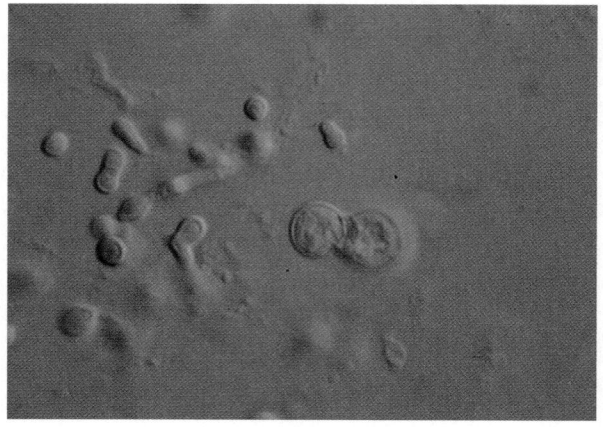

Figure 23-31

Conversion of the mold phase of *Blastomyces dermatitidis* to the "broad-based bud" yeast form (Nomarski optics, ×1250).

TABLE 23-9
Mold to Yeast Conversion in Dimorphic Fungi*

Fungus	Culture Media and Temperature	Yeast Form
B. dermatitidis	Blood agar, 37° C	Large yeast (8–12 μm) Blastoconidia attached by broad base
H. capsulatum	Pines medium, glucose-cysteine-blood, or BHI-blood, 37° C	Small, oval yeast (2–5 μm)
P. brasiliensis	BHI-blood, 37° C	Multiple blastoconidia budding from single, large yeast (15–30 μm)

**Coccidioides immitis* may be converted to the spherule phase in a modified Converse medium at 40° C in 5%-10% CO_2. Exoantigen testing is preferred to this procedure in the routine clinical laboratory.

TABLE 23-10
Exoantigens Identified in Dimorphic Fungal Pathogens*

Fungus	Exoantigen(s)
Blastomyces dermatitidis	A
Histoplasma capsulatum	H, M
Coccidioides immitis	F, HL, HS
Paracoccidioides brasiliensis	1, 2, 3

*Exoantigens are identified by forming lines of identity with reference antigen-antibody complexes (see Figure 23-33).

phase is susceptible to cycloheximide, nonselective media such as Sabouraud dextrose agar or brain-heart infusion should be employed. Heavily contaminated material should be plated on similar media containing antibacterial agents such as chloramphenicol, gentamicin, streptomycin, or penicillin. Two sets of cultures are set up, one to be incubated at 25° C and the other at 37° C.

Characteristics at room temperature In culture at 25° C, the organism may produce a variety of colonial morphologies. Colonies may be white, tan, or brown and may be fluffy to glabrous, growing in concentric rings. Frequently, raised areas termed *spicules* or *prickles* are seen in the centers of the colonies.

Microscopically, the anamorphic or asexual form of the fungus produces conidia borne on short lateral branches that are ovoid to dumbbell shaped and vary in diameter from 2 to 10 μm. They often resemble the microconidia of *H. capsulatum* var. *capsulatum* (Figure 23-32).

The teleomorph or sexual form of *B. dermatitidis* was described in 1967 and named *Ajellomyces dermatitidis*. It occurs only in rigidly controlled environments by mating of isolates with tester strains to produce gymnothecia containing ascospores. This teleomorph does not occur in the routine laboratory because the species is heterothallic (requires two mating strains to produce the sexual form).

Characteristics at 37° C When grown at 37° C on suitable media (Table 23-9), *B. dermatitidis* pro-

duces characteristic broad-based yeast cells (see Figure 23-31). This conversion process is necessary to identify this dimorphic fungus. The organism may also be identified by utilizing the exoantigen technique of Kaufman and Standard (1987). Exoantigens, cell-free antigens produced by the mycelial forms of dimorphic fungi (Table 23-10), are detected by precipitin lines of identity in immunodiffusion tests (Figure 23-33).

Histoplasma capsulatum var. *capsulatum*
Epidemiology
Histoplasma capsulatum var. *capsulatum* causes histoplasmosis, also known as reticuloendothelial cytomycosis, cave disease, spelunker's disease, and Darling's disease. Histoplasmosis occurs worldwide. The highest endemicity in the United States occurs in the Ohio, Missouri, and Missis-

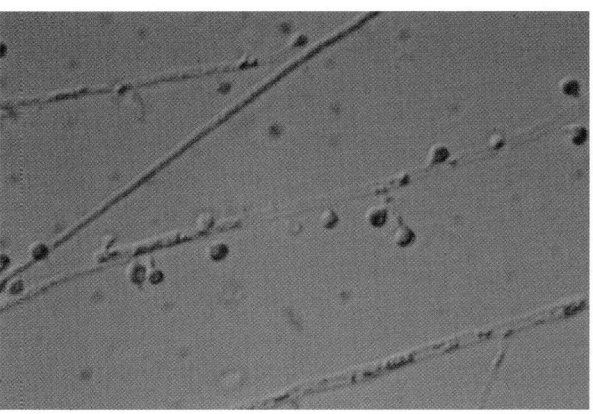

Figure 23-32
Mold phase of *Blastomyces dermatitidis* grown on potato flakes agar (Nomarski optics, ×1250).

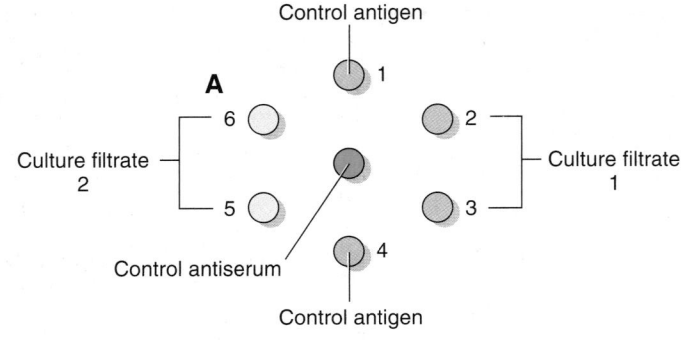

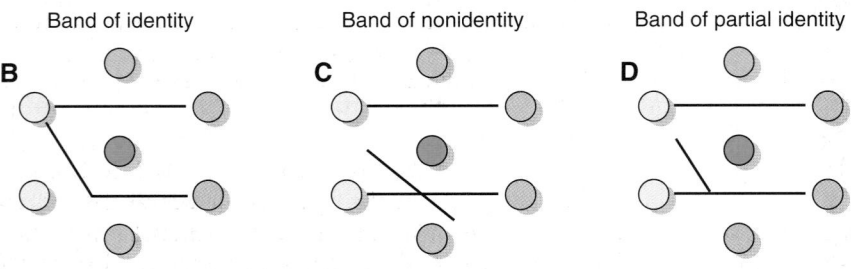

Figure 23-33

How the exoantigen immunodiffusion test is set up **(A)**; a band of identity **(B)**; a band of nonidentity **(C)**; and a band of partial identity **(D)**.

sippi river deltas. This organism resides in soil containing a high nitrogen content, particularly in areas heavily contaminated with bat and bird guano. Skin testing of long-term residents in endemic areas indicates that approximately 80% of the population have been infected. *Histoplasma capsulatum* var. *duboisii,* which is endemic in Central Africa, causes a clinically distinct form of disease. Another variant, *H. capsulatum* var. *farciminosum,* causes epizootic lymphangitis in horses and mules. These two forms of the organism are not discussed in this chapter. *H. capsulatum,* like *B. dermatitidis,* is also a heterothallic ascomycete, which produces the teleomorph state, *A. capsulatus,* when mated with appropriate tester strains.

Clinical infections

Histoplasmosis is acquired by the inhalation of the microconidia of *H. capsulatum* var. *capsulatum.* The microconidia are phagocytized by macrophages present in the pulmonary parenchyma. In the host with intact immune defenses, the infection is limited and is usually asymptomatic, the only sequelae being areas of calcification in the lungs, liver,

and spleen. With heavy exposure, however, acute pulmonary disease may occur. In the mild form of the disease, viable organisms remain in the host, quiescent for years; this is the presumed source of reactivation in individuals with abrogated immune systems. In immunocompromised individuals, *H. capsulatum* may cause a progressive and potentially fatal disseminated disease. Chronic pulmonary histoplasmosis in patients with chronic obstructive pulmonary disease may also occur. Other various manifestations of the disease are mediastinitis, pericarditis, and mucocutaneous lesions.

Laboratory diagnosis

Unlike blastomycosis, serologic procedures for the diagnosis of histoplasmosis may be an adjunct to culture methods. Tests that may be employed include skin tests (delayed or immediate sensitivity reactions), complement fixation, immunodiffusion, latex agglutination, counterimmunoelectrophoresis, radioimmunoassay (detection of circulating antibody), and fluorescent antibody (FA) microscopy (to detect either viable or nonviable fun-

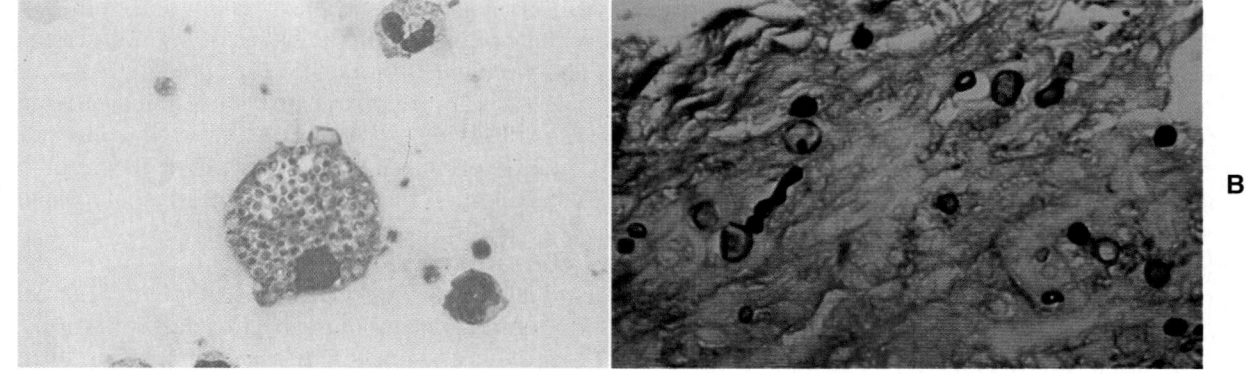

Figure 23-34

A, Bone marrow aspirate stained with Giemsa, showing the yeast cells of *Histoplasma capsulatum* var. *capsulatum* inside the monocytes (×1200). **B,** Tissue phase of *Histoplasma capsulatum* var. *capsulatum*. (GMS stain, ×1200).

gal elements in tissue sections). Currently, the most useful serologic applications for the diagnosis of histoplasmosis appears to be the combination of complement fixation and immunodiffusion tests, in which rising titers in serial dilutions are considered significant.

SPECIMEN COLLECTION

A variety of specimens, such as centrifuged sputum and bronchoscopic fluids from patients with cavitary disease, may yield *H. capsulatum*. In AIDS patients, the organisms are usually numerous in bone marrow aspirates and are frequently even present in peripheral blood smears. Exudates from mucocutaneous lesions, liver, and spleen may also be submitted for recovery of the organism. Clinical specimens are inoculated on two sets of Sabouraud dextrose agar, brain-heart infusion agar, or inhibitory mold agar media and incubated 25° C and 37° C.

DIRECT MICROSCOPIC EXAMINATION

Careful examination of direct smear preparations of specimens for histoplasmosis frequently reveals the small yeast cells of *H. capsulatum,* particularly in the opportunistic infections seen in the immunodeficient host. The yeast cells measure 2 to 3 μm by 4 to 5 μm. When smears are stained with Giemsa or Wright stain, the yeast cells are commonly seen within monocytes and macrophages occurring in significant numbers, as shown in Figure 23-34, *A,* bone marrow smear stained with Giemsa. These small cells, when found in tissue

(Figure 23-34, *B*), resemble the blastoconidia of *Torulopsis glabrata* but may be differentiated by FA techniques or culture. Yeast cells of *H. capsulatum* should also be distinguished from the small yeast form of *B. dermatitidis,* yeast cells of *Cryptococcus neoformans,* and the released endospores from spherules of *Coccidioides immitis.*

CULTURE

Histoplasma capsulatum grows as a white to brownish mold. Early growth of the mycelial culture produces round to pyriform microconidia measuring 2 to 5 μm. As the colony matures, large echinulate or tuberculate macroconidia, a characteristic of the species, are formed (Figure 23-35). Although

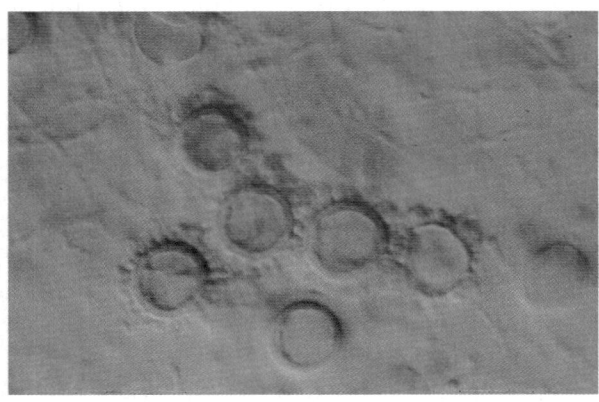

Figure 23-35

Large tuberculate macroconidia of *Histoplasma capsulatum* var. *capsulatum* (Nomarski optics, ×1250).

microconidia may resemble *Chrysosporium* spp. and the macroconidia resembles *Sepedonium* spp., neither saprobe produces two types of conidia, nor are they dimorphic. Conversion of the mold form to the yeast form, utilizing brain-heart infusion agar incubated at 37° C, is confirmation for *H. capsulatum*. Although complete conversion is seldom noted, a combination of forms is sufficient for identification. Identification of the isolates is confirmed by exoantigen procedures detecting two exoantigens (see Table 23-9) produced by this species, H and M antigens. Demonstration of these exoantigens is necessary for identification of isolates that fail to produce characteristic conidia.

Coccidioides immitis

Epidemiology

Coccidioides immitis causes coccidioidomycosis, also called Posada-Wernicke disease, coccidioidal granuloma, valley fever, desert rheumatism, valley bumps, and California disease. It resides in a narrow ecologic niche known as the Lower Sonoran Life Zone, characterized by low rainfall and semiarid conditions. Highly endemic areas include the San Joaquin Valley of California, the Maricopa and Pima counties of Arizona, and southwestern Texas. Outside the United States, high areas of endemicity are found in northern Mexico, Guatemala, Honduras, Venezuela, Paraguay, Argentina, and Columbia.

Clinical infections

C. immitis is probably the most virulent of all human mycotic agents. The inhalation of only a few arthroconidia produces primary coccidioidomycosis. Clinical infections include asymptomatic pulmonary disease and allergic manifestations. Allergic manifestations may manifest as toxic erythema, erythema nodosum (desert bumps), erythema multiforme (valley fever), and arthritis (desert rheumatism). Primary disease usually resolves without therapy and confers a strong, specific immunity to reinfection, which is detected by the coccidioidin skin test.

In symptomatic patients, fever, respiratory distress, cough, anorexia, headache, malaise, and myalgias may manifest for 6 weeks or longer. The disease may then progress to secondary coccidioidomycosis, which can include nodules, cavitary disease, or progressive pulmonary disease. Single or multisystem dissemination follows in approximately 1% of this population. Filipinos and African Americans run the highest risk of dissemination, with meningeal involvement as a common sequela. The sex distribution ratio for clinically apparent disease is approximately 9:1 (male/female), which also holds true for other classic systemic diseases. The exception is in pregnant women, in whom the dissemination rate equals or exceeds that for men.

Laboratory diagnosis

Several serologic procedures exist for initial screening, confirmation, and prognostic evaluation of coccidioidomycosis. The combined use of the immunodiffusion test and the latex particle agglutination test detects approximately 93% of the cases. The complement fixation (CF) and tube precipitin tests may also be employed for diagnosis as well as for confirmation. Prognostic studies commonly employ serial CF titers.

SPECIMEN COLLECTION

Respiratory specimens such as sputum, tracheal aspirates, and lung biopsy tissue may be submitted for suspected cases. CSF and blood cultures are performed for patients suspected of having disseminated forms.

DIRECT MICROSCOPIC EXAMINATION

After inhalation, the barrel-shaped arthroconidia, which measure 2.5 to 4 μm by 3 to 6 μm, round up as they convert to spherules. At maturity, the spherules (30 to 60 μm) produce endospores by a process known as *progressive cleavage*: rupture of the spherule wall releases the endospores, which in turn form new spherules (Figure 23-36). Direct smear examination of secretions may reveal the

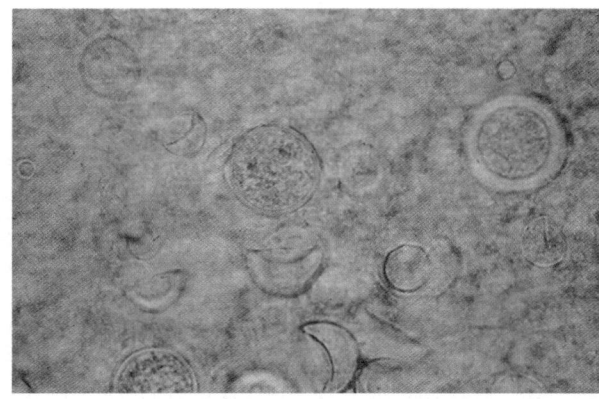

Figure 23-36 —————————————————

Spherules of *Coccidioides immitis* in tissue (×300).

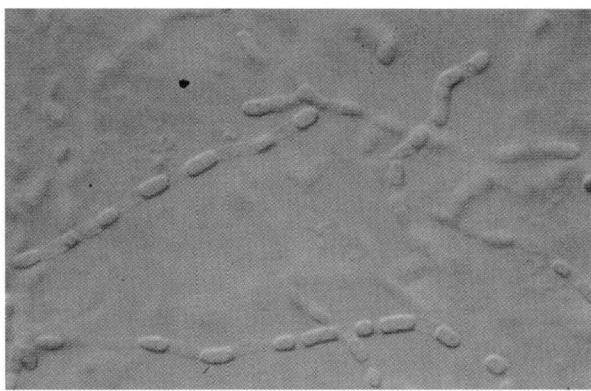

Figure 23-37

Mold phase of *Coccidioides immitis,* 25° C (Nomarski optics, ×1250).

spherules containing the endospores. Caution must be exercised, however, when diagnosis is made by histopathologic means only. Small, empty spherules may resemble the yeast cells of *B. dermatitidis,* and the endospores can be confused with the cells of *C. neoformans, H. capsulatum,* and *P. brasiliensis.*

CULTURE

Although *C. immitis* does not readily convert to the spherule stage at 37° C in the laboratory, it does produce a variety of mold morphologies at 25° C. Initial growth, which occurs within 3 to 4 days, is white to gray, moist, and glabrous. It rapidly develops abundant aerial mycelium, and the colony appears to enlarge in a circular "bloom." Mature colonies usually become tan to brown to lavender. Microscopically, fertile hyphae arise at right angles to the vegetative hyphae produce alternating (separated by a disjunctor cell), hyaline arthroconidia. When released, conidia have an annular frill at both ends. As the culture ages, the vegetative hyphae also fragment into arthroconidia (Figure 23-37). *Malbranchea* spp. resemble *C. immitis* but fail to convert to spherules in infected animals or special culture media. *Malbranchea* spp. also lack lines of identity in the exoantigen tests, which are specific for *C. immitis.*

Paracoccidioides brasiliensis
Epidemiology

Paracoccidioides brasiliensis is the causative agent of paracoccidioidomycosis (South American blastomycosis, Brazilian blastomycosis, Lutz-Splendore-Almeida disease, paracoccidioidal granuloma), a chronic, progressive fungal disease that is endemic in Central and South America. Geographic areas of highest incidence are typically humid, high-rainfall areas with acidic soil conditions. As with other systemic mycoses, the sex distribution for clinically significant disease is approximately 9:1 (male/female).

Clinical infections

Although the primary route of infection is pulmonary, and is usually inapparent and asymptomatic, subsequent dissemination leads to the formation of ulcerative granulomatous lesions of the buccal, nasal, and occasionally, gastrointestinal mucosa. A concomitant striking lymph node involvement is also evident. Although *P. brasiliensis* has a rather narrow range of temperature tolerance, as evidenced by its predilection for growth in cooler areas of the body (nasal and oropharyngeal), dissemination to other organs, particularly the adrenals, occurs with diminished host defenses.

Laboratory diagnosis

A wide variety of samples may be submitted to the laboratory for recovery of *P. brasiliensis.* They include sputum, bronchoalveolar lavage, pus from draining lymph nodes, scrapings from ulcers and biopsy tissue. Direct microscopic examination of cutaneous and mucosal lesions demonstrates the characteristic yeast cells. The typical budding yeast measures 15 to 30 μm in diameter with multipolar budding at the periphery, resembling a mariner's wheel (Figure 23-38). These "daughter"

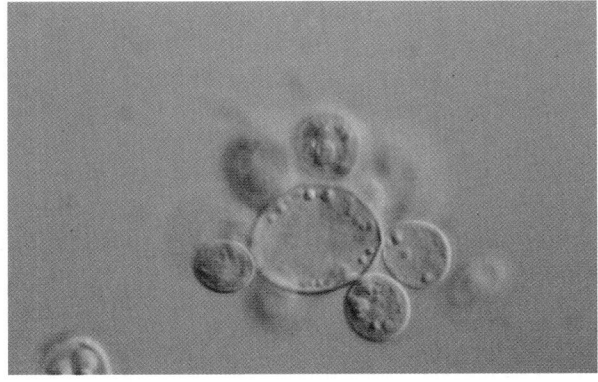

Figure 23-38

Yeast phase ("mariner's wheel") of *Paracoccidioides brasiliensis* with multipolar budding (Nomarski optics, ×1250).

cells (2 to 5 μm) are connected by a narrow base, unlike the broad-based attachment in *B. dermatitidis*. Many buds of various sizes may occur, or there may be only a few buds, giving the appearance of a "Mickey Mouse cap" to the yeast cell.

P. brasiliensis produces a variety of mold morphologies when grown at 25° C. Flat colonies are glabrous to leathery, wrinkled to folded, floccose to velvety, pink to beige to brown with a yellowish-brown reverse, resembling those of *B. dermatitidis*. Microscopically, the mold form produces small (2 to 10 μm in diameter), one-celled conidia, generally indistinguishable from those observed with the mold phase of *B. dermatitidis* or the microconidia of *H. capsulatum*. On BHI-blood agar at 37° C, the mycelial phase rapidly converts to yeast phase. Both complement fixation and agar gel immunodiffusion procedures are available for serodiagnosis.

Recently, DNA probe technology has permitted rapid identification of many systemic fungal isolates.

AGENTS OF OPPORTUNISTIC FUNGAL INFECTIONS: THE SAPROBES

Saprobe and *saprophyte* have been used to describe free-living microorganisms in the environment that are not of concern as agents of human disease. Toward the end of this century, the line between saprobic and parasitic or pathogenic organisms is increasingly blurred. The major reason for this development is the growing number of persons with minor or major defects in their immune systems. For several decades, medical science has made advances in life-sustaining and life-lengthening treatments. A serious side effect of procedures such as organ transplants and cancer chemotherapy is the short- or long-term insult to the host defenses. Magnifying the problem greatly during the last two decades has been the spread of acquired immune deficiency syndrome (AIDS). All these persons constitute the prime targets for infection by a wide variety of microorganisms, including the recognized pathogenic fungi and a growing list of fungi heretofore regarded as harmless.

The types of disease caused by these fungi are as varied as the species, and sometimes more so, because a given fungus may cause multiple disease forms. Various wounds from surgical proce-

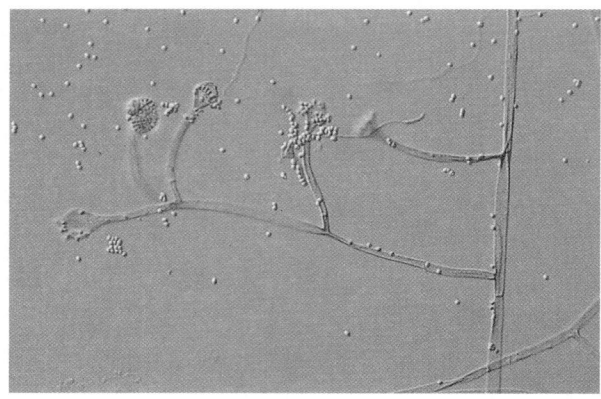

Figure 23-39
Absidia species.

dures are ideal points of inoculation for these saprobes to become opportunistic agents of disease, especially in the compromised host. Skin and nail bed infections as well as severe respiratory infections may be caused by a variety of fungi in the AIDS patient. What follows is a discussion of the most common saprobes that have been associated with opportunistic infections at different body sites. Characteristic morphologic features of each fungal species are described.

- *Absidia* species (Figure 23-39): Rapid-growing zygomycete with erect sporangiophores that terminate in a columella surrounded by a sporangium. Sporangiophores are formed in clusters on the intermediate portion of the stolons, and rhizoids are formed at the ends of the stolons.
- *Alternaria* species (Figure 23-40): Dematiaceous, rapid-growing fungus. Short conidiophores bear conidia in chains that lengthen in acropetal fashion. Multicelled conidia have angular cross-walls and taper toward the distal end.
- *Aureobasidium* species: Moderately rapid-growing, yeastlike fungus. Young cultures are off-white to pink, but with age, many cells become enlarged, thick-walled and very darkly pigmented. Short hyphae may be formed and may give rise to buds, both synchronously and asynchronously. Many of these cells become pigmented and usually result in black colonies.

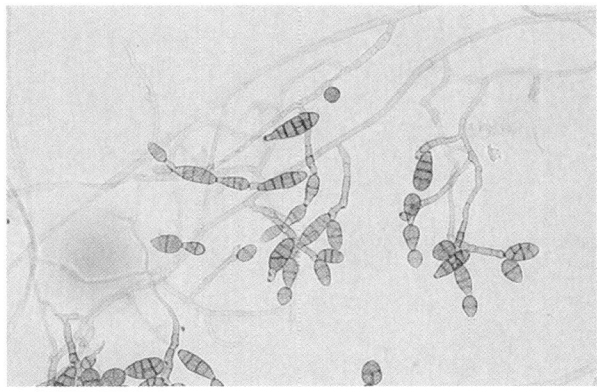

Figure 23-40 _____

Alternaria species.

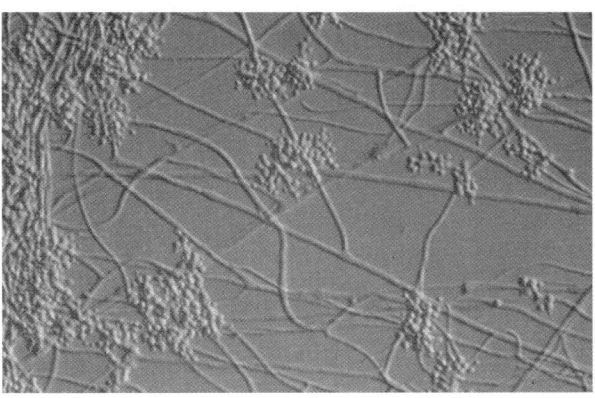

Figure 23-42 _____

Beauveria species.

▪ *Aspergillus* species (Figure 23-41): Perhaps the most commonly encountered genus of fungi in the clinical laboratory. Many species exist, and they are differentiated by their conidial and conidiophore morphology and color. The erect conidiophore arises from a "foot cell" within a vegetative hypha and terminates in a swelling or vesicle on which are borne phialides in a distinctive pattern. These produce phialoconidia in long chains. Conidia of some species are separated easily, whereas others remain in chains, these chains may align in very straight, parallel columns. Most of the colony color in *Aspergillus* species lies in the conidia. Color ranges from black to white, and includes yellow, brown, green, gray, pink,

beige, and tan. Some species also form diffusible subsurface pigments on a variety of media.

▪ *Beauveria* species (Figure 23-42): Hyaline, moderately rapid-growing, fluffy colonies, sometimes developing a powdery surface reminiscent of *Trichophyton mentagrophytes*. Abundant, single-celled, tear-shaped sympoduloconidia are formed on sympodulae, which taper extremely from a rather swollen base. Conidiophores may cluster in some isolates to form radial tufts.

▪ *Chaetomium* species (Figure 23-43): Moderately rapid-growing, dematiaceous ascomycete. Young colonies may be dirty gray; with age, they develop numerous perithecia, which

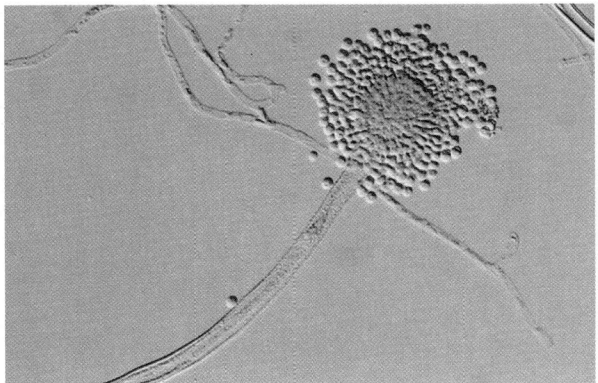

Figure 23-41 _____

Aspergillus species.

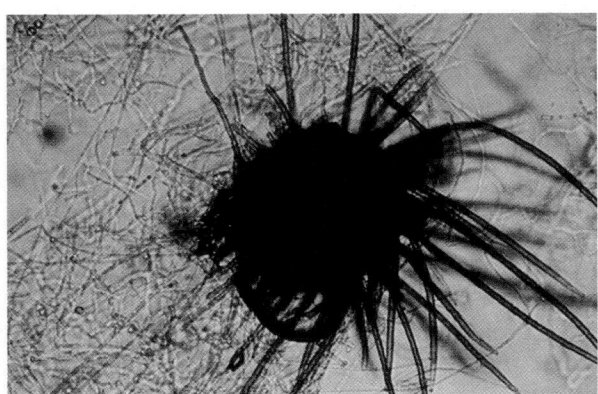

Figure 23-43 _____

Chaetomium species.

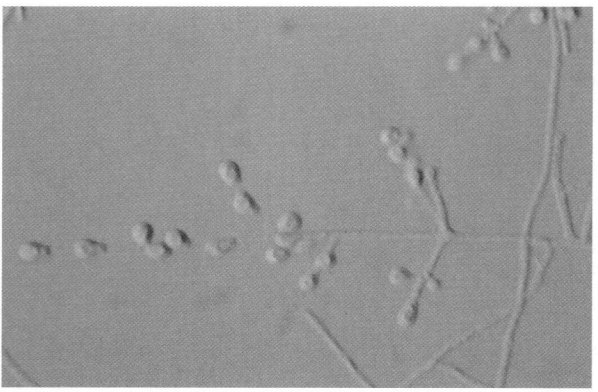

Figure 23-44 _____

Chrysosporium species.

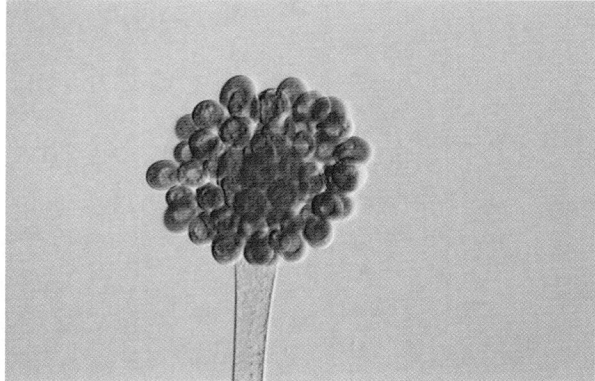

Figure 23-46 _____

Cunninghamella species.

are ornamented with straight or curled elaters. The asci are evanescent, so at maturity, the pigmented, lemon-shaped ascospores are released within the perithecium.

- *Chrysosporium* species (Figure 23-44): Hyaline fungus with moderate growth rate that, with age, may develop light shades of pink, gray, or tan pigment. Simple, wide-based, single-celled conidia are produced on nonspecialized cells. The conidiogenous cell disintegrates or breaks to release the conidia.
- *Cladosporium* species (Figure 23-45): Slow-growing to moderately rapid-growing dematiaceous fungus. Brown to olive to black hyphae and conidia. Conidiophores are erect and may branch into several conidiogenous cells. Spherical to ovoid conidia form blastically on

the end of each previously formed conidium. Branched conidium-bearing cells may dislodge, and the three scars on each of these cells give them somewhat the appearance of a shield. Generally, conidial chains of the saprophytic species break up easily, whereas those of pathogenic species remain connected.

- *Cunninghamella* species (Figure 23-46): Rapid-growing zygomycete that forms a cottony colony. Sporangiophores are erect, branching into several vesicles that bear sporangioles. These may be covered with long, fine spines.
- *Curvularia* species (Figure 23-47): Rapid-growing dematiaceous fungus that forms a cottony, dirty gray to black colony. The multicelled conidia are produced on sympodulae.

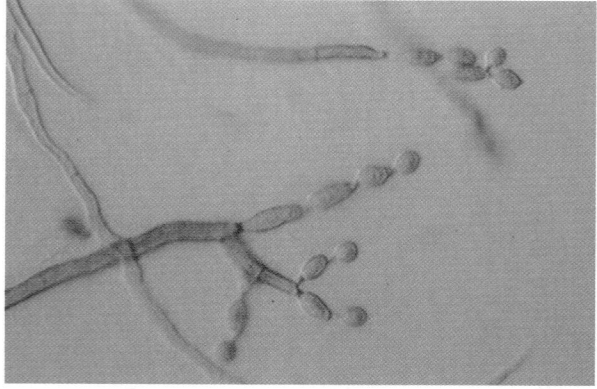

Figure 23-45 _____

Cladosporium species.

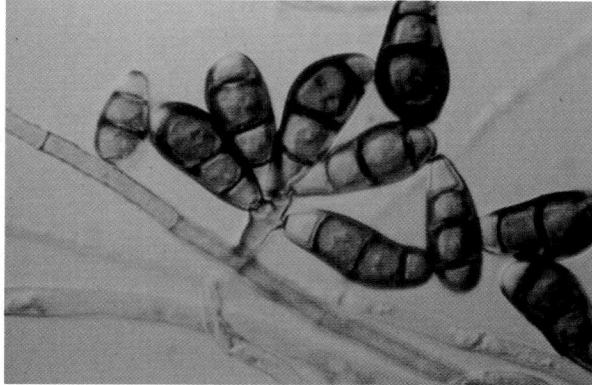

Figure 23-47 _____

Curvularia species.

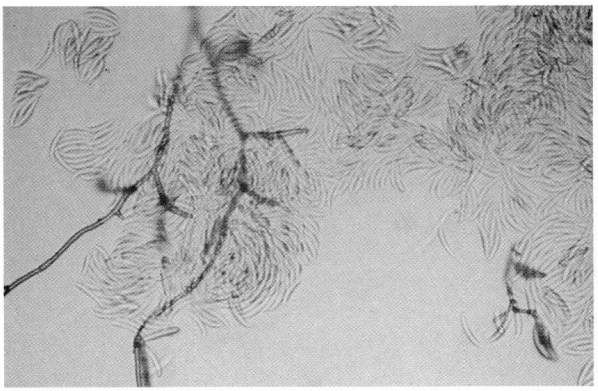

Figure 23-48 _____
Fusarium species.

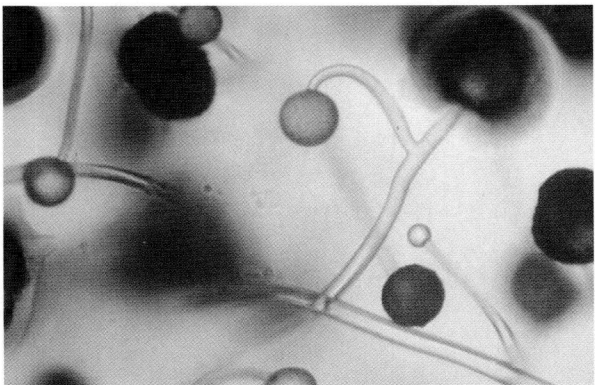

Figure 23-50 _____
Mucor species.

This genus is among the easier to identify because of the frequently crescent-shaped conidia with three to five cells of unequal sizes and usually slight pigmentation differences.

- *Epicoccum* species: Moderately rapid-growing dematiaceous fungus with yellow to orange hyphae that give rise to brown to black multicelled conidia in sporodochial clusters. The conidial cross-walls lie in diverse planes.
- *Fusarium* species (Figure 23-48): Rapid-growing hyaline fungus that may develop various colors with age, ranging from rose to mauve to purple to yellow. Normally abundant macroconidia and microconidia are produced on vegetative hyphae. These may cluster in sporodochia or may be formed singly. Macroconidia typically are multicelled and crescent-shaped.

- *Geotrichum* organisms (Figure 23-49): Rapid-growing, yeast-like, hyaline fungus that forms arthroconidia from vegetative hyphae.
- *Mucor* species (Figure 23-50): Rapid-growing zygomycete that forms cottony, dirty white colonies. Sporangiospores are formed in sporangia on erect sporangiophores. Rhizoids, typical of some zygomycetes, are not found in *Mucor*.
- *Nigrospora* species: Rapid-growing fungus with hyaline hyphae that turn gray to black with age. Conidia are dense, black ovoid cells formed on slightly swollen conidiophores.
- *Paecilomyces* species (Figure 23-51): Rapid-growing, usually very flat colony covered with conidia that are pastel tan, brownish-gold, or

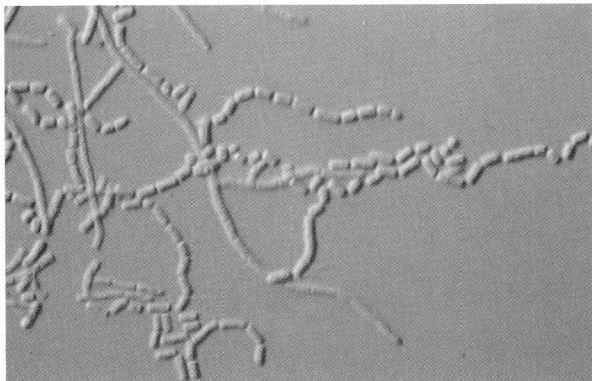

Figure 23-49 _____
Geotrichum species.

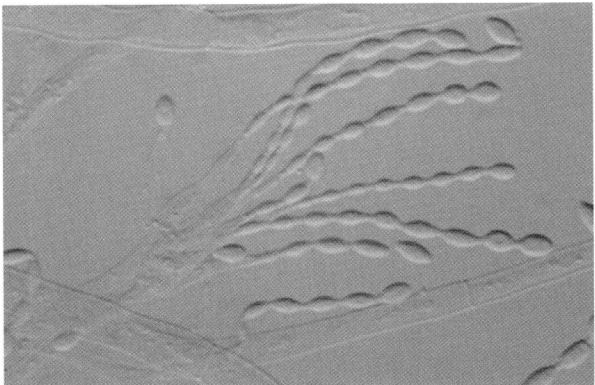

Figure 23-51 _____
Paecilomyces species.

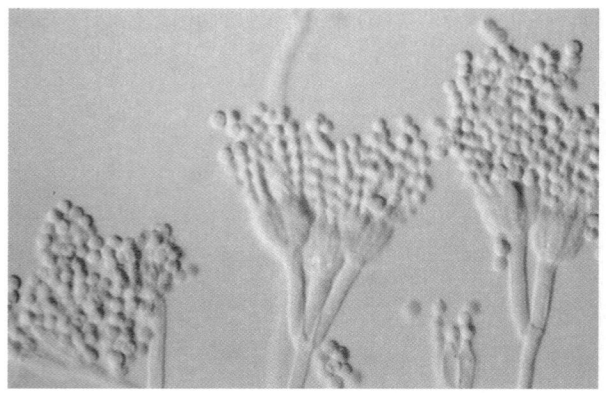

Figure 23-52 ───────────
Penicillium species.

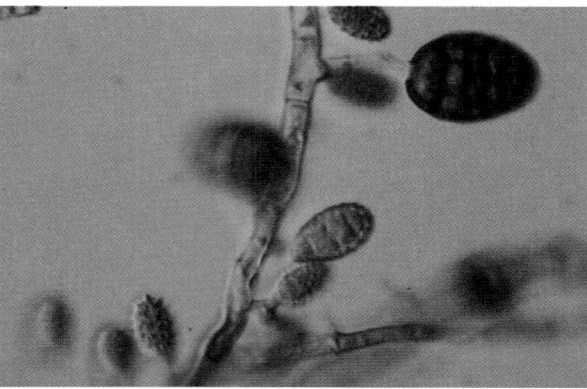

Figure 23-54 ───────────
Pithomyces species.

lavender. Green or blue-green colors are not seen. Care must be taken to avoid confusion between *Paecilomyces* and *Penicillium* species. Phialides of *Paecilomyces* are generally longer and more obviously tapered, and they may be singly formed or arranged in a verticillate pattern, on which long chains of spindle-shaped or somewhat cylindrical conidia are formed.

▪ *Penicillium* species (Figure 23-52): Rapid-growing, commonly seen fungus with colonies most often in shades of green or blue-green. Conidiophores are erect, sometimes branched, with metulae bearing one or several phialides on which oval to ovoid conidia are produced in long, loose chains.

▪ *Phoma* species (Figure 23-53): Moderately rapid-growing gray to brown colony that produces pycnidia-organized black fruiting bodies that are globose and lined inside with short conidiophores. Large numbers of hyaline conidia are generated in the pycnidium and flow out a small apical papilla.

▪ *Pithomyces* species (Figure 23-54): Rapid-growing dematiaceous colonies that produce dark, somewhat barrel-shaped conidia singly on simple short conidiophores. Conidia have both transverse and longitudinal cross-walls and often echinulate surfaces.

▪ *Rhizopus* species (Figure 23-55): Rapid-growing zygomycetous fungus with erect spo-

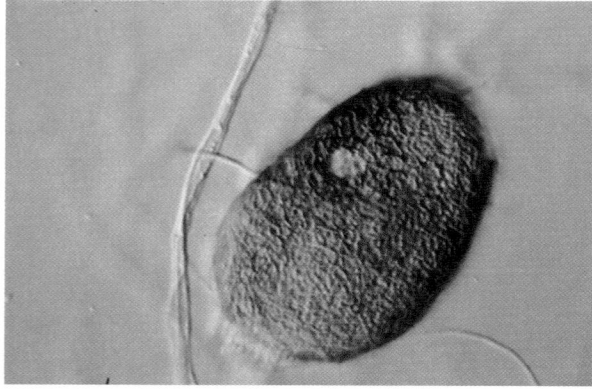

Figure 23-53 ───────────
Phoma species.

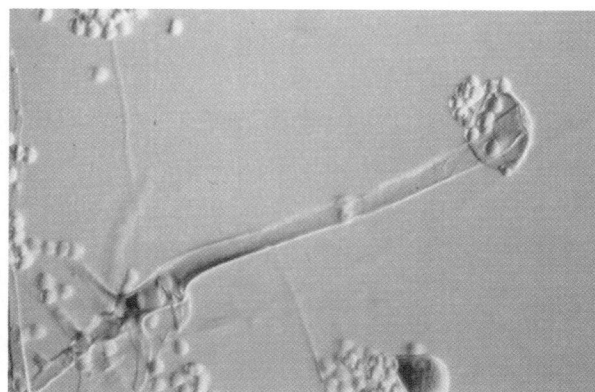

Figure 23-55 ───────────
Rhizopus species.

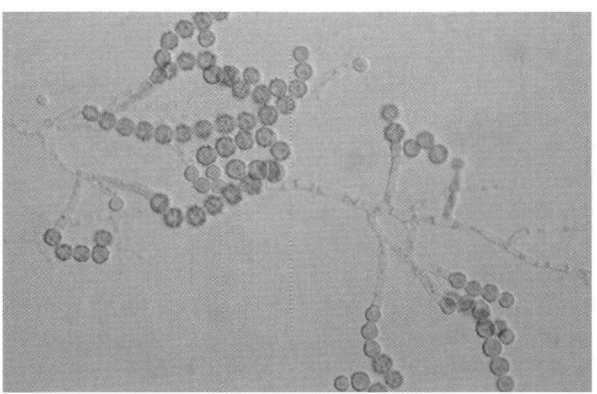

Figure 23-56 _____

Scopulariopsis species.

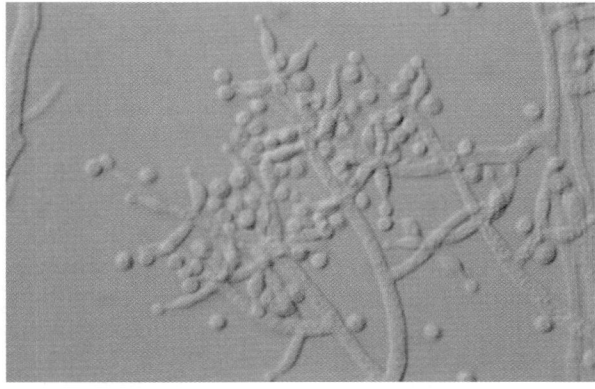

Figure 23-58 _____

Trichoderma species.

rangiophores terminated by dark sporangia and sporangiospores. At the base of the sporangiophore are brown rhizoids. Separate clusters of sporangiophores are joined by stolons, arching filaments that terminate at the rhizoids.

- *Scopulariopsis* species (Figure 23-56): Moderately rapid-growing colonies covered by tan to buff conidia. The clusters of conidiophores are annellides that increase in length as conidia are formed. The truncate-based conidia tend to remain in chains on the annellides.
- *Syncephalastrum* species (Figure 23-57): Rapid-growing zygomycete with erect spo-

rangiophores. Each sporangiophore has a large columella on which merosporangia, containing stacks of sporangiospores, are formed.

- *Trichoderma* species (Figure 23-58): Rapid-growing hyaline hyphae that give rise to yellow-green to green patches of conidia formed on clusters of tapering phialides. Conidia may remain clustered in balls at the phialide tips.
- *Ulocladium* species (Figure 23-59): Rapid-growing dematiaceous fungus bearing dark, multicelled conidia on sympodulous conidiophores. Conidia have angular cross-walls and, in some species, echinulate surfaces.

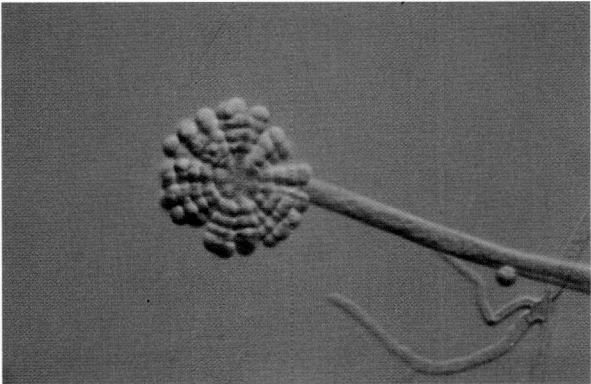

Figure 23-57 _____

Syncephalastrum species.

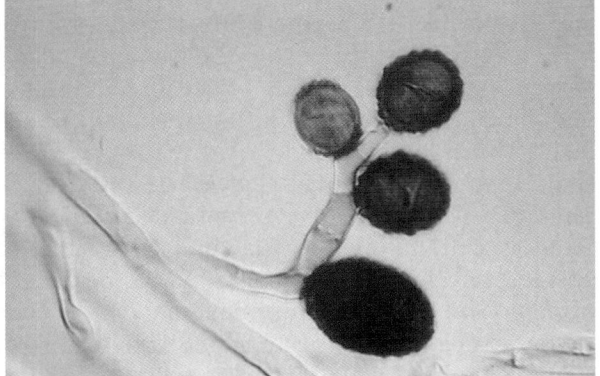

Figure 23-59 _____

Ulocladium species.

AGENTS OF YEAST INFECTIONS

The escalating incidence of yeast and yeastlike fungi isolated from patient specimens has increased the importance of identifying yeast isolates to the species level. With greater immunosuppression, the variety of organisms implicated in disease also expands. *Candida albicans* has become the fourth most common cause of blood-borne infection in the United States today. Isolation of other yeasts from clinical samples, including *Candida tropicalis, Candida parapsilosis,* and *Candida krusei,* is also increasing. Infections caused by these yeasts are extremely aggressive and difficult to treat.

Yeast fungi can be classified in one of two groups—yeasts and yeastlike fungi. Isolates that reproduce sexually, either by forming ascospores or basidiospores, are termed *yeasts.* The majority of isolates that are not capable of sexual reproduction or whose sexual state has not yet been discovered are correctly called *yeastlike fungi.* For ease of discussion, all isolates are referred to here as *yeasts.*

General Characteristics

Molds and yeasts are very different morphologically, but some of the macroscopic characteristics used as aids in identifying molds can also be used to identify yeasts. The most common characteristics noted are color and colony texture. The color of a yeast colony ranges from white to cream or tan, with a few species in the pink to salmon spectrum. Some yeast isolates referred to as *dematiaceous* yeasts, are darkly pigmented owing to melanin in their cell walls. Dematiaceous yeasts are associated with several species of the polymorphic fungi and are discussed elsewhere in this chapter.

The actual texture of the yeast colonies also varies. For example, *Cryptococcus* spp. tend to be very mucoid and may flow across the plate, a trait shared by some bacterial isolates, such as *Klebsiella* spp. Some yeasts are butterlike, and others range in texture from velvety to wrinkled. Strain-to-strain variation in texture may be noted within a species, but the microbiologists should be aware of *phenotypic switching;* this phenomenon is noted when two colony types occur upon subculture. Further DNA testing proves the two types to be the same organism. Switching occurs most often with *T. beigelii* but may also be seen in other isolates.

Clinically Significant Yeast Species

C. albicans and *Cryptococcus neoformans* are two of the more widely recognized clinically significant yeasts. A number of other organisms, however, including other *Candida* spp., *Rhodotorula* organisms, and *Torulopsis* sp., have also been implicated in clinical infections.

Candida species

Candida spp. not only are commonly present as normal flora of the mucosa, skin, and digestive tract but also are the most notorious agents of yeast infection. Clinical disease ranges from superficial skin infections to disseminated disease.

C. albicans currently reigns as the premier cause of yeast infection in the world. This isolate may be recovered as normal host flora from a variety of sites, including skin, oral mucosa, and vagina. When host conditions are altered, however, this isolate is capable of causing disease in virtually any site. One of the most widely recognized manifestations of *C. albicans* infection is thrush. In individuals with an intact immune system, infections are localized and limited. Thrush is also recognized as an indicator of immunosuppression. Among individuals infected with human immunodeficiency virus (HIV) as well as those receiving prolonged antimicrobial therapy or other chemotherapeutic agents, thrush manifests as a serious and, in some cases, disseminated infection.

C. glabrata is probably the second most common *Candida* species to incite disease. Infections associated with *C. glabrata* tend to be aggressive and difficult to treat with traditional antifungal therapy. This organism has different sugar assimilation patterns from those of *C. albicans* and therefore can easily be differentiated.

Other notable species of *Candida* are *Candida parapsilosis, Candida tropicalis,* and *Candida lusitaniae. Candida parapsilosis* has become a major cause of hospital outbreaks of nosocomial infections. This organism, like *C. tropicalis* and *C. glabrata,* is refractory to traditional antifungal therapy. These two isolates are identified by the differences in their carbohydrate assimilation patterns and other secondary testing procedures. Table 23-11 shows important differentiating characteristics among *Candida* species and other yeasts.

TABLE 23-11

Differentiating Characteristics of Yeast Isolates

| | Temperature Growth at | | | Cornmeal Agar | | | | | |
	37° C	42° C	45° C	Pseudohyphae	True Hyphae	Arthroconidia	Cyclohexamide	Urea	Nitrate
Candida									
C. albicans	+	+	+	+	+	−	+	−	−
C. guilliermondi	+	+	−	+	−	−	+	−	−
C. krusei	+	+	−	+	−	−	−	v	−
C. lusitaniae	+	+	+	+	−	−	v	−	−
C. parapsilosis	+	−	−	+	−	−	−	−	−
C. stellatoidea	+	+	+	+	+	−	−	−	−
C. tropicalis	+	+	+	+	−	−	v	−	−
Cryptococcus									
C. albidus	−	−	−	−	−	−	−	+	+
C. neoformans	+	−	−	−	−	−	−	+	−
Trichosporon									
beigelii	+	v	−	+	+	+	+	+	−
Torulopsis glabrata	+	+	+	−	−	−	−	−	−

+, Positive; −, negative; v, variable.

Cryptococcus species

Cryptococcus spp. are important causes of meningitis and pulmonary disease. *Cryptococcus neoformans,* the most noted pathogen in this group, has become one of the major causes of opportunistic infection in AIDS patients. The organism is commonly found in soil contaminated with pigeon droppings and is most likely inhaled prior to clinical infections. Common manifestations include meningitis, pneumonia, and bacteremia.

Cryptococcus spp. are surrounded by a capsule that produces the characteristic mucoid colonial appearance. The capsule can be detected surrounding the budding yeast in spinal fluid with the aid of India ink (see Figure 23-11). The ink stains the CSF while leaving clear halos around individual yeast cells. The use of India ink preparation is being replaced by the latex agglutination test for cryptococcal antigen, because of the former's low sensitivity and rate of detection. The latex agglutination test is being recommended for routine use in most clinical microbiology laboratories.

Cryptococcus spp. are noted for not producing true hyphae or **pseudohyphae** on cornmeal agar. Although all species of the genus are urease positive, nitrate reaction varies. Production of phenol oxidase is a feature differentiating *C. neoformans* from other *Cryptococcus* species. Sugar assimilations also vary for each species. *Cryptococcus neo-* *formans* may be differentiated by using the characteristics described in Table 23-11.

Rhodotorula species

Rhodotorula spp. are noted for their bright, salmonpink color. They are closely related to the cryptococci in that they bear a capsule and are urease positive. Some species are also nitrate positive. They are not common agents of disease but have been known to cause opportunistic infection.

Trichosporon beigelii

Trichosporon beigelii is most commonly regarded as a cause of white piedra—a yeast overgrowth on the hair shafts of individuals lacking proper personal hygiene. It is also an emerging agent of disseminated infection that has occurred in major outbreaks among cancer patients. Treatment is complicated by the fact that *T. beigelii* tends to be resistant to amphotericin B (AMB), the choice for treatment of life-threatening fungal infection. *Trichosporon* sp. are noted for their production of arthroconidia as well as blastoconidia on cornmeal agar.

Methods of Yeast Identification

Tests used in the identification of yeast range from simple tests, such as production of germ tubes, urease, and characteristic structures on cornmeal agar, to carbohydrate assimilation.

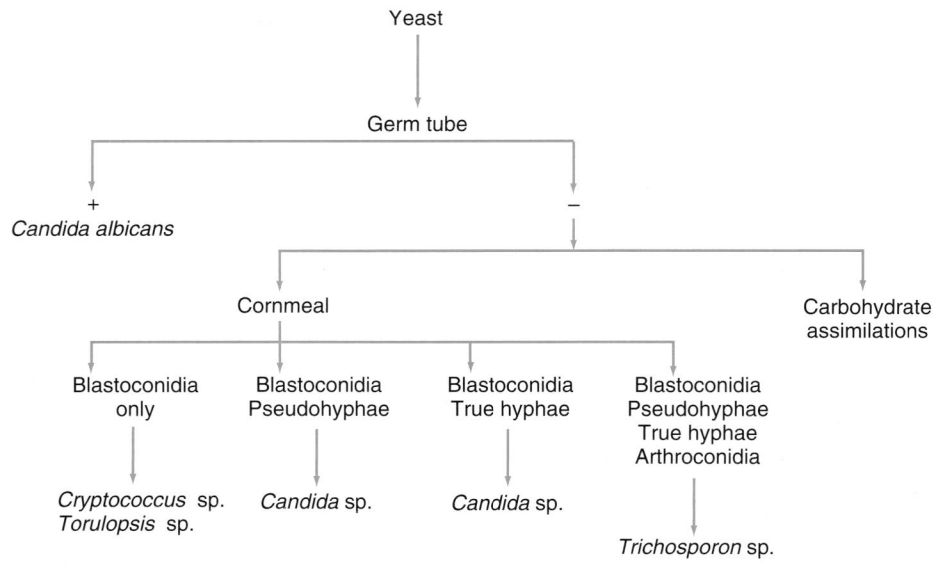

Figure 23-60
Schematic diagram showing how the germ tube test may be used to presumptively identify yeasts.

Germ tube production

The **germ tube** test is probably the most basic and easiest test to perform for identification of yeasts. Figure 23-60 shows a schematic diagram of how the germ tube test may be used to presumptively identify yeasts species. *C. albicans* is identified by its germ tube production (Figure 23-61). The standard procedure as described in Procedure 23-2 requires the use of serum or plasma. Expired fresh-frozen plasma, negative for both hepatitis B and HIV, from the blood bank is useful in this test and can be stored at 4° C indefinitely. Many other liquid media (e.g., brain heart infusion, trypticase soy broth, or nutrient broth) have been used successfully as al-

ternative media. See Procedure 23-2, Germ Tube Production. Care must be taken not to over-incubate the tube, because other agents are capable of forming germ tubes with extended incubation.

After the incubation period, an accurate identification of *C. albicans* can be made when true germ tubes are present. True germ tubes lack constriction at their bases, where they attach to the mother cell. If a constriction is present at the base of a germ tube, the yeast is not *C. albicans.* Such constricted germ tubes are more in keeping with *C. tropicalis* (Figure 23-62). *Candida stellatoidea* and *Candida dubliniensis* are also capable of germ tube production. *C. stellatoidea* is differentiated from

---

PROCEDURE 23-2. Germ Tube Production

1. Suspend one yeast colony onto a 0.5 ml of serum. Germ Tube Solution (Remel, Lenexa, Kan.), composed of fetal bovine serum and trypticase soy broth, may be used as an alternative. This alternative eliminates need for HIV and hepatitis testing of human serum.

2. Incubate at 35° C for 2.5 to 3 hours.

3. Place one drop of suspension on a microscopic glass slide and coverslip.

4. Observe for presence of germ tubes under the microscope.

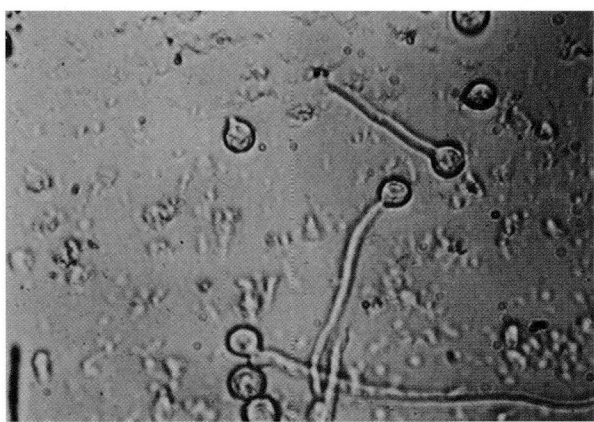

Figure 23-61 _____

Germ tube production by *Candida albicans.* A positive germ tube has no constriction at its base.

C. albicans by its inability to assimilate sucrose whereas *C. dubliniensis* is differentiated by its inability to grow at 45° C.

Negative germ tube results should lead the technologist to other procedures for identification. It should be noted that only rarely do *C. albicans* isolates yield a negative germ tube test result.

Positive and negative controls should be set up in conjunction with all testing. A known germ tube–positive isolate of *C. albicans* can serve as the positive control; *Cryptococcus* sp. works well as a negative control.

Carbohydrate assimilation

Sugar fermentation tests, although valuable, are time and labor intensive, thus making them impractical for the routine microbiology laboratory. Carbohydrate assimilation tests, however, can be readily performed as part of the routine bench procedures. Assimilation tests identify which carbohydrates a yeast can utilize as a sole source of carbon. Assimilation patterns may be determined from methods as sophisticated as the automated identification system or as simple as the various manual procedures and commercial kits. The individual laboratory should adopt the method that can be practically implemented into its particular working environment.

API 20C

Although many such kits are available for yeast identification, the API 20C yeast identification sys-

tem remains the gold standard for assimilation testing. In this method, a series of freeze-dried sugars are placed into wells on a plastic strip. Unknown yeast isolates are suspended in an agar basal medium, pipetted into the wells, and incubated at 30° C for 72 hours. As sugars are assimilated, the wells become turbid with growth. Wells remain clear when the sugar is not assimilated. A code is derived from the assimilation patterns and matched against a computerized database. Identifications are accompanied by a percentage, which indicates the probability that the identification is correct. Although this test is very reliable, other auxiliary testing should accompany assimilation results before a final identification is made.

Automated systems are also available for yeast identification. Many of these systems use enzyme reactions as well as assimilation reactions to aid in yeast identification.

Cornmeal agar morphology

Yeast morphology on cornmeal agar is second in importance to sugar assimilations in determining proper yeast identification. Procedure 23-3, Procedure to Inoculate a Cornmeal Agar, tests for production of hyphae.

Recognition of one of these four different types of morphology is a very important clue to yeast identification. Blastoconidia are the characteristic budding yeast forms most often seen on di-

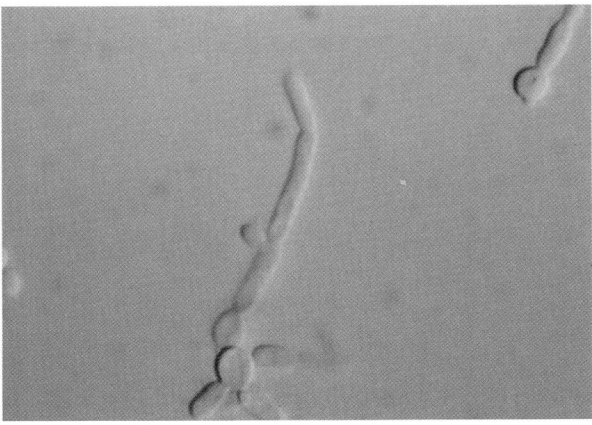

Figure 23-62 _____

Candida tropicalis shows constriction at the base of the germ tube.

PROCEDURE 23-3. Procedure to Inoculate a Cornmeal Agar

1. Pick up a small amount of a yeast colony with inoculating needle.

2. Make two parallel 1-cm streaks of inoculum on the agar surface.

3. Streak the agar between the two parallel inocula, being careful not to cut into the agar.

4. Coverslip and incubate for 48 hours at room temperature.

5. Observe the petri dish under the low- and high-power objectives for the presence of hyphae, pseudohyphae, arthroconidia, or chlamydoconidia or blastoconidia.

rect mounts. *C. albicans* produces chlamydoconidia along with hyphae, as shown in Figure 23-63. Pseudohyphae (Figure 23-64) occur when the blastoconidia germinate to form a filamentous mat. The cross-walls help determine whether the structures are true hyphae or pseudohyphae. Cross-walls of pseudohyphae are constrictions, not true septations, whereas true hyphae remain parallel at cross-walls, with no indentation. The fourth morphology type is arthroconidia. These begin as true hyphae but break apart at the cross-walls with maturity. Rectangular fragments of hyphae should be accompanied by blastoconidia in order for an isolate to be considered a yeast.

Potassium nitrate assimilation

Potassium nitrate assimilation patterns provide additional valuable information for separating the clinically significant yeasts. Use of the modified KNO_3 agar described by Pincus et al (1988) is a fairly rapid, easy, and accurate method to determine nitrate assimilations. A positive KNO_3 assimilation result turns the agar medium blue, and a negative result turns the medium yellow. Control organisms that may be used are *C. albidus* (positive) and *C. albicans* (negative).

Urease test

Yeast isolates producing the enzyme urease can easily be detected with a simple urea agar. This fairly rapid, easily read test aids in differentiation between *Cryptococcus* and *Rhodotorula* species. Media for detecting urea hydrolysis may be obtained commercially. Positive test results turn the media bright fuchsia pink, whereas negative results cause little if any change. *C. albidus* can be used as a positive control, and *C. albicans* as a negative control.

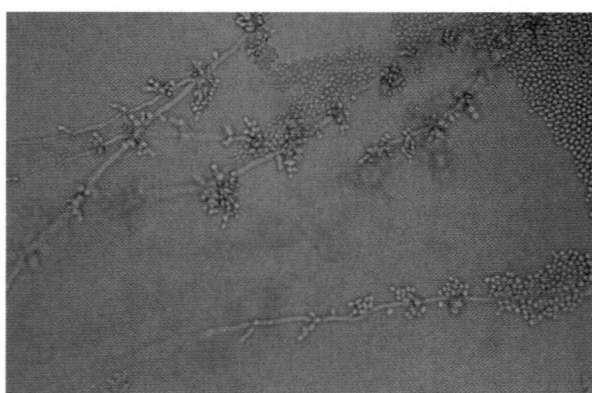

Figure 23-63 _____

Candida albicans on cornmeal agar showing typical chlamydospores.

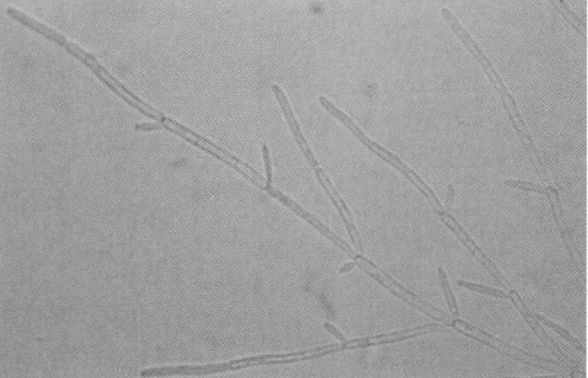

Figure 23-64 _____

Pseudohyphae occur when the blastoconidia germinate and form a filamentous mat.

Temperature

Temperature studies also offer additional information for yeast identification. *Cryptococcus* spp. have weak growth at 35° C and no growth at 42° C. Several *Candida* spp. have the ability to grow well at temperatures as high as 45° C.

Any one of these tests alone, with the exception of the germ tube test, is not sufficient for proper identification, but when they are used in concert, proper identification is often easily accomplished. Armed with the foregoing procedures, the laboratory professional should be able to identify the most commonly encountered yeast isolates.

Bibliography

Ajello L, editor: *Coccidiodomycosis: current clinical and diagnostic status,* New York, 1977, Stratton Intercontinental Medical Book Corp.

Ajello L, et al: A case of phaeohyphomycosis caused by a new species of *Phialophora, Mycologia* 66:490, 1974.

Bonner JR et al: Disseminated histoplasmosis in patients with acquired immune deficiency syndrome, *Arch Intern Med* 144:2178, 1984.

Cooper BH, Silva-Hutner M: Yeast of medical importance. In Lennette EH et al, editors: *Manual of clinical microbiology,* ed 4, Washington, DC, 1985, American Society for Microbiology.

Denton JF, DiSalvo AF: Isolation of *Blastomyces dermatitidis* in soil associated with a large outbreak of blastomycosis in Wisconsin, *N Engl J Med* 31:529, 1964.

Einstein HE, Cantanzara A: *Coccidioidomycosis.* Proceedings of the Fourth International Conference of the National Foundation of Infectious Diseases, Washington, DC, 1985.

Ellis MB: *Dematiaceous hyphomycetes,* Kew, Surrey, England, 1971, Commonwealth Mycological Institute.

Fuchs PC: Fungal infection in the patient with compromised defenses, *Lab Med* 27:284: 1996.

Goodman NL, Larsh HW: Environmental factors and growth of *Histoplasma capsulatum* in soil, *Mycopathol Mycol Appl* 33:145, 1967.

Greer DL, Restrepo A: The epidemiology of paracocciioidomycosis. In Al-Doory Y, editor: *The epidemiology of human mycotid diseases,* Springfield, Ill, 1975, Charles C Thomas.

Holdane DJ, Robart E: A comparison of caldofluor white, potassium hydroxide and culture for the laboratory diagnosis of superficial fungal infections, *Diagn Microbiol Infect Dis* 13:337, 1990.

Huppert M: Serology of *Coccidiodomycosis, Mycopathologia* 41:107, 1970.

Kaufman L, Standard PG: Improved version of the exoantigen test for identification of *Coccidioides immitis* and *Histoplasma capsulatum* cultures, *J Clin Microbiol* 8:42, 1978.

Kaufman L, Standard PG: Specific and rapid identification of medically important fungi by exoantigen detection, *Ann Rev Microbiol* 41:209, 1987.

Kedes LJ, Siemski J, Braude AI: The syndrome of the alcoholic rose gardener: sporotrichosis of radial tendon sheath— report of a case with amphotericin B, *Ann Intern Med* 61:1139, 1964.

Klein BS et al: Isolation of *Blastomyces dermatitidis* in soil associated with a large outbreak of blastomycosis in Wisconsin, *N Engl J Med* 31:529, 1986.

Kwon-Chung KJ, Bennett JE: *Medical mycology,* Malvern, Penn, 1992, Lea & Febiger.

Manos NE, Ferebee SH, Kerschbaum WF: Geographic variation in the prevalence of histoplasmin sensitivity, *Dis Chest* 29:649, 1956.

Matsumoto T et al: Critical review of human isolates of *Wangiella dermatitidis, Mycologia* 76:232, 1984.

McDonough ES, Lewis AL: *Blastomyces dermatitidis:* production of the sexual stage, *Science* 156:528, 1969.

McGinnis MR: Chromoblastomycosis and paeohyphomycosis: new concepts, diagnosis and mycology, *J Am Acad Dermatol* 8:1, 1983.

McGinnis MR: *Laboratory handbook of medical mycology,* New York, 1980, Academic Press.

McManus EJ, Jones JM: Detection of a *Trichosporon beigelii* antigen cross-reactive with *Cryptococcus neoformans* capsular polysaccharide in serum from a patient with disseminated *Trichosporon* infection, *J Clin Microbiol* 21:681: 1985.

Pincus DH et al: Modification of potassium nitrate assimilation test for identification of clinically important yeasts, *J Clin Microbiol* 26:366, 1988.

Rebell G, Taplin D: *Dermatophytes, their recognition and identification,* Coral Gables, Fla, 1970, University of Miami Press.

Restrepo MA et al: The gamut of paracoccidioidomycosis, *Am J Med* 61:33, 1976.

Rippon JW: *Medical mycology: the pathogenic fungi and the Actinomycetes,* ed 3, Philadelphia, 1988, WB Saunders.

Sekhon AS et al: Blastomycosis: report of three cases from Alberta and a review of Canadian cases, *Mycopathologica* 65:53, 1979.

Stevens D: *Coccidiodomycosis: a test,* New York, 1981, Plenum Press.

Walsh et al: Disseminated trichosporonosis resistant to amphotericin B, *J Clin Microbiol* 28:1616, 1990.

Wheat LJ et al: The diagnostic laboratory tests for histoplasmosis: analysis of experience in a large urban outbreak, *Ann Intern Med* 97:680, 1982.

LEARNING ASSESSMENTS

1. For each of the following dimorphic fungi, describe the characteristic microscopic appearance at 37° C or in vivo and when grown at 25° C:
   Blastomyces dermatiditis
   Coccidioides immitis
   Histoplasma capsulatum var. *capsulatum*
   Sporothrix schenkii

2. Describe the microscopic morphology for each of the following organisms. Compare the results of the urease test and the hair perforation test for *T. rubrum* and *T. mentagrophytes:*
   Microsporum gypseum
   Microsporum canis
   Trichophyton rubrum
   Trichophyton mentagrophytes

3. Describe the significance of isolating a saprobe from an infection in an immunocompromised patient.

4. Compare the macroscopic and microscopic morphology of the following saprobes: *Penicillium* sp., *Aspergillus fumigatus, Fusarium* sp., and *Curvularia* sp.

5. You suspect a yeast isolated from the oral cavity of a patient with HIV is *Candida albicans*. Describe the results of the germ tube test. What morphology would you see if you inoculated the colony onto cornmeal agar?

CHAPTER 24

Diagnostic Parasitology

Linda A. Smith

GENERAL CONCEPTS IN PARASITOLOGY
LABORATORY METHODS
Fecal Specimens
Collection, handling, and transport
Preservation
Examination of the fecal specimen
Procedures for detection of specific parasites
Other Specimens Examined for Intestinal Parasites
Duodenal aspirates
Sigmoidoscopy specimens
Urine, vaginal, or urethral specimens
Sputum
Examination of Specimens for Blood and Tissue
Parasites
Blood smears
Biopsy specimens
Cerebrospinal fluid
Immunologic Diagnosis
Enzyme immunoassay
Fluorescent antibody techniques
Quality Assurance in the Parasitology Laboratory
Ocular micrometer

MEDICALLY IMPORTANT PARASITIC AGENTS
Protozoa
Intestinal amebae
Tissue amebae
Ciliates
Pathogenic intestinal and urogenital flagellates
Nonpathogenic intestinal flagellates
Blood and tissue flagellates
Apicomplexa
Plasmodium spp.
Babesia microti
Toxoplasma gondii
Pneumocystis carinii
Opportunistic intestinal apicomplexa
Microsporidia
Clinical infection
Life cycle
Laboratory diagnosis
Helminths
Flukes
Tapeworms
Tissue infections with cestodes
Roundworms
Blood and tissue infections with roundworms

OBJECTIVES

1. Cite the major considerations in the collection and handling of specimens for identification of intestinal and blood and tissue parasites.

2. Describe the general procedure for performing the direct wet mount, concentration procedures, and permanent stained smears.

3. List the stages of parasites found with each of the following: direct wet mount, concentration, and permanent stained smears.

4. Identify the general characteristics of major phyla of parasites.

5. For the major human pathogens, describe the mechanism of pathogenesis, method of infection, clinical symptoms, prevention, and treatment.

6. For each organism, describe the morphology, the life cycle, including the infective stage and the diagnostic stage, and the usual procedure for identification.

KEY TERMS

Etiologic agent	Diagnostic stages	Sporogony	Cercaria
Karyosomes	Amastigote	Schizogony	Metacercaria
Chromatoidal bars	Trypomastigote	Exoerythrocytic phase	Proglottid
Pathogen	Zoonotic	Oocyst	Scolex
Nonpathogens	Definitive host	Tachyzoite	Hexacanth embryo
Trophozoite	Sexual reproduction	Bradyzoite	(oncosphere)
Cyst	Asexual reproduction	Congential transmission	Cysticercus
Intermediate hosts	Schizont	Sporoblast	Rhabditiform larva
Pathogenicity	Merozoites	Sporocysts	Filariform larva
Peripheral chromatin	Sporozoites	Worm burden	
Vectors	Gametocytes		

CASE STUDY

A 24-year-old man consulted his physician about the following symptoms: abdominal cramping, loss of appetite, and liquid stools (up to eight a day) with no evidence of blood. The symptoms had been present for about 1 week. The man's history included extensive travel over the past 2 years in Europe and Africa, and, most recently, in Central and South America, from which he had returned about 3 weeks ago. He had said that he often ate and drank whatever the local people did. He had a medical history of malaria and hepatitis A but no other known infectious diseases. The physician ordered a bacterial culture for pathogens and an ova and parasite (O&P) examination.

Parasites have always contributed to human morbidity and mortality. In the United States and other developed countries, they seldom are regarded as major causes of disease. In the past few years, however, practitioners have become increasingly aware that parasites must be considered as a possible **etiologic agent** in a patient's clinical condition. Factors that have led to this greater awareness include the rising number of immunocompromised patients who are susceptible to infections caused by known pathogens and opportunistic organisms, the increasing number of people who travel to countries that have less than ideal sanitation and a large number of endemic parasites, and the growing population of immigrants from areas with endemic parasites.

When a clinician is confronted with an infection that may be due to an intestinal or a blood and tissue parasite, the patient's symptoms and clinical history, including travel, are significant data to be gathered and shared with the clinical laboratory scientist. The laboratorian and clinician should collaborate to make sure that the appropriate specimen is properly collected and handled before and during the clinical workup. A knowledge of common pathogens and of nonpathogens that exist in specific geographic regions and for a given body site is necessary to ensure identification and, if necessary, therapy.

Parasitic infections can be difficult to diagnose because patients often have nonspecific clinical symptoms that can be attributed to a number of disease agents. Detection and identification of a parasite depend not only on the adequacy of the submitted specimen but also on the procedures established by the clinical laboratory, including the criteria for specimen collection, handling, and transport, and for the laboratory methods used. The purpose of this chapter is to:

- Present a general overview of sample collection, handling and transport, and quality assurance
- Describe procedures, such as the preparation of blood films, wet mounts, concentration methods, and staining methods
- Discuss the major medically important parasites, their epidemiology and life cycle, and the clinical infections they cause
- Present the diagnostic features that characterize these agents and explain their differentiation from nonpathogens

Readers are referred to standard parasitology references for detailed procedures, reagent preparation, and a comprehensive description of parasites that have been implicated in human disease.

GENERAL CONCEPTS IN PARASITOLOGY LABORATORY METHODS

Fecal Specimens

Collection, handling, and transport

A single stool specimen may not be sufficient to isolate an intestinal parasite, because many intestinal organisms shed eggs or cysts on an irregular schedule. It traditionally has been recommended that for optimal detection of intestinal parasites, a series of three stool specimens should be collected within 10 days but spaced a day or two apart. This procedure of examining each specimen submitted is very time-consuming and labor-intensive. Recent articles suggest that in some circumstances, pooling of the three formalin-preserved specimens gives a recovery rate comparable to that of individual examination of formalin-preserved stools. In addition, whether the cases are inpatient or outpatient and the presence of symptoms should dictate whether three specimens are needed.

The appropriate collection container is clean, dry, and waterproof, such as a half-pint waxed cardboard or plastic container with lid. Commercial systems that incorporate collection container and preservatives are also available. Stool specimens should never be collected from bedpans or the toilet bowl; such a practice might contaminate the specimen with urine or water, resulting in the destruction of trophozoites or introduction of free-living protozoa. As an alternative, the specimen should be collected on a clean piece of waxed paper or newspaper and transferred to the container. Another alternative is to use one of the disposable collection containers that can be fitted under the toilet bowl rim. The specimen should be submitted as soon as possible after passage. Identification noted on the container should include the patient's name and the date and time the stool was collected. The laboratory requisition should include the same information and any additional pertinent clinical data, such as the suspected diagnosis.

Stool specimens for parasites should be collected before a barium series or before the start of antimicrobial therapy. Antimicrobials can reduce the number of organisms present. If the patient has undergone a barium series, stool examination should be delayed for 7 to 10 days, because barium obscures organisms. If a purged specimen is to be collected, it is recommended that a saline or phosphosoda purgative be used, because mineral oil droplets interfere with identification of parasites, especially protozoan cysts. The second or third specimen after the purge is more likely to contain trophozoites that inhabit the cecum.

Preservation

Several methods are available for stool preservation if the specimen will not be delivered immediately to the laboratory. The preservative to be used is determined by the procedure to be performed on the fecal sample. Regardless of the preservative used, the ratio of three parts fixative to one part feces should be maintained for optimal fixation. Table 24-1 presents some of the more common preservatives, their appropriate use, and the organism stages preserved. The time that the stool was passed and the time that it was placed in the fixative should be written on the laboratory requisition and the container. A commercially available two-vial system using polyvinyl alcohol (PVA) fixative in one vial and 10% formalin in the other vial is the most commonly used system. The system comes with patient instructions and a self-sealing plastic bag for transport. PVA fixative, which consists of mercuric chloride (for fixation) and polyvinyl alcohol (a resin to increase adhesion of the stool to the slide) is used when a permanently stained smear will be made. Concern about disposal of hazardous mercury compounds has led to development and evaluation of a zinc sulfate–based compound for PVA. Evaluation of stains made from stools preserved with the zinc-based compound showed a less sharp morphology but overall good agreement with identifications made from trichrome-stained smears using traditional PVA preservative.

Formalin (10%) can be used when either a wet mount or concentration procedure (either sedimentation or flotation) will be performed. The fixative sodium acetate–acetic acid–formalin (SAF) can be used for the preservation of fecal specimens when both concentration procedures and permanent stains will be used. Vials of Merthiolate-iodine-formalin (MIF) can also be used to preserve trophozoites, cysts, larvae, and helminth eggs for wet mount or concentration procedures. This preservative, however, is not routinely used for permanently stained smears.

Examination of the fecal specimen

Any stool specimen submitted to the microbiology laboratory should be handled carefully because it is a potential source of infection. Specimens should be opened and handled in designated areas that provide protection for the technologist.

MACROSCOPIC EXAMINATION

The examination of an unpreserved stool specimen should include macroscopic (gross) and microscopic procedures. The initial laboratory procedure is the macroscopic examination. During gross examination, intact worms or proglottids may be identified on the surface of the stool.

Gross examination of the specimen reveals the consistency (liquid, soft, formed) of the stool sample. Consistency may help determine the type of preservation to be used, may indicate the forms of parasites that may be expected to be present, or may dictate the immediacy of examination. Figure 24-1 shows the relationship between stool consistency and protozoan stage. For example, a soft or liquid stool specimen or a purged specimen primarily contains motile protozoan trophozoites; hence, purged specimens should be examined immediately after passage. Soft or liquid specimens should be examined within one-half hour of passage to ensure motility of the organisms. If examination will be delayed, a portion should also be placed in a fixative such as PVA, so that permanent stained smears for definitive identification can be made.

Gross examination also reveals the color of the stool specimen. A normal stool sample usually appears brown. Stool that appears black may indicate bleeding in the upper gastrointestinal tract, whereas the presence of fresh blood may indicate bleeding in the lower portion of the intestinal tract.

TABLE 24-1

Preservatives Commonly Used for Fecal Samples

Preservative	Laboratory Examination Method	Organism Stages Preserved
Polyvinly alcohol (PVA)	Permanently stained smear	Protozoan cysts and trophozoites
10% Formalin	Formalin–ethyl acetate (FEA) concentration or direct wet mount	Helminth eggs and larvae Protozoan cysts
Sodium acetate–acetic acid–formalin (SAF)	Permanently stained smears or concentration	Permanent stain: protozoan cysts and trophozoites Concentration: helminth eggs and larvae, protozoan cysts
Merthiolate-iodine-formalin (MIF)	Concentration or direct wet mount	Helminth eggs and larvae, protozoan cysts

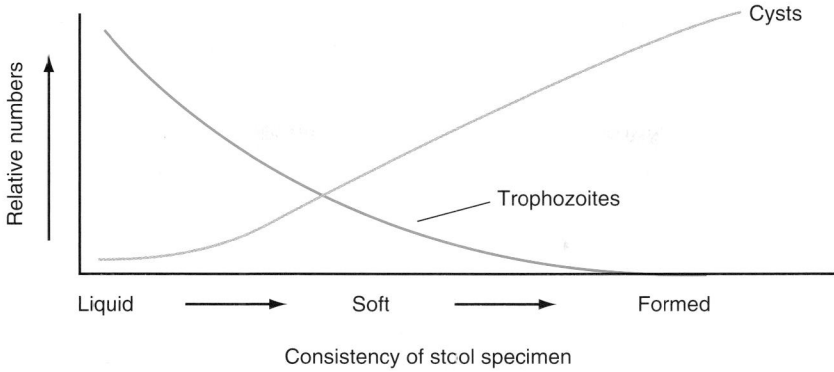

Figure 24-1

Relationship of stool consistency to protozoan stage.

Any portion of the stool that contains blood or blood-tinged mucus should be selected for wet mount preparations and be placed in preservative.

A formed stool specimen should be examined within 2 to 3 hours of passage if held at room temperature; however, examination may be delayed up to 24 hours after passage if the specimen is placed in the refrigerator. A portion of the formed stool should be placed in formalin for concentration procedures and another portion placed in PVA for permanently stained smears. The specimen should not be placed in a 37° C incubator, which will increase the rate of disintegration of organisms present and enhance overgrowth by bacteria.

MICROSCOPE EXAMINATION

Several diagnostic methods can be used in the microscopic examination of a fecal specimen:

- Direct wet mount examination (stained and unstained) of fresh stool specimens
- Concentration procedures with wet mount examination of the concentrate
- Preparation of permanently stained smears

In general, the concentration and permanent staining procedures should be performed on all specimens.

Direct wet mount The direct wet mount of unpreserved fecal material is primarily used to detect the presence of motile protozoan trophozoites in a fresh liquid or soft stool or from sigmoidoscopy material. A direct wet mount of a formalin-preserved stool specimen or a formed stool specimen may demonstrate helminth eggs or larvae and proto-zoan cysts. Because of the low diagnostic yield and labor-intensiveness of a wet mount from stool specimens, however, it has been suggested that routine use of this practice be discontinued on formed specimens.

The direct wet mount procedure uses a 3 × 2-inch glass slide on which a drop of physiologic saline (0.85%) has been placed at one end and a drop of iodine (Dobell and O'Connor solution, D'Antoni solution, or a 1:5 dilution of Lugol solution) at the other end. A small amount (2 mg) of feces is added to each drop and mixed well. Each preparation should be covered with a No. 1, 22-mm square coverslip. The preparation should be thin enough so that newsprint can be read through it and should not overflow beyond the edges of the coverslip. If the specimen has been preserved in 10% formalin, the drop of saline may be omitted from the unstained preparation.

PVA-preserved specimens are not acceptable for wet mounts, because the PVA becomes cloudy when exposed to air.

The saline preparation is useful for detection of helminth eggs or larvae and refractile protozoan cysts. Iodine emphasizes nuclear detail and glycogen masses. Stains such as buffered methylene blue have been used to enhance nuclear morphology in trophozoites but may inhibit motility and cause the organism to round up.

Reading the wet mount involves thorough examination of each coverslipped preparation at low power, starting at one corner and following a systematic vertical or horizontal pattern until the entire preparation has been examined. A high-power objective is used to identify any suspicious structures. Oil immersion should not be used on a wet preparation unless the preparation has been sealed with either clear nail polish or Vaspar (50-50 mixture of petroleum jelly and paraffin). Sealing the preparation also prevents rapid drying out and allows further examination.

Concentration techniques Concentration techniques are designed to concentrate the parasites present into a small volume of fluid and remove as much debris as possible. Either fresh or formalin–preserved stool specimens may be used. The concentrate may then be examined either unstained or stained with iodine. Protozoan trophozoites do not survive the procedure; protozoan cysts, helminth larvae, and helminth eggs are usually detected using this method.

Sedimentation and flotation methods, both of which are based on the difference in specific gravity between the parasites and the concentrating solution, are used to concentrate parasites into a small volume for easier detection. In sedimentation methods, the organisms are concentrated in sediment at the bottom of the centrifuge tube. In flotation methods, the organisms are suspended at the top of a high-density fluid. Overall, sedimentation methods concentrate a greater diversity of organisms, including cysts, larvae, and eggs.

The formalin-ether method, once the classic sedimentation procedure, has been replaced by the formalin–ethyl acetate (FEA) method to avoid the safety hazards associated with use of ether. A number of manufacturers now market self-contained fecal concentration kits. Although these kits offer disposability and a cleaner preparation owing to the filtration used, initial studies indicate that their use is more expensive and time consuming than the traditional formalin-ether technique.

The zinc sulfate method is the usual flotation procedure. Although the zinc sulfate method yields less fecal debris in the finished preparation than the FEA method, the zinc sulfate causes operculated eggs to open or collapse. It also tends to distort protozoan cysts. Infertile *Ascaris lumbricoides* eggs and *Schistosoma* sp. eggs may be missed if this procedure is used. Owing to their high density, these eggs sink to the bottom of the tube. Most organisms also tend to settle after about 30 minutes. Therefore, the examination should be made as soon as possible after the pro-

cedure has been completed to ensure optimum recovery of organisms.

Special flotation procedures, such as the Sheather sugar flotation method, have been used in detection of specific organisms such as *Cryptosporidium* sp. Although oocysts of *Cryptosporidium* sp. can be detected with either the formalin–ethyl acetate or the zinc sulfate method, Sheather flotation allows for better visibility of the oocysts because of the greater refractility of the oocyst against the background solution. Fresh or formalin-fixed feces can be used in this procedure. A new concentration method that involves laying sediment from an FEA concentration procedure over saturated sodium chloride has been described. This method increases separation of oocysts from fecal debris and enhances detection. It has particular application for oocysts of organisms such as *Cryptosporidium* spp.

Permanently stained smears Permanently stained smear preparations should be made of all stool specimens to detect and identify protozoan trophozoites and cysts. Characteristics needed for identification of the protozoa, including nuclear detail, size, and internal structures, are visible in a well-made and properly stained smear. Permanent stains commonly used include iron hematoxylin and trichrome (Wheatley modification of the Gomori stain). The stain of choice in most laboratories is the trichrome stain, because results are somewhat less dependent on technique and the procedure is less time-consuming. A trichrome stain can be performed on a smear made from a fresh stool specimen fixed in Schaudinn fixative or from one that has been preserved in PVA. Although laboratories have traditionally prepared the stain in-house, some manufacturers now provide prepared, prepackaged stains and reagents for this procedure. Specimens preserved in SAF do not stain well with trichrome and should be stained with iron hematoxylin.

To prepare a trichrome-stained smear on a fresh specimen, applicator sticks are used to smear a thin film of stool across a 1×3-inch slide, with care taken to ensure that the stool extends to the sides of the slide. The smear is placed immediately in Schaudinn fixative; it must not be allowed to dry before fixation. For PVA-fixed specimens, several drops of specimen are placed on a paper towel to drain excess fluid; the material on the paper towel is collected to prepare the smear in the same way as for a fresh specimen. This specimen is allowed to air dry thoroughly before staining.

In a well-stained trichrome smear, the cytoplasm of protozoan cysts and trophozoites stains a blue-green, although *Entamoeba coli* often takes on a purple color. Nuclear chromatin, **karyosomes, chromatoidal bars,** and red blood cells stain a dark red-purple. Eggs and larvae stain red; background debris and yeasts stain green. In an iron hematoxylin stain, the organisms stain gray-black, nuclear material stains black, and background material is light blue-gray. With either stain, poor fixation of fecal material results in poorly staining or nonstaining organisms. A number of modifications of the trichrome staining procedure have been developed to allow detection of newly identified pathogens, such as microsporidia.

Smears should be examined by first scanning for thick and thin areas using lower power of magnification (10× or 40× objective). Thin areas should be selected and observed under oil immersion (100× objective) for examination and identification of organisms. It should take approximately 10 to 15 minutes to adequately examine selected areas. Organisms that stain lightly and may be difficult to identify are *Entamoeba hartmanni, Dientamoeba fragilis, Endolimax nana, Chilomastix mesnili,* and *Giardia lamblia.*

Procedures for detection of specific parasites

CELLOPHANE TAPE PREPARATION FOR PINWORM

The life cycle of the pinworm *(Enterobius vermicularis)* includes migration of the female from the anus at night to lay eggs in the perianal area. Therefore, a fecal specimen is not the optimal specimen for detection of infection with this organism. Instead, the cellophane tape preparation is routinely used for detection of suspected pinworm infections. This procedure involves swabbing the child's perianal area with a tongue blade covered with cellophane tape (sticky side out). The sampling should take place first thing in the morning, before the child uses the bathroom or is bathed. After the sample has been taken, the sticky side of the tape is placed on a microscope slide and scanned at low- and high-power fields of magnification for the characteristically shaped eggs. Commercial kits are now available to reduce manipulation of the specimen by caregivers.

MODIFIED ACID-FAST PROCEDURE FOR *CRYPTOSPORIDIUM* SP.

Use of a Kinyoun modified acid-fast stain enhances detection of oocysts of *Cryptosporidium parvum, Isospora belli,* and *Cyclospora cayetanensis.* With this procedure, the oocysts appear as magenta-stained organisms against a blue background. The use of a stain combining iron hematoxylin with carbol fuchsin for simultaneous staining of *Isospora* sp., *Cryptosporidium* sp., and protozoa has been reported.

STAINS FOR *PNEUMOCYSTIS CARINII*

Stains that are used in identification of *Pneumocystis carinii* include Gomori methenamine silver and Giemsa stains. The silver stain is used to identify cysts of the organism, which appear as black, rounded or punched-in balls against a greenish background. The Giemsa stain demonstrates the trophozoites and intracystic bodies within the cyst, but the outside wall of the cyst will not stain. Nonspecific fluorescent stains, such as calcofluor white, can also be used. This type of stain detects any organism that contains chitin in its cell wall. Fungi and yeast *Pneumocystis carinii* will fluoresce with a blue-white color when stained and viewed under ultraviolet (UV) light.

Other Specimens Examined for Intestinal Parasites

Duodenal aspirates

Material obtained from the Enterotest (HDC Corp., San Jose, Calif.) or from duodenal aspirates may be submitted in cases of suspected giardiasis or strongyloidiasis when clinical symptoms are suggestive but routine stool examination results are negative. This material may be examined by direct wet mount for trophozoites or may be placed in PVA for preparation of permanently stained smears. Eggs of *Fasciola hepatica* or *Opisthorchis sinensis,* as well as oocysts of *Cryptosporidium* spp. or *I. belli,* may also occasionally be recovered.

Sigmoidoscopy specimens

Scrapings or aspirates obtained by sigmoidoscopy may be used to diagnose amebiasis or cryptosporidiosis. These specimens are examined immediately for motile trophozoites, and a portion of the sample is placed in PVA fixative so that permanently stained smears can be prepared for examination.

Urine, vaginal, or urethral specimens

Eggs of *Schistosoma haematobium,* eggs of *E. vermicularis,* and trophozoites of *Trichomonas vaginalis* can be detected in the sediment of a urine specimen. *T. vaginalis* can also be detected in a wet mount of vaginal or urethral discharge. A plastic envelop method for culturing *T. vaginalis* has been developed. Dry ingredients in the culture bag are rehydrated, the specimen is added, and growth of the organism can be observed within 3 days.

Sputum

In cases of *Strongyloides stercoralis* hyperinfection, the filariform larvae may be seen in a direct wet mount of sputum. Eggs of the lung fluke *Paragonimus westermani* can also be identified in a sputum wet mount. If the patient is suspected of having a pulmonary abscess caused by *Entamoeba histolytica,* the sputum specimen should be examined as a permanently stained smear.

Examination of Specimens for Blood and Tissue Parasites

Blood smears

Examination of a blood smear stained with Giemsa or Wright stain is the most common method of detecting malaria, *Babesia* sp., *Trypanosoma* spp., and some species of microfilaria. Although motile organisms such as *Trypanosoma* spp. and microfilariae can be detected on a wet preparation of a fresh blood specimen under low- and high-power magnification, identification is made on the basis of characteristics seen on a permanently stained smear. Concentration methods using membrane filters can be used to detect *Trypanosoma* sp. or microfilariae but are rarely performed in the clinical laboratory. Tissue parasites such as *Trichinella spiralis, Leishmania* spp., *P. carinii,* and *Toxoplasma gondii* can be identified by examination of tissue biopsy or by serologic methods.

COLLECTION AND PREPARATION OF THE BLOOD SPECIMEN

Blood taken directly from a finger stick should be used for a malarial smear because it tends to give the best staining characteristics. Blood collected in ethylenediaminetetraacetic acid (EDTA) gives adequate staining if processed within 1 hour. With Giemsa stain, the cytoplasm of the parasite stains bluish and the chromatin red to purple-red. If malarial stippling is present, it appears as discrete pink-red dots. Giemsa staining gives the best morphologic detail but is a time-consuming procedure. Wright stain has a shorter staining period, but the color intensity for differentiation of parasites is not as good as that with Giemsa stain.

PROCEDURE FOR IDENTIFICATION OF THE ORGANISM

For suspected cases of blood parasites, both a thick film and a thin film should be made. Both preparations can be made on the same slide or on separate slides. Because the two preparations are treated differently before staining, however, use of two slides is more efficient. Giemsa stain provides the best staining of the organisms and should be used on both thick and thin films. Wright stain cannot be used for a thick film because the methanol content will fix red cells.

A thick film is best for detection of parasites, because organisms are concentrated in a relatively small area. The thick film is made by pooling several drops of blood on the slide and then spreading it into a 1.5-cm area. A too thick film peels from the slide; thickness is optimal when newsprint is barely visible through the drop of blood before it dries. The blood should be allowed to dry for at least 6 hours before staining. It should not be fixed with methanol before staining; fixing prevents hemoglobin from being released from the red cell. Use of Giemsa stain automatically lakes hemoglobin from unfixed red cells. Initial scanning of the stained smear at 10× detects microfilariae. At least 100 oil immersion fields should be examined before a negative result is reported.

Species identification should be made from a thin film, because the characteristics of the parasite and the red blood cells can be seen. The thin film is made in the same way as that for a differential count. It should be fixed in methanol for 1 minute and air dried before staining with Giemsa stain. The entire smear should be scanned at 10× for detection of large organisms such as microfilariae; then at least 100 oil immersion fields must be examined for the presence of organisms such as *Trypanosoma* sp. or for intracellular organisms such as *Plasmodium* sp. or *Babesia* sp. For a symptomatic patient, several blood smears from samples collected at approximately 6-hour intervals over 36 to 48 hours should be examined before a final negative diagnosis is made.

Biopsy specimens

Biopsy specimens are usually needed to diagnose infections with *Leishmania* spp. because the organisms are intracellular. Depending on the species present, the amastigote stage can be detected in tissues such as skin, liver, spleen, and bone marrow. Cutaneous lesions should be sampled below the edges of the ulcer; surface samples do not yield infected cells.

Cerebrospinal fluid

Viable organisms in suspected cases of amebic meningitis or sleeping sickness can occasionally be seen in a cerebrospinal fluid (CSF) specimen. The trypomastigote is visible because of the motion of the flagellum and undulating membrane. It requires a skillful microscopist, however, to discern amebic motility in a field of neutrophils. If amebic meningoencephalitis caused by *Naegleria fowleri* is suspected, the CSF can be cultured. Nonnutrient agar is seeded with an *Escherichia coli* overlay, and the spinal fluid sediment is inoculated onto the media. The specimen is sealed and incubated at 35° C. The medium is examined daily for thin tracks in the bacterial growth, which indicate that amebae have been feeding on the bacteria.

Immunologic Diagnosis

Parasites that invade tissue are the primary organisms that stimulate antibody production. Many serologic tests are useful if invasive methods cannot be used for identification. In most cases, however, tests for antibody serve only as epidemiologic markers. Current tests detect antibody that may persist after acute infection and are not useful in endemic areas. They may, however, be useful for diagnosis in a person who has traveled to an endemic area and is now symptomatic. Another disadvantage of antibody tests is that they may have a large number of cross-reactions, which limit their diagnostic usefulness. In addition, serologic tests used by reference laboratories such as the Centers for Disease Control and Prevention (CDC) are not commercially available. Immunoassay or fluorescent antibody tests for antibodies to *T. gondii* or *E. histolytica* (extraintestinal infections) are available for use in clinical laboratories. In contrast, tests for parasitic antigens provide information about current infection.

The parameters that should be considered by a laboratory in selecting methods to be used include not only cost but also diagnostic yield, patient population, relative incidence of the parasite in the area, and number of specimens to be processed.

Enzyme immunoassay

Enzyme immunoassay (EIA) methods for the detection of antibody to intestinal parasites are rarely used in the clinical laboratory because of the difficulty in obtaining antigen, cross-reactivity of antibodies, and poor sensitivity and specificity. The major use of the enzyme immunoassay has been to detect antigens from specific parasites. Giardiasis is often difficult to detect because the cysts are shed irregularly. Enzyme immunoassays to detect the presence of *Giardia*-specific antigen in stool and adhesion proteins of *E. histolytica* are available. Tests using monoclonal antibody to detect both *Giardia* and *Cryptosporidium* organisms are also available.

Fluorescent antibody techniques

Fluorescent antibody (FA) techniques using monoclonal antibodies have been developed to detect *Cryptosporidium* oocysts in fecal specimens. These methods are more expensive than the modified acid-fast procedure but demonstrate greater sensitivity, especially when only rare oocysts are present. An FA combination reagent for *G. lamblia* and *Cryptosporidium* antigens has been developed. The monoclonal antibodies eliminate false-positive and false-negative results. Such procedures are useful in screening large numbers of specimens during epidemiologic studies. Fluorescent antibody techniques for *P. carinii* are also available.

Quality Assurance in the Parasitology Laboratory

Quality assurance procedures in the parasitology laboratory are similar to those in other sections of the laboratory. An updated procedure manual, controls for staining procedures, records of centrifuge calibration, ocular micrometer calibration, and re-

---

PROCEDURE 24-1. Calibration of the Ocular Micrometer

1. Insert the ocular micrometer in the eyepiece of the microscope so that the zero of the scale is on the left side. The etched side of the micrometer should be facing you.

2. Place the calibrated stage micrometer on the stage and focus on low power (10×).

3. While using low power, align the left-hand zero of the stage micrometer with the left-hand zero of the ocular micrometer. Do not move the stage micrometer after this point.

4. Scan the two scales until a division line on the ocular micrometer directly aligns with a division line on the stage micrometer.

5. Count the number of stage units and ocular units at this point. Divide the number of stage units by the number of ocular units, and multiply the result by 1000. This gives the value (in micrometers) for one ocular unit on low power.

6. Repeat the procedure at high power and with oil immersion to get the value of one ocular unit at each of those magnifications.

To calculate the size of an organism, count the number of ocular units, multiply by the value for an ocular unit at that magnification, and report the value in micrometers.

---

frigerator and incubator temperatures should be available. Reagents and solutions should be properly labeled.

In addition, the parasitology laboratory should have the following:

- A textbook collection, including reference texts and atlases
- A set of 2 × 2 Kodachrome slides of common parasites
- A set of clinical reference specimens, including permanently stained smears and formalin-preserved feces

The department should also be enrolled in an external proficiency testing program. An ongoing internal proficiency testing program should be used to enhance identification skills of the technologists, especially if a full-time parasitologist is not employed. It has been shown that approximately twice as many parasites are detected when a single technologist staffs the parasitology department as when technologists rotate through the department.

Ocular micrometer

Size is an important diagnostic criterion for parasites, and use of a properly calibrated ocular micrometer ensures accurate measurement of or-

ganisms. The micrometer should be calibrated for each objective on the microscope.

The micrometer consists of two separate parts: the stage micrometer, a 0.1-mm line, which is ruled in 0.01-mm units, and the ocular micrometer, which is ruled in 100 units but has no value assigned to the units. Values for each ocular unit can be calculated by using the stage micrometer according to Procedure 24-1.

MEDICALLY IMPORTANT PARASITIC AGENTS

Medically important parasites can be found in phyla representing single-celled organisms such as the protozoa and complex, multicelled organisms such as tapeworms and roundworms. Table 24-2 lists the characteristics of the classes in which most medically important human parasites are found; they are described in the remainder of this chapter.

Protozoa

Intestinal amebae

In general amebae present the most difficult challenge with regard to identification. Their average size range is smaller than that of most other parasitic organisms, and they must be distinguished from artifacts and cells that appear in the clinical specimen. The intestinal amebae discussed in this section are:

- *Entamoeba histolytica*
- *Entamoeba dispar*
- *Entamoeba hartmanni*
- *Entamoeba coli*

TABLE 24-2
Characteristics of Phyla of Medically Important Parasites

Organisms	Characteristics
Phylum: Sarcomastigophora	
Subphylum: Sarcodina (ameba)	Single celled
	Move by pseudopodia
	Trophozoite and cyst stages
	Asexual reproduction
Subphylum: Mastigophora (flagellates)	Single celled
	Most move by action of flagella
	Trophozoite and cyst stages for intestinal organisms
	Asexual reproduction
	Some blood flagellates
Phylum: Ciliaphora (ciliates)	Single celled
	Move by action of cilia
	Trophozoite and cyst stages
	Asexual reproduction
Phylum: Apicomplexa (sporozoa)	Single celled
	Usually inhabit tissue and blood cells
	Insects and other mammals are involved as part of life cycle
	May have both sexual and asexual life cycles
Phylum: Platyhelminthes (flatworms)	
Class: Trematoda (flukes)	Multicelled and bilaterally symmetric
	Most are hermaphroditic
	Egg, miracidium, cercaria, and adult are life cycle stages
	Fish, snails, crabs are involved as intermediate hosts in life cycle
Class: Cestoda (tapeworms)	Multicellular, ribbonlike body
	Hermaphroditic
	Egg, larva, and adult worm are life cycle stages
	Mammals and insects are involved as intermediate hosts in life cycle
Phylum: Aschelminthes	
Class: Nematoda (roundworms)	Adults of both sexes
	Egg, larva, and adult worm are life cycle stages
	May have free-living form or may require intermediate host

- *Endolimax nana*
- *Iodamoeba bütschlii*

Entamoeba histolytica is recognized as a true **pathogen;** the remainder of the organisms listed are considered **nonpathogens.** *Entamoeba polecki,* which is rarely isolated in the United States, is not discussed. The organism *Blastocystis hominis* is included in this section, although it is not recognized as a true ameba.

GENERAL CHARACTERISTICS OF AMEBAE
Species identification, whether in the cyst or trophozoite stage, often rests on the following characteristics: size, number of nuclei, nuclear structure, and presence of specific internal structures. In a wet preparation, the motility of the trophozoite may aid in presumptive identification. Overall, however, the permanently stained smear is the best preparation for identification of the amebae.

All the organisms discussed live in the large intestine. With the possible exception of *B. hominis,* all possess both a trophozoite stage and a cyst stage. The **trophozoite** is the motile, feeding stage that reproduces by binary fission. The **cyst** is a resistant stage that is infective for humans. Multiplication of nuclei in the cyst stage also serves a reproductive function.

TREATMENT
Treatment is given only for *E. histolytica* infections; treatment for nonpathogens is not usually indicated. Luminal amebicides such as metronidazole are given to carriers in nonendemic areas to prevent the invasive phase and to reduce the risk of transmission. In endemic areas with a high risk of reinfection, treatment may not be indicated. Patients with invasive amebiases are treated with systemic drugs as well as luminal amebicides.

LIFE CYCLE
The life cycle of amebae is relatively simple, with no **intermediate hosts** and direct fecal-oral transmission in food or water via the cyst stage. Humans ingest the infective cyst, and organisms excyst in the intestinal tract and multiply by binary fission. Trophozoites colonize the cecal area. Figure 24-2 illustrates a generalized life cycle for amebae, as well as the extraintestinal phase of *E. histolytica.*

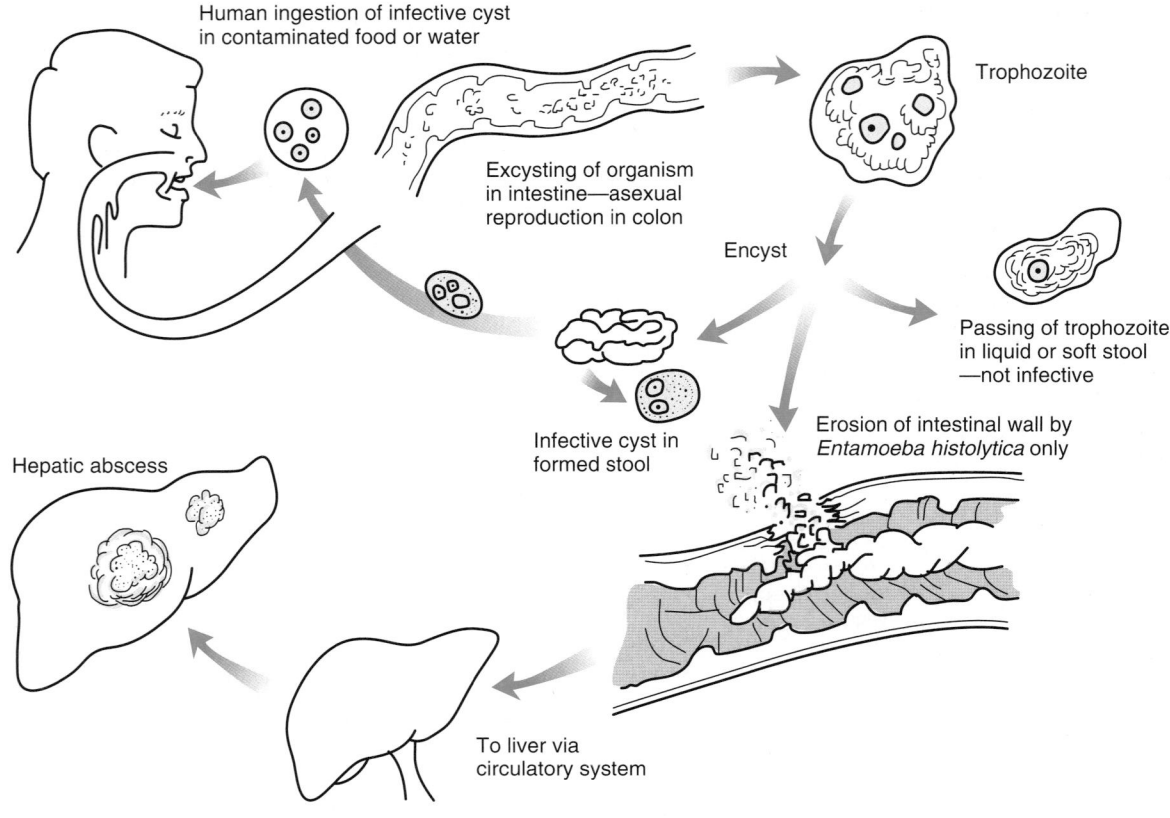

Human ingestion of infective cyst
in contaminated food or water

Trophozoite

Excysting of organism
in intestine—asexual
reproduction in colon

Encyst

Passing of trophozoite
in liquid or soft stool
—not infective

Infective cyst in
formed stool

Erosion of intestinal wall by
Entamoeba histolytica only

Hepatic abscess

To liver via
circulatory system

Figure 24-2

Generalized life cycle of intestinal amoeba.

ENTAMOEBA HISTOLYTICA
Entamoeba histolytica is found worldwide but especially in the tropics and subtropics. It is the major amebic pathogen for human beings and ranks third behind malaria and schistosomiasis as a cause of death, accounting for an estimated 40,000 to 100,000 deaths per year. The prevalence varies according to socioeconomic levels and sanitary practices; infection is more common in poorly developed areas or crowded institutions. The organism has also been identified as a sexually transmitted agent in the homosexual population.
Clinical infection The **pathogenicity** of *E. histolytica* is reflected in its ability to cause invasive intestinal amebiasis and extraintestinal amebic infections. The mechanism of invasion consists of the following steps:

▪ Adherence to the mucous layer of the intestine, which is mediated by an adherence lectin (*N*-acetyl *D*-galactosamine)

▪ Disruption of the intestinal barrier by secretion of proteolytic enzymes
▪ Invasion of the epithelial cells
▪ Lysis of intestinal epithelial cells

The organism also demonstrates resistance to host immune defense mechanisms, including phagocytosis and complement-mediated cell lysis.

Individuals infected with *E. histolytica* may be asymptomatic, but this generally occurs when only the lumen of the intestine is colonized. A symptomatic clinical infection may appear as an acute or chronic form. In acute infections the patient may experience vague abdominal symptoms such as tenderness, cramping, fever, and up to 20 diarrheic stools per day that contain the trophozoite form, blood, and mucus. In severe cases the patient may shed pieces of intestinal mucosa.

In chronic infections, on the other hand, the patient usually is asymptomatic. The cyst form is passed, hence these patients are referred to as cyst passers, although the trophozoite may be passed in the stool during diarrheal episodes.

The characteristic lesion in the intestinal mucosa, referred to as the "flask-shaped" ulcer of *E. histolytica,* is a result of lysis of the intestinal mucosa. The lesion shows a pinpoint ulceration on the mucosal surface and a gradual widening in the submucosal areas as the parasite invades the tissue. The organism may completely erode the intestinal mucosa and enter the circulation. When this occurs, the organ most commonly colonized is the right lobe of the liver, because organisms are trapped in the venules of the liver.

Some patients with *E. histolytica* develop an ameboma (amebic granuloma), a tumorlike lesion that forms in the submucosa of the intestine. This represents an area of chronic lysis and infiltration with neutrophils, lymphocytes, and eosinophils.

Patients with hepatic abscesses may have symptoms such as fever and pain in the upper right quadrant or may be asymptomatic. Fever, weight loss, increased white blood cell counts or elevated liver enzymes may be present.

Lung abscesses may be seen as the result of penetration of the diaphragm by amebae from hepatic abscesses or from hematogenous spread. Invasion of the lung may cause the patient to have chest pain, dyspnea, and a productive cough.

Other sites, such as the perianal area or bladder, also may be colonized, with resulting tissue destruction.

In recent years the pathogenicity of *E. histolytica* and its ability to cause extraintestinal infections have been investigated. Recent studies using electrophoretic isoenzyme patterns show that pathogenic strains differ from noninvasive strains. Zymodemes of pathogenic and nonpathogenic *E. histolytica* have been identified. Initial studies show that strains in cyst passers and in most homosexual patients are nonpathogenic, whereas several strains from areas with high rates of endemic disease are pathogenic. These zymodeme studies have led to identification of *Entamoeba dispar* (formerly known as nonpathogenic *E. histolytica*), a newly named species that is discussed at the end of the section.

Laboratory diagnosis Patients with diarrhea are most likely to have trophozoites in the stool specimen, which may be seen in wet mounts or trichrome-stained smears. Sigmoid biopsies may be used to demonstrate the characteristic morphology of the intestinal ulcers or to identify trophozoites in tissue when none can be isolated from the stool specimen.

Characteristics of the trophozoite. Table 24-3 summarizes the characteristics of the *E. histolytica* trophozoite and cyst and compares *E. histolytica* with other amebae. In a direct saline wet mount of a *diarrheic stool,* the trophozoite of *E. histolytica* may exhibit a progressive, directional motility by extending long, thin pseudopods. The size of the organism ranges from 10 to 50 μm, averaging 15 to 25 μm. The organism is refractile, and the characteristic bull's-eye nucleus, consisting of a small central karyosome and even, fine **peripheral chromatin,** may be only slightly visible. In a trichrome-stained smear, the cytoplasm of the organism appears clean and free of ingested bacteria and vacuoles. Finely granular nuclear chromatin, which is evenly distributed on the nuclear membrane, and the small central karyosome stain a dark purple-red. Ingested red cells are diagnostic for *E. histolytica* trophozoites but may not be seen in all organisms. Figure 24-3 shows trichrome-stained trophozoites of *E. histolytica,* with the trophozoite in Figure 24-3, *B* demonstrating an ingested red blood cell.

Characteristics of the cyst. The average size of the cyst is 10 to 20 μm (Figure 24-4). Cysts of the organism may have one to four nuclei each with a small central karyosome and fine, evenly distributed peripheral chromatin. The cytoplasm may contain cigar-shaped chromatoidal bars with rounded ends. These bars are composed of ribonucleic acid. In an iodine wet mount, the nuclei appear as yellowish refractile bodies within the cyst; chromatoidal bars do not take up stain and appear as colorless areas. With trichrome stain, the cyst is light green-gray; nuclear material and chromatoidal bars stain a dark purple-red. Young cysts may show discrete glycogen masses that stain light brown in an iodine wet mount, but in the more mature cyst, the glycogen is diffuse. Cysts may be killed by drying, temperatures over 55° C, superchlorination, or addition of iodine to drinking water.

Amebic ulcers of the liver often are detected by ultrasonographic or radiographic tests. Subsequent aspiration of the abscess may yield motile trophozoites and necrotic material composed of lysed

TABLE 24-3
Comparison of Amebae

Organism	Trophozoite				Cyst				
	Size (μm)	Motility	Cytoplasm	Trophozoite and Cyst Nuclear Structure	Size (μm) and Shape	Number of Nuclei in Mature Cyst	Chromatoidal Bars	Glycogen Vacuole	
Entamoeba histolytica	15-25	Progressive, directional	Finely granular May contain ingested red blood cells	Small, central karyosome Fine, evenly distributed peripheral chromatin	10-20, round	4	Rounded Elongated Usually seen	Not usually seen Diffuse in young cyst	
Entamoeba coli	15-50	Nondirectional	Vacuolated Ingested bacteria	Large, eccentric karyosomes Coarse, uneven peripheral chromatin	15-25, round	8	Elongated Splintered ends Not always seen	Not seen	
Entamoeba hartmanni	4-12	Nondirectional	Finely granular	Small, central karyosomes Fine, evenly distributed peripheral chromatin	5-10, round	4	Rounded ends Elongated Not always present	Not seen	
Endolimax nana	5-12	Nondirectional	Vacuolated May contain ingested bacteria	Large, irregularly shaped karyosome No peripheral chromatin	5-12, oval	4	Not present	Not seen	
Iodamoeba bütschlii	6-20	Nondirectional	Vacuolated May contain ingested bacteria	Large karyosome surrounded by achromatic granules No peripheral chromatin	6-15, oval or irregular	1	Not present	Single, defined	

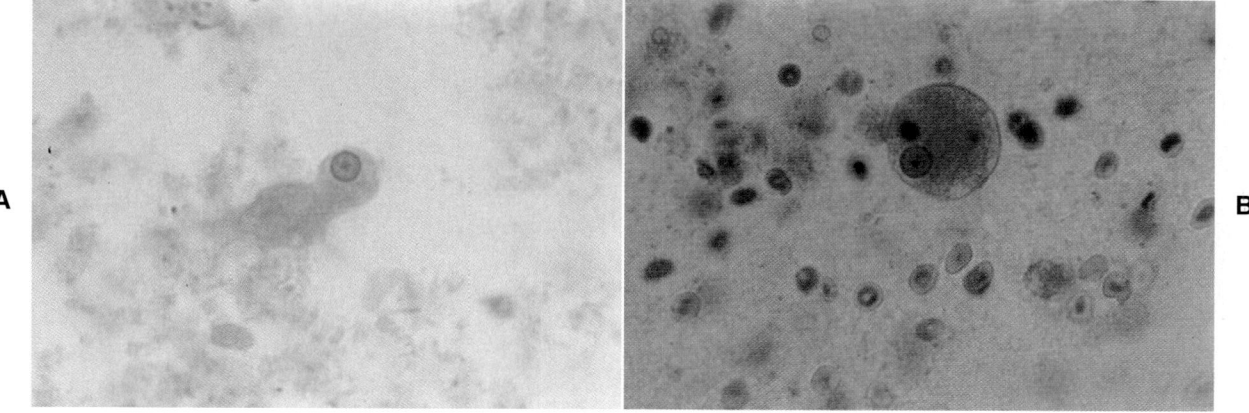

Figure 24-3

A, *Entamoeba histolytica* trophozoite (trichrome stain). **B,** *E. histolytica* trophozoite. Notice darkly staining, ingested red blood cell near nucleus (trichrome stain).

cells. Serologic methods of detecting antibody to *E. histolytica* are available, and the results are positive in more than 90% of patients with extraintestinal disease. These antibody levels rise after tissue invasion but are not protective. Tests for antibody, however, are not particularly useful in distinguishing between past and current infection, because antibodies may persist for years after an infection has cleared up. In addition, these tests provide limited information in patients from endemic areas. Tests that detect *E. histolytica* antigen in stool provide evidence of current infection. These tests involve enzyme-linked immunosorbent assay (ELISA) methodology using monoclonal antibodies to proteins or adhesion lectins, and they can be used in a clinical laboratory to distinguish infection by *E. histolytica* from that caused by *E. dispar.*

ENTAMOEBA DISPAR
As was mentioned previously, a large number of people have been infected with an organism that was identified morphologically as *E. histolytica*. However, only about 10% of these individuals developed clinical symptoms or invasive disease. The initial clinical studies provided evidence to explain this discrepancy by identifying differing zymodeme patterns. Further immunologic and DNA probe studies supplied additional evidence, such as differences in epitopes of the galactose-specific binding lectin and differences in surface antigens. Based on this evidence, the noninvasive organism, for-

merly referred to as nonpathogenic *E. histolytica,* has been named *Entamoeba dispar.* The pathogenic organism still is identified as *E. histolytica.*

ENTAMOEBA HARTMANNI
Entamoeba hartmanni, once known as "small race" *Entamoeba histolytica,* is a nonpathogen. It generally resembles *E. histolytica* in a trichrome-stained smear but is more likely to have an eccentric karyosome or uneven peripheral chromatin resembling that of *Entamoeba coli.* Size is a major determinant in differentiating *E. histolytica* and *E. hartmanni.* The average size of the trophozoites

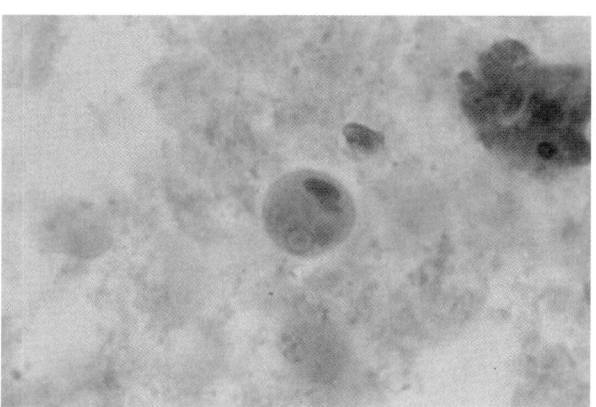

Figure 24-4

Entamoeba histolytica cyst with round-end chromatoidal bars. Two nuclei are visible (trichrome stain).

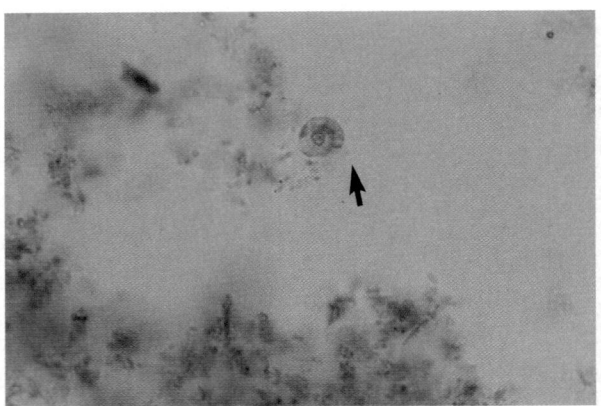

Figure 24-5 _____

Entamoeba hartmanni trophozoite (trichrome stain).

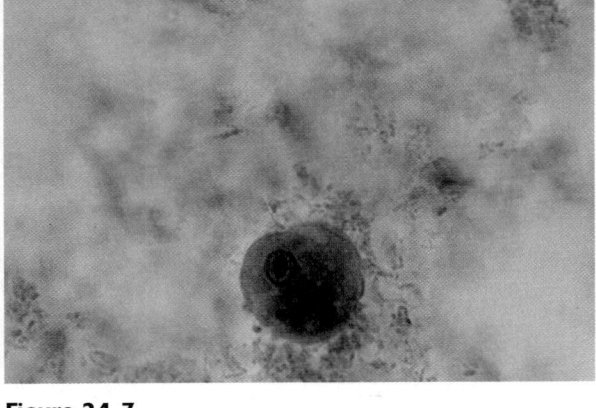

Figure 24-7 _____

Entamoeba coli trophozoite. Notice dark staining, highly vacuolated cytoplasm (trichrome stain).

of *E. hartmanni* is 4 to 12 μm; trophozoites with an average size measuring greater than 12 μm are identified as *E. histolytica*. *E. hartmanni* cysts measure 5 to 10 μm; those of 10 μm or more are identified as *E. histolytica*. Figure 24-5 shows the trichrome-stained trophozoite, and Figure 24-6 shows the cyst of *E. hartmanni* with three nuclei visible.

ENTAMOEBA COLI

Entamoeba coli is a commonly found intestinal commensal transmitted by ingestion of cysts in fecally contaminated food or water. The average size of the trophozoite is 15 to 50 μm with most measuring 25 μm (Figure 24-7). The nuclear structure is characterized by a large, eccentrically placed karyosome and coarse, uneven peripheral chromatin on the nuclear membrane. The motility of the trophozoite in a wet preparation is sluggish and nondirectional. In a permanently stained preparation, the cytoplasm of the trophozoite may stain a purplish gray; it contains vacuoles and ingested materials.

The mature cyst has eight nuclei; the immature cyst may have one or two large nuclei with a large glycogen vacuole. Chromatoidal bars, when present, have a pointed, splintered appearance. The average size of the cyst is 15 to 25 μm. Figure 24-8, *A*, shows a Merthiolate-iodine-formalin (MIF) wet mount of a cyst of *E. coli*, and 24-8, *B*, shows a trichrome-stained cyst.

ENDOLIMAX NANA

The trophozoite of *Endolimax nana* has a large karyosome with no peripheral chromatin on the nuclear membrane. The trophozoite ranges in size from 5 to 12 μm with the average being less than 10 μm (Figure 24-9). The cytoplasm is granular and vacuolated. In a wet preparation, the motility is sluggish. In a wet mount it may be difficult to distinguish the large karyosome of *E. nana* from the karyosome of *E. hartmanni*, and the organisms may be misidentified. The cyst of *E. nana* is oval or spherical, 5 to 12 μm, and has up to four large karyosomes (Figure 24-10).

IODAMOEBA BÜTSCHLII

Iodamoeba bütschlii is less commonly encountered than *E. coli* or *E. nana*. The nucleus is composed of a single, irregularly shaped karyosome sur-

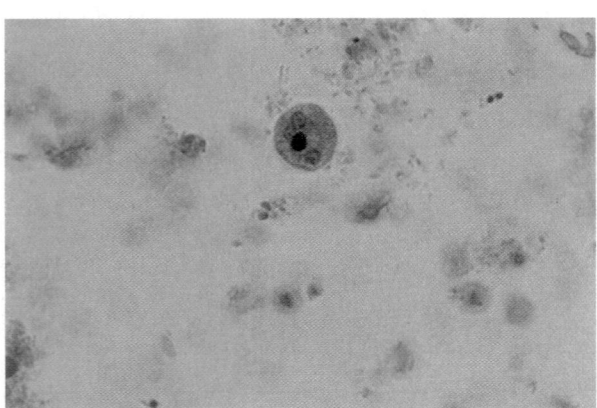

Figure 24-6 _____

Entamoeba hartmanni cyst (trichrome stain).

Figure 24-8 _____

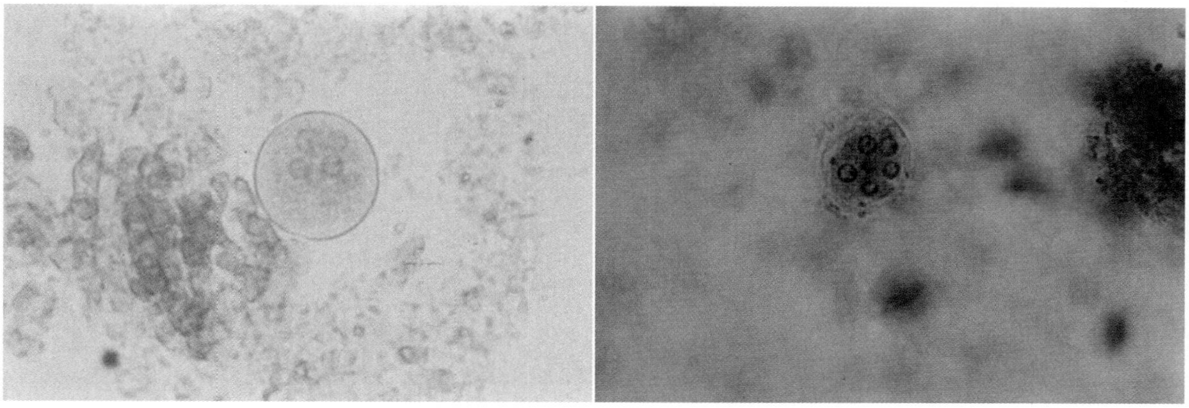

A, *Entamoeba coli* cyst (Merthiolate-iodine-formalin [MIF]) wet mount. **B,** *E. coli* cyst with five nuclei visible (trichrome stain).

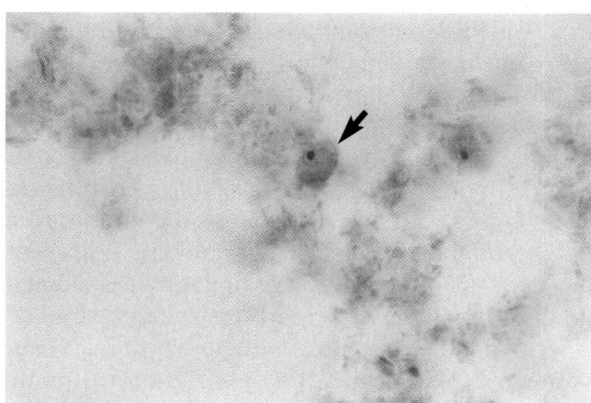

Figure 24-9 _____

Endolimax nana trophozoite (trichrome stain).

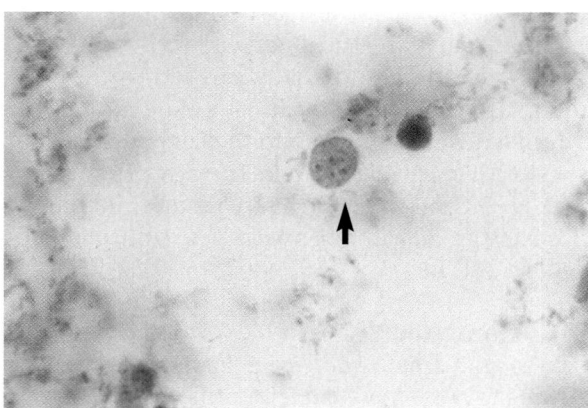

Figure 24-10 _____

Endolimax nana cyst (trichrome stain).

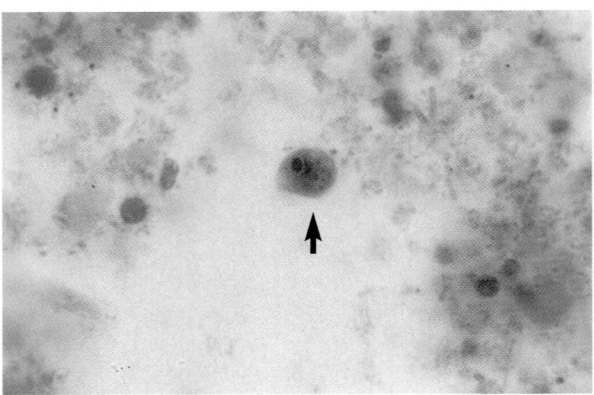

Figure 24-11
Iodamoeba butschlii trophozoite (trichrome stain).

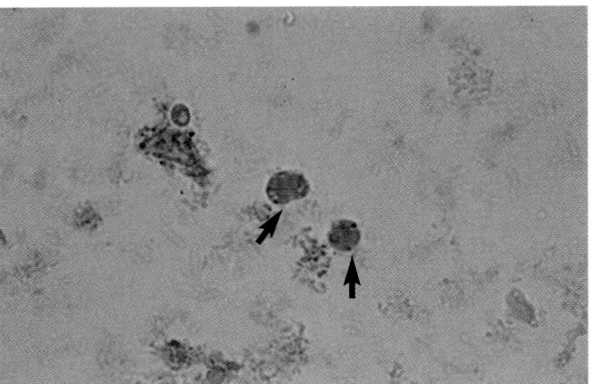

Figure 24-13
Blastocystis hominis spherical form (trichrome stain).

rounded by achromatic granules and a thin nuclear membrane with no peripheral chromatin. The trophozoites of *I. bütschlii,* which are 6 to 20 μm, show a vacuolated cytoplasm in a permanently stained smear (Figure 24-11). The oval cyst is 6 to 15 μm (average 9 to 10 μm) and contains a single large karyosome and a large, well-defined glycogen vacuole. The vacuole stains dark brown in an iodine wet mount and appears empty in a permanently stained smear. Figure 24-12 demonstrates a trichrome-stained cyst of *I. bütschlii.*

BLASTOCYSTIS HOMINIS
Blastocystis hominis, a protozoan once thought to be a yeast, also has come to prominence as a pos-

sible cause of diarrhea in humans, although controversy concerning its pathogenicity still exists. Not considered a common cause of diarrheal disease, this organism nevertheless has been found in patients with diarrhea who have no other intestinal pathogens. These patients often have a history of travel abroad. Some authors suggest that *B. hominis* has no role as a pathogen, but others suggest that the organism be considered a pathogen in symptomatic patients if it is present in a count of more than 5 per high-power field and no other known enteric pathogens can be found.

The organism exists in ameboid, granular, and spherical forms, with the spherical form being most commonly identified. *B. hominis* has no identifiable cyst stage. The average size for the spherical form is 5 to 15 μm, but up to 20% of organisms are smaller than 5 μm. The organism has a layer of cytoplasm lining the inner wall with as many as four nuclei present, usually pushed to the side, and a large central body. In an iodine mount, the cytoplasm stains brown and the central area does not stain. On trichrome stain, the cytoplasm stains dark green and the central area may stain pale to intensely green with the nuclei a dark purple-black (Figure 24-13).

Tissue amebae
Two organisms, *Naegleria fowleri* and *Acanthamoeba* spp., have been identified as the organisms most commonly associated with tissue invasion in humans. The ameboflagellate *N. fowleri* is the etiologic agent of primary amebic menin-

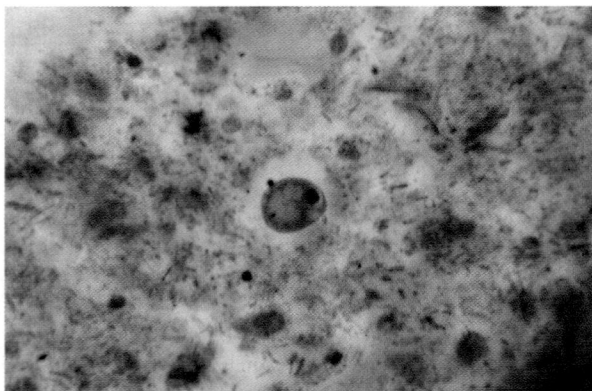

Figure 24-12
Iodamoeba bütschlii cyst with prominent glycogen vacuole (trichrome stain).

goencephalitis, a rapidly fatal condition involving the central nervous system. *Acanthamoeba* spp. have been associated with a more chronic condition, granulomatous amebic encephalitis, and with amebic keratitis. A comparison of the central nervous system (CNS) infections caused by tissue amebae is given in Table 24-4.

NAEGLERIA FOWLERI
Primary amebic meningoencephalitis (PAM) has been reported from countries all over the world. It occurs in children and young adults with no predisposing condition. A common factor is the report of recent swimming or other water-related activities in warm, artificial lakes or brackish or muddy water. The life cycle of *N. fowleri* is relatively simple, consisting of three stages: a free-living amebic trophozoite, a transient flagellate form, and an environmentally resistant cyst.

The organism enters the nasal cavity, colonizes in the amebic form within the nasal cavity, penetrates the cribriform plate, moves along the olfactory nerve, and invades the central nervous system. **Clinical infection** The incubation period is usually 2 to 3 days but may range up to 2 weeks. Clinically, the disease cannot be distinguished from bacterial meningoencephalitis. Initial symptoms include severe bifrontal headache, fever, stiff neck, and nausea and vomiting. The organism multiplies within brain tissue, and within 2 to 4 days, the patient may suffer drowsiness, confusion, and seizures, and progress into a coma. The disease

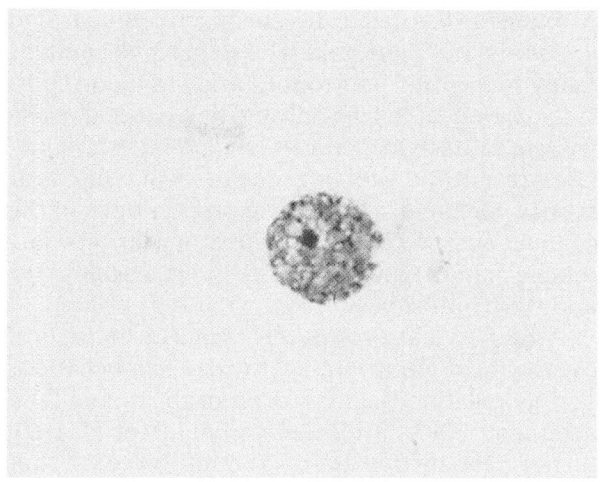

Figure 24-14
Naegleria fowleri trophozoite (Wright's stain).

usually is fatal within 1 week of the appearance of clinical symptoms. The possibility of cure depends on early diagnosis. Aggressive therapy with intravenous and intrathecal amphotericin B has been used. Rifampin, miconazole, and tetracycline have been used in addition to amphotericin B.
Laboratory diagnosis Diagnosis can be made by finding motile trophozoites in the spinal fluid. The trophozoite is 10 to 12 μm and moves by extending large, broad pseudopods. The nucleus contains a large central karyosome that may be surrounded by a halo. Figure 24-14 shows a trophozoite of

TABLE 24-4
Comparison of Central Nervous System Infections Caused by Amebae

	Primary Amebic Meningoencephalitis	Granulomatous Amebic Encephalitis
Etiologic agent	*Naegleria fowleri*	*Acanthamoeba* spp.
Stages in		
Cerebrospinal fluid	Trophozoite	Trophozoite
Brain biopsy	Trophozoite	Trophozoite and cyst
Characteristics	Trophozoite 10-12 μm	Trophozoite 10-45 μm
	Large karyosome	Spinelike pseudopod
	Broad pseudopods	Cyst
		15-20 μm
		Wrinkled double wall
Entry	Nasal passage olfactory nerve to central nervous system (CNS)	Lungs and skin with hematogenous spread to CNS
Clinical course	Fulminant (death within 1 week of onset)	Slow and chronic
Population at risk	Children to young adults, healthy (history of water activities in stagnant, warm water)	Immunocompromised

N. fowleri as it appears in a specimen of spinal fluid stained with Wright stain. The spinal fluid contains many segmented neutrophils and red blood cells; it also has elevated protein and decreased glucose values. Cysts, which are 10 μm and have a round, smooth double wall, are not seen in clinical or biopsy specimens. Histologic preparations of the brain at autopsy show inflammatory lesions containing many segmented neutrophils, eosinophils, and the trophozoites.

A method that isolates this organism consists of overlaying nonnutrient agar with *Escherichia coli* and inoculating it with a drop of the spinal fluid sediment. Plates are examined daily for clearing of the agar in thin tracks, which indicate that trophozoites have fed on the bacteria. The trophozoite stage can be converted to the flagellate stage by adding one drop of spinal fluid sediment to 1 ml of distilled water and incubating at 37° C. Conversion to the flagellate form occurs in 2 to 20 hours.

ACANTHAMOEBA SPP.

Acanthamoeba spp., also soil and water organisms, cause granulomatous amebic encephalitis (GAE), which occurs primarily in immunosuppressed or debilitated patients. Unlike PAM, this condition is characterized by hematogenous spread to the central nervous system from a primary inoculation site in either the lungs or the skin. The incubation time is unknown but may range from months to years. Symptoms include drowsiness, seizures, hemiparesis, headache, stiff neck, and personality disorders. The trophozoite is rarely seen in spinal fluid; brain biopsy demonstrates both cyst and trophozoite. Histologic preparations of the brain at autopsy show inflammatory lesions containing many segmented neutrophils, eosinophils, and trophozoites. Therapeutic agents for GAE are generally not established because most infections have been diagnosed at autopsy.

Amebic keratitis is another condition associated with *Acanthamoeba* spp. that has been identified since the 1980s. The primary group at risk for developing this condition are individuals who wear contact lenses, especially the soft and extended-wear types. A common factor in these infections is the preparation of homemade saline solution, although some patients also report a history of corneal trauma or of wearing the contact lenses during swimming. Patients experience photophobia, blurred vision, inflammation, ring infiltrates, and pain. Because of the similarity in tissue damage, the infection may initially be confused with herpes simplex viral infection. Phase microscopy of direct wet mount preparations of corneal scrapings may show the cyst. Permanent stains such as trichrome and Giemsa may also demonstrate the trophozoite in clinical specimens. Isolation of *Acanthamoeba* may be performed in a manner similar to that for *N. fowleri,* except that corneal scrapings serve as the inoculum. Amebic keratitis has been treated with propamidine isethionate, neomycin–polymyxin B, gramicidin, and clotrimazole. Corticosteroids are used to reduce inflammation. Many patients lose the sight in the affected eye despite treatment.

Acanthamoeba spp. have only two stages, the resistant cyst and the motile trophozoite. The cyst is approximately 15 to 20 μm, spherical, and double walled, with the walls having a wrinkled appearance. The trophozoite ranges from 10 to 45 μm (average size 20 μm) and has a single nucleus with a central prominent endosome. Blunt pseudopods and characteristic spinelike projections of the cytoplasm (acanthopodia) may also be seen on a wet mount. The method described to recover *N. fowleri* organisms in culture may also be used to recover *Acanthamoeba* spp. from corneal scrapings.

Ciliates

BALANTIDIUM COLI

Only one ciliate, *Balantidium coli,* is considered a pathogen for humans. The true host for this organism is the hog, and human beings serve as accidental hosts. The organism lives in the large intestine, where it may cause mucosal lesions but not extraintestinal infections. Most people with this infection are asymptomatic, but the organism may cause a self-limiting diarrhea with nausea, vomiting, and abdominal tenderness.

Life cycle and morphology The life cycle is similar to that of the amebae, with the cyst being the infective stage for human beings. The organism is quite large and covered with short cilia (Figure 24-15). The oval trophozoite demonstrates two size ranges: 45 to 60 by 30 to 40 μm and 90 to 120 by 60 to 80 μm. The cilia-lined cytostome is located at the slightly pointed anterior end. The cytoplasm contains food vacuoles. A small opening at the posterior, the cytopyge, is used to expel the

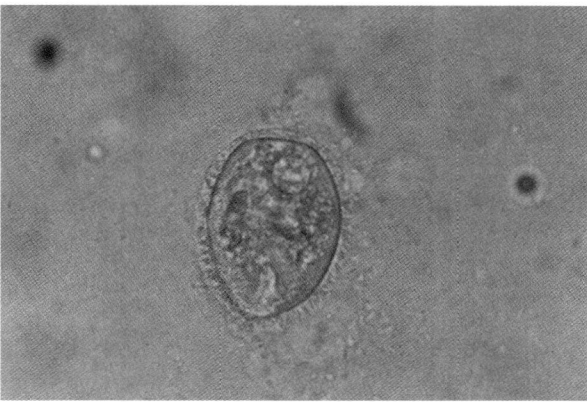

Figure 24-15 _____

Balantidium coli trophozoite (wet mount).

contents of food vacuoles. In a wet mount, the cilia are seen propelling the organism with a rotary motion.

The rounded, thick-walled cyst averages 45 to 75 μm. Cilia may be seen retracted within the cyst wall. Both stages are characterized by the presence of two nuclei: a kidney bean–shaped macronucleus and a small, round micronucleus that usually is situated in the small curvature of the macronucleus.

Pathogenic intestinal and urogenital flagellates

The flagellates constitute another major group of parasites that may inhabit the intestinal tract. The life cycle is relatively simple, resembling that of the amebae (Figure 24-16). Most flagellates have both cyst and trophozoite stages. *Dientamoeba fragilis, Trichomonas vaginalis,* and *Trichomonas hominis* lack a cyst stage, however, and the trophozoite of these organisms serves as the infective stage.

The intestinal organisms covered in the section are:

- *Giardia lamblia*
- *Dientamoeba fragilis*
- *Chilomastix mesnili*
- *Trichomonas hominis*

Giardia lamblia originally was considered the only pathogenic intestinal flagellate. In recent years, however, *D. fragilis* has been identified as a potential pathogen. *T. vaginalis,* an inhabitant of the genitourinary tract in both men and women, is also

discussed in this section. Table 24-5 shows the characteristics of the trophozoite and cyst stages of the intestinal and genitourinary flagellates.

Nonpathogenic organisms, such as *Retortomonas intestinalis* and *Enteromonas hominis,* that have low infection or detection rates are not discussed. Readers are referred to a standard parasitology text for information on such organisms.

GIARDIA LAMBLIA

Giardia lamblia has a worldwide distribution and is often the etiologic agent of outbreaks of gastroenteritis and traveler's diarrhea. In the United States it is the most commonly reported intestinal parasite. Animals such as the beaver may serve as reservoirs and may be a source of infection for backpackers who drink from streams or rivers. *Giardia lamblia* has also been isolated in outbreaks of diarrhea in nurseries and day care centers as a

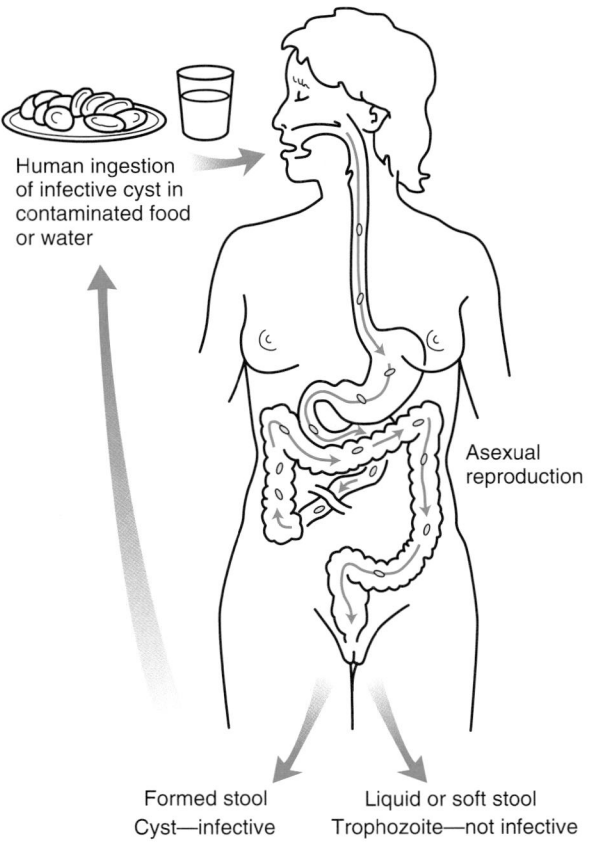

Human ingestion of infective cyst in contaminated food or water

Asexual reproduction

Formed stool
Cyst—infective

Liquid or soft stool
Trophozoite—not infective

Figure 24-16 _____

Generalized life cycle for intestinal flagellates.

TABLE 24-5
Comparison of Intestinal and Urogenital Flagellates

Organism	Trophozoite				Cyst		
	Size (μm)	Motility	Number of Nuclei	Other Features	Size (μm) and Shape	Number of Nuclei	Other Features
Giardia lamblia	9-21 × 5-15	"Falling leaf"	2	Sucking disk, ventral surface Parabasal bodies and axonemes	8-12, oval	4	Cytoplasm retracted from cyst wall Fibrils and flagella inside cyst
Chilomastix mesnili	10-20 × 3-10	Rotary	1	Spiral groove Cytostome	6-10, lemon-shaped	1	Anterior of cyst has nipplelike protrusion
Trichomonas hominis	6-14	Jerky	1	Undulating membrane the entire length of the organism Axostyle through body			No cyst stage
Dientamoeba fragilis	5-12	Nondirectional	2 (20% have 1)	Nucleus made of 4 to 8 clustered granules Resembles ameba			No cyst stage
Trichomonas vaginalis	7-23 × 5-12; average, 15-18	Jerky, nondirectional	1	Undulating membrane half the length of the body Found in urine			No cyst stage

result of person-to-person contact as well as in food-borne and waterborne infections. Along with *E. histolytica*, *G. lamblia* has been identified as a sexually transmitted pathogenic protozoan in the male homosexual population.

Clinical infection *Giardia lamblia* lives in the duodenal area of the small intestine. Although it does not invade the mucosal surface, it does attach to the surface of columnar epithelial cells. Possible pathologic mechanisms associated with the organism are adherence and damage to the intestinal mucosa, interference with absorption of nutrients, and irritation. There is no enterotoxin activity, but atrophy of the intestinal villi can be seen in heavy infections. Patients with deficiencies in secretory immunoglobulin A (IgA) often have a more severe infection.

In most patients, the acute infection manifests as a self-limiting diarrhea with malaise, cramps, nausea, and abdominal tenderness after an incubation period of 12 to 14 days. Explosive, foul-smelling diarrhea is present. Patients with secretory IgA deficiency or achlorhydria seem not only to be more prone to the infection but also to develop chronic infection. In these cases, there may be a malabsorption-like syndrome with weight loss, fatigue, anorexia, and steatorrhea with large amounts of gas. Metronidazole is the drug given for infection.

Laboratory diagnosis Feces serve as the usual diagnostic specimen, but shedding of the cysts is irregular, and multiple specimens often fail to reveal the organism. In cases in which clinical symptoms persist and the organism cannot be demonstrated, a duodenal aspirate or the Enterotest (HDC Corp., San Jose, Calif.) may be used to isolate the organism. In the Enterotest, the patient swallows a gelatin capsule containing a weighted string. One end of the string has been taped to the side of the patient's mouth; the weighted end is carried into the upper small intestine. After about 4 hours, the string is brought up, and part of the mucus adhering to the surface is stripped off and examined on a wet mount for motile trophozoites. The remainder of the specimen is placed in a fixative for a permanently stained smear. Serologic tests using monoclonal antibodies to detect *G. lamblia* antigens in stool have also been developed.

Characteristics of the trophozoite. Table 24-5 summarizes the characteristics of *G. lamblia* and compares them with those of other flagellates. The trophozoites of *G. lamblia* are pear shaped, bilaterally symmetric, and measure approximately 9 to 21 by 5 to 15 μm. They show a characteristic "falling leaf" motility in a wet mount. In a permanently stained smear, the binucleate organism has been described as having an "old man" appearance (Figure 24-17). Two oval nuclei, each with a large central karyosome, are on each side of the midline. Four pair of flagella, midline axonemes, and two median bodies posterior to the nuclei are also present. A large ventral sucking disk is used by the organism to attach to the intestinal wall. The organism often stains faintly with trichrome stain.

Cysts. Cysts of *G. lamblia* are oval and approximately 8 to 12 by 7 to 10 μm. There are up to four nuclei, and the cytoplasm often is pulled away from the cyst wall. On a permanently stained smear, the retracted flagella and other internal structures give the cyst a cluttered appearance (Figure 24-18).

DIENTAMOEBA FRAGILIS
Dientamoeba fragilis is another flagellate organism of the large intestine that is now recognized as a cause of gastrointestinal illness. Patients infected with the organism are usually asymptomatic but may have abdominal pain or tenderness and diarrhea. The organism lacks a cyst stage; it appears that the trophozoite may be transmitted to human beings by being ingested on a helminth egg, especially that of *E. vermicularis*.

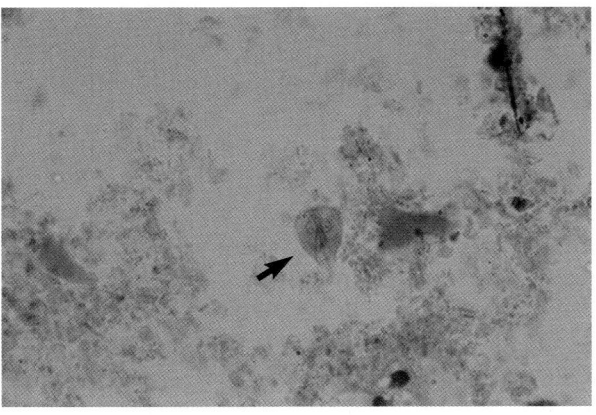

Figure 24-17
Giardia lamblia trophozoite (trichrome stain).

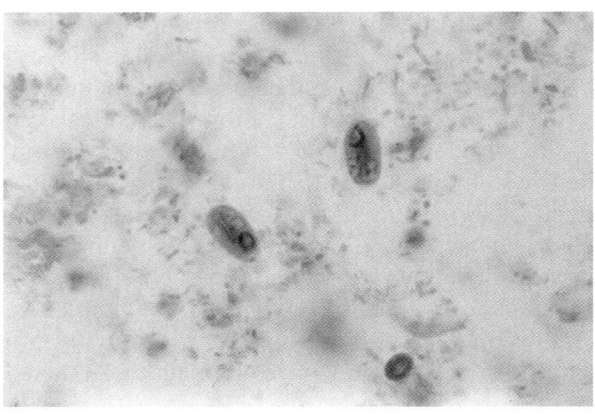

Figure 24-18 ————————————————

Giardia lamblia cyst (trichrome stain).

The morphology of *D. fragilis* closely resembles that of the amebae, but studies of ultrastructure indicate that it belongs to the subphylum Mastigophora. The organism is characteristically described as being binucleate, with 50% to 80% of the organisms demonstrating this characteristic. The nuclear membrane has no peripheral chromatin, and the karyosome consists of four to eight discrete granules. The size of the trophozoite ranges from 5 to 12 μm, and the cytoplasm contains many food vacuoles and bacteria (Figure 24-19). This organism can be difficult to see on a trichrome-stained smear, because its outline often is indistinct and blends into the background.

TRICHOMONAS VAGINALIS

Trichomonas vaginalis, a pathogen of the urogenital tract in men and women, causes trichomoniasis, one of the most common sexually transmitted diseases. The organism lacks a cyst stage, and the trophozoite stage is infective through sexual contact.

Clinical infection In women, the infection is primarily localized in the vagina, resulting in itching and the production of a frothy, creamy vaginal discharge as well as dysuria. Men infected with *T. vaginalis* are usually asymptomatic and serve as carriers, although they may develop nonspecific urethritis with a milky discharge that lasts up to 4 weeks. Infections in either sex are usually treated with metronidazole. Treatment of both sexual partners is suggested to obtain optimum cure.

Long-term immunity is not developed after an acute infection, and reinfection can occur.

Laboratory diagnosis In women the diagnosis may be made by finding the trophozoite in urine or vaginal discharge; in men the trophozoite is seen in urine or prostatic secretions. The organism has four free anterior flagella and an undulating membrane that extends half the length of the body. In a wet mount the trophozoite has a characteristic jerky motility, and the motion of the flagella and undulating membrane may be seen. In a stained preparation the pear-shaped organism shows the presence of an axostyle, single nucleus, and chromatic granules extending the length of the axostyle. The average size of *T. vaginalis* is 5 to 18 μm. Although most clinicians rely on wet mount preparations, the method has relatively low sensitivity. Culture is the most sensitive and definitive method of detection, although specimens must be held for up to 7 days for results. There are no commercially available kits for serologic diagnosis of trichomoniasis.

Nonpathogenic intestinal flagellates

Chilomastix mesnili and *Trichomonas hominis* are intestinal nonpathogens that must be differentiated from pathogenic flagellates. *Chilomastix mesnili* trophozoites are pear shaped and approximately 10 to 20 μm long by 3 to 10 μm wide. The cytostome and nucleus are prominent in the anterior of the organism, and a spiral groove encircles the body of the organism. The nucleus has a

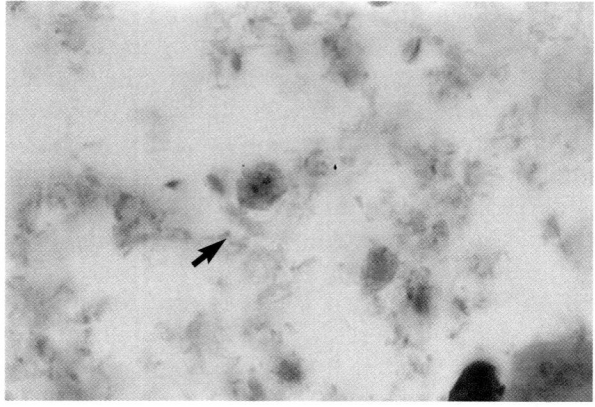

Figure 24-19 ————————————————

Dientamoeba fragilis binucleate trophozoite (trichrome stain).

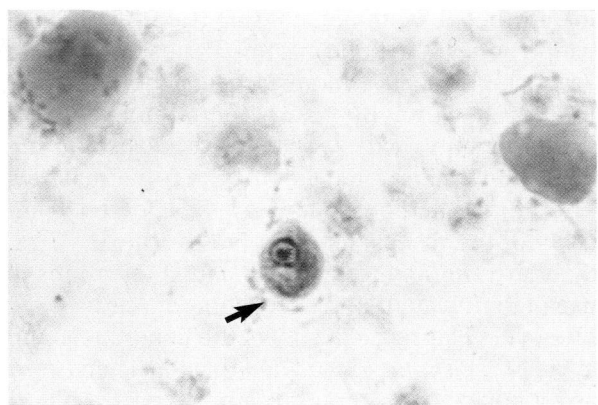

Figure 24-20 _____

Chilomastix mesnili cyst (trichrome stain).

small central karyosome and is surrounded by fibrils that curl around the cytostome to give a "shepherd's crook" appearance. The cytostome is elongate and rounded at the anterior and posterior. The cyst of *C. mesnili,* which measures 6 to 10 μm, is lemon shaped with an anterior nipple. The nucleus, cytostome, and curved fibrils are visible in a stained smear (Figure 24-20).

T. hominis is a small organism not usually identified in the stool. The trophozoite is 6 to 14 μm long with a prominent axostyle extending through the posterior of the organism, four anterior flagella, and an oval nucleus with a small karyosome. The undulating membrane extends the length of the organism and is joined to the body along the costa.

Blood and tissue flagellates

The hemoflagellates in the genera *Leishmania* and *Trypanosoma* differ in several ways from the intestinal flagellates. First, they are transmitted by insect **vectors,** which are necessary for completion of the life cycle. Second, these organisms have different life cycle stages for diagnosis. Figure 24-21 shows the four life cycle stages of the hemoflagellates. The trypomastigote and the amastigote are the **diagnostic stages** found in human beings. The **amastigote** is an obligate intracellular organism, 2 to 3 μm, found within macrophages, liver or spleen cells, or bone marrow in diseases caused by the *Leishmania* spp. The **trypomastigote,** a flagellated form measuring 15 to 20 μm, is found in the blood, lymphatic fluid, and cere-

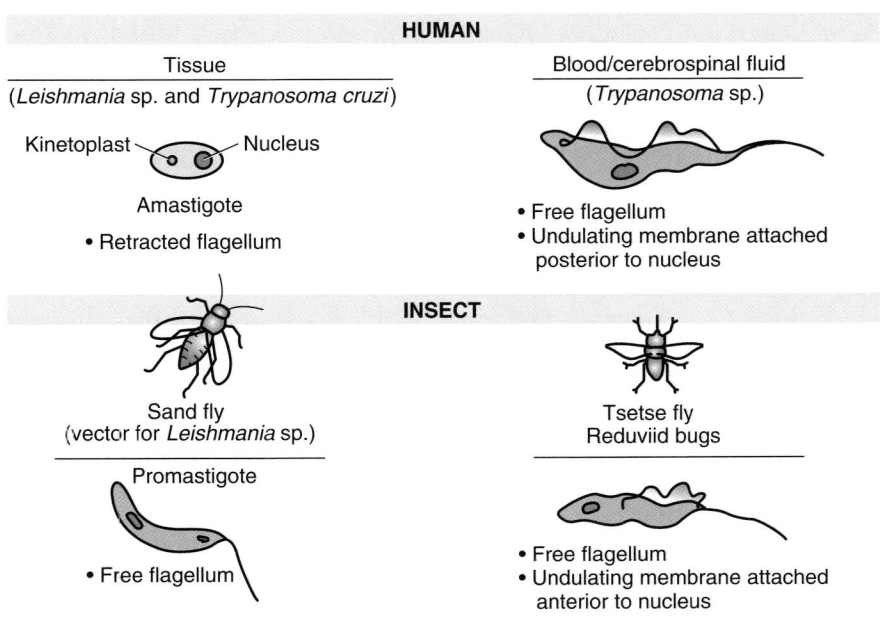

Figure 24-21 _____

Life cycle stages of the blood and tissue flagellates.

brospinal fluid of patients infected with *Trypanosoma* organisms. In addition, the amastigote stage may be seen in cells of patients infected with *Trypanosoma cruzi.* The epimastigote and promastigote stages are seen in the insect vectors.

LEISHMANIA

The genus *Leishmania* contains several complexes of species that cause disease in human beings. These complexes are:

- *Leishmania tropica* complex
- *Leishmania braziliensis* complex
- *Leishmania mexicana* complex
- *Leishmania donovani* complex

Dogs and rodents serve as the primary reservoir hosts for all species. The insect vectors are sandflies of the genera *Phlebotomus* and *Lutzomyia.*

Clinical infections *L. tropica* complex, the cause of cutaneous leishmaniasis or Oriental sore, is found primarily in the Orient and North Central Africa. *L. mexicana* complex, the cause of New World leishmaniasis, is found in South and Central America. The condition is characterized by the presence of a crusted circular lesion on any of the exposed body surfaces, especially the face and extremities. The lesion begins as a small red papule and progresses to a lesion with an elevated, indurated margin that may reach 8 cm. Another form of the disease, chiclero ulcer, is characterized by lesions on the ear. The infection is self-limiting and does not invade mucosal surfaces, but secondary bacterial infection may occur.

    L. braziliensis complex is the causative organism of mucocutaneous leishmaniasis or espundia. This infection manifests as an initial lesion that may increase in size, invading and destroying the mucosal surfaces of the nose and mouth. It may also destroy cartilage, leaving the patient with significant disfigurement. *L. braziliensis* complex is primarily found in Mexico, South America, and Central America.

    The most severe infection, visceral leishmaniasis or Kala-azar, is endemic in parts of South America, Africa, Southern Europe, and Asia. The etiologic agents are organisms of the *L. donovani* complex. In this disease, organisms spread through the lymphatics and invade organs of the reticuloendothelial system, including the liver, spleen, lymph nodes, and bone marrow. Patients with Kala-azar exhibit malaise, anorexia, headache, and fever. In addition, they may show hepatomegaly and splenomegaly with invasion of *Leishmania*-containing macrophages into the bone marrow. The kidneys and heart may also be affected. If untreated, the disease is often fatal within 2 years. Standard therapy for all leishmanial infections is use of pentavalent antimony compounds.

Life cycle Figure 24-22 shows the generalized life cycle for *Leishmania* sp. The organism is ingested as an amastigote when the insect takes a blood meal. It develops as a promastigote in the gut of the insect and migrates to the salivary glands when mature. The promastigote is transmitted to the human being through the salivary glands of the insect when it takes a blood meal. The promastigote is taken up by a macrophage, converts to the amastigote stage, and multiplies within the cell.

Laboratory diagnosis The amastigote is the diagnostic stage in human beings. It is a small intracellular stage found in macrophages or histiocytes around the periphery of the skin lesions (*L. tropica* or *L. braziliensis*) or within cells of a bone marrow aspirate or liver or spleen biopsy specimen (*L. donovani*). Wright stain shows an oval organism 2 to 5 μm long, with pale blue cytoplasm, a large red nucleus, and rodlike kinetoplast within the cytoplasm (Figure 24-23).

TRYPANOSOMA

Trypanosomes are blood and CSF flagellates that require an insect vector for transmission. *Trypanosoma brucei rhodesiense* and *Trypanosoma brucei gambiense* are the causative agents of sleeping sickness, which is seen primarily in Central Africa. *Trypanosoma cruzi,* the agent of American trypanosomiasis or Chagas disease, is discussed in the next section.

    West African sleeping sickness, caused by *T. brucei gambiense,* is the milder and more chronic of the two diseases. East African sleeping sickness, caused by *T. brucei rhodesiense,* is characterized by a rapid course often resulting in death within 1 year. In addition, game animals serve as important reservoir hosts of *T. rhodesiense.*

Clinical infection Initial symptoms include a local reaction at the site of the insect bite within 2 to

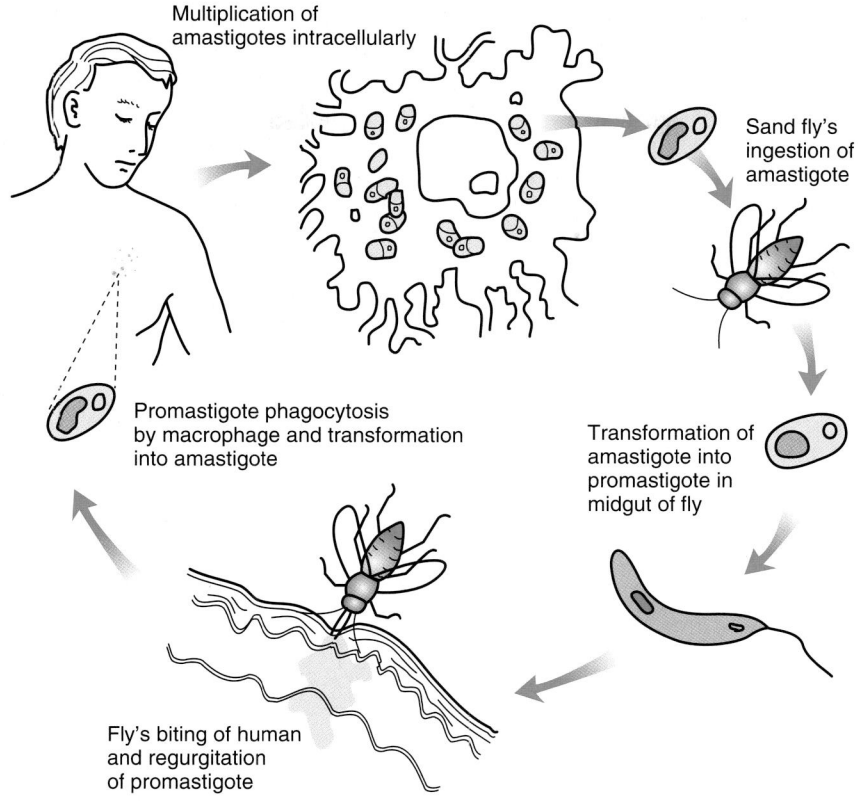

Figure 24-22 _____

Life cycle of *Leishmania* spp.

3 days. As the trypomastigotes enter the blood and lymphatics, the patient experiences fever, headache, joint and muscle pain, enlarged lymph nodes, especially in the posterolateral triangle of the neck (Winterbottom's sign). Edema in the legs and arms and around the eyes is possible. As the trypomastigotes invade the central nervous system, the patient develops severe headaches, mental dullness, and apathy and may experience coordination problems, altered reflexes, and paralysis.

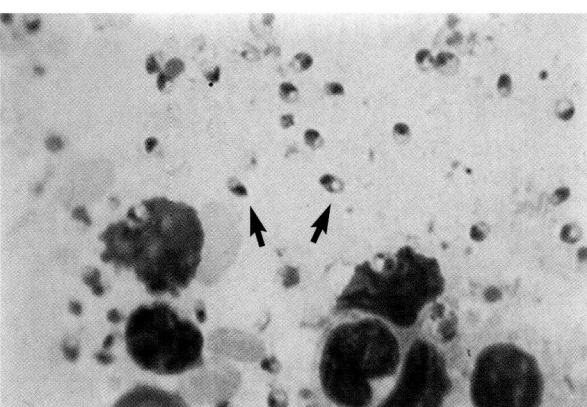

Figure 24-23 _____

Amastigotes of *Leishmania* spp.

Eventually, the patient has convulsions, lapses into a coma, and dies.

Life cycle The tsetse fly (*Glossina* sp.) is the biologic vector for agents of sleeping sickness. Figure 24-24 shows a generalized life cycle for these agents. The fly ingests the trypomastigote stage when it takes a blood meal from a human being. The organisms migrate to the insect gut and develop into an epimastigote, which, when mature, migrates to the salivary gland. There it develops into an in-fective metacyclic trypomastigote, which is trans-mitted to human beings in saliva when the fly bites.

Laboratory diagnosis The diagnostic stage in hu-man beings is the trypomastigote, which is usually seen in a Wright-stained blood smear. The organ-ism, however, can also be isolated from lymphatic fluid and cerebrospinal fluid. The trypomastigote is 15 to 20 μm with a single large nucleus and a pos-terior kinetoplast to which is attached the flagellum of the undulating membrane (Figure 24-25). *Try-*

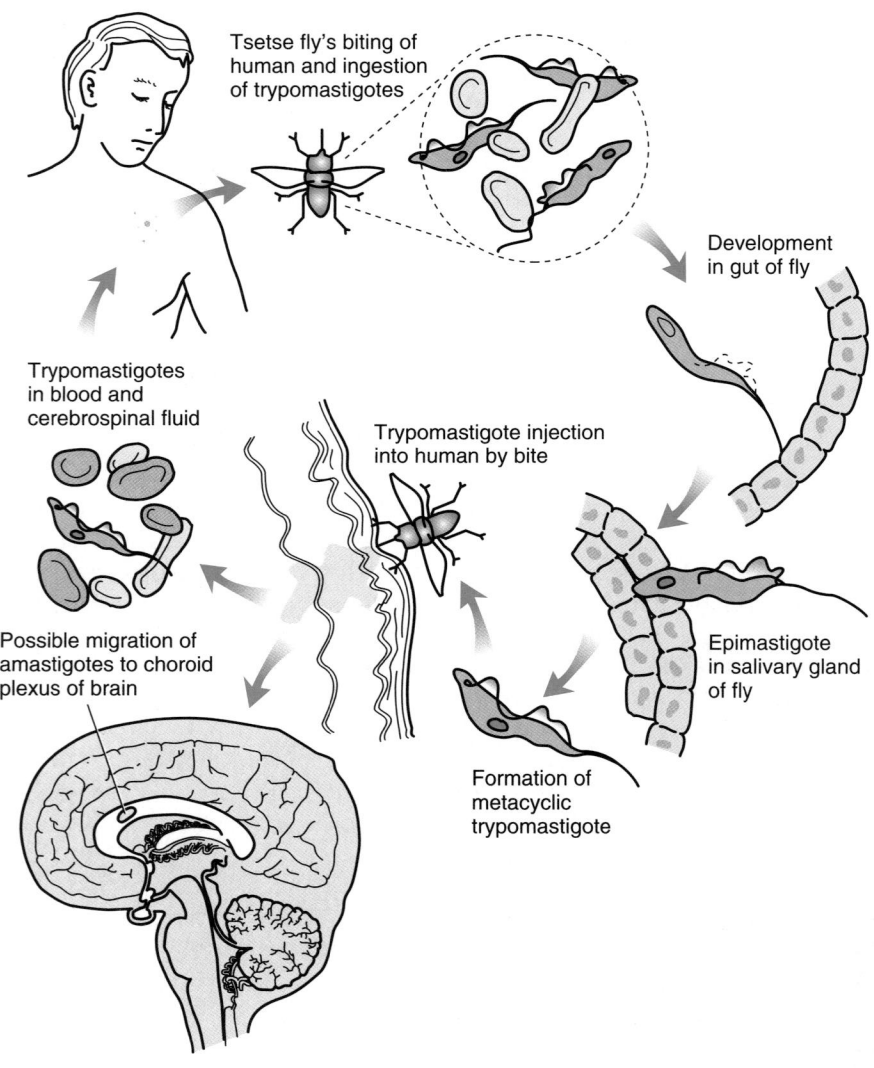

Tsetse fly's biting of human and ingestion of trypomastigotes

Development in gut of fly

Trypomastigotes in blood and cerebrospinal fluid

Trypomastigote injection into human by bite

Epimastigote in salivary gland of fly

Possible migration of amastigotes to choroid plexus of brain

Formation of metacyclic trypomastigote

Figure 24-24

Life cycle of the agents of sleeping sickness (*Trypanosoma gambiense* and *Trypanosoma rhodesiense*).

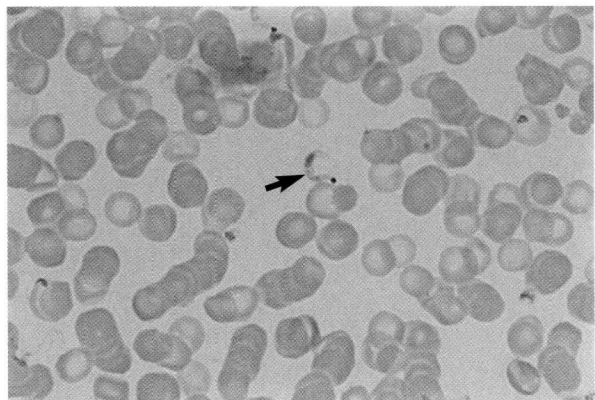

Figure 24-25 ————————————————

Trypanosoma trypomastigote in a blood smear.

panosoma species cannot be differentiated on a blood smear; diagnosis is based on clinical symptoms as well as the geographic area.

TRYPANOSOMA CRUZI

Chagas disease is a **zoonotic** infection found primarily in rural areas of Mexico, Central America, and South America. It is caused by *T. cruzi,* which is transmitted by the insect known as the triatomid bug, reduviid bug, or kissing bug (*Triatoma* sp. or *Panstrongylus* sp.). These insects live within mud or thatch walls of a dwelling during the day and come out at night to take a blood meal from the human inhabitants. Although insect transmission is most common, the organism has been transmitted by blood transfusion and congenital infection.

Clinical infection Acute infection with this organism usually occurs in children and may involve multiple organ systems. The incubation period ranges from 2 to 4 weeks. Symptoms during the acute stage vary and may include the presence of a chagoma (ulcerative skin lesion), fever, a unilateral edema around the eye (Romaña's sign), lymphadenitis, hepatosplenomegaly, malaise, muscular pains, and diarrhea and vomiting. Acute myocarditis, which progresses into a chronic form, also develops in many cases and may progress to congestive heart failure. Chronic disease in some patients may manifest as megacolon, megastomach, or megaesophagus.

Life cycle Transmission of the organism to human beings occurs when the insect defecates in the area surrounding its bite. Organisms in the feces are scratched into the bite and invade the blood stream as trypomastigotes. The trypomastigote enters a cell, transforms into an amastigote, multiplies, breaks out of the cell, and invades other cells. Cells of the cardiac muscle and skeletal muscle are most commonly infected. Figure 24-26 shows the life cycle of *T. cruzi.*

Laboratory diagnosis The primary diagnostic stage in the blood is the trypomastigote. It is an elongate structure 15 to 20 μm long that often appears in a C or U shape. Like the other trypomastigotes, it shows a single large nucleus midbody and a posterior kinetoplast to which is attached the undulating membrane. Occasionally, the suggestion of a flagellum can be seen at the anterior end. In a cardiac or other tissue biopsy specimen, the organism can be seen in the amastigote stage. The morphology of all trypomastigotes is similar; therefore, a complete patient history is necessary to determine the species present.

Xenodiagnosis is used in Central and South America as a diagnostic method. A laboratory-raised triatomid bug is allowed to feed on patients suspected of harboring *T. cruzi.* When the insect is returned to the laboratory, its feces is examined on a regular basis for the presence of trypomastigotes. Presence of this stage in the insect's feces indicates that the patient was infected.

Apicomplexa

The phylum Apicomplexa includes blood and tissue parasites that represent both age-old pathogens and newly recognized agents of opportunistic infection. This group of organisms shows a diversity of morphology and transmission methods. Life cycles are complex and are characterized by sexual and asexual reproduction phases. In addition, some may require an insect vector or intermediate host for completion of the life cycle. A human being may serve as a **definitive host** when **sexual reproduction** takes place in human tissues and as an intermediate host when **asexual reproduction** occurs. Organisms in this group infect many different body sites:

- *Plasmodium* spp. and *Babesia* sp. infect red blood cells

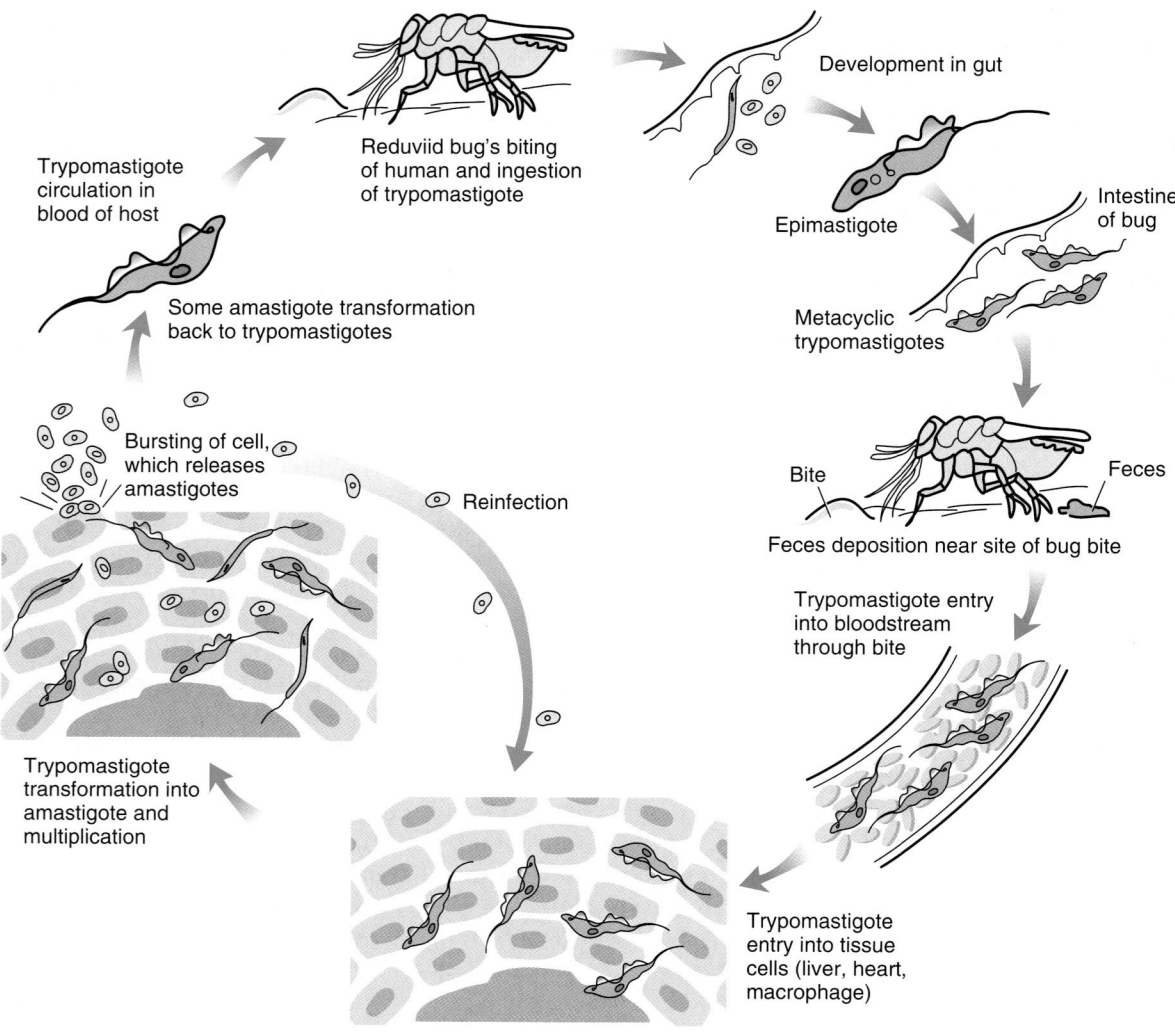

Figure 24-26

Life cycle of *Trypanosoma cruzi.*

- *Cryptosporidium parvum, Isospora belli,* and *Cyclospora cayetanensis* infect cells of the intestinal tract
- *Pneumocystis carinii* is found in the lung
- *Toxoplasma gondii* infects a variety of organs

Plasmodium spp.

Plasmodium spp., which cause malaria, remain endemic throughout the world in tropical and subtropical countries. Along with schistosomiasis and amebiasis, malaria is a major cause of mortality in people in underdeveloped countries. Between 1 million and 2 million deaths are caused by malaria each year. *Plasmodium vivax, Plasmodium ovale, Plasmodium malariae,* and *Plasmodium falciparum* are the etiologic agents of human malaria. *P. vivax* has the widest geographic distribution and is the one most likely to be found in temperate climates. *P. ovale* is confined to Africa; *P. falciparum* and *P. malariae* have similar distributions throughout Africa and tropical countries. In general, infections caused by *P. vivax, P. ovale,* and *P. malariae* are less severe than those caused by *P. falciparum.* The Centers for Disease Control Malaria Surveillance document (1990) noted that the number of malarial infections increased 8% in the United States from

1989 to 1990. Of the 1102 reported cases, *P. vivax* was the etiologic agent in 48%; *P. falciparum* in 41%. Most cases, however, were imported.

Although malaria most commonly is transmitted through insects, transmission through blood transfusion and infected needles has been reported. Transplacental infection also has been documented.

Before the life cycle of malaria is detailed, the characteristics that distinguish the erythrocytic stages in a Giemsa-stained smear should be discussed (Figure 24-27). The earliest stage is the *ring form trophozoite,* in which the organism has a prominent red-purple chromatin dot and a small blue ring of cytoplasm surrounding a vacuole. The *growing trophozoite* is characterized by an increase in cytoplasm, the disappearance of the vacuole, and the appearance of malarial pigment in the organism's cytoplasm. The *immature* **schizont** is characterized by a splitting of the chromatin mass. The *mature schizont* contains **merozoites,** which are individual chromatin masses, each surrounded by cytoplasm. *Microgametocyes* (male) have pale blue cytoplasm and a diffuse chromatin mass that stains pale pink-purple. The chromatin may be surrounded by a clear halo. *Macrogametocytes* (female) show a well-defined, compact chromatin mass that stains dark pink, and the cytoplasm stains a darker blue than in microgametocytes. The chromatin mass often is set eccentrically in the organism. Pigment is distributed throughout the cytoplasm except in *P. falciparum,* in which it often is clumped near the chromatin mass.

CLINICAL INFECTIONS

The malarial paroxysm is the primary symptom associated with the erythrocytic cycle. It is linked to rupture of the red cell and release of merozoites, malarial metabolites, and endotoxin-like substances into the bloodstream. The prodromal phase of the paroxysm involves headache, bone pain, nausea, or flulike symptoms. A shaking chill (10 to 15 minutes) initiates the paroxysm and is followed by a fever of up to 40° C. The paroxysm can last from 2 hours up to 20 hours. When the fever finally breaks, the patient begins to sweat profusely. This cycle repeats itself at regular intervals, depending on the species of malarial organism present. Long-term infection with any malarial organism may result in damage to the liver and spleen caused by deposits of malarial pigment (hemozoin).

P. vivax and *P. ovale* infections generally do not have the range of complications seen with other species. *P. malariae* infections may lead to nephrotic syndrome, which arises from deposition of circulating immune complexes of malarial antigen and antibody on the basement membrane of the glomerulus, causing an autoimmune reaction against the basement membrane.

The most severe form of malaria is caused by *P. falciparum,* with the primary complication being the development of cerebral malaria. Between 20% and 50% of deaths caused by *P. falciparum* are the result of this CNS complication. The parasite-infected red blood cell develops sticky knobs that mediate adhesion to the endothelial cells of the capillary walls. Blood flow is slowed, reducing oxy-

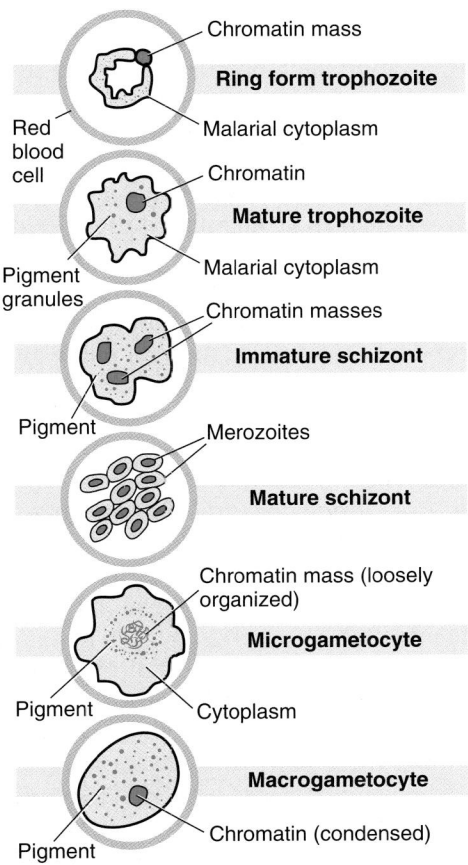

Figure 24-27 _____

Life cycle stages of malaria.

gen delivery to the tissues, with resultant tissue anoxia. The patient has severe headaches, may be confused, and ultimately lapses into a coma. Renal failure results from the tubular necrosis caused by the diminished blood flow.

A second but less common complication of infection with *P. falciparum* is *blackwater fever.* It usually develops in patients with repeated infections and those undergoing quinine therapy. Blackwater fever may be mediated by an antigen-antibody reaction caused by the development of an autoantibody to the red cell. The black appearance of the urine is the result of massive intravascular hemolysis and resulting hemoglobinuria.

Although complete immunity to malaria does not exist, patients in endemic areas develop antibodies against asexual stages, which helps reduce the parasite load and the severity of illness. In addition, reports of antibodies directed against **sporozoites** and gametes indicate that these also may help reduce the rate of infection and the severity of illness. Patients with hemoglobinopathies, such as sickle cell disease, are somewhat protected against severe malaria because the parasite cannot exist in these cells.

Treatment Chloroquine remains the primary drug for prophylaxis and treatment of malaria. It is effective against all asexual stages of malarial organisms and all **gametocytes** except those of *P. falciparum*. In addition, some strains of *P. falciparum* have become resistant to the drug. Recent reports indicate that strains of *P. vivax* in Southeast Asia and Papua New Guinea show diminished response to treatment with the drug.

Pyrimethamine/sulfadoxine can be given along with chloroquine to individuals traveling to areas with endemic *P. falciparum*–resistant strains. However, some strains of *P. falciparum* and *P. vivax* also have become resistant to this drug combination. Mefloquine may be used as prophylaxis and in the treatment of multidrug-resistant strains of *P. falciparum,* although some evidence indicates that resistance to this drug is developing in the malarious areas of Southeast Asia and Africa. Quinine use has been reestablished in some cases of multidrug-resistant *P. falciparum.*

Primaquine, which is effective against hypnozoites that persist in the liver, is used to treat individuals infected with *P. vivax* and *P. ovale* to prevent relapses of these infections. There is also evidence that some strains of *P. vivax* in the geographic areas where it is chloroquine resistant may be refractory to primaquine. Alternative drugs for treating these strains must be evaluated in clinical studies.

LIFE CYCLE

The life cycle of *Plasmodium* involves both sexual reproduction **(sporogony)** and asexual reproduction **(schizogony),** as shown in Figure 24-28. The *Anopheles* mosquito serves as biologic vector and definitive host.

Asexual reproduction Asexual reproduction, which occurs in the human being, has an **exoerythrocytic phase** that takes place in the liver and an erythrocytic phase that takes place in red blood cells.

Exoerythrocytic phase. The human being serves as intermediate host and acquires the infection when the female mosquito takes a blood meal and injects the infective sporozoites with salivary secretions. At this time, sporozoites enter the human circulation and initiate schizogony. Sporozoites take approximately 30 to 60 minutes to reach the liver, where they begin the exoerythrocytic cycle by penetrating parenchymal cells. Maturation through the trophozoite and schizont phases results in production of merozoites. Each schizont contains 10,000 to 30,000 merozoites. Release of mature merozoites from liver cells and invasion of red blood cells signal the beginning of the erythrocytic phase. Generally, only one cycle of merozoite production occurs in the liver before red cells are invaded. Organisms such as *P. vivax* and *P. ovale,* however, may persist in the liver in a dormant stage known as hypnozoites, which accounts for the relapse of the disease after many years. Neither *P. malariae* nor *P. falciparum* has a persistent liver phase, although recrudescence in untreated individuals with either of these organisms may be the result of a continued subclinical erythrocytic infection.

Erythrocytic phase. Merozoites have structures that are selectively adhesive for the red blood cell membrane and that attach to receptors on the membrane. Once merozoites have attached, endocytic invagination of the red cell membrane allows the organism to enter the red cell within a vacuole. *P. vivax* may use antigens of specific blood groups such as those in the Duffy system as receptors, whereas *P. falciparum* may simply attach

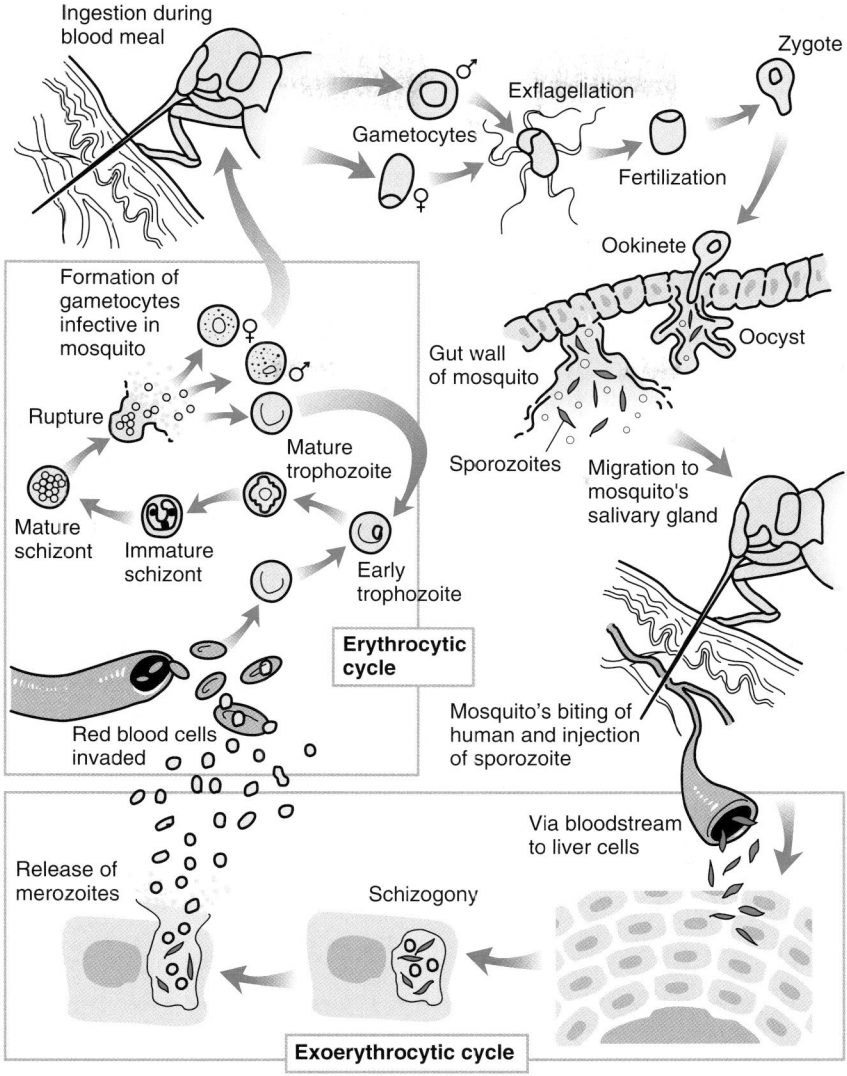

Figure 24-28

Life cycle of *Plasmodium* sp.

to receptors that are integral parts of the red cell membrane itself.

Once inside the cell, the organism feeds on hemoglobin and goes through a maturation sequence—ring form trophozoite to mature trophozoite. Malarial pigment is formed in the growing trophozoite as a result of incomplete metabolism of the hemoglobin. Unutilized hematin is combined with protein and deposited in the cytoplasm of the organism. Once the organism has reached the mature trophozoite stage, the chromatin begins to divide (schizont). When the chromatin split has been completed, each chromatin mass is surrounded by its own bit of malarial cytoplasm (merozoite). Each malarial species, has a typical number of merozoites, which may be used as an identifying characteristic. When the red cell ruptures, merozoites are released to invade other red cells. At this point, two outcomes are possible: one is that the merozoite enters a cell and repeats development into a schizont; the other is that it enters a cell and develops into one of the sexual stages—either the microgametocyte or the macrogametocyte.

Sexual reproduction Sporogony, which takes place in the mosquito, results in production of sporozoites infective for human beings. Both microgametocyte and macrogametocyte are infective for the female mosquito when she takes a blood meal. In the insect's stomach, exflagellation by the male and subsequent fertilization of the female result in formation of an ookinete that migrates through the gut wall and forms an **oocyst** on the exterior gut wall. Sporozoites are produced within the oocyst. Mature sporozoites are released into the body cavity of the mosquito and migrate to the salivary glands. The cycle is repeated when the female injects sporozoites into a human as she takes her blood meal.

LABORATORY DIAGNOSIS

A history of travel to an endemic area and the presence of classic clinical symptoms, including the malarial paroxysm of fever and chills, should alert a clinician to request Giemsa-stained thick and thin smears for malaria. Examination of these blood smears remains the classic method of diagnosing malaria. Laboratory identification of malarial species involves examination both of the red cell morphology and of the characteristic morphology of the parasite. In the thick film, which is used to detect malarial parasites, the red blood cells (RBCs) are destroyed, so that only white cells, platelets, and malarial parasites are visible. Dis-

tortions of morphology and the lack of red cells require that a thin smear be examined to determine the actual species present. The thin smear is used for species identification because the morphology of the red cells, as well as that of the organism, can be seen. Trophozoites, schizonts, and gametocytes may be seen in the blood smear. Table 24-6 gives the general characteristics of trophozoites and schizonts of the malarial species.

Several articles have described a procedure using a modified microhematocrit tube coated with acridine orange for the detection and identification of malarial species. This method, the quantitative buffy coat (QBC) system, demonstrates the presence of parasites, but a thin smear must still be made for definitive identification. DNA probes have been proposed as another method for diagnosing malaria. However, the extended time and costly equipment required do not make the procedure cost-effective or efficient, especially for field work. A dipstick method has been described that may be used in field studies to detect *P. falciparum* infection. The dipstick uses an antigen-capture ELISA principle to detect soluble proteins from *P. falciparum* in the blood. Additional studies have shown it may be used to screen units of blood from donors who may have been exposed to malaria.

Serologic tests for antibody to malaria are not useful in an endemic area but may be useful in in-

TABLE 24-6

Comparison of Malarial Species

Plasmodium Species	Red Blood Cell Morphology	Trophozoite	Number of Merozoites in Schizont	Reproductive Cycle (Hours)	Other Characteristics
P. vivax	Enlarged (½ to 2×) Schüffner stippling	Ameboid Large vacuoles Golden-brown pigment	12-24 Average: 16	48	Wide range of stages in peripheral blood
P. malariae	Normal size May have dark hue Ziemann dots (rare)	Compact May assume "band form" across cell Coarse, dark brown pigment	6-12 Average: 8 with daisy petal–like arrangement around clumped pigment	72	—
P. ovale	Enlarged, oval Fringed edge Schüffner stippling	Compact Coarse, dark pigment (resembles *P. malariae*)	6-16 Average: 8	48	—
P. falciparum	Normal size Multiple infections	Small, delicate Double chromatin dots Appliqué forms Dark pigment	12-36 Average: 20-24	Irregular, 36-48	Crescent-shaped gametocyte Ring and gametocyte stages only in peripheral blood

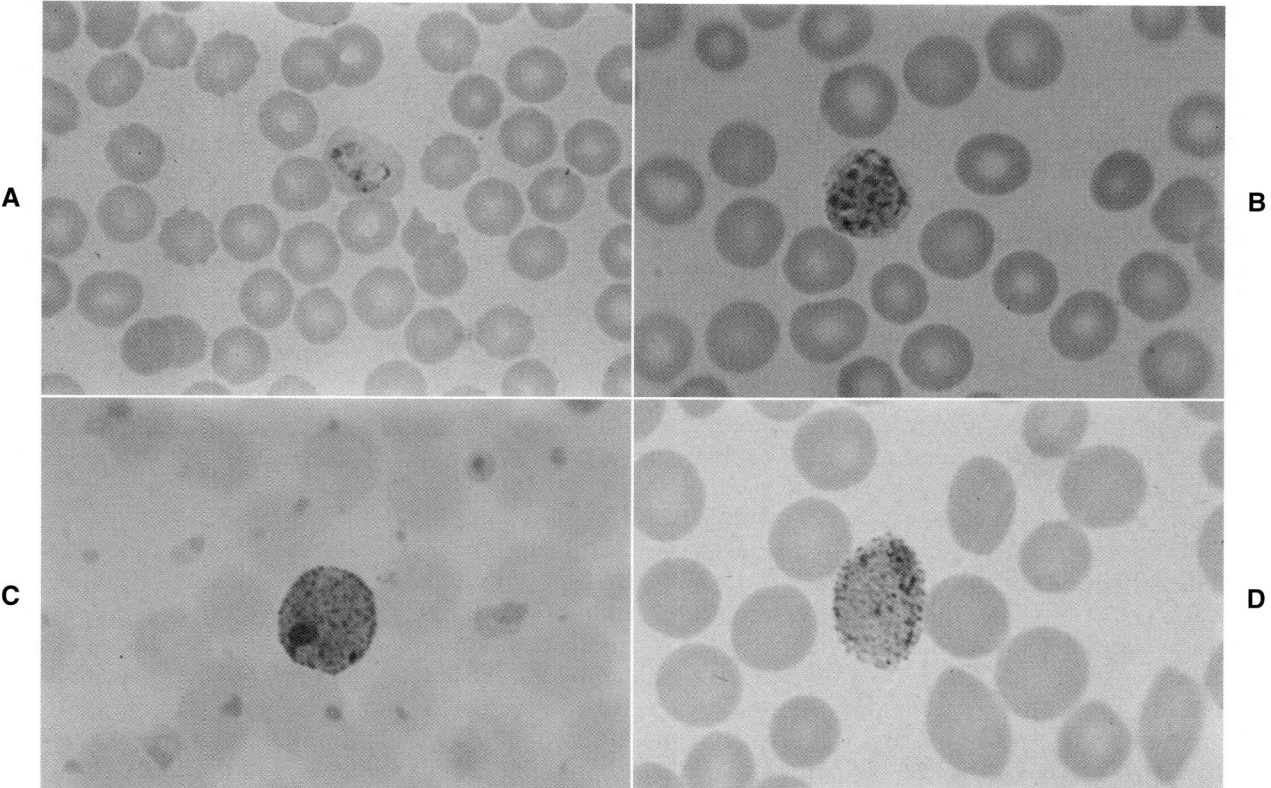

Figure 24-29

A, *Plasmodium vivax* trophozoite. **B,** *P. vivax* immature schizont. **C,** *P. vivax* macrogametocyte. **D,** *P. vivax* microgametocyte.

dividuals who have traveled to an endemic area and who have clinical symptoms of malaria.

Plasmodium vivax *P. vivax* has a tertian life cycle pattern—that is, it takes approximately 48 hours for the life cycle to complete itself. The invasion of a new group of red cells begins on the third day. *P. vivax* usually invades young RBCs (reticulocytes) and therefore is characterized by enlarged red cells, often 1½ to 2 times normal. A fine pink stippling known as *Schüffner stippling* may be present in the cell. The young trophozoite is characterized by its ameboid appearance; by maturity, it usually fills the RBC, and golden brown malarial pigment is present. The mature schizont contains 12 to 24 merozoites, with an average of 16. Gametocytes are rounded and fill the cell. Macrogametocytes are often difficult to differentiate from mature trophozoites. Figure 24-29, shows the stages of *P. vivax*.

Plasmodium malariae *P. malariae,* on the other hand, usually invades older red cells, perhaps ac-

counting for the occasional darker appearance of the invaded red cell. The life cycle is characterized as quartan, with reproduction occurring every 72 hours and invasion of new red cells every fourth day. The trophozoite is compact and may assume a characteristic "band" appearance, in which it stretches across the diameter of the red cell (Figure 24-30, *A*). Dark, coarse brown-black pigment is present. Occasionally, a few pink cytoplasmic dots, called Ziemann dots, may be seen. The mature schizont contains 6 to 12 merozoites (Figure 24-30, *B*), with an average of 8. Merozoites may be arranged in a characteristic loose "daisy petal" arrangement around the clumped pigment; however, they may also be randomly arranged.

Plasmodium ovale *P. ovale,* the least commonly seen of the species, looks like a *P. malariae* but cells infected with *P. ovale* exhibit the characteristics of cells infected by *P. vivax*. In *P. ovale* infections, the RBC is enlarged and may assume an oval shape with fimbriated or fringelike edges. Schüffner stippling is less common than with *P. vivax.* The parasite remains compact, has dark brown pigment, and has a range of 6 to 12 merozoites in the mature schizont. It also exhibits a tertian life cycle. Figure 24-31 shows a trophozoite of *P. ovale.*

Plasmodium falciparum Although identified as having a tertian life cycle, *P. falciparum* usually demonstrates an asynchronous life cycle, with rupture of the red cells taking place at irregular intervals ranging from 36 to 48 hours. The life cycle stages seen in peripheral blood are usually limited to the ring form trophozoite and the gametocyte. Other stages mature in the venules and capillaries of the major organs. *P. falciparum* invades red cells of any age and, for this reason, often exhibits the highest parasitemia—reaching 50% in some cases. Wedge-shaped dots, known as Maurer clefts, may be present, but they are uncommon and require excellent staining to be visualized. The ring forms of *P. falciparum* (Figure 24-32, *A*) are more delicate than those of other species and often have two chromatin dots. Appliqué forms of the parasite appear to be external to the RBC membrane, and multiple ring forms in a single cell are common. The mature trophozoite is small and compact and may have dark brown pigment. The schizont has 8 to 36 merozoites, with an average of 20 to 24. Gametocytes have a characteristic banana or crescent shape (Figure 24-32, *B*).

Babesia microti

Babesia microti is another intraerythrocytic human parasite. *Babesia* spp. have been known to infect

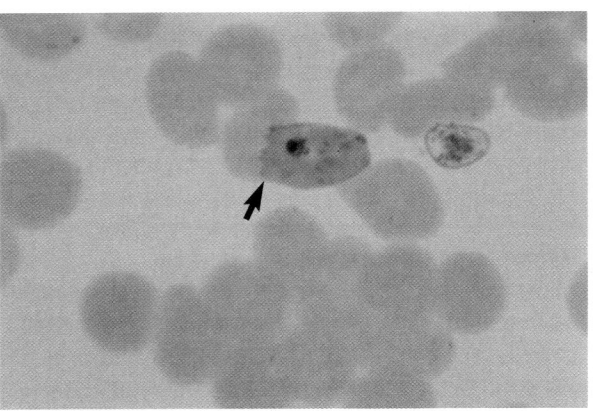

Figure 24-31 _____

Plasmodium ovale trophozoite.

cattle and other animals, but the first cases to be reported in human beings occurred in the 1950s. These initial cases were limited to patients who had undergone splenectomy, but since then, cases of babesiosis have been reported in patients who are not asplenic. The first documented cases in the United States were in the Martha's Vineyard and Nantucket Island area, where a hard tick *(Ixodes dammini)* served as the vector. As with malaria, cases of perinatal and transfusion-transmitted babesiosis have been reported.

There also have been reports indicating simultaneous transmission of babesiosis and Lyme borreliosis, because the tick vectors are the same for the two causative organisms. Patients manifest clinical symptoms of one disease but show a concurrent rise and fall in antibody titers to both the *Babesia* and the Lyme borreliosis organisms.

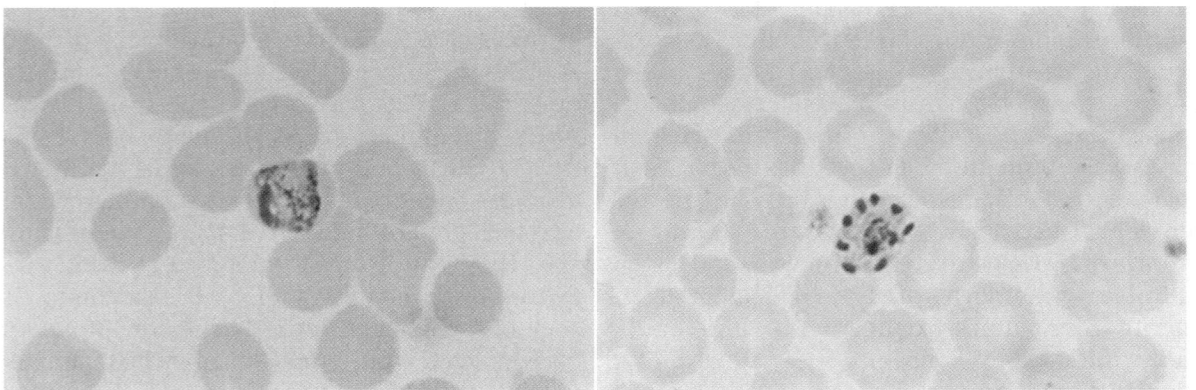

Figure 24-30 _____

A, *Plasmodium malariae* band form trophozoite. **B,** *P. malariae* schizont.

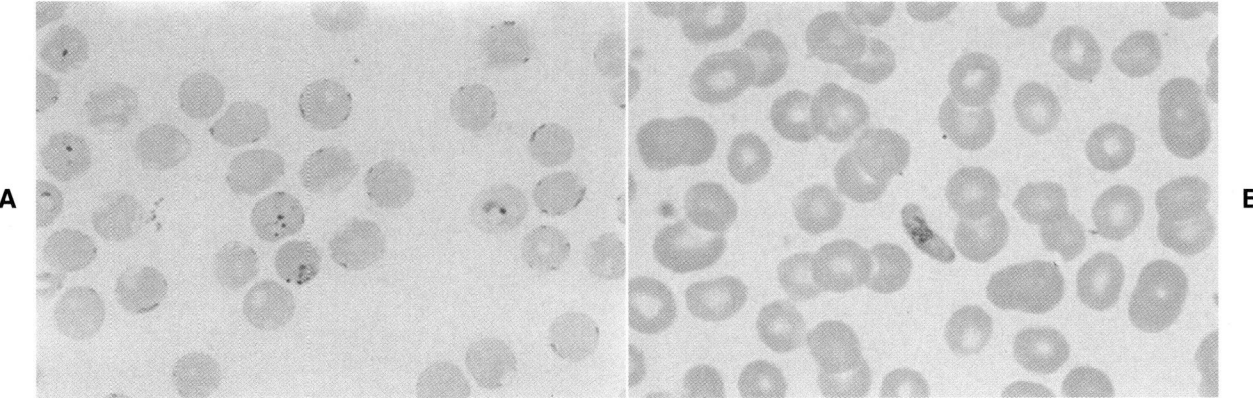

Figure 24-32

A, *Plasmodium falciparum* ring form trophozoites. **B,** *P. falciparum* gametocyte.

CLINICAL INFECTIONS

Patients with babesiosis may have malaria-like symptoms such as fever, chills, sweating, and myalgia. Many cases are asymptomatic, however. Anemia may develop if hemolysis is severe or prolonged. The clinical course tends to be more severe if the patient has undergone splenectomy. Treatment with quinine sulfate and clindamycin is effective in eliminating the infection.

LIFE CYCLE

As with *Plasmodium* spp., the life cycle of *Babesia* has alternating sexual and asexual reproduction stages. Production of the infective stage (sexual reproduction) takes place in the tick, and schizogony (asexual reproduction) in the red blood cells of human beings. There is no exoerythrocytic cycle in human beings and no identifiable gametocyte stage in the red cell. Transovarian transmission can occur in the tick, allowing the life cycle to persist without an intermediate host.

LABORATORY DIAGNOSIS

The diagnosis of babesiosis is made from a Wright- or Giemsa-stained thin blood smear. The organisms appear as small, delicate, ring form trophozoites, about 1 to 2 μm, with a prominent chromatin dot and faintly staining cytoplasm. More mature trophozoites may appear as pyriform organisms in single, double, or the classic tetrad (Maltese cross) formation within the red cell. The morphology initially may be confused with that of *P. falciparum*. Unlike with malaria, however, extracellular organisms are seen. Lack of pigment and absence of other life cycle stages serve as additional keys to differentiate *Babesia* from *P. falciparum*. Serologic studies can be used to quantitate antibody titers. Although transfusion-transmitted babesiosis has been reported, there is no screening test for blood donors. Figure 24-33, *A*, shows the small, compact, ringlike trophozoites of *B. microti;* Figure 24-33, *B*, demonstrates the tetrad formation characteristic of the organism.

Toxoplasma gondii

Toxoplasmosis can manifest with a wide range of clinical symptoms and complications. The organism, *T. gondii*, is found worldwide, and serologic studies indicate that more than 50% of people in the United States have antibodies to this organism.

CLINICAL INFECTION

Patients with acute infections may be asymptomatic or may have mild flulike or mononucleosis-like symptoms, including low-grade fever, lymphadenopathy, malaise, and muscle pain. Once the acute infection has resolved, the organism enters a relatively inactive stage in the tissues.

The organism may also be transmitted congenitally. Children who acquire *T. gondii* this way may have a range of serious complications, including mental retardation, microcephaly, seizures, hydrocephalus, retinochoroiditis, and blindness. If the fetus is exposed to the infection early in the pregnancy, severe complications are more likely to result. Infections acquired later in pregnancy may result in the child's being asympto-

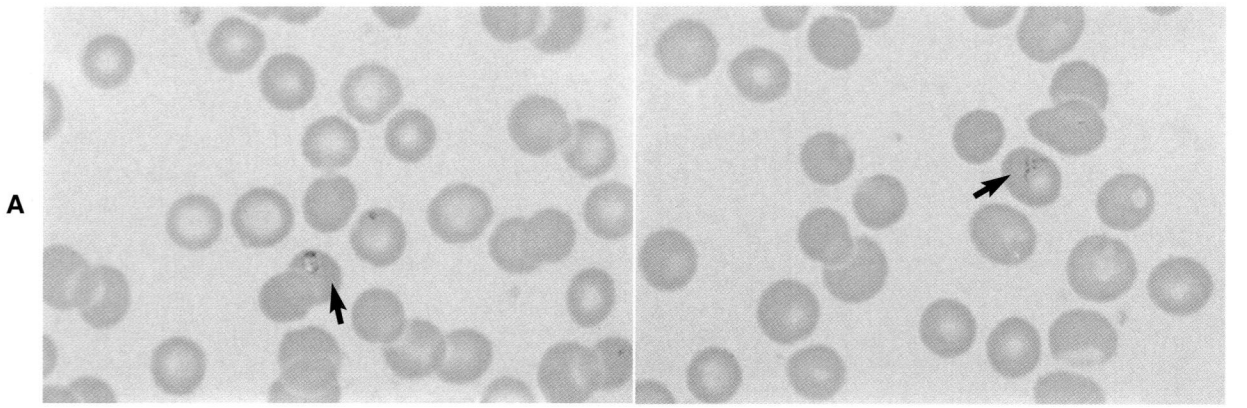

Figure 24-33

A, *Babesia microti* trophozoite. **B,** *B. microti* tetrad form.

matic at birth but developing complications later in childhood.

Immunosuppressed patients, particularly those with leukemia or lymphoma and those undergoing chemotherapy, may suffer from a primary infection or reactivation of a latent infection. Either may manifest as a fulminating encephalitis and result in rapid death. There are also a number of reports of the death of patients with acquired immunodeficiency syndrome (AIDS) caused by disseminated toxoplasmosis. These infections also show CNS symptoms as primary evidence of infection. Computed tomography scans may demonstrate lesions in the brain that represent *Toxoplasma* cysts. Pulmonary toxoplasmosis may be present in conjunction with the CNS infections.

LIFE CYCLE

There are two life cycle stages in human beings—the **tachyzoite** and the **bradyzoite.** Actively motile and reproducing forms are referred to as tachyzoites. They are crescent shaped, are 4 to 6 μm long, and have a prominent nucleus (Figure 24-34, *A*). Figure 24-34, *B*, shows lung tissue containing free tachyzoites as well as a number of intracellular forms. Bradyzoites are the slowly growing and reproducing forms found within a cystlike structure during the dormant phase of the infection.

The household cat and other members of the family Felidae serve as definitive hosts for the organism. Sexual and asexual reproduction occur in the intestine of the cat; only asexual reproduction occurs in human beings and other intermediate hosts. The

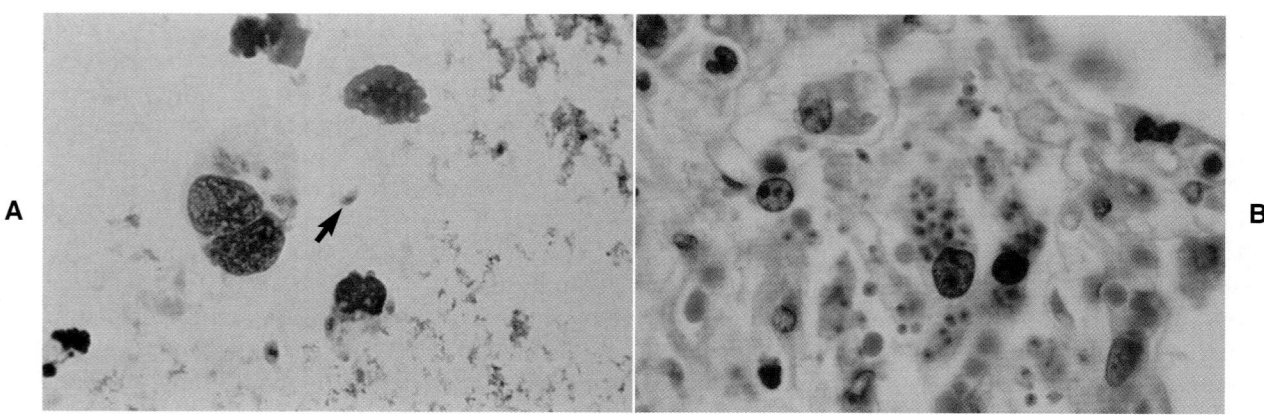

Figure 24-34

A, *Toxoplasma gondii* tachyzoites. **B,** *T. gondii* tachyzoites in lung tissue.

result of sexual reproduction is the oocyst, which is passed in cat feces. The oocyst requires 2 to 5 days in the environment to mature and become infective.

There are basically three ways in which human beings can acquire infection with *T. gondii,* as shown in the life cycle illustrated in Figure 24-35:

- Ingestion or inhalation of the oocyst, which is shed in cat feces
- Ingestion of undercooked meat containing the cyst with bradyzoites
- Congenital transmission

When a human being ingests the infective oocyst, sporozoites present in the oocyst are liberated in the intestine, penetrate the intestinal wall, gain access to the circulation, and migrate to the organs. These tachyzoites, as they are now called, invade cells, multiply, and eventually cause cells to rupture and release tachyzoites to invade other cells. The immune system, in particular the T cells, respond when tachyzoites invade the tissues. This immune response results in formation of a large cystlike structure that contains the slowly growing and reproducing bradyzoites. At this point

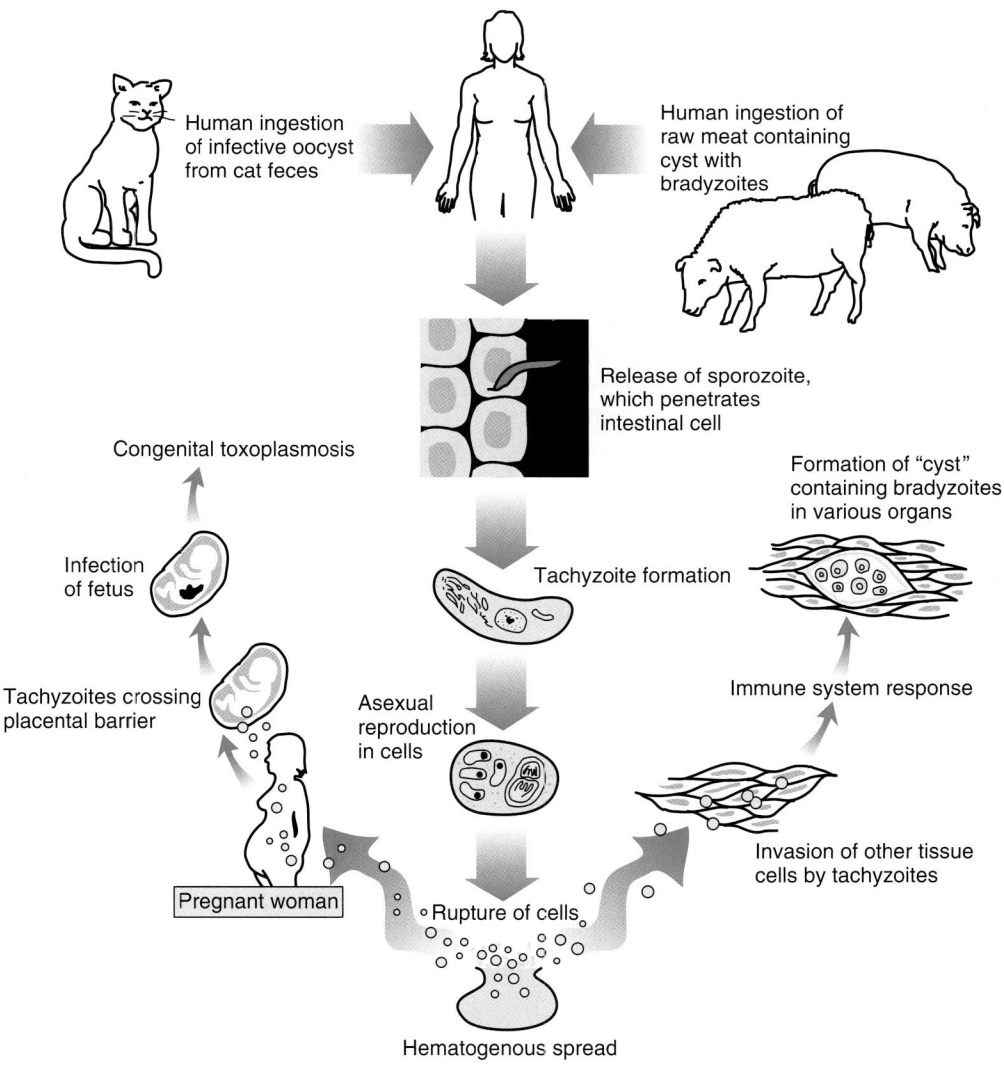

Figure 24-35

Life cycle of *Toxoplasma gondii.*

the infection remains in a dormant state, unless the immune system is compromised. In the immunocompromised patient, the bradyzoites are released from the cyst and become active tachyzoites that invade multiple organs, resulting in disseminated infection.

In the second method of infection, a human being ingests raw or undercooked meat containing the cyst with bradyzoites. The cyst wall is dissolved, and bradyzoites are liberated. Studies show that these organisms are resistant to digestive tract enzymes for about 6 hours, during which time they convert to tachyzoites and invade the intestinal wall. They then gain access to the circulation and subsequently invade various organs.

Congenital transmission occurs when tachyzoites in the maternal circulation cross the placenta and enter the fetal circulation and tissues.

LABORATORY DIAGNOSIS

Identification of the tachyzoite or pseudocysts with bradyzoites in tissue is very difficult, because no single organ is invaded. Antibodies to the organism show a rapid rise during infection, and tests for antibodies are most commonly used for diagnosis. The Sabin-Feldman dye test was the first antibody test developed. It is not used in clinical laboratories because it requires live organisms. Indirect fluorescent antibody tests and enzyme immunoassay tests using *T. gondii* organisms as antigen are routinely used for diagnosis. Because most people have an antibody titer to the organism, interpretation of the titer must be linked to clinical symptoms and the patient's history. A rise in titer between acute and convalescent specimens may indicate acute infection. An IgM-specific test may also be used to diagnose acute infections and may be useful in the diagnosis of toxoplasmosis in pregnant women suspected of having been exposed to the organism or in neonates in whom congenital infection is suspected. IgM titers usually peak within the first month of infection. In disseminated toxoplasmosis, histologic stains of biopsy materials may demonstrate the cyst with bradyzoites, or, in some cases, the tachyzoites. Noninvasive technology, such as magnetic resonance imaging and computed tomography, may be used in the diagnosis of patients suspected of having disseminated toxoplasmosis. Antibody titers may be unreliable in immunocompromised patients, because these patients lack the ability to produce sufficient antibody to cause a significant rise in titer.

Pneumocystis carinii

Pneumocystis carinii originally was believed to be a yeast, was then classified with the protozoa, and now is being reevaluated for classification as a fungus. It initially was identified as the etiologic agent in interstitial plasma cell pneumonia seen in malnourished or premature infants. Since the early 1980s, it has been one of the primary opportunistic infections found in patients with AIDS. The higher incidence also is the reuslt of the use of immunosuppressive drugs in patients with malignancies or organ transplants. Underlying defects in cellular immunity apparently make patients susceptible to clinical infection with the organism.

CLINICAL INFECTION

Patients infected with *P. carinii* may have fever, nonproductive cough, and shortness of breath. Chest radiographs show a diffuse interstitial infiltrate. The immune response to the organism after it attaches to and destroys alveolar cells is partly responsible for this radiographic pattern. When the infiltrate is examined, it is found to contain cells from the alveoli and plasma cells.

Treatment includes the use of trimethoprim-sulfamethoxazole or pentamidine. Some patients with AIDS have been given aerosolized pentamidine as a prophylactic treatment. However, there have been reports of disseminated *P. carinii* infection in such patients.

LIFE CYCLE

The life cycle of *P. carinii* has two stages—the trophozoite, which is 1 to 4 μm in size and is irregularly shaped, and the cyst, which is a thick-walled sphere of 6 to 8 μm containing up to eight intracystic bodies. Transmission of the organism is known to occur through the respiratory route, with the cyst being the infective stage. The intracystic bodies are released from the cyst in the lung and multiply on the epithelial cells lining the lung.

LABORATORY DIAGNOSIS

Traditionally, diagnosis was made by finding the cyst or trophozoite in tissue obtained through open lung biopsy. Specimens now used include those from bronchoalveolar lavage or transbronchial biopsy, and induced sputum. Sputum, however, is the least productive specimen. Lavage and sputum specimens are often prepared using the cytocentrifuge.

Histologic stains such as Giemsa and Gomori methenamine silver are used. With the methenamine silver stain, the cyst wall stains black. Cysts often having a punched-out, "Ping-Pong ball" appearance. With the Giemsa stain, the organism appears round and the cyst wall is barely visible. Intracystic bodies are seen around the interior of the organism. Figure 24-36, *A,* shows the characteristic black-staining cyst of *P. carinii* with methenamine silver stain. Figure 24-36, *B,* shows the cyst as stained with Giemsa stain. The exterior of the cyst does not pick up stain, but the intracystic bodies can be demonstrated as a circular arrangement within the cyst. Calcofluor white stain can be used to screen specimens for *P. carinii* and other fungi or yeast. A fluorescent monoclonal antibody stain has also gained wide use.

Opportunistic intestinal apicomplexa

Cryptosporidium parvum and *Isospora belli* have been recognized as organisms that cause self-limiting gastrointestinal infection in the immunocompetent host. Both organisms, however, have also been identified as opportunistic pathogens in immunocompromised hosts, particularly those with AIDS. The organisms are transmitted by the fecal-oral route, and sexual and asexual reproduction occurs in the human intestinal tract.

Cyclospera cayetanensis, on the other hand, is primarily seen in immunocompetent hosts with a history of travel to specific areas in which the organism is endemic.

CRYPTOSPORIDIUM PARVUM
Cryptosporidium spp. are recognized animal parasites that were initially seen in human beings as zoonotic infections in veterinarians and other animal handlers. Outbreaks in day care centers and from environmental contamination of municipal water supplies, as well as in the general population, have been reported. They are obligate intracellular parasites transmitted by ingestion of the infective oocyst. In the 1980s, cryptosporidiosis was identified as a major opportunistic infection in patients with AIDS. The primary organism associated with human outbreaks is *C. parvum.*

Clinical infection In immunocompetent patients, *C. parvum* causes a profuse, watery diarrhea along with mild to severe nausea and vomiting, headache, and cramps. The onset is rapid, but the infection is self-limiting, and symptoms resolve in several weeks owing to a cell-mediated immune response. In patients with AIDS, the infection may be life-threatening. The organism alters osmotic pressure in the gut, with a resulting influx of fluid. The diarrhea is cholera-like, with bits of mucus and little fecal material. Fluid loss has been reported to range from 3 to 6 L/day to as much as 17 L/day. In addition to weight loss, patients show signs of dehydration and electrolyte imbalance. In

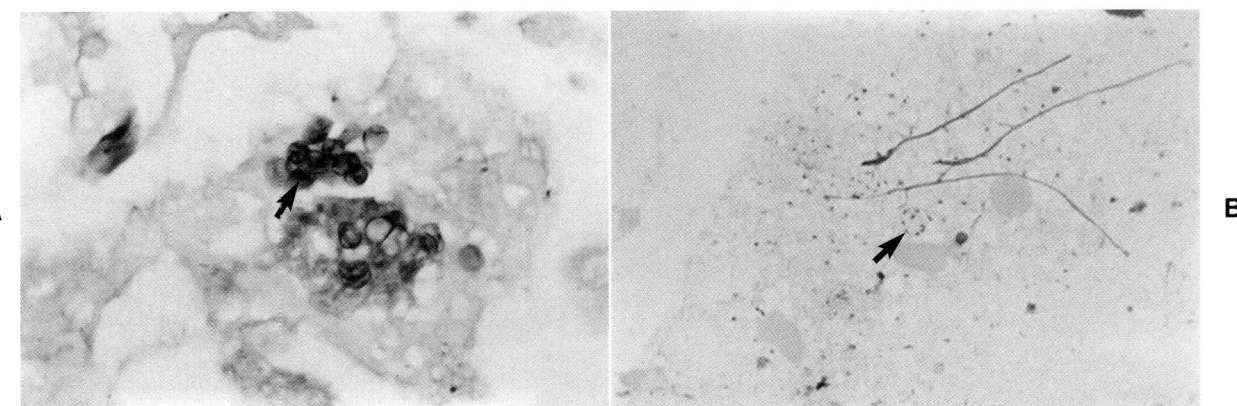

Figure 24-36

A, *Pneumocystis carinii* cysts (silver stain). **B,** *P. carinii* (Giemsa stain). Notice circular arrangement of intracystic bodies within faint outline of cyst wall in center of field.

chronic cases, the intestinal villi may be injured or destroyed, and the patient shows signs of malabsorption syndrome. No antimicrobial is completely effective for this infection. Spiramycin, paromomycin, and azithromycin have been used with mixed results.

Life cycle The sexual and asexual life cycles of *C. parvum* occur in the same host. Life cycle stages, as shown in Figure 24-37, develop under the brush border of the intestinal mucosal epithelial cells. Infective oocysts may be ingested in contaminated water or food or passed by person-to-person contact. Ingestion of the infective oocyst initiates the asexual cycle (merogony) with release of sporozoites. These attach to and penetrate the intestinal mucosal border and mature into trophozoites.

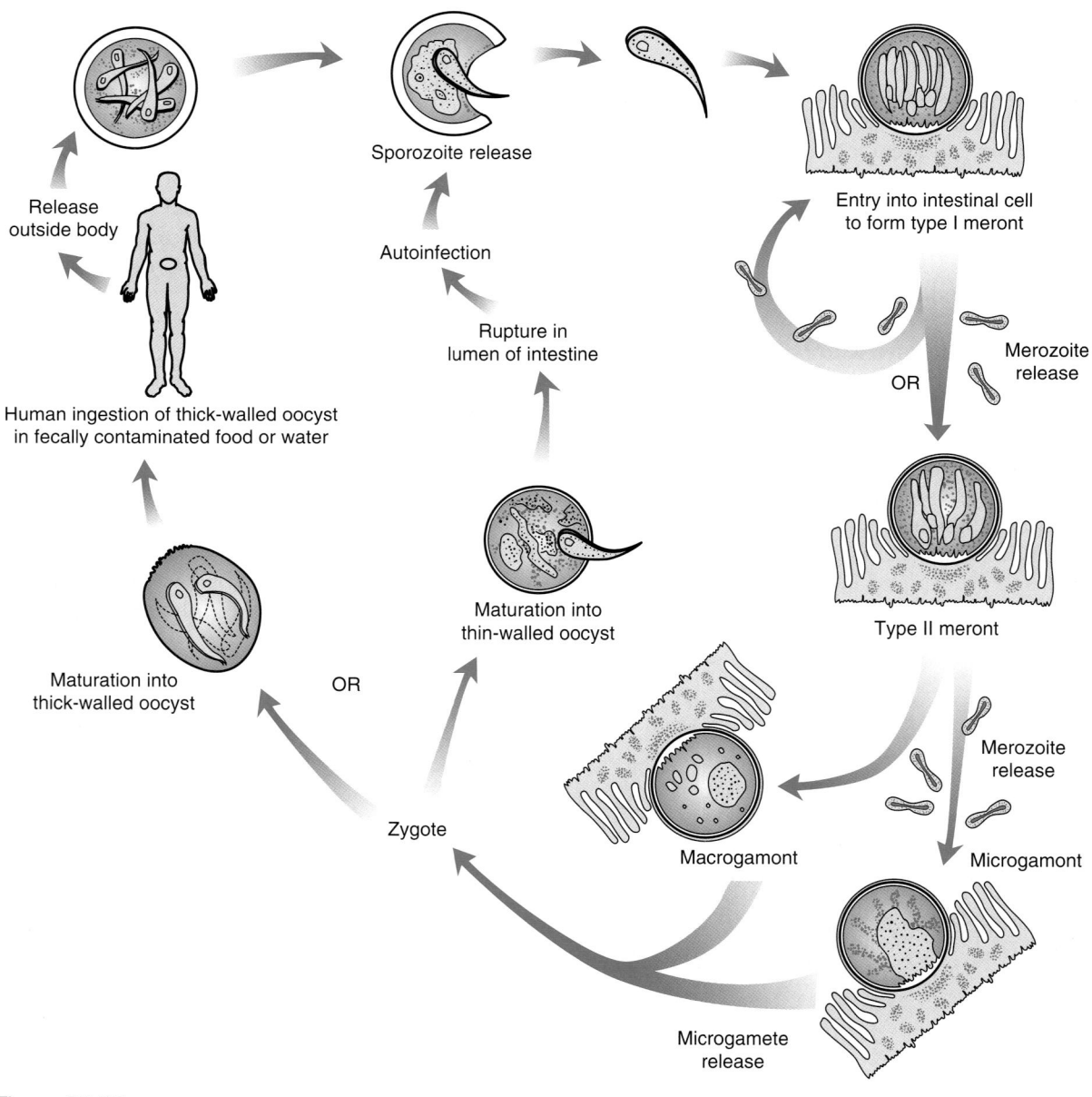

Figure 24-37

Life cycle *Cryptosporidium* sp.

Once trophozoites have matured, the development of meronts with merozoites begins. The nucleus and cytoplasm divide to form individual organisms known as merozoites. When the meront ruptures, merozoites are released and penetrate other cells, either to continue asexual reproduction or to transform into microgametes or macrogametes of the sexual reproductive cycle (gametogony). Fertilization of the macrogamete results in formation of the oocyst, which contains four sporozoites. Two types of oocysts may be formed—the thin-walled oocyst, which ruptures within the intestine and results in autoinfection, and the thick-walled oocyst, which is infective when passed in the stool.

Key factors in the life cycle of this organism that contribute to its pathogenicity are as follows:

1. The oocysts are infective when passed.
2. Rupture of thin-walled oocysts in the intestine creates the potential for continual autoinfection.
3. Patients may remain infective and continue to shed oocysts for a time after the diarrhea ceases.

Laboratory diagnosis The small size (4 to 6 μm), refractile appearance, and round shape of the oocyst make detection difficult with routine concentration procedures because the organism may resemble a yeast or red cell. More oocysts are seen in a liquid stool; fewer in a formed stool. One of the first alternate concentration methods, the Sheather sugar flotation method, improved detection of *C. parvum,* but other intestinal parasites are not easily identified using this method. In addition, one study showed that concentration of a stool by the formalin–ethyl acetate method may lead to a significant decrease in the number of oocysts seen. Another concentration method involving use of traditional formalin–ethyl acetate and subsequent overlay of sediment with saturated sodium chloride has been described. This method improves the recovery rate of oocysts.

Trichrome and iron hematoxylin are not useful permanent stains for identification of *Cryptosporidium* sp. The recommended detection methods when *Cryptosporidium* infection is suspected are the modified Ziehl-Nielsen acid-fast stain and an indirect fluorescent antibody test using a monoclonal antibody directed against *Cryptosporidium* sp. With the acid-fast stain, the organism stains as

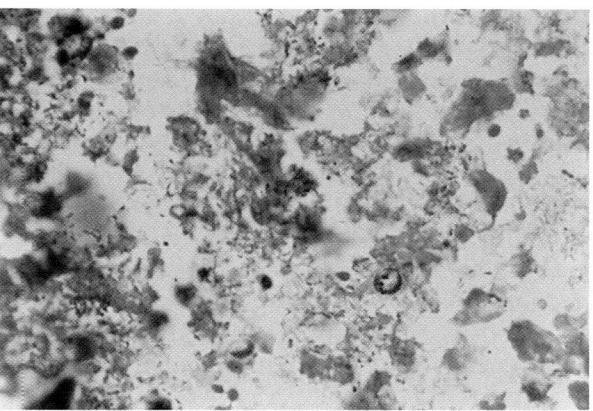

Figure 24-38

Cryptosporidium oocysts (modified acid-fast stain).

a bright red sphere, which distinguishes it from yeasts, which stain green. Figure 24-38 shows an acid-fast stain of *Cryptosporidium* sp. Studies indicate that the monoclonal antibody test demonstrates greater sensitivity and specificity than the modified acid-fast stain. Although biopsy specimens initially were required to identify life cycle stages, they are not routinely used for laboratory diagnosis.

ISOSPORA BELLI

Isospora belli is seen less often than *C. parvum,* and acute infections with *I. belli* are usually clinically indistinguishable from infections with *Cryptosporidium* spp.

Clinical infection Most patients infected with *I. belli* are asymptomatic, but symptoms such as low-grade fever, headache, diarrhea, and abdominal pain may be present. The infection is self-limiting and usually resolves in several weeks. The immunocompromised patient infected with *I. belli* may have watery diarrhea and concurrent weight loss. Treatment with trimethoprim-sulfamethoxazole has been effective in eliminating diarrhea, but patients often show recurrence of infection when therapy is discontinued.

Life cycle The life cycle of *I. belli* is similar to that of *Cryptosporidium* sp. but occurs within the cytoplasm of epithelial cells of the small intestine. The oocyst of this organism is not infective when passed in the feces and requires 24 to 48 hours of existence outside the body before it is infective.

Laboratory diagnosis The mature oocyst of *I. belli* is oval, 20 to 33 by 10 to 19 μm with a hyaline cell wall. The immature oocyst usually shows a single **sporoblast;** the mature oocyst has two **sporocysts,** with four elongated sporozoites within each. Both may be seen in wet mounts. The modified acid-fast stain has been used to increase identification capabilities. The oocyst wall does not stain but often shows a faint outline owing to precipitated stain, and the sporoblasts or sporocysts stain dark red. Figure 24-39 shows the characteristic appearance of an acid-fast stain of the oocyst of *I. belli.*

CYCLOSPORA CAYETANENSIS

Cyclospora cayetanensis is another organism recently implicated as a cause of diarrheal disease. This protozoan had been identified in animals for a number of years but had not been linked with human illness until the mid-1990s. When the organism was first seen in human stool specimens, it was originally thought to be a Cyanobacterium-like body, blue-green algae, or large *C. parvum.* It is now classified as a member of the Apicomplexa. The organism is endemic in Nepal, Peru, and Haiti, but outbreaks have been reported in many countries, including those in Central and South America, parts of the Caribbean, India, and Europe. Initial reports linked the disease to travel to these and other underdeveloped countries. The usual mode of transmission is ingestion of fecally contaminated water or food. Most outbreaks in endemic areas occur during the rainy season.

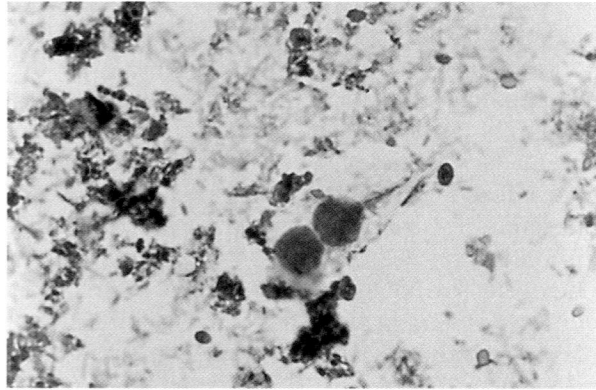

Figure 24-39 _____

Isospora belli oocysts (modified acid-fast stain).

In 1996 there were almost 1000 confirmed cases of diarrhea caused by *Cyclospora* sp., most of them associated with the consumption of contaminated fresh fruit, especially raspberries and strawberries imported from endemic areas of Central America. Although the organism is most commonly encountered in immunocompetent patients, it may be considered an opportunistic infection in patients with AIDS.

Clinical infections *C. cayetanensis* may cause prolonged but self-limiting diarrhea in both immunocompetent and immunocompromised hosts. The incubation period is approximately 1 week. The organism infects cells in the small intestine and causes frequent, watery, but nonbloody stools that may alternate with bouts of constipation. Symptoms, which may mimic those of cryptosporidiosis or isosporiasis, include anorexia, weight loss, abdominal cramping, vomiting, low-grade fever, and nausea. Patients often report a flulike syndrome before the onset of diarrhea. Symptoms persist for several weeks but may occur in a relapsing pattern for up to 2 months. Immunocompromised patients suffer a prolonged course and may be symptomatic for as long as 4 months. Some cases of malabsorption have been associated with *C. cayetanensis.* Trimethoprim-sulfamethoxazole is used to treat the infection, and once treatment is started, symptoms usually abate within several days.

Life cycle Details of the life cycle of *C. cayetanensis* have not been fully described in human beings, but the organism most likely shares the general characteristics of other intestinal Apicomplexa. The result of sexual reproduction is the immature oocyst, which is shed in feces. Unlike with *C. parvum,* however, immediate person-to-person transmission is unusual because these oocysts require several days to a week outside body to mature and become infective.

Laboratory diagnosis The oocyst is similar to that of *C. parvum* but larger, with an average size of 8 to 10 μm. In wet mounts the oocyst appears nonrefractile, spherical, and unsporulated with multiple internal globules or granules. Sporulation occurs after several days, resulting in the production of two sporocysts with two sporozoites each. The organism does not stain with traditional trichrome or iron hematoxylin stains. The modified acid-fast stain demonstrates variably staining organisms, from dark pink to almost colorless, with no visi-

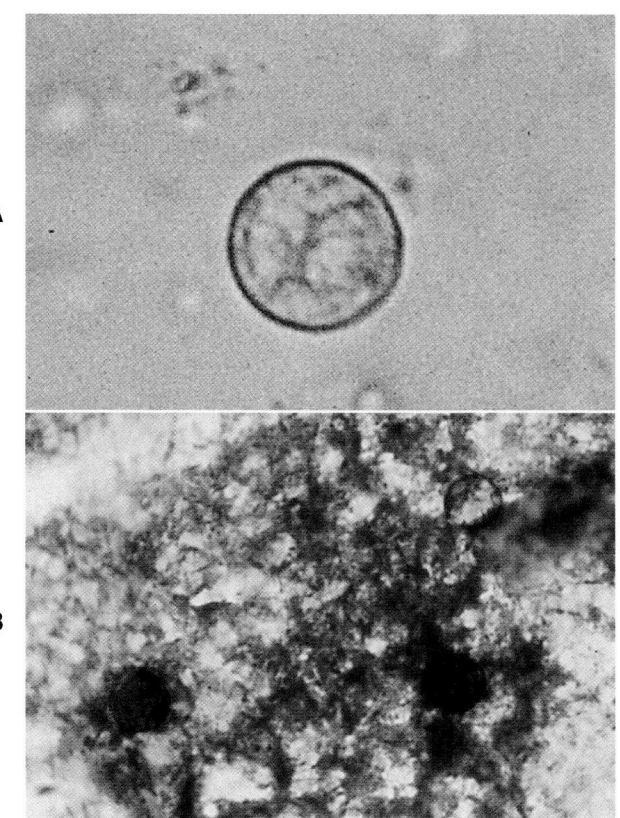

Figure 24-40

Cyclospora cayetanensis oocyst. **A,** Wet mount. **B,** Modified acid-fast stain.

ble internal structures. One distinguishing characteristic of *C. cayetanensis* is its autofluorescence. *C. cayetanensis* shows a bright blue fluorescence under ultraviolet light. Figure 24-40, *A,* shows an oocyst of *C. cayetanensis* in a wet mount, and Figure 24-40, *B,* shows an acid-fast preparation.

Microsporidia

A newly described group of organisms in the phylum Microspora have been linked to infections in patients who are infected with the human immunodeficiency virus (HIV). These organisms, collectively referred to as microsporidia, are obligate intracellular parasites common to invertebrates and other animals. A number of genera, including *Nosema, Encephalitozoon, Pleistophora, Septata,* and *Enterocytozoon,* have been implicated in human infections. Unclassified organisms usually are referred to with the encompassing term of microsporidia. These organisms most frequently have been associated with intestinal infections but have been reported to cause infections in the eyes, CNS, and liver. Disseminated infections have also been reported. The symptoms of intestinal infections are similar to those of cryptosporidiosis and are most often caused by *Enterocytozoon* or *Encephalitozoon* organisms.

Clinical infection

Chronic diarrhea with dehydration and weight loss are the predominant symptoms. Infected patients have four to eight liquid or loose stools a day, and symptoms may persist up to 8 months with spontaneous exacerbations and remissions. In some patients with AIDS the diarrhea may persist several years, with high mortality rates. In addition, *Septata intestinalis* and *Enterocytozoon bieneusi* have been linked to chronic malabsorptive diarrhea. Albendazole has been used to treat infections with *Encephalitozoon* sp., but most other microsporidial organisms are resistant to this and other drugs. Metronidazole may provide some relief, but the symptoms recur once the drug is discontinued.

Life cycle

The organisms reproduce by a combination of asexual and sexual methods. Once the infective spore is ingested, it gains access to host cells by inserting a coiled tube (polar filament) through the cell membrane. The contents of the spore (sporoplasm) are then transferred into the new cell. Within the cell binary fission (schizogony) and a sexual cycle may occur, resulting in the production of spores. The host cell ruptures, and spores are released into the stool or can penetrate other host tissue cells to repeat the reproductive cycle in the host.

Laboratory diagnosis

Initially, identification methods were limited to finding the small one or two spores in Giemsa-stained tissue sections or in electron microscopic examination of biopsy specimens. Electron microscopy must be used to identify the species of the organism. Speciation is based on the number of coils in the polar tubule, septations in the spore, and size. Routine ova and parasite examination will not detect the spores in a fecal specimen. However, staining of formalin-preserved feces using modified trichrome procedures allows identification in the clinical laboratory. The Weber modification of the trichrome stain and the Ryan trichrome blue stain can be used to detect microsporidial spores in stool specimens. Figure 24-41 shows the spores in a chromotrope stain of a fecal specimen. Spores stain pink-red and may have a diagonal or equatorial band that helps distinguish them from bacteria or yeast. Background staining in Weber stain is pale green, whereas in Ryan stain it is blue. A thin smear of feces must be used so that debris does not obscure the small, faintly staining spores. Calcofluor white, a stain used for fluorescent detection of yeast and fungi, can also be used to screen for microsporidia spores. The stain is nonspecific, and the presence of spores should be confirmed using one of the modified trichrome stains. Polymerase chain reaction (PCR) amplification methods, as well as monoclonal and polyclonal antibodies for fluorescent staining procedures, are under development.

Helminths

Helminth infections in human beings are caused by flukes, tapeworms, or roundworms. Human beings may become infected by directly ingesting the egg, by ingesting larvae in an intermediate host, or through direct larval penetration of skin. Adult forms do not multiply in the human body; therefore, the number of adult worms present is related to the number of egg or larvae ingested. The pathologic consequences and severity of infec-

tion are related to the number of adults present, commonly referred to as the **worm burden.** The patient with only a few adults is usually asymptomatic, whereas a patient with a large number of adults shows clinical symptoms. Most of the parasites are in the intestinal tract, but species also inhabit the liver, lungs, lymphatics, and blood vessels. Because of the variety of body sites that can be infected, clinical symptoms are described with each organism.

Flukes

Flukes (trematodes) are members of the phylum Platyhelminthes, or flatworms. Most infections are seen in people from the Orient, Africa, South America, and some areas of the Caribbean. Adults can range in size from several millimeters to almost 8 cm. With the exception of the blood flukes, adult flukes are dorsoventrally flattened and have an oral sucker at the anterior end and a ventral sucker located midline, posterior to the anterior sucker. Also except for the blood flukes, flukes are hermaphroditic. In all species eggs must reach water to mature, and all have a snail species as the first intermediate host.

LIFE CYCLE
Figure 24-42 shows a generalized life cycle of the liver, lung, and intestinal flukes. The miracidium (first-stage larva) is ingested by a snail while within the egg or is released from eggs and penetrates the snail, which serves as the first intermediate host. Within the snail tissue, a complex development of germinal tissue occurs resulting first in sporocysts, which contain undifferentiated germinal structures, and then in rediae, which contain partially differentiated germinal material. The **cercaria** (second-stage larva) develops within the redia and is released into the water. The cercaria then attaches to aquatic vegetation or invades the flesh of aquatic organisms. At this stage the organism is referred to as a **metacercaria** and is infective for human beings. With the exception of the schistosomes, which infect human beings by direct cercarial penetration, infection occurs when a person ingests the metacercaria in raw or undercooked aquatic animals or on water vegetation. Prevention includes adequate cooking of water vegetation, fish, and crustaceans. In the case of the blood flukes, people should wear clothing and

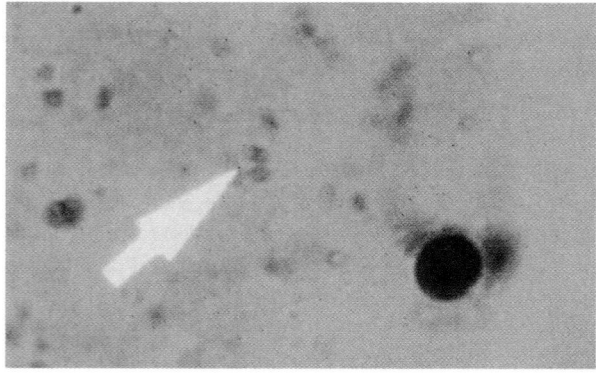

Figure 24-41
Microsporidia spores (chromotrope stain). (Courtesy Texas Department of Health.)

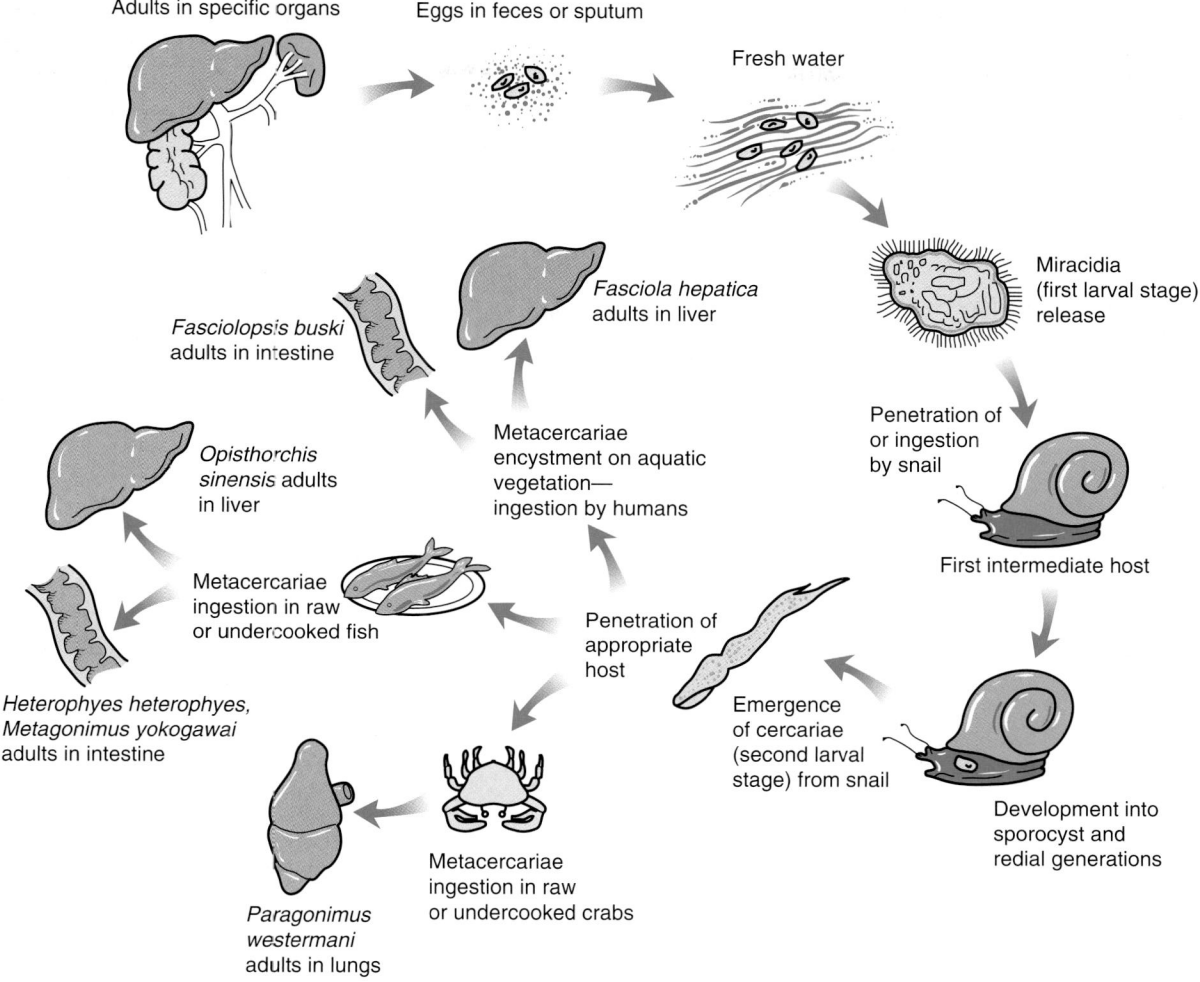

Adults in specific organs

Eggs in feces or sputum

Fresh water

Miracidia
(first larval stage)
release

Fasciola hepatica
adults in liver

Penetration of
or ingestion
by snail

Fasciolopsis buski
adults in intestine

First intermediate host

Metacercariae
encystment on aquatic
vegetation—
ingestion by humans

*Opisthorchis
sinensis* adults
in liver

Metacercariae
ingestion in raw
or undercooked fish

Penetration of
appropriate
host

Emergence
of cercariae
(second larval
stage) from snail

*Heterophyes heterophyes,
Metagonimus yokogawai*
adults in intestine

Development into
sporocyst and
redial generations

Metacercariae
ingestion in raw
or undercooked crabs

*Paragonimus
westermani*
adults in lungs

Figure 24-42
Life cycle of liver, lung, and intestinal flukes.

shoes to prevent cercarial penetration. The drug of choice for treating fluke infections, regardless of body site, is praziquantel.

LABORATORY DIAGNOSIS
The egg is the primary diagnostic stage. It is best detected on a wet mount of a concentrated specimen. Routine concentration procedures such as formalin–ethyl acetate may be used. The zinc sulfate method is not satisfactory, however, because all eggs except those of schistosomes are operculated. With the zinc sulfate method, the operculum may open and release the contents or sink. Table 24-7 shows a comparison of the characteristics of the fluke eggs.

INTESTINAL FLUKES
Fasciolopsis buski, known as the giant intestinal fluke, is found in the Far East, including China, Vietnam, and India. Dogs and pigs may serve as reservoir hosts. Human beings acquire the infection by ingesting metacercaria on freshwater vegetation such as bamboo shoots and water chestnuts. Adults of *F. buski* live in the duodenum, where they cause mechanical and toxic damage. Inflammation and ulceration of the mucosa may be present. Heavy infections may result in persistent diarrhea, anorexia, edema, ascites, nausea and vomiting, or intestinal obstruction.

Finding the adult or egg is diagnostic, although the egg is more commonly seen. The adult is flat-

TABLE 24-7

Comparison of Fluke Eggs

Organism	Average Size (μm) and Shape	Other Identifying Features
Fasciola hepatica	130 × 60-90 Ellipsoidal	Small, indistinct operculum Yellow-brown color Unembryonated when passed
Fasciolopsis buski	130 × 80-85 Ellipsoidal	Cannot be distinguished from *F. hepatica* Unembryonated when passed
Paragonimus westermani	80-118 × 48-60 Oval	Brown, thick shell Slightly flattened operculum Shoulders at operculum Unembryonated when passed
Opisthorchis sinensis	29-35 × 12-19 Vase shaped	Domed operculum Prominent shoulders Knob at end opposite operculum Embryonated when passed
Heterophyes heterophyes and *Metagonimus yokogawai* **Note:** These two species are virtually indistinguishable.	28-30 × 15-17 Vase shaped	Operculated Shoulders not distinct Small knob Embryonated Similar to *O. sinensis*
Schistosoma mansoni	115-175 × 45-75 Oval	Lateral spine No operculum Embryonated when passed
Schistosoma haematobium	110-170 × 40-70 Oval	Rounded anterior Terminal spine Embryonated when passed
Schistosoma japonicum	60-95 × 40-60 Round to slightly oval	Small, inconspicuous, hooked lateral spine Embryonated when passed

tened, is 2 to 7 cm long, and lacks the cephalic cone seen in *Fasciola hepatica.* Adults are usually not seen in a stool specimen unless it is a purged specimen. Eggs are yellow-brown, average 130 to 140 by 80 to 85 μm, and have a small, relatively in-conspicuous operculum. They are unembryonated when passed (Figure 24-43).

Metagonimus yokogawai and *Heterophyes heterophyes* are two small flukes found in the Far East and Mideast. Human beings acquire infection with

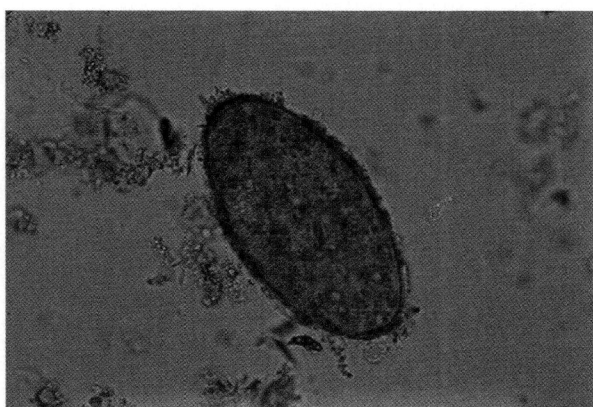

Figure 24-43 _____

Fasciola hepatica/Fasciolopsis buski egg.

these organisms by ingesting the metacercaria in undercooked or raw fish. Adults live in the small intestine and produce few symptoms. A patient with a heavy worm burden may have diarrhea, colic, and stools with a large amount of mucus. Adults of both species are small (1 to 2 mm) and delicate. Eggs serve as the primary diagnostic stage. They are 28 to 30 μm long and have a vase or flask shape. They are embryonated and operculated with inconspicuous shoulders at the operculum. Eggs of these species resemble each other as well as those of *Opisthorchis sinensis.*

LIVER FLUKES

Fasciola hepatica, the sheep liver fluke, is seen in the major sheep-raising areas of the world, including parts of the southwestern United States. In sheep, the organism causes a disease known as liver rot, which is characterized by destruction of the liver. Human beings acquire the infection by ingesting metacercaria on raw water vegetation, especially watercress. The larvae reach the liver by migrating through the intestinal wall and peritoneal cavity. Adults live in the biliary passages and gallbladder and rarely cause overt symptoms because infections are light. Tissue damage during migration through the liver may result in an inflammatory reaction, secondary infection, and fibrosis in the biliary ducts. Heavy infections may induce diarrhea, abdominal pain, hepatomegaly, cirrhosis, and liver obstruction, with resulting jaundice.

Adults are approximately 3 cm long and have a prominent cephalic cone. The unembryonated and

operculated eggs are carried in the bile to the intestinal tract and are passed in the feces. The size range is 130 to 150 by 60 to 90 μm. They are virtually indistinguishable from eggs of *F. buski* (see Figure 24-43). Eggs that have these characteristics should be reported as "*F. buski/F. hepatica* eggs seen."

The Chinese liver fluke, *Opisthorchis sinensis,* is geographically limited to the Far East, where dogs and cats serve as reservoir hosts. The adults live in the distal bile ducts. As with *F. hepatica,* light infections produce few or no symptoms. Repeated or heavy infections may cause inflammation due to mechanical irritation, fever, diarrhea, pain, fibrotic changes, or obstruction of the bile duct. Humans acquire the infection by ingesting the metacercaria in raw, undercooked, or pickled fish. The diagnosis is made by finding the egg in a stool specimen or, occasionally, in duodenal aspirates. Adults are thin, tapered at both ends, and 1 to 2.5 cm long. The egg is 29 to 35 μm long, embryonated when passed, flask shaped, and operculated with prominent shoulders at the operculum and a knob at the opposite end (Figure 24-44).

LUNG FLUKE

Organisms of the genus *Paragonimus* usually infect tigers, leopards, dogs, and foxes. *Paragonimus westermani,* the lung fluke, is primarily found in the Orient, where human beings acquire the infection by ingesting metacercaria in raw, pickled, or undercooked freshwater crabs or crayfish. The metacercaria excysts in the intes-

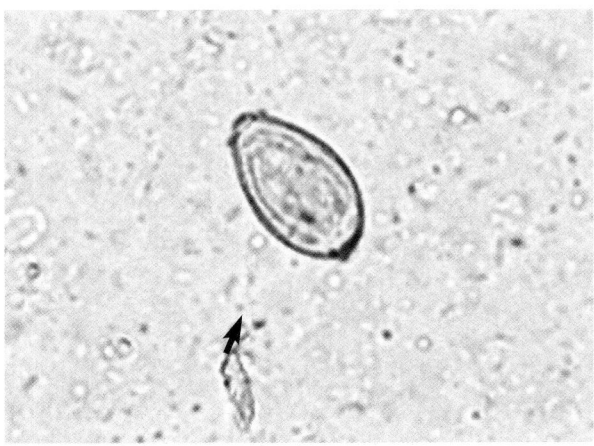

Figure 24-44 _____

Opisthorchis sinensis egg.

tine and burrows through the intestinal wall and diaphragm, eventually entering the lung. The host shows few symptoms during this migration. Major symptoms associated with lung habitation are nonspecific and may include an inflammatory response, persistent cough, chest pain, and hemoptysis. Adults, which are reddish brown and approximately 1 cm long, live within capsules in the bronchioles.

Sputum is the primary diagnostic specimen. Eggs are expelled from the capsule into the bronchioles and carried upward in the sputum. Eggs may be found in the feces if they have been coughed up and subsequently swallowed. Eggs are broadly oval, 80 to 118 by 48 to 60 μm, with a flattened operculum and slight shoulders. They are unembryonated when passed. The shell thickens at the end opposite the operculum (Figure 24-45). These eggs can appear similar to those of *Diphyllobothrium latum* and must be carefully examined when seen in the feces. A wet mount of sputum demonstrates the egg in some patients.

BLOOD FLUKES

The blood flukes, *Schistosoma* spp., differ from other flukes in that:

- There is both a male and a female. (The female lives in an involuted chamber, the gynecophoral canal, that extends the length of the male.)
- The eggs are unoperculated.

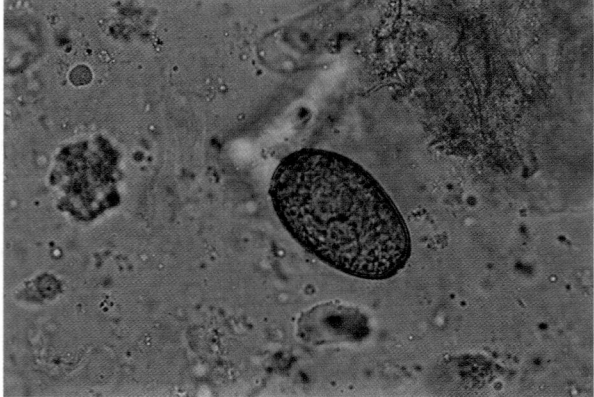

Figure 24-45 _____

Paragonimus westermani egg.

- Human beings are infected by direct cercarial penetration of the skin.
- They have a cylindric shape rather than being dorsoventrally flattened.

The three primary species of schistosomes pathogenic to human beings are *S. mansoni, S. haematobium,* and *S. japonicum. S. mansoni,* which is most commonly found in Africa, parts of South America, the West Indies, and Puerto Rico, lives in venules of the large intestine. *S. japonicum,* which is commonly found in the Far East, including Japan, China. and the Philippines, lives in venules of the small intestine. This species, unlike the other two, has many mammalian reservoir hosts. *S. haematobium,* which is primarily found in the Nile Valley, the Mideast, and East Africa, lives in the veins surrounding the bladder. Adults measure 7 to 20 mm for males and 7 to 26 mm for females.

Clinical infection Schistosomiasis (bilharziasis), has a prevalence of about 200 million cases worldwide. The term is used to describe symptoms caused by any of the schistosomes. Symptoms are related to the phases of the fluke's life cycle. Cercarial penetration may cause local dermatitis, including irritation, redness, and rash, that persists for about 3 days. Larval migration through the body causes generalized symptoms such as urticaria, fever, and malaise, which may last up to 4 weeks. Adults in and of themselves cause little inflammatory damage because they acquire host antigens on their surface that diminish the host's immune response. Egg production and migration through the tissues are responsible for the most acute damage. After the adult female dilates the vein to lay eggs, the vein contracts, and aided by secretion of enzymes, the eggs begin to penetrate vessel walls and tissue. Eggs subsequently find their way into the lumen of the intestine or bladder. The egg spines cause trauma to the tissues and walls of the vessels during the early stage of acute infections and may result in hematuria *(S. haematobium)* or diarrhea *(S. mansoni* and *S. japonicum).*

In chronic infections, the eggs remaining in the tissue induce granuloma formation, which leads to thickening and fibrotic changes. Scarring of the veins, development of ascites, pain, anemia, hypertension, hepatomegaly, and splenomegaly are also seen. In urinary schistosomiasis, microscopic bleeding into the urine is present during the acute

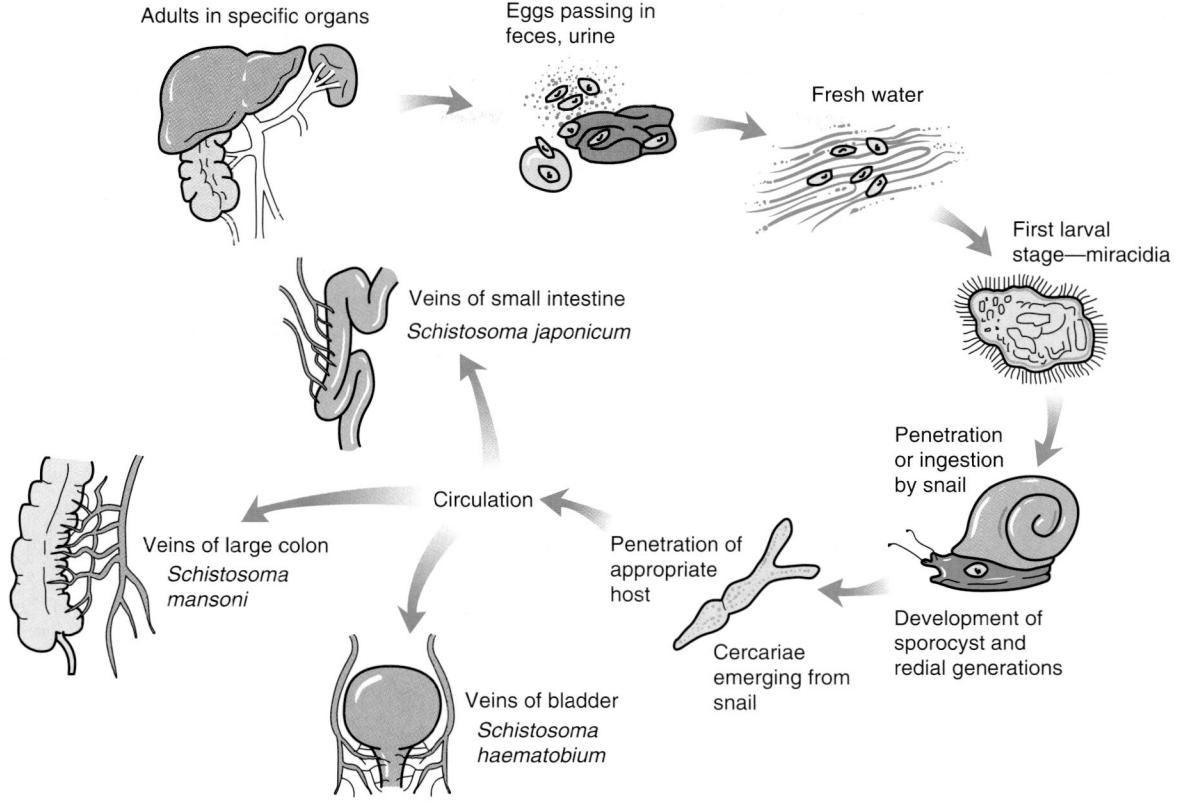

Figure 24-46

Life cycle of blood flukes (*Schistosoma* spp.).

phase. In chronic stages, dysuria, urine retention, and urinary tract infections are present.

Life cycle The life cycles of all three schistosomes are identical (Figure 24-46). The eggs are embryonated when passed, and the miracidium is released when the egg reaches water. After penetrating the snail (first intermediate host), sporocysts and then cercaria are produced during a 6-week period. Cercaria migrate from the snail into water. When the cercaria encounter the skin of a human being, they shed their forked tails, secrete enzymes, and begin penetration. Once in the veins, they are referred to as schistosomula. They circulate until they reach the lungs or enter the liver, where maturation is completed. The paired adult flukes use the portal system to reach veins of the intestine or bladder.

Laboratory diagnosis Diagnosis is made by finding embryonated eggs in the feces *S. mansoni* and *S. japonicum)* or in the urine *(S. haematobium)*. The egg of *S. mansoni* (Figure 24-47, *A*) is yellowish, elongated, and 115 to 175 by 45 to 75 μm, and has a prominent lateral spine. *S. haematobium* eggs (Figure 24-47, *B*) are elongated and 110 to 170 by 40 to 70 μm, and have a terminal spine. *S. japonicum* eggs (Figure 24-47, *C*) are round and 60 to 95 by 40 to 60 μm, and have a small, curved, rudimentary spine. The best time to collect eggs in urinary schistosomiasis is during peak excretion time in early afternoon (12 PM to 2 PM). Hatching tests and biopsies may also be used in the diagnosis of schistosomiasis. Serodiagnosis may be useful to diagnose infection in patients from nonendemic countries who develop symptoms after visiting endemic areas.

SCHISTOSOMAL DERMATITIS

Penetration of human beings by cercaria of the flukes of birds and other mammals causes a dermatitis commonly referred to as *swimmer's itch*. Foreign proteins from these cercaria elicit a tissue

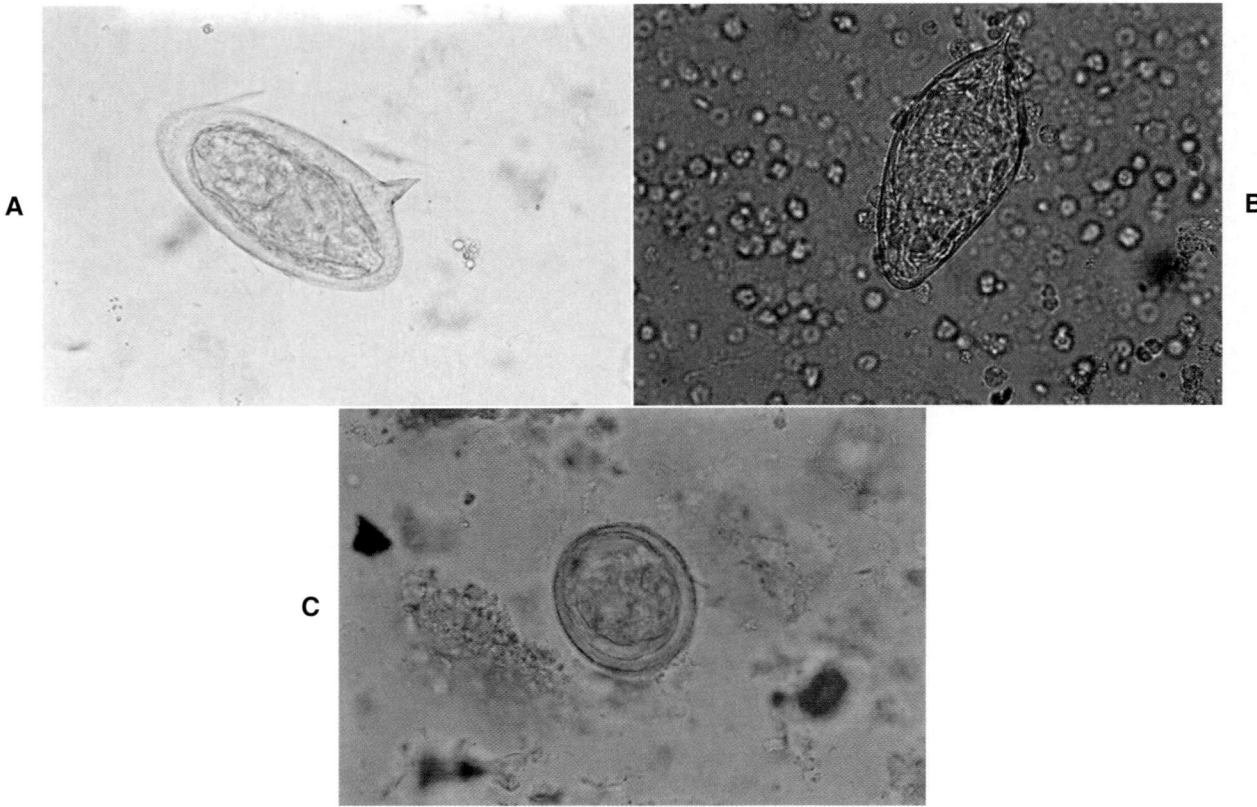

Figure 24-47

A, *Schistosoma mansoni* egg. **B,** *Schistosoma haematobium* egg. Notice red blood cells in background. **C,** *Schistosoma japonicum* egg.

reaction characterized by small papules 3 to 5 mm in diameter, edema, erythema, and intense itching. Symptoms last about a week and disappear as cercaria die and degenerate.

Tapeworms

Tapeworms (cestodes) are the second group of human parasites in the phylum Platyhelminthes. They show a wide range of sizes, from 3 mm to 10 m, generally require intermediate hosts in their life cycle, and are hermaphroditic. They are ribbonlike organisms whose method of growth involves the addition of segments, called proglottids. Each **proglottid,** when mature, produces eggs that are infective for the intermediate host. Figure 24-48 shows a general diagram of the tapeworm. The **scolex,** or head, has suckers and, in some species, hooklets as a means of attachment to the intestinal mucosa. The neck is

directly behind the scolex. Treatment is targeted at detaching the scolex from the mucosa, because the neck area is the origin of proglottid production. Gravid proglottids at the distal end of the organism contain eggs to be discharged into the feces.

Eggs of most of the tapeworms contain a **hexacanth embryo (oncosphere)** that is infective for the intermediate host. Transmission to human beings involves ingestion either of a larval stage, called the **cysticercus,** cysticercoid, or plerocercoid larva in raw or undercooked meat or fish or of insects harboring the larval stage. This larval stage contains an invaginated scolex of the tapeworm inside a protective membrane. The diagnosis of tapeworm infection is usually made by finding the eggs in feces, although proglottids can be used if passed intact. Table 24-8 presents a comparison of the characteristics of tapeworm eggs.

DIPHYLLOBOTHRIUM LATUM

Diphyllobothrium latum, the fish tapeworm, is found worldwide in areas where the population eats pickled or raw freshwater fish. In the United States, it is primarily seen in the areas around the Great Lakes. Fish-eating mammals in endemic areas may also be infected.

Clinical infection Human beings usually harbor only a single worm, which attaches in the jejunum and may reach a length of up to 10 m. Most infected individuals demonstrate no clinical symptoms; others have vague gastrointestinal symptoms, including nausea and vomiting and intestinal irritation. The organism competes with the host for vitamin B_{12}, and long-term infection may lead to a megaloblastic anemia. The treatment of choice is niclosamine, although quinacrine hydrochloride has been used.

Life cycle The life cycle of *D. latum* is somewhat of a hybrid between that of the flukes and that of the tapeworms. The operculated, unembryonated egg, which is passed in human feces, must reach water to mature. The first larval stage (coracidium) is ingested by a copepod and develops into

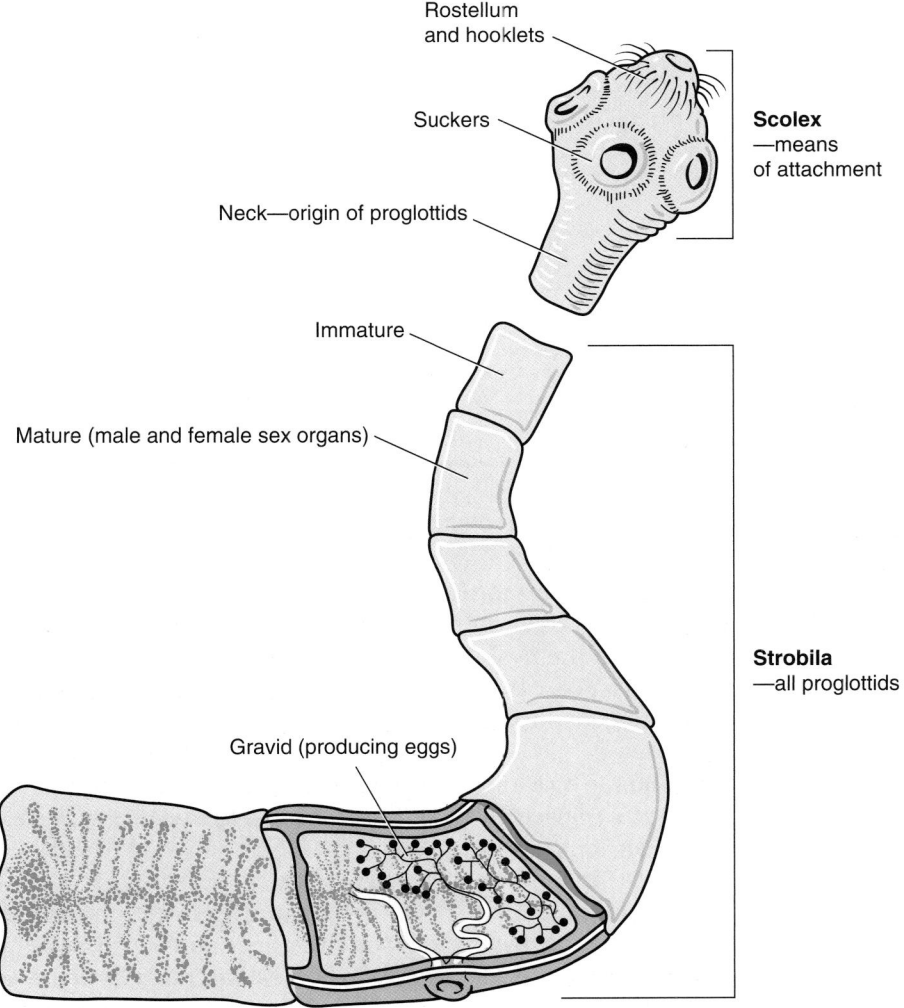

Figure 24-48

Diagram of a tapeworm.

TABLE 24-8

Comparison of Tapeworm Eggs

Organism	Average Size (μm) and Shape	Other Identifying Features
Diphyllobothrium latum	58-76 × 40-50 Oval	Inconspicuous operculum Small knob at end opposite operculum Unembryonated when passed
Taenia spp.	30-45 Round	Thick, brown, radially striated shell Embryonated with six-hooked oncosphere when passed
Hymenolepis nana	30-47 Oval	Two membranes—inner has two polar knobs, from which four polar filaments extend into space between inner and outer membranes Embryonated with six-hooked oncosphere when passed
Hymenolepis diminuta	50-75 Round to slightly oval	Two membranes—inner has very slight polar knobs No polar filaments Embryonated with six-hooked oncosphere when passed
Dipylidium caninum	20-40 (each egg) Round Resembles *Taenia* spp.	Eggs passed in a packet of 15-25 Eggs embryonated with six-hooked oncosphere when passed

a procercoid larva within the copepod. When the infected copepod is ingested by a fish, the larva leaves the fish's intestine and invades the flesh, where it develops into a plerocercoid larva, which consists of a scolex with a thin, ribbonlike portion of tissue.

Humans ingest the plerocercoid larvae by eating raw or undercooked fish. The scolex is released in the intestine, where it develops into an adult worm. Figure 24-49 shows the life cycle of *D. latum*.

Laboratory diagnosis The scolex, proglottid, or egg may be used as a diagnostic finding in a fecal specimen. The egg is unembryonated when passed, operculated, and yellow-brown (Figure 24-50). It is about 58 to 76 by 40 to 50 μm and has a small, knoblike protuberance at the end opposite the operculum. The knob may not be seen on all eggs, so size and lack of shoulders must be used to distinguish the egg from that of *P. westermani*. The proglottid is wider than it is long, with a characteristic rosette-shaped or coiled uterus. The scolex, which is 2 to 3 mm long, is elongated and has two sucking grooves, one located on the dorsal surface and the other on the ventral surface.

TAENIA SPECIES

Two *Taenia* species infect human beings—*Taenia saginata,* the beef tapeworm, which is found primarily in beef-eating countries of the world, and *Taenia solium,* the pork tapeworm, which is found in those areas of the world, such as Latin America, with a high consumption of pork. Both organisms attach

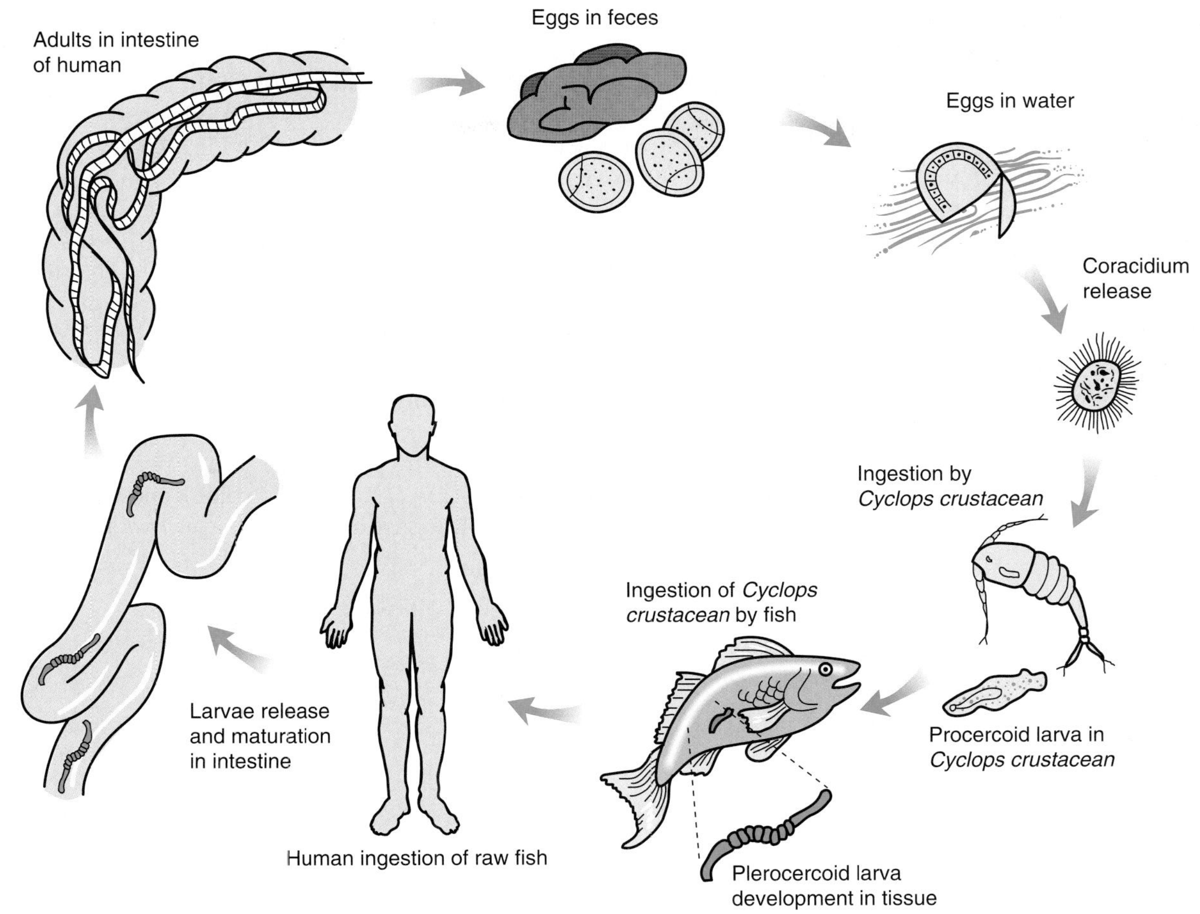

Adults in intestine of human

Eggs in feces

Eggs in water

Coracidium release

Ingestion by *Cyclops crustacean*

Procercoid larva in *Cyclops crustacean*

Ingestion of *Cyclops crustacean* by fish

Plerocercoid larva development in tissue

Human ingestion of raw fish

Larvae release and maturation in intestine

Figure 24-49

Life cycle of *Diphyllobothrium latum*.

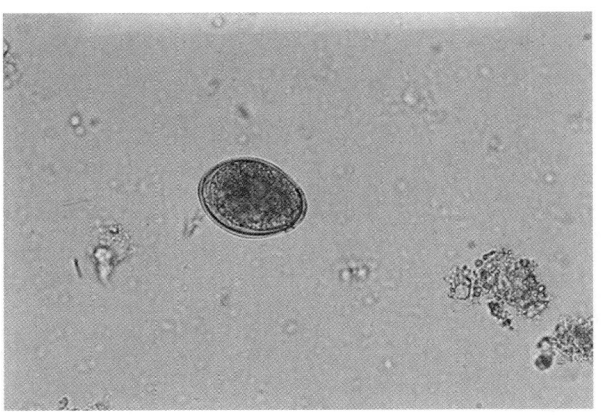

Figure 24-50

Diphyllobothrium latum egg.

to the intestinal mucosa of the small intestine. Adults of *T. saginata* may reach a length of 10 m, whereas those of *T. solium* may reach only 7 m.

Clinical infection Infection with the adult tapeworm of either species usually causes few clinical symptoms, although vague abdominal pain, indigestion, and loss of appetite may be present. The proglottids are motile and, if broken off in the intestinal tract, may actively migrate out the anus.

The major complication of infection with *T. solium* is cysticercosis, in which the human being becomes the intermediate host and harbors the larvae in tissues. This infection is discussed in the section on tissue infections.

Life cycle As previously mentioned, the life cycles of the two *Taenia* organisms are identical except for the fact that human beings may also serve as

intermediate hosts for *T. solium.* Embryonated eggs are passed in human feces and ingested by the intermediate host. The oncosphere is freed in the intestinal tract, migrates through the intestinal wall, and gains access via the circulatory system to the muscles of the host, where it transforms into a cysticercus. When human beings ingest raw or undercooked meat, the scolex within the cysticercus is freed, attaches in the human small intestine, and matures into the adult tapeworm within 10 weeks. Figure 24-51 shows the life cycle of *Taenia* spp.

Laboratory diagnosis Diagnosis of *Taenia* sp. infection can be made by finding the egg, scolex, of proglottid in the feces. The egg is yellow-brown, round, and surrounded by a thick wall with radial striations; it measures 30 to 43 μm. The egg is em-

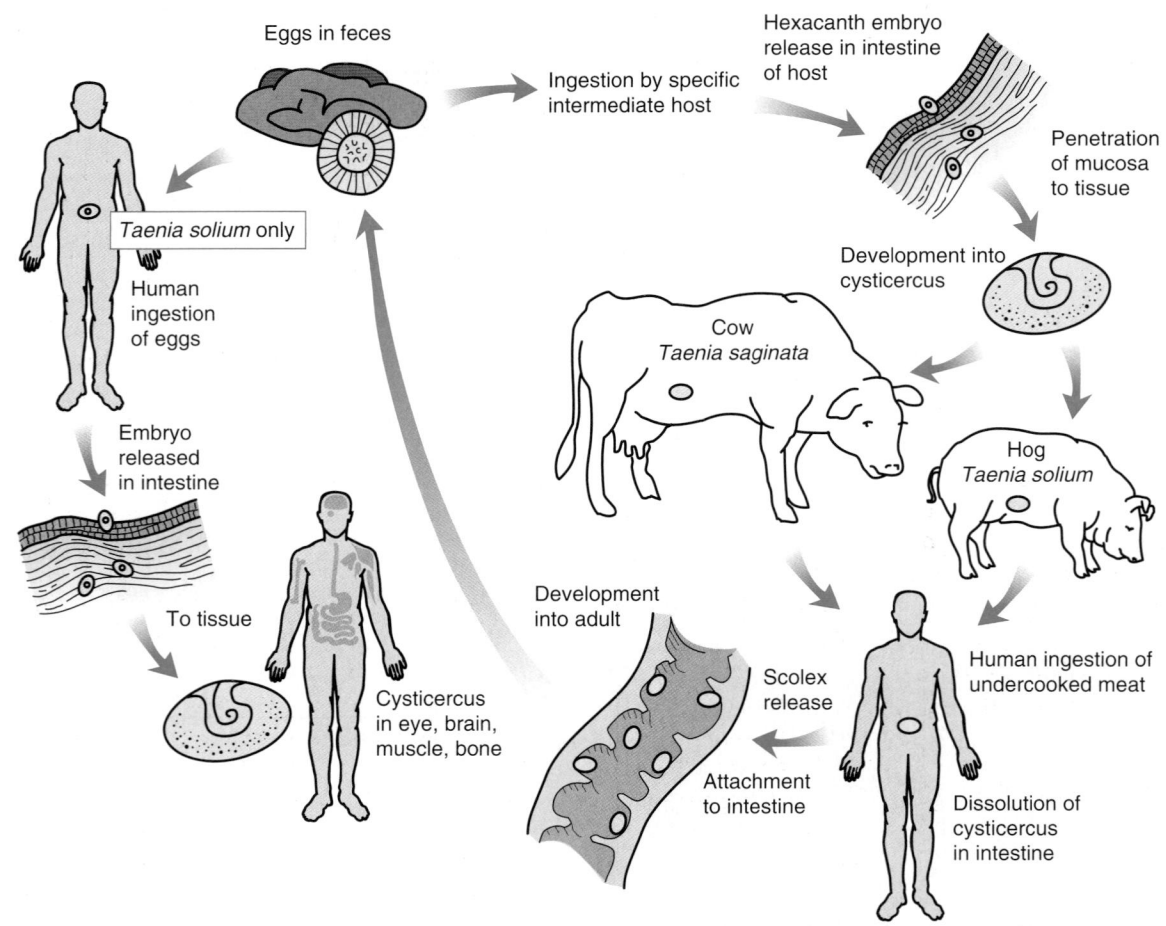

Figure 24-51 _____

Life cycle of *Taenia* spp.

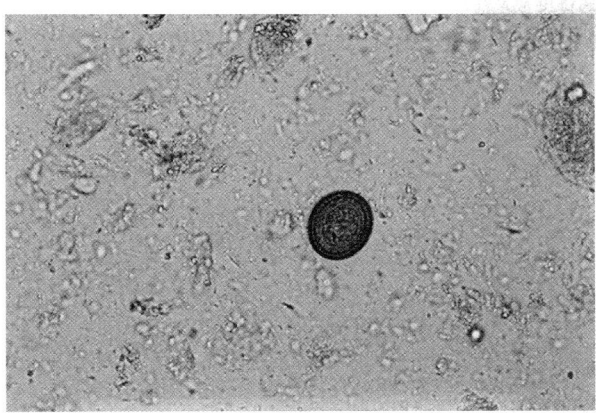

Figure 24-52
Taenia sp. egg.

bryonated with a six-hooked oncosphere (hexacanth embryo) when passed in the feces (Figure 24-52). Eggs of these species are indistinguishable and must be reported as "*Taenia* sp. eggs." Gravid proglottids may be seen in the stool specimen and can be used to differentiate the two organisms. Proglottids of *T. solium* show 7 to 13 primary uterine branches on each side of the main uterine trunk, whereas proglottids of *T. saginata* show 15 to 20 per side. The scolex, if found, can also be used to distinguish the organisms. The scolex of *T. saginata* is less than 5 mm long and has four suckers, whereas that of *T. solium* has a rostellum with a double row of 25 to 30 hooklets in addition to the four suckers.

HYMENOLEPIS SPP.
The dwarf tapeworm, *Hymenolepis nana,* is found worldwide and is a common tapeworm in children whereas *Hymenolepis diminuta,* the rat tapeworm, is less frequently seen. Light infections are usually asymptomatic; large numbers of worms may cause abdominal pain, diarrhea, irritability, and headache. Infections with *H. nana* are easily transmitted among children, because an intermediate host is not required. Direct fecal-oral transmission of the egg, development of the cysticercoid in the intestinal tissue of the host, and reentry into the lumen for development into an adult characterize the life cycle (Figure 24-53). An insect vector may serve as intermediate host.
Laboraotry diagnosis The adult of *H. nana* is 40 mm long and has a small scolex with four suckers and a rostellum with spines. The primary

method of diagnosis is finding the egg in a stool specimen. The egg is spherical to oval, measures 30 to 47 μm, and has a grayish color. The hexacanth embryo is contained within an inner membrane, and the area between the inner membrane and egg wall contains two polar thickenings from which four to eight polar filaments extend (Figure 24-54).

Infection with *H. diminuta* is acquired by ingesting fleas that contain the infective cysticercoid. The adult is 20 to 60 cm long. The egg, which must be distinguished from that of *H. nana,* is 50 to 75 μm, gray or straw colored, and oval. An inner membrane with inconspicuous polar thickenings but no polar filaments surrounds the oncosphere (Figure 24-55).

DIPYLIDIUM CANINUM
The human being serves as an accidental host for *Dipylidium caninum,* the dog tapeworm. Children are most often infected by ingesting fleas containing the larval stage. The infections are usually asymptomatic. The proglottid may be seen in human feces and is characterized by its pumpkin seed shape, twin genitalia, and the presence of two genital pores, one on each side of the proglottid. The eggs are characteristically seen in packets of 15 to 25 eggs. Individual eggs are 20 to 40 μm and may resemble those of *Taenia* spp. (Figure 24-56).

Tissue infections with cestodes
Cysticercosis, sparganosis, and hydatid cyst disease are the major diseases caused by the tissue stage of the tapeworm. They originate when a human being accidentally becomes the intermediate host for the parasite.

CYSTICERCOSIS
Cysticercosis results when a human ingests the eggs of *T. solium,* the pork tapeworm. The hexacanth embryo is released in the intestine, penetrates the intestinal wall, and enters the circulation to develop as a cysticercus in any tissue or organ. The living organism may elicit a host-tissue reaction, resulting in production of fibrous capsule. Once the larva has died, an increased inflammatory reaction and eventual calcification occur. The most commonly infected sites are striated muscle, the eye, and the brain.

Light infections usually cause no clinical symptoms. When present, symptoms depend on the or-

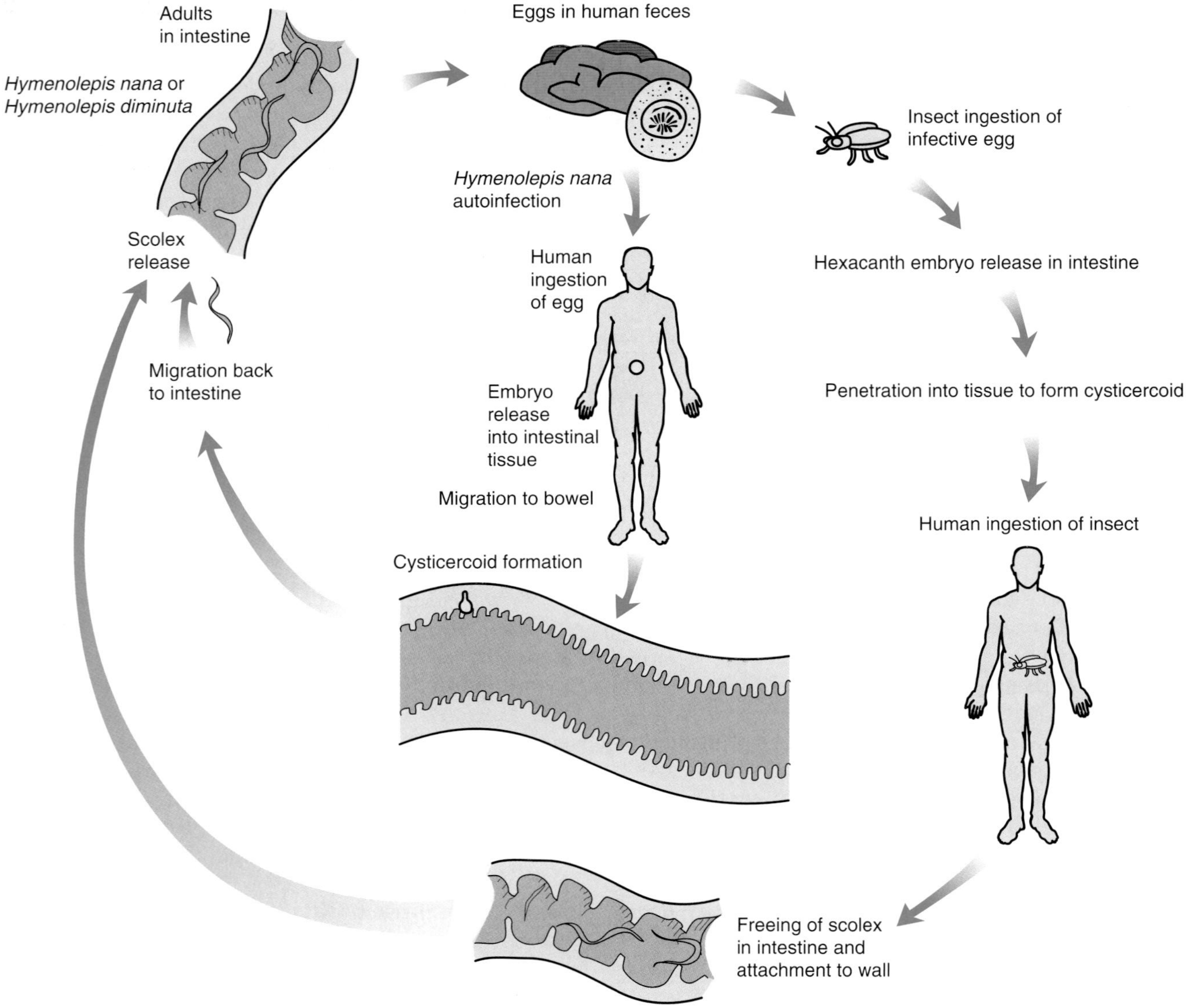

Adults
in intestine

Hymenolepis nana or
Hymenolepis diminuta

Scolex
release

Eggs in human feces

Insect ingestion of
infective egg

Hymenolepis nana
autoinfection

Human
ingestion
of egg

Hexacanth embryo release in intestine

Migration back
to intestine

Embryo
release
into intestinal
tissue

Penetration into tissue to form cysticercoid

Migration to bowel

Human ingestion of insect

Cysticercoid formation

Freeing of scolex
in intestine and
attachment to wall

Figure 24-53 _____

Life cycle of *Hymenolepis nana*.

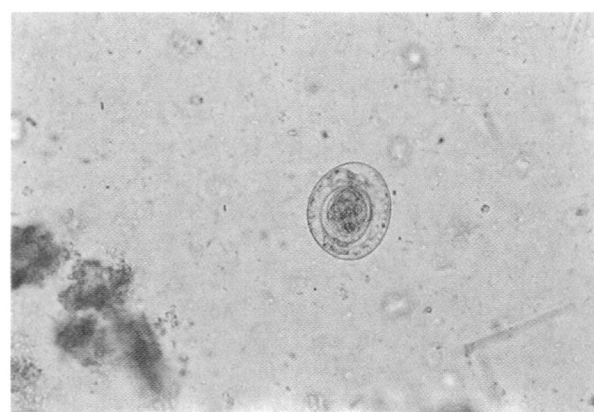

Figure 24-54 _____

Hymenolepis nana egg.

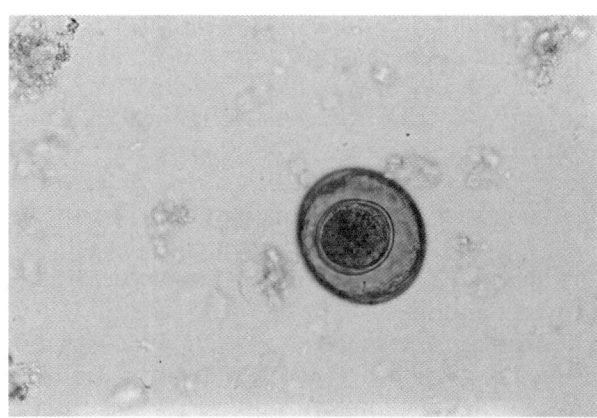

Figure 24-55 _____

Hymenolepis diminuta egg.

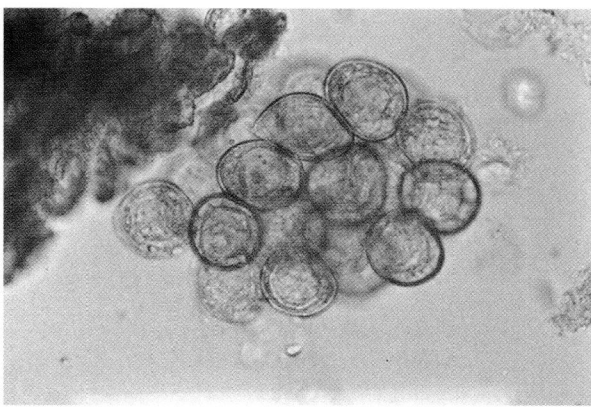

Figure 24-56

Dipylidium caninum egg packet.

gan affected. Muscular pain, weakness, and cramps characterize infections of the striated muscle. Neurocysticercosis may be manifested by headaches, symptoms resembling those seen with meningitis or a brain tumor, convulsions, or a variety of motor and sensory problems. In the eye, a cysticercus forms in the vitreous or supretinal space. Retinal detachment, intraorbital pain, flashes of light, and blurred vision may occur.

The cysticercus is oval, translucent, and about 2 to 5 mm in size. It contains an invaginated scolex containing four suckers and a circle of hooklets on the rostellum. Diagnosis of the infection may be made by a variety of methods, including:

- Radiography to detect calcified cysts
- Examination of the eye with the ophthalmoscope to detect cysticerci
- Imaging techniques to locate larva in the brain
- Biopsy and histologic staining of tissue

SPARGANOSIS

Human infection with the plerocercoid larva (sparganum) of a dog or cat tapeworm can result in sparganosis. Human beings acquire the infection by ingesting a copepod containing the procercoid larva, by ingesting reptiles, amphibians, or other animals containing the plerocercoid larva, or through invasion by the plerocercoid larva when the raw tissue from the second intermediate host is used as a poultice. The disease is most common in Southeast Asia. An infection is often seen in the eye after a poultice has been applied to relive an infection. The organism may also cause migratory subcutaneous nodules, itching, and pain. The diagnosis of sparganosis is made by finding a small, white, ribbonlike organism with a rudimentary scolex. Size varies from a few millimeters to 40 cm. The organism may be removed surgically.

ECHINOCOCCOSIS

Echinococcosis (hydatid cyst disease) is an infection by *Echinococcus granulosus* that normally involves the dog or other member of the family Candidae as the definitive host. Sheep and other herbivores are the usual host of the larval stage (hydatid cyst). The disease is primarily seen in sheep-raising areas of the world, including Australia, southern South America, and parts of the southwestern United States.

The adult worm is about 5 mm long and contains only three proglottids. The eggs are found in the feces of the dog or other definitive host and resemble those of *Taenia* sp.

A human being becomes an intermediate host by accidentally ingesting the eggs of *E. granulosus* containing the hexacanth embryo. The oncosphere is liberated in the intestine, penetrates the mucosa, enters the circulation, and usually lodges in the liver. The embryo develops a central cavity–like structure lined with a germinal membrane, from which blood capsules and protoscolices (hydatid sand) develop. The hydatid cyst's size is limited by the organ in which it develops. In bone, a limiting membrane never develops, so the cyst fills the marrow and eventually erodes the bone.

Symptoms vary according to the organ infected. Pressure from the increasing size of a cyst may cause necrosis of surrounding tissue. Rupture of the cyst liberates large amounts of foreign protein that may elicit an anaphylactic response. In addition, freed germinal epithelium may serve as a source of new infection.

The diagnosis may be made by radiologic examination, ultrasound, or other imaging techniques. Aspiration of the cyst contents usually reveals the presence of protoscolices.

Roundworms

Roundworms that infect human beings include those that occupy the intestinal tract and those that occupy blood and tissue. These organisms, found worldwide, may be transmitted by ingestion of the embryonated egg or by direct penetration of the

TABLE 24-9

Comparison of Intestinal Roundworm Eggs and Larvae

Organism	Average Size (μm) and Shape	Other Identifying Features
Ascaris lumbricoides Fertile	45-75 × 35-50 Oval	Bile-stained shell Bumpy, mammillated In one-cell stage when passed Some eggs may be decorticated (lack mammillated coat)
Infertile	85-95 × 43-47 Oval (some bizarrely shaped)	Mammillated Thin shell Undifferentiated internal granules
Enterobius vermicularis	50-60 × 20-30 Oval, flattened on one side	Colorless shell Usually embryonated with C-shaped larva
Trichuris trichiura	50-55 × 22-23 Barrel shaped	Bile-stained, thick shell Hyaline polar plugs Unembryonated when passed
Hookworm Egg	50-60 × 35-40 Broadly oval	Thin shell, colorless In four- to eight-cell stage when passed
Rhabditiform larva	250-300	Long buccal capsule Inconspicuous genital primordium
Filariform larva	500	Pointed tail Esophageal-intestinal ratio 1 : 4
Strongyloides stercoralis	Egg rarely seen—resembles that of hookworm	
Rhabditiform larva	200-250	Short buccal capsule Prominent genital primordium
Filariform larva	500	Notched tail Esophageal-intestinal ratio 1:1

skin by larvae in the soil, or they may require an insect vector. Intestinal roundworms are the most common of all the helminths that infect human beings in the United States. Infected individuals are found in highest numbers in the warm, moist area of the Southeast and in areas with poor sanitation. These organisms are characterized by the presence of two sexes and a life cycle that may involve larval migration throughout the body. The adults obtain nourishment by absorbing nutrients from partly digested intestinal contents or by sucking blood. Patients may be asymptomatic or symptomatic, and the severity of the symptoms is related to the worm burden, the host's nutritional status and age, and the duration of infection. The roundworms discussed in this section are *Enterobius vermicularis, Trichuris trichiura, Ascaris lumbricoides,* hookworm, and *Strongyloides stercoralis.* Blood and tissue roundworms are discussed in a separate section. Table 24-9 gives a comparison of diagnostic characteristics of the eggs and larvae of intestinal roundworms.

ENTEROBIUS VERMICULARIS

Enterobius vermicularis, commonly called the pinworm, is a worldwide parasite commonly detected in children, especially those 5 to 10 years old. Enterobiasis is often found in families or in crowded conditions where the eggs may be easily transmitted. The eggs are resistant to drying and are easily spread in the environment. Adult worms live in the large intestine, although they have occasionally been found in the appendix or vagina.

Clinical infection Although infection with *E. vermicularis* is often asymptomatic, the patient may experience loss of appetite, abdominal pain, loss of sleep, and nausea and vomiting. Anal pruritus is caused by migration of the female to the perianal area. Treatment, if given, is usually pyrantel pamoate, mebendazole, or piperazine citrate. The treatment is repeated in 2 weeks to eliminate organisms that matured as a result of ingestion of eggs remaining in the environment.

Life cycle The life cycle of this organism (Figure 24-57) is characterized by migration of the female out the anus during the night to lay eggs in the perianal area. The eggs are infective with a third-stage larva within several hours of being laid. Transmission involves inhalation or ingestion of the infective egg. Direct anal-mouth transmission is common in children. Retroinfection, in which the hatched larva reenters the intestine to mature into an adult, may also occur.

Laboratory diagnosis A fecal specimen is unsatisfactory, because eggs are laid outside the body

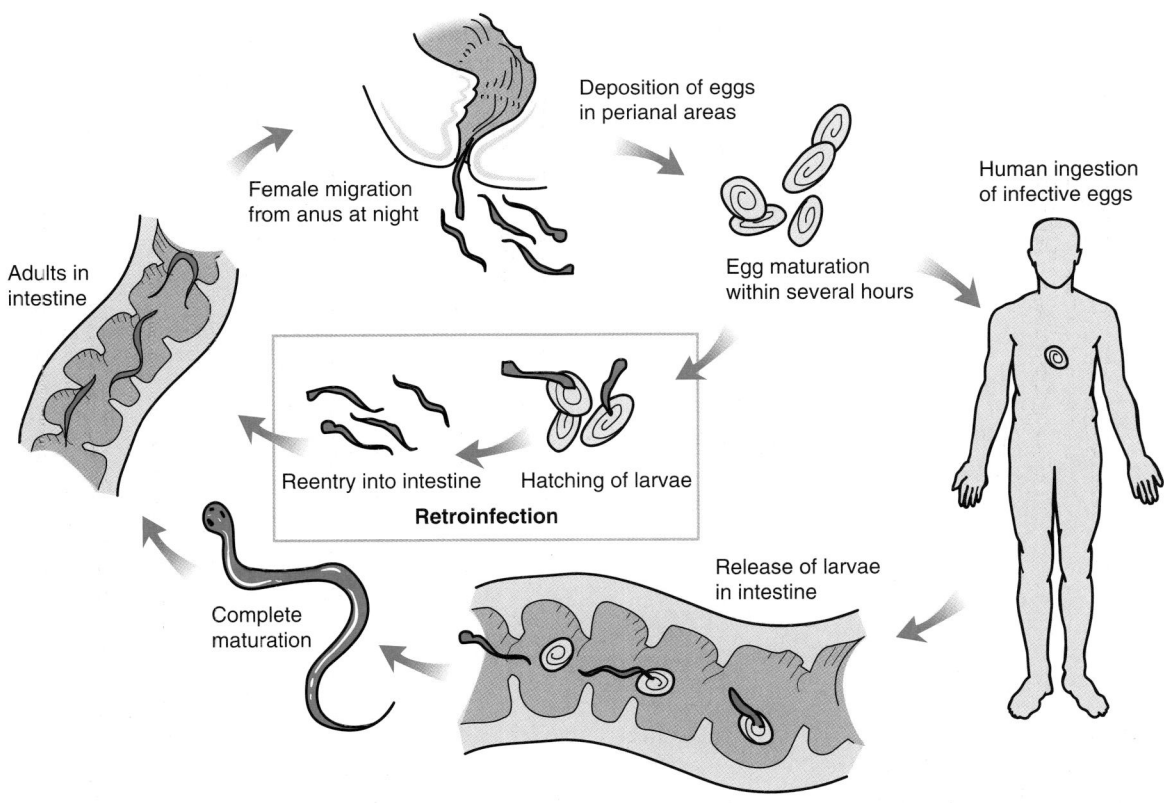

Figure 24-57

Life cycle of *Enterobius vermicularis.*

in the perianal area and are rarely present in the stool. The cellophane tape preparation is considered the diagnostic method of choice. The procedure must be done as soon as the child arises in the morning—before going to the bathroom or bathing—in order to recover eggs. A piece of cellophane tape is placed sticky side out over the edge of a tongue blade. The perianal area is touched with the sticky side of the tape, and then the tape is placed on a glass slide. Adaptations of this procedure using paddles with a sticky surface are available commercially. The adult female occasionally may be seen in this preparation. Eggs may also be seen in a first morning urine specimen if they drop from the perianal area.

The adult female measures 8 to 13 mm long and has a long, pointed tail and three cuticle lips with alae at the anterior end. The less commonly seen male is 2 to 5 mm long with a curved posterior. The egg is oval, colorless, and slightly flattened on one side. It measures approximately 50 to 60 by 20 to 30 μm. The egg is usually seen embryonated with a C-shaped larva (Figure 24-58).

TRICHURIS TRICHIURA

Trichuris trichiura, commonly referred to as the whipworm, is found worldwide, especially in areas with a moist, warm climate. It occurs in the southeastern United States, often as a co-infection with *A. lumbricoides.*

Clinical infections Light infections with *T. trichiura* rarely cause symptoms; heavy infections result in

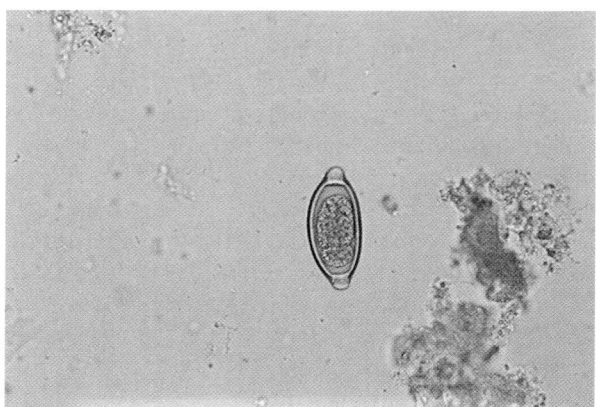

Figure 24-59

Trichuris trichiura egg.

bleeding, weight loss, abdominal pain, nausea and vomiting, and chronic diarrhea. Inflammation of the mucosa occurs as the adults thread themselves through it. Prolonged, heavy infection may result in diarrhea with blood-tinged stools. Rectal prolapse is the result of repeated heavy infections in undernourished children. Hypochromic anemia may occur with inadequate iron and protein intake in the presence of constant, low-level bleeding in chronic infection. Infection usually is treated with mebendazole.

Life cycle Eggs are passed in the feces and require at least 14 days in warm, moist soil for embryonation to occur. Human beings acquire infection by ingesting the infective egg. The larva is released in the small intestine and undergoes several molts before maturing into an adult worm in the cecum.

Laboratory diagnosis The egg and occasionally the adult of *T. trichiura* may be seen in the fecal specimen. The adult male measures 30 to 45 mm and has a thin anterior and a thick, coiled posterior. The female is 30 to 50 mm with a thin anterior and thick, straight posterior. The brown barrel-shaped egg is unembryonated when passed, 50 to 55 by 22 to 23 μm, and has a thick wall and hyaline polar plugs at each end (Figure 24-59).

ASCARIS LUMBRICOIDES

Up to 1 billion people worldwide are infected with *A. lumbricoides.* The organism can be found in tropical as well as temperate areas, and children are most commonly infected. Transmission is primar-

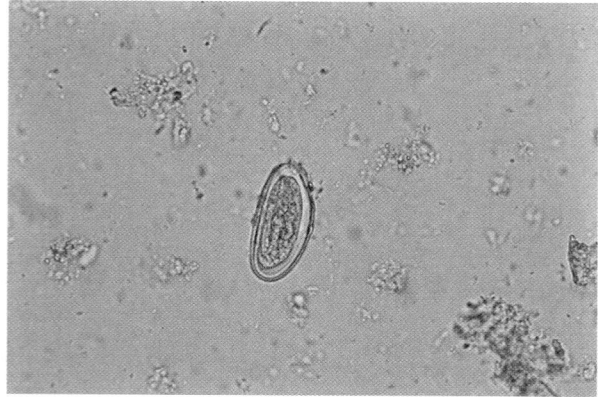

Figure 24-58

Enterobius vermicularis egg.

ily fecal-oral, and clinical symptoms may be related to the different phases of the life cycle. The organism is often found concurrently with whipworm.

Clinical infection Abdominal discomfort, loss of appetite, and colicky pains are caused by the presence of adults in the intestine. Large numbers of adult worms may cause intestinal obstruction. Chronic infection with *A. lumbricoides* in children may hamper growth and development, because the worms feed on liquid intestinal contents. Larva migrating through the lungs may cause an immune response in the host referred to as Löffler syndrome, which is characterized by asthma, edema, pneumonitis, and eosinophilic infiltration. On some occasions, fever or other disease conditions may cause the adults to migrate from the intestine and invade other organs, resulting in peritonitis, liver

abscess, or secondary infection in the lungs. The infection is treated with piperazine citrate, which relaxes the worm and allows peristalsis to carry it out of the intestinal tract.

Life cycle Figure 24-60 shows the life cycle of *A. lumbricoides*. Eggs that are deposited in warm, moist soil become infective within about 2 weeks. After the egg is ingested, larvae hatch in the duodenum, penetrate the intestinal wall, and gain access to the circulatory system. They break out from capillaries into the lungs, travel up the bronchial tree and trachea and over the epiglottis, and are swallowed. Maturation is completed in the intestine. The life cycle takes about 30 days from infection until adults are mature.

Laboratory diagnosis The usual diagnostic stage is the egg. Fertile *Ascaris* eggs are oval, measure

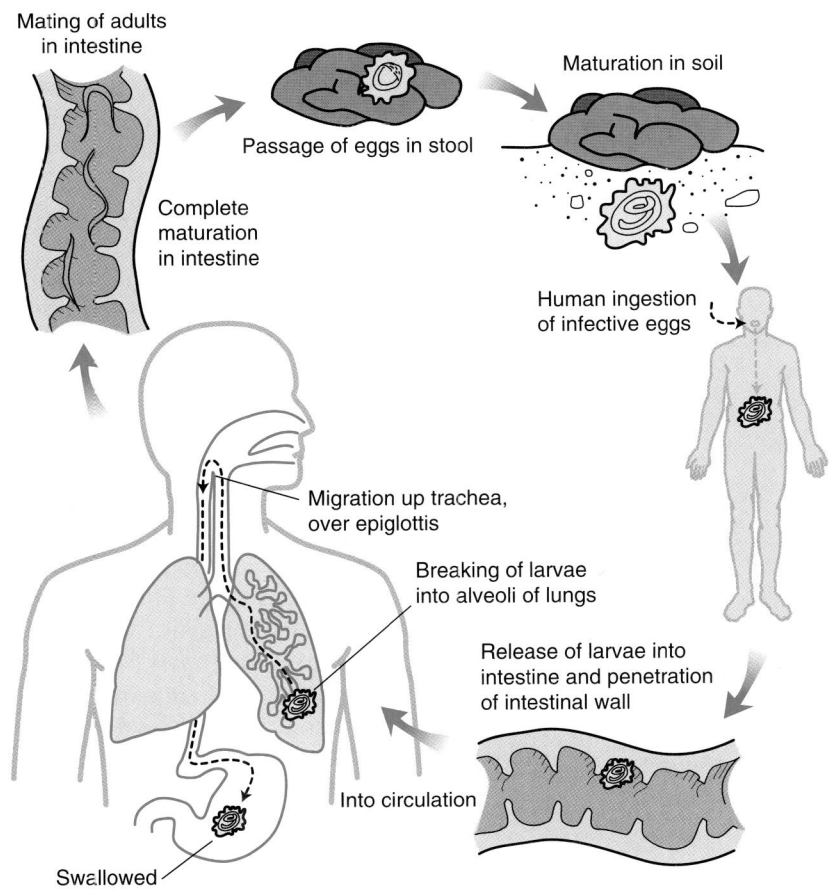

Figure 24-60

Life cycle of *Ascaris lumbricoides.*

45 to 75 by 35 to 50 μm, and have a thick hyaline wall surrounding a one cell–stage embryo. Most eggs have a brown, bile-stained, mammillated outer layer (Figure 24-61). Some eggs, referred to as decorticated, lack the mammillated outer coat. Infertile eggs, whose size may range up to 90 μm, are often elongated or bizzarely shaped and contain a mass of highly refractile granules. Adults measure 15 to 35 cm long and about the diameter of a lead pencil may be seen in a stool sample. The female has a straight posterior, and the male has a curved posterior. Both have three anterior lips with small, toothlike projections.

HOOKWORM

Two species of hookworm, *Necator americanus* (New World) and *Ancylostoma duodenale* (Old World), infect human beings. *A. duodenale* is seen in southern Europe and northern Africa along the Mediterranean, as well as in parts of Southeast Asia and South America. *N. americanus* has a geographic distribution in Africa, Southeast Asia, and South and Central America and is endemic in rural areas of southeastern United States. Adults of the two species can be differentiated by the morphology of the buccal capsule or, in the male, the copulatory bursa. The eggs, however, are identical. These worms live in the small intestine and attach to the mucosa by means of teeth (*A. duodenale*) or cutting plates (*N. americanus*). Once attached, they secrete anticoagulants and ingest blood as a source of nourishment. There seems to be a racial distribution, with infections more prevalent in whites than in African Americans.

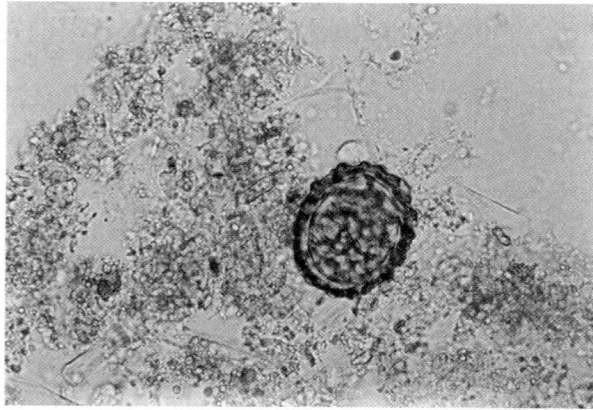

Figure 24-61

Ascaris lumbricoides egg, fertile.

Clinical infection Clinical symptoms vary according to the phase of the life cycle and worm burden. A small, red, itchy papule, referred to as ground itch, develops at the site of larval penetration. If large numbers of larvae are present during the lung phase of migration, the patient may have bronchitis, but no host sensitization occurs, unlike with *Ascaris* larva. The most severe symptoms are associated with the adult, including nonspecific symptoms such as diarrhea, fever, and nausea and vomiting. Blood loss, ranging from 0.03 to 0.2 ml per worm per day, is primarily the result of the ingestion of blood as a source of nourishment for the adult worm. Hemorrhages at the site of attachment, however, also contribute to total blood loss. Chronic heavy infection with hookworm may lead to microcytic hypochromic anemia, especially in children whose diet is inadequate in iron and protein. The mental and physical development of a child may be affected by chronic heavy infections. Infection usually is treated with mebendazole, which blocks glucose uptake by the organism, or with pyrantel pamoate, which paralyzes the worm so that it can be expelled. Supportive therapy, including iron and protein supplements, may be needed in severe cases.

Life cycle Figure 24-62 shows the life cycle of the hookworm. Once the eggs have been deposited in warm, moist soil, the first-stage **rhabditiform larva** develops within 1 to 2 days and feeds on bacteria in the soil. A nonfeeding infective **filariform larva** forms within a week. Human beings are infected when the filariform larvae penetrate their skin. The organisms enter the circulation and break out of the capillaries into the lung, then migrate up the bronchial tree, over the epiglottis, and into the digestive tract. After additional larval molts, the worms attach to the mucosa in the small intestine. Eggs are produced about 5 weeks after skin penetration by the filariform larva.

Laboratory diagnosis Adult hookworms are rarely seen in the stool specimen; the egg and the rhabditiform larva are considered the usual diagnostic stages. As mentioned before, adult males may be distinguished and speciated by examination of the copulatory bursa in the posterior. The eggs and rhabditiform larvae of the two species are indistinguishable; therefore, the laboratory can report only "hookworm" when a characteristic egg or larva is found in a stool specimen. The egg is

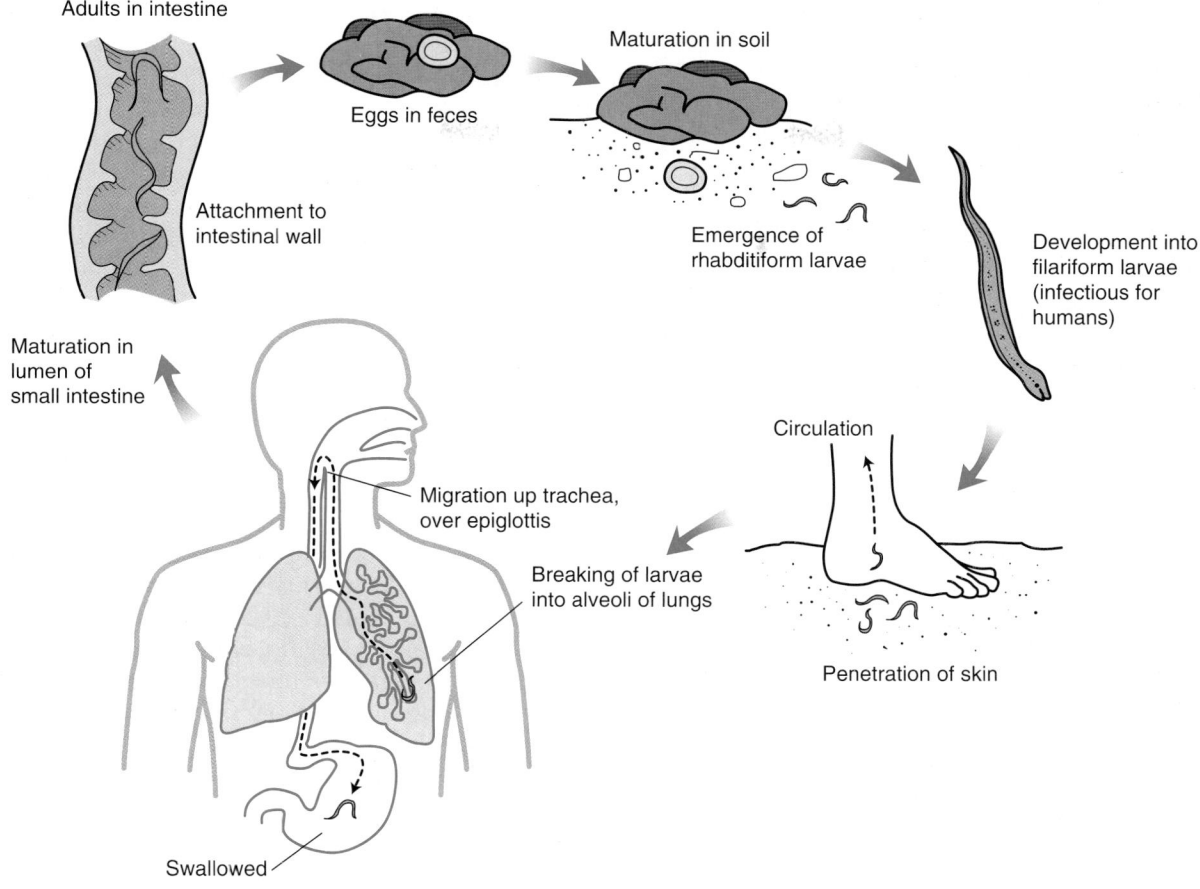

Figure 24-62

Life cycle of hookworm.

---

oval, colorless, thin shelled, and 50 to 60 μm and usually contains an embryo in the four- to eight-cell stage of cleavage (Figure 24-63). The rhabditiform larva must be differentiated from that of *S. stercoralis.* The hookworm rhabditiform larva is 250 to 300 μm long and has a long buccal capsule and small, inconspicuous genital primordium (Figure 24-64, *A*). Figure 24-64, *B* shows a close-up of the buccal capsule. The filariform larva also must be distinguished from that of *S. stercoralis.* Hookworm filariform larvae are about 500 μm, with a pointed tail and an esophageal-intestinal ratio of 1:4.

STRONGYLOIDES STERCORALIS

Strongyloides stercoralis, known as the threadworm, inhabits the small intestine but is also capable of existing as a free-living worm. It is endemic in the tropics and subtropics and has been identified in a number of U.S. military veterans who served in Vietnam and other Southeast Asian countries. In the United States, most cases are found in people living in Appalachia or in rural areas of the Southeast.

Clinical infection Although many people with *S. stercoralis* are asymptomatic, patients may have nausea and vomiting and sharp, stabbing pains that resemble those of an ulcer. Chronic mild diarrhea may be present. Unlike with the hookworm, *S. stercoralis* larval penetration of the skin does not cause a prominent papule, and migration through the lungs rarely elicits pneumonitis.

In contrast to the mild symptoms in an immunocompetent host, immunocompromised patients may develop severe infections, referred to as disseminated strongyloidiasis or hyperinfection. In this population, large numbers of the

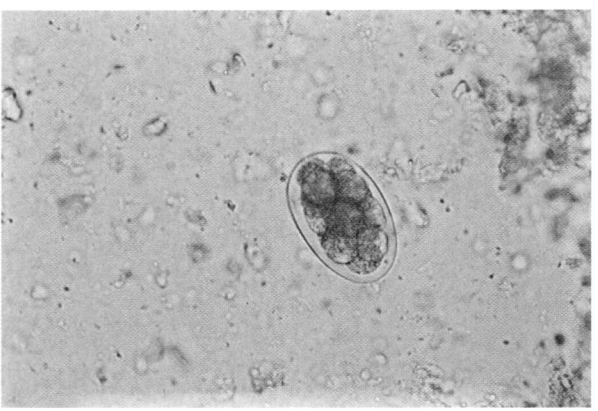

Figure 24-63
Hookworm egg.

filariform larvae develop in the intestine and migrate from the intestine into other organs, such as the liver, heart, and central nervous system, causing a fulminating, often fatal infection. Death is caused by complications resulting in respiratory failure. Respiratory failure has been reported in patients undergoing chemotherapy or who have malignancies, chronic debilitating disease, or lymphoma, but is not yet commonly encountered in patients with AIDS.

Life cycle The life cycle of *S. stercoralis* can take one of three forms—direct, which is similar to that of hookworm; indirect, which involves a free-living phase; or autoinfection (Figure 24-65). In the direct life cycle, the fertile egg hatches in the intes-

tine and develops into the rhabditiform larva, which is passed in the stool. This larval form develops into a filariform larva, which is infective for human beings by direct penetration. Once the larva has penetrated the skin, it enters the circulation, breaks out from capillaries in the lung, migrates up the bronchial tree and over the epiglottis, and enters the digestive tract, where it matures into the adult worm. In some patients, development into the filariform larva occurs in the intestine. These filariform (infective) larvae then penetrate the mucosa, enter the circulation, and return to the intestine to develop into adults. This part of the life cycle, called autoinfection, may allow an initial infection to persist for years. In the indirect life cycle, the rhabditiform larvae develop into free-living male and females that produce eggs. At any point, the free-living cycle may revert and result in production of infective filariform larvae.

Laboratory diagnosis The parasitic female threadworm is small (2.5 mm) and rarely seen in a stool specimen. No male has been identified in the intestinal infection. The primary diagnostic stage in human beings is the rhabditiform larva. It is 200 to 250 μm long with a short buccal capsule, large bulb in the esophagus, and a prominent genital primordium located in its posterior half to posterior third (Figure 24-66, *A*). Figure 24-66, *B*, shows a close-up of the buccal capsule. The egg, which is rarely seen except in cases of severe diarrhea, resembles that of a hookworm. It is thin shelled, measures 54 by 32 μm, and often is segmented. The

A 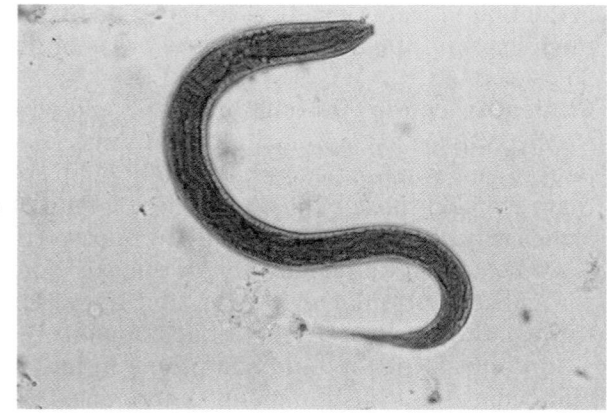 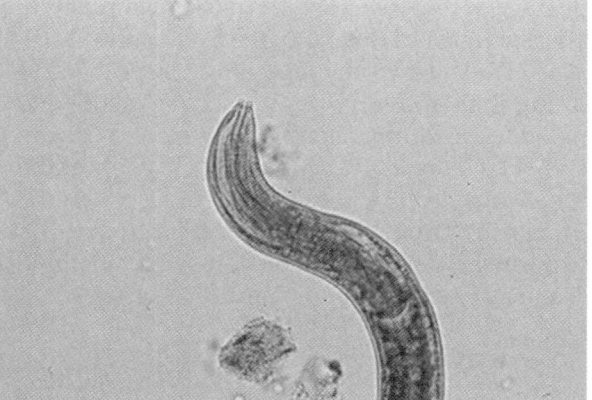 B

Figure 24-64
A, Hookworm rhabditiform larva. Notice long buccal capsule and lack of genital primordium. **B,** Hookworm rhabditiform larva, buccal capsule.

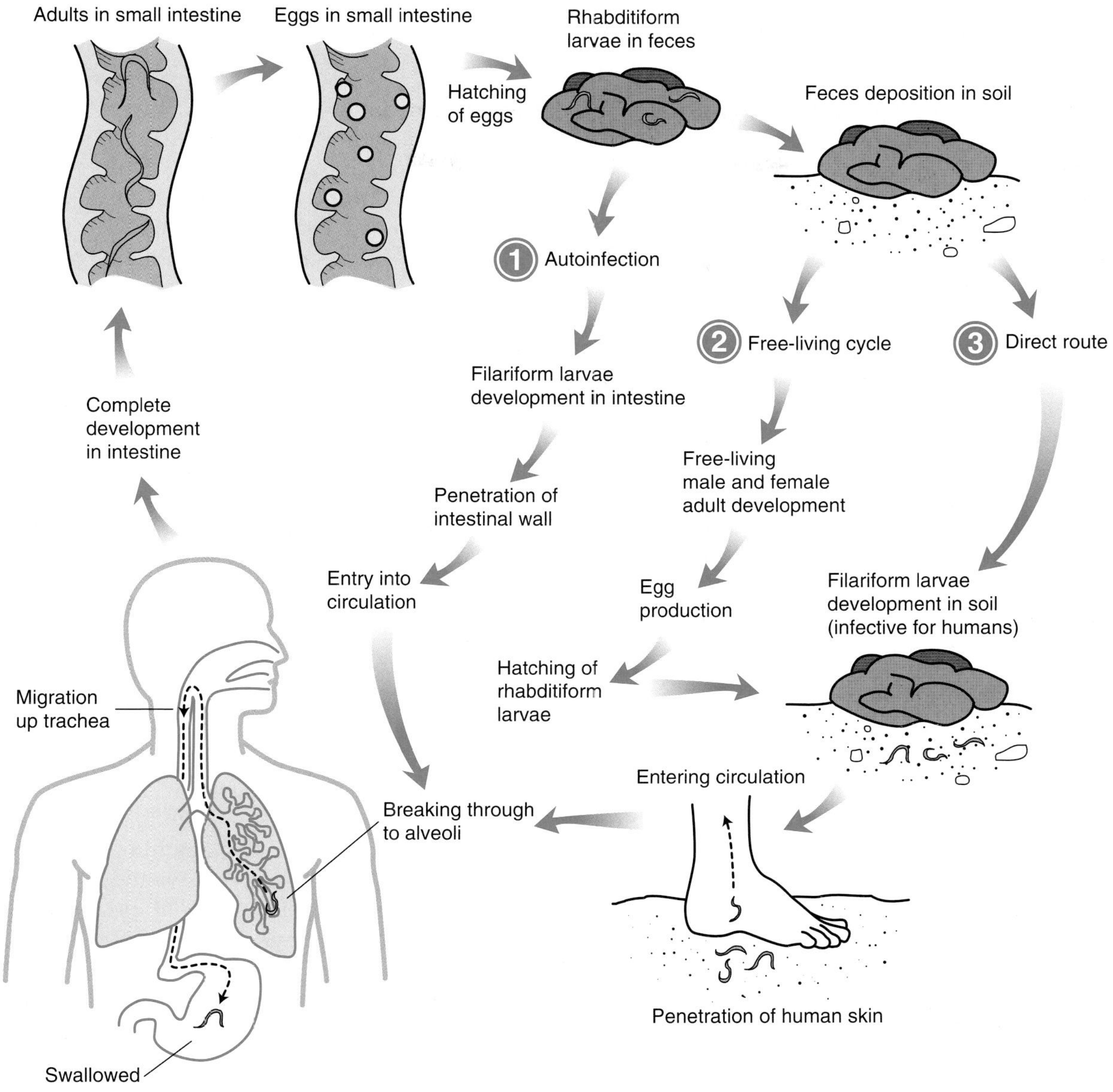

Adults in small intestine   Eggs in small intestine   Rhabditiform
                                                        larvae in feces

                                                                          Feces deposition in soil
                              Hatching
                              of eggs

                                        (1) Autoinfection

                                                            (2) Free-living cycle   (3) Direct route

Complete   Filariform larvae
development   development in intestine
in intestine
                                                    Free-living
                                                    male and female
                          Penetration of   adult development
                          intestinal wall
                                                                          Filariform larvae
              Entry into   Egg   development in soil
              circulation   production   (infective for humans)

                                            Hatching of
                                            rhabditiform
Migration   larvae
up trachea

                                                                          Entering circulation

                                  Breaking through
                                  to alveoli

                                                                Penetration of human skin

Swallowed

Figure 24-65 _____

Life cycle of *Strongyloides stercoralis*.

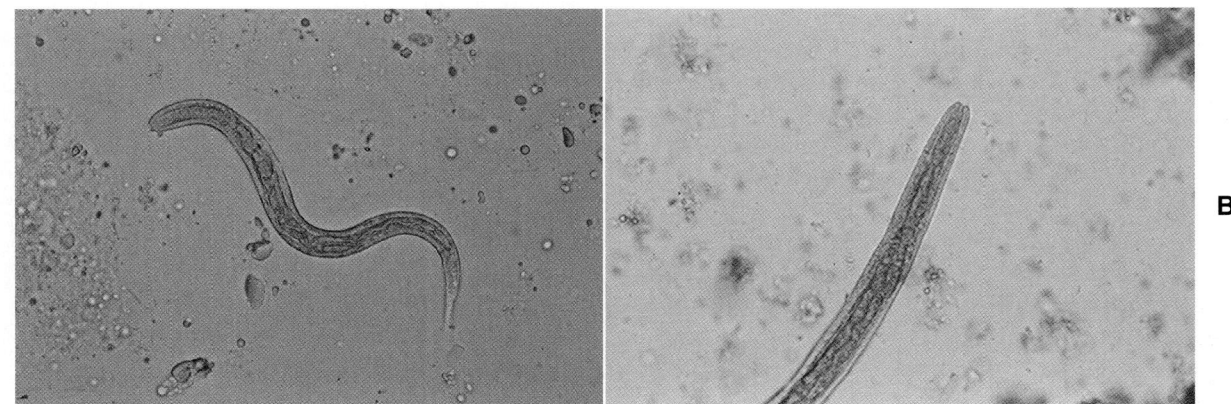

Figure 24-66 _____

A, *Strongyloides stercoralis* rhabditiform larva. Notice short buccal capsule and prominent genital primordium. **B,** *S. stercoralis*
rhabditiform larva, buccal capsule.

filariform larva has a notched tail, is 500 μm long, and has an esophageal-intestinal ratio of 1:1. Filariform larvae may be identified in the sputum of patients with hyperinfection.

If clinical symptoms suggest *Strongyloides* infection but multiple stool specimens test negative for the larvae, a duodenal aspirate or the Enterotest (HDC Corp., San Jose, Calf.) may be used for diagnosis. Treatment to eliminate the worm usually requires albendazole. Mebendazole can be used but requires a longer course of treatment, because it is not as effective against the larval stage.

Blood and tissue infections with roundworms

TRICHINELLA SPIRALIS

Trichinosis is the infection of muscle tissue with the larval form of *Trichinella spiralis,* a helminth whose adult stages live in the human intestine.

Clinical infection During the intestinal phase the individual has few symptoms, although diarrhea and abdominal discomfort may be present. Most symptoms occur during the migration and encapsulation period, and the severity of the symptoms depends on the number of parasites, the tissues invaded, and the person's general health. Symptoms that occur during the larval phase are the result of an intense inflammatory response by the host. Common symptoms include periorbital edema, fever, muscular pain or tenderness, headache and general weakness. Splinter hemorrhages beneath the nails may be seen in many patients. Eosinophilia of 40% to 80% is common. Patients with symptoms should be treated with analgesics and general supportive measures. Steroids are given only in rare cases.

Life cycle Human beings acquire the infection by eating undercooked meat, particularly pork, that contains the larval forms. The larvae are released from the tissue capsule in the intestine and mature into adults. The female produces liveborn larvae that penetrate the intestinal wall, enter the circulation, and are carried to all areas of the body. Once the larvae enter the striated muscle, they begin a maturation cycle that is completed in about 1 month. The larvae coil and become encapsulated. Although larvae may remain viable for many years, eventually the capsules calcify and the larvae die.

Laboratory diagnosis Because it is difficult to recover adults or larvae in a stool specimen, the diagnosis often is based on clinical symptoms and the patient's history. Biopsy of muscle tissue and identification of the encapsulated, coiled larva is the definitive diagnostic method. Figure 24-67 shows a biopsy specimen of a muscle containing the larva of *T. spiralis.* Specimens from large muscles, such as the deltoid and gastrocnemius muscles, should be examined for viable larvae and stained for histologic examination. The presence of calcified larvae on a radiographic film indicates previous infection. Serologic tests are available. An intradermal skin test yields a positive reaction within 3 weeks of infection.

LARVA MIGRANS

Two forms of larva migrans exist in human beings— cutaneous (creeping eruption) and visceral. Both are the result of infection with nonhuman nematode larvae that are unable to compete their life cycle in human beings.

In cutaneous larva migrans, the infecting organism is commonly the filariform larva of the dog or cat hookworm *(Ancylostoma braziliense).* Once the larva penetrates the skin of a human being, it cannot enter the circulation. It wanders through the subcutaneous tissue, creating long, winding tunnels that itch intensely. The infection resolves within several weeks when the larva dies. The diagnosis is based primarily on clinical symptoms.

In visceral larva migrans, a human being accidentally ingests the eggs of the dog roundworm

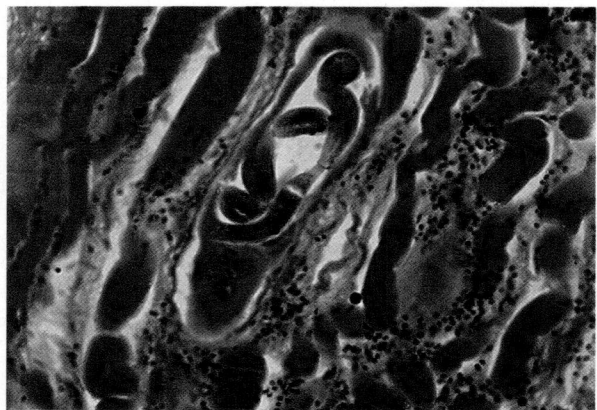

Figure 24-67 ————————————————————

Trichinella spiralis larva (biopsy specimen).

(Toxocara canis) or cat roundworm *(Toxocara cati).* The larvae hatch in the intestine, penetrate the gut, wander through the abdominal cavity, and may penetrate lungs, eye, liver, or brain. The infection is seen primarily in children 1 to 4 years old. Clinical symptoms include fever, pneumonitis, and hepatomegaly. Eosinophilia of 30% to 50% is common. CNS complications may develop. The diagnosis usually is made on the basis of clinical findings and the results of serologic tests.

FILARIAL WORMS
Filarial worms are roundworms of blood and tissue that give birth to larvae referred to as microfilariae. A number of species infect human beings. Those considered most pathogenic are *Brugia malayi, Wuchereria bancrofti, Onchocerca volvulus,* and *Loa loa.* In addition, the nonpathogens *Mansonella ozzardi, Mansonella perstans,* and *Mansonella streptocerca* may be seen. Identification of the various species depends on the morphology of the microfilaria, its periodicity, and its location in the host. The morphologic characteristics that are considered include the presence or absence of a sheath (the remnant of the egg from which the larva hatched) and the presence and arrangement of nuclei in the tail. Table 24-10 presents a comparison of the tail morphology, periodicity, insect vector, and location for the species of microfilariae commonly found in human beings.
Life cycle Adults, which may range in size from 2 to 50 cm, live in human lymphatics, muscles, or connective tissues. Mature females produce live-born larvae (microfilariae) that are the infective stage for the insect during the insect's blood meal. Once ingested, microfilariae penetrate the insect's gut wall and develop into infective third-stage (filariform) larvae. These enter the insect proboscis and are introduced into human circulation when the insect feeds. Figure 24-68 shows a generalized life cycle for microfilariae.

WUCHERERIA BANCROFTI
The causative agent of bancroftian filariasis and elephantiasis, *W. bancrofti* is primarily limited to the tropical and subtropical regions. The insect vector is a mosquito, either *Culex* or *Aedes* sp.
Clinical infection The adult filarial worm lives in the lymphatics and lymph nodes, especially those in the lower extremities. Presence of the adults initiates an immunologic response consisting of cellular reactions, edema, and hyperplasia. A strong granulomatous reaction with production of fibrous tissue around the dead worms ensues. The end result of the reaction is that small lymphatics may be narrowed or closed, with subsequent development or collateral lymphatics. During this period, the patient may experience generalized symptoms such as fever, headache, and chills as well as localized swelling, redness, and lymphangitis, primarily at sites in the male and female genitalia and the extremities. Elephantiasis, a debilitating and deforming complication, occurs in less than 10% of infections, usually after many years of continual filarial infection. Chronic obstruction in the lymphatic flow results in lymphatic varices, fibrosis, and proliferation of dermal and connective tissue. The enlarged areas eventually develop a hard, leathery appearance.
Laboratory diagnosis Diagnosis of *W. bancrofti* should include the examination of a blood specimen obtained at night (10 PM to 2 AM) for the presence of microfilariae. The blood may be examined immediately for live microfilariae or may be pooled on a slide and stained. Filtration of up to 5 ml of blood through a 5 μm Nucleopore filter (Nucleopore Corp., Pleasanton, Calif.) may detect light infections. The microfilariae of *W. bancrofti* are sheathed, and the nuclei do not extend to the tip of the tail (Figure 24-69).
Brugia malayi Brugia malayi, another nocturnal microfilarial species, is limited to the Far East, including Korea, China, and the Philippines. Mosquitoes of the genera *Mansonia, Anopheles,* and *Aedes* have been shown to transmit the organism. The pathology of the disease and the clinical symptoms are the same as those seen with *W. bancrofti* infections. The distinguishing characteristic of the microfilaria is the presence of a sheath and the arrangement of tail nuclei—the nuclei extend to the tip, but a space separates the two terminal nuclei.

LOA LOA
Infection with *Loa loa,* the eye worm, is limited to the African equatorial rain forest, where the fly vector *(Chrysops* sp.) breeds. Adults migrate through the subcutaneous tissue, causing temporary inflammatory reactions, called Calabar swellings. These characteristic swellings may cause pain and pruritus that last about a week before

TABLE 24-10

Comparison of Microfilariae

Organism	Arthropod Vector	Periodicity	Location of Adult/Microfilaria	Tail Morphology	
Wuchereria bancrofti	Mosquito (*Culex, Aedes, Anopheles* spp.)	Nocturnal	Lymphatics, blood	Sheathed Nuclei do not extend to tip of tail	
Brugia malayi	Mosquito (*Aedes* sp.)	Nocturnal	Lymphatics, blood	Sheathed Terminal nuclei separated	
Loa loa	Fly (*Chrysops* sp.)	Diurnal	Subcutaneous tissue, blood	Sheathed Nuclei extend to tip of tail	
Onchocerca volvulus	Fly (*Simulium* sp.)	Nonperiodic	Subcutaneous nodule, subcutaneous tissue	Unsheathed Nuclei do not extend to tip of tail	
Mansonella ozzardi	Midge (*Culicoides* sp.)	Nonperiodic	Body cavity, blood, skin	Unsheathed Nuclei do not extend to tip of tail	
Mansonella perstans	Midge (*Culicoides* sp.)	Nonperiodic	Mesentery, blood	Unsheathed Nuclei extend to blunt tip of tail	
Mansonella streptocerca	Midge (*Culicoides* sp.)	Nonperiodic	Subcutaneous, skin	Unsheathed Nuclei extend to tip of hooked tail	

disappearing, only to reappear in another part of the body. The adult worm can often be seen as it migrates across the surface of the eye.

Diagnosis may be based on the presence of Calabar swellings or of the adult worm in the conjunctiva of the eye. Microfilariae may be seen in a blood specimen if it is taken during the day, especially around noon, when migration peaks. The microfilaria is sheathed, and nuclei extend to the tip of the tail.

ONCHOCERCA VOLVULUS
Infection with *Onchocerca volvulus* is referred to as onchocercosis or river blindness. The organism

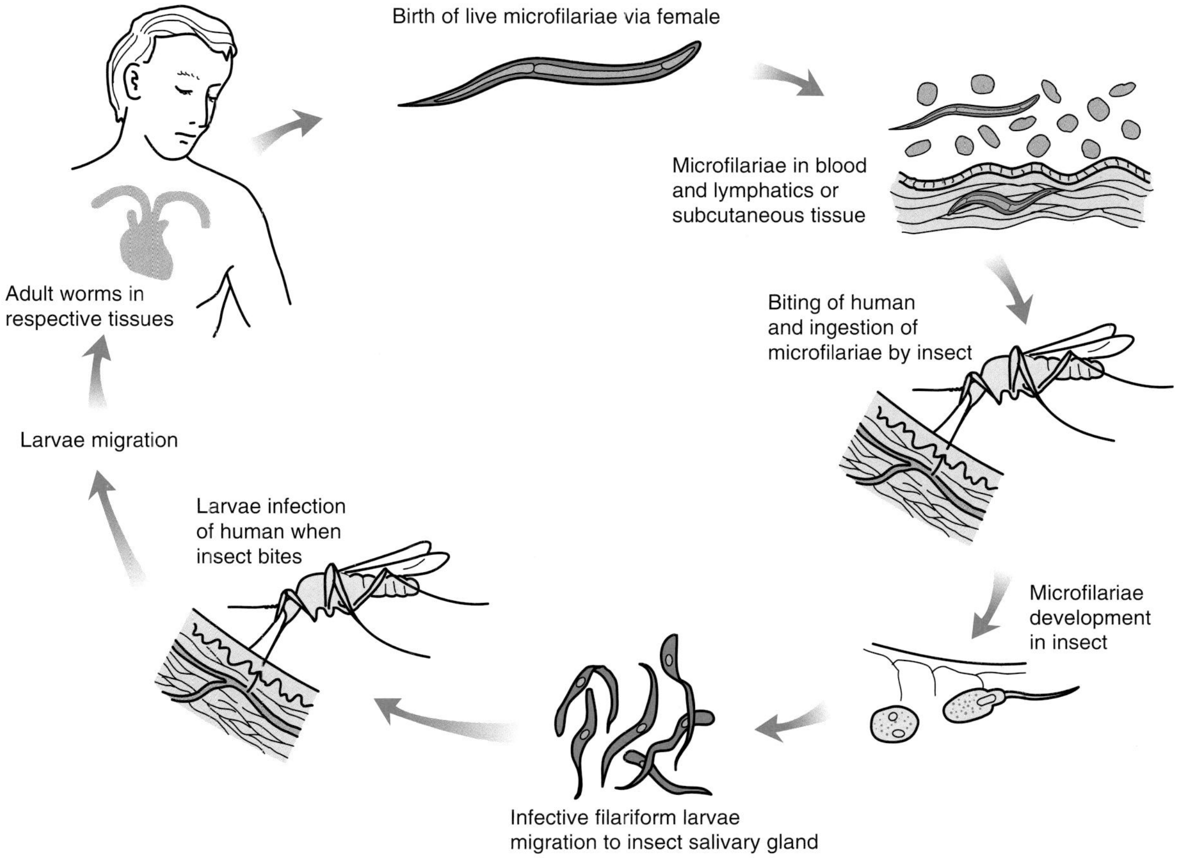

Birth of live microfilariae via female

Microfilariae in blood
and lymphatics or
subcutaneous tissue

Adult worms in
respective tissues

Biting of human
and ingestion of
microfilariae by insect

Larvae migration

Larvae infection
of human when
insect bites

Microfilariae
development
in insect

Infective filariform larvae
migration to insect salivary gland

Figure 24-68 _____

Generalized life cycle microfilaria.

may be found in Africa and South and Central America; transmission occurs by the bite of the black fly (*Simulium* sp). Adults are encapsulated in fibrous tumors in human subcutaneous tissues. Microfilariae may be isolated from the subcuta-neous tissue, skin, and the nodule itself but are rarely found in blood or lymphatic fluid.

The nodules in which adults live may measure up to 25 mm and can be found on most parts of the body. They are the result of an inflammatory and

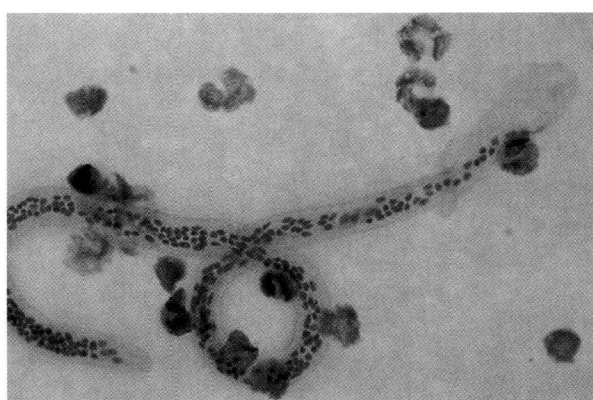

Figure 24-69 _____

Wucheraria bancrofti microfilaria. Notice faintly staining sheath extending from both ends of organism.

granulomatous reaction around the adult worms. Figure 24-70 shows a cross-section of tissue containing these organisms. Blindness, the most serious complication, results when microfilariae collect in the cornea and iris, causing keratitis and atrophy of the iris.

Diagnosis involves clinical symptoms, such as the presence of nodules, and microscopic identification of microfilariae. The diagnostic method used is the skin snip, in which a small slice of skin is obtained and placed on a saline mount. Microfilariae with no sheath and with nuclei that do not extend into the tip of the tail are characteristic of this organism.

MANSONELLA SPECIES
Mansonella ozzardi, M. streptocerca (Dipetalonema streptocerca), and *M. perstans (Dipetalonema perstans)* are filarial worms not usually associated with serious infections. They are transmitted by midges belonging to the genus *Culicoides.* The microfilariae of *M. streptocerca* are found in the skin. They are unsheathed and have nuclei that extend to the end of the "shepherd's crook" tail. Microfilariae of *M. ozzardi* and *M. perstans* are found in the blood as unsheathed organisms. *M. ozzardi* microfilariae have tails with nuclei that do not extend to tips, whereas the nuclei in the tail of an *M. perstans* microfilaria extend to the tip.

DRACUNCULUS MEDINENSIS
Dracunculus medinensis (guinea worm, fiery serpent of the Israelites) causes serious infections in the Middle East, parts of Africa, and India. It is often found in areas in which "step-down" wells are used.

Clinical infection Initially a painful, blisterlike, inflammatory papule appears on the leg in the area of the gravid female. The papule ulcerates, and when the person's body comes in contact with water, the female worm exposes her uterus through the ulceration and releases larvae into the water. Patients may have nausea and vomiting, urticaria, and dyspnea before the rupture of the worm's uterus. If the worm is broken during an attempt to remove it, the patient may experience a severe inflammatory reaction and secondary bacterial infection.

Life cycle Human beings acquire the infection by ingesting a copepod (*Cyclops* sp.) that contains an infective larva. The larva is released in the intestine, penetrates the intestinal wall, and migrates to the body cavity, where males and females mature. When mature and gravid, the female migrates through the subcutaneous tissues to the arm or leg to release liveborn larvae into the water. The rhabditiform larvae are then ingested by the copepod.

The diagnosis is made from the typical appearance of the lesion. Metronidazole is given to treat the infection. The ancient method of removal by rolling the worm a few inches at a time onto a stick is still practiced in some areas of the world.

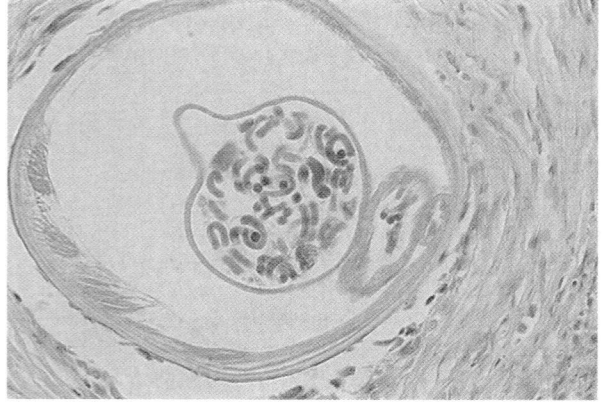

Figure 24-70 _____
Cross-section of tissue infected with *Onchocerca volvulus.*

Bibliography

Acuno-Soto R et al: Application of the polymerase chain reaction to the epidemiology of pathogenic and nonpathogenic *Entamoeba histolytica, Am J Trop Med Hyg* 48:58, 1993.

Addiss DG et al: Evaluation of a commercially available enzyme-linked immunosorbent assay for *Giardia lamblia* antigen in stool, *J Clin Microbiol* 29:1137, 1991.

Ahmed M et al: Systemic manifestations of invasive amebiasis, *Clin Infect Dis* 15:974, 1992.

Aikawa M: Human cerebral malaria, *Am J Trop Med Hyg* 39:3, 1988.

Aldeen WE et al: Comparison of pooled formalin-preserved fecal specimens with three individual samples for detection of intestinal parasites, *J Clin Microbiol* 31:144, 1993.

Allason-Jones E et al: *Entamoeba histolytica* as a commensal intestinal parasite in homosexual men, *N Engl J Med* 315:353, 1986.

Allason-Jones E et al: Outcome of untreated infection with *Entamoeba histolytica* in homosexual men with and without HIV antibody, *Br Med J* 297(6649):654-7, 1988.

Anthony RL et al: On-site diagnosis of *Plasmodium falciparum, P. vivax,* and *P. malariae* by using the quantitative buffy coat system, *J Parasitol* 78:994, 1992.

Baron EJ, Schenone C, Tanenbaum: Comparison of three methods for detection of *Cryptosporidium* oocysts in a low-prevalence population, *J Clin Microbiol* 27:223, 1989.

Baselski VS et al: Rapid detection of *Pneumocystis carinii* in bronchoalveolar lavage samples by using cellufluor staining, *J Clin Microbiol* 28:393, 1990.

Beadle C et al: Diagnosis of malaria by detection of *Plasmodium falciparum* HRP-2 antigen with a rapid dipstick antigen-capture assay, *Lancet* 343:564, 1994.

Beal C et al: The plastic envelope method: a simplified technique for culture diagnosis of trichomoniasis, *J Clin Microbiol* 30:2265, 1992.

Berger ST et al: Successful medical management of *Acanthamoeba* keratitis, *Am J Opthalmol* 110:395, 1990.

Blumenfield W, Kovacs JA: Use of a monoclonal antibody to detect *Pneumocystis carinii* in induced sputum and bronchoalveolar lavage fluid by immunoperoxidase staining, *Arch Pathol Lab Med* 112:1233, 1988.

Bottone EJ: Diagnosis of acute pulmonary toxoplasmosis by visualization of invasive and intracellular tachyzoites in Giemsa-stained smears of bronchoalveolar lavage fluid, *J Clin Microbiol* 29:2626, 1991.

Brennan MK et al: Cyclosporiasis: a new cause of diarrhea, *Can Med Assoc J* 155:1293, 1996.

Brown RL: Successful treatment of primary amebic meningoencephalitis, *Arch Intern Med* 151:1201, 1991.

Carr JM et al: Babesiosis: diagnostic pitfalls, *Am J Clin Pathol* 95:774, 1991.

Casemore DP, Roberts C: Guidelines for screening for *Cryptosporidium* in stools: report of a joint working group, *J Clin Pathol* 46:2, 1993.

Chan FTH, Guan MX, Mackenzie AMR: Application of indirect immunofluorescence to detection of *Dientamoeba fragilis* trophozoites in fecal specimens, *J Clin Microbiol* 31:1710, 1993.

Chiodini PL et al: Evaluation of a malaria antibody ELISA and its value in reducing potential wastage of red cell donations from blood donors exposed to malaria, with a note on a case of transfusion-transmitted malaria, *Vox Sang* 73:143, 1997.

Chulay JD, Ockenhouse CF: Host receptors for malaria-infected erythrocytes, *Am J Trop Med Hyg* 43(suppl 2):6, 1990.

Clarridge JE et al: Quantitative light microscopic detection of *Entercytozoon bieneusi* in stool specimens: a longitudinal study of human immunodeficiency virus–infected microsporidiosis patients, *J Clin Microbiol* 34:520, 1996.

Couroux P, Schieven BC, Hussain Z: *Pneumocystis carinii, ASM News* 59:179, 1993.

Cregan P et al: Comparison of four methods for rapid detection of *Pneumocystis carinii* in respiratory specimens, *J Clin Microbiol* 28:2432, 1990.

Current WL: The biology of *Cryptosporidium.* In Leech JH, Sande MA, Root RK, editors: *Contemporary issues in infectious diseases,* vol 7, Parasitic infections, New York, 1988, Churchill Livingstone.

Diamond LA, Clark CG: A redescription of *Entamoeba histolytica* Schaudinn, 1903 (emended Walker, 1911) separating it from *Entamoeba dispar* Brumpt, 1925, *J Eukaryot Microbiol* 40:340, 1993.

Didier ES et al: Comparison of three staining methods for detecting Microsporidia in fluids, *J Clin Microbiol* 33:3138, 1995.

Doyle PW et al: Epidemiology and pathogenicity of *Blastocystis hominis, J Clin Microbiol* 28:116, 1990.

Draper D et al: Detection of *Trichomonas vaginalis* in pregnant women with the InPouch TV culture system, *J Clin Microbiol* 31:1016, 1993.

Esernio-Jenssen D et al: Transplacental/perinatal babesiosis, *J Pediatr* 110:570, 1987.

Estevez EG, Levine JA: Examination of preserved stool specimens for parasites: lack of value of the direct wet mount, *J Clin Microbiol* 22:666, 1985.

Fedorko DP, Hijazi YM: Application of molecular techniques to the diagnosis of microsporidial infection, *Emerging Infectious Diseases* 2:183, 1996.

Flores BM et al: Differentiation of *Naegleria fowleri* from *Acanthamoeba* species by using monoclonal antibodies and flow cytometry, *J Clin Microbiol* 28:1999, 1990.

Garcia LS, Shimizu RY, Bruckner DA: Detection of microsporidial spores in fecal specimens from patients diagnosed with cryptosporidiosis, *J Clin Microbiol* 32:1739, 1994.

Garcia LS, Schum AC, Bruckner DA: Evaluation of a new monoclonal antibody combination reagent for direct fluorescence detection of *Giardia* cysts and *Cryptosporidium* oocysts in human fecal specimens, *J Clin Microbiol* 30:3255, 1992.

Garcia LS et al: Evaluation of intestinal protozoan morphology in polyvinyl alcohol preservative: comparison of zinc sulfate– and mercuric chloride–based compounds for use in Schaudinn's fixative, *J Clin Microbiol* 31:307, 1993.

Garcia LW et al: Acquired immunodeficiency syndrome with disseminated toxoplasmosis presenting as an acute pulmonary and gastrointestinal illness, *Arch Pathol Lab Med* 15:459, 1991.

Gelbart SM et al: Growth of *Trichomonas vaginalis* in commercial culture media, *J Clin Microbiol* 28:962, 1990.

Gellin BG, Soave R: Coccidian infections in AIDS: toxoplasmosis, cryptosporidiosis, and isosporiasis. In Medical management of AIDS patients, *Med Clin North Am* 76:205, 1992.

Genta RM: Global prevalence of strongyloidiasis: critical review with epidemiologic insights into the prevention of disseminated disease, *Rev Infect Dis* 11:755, 1989.

Genta RM et al: Strongyloidiasis in US veterans of the Vietnam and other wars, *JAMA* 258:49, 1987.

Gill VJ et al: Optimal use of the cytocentrifuge for recovery and diagnosis of *Pneumocystis carinii* in bronchoalveolar lavage and sputum specimens, *J Clin Microbiol* 26:1641, 1988.

Gonzalez-Ruiz A et al: A monclonal antibody for distinction of invasive and noninvasive clinical isolates of *Entamoeba histolytica, J Clin Microbiol* 30:2807, 1992.

Goodgame RW et al: Intensity of infection in AIDS-associated cryptosporidiosis, *J Infect Dis* 167:704, 1993.

Goodman PC, Schnap LM: Pulmonary toxoplasmosis in AIDS, *Radiology* 184:791, 1992.

Haque R et al: Diagnosis of pathogenic *Entamoeba histolytica* infection using a stool ELISA based on monoclonal antibodies to the galactose-specific adhesion, *J Infect Dis* 167:247, 1993.

Haque R et al: Rapid diagnosis of *Entamoeba* infection by using *Entamoeba* and *Entamoeba histolytica* stool antigen detection kits, *J Clin Microbiol* 33:2558, 1995.

Harcourt-Webster JN, Scaravilli F, Darwish AH: *Strongyloides stercoralis* hyperinfection in an HIV-positive patient, *J Clin Pathol* 44:346, 1991.

Ho M et al: Clinical correlates of in vitro *Plasmodium falciparum* cytoadherence, *Infect Immun* 59:873, 1991.

Hogle CW et al: Prevalence of *Cyclospora* species and other enteric pathogens among children less than 5 years of age in Nepal, *J Clin Microbiol* 33:3058, 1995.

Huang P et al: The first reported outbreak of diarrhea illness associated with *Cyclospora* in the United States, *Ann Intern Med* 123:409, 1995.

Institute of Medicine: *Malaria: obstacles and opportunities,* Washington, DC, 1991, National Academy Press.

Irusen EM, Jackson TF, Simjee AE: Asymptomatic intestinal colonization by pathogenic *Entamoeba histolytica* in amebic liver abscess: prevalence, response to therapy, and pathogenic potential, *Clin Infect Dis* 14:889, 1992.

Janoff EN, Reller LB: *Cryptosporidium* species: a protean protozoan, *J Clin Microbiol* 25:967, 1987.

Joiner KA, Dubremetz JF: *Toxoplasma gondii:* a protozoan for the nineties, *Infect Immun* 61:1169, 1993.

Kilvington S et al: Laboratory investigation of *Acanthamoeba* keratitis, *J Clin Microbiol* 28:2722, 1990.

Kokoskin E et al: Modified technique for efficient detection of Microsporidia, *J Clin Microbiol* 32:1974, 1994.

Krause PJ et al: Geographical and temporal distribution of babesial infection in Connecticut, *J Clin Microbiol* 29:1, 1991.

Lanar DE et al: Leishmaniasis: another threat to Persian Gulf veterans, *Postgrad Med* 90:213, 1991.

Lindquist TD, Sher NA, Doughman DJ: Clinical signs and medical therapy of early *Acanthamoeba* keratitis, *Arch Ophthalmol* 106:73, 1988.

List PJ et al: Monocloncal antibody–based enzyme-linked immunosorbent assay for *Trichomonas vaginalis, J Clin Microbiol* 26:1684, 1988.

Lotter H et al: Sensitive and specific serodiagnosis of invasive amebiasis by using a recombinant surface protein of pathogenic *Entamoeba histolytica, J Clin Microbiol* 30:3163, 1992.

Ma P et al: *Naegleria* and *Acanthamoeba* infections: review, *Rev Infect Dis* 12:490, 1990.

MacPherson DW, McQueen R: Cryptosporidiosis: multiattribute evaluation of six diagnostic methods, *J Clin Microbiol* 31:198, 1993.

MacPherson DW, McQueen WM: Morphological diversity of *Blastocystis hominis* in sodium acetate–acetic acid—formalin–preserved stool samples stained with iron hematoxylin, *J Clin Microbiol* 32:267, 1994.

Markell EK, Udkow MP: *Blastocystis hominis:* pathogen or fellow traveler? *Am J Trop Med Hyg* 35:1023, 1986.

Marti H, Koella JC: Multiple stool examinations for ova and parasites and rate of false-negative results, *J Clin Microbiol* 31:3044, 1993.

Martinez-Palomo A et al: Ultrastructure of experimental intestinal invasive amebiasis, *Am J Trop Med Hyg* 41:273, 1989.

Mattia AR, Wladron MA, Sierra LS: Use of the quantitative buffy coat system for detection of parasitemia in patients with babesiosis, *J Clin Microbiol* 31:2818, 1993.

McDougall RJ et al: Incidental finding of a microsporidian parasite from an AIDS patient, *J Clin Microbiol* 31:436, 1993.

Meredith JT: Toxoplasmosis of the central nervous system, *Am Fam Physician* 35:113, 1987.

Centers for Disease Control and Prevention: Outbreaks of *Cyclospora cayetanensis* infection: United States, 1996, *JAMA* 276:183, 1996.

Mohr E, Mohr I: Statistical analysis of the incidence of positives in the examination of parasitlogical specimens, *J Clin Microbiol* 30:1572, 1992.

Morris AJ, Wilson M, Reller LB: Application of rejection criteria for stool ovum and parasite examinations, *J Clin Microbiol* 30:3213, 1992.

Murphy GS et al: *Vivax* malaria resistant to treatment and prophylaxis with chloroquine, *Lancet* 341:96, 1993.

Namsiripongpun V et al: Field study of an antigen detection ELISA specific for *Plasmodium falciparum* malaria, *Trans R Soc Trop Med Hyg* 87:32, 1993.

Neimeister R et al: Evaluation of direct wet mount parasitological examination of preserved fecal specimens, *J Clin Microbiol* 28:1082, 1990.

Neva FA: Biology and immunology of human strongyloidiasis, *J Infect Dis* 153:397, 1986.

Newman RD et al: Evaluation of an antigen capture enzyme-linked immunosorbent assay for detection of *Crytosporidium* oocysts, *J Clin Microbiol* 31:2080, 1993.

Ng VL et al: Rapid detection of *Pneumocystis carinii* using a direct fluorescent monoclonal antibody stain, *J Clin Microbiol* 28:2228, 1990a.

Ng VL et al: Evaluation of an indirect fluorescent antibody stain for detection of *Pneumocystis carinii* in respiratory specimens, *J Clin Microbiol* 28:975, 1990b.

Norton SA, Frankenburg S, Klaus SN: Cutaneous leishmaniasis acquired during military service in the Middle East, *Arch Dermatol* 128:83, 1992.

Ortega YR et al: *Cyclospora* species: a new protozoan pathogen of humans, *N Engl J Med* 328:1308, 1993.

Pape JW et al: *Cyclospora* infection in adults infected with HIV, *Ann Intern Med* 121:654, 1994.

Parisi MT, Tierno PM: Evaluation of new rapid commercial enzyme immunoassay for detection of *Cryptosporidium* oocysts in untreated stool specimens, *J Clin Microbiol* 33:1963, 1995.

Pawlowski ZS, Schad GA, Stott GJ: *Hookworm infection and anemia: approaches to prevention and control,* Geneva, 1991, World Health Organization.

Peiris JS et al: Monoclonal and polyclonal antibodies both block and enhance transmission of human *Plasmodium vivax* malaria, *Am J Trop Med Hyg* 39:26, 1988.

Perry JL, Matthews JS, Miller GR: Parasite detection efficiencies of five stool concentration systems, *J Clin Microbiol* 28:1094, 1990.

Petri WA: Invasive amebiasis and the galactose-specific lectin of *Entamoeba histolytica, ASM News* 57:299, 1991.

Petri WA et al: Pathogenic and nonpathogenic strains of *Entamoeba histolytica* can be differentiated by monoclonal antibodies to the galactose-specific adherence lectin, *Infect Immun* 58:1802, 1990.

Pomery C, Filice GA: Pulmonary toxoplasmosis: a review, *Clin Infect Dis* 14:863, 1992.

Porter JD et al: *Giardia* transmission in a swimming pool, *Am J Public Health* 78:659, 1988.

Qadri SMH, Al-Okaili GA, Al-Dayel F: Clinical significance of *Blastocystis hominis, J Clin Microbiol* 27:2407, 1989.

Rabeneck L et al: The role of Microsporidia in the pathogenesis of HIV-related chronic diarrhea, *Ann Intern Med* 119:895, 1993.

Ravdin JI: Amebiasis now, *Am J Trop Med Hyg* 41(suppl):40, 1989a.

Ravdin JI: *Entamoeba histolytica:* from adherence to enteropathy, *J Infect Dis* 159:420, 1989b.

Ravdin JI: *Entamoeba histolytica:* pathogenic mechanisms, human immune response, and vaccine development, *Clin Res* 38:215, 1990.

Raviglione MC: Extrapulmonary pneumocystosis: The first 50 cases, *Rev Infec Dis* 12:1127, 1990.

Recommendations for the prevention of malaria in travelers, *MMWR* 39:No RR-3, 1990.

Reed SL; Amebiasis: an update, *Clin Infect Dis* 14:385, 1992.

Rickman LS et al: Rapid diagnosis of malaria by acridine orange staining of centrifuged parasites, *Lancet* 58:69, 1989.

Rieckman KH, Davis DR, Hutton DC: *Plasmodium vivax* resistance to chloroquine? *Lancet* 2:1183, 1989.

Rosenblatt JE, Sloan LM, Bestrom JE: Evaluation of an enzyme-linked immunoassay for the detection in serum of antibodies to *Entamoeba histolytica, Diagn Microbiol Infect Dis* 22:2775, 1995.

Rosenblatt JE, Sloan LM: Evaluation of an enzyme-linked immunosorbent assay for detection of *Cryptosporidium* spp. in stool specimens, *J Clin Microbiol* 31:1468, 1993.

Rosoff JD et al: Stool diagnosis of giardiasis using a commercially available enzyme immunoassay to detect *Giardia*-specific antigen 65 (GSA 65), *J Clin Microbiol* 27:1997, 1989.

Rusnak J et al: Detection of *Cryptosporidium* oocysts in human fecal specimens by an indirect immunofluorescence assay with monoclonal antibodies, *J Clin Microbiol* 27:1135, 1989.

Ryan NJ et al: A new technique for detection of microsporidial species in urine, stool, and nasopharyngeal specimens, *J Clin Microbiol* 31:3264, 1993.

Samuelson J et al: DNA hybridization probe for clinical diagnosis of *Entamoeba histolytica, J Clin Microbiol* 27:671, 1989.

Sargeaunt PG, Williams JE: The differentiation of invasive and noninvasive *Entamoeba histolytica* by isoenzyme electrophoresis, *Trans R Soc Trop Med Hyg* 72:519, 1978.

Sargeaunt PG, Williams JE: Electrophoretic isoenzyme patterns of the pathogenic and nonpathogenic intestinal amoebae of man, *Trans R Soc Trop Med Hyg* 73:225, 1979.

Scheffler EH, Van Etta LL: Evaluation of rapid commercial enzyme immunoassay for detection of *Giardia lamblia* in formalin-preserved stool specimens, *J Clin Microbiol* 32:1807, 1994.

Schnapp LM et al: *Toxoplasma gondii* pneumonitis in patients infected with the human immunodeficiency virus, *Arch Intern Med* 152:1073, 1992.

Senay H, MacPherson D: *Blastocystis hominis:* epidemiology and natural history, *J Infect Dis* 162:987, 1990.

Shandera WX: From Leningrad to the day care center: the ubiquitous *Giardia lamblia, West J Med* 153:154, 1990.

Sheehan DJ, Raucher BG, McKitrick JC: Association of *Blastocystis hominis* with signs and symptoms of human disease, *J Clin Microbiol* 24:548, 1986.

Soave R, Johnson WD: *Cryptosporidium* and *Isospora belli* infections, *J Infect Dis* 157:225, 1988.

Sorvillo FJ et al: Swimming-associated cryptosporidiosis, *Am J Public Health* 82:742, 1992.

Spielman et al: Malaria diagnosis by direct observation of centrifuged samples of blood, *Am J Trop Med Hyg* 39:337, 1988.

Stanley SL et al: Serodiagnosis of invasive amebiasis using a recombinant *Entamoeba histolytica* protein, *JAMA* 266:1984, 1991.

Stibbs HH: Monoclonal antibody–based enzyme immunoassay for *Giardia lamblia* antigen in human stool, *J Clin Microbiol* 27:2582, 1989.

Strachan WD et al: Immunological differentiation of pathogenic and nonpathogenic isolates of *Entamoeba histolytica, Lancet* 1:561, 1988.

Sullivan PB et al: Prevalence and treatment of giardiasis in chronic diarrhoea and malnutrition, *Arch Dis Child* 65:304, 1990.

Tangermann RH et al: An outbreak of cryptosporidiosis in a day care center in Georgia, *Am J Epidemiol* 133:471, 1991.

Travis WD et al: Respiratory cryptosporidiosis in a patient with malignant lymphoma: report of a case and review of the literature, *Arch Pathol Lab Med* 114:519, 1990.

Tschirhardt D, Klatt EC: Disseminated toxoplasmosis in the acquired immunodeficiency syndrome, *Arch Pathol Lab Med* 112:1237, 1988.

Wahlquist SP et al: Use of pooled formalin-preserved fecal specimens to detect *Giardia lamblia, J Clin Microbiol* 29:1725, 1991.

Walker J et al: Giemsa staining for cysts and trophozoites of *Pneumocystis carinii, J Clin Pathol* 42:432, 1989.

Walsh JA: Problems in recognition and diagnosis of amebiasis: estimation of the global magnitude of morbidity and mortality, *Rev Infect Dis* 8:228, 1988.

Wanke C et al: *Toxoplasma* encephalitis in patients with acquired immunodeficiency syndrome: diagnosis and response to therapy, *Am J Trop Med Hyg* 36:509, 1987.

Watson B et al: Direct wet mounts versus concentration for routine parasitological examination: are both necessary? *Am J Clin Pathol* 89:389, 1988.

Weber R, Bryan RT, Juranek DD: Improved stool concentration procedure for detection of *Cryptosporidium* oocysts in fecal specimens, *J Clin Microbiol* 30:2869, 1992.

Weber R et al: Threshold of detection of *Cryptosporidium* oocysts in human stool specimens: evidence for low sensitivity of current diagnostic methods, *J Clin Microbiol* 29:1323, 1991.

Weinke T et al: Prevalence and clinical importance of *Entamoeba histolytica* in two high-risk groups: travelers returning from the tropics and male homosexuals, *J Infect Dis* 161:1029, 1990.

Whitby M: Drug-resistant *Plasmodium vivax* malaria, *J Antimicrob Chemother* 40:749, 1997.

Wijdicks EFM et al: Fatal disseminated hemorrhagic toxoplasmic encephalitis as the initial manifestation of AIDS, *Ann Neurol* 29:683, 1991.

Wilson M, Ware DA, Walls KW: Evaluation of commercial serodiagnosis kits for toxoplasmosis, *J Clin Microbiol* 25:2262, 1987.

Wilson RJM: Biochemistry of red cell invasion, *Blood Cells* 16:237, 1990.

Wongrichanalai C et al: Acridine orange fluorescent microscopy and the detection of malaria in populations with low-density parasitemia, *Am J Trop Med Hyg* 44:17, 1991.

World Health Organization: *Drugs used in parasitic diseases,* Geneva, 1990, World Health Organization.

World Health Organization: *Prevention and control of intestinal parasitic infections,* Report of a WHO expert committee, World Health Organization Technical Report Series #749, Geneva, 1987, World Health Organization.

Wyler DJ: Malaria chemoprophylaxis for the traveler, *N Engl J Med* 329:31, 1993.

Xaio L, Herd RP: Quantitation of *Giardia* cysts and *Cryptosporidium* oocysts in fecal samples by direct immunofluorescence assay, *J Clin Microbiol* 31:2944, 1993.

Yeoh R, Warhurst DC, Falcon MG: *Acanthamoeba* keratitis, *Br J Opthalmol* 71:500, 1987.

Zierdt CH: *Blastocystis hominis:* past and future, *Clin Microbiol Rev* 4:61, 1991.

Zierdt CH, Gill VJ, Zierdt WS: Detection of microsporidian spores in clinical samples by indirect fluorescent antibody assay using whole cell antisera to *Encephalitozoon cuniculi* and *Encephalitozoon hellem, J Clin Microbiol* 31:3071, 1993.

Zimmerman SK, Needham CA: Comparison of conventional stool concentration and preserved-smear methods with Merifluor *Cryptosporidium/Giardia* direct immunofluoresence assay and Prospect *Giardia* EZ microplate assay for detection of *Giardia lamblia, J Clin Microbiol* 33:1942, 1995.

LEARNING ASSESSMENT

1. A trichrome-stained smear of a patient's fecal specimen shows the presence of cysts that are oval, approximately 11 μm in size, have 4 nuclei characterized by large karyosomes with no peripheral chromatin, and a "cluttered" appearance in the cytoplasm.
   a. What is the most likely identification of the organism?
   b. Is the organism classified as a pathogen? If yes, describe the typical patient symptoms and possible complications.
   c. Why would these complications occur?

2. A patient with a history of travel to Africa has fever and chills. The physician suspects malaria and orders a blood smear for examination.
   a. Why might you do both a thin film and a thick film? Why would final species identification be made from the thin smear?
   b. What characteristics would you use to identify the species of malarial organism present? For each species give the major characteristics.
   c. What are the complications of infection with *Plasmodium falciparum?* Explain why or how these occur.

3. Give the major characteristics (including size) that you would use to identify eggs of the following organisms:
   Taenia sp.
   Ascaris lumbricoides
   Trichuris trichiura
   Enterobius vermicularis
   Hookworm
   Schistosoma mansoni

4. Describe the diagnostic method you would use to detect *Enterobius vermicularis* eggs that would not be used with the other types of eggs. Explain why.

CHAPTER 25

Clinical Virology

William F. Nauschuetz

VIRUSES
  Structure
  Taxonomy

LABORATORY DIAGNOSIS OF VIRAL
  INFECTIONS
  Specimen Collection and Transport
  Appropriate Specimens for Maximum Recovery
  Methods in Diagnostic Virology
    Direct detection
    Serologic assays
    Viral isolation

CELL CULTURE FOR VIRAL ISOLATION
  Cytopathic Effect on Cell Cultures for
    Presumptive Identification of Viral Agents
  Centrifugation-Enhanced Shell Vial Culture

RESPIRATORY VIRUSES
  Influenza Viruses
  Parainfluenza Viruses
  Respiratory Syncytial Virus
  Adenoviruses
  Rhinoviruses
  Coronaviruses

EXANTHEMAS
  Mumps
  Measles (Rubeola)
  Rubella
  Hand, Foot, and Mouth Disease
  Parvovirus B19

IMMUNODEFICIENCY VIRUSES: HUMAN
  IMMUNODEFICIENCY VIRUS TYPE 1

CENTRAL NERVOUS SYSTEM VIRUSES:
  ENTEROVIRUSES

AGENTS OF GASTROINTESTINAL INFECTIONS
  Rotaviruses
  Norwalk and Norwalk-Like Agents

Enteric Adenoviruses
Other Viruses

ARBOVIRUSES
  Family Bunyaviridae
  Family Togaviridae
  Family Flaviviridae
  Family Reoviridae
  Laboratory Diagnosis of Arboviral Infections

FAMILY ARENAVIRIDAE

GENUS HANTAVIRUS

FAMILY FILOVIRIDAE

RABIES

HUMAN PAPILLOMAVIRUSES

HEPATITIS VIRUSES
  Hepatitis A
  Hepatitis B
  Hepatitis D (Delta Hepatitis)
  Hepatitis C
  Hepatitis E

HERPESVIRUSES
  Herpes Simplex Virus
  Human Cytomegalovirus
  Epstein-Barr Virus
  Varicella-Zoster Virus
  Human Herpesvirus 6
  Human Herpesvirus 7
  Human Herpesvirus 8

ANTIVIRAL THERAPY
  Absorption
  Penetration
  Uncoating
  Eclipse/Synthesis
  Maturation/Release

OBJECTIVES

1. Describe the characteristics of viruses, and differentiate these organisms from bacteria.
2. Describe how viruses multiply.
3. Describe the proper procedures for collection and transport of viral specimens.
4. Name the appropriate specimen for maximum recovery of the suspected viral agent.
5. Describe the different methods used in the diagnosis of viral infections.
6. Explain the advantages and limitations of conventional tissue cultures.
7. Explain the advantages and limitations of rapid viral antigen detection methods.
8. Discuss the indications and limitations of serologic assays in the diagnosis of viral infections.
9. Define *cytopathic effect (CPE)* and describe how it is used to presumptively identify viral agents.
10. For each of the viral agents presented in this chapter, discuss how the virus is transmitted or acquired, the infection the virus produces, and the effective method of laboratory diagnosis.

KEY TERMS

Obligate intracellular parasites
Cell cultures
Viral genome
Capsid
Virion
Enveloped viruses
Replication
Cytopathic effect (CPE)
Tissue culture, organ culture
Primary cell cultures

Diploid cell cultures
Continuous (heteroploid) cell cultures
HEp2
A549
Vero
Hemagglutinin (H)
Antigenic drift
Amantadine
Ribavirin
Rubeola

Exanthem
Koplik's spots
Rubella
Erythema infectiosum (EI), fifth disease
Acquired immune deficiency syndrome (AIDS)
Zidovudine
Enteroviruses
Enteric adenoviruses

Arboviruses
Dengue virus
Sin Nombre
Infectious hepatitis
Serum hepatitis
HBsAg
HBcAg
HBeAg
Delta hepatitis (HDV)
Coinfection
Superinfection

VIRUSES

Viruses are **obligate intracellular parasites.** Full-service virology laboratories have several different mammalian **cell cultures** to support the growth of clinically significant viruses; they then identify viruses grown in culture. Many laboratories still do not have the space, funds, and expertise to provide viral culturing services. However, these laboratories can still provide laboratory professionals information about viral infections using a variety of rapid tests that detect specific viruses in clinical specimens. These rapid tests can involve either fluorescent antibody detection or detection of viral antigens with either an enzyme immunoassay (EIA) or optical immunoassay (OIA) test. Some tests are even

Clinical Laboratory Improvement Act (CLIA) waived, bringing viral identification services into physicians' offices and clinics. Other laboratories may limit their virology services to viral serology—determining the patient's immune response to viruses—rather than searching for the viruses directly.

Structure

At a minimum, viruses contain a **viral genome** (of either RNA or DNA) and a protein coat (the **capsid**). The genome can be either double stranded (ds) or single stranded (ss). The genome and its protein coat is a **virion.** Some viruses also have a phospholipid envelope surrounding the virion. **Enveloped viruses** are often more susceptible to inactivation by temperature, pH, and chemicals than

CASE STUDY

A 36-year-old man was admitted to the hospital after going to the emergency room and stating that for 7 months he had been experiencing numbness and weakness in his right leg. He had lost 25 lb, was experiencing bowel incontinence, and had been unable to urinate for 3 days. Two years previously, the patient had been diagnosed as having the human immunodeficiency virus (HIV). A physical examination demonstrated bilateral lower extremity weakness, and his reflexes were slower throughout his body. Kaposi's lesions were noted, especially on the lower extremities. Recurrent thrush and herpes lesions in the perianal region were also observed. A magnetic resonance imaging (MRI) examination was performed to rule out spinal cord compression and was negative. The patient was afebrile.

The patient had history of intravenous (IV) drug use, as well as a history of chronic diarrhea for 1½ years, Kaposi's sarcoma for 2 years, and pancytopenia for several weeks. The patient had large, right arachnoid cysts of congenital origin. No previous reports indicated infectious agents in the cerebrospinal fluid (CSF). Meningitis was suspected, and the patient was admitted with a diagnosis of polyradiculopathy secondary to acquired immunodeficiency syndrome (AIDS). Acyclovir was administered after culture results were received. Blood and CSF were taken. The CSF produced no growth on a routine bacteriological culture, although numerous white blood cells were found.

on genome type (RNA or DNA), the number of strands in the genome (ds or ss), morphology, and presence or absence of an envelope. The International Committee on Taxonomy of Viruses classifies viruses into 71 families, 9 subfamilies, 164 genera, and 3600 species. However, as many as 30,000 different strains and subtypes may exist. A summary of the clinically significant viruses is shown in Tables 25-1 and 25-2.

Viral reproduction, or **replication,** is unique to viruses. The virus attaches to the surface of a susceptible cell by means of specialized structures on its surface and specific receptors on the surface of the cell. The virus enters the cell by endocytosis—fusion of the viral membrane and cell membrane—or lysis of the cell's membrane. Once inside the cell, the virus loses its coat, removing the capsid from the genome. The viral genome then directs the host cell to make viral proteins and genome. Depending on the virus, the metabolism of the host cell may be shut off completely (as with polioviruses), or it may continue on a restricted scale (as with influenza viruses and papovaviruses). The virus-encoded proteins and genome then reassemble in the host cell. The new virions are then released by lysis of the cell (if infected with a virus such as poliovirus) or by budding through the cell membrane (if infected by viruses such as influenza and parainfluenza viruses).

LABORATORY DIAGNOSIS OF VIRAL INFECTIONS

Specimen Collection and Transport

Viral shedding is usually greatest during the early stages of infection, so the best specimens are those collected as early as possible. The sensitivity of viral culture may decrease rapidly 3 days after onset of symptoms. Specimens should be collected as aseptically as possible. Aspirated secretions are often preferable, but swabs are easier to use for collection. Swabs must be made of cotton, Dacron, or nylon. Calcium alginate swabs inhibit the growth of some viruses. Tissue samples must be kept moist. Viral transport medium, saline, or trypticase soy broth can be added to sterile containers to keep tissues from drying out.

Several viral transport systems are commercially available. Most transport media consist of a buffered isotonic solution with some type of pro-

nonenveloped viruses. The envelopes are of host origin, but they contain virus-encoded proteins. The viruses acquire the lipid membrane as they bud off host cells.

The morphology of virions is either helical, icosahedral (a geometric shape with 20 faces), or complex. The envelope masks the shape of the virion, so most enveloped viruses are *pleomorphic,* or variably shaped. The poxviruses are the largest viruses (250 by 350 nm), and the smallest human virus is the poliovirus, which is 25 nm in diameter.

Taxonomy

Originally, viruses were classified by their host range and the type of diseases they caused. Now viruses are classified in families and genera based

TABLE 25-1

Clinically Significant DNA Viruses

Genome	Envelope	Family	Subfamily	Genus	Significant Members
dsDNA	Yes	Herpesviridae	Alphaherpesvirinae	*Simplexvirus*	Herpes simplex viruses (types 1 and 2)
				Varicellovirus	Varicella-zoster virus
			Betaherpesvirinae	*Cytomegalovirus*	Cytomegalovirus (human herpesvirus 3)
			Gammaherpesvirinae	*Lymphocryptovirus*	Human herpesvirus 4
		Poxviridae	Chordopoxvirinae	*Orthopoxvirus*	Vaccinia
					Variola
				Molluscipoxvirus	Molluscum contagiosum virus
	No	Adenoviridae		*Mastadenovirus*	Human adenovirus
		Papovaviridae		*Papillomavirus*	Human papillomavirus
ssDNA	No	Parvoviridae	Parvovirinae	*Erythrovirus*	B19
ss/dsDNA	Yes	Hepadnaviridae		*Orthohepadnavirus*	Hepatitis B virus

TABLE 25-2

Clinically Significant RNA Viruses

Genome	Envelope	Family	Genus	Significant Members
dsRNA (positive, segmented)	No	Reoviridae	*Orthoreovirus*	Human reovirus
			Rotavirus	Human rotavirus
			Coltivirus	Colorado tick fever virus
ssRNA (positive)	Yes	Flaviviridae	Yellow fever virus group	Yellow fever virus
			Dengue virus group	Dengue virus
			Japanese encephalitis group	Japanese encephalitis virus
			Tick-borne encephalitis group	
		Hepatitis C–like viruses		Hepatitis C virus
		Coronaviridae	*Coronavirus*	Human coronavirus
		Togaviridae	*Alphavirus*	Sindbis virus
				Eastern encephalitis virus
				Western encephalitis virus
				Semliki Forest virus
				Ross River virus
			Rubivirus	Rubella virus
		Retroviridae	BLV-human T-cell leukemia retroviruses	Human T-cell leukemia virus
			Lentivirus	Human immunodeficiency virus type 1
				Human immunodeficiency virus type 2
				Simian immunodeficiency virus
	No	Caliciviridae	*Calicivirus*	Norwalk virus
				Hepatitis E virus
		Picornaviridae	*Enterovirus*	Human poliovirus
				Coxsackie A virus
				Coxsackie B virus
				Echovirus
				Enterovirus
			Rhinovirus	Human rhinovirus
			Hepatovirus	Hepatitis A virus
			Cardiovirus	Encephalomyocarditis virus
			Aphthovirus	Foot and mouth disease virus
ssRNA (negative)	Yes	Orthomyxoviridae	*Influenzavirus A, B*	Influenza A virus
				Influenza B virus
			Influenzavirus C	Influenza C virus
		Filoviridae	*Filovirus*	Ebola virus
				Marburg virus
		Rhabdoviridae	*Lyssavirus*	Rabies virus
ssRNA (negative)	Yes	Arenaviridae	*Arenavirus*	Lassa virus
			Deltavirus	Hepatitis delta virus
		Bunyaviridae	*Hantavirus*	Hantavirus
				Hantaanvirus

tein such as albumin, gelatin, or serum to protect less stable viruses. Antibiotics are added in some transport systems to inhibit contaminating bacterial flora. It is also important for the transport container to be unbreakable and able to withstand freezing and thawing.

It is optimal to process viral specimens for culture immediately. Some viruses, such as respiratory syncytial virus (RSV), become more difficult to recover even a few hours after collection. However, if specimens cannot be processed immediately after collection, they should be stored at 4° C. Specimens should not be frozen unless a significant delay (greater than 4 days) in processing occurs. In that case, specimens should be frozen and held in a −70° C freezer. Do not freeze specimens at −20° C. This temperature facilitates the formation of ice crystals, which disrupt the host cells and result in significant loss of viral viability.

Appropriate Specimens for Maximum Recovery

A common sense approach in selecting specimens for isolation is to collect the specimens from the affected site. For example, secretions from the respiratory mucosa are most appropriate for viral diagnosis of respiratory infections. Aspirates (or surface swabs) are usually appropriate for lesions. If the intestinal mucosa is involved, a stool specimen is most appropriate. However, if systemic, congenital, or generalized disease is involved, then specimens from multiple sites, including blood (huffy coat) and CSF, as well from the portals of entry (oral or respiratory tract) or exit (urine or stool) are appropriate. Enteroviruses may cause respiratory infections and may be recovered from the stool after the respiratory shedding has ceased. Because enteroviruses have been associated with congenital infections, the stool may be an appropriate specimen for congenital infections. In addition, enteroviruses are a major cause of aseptic meningitis and may be isolated from urine specimens. Table 25-3 lists suggested specimens to be collected for viral diagnosis according to the affected body site.

Methods in Diagnostic Virology

The laboratory uses three major methods to diagnose viral infections:

- Direct detection of the virus in the clinical specimen
- Serologic antibody assays to detect viral antibodies
- Isolation of the virus in culture

Each laboratory must decide which of these methods fulfills the spectrum of infections encountered. In most circumstances a combination of these assays is used to determine the viral agent responsible for an infection. Table 25-3 also lists various tests available to detect viral infectious agents.

Direct detection

Direct detection methods are generally not as sensitive as culture methods, but they can offer valuable assistance to the laboratory professional. Many of these tests can be run in a few minutes. Box 25-1 shows the advantages and disadvantages of direct detection methods. Rapid testing can include the methods described in the following paragraphs.

IMMUNOSTAINING
Immunofluorescence (IF) can be a flexible tool used to detect various viral agents directly in clinical specimens. Some tests use direct fluorescent antibody (DFA), in which fluorescence-labeled antibodies are incubated on fixed smears of host cells. A more specific test is the indirect immunofluorescent antibody (IFA) test, which uses an unlabeled antibody to the virus that is then detected by a second immunolabeled antibody. These tests can be used to detect adenovirus, influenza viruses A and B, measles, parainfluenza viruses 1 through 4, and RSV from respiratory specimens; herpes simplex virus types 1 and 2 (HSV-1 and HSV-2) and varicella-zoster virus (VZV) from cutaneous lesion material, and cytomegalovirus (CMV) antigen from blood.

ENZYME IMMUNOASSAY (EIA)
Many EIA tests for viral detection are available. Many are packaged as microtiter plate assays. These tests can be used to detect RSV and influenza A from respiratory specimens, hepatitis B virus (HBV) and HIV type 1 (HIV-1) from serum or plasma, the enteric adenoviruses from stool, and HSV from cutaneous lesions and conjunctival swabs. Other tests are packaged in single-test platforms, with colorimetric detection on membrane surfaces. These tests can be used to detect RSV, influenza viruses A and B from respiratory specimens, and rotavirus and enteric adenovirus from rectal swabs. EIA tests are often less sensitive than

TABLE 25-3

Tests Available for Common Viral Pathogens and Specimens for Culture

Body System Affected	Antigen Detection	Virus Isolation	Serology	Culture Specimens
Respiratory tract	Adenovirus, herpes simplex virus (HSV), cytomegalovirus (CMV), influenza virus types A and B, parainfluenza virus, respiratory syncitial virus (RSV)	Adenovirus, Coxsackie A, Coxsackie B, echovirus, HSV, CMV, influenza virus types A and B, parainfluenza virus, RSV, reovirus, rhinovirus	Adenovirus, coxsackie A virus, coxsackie B virus, Echovirus, HSV, CMV, Influenza virus types A and B, parainfluenza virus, RSV	Nasal aspirate, nasopharynx (NP) or throat swabs, bronchoalveolar lavage, lung biopsy
Gastrointestinal	Adenoviruses 40 and 41, rotavirus	Adenovirus 40 and 41, coxsackie A, reovirus	Adenoviruses 40 and 41, coxsackie A	Stool, rectal swab
Hepatitis			Hepatitis A virus (HAV), hepatitis B virus (HBV), hepatitis C virus (HCV), hepatitis D virus (HDV), hepatitis E virus (HEV), Epstein-Barr virus (EBV)	
Cutaneous	HSV, adenovirus, varicella-zoster virus	HSV, adenovirus, coxsackie group A virus, coxsackie group B virus, echovirus, enterovirus, measles virus, VZV, reovirus, rubella virus, vaccinia virus	HSV, adenovirus, coxsackie group B virus, dengue virus, echovirus, human herpes virus 6 (HHV-6), measles virus, VZV, parvovirus B19, rubella virus, vaccinia virus	Vesicle aspirate, NP aspirate and stool, lesion swab
Central nervous system	HSV, mumps virus	Coxsackie group A virus, coxsackie group B virus, echovirus, enterovirus, poliovirus, HSV, mumps virus	Coxsackie group A virus, Coxsackie group B virus, echovirus, poliovirus, HSV, HHV-6, mumps virus	CSF, brain biopsy, NP swabs, stool
Ocular	Adenovirus, HSV	Adenovirus, HSV, coxsackie group A, Enterovirus	HSV, coxsackie group A virus	Corneal swabs, conjunctival scrapings
Genital	HSV	HSV	HSV	Vesicle aspirate, vesicle swab

Box 25-1

Advantages and Disadvantages of Direct Detection

Advantages

Potential for rapid diagnosis
Detection of nonculturable viruses
No need for culture

Disadvantages

Confined to the specific antibody used
Costly and labor intensive (immunofluorescent antibody methods)
Dependent on specimen adequacy and quality; no assessment of specimen quality in enzyme immunoassay methods

Modified from Costello MJ, Morrow S et al: Guidelines for specimen collection, transportation, and test selection, *Lab Med* 24:19, 1993.

---

culture or FA, so negative results are confirmed with culture, FA, or gene amplification.

OPTICAL IMMUNOASSAY (OIA)

OIAs use silicon wafers coated with antibody as a means of viral detection. Viruses combine with antibodies on the wafer and produce a reflection change in the silicon wafer (Figure 25-1). These tests can detect influenza viruses A and B from respiratory specimens.

NUCLEIC ACID PROBES

Nucleic acid hybridization tests can detect viruses from various clinical specimens. One of the tests can detect the human papillomavirus (HPV) from endocervical specimens and classify them into high-risk and low-risk HPV types. Other hybridization tests can detect CMV from blood and HBV from plasma and serum.

GENE AMPLIFICATION ASSAYS

Numerous gene amplification techniques are available for the amplification and detection of viruses, primarily of the blood-borne pathogens such as HIV-1, HBV, and hepatitis C virus (HCV). Different technologies include branched DNA (bDNA), nucleic-acid sequence-based amplification (NASBA), and polymerase chain reaction (PCR) technologies.

ELECTRON MICROSCOPY

Electron microscopy is becoming an increasingly rare asset in clinical laboratories, yet it can detect noncultivable viruses, such as the Norwalk viruses in stool filtrates.

LIGHT MICROSCOPY

Many viruses form characteristic inclusion bodies in infected cells. These inclusions can be detected in cell scrapings from infected sites. For instance, a Tzanck smear can detect Cowdry type A bodies from HSV and VZV lesions, and Papanicolaou's (Pap) smears detect HPV-associated koilocytosis, a **cytopathic effect (CPE)** in which squamous cells have an enlarged nucleus surrounded by a nonstaining halo. Rabies is often diagnosed by detecting Negri bodies, which are eosinophilic cytoplasmic inclusions, in neurons.

Serologic assays

Viral serology provides limited information, and certain problems are inherent in the methods. First, serologic assays measure host response rather than detect the virus. Second, the antibody-producing capabilities of human hosts varies widely. Third, the antibody level does not necessarily correlate with the acuteness or activity level of the of infection.

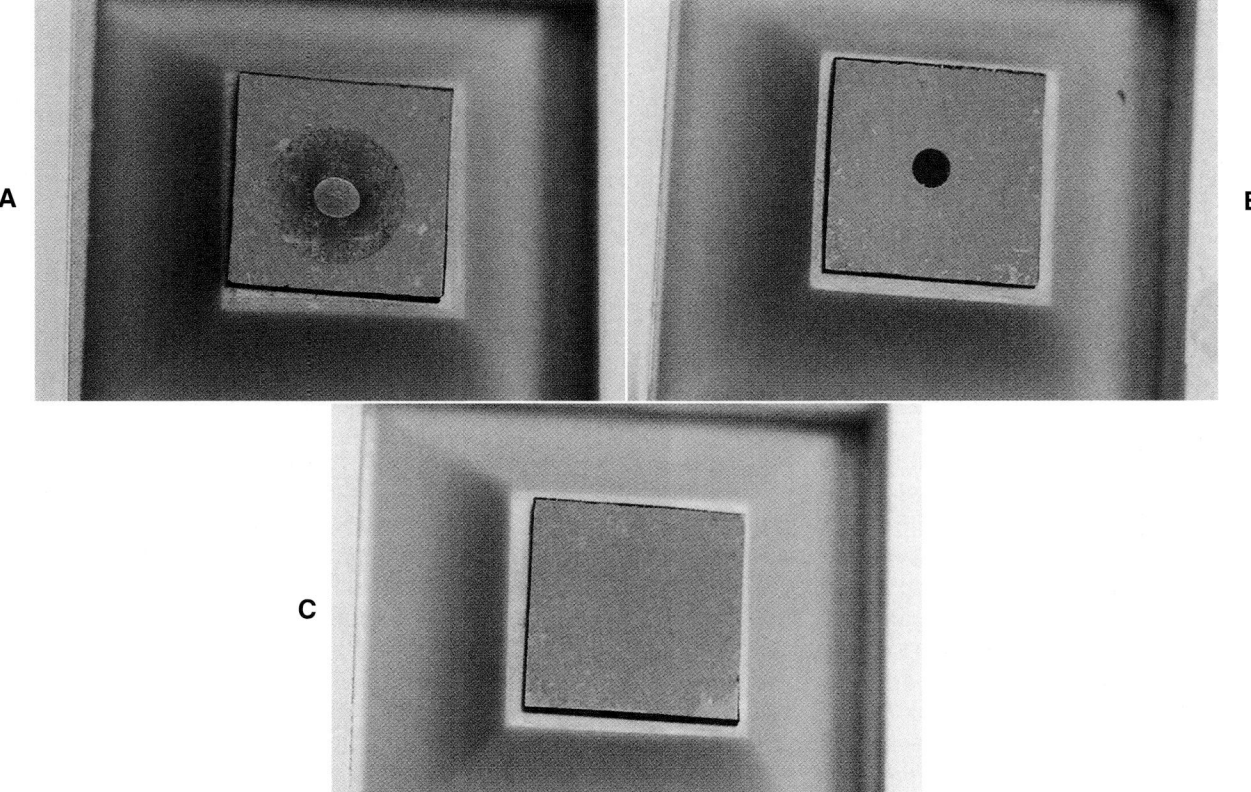

Figure 25-1

Optical immunoassay (OIA). **A,** Positive reaction. **B,** Negative reaction. **C,** Invalid reaction. (From Forbes B, Sahm D, Weissfeld S: *Bailey and Scott's diagnostic microbiology,* ed 10, St Louis, 1998, Mosby and courtesy BioStar, Inc, Boulder Colo.)

With few exceptions, paired sera (acute and convalescent) demonstrating seroconversion or a fourfold rise in titer are required to establish a diagnosis of recent infection. Serologic studies are also usually retrospective because of the need for paired sera. In addition, cross-reactions with nonspecific antibodies produced by the host may be detected, which makes interpretation of results obscure. Interpretation is also difficult in passive transfer of antibodies, such as in transplacental or transfusion transmission. Indications for serology are as follows:

- Diagnosis of infections with nonculturable organisms such as hepatitis viruses
- Determination of immune status in regards to rubella, measles, VZV, and HBV
- Monitoring of patients who have immunosuppression or have had transplants
- Epidemiologic or prevalence studies

Viral isolation

In clinical virology, isolating virus is still the gold standard against which all other methods are compared. Traditionally, three methods are used for isolation of viruses in diagnostic virology: cell culture, animal inoculation, and embryonated eggs. Of these three methods, the most commonly used is cell culture. Animal inoculation is extremely costly and used only as a special resource and in reference or research laboratories. For example, certain coxsackie A viruses require suckling mice for isolation of the virus. Embryonated eggs are rarely used; isolation of influenza viruses is enhanced in embryonated eggs, but this is generally much more easily accomplished in cell culture.

Establishing at least a limited clinical virus isolation capability in routine laboratories is amply justified. The majority of the clinical workload focuses in the detection of HSV and genital specimens and respiratory viruses. A significant percentage of common clinical viruses can often be identified within 48 hours of inoculation, including HSV, influenza A and B viruses, parainfluenza viruses 1 through 4, RSV, adenovirus (using shell vial cultures), and many enteroviruses (using shell vial cultures). Detection allows physicians to make relevant decisions about therapy and hospitalization. Sometimes situations, virology results may be available before routine bacteriology culture results.

CELL CULTURE FOR VIRAL ISOLATION

The term *cell culture* is technically used to indicate culture of cells in vitro; the cells are not organized into a tissue. The term **tissue culture** or **organ culture** is used to denote growth of tissues or an organ in a way that preserves the architecture or function of the tissue or organ. However, for practical purposes, most clinical virology laboratory professionals use the terms *cell culture* and *tissue culture* interchangeably.

Cell cultures can be divided into three categories: primary, diploid, and continuous (heteroploid). **Primary cell cultures** are obtained from tissue removed from an animal. The tissue is finely minced and then treated with an enzyme such as trypsin to further disperse individual cells. The cells are then seeded onto a surface to form a monolayer. With primary cell lines, only very minimal cell division occurs. An example of a commonly used primary cell culture is primary monkey kidney (PMK).

Diploid cell cultures can divide (passage), but passage is limited to 50 generations. With increasing passage, diploid cells become more insensitive to viral infection. Human neonatal lung (HNL) is an example of a standard diploid cell culture used in diagnostic virology.

Continuous (heteroploid) cell cultures have variable numbers of chromosomes and are capable of indefinite passage. **HEp2** (which is derived from a human laryngeal carcinoma), **A549** (which is derived from a human lung carcinoma), and **Vero** (which is derived from monkey kidney) are examples of continuous cell lines used in diagnostic virology. Each laboratory must decide which cell lines to use based on the spectrum of viral sensitivity, availability, and cost. Table 25-4 lists some cell culture lines commonly used in clinical virology. Box 25-2 describes briefly the advantages and disadvantages of viral isolation.

Cytopathic Effect on Cell Cultures for Presumptive Identification of Viral Agents

Cell cultures can be used for presumptive identification because of a characteristic CPE that viruses produce on certain cells. For example, HSV grows rapidly on many different types of cell cultures and

Box 25-2

Advantages and Disadvantages of Viral Isolation

Advantages

Is sensitive (general "gold standard")
Detects broad spectrum of viruses
Is flexible, adaptable to viral variation
Can use spin amplification (shell vial)
Can use susceptibility testing possible*
Involves confirmation and cross-checks
Involves comprehensive quality
Uses skilled personnel

Disadvantages

Time required for isolation and identification:
   HSV, 1 to 3 days
   Enterovirus, 2 to 5 days
   Respiratory viruses, 2 to 5 days
Viable organism required
Facility required
Skilled personnel required

*Still rarely performed; expensive and limited.

frequently produces a CPE within 24 hours. A predominantly cell-associated virus, HSV produces a focal CPE (in which adjacent cells become infected) and plaques (or clusters of infected cells). The combination of rapid growth, plaque formation, and growth on many different cell types (such as PMK, human fibroblasts, Vero, HEp2, mink lung, and primary human kidney) is presumptive evidence for the diagnosis of HSV. HSV is one of the few viruses that grows on rabbit kidney cells (Figure 25-2), therefore it is a useful cell line in herpes detection programs.

CMV also has an HSV-like CPE (Figure 25-3) but grows much more slowly and only on diploid fibroblasts. VZV grows on several types of cells, including diploid fibroblasts, A549, and Vero cells. Enteroviruses characteristically produce rather small, round cells that spread diffusely on PMK, diploid fibroblasts, human embryonal rhabdomyosarcoma (RD) cells, and A549 cells. Adenoviruses also produce cell rounding (Figure 25-4) (that is usually larger than that caused by enteroviruses) on a number of cell types, including diploid fibroblasts, HEp2, A549, and monkey kidney cells (PMK). The rounding may be diffuse or focal (appearing like a cluster of grapes).

The respiratory viruses may not produce a characteristic CPE. RSV may produce a classic syncytial formation in HEp2 cells or even monkey kidney cells. Parainfluenza type 2 (and to a lesser extent, parainfluenza type 3) viruses may also produce syncytia. Influenza virus commonly does not exhibit a well-defined CPE. Specimens submitted for influenza virus cultures are usually inoculated onto primary rhesus monkey kidney, LLC-MK2 (a continuous line derived from rhesus monkey kidney) or MDCK (canine kidney) cells. Because influenza CPEs are usually not detected, a hemagglutination or hemadsorption test is done to detect these viruses. Cells infected with influenza virus have a viral **hemagglutinin (H)** that binds to red blood

TABLE 25-4

Cell Cultures Commonly Used in the Clinical Virology Laboratory

Virus	PMK	HDF	Hep2	RK	A549	CPE
Herpes simplex virus	−	+++	+++	+++	+++	Large, rounded cells
Cytomegalovirus	−	+++	−	−	−	Large, rounded cells
Varicella-zoster virus	−	+++	−	−	+/−	Foci or rounded cells; possible syncytia
Enterovirus	+	+	+++	−	+	Refractile, round cells in clusters
Adenovirus	+	++	+++	−	++	Large, rounded cells in clusters
Respiratory syncitial virus	+/−	+	+++	−	++	Syncytia
Influenza/parainfluenza	+++	+/−	−	−	−	Variable–none to granular appearance

Modified from Costello MJ et al: Guidelines for specimen collection, transportation, and test selection, *Lab Med* 24:19, 1993. *A549,* Human lung carcinoma cell line; *HDF,* human diploid fibroblasts; *Hep2,* human laryngeal carcinoma cell line; *PMK,* primary monkey kidney; *RK,* rabbit kidney; *CPE,* cytopathic effect.

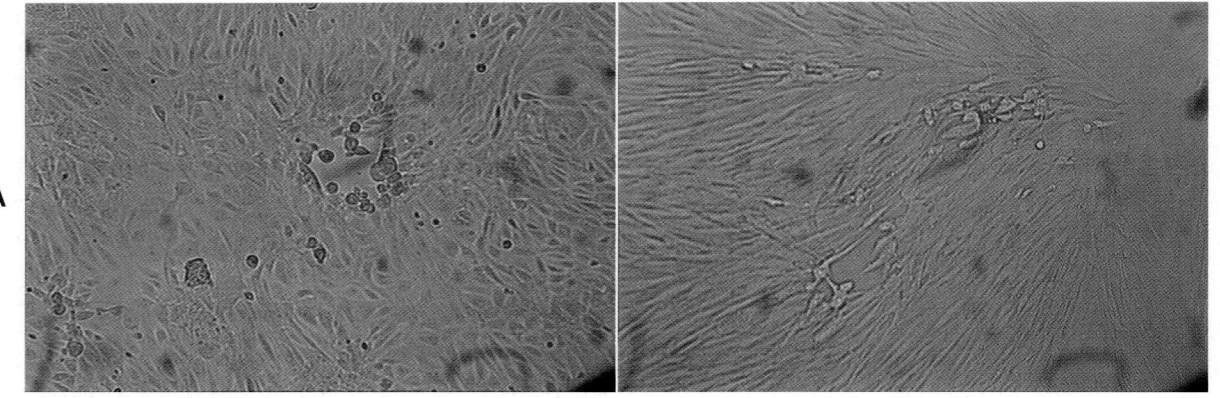

A

B

Figure 25-2 _____

A, Herpes simplex virus (HSV) from the skin, showing a cytopathic effect (CPE) in less than 1 day on rabbit kidney cells.
B, HSV showing a cytopathic effect in less than 1 day on Hela.

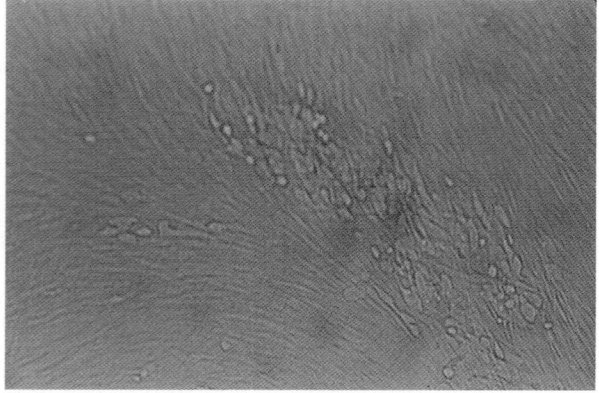

Figure 25-3 _____

Cytomegalovirus (CMV) from cerebrospinal fluid forming cytopathic effect (CPE) on diploid fibroblast cells.

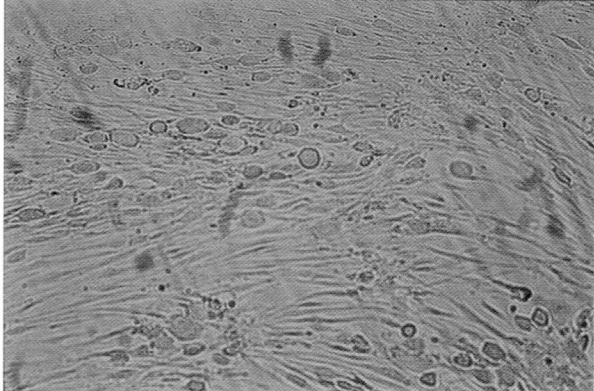

Figure 25-4 _____

Cytopathic effect (CPE) of adenovirus on Hela.

cells. Fluorescent antibody stains can also be used to screen the cell cultures before a final negative result is reported.

Centrifugation-Enhanced Shell Vial Culture

The shell vial culture technique is a simple method that more rapidly identifies the virus than the traditional viral culture method. Cells are grown on a round coverslip in a shell vial. The shell vial is inoculated with the clinical sample and then centrifuged to promote viral absorption. The shell vial is incubated for 24 to 48 hours, after which the cells are scraped from the coverslip, and the DFA technique is performed using a variety of antibodies.

RESPIRATORY VIRUSES

Influenza Viruses

Influenza virus A remains one of the most crucial health problems throughout the world. In the pandemic of 1918 and 1919, influenza killed 20 million people, more than 500,000 of which were Americans. Yet in the past 80 years, the world has only been able to react to the threat of influenza rather than vanquish it. Even now, a "mild" influenza outbreak may kill 20,000 Americans. In 6 different years from 1972 to 1995, influenza deaths in the United States exceeded 40,000.

The key to the persistence of the influenza virus is its genetic material and antigenic composition. Influenza viruses are enveloped and have eight segments of ssRNA. Their major surface antigens are hemagglutinin (H) and neuraminidase (N). The H antigen is used to bind to host cells, and neuraminidase cleaves budding viruses from infected cells. Hemagglutinin has four subtypes (H1, H2, H3, and H5) and the N antigen has two (N1 and N2) that have caused human disease. The surface antigens can change, or *shift,* over time. Three major shifts occurred during the twentieth century: influenza (H1N1) appeared in 1918 and 1919 (the "swine flu"), shifted to influenza A (H2N2) in 1957 and 1958 (the "Asian flu"), and shifted to H3N2 in 1968 and 1969 (the "Hong Kong flu").

The dominant strains of influenza A since 1977 have been influenza A (H1N1) and influenza A (H3N2). In early 1998 an outbreak of human influenza A (H5N1) appeared in Hong Kong (the "avian flu"). Sixteen patients had evidence of infection, and six of them died. Public health officials flocked to Hong Kong to determine whether another major worldwide shift would occur. In this case, influenza A (H5N1) did not transmit from human-to-human efficiently enough to cause a widespread outbreak.

The H and N antigens of the influenza A virus change continuously, reflecting mutations in their genetic material. **Antigenic drift** describes subtle changes in the H and N antigens. However, antigenic *shift* occurs when a *major* change occurs in the antigens. Antigenic shift often triggers a pandemic, because humans often have little preexisting immunity to the new strain. The World Health Organization makes recommendations regarding composition of the trivalent influenza vaccine several months before influenza season begins. The vaccine contains one strain of influenza virus B and two different strains of influenza virus A.

Influenza viruses are spread by aerosols. The incubation period is 1 to 4 days. Although asymptomatic infections can occur, infections are usually characterized by a rapid onset of malaise, fever, myalgia, and often a nonproductive cough. The fever can be as high as 41° C. Vomiting is more likely to occur in children than adults. Infected patients are often ill for days and often require a lengthy convalescence. Influenza can also cause a fatal viral pneumonia.

The viruses attack the ciliated epithelial cells lining the respiratory tract, causing necrosis and sloughing of the cells. Complications include secondary bacterial pneumonia. The antiviral drugs **amantadine** and rimantadine can prevent infection or reduce the severity of symptoms if administered within 48 hours of onset. These antiviral drugs are effective only against influenza A.

Influenza viruses have a worldwide distribution and originate as zoonotic infections, being carried by different species of birds and mammals. Influenza season in the southern hemisphere is from May to October and in the northern hemisphere is from November to April.

Nasopharyngeal swabs, washes, or aspirates of specimens taken early in the course of the disease are the best specimens. The viruses are fragile and need to be handled carefully; specimens should never be frozen. Influenza virus can be identified in respiratory secretions by DFA, EIA, and OIA. Influenza viruses grow in the amniotic cavity of embryonated chicken eggs, PMK cells, and MDCK cells with trypsin added. Hemagglutination inhibition (HI) can be used to identify and type the viruses.

Parainfluenza Viruses

Four types (1 through 4) of parainfluenza viruses can cause disease in humans. The parainfluenza viruses are enveloped RNA viruses with two surface antigens: the hemagglutinin-neuraminidase, or HN, antigen and the fusion, or F, antigen. The HN antigen gives the viruses specificity, and the F antigen is responsible for the fusion of the virus to the cell and of one infected cell to another infected cell.

Parainfluenza viruses are the major cause of respiratory disease in young children. Types 1 and 2 cause the most serious illnesses in children between 2 and 4 years of age. Parainfluenza type 3 causes bronchiolitis and pneumonia in infants. The viruses are spread through respiratory secretions, aerosols, and direct contact. Infection of the cells in the respiratory tract leads to cell death and an inflammatory reaction in the upper and lower respiratory tract. Rhinitis, pharyngitis, laryngotracheitis, tracheobronchitis, bronchiolitis, and pneumonia may result.

Parainfluenza viruses are found worldwide. Aerosolized **ribavirin** can be used to treat them. No vaccines are available.

Parainfluenza viruses are fragile. The best specimens for viral culture are from aspirated secretions and nasopharyngeal washes. Specimens for viral isolation should be taken as early in the illness as possible, kept cold, and inoculated into PMK cells or LLC-MK2 cells. The viruses can be identified by hemadsorption, FA, neutralization, or EIA techniques. Direct examination of nasopharyngeal secretions by FA can give rapid results. Serologic studies are more valuable for epidemiology studies than for diagnostic purposes.

Respiratory Syncytial Virus

RSV is the most common virus isolated from infants with lower respiratory tract infections and causes croup, bronchitis, bronchiolitis, or interstitial pneumonia. Almost half of all infants are infected with RSV during their first year of life, and by the age of 2 years almost all have been exposed to RSV. Because infection does not confer complete immunity, multiple infections can occur throughout life. More than 90,000 children are admitted into hospitals each year with RSV lower respiratory tract infections. For that reason, nosocomial RSV is a problem in many medical treatment facilities. The virus spreads mostly through large particle droplets and contact with fomites rather than through inhalation of small particle aerosols.

RSV occurs in yearly outbreaks that last 2 to 5 months and usually appear during the winter or early spring in the temperate zones. The virus may be carried in the nares of asymptomatic adults. Testing hospital personnel and infants for RSV, isolating RSV-infected infants, following good handwashing practices, and organizing patients and staff into cohorts can reduce the risk of nosocomial spread.

RSV may also be a significant cause of morbidity and mortality in the elderly as well. Retrospective data suggest that RSV may cause 2% to 9% of the 687,000 pneumonia hospital admissions and 74,000 pneumonia deaths for elderly patients.

RSV can be identified in specimens from nasopharyngeal swabs and washes directly by FA or EIA methods. Because the virus is extremely fragile, recovering it from cultures is a major problem. Specimens must be kept cold but cannot be frozen. Once inoculated into cells, RSV grows readily in continuous epithelial cell lines such as HEp2 to form large, multinucleated cells (Figure 25-5). It also grows in PMK and human diploid fetal cells. Once CPEs are detected, RSV can be identified using FA, EIA, and serum neutralization tests.

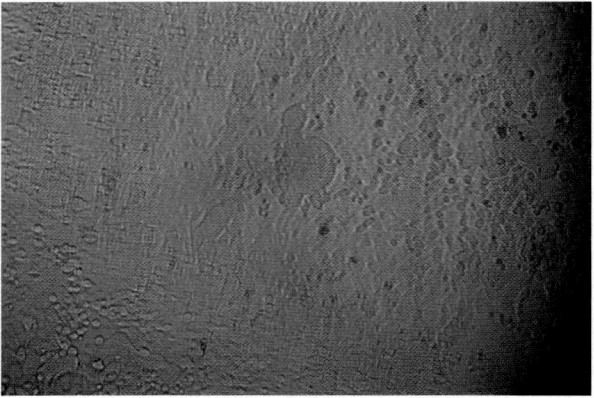

Figure 25-5

Cytopathic effect (CPE) of respiratory syncitial virus (RSV) on HEp2.

The antiviral compound ribavirin was approved in 1986 as a treatment for patients with RSV. Recently some controversy has developed regarding the efficacy of ribavirin therapy. In 1996, RSV immune globulin (RSVIG) was released for prophylaxis of susceptible patients.

Adenoviruses

Adenovirus has more than 45 serotypes, and the different serotypes are associated with varying clinical manifestations. Although half of all adenovirus infections are asymptomatic, the virus causes about 10% of all pneumonia and 5% to 15% of all gastroenteritis in children. The virus causes upper respiratory tract infections, acute respiratory distress (ARD), epidemic keratoconjunctivitis, acute hemorrhagic cystitis, and pharyngoconjunctival fever. Adenovirus infections occur throughout the year and strike every age group. The virus is shed in secretions from the eyes and respiratory tract. Viral shedding in stool and urine can occur for days after the disease has disappeared. The viruses are spread by aerosols, fomites, the oral-fecal route, and personal contact.

Adenoviruses are naked icosahedral viruses with dsDNA. Adenoviruses have a common group antigen that is detectable by EIA and complement fixation (CF). The most common serotypes are 1 to 8, 11, 21, 35, 37, and 40.

Adenoviruses are quite stable and can be isolated in human embryonic kidney, continuous epithelial cell lines, and Graham 293 transformed cell lines. They have a characteristic CPE, with swollen cells in grapelike clusters. Isolates can be identified by FA, EIA, and CF methods. Serotyping is accomplished with serum neutralization or HI.

Rhinoviruses

Rhinoviruses are the major cause of the common cold. Most people experience 2 to 5 colds each year, and about half of these colds are caused by the rhinovirus. Rhinoviruses infect the nasal epithelial cells and activate inflammatory mediators. Symptoms include a profuse watery discharge, nasal congestion, sneezing, headache, sore throat, and cough. In severe cases, bronchitis and asthma may result. Rhinovirus infections occur throughout the year, but incidences increase in the winter and spring. Transmission is primarily via aerosols, but contact with secretions and fomites can also cause infection.

Small, naked ssRNA viruses, rhinoviruses are closely related to the enteroviruses. Rhinoviruses are resistant to detergents, lipid solvents, and temperature extremes but are sensitive to pHs of less than 6. More than 100 serotypes exist.

Rhinoviruses grow best on human diploid fibroblast cells. They do not have a group antigen and there are too many to serotype, so the best method of identifying a rhinovirus is to incubate it at pH 3 with a lipid solvent. Only rhinoviruses are resistant to lipid solvents and sensitive to pH 3.

Unfortunately, no cure has been found for the common cold. Treatment with interferon does block the rhinovirus infection but has undesirable side effects such as nose bleeds.

Coronaviruses

Coronaviruses are enveloped viruses with helical ssRNA and have distinctive club-shaped projections on their surfaces. They may be responsible for 15% of coldlike infections in adults, but higher seroconversion rates are seen in children. Coronaviruses are extremely fragile and difficult to culture, but it is possible to test specimens directly by FA and EIA methods.

EXANTHEMAS

Mumps

Mumps is an acute, usually self-limiting systemic illness marked by unilateral or bilateral swelling of the parotid glands, although other glands such as the testes, ovaries, and pancreas can be infected. The primary infection of the ductal epithelial cells in the glands results in cell death and inflammation. The salivary glands recover, but the testes and ovaries may be permanently impaired. Orchitis occurs in 5% of all males, with men having a higher infection rate (18%) than boys. Oophoritis occurs rarely in females (5%), and encephalitis is even less common (0.5% to 2%).

The mumps virus is related to the parainfluenza viruses; it is an enveloped ssRNA virus with the HN and F surface antigens. Mumps is spread by droplets of infected saliva and has a worldwide distribution. Fortunately, an effective vaccine is available.

The mumps virus can be isolated from infected saliva and swabs rubbed over the Stensen duct from 9 days before onset of symptoms until 8 days after parotitis appears. The virus can also be recovered from the urine. The mumps virus is relatively fragile. Specimens may be examined directly by FA and EIA methods. The virus can be isolated in the amniotic cavity of embryonated chicken eggs as well as PMK and human embryonic kidney cell cultures.

Isolates can be identified by hemadsorption inhibition, HI, FA, and EIA tests; paired sera can be tested for mumps antibody by enzyme-linked immunosorbent assay (ELISA), FA, and HI tests. Paired sera taken as little as 4 to 5 days apart can demonstrate diagnostic or fourfold rise in titer when tested by EIA or HI. Paired sera for CF tests should be taken at least 10 days apart. Cross-reactions between soluble and viral antigens can confuse interpretation of serologic results. Virus isolation is preferable, although physicians rarely have trouble recognizing mumps.

Measles (Rubeola)

Measles **(rubeola)** was once the most common viral disease in children. An average of 500,000 cases of measles were reported annually in the 1950s, with an average mortality of 500. Immunization programs began in the United States in 1963, and the reported number of cases dropped to less than 1500 by 1983. A reemergence of measles occurred in 1989 through 1991. A decision to administer a second dose of vaccine to school-age children has drastically reduced the incidence of measles in the United States. In 1997, 135 cases of measles were reported; in 1998, 89 cases of measles were reported in the United States, 26 of which were imported from other countries.

Measles is highly contagious and spreads by aerosol. Measles causes a generalized infection characterized by a maculopapular rash and fever. Initial replication takes place in the mucosal cells of the respiratory tract; it then replicates in the local lymph nodes and spreads systemically. The virus circulates in the T and B cells and monocytes until eventually the lungs, gut, bile duct, bladder, skin, and lymphatic organs are all involved.

Measles has an abrupt onset, with symptoms of sneezing, a runny nose and cough, red eyes, and rapidly rising fever. Approximately 2 to 3 days later, a maculopapular rash appears on the head and trunk. The rash, or **exanthem,** consists of white spots **(Koplik's spots)** on a red background. Complications such as otitis, pneumonia, and encephalitis may occur. A progressive, highly fatal form of encephalitis may occur but is rare. In third world countries with malnutrition and poor hygiene, measles can be fatal.

The measles virus is an enveloped ssRNA virus, and is found worldwide. In the temperate zones, epidemics occur during the winter and spring. Infection confers lifelong immunity. An effective attenuated vaccine should be given to all children.

Measles is easily diagnosed clinically, so few requests for laboratory identification are made. The virus is fragile and must be handled carefully. The specimens of choice are from the nasopharynx and urine, but the virus can only be recovered from these sources in the early stages of infection. The virus grows on primary human kidney or PMK cells, causing formation of distinctive spindle-shape or multinucleated cells. The virus isolates can be identified using serum neutralization, EIA, or FA tests. Serologic diagnosis of measles is accomplished by demonstrating measles-specific immunoglobulin M (IgM) in the specimens collected during the acute phase of the disease.

Rubella

The disease **rubella** is a mild febrile illness accompanied by an erythematous, maculopapular, discrete rash with postauricular and suboccipital lymphadenopathy. The rash starts on the face and spreads to the trunk and limbs. No rash appears on the palms and soles. As many as 50% of individuals with rubella are asymptomatic. Transient polyarthralgia and polyarthritis may occur in children and are common in adults. Rubella would be of little concern if it did not cross the placentas of pregnant women and disseminate to all fetal tissues. The results range from the birth of a normal baby to the birth of a severely impaired infant to fetal death and spontaneous abortion. The impact on the embryo is worst when the infection develops in the earliest stages of pregnancy, because the rubella virus halts or slows the growth of the cells it infects. An effective attenuated vaccine is available and should be administered to all children, particularly to young women before they become sexually active. Fewer than 350 cases of rubella were reported in the United States in 1998.

The rubella virus is an enveloped ssRNA virus and is transmitted by droplets. Like measles, rubella occurs in the winter and spring. The virus is present in nasopharyngeal specimens or any secretions or tissues of infected infants, who shed the virus in large amounts for long periods. Direct examination of the specimens by FA or EIA is recommended because isolation procedures are cumbersome and involve a second, or challenge, virus. Serologic procedures are effective because any rubella antibody is presumed to be protective. The most sensitive assays are the solid-phase assays and passive hemagglutination tests. Latex agglutination and antigen-coated red blood cell tests are useful but less sensitive.

Hand, Foot, and Mouth Disease

Hand, foot, and mouth disease (HFMD) is caused primarily by coxsackievirus types A5, 10, and 16 and occasionally enterovirus type 71. These viruses are naked ssRNA viruses. HFMD is generally a disease that occurs in young children. It is spread by fomites or the oral-fecal route. A mild prodromal phase may develop, with malaise, headache, and abdominal pains. Suddenly, small, painful sores appear on the tongue, buccal mucosa, and soft palate. Simultaneously, a maculopapular rash appears on the hands, feet, and buttocks, followed by bullae on the soles of the feet and palms of the hands. The lesions regress in about a week. If a rash develops it is transient. The virus can be isolated from specimens from swabs of the mouth and bullae. Coxsackievirus A16 grows in PMK and human diploid fibroblast cells and can be identified by serum neutralization tests.

Parvovirus B19

Parvovirus B19, a small, nonenveloped ssDNA virus, causes infections ranging from asymptomatic to potentially fatal infections. The most commonly recognized syndrome is **erythema infectiosum (EI),** which also has the curious name **fifth disease,** derived from the fact that it is the fifth infectious rash characterized by physicians (after rubeola, rubella, varicella, and roseola). Patients with EI experience a prodrome of fever, headache, malaise, and myalgia with respiratory and gastrointestinal symptoms (nausea, vomiting). The prodromal phase lasts a few days, after which a rash often appears. The rash gives a "slapped-cheek" appearance and then spreads to the trunk and limbs. The rash occurs more commonly in children than adults. The rash may last up to 2 weeks and can recur after heat and sunlight exposure. Adults may also experience arthralgia or arthritis or both. In some cases, this connective tissue manifestation may occur without the prodrome or rash stage.

Parvovirus B19 viremia can cause hematologic manifestations. Red blood cells contain a receptor for the virus. The infection of reticulocytes causes a decrease in red blood cell production in the bone marrow. In normal patients, this decrease results in a short-lived anemia. However, patients with chronic hemolytic conditions, such as sickle cell disease and thalassemia, may experience transient aplastic crisis. Within about a week, reticulocytosis occurs and the patient recovers.

The viremia of parvovirus B19 creates a risk for fetuses. In utero infection can cause hydrops fetalis, resulting from anemia. Although the most vulnerable period for the fetus is the third trimester, most women exposed to the virus do not develop an acute disease, and very few infections result in loss of the fetus.

IMMUNODEFICIENCY VIRUSES: HUMAN IMMUNODEFICIENCY VIRUS TYPE 1

Of all the viruses discussed in this chapter, none has the worldwide impact of HIV-1. As seen in Table 25-5, the burden of this virus is staggering. HIV-1 causes **acquired immune deficiency syndrome (AIDS).** HIV-1 is a spherical virus with a three-layer structure (Figure 25-6). In the center are two identical copies of ssRNA associated with reverse transcriptase and surrounded by an icosahedral capsid. The genome is enclosed by a viral envelope with viral glycoprotein (gp) spikes. The diagnostically important HIV antigens are the structural proteins p24, gp4l, gpl20, and gpl60 (Figure 25-7).

The virus is transmitted by blood (especially through transfusions) and exchange of other body fluids. HIV is cell associated, so less virus is found in cell-free plasma than in whole blood, and even less virus is found in saliva, tears, urine, or milk. HIV is not highly contagious, and normal, social, nonsexual contact poses no threat.

TABLE 25-5
World Health Organization Data on Impact of HIV and AIDS

	Estimated Child Deaths through 1997	Estimated Child and Adult Deaths through 1997	Estimated Child Deaths from AIDS during 1997	Estimated Newly-Infected Adults and Children during 1997
North America	5000	420,000	<400	44,000
Caribbean	14,000	110,000	2100	47,000
Latin America	23,000	470,000	3600	180,000
Western Europe	2800	190,000	<200	30,000
North Africa and the Middle East	4400	42,000	1000	19,000
SubSaharan Africa	2,500,000	9,700,000	430,000	4,000,000
Eastern Europe and Central Asia	4200	4500	<200	100,000
East Asia and the Pacific	1700	12,000	700	180,000
South and Southeast Asia	100,000	740,000	29,000	1,300,000
Australia and New Zealand	<100	7100	<10	600
TOTAL	~2,700,000	~11,700,000	~460,000	~5,800,000

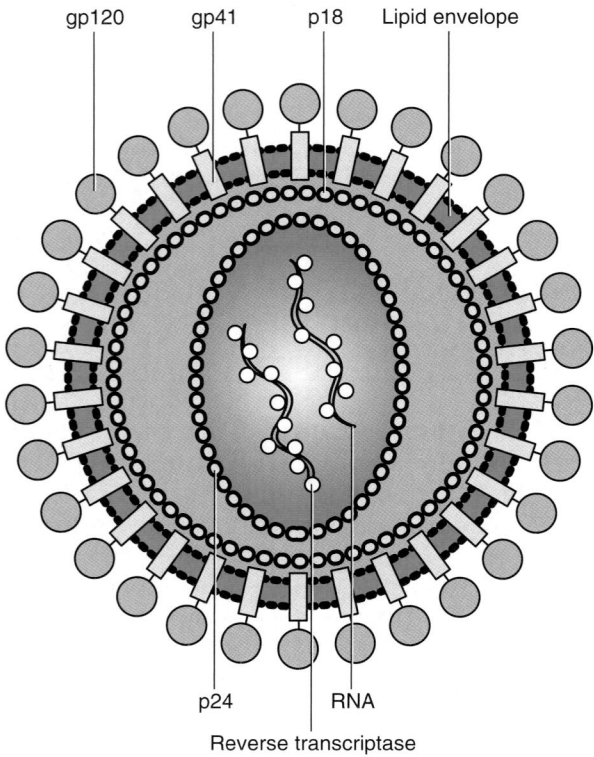

Figure 25-6

Human immunodeficiency virus (HIV).

The patients at greatest risk for contracting the virus are individuals who have received transfusions of blood and blood products, intravenous drug addicts, individuals who have had sex with infected individuals, and children of infected mothers. Individuals with ulcerative sexually transmitted infections (e.g., syphilis, genital herpes, chancroid) are also at increased risk. Today, all blood is screened for the HIV virus, and blood products are screened and treated.

From 1995 to 1997, new cases of HIV in the United States were associated with the following:

- Heterosexual contact (18%)
- Homosexual contact (48%)
- Intravenous drug use (32%)
- Transfusions or mother-to-infant transmission (2%)

For adults living in developed countries, the average length of time from infection with HIV to development of AIDS is approximately 10 years. Approximately 20% develop AIDS within 5 years, and

less than 5% have an asymptomatic HIV infection for periods longer than 10 years. The rate at which the virus multiplies in the host is related to the development of AIDS. This rate can be measured with an HIV viral load technique, a quantitative gene amplification technique that measures the amount of HIV-1 RNA in the plasma of the patient.

AIDS is a global pandemic. It is spreading in the United States and Europe and is wiping out the population in some areas of central Africa. In Africa the disease is evenly distributed between males and females. In these areas, severe, chronic diarrhea caused by AIDS is so common that AIDS is called the "slim disease." The prevalence of internal parasites in these areas may play a role in the

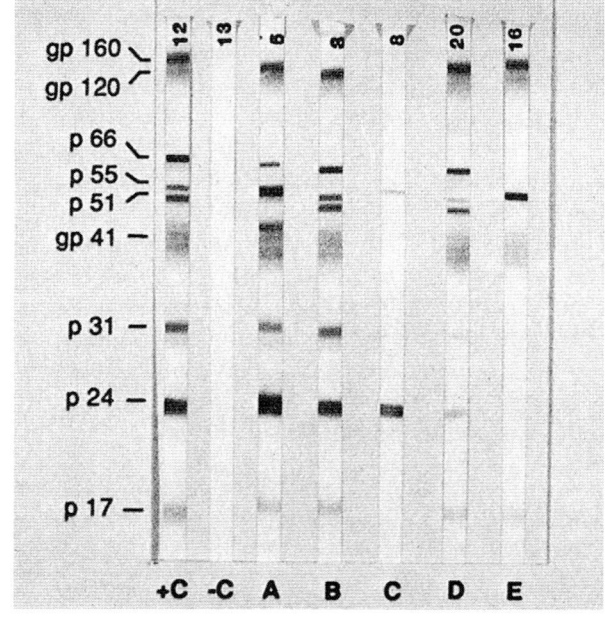

Figure 25-7

Human immunodeficiency (HIV) immunoblot. Reactive protein *(p)* bands appear as purplish lines across the strip. Proteins with higher molecular weights appear at the top of the strip. Structural and nonstructural proteins are given RNA structural genome codes: *GAG*—group-specific antigens, *POL*—polyermerase, and *ENV*—envelope. ENV codes for glycoprotein precursors (gp)—gp160, gp120, and gp41 through gp43. POL codes for p65, p51, and p31. GAG codes for p55, p24, and p17. Results are negative, indeterminate, or positive based on the pattern on the strip. *Positive:* reactivity with a score of + or greater to GAG p24 or ENV gp120/gp160 or gp41. *Indeterminate:* the appearance of one or more bands in a pattern that does not satisfy the positive criteria. *Negative:* the absence of any band on the strip. (Courtesy Patricia A. Cruse.)

chronic diarrhea. The major risk groups everywhere are indiscriminate homosexual and bisexual men, prostitutes, intravenous drug users, blood transfusion recipients (especially hemophiliacs), the sexual contacts of the at-risk groups, and newborn infants born to infected mothers.

Once HIV enters the body, the target cells are the CD4+ T cells, monocytes, macrophages, regional lymph nodes, and cells of macrophage derivation in the brain. Eventually, lymphopenia results, with the greatest losses being in the CD4+ T-cell population. Lymph nodes become enlarged and hyperplastic. Encephalitis and vacuolar myelopathy are common. The virus destroys the cells that are the major defense against viral, fungal, and protozoan infections. Death usually occurs from the resulting opportunistic infections, although HIV-1 itself can directly cause encephalitis and dementia.

The immunologic markers of AIDS are the following:

- Steady decline in number of the CD4+ T cells
- Depression of the T4:T8 cell ratio to less than 0.9 (with normal being more than 1.5)
- Functional impairment of monocytes and macrophages
- Decreased natural killer cell activity
- Anergy to recall antigens in skin tests

Another marker of AIDS is the presence of the following opportunistic infections or conditions:

- Burkitt's lymphoma
- Candidiasis of the respiratory tree
- Coccidiomycosis
- Cryptococcal meningitis
- Cryptosporidiosis with persistent diarrhea
- CMV infections of organs other than the liver, spleen, or lymph nodes
- Histoplasmosis
- Persistent HSV infections
- Kaposi's sarcoma or lymphoma of the brain in patients less than 60 years
- Lymphoid interstitial pneumonia or pulmonary lymphoid hyperplasia or both in children less than 13 years
- *Mycobacterium avium, Mycobacterium kansasii,* or *Pneumocystis carinii* pneumonia
- Progressive multifocal leukoencephalopathy
- Recurrent pneumonia

- *Salmonella* sp. septicemia
- Toxoplasmosis of the brain in infants more than 1 month
- Wasting disease

HIV-1 is fragile. The virus can be isolated from peripheral blood mononuclear cells (PBMCs) of infected patients. Once purified, the PBMCs are stimulated with interleukin-2 and inoculated into cultures of PBMCs from healthy donors that have been grown in the presence of phytohemagglutinin (PHA) or into cell lines that allow growth of HIV. Periodically the culture fluid can be tested for HIV-specific reverse transcriptase or viral antigens, or the cells can be examined using FA tests. Serologic tests for HIV are more practical in the average laboratory. The EIA test for donated blood is one of the most sensitive tests. A positive specimen should be retested and if positive the second time tested by another method such as an immunoblot (Western blot) or FA. The immunoblot methods test for antibodies to specific viral antigens such as p24, p31, gp41, and gpl20/gpl60 (see Figure 25-7). The presence of HIV antibodies is diagnostic, but a negative result simply means that no antibody is present. It may take 6 weeks after infection before antibodies appear, and they disappear as immune complexes form in the late stages of the disease.

Antiviral therapy for HIV-1 currently includes a combination of three antiviral compounds used to suppress HIV replication. The three drugs usually include two nucleoside analog reverse transcriptase inhibitors (e.g., **zidovudine,** didanosine, zalcitabine, lamivudine) combined with a protease inhibitor (e.g., ritonavir, saquinavir). HIV viral load techiques can predict therapy efficacy. In different studies, suppression of HIV RNA levels to less than 5000 copies of RNA per milliliter for up to 2 years was correlated with an increase in CD4+ cells up to 90 cells/mm^3. In contrast, patients with HIV RNA loads of more than 5000 copies of RNA per milliliter generally showed declines in CD4+ cell counts.

CENTRAL NERVOUS SYSTEM VIRUSES: ENTEROVIRUSES

The **enteroviruses** include the following:

- Polioviruses 1 through 3
- Coxsackieviruses A 1 through 23

- Coxsackieviruses B 1 through 6
- Echoviruses l through 32
- Enteroviruses 68 through 72

These small, nonenveloped, ssRNA viruses cause various infections and conditions, including the following:

- Fever of unknown origin (FUO)
- Aseptic meningitis
- Paralysis
- Sepsislike illness
- Myopericarditis
- Pleurodynia
- Conjunctivitis
- Exanthemas
- Pharyngitis
- Pneumonia

Enteroviruses have also been implicated in early-onset diabetes, cardiomyopathy, and fetal malformations.

The portal of entry is the alimentary canal via the mouth. The viruses replicate initially in the lymphoid tissue of the pharynx and gut. Viremia can result in the virus spreading to the spinal cord, heart, and skin. Enterovirus infections often cause nausea and diarrhea. The viruses destroy their host cells. In the intestines the damage is temporary because the cells lining the gut are rapidly replaced. In contrast, neurons are not replaced, so neuron death can result in permanent paralysis.

Most serotypes of the enteroviruses are distributed worldwide. In the temperate zones, enterovirus epidemics occur in the summer and early fall. Enterovirus infections are more prevalent in areas with poverty, overcrowding, and poor hygiene and sanitation. Viruses are spread via aerosol, the oral-fecal route, and fomites.

Excellent poliovirus vaccines of either attenuated viruses or killed viruses are available. No other vaccines are available for enteroviruses; good personal and nosocomial hygiene and good sanitation can reduce the incidence of enterovirus infections.

Enteroviruses can be cultured from the pharynx immediately before the onset of symptoms and for 1 to 2 weeks afterward; they can be isolated from the feces for as long as 6 weeks afterward. However, obtaining specimens early in the infection is ideal. Specimens from throat cultures, feces, rectal swabs, CSF, and conjunctival swabs are recommended.

Polioviruses, type B coxsackieviruses, and echoviruses grow readily in a number of cell lines, including PMK, continuous human and primate, and human fetal diploid fibroblast lines. The high-numbered enteroviruses (68 to 72) require special handling. The CPEs appear quickly and are readily identifiable. Enteroviruses have no group antigen, so they must be identified individually by a serum neutralization test. The World Health Organization distributes pools of enterovirus antisera that allow identification by neutralization patterns in the pools. The CPE and resistance to detergent, acid, and solvents constitute a presumptive diagnosis of enterovirus infection.

AGENTS OF GASTROINTESTINAL INFECTIONS

Rotaviruses
Rotaviruses are naked, isometric dsDNA viruses with a double-layer protein capsid. Rotaviruses are the most common cause of gastroenteritis in infants, children, and the elderly. Gastroenteritis is a major cause of infant mortality and the failure of young children to thrive. Rotaviruses have a worldwide distribution. Outbreaks occur primarily in the winter months in the temperate zones and year round in the tropics.

Rotaviruses are spread by the oral-fecal route and have an incubation period of 1 to 2 days. The sudden onset of symptoms includes vomiting, diarrhea, fever, and in some cases abdominal pain and respiratory symptoms. The vomiting and diarrhea can cause fatal dehydration. The rotavirus replicates in the epithelial cells in the tips of the microvilli of the small intestine. The microvilli are stunted and adsorption is reduced. The virus is shed in large quantities in the stool and can cause nosocomial outbreaks in the absence of good hygiene.

Although the rotavirus is present in large numbers in the stools, it can be isolated only with special procedures. ELISA and latex agglutination tests detect the virus in fecal material. Rapid, membrane-bound colorimetric tests are also available.

Norwalk and Norwalk-Like Agents
The Norwalk family of agents includes small, round viruses of 27 to 30 nm in diameter. They are most commonly associated with gastroenteritis in older

children and adults in developed countries. They have caused outbreaks of acute gastroenteritis in schools, in colleges, in camps, on cruise ships, in communities, in nursing homes, and in families. These viruses have been found in drinking water, swimming areas, and contaminated food. The incubation period is 24 to 48 hours, and the onset of severe nausea, vomiting, diarrhea, and low-grade fever is abrupt. The infection rate can be as high as 50%. The illness usually subsides within 72 hours, and immunity wanes after 4 years. The viruses cannot be grown in culture, so diagnosis is usually accomplished by examination of suspect fecal material by electron microscopy. A few laboratories specializing in Norwalk agents can perform serologic procedures.

Enteric Adenoviruses

Adenoviruses type 40 and 41 are called **enteric adenoviruses** because they cause epidemics of gastroenteritis in young children. Diarrhea is a prominent feature of the illness, but less vomiting and fever occurs than with rotaviruses. Enteric adenoviruses have a worldwide, endemic distribution, and numbers of cases increase during the warmer months. These adenoviruses can be identified but not serotyped by EIA. Kits are available for adenovirus detection.

Other Viruses

Coronaviruses are described in the previous discussion of respiratory viruses. They were first recovered from a case of upper respiratory infection, but they are also responsible for a small percentage of pediatric diarrhea cases. The illness lasts for about a week, and blood may appear in the stool.

Caliciviruses are small (30 to 35 nm in diameter) and distinguished by 32 cup-shape structures on their surfaces. They cause minor outbreaks of pediatric gastroenteritis worldwide in children from 1 to 24 months of age. The outbreaks can be endemic or epidemic and peak in the winter. Vomiting may occur, and the illness lasts about 4 days.

Astroviruses are smaller viruses (28 to 30 nm) with a five-point or six-point starlike configuration on their surfaces. These viruses are ubiquitous and cause relatively mild infections in children up to 7 years of age.

Generally the viruses causing gastroenteritis are extremely small, are hard to see, and do not grow in culture. They are associated with gastroenteritis because they have been seen by electron microscopy in large numbers in stool from patients involved in gastroenteritis outbreaks. When convalescent serum from a diarrheal patient is added to a suspension of the patient's stool specimen, the viruses clump together. This procedure is called *immune electron microscopy*.

Gastroenteritis viruses are usually fatal only in malnourished or dehydrated children. The best treatment is oral rehydration with parenteral fluids administration when needed. Prevention requires proper sanitation, clean water supplies, uncontaminated food, and good hygiene.

ARBOVIRUSES

The group of viruses formerly known as the **arboviruses** (*ar*thropod *bo*rne) obtained its name because the viruses were usually transmitted by blood-feeding arthropods, such as mosquitoes, ticks, sandflies, and fleas. The arboviruses have been reclassified into the following four families (Table 25-6):

Family Bunyaviridae
- Genus *Phlebovirus* (including the Rift Valley fever virus)
- Genus *Nairovirus* (including the Crimean-Congo hemorrhagic fever virus)

Family Flaviviridae
- Genus *Flavivirus* (including the yellow fever virus, St. Louis encephalitis virus, Japanese encephalitis virus, and dengue virus)

Family Reoviridae
- Genus *Coltivirus* (including Colorado tick fever)

Family Togaviridae
- Genus *Alphavirus* (including Eastern encephalitis virus, Western encephalitis virus, Venezuelan encephalitis virus, and Ross River virus)

Many of the viruses in this group are referred to as *emerging viruses,* reflecting the fact that the vectors of these diseases are spreading into new regions, bringing the risk of disease to countries that were previously not at risk.

In most of these infections, humans are dead-end hosts, meaning that human-to-arthropod-to-

TABLE 25-6

New Classifications of the Arboviruses

Family	Genus	Virus	Disease	Vector	Reservoir	Geographic Location
Bunyaviridae	*Phlebovirus*	Rift Valley Fever birus	Fever, encephalitis, hemorrhagic fever	*Aedes* sp. mosquitoes	Sheep, cattle, goats	South Africa, Uganda, Kenya, Sudan, Egypt, Mauritania
	Nairovirus	Crimean-Congo hemorrhagic fever virus	Hemorrhagic fever	*Hyalomma* sp. tick	Rodents	Eastern Europe, Russia, China, Middle East, subSaharan Africa
	Bunyavirus	LaCrosse virus	Encephalitis	*Aedes triseriatus* mosquitoes	Squirrels, chipmunks	Midwest and midAtlantic United States, Canada
Flaviviridae	*Flavivirus*	Yellow fever virus	Fever, hemorrhagic fever	*Aedes* sp. mosquitoes	Monkeys	Africa, South America, Caribbean
		St. Louis encephalitis virus	Encephalitis	*Culex* sp. mosquitoes	Birds	North America
		Japanese encephalitis virus	Encephalitis	*Culex* sp. mosquitoes	Birds, pigs	Asia, Australia, Pacific Rim
		Dengue virus	Fever, hemorrhagic fever	*Aedes* sp. mosquitoes	—	Asia, Pacific, South America, Caribbean
Togaviridae	*Alphavirus*	Eastern encephalitis virus	Encephalitis	*Aedes and Culex* mosquitoes	Birds, horses	Eastern, southeastern, and midwestern United States
		Western encephalitis virus	Encephalitis	*Culex and Aedes* spp. mosquitoes	Birds, horses	Western United States and Canada
		Venezuelan encephalitis virus	Encephalitis, flulike illness	Mosquitoes	Rodents	South and Central America, Texas
Reoviridae	*Coltivirus*	Colorado tick fever	Fever, hemorrhagic fever	Tick *(Dermacentor)*	Rodents	Western and northwestern United States, Canada

human transmission does not occur. Two important exceptions to this rule exist: humans with dengue fever and humans with yellow fever can have so much virus circulating in the bloodstream that a human-mosquito-human transmission can occur.

These viruses are fragile in the environment, making them dependent on vector-borne transmission.

Family Bunyaviridae

The arboviruses in the Bunyaviridae family replicate initially in the gut of the arthropod vector and eventually appear in the saliva. The arthropod transmits the virus by feeding on the blood of the vertebrate hosts, which include humans. After a few days the infected host usually develops an asymptomatic viremia. In less common cases, the host becomes febrile. Some of the viruses in this family cause diseases that reflect damage to target organs. For instance, Rift Valley fever (RVF) virus targets the brain and liver to cause encephalitis and hepatitis. LaCrosse (LAC) virus targets the brain, causing encephalitis, and the Crimean-Congo hemorrhagic fever (CCHF) virus targets the vascular endothelium and liver.

Members of the Bunyaviridae family cause a basic fever, hemorrhagic fever, or encephalitis. CCHF virus causes a high-mortality infection in humans. Infection begins with fever, myalgia, arthralgia, and photophobia. Patients develop mental status changes, ranging from confusion and agitation to depression and drowsiness. Petechia and ecchymoses can form on mucosal surfaces and on skin. The patient may bleed from the bowel, nose, and gums. Approximately 30% of the patients die. Others begin recovering after about 10 days of illness. Nosocomial transmission of CCHF has been reported.

RVF virus can cause epizootics in grazing animals such as sheep, cattle, buffalo, goats, and camels. One such epizootic in 1950 killed 100,000 sheep. Humans are usually at risk for RVF during periods of excessive rainfall, when the vectors are plentiful. In humans, RVF virus causes a range of clinical manifestations, from asymptomatic infection to mild febrile disease. However, some patients progress to hemorrhagic fever or encephalitis. Mortality in humans is about 1%, but as many as 10% of the patients develop sequellae such as blindness.

Usually fewer than 100 cases of encephalitis are caused by the LAC virus in the United States each year. The incidence is probably underestimated because the disease manifests as a nonspecific fever, headache, nausea, vomiting, and lethargy. The disease is commonly found in children, and most often develops in the summer. Patients are usually tested for HSV or enterovirus aseptic meningitis. Because serology tests for LAC virus are not offered in most laboratories and because this disease has very low mortality (approximately 1%), definitive diagnosis does not occur often.

Family Togaviridae

Similar to LAC virus, the alphaviruses of the Togaviridae family also cause encephalitis. However, mortality in patients with Eastern equine encephalitis (EEE) is as high as 30%. Many survivors of the infection suffer permanent central nervous system damage. Because horses and humans are dead-end hosts of infection, equine EEE disease can be a predictor of human EEE cases. The Western equine encephalitis (WEE) virus also causes disease in humans and horses. WEE virus causes a milder disease than EEE virus, and patients develop either an asymptomatic infection or fever, headache, nausea, and mental status changes. As many as 30% of the infected young children and infants may suffer permanent central nervous system damage. Mortality is approximately 3%. Venezuelan equine encephalitis (VEE) has caused large outbreaks of human and equine encephalitis in the Americas. During an outbreak that lasted from 1969 to 1971, 200,000 horses died from VEE. Much more recently, VEE caused encephalitis in 90,000 patients in Venezuela and

Colombia. Mortality is much less common in patients with VEE than with WEE and EEE. Infected adults often develop an influenzalike illness, whereas encephalitis is more commonly seen in VEE-infected children.

Family Flaviviridae

The Flaviviridae Japanese encephalitis (JE) virus is endemic in Asia and is the most common cause of arboviral encephalitis in the world. JE virus is considered an emerging pathogen because it is being reported in regions previously free of JE including Australia. Currently 30,000 to 50,000 cases of JE are reported each year. Most infections are asymptomatic. Disease may range from influenzalike illness to acute encephalitis. Children assume the major burden of this infection as well, with a mortality as high as 30%; mortality in adults is much lower.

Another important emerging virus in the family Flaviviridae is **dengue virus.** This virus causes two distinct diseases—classic dengue fever (DF) and dengue hemorrhagic fever (DHF). Worldwide, tens of millions of cases of DF and approximately 500,000 cases of the more serious DHF exist. The average mortality associated with DHF is 5%, accounting for 24,000 deaths each year. Most deaths occur in children less than the age of 15 years. The virus is transmitted by *Aedes* spp. mosquitoes, including *Aedes aegytpi* and *Aedes albopictus*. These mosquitoes infest more than 100 countries and bring the risk of DF to 2.5 billion people. Dengue virus has four serotypes: 1 through 4. Dengue fever, which is a relatively mild infection, occurs when patients are bitten by mosquitoes carrying the virus. Patients with DF develop fever, headache, myalgia, and bone pain (resulting in the virus' nickname, "breakbone fever"). Some patients may also develop a rash. The disease is self-limiting, is not fatal, and resolves in 1 to 2 weeks. Although classic DF is a mild disease, DHF is not. Patients develop DHF after they have already been exposed to one serotype of dengue virus and are then exposed to one of the other three serotypes. Exposure to two different serotypes of dengue virus is necessary for developing DHF. Patients with DHF develop the symptoms of classic DF, along with thrombocytopenia, hemorrhage and shock, and sometimes death. Until recently, most of the United States was not considered to be at risk for contracting dengue fever because *A. aegypti* generally was not able to survive winters in most of the country; two factors changed that fact. First, global warming is allowing the mosquito to survive winters in states once too cold for survival. Second, in the late 1980s a new mosquito was introduced to the United States from Asia. The Asian tiger mosquito, *A. albopictus,* was transported from China into Houston, Texas in the wells of old tires containing mosquito larvae. These mosquitoes have spread throughout the southeastern portion of the United States and continue to spread to new states. This mosquito is less domesticated than *A. aegypti* and is able to survive winters better than *A. aegypti.* Although the number of autochthonous cases of dengue fever is currently low in the United States, the mosquito vectors are bringing risk of infection to many states.

Yellow fever is also considered an emerging infection. Although a safe vaccine has been available for decades, approximately 200,000 cases of yellow fever and 30,000 resulting deaths are reported annually. Actual incidence may greatly exceed these numbers. The emergence results from increased spread of the mosquito vectors, deforestation of Africa and South America, and increased travel by people in the endemic regions. The vaccine has greatly reduced or eliminated the transmission of yellow fever in some countries. However, yellow fever is still an epidemic in parts of Africa and South America, where about 80% of the population must be vaccinated to reduce the impact of the disease.

Patients bitten by mosquitoes carrying the yellow fever virus may develop an asymptomatic infection or an acute infection involving fever, myalgia, backache, headache, anorexia, nausea, and vomiting. Most patients experiencing this acute disease recover after about 4 days. However, about 15% enter a systemic toxic phase in which fever reappears. The patient develops jaundice (thus the name "yellow" fever) and hemorrhages and bleeds from the mouth, eyes, nose, or stomach or all areas. The kidneys may fail, and about 50% of the patients in the toxic phase die. The other 50% recover without serious sequellae.

The three different transmission cycles for the yellow fever virus are the sylvatic, urban, and intermediate cycles. In the sylvatic cycle, yellow fever is maintained in monkey populations and transmitted by mosquitoes. Monkeys become sufficiently viremic to pass the virus to other mosquitoes as the mosquitoes feed on the monkeys, thus keeping the transmission cycle active. Humans are not the usual hosts when they enter jungle areas in which the sylvatic cycle exists.

The urban cycle occurs in larger towns and cities, with infected *A. aegypti* mosquitoes transmitting the infection to people. Because infected humans can continue the transmission when bitten by uninfected mosquitoes, large outbreaks can occur from a single case of infection. The intermediate transmission cycle of yellow fever occurs in smaller villages in Africa. In the intermediate cycle, humans, monkeys, and semidomesticated mosquitoes are the vectors and reservoirs for the high-morbidly, low-mortality outbreaks. In the intermediate cycle, mosquitoes can transmit the yellow fever virus from monkeys to humans and vice versa. If patients who develop yellow fever from the intermediate cycle travel to larger cities and if they are bitten by domestic mosquitoes, they can trigger an outbreak of urban yellow fever.

In the United States the most common flavivirus infection is St. Louis encephalitis (SLE). During the past 35 years, an average of 193 cases of SLE have been reported annually in the United States. Epidemics are more likely to occur in midwestern or southeastern states, but cases have been reported in all of the lower 48 states. Patients with SLE are most likely to have an asymptomatic infection. Symptomatic patients may develop a fever only, whereas some patients develop meningoencephalitis. The mortality rate of symptomatic patients is 3% to 20%. Unlike many of the arboviral infections, SLE is milder in children than adults, with the elderly having the greatest risk of serious illness and death. SLE is transmitted to humans by the bird-biting *Culex* mosquitoes. Most infections occur in the summer months.

Family Reoviridae

Colorado tick fever causes a denguelike infection in the western United States and Canada. Because it is not a reportable infection, actual numbers of cases are difficult to calculate, but Colorado tick fever may be one of the most common diseases transmitted by ticks in the United States. Patients develop a fever, photophobia, myalgia, arthralgia, and chills. Similar to dengue symptoms, patients may also have a biphasic fever with a rash, and children may experience hemorrhagic fever.

The vector of the infection is *Dermacentor andersoni,* which has many reservoirs in nature including deer, squirrels, and rabbits.

Laboratory Diagnosis of Arboviral Infections

Arboviruses are very fragile and must be handled with care. Identification procedures are difficult and not practical for use by the average clinical laboratory. For information on isolation and identification of arboviruses, contact the World Health Organization for Arbovirus Reference and Research at the Division of Vector-Borne Infectious Diseases of the Centers for Disease Control and Prevention (PO Box 2087, Fort Collins, CO 80521) or the Yale Arbovirus Research Unit (Box 333, New Haven, CT 06510). Some state public health laboratories also perform arbovirus studies. Serology tests are available for some arboviral infections, but they are not currently FDA approved. Several commercial reference laboratories offer serology tests for the encephalitides and other arboviral infections.

FAMILY ARENAVIRIDAE

The name *Arenavirus* is derived from the Latin term *arena,* meaning sand. Under an electron microscope, arenaviruses appear sandy and granular, almost as if they had ribosomes. The viruses in the family Arenaviridae include many species that cause hemorrhagic fever (Table 25-7). The first arenavirus to be described was the lymphocytic choriomeningitis (LCM) virus in 1933. The Tacaribe virus was discovered in 1956, and since then several arenaviruses have been detected each decade. The first of the arenaviruses discovered to cause hemorrhagic fever was the Junin virus, which causes Argentine hemorrhagic fever. The Machupo virus, another hemorrhagic fever virus, was isolated from a viral outbreak in Bolivia in 1963. In 1969 the Lassa virus was isolated in Africa, which triggered a novel entitled *Fever,* written by John Fuller. The book details the emergence of Lassa fever, which in retrospect is eerily similar to the emergence of other hemorrhagic fevers that would be discovered later in Africa, including that of the Ebola virus.

The arenaviruses infect rodents, and humans are then exposed to the disease by zoonotic transmission. The rodents are infected for long periods and typically do not become ill from the viruses, which they shed in urine, feces, and saliva.

In some parts of the United States, as many as 20% of the *Mus musculus* mice carry the LCM virus. Pet hamsters are also reservoirs. Humans become infected when they inhale the aerosolized virus or come in contact with fomites. The LCM virus causes an influenzalike illness. About 25% of infected patients develop meningitis from the virus.

Lassa virus is the most well-known of the arenaviruses. One recent outbreak in Sierra Leone resulted in 823 cases and 153 deaths (18.6% of the patients). Most patients develop an asymptomatic infection, but some patients experience fever, headache, pharyngitis, myalgia, diarrhea, and vomiting. Some patients develop pleural effusions, hypotension, and hemorrhaging. Central nervous system involvement includes seizures and encephalopathy. The mortality rate is about 15% for patients ill enough to require hospitalization.

Most cases of Lassa fever are community acquired, primarily by contact with excretions from the multimammate rat *Mastomys natalensis,* which

TABLE 25-7
Summary of Arenaviridae Family

Arenavirus	Disease	Animal Reservoir	Geographic Location
Lymphocytic choriomeningitis virus	Lymphocytic choriomeningitis (aseptic meningitis)	*Mus* sp. (mouse), hamsters	Worldwide
Lassa virus	Lassa fever (hemorrhagic fever)	*Mastomys natalensis* (rat)	West Africa
Machupo virus	Bolivian hemorrhagic fever	*Calomys callosus* (mouse)	Bolivia
Guanarito virus	Venezuelan hemorrhagic fever	*Zygodontomys brevicauda* and *Sigmodon alsoni* (rats)	Venezuela
Sabia	Brazilian hemorrhagic fever	Unknown	Brazil
Junin virus	Argentinian hemorrhagic fever	*Calomys* sp.	Argentina

sheds the virus throughout its life once infected. Humans either inhale the aerosolized virus or contract the virus directly through breaks in the skin. Lassa fever can also be transmitted from human to human. The virus is present in throat secretions. It can be transmitted through sexual contact and nosocomially. Lassa virus can be treated effectively with ribavirin if therapy begins within the first 6 days of exposure.

GENUS *HANTAVIRUS*

The genus *Hantavirus* is included in the Family Bunyaviridae. It is one of the most rapidly growing genera of viruses. In the early 1990s, several viruses caused a disease referred to as *hemorrhagic fever with renal syndrome* (HFRS). The causative viruses were Hantaan virus, Seoul virus, Puumala virus, and Dobrava virus. All are in the genus *Hantavirus*. Most cause HFRS only in Asia and Europe, except for the Seoul virus, which is found worldwide.

In May, 1993, a man and woman living in the same house in New Mexico died from an unusual respiratory illness. Public health officials quickly ruled out common infectious diseases as the cause of death. Sera from the patients were sent to the Centers for Disease Control (CDC) and were compared with pools of known antisera. Oddly enough the serology tests indicated that the patients had been exposed to an unknown agent that was antigenically related to one of the Asian hantaviruses; regardless, it was clear that the patients had a pulmonary syndrome, not a renal syndrome. Public health officials conducted surveys on rodents and found that 30% of the deer mice in the New Mexico area were seropositive for the same unknown virus associated with the patients' deaths. Using PCR, the CDC was able to deduce that the patients had been exposed to a new hantavirus carried by deer mice. The virus was named **Sin Nombre** ("no name") virus (SNV), and the disease caused by the virus was named *hantavirus pulmonary syndrome (HPS)*. The same technology used to detect and describe SNV has been used to detect many new hantaviruses in the Americas (Table 25-8). These are sometimes called the "New World" hantaviruses.

Hantaviruses endemic to Europe and Asia are called "Old World" hantaviruses. The Puumala hantavirus is the most common species in Europe and

TABLE 25-8

Hantaviruses that Cause Hantavirus Pulmonary Syndrome

Hantavirus	Host	Location
Sin Nombre	*Peromyscus maniculatis* (deer mouse)	United States, and western Canada
Black Creek Canal	*Sigmodon hispidus* (cotton rat)	United States, South America
Bayou	*Oryzomys palustris* (rice rat)	Southeastern United States
Monongahela	*Peromyscus maniculatis* (deer mouse)	Eastern United States
New York	*Peromyscus leucopus* (white-foot deer mouse)	New York
Oran	*Oligoryzomys longicaudatus*	Argentina
Andes	*Oligoryzomys longicaudatus*	Argentina, Chile
Lechiguanas	*Oligoryzomys flavescens*	Argentina
Laguna Negra	*Calomys laucha*	Paraguay, Bolivia

causes a mild form of HFRS called *nephropathia epidemica*.

It seems that not all hantaviruses are pathogenic to humans. Several species of hantavirus have been described that have no human disease associated with them. These include the Prospect Hill and El Moro Canyon viruses.

Patients with HPS have a 3- to 5-day febrile prodrome, with fever, chills, and myalgia. The patient then enters a phase of hypotensive shock and pulmonary edema. Laboratory tests indicate hemoconcentration and thrombocytopenia because as platelet counts may drop to less than 150,000. The patient develops tachycardia, hypoxia, and hypotension. In severe cases, the patient may develop disseminated intravascular coagulation (DIC). The mortality of HPS is approximately 50%.

Patients with HFRS have generally the same course of illness as patients with HPS, but the target organ is the kidney instead of the lung. The patients then develop a febrile prodrome and enter a phase of fever and shock accompanied with oliguria. The kidneys then regain function as the patient recovers. The mortality of HFRS is 1% to 15%.

Some evidence shows that the incidence of HPS, particularly when caused by the Sin Nombre virus, increases dramatically after an El Niño year. The El Niño weather pattern brings rain to the deserts of the southwestern United States, causing abundant growth of vegetation and increases in the number of deer mice (and therefore human-mouse contact). The virus, which is shed in mouse urine, saliva, and feces, is inhaled by humans in aerosolized virus particles. Generally, person-to-person transmission does not occur with hantaviral infections. However, strong evidence indicates that the Andes hantavirus has caused HPS in patients as a result of person-to-person transmission.

No FDA-approved laboratory tests are available for the identification of a hantavirus infection. Some state health laboratories and the CDC run ELISAs to detect anti-SNV IgM and IgG. Immunohistochemistry is a sensitive method that is used to detect hantaviral antigens in capillary endothelium, with an increased concentration of antigens in capillary tissue from the lung.

Treatment for HPS is primarily supportive care. Ribavirin may be effective in patients with HFRS but not in patients with HPS.

FAMILY FILOVIRIDAE

The genus *Filovirus* family Filoviridae includes two of viruses: Ebola and Marburg. These viruses have some striking similarities, including the following:

- They rarely cause human infections.
- Human infections may result from contact with infected monkeys.
- They both cause infections with high mortality rates.
- They both have unknown reservoirs in nature.

Marburg hemorrhagic fever was named after one of the first places an outbreak occurred—Marburg, Germany. In 1967, 37 people from Marburg and Frankfurt, Germany and Belgrade, Yugoslavia contracted an unknown infection. Seven people died. Epidemiologists noted that the deceased individuals all worked in vaccine-producing facilities and had contact with monkeys that had recently arrived from Uganda. The virus had been transmitted to 24 other people through nosocomial transmission, casual contact, and sexual contact. Patients with this secondary infection had a more mild illness, and all survived the infection. Another outbreak occurred in 1975 when two adults from Australia were hiking in Rhodesia. The man developed Marburg hemorrhagic fever and transmitted it to his female friend and a nurse while in the hospital. All three individuals died. Similar cases occurred in 1980, when a patient and his physician died in Kenya, and in 1987, when a young man travelling through Kenya died.

Marburg hemorrhagic fever begins with a febrile prodrome. The fever can last 12 to 22 days. At the end of the first week of infection, a maculopapular rash appears on the trunk and extremities. Patients begin bleeding from the nose, gums, and gastrointestinal tract during the latter part of the first week. Liver hemorrhaging, myocarditis, kidney damage, and mental status changes occur and are often followed by death.

The infection can be diagnosed using PCR, immunohistochemistry, and IgM-capture ELISA. Treatment of infected patients is primarily supportive and includes replacement of blood and clotting factors.

The Ebola virus is named after the Ebola river in Zaire, where the infection first emerged in 1976, although the virus emerged almost simultaneously in Sudan. In Zaire a patient treated at a village hospital for a bloody nose probably introduced the virus into the hospital, where it was then transmitted both nosocomially and via contact with infected patients at home. Nuns in the hospital routinely reused syringes without sterilizing them. Therefore the hospital amplified the number of cases. Infections were passed to the victim's families, often during a process in which intestines of infected deceased males were cleaned out to prepare the bodies for funerals.

Even though the two outbreaks of Ebola occurred simultaneously, they were caused by two different strains—Ebola-Zaire and Ebola-Sudan. Ebola-Zaire is the more virulent strain. Its initial outbreak infected 318 patients in Zaire and had an 88% mortality. The outbreak in Sudan infected 284 people and had a 53% mortality. After the initial two large outbreaks, smaller outbreaks occurred. In Sudan, 34 cases occurred in 1979, and 65% of the 34 patients died. The virus seemed to retreat back into the jungles for the next 15 years. However, an unusual sequence of events occurred in 1989, when monkeys imported to Reston, Virginia from the Phillipines experienced an epidemic of what eventually became the fourth type of Ebola,

Ebola-Reston. Four workers in the animal facility developed antibodies to Ebola-Reston but did not develop the disease. One of the workers had Ebola-Reston isolated from his bloodstream. Another outbreak of Ebola-Reston occurred in monkeys at a Texas quarantine facility in 1996.

In 1994, Ebola again appeared in Africa, when a scientist observing wild chimpanzees performed a necropsy on one chimpanzee after it died. The scientist soon developed symptoms but survived her infection. However, her isolate of Ebola virus was different from the Zaire and Sudan strains. It was named *Ebola-Ivory Coast.* A few months later, Ebola-Zaire struck Kikwit, Democratic Republic of the Congo (formerly Zaire). Much like the first outbreak in Zaire, 81% of the 315 infected patients died. In 1996, two separate outbreaks of Ebola-Zaire occurred in Gabon, with 65 of the 95 infected patients (68%) dying.

Symptoms of Ebola hemorrhagic fever include fever, chills, myalgia, and anorexia 4 to 16 days after infection. Patients develop a sore throat, abdominal pain, diarrhea, and vomiting and also start to bleed from injection sites and the gastrointestinal tract. Hemorrhaging in the skin and internal organs may occur as well.

Because no treatment or vaccine exists for Ebola, all laboratory work is done in a BSL-4 facility. Diagnosis of the infection can be made using PCR, FA, or viral culture methods.

RABIES

Rabies is caused by several strains of viruses belonging to the family Rhabdoviridae and genus *Lyssavirus.* The fear associated with the rabies virus is well-deserved. Estimates of annual worldwide human deaths from rabies vary from 30,000 to 100,000. In the United States, human rabies is rare, with approximately two cases per year. However, rabies is an emerging infection in animals. Forty years ago the majority of rabies infections occurred in dogs, with some infections also occurring in cats, foxes, and skunks. Programs to vaccinate domestic animals reduced the number of rabid dogs and cats. In contrast, current annual rabies infections are distributed as follows:

- Raccoons (4000 cases per year)
- Skunks (1800 cases per year)
- Bats (800 cases per year)
- Foxes (500 cases per year)
- Cats (300 cases per year)
- Dogs (250 cases per year)
- Cattle (150 cases per year)
- Coyotes (100 cases per year)

Currently in the United States, rabid raccoons are found in the eastern part of the country, from Georgia into New England. Rabid skunks are found in California, the central United States, and in New England. Rabid bats are found in all states but Alaska and Hawaii. Fox and coyotes infected with rabies are found in an area that stretches from Arizona to Texas. Rabid coyotes may have been shipped accidentally from Texas to Florida, resulting in rabies outbreaks in dogs and cats.

Humans acquire the rabies virus when they are bitten or scratched by rabid animals. With the number of endemic areas increasing for wildlife, the risk of human exposure to rabies increases because of the increased likelihood of encountering a rabid animal or a domestic animal that has contracted rabies from the wildlife.

Humans infected with rabies experience a brief prodrome of pain in the exposure site and have vague, flulike symptoms. Mental status changes, such as anxiety, irritability, and depression, may also become evident. After the prodrome, patients suffer additional central nervous system changes, including hallucinations, paralysis, excessive salivation, hydrophobia, bouts of terror, seizures, respiratory and cardiac abnormalities, and hypertension. These symptoms are followed ultimately by coma and death.

Laboratory diagnosis of rabies involves determining whether an animal that has bitten a human has rabies. The animal is killed quickly, and its head is removed and sent to a reference laboratory. The fastest and most sensitive method of identifying rabies viruses in a specimen is by using direct FA techniques. Impression smears should be made from various areas of the brain, primarily the hippocampus, pons, cerebella, and medulla oblongata. In living patients suspected of having rabies, biopsies of skin (especially at the hairline) and impressions of the cornea can be made. The presence of rabies virus in such specimens is diagnostic, but its absence merely means that no virus is present in those particular specimens, not that the patient does not have rabies. Rabies viruses can be grown in suckling or young adult mice, murine neuroblastoma, or related cell lines. ELISAs are currently the most sensitive assays to use for serologic tests.

Rabies cannot be treated once symptoms appear. However, postexposure prophylaxis (PEP) is 100% effective in preventing the disease if the patient is treated early enough. PEP includes vigorously cleaning the wound site, providing therapy with human rabies immune globulin, and administering the human diploid cell rabies vaccine. A vaccine can be given to persons who may be exposed to rabies, such as veterinarians, laboratory personnel, people who explore caves, and people visiting high-risk countries for more than 30 days.

HUMAN PAPILLOMAVIRUSES

Papillomas, or warts, are caused by the human papillomaviruses (HPVs). Although associated with the common wart, some of the HPV types are associated with cancer. More than 70 types of these small, dsDNA viruses exist, and certain types are characteristically associated with certain diseases.

- HPVs 1 through 4 are associated with common and plantar warts.
- HPVs 5 and 8 are associated with a rare autosomal disease called *epidermodysplasia verruciformis.*
- HPVs 6 and 11 are associated with condylomata acuminata (genital warts) and are transmitted sexually.
- HPVs 16 and 18 are associated with flat condylomas and cervical cancer. They are transmitted sexually.

Laboratory diagnosis of HPV infection primarily involves cytology sections. Cytotechnologists and cytopathologists read Pap smears and look for koilocytic cells, which are indicative of HPV infection. DNA probe tests can detect HPV in endocervical cells and group the HPV into a high-risk or low-risk cancer category. PCR techniques have shown that HPV is present in as many as 80% to 90% of invasive cervical cancers, but the presence of the virus alone is not the sole factor in cancer development. As many as one third of all college-age women are infected with HPV, and most never develop anything beyond subclinical infections.

Because finding HPV in cervical tissue is not the sole predictor of invasive disease, some doubt surrounds whether it is useful to routinely look for the virus in cervical specimens.

Cervical HPV lesions consist of flat areas of dysplasia and can be visualized by rinsing the area with 5% acetic acid, which turns the lesion white. Lesions can then be removed by surgery, cryotherapy, or laser.

HEPATITIS VIRUSES

Before the 1960s and 1970s, patients with hepatitis were classified as having either **infectious hepatitis** or **serum hepatitis.** Infectious hepatitis was transmitted from person to person via the fecal-oral route, and serum hepatitis resulted from transfusion of infected blood and blood products. During the past 30 years at least five different hepatitis viruses have been recognized: hepatitis A (HAV), hepatitis B (HBV), hepatitis C (HCV), delta hepatitis (HDV), and hepatitis E (HEV) (Table 25-9). HAV and HEV are transmitted by the fecal-oral route, and HBV, HCV, and HDV are transmitted by infected blood and blood products. The viruses are unrelated viruses and biologically and morphologically disparate (Figure 25-8). Many of the clinical symptoms caused by the different hepatitis viruses are similar, so differentiation on the basis of clinical findings is not reliable. Common symptoms are fatigue, headache, anorexia, nausea, vomiting, abdominal pain (right upper quadrant or diffuse), and jaundice and dark urine, which are the most characteristic symptoms.

Hepatitis A

HAV is a small, enveloped ssRNA virus in the picornavirus group. HAV infects people of all ages. In the United States, children between the ages of 5 and 14 have the highest rate of infection. Nearly 30% of all cases occur in children under the age of 15 years. In the United States, epidemics occur every 10 to 15 years; the last epidemic occurred in 1989.

Approximately 25% of the people who contract HAV do so via personal contact (sexual or household) with an HAV-infected person. Many patients are exposed in daycare settings. Outbreaks are caused most commonly by oral-fecal transmission. The virus is shed in large amounts in the feces during the incubation period and early prodromal stage, and food and water contamination can re-

TABLE 25-9

Clinical and Epidemiologic Differences of HAV, HBV, HDV, and NANBH

Clinical Features	Hepatitis A (HAV)	Hepatitis B (HBV)	Delta Hepatitis (HDV)	Non–A, Non–B Hepatitis (NANB)
Incubation (days)	15-45	30-120	21-90	40-120
Type of onset	Acute	Insidious	Usually acute	Insidious
Mode of transmission				
Fecal/oral	Usual	Infrequent	Infrequent	Usual for Hepatitis E virus (HEV)
Parenteral	Increasing	Usual	Usual	Usual for Hepatitis C virus
Other	Food borne, water-borne	Intimate contact, transmucosal transfer	Intimate contact, less efficient than for HBV	Unknown
Sequellae				
Carrier	No	5%-10%	Yes	Yes
Chronic hepatitis	No	Yes	Yes	Yes
Mortality (%)	0.1-0.2	0.5-2.0	30 (chronic form)	Uncertain

sult. About 45% of patients with HAV do not have any obvious risk factors, although undocumented exposure to infected children may account for many of these cases.

The incubation for HAV is approximately 1 month. After the patient is inoculated with the HAV, the patient experiences a transient viremia, after which the virus reaches the liver and replicates in liver cells. The virus passes into the intestine, and viral shedding begins. The onset is abrupt and patients experience fever, chills, fatigue, malaise, aches, pains, and in some cases jaundice. The infection is self-limiting, with convalescence possibly lasting weeks. Complete re-

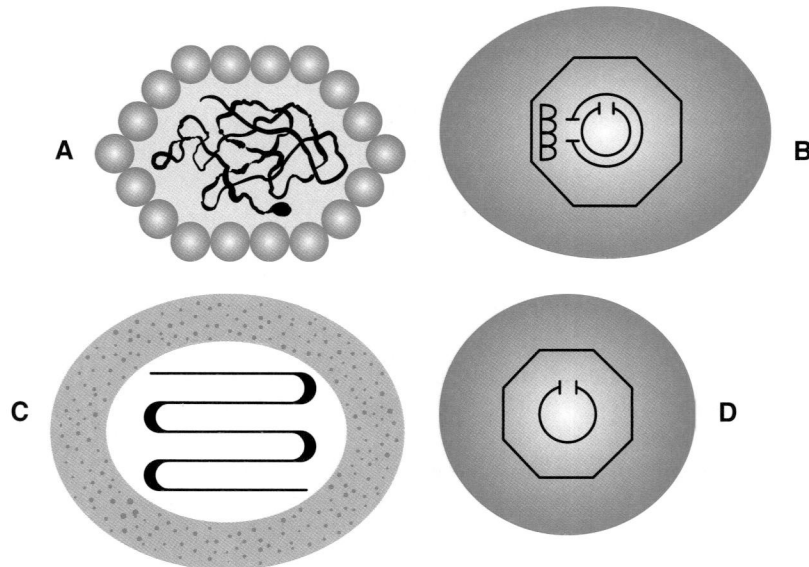

Figure 25-8

A, Hepatitis A virus (HAV). **B,** Hepatitis B virus (HBV). **C,** Hepatitis C virus (HCV). **D,** Hepatitis D, or delta hepatitis, virus (HDV).

covery can take months. HAV has a low mortality, no persistence, and does not cause chronic liver damage.

The best method for laboratory diagnosis of HAV is to demonstrate IgM to HAV (Figure 25-9). Isolation of HAV is not practical, but the virus can be detected in fecal samples.

Safe and effective vaccines for HAV are now available in the United States. Vaccination of children has the potential to reduce the incidence of HAV. Other vaccination target groups include people who travel to countries with endemic HAV, sexually active males, drug abusers, and patients with chronic liver disease. Persons who have not been vaccinated and have been exposed to HAV can receive PEP with immune globulin, which is 80% to 90% effective in preventing infection when administered in a timely fashion. Immune globulin can also be used as preexposure prophylaxis.

Hepatitis B

HBV is a hepadnavirus, which has a partially dsDNA genome. The virus contains surface antigens **(HBsAg)** that circulate in the bloodstream as 22-nm particles. The virion also contains a core antigen **(HBcAg)**—the hepatitis B e antigen **(HBeAg).**

Almost half of the world's population lives in areas with endemic HBV, and more than 8% of the population is positive for HbsAg. Approximately 200 million people are chronic carriers of the virus.

HBV is a blood-borne pathogen. Infected patients can have up to one million infectious particles per milliliter of blood. Lower concentrations of virus appear in semen, vaginal fluid, and saliva. Many other body fluids (e.g., tears, urine, sweat, breast milk) contain HbsAg but do not seem to be infective. The main modes of transmission are through sexual, perinatal, and parenteral routes. In the United States, heterosexual and homosexual sexual contact are the most common transmission routes. High-risk groups include IV drug abusers, homosexuals, individuals from endemic areas, persons who have household or sexual contacts with HBV carriers, health care personnel, people who have tattoos or body piercing, and infants born to HBV-positive mothers.

Once HBV enters the host, it travels from the blood to the liver, and cytotoxic T cells attack the

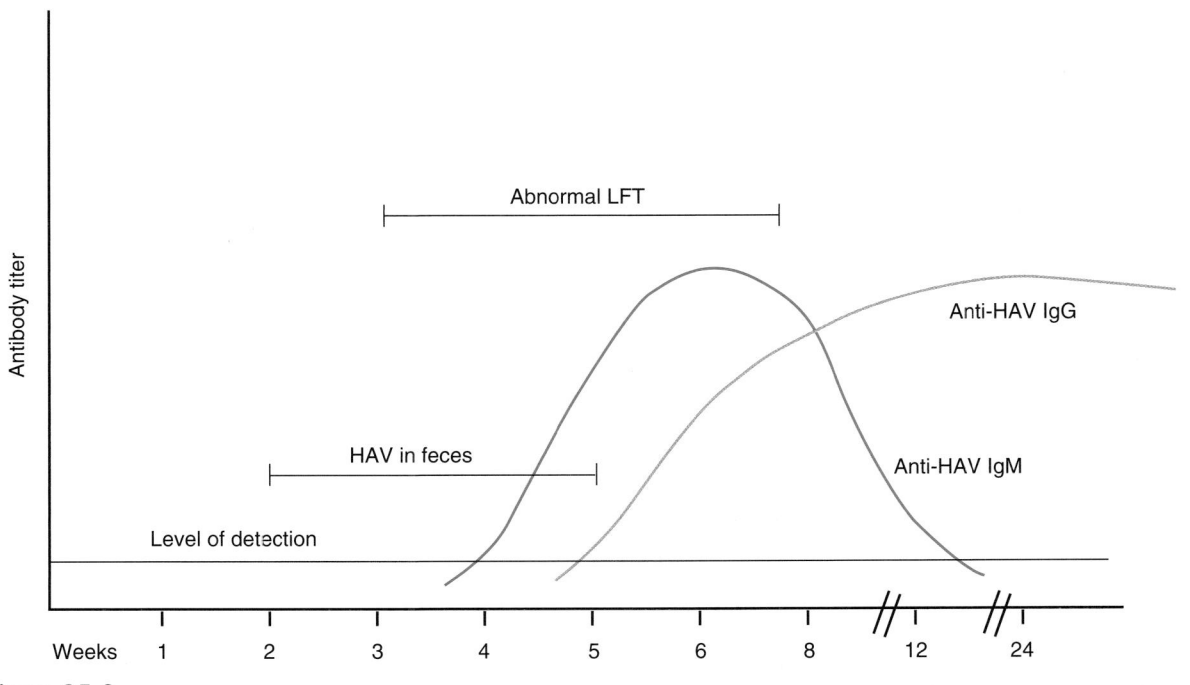

Figure 25-9

Serologic evaluation of hepatitis A virus (HAV) infection showing the rise and fall of detectable antibodies. *LFT,* Liver function test.

TABLE 25-10

Interpretation of Hepatitis B Serology Markers

HBsAG	HBeAg	Anti-HBc	Anti-HBc IgM	Anti-HBs	Anti-HBe	Interpretation
−	NA	−		−	NA	No previous infection with HBV or early incubation
−	NA	+	−	+/−	NA	Convalescent or past infection
−	NA	−	−	±	NA	Immunization to HBsAg
+	−	−	+/−	−	−	Acute infection
+	+	+/−	+	−	−	Acute infection, high infectivity
+	−	+/−	+	−	+	Acute infection, low infectivity
+	+	+			−	Chronic infection, high infectivity
+	−	+	−	−	+	Chronic infection, low infectivity

+, Positive; −, negative; +/−, positive or negative; *NA,* not applicable.

HBV-infected liver cells. The incubation period for HBV infection varies from 2 to 6 months, with an insidious onset that includes symptoms of fever, anorexia, and hepatic tenderness. Jaundice only occurs in about 10% of children who are less than the age of 5 years and is more common in older children and adults (30% to 50%). Serum aminotransferase levels elevate in infected patients. As the immune response activates, the virus is slowly cleared from the system, and the majority of patients become noninfectious. Approximately 50% to 70% of infections are asymptomatic; another 20% to 30% of the patients have clinical jaundice but have a benign resolution of the infection. Therefore approximately 90% of infections do not cause serious sequellae. Nevertheless, about 10% of infected individuals are chronic carriers for more than 6 months. Many of these individuals may develop a chronic infection and have a higher risk of liver disease such as cirrhosis or hepatic carcinoma.

Diagnosis of hepatitis B infections is based on clinical presentation and demonstration of specific serologic markers for HBV. Numerous hepatitis B antigens and their corresponding antibodies have been identified and characterized:

- **HBsAg:** Hepatitis B surface antigen, the covering surface of the virion
- **Anti-HBs:** Antibody to hepatitis B surface antigen
- **Anti-HBc:** Total antibody to hepatitis B core antigen
- **IgM anti-HBc:** IgM antibody to hepatitis B core antigen
- **HBeAg:** A part of the core; related to the potential for infectivity
- **Anti-HBe:** Antibody to hepatitis B e antigen.

The presence of HBsAg in a patient's serum indicates that the patient has an active HBV infection, is a chronic carrier, or is in an incubation period. IgM anti-HBc appears early in the course of the disease and indicates an acute infection. In cases in which HBsAg is not detected and anti-HBs has not appeared, detection of IgM anti-HBc confirms the diagnosis of acute HBV infection. The detection of anti-HBs in the serum indicates a convalescent or immune status. When the infection resolves, IgG anti-HBc and anti-HBs become detectable in the patient's serum. The presence of HBsAg after 6 months of acute infection is a strong indication that the patient is a chronic carrier; the appearance of HBeAg in this case is indicative of a chronic infection and high infectivity. Table 25-10 shows the interpretation of HBV serologic markers. Figure 25-10 shows the rise and fall of detectable antibodies during an acute hepatitis B infection and resolution and of chronic hepatitis B infection.

The safe and effective vaccine for HBV plays a large role in the strategy to eliminate HBV transmission in the United States. The strategy involves the following:

- Screen pregnant women for HBsAg and give hepatitis B immune globulin and HBV vaccine to children of HBsAg mothers.
- Vaccinate all infants.
- Provide "catch-up" vaccinations for older high-risk children and adults.

Hepatitis D (Delta Hepatitis)

Delta hepatitis (HDV) is a defective ssRNA virus that requires HBV for replication. HDV uses the HBV HBsAg as its own envelope. HDV is primarily

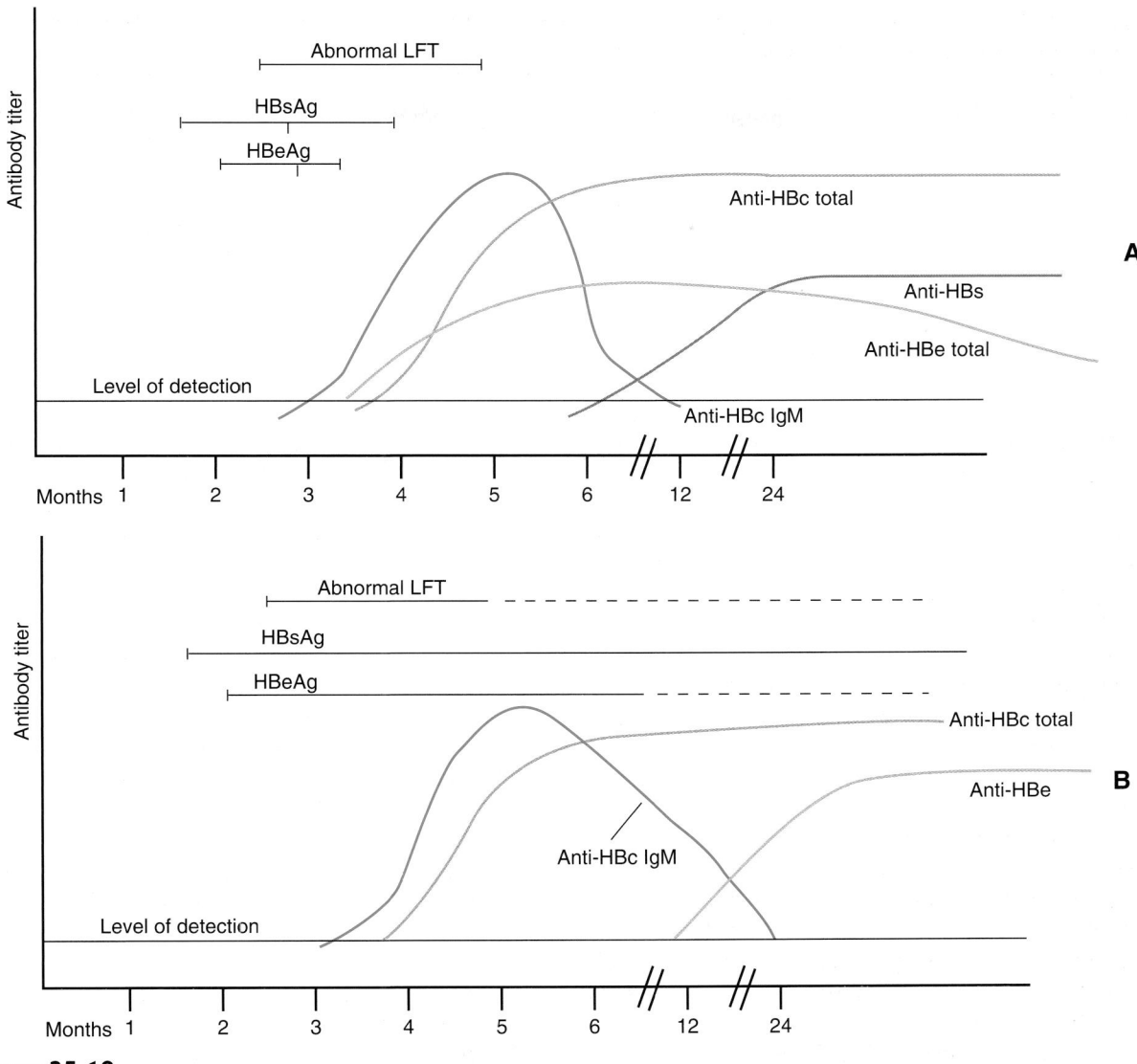

Figure 25-10

Serologic evaluation of hepatitis B virus (HBV) infection showing the rise and fall of detectable antibodies. **A,** Serologic presentation in acute hepatitis infection with resolution. **B,** Serologic presentation of chronic hepatitis infection with late seroconversion. *LFT,* Liver function test.

transmitted by parenteral means, although transmission by mucosal contact has been implicated in epidemics in endemic areas. At-risk groups in the United States are primarily IV drug users, although limited numbers of homosexual individuals in certain parts of the country are also at risk. Because of overlaps in the clinical presentation, a presumed low incidence of infection, and lack of an effective surveillance mechanism, the current epidemiology of delta hepatitis is minimal.

HDV is commonly severe and results in either acute or chronic symptoms. The viral infection can occur in one of two clinical variants: **coinfection** or **superinfection.** In a coinfection, the patient is simultaneously infected by HBV and HDV. In a superinfection a chronic HBV carrier is infected with delta hepatitis; that is, an HDV infection develops in a patient with a chronic HBV infection.

Patients with a coinfection suffer a more severe acute infection and have a higher risk of fulminant hepatitis than patients with a superinfection. However, chronic carriers of HBV who become superinfected with HDV also develop chronic HDV, which increases their chance of developing cirrhosis.

Diagnosis of delta hepatitis infections requires serologic testing for specific HDV antibody markers. Commercial tests are available for HDV IgG. Reference laboratories may offer IgM and HDVAg testing, as well as and PCR for HDV. Table 25-11 shows interpretation of HDV serologic markers, and Figure 25-11 shows serologic presentations of delta hepatitis coinfection and superinfection.

Hepatitis C

After methods for the diagnosis of HAV and HBV became available, it was apparent that they were not responsible for transfusion-related hepatitis. The resulting disease was merely called non-A, non-B hepatitis (NANB). The diagnosis of NANB hepatitis was primarily one of exclusion. In 1974, without any direct evidence, scientists predicted that a "hepatitis virus type C" must exist. Fifteen years later, with the aid of cloning techniques, the genomic sequence of HCV was determined before the virus was ever seen with an electron microscope. HCV is a parenterally transmitted virus. It is a ssRNA virus belonging to the family Flaviviridae and accounts for about 90% of all previous cases of NANB hepatitis. Currently, estimates in the United States are that approximately 150,000 to 170,000 acute infections occur per year. Throughout the 1980s, the incidence of acute infections was 12 to 18 cases per 100,000 individuals. A combination of factors, such as safer use of needles by IV drug abusers and reduction of posttransfusion infections because of better testing, has dropped the incidence to approximately 5 cases per 100,000 people in the United States. Worldwide, up to 170 million new cases may develop each year.

Although perinatal and sexual transmission of infection do occur, and parenteral transmission has been identified as a major route for infection, the HCV antibody has been detected in patients in whom the routes of transmission are poorly or who have no evidence of identifiable risk factors.

Gene amplification tests prove that HCV RNA appears in newly infected patients in as little as 2 weeks. However, most virus detection is accomplished by serology testing, not gene amplification. Antibodies to HCV appear in about 6 weeks in 80% of patients and within 12 weeks in 90% of patients. Symptoms may be very subtle and take time to become apparent. Approximately 50% of HCV-positive patients become chronic carriers; about 20% of patients with chronic infections develop cirrhosis within 20 to 30 years. Cirrhosis is a major risk factor for hepatocellular carcinoma (cancer of the liver). Approximately 3.5 million people are chronic carriers of HCV in the United States.

ELISA tests that detect serum antibodies to proteins c100, c33, and c22 are available as standard screening tests. Two generations of serology tests exist, with the current test being the most sensitive. A recombinant immunoblot assay (RIBA) can be performed to confirm positive tests. The "blot" or "strip" contains separate bands of proteins 5-1-1, cl00, c33, and c22 (in additiion to controls) to detect antibodies to these proteins by ELISA.

Interpretation of the RIBA is as follows:

- No bands present: negative
- One band or 5-1-1 and cl00 present: indeterminant
- Two or more bands (with 5-1-1 and c100 counting as one band) present: positive

HCV is less immunogenic than HBV. Hepatitis C infection does not produce persistent, lifelong levels of antibody; rather, persistence of anti-HCV is linked to the presence of replicating HCV. Figure 25-12 shows a representation of HCV infection.

Patients with a chronic HCV infection can be treated with interferon with or without ribavirin. Some laboratories offer HCV viral loads to help monitor efficacy of treatment in patients.

Hepatitis E

Hepatitis E (enterically transmitted hepatitis) virus (HEV) is a small (32 to 34 nm), nonenveloped, ssRNA virus that is classified as a member of the family Caliciviridae. With HCV, HEV is the other historic NANB hepatitis virus. Unlike

TABLE 25-11

Interpretation of Delta Hepatitis Infection Serologic Markers

Clinical Variant	Serologic Markers			
	Anti-HBc IgM	HBsAg	Anti-HDV	Anti-HDV IgM
Coinfection	+	+	+	+
Superinfection	−	+	+	NA

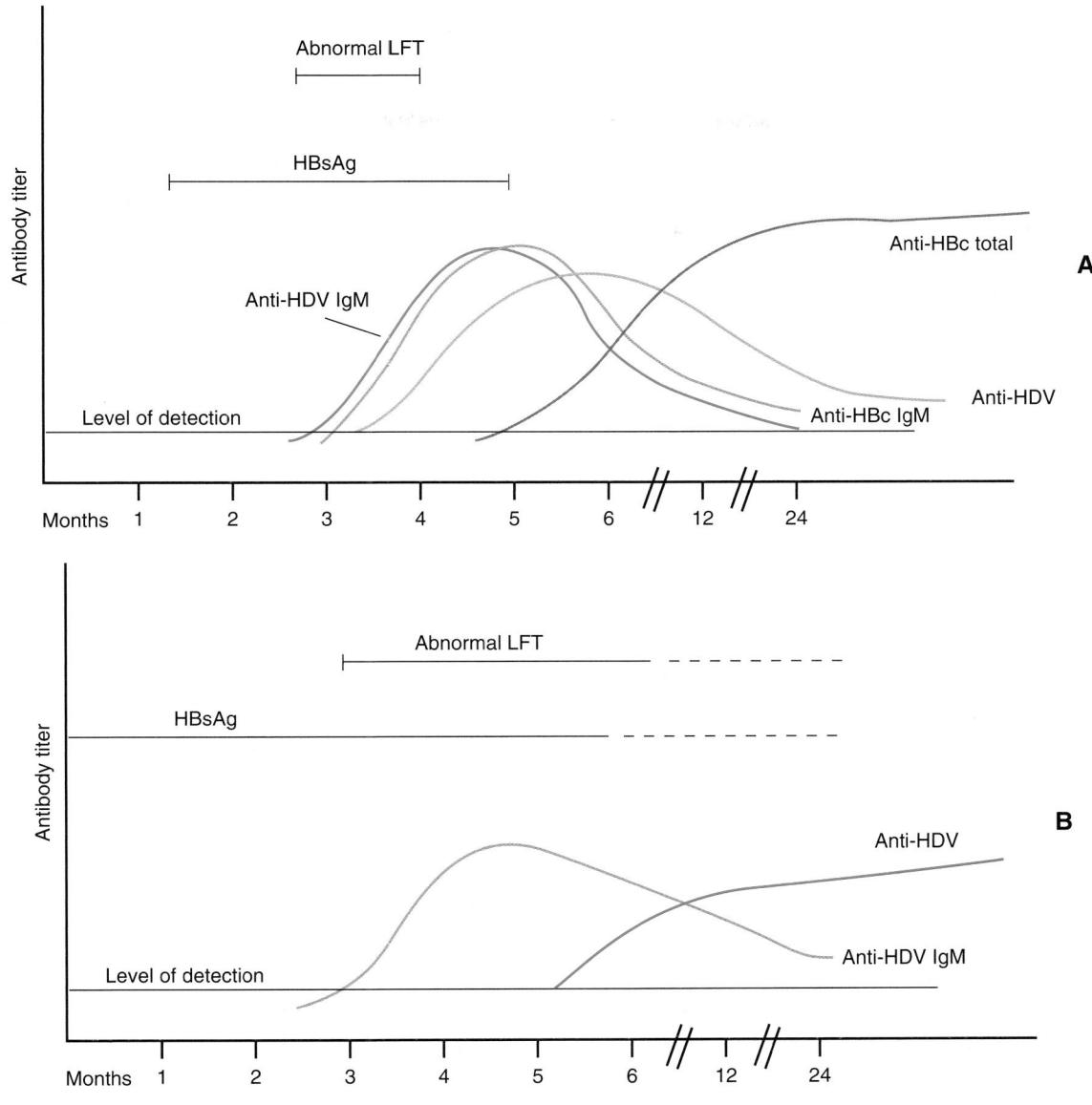

Figure 25-11
Serologic evaluation of hepatitis D virus (HDV) infection showing the rise and fall of detectable antibodies. **A,** Serologic presentation in HDV coinfection. **B,** Serologic presentation of HDV superinfection. *LFT,* Liver function test.

HCV, HEV is a water-borne enteric agent, caused primarily by fecally-contaminated drinking water. HEV has been identified as a cause of epidemics of enterically transmitted hepatitis in developing countries in Asia, Africa, and Central America. Although the virus has not been associated with outbreaks in the United States, it has been linked to sporadic cases in travelers returning from endemic areas.

Hepatitis E is an acute, self-limiting disease with clinical symptoms that are similar to those of HAV. The incubation period of the virus is 2 to 9 weeks. Symptoms and signs of HEV include fever, malaise, nausea, vomiting, jaundice, and dark urine. The mortality rate of HEV is 1% to 3% overall, with a higher likelihood of death in pregnant women (15% to 25%). The epidemics affect primarily young to middle-age adults.

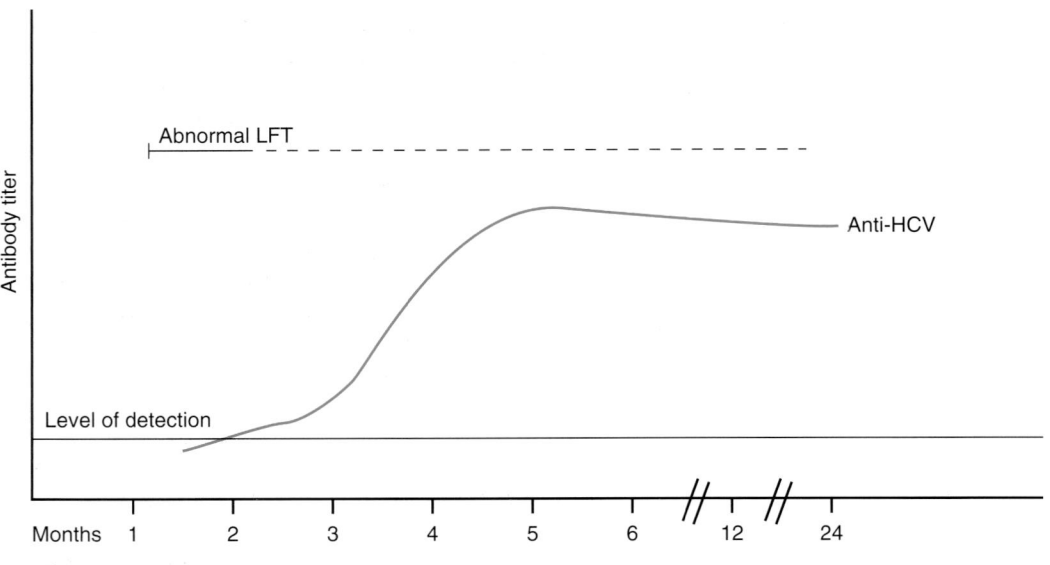

Figure 25-12

Serologic evaluation of hepatitis C virus (HCV) infection showing persistence of detectable antibodies indicating the presence of replicating HCV. *LFT,* Liver function test.

An ELISA test has been developed to detect IgG and IgM antibodies to HEV, although HEV testing is not currently performed in diagnostic laboratories in the United States.

HERPESVIRUSES

The herpesviruses have a core of linear dsDNA, a capsid surrounding the core, an amorphous integument surrounding the capsid, and an outer envelope. In addition, all herpesviruses share the property of being able to achieve latency and lifelong persistence in their hosts. The following eight species of human herpesviruses (HHV) currently are known:

- Herpes simplex virus type 1 (HSV-1, also known as HHV-1)
- Herpes simplex virus type 2 (HSV-2, also known as HHV-2)
- Varicella-zoster virus (VZV, also known as HHV-3)
- Epstein-Barr virus (EBV, also known as HHV-4)
- Cytomegalovirus (CMV, also known as HHV-5)
- Herpesvirus 6 (HHV-6)
- Human herpesvirus 7 (HHV-7)
- Human herpesvirus 8 (HHV-8)

Herpesvirus infections last for life. The virus is latent between acute infections. Certain stimuli, including stress, caffeine, and sunlight, can activate the virus. Activation can cause lesions to reappear.

Herpes Simplex Virus

HSV infections are very common. By adulthood, approximately 80% of Americans have been infected with HSV-1. Approximately 45 million Americans (20%) have HSV-2 infections. Most infections with HSV are asymptomatic. Disease caused by HSV infection is classically divided into two categories: primary (first or initial infection) and recurrent (reactivation of the latent virus).

Infections are spread by contaminated secretions. Lesions usually occur on mucous membranes, with an incubation period of 2 to 11 days. Infected individuals are most infectious during the early days of a primary infection. Virus-infected cells are usually found at the edge and in the base of lesions. However, the virus can be transmitted from older lesions and asymptomatic patients.

Although usually asymptomatic, HSV infections can cause a wide spectrum of clinical manifestations, including the following:

- **Oral herpes.** Oral herpes infections are usually but not exclusively caused by HSV-1. The incubation period varies from 2 days to 2 weeks. Primary infections are usually asymptomatic but when apparent commonly manifest as intraoral mucosal vesicles (which are rarely seen) or ulcerations that may be quite widespread and involve the buccal mucosa, posterior pharynx, and gingival and palatal mucosae. In young adults, a primary herpes simplex infection may involve the posterior pharynx and appear as acute pharyngitis. Recurrent, or reactivation, herpes simplex usually occurs on the border of the lip at the junction of the oral mucosa and skin. A prodrome of burning or pain followed by vesicles, ulcers, and crusted lesions is the typical pattern.
- **Genital herpes.** Genital herpes infections are usually caused by HSV-2, although HSV-1 virus can cause as many as one third of the infections. As with oral infections, genital primary infections are usually asymptomatic. When the infection manifests, it appears in the female as vesicles on the mucosa of the labia, vagina, or both. Cervical and vulvar involvement is not uncommon. In the male the shaft, glans, and prepuce of the penis are the commonly affected sites. The urethra is commonly involved in both sexes. Recurrent herpes infections involve the same sites as primary infections, but the urethra is less commonly involved. The symptoms are usually less severe in recurrent disease.
- **Neonatal herpes.** Transmission of HSV from infected mothers to neonates is less common than might be expected. However, mortality associated with disseminated neonatal disease is approximately 60% in treated patients. Infection may be acquired in utero, intrapartum (during birth), or postnatally (after birth). The infection is most commonly transmitted during a vaginal delivery. Transmission is approximately 50% for a mother who has a primary infection. Most newborns are infected by mothers who are asymptomatically shedding the virus during a primary infection. The risk of transmission is very low when the mother has recurrent herpes. Cesarean sections significantly reduce the risk of transmission.
- **HSV encephalitis.** HSV encephalitis is a rare but devastating disease, with a mortality of approximately 70%. Encephalitis is usually caused by HSV-2 in neonates and HSV-1 in older children and adults.
- **Ocular herpes.** A herpes simplex infection of the conjunctiva may manifest as swelling of the eyelids associated with vesicles. Corneal involvement may result in destructive ulceration and even perforation of the cornea.

Diagnosis of HSV infections is best made by viral isolation or antigen detection. The best specimens for culture are aspirates from vesicles or open lesions and other materials from infected sites. Culture of CSF is usually not productive. To get a culture-confirmed diagnosis of encephalitis, brain biopsy material is required. Alternatively, CSF can be sent to a reference laboratory for PCR detection of HSV. In some studies, gene amplification for HSV in CSF approaches 100% sensitivity.

In culture, HSV replicates rapidly, and a CPE can be seen within 24 hours (see Figure 25-2). Therefore diagnosis and appropriate therapy can be readily accomplished. An indiscriminate virus, herpes simplex can be isolated by using numerous cell lines, including human embryonic lung, rabbit kidney, HEp2, and A549. Once isolated, monoclonal antibodies can be used to type the virus. Typing genital lesion isolates can be prognostic in that HSV-2 reactivation occurs more readily than HSV-1. In additiion, typing genital lesions from children might provide medicolegal evidence supporting potential sexual abuse.

Serology has traditionally provided very limited information to aid in the diagnosis of HSV infections. Reagents that could distinguish between antibodies to HSV-1 and to HSV-2 were not previously available. This was problematic because most adult patients have antibodies to HSV-1. One new assay, a glycoprotein G-based EIA, has been sensitive and specific when differentiating antibodies to HSV-1 and HSV-2.

Human Cytomegalovirus

CMV is a typical herpesvirus but replicates only in human cells and much more slowly than herpes simplex or varicella-zoster. CMV is spread by close contact with an infected person. Most adults demonstrate antibody against the virus, and those who live in overcrowded living conditions may acquire CMV at an early age. The virus is shed in saliva, tears, urine, stool, and breast milk. CMV infection can also be transmitted sexually via semen and cervical and vaginal secretions. The virus can also be transmitted through blood and blood products. CMV is the most common congenital infection in the United States.

The vast majority of CMV infections are asymptomatic. Occasionally, in immunocompetent patients the infection may manifest as a self-limiting, infectious mononucleosislike illness with fever and hepatitis. Congenital infections and infections in immunocompromised patients may be symptomatic and serious. A congenital infection is unlikely to occur if the mother was seropositive at the time of conception. Serious clinical manifestations may develop if the mother acquires the primary infection during pregnancy. Symptomatic congenital infection is characterized by petechiae, hepatosplenomegaly, microcephaly, and chorioretinitis. Other manifestations are low birth weight, central nervous system involvement, mental retardation, and death.

In immunocompromised hosts, such as transplant recipients and HIV-infected patients, a CMV infection may become a life-threatening disseminated disease involving almost any organ, including the lungs, liver, intestinal tract, retina, and central nervous system.

The diagnosis of CMV infection is best confirmed by isolation of the virus from normally sterile body fluids or tissues such as the buffy coat of blood or other internal fluids or tissue. The virus can also be cultured from urine or respiratory secretions, but because shedding of CMV from these sites is common in normal hosts, isolation from such sources must be interpreted with some caution.

A congenital infection is best confirmed by isolation of CMV from the infant within the first 2 weeks of life. Isolation after the first 2 weeks of life does not confirm congenital infection. Urine is the most common source utilized. As with HSV, serology is not as helpful in diagnosing the infection as a culture.

CMV can be isolated only by using human diploid fibroblasts, such as human embryonic lung or human foreskin fibroblasts (see Figure 25-3). The virus replicates slowly, so it may take up to 3 weeks for a CPE to appear in culture. However, shell vials can reduce the time of detection to as little as 1 day. Commercial tests to detect CMV antigenemia are available and may prove helpful in assessing the efficacy of antiviral therapy.

Epstein-Barr Virus

Epstein-Barr virus (EBV) causes infectious mononucleosis (IM). Symptoms and signs of IM include sore throat, fever, lymphadenopathy, hepatomegaly, splenomegaly, and general malaise. The signs and symptoms usually resolve within a few weeks, although malaise may be prolonged. EBV can be recovered from the oropharynx of symptomatic and healthy persons, who can transmit the virus to susceptible persons via infected saliva.

The incubation period for EBV varies from 2 weeks to 2 months. As with the other herpes group viruses, infection is very common and most adults demonstrate antibody against the virus. Infection in young children is almost always asymptomatic. As age increases to young adulthood, a corresponding increase occurs in the ratio of symptomatic to asymptomatic infections.

EBV has been associated with some cancers, including Burkitt's lymphoma and nasopharyngeal carcinoma (NPC). Burkitt's lymphoma is a malignant disease of the lymphoid tissue seen most commonly in African children. The virus is also increasingly being recognized as an important viral agent in transplant recipients. The most significant clinical effect of EBV infection in these patients is the development of a B-cell lymphoproliferative disorder or lymphoma.

Other complications of EBV infections are splenic hemorrhage and rupture, frank hepatitis, thrombocytopenia purpura with hemolytic anemia, Reye's syndrome, encephalitis, and other neurologic syndromes.

A viral culture for EBV requires human B lymphocytes, which is beyond the capabilities of most clinical virology laboratories. Diagnosis of EBV is done with serologic tests. EBV infects circulating

TABLE 25-12

Interpretation of Epstein-Barr Virus Serologic Markers

PB	Anti–VCA-IgM	Anti–VCA-IgG	Anti–EA-IgG	Anti-EBNA	Interpretation
−	−	−	−	−	No previous exposure to Epstein-Barr virus
+	+	+	+/−	−	Acute infectious mononucleosis
+/−	+/−	+	+/−	+	Recent infection
−	−	+	−	+	Remote infection

PB, Paul Bunnell; *anti-VCA-IgM,* IgM antibodies against the viral capsid antigen; *anti-VCA-IgG,* IgG antibodies against the viral capsid antigen; *anti-EA-IgG,* antibody to early antigen; *anti-EBNA,* antibodies to the nuclear antigen.

B lymphocytes and stimulates them to produce multiple (heterophil) antibodies, including antibodies to sheep and horse red blood cells and to *Proteus* OX19. The Paul-Bunnell heterophil antibody test is an excellent screen for these antibodies, although some false-positive reactions occur. Some false-positive tests represent patients who have had IM and still have low levels of antibody. Young children may have false-negative results with the heterophil test; running an EBV-specific antibody test on these individuals is appropriate (Table 25-12).

EBV-specific serologies (Figure 25-13) measure the presence or absence of the following:

- *Anti–VCA-IgM (IgM antibodies against the viral capsid antigen):* The IgM to the viral capsid antigen occurs early in the infection, so its presence indicates current infection.

- *Anti–VCA-IgG (IgG antibodies against the viral capsid antigen):* The viral capsid antigen IgG appears during the acute phase, and the patient will be seropositive from then on.
- *Anti–EA-IgG (antibody to early antigen):* The IgG to EA may appear in the acute phase, and its presence indicates either current or recent infection. The antibody usually cannot be detected after 6 months.
  Anti-EA/D (diffuse): The EA/D is elevated in patients with NPC.
  Anti-EA/R (rough): The EA/R is elevated in patients with BL.
- *Anti-EBNA (antibody to the nuclear antigen)*
  Anti–EBNA-1: is elevated in patients with NPC, and its presence indicates recent, past, or reactivated infection.
  Anti–EBNA-2: is seen in acute, recent, past and reactivated infection.

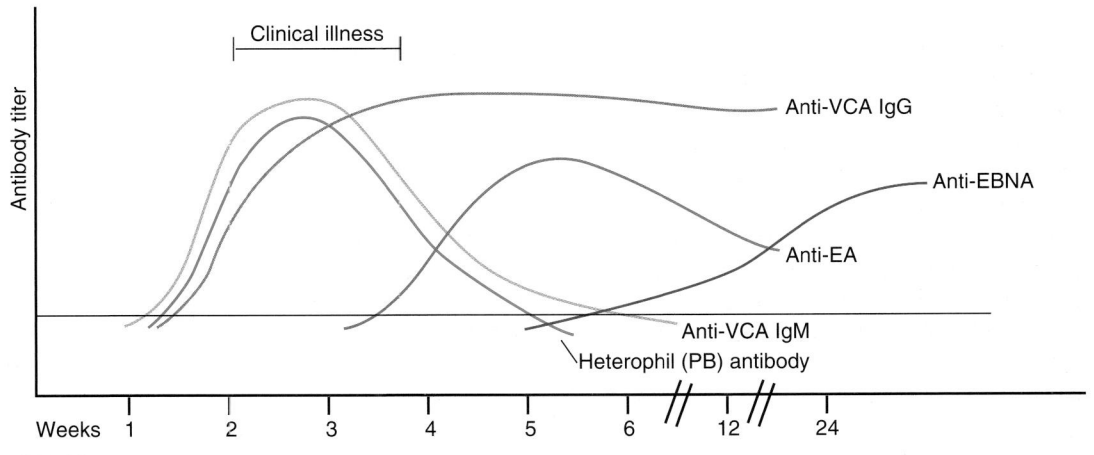

Figure 25-13

Serologic evaluation of Epstein-Barr virus (EBV) infection (infectious mononucleosis) showing the rise and fall of detectable antibodies.

Varicella-Zoster Virus

VZV has the typical structure of the herpesvirus group. It spreads by droplet inhalation or direct contact with infectious lesions. The virus causes two different clinical manifestations: varicella (chickenpox) and zoster (shingles). More than 90% of adults have antibody to VZV.

Varicella, or chickenpox, is the primary infection and is highly contagious. In contrast to infections with the other herpes group viruses, which are usually asymptomatic, varicella is usually clinically apparent. It commonly appears in childhood and includes symptoms such as a mild febrile illness, rash, and vesicular lesions. Usually the lesions appear first on the head and trunk and then spread to the limbs. The lesions dry, crust over, and heal in 1 to 2 weeks. Painful oral mucosal lesions may develop, particularly in adults.

Zoster is the clinical manifestation reactivated by VZV and usually occurs in adults. It is thought that the virus remains latent in the dorsal root or cranial nerve ganglia after primary infection with chickenpox. In a small proportion of patients the virus becomes reactivated, travels down the nerve and causes zoster. The most common presentation is rash, followed by vesicular lesions in a unilateral dermatome pattern. These lesions may be associated with prolonged disabling pain that can remain for months, long after the vesicular lesions disappear.

VZV is usually diagnosed on the basis of characteristic clinical findings. In atypical cases, such as in immunosuppressed patients, the diagnosis may be more difficult or questionable. In such patients, culture of fresh lesions (vesicles) or use of fluorescent-tagged monoclonal antibodies against VZV confirms the diagnosis. VZV can be cultured on human embryonic lung or Vero cells. Cytopathic changes may not be evident for 3 to 7 days.

Human Herpesvirus 6

HHV-6 is a common pathogen, with about 95% of young adults being seropositive. Inhalation of respiratory droplets from and close contact with infected individuals are probably the means of transmission.

Most infections are asymptomatic. HHV-6 has been associated with the childhood disease *exanthem subitum* (which is also called *roseola infantum* and *fourth disease*). Children are protected by maternal antibodies until approximately age 6 months. Seroconversion occurs in 90% of the children between the age of 6 months and 2 years. The disease is acute, febrile, and mild. A maculopapular rash appears as the fever resolves. Approximately 30% to 40% of the infected children with symptoms experience seizures.

The diagnosis of HHV-6 infection is usually made clinically. Isolation of virus requires a lymphocyte culture, which is not practical for routine diagnoses. Serology may not be helpful unless paired sera are available. Patients do not usually have a positive IgM until approximately the fifth day; IgG appears several days later. PCR and viral load testing may offer sensitive and specific means of diagnosing primary HHV-6 infection.

Human Herpesvirus 7

HHV-7 was first isolated from peripheral blood monocytes of infected patients in 1989. The virus infects CD4+ lymphocytes at the same site HIV uses for infection. HHV-7 is similar to HHV-6 and is classified as a beta herpesvirus with HHV-6 and CMV. Like HHV-6, HHV-7 is extremely common and shed in the saliva of 75% of adults. The virus causes exanthem subitum that is clinically identical to that of HHV-6. Despite the similarities between HHV-6 and HHV-7, their antigenic diversity is such that antibodies to one virus do not protect against infection from the other. In addition, exposure to HHV-7 seems to occur later than with HHV-6. Most 2 year olds are seronegative for HHV-7, but most children are seropositive by the age of 6 years.

Like HHV-6, HHV-7 can be isolated in culture in peripheral blood lymphocytes or cord blood lymphocytes. PCR can detect the virus, but the ubiquitous nature of the virus can lead to difficulties in interpreting the results. Serologies can be confusing because of cross-reactions, but patients with rising antibody levels to HHV-7 but not to HHV-6 may have an active HHV-7 infection.

Human Herpesvirus 8

HHV-8 can be detected in all forms of Kaposi's sarcoma including AIDS-related, Mediterranean, HIV-1–negative endemic to Africa, and posttransplantation Kaposi's sarcoma. The virus is probably transmitted sexually, and the pattern of infection is similar to that of HSV-2. About 20% of normal adults have antibodies to HHV-8, as well as 27% of patients with HIV-1 who do not have Kaposi's sarcoma and 60% of patients with HIV and Kaposi's sarcoma.

The virus cannot currently be recovered from culture. Serologic tests are being evaluated, but testing is not standardized. PCR is currently the most sensitive and specific test for the detection of HHV-8 and can detect the virus in various specimens, including tissues, blood, bone marrow, saliva, and semen.

ANTIVIRAL THERAPY

Clinical virology is more relevant today than ever. Some viral infections are treatable, especially if a laboratory can rapidly identify the pathogen. Antiviral compounds must target an essential viral replicative mechanism without destroying or damaging the host cell. Several antivirals comprise nucleosides used in viral replication. The viruses insert these "counterfeit" nucleoside analogs into their own nucleic acid, resulting in a disruption of viral replication. Other antiviral compounds inhibit viral replication by targeting key viral proteins. For instance, phosphonoformic acid (foscarnet) is an analog of pyrophosphate that acts directly as a DNA polymerase inhibitor. Examples of some of the more commonly used antiviral agents are listed in Table 25-13.

Just as antibiotic use increases the risk of antibiotic resistance in bacteria, the use of antivirals can result in viruses that are resistant to therapy. As more antiviral agents become available, antiviral susceptibility testing will become increasingly important. For example, foscarnet is being used to treat infections caused by HSV strains that are resistant to acyclovir and to treat CMV strains that are resistant to ganciclovir.

The viral infection cycle occurs in five steps, or phases, which are potential targets for antiviral compounds.

Absorption

For infection of a cell to occur, virions must absorb or attach to the cell. Absorption is usually specific for certain cell receptors. Most host cell receptors are glycoproteins, some of which include the following:

- Immune globulin superfamily molecules (for poliovirus)
- Acetylcholine (for rabies virus)
- Sialic acid (for influenza virus)
- CD4 (forHIV)
- Complement receptor C3d (for EBV)

TABLE 25-13
Antiviral Compounds

Antiviral	Inhibits	Active Against
Acyclovir	DNA polymerase	Herpes simplex virus (HSV), varicella-zoster virus
Cidofovir	DNA polymerase	Cytomegalovirus (CMV) (retinitis)
Famciclovir	DNA polymerase	HSV-2
Ganciclovir	DNA polymerase	CMV (retinitis)
Valacyclovir	DNA polymerase	HSV-2
Idoxuridine, trifluridine	DNA synthesis (DNA base analog)	HSV (keratitis)
Amantadine, rimantadine	Uncoating	Influenza A (treatment and prophylaxis)
Inferferon-alpha	Viral replication (multiple mechanisms)	Human papillomavirus (HPV) (genital warts); chronic hepatitis C virus (HCV), Kaposi's sarcoma
Ribavirin	Viral replication (multiple mechanisms)	Respiratory syncitial virus (RSV)
ddl	Reverse transcriptase	Human immunodeficiency virus (HIV)
3TC	Reverse transcriptase	HIV
d4T	Reverse transcriptase	HIV
ddC	Reverse transcriptase	HIV
ZDV	Reverse transcriptase	HIV
Indinavir	Proteases	HIV
Nelfinavir, ritonavir	Proteases	HIV
Saquinavir	Proteases	HIV

Penetration

Nonenveloped virions may directly penetrate the cell membrane. Once the virus is in the cell, the viral capsid is removed, releasing the genome. Enveloped viruses may enter the cell by fusion with the cell membrane. Another method of penetration is endocytosis, whereby the virus enters the cell in a cytoplasmic vacuole that fuses with cytoplasmic lysosomes.

Uncoating

After entry into the host cell, the genome is uncoated. RNA viruses usually release the genome into cytoplasm, whereas most DNA viruses release the genome into the host nucleus.

Eclipse/Synthesis

The eclipse phase is the time from infection until the time of progeny virus production. In most infections, this period lasts several hours.

Maturation/Release

The capsid protein subunits aggregate to form capsomers and associate with the genome to form the nucleocapsid. The virion is released from the cell by budding or lysis.

Bibliography

Anonymous: Hantavirus pulmonary syndrome in the Americas, *Week Epidemiolog Rec* 72(41):305, 1997.

Belshe RB: *Textbook of human virology,* ed 2, St Louis, 1991, Mosby.

Costello MI et al: Guidelines for specimen collection, transportation, and test selection, *Lab Med* 24:t9, 1993.

Creager JG, Black JG, Davison VE: *Microbiology: principles and applications,* Englewood Cliffs, NJ, 1990, Prentice-Hall.

Fields BN, Knipe DM, editors: *Fields virology,* ed 2, New York, 1990, Raven Press.

Galasso GJ, Whitley RJ, Merigan TC, editors: *A practical diagnosis of viral infections,* New York, 1993, Raven Press.

Gold E: Current progress in measles eradication in the United States, *Infect Med* 14:297, 1997.

Han LL, Alexander JP, Anderson LJ: Respiratory syncytial virus pneumonia among the elderly: an assessment of disease burden, *J Infect Dis* 179:25, 1999.

Haukenes G, Haaheim LR, Pattison JR, editors: *A practical guide to clinical virology,* New York, 1989, John Wiley & Sons.

Henig RM: *A dancing matrix: voyages along the viral frontier,* New York, 1993, Alfred A Knopf.

Koneman EW et al, editors: Diagnosis of infections caused by viruses, *Chlamydia, Rickettsia,* and related organisms. In *Color atlas and textbook of diagnostic microbiology,* ed 5, Philadelphia, 1997, Lippincott.

LeDuc JW et al: Hantaan (Korean hemorrhagic fever) and related rodent zoonoses. In Morse SS, editor: *Emerging viruses,* New York, 1993, Oxford University Press.

Lennette DA, Smith TF, Waner JL, editors: Virology. In Murray PR et al, editors: *Manual of clinical microbiology,* ed 7, Washington, DC, 1999, American Society for Microbiology.

Lennette EH, Halonen P, Murphy FA editors: *Laboratory diagnosis of infectious diseases principles and practice,* vol 2, New York, 1988, Springer-Verlag.

Levine PH, Ablashi DV: An etioloic perspective of the new herpesviruses: HHV-7 and HHV-8, *Infect Med* 16:24, 1999.

Nesher G, Moore TL: Human parvovirus infection, *Infect Med* 14:637, 1997.

Ottolini MG, Hemming VG: Prevention and treatment recommendations for respiratory syncytial virus infection. Background and clinical experience 40 years after discovery, *Drugs* 54:867, 1997.

Roizman B, Whitley RI, Lopez C: *The human herpes viruses,* New York, 1993, Raven Press.

Skidmore SI, Yarbough PO et al: Hepatitis E virus: the cause of a waterborne hepatitis outbreak, *J Med Virol* 37:58, 1992.

Spector S, Lancz G: *Clinical virology manual,* ed 2, New York, 1992, Elsevier.

Yarbough PO: Hepatitis E: diagnosis of infection, *Microbiol Newsl* 15:113, 1993.

Zapikan AZ: Viral gastroenteritis. In Notkins AL, Oldstone MB, editors: *Concepts in viral pathogenesis,* New York, 1984, Springer-Verlag.

Zuckerman M, Banatvala JE, Pattison JR: *Principles and practice of clinical virology,* ed 2, New York, 1990, John Wiley & Sons.

LEARNING ASSESSMENT

1. Which clinical manifestations of the patient described in the case study at the beginning of the chapter indicate that he has acquired immune deficiency syndrome (AIDS)?

2. Which opportunistic infections or conditions are used as indicators of AIDS?

3. Which immunologic markers are used to diagnose a human immunodeficiency virus (HIV) infection?

4. Which viral agent is suspected to cause meningitis in patients who have AIDS or have had transplants?

5. Which infections do Epstein-Barr virus (EBV) produce? Which complications may result from EBV infections?

6. How is an acute viral hepatitis B infection differentiated from a chronic infection? Which markers indicate resolution of the infection?

7. What are the differences between classic dengue fever and dengue hemorrhagic fever?

8. What is the method used to identify the rabies virus?

9. What is fifth disease? What is the cause of this disease?

10. Which viruses comprise the enteroviruses?

11. What are arenaviruses?

Continued

LEARNING ASSESSMENT—cont'd

12. Which types of infections do papillomaviruses produce?

13. Which virus has the potential for latency?

14. Why are vaccines for influenza not always effective?

15. Which antiviral agents have been developed, and which specific viral agents are they used against?

PART III

Laboratory Diagnosis of Infectious Diseases: an Organ System Approach to Diagnostic Microbiology

CHAPTER 26

Upper and Lower Respiratory Tract Infections

James L. Cook

GENERAL CONCEPTS OF INFECTIOUS DISEASES
OF THE RESPIRATORY TRACT
  The Role of Normal Flora
  The Immune Status of the Host
  Seasonal and Community Trends in Infections
  Empiric Antimicrobial Therapy

ANATOMIC CHARACTERIZATION
OF THE RESPIRATORY TRACT
  Anatomy of the Respiratory Tract
  Barriers to Infection

VIRULENCE FACTORS OF PATHOGENIC
ORGANISMS
  Adherence
  Toxin Elaboration
  Evasion of Host Defenses

UPPER RESPIRATORY TRACT INFECTIONS
  Pharyngitis
  Sinusitis

  Otitis Media
  Epiglottitis
  Pertussis

LOWER RESPIRATORY TRACT INFECTIONS
  Bronchitis and Bronchiolitis
  Acute Pneumonia
  Aspiration Pneumonia
  Chronic Pneumonia
  Empyema

OPPORTUNISTIC INFECTIONS OF THE
RESPIRATORY TRACT
  Granulocytopenic Patients
  Patients with Defects in Cellular Immunity
  Patients with Defects in Humoral Immunity
  Diagnosis

OBJECTIVES

1. Describe the basic anatomy of the respiratory tract and explain the mechanical defenses of each anatomic site and how alterations of these defenses may lead to infectious diseases.

2. Define the importance of normal flora in the respiratory tract and explain how alterations in the normal flora may lead to infectious diseases.

3. Discuss the basic pathogenic mechanisms of infectious diseases of the respiratory tract and associate the virulence factors of the organisms that cause that disease.

4. Given the clinical picture presented and the symptoms, associate the most probable organisms that cause upper and lower respiratory tract infections.

5. Describe the pathogenesis, risk factors, and complications associated with respiratory tract infections as well as the types of specimens collected for diagnosis.

6. Determine the risk factors in immunocompromised hosts that predispose to infections and provide examples of respiratory tract diseases in different types of immunocompromised hosts.

7. Describe the principles and methods of proper specimen collection and transport of respiratory secretions.

8. Discuss the importance of visual examination and proper culturing of respiratory samples and determine the acceptability for culture of respiratory secretions.

9. Appraise the important aspects of diagnosis of infections of the respiratory tract through case studies.

KEY TERMS

Normal flora	Nosocomial infection	Pertussis	Aspiration pneumonia
Pathogenic microorganisms	Bacterial pharyngitis	Bronchitis	Empyema
	Acute sinusitis	Acute bronchiolitis	Opportunistic infections
Empiric antimicrobial therapy	Otitis media	Pneumonia	
	Acute epiglottitis	Atypical pneumonia	

This chapter describes respiratory tract infections from the perspective of the clinical microbiologist working with the clinician who must make the differential diagnosis of these infections. The chapter includes the following:

- An overview of the anatomy of the upper and lower compartments of the respiratory tract to show how infections are established after mechanical and functional changes in these areas occur
- The importance of the normal flora of the respiratory tract in preventing colonization by potential pathogens and how alterations in the normal flora as well as colonization of normally sterile areas may lead to infection

- An explanation of how microorganism virulence factors relate to the mechanisms of establishment and progression of infection
- Clinical syndromes of patients with upper and lower respiratory tract infections to provide the clinical aspects of the microbiology of the respiratory tract
- Pathogenesis, risk factors, and complications of specific disease states
- Infections in normal hosts, risk factors that predispose immunocompromised hosts to respiratory tract infections, and how presentations of these infections differ in immunodeficient patients
- Case studies that illustrate and integrate concepts presented in the chapter

GENERAL CONCEPTS OF INFECTIOUS DISEASES OF THE RESPIRATORY TRACT

General concepts apply to the infectious diseases of each organ system. A brief introductory discussion of some of these concepts provides a better understanding of the different disease entities related to infections of the respiratory tract. These concepts include the following:

- The role of the normal microbial flora
- The immune status of the host
- Seasonal and community trends in communicable respiratory diseases
- The role of empiric antimicrobial therapy

The Role of Normal Flora

In the diagnostic approach to all types of infections, laboratory professionals must consider the types of organisms normally found at the site to be able to determine whether diagnostic microbiology data indicate the presence of a pathogen. This requires a knowledge of the **normal flora,** the clinical setting, and the patient's presentation.

The normal microbial flora exists in a symbiotic relationship with the host. These organisms are isolated from the host in the absence of disease; this is referred to as colonization. The normal flora of the respiratory tract plays an important role in protecting the host from infection with **pathogenic microorganisms.** The normal flora can prevent proliferation and invasion of pathogenic organisms through competition for the same nutrients and the same receptor sites on host cells. In addition, these organisms produce bacteriocins, bacterial products that are toxic to other organisms. The presence of these organisms keeps the immune system primed for a rapid response to invading organisms and stimulates cross-protective immune factors known as natural antibodies. Under normal conditions, a balance is maintained that limits the quantity or dominance of any one organism.

Discriminating between normal flora and pathogenic microorganisms

Although a standard list of organisms can be routinely cultured from the upper respiratory tract (Box 26-1), it is interesting that the consensus concerning what is considered "normal flora" can

---

Box 26-1

Common Nasopharyngeal and Oropharyngeal Organisms Isolated in the Normal Host

Bacteria

Usually present

Streptococcus mitis and other α-hemolytic streptococci
Non–group A β-hemolytic streptococci
Streptococcus pneumoniae
Streptococcus pyogenes
Streptococcus salivarius
Veillonella spp.
Bacteroides spp.
Fusobacterium spp.
Prevotella spp.
Porphyromonas spp.
Coagulase-negative staphylococci
Neisseria spp.
Nonhemolytic streptococci
Diphtheroids
Micrococcus spp.
Eikenella spp.
Capnocytophaga spp.

Occasionally present

Haemophilus influenzae
Haemophilus parainfluenzae
Peptostreptococcus
Actinomycetes
Staphylococcus aureus
Mycoplasma

Fungus
Candida spp.

Virus
Herpes simplex

---

change with time as new associations between organisms and disease states are recognized. For example, in past years, *Moraxella catarrhalis* was considered part of the upper respiratory tract flora that was only rarely associated with serious infections. However, since the early 1970s, awareness is increasing that these organisms can be associated with complicated infections of the respiratory tract in children and in adults with chronic lung diseases. This indicates the importance of periodic reevaluation of the pathogenicity of all organisms.

Familiarity with the normal flora of respiratory tract compartments is also important in determining the clinical relevance of an isolate. For example, isolation of α-hemolytic colonies from a pharyngeal culture from a patient with pharyngitis arouses little clinical interest, because α-hemolytic streptococci are normal flora in the oropharynx. In contrast, isolation of α-hemolytic colonies from a properly collected sputum specimen or bronchial aspirate in the clinical setting of lobar pneumonia should prompt full identification of the organism and perhaps initiation of empirical therapy for possible pneumococcal infection.

Normal upper respiratory tract flora in an asymptomatic patient may change depending on the clinical setting. Patients who have previously received broad-spectrum antibiotics, have been hospitalized recently, or have chronic illnesses may have different pharyngeal flora. Gram-negative bacilli are commonly isolated from the pharynx in such patients in the absence of clinical signs of infection. Therefore it is important to distinguish between a positive culture for an organism that is a potential pathogen and a clinical disease state caused by that pathogen. Table 26-1 lists organisms that are considered primary pathogens. This table also shows a number of organisms that can be pathogens in the correct clinical setting (possible pathogens). In this case, as in many others, proper communication between the clinical microbiologist and the clinician is essential.

Differentiating colonization from infection

The isolation of certain organisms from respiratory specimens may represent either colonization or disease, depending on the circumstances. An interpretation must be based on several factors. The method and site of collection of the specimen can influence the risk of contamination with organisms that are part of the normal flora. Characteristics of the specimen such as the presence of white blood cells and the number of organisms in the specimen can help distinguish between colonization and infection. Most important, a compatible clinical syndrome should be present to determine whether the presence of a potential pathogen is clinically relevant. For example, the isolation of a few colonies of *Staphylococcus aureus* from a sputum specimen with many epithelial cells does not represent *S. aureus* pneumonia but is more likely to be contamination with an organism that is part of the normal flora of the patient. In contrast, heavy growth of the same organism from a respiratory specimen with many white blood cells from an elderly man with post-influenza pneumonia is highly suggestive of *S. aureus* pneumonia, especially if the sputum culture is accompanied by a positive culture from a normally sterile site such as blood or pleural fluid.

Other organisms are potentially pathogenic and cause disease only when some interruption occurs in the pulmonary defense mechanisms. *Streptococcus pneumoniae* has been isolated from 5% to 70% of the normal adult population, yet only a very small proportion of these carriers will develop pneumococcal pneumonia. Pneumonia may also result from aspiration of upper respiratory tract secretions in patients with impaired pulmonary defenses, such as those with alcoholism or congestive heart failure.

Other organisms are always considered pathogenic when isolated, even in small numbers. Isolation of *Mycobacterium tuberculosis* in any amount is significant because of the virulence of the organism and the contagiousness of the infected patient.

The Immune Status of the Host

The defenses of the host with a suspected infection must be evaluated when determining whether the

---

TABLE 26-1

Selected Nonviral Pathogens in the Respiratory Tract

Primary Pathogens	Possible Pathogens
Streptococcus pneumoniae	*Acinetobacter* spp.
Group A β-hemolytic streptococci	Enterics and other gram-negative bacilli
Neisseria meningitidis	Fungi
Neisseria gonorrhoeae	*Nocardia* spp.
Bordetella pertussis	*Staphylococcus aureus*
Mycobacterium kansasii	*Haemophilus influenzae*
Mycobacterium tuberculosis	β-Hemolytic streptococci, non–group A
Legionella pneumophila	*Moraxella catarrhalis*
Toxin-producing *Corynebacterium diphtheriae*	Anaerobes
Mycoplasma pneumoniae	*Mycobacterium* spp.
Chlamydia trachomatis	Actinomycetes
Chlamydia pneumoniae	
Pneumocystis carinii	

identification of a specific microorganism is likely to be significant in causing disease. When considering the likelihood that a microorganism will cause infection in a given host, the laboratory professional must consider both the virulence of the organism and the defenses available to the host to counteract establishment and progression of infection. At one end of the spectrum of organisms are the normal flora of the respiratory tract that usually exist as commensals for the life of the normal host without causing disease. At the other end are organisms that often establish infection and cause disease in the normal host when present in numbers above a certain threshold. For these purposes, a normal host is considered to be one with mature immunologic defenses but without specific immunity against the microorganism in question. Examples of microorganisms that cause respiratory tract infections in normal hosts are the common respiratory viruses of childhood. In normal children, these viral infections occur at a high incidence but are relatively benign. The clinical outcomes of these and other respiratory tract infections in normal hosts depend on both the injurious effects of the microorganism and its products at the site of infection and the host immune response to infection.

Previous exposure of a normal host to pathogens such as the respiratory tract viruses is one example in which the host usually develops immunity to reinfection with the same organism. Organism-specific immune responses may prevent or alter the course of subsequent infection. For example, adults previously infected with a given virus serotype as children usually do not manifest the same severity of infection when reexposed to the same pathogen. Evidence of infection may not be present, or clinical signs and symptoms of infection are greatly reduced.

In an immunocompromised host, however, microorganisms that are usually not pathogens in a normal host may cause serious infection. This type of infection is referred to as an "opportunistic" infection to indicate that a combination of a reduced host response and a pathogen of low virulence has resulted in the establishment of infection. Of course, organisms exhibiting high levels of virulence also cause disease in immunocompromised hosts. Because the host response is diminished, infections with virulent pathogens are usually more severe and more rapidly progressive than in the normal host.

Age as a risk factor

Immunocompromise by reason of age is a form of "functional immunodeficiency." Infants and the elderly are more susceptible to certain respiratory tract infections and are more likely to develop complications of these infections. For example, respiratory tract infections with *Haemophilus influenzae* are more commonly complicated by meningitis in infants than in older children or adults. Similarly, in the elderly, complications of common respiratory tract infections occur more frequently than in the younger adult population. One hallmark of seasonal outbreaks of influenza virus infection of the respiratory tract is the increased incidence of death from complicating bacterial pneumonias in the elderly.

It is apparent from these observations that one cannot determine the significance of a respiratory tract microbial isolate without considering the source of the specimen, the age and immunologic status of the host, and the clinical setting of the patient. The isolation of an organism that has great potential to cause disease may represent either simple colonization of the upper respiratory tract or life-threatening disease. In contrast, isolation of a "nonpathogenic" organism that may be part of the normal flora of the upper respiratory tract may be an indication of serious disease if it is found in an unusual location or in a host with decreased defenses against infection. Availability of proper clinical data in these cases facilitates planning by the clinical microbiologist of proper evaluation of the respiratory tract specimen.

Reduced clearance of secretions

In addition to age as a compromising factor, reduced clearance of secretions or obstruction of an area in either the upper or the lower respiratory tract predisposes to infection and can, on occasion, seriously compromise respiratory tract function. Infection behind an obstruction is a common theme in the study of infectious diseases of many organ systems. Obstruction prevents the mechanical clearance that is important in limiting both the numbers of potential pathogens and the associated inflammatory response at a specific site. Decreased clearance of respiratory secretions may result from the following:

▪ Immature anatomic development (e.g., eustachian tube anatomy in young children)

- Transient reduction in function of the mucociliary mechanism (e.g., after a viral infection)
- Obstruction by a foreign body (e.g., aspirated food or foreign object)
- Previous disease that alters the normal respiratory tract anatomy (e.g., bronchiectasis; obstructing lymph node or tumor)
- Alterations in the viscosity of mucus (e.g., cystic fibrosis)

Infection-induced airway obstruction

Another way in which respiratory tract obstruction can be a factor in infectious disease involves compromise of respiration. In these cases, the obstruction may be a consequence of, rather than the factor that precipitates, infection. The anatomy of the area, rather than the type of pathogen, dictates the urgency with which treatment is initiated. An example of this type of respiratory tract infection is acute epiglottitis caused by infection with *H. influenzae.* This inflammatory response to bacterial infection can cause life-threatening upper airway obstruction if it is not recognized and treated early in the course of the disease. This is a medical emergency. In contrast, other infections caused by the same pathogen, such as sinusitis or cellulitis, can be treated more deliberately. In summary, these conditions warrant a search for factors that predispose the host to infection, such as anatomic obstruction or altered clearance of secretions in the respiratory tract.

Seasonal and Community Trends in Infections

Awareness of the patterns of respiratory tract infections at different times of the year and within the community where the patient resides is important for the efficient use of diagnostic microbiology resources. Certain types of respiratory tract infections have peak seasonal incidences and may occur in epidemics in the community. Other infections are observed throughout the year without major seasonal variations. For example, viral respiratory tract infections are more common in the fall and winter months than during other seasons, a fact that can be useful in diagnostic and therapeutic decisions. Therefore if influenza virus infection is epidemic in the community and a patient presents with symptoms and signs compatible with this viral illness, the likelihood is very high that influenza is the cause of the infection. In such cases, performing extensive bacterial cultures to define the cause of the respiratory tract infection is both wasteful of resources and unnecessarily expensive. In contrast, diseases associated with *Mycoplasma pneumoniae* typically occur throughout the year, without marked seasonal variability. The incidence of viral infections and secondary bacterial pneumonias is reduced during the summer months; therefore *M. pneumoniae* may cause up to 50% of all pneumonias in the summer months. Communication among clinical microbiologists, physicians interested in infectious diseases, and state health department personnel to share information on community trends in the pathogens causing respiratory tract infections helps focus diagnostic and therapeutic efforts. Periodic review of publications such as the *Morbidity and Mortality Weekly Report* from the Centers for Disease Control and Prevention is another means by which clinical microbiologists can review patterns of respiratory tract infections in the community and national setting.

Empiric Antimicrobial Therapy

To properly position the diagnostic microbiology laboratory in the scheme of the patient's care plan, it is important to understand the role of **empiric antimicrobial therapy** in the care of patients with respiratory tract infections. Although basing antimicrobial therapy on the results of diagnostic microbiologic studies is desirable, certain circumstances dictate that therapy be initiated before obtaining these results or without submitting specimens for culture even though an infectious cause is suspected. For example, antimicrobial therapy should be initiated before obtaining microbial identification and susceptibility testing results in patients who are seriously ill with pneumonia. In other cases, cultures should be obtained from the primary site of involvement, if possible (as well as from the blood if bacteremia is suspected), before initiating empiric antimicrobial therapy. In some types of respiratory tract infections, however, it is standard to initiate antimicrobial therapy without obtaining any specimens for culture. This is the procedure in the case of a child who has signs of a middle ear infection (otitis media). It can be predicted that the pathogen will usually be *S. pneumoniae, H. influenzae,* or *M. catarrhalis.* Considering the difficulty in obtaining cultures directly from the middle ear and the knowledge of the likely pathogens, treatment without obtaining cultures is reasonable. If treatment fails, it may be necessary to do an invasive procedure to obtain specimens to test for resistant or unexpected pathogens. This same rationale applies to other respiratory tract sites that are difficult to culture directly, such as the sinuses.

When empiric antimicrobial therapy is necessary, it is important to have a working knowledge of the organisms most likely to cause the type of infection observed and of the antibiotics that are most likely to be effective. If the infection is hospital-acquired (so-called **nosocomial infection**), it is important to know whether the antimicrobial susceptibility patterns of the infectious agent in question as determined in that institution's microbiology laboratory differ from those reported in general. Annual reviews of bacterial antibiotic susceptibility patterns are published by clinical microbiology services to facilitate this type of decision-making process. The empiric use of antibiotics and the adjustment of therapy based on the results of subsequent microbiologic data rep-resent another important interaction between the clinician and the clinical microbiologist.

ANATOMIC CHARACTERIZATION OF THE RESPIRATORY TRACT

Anatomy of the Respiratory Tract

The function of the respiratory tract is not only to perform respiration (i.e., the exchange of oxygen and carbon dioxide) but also to deliver air from the outside of the body to the alveoli where the gas exchange occurs. Consideration of the anatomy of the respiratory tract (Figure 26-1) must include the entire course that the air must travel: from the mouth and nose past the sinuses, into the pharynx, past the epiglottis, through the larynx, into the trachea and bronchi, and eventually into the alveoli. In addition to a role in air transport, each of these areas also plays an important role in defending the respiratory tract from infection.

Barriers to Infection

The respiratory tract has many natural barriers to infection that inhaled particles must penetrate

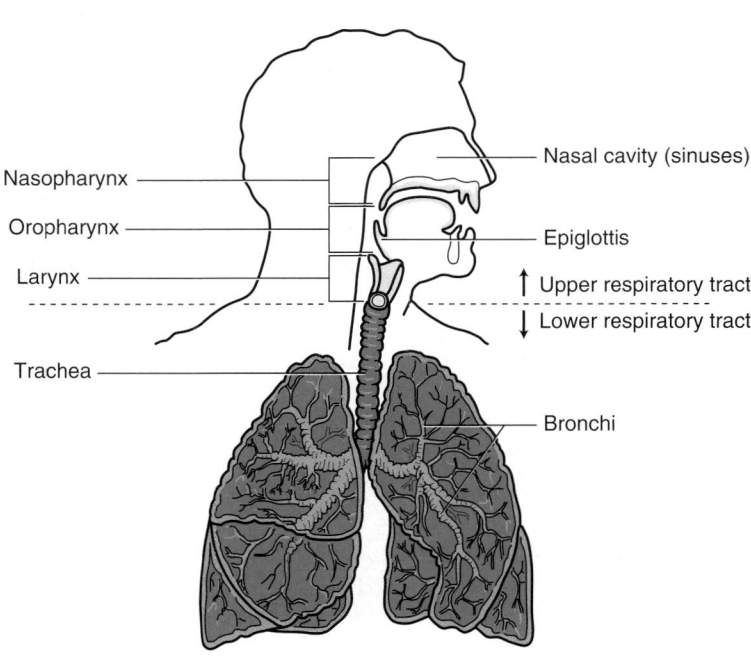

Figure 26-1

Anatomy of the respiratory tract.

to cause disease. These mechanisms that normally maintain a sterile environment below the larynx include nasal hair; mucociliary cells that line mucosal surfaces; coughing; normal flora; and phagocytic inflammatory cells.

In the nasopharynx and oropharynx, turbulent air flow causes large particles to impact on mucosal surfaces. Nasal hairs filter air as it passes through the nasal passages. Humidification of the air causes hygroscopic organisms to increase in size, making it more difficult for them to pass to the lower respiratory tract and easier for them to be phagocytosed. The normal flora of the nasopharynx and oropharynx helps protect the host by preventing colonization by pathogenic organisms, and the mucociliary blanket of the sinuses, middle ear, and tracheobronchial tree clears particulate matter and secretes immunoglobulin and other antimicrobial substances.

In addition, coughing can aid in the expulsion of particulate matter. If the particles reach the alveoli, macrophages ingest organisms; polymorphonuclear leukocytes and monocytes are called in once the lung becomes inflamed.

Alterations in these barriers may lead to infection. For example, cigarette smoking impairs the ability of the mucociliary blanket to clear particulate matter and interferes with macrophage activity. Structural abnormalities of the bronchial tree such as bronchiectasis or extrinsic compression of the bronchus by a malignancy can alter clearance of mucus that may contain infectious agents.

VIRULENCE FACTORS OF PATHOGENIC ORGANISMS

The disease-producing capability of an organism is the clinical manifestation of its virulence. Microorganisms infect the host by entering the host, interacting with specific target tissues, evading the host's defenses, proliferating, damaging the host, and disseminating or elaborating products that cause systemic disease. Virulence factors involved in disease-producing mechanisms, such as adherence, toxin elaboration, and host evasion, enable the microorganism to complete this process.

Adherence

Attachment of the microorganism to the host tissue is a primary step in the pathogenic process of infection. This is accomplished by adhesions, microbial surface molecules or organelles that bind the organism to a host surface. Specific bacterial adhesions interact with specific cellular receptors. The following are some examples. Streptococci possess fimbriae, which are fine, irregular structures that are composed of M protein and lipoteichoic acid and bind to epithelial cells. Group A streptococci release their surface lipoteichoic acid in the presence of sublethal doses of penicillin and lose their ability to bind to epithelial cells. Enterobacteriaceae such as *Escherichia coli* use fimbriae, nonflagellar filamentous structures, to adhere to host cells.

Toxin Elaboration

Microorganisms may elaborate toxins that produce different pathogenic effects, depending on the activity of the toxin and the target cell it interacts with in the host. For example, *Corynebacterium diphtheriae* produces an ADP-ribosylating toxin that interferes with protein synthesis. Locally, the toxin induces necrosis, resulting in a "pseudomembrane" composed of necrotic respiratory epithelial cells, leukocytes, and organisms. Systemically, the toxin preferentially adheres to myocardial, nerve, and kidney tissue, causing myocarditis, neuritis, and renal tubular necrosis. *Pseudomonas* exotoxin A's mechanism of action is similar to that of diphtheria toxin, but it has a different pathogenic effect because of the different target tissue and the involvement of other virulence factors. Another example of the role of toxins is provided by those produced by *Bordetella pertussis.* One is an adenylate cyclase toxin that enters target cells and increases intracellular cAMP levels, causing cell damage or cell death. Another is the pertussis toxin, which interrupts the transduction of signals from cell surface receptors to intracellular systems. During the paroxysmal phase of the illness when patients develop the characteristic whooping cough, the clinical signs and symptoms are attributed to toxin elaborated by the organism.

Evasion of Host Defenses

Evasion of host defenses enables microorganisms to proliferate and cause damage to the host. Certain respiratory pathogens, such as *S. pneumoniae, H. influenzae,* and mucoid *Pseudomonas aeruginosa,* evade host defenses by expressing polysaccharide capsules that prevent phagocytosis by host leukocytes. *Chlamydia* are obligate intracellular parasites that are taken up by host cells, where they are protected from the host immune system. *Mycobacterium tuberculosis,* another intracellular pathogen, survives by inhibiting phagosome-lysosome fusion. Other respiratory pathogens are able to cleave host secretory antibody by producing IgA-specific proteases.

UPPER RESPIRATORY TRACT INFECTIONS

Pharyngitis

CASE STUDY

An 8-year-old girl was brought to an emergency room by her mother because the child was complaining of a sore throat and a low-grade fever. The mother stated that the girl had had a runny nose and cough for the last few days. On examination, the patient had a temperature of 99° F. Her pharynx was red and her tonsils were slightly swollen, but no exudates were present. A neck examination revealed no tender lymph nodes.

Etiology

Table 26-2 summarizes the clinical syndromes encountered in the upper respiratory tract and the associated etiologic agents. The most commonly encountered etiologic agent of **bacterial pharyngitis** is group A streptococci. Identified in 30% to 40% of microbial isolates in school-age children who present with pharyngitis, the isolation of group A streptococci is much lower (less than 10% of microbial isolates) in adults with a similar presentation. Most cases of pharyngitis as described in the above case, are viral in origin and occur as part of the symptom complex of a common cold or an early case of influenza. The presence of exudates in the pharynx, fever, and painful adenopathy, or the lack of a cough, would be suggestive of pharyngitis caused by *Streptococcus pyogenes.* This can be diagnosed by throat culture or rapid antigen tests. In certain cases of presumed viral pharyngitis, a specific pathogen can be isolated. However, many cases of pharyngitis do not have an identifiable pathogen.

Cases of pharyngitis caused by unusual pathogens such as *Neisseria gonorrhoeae, Corynebac-terium diphtheriae,* or other bacterial pathogens are suspected in patients with suggestive histories or in cases of pharyngitis refractory to conventional therapy.

Epidemiology

Most pharyngeal infections associated with viral and streptococcal infections occur during the winter and early spring. The increase in person-to-person contact during these seasons favors transmission of the causative pathogens. The pathogens are usually inoculated by contamination of the hands and then gain entrance into the upper respiratory tract.

Clinical manifestations

Clinically, differentiation between viral and streptococcal pharyngitis is difficult. With most cases of viral pharyngitis, symptoms of a common cold, including rhinorrhea, are present, which is uncommon with streptococcal pharyngitis. Pharyngitis associated with influenza virus infection is accompanied by more numerous and more severe systemic symptoms, including fever, myalgias, and more profound fatigue. In contrast, other forms of viral pharyngitis that are associated with infectious mononucleosis are more commonly accompanied by cervical and generalized lymphadenopathy and enlargement of the spleen.

Streptococcal pharyngitis is associated with marked pharyngeal pain and difficulty in swallowing. Fever is more commonly a major component of the illness with streptococcal than with viral infection. In typical cases, a thick exudate covers the tonsils and posterior pharynx, which is uncommon in viral pharyngitis. It is important to realize, however, that documented streptococcal pharyngitis may also present in a manner that is indistinguishable from that of viral pharyngitis.

Another form of pharyngitis that is uncommon in most clinical practices today is that caused by *C. diphtheriae,* the primary clinical presentation of diphtheria. This bacterial pharyngitis is classically associated with the presence of a tightly adherent pharyngeal membrane. Diphtheria is now uncommon in the United States, and it should be suspected only in patient populations in which children have not received DPT (diphtheria/pertussis/tetanus) vaccination. The importance of a good vaccination history in children with pharyngitis is obvious.

TABLE 26-2
Upper Respiratory Tract Infections

Clinical Syndrome	Causative Agents	Specimen Collection	Other
Pharyngitis	Group A *Streptococcus* (children), viral (adults)	Swab tonsils and posterior pharynx, and place in transport media; do not allow to dry; viral cultures not necessary	Culture for *N. gonorrhoeae* or *C. diphtheria* if clinically indicated

Sinusitis	Most common:
	  S. pneumoniae
	  H. influenzae
	Less common:
	  S. pyogenes
	  M. catarrhalis
	  S. aureus
		Direct sinus sampling or nasal culture of sinus ostium	Direct sampling more reliable, indicated for patients who fail empiric therapy or who are severely ill or immunocompromised, or if unusual pathogen is suspected

Otitis media	Most common:
	  S. pneumoniae
	  H. influenzae
	Less common:
	  S. pyogenes
	  M. catarrhalis
	  S. aureus
		Direct culture by tympanocentesis	Direct culture indicated for patients who are severely ill or immunocompromised, or if unusual pathogen is suspected

Epiglottitis	*H. influenzae* type B	Direct swab of epiglottis, blood cultures	Direct swab should be performed only if airway is secure

Pertussis	Most common:
	  B. pertussis
	  B. parapertussis
	Less common:
	  B. bronchiseptica
	  Adenovirus
		Nasopharyngeal swab:
		  a. plate directly onto Bordet-Gengou medium
		  b. direct fluorescent antibody stain
		  c. adenovirus shell vial culture for antigen detection
			—

Pathogenesis

The reasons for the symptom complex in patients with viral or streptococcal pharyngitis are incompletely understood. Some viruses (e.g., adenoviruses) that infect the pharyngeal mucosa cause cellular destruction (cytopathology) and all such agents elicit inflammatory cell responses. The combination of these events is responsible for the pharyngeal pain and swelling experienced by patients with pharyngitis. However, in other cases, the viral pathogens (e.g., rhinoviruses) cause symptoms of pharyngitis with little mucosal cell destruction. In some cases, these noncytophatic viruses have been shown to elicit production of inflammatory mediators that can reproduce the symptoms of pharyngitis.

The pathogenesis of streptococcal pharyngitis may be due predominantly to the inflammatory effects of a variety of extracellular products elaborated by the streptococci. These products exhibit a variety of activities, including toxicity to a variety of cells, pyrogenicity, and enhancement of the spread of streptococci through infected tissues.

Complications

Other than the infrequent problem of upper airway obstruction associated with severe soft-tissue swelling, few complications can be attributed directly to either bacterial or viral pharyngitis. The occasional complications of viral infections associated with pharyngitis usually are due to systemic manifestations of the infections or to secondary bacterial infections such as sinusitis, otitis media, or pneumonia. Displacement of either or both of the tonsils or asymmetric swelling of the soft tissues of the pharynx following pharyngitis should raise suspicion of peritonsillar or pharyngeal abscess. Although group A streptococci have often been associated with these soft-tissue infections, oral anaerobic bacteria should also be considered in the differential diagnosis.

The goals of antibiotic treatment of streptococcal pharyngitis include amelioration of the symptoms, limitation of transmission of the infection to contacts (especially in school-age children), and prevention of the serious complications of acute rheumatic fever and acute glomerulonephritis.

Laboratory diagnosis

SPECIMEN COLLECTION

The primary goal of obtaining cultures in most cases of acute pharyngitis is to differentiate streptococcal pharyngitis from more common cases of viral pharyngitis. A secondary goal is to be able to detect the uncommon causes of bacterial pharyngitis (e.g., diphtheria, gonorrhea) in cases in which the clinical history is suggestive or symptoms are persistent.

In collecting pharyngeal specimens for streptococcal cultures (Figure 26-2), it is important, using adequate lighting, to vigorously swab the tonsillar areas and the posterior pharynx. It is not uncommon for negative streptococcal cultures to be obtained from specimens collected by personnel who did not swab these areas well because of the discomfort of patients with severe pharyngitis; second cultures by more experienced personnel have been positive. The tongue and other oral structures should be avoided with the swab to minimize contamination with oral flora and dilution of the specimen. If any tonsillar exudate is seen, specific efforts should be made to directly swab the areas where it is present. After collecting the specimen, swabs may be placed in transport medium.

DIRECT MICROSCOPIC EXAMINATION

Direct microscopic examination of pharyngeal secretions is not useful for clinical or laboratory diagnosis. Because respiratory exudates contain a wide variety of organisms, a direct Gram stain will not differentiate suspected pathogens from normal microbial flora.

CULTURE

Culture of the pharyngeal area will isolate bacterial pathogens such as β-hemolytic group A streptococci. A nonselective medium such as sheep's blood agar (SBA) is commonly used. The addition of a selective medium with an antimicrobial, such as sulfamethoxazole trimethoprim, may enhance the isolation of β-hemolytic streptococci.

OTHER METHODS

Latex agglutination, coagglutination tests, and enzyme immunoassays have been introduced into the clinical practice to detect group A streptococci directly from throat swabs. Although these tests are highly specific, problems with the sensitivities of these assays have required follow-up culture on blood agar plates. The increased sensitivity of recent optical immunoassays may have reduced this need for routine, confirmatory cultures. Therefore negative results should be followed with a conventional culture.

Sinusitis

CASE STUDY

A 40-year-old woman went to the doctor's office complaining of fever and nasal drainage. She stated that she had developed cold symptoms approximately 1 week earlier and had been treating herself with over-the-counter medicines with little improvement. In fact, she had gotten worse over the last 48 hours, with increasing headache.

The physical examination was notable for low-grade fever and tenderness over the left maxillary sinus as well as purulent drainage in the left side of the nose. Sinus radiographs showed an air-fluid level in the left maxillary sinus.

Etiology

S. pneumoniae and *H. influenzae* are the pathogens identified in approximately half the cases of sinusitis in which a culture is performed. In community-acquired infections, *S. pyogenes, M. catarrhalis,* and *S. aureus* account for most of the other pathogens commonly associated with sinusitis. In hospital-acquired infections, *S. aureus* and gram-negative bacilli are recovered more frequently. The incidence of *M. catarrhalis* as a pathogen in **acute sinusitis** is much higher in children than in adults, approaching the incidence of *H. influenzae.*

The role of viruses in the direct cause of sinusitis is not as clear as with the major bacterial pathogens. Pathogenic viruses that are isolated alone in the setting of acute sinusitis are the most compelling evidence for their role in the disease. Although common respiratory viruses can be recovered from infected sinuses, they are often isolated along with potential bacterial pathogens. This observation raises the possibility that the viral infection preceded a secondary bacterial infection. With the increasing availability of more sensitive and rapid means of viral diagnosis, further evaluation of the association between viruses and acute sinusitis may be possible.

Acute fungal sinusitis is uncommon in normal

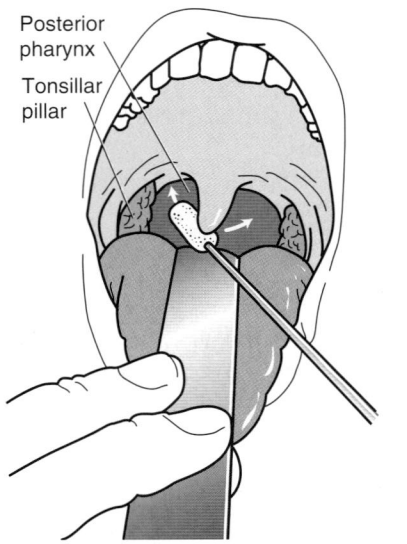

Posterior pharynx

Tonsillar pillar

Figure 26-2

Specimen collection from the throat.

patients; it occurs predominantly in immunosuppressed hosts treated with cytotoxic or immunosuppressive drugs or in patients with severe underlying illnesses such as uncontrolled diabetes mellitus. In contrast, chronic fungal colonization or sinusitis usually occurs in immunocompetent hosts in the clinical setting of other forms of chronic sinusitis (e.g., allergic sinusitis).

Epidemiology

The incidence of acute sinusitis follows that of other upper respiratory tract infections occurring predominantly in the winter and spring months. The clinical diagnosis of acute sinusitis is less common in children than in adults, in part because of the incomplete development of most of the paranasal sinuses until adolescence.

Clinical manifestations

The presentation of acute sinusitis in older children and adults is often that of a prolonged respiratory tract infection that involves a set of symptoms that are subtly different from those present early in the course of the illness. The most constant features include purulent nasal discharge and pain in the face. When the maxillary sinus is involved, facial pain is worse when leaning forward or when a jarring force is experienced, such as walking down stairs. Patients with maxillary si-

nusitis may also experience headache and pain that is perceived to come from the upper teeth. Fever is present in only about half the patients with acute sinusitis. In hospitalized patients, sinusitis can result from obstruction of the sinus openings (ostia) by indwelling nasal tubes.

In young children, the only symptoms observed may be persistent rhinorrhea and cough either directly after a viral upper respiratory tract infection or following a brief period of clinical improvement after such an infection. Ear examination is frequently abnormal in these children, with either middle ear infection or sterile fluid behind the tympanic membrane (serous otitis media). This involvement of the middle ear in young patients with sinusitis probably reflects the common problem of drainage obstruction in these two anatomic areas. In young children with signs and symptoms of persistent sinusitis, foreign bodies in the nose must always be considered.

The most sensitive test for the routine diagnosis of acute and chronic sinusitis in adult (adolescent or older) patients is the sinus radiograph; air-fluid level seen in a sinus is the most specific indicator of acute sinusitis. Complete sinus opacification is also seen frequently. A debate is evolving over the role of computed tomography in the initial diagnosis of sinusitis. Computed tomography (Figure 26-3) and magnetic resonance imaging are clearly superior to plain radiographs for detailed analysis of the anatomy of the paranasal sinuses and are especially useful for studies of the ethmoid and sphenoid sinuses, which are difficult to image using plain films.

Pathogenesis

Acute sinusitis is usually a complication of common colds or other viral infections of the upper respiratory tract. Respiratory allergies also predispose individuals to acute sinusitis. When recurrent infectious sinusitis occurs, associated with recurrent pulmonary infection over prolonged periods, it should suggest the possibility of cystic fibrosis, hypogammaglobulinemia, or ciliary dysfunction.

Obstruction is another predisposing factor in sinusitis. The sinuses normally undergo a continuous cleansing process through the action of ciliated epithelial cells. These ciliated epithelial cells move the mucous layer lining these areas toward the sinus ostia. This process normally clears the sinuses of bacteria from the adjacent nasopharynx. During acute rhinosinusitis, whether of viral or allergic origin, mucosal swelling may cause partial or complete obstruction of these sinus ostia, interrupting the flow of secretions and predisposing to bacterial overgrowth behind the obstruction. The function of the normal ciliated epithelial cells (altered by viral infection and bacterial toxins) and the viscosity of the mucous layer (which may be increased by the exudation and inflammation associated with infection or allergic reactions) may also be altered so that the clearance of sinus secretions is less efficient.

Other processes that may limit normal drainage from the sinuses include foreign bodies, tumors, and congenital structural abnormalities of the nasopharynx. Nasotracheal tubes in hospitalized patients in respiratory failure and packing materials used during surgical procedures provide other forms of obstruction to normal sinus drainage that predispose to infection.

Falling oxygen concentration has also been implicated in the pathogenesis of infectious sinusitis. With obstruction of the sinus ostium, the partial pressure of oxygen in the sinus cavity falls, impairing the function of inflammatory cells and facilitating the growth of facultative and true anaerobic bacteria.

After repeated bouts of acute sinusitis, the ciliated epithelium may be replaced by squamous epithelium, compromising the normal movement of the sinus mucous layer. This usually results in colonization of the chronically inflamed sinus with aerobic and anaerobic bacteria that are not present in the healthy sinus. The importance of this colonization in chronic sinusitis remains uncertain. It is generally believed that the presence of this colonization does not warrant treatment and that acute flare-ups of chronic sinusitis should be managed essentially the same as acute sinusitis in patients without chronic disease.

Complications

Complications of acute sinusitis result from extension of the infection to adjacent areas or structures. These complications include orbital cellulitis, osteomyelitis, meningitis, brain abscess, and cavernous sinus thrombosis.

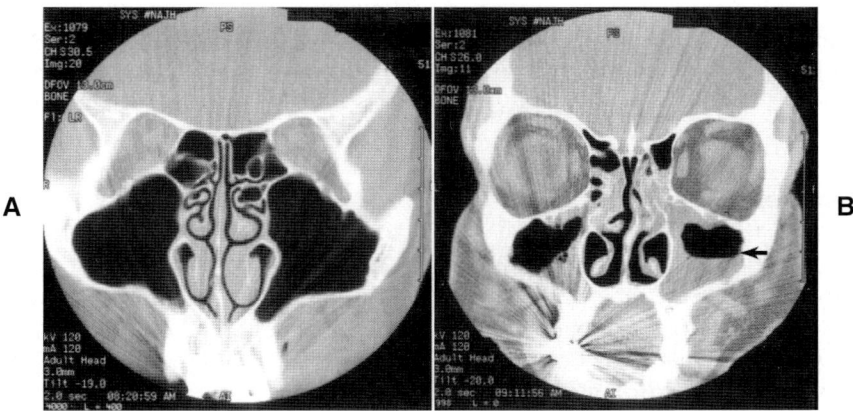

Figure 26-3

Computed tomography of the paranasal sinuses in a patient with normal maxillary sinuses **(A)** and in a patient with bilateral maxillary sinusitis **(B)**. In **A,** the large *(black)* cavities on either side of the lobulated midline structures of the nasopharynx are the normal maxillary sinuses in this patient who does not have sinusitis. Of note is the absence of thickening of the mucosal lining of the maxillary sinuses and the absence of opacity within the sinus. In **B,** a tomogram from another patient was taken at a slightly different orientation through the skull. This difference in orientation results in sampling of a smaller cross-section of the maxillary sinuses. The significant difference in the maxillary sinuses between the study in **B** and that in **A** is the presence of a large amount of opacity in both maxillary sinuses. This bilateral partial opacification represents both mucosal thickening and pus within the maxillary sinuses. The maxillary sinus on the right side of the figure also demonstrates an air-fluid level (the relatively straight, horizontal line between the air-filled black space above and the gray, fluid-filled space below; *arrow*) that is characteristic of acute, purulent sinusitis.

Orbital cellulitis or retroorbital abscess can result from direct extension of infection from adjacent sinuses to the area around and behind the eye. Protrusion of the eye (proptosis) or limitation of ocular movements should suggest the possibility of extension of the infection to the retroorbital space. This is a serious complication that requires aggressive diagnosis and emergency management.

Extension of frontal sinusitis can cause cellulitis in the area of the forehead overlying these sinuses. Osteomyelitis of the frontal bone, referred to as *Pott's puffy tumor,* may also develop. Further extension of frontal sinusitis may cause an abscess of the frontal lobes of the brain, a serious complication that is difficult to diagnose. Extension of infection from other sinuses (e.g., ethmoid, sphenoid) to the central nervous system in the form of meningitis, brain abscess, or cavernous sinus thrombosis is difficult to diagnose because of the deep location of these sinuses. Suspicion of such severe complications must remain high in patients who appear to have refractory sinusitis in the setting of altered mental status.

In cases in which the adjacent bone is involved (osteomyelitis), active sinusitis can complicate the interpretation of diagnostic radiologic studies. These complications can make the diagnosis difficult. It is usually necessary to follow serial studies of bone inflammation and integrity during therapy of sinusitis to establish the diagnosis of this complication.

Laboratory diagnosis

SPECIMEN COLLECTION

Cultures of nasal secretions or of nasal swabs are unreliable indicators of the pathogen causing acute infection within the sinus. Most clinicians caring for adult patients with acute sinusitis believe that the only cultures useful in the etiologic diagnosis of acute sinusitis are those cultures that are obtained through direct sinus puncture and aspiration. This is another example in diagnostic microbiology of normal flora interfering with etiologic diagnosis.

The pediatric infectious diseases literature demonstrates a subtle difference of opinion, however, about the value of doing nasal cultures instead of direct sinus punctures for diagnosis of acute sinusitis in children. Because studies have shown that *S. pneumoniae, H. influenzae,* and *S. pyogenes* (three of the most common etiologic agents in acute sinusitis in children) are only rarely isolated from nasal cultures from normal children, identification of these agents in cultures of the nose should suggest the etiology of paranasal sinusitis in pediatric patients. It has therefore been suggested that properly collected nasal cultures taken from the area of the sinus ostium are useful in establishing the cause of acute sinusitis. However, professionals generally agree that randomly collected cultures from the nasopharynx of either adult or pediatric patients are of no value in defining the bacterial cause of this disease.

In most cases of acute sinusitis in a normal host, studies have shown that the infection is caused by only a few well-known pathogens; therefore sinus puncture is not indicated before initiation of treatment. Because most cases of acute sinusitis are caused by *Streptococcus pneumoniae* or *Haemophilus influenzae,* empiric antibiotic therapy can be used to treat these patients.

However, in patients who fail empiric antimicrobial therapy, direct sinus cultures are indicated to investigate the possibility of antibiotic-resistant strains of bacteria or unusual pathogens. Direct culture by sinus puncture is also indicated early in the diagnostic evaluation of severely ill or immunocompromised patients or in cases in which an unusual pathogen is suspected, such as a hospital-acquired infection.

DIRECT MICROSCOPIC EXAMINATION

Gram stain preparations are useful only for sinus specimens obtained by direct aspiration from the sinus ostia or from sinus puncture. In these cases, finding a predominant bacterial type can be of diagnostic and therapeutic value.

CULTURE

As mentioned previously, culture of sinus aspirations is useful only when performed on specimens obtained by sinus puncture or by direct aspiration of purulent secretions from sinus ostia. In these cases, samples are inoculated on culture media such as sheep's blood agar, chocolate agar, and MacConkey agar, which are routinely used to isolate respiratory tract pathogens.

Otitis Media

Etiology

As in the case of acute sinusitis, the microbial etiology of the average case of acute **otitis media** has been clearly defined by cultures of infected middle ear specimens obtained by direct aspiration from the area. Considering the similarities in their pathogenesis, it is not surprising that the same group of pathogens is involved in both acute otitis media and acute sinusitis. *S. pneumoniae* and *H. influenzae* account for more than 50% of the isolates from cases of acute otitis media. *S. pyogenes, M. catarrhalis,* and *S. aureus* have also been implicated in this disease. In patients who have received multiple courses of broad-spectrum antibiotics for acute otitis media, those who have tympanic membrane perforations, or those with severe underlying disease associated with pharyngeal colonization with gram-negative bacilli, acute otitis media is more likely to be caused by gram-negative pathogens.

The analogy with the etiology of acute sinusitis also extends to the role of viruses in acute otitis media. Because most cases of acute otitis media occur on the heels of a viral infection of the upper respiratory tract, it is not surprising that viruses can be isolated from cultures taken from the middle ears of these patients. The exact role of these viruses in the pathogenesis of acute otitis media, other than inducing inflammation and thereby reducing eustachian tube drainage of the middle ear, remains to be determined. The availability of more sensitive and rapid viral diagnostic studies may allow a clearer definition of the frequency with which viruses can be identified as primary pathogens in cases of acute otitis media. Such data will be necessary before predominant or cofactor involvement of concomitantly isolated bacteria can be clearly dissected.

Other possible causes of acute otitis media should be considered in unusual cases or circumstances. Theoretically, other pathogens that infect the upper and lower respiratory tract, such as *Mycoplasma pneumoniae* and *Chlamydia trachomatis,* can cause acute otitis media. However, the association between these potential pathogens and the average case of middle ear infection is not clear. In newborns, group B streptococci and gram-negative bacilli can be added to *S. pneumoniae* and *H. influenzae* as causes of occasional cases of acute otitis media. Acute otitis media occurs less often than acute sinusitis in the presence of nasal tubes in hospitalized patients with eustachian tube obstruction. Gram-negative bacillary pathogens are isolated more often in this setting than in community-acquired acute otitis media.

Epidemiology

Otitis media is the most common localized infection of the upper respiratory tract in preschool-age patients. One study showed that almost a third of all visits by preschool children to pediatricians involved diseases of the middle ear. The increased incidence of these infections in preschoolers has been attributed to the crowding of susceptible hosts in day-care centers. In older children and adults, the syndrome of middle ear infection, although less common, is still a major precipitant of outpatient office visits during the winter and spring seasons, when viral respiratory infections are common.

Clinical manifestations

Early signs and symptoms of acute otitis media may be nonlocalized, especially in young children. In these cases, fever and irritability may be the only signs of illness. In older children, tugging at the involved ear may be noticed during or at the end of the course of an upper respiratory tract infection. Other symptoms include ear pain, changes in hearing, and, late in the course of the infection, drainage of purulent secretions from the ear canal, associated with perforation of the tympanic membrane. On direct examination of the tympanic membrane, the presence of acute otitis media may be indicated by a red, bulging membrane. However, the changes in the membrane are often more subtle. In these cases, it is important to perform pneumatic otoscopy to identify any evidence of fluid or pus behind the tympanic membrane, as evidenced by its reduced or absent movement in response to changes in air pressure in the canal.

Pathogenesis

The eustachian tube, which is the canal that links the middle ear to the nasopharynx, is shorter and travels a more direct course from the nasopharynx to the middle ear in young children than in older children and adults. This anatomic immaturity appears to predispose young patients to easier contamination of the middle ear with nasopharyngeal bacteria. This factor, coupled with the greater incidence of viral respiratory tract infections in preschool-age children, may explain the greater incidence of acute otitis media in this population.

Both the eustachian tube and the middle ear are lined with ciliated epithelium and mucus-secreting cells. This creates a situation similar to that seen in the paranasal sinuses, where a mucous layer clearance mechanism can defend against invasion and overgrowth of nasopharyngeal organisms. When this function is altered or impaired, infection may develop. Suppurative otitis media may result from relative or absolute obstruction of this drainage mechanism as a consequence of obstruction of the eustachian tube. Edema of the eustachian tube mucosa resulting from viral infections is much like the swelling that is induced around the ostia of the sinuses. Similarly, viral infections can cause impairment of the cleansing function of the ciliated epithelium of the eustachian tube–middle ear complex. In a manner similar to that associated with viral infection, the eustachian tube edema associated with allergic nasopharyngitis can cause obstruction and predispose to postobstructive infection of the middle ear. Infection behind the obstruction, irrespective of the nature of the precipitating cause, can cause tissue damage that may affect hearing and can, if therapy is inadequate, lead to progressive infection of adjacent structures.

Complications

Progression of acute otitis media may lead to damage of the tympanic membrane and other associated problems that follow this destructive process. Tympanic membrane damage with subsequent hearing loss can have devastating effects on the speech development and education of young children, but it may be of less consequence in adults. A membrane perforation may heal without long-term effects on hearing or may become chronic, depending on the size of the perforation and the frequency of reinfection. If the perforation destroys crucial areas in the membrane, surgical correction may be necessary to close the perforation and restore membrane function. The necessity of such a procedure depends on multiple factors, the most

important of which is the age of the patient. Unfortunately, most such complications occur in children who do not obtain adequate early medical care. Similar considerations apply when considering the approach to chronic adhesive changes in the repeatedly infected, but intact, tympanic membrane and chronic middle ear effusions (serous otitis media).

Acute mastoiditis is an uncommon complication of acute otitis media in the antibiotic era. As a result, surgical treatment (mastoidectomy) to prevent progressive disease and extension to the central nervous system is a rare procedure in modern practice.

All the considerations discussed under acute sinusitis concerning the spread of infection to adjacent areas also apply to acute otitis media that goes untreated. Local extension of infection and spread to the central nervous system are potential problems. These problems are encountered less commonly in the antibiotic era in most clinical settings. However, in situations in which access to health care is limited for any reason, such severe late complications of middle ear infection must be considered.

Laboratory diagnosis

Because the predominant pathogens for acute otitis media are known, obtaining specimens for culture before initiating therapy is unnecessary in the average case. If the patient is seriously ill or immunocompromised and likely to have rapidly progressive disease or if, for some reason, an unusual or drug-resistant organism is suspected, direct culture by tympanocentesis is indicated. As with acute sinusitis, probably no value exists in culturing the nasopharynx as an indicator of the type of pathogen that may be present in the middle ear.

Epiglottitis

CASE STUDY

A 4-year-old boy was brought to the pediatrician's office with a 6-hour history of fever and trouble swallowing. Inspiratory stridor was noted by the pediatrician. The patient was immediately taken to the emergency room, where the epiglottis was visualized and noted to be red and edematous.

Etiology

H. influenzae type b is uniquely associated with epiglottitis. This organism is isolated from pharyngeal cultures in most children with this syndrome and from one fourth of adult cases. Positive blood cultures for *H. influenzae* are common in both children and adults with **acute epiglottitis.** Association of this syndrome with other bacteria such as staphylococci, pneumococci, and other streptococci has been reported but is rare. Viral pathogens have not clearly been implicated in this problem.

Epidemiology

Most cases of epiglottitis occur in preschool-age children. Although an uncommon occurrence in the average clinical practice, the fact that it is a potentially life-threatening infection that is almost uniquely associated with a single pathogen, *H. influenzae* type b, warrants familiarity with the syndrome.

Clinical manifestations

The epiglottis is a structure positioned at the anterior aspect of the opening of the trachea. It normally protects the airway from aspiration of secretions and food during swallowing. Acute epiglottitis is a rapidly progressive infection of this structure and the adjacent soft tissues in the upper airway. The presence of severe symptoms of pharyngitis and pain on swallowing in the absence of signs of pharyngitis on physical examination should suggest the diagnosis of epiglottitis. In the case study presented, visualization of the epiglottis is the most important step in the diagnosis of acute epiglottitis. However, this must be done in a setting where intubation or tracheostomy can be performed immediately because of the risk of airway obstruction during manipulation of the pharynx and the associated edema of epiglottitis. Generally, an endotracheal tube is inserted at the time of diagnosis to secure the airway until the inflammation and infection subside with treatment. Blood cultures and cultures of the epiglottis should be obtained, and intravenous antimicrobial therapy should be initiated immediately. The associated edema of the epiglottis can also cause the sudden onset of upper airway obstruction and respiratory arrest.

Early manifestations of epiglottitis include fever associated with severe sore throat and difficulty swallowing. Patients often prefer to lean forward and drool rather than to swallow their secretions, because of the extreme pain experienced. The speed with which symptoms may proceed to involve respiratory difficulty and eventually complete airway obstruction is what makes this diagnosis one to remember. A rapid downhill course is more likely in children than in adults with epiglottitis. However, caution is warranted in the diagnostic approach to any patient suspected of having this disease. In small children, signs of upper airway obstruction should always prompt consideration of a foreign body lodged in the upper airway in the differential diagnosis of epiglottitis.

The syndrome of croup associated with viral respiratory tract infections is the main condition to differentiate from epiglottitis in children. The viral illness that precedes and accompanies croup syndrome is not observed in patients with epiglottitis, and the cough typical of croup syndrome is not common in epiglottitis. In contrast, patients with epiglottitis usually have a relatively short history of illness. Patients with croup typically have predominant inflammation and airway narrowing below the epiglottis.

As discussed in the section on the complications of pharyngitis, other soft-tissue infections of the upper respiratory tract are associated with narrowing of the upper airway, such as retropharyngeal abscess. However, these processes usually do not exhibit the same symptom complex and fulminant course seen with *H. influenzae*–induced epiglottitis. In distinction from bacterial pharyngitis (e.g., streptococcal or, rarely, diphtheria pharyngitis), patients with epiglottitis usually do not have tonsillar or pharyngeal exudates.

Pathogenesis

The soft tissues of the epiglottis and the surrounding structures appear to be susceptible to significant accumulation of edema fluid during the inflammatory process incited by *H. influenzae* infection. Combined with the critical location of the epiglottis at the opening of the trachea, this creates the danger of complete airway obstruction as the disease progresses. The reason that *H. influenzae* is so commonly associated with this syndrome, whereas other common respiratory pathogens are not, is unknown. Similarly, it is unclear why inflammation in the area above and including the epiglottis should be prevalent in this condition.

Complications

The main complication is respiratory compromise associated with the sudden onset of airway obstruction. Although bacteremia is common in these patients, development of infections at sites other than the epiglottis is uncommon. Some patients with epiglottitis have simultaneous pneumonia. However, the clinical significance of the lower respiratory tract involvement is relatively minor compared to the potential problems with upper airway obstruction early in the course of this infection.

Laboratory diagnosis

SPECIMEN COLLECTION

Direct swab cultures from the area of the epiglottis are useful in establishing the etiologic diagnosis, but they should be taken only when the airway is secure. Blood cultures should also be performed in all patients in whom epiglottitis is suspected. The incidence of positive blood cultures is high, and a positive culture confirms the diagnosis and justifies antibiotic therapy focused on *H. influenzae* type b infection.

DIRECT MICROSCOPIC EXAMINATION

A direct smear from exudates for microscopic examination is a rapid method for early diagnosis. Exudates taken from the epiglottal area may reveal numerous white blood cells and pleomorphic gram-negative bacilli characteristic of *H. influenzae* (Figure 26-4).

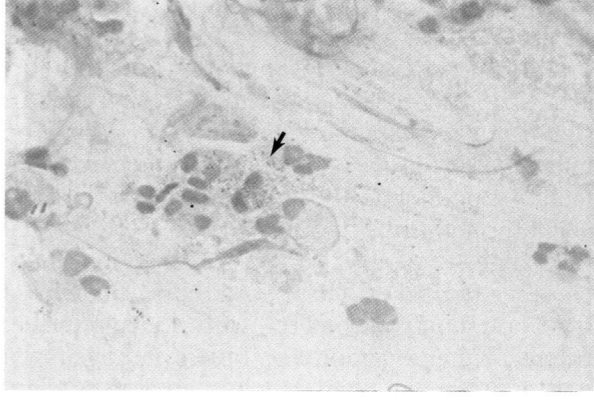

Figure 26-4 _____

Gram-stained smear of sputum/exudate with *Haemophilus* organisms *(arrow)*.

CULTURE

H. influenzae are isolated from blood cultures and from exudates. An enriched medium such as chocolate agar is required to recover this organism. An environment with an enhanced concentration of carbon dioxide (5% to 10%) is also required for recovery. The organism is identified by determining the X and V factor requirements, porphyrin test, and hemolysis on Casman blood agar.

Pertussis

Etiology

Bordetella pertussis and *Bordetella parapertussis* are most frequently associated with the pertussis syndrome. *Bordetella bronchiseptica* has also been associated with a similar clinical syndrome. Low-serotype adenoviruses (types 1, 2, 3, and 5) have been isolated from patients with an illness that can be indistinguishable from pertussis. The recent availability of rapid viral diagnostic tests makes it feasible to distinguish adenovirus infection based on culture data from *B. pertussis* during the acute illness. Formerly, this distinction between pertussis and viral illness required serologic studies that were useful only in retrospect.

Epidemiology

Pertussis is a highly transmissible respiratory illness in susceptible patient populations that occurs with little seasonal variation. The infection occurs more commonly in infants and young children, and serious complications are seen more often in this age group. In recent years, the incidence of this illness has increased in the teenage population. Adolescents and adults with unusual manifestations of the illness may serve as reservoirs for transmission of the infection to susceptible children.

Clinical manifestations

In the early phase of the illness, the symptom complex of pertussis is similar to that of a viral upper respiratory tract infection, and the differential diagnosis is difficult. Fever is uncommon throughout the course of the illness unless a secondary bacterial infection has occurred. Following the early phase of the illness, the patient experiences exhausting paroxysms of coughing, often with multiple coughs during one expiratory cycle, which are typically worse at night. The cycle classically ends with an episode of vomiting resulting from the extreme nature of the cough. The "whooping" sound associated with the forceful inspiration through a narrowed airway after a prolonged episode of coughing is the source of the term "whooping cough," which has been used in common reference to *B. pertussis* infection. The whooping characteristic of the inspiratory cycle is not uniformly present during pertussis infection, however. Therefore it should not be used as a diagnostic criterion.

A major public health problem associated with the diagnosis of this infection in a child is limiting its spread within susceptible close contacts. Careful vaccination histories from contacts will allow the formulation of a plan for their protection by active immunization and antibiotic prophylaxis.

Pathogenesis

Although the pathogenesis of pertussis is incompletely understood, numerous studies suggest a significant role for pertussis toxin in the clinical presentation of this infection. Factors produced by these organisms have been implicated in several stages in the disease process, including damage to tracheal epithelial cells, impairment of host immunity, and induction of systemic symptoms of pertussis. It is apparent that pertussis is not a disease that is caused by the effects of a single toxin, as is the case in some other bacterial infections. Rather, it appears that the clinical syndrome may be a manifestation of the sum of several toxins produced by the pathogen and the host response that is elicited.

Complications

The most common complication of pertussis is the pneumonia that occurs in young children. These lower respiratory tract infections are commonly caused by secondary infections with other bacteria, although *B. pertussis* itself may cause pneumonia. Other secondary bacterial infections such as otitis media also occur.

Many of the complications associated with pertussis are a consequence of the severe and forceful coughing episodes that occur during this illness. Alveolar rupture may induce interstitial and subcutaneous emphysema. Forceful coughing has also been associated with subconjunctival (and other superficial) hemorrhages, epistaxis, rupture of the diaphragm, umbilical and inguinal hernias, and rectal prolapse.

Among the most serious complications of pertussis are those that affect the central nervous system. These problems are most dangerous in infants with pertussis. Seizures during pertussis have been related to fever, cerebral hypoxia, and toxic encephalopathy.

This infection has been implicated as a cause of bronchiectasis later in life. However, the decreasing incidence of pertussis and the increased use of antibiotics for respiratory tract infections in general probably make this infection an uncommon cause of bronchiectasis in the modern era.

Laboratory diagnosis
SPECIMEN COLLECTION
Recovery of *B. pertussis* depends to a large extent on proper specimen collection and processing. Pernasal nasopharyngeal swabs using calcium alginate are preferred. Specimens should be plated directly onto selective media such as Bordet-Gengou or Regan-Lowe (RL). If delay is expected, a transport medium such as RL transport medium should be used.

DIRECT MICROSCOPIC EXAMINATION
Complementary data may be obtained by performing direct fluorescent antibody (DFA) staining of secretions from such swabs. Although DFA has limitations regarding false-negative and false-positive results, it can provide a rapid indicator that may be useful in initiating empiric therapy.

CULTURE
Immunofluorescence studies should not be used in place of culture data. At the same time that nasopharyngeal cultures are being collected for *B. pertussis* culture, specimens should be submitted for adenovirus culture using a rapid diagnostic assay such as the shell vial culture/antigen detection method. Specimens for viral culture are either inoculated directly or placed in a viral carrier medium containing antibiotics to suppress bacterial contamination.

LOWER RESPIRATORY TRACT INFECTIONS

Infections in the lower respiratory tract usually occur when infecting organisms reach the lower airways or pulmonary parenchyma by bypassing the mechanical and other nonspecific barriers of the upper respiratory tract. Infections may result from inhalation of infectious aerosols, aspiration of oral or gastric contents, or hematogenous spread.

A series of host defenses must be overcome before a potential pathogen can establish infection in the lower respiratory tract. The sequence of events is somewhat different for respiratory viruses than for bacterial pathogens. The progression of viral pathogens from the upper to the lower respiratory tract is a process that involves both spread among adjacent cells and distant inoculation of susceptible cells by aspiration of infectious secretions and, to a lesser extent, by bloodborne (hematogenous) transmission of the virus. Lung infections by bacterial pathogens usually occur via direct inoculation of organisms through aspiration from the upper respiratory tract. The ways in which mechanical host defenses are bypassed or suppressed, leading to lower respiratory tract infection, have been considered previously. Table 26-3 summarizes clinical syndromes encountered in the lower respiratory tract and the associated etiologic agents.

Bronchitis and Bronchiolitis
Etiology
Any of the respiratory viruses that cause upper respiratory tract infection can cause cough as a manifestation of acute **bronchitis.** The severity of the bronchial involvement varies with the different viral respiratory tract pathogens and, to some extent, with the patient population being studied. For example, during seasons when influenza is epidemic in the community, this viral respiratory pathogen is the most common cause of acute bronchitis and bronchiolitis in the general population. Respiratory syncytial virus (RSV) also causes community-wide seasonal outbreaks of bronchiolitis in infants. During nonepidemic periods, other respiratory viral pathogens such as rhinovirus, coronavirus, and parainfluenza virus are more likely to be isolated. In populations of young military recruits, adenovirus infections were the primary cause of acute bronchitis prior to the use of adenovirus vaccine. During the summer months, patients with enterovirus infection may exhibit acute bronchitis as part of the clinical syndrome, although this is not a major part of the illness in most cases.

Nonviral respiratory tract pathogens including *M. pneumoniae, Chlamydia pneumoniae,* and *B. pertussis* can also induce the syndrome of acute bronchitis. Therefore the clinical presentation of these infections may be indistinguishable from cases of acute bronchitis caused by viral pathogens.

Epidemiology
Acute bronchitis can be viewed as the lower respiratory tract extension of many of the same viral infections that cause seasonal upper respiratory tract infections. The peak season for acute bronchitis is the winter months, which matches the peak incidence of these viral respiratory tract infections. It is somewhat artificial to separate the clinical syndromes of viral upper respiratory tract infections and acute bronchitis, because in many instances these represent a continuum of the same infection. The difference in the clinical presentations of these two conditions is often simply one of degree.

Clinical manifestations
Patients with acute bronchitis often begin their illness with a syndrome typical of a nonbacterial upper respiratory tract infection. The course of the illness may exhibit a fairly rapid progression to lower respiratory tract involvement or, after several days of an upper respiratory tract syndrome, may evolve to symptoms of bronchitis. The typical patient with acute bronchitis has cough and fever as the primary manifestations of the illness. The amount of sputum produced with coughing varies with the individual, with the pathogen causing the illness, with the stage of the illness (the cough usually becomes more productive later in the course), and with the incidence of secondary bacterial infections that may follow nonbacterial acute bronchitis. Systemic symptoms such as diffuse myalgias and fatigue associated with viremic illnesses may also be seen early in the course of infection.

ACUTE VERSUS CHRONIC BRONCHITIS
The distinction between acute and chronic bronchitis is one of both definition and pathogenesis. For purposes of definition, chronic bronchitis is evidenced by the presence of a cough productive of sputum on most days for at least 3 months of the year for a minimum of 2 years in succession.

TABLE 26-3

Lower Respiratory Tract Infections

Clinical Syndrome	Causative Agents	Specimen Collection	Other

Bronchitis, bronchiolitis	Most common:
	  Respiratory viruses
	Less common:
	  M. pneumoniae
	  C. pneumoniae
	  B. pertussis
	  Simkania Z
		Nasopharyngeal or lower respiratory culture if influenza type A or respiratory syncytial virus infection of the lower respiratory tract is suspected	Diagnostic cultures not indicated in uncomplicated cases

Community-acquired pneumonia	Children:
	  Most common:
	    Respiratory syncytial virus
	    Parainfluenza
	    Adenovirus
	    M. pneumoniae
	  Less common:
	    S. pneumoniae
	    H. influenzae
	    Group B *Streptococcus*
	    (neonates)
	Adults:
	  Most common:
	    S. pneumoniae
	    M. pneumoniae
	  Less common:
	    H. influenzae
	    Gram-negative bacilli
	    S. aureus
	    Legionella spp.
		"Deep" expectorated sputum (see text)	Avoid contamination with oropharyngeal flora; specimen collection via fiber-optic bronchoscopy or open lung biopsy may be indicated in some circumstances

Nosocomial pneumonia	Gram-negative bacilli (60%) Gram-positive organisms (16%) Anaerobes *Legionella* spp.	"Deep" expectorated sputum	Avoid contamination with oropharyngeal flora; specimen collection via fiber-optic bronchoscopy or open lung biopsy may be indicated in some circumstances
Aspiration pneumonia	Mixed anaerobes and aerobes (50%), anaerobes alone (50%)	Expectorated sputum is of little value; bronchoscopic techniques required for specific diagnosis	Pleural fluid cultures may be useful with anaerobic empyema
Chronic pneumonia	Mycobacteria, fungi	Early morning "deep" expectorated sputum; bronchoscopy or open lung biopsy may be required to identify pathogen	—

Empyema	Community-acquired:
	  S. aureus
	  S. pneumoniae
	  S. pyogenes
	Nosocomial:
	  Gram-negative bacilli
		Pleural fluid should be aspirated directly into a sterile syringe, with excess air removed from syringe immediately	Aliquots of specimen should be distributed to hematology and chemistry labs for other studies

Whereas acute bronchitis is usually of infectious etiology, chronic bronchitis is usually caused by long-term cigarette smoking and occasionally other toxic exposures. From the perspective of infectious diseases of the respiratory tract, the main point to remember is that acute exacerbations of chronic bronchitis are usually initiated by the same pathogens that cause acute bronchitis in patients of the same age without underlying chronic respiratory tract disease. The difference is that patients with chronic bronchitis who experience an acute exacerbation of their illness resulting from intercurrent infection are more likely to have a severe primary illness or a prolonged illness associated with secondary bacterial infection than are otherwise healthy patients with acute bronchitis.

ACUTE BRONCHIOLITIS

Acute bronchiolitis is a term reserved for an infectious disease of infants that is associated with a typical clinical picture. This syndrome is usually caused by respiratory syncytial virus infection, although other respiratory viruses (e.g., parainfluenza virus) can cause the same clinical picture. In addition to signs of a febrile upper respiratory tract infection, these patients present with signs of lower respiratory tract airway obstruction such as wheezing, respiratory distress, and air trapping. Chest radiographs do not usually show typical signs of pneumonia. Increased lucency and areas of lung that are underaerated resulting from airway obstruction (atelectasis) are more common.

Pathogenesis

As mentioned, evidence almost always exists of antecedent or coexistent upper respiratory tract infection in patients with acute bronchitis. The spread of these upper respiratory tract infections to the lower airways, manifested as acute bronchitis, represents infection and damage of respiratory epithelial cells by the same (usually viral) pathogens. The extent of destruction of the respiratory epithelium varies with the pathogen causing the illness. Viruses such as influenza and adenovirus are highly cytopathic and cause significant epithelial cell destruction; other viral infections such as rhinovirus cause epithelial cell dysfunction without inducing much cytopathology.

The inflammatory response, necrotic debris from epithelial cell destruction, and edema of the lower respiratory tract also contribute to the airway abnormalities and symptoms in these infections. In probably no clinical syndrome is this potential for airway obstruction more important than in bronchiolitis in infants. The resulting obliteration of the lumen of small airways appears to be the primary pathogenetic mechanism in this infection. Indirect effects of viral infection on airway function are probably also important in the pathogenesis of some forms of acute bronchitis. The results of several studies suggest that alterations in airway β-adrenergic receptors and the production of inflammatory mediators during viral infections

of the respiratory tract may be involved in many of the signs and symptoms associated with these infections.

Complications

A complication that is apparent in some patients with acute viral bronchitis is the development of secondary bacterial infections. These secondary infections can present in several ways. Some patients experience persistent or increasing symptoms of bronchitis, with an increase in the volume and purulence of the sputum produced. This usually occurs at a time in the course of the illness when most cases of acute bronchitis would be resolving. A further extension of this scenario is secondary bacterial infection presenting as acute or evolving pneumonia after an episode of acute bronchitis. These secondary bacterial infections of the lower respiratory tract are usually associated with the common pathogens that are found in community-acquired pneumonia (e.g., *S. pneumoniae, H. influenzae*), although other bacterial pathogens (e.g., *M. catarrhalis,* gram-negative bacilli) may be secondary pathogens in selected patient populations (e.g., patients with underlying respiratory diseases or who are hospitalized).

The long-term consequences of acute bronchitis continue to be debated. Several epidemiologic studies suggest an association between acute viral infections of the lower respiratory tract and subsequent asthma. Whether the infectious agents that caused acute bronchitis in these patients actually induced a permanent change in their airways that resulted in future airway hyperreactivity, or whether these infections occurred in patients who would have eventually developed asthma irrespective of intercurrent episodes of acute bronchitis, remains an interesting puzzle. Speculation also exists that certain viruses that cause acute bronchitis can cause bronchiectasis. This is an abnormality in which inadequate drainage of respiratory secretions results from airway wall destruction, dilatation, and scarring that are associated with recurrent lower respiratory tract infections. Considering the cytopathic nature of some viral (e.g., adenovirus) infections that can cause acute bronchitis, the suggested association between these pathogens and long-term development of bronchiectasis seems reasonable.

Laboratory diagnosis

The collection of specimens for culture in cases of acute bronchitis largely follows the procedures outlined in the section on viral pharyngitis. Because acute bronchitis is an extension of a syndrome of nonbacterial upper respiratory tract infection, diagnostic cultures are not indicated in uncomplicated cases that follow the expected, self-limited course. If, however, patients develop signs of secondary bacterial bronchitis or pneumonia, culture data may be useful in designing therapy. When such cultures are used to guide the design of a treatment plan, it is important to attempt to obtain lower respiratory tract secretions that are minimally contaminated with oral flora.

In practice, collection of an adequate specimen is usually not difficult in patients with secondary bacterial bronchitis, because a marked increase exists in both the volume and the purulence of sputum. The issue of proper collection of lower respiratory tract secretions for the diagnosis of pneumonia is covered in the section on pneumonia.

Other situations in which cultures might be indicated in cases of acute bronchitis or acute bronchiolitis are those in which effective antiviral agents are available against the viral pathogens suspected. For example, in cases of suspected influenza type A or respiratory syncytial virus infection of the lower respiratory tract, the identification of these agents in respiratory tract secretions may be useful in guiding early antiviral therapy. As rapid viral diagnostic techniques become more widely available in diagnostic microbiology laboratories, and as more effective antiviral agents become available to treat these respiratory tract infections, such studies will become a more important part of the daily practice in diagnostic virology laboratories.

Acute Pneumonia

The distinction between acute bronchitis and acute pneumonia may be a subtle one. Both of these conditions are lower respiratory tract infections. The differentiation between acute bronchitis and **pneumonia** depends on the degree and extent of involvement of the lower respiratory tract with the infectious process. By definition, patients who have bronchitis do not present the physical and chest radiograph findings of pulmonary parenchyma involvement of the infectious and inflammatory process. Such detectable lung tissue involvement defines pneumonia.

Pneumonia can be subdivided into diagnostic categories based on the clinical setting, presentation of the illness, exposure to specific pathogens, and age and type of host infected. The importance of using such a strategy to make a presumptive determination of the infectious etiology of pneumonia is evident when one considers the long list of possible pathogens that can cause this type of infection. Table 26-4 lists the most common etiologic agents of lower respiratory tract infections and the usual affected patient populations. It is important to focus the clinical diagnosis on a subgroup of likely pathogens to allow the institution of reasonable empirical therapy while awaiting a specific etiologic diagnosis and to make optimal use of the diagnostic microbiology laboratory in planning the diagnostic approach.

To begin this process of presumptive etiologic diagnosis in pneumonia, one must consider those pneumonias that develop in patients in their normal setting in the community (community-acquired pneumonia) and those that develop in hospitalized patients (nosocomial pneumonia). The highest incidence of both community-acquired and nosocomial pneumonias occurs in very young and very old patients. However, the types of etio-

TABLE 26-4

Most Common Pathogens of Lower Respiratory Infections by Age

Age	Etiology
Neonates	C. trachomatis
Children	
Infants	Respiratory syncytial virus
	Influenza virus
5–18 months	S. pneumoniae
	H. influenzae
3 months–teens	Viruses
	S. aureus
	M. pneumoniae
Young adults (18–45 years)	M. pneumoniae
Older adults	S. pneumoniae
	Legionella spp.
Institutionalized adults	Gram-negative rods
	S. pneumoniae
	S. aureus

logic agents that are most likely to cause pulmonary infections in these two groups are different. In infants and children, respiratory viruses cause the majority of pneumonias; in elderly adults, bacterial pathogens are more likely to be implicated.

Community-acquired pneumonia

CASE STUDY

A 52-year-old, previously healthy woman came to the emergency room complaining of right-sided chest pain with each breath, a cough that produced rust-colored sputum, and fever. She reported that her symptoms had begun abruptly the day before with the onset of shaking chills.

Examination revealed that the patient had a fever of 102° F and coarse breath sounds in the right anterior chest. The chest radiograph (Figure 26-5) showed a right upper lobe infiltrate; the laboratory analysis included a white blood cell count, which was elevated.

ETIOLOGY

Respiratory syncytial virus is the most commonly identified cause of viral pneumonias in children, especially in infants, in most communities. This pathogen has also been recognized in infections among the elderly, those being cared for in nursing homes, and those who are immunosuppressed. Parainfluenza is the second most commonly recognized viral pathogen to cause childhood pneumonias. Other etiologic agents to consider in pneumo-

nias in this age group are low-serotype adenoviruses and mycoplasma. Viral pneumonias caused by influenza type A and B viruses are prevalent in communities only during epidemic periods.

Although less common than viral pneumonias, bacterial pneumonias also occur in children and must be considered in the differential diagnosis. *S. pneumoniae* and *H. influenzae* type B are by far the most common pathogens isolated in childhood bacterial pneumonia. Other bacterial pathogens must also be considered, depending on the clinical situation. For example, group B streptococci are more likely to be associated with pneumonia in neonates than in older children.

In adults, *S. pneumoniae* remains the most common cause of community-acquired bacterial pneumonia in the general population. In addition, depending on the severity of the illness, the season of the year, and whether the community is experiencing an epidemic respiratory infection such as influenza, other pathogens such as respiratory viruses and *M. pneumoniae* are seen in community-acquired pneumonias in adolescents and adults and are responsible for the **atypical pneumonia** syndrome. It is "atypical" in that typical signs and symptoms of bacterial pneumonias that are more common in these age groups are absent or less impressive.

The type of patient involved may also help determine which bacterial pathogens are more likely causes of community-acquired pneumonia. For example, in adult patients with chronic lung disease, *H. influenzae* and *S. pneumoniae* are frequent colonizers. *H. influenzae* pneumonia is seen more fre-

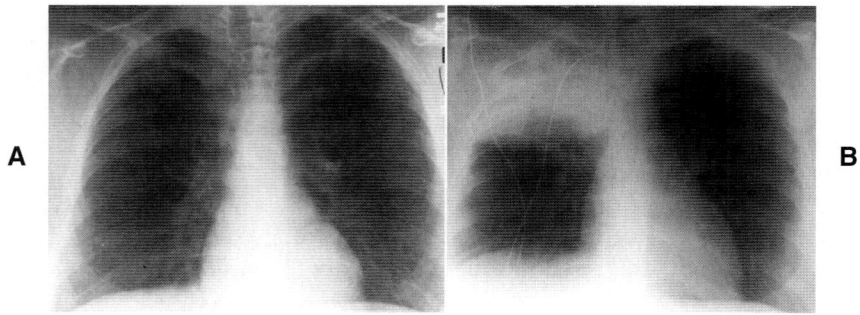

Figure 26-5

Chest radiographs before **(A)** and after **(B)** development of an acute, community-acquired, pneumococcal pneumonia. The patient is facing toward the reader. In **B,** consolidation of the right upper lobe of the lung is evidenced by the dense, whitish opacification of this lobe, which contrasts with the normal air *(black)* density of the remainder of the lung.

quently in these patients than in the general population. Patients with alcoholism and patients who have recently been hospitalized or treated with broad-spectrum antibiotics have an increased risk of being colonized with gram-negative bacillary pathogens that may cause pneumonia. Patients with recent influenza infection are at increased risk of developing pneumonia caused by *S. aureus* as well as by *S. pneumoniae*. These types of associations provide general guidelines that are useful for initiating empiric antibiotic therapy and for focusing diagnostic efforts.

Another group of pathogens that has emerged in recent years as a cause of both atypical pneumonia and typical bacterial pneumonia is *Legionella* species. These cases can be difficult to diagnose because unusual laboratory efforts are required to identify the organism in the sputum or bronchial aspirate specimen. *Legionella* species do not stain well with Gram stain (Figure 26-6) and are often missed in sputum or other types of respiratory secretions. Although patients may initially present with symptoms and signs typical of a viral respiratory tract syndrome, both pulmonary and systemic signs of infection may rapidly progress. Chest radiographs may show progressive involvement of multiple areas of the lung, with increasing patchy and lobar consolidation. Other signs and symptoms such as electrolyte abnormalities and gastrointestinal symptoms have also been associated with this infection, but it is usually not possible to distinguish *Legionella* pneumonia from other forms of bacterial pneumonia without specific diagnostic studies. Of primary importance is the consideration of this diagnosis in atypical cases of pneumonia in which the pathogen is not defined early in the course of investigation, so that specific diagnostic studies can be planned to address the possibility of *Legionella* infection.

EPIDEMIOLOGY

Community-acquired pneumonias in children are usually attributable to viral pathogens that cause respiratory tract infections in the community during the winter months. It is useful during such epidemic periods to contact the local state health department virology laboratory to inquire about the prevalent viral pathogen in the community, because seasonal viral respiratory infections often pass through the community in waves.

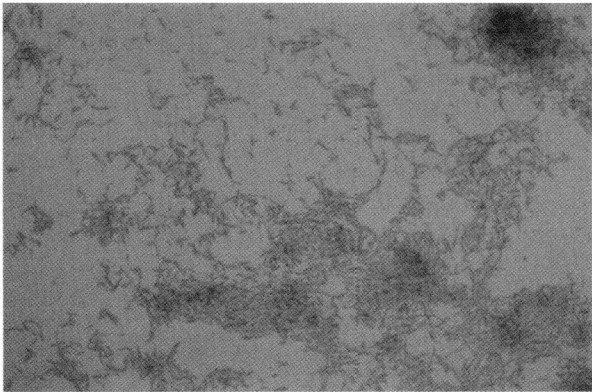

Figure 26-6 _____

Gram-stained smear of *Legionella* species taken from culture.

Unlike those seen in children, the majority of community-acquired pneumonias in adults are caused by bacterial infections. Although a patient with no other known medical problems can present with an acute bacterial pneumonia, the typical adult patient with community-acquired pneumonia either is elderly or has an underlying disease, such as chronic lung disease, cardiovascular disease, diabetes mellitus, or alcoholism, that predisposes to lower respiratory tract bacterial infection. These patients may either present with a primary pneumonia or develop pneumonia as a secondary infection complicating a primary viral infection. This predisposition to bacterial pneumonias is the reason that the elderly and patients with underlying chronic illnesses are the major targets for influenza and pneumococcal vaccination programs. In the community, the major cause of death in patients with influenza virus infection is secondary bacterial pneumonia. Based on this observation, it has been reasoned that prevention of influenza by vaccination of these high-risk patients will also prevent the serious bacterial pneumonias that may follow.

CLINICAL MANIFESTATIONS

The usual onset of nonbacterial pneumonias in children is indistinguishable from an average viral upper respiratory tract infection. However, instead of resolving in the time expected for upper respiratory tract infections, the clinical course proceeds toward increasing severity of illness, with signs of respiratory distress. Few other signs may be seen in young children with viral pneumonia.

In older children and adolescents, the typical signs of systemic viral infection include general fatigue and myalgias associated with early signs of upper respiratory tract infection. The cough usually does not produce sputum early in the course of the illness. Low-grade fever is common. The findings on physical examination are variable, and the chest radiograph may show diffuse interstitial changes, patchy infiltrates, or lobar consolidation (dense localized changes restricted to one lobe of the lung; see Figure 26-5). Lobar consolidation should always prompt an evaluation for a bacterial pathogen, because this radiographic presentation is atypical for viral pneumonia but common with bacterial infection. Routine laboratory studies are rarely helpful in making the clinical diagnosis of viral pneumonia in either children or adults.

In adolescents and adults, the atypical pneumonia syndrome, represented by *M. pneumoniae*, has a symptom complex and clinical presentation that are not dramatically different from those of other nonbacterial pneumonias. Its onset is like that of other nonbacterial upper respiratory tract infections but progresses to produce symptoms and signs of lower tract involvement. Chest radiograph abnormalities are classically more dramatic than would be expected based on the physical examination. The time of the year during which the infection is seen may be helpful in narrowing the list of choices for the etiologic diagnosis. During the winter months, a nonbacterial pneumonia syndrome is often caused by a viral pathogen that is prevalent in the community, for example, influenza. During the summer months, however, when pneumonia caused by most other nonbacterial respiratory pathogens is uncommon, the likelihood that an atypical pneumonia will be caused by *M. pneumoniae* approaches 50%.

The clinical presentation of community-acquired pneumonia in adults varies with the age and immunocompetence of the host. Most patients with bacterial pneumonia note a relatively sudden onset of fever associated with chills. In fact, they are often able to report the exact time their illness started. Cough productive of purulent sputum that may be blood-tinged is typical of this type of infection. Chest examination and radiographs typically show a localized area of infiltration in the lung, described as lobar consolidation (see Figure 26-5). This abnormality in the lung parenchyma is often associated with reduced oxygenation as mea-

sured by arterial blood gas monitoring. Routine laboratory studies will usually show a neutrophilic leukocytosis with an increased percentage of immature forms of granulocytes in the differential white blood cell count.

Such is the presentation of the patient described in the case study. This presentation is classic for pneumococcal pneumonia. Sputum Gram stain should show gram-positive lancet-shaped diplococci. Sputum culture should also grow *S. pneumoniae* if significant overgrowth from oral contaminants does not exist. In 25% to 30% of cases of pneumococcal pneumonia, patients demonstrate positive blood cultures for this organism (Figure 26-7).

The differential diagnosis should include other common causes of community-acquired pneumonia such as *H. influenzae, M. catarrhalis,* or *Legionella* organisms. *S. aureus* must be considered if a recent history of influenza exists. In cases of atypical pneumonia, patients have more constitutional symptoms and less sputum production. The chest radiograph is more likely to show patchy infiltrates rather than lobar consolidation. *Mycoplasma, Chlamydia,* and *Legionella* organisms, and viruses are potential causes of atypical pneumonia.

In elderly or immunocompromised patients, the clinical presentation may be less impressive than in patients who are able to mount a normal immune response to pulmonary bacterial infection. These immunologically compromised patients may

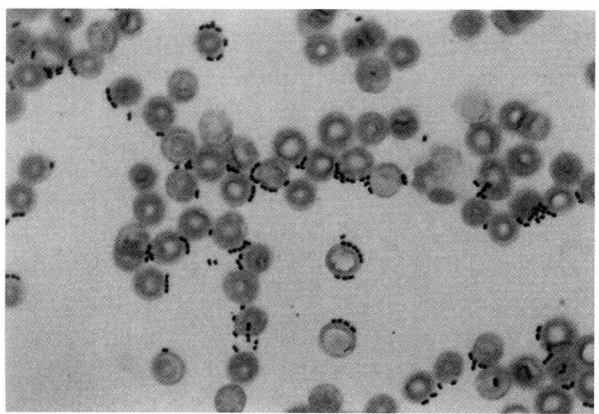

Figure 26-7

Gram-stained smear of *Streptococcus pneumoniae* isolated from the blood culture of a patient with pneumococcal pneumonia.

have few respiratory tract complaints and little or no fever. Nonspecific symptoms such as weakness, loss of appetite, and a minor cough may be the only manifestations of a progressive pneumonia. It is important to maintain a high index of suspicion in these patients and to routinely pursue changes in patterns of behavior with complete evaluations to avoid missing the diagnosis of pneumonia. These patients are also at increased risk for developing pneumonia after influenza infections. Therefore during influenza epidemics in the community, clinicians should have a heightened awareness of changes in respiratory symptoms that could be compatible with pneumonia in the elderly patient population.

Nosocomial pneumonia

CASE STUDY

A 60-year-old man with a history of emphysema and chronic bronchitis was admitted to the hospital to have his gallbladder removed. He was given perioperative antibiotic prophylaxis with cefoxitin. Because of his underlying lung disease, he could not be weaned from the ventilator postoperatively. His antibiotics were continued for a few more days. Seven days after surgery, he developed a high fever, increased secretions from his endotracheal tube, and a new infiltrate on his chest radiograph.

ETIOLOGY

Statistics from the Centers for Disease Control and Prevention show that almost 60% of nosocomial (hospital-acquired) lower respiratory tract infections are caused by gram-negative bacilli, including *Klebsiella* spp., *Enterobacter* spp., *Escherichia* spp., *Serratia marcescens,* and *Pseudomonas* spp. A smaller percentage (16%) of cases are associated with gram-positive isolates. Other comparisons of etiologic agents in nosocomial pneumonias have shown that the incidence with which anaerobic bacteria can be isolated varies greatly from study to study, apparently because of differences in sampling techniques and laboratory techniques used to isolate these organisms.

EPIDEMIOLOGY

Development of pneumonia in the hospital setting has different implications for both the diagnosis and the potential outcome of the infection. Colonization of the oropharynx with gram-negative bacillary pathogens is relatively uncommon in otherwise healthy patients but is common in hospitalized patients, especially those with severe underlying illnesses.

Epidemiologic studies have shown that gram-negative bacterial pneumonia is the leading cause of fatal hospital-acquired infections. An aggressive approach to early diagnosis and treatment of these pneumonias is therefore essential. An awareness of risk factors that predispose patients to nosocomial pneumonias sensitizes both the clinician and the clinical microbiologist to this problem so that an etiologic diagnosis can be established as early as possible in the course of the illness. These risk factors can be subdivided into two general categories:

1. Increased colonization of the upper respiratory tract with bacterial pathogens
2. Compromise of the barriers that normally protect the lower respiratory tract from infection with these pathogens

Increased oropharyngeal colonization Increased patient age, more severe illness, previous treatment with antibiotics, and manipulations that increase the gastric pH are all associated with increased oropharyngeal colonization with gram-negative bacilli. Such pathogens may be acquired from the patient's own gastrointestinal tract, but exposure of patients to the microbial flora encountered during hospitalization provides an exogenous source of colonization that can also be involved in subsequent nosocomial pneumonia.

In the case study described, previous antibiotic therapy, the presence of an endotracheal tube, and the patient's underlying lung disease, favored colonization with pathogenic (especially gram-negative) bacteria, invasion of the lower respiratory tract with these potential pathogens, and decreased lung defenses against the establishment of infection. Cases such as these warrant suspicion that a gram-negative bacillus (e.g., *Pseudomonas aeruginosa*) is the cause of the pneumonia and that it may be a drug-resistant organism. Gram stain and culture should be performed from the endotracheal secretions, and blood cultures should be done. It is often difficult to distinguish between colonization and infection in patients with endotracheal tubes. In addition to a positive sputum culture, other evidence, such as a new infiltrate on the chest radiograph or positive blood cultures, should be sought. If empyema fluid is present, it should be Gram stained and cultured.

Compromised normal barriers Compromise of normal barriers that prevent invasion of the usually sterile lower respiratory tract with pathogens colonizing the oropharynx predispose hospitalized patients to nosocomial pneumonia. Hospitalized patients with altered levels of consciousness aspirate pharyngeal contents into the lung more often than normal volunteers (70% versus 45%). In addition, intubation of the lower airway, which is commonly used in the intensive care setting for respiratory support of seriously ill patients, greatly increases the risk of developing nosocomial pneumonia by bypassing the normal mechanical defenses provided by the glottis and cough reflex. The longer such intubation is continued, the greater the risk of acquiring an associated nosocomial pneumonia. Nasogastric intubation also increases the risk of aspiration resulting from interference with glottic function and increased reflux of gastric secretions into the oropharynx.

Antibiograms of nosocomial pathogens In addition to an appreciation of the risk factors for colonization with and aspiration of hospital-acquired pathogens, the clinician needs a working knowledge of the antibiotic susceptibility patterns of the common nosocomial pathogens in the institution. Annual reviews of patterns of antibiotic susceptibility of the most common pathogens in nosocomial pneumonias should be performed at each institution by the clinical microbiologist in conjunction with the hospital infection control coordinator. The availability of data provides two important strengths to the institution. The clinician can design the best empiric antibiotic regimen while awaiting the results of specific antibiotic susceptibility testing. The infection control coordinator can also use the information to define changing trends in susceptibility patterns of hospital pathogens.

Nosocomial *Legionella* sp. pneumonia Hospitals are also among the institutional settings in which contaminated water supplies have been associated with *Legionella* sp. pneumonia. The exact mode of transmission of infections to patients is debatable. A higher incidence of these infections has been observed among patients with underlying lung disease and among immunocompromised pa-

tients (e.g., immunosuppression associated with solid organ transplants or corticosteroid therapy for various underlying conditions). Because the clinical presentation of patients with nosocomial *Legionella* sp. pneumonia is usually not distinct from that of other nosocomial pneumonias, early diagnosis depends on a high index of suspicion and specific diagnostic studies.

Aspiration Pneumonia
Etiology
Aspiration pneumonia, which occurs in both children and adults, follows aspiration of oropharyngeal or gastric contents into the lower respiratory tract. Among patients with aspiration pneumonia, 50% have mixed aerobic and anaerobic bacteria isolated, and 50% have only anaerobic bacteria isolated. The primary anaerobes isolated in these cases are usually *Peptostreptococcus* sp., *Fusobacterium* sp., and *Bacteroides* sp.; the primary aerobes isolated are usually *Streptococcus* sp., *Eikenella corrodens,* *S. aureus,* Enterobacteriaceae, and *P. aeruginosa.*

Patients with nosocomial aspiration pneumonia are more likely to have aerobic pathogens (predominantly gram-negative bacilli) than are patients with community-acquired aspiration pneumonia. Seriously ill hospitalized patients have an increased risk of lower respiratory tract infection with aerobic gram-negative bacilli because of increased colonization with these organisms. Patients who are immunosuppressed by preexisting disease or by chemotherapy and patients with altered lung defenses (e.g., chronic lung disease, cigarette smoking, advanced age) are at increased risk for the development of infection after aspiration of a bacterial inoculum.

In community-acquired aspiration pneumonia, the presence of periodontal disease, associated with an increased burden of oral anaerobic bacteria, increases the risk for the establishment of infection after aspiration.

Epidemiology
Aspiration of oropharyngeal secretions is common in the general population and hospitalized patients. The likelihood of developing infectious pneumonia after aspiration depends on the frequency of aspiration, quality and quantity of material aspirated, and host defenses.

It is useful for diagnosis and treatment planning to attempt to discriminate between chemical aspiration and aspiration of material contaminated with bacteria. Chemical aspiration (Mendelson's syndrome) resulting from aspiration of low-pH gastric contents not contaminated with large numbers of bacteria does not require initial antibiotic treatment. Because the injured lung is at increased risk of secondary bacterial infection, one must watch for signs of bacterial superinfection in the setting of "pure" chemical aspiration pneumonia.

Clinical manifestations

The typical clinical presentation of patients with aspiration pneumonia and its complications may vary from an acute pneumonitis to a chronic, indolent respiratory condition presenting as chronic productive cough. If treatment fails, aspiration pneumonia may progress to a necrotizing pneumonia and lung abscess.

Patients with anaerobic lung abscess usually have a longer history of illness (weeks) with a more subtle onset than patients with common acute bacterial pneumonia whose illness has typically been present for hours to days before they seek medical attention. Patients with lung abscess are also more likely to have putrid sputum and to complain of halitosis resulting from the involvement of anaerobic bacteria in the lung infection.

On chest radiographs, areas of necrotizing pneumonia and lung abscess resulting from aspiration are more likely to involve parts of the lung that are dependent in the supine position (superior segments of the lower lobes and posterior segments of the upper lobes), because this is the most common position in which aspiration into the lung occurs. Right-sided lung involvement is twice as common as left-sided involvement because the right main-stem bronchus has a more direct course into the lower lobe of the lung than the left main-stem bronchus.

Pathogenesis

Once bacterial pathogens are established in the lung, the outcomes of interactions between the infectious agent and the host's response to infection determine the nature of the pneumonia and depend to some extent on the virulence of the organisms. For example, in pneumonias caused by *P. aeruginosa,* extensive tissue destruction may occur as a result of the production of proteases and cytotoxins by the organism, causing necrotizing pneumonias.

Complications

Patients with extensive viral or bacterial pneumonias may have insufficient ventilation to the involved lung to adequately support respiration. In rapidly progressive, multilobe pneumonias, ventilatory support may be needed as a result of overwhelming infection or an injury response of the lung termed "respiratory distress syndrome." In these cases, mechanical support of ventilation and other supportive measures are used to provide time for antimicrobial therapy to control the pneumonia and to allow recovery of lung function. An example of tissue destruction caused by pneumonia is the development of a lung abscess cavity. In this case, the pulmonary infection, usually an anaerobic infection of the lung associated with aspiration pneumonia, results in destruction of the lung parenchyma in the area of a necrotizing bacterial infection. These infections usually can be treated with antibiotic therapy alone. If the abscess cavity is large and refractory to therapy, surgery may be required.

An example of local extension of a lung infection is **empyema,** an infection of the pleural space between the lung and the chest wall. Because of the limited ability to deliver antimicrobial agents to this type of space (limited blood supply), bacterial empyema usually requires a drainage procedure, such as insertion of a chest tube, to promote resolution of the infection. Extension of the infection beyond the chest occurs most commonly when bacterial invasion of the blood stream occurs (bacteremia). The same type of spread is possible with viral pneumonias (viremia), although the consequences of viremia are usually much less severe than those of bacteremia. Patients with bacteremia as a complication of pneumonia have an increased mortality compared with patients with pneumonia without bacteremia. In some cases, this may simply be a reflection of the bacterial burden and the difficulty in controlling the infection. In other cases, such as gram-negative bacillary bacteremia, the presence of bacteria and their constituents (e.g., endotoxin) may be associated with severe shock, further complicating the care of the patient and increasing the likelihood of a fatal outcome. In addition to the direct consequences of bacteremia, in some instances an infection originally established in the lung may spread via the blood stream to other sites, such as the central nervous system—a so-called metastatic infection.

Laboratory diagnosis

SPECIMEN COLLECTION

The lower respiratory tract is exposed to a constant risk of contaminating the clinical specimen with the normal flora from the upper respiratory tract. Despite the limited usefulness of this type of specimen from the lower respiratory tract, expectorated sputum specimens can be useful in the diagnosis of pneumonia. In addition, expectorated sputum, when compared with other procedures, involves no risk to the patient.

Using both the Gram stain and culture, expectorated sputum specimens yield an etiologic diagnosis in almost half the cases of bacterial pneumonia. However, care must be taken to avoid contamination of the specimen with oropharyngeal flora. Patients should be instructed to rinse out their mouths and collect a "deep" sputum specimen. Such communication with patients can be rewarding. It is important that they understand that the purpose of the exercise is to collect lung secretions and not saliva or drainage from the nasopharynx. In addition, patients should remove dentures during the specimen collection.

The expectorated sputum specimen should be examined for its character, which provides a preliminary indication about the type of pneumonia. A patient with typical bacterial pneumonia (e.g., pneumococcal pneumonia) will produce purulent sputum that may be streaked with small amounts of blood or may be rusty in color. In contrast, patients with nonbacterial pneumonia (e.g., mycoplasma pneumonia) may produce no sputum or small amounts of sputum that is relatively clear.

OTHER SPECIMEN COLLECTION METHODS

In some cases of pneumonia, expectorated sputum specimens may be either unavailable or of unsatisfactory quality. Early attempts to sample lower respiratory tract secretions more directly involved transtracheal aspiration and transthoracic needle aspiration directly from the site of pneumonia. Although both these techniques were more successful diagnostic tools than the use of expectorated sputum, the morbidity associated with these invasive procedures (e.g., bleeding and pneumothorax)

significantly increased. Therefore the recent trend has been toward the use of the flexible, fiber-optic bronchoscope when direct specimen collection from the lower respiratory tract is required. Proper use of a protected brush extended from the end of the bronchoscope to collect specimens from the area of pneumonia has been valuable for diagnosing both aerobic and anaerobic infections of the lung.

The same general approach used to process expectorated sputum specimens is used to process specimens collected using this method. In addition, quantitative cultures may be performed to provide a further check against the possibility that the pathogen isolated is a contaminant from the upper respiratory tract.

Immunocompromised patients produce minimal secretions as a result of a weak inflammatory response to infection; in these patients bronchoalveolar lavage adds an extra dimension that increases the diagnostic yield. The segment of the lung suspected of being involved in a pneumonic process is lavaged with sterile fluid; this fluid is then collected after aspiration through the bronchoscope and is concentrated before processing. This technique has been highly useful in diagnosing *P. carinii,* cytomegalovirus, and other opportunistic infections in patients with AIDS. In occasional cases an infectious pneumonia is strongly suspected (or must be differentiated from a lung abnormality of another type) and in which the procedures mentioned to this point are unsuccessful in establishing an etiologic diagnosis. In such instances, it may be necessary to proceed to a lung biopsy to obtain tissue for culture and histologic study. Transbronchial biopsy can be performed through the flexible bronchoscope. However, the size of the specimen taken is small and may be insufficient for diagnosis. Video-assisted thoracoscopic (VATS) lung biopsy has been introduced as a means of sampling pleural-based lung lesions. As a final option, an open lung biopsy performed during a surgical procedure may be necessary to obtain a larger tissue specimen for analysis.

DIRECT MICROSCOPIC EXAMINATION

The quality of the specimen is determined by a direct Gram-stained smear. The goal of this evaluation is to eliminate specimens that are contaminated with oropharyngeal contents. Gram-stained smears of sputum samples show the relative numbers of neutrophils and epithelial cells, which should be

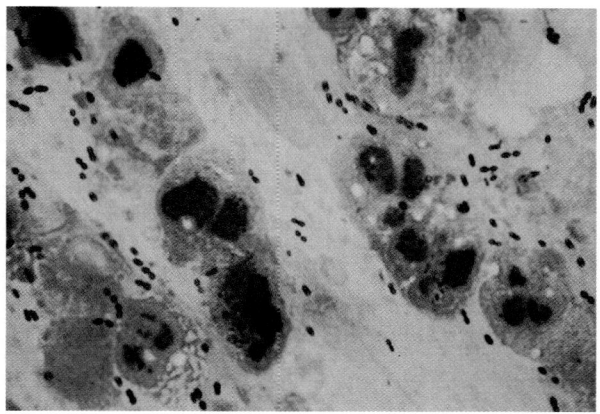

Figure 26-8

Gram-stained smear with white blood cells and gram-positive diplococci—acceptable for culture.

quantitated under low-power magnification (10×). As a general guideline, samples with greater than 25 neutrophils and fewer than 10 epithelial cells per field are considered to be relatively free of such contamination (Figure 26-8); samples containing more than 25 squamous epithelial cells per field (Figure 26-9, *A*) should not be cultured.

Gram stain of samples collected by invasive procedures can produce more meaningful results. In addition to the presence or absence of microor-ganisms and inflammatory cells, the microscopic morphology of the organisms present may lead to a presumptive diagnosis (Figure 26-9, *B*).

CULTURE

Only high-quality specimens should be processed for culture. The protocol should include culture media such as sheep's blood agar, MacConkey, and chocolate agar plates to recover all the agents that may be suspected. Samples collected by invasive procedures—and therefore unlikely to be contaminated with upper respiratory flora—should be processed for anaerobic culture, particularly if the patient is suspected of having aspiration pneumonia, lung abscess, or empyema.

Chronic Pneumonia

Bacterial pneumonias usually resolve completely over a period of many weeks. On occasion, however, resolution of pneumonia is delayed, with radiographic lung abnormalities persisting far beyond the improvement of clinical symptoms. Some bacteria that typically cause acute pneumonias induce necrotizing processes in the lung that are generally slow to resolve despite a clinical cure. Examples of such infections include anaerobic infections of the lung, gram-negative bacillary pneumonias, and pneumonias caused by *S. aureus*.

A 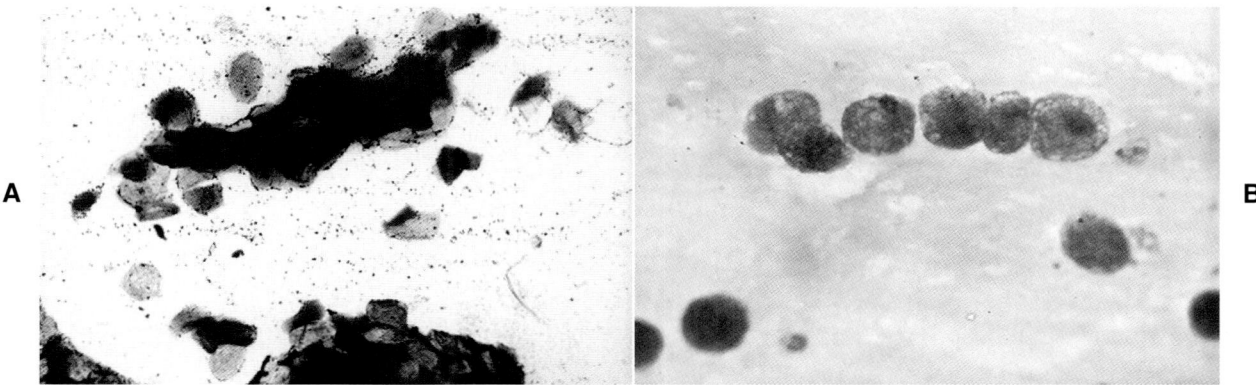 B

Figure 26-9

A, Expectorated sputum, smear, Gram stain, light microscopy, low-power view (LPV). Purulence none. Contaminating bacteria and epithelial cells heavy. No pathogens seen. Please submit carefully collected sample of lower respiratory tree material. The sample is saliva, not sputum. There could be several reasons for submission of this sample to the laboratory. The patient could have been poorly directed and simply "spit" into the collection container, or the patient's cough may not be productive of sputum. **B,** Aspirated sputum, smear, Gram stain, light microscopy, high-power view (HPV). Purulence none. Local materials moderate. No organisms seen. The alveolar macrophages and mucus (pink-stained background) are the local materials from the surface of the tracheobronchial tree. This smear confirms that sputum was sampled and that there is no suspicion for infection and no evidence of significant contamination. Routine bacterial culture of this specimen will still grow insignificant oral flora because culture is more sensitive than direct examination.

When abnormalities in the lung persist, the clinician is faced with several questions regarding diagnosis and therapy. Is the process the result of a slowly resolving necrotizing pneumonia or a slowly progressing chronic pneumonia? Is an unsuspected pathogen causing progressive infection in the lung? Is an underlying noninfectious problem in the lung causing chest radiograph abnormalities?

CASE STUDY

A 60-year-old man came to an emergency room complaining of cough and fever lasting several weeks. He reported night sweats and weight loss over the last few months. He admitted to drinking alcohol heavily on weekends and to staying in a shelter for the homeless most of the previous winter.

The patient had a fever and appeared very thin. He coughed frequently during the examination. His chest radiograph revealed a right upper lobe infiltrate.

Etiology

Among the pathogens that cause clinically apparent chronic pneumonias, mycobacteria are the most common in immunologically intact hosts.

The annual incidence of *M. tuberculosis* infection has resumed its downward trend after the increases that were observed in the late 1980s and early 1990s. However, tuberculosis (TB) continues to be a major cause of chronic pneumonia in certain regions of the country. An increasing percentage (now nearly 40%) of all TB cases are diagnosed among recent immigrants to the United States. The remainder of cases continue to occur among socially disadvantaged, elderly, and immunocompromised (e.g., those with AIDS) subpopulations of our society. Infections with nontuberculous mycobacteria—so-called NTM—(e.g., *Mycobacterium kansasii, Mycobacterium avium* complex, *Mycobacterium fortuitum-chelonei*) can present in a fashion that is indistinguishable from tuberculosis.

Opportunistic fungal pathogens, including *Candida, Aspergillus* (Figure 26-10) and *Cryptococcus* organisms, can also cause chronic pneumonia. They rarely cause invasive disease in immunologically intact hosts but can cause acute and chronic pneumonias in immunosuppressed patients. In contrast, true fungal pathogens such as *Histoplasma capsulatum, Coccidioides immitis,* and *Blastomyces dermatitidis* organisms, when acquired in a sufficient inoculum, can cause chronic pneumonias in normal hosts.

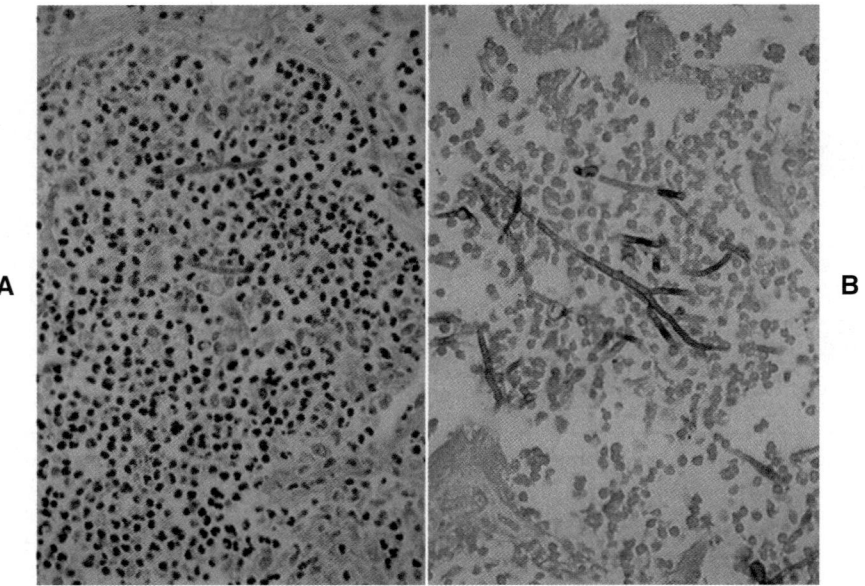

Figure 26-10 ───

Lung exudate from a patient with hematologic disorder, showing alveoli containing branching fungal elements. **A,** Hematoxylin and eosin stain; **B,** GMS stain. (Courtesy Shirlyn B. McKenzie, PhD.)

Clinical manifestations

Some infections of the lung are inherently slow in their progress and are chronic in nature. The most common examples of these types of infections are mycobacterial and fungal infections of the lung. Although some of the symptoms seen in the setting of acute pneumonia (e.g., fever, chills, and general weakness) are also observed in patients with chronic pneumonias, these and other symptoms may be less dramatic in their onset and less intense in these cases. As a result, often a longer delay occurs between the onset of symptoms and seeking of medical attention. Because of the prolonged period of illness associated with chronic pneumonias, the patient may also exhibit other signs that are not typically seen with acute infections, such as marked weight loss.

In immunocompromised patients, mycobacterial or fungal infections may be unusually severe, with either local or disseminated infection causing life-threatening complications. For example, *Aspergillus* ssp. may cause overwhelming pneumonia in neutropenic leukemia patients, and *Cryptococcus* infections acquired by the respiratory route may cause fatal infections after dissemination to the central nervous system in patients who are immunosuppressed following chemotherapy. Immunosuppressed patients may also have nonspecific symptoms of fever and weakness as manifestations of low-grade chronic pneumonias.

The physical examination of patients with chronic pneumonia usually shows few specific signs other than those associated with general debility. Routine laboratory studies are rarely of help in making a specific diagnosis. In addition to the history, a chest radiograph and, in selected cases, computed tomography of the chest are the most important initial diagnostic studies in establishing a presumptive diagnosis of chronic pneumonia. For example, upper lobe cavitary lung disease is suggestive of tuberculosis or related mycobacterial infection. However, because many infections that cause chronic pneumonia can cause similar radiologic abnormalities, further studies must be planned for a specific diagnosis.

Pathogenesis

Chronic pneumonias caused by mycobacterial or fungal pathogens typically elicit a granulomatous response in the lung that is distinct from the acute inflammatory response seen with most acute bacterial pneumonias. The interactions between components of the infecting organism and the host immune response that lead to this granulomatous response are still being characterized. Both humoral (e.g., production of a specific antibody) and cellular (e.g., delayed type hypersensitivity) responses are elicited by these pathogens. However, it seems clear that the cellular immune response to infection is primarily involved in both protective and tissue-destructive aspects of these illnesses. One goal of the study of the immunobiology of the infections that can cause chronic pneumonias is to dissect these two general types of cellular immune responses to allow the development of approaches that favor protective cellular immunity while minimizing the potential for lung tissue destruction.

Complications

The complications of chronic infectious pneumonias depend on the extent of the local and systemic spread of the infection and the immunologic status of the host. Patients who develop extensive lung involvement with a chronic infection resulting from late or inadequate medical intervention or failed therapy may eventually suffer from respiratory insufficiency. This is usually the result of progressive lung tissue destruction and progression of the fibrotic process that can accompany these chronic pneumonias. When the infection extends beyond the lung (e.g., in immunocompromised patients), other vital organs may be involved, such as central nervous system infection with *Cryptococcus* organisms in an immunosuppressed host. Patients with chronic pneumonias for prolonged periods commonly become cachectic. This is a maladaptive response of components of the host cellular immune response to chronic infection that results from production of cytokines (e.g., cachectin/tumor necrosis factor α), that interfere with nutrient metabolism.

Laboratory diagnosis

Among the chronic pneumonias, tuberculosis is usually the easiest cause to diagnose. With the proper clinical picture, the presence of *M. tuberculosis* in an expectorated sputum specimen is diagnostic of infection. Similarly, the discovery of *M. kansasii* in the expectorated sputum of a patient with a clinical picture of chronic cavitary pneumonia is sufficient to establish the etiologic diagnosis. In patients with chronic pneumonia caused by nontuberculous mycobacteria (NTM), repeated sputum specimens in the context of progressive pneumonia and in the absence of another definable pathogen may be needed to establish an association between the pathogen and the illness. This is true because these pathogens can colonize the respiratory tract in the absence of apparent infection. Therefore the isolation of an organism (e.g., *M. avium*) from a single sputum specimen is insufficient to establish an etiologic diagnosis.

In the case study the clinician must suspect the diagnosis of tuberculosis and other types of pneumonia so that appropriate diagnostic studies can be performed. Because of the public health implications of *M. tuberculosis* infections, which can be highly contagious, any positive stain or culture for mycobacteria should be reported, and proper respiratory isolation should be established until the organism is identified. Until the acid-fast bacilli studies are completed, other etiologies that should be included in the differential diagnosis are community-acquired bacterial pneumonia and aspiration pneumonia.

With chronic pneumonias of fungal etiology, it is typically difficult to isolate the pathogen from expectorated sputum. As a result, invasive procedures to obtain either bronchoscopic, thoracoscopic, or open lung biopsies are often required to establish the identity of the pathogen. Depending on the severity of the clinical illness, empiric therapy may be initiated based on a presumptive diagnosis from the results of histopathologic studies while awaiting culture confirmation from the diagnostic microbiology laboratory.

DIRECT MICROSCOPIC EXAMINATION

Smears prepared from concentrated sputum samples for mycobacterial cultures should be stained with acid-fast stains (Figure 26-11) such as Kinyoun, Ziehl-Neelsen, or any of the fluorochrome stains. Although the sensitivity of acid-fast smears is approximately 50%—maybe higher with fluorochrome stains—finding mycobacterial organisms on the smear indicates the patient's possible infectiousness. Rapid diagnosis and initiation of empiric treatment may be established prior to the availability of culture results, which take several weeks.

Direct microscopic examination of respiratory secretions should also include preparations to detect fungal agents. Potassium hydroxide and cal-

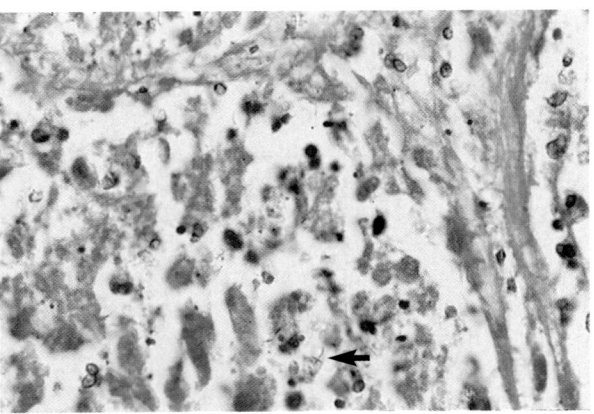

Figure 26-11

Acid-fast bacillus (AFB) stain of sputum containing mycobacteria (red-stained organisms).

cofluor white are commonly used to detect yeast cells and hyphal elements.

CULTURE

Culture studies in patients with chronic pneumonias require close communication between the clinician and the clinical microbiologist. It is necessary to use special techniques to process respiratory secretions and lung tissue specimens for identification of mycobacterial and fungal pathogens. Furthermore, in some occasions (e.g., in cases of pulmonary tuberculosis and coccidioidomycosis) isolation of the pathogen creates a potential biohazard in the diagnostic laboratory. Therefore laboratory personnel must use special precautions when culturing these specimens.

RAPID DIAGNOSTIC TESTS FOR TUBERCULOSIS

In addition to conventional smear and culture techniques, nucleic amplification tests are gaining increased acceptance for the rapid diagnosis of *M. tuberculosis* infections of the lung (and also of extrapulmonary infections). Current data indicate that these assays are highly sensitive (usually greater than 90%) for smear positive sputum specimens but are less sensitive (40% to 60%) for smear negative sputum specimens. Specificity has been high under both circumstances in most reports. These rapid assays require skilled personnel and are relatively costly compared with conventional diagnostic methods. However, the rapid assays offer the real possibility of a greatly increased speed of diagnosis for active tuberculosis cases. It is likely that the first area of general acceptance of these new methods will be for diagnosis of smear positive cases. The most clinically useful and cost-effective use of these assays for smear negative cases will require further study.

Empyema

Empyema is defined as a collection of purulent fluid in the pleural space between the lung and the chest wall. Although the accumulation of pleural fluid is fairly common in association with acute bacterial pneumonia, most such accumulations are sterile, and only a small percentage qualify as empyemas. The distinction between a sterile pleural effusion and an empyema depends on the presence of a pathogen and an inflammatory response and is made using chemical and cellular parameters of the fluid.

Etiology

In patients with community-acquired pneumonia, *S. aureus, S. pneumoniae,* and *S. pyogenes* are the most common causes of empyema. Anaerobic bacteria are being isolated with increasing frequency from empyema fluids in patients with a history of aspiration pneumonia and lung abscess. Empyema among hospitalized patients is caused primarily by aerobic gram-negative bacilli—the cause of the majority of nosocomial pneumonias. In patients with chronic pneumonia caused by *M. tuberculosis,* empyema may occur as a result of rupture of an underlying cavity into the pleural space.

Clinical manifestations

The clinical presentation of a patient with empyema is usually an extension of the illness of the underlying lung (e.g., bacterial pneumonia or lung abscess). Patients may have chest pain on the affected side, fever, chills, and night sweats. If the empyema is large, it may be detected during the physical examination. If empyema is not suspected based on the physical examination, the first evidence of it usually comes from chest radiographic studies. Computed tomography of the chest may be necessary to differentiate empyema from underlying lung abscess or lung consolidation.

Empyema may complicate chest surgery or chest trauma, both of which provide a potential route of infection directly from the exterior to the pleural space. Less commonly, empyema results from direct contamination of the pleural space as a result of peritoneal or gastrointestinal disease. Infection may extend to the pleural space from a pyogenic process beneath the diaphragm. Rarely, empyema results from infection of the pleural (and mediastinal) space after esophageal rupture.

Pathogenesis

Once organisms gain access to the pleural space, the resulting inflammatory response to this infection, along with the pleural response to the underlying process that seeded the pleural space, stimulates the exudation of fluid into this area. Typically, accumulation of large numbers of neutrophilic leukocytes occurs, resulting in the purulent appearance of most empyemas. Toward the later (or organizing) stages of an empyemic process, fibroblast infiltration into the area is associated with organization of the contents of the pleural space into a thick capsule that adheres to the lung and chest wall surfaces. If the empyema is not treated before this stage, the process may encase and limit the motion and function of the underlying lung.

Characteristics of the empyema fluid create an environment in which elimination of the offending pathogen is compromised. Opsonins and complement activity, which are necessary for the proper phagocytosis of bacteria by infiltrating granulocytes, are present in reduced concentrations in empyema fluid. In addition to this limitation of the host response, the usefulness of antibiotics in treating empyema is limited by the minimal blood supply to this area, resulting in reduced drug delivery, and by the low pH of empyema fluid, which can reduce the antimicrobial activity of antibiotics.

Complications

The complications associated with empyema depend primarily on the nature of the underlying disease. The main consequence of empyema per se is persistence of infection. If the empyema is not drained properly and treated with appropriate antibiotics, the infection causing the empyema may be difficult to eliminate. Persistent, poorly controlled infection may lead to the multiple complications associated with unresolved sepsis. A long-term complication of empyema is encasement of the lung in a thick capsule, which may alter lung function. This complication may necessitate removal of the thickened pleural lining (decortication), which may or may not restore the function of the underlying lung, depending on the duration of the dysfunction.

Laboratory diagnosis

Pleural fluid should be aspirated directly into an evacuated sterile syringe. If the volume of the pleural fluid is relatively large (greater than 500 mL) as estimated by chest radiograph, this procedure can usually be performed at the patient's bedside. If the volume is smaller or if the space is loculated, pleural fluid aspiration may have to be done in the radiology suite guided by ultrasound. Because the volume of pleural fluid needed for diagnostic studies is small (a few milliliters), it is not necessary to remove the majority of the effusion for this purpose. Any excess air in the syringe should be expelled promptly to improve the yield of anaerobic bacteria.

The syringe containing the fluid should be transported directly to the diagnostic microbiology laboratory so that Gram stain and processing for anaerobic and other bacteria can be performed promptly. The character (i.e., purulence, odor, presence of blood) of the fluid should be recorded. Aliquots of the remaining fluid should be distributed to the hematology and chemistry laboratories for studies of cell count and differential count, total protein and lactic dehydrogenase concentration, and pH. These measurements provide parameters that are useful in differentiating an empyema from a transudative effusion.

An aliquot of the pleural fluid should be saved in case special studies are required to detect capsular polysaccharide antigens of pathogenic bacteria such as *S. pneumoniae* or *H. influenzae*. If malignancy is in the differential diagnosis, a fluid specimen should also be submitted for cytology. Because it is usually desirable to submit a large specimen for cytology when a malignant pleural effusion is suspected, a larger sample may have to be collected specifically for this purpose. If a diagnosis of tuberculous pleural effusion is suspected, it is usually useful to obtain a pleural biopsy to complement the pleural fluid sample for mycobacterial culture. The combined data from culture of these two specimens can be diagnostic in approximately 85% of cases, whereas culture of pleural fluid alone is positive in less than 25% of confirmed cases of tuberculous empyema.

OPPORTUNISTIC INFECTIONS OF THE RESPIRATORY TRACT

Opportunistic pathogens ordinarily do not cause disease in normal hosts but require an impairment of host defense mechanisms to exhibit pathogenicity. Patients who are susceptible to **opportunistic infections** are called immunocompromised hosts. Impairment of different components of the immune response can render a host susceptible to infection with different types of microorganisms. To consider the associations between the commonly observed immunodeficiency states, it is convenient to consider three categories of defects: granulocytopenia, cellular immune deficiency, and humoral immune deficiency. It is important, however, to realize that in many conditions in which the function of more than one component of the immune response is altered.

Granulocytopenic Patients

Severe granulocytopenia is defined as a reduction of the absolute granulocyte count to 500/mm^3 or less. This state is usually observed in patients with leukemia or those who have been treated with a variety of chemotherapeutic agents. Granulocyte dysfunction associated with conditions such as diabetes mellitus, azotemia, and alcoholism also appears to increase the risk of infection. The linkage between severe infection and secondary granulocyte dysfunction of this type is less clear, however, than the risk observed with severe granulocytopenia.

Granulocytopenic patients are highly susceptible to bacterial infections (e.g., encapsulated bacteria) and to some fungal infections (e.g., invasive *Aspergillus* disease), especially if the granulocytopenia is prolonged. Such patients may present with rapidly progressive sinusitis or otitis media. Diabetic patients with ketoacidosis (and associated granulocyte dysfunction) and leukemic patients with prolonged neutropenia who have been treated with broad-spectrum antibiotics are at risk for both severe bacterial and fungal sinusitis. Nasal and sinus infections with fungal agents such as Zygomycetes can progress rapidly into the orbit and even the brain and can result in death.

In addition to causing granulocytopenia, chemotherapeutic agents can damage the mucosal membranes of the mouth and pharynx. This breakdown of normal barriers predisposes the patient to stomatitis and pharyngitis and to damage of the tracheal mucosa and cilia, increasing the risk of both upper respiratory tract infection and pneumonia. In these circumstances, respiratory pathogens colonize the oropharynx and nasopharynx of these patients prior to the development of pneumonia. Because the patients are immunologically compromised, organisms that constitute part of the normal flora that are not pathogenic in normal hosts may also become invasive pathogens. Furthermore, exposure of these patients to prolonged hospitalization and to repeated courses of broad-spectrum antibiotics often results in increased colonization with virulent or drug-resistant microorganisms. Some of these colonizing pathogens, such as *Pseudomonas aeruginosa*, have a high propensity to progress from colonization to invasive disease in immunologically compromised patients. These infections have the potential for rapid progression to sepsis and death. Therefore empiric therapy is usually initiated at the first sign of infection while awaiting the results of specific diagnostic studies.

Patients who have had bone marrow or organ transplants are also at increased risk for serious pneumonias. During the initial period of severe neutropenia after bone marrow transplantation, the same types of infections seen in other neutropenic states may be observed in these patients. After neutropenia resolves in bone marrow transplant patients, the risk is increased of cytomegalovirus and *Aspergillus* infections associated with ongoing immunosuppression. The incidence of *P. carinii* pneumonia as a complication of bone marrow transplantation has decreased with the introduction of antibiotic prophylaxis with trimethoprim and sulfamethoxazole. In bone marrow transplant patients being treated for chronic graft versus host disease, the rate of late *S. pneumoniae* infection is unusually high. Similar infections occur in immunosuppressed recipients of solid organ transplants, with the addition of *S. aureus* and *Legionella* spp. to the list of potential pathogens. Pneumonia with either of these organisms or with gram-negative bacilli has a 60% mortality in solid organ transplant recipients. *Nocardia, Strongyloides,* and mycobacterial respiratory infections also occur with significant morbidity and mortality in these patients.

Patients with Defects in Cellular Immunity

CASE STUDY

A 30-year-old homosexual man presented to an emergency room with a 2-week history of shortness of breath. He first noticed having difficulty in climbing stairs at work, but more recently he has felt short of breath even at rest. On questioning, he reported some subjective fever but denied weight loss or a productive cough. The patient denied ever having been tested for human immunodeficiency virus (HIV) and had been monogamous for the last 4 years.

The patient's temperature was slightly elevated, and he appeared mildly short of breath. His lung examination was normal, but his chest radiograph showed hazy infiltrates in both lower lung fields. Arterial blood gas sampling showed hypoxia.

Defects in the network of T-lymphocyte and mononuclear-macrophage interactions can lead to cellular immune dysfunction and increased susceptibility to certain types of infections. These defects may be either congenital or acquired.

Acquired immunologic defects are much more common and are usually caused by immunosuppressive therapy used for cancer chemotherapy or for bone marrow or organ transplantation. A variety of underlying diseases, including lymphomas, other malignancies, and collagen vascular diseases, also appear to impair cellular immune responses independently of chemotherapy.

The types of opportunistic infections observed in patients with defects in cellular immune responses, such as those with acquired immunodeficiency syndrome (AIDS), are typically viral (e.g., herpesvirus, cytomegalovirus), mycobacterial (e.g., tuberculosis, *M. avium*), fungal (e.g., *Cryptococcus, Aspergillus,* and *Histoplasma* organisms), or parasitic (e.g., *P. carinii*) in origin. In patients with AIDS resulting from HIV infection, *P. carinii* pneumonia is the most common cause of death.

As in the case study presented, *P. carinii* pneumonia is often the first manifestation of HIV infection. Therefore the clinician must consider this diagnosis in high-risk patients even if no history of previous opportunistic infection exists. Patients may have severe disease despite a paucity of symptoms and signs. Induced sputum is stained with Giemsa or methenamine silver stain and examined for the presence of pneumocystis cysts. In experienced laboratories, the diagnosis can be made quickly and with excellent sensitivity, eliminating the need for more invasive diagnostic procedures in most cases.

Other potential but less likely causes of pneumonia in patients with HIV infection are community-acquired bacterial pneumonia (e.g., *S. pneumoniae*), fungal pneumonia (e.g., *Cryptococcus neoformans* or *Histoplasma capsulatum*), or noninfectious causes (e.g., Kaposi's sarcoma or lymphoma).

Tuberculosis tends to occur earlier in the course of HIV infection than do most of the other opportunistic pneumonias seen in these patients. Later in the course of AIDS, tuberculosis may have an atypical presentation, increasing the probability that the diagnosis will be missed and that more contacts will become infected. As AIDS progresses, the likelihood that a mycobacterial infection will be caused by *M. avium* rather than *M. tuberculosis* increases. Encapsulated bacteria, *C. neoformans* and other fungi, and cytomegalovirus are other significant respiratory pathogens in the later phase of AIDS.

The oropharynx is susceptible to infection with *Candida* spp. and herpes simplex virus in patients with AIDS and in patients receiving immunosuppressive chemotherapy. Damage to the oral mucosa from chemotherapeutic agents can cause mucositis followed by secondary bacterial and fungal infections or reactivation of a latent viral infection. The appearance of the mucosa can be misleading, and diagnosis may require culture or biopsy.

Another acquired immunodeficiency state that can be classified loosely with the cellular immune defects is splenic insufficiency. The spleen is an important part of the reticuloendothelial system. In addition to the numerous immunologic responses provided by the cells of the spleen, it appears that a key splenic activity involves clearance of pneumococci *(S. pneumoniae)* from the blood. Patients with either splenic dysfunction or who lack a spleen (usually from surgical removal after traumatic rupture) have a greatly increased incidence of serious pneumococcal infections.

Patients with Defects in Humoral Immunity

The humoral arm of the immune response to infection consists primarily of the production of spe-

cific opsonizing and neutralizing antibodies. The serum complement system also plays a role in humoral immune responses to infection. As with other types of immunodeficiency disease, most defective humoral immune responses are acquired as a result of specific immunosuppressive therapy or underlying disease states (e.g., multiple myeloma, chronic lymphocytic leukemia). Less commonly, congenital defects in both antibody production (hypogammaglobulinemia) and complement synthesis (classical and alternative complement pathway defects) are observed.

Pneumonias in patients with hypogammaglobulinemia are usually caused by encapsulated bacteria (e.g., *S. pneumoniae, H. influenzae*) resulting from the lack of specific opsonizing antibodies to enhance phagocytosis of these organisms by granulocytic cells. Viral, mycobacterial, and fungal respiratory tract infections are not more of a problem than usual in patients with humoral immunodeficiency states, unless some component of the cellular immune response is also defective. In addition to problems with other encapsulated bacteria, patients with complement defects may have serious infections with *N. meningitidis*. These pneumonias are often more severe in these patients and may be accompanied by bacteremia in a higher percentage of patients compared to normal hosts. Most episodes of fatal bacteremia in patients with leukemia originate with infections in the lung. Gram-negative bacilli account for most of these infections, with *K. pneumoniae, E. coli,* and *P. aeruginosa* being the most common.

Diagnosis

Diagnosis of opportunistic infections in patients with immunodeficiency diseases requires a high index of suspicion in addition to a working knowledge of the likely pathogens. Pneumonias may be difficult to diagnose because of the broad range of potential pathogens, the atypical presentation of the illness, and the noninfectious conditions that can mimic pneumonia.

In patients with underlying malignancy, open lung biopsy is required in many cases to establish a specific etiologic diagnosis. The current trend is toward using bronchoscopy and bronchoalveolar lavage as the first step in the diagnostic strategy, resulting from the experience with AIDS patients. Bronchoalveolar lavage is diagnostic in most of these patients. Transbronchial biopsy may be required for diagnosis in some cases, and video-assisted thoracoscopic (VATS) lung biopsy is increasingly used as the next diagnostic step short of open lung biopsy. Establishment of a specific etiologic diagnosis can be complicated by the presence of more than one potential pathogen in a specimen or by the coexistence of malignancy and infection.

It has been possible to diagnose cases of *P. carinii* pneumonia in some patients with AIDS by direct examination of expectorated sputum for the presence of cysts. This may be due to the presence of large numbers of organisms in these immunocompromised patients. The specimen must be digested, centrifuged, smeared, and fixed and then stained with Giemsa, methenamine silver, or a fluorescent antibody stain. Yield is higher if the sputum is collected in the morning after an overnight fast. Examination of induced sputum is 80% sensitive, whereas bronchoalveolar lavage (Figure 26-12) increases sensitivity to 85% to 95%, and the addition of transbronchial biopsy increases the diagnostic yield to nearly 100%. Currently, *P. carinii* cannot be cultured in the laboratory and must be diagnosed by histologic or immunofluorescent techniques. Reports exist of successful detection of *P. carinii* using polymerase chain reaction assays. However, these methods are currently restricted to the research setting.

The common theme in these and other invasive infections of the lower respiratory tract in immunocompromised patients is that an aggressive approach to diagnosis and empirical therapy is essential. It is important to make an etiologic diagnosis as frequently as possible to allow antimicrobial therapy to be focused on the specific pathogen.

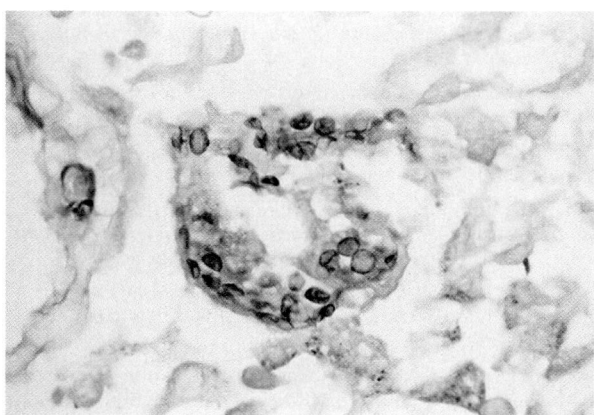

Figure 26-12

GMS stain of bronchoalveolar lavage (BAL) with *P. carinii* cysts.

Bibliography

Alkan ML, Beachey EH: Excretion of lipoteichoic acid by group A streptococci: influence of penicillin on secretion and loss of ability to adhere to human oral epithelial cells, *J Clin Invest* 61:671, 1978.

Axelsson A, Brorson JE: The correlation between bacteriological findings in the nose and maxillary sinus in acute sinusitis, *Laryngoscope* 83:2003, 1973.

Bartlett JG, Finegold SM: Anaerobic infections of the lung and pleural space, *Am Rev Respir Dis* 110:56, 1974.

Beachey EH: Bacterial adherence: adhesin-receptor interactions mediating the attachment of bacteria to mucosal surfaces, *J Infect Dis* 143:325, 1981.

Beachey EH, Ofek I: Epithelial cell binding of group A streptococci by lipoteichoic acid on fimbriae denuded of M protein, *J Exp Med* 143:759, 1976.

Bennedsen J et al: Utility of PCR in diagnosing pulmonary tuberculosis, *J Clin Microbiol* 34:1406, 1996.

Betts RF, Reese RE: Lower respiratory tract infections. In Reese RE, Douglas RG, editors: *A practical approach to infectious diseases,* ed 2, Boston, 1986, Little Brown, p 202.

Beutler B, Cerami A: Cachectin: more than a tumor necrosis factor, *N Engl J Med* 316:379, 1987.

Bodey GP, Buckley M, Sathe YS: Quantitive relationships between circulating leukocytes and infection in patients with acute leukemia, *Ann Intern Med* 64:328, 1966.

Brien JH, Bass JW: Streptococcal pharyngitis: optimal site for throat culture, *J Pediatr* 106:781, 1985.

Broaddus C et al: Bronchoalveolar lavage and transbronchial biopsy for the diagnosis of pulmonary infections in the acquired immunodeficiency syndrome, *Ann Intern Med* 102:747, 1985.

Broughton WA et al: Bronchoscopic protected specimen brush and bronchoalveolar lavage in the diagnosis of bacterial pneumonia, *Infect Dis Clin North Am* 5:437, 1991.

Brubaker RR: Mechanisms of bacterial virulence, *Annu Rev Microbiol* 39:21, 1985.

Buckner CK et al: Parainfluenzae 3 infection blocks the ability of a beta adrenergic receptor agonist to inhibit antigen-induced contraction of guinea pig isolated airway smooth muscle, *J Clin Invest* 67:376, 1981.

Caplan ES, Hoyt NJ: Nosocomial sinusitis, *JAMA* 247:639, 1982.

Carenfelt C, Lundberg C: Purulent and nonpurulent maxillary sinus secretions with respect to pO_2, pCO_2, and pH, *Acta Otolaryngol* (Stockh) 84:138, 1977.

Centers for Disease Control: Cases of specified notifiable diseases—United States, weeks ending December 29, 1990, and December 30, 1989 (52nd week) 39:944, 1991.

Chapman SW, Wilson JP: Nocardiosis in transplant recipients, *Semin Respir Infect* 5:74, 1990.

Cherry JD, Dudley JP: Sinusitis. In Feigin RD, Cherry JD, editors: *Textbook of pediatric infectious diseases,* ed 2, Philadelphia, 1987, WB Saunders, p 161.

Daum RS, Smith AL: Epiglottitis (supraglottitis). In Feigin RD, Cherry JD, editors: *Textbook of pediatric infectious diseases,* ed 2, Philadelphia, 1987, WB Saunders, p 224.

Dobie RA, Tobey DN: Clinical features of diphtheria in the respiratory tract, *JAMA* 242:2197, 1979.

Douglas RG Jr, Alford BR, Couch RB: Atraumatic nasal biopsy for studies of respiratory virus infection in volunteers, *Antimicrob Agents Chemother* 8:340, 1968.

Epstein JB, Gangbar SJ: Oral mucosal lesions in patients undergoing treatment for leukemia, *J Oral Med* 42:132, 1987.

Fishman JA: Diagnostic approach to pneumonia in the immunocompromised host, *Semin Respir Infect* 1:133, 1986.

Foy HM et al: Long-term epidemiology of infections with *Mycoplasma pneumoniae, J Infect Dis* 139:681, 1979.

Friend PA: Pulmonary infection in cystic fibrosis, *J Infect* 13:55, 1986.

Gerber MA et al: Optical immunoassay test for group A beta-hemolytic streptococcal pharyngitis: an office-based, multicenter investigation, *JAMA* 278:23, 1997.

Goldman WE, Klapper DG, Baseman JB: Detection, isolation and analysis of a released *Bordetella pertussis* product toxic to cultured tracheal cells, *Infect Immun* 36:782, 1982.

Good JA et al: The diagnostic value of pleural fluid pH, *Chest* 78:55, 1980.

Goren MB: Phagocyte lysosomes: interactions with infectious agents, phagosomes, and experimental perturbations in function, *Annu Rev Microbiol* 31:507, 1977.

Green GM: In defense of the lung, *Am Rev Respir Dis* 102:691, 1970.

Green GM, Carolin D: The depressant effect of cigarette smoke on the in vitro antibacterial activity of alveolar macrophages, *N Engl J Med* 276:421, 1967.

Gross PA: Epidemiology of hospital-acquired pneumonia, *Semin Respir Infect* 2:2, 1987.

Gwaltney JM Jr: Sinusitis. In Mandell GL, Douglas RG Jr, Bennett JE, editors: *Principles and practice of infectious diseases,* ed 3, New York, 1990, Wiley & Sons, p 510.

Hawkins DB et al: Acute epiglottitis in adults, *Laryngoscope* 83:1211, 1973.

Hays GC, Mullard JE: Can nasal bacterial flora be predicted from clinical findings? *Pediatrics* 49:596, 1972.

Hendley JO et al: Spread of *Streptococcus pneumoniae* in families. I. Carriage rate and distribution of types, *J Infect Dis* 132:55, 1975.

Hooton RW et al: The joint associations of multiple risk factors with the occurrence of nosocomial infection, *Am J Med* 70:960, 1981.

Hopewell PC: Tuberculosis and human immunodeficiency virus infection, *Semin Respir Infect* 4:111, 1989.

Hopewell PC, Luce JM: Pulmonary involvement in the acquired immune deficiency syndrome, *Chest* 87:104, 1984.

Huxley EJ et al: Pharyngeal aspiration in normal adults and patients with depressed consciousness, *Am J Med* 64:564, 1978.

Ida S et al: Enhancement of IgE-mediated histamine released from human basophils by viruses: role of interferon, *J Exp Med* 145:892, 1977.

Johanson WG, Pierce AK, Sanford JP: Changing pharyngeal bacterial flora of hospitalized patients, *N Engl J Med* 281:1137, 1969.

Johnston RB: Monocytes and macrophages, *N Engl J Med* 318:747, 1988.

Kasupski GJ, Leers WD: Presumed respiratory syncytial virus pneumonia in three immunocompromised adults, *Am J Med Sci* 285:28, 1983.

Kendrick PL, Eldering G, Eveland WC: Fluorescent antibody techniques. Methods for identification of *Bordetella pertussis, Am J Dis Child* 101:149, 1961.

Klein JO: Otitis externa, otitis media, mastoiditis. In Mandell GL, Douglas RG Jr, Bennett JE, editors: *Principles and practice of infectious diseases,* ed 3, New York, 1990, Wiley & Sons, p 505.

Lang WR et al: Bronchopneumonia with serious sequalae in children with evidence of adenovirus type 21 infection, *BMJ* 1:73, 1969.

Levy M et al: Community-acquired pneumonia: importance of initial non-invasive bacteriologic and radiographic investigations, *Chest* 92:43, 1988.

Lew P, Zubler R, Vaudaux P: Decreased heat-labile opsonic activity and complement levels associated with evidence of C3 breakdown products in infected pleural effusions, *J Clin Invest* 63:326, 1979.

Linden BE, Aguilar EA, Allen SJ: Sinusitis in the nasotracheally intubated patient, *Arch Otolaryngol Head Neck Surg* 114:860, 1988.

Linneman CC Jr, Nasenbeny J: Pertussis in the adult, *Annu Rev Med* 28:179, 1977.

Lorber B, Swenson RM: Bacteriology of aspiration pneumonia. A prospective study of community and hospital acquired cases, *Ann Intern Med* 181:329, 1974.

Luce JM, Clement MJ: Pulmonary diagnostic evaluation in patients suspected of having an HIV-related disease, *Semin Respir Infect* 4:93, 1989.

Mackowiak PA: The normal microbial flora, *N Engl J Med* 307:83, 1982.

Maki DG: Control of colonization and transmission of pathogenic bacteria in the hospital, *Ann Intern Med* 89:777, 1978.

Male CJ: Immunoglobulin A_1 protease production by *Haemophilus influenzae and Streptococcus pneumoniae, Infect Immun* 26:254, 1979.

McDonald CJ et al: A controlled trial of erythromycin in adults with nonstreptococcal pharyngitis, *J Infect Dis* 152:1093, 1985.

McMillian JA et al: Viral and bacterial organisms associated with acute pharyngitis in a school-aged population, *J Pediatr* 109:747, 1986.

Mermel LA, Maki DG: Bacterial pneumonia in solid organ transplantation, *Semin Respir Infect* 5:10, 1989.

Meyers BR, Wormser G, Hirschman SZ: Rhinocerebral mucormycosis. Premortem diagnosis and therapy, *Arch Intern Med* 139:557, 1979.

Murray PR, Washington JA: Microscopic and bacteriologic analysis of expectorated sputum, *Mayo Clin Proc* 50:339, 1975.

Mustoe T, Strome M: Adult epiglottitis, *Am J Otolaryngol* 4:393, 1983.

Pappenheimer AM: The diphtheria bacillus and its toxin: a model system, *J Hygiene* 93:397, 1984.

Pearson RD et al: Inhibition of monocyte oxidative responses by *Bordetella pertussis* adenylate cyclase toxin, *J Immunol* 139:2749, 1987.

Pittman M, Furman BL, Wardlaw AC: *Bordetella pertussis:* respiratory tract infection in the mouse: pathophysiological responses, *J Infect Dis* 142:56, 1980.

Proud D et al: Nasal provocation with bradykinin induces symptoms of rhinitis and a sore throat, *Am Rev Respir Dis* 137:613, 1988.

Root RK, Sande MA: *New dimensions in antimicrobial therapy,* New York, 1984, Churchill Livingstone.

Sakakura Y et al: Mucociliary function during experimentally induced rhinovirus infection in man, *Ann Otol Rhinol Laryngol* 82:203, 1973.

Scharer L, McClement JH: Isolation of tubercle bacilli from needle biopsy specimens of parietal pleura, *Am Rev Respir Dis* 97:466, 1968.

Schimpff SC, Young VM, Greene WH: Origin of infection in acute nonlymphocytic leukemia: significance of hospital acquisition of potential pathogens, *Ann Intern Med* 77:707, 1972.

Schneerson R, Robbins JB: Induction of serum *Haemophilus influenzae* type b capsular antibodies in adult volunteers fed cross reacting *Escherichia coli* 075:K100:H5, *N Engl J Med* 292:1093, 1975.

Schuller DE, Birch JG: The safety of intubation in croup and epiglottitis: an eight-year follow-up, *Laryngoscope* 85:33, 1975.

Shapiro ED: Milmoe GJ, Wald ER: Bacteriology of the maxillary sinuses in patients with cystic fibrosis, *J Infect Dis* 146:589, 1982.

Simmons BP, Wong ES: CDC guidelines for the prevention and control of nosocomial infections: guideline for prevention of nosocomial pneumonia, *Am J Infect Control* 11:230, 1983.

Sinnott JT, Emmanuel PJ: Mycobacterial infections in the transplant patient, *Semin Respir Infect* 5:65, 1990.

Sorvillo FJ et al: An outbreak of respiratory syncytial virus pneumonia in a nursing home for the elderly, *J Infect* 9:252, 1984.

Stiehm ER et al: Deficient antigen expression on human cord blood monocytes. Reversal with lymphokines, *Clin Immunol Immunopathol* 30:430, 1984.

Stone WJ, Schaffner W: *Strongyloides* infection in transplant recipients, *Semin Respir Infect* 5:58, 1990.

Teele DW et al: Middle ear disease and the practice of pediatrics, *JAMA* 249:1026, 1983.

Todd JK: Throat cultures in the office laboratory, *Bull NY Acad Med* 1:265, 1982.

Uchida T: Diphtheria toxin. In Dorner F, Drews J, editors: *Pharmacology of bacterial toxins,* Tarrytown, N.Y., 1986, Pergamon, p 693.

Vianna NJ: Nontuberculous bacterial empyema in patients with and without underlying disease, *JAMA* 215:69, 1971.

Wald ER et al: Acute maxillary sinusitis in children, *N Engl J Med* 304:749, 1981.

Weiss AA, Hewlett EL: Virulence factors of *Bordetella pertussis,* *Annu Rev Microbiol* 40:661, 1986.

Welliver RC et al: The development of respiratory syncytial virus-specific IgE and the release of histamine in nasopharyngeal secretions after infection, *N Engl J Med* 305:841, 1981.

Wells RG, Sty JR, Landers AD: Radiological evaluation of Pott puffy tumor, *JAMA* 255:1331, 1986.

Winston DJ, Schiffman G, Wang DC: Pneumococcal infections after human bone-marrow transplantation, *Ann Intern Med* 91:835, 1979.

LEARNING ASSESSMENTS

1. Why is it important to distinguish between a positive culture and an infection?

2. Why is it important to assess the clinical history and the patient's immunologic status when considering the potential pathogenicity of a microorganism detected in the diagnostic microbiology laboratory?

3. Why is obstruction of an area of the respiratory tract a risk for infection?

4. Why should the microbiologist maintain awareness of seasonal trends in respiratory tract infections?

5. What are some example situations in which empirical therapy of respiratory tract infections is indicated instead of antibiotic treatment based upon culture and susceptibility testing data?

6. Why are calcium alginate swabs recommended for nasopharyngeal cultures in the diagnosis of *Bordetella pertussis* infection?

7. What is the key clinical difference between bronchitis and pneumonia?

8. For the microbiologist what is the significance of the difference between community-acquired and nosocomial pneumonia?

9. What constitutes a "good sputum specimen" from the perspective of the microbiologist screening a submitted sputum for culture of bacterial respiratory pathogens?

10. Why is it important for the microbiologist to recommend that the clinician expel all air from the syringe and bring it to the lab immediately when aspirating a specimen from an infected space (e.g., empyema fluid)?

CHAPTER 27

Skin and Soft-Tissue Infections

Raymond A. Smego, Jr.

SKIN AND SKIN STRUCTURES
  Anatomy of the Skin
  Usual Skin Flora

CLINICAL INFECTIONS
  Bacterial Skin Infections
    Primary pyodermas
    Secondary bacterial skin infections
    Cutaneous manifestations as a result of toxin
      production
    Miscellaneous bacterial skin infections
    Mycobacterial skin infections
    Actinomycetes and the skin
    Laboratory diagnosis of bacterial skin and
      soft-tissue infections
  Cutaneous Infections Caused by Miscellaneous
    Agents
  Spirochetal Infections
  Mycoplasmal Infections

Viral Skin Diseases
  Warts
  Varicella and zoster
  Herpes simplex
  Other herpesviruses
  Molluscum contagiosum and orf
  Rubeola
  Rubella
  Erythema infectiosum
  Roseola
  Enteroviruses
  Hemorrhagic fever viruses
Fungal Skin Infections
  Dermatophytoses
  Candidiasis
  Subcutaneous mycoses
  Systemic mycotic infections
Parasitic Skin Infections

OBJECTIVES

1. Describe the function of the skin as a host defense mechanism.
2. Discuss the role of the microbial skin flora.
3. List the organisms that compose the skin flora.
4. Name the causative agents of primary bacterial infections.
5. Characterize each of the following pyodermas:
   - Impetigo
   - Folliculitis
   - Furuncle and carbuncle
   - Cellulitis and erysipelas
   - Myonecrosis
   - Paronychia
   - Erysipeloid
   - Erythrasma
6. Describe how each of these infections are diagnosed in the laboratory.
7. Discuss how other agents, such as fungal, parasitic, and viral agents, cause skin infections.
8. Name the mycobacterial species that cause skin infections and describe how the infection is acquired.

KEY TERMS

Impetigo
Pyoderma
Vesicles
Folliculitis
Furuncle
Carbuncle
Cellulitis
Erysipelas
Myonecrosis
Gas gangrene
Paronychia
Erysipeloid
Erythrasma
Hidradenitis
  suppurativa
Ecthyma gangrenosum
Meningococcemia
Petechiae

Purpura
Staphylococcal scalded
  skin syndrome
Toxic shock syndrome
Intertrigo
Buruli ulcer
Leprosy
Cervicofacial
  actinomycosis
Syphilitic chancre
Dermatophytosis
Tinea
Mycetoma
Chromomycosis
Swimmer's itch
River blindness
"Creeping eruption"

SKIN AND SKIN STRUCTURES

The skin is the body's first line of defense against microbial invasion. As a dynamic physical barrier, it continually undergoes epithelial cell turnover, removing substances as well as potentially pathogenic microorganisms that are present on its sur-

face. In addition, the skin is colonized with a variety of resident microbes that perform a protective function.

This chapter discusses the following:

- The role of the indigenous skin flora in the pathogenesis of skin infections
- The wide variety of skin and soft-tissue infections
- The etiology of each of these infections

Anatomy of the Skin

The skin consists of three layers: epidermis, dermis, and subcutaneous layer (Figure 27-1). The epidermis is the outermost layer and is composed of several layers of epithelial cells. The stratum corneum, which is the outermost layer of the epidermis, contains dead cells consisting of a protein called *keratin*. The second skin layer, the dermis, is a thick layer composed of connective tissue. Sweat gland ducts, hair follicles, and oil gland ducts are found in the dermis and penetrate into the subcutaneous layer. These structures also provide potential passageways through which microbes can enter the skin. Sebum and perspiration are able to provide moisture and nutrients necessary for the growth of certain microbes. However, proliferation of other pathogenic mi-

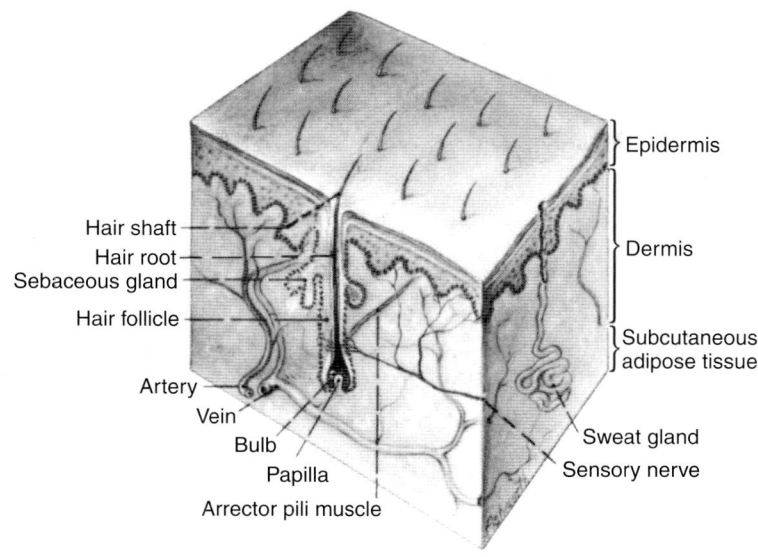

Figure 27-1

Anatomy of the skin. (From Jacob SW, Francone CA: *Elements of anatomy and physiology,* ed 2, Philadelphia, 1989, WB Saunders.)

croorganisms can be inhibited by salt and lysozymes contained in perspiration and in the fatty acids found in sebum.

Usual Skin Flora

Usual flora of the skin consists of those microbes able to adapt to the high salt concentration and drying effects of the skin. Important microflora includes gram-positive cocci such as staphylococci and streptococci. Coagulase-negative staphylococci such as *Staphylococcus epidermidis* are permanent skin residents; coagulase-positive *Staphylococcus aureus* is a transient colonizer. Other normal flora includes diphtheroids, such as *Propionibacterium acnes* and *Corynebacterium xerosis,* and the yeasts *Candida* and *Pityrosporum.* Although vigorous washing reduces the amount of surface skin flora, it does not eliminate resident flora colonization.

| CLINICAL INFECTIONS

There are many infectious diseases of the skin. These can be classified in various ways: according to etiologic organisms (e.g., bacterial, viral, mycobacterial, fungal, parasitic); whether they occur as primary entities, secondary to preexisting skin lesions, or manifestations of systemic disease; or according to the morphology of the skin lesion

(Table 27-1). This section examines each classification and describes some clinically important and prevalent infections of skin and soft tissues.

Bacterial Skin Infections

CASE STUDY

A 37-year-old Haitian woman presented with complaints of a swollen, painful, right breast for 1 week, associated feverishness, and general malaise. She was actively breastfeeding a 2-year-old child. On examination, the woman had a low-grade fever of 100.4° F and there was a 4.5 × 4 cm warm, tender, fluctuant mass involving the medial aureola of the right breast. A small 20-gauge needle was inserted at the point of maximal softening (fluctuance) and 17 ml of pus was aspirated. The lesion resolved with warm compresses and 10 days of dicloxacillin treatment.

Primary pyodermas

IMPETIGO

Impetigo is a common **pyoderma** most often caused by group A streptococci (*Streptococcus pyogenes*) (Table 27-2). Less than 10% of cases are caused by *S. aureus.* Group B streptococci may oc-

TABLE 27-1

Morphologic Types of Skin Lesions and Some Associated Infectious Diseases

Macular, Papular, or Maculopapular Rashes

Rubeola (measles)
Rubella (German measles)
Roseola
Other viral exanthems
Scarlet fever
Toxic shock syndrome
Secondary syphilis

Smooth Papules

Molluscum contagiosum
Condyloma latum (secondary syphilis)

Verrucous Papules or Plaques

Condyloma acuminata (venereal warts)
Viral warts
Cutaneous tuberculosis
Blastomycosis
Coccidioidomycosis
Chromomycosis
Wheals
Urticaria
Scabies
Cercarial dermatitis (swimmer's itch)
Pruritic Papules
Scabies
Folliculitis
Erythematous patches or nodules
Erythema infectiosum (fifth disease)
Bacterial cellulitis
Necrotizing (gangrenous) cellulitis, fasciitis, myonecrosis
Disseminated mycoses

Serpiginous or Annular Plaques

Erythema multiforme
Erythema chronicum migrans (Lyme borreliosis)
Cutaneous larval migrans (creeping eruption)

Vesicles or Bullae

Herpes simplex
Herpes zoster
Varicella (chickenpox)
Hand-foot-mouth disease
Herpangina
Staphylococcus scalded skin syndrome

Pustules

Folliculitis
Impetigo
Acne
Disseminated gonococcal infection
Furuncles, carbuncles
Kerion
Herpetic whitlow
Ecthyma contagiosum (orf)
Milker's nodule
Hidradenitis suppurativa

Petechiae, Purpura, and Ecchymoses

Rocky Mountain spotted fever
Other rickettsial infections
Meningococcemia
Gonococcemia
Infective endocarditis
Plague
Dengue and other hemorrhagic fever viruses
Enteroviral infections
Leptospirosis

Ulcers or Necrosis

Primary syphilis
Herpes simplex
Chancroid
Lymphogranuloma venereum
Granuloma inguinale
Impetigo
Ecthyma gangrenosum
Sporotrichosis
Atypical mycobacteria
Nocardiosis
Histoplasmosis
Anthrax
Ecthyma contagiosum (orf)
Tularemia
Leishmaniasis

casionally cause impetigo in a newborn infant, secondary to acquisition of colonizing vaginal flora from the mother. Initially, lesions of impetigo begin as small **vesicles** that pustulate and rupture, creating a thick, yellow, encrusted appearance. The lesions are superficial and painless but pruritic and easily spread by scratching. A bullous form of impetigo is caused by phage group II strains of *S. aureus* that produce an exfoliative toxin. The localized and discrete lesions produced are thin-walled and blister-like and contain a clear yellow fluid (Figure 27-2). When the bullae rupture, they dry to form a transparent, varnish-like crust.

Impetigo is common in hot and humid climates and is highly contagious. Prompt treatment of impetigo is especially important in infants and children to prevent the development of immune complex–related acute glomerulonephritis, a serious nonsuppurative complication of *S. pyogenes* infections. Oral penicillin or dicloxacillin are the drugs of choice, or erythromycin if the patient is allergic to penicillin. Older topical antibiotic-containing ointments were ineffective in the treatment of impetigo. However, a relatively new topical agent, mupirocin, has proved to be clinically useful and as effective as oral systemic therapy.

TABLE 27-2

Most Common Primary Pyodermas

Infection	Organism	Comments
Impetigo	*Streptococcus pyogenes,* occasionally; *Staphylococcus aureus,* if bullous	Children affected most; communicable; no fever
Erysipelas	*S. pyogenes,* occasionally; other β streptococci or *S. aureus*	Distinct raised borders; fever common
Cellulitis	*S. pyogenes, S. aureus; Haemophilus influenzae* in children	Erythema, tenderness, pain, edema, warmth; fever common
Folliculitis	*S. aureus;* gram-negative bacilli or *Candida* if predisposing conditions	Papules around hair follicles; areas exposed to whirlpool bath (*Pseudomonas aeruginosa*)
Furuncle	*S. aureus*	Fluctuant, painful nodules often in intertriginous areas
Carbuncle	*S. aureus*	Multiple abscesses
Paronychia	*S. aureus,* gram-negative bacilli, *Candida*	Periungual swelling

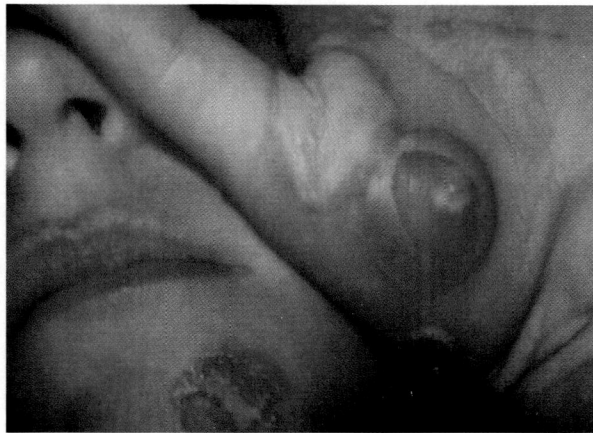

Figure 27-2

Bullous impetigo caused by *Staphylococcus aureus*.

Application of mupirocin to minor abrasions and insect bites in day-care centers may help prevent the spread of impetigo. Healing generally occurs without scarring. Effective treatment of bullous impetigo consists of an oral penicillinase-resistant penicillin, cephalosporin, or erythromycin.

FOLLICULITIS

Folliculitis is an inflammation and infection of hair follicles. *S. aureus* is the most common etiologic agent of folliculitis, although *Pseudomonas aeruginosa* has been implicated in cases acquired from contaminated swimming pools or whirlpools. Lesions appear as small, erythematous papules and often evolve to form pustules with a whitish or yellowish central zone. Common sites for folliculitis include points of friction, such as the hips, buttocks, axillae, and scalp. Infection within the ear canal may lead to otitis externa. Scarring rarely develops. Sycosis barbae is a form of folliculitis occurring in bearded men. A folliculitis caused by *Candida* species or gram-negative bacteria, including *P. aeruginosa,* may occur in immunocompromised hosts.

FURUNCLES AND CARBUNCLES

Lesions of folliculitis may develop into a deeper inflammatory nodule called a **furuncle.** The lesion in Figure 27-3 is a furuncle of the breast described in the case study, perhaps developing secondary to trauma and mastitis related to breastfeeding a toddler. If facilities had been available, Gram stain

of the purulent aspirate would likely have demonstrated gram-positive cocci in clusters and short chains indicative of *S. aureus.* A **carbuncle** is an abscess that extends even more deeply into the subcutaneous fat and may have multiple draining sites. *S. aureus* is the most common causative pathogen. Furuncles are initially red and firm but soon become painful and fluctuant. They generally drain spontaneously. Systemic symptoms such as fever, chills, and malaise may accompany a carbuncle. Carbuncles commonly occur at the nape of the neck and on the back of the thighs. If a carbuncle or furuncle is associated with cellulitis or constitutional symptoms, it should be treated with an oral penicillinase-resistant penicillin or cephalosporin, erythromycin, or clindamycin. Furuncles usually can be managed by the application of moist heat and antimicrobial therapy. Surgical drainage is generally needed for most carbuncles. In cases of recurrent furunculosis, nasal application of mupirocin ointment and orally-administered antibiotics such as ciprofloxacin and rifampin may be useful in reducing or eliminating the nasopharyngeal carriage of *S. aureus.*

CELLULITIS AND ERYSIPELAS

Cellulitis is a diffuse inflammation and infection of the superficial skin layers. It appears as a localized area of mildly painful erythema, warmth, and swelling of the skin with poorly demarcated margins. Depending on its extent and severity, cellulitis may or may not be accompanied by fever and other clinical or laboratory features of sys-

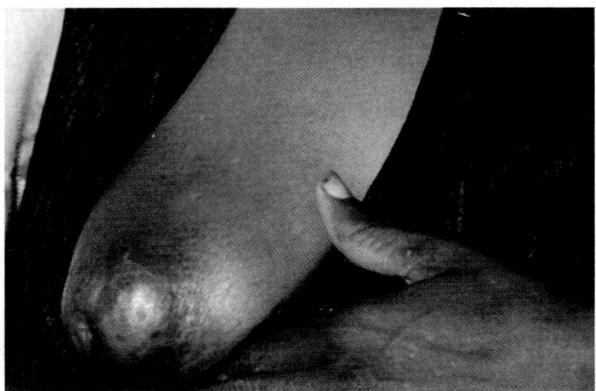

Figure 27-3

Staphylococcus aureus furuncle of the breast.

temic infection (e.g., malaise, rigors, headache, elevated white blood cell count).

In contrast, **erysipelas** is a deeper form of cellulitis that involves not only the superficial epidermis but also the underlying dermis and lymphatic channels. Erysipelas is characterized as a painful, indurated area of cellulitis with a raised, sharply demarcated border and a typical deep crimson hue. Patients generally have fever and leukocytosis. Most uncomplicated cases remain confined to the dermis and lymphatics, but the potential for bacteremia makes erysipelas a potentially life-threatening infection. Erysipelas has a strong predilection for involvement of the face and, to a lesser extent, the lower extremities (Figure 27-4). The majority of cases are caused by group A streptococci, although *S. aureus* can be implicated in roughly 10% of cases. Factors predisposing to erysipelas include diabetes mellitus, venous stasis, alcohol abuse, and lymphatic obstruction. Diagnostic aspiration of the advancing margins of the erysipelas lesion, as described above, may be useful. With bacteremic disease, the causative organism may be recovered from blood cultures. Intramuscular or oral penicillin or oral erythromycin may be effective in very mild cases. In most cases, however, because of the involvement of lymphatics and the potential for blood stream invasion, intravenous therapy with penicillin G or an antistaphylococcal agent should be given.

MYONECROSIS

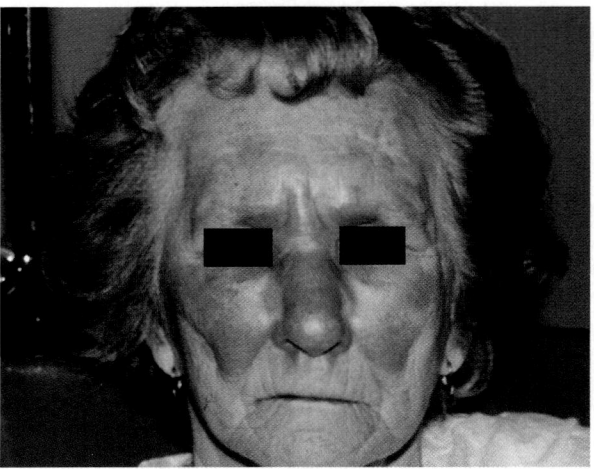

Figure 27-4

Erysipelas due to *Streptococcus pyogenes.*

CASE STUDY

An 18-year-old man suffered a severe crush injury to his right forearm in a dune buggy accident on the beach. He was admitted to a local hospital where within 18 hours he developed high fever and systemic toxicity, with rapidly progressive areas of necrosis, crepitus, and hemorrhagic bulla formation on the arm to the midshoulder. Broad-spectrum antibiotics were begun, and he was transferred by life-flight helicopter to the university hospital for hyperbaric oxygen therapy and surgery. Immediately on transfer he was taken to the operating room for extensive soft tissue débridement.

Clostridial **myonecrosis** is known as **gas gangrene** caused by histotoxic clostridia, which include *Clostridium septicum, Clostridium perfringens, Clostridium novyi, Clostridium histolyticum* and *Clostridium sordelii.* Histotoxic clostridia are anaerobic, gram-positive, sporeforming bacilli found in the soil and are part of the normal flora of the large intestine. Contamination of injured tissue with spore from soil containing these organisms or from bowel flora is the usual means of transmission. For myonecrosis to develop, a lowered oxidation-reduction potential must be present. This is a result of a drop in pH due to the reduction of pyruvate to lactate.

Most infections are polymicrobial, with mixed aerobic-anaerobic, gram-positive and gram-negative bacterial flora being recovered. Anaerobes are the most important gas-producing organisms, with gas being detectable by palpation of the infected area or by soft-tissue radiograph (Figure 27-5). Other bacteria, however, are capable of gas production, including Escherichia coli, Proteus, Klebsiella, Aeromonas, and hemolytic strains of *S. aureus.*

Clinical manifestations of myonecrosis include severe pain, edema, cellulitis, production of gas, and foul-smelling purulent discharge, all leading to tissue death. Treatment is extensive surgical débridement and the administration of polyvalent antitoxin and antimicrobials. The use of a hyperbaric chamber also has proved to be effective.

Infections that produce tissue necrosis and soft-tissue gas represent an important subset of cellulitis cases. Serious and frequently life-threatening, these gangrenous and crepitant soft-tissue infections can be classified according to their level of soft-tissue involvement (e.g., superficial epidermal or dermal structures, fascia, or muscle) and according to the causative microbiologic agent or agents.

As infection progresses from superficial gangrene to deeper necrotizing fasciitis to still deeper myonecrosis, patients appear more acutely ill and toxic, have more soft-tissue pain, and can exhibit a progressive and fulminant downhill course. Gangrenous and crepitant cellulitis represent true medical-surgical emergencies; surgical exploration is invariably required to determine the degree and level of soft-tissue spread, excise all devitalized tissue, and obtain useful deep-tissue specimens for accurate microbiologic processing.

In the case described, superficial, fascial, and muscle compartments of the lower and upper arm were found to be involved by infection during surgery. Gram-staining of bulla fluid and operative specimens revealed fat, spore-forming gram-positive rods with few polymorphonuclear leukocytes, and a diagnosis of clostridial myonecrosis was made. A high amputation of the humerus was performed. Three postoperative treatments with

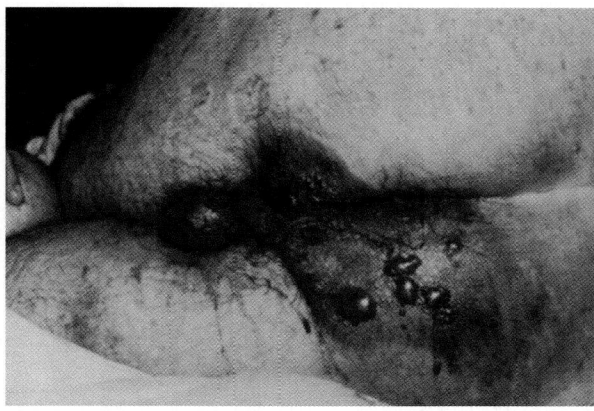

Figure 27-5

Clostridial myonecrosis ("gas gangrene"). (From Upjohn monogram: *Anaerobic infections,* Kalamazoo, Mich, 1986, The Upjohn Co.)

hyperbaric oxygen were administered, and high-dose penicillin G was continued for 14 days. Biochemical testing of anaerobic organisms in pure culture revealed *Clostridium perfringens.*

Aside from cases of infection caused by a single organism (e.g., *C. perfringens* myonecrosis [see Figure 27-5] or *S. pyogenes* necrotizing fasciitis), most of these infections can be treated with a combination of agents active against aerobic gram-positive cocci, Enterobacteriaceae, *Pseudomonas,* and anaerobes.

PARONYCHIA

Paronychia is an infection of the cuticle surrounding the nail bed. Cases generally follow minor trauma, such as removing a hangnail. The involved part of the finger at the nail margin becomes painful, red, warm, and swollen, and pus may be expressed from around the nail bed. Staphylococci usually are the causative organisms. Paronychia usually responds to warm soaks, which often lead to spontaneous drainage of pus and resolution. Systemic antimicrobials and surgery typically are not required.

ERYSIPELOID

Erysipeloid is a superficial soft-tissue infection caused by *Erysipelothrix rhusiopathiae.* It typically occurs as an occupational hazard among handlers of animals, meat, poultry, and fish. The organism is difficult to Gram stain but may be isolated in culture. Mimicking erysipelas, the erysipeloid lesion is red and painful, with raised borders. The finger and the dorsum of the hand are the most common sites of infection. Penicillin G is the preferred treatment.

ERYTHRASMA

Erythrasma is a chronic, pruritic, reddish-brown macular infection found most commonly in men and obese patients with diabetes mellitus. The infection typically is located in intertriginous areas such as the groin, toe web, axilla, and inframammary folds. The lesion tends to be finely scaled and wrinkled. *Corynebacterium minutissimum* is the causative organism and is easily observed with a Gram stain of the stratum corneum. The lesions produce a coral-red fluorescence when examined under a Wood's lamp. Topical clindamycin and oral erythromycin are useful in the management of erythrasma.

TABLE 27-3

Infections Secondary to Preexisting Lesions

Infection	Major Pathogen
Surgical wound infection	
Clean	*Staphylococcus aureus,* gram-negative bacilli
Contaminated, such as colon	Plus anaerobes, streptococci
Intravenous infusion sites	*S. aureus,* coagulase-negative staphylococci
Trauma	
Soil contamination	*Pseudomonas aeruginosa,* clostridia
Freshwater contamination	*Aeromonas, Plesiomonas*
Saltwater contamination	*Vibrio vulnificus*
Bites	
Human	Oral aerobes and anaerobes, *S. aureus*
Dog, cat	*Pasteurella multocida, S. aureus,* anaerobes
Rat	*Streptobacillus moniliformis, Spirillum minus (minor)*
Decubitus ulcer	Streptococci, *S. aureus,* coliforms, *Pseudomonas,* anaerobes including *Bacteroides fragilis*
Foot ulcer in diabetic patients	*S. aureus,* streptococci, coliforms, *P. aeruginosa,* anaerobes
Hidradenitis suppurativa	*S. aureus,* streptococci, coliforms, *Pseudomonas,* anaerobes
Burns	*S. aureus, Candida, P. aeruginosa*

Secondary bacterial skin infections

Table 27-3 lists some common secondary bacterial skin infections that complicate preexisting dermatologic lesions. Etiologic organisms and important epidemiologic associations are also shown. Table 27-4 lists several systemic bacterial infections that have important cutaneous manifestations.

The syndrome **hidradenitis suppurativa** is associated with a genetic defect of the apocrine sweat glands. Chronic obstruction of these glands, especially in the axillae and groin, predisposes to mixed bacterial superinfection of skin and skin structures, often accompanied by fever and tender lymphadenitis. Multiple recurrences of infection led to tissue fibrosis, sinus tract formation, and scarring and disfigurement. Individual episodes of infection are treated with local moist heat, broad-spectrum antibiotics, and frequently with surgical incision and drainage.

CUTANEOUS MANIFESTATIONS OF SYSTEMIC BACTERIAL INFECTIONS

CASE STUDY

A 55-year-old Hispanic man with non–insulin-dependent diabetes came to an emergency room with complaints of fever, pain, and swelling of the right lower leg (Figure 27-6). The patient gave a history of alcohol abuse and hepatitis as a child. Four weeks before admission the patient had eaten raw oysters, and he had experienced diarrhea for the past 2 to 3 weeks. On examination, the patient was acutely ill with tachycardia, hypotension, a slightly enlarged liver, and a right pleural effusion. An ulcerative cellulitis of the right lower leg was present with overlying exudate. The admitting diagnosis was severe soft tissue infection with sepsis syndrome.

Bacteremia with particular organisms can result in various morphologic rashes or lesions. *Vibrio vulnificus,* a halophilic vibrio, has been recognized as a virulent pathogen since 1976, when it was first described. The organism is known to

TABLE 27-4

Cutaneous Involvement in Systemic Bacterial Infections

Infective endocarditis
Bacteremia and sepsis
Scarlet fever
Toxic shock syndrome
Staphylococcal scalded skin syndrome
Enteric fever

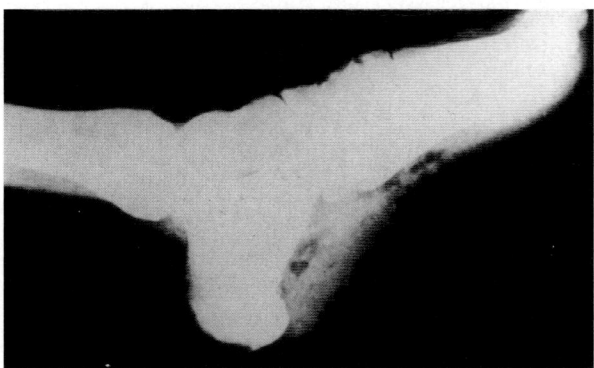

Figure 27-6

Diabetic foot infection with soft-tissue gas formation.

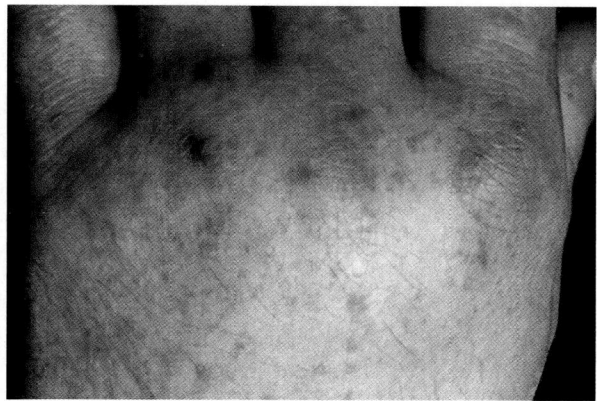

Figure 27-7

Petechial lesion in meningococcemia.

cause severe necrotic cellulitis and primary sepsis. Infections usually are acquired when wounds are exposed to marine water or direct contact with raw shellfish. Ingestion of raw oysters also has been associated with primary septicemia due to *V. vulnificus.* In the case presented, cultures of blood, stool, and urine showed no pathogenic growth. A smear made from the soft tissue exudate showed many gram-negative bacilli, and culture yielded *V. vulnificus.* This isolate was differentiated from *Aeromonas hydrophila. A. hydrophila* has been isolated from cellulitis infections from patients with history of liver disorders. The patient was placed on antimicrobial therapy with ampicillin, gentamicin, and clindamycin; however, the cellulitis continued to worsen and became gangrenous. Surgical exploration revealed necrotizing cellulitis, and an above-the-knee amputation was performed. The patient ultimately had a successful recovery and was discharged from the hospital in stable condition.

Other organisms such as *Pseudomonas aeruginosa* may produce vesicles and bullae in some circumstances. Infection with this organism may cause a macular or maculopapular rash, as in Shanghai fever, a *Pseudomonas* sepsis syndrome seen in the tropics and associated with fever and diarrhea. Also associated with *Pseudomonas* bacteremia are **ecthyma gangrenosum;** a characteristic lesion appears as a painless ulcer with a central black eschar and gangrenous cellulitis. Both of these latter syndromes are encountered most frequently in neutropenic patients.

Bacteremic infections with *Staphylococcus aureus, Streptococcus pneumoniae,* and *Haemophilus influenzae* can cause a rapidly progressive, frequently fatal syndrome called *purpura fulminans,* which results in intracutaneous bleeding. Similarly, the initial skin lesions of **meningococcemia** are erythematous macules, **petechiae,** and **purpura** located on the trunk and extremities (Figure 27-7). They progress to gray, hemorrhagic, necrotic areas. The rash of disseminated *Neisseria gonorrhoeae,* on the other hand, consists of a few painful pustules with a thin zone of purpura. There can be macules, papules, or bullae and occasionally purpuric infarcts. Cutaneous infections due to candidemia are characterized by multiple pink maculopapules or subcutaneous nodules on the trunk or extremities. These lesions are typically seen in immunosuppressed hosts such as neutropenic cancer patients and tissue transplant recipients.

Cutaneous manifestations as a result of toxin production

CASE STUDY

A 48-year-old diabetic man sustained a minor blunt injury to his biceps region. Within 24 hours he developed pain and swelling of the arm, with delirium and high fever, and he was brought to a local emergency room. He appeared acutely ill, and there was edema and tenderness of the upper arm, with several areas of broken skin and black tissue necrosis. No soft-tissue gas was detectable by examination or radiography. The patient underwent immediate surgical exploration, and the infection was noted to have tracked extensively along the fascial planes of the arm, from elbow to shoulder. All devitalized tissue was débrided, and antibiotics begun, but the patient expired 12 hours later.

Certain organisms are capable of producing toxins that affect the skin and result in distinct clinical syndromes. In **staphylococcal scalded skin syndrome** (SSSS), *S. aureus* produces an exfoliative toxin that results initially in fever, skin tenderness, and a scarlatiniform rash, followed by extensive bullae formation and exfoliation similar to that seen in burn patients. Large flaccid blisters form and rupture, causing skin to denude and peel off in sheets and leaving areas of bright-red underlying skin exposed. Nosocomial epidemics of SSSS have been reported in newborn nurseries. Scarring generally does not occur. SSSS requires intravenous administration of antistaphylococcal agents.

In **toxic shock syndrome,** cutaneous desquamation may occur in the late stage as a result of exotoxin F, produced by *S. aureus.* A diffuse sunburn-like erythroderma appears early in the course and is accompanied by fever, hypotension, and evidence of multiorgan dysfunction. Desquamation of skin, especially on the palms and soles, occurs during the convalescent stage of the illness. Although originally described in women in epidemiologic association with superabsorbent tampons colonized with *S. aureus,* toxic shock syndrome occurs in many different clinical settings. Examples are surgical wound infections and contaminated nasal packing in patients with nosebleeds. Treatment consists of supportive measures and antistaphylococcal antibiotic therapy.

A streptococcal toxic shock syndrome caused by *Streptococcus pyogenes* also has been well-described, especially in recent years, with the resurgence of invasive and complicated streptococcal infections. Like its staphylococcal counterpart, streptococcal toxic shock syndrome may occur whenever exotoxin-producing strains of group A streptococci cause infection or colonization of the skin or mucous membranes. In the case presented, Gram stain of the operative deep-tissue specimens revealed gram-positive cocci in chains, and all cultures grew β-hemolytic *Streptococcus pyogenes,* confirming the diagnosis of group A streptococcal necrotizing fasciitis.

Scarlet fever is a characteristic form of group A streptococcal disease that occurs when the infecting strain produces a scarlatiniform or erythrogenic toxin. Clinical characteristics may include those symptoms occurring with a streptococcal sore throat (or the disease may be associated with a wound, skin, or puerperal infection) as well as an erythroderma and a "strawberry tongue" with prominent papillae. The bright red, sandpaper-textured rash is often felt better than seen and appears most often on the neck and chest and in skin folds. Typically, the rash does not involve the face, but there is a flushing of the skin with circumoral pallor. During convalescence, desquamation of the skin occurs, especially on the hands and feet.

Infective endocarditis may cause a number of secondary skin manifestations. Immunologically mediated painful skin lesions located on the pads of the fingers and toes and on the thenar eminence are called *Osler's nodes.* These lesions reflect soft-tissue immune complex deposition. On the other hand, *Janeway lesions* are flat, painless lesions located on the palms and soles that represent microembolic seeding of the skin. Hemorrhagic, vasculitic skin lesions may also be seen in endocarditis (Figure 27-8). Staphylococci and streptococci are typically associated with the above-mentioned skin manifestations, although gram-negative bacteria and *Candida* may produce similar lesions.

The rose spots of typhoid fever, caused by *Salmonella typhi,* are erythematous maculopapular lesions measuring 2 to 4 mm that blanch on pressure. They appear characteristically on the upper abdomen in crops of approximately 10 lesions. The lesions are transient and resolve within hours to days. Rose spots are observed in less than 50% of patients with typhoid fever.

Miscellaneous bacterial skin infections

Cutaneous diphtheria is rare in developed countries but may be seen in tropical climates, especially in areas of overcrowding and where immunization of susceptible populations is inadequate or incomplete. Access is gained through wounds or insect bites. The disease appearance of cutaneous diphtheria is variable and may be indistinguishable from impetigo.

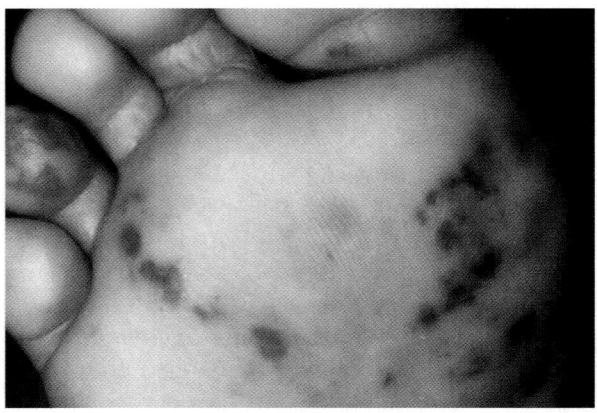

Figure 27-8

Hemorrhagic vasculitic lesion of *Staphylococcus aureus* endocarditis.

Intertrigo is a cutaneous infection occurring in body areas of heat and moisture. As a result of erythema and maceration, skin breakdown may result. This occurs most frequently in the skin folds of obese adults and infants. The most likely organisms include *S. aureus, Candida,* and coliforms.

Melioidosis and *glanders* are diseases caused by *Burkholderia (Pseudomonas) pseudomallei* and *B. mallei,* respectively. Localized infection with lymphangitis and lymphadenitis may be the result of primary inoculation of organisms into the skin. A generalized papular or pustular rash may be seen in the septicemic form of these diseases. Glanders is rare but is often zoonotic in nature.

Francisella tularensis, a gram-negative bacterium, causes several forms of tularemia, including glandular, oculoglandular, pulmonic, and septicemic or typhoidal forms. The ulceroglandular type, however, is most frequently seen and presents as an indolent ulcer, often on the hand, accompanied by painful swelling of the regional lymph nodes. The disease is zoonotic, and human transmission occurs by direct inoculation of skin through handling of infected rabbits and other wild or, less commonly, domestic animals or by the bite of infected fleas, ticks, deerflies, and mosquitoes. Diagnosis of tularemia is most commonly made by a rise in specific antibodies in the patient's serum, although cross-agglutinations with *Brucella, Proteus,* and heterophile antibodies occur. Examination of ulcer exudates, lymph node aspirates, and other clinical specimens using a fluorescent antibody test may provide a rapid diagnosis. The infectious organism can be identified by culture on special media or by inoculation of laboratory animals with material from lesions, blood, or sputum; great care must be exercised with this approach, however, as this highly infectious agent poses an occupational hazard for laboratory workers. Streptomycin with or without tetracycline is the usual treatment.

Two bacterial diseases, rare in the United States, are included under the general term *rat-bite fever;* streptobacillosis is caused by *Streptobacillus moniliformis,* and spirillosis is caused by *Spirillum minus (minor).* They share several clinical and epidemiologic characteristics. An abrupt onset of fever and chills, headache, and muscle pain is followed shortly by a maculopapular or sometimes petechial rash that is most marked in the extremi-

ties. One or more joints then become swollen, red, and painful. There is typically a history of a rat bite within 10 days that healed normally. Laboratory confirmation is made by isolation of the causative organism after inoculating material from the primary lesion, lymph node, blood, joint fluid, or pus into culture media or laboratory animals. Serum antibodies may be detected by agglutination tests. Penicillin G is the treatment of choice.

Bartonellosis is a disease geographically restricted to the high-altitude valleys of Peru, Ecuador, and southwest Colombia. This disease, also called *verruca peruana,* is caused by the aerobic, pleomorphic, poorly staining gram-negative bacterium *Bartonella bacilliformis* and is transmitted to humans by the bite of infected sandflies. Bartonellosis is a febrile systemic infection with associated hepatosplenomegaly, generalized lymphadenopathy, severe anemia, and cutaneous manifestations. The dermal eruption may be miliary, with widely disseminated small, hemangiomatous nodules, or it may be nodular, with fewer but larger deep-seated lesions that are most prominent on the extensor surfaces of the limbs. Individual nodules may develop into tumor-like masses with an ulcerated surface. *Salmonella* infection frequently complicates bartonellosis. The organism may be cultured from the skin and subcutaneous lesions or occasionally from the blood. Diagnosis can also be made by histopathologic demonstration of organisms in tissue specimens using Giemsa staining.

Mycobacterial skin infections

Several *Mycobacterium* species are capable of causing skin infections. Primary or secondary infection with *Mycobacterium tuberculosis* can cause a morphologic array of localized skin lesions, appearing as inflammatory nodules or papules, with lymphangitis and lymphadenitis. Extension from the lymph nodes or bones into the skin is called *scrofuloderma.* Multiple, diffuse skin lesions may result from hematogenous, or bloodborne, seeding to the skin.

Infection with the marine organism *Mycobacterium marinum* develops in individuals with a history of cleaning fish tanks or using swimming pools. The microorganism enters through an open wound or through traumatic inoculation of intact skin. The lesions are generally solitary and appear as a tuberculoid granuloma. Alternatively, the organism may produce a lymphocutaneous syndrome characterized by the initial lesion (ulcer or nodule) followed by satellite lesions and nodular lymphangitis.

Mycobacterium ulcerans infection usually occurs as a single painless ulcer with undermined edges (the so-called **Buruli ulcer** of the tropics). The disease is associated with swamps and may be a chronic infection in tropical climates. *Mycobacterium chelonei* can produce subcutaneous nodules as part of either a local or a disseminated infection, the latter being seen most commonly in patients receiving corticosteroids (Figure 27-9).

The classic skin manifestation of **leprosy,** caused by *Mycobacterium leprae,* is a circumscribed, hypopigmented, or, less commonly, hyperpigmented macule. Lesions can occur singly or multiply, and because peripheral nerves are involved and infiltrated with organisms, these lesions are painless. Acid-fast bacilli and granulomas can be seen in variable numbers in tissue biopsy examinations from persons with leprosy. Disfigurement and deformity of the hands, feet, and cooler parts of the

body, such as the ears and nose, are frequently seen. This is the result of repeated trauma and secondary bacterial infection of neuropathic and anesthetic body parts. Effective treatment usually involves protracted combination chemotherapy (2 years or more) with agents such as rifampin, dapsone, and clofazimine.

Actinomycetes and the skin

Actinomycosis is a chronic disease characterized by the formation of abscesses, fibrosis of tissues, and draining sinuses that discharge sulfur granules. It is caused by non–spore-forming anaerobic or microaerophilic bacterial species (especially *Actinomyces israelii*) of the genus *Actinomyces,* order Actinomycetales. Once thought to be fungi because of their branching, *Actinomyces* species and the closely related *Nocardia* species are classified as higher prokaryotic bacteria. *Actinomyces* species are gram-positive, pleomorphic, and diphtheroidal or, more commonly, delicately filamentous. Although there are thoracic, abdominopelvic, and central nervous system forms of the disease, involvement of the face and neck is the most common manifestation and often follows dental sepsis or manipulation, trauma, tonsillitis, otitis, or mastoiditis. **Cervicofacial actinomycosis** may extend to the underlying mandible or facial bones, leading to osteomyelitis. Penicillin is the preferred treatment.

Nocardia brasiliensis is primarily a cause of skin and soft-tissue infection. Clinical forms of the disease include subcutaneous abscesses, cellulitis, mycetoma, and the lymphocutaneous syndrome. *Nocardia* species can be differentiated from *Actinomyces* by their aerobic growth and partial acid-fastness using a modified Kinyoun stain.

Laboratory diagnosis of bacterial skin and soft-tissue infections

In the management of bacterial infection of the skin, the surface of intact or ulcerated skin is often swabbed for purposes of Gram staining and culture. In most cases, however, this provides little or no clinically useful information because of the lack of correlation between surface colonization and below-the-surface infection. Deep aspirates of involved tissue or specimens taken from closed skin lesions are more interpretable. For example, if pustules or vesicles are present, the roof or crust should be removed

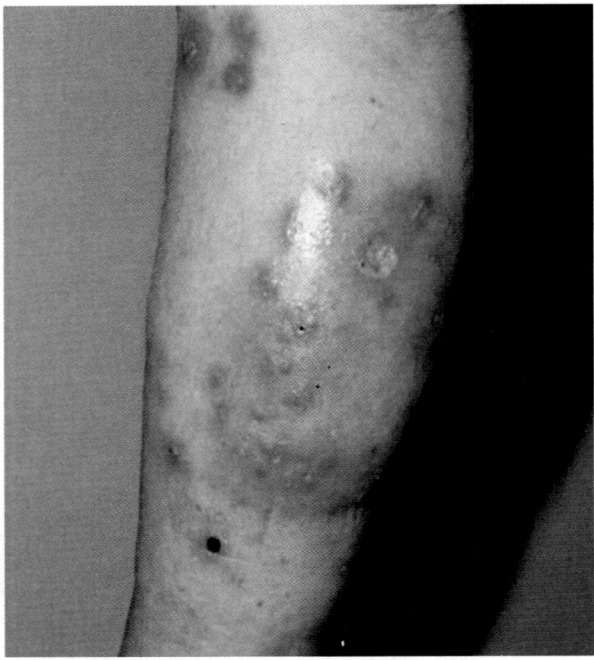

Figure 27-9 _____

Subcutaneous nodules and cellulitis due to disseminated *Mycobacterium chelonei.*

with a sterile blade, and any pus or exudate should be examined, Gram stained, and cultured. Obtaining a specimen in a patient with erysipelas or gangrenous or crepitant cellulitis may involve injecting a small amount (about 3 cc) of preservative-free physiologic saline into the advancing margin of the affected skin, aspirating back, and culturing the fluid that is withdrawn. Exuded pus or wound dressings should always be examined for the presence of granules and branching filaments, suggestive of infections with actinomycetes or fungi.

Laboratory diagnosis of bacterial skin infections may consist of direct smear examination and culture of the affected site, which usually reveal the causative agents. Smears prepared from exudative material and subsequently Gram stained may show the presence of inflammatory cells as well as characteristic morphology that may lead to an initial diagnosis, particularly if the infecting agents are gram-positive bacteria. Myonecrosis infections reveal a mixture of gram-positive and gram-negative bacteria. Results of the direct smear examination are especially important to the clinician, particularly if anaerobic organisms such as *Clostridium* spp. are suspected.

Culture is still the most sensitive method of diagnosing cutaneous infections. Agents of primary infections are recovered in routine culture using primary nonselective media such as blood and chocolate agars and selective media such as MacConkey agar. Additional selective media such as PEA (phenylethyl alcohol) or CNA (Columbia colistin-nalidixic acid) must be included if a mixed infection with gram-positive cocci and gram-negative bacilli is suspected. Samples taken from sites suspected of anaerobic organisms must be transported properly, using an anaerobic transport medium or container to maximize recovery. Since most anaerobic infections are polymicrobial, samples must be inoculated on culture media that are selective for gram-positive and gram-negative bacteria. Identification of isolates is performed using a variety of methods, both conventional and automated.

Antimicrobial susceptibility testing is performed on isolates to demonstrate variable susceptibility patterns. In other cases, such as group A streptococcus in impetigo, the infection is treated empirically.

Agents of cutaneous infections that manifest secondary to systemic bacterial invasion, as in the case of meningococcemia, may or may not be isolated from blood cultures or the site of manifestation. With skin infections that manifest as a result of toxins produced by the invading organism, such as in cases of scalded skin syndrome, toxic shock syndrome, and scarlet fever, the invading organism may not be recovered from the blood or desquamated skin. In most of these cases, the invading organisms are colonizing at a distant focus.

Cutaneous Infections Caused by Miscellaneous Agents

Rickettsiae are gram-negative pleomorphic intracellular pathogens, classified as higher bacteria, that reside within endothelial cells and macrophages. Rickettsial infections are zoonoses; they have various types of animal reservoirs and are transmitted to humans through a number of species-specific insect vectors (e.g., ticks, mites, lice, fleas). Clinical symptoms common to rickettsial infections include high fever, chills, malaise, headache, myalgias, skin rash, and conjunctival injection. Systemic and cutaneous disease manifestations are the pathophysiologic result of diffuse small-vessel vasculitis. Dermatologically, individual rickettsial infections are characterized by the type and distribution of the associated skin rash (e.g., petechial or vesicular, centripetal or centrifugal) and the presence or absence of a black eschar at the insect bite inoculation site.

In Rocky Mountain spotted fever (RMSF), the most frequently seen rickettsial infection in the United States, a maculopapular rash appears on the extremities around the third day. It usually includes the palms and soles and spreads rapidly to most of the body. Petechia and purpura represent extravasation of blood out of blood vessels and into the skin and evolve commonly as a result of the cutaneous vasculitis. The clinical syndrome of RMSF may be confused with atypical measles, meningococcemia, other bacterial sepsis, enteroviral infection, and leptospirosis. The infection is generally successfully treated with either a tetracycline or chloramphenicol.

Spirochetal Infections

Syphilis is an acute and chronic, venereally transmitted treponemal disease. It is characterized clinically by a primary lesion, a secondary eruption involving skin and mucous membranes, long periods of latency, and late tertiary lesions of the skin, bone, central nervous and cardiovascular systems, and other viscera.

The primary lesion usually appears as a papule at the inoculation site about 3 weeks after the initial exposure. Erosion and ulceration then occur, forming the characteristic indurated, painless **syphilitic chancre** (Figure 27-10) (in contrast to the painful "soft chancre" or chancroid caused by *Haemophilus ducreyi*). Firm, enlarged, nonfluctuant regional lymph nodes, called *buboes,* commonly follow. Spontaneous resolution of the primary lesion occurs in 4 to 6 weeks, only to be followed by a secondary eruption involving skin, mucous membranes, and internal viscera such as the liver. Mild systemic complaints, including fever and malaise, commonly accompany secondary syphilis. Both primary and secondary lesions are typically teeming with spirochetes and thus are infectious. Secondary manifestations also disappear spontaneously within weeks. Subsequently, the infection remains clinically latent for weeks to years. Within the first few years, latent syphilis may revert to form infectious mucocutaneous lesions.

Yaws (caused by *Treponema pallidum* spp. *pertenue*), pinta *(Treponema carateum),* and bejel (*T. pallidum;* endemic syphilis) are three other important human treponemal diseases. These diseases differ notably from syphilis in certain respects, such as their geographic occurrence (all rural and outside of the United States), mode of

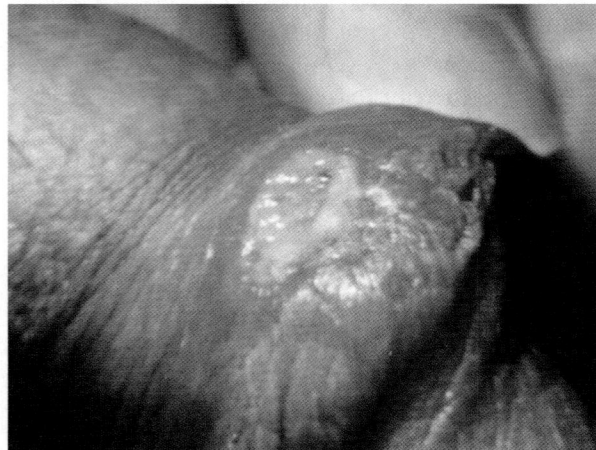

Figure 27-10 _____

Penile syphilitic chancre caused by *Treponema pallidum.*

transmission (all nonvenereal by direct contact), and tissue involvement (skin and/or mucous membrane and bone). They all exhibit clinical latency, share serologic cross-reactivity, and respond to penicillin.

The tick-borne spirochete of Lyme disease, *Borrelia burgdorferi,* characteristically produces a distinctive serpiginous skin lesion called *erythema chronicum migrans* (ECM) at the inoculation site. ECM is the most useful clinical diagnostic marker of Lyme disease. Later manifestations include joint, central nervous system, and cardiovascular system involvement. Various antibiotics, including ceftriaxone, penicillin G, amoxicillin, erythromycin, tetracycline, and cefuroxime axetil, are useful in the treatment of Lyme disease; selection of the most appropriate agent depends on the stage and site of infection.

A nonspecific petechial, macular, or papular skin rash is commonly seen during the primary febrile episode of relapsing fever caused by *Borrelia recurrentis.* The disease can be either epidemic and louse-borne or endemic and tickborne. Diagnosis of relapsing fever is made by demonstration of borreliae in the peripheral blood of febrile patients using darkfield microscopy or Giemsa- or Wright-stained thick and thin blood smears.

Leptospirosis, a zoonotic disease caused by pathogenic leptospires belonging to the species *Leptospira interrogans,* has protean multisystem disease manifestations that may include a nonspecific maculopapular, or at times hemorrhagic, skin rash. The most common mode of transmission of leptospirosis is through contact of intact or broken skin or mucous membranes with water, moist soil, or vegetation contaminated with the urine of infected animals. Many species of domestic and wild animals, rodents, reptiles, and amphibians may be infected. Diagnosis of leptospirosis is made culturally or serologically; penicillin G and doxycycline have some clinical efficacy for this disease.

Mycoplasmal Infections

Although a primary pathogen of the respiratory tract, *Mycoplasma pneumoniae* can cause maculopapular and vesicular rashes, urticaria, and immunologically mediated erythema nodosum and erythema multiform. The major (Stevens-Johnson syndrome) and minor clinical variants of erythema multiforme involve skin plus mucous membranes or skin only, respectively. Mycoplasma-associated erythema multiforme lesions have been reported both with and without apparent respiratory disease.

Viral Skin Diseases

Warts

Warts can manifest in a variety of skin and mucous membrane lesions. These include common warts (circumscribed, hyperkeratotic, rough-textured, painless papules varying in size from a pinhead to large masses), filiform warts (delicate elongated and pointed lesions that may reach 1 cm in length), laryngeal papillomas (located on the vocal cords and epiglottis of children), flat warts (smooth, slightly elevated, usually multiple lesions varying in size from 1 mm to 1 cm), venereal warts or condyloma acuminata (cauliflower-like fleshy growths seen most often in the moist genital and perianal regions—to be differentiated from condyloma lata of secondary syphilis), flat papillomas of the cervix, and plantar warts (flat, hyperkeratotic lesions of the plantar surface of the feet, which are frequently painful).

Warts are caused by several different types of papillomaviruses. Lesions are the result of an uncontrolled but generally benign growth of skin cells. Some forms of cancer, however, namely skin and cervical cancers, may be associated with oncogenic types of papillomavirus.

Varicella and zoster

Varicella infection, or *chickenpox,* is a common childhood illness acquired by respiratory inhalation of the varicella-zoster virus. The skin lesions of primary varicella infection become apparent approximately 2 weeks after initial exposure. The lesions begin as vesicles or small blisters but quickly rupture, pustulate, and begin to scab in 3 to 4 days. The distribution of the rash is centripetal, starting on the trunk and face and later extending to the extremities. A hallmark of the early stages of chickenpox is the appearance of lesions at all of these stages. When primary varicella infection occurs in adults, it tends to be more severe and systemic, involving lungs, central nervous system, and liver. Treatment with the antiviral agent acyclovir is recommended in adults and immunosuppressed individuals.

Varicella-zoster virus is a herpesvirus that exhibits, like other members of the family Herpesviridae, lifelong latency in the human host. After primary infection, the virus enters peripheral nerves and establishes persistence within the dorsal root ganglia. The virus may be reactivated by imbalances between host and virus that are induced by diverse phenomena such as sunlight, emotional and physiologic stress, intercurrent infection, or immunosuppression associated with age, certain diseases, or drug therapies (e.g., corticosteroids and cytotoxics). With reactivation, the virions move along peripheral sensory nerves of the skin, leading to the appearance of a vesicular eruption in a unilateral dermatomal distribution. The resulting condition is called *shingles.* The vesicles are similar to those of chickenpox but remain localized along specific sensory nerves. The disease generally heals in a benign fashion, but with facial involvement, it may spread contiguously along the ophthalmic branch of the trigeminal nerve to the eye (zoster ophthalmicus), resulting in severe pain and threatening sight. In immunosuppressed patients, the virus may disseminate widely to the skin and to internal viscera such as lungs, meninges, brain, and liver. In some elderly patients, a chronic pain syndrome called *postherpetic neuralgia* may follow the acute infection. Acyclovir is the drug of choice for treatment of complicated zoster or to prevent dissemination of localized disease in immunosuppressed hosts.

Herpes simplex

Herpes simplex is a viral infection characterized by a local primary lesion, latency, and the tendency for localized recurrence. The herpes simplex virus, a DNA virus of the herpesvirus family, causes some of the most common skin, and mucous membrane infections affecting humans. Direct contact, with transmission through infected secretions, is the principal mode of spread of herpes simplex.

Primary HSV-1 infection is frequently asymptomatic but may present as severe ulcerative gingivostomatitis and pharyngitis in children under 5 years of age. This initial bout of infection is often accompanied by fever and systemic toxicity. Oral vesicles involving the soft palate, buccal mucosa, tongue, and floor of the mouth quickly ulcerate and may coalesce. Gums are tender and bleed easily, and lesions may spread to the lips and cheek. The breath is fetid, and tender cervical adenopathy is usually present. The differential diagnosis of primary herpetic gingivostomatitis is strepto-coccal pharyngitis, diphtheritic pharyngitis, herp-angina caused by Coxsackie A virus, aphthous stomatitis, erythema multiforme major (Stevens-Johnson syndrome), Vincent's angina (necrotizing gingivitis), and infectious mononucleosis. Herpetic keratitis can be a serious and sight-threatening oc-ular complication of HSV-1 infection, with the de-velopment of punctate, dendritic epithelial opac-ities of the cornea.

Herpes simplex type 1 is the most frequent eti-ologic agent for herpes labialis, a condition com-monly known as *fever blisters* or *cold sores*. Lesions begin as superficial clear vesicles on an erythe-matous base and occur on the lips or in the oropharynx. The lesions heal spontaneously, but because of the property of viral latency and en-dogenous reactivation, they can recur in the same area. Recurrent herpes labialis is generally unac-companied by systemic complaints.

Cutaneous herpes simplex lesions are indistin-guishable from those caused by varicella-zoster virus, although generally they are not as dermatomal in their distribution. In severely immunosuppressed hosts, such as patients with hematologic and lym-phoreticular malignancies and tissue transplant re-cipients, a disseminated and life-threatening form of herpes simplex is associated with diffuse cuta-neous lesions and visceral organ involvement. Eczema herpeticum is a generalized vesicular erup-tion complicating chronic eczema (Figure 27-11). Up to 75% of cases of erythema multiforme, including Stevens-Johnson syndrome, are preceded by an at-tack of herpes simplex, either type 1 or type 2. HSV antigen has been identified in skin biopsy specimens from affected lesions.

Primary herpetic lesions of the finger, called *her-petic whitlow,* can be caused by either HSV-1 or HSV-2. Usually a single digit is involved, with the appearance of one or multiple deep vesicles that may coalesce. Fever and intense local pain are of-ten present. The condition may be misdiagnosed as bacterial paronychia, and unnecessary incision may be performed. Recurrent herpetic whitlow, usually caused by HSV-2, can be a difficult occu-pational problem among medical, paramedical, and dental personnel. Herpetic whitlow in new-borns following fingersucking and serious dis-seminated infection are two important neonatal herpes syndromes. Infants are infected during pas-sage through the infected maternal genital tract.

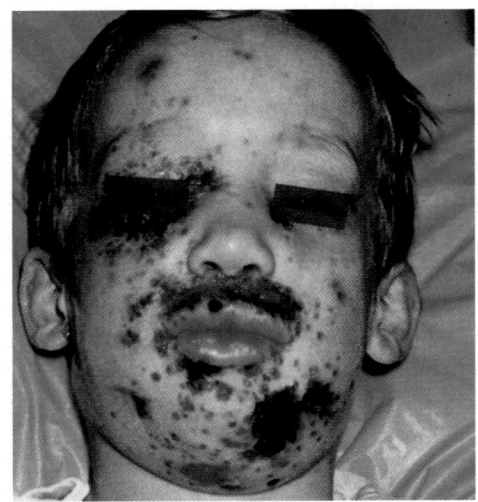

Figure 27-11

Eczema herpeticum due to herpes simplex.

HSV-2 in adults is transmitted primarily by sexual contact, resulting in primary and recurrent her-pes genitalis and perirectal infections. Acyclovir is the drug of choice for herpes simplex infections re-quiring treatment.

Other herpesviruses

Petechial rashes may be observed in congenital cytomegalovirus (CMV) disease. Rubelliform or maculopapular rashes may occur in CMV-induced mononucleosis in both normal adults and im-munosuppressed hosts. Vesicular lesions are dis-tinctly unusual in congenital or acquired CMV in-fection. Epstein-Barr virus (EBV), the cause of heterophile-positive infectious mononucleosis, may produce a rash that can be macular, petechial, scar-latiniform, urticarial, or erythema multiforme–like in about 5% of patients. Administration of ampi-cillin results in a pruritic, maculopapular eruption in 90% to 100% of EBV mono patients, although the mechanism is unclear; the rash disappears after cessation of the drug. This phenomenon has been used by some as a clinical marker of the illness.

Molluscum contagiosum and orf

Molluscum contagiosum is a common skin disease caused by a poxvirus and is characterized by small, firm, waxy papules, often with umbilicated centers; occasionally giant lesions may be seen (Figure 27-12). Molluscum contagiosum is transmitted from person to person by direct contact, in many instances by venereal spread. The disease most often appears on the genitalia, face, or perirectal area. It tends to be self-limited and benign, although lesions can be removed by curettage or cryotherapy using liquid nitrogen for cosmetic reasons.

Human orf is another proliferative cutaneous viral disease caused by a poxvirus of the family Poxviridae. The disease is zoonotic, and humans become infected through contact with infected sheep and goats. The skin lesion is usually solitary and located on the hands, arms, or face; it appears maculopapular or, if secondarily infected with bacteria, may become pustular and be confused with human anthrax. Orf virus, a DNA virus, is closely related to several other parapoxviruses that can be transmitted to humans as occupational diseases (e.g., milker's nodule virus and bovine papular stomatitis virus of cattle). Person-to-person spread is rare, and there is no specific treatment.

Rubeola

Rubeola, or *measles,* is caused by a paramyxovirus and is spread by direct contact with respiratory secretions of infected persons. Measles is one of the most communicable of all infectious diseases. After an incubation period of 10 to 14 days, the clinical features of coryza, conjunctivitis, and cough develop, followed soon thereafter by a maculo-

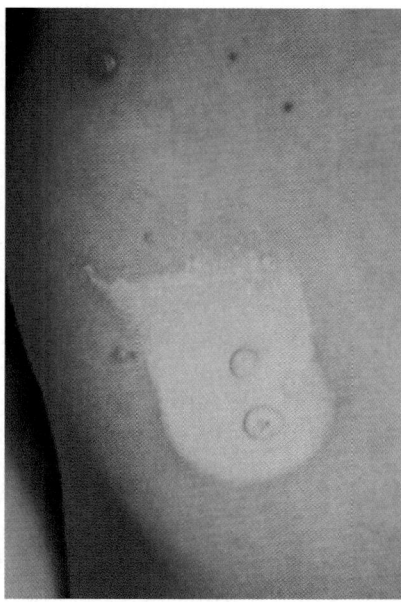

Figure 27-12 _____

Giant molluscum contagiosum.

papular rash. The rash extends from the face to the trunk and extremities. Small red patches with central white specks, called *Koplik's spots,* are characteristically found on the buccal mucosa. Patients with measles are most infectious during the late prodromal phase of the illness, when cough and coryza are at their peak. However, the disease is probably contagious from several days before the onset of the rash to several days after its onset.

Measles can be complicated by secondary bacterial pneumonia, otitis media, or meningoencephalitis. A chronic degenerative neurologic disease called *subacute sclerosing panencephalitis* (SSPE) has been associated with latent measles infection. This condition occurs more often in immunosuppressed children who had measles in early childhood, usually before 2 years of age. Patients with SSPE have unusually high antibody titers to measles virus in their cerebrospinal fluid and blood, and measles virus has been isolated from brain and lymph nodes of patients with SSPE.

Rubella

Rubella (German measles) is an acute exanthematous viral infection of children and adults caused by an RNA agent of the Togaviridae family. Rubella virus is spread in droplets shed from the respiratory secretions of infected persons. The period of contagion extends from about 10 days before the appearance of the rash to 15 days after its onset. Many or most rubella infections are subclinical. For symptomatic persons, the nonspecific maculopapular rash of rubella begins on the face and moves down the body often is accompanied by cervical and occipital lymphadenopathy and, at times, splenomegaly. The disease is clinically milder than measles, although arthritis and encephalitis can be complications. Maternal infection during the first trimester of pregnancy is associated with a congenital rubella syndrome characterized by serious birth defects in the brain, eyes, ears, and heart. Vaccination is highly effective in preventing rubella in susceptible individuals.

Erythema infectiosum

Erythema infectiosum, or *fifth disease,* is one of the common viral exanthematous diseases of childhood. Caused by the human parvovirus B19, epidemic or sporadic disease is characterized by a striking erythema of the face (the so-called "slapped cheek appearance"), followed in 1 to 4 days by a fine, lacelike rash on the trunk or extremities. The rash may fade quickly only to recur during the ensuing 2 to 3 weeks upon exposure to sunlight or heat. Infection is generally not associated with fever, although mild constitutional symptoms may precede the rash. Scarlet fever and rubella are other childhood diseases to be distinguished from fifth disease.

Roseola

Another acute viral infection of childhood is *roseola infantum,* also called *exanthem subitum,* caused by human herpesvirus-6. Infection is most common in children aged 2 to 4 years and is associated with a high fever and a centrifugal maculopapular rash, which ordinarily follows lysis of the fever. Symptoms are generally mild, but febrile seizures have been reported. Subclinical infection occurs commonly, and full immunity follows.

Enteroviruses

Coxsackieviruses and echoviruses cause a variety of exanthems, sometimes associated with enanthems of the mucous membranes of the oropharynx. Mucocutaneous features occur more commonly in infants and children than in adults. With the exception of hand-foot-and-mouth disease, these rashes are not sufficiently distinctive to permit reliable etiologic diagnosis on clinical grounds alone. Rashes caused by enteroviruses therefore may be grouped according to the type of exanthem they mimic: morbilliform or rubelliform (maculopapular) (Coxsackie group A, echoviruses); roseoliform (Coxsackie group A, echoviruses); and herpetiform (Coxsackie group A, herpangina and hand-foot-and-mouth disease). At times, enteroviruses may produce a nonblanching petechial or purpuric rash resembling meningococcemia.

Hemorrhagic fever viruses

A number of viruses of the Togaviridae (e.g., yellow fever and dengue virus), Arenaviridae (e.g., Junin and Machupo viruses), and Bunyaviridae (e.g., Hantavirus) families, as well as several ungrouped viruses (e.g., Ebola, Marburg, and Lassa fever viruses), may cause a characteristic viral syndrome (fever, headache, myalgias, nausea and vomiting, abdominal pain, prostration) accompanied by severe bleeding manifestations (e.g., gastrointestinal bleeding, hematuria). Bleeding into the skin results in petechiae, purpura, and ecchy-

moses. Many of these hemorrhagic fever viruses are zoonotic, having a rodent reservoir and/or an arthropod vector, with humans as accidental hosts. Treatment is supportive only, and preventive measures include rodent vector control and isolation for those illnesses in which person-to-person transmission occurs, such as Lassa fever, Congo-Crimean hemorrhagic fever, and Marburg and Ebola viruses.

Fungal Skin Infections
Dermatophytoses

Dermatophytes are fungi that colonize keratinized hair, nails, and skin. **Dermatophytosis** and **tinea** are general terms, essentially synonymous, used to denote superficial fungal diseases of various parts of the body. *Ringworm* is another term often applied to these infections and reflects the tendency of some lesions to expand annularly. The mode of transmission is generally through direct skin-to-skin contact or indirect contact through fomites or environmental surfaces. Various genera and species of fungi known collectively as dermatophytes are the causative agents. For most dermatophytoses, humans are the primary reservoir; occasionally, infections may be acquired from infected domestic animals. The various tinea infections generally have an appellation to describe the site of occurrence. For example, *tinea cruris* (jock itch) is ringworm of the groin and perianal region; *tinea pedis* (athlete's foot) is ringworm of the feet; *tinea corporis* is ringworm of the body (Figure 27-13); *tinea capitis* is ringworm of the scalp (Figure 27-14); and *tinea unguium,* or *onychomycosis,* is ringworm of the nails. Three genera and more than 30 species of dermatophytes cause infection; superficial fungal species that most often cause dermatophytoses include *Trichophyton,* which infects hair, skin, and nails, *Epidermophyton,* which infects skin and nails, and *Microsporum,* which generally infects only the hair and skin.

Tinea versicolor, or *pityriasis versicolor,* is an extremely common dermatophytosis that occurs worldwide. The disease is caused by *Malassezia furfur,* a lipophilic yeast and normal skin commensal. The characteristic skin manifestation of tinea versicolor is a diffuse distribution of hypopigmented or, less commonly, hyperpigmented macules principally located on the trunk and proximal portions of the extremities (Figure 27-15, *A* and *B*). The le-

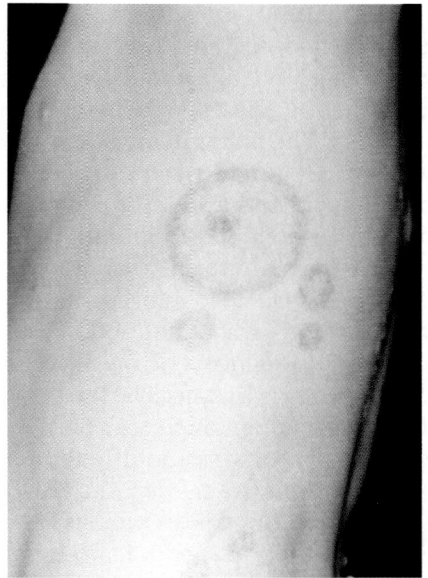

Figure 27-13
Tinea corporis.

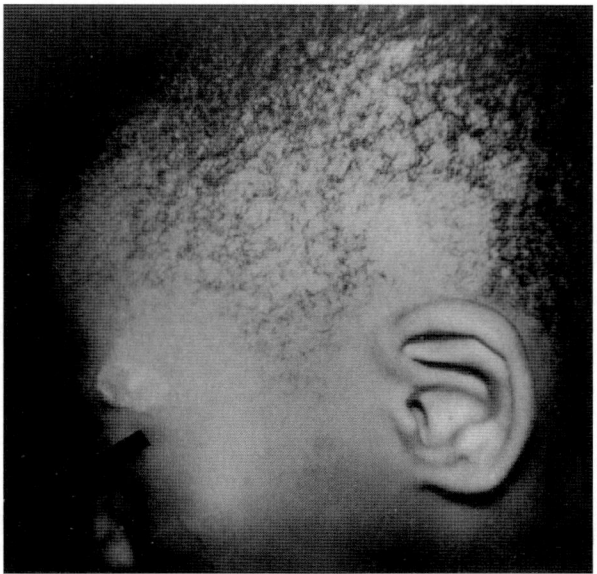

Figure 27-14
Tinea capitis.

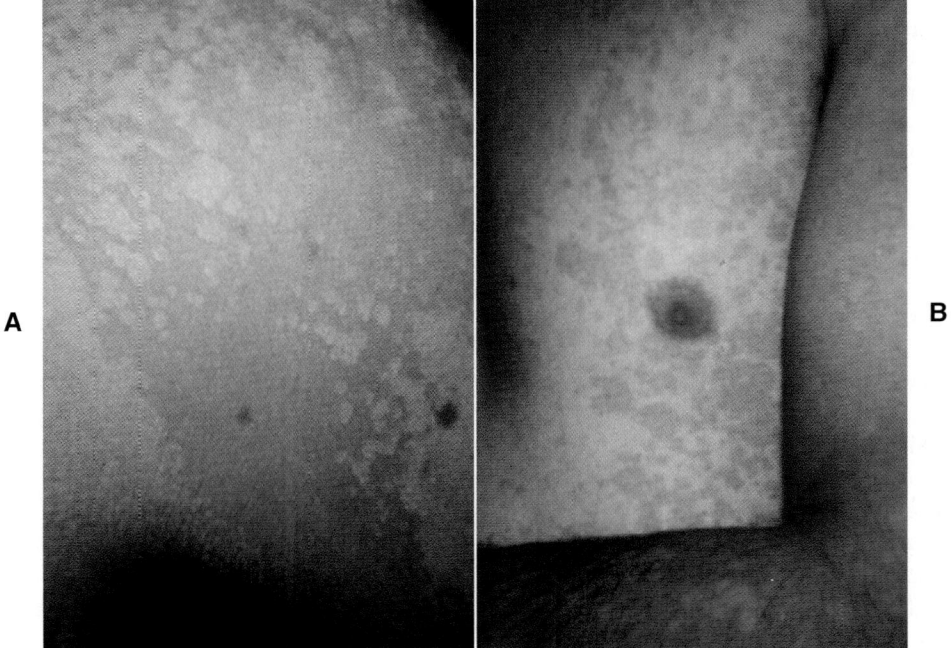

Figure 27-15
Hypopigmented **(A)** and hyperpigmented **(B)** rash of tinea versicolor.

sions are usually nonpruritic and often coalesce to form scaly plaques. Spontaneous remission may occur in some patients; for others, topical ketoconazole cream or selenium sulfide lotion is usually curative.

The diagnosis of dermatophytosis and the identification of its etiologic agents can generally be accomplished by microscopic examination of 10% potassium hydroxide (KOH) preparations of involved skin, hair, and nails or detritus beneath the nails. Skin or nails can be scraped with a scalpel blade, or nails can be clipped to obtain material for identification. Any deep or suppurative lesions should be aspirated. Precise mycologic etiology is confirmed by culture on Sabouraud agar.

Effective antifungal therapy in managing these superficial infections consists of topical powders, ointments, and creams. Useful preparations contain zinc undecylenate, tolnaftate, miconazole, or clotrimazole. Griseofulvin and ketoconazole, two oral agents, are used to treat more deep-seated nail infections.

Candidiasis

Candidiasis is a superficial mycosis caused by *Candida albicans* and other species. It is generally confined to the superficial layers of the skin or mucous membranes. The term *thrush* is applied to a specific form of oral candidiasis characterized by white, curd-like patches on the tongue or elsewhere on the mucosal surface of the oropharynx. These lesions are typically adherent but can be removed by scraping, leaving a raw, bleeding, and painful surface. Other mucocutaneous candidal syndromes are *intertrigo* (including diaper rash), an inflammation of the webs of the toes, axillae, umbilicus, groin, and inter- or inframammary and gluteal folds; *paronychia,* an inflammation of the folds of the skin bordering the nail beds; *onychia,* an inflammation of the matrix that may lead to loss of the nail; *folliculitis,* an inflammation of the hair follicles; *balanitis,* an inflammation of the glans penis; and vulvovaginitis.

Cutaneous lesions of bloodborne disseminated candidiasis can be polymorphic in appearance, but they are most commonly found as macronodules, petechiae, purpura, and ecthyma gangrenosum. These lesions are most commonly seen in immunosuppressed individuals, such as neutropenic cancer patients. *Chronic mucocutaneous candidiasis* is a term used to describe a heterogeneous group of *Candida* infections of the skin, mucous membranes, hair, and nails that have a protracted and persistent course despite what is usually adequate therapy. The major manifestations are disfiguring lesions of the face, scalp, and hands. These infections have been associated with defects in T-cell lymphocyte-mediated immunity and with endocrinopathies such as hypoparathyroidism and Addison's disease. Most forms of this disease begin in infancy or early childhood.

A presumptive diagnosis of any of the mucocutaneous *Candida* syndromes is based on the characteristic clinical appearance of the lesions and is supported by demonstration of pseudohyphae and/or yeast cells in Gram-stained or KOH preparations of swabs, scrapings, or biopsies of infected tissue. Culture on blood agar or Sabouraud agar is confirmatory. Gentian violet, topical nystatin, and imidazoles such as clotrimazole and miconazole are effective in many forms of superficial candidiasis. Systemic agents such as ketoconazole, fluconazole, and amphotericin B may be needed for more severe or systemic infections.

Subcutaneous mycoses

The subcutaneous mycoses include a number of infections of skin and soft tissues caused by diverse fungi. These infections include mycetoma, chromomycosis, sporotrichosis, phaeohyphomycosis, subcutaneous phycomycosis, rhinosporidiosis, rhinoentomophthoromycosis, and Lobo's disease (Table 27-5). Typically, causative organisms present in soil and vegetation are traumatically inoculated into the skin and slowly spread to surrounding tissues. As a rule, there are no spontaneous remissions. Mycetoma, chromomycosis, and sporotrichosis are discussed below in some detail.

MYCETOMA

Mycetoma (also called *Madura* foot or *maduromycosis*) is a clinical syndrome caused by a variety of aerobic actinomycetes (actinomycetoma) and fungi (eumycetoma) (see Table 27-5). It is characterized by swelling and suppuration of subcutaneous tissues and formation of sinus tracts, with visible granules in the pus draining from these fistulae. The disease process is slowly progressive and destructive, with extension to muscle and

TABLE 27-5
Major Etiologic Agents of Subcutaneous Mycoses

Disease	Principal Organism(s)
Mycetoma	*Madurella mycetomatis, Madurella grisea, Scedosporium apiospermum, Leptosphaeria senegalensis, Exophiala jeanselmei, Pyrenochaeta romeroi, Fusarium* spp., *Acremonium* spp., *Pseudoallescheria boydii, Aspergillus nidulans, Neotestadina rosatii, Actinomadura madurae, Actinomadura pelletieri, Nocardia brasiliensis, Nocardia asteroides, Nocardia caviae, Streptomyces somaliensis*
Chromomycosis	*Phialophora verrucosa, Fonsecaea pedrosoi, Fonsecaea. compacta, Cladophialophora carrionii, Rhinocladiella aquaspersa*
Subcutaneous phycomycosis	*Basidiobolus haptosporus*
Phaeohyphomycosis	Dematiaceous fungi
Sporotrichosis	*Sporothrix schenckii*
Rhinosporidiosis	*Basidiobolus seeberi*
Rhinoentomoph- thoromycosis	*Conidiobolus*
Lobo's disease	*Loboa loboi*

bone. Soil and decaying vegetation are reservoirs for the etiologic organisms. The disease develops through subcutaneous implantation of conidial, hyphal, or filamentous elements from a saprophytic source by penetrating trauma (e.g., thorns, splinters). There is no person-to-person transmission. Lesions usually appear on the lower leg or face, sometimes on the hand, shoulder, and back, and rarely at other sites.

Mycetoma is rare in the continental United States but common in tropical and subtropical parts of the world, especially where people go barefoot. Actinomycetoma frequently responds to combination antimicrobial treatment with sulfones and streptomycin or trimethoprim-sulfamethoxazole plus streptomycin or rifampin. Eumycetoma is generally refractory to drug therapy, and radical surgery is usually required.

Mycetoma may be difficult to distinguish from chronic osteomyelitis and botryomycosis, the latter being a clinically and pathologically similar entity caused by a variety of bacteria, including staphylococci and gram-negative bacteria. Specific diagnosis depends on visualizing the granules in fresh preparations or histopathologic sections and isolating the causative actinomycete or fungus in culture.

CHROMOMYCOSIS

Chromomycosis, or *chromoblastomycosis,* is a chronic spreading mycosis of the skin and subcutaneous tissues, usually of a lower extremity and, less commonly, the hand or back. The geographic occurrence and mode of transmission are similar to those of mycetoma. Progression to contiguous soft tissue is slow, over a period of years, with eventual large verrucous or even cauliflower-like masses and lymphatic stasis. Unlike the case with mycetoma, muscle and bone are generally not involved.

Infectious agents of chromomycosis include *Phialophora verrucosa, Fonsecaea pedrosoi, Cladophialophora carrionii,* and *Rhinocladiella aquaspersa.* Microscopic examination of scrapings or biopsies from lesions reveals characteristic brown, thick-walled, rounded cells that divide by fusion in two planes. Confirmation of the diagnosis is made by biopsy and culture of the causative fungus.

SPOROTRICHOSIS

Sporotrichosis is caused by a dimorphic fungus called *Sporothrix schenckii,* which is capable of existing in both yeast (in human tissue) and hyphal (in the environment) forms. Introduction of the fungus through the skin occurs by pricks of thorns or barbs, the handling of sphagnum moss, or slivers from wood, lumber, and other material contaminated with the organism. Worldwide in distribution but characteristically sporadic in occurrence, sporotrichosis is most often an occupational disease of gardeners, farmers, and horticulturalists.

The disease begins as a nodule at the inoculation site, which may ulcerate and remain confined (cutaneous form) or grow and develop surrounding satellite nodules and involve draining lymphatic channels as nodular lymphangitis (lymphocutaneous form). Internal visceral spread is rare. Other microorganisms capable of causing a lymphocutaneous syndrome are listed in Table 27-6.

Laboratory confirmation of sporotrichosis is made by culture of pus or exudate, preferably aspirated from an unopened lesion. Organisms are rarely visualized by direct smear of these materials, but Gomori methenamine silver and other fungal stains of biopsied tissue often reveal the causative agent. Oral potassium iodide is an effective treatment in many cases of soft-tissue sporotrichosis; more extensive or refractory in-

TABLE 27-6
Microbiologic Causes of Lymphocutaneous Syndrome

Fungi	Mycobacteria
Sporothrix schenckii	*Mycobacterium marinum*
Blastomyces dermatitidis	*Mycobacterium kansasii*
Histoplasma capsulatum	*Mycobacterium chelonae*
Coccidioides immitis	
Scopulariopsis blochi	**Spirochetes**
	Treponema pallidum
Actinomycetes	
Nocardia brasiliensis	**Bacteria**
	Staphylococcus aureus
Parasites	*Francisella tularensis*
Leishmania braziliensis ssp.	**Viruses**
braziliensis ssp. *panamensis*	Herpes simplex
Leishmania major	

fections may be treated with intravenous amphotericin B or oral itraconazole.

Systemic mycotic infections

Although the respiratory tract is their portal of entry into the body, almost all systemic mycoses can produce secondary skin lesions through hematogenous seeding to skin. Lesions most commonly appear as macronodules (e.g., caused by *Candida, Cryptococcus,* or dimorphic fungi), verrucous papules or plaques *(Blastomyces, Coccidioides),* ulcers *(Histoplasma),* or areas of black tissue necrosis (due to *Aspergillus,* Zygomycetes, or dematiaceous and other opportunistic fungi).

Parasitic Skin Infections

A number of parasites have minor dermatologic manifestations. The larvae of certain schistosomes of birds and mammals may penetrate the human skin and cause a dermatitis, sometimes known as **swimmer's itch.** Infection is acquired from water containing free-living larvae, or *cercariae,* that have developed in snails. These nonhuman schistosomes do not mature in humans. Such infections may be prevalent among bathers in lakes in many parts of the world, including the Great Lakes region of North America and certain coastal beaches.

The intestinal helminth *Strongyloides stercoralis* may also cause a transient dermatitis when larvae of the parasite penetrate the skin on initial infection. The usual permanent habitat of adult *Strongy-*

loides worms is the large intestine. With chronic infection, an intensely pruritic dermatitis radiating from the anus may occur. Stationary urticarial wheals lasting 1 to 2 days may appear, as well as a migrating serpiginous rash. Penetration of skin, usually of the feet, by hookworm larvae may cause a "ground-itch" dermatitis.

Onchocerciasis is a chronic, nonfatal filarial disease caused by the tissue nematode *Onchocerca volvulus.* Confined geographically to parts of West Africa, Mexico, Central and South America, and the Middle East, the disease is spread to humans by the bite of infected blackflies. Infective larvae injected by the bite develop into adult worms and form nodules in subcutaneous tissues (Figure 27-16), particularly in the head and shoulders, pelvic girdle, and lower extremities. Adult female worms discharge microfilariae, which migrate through the skin, often accompanied by an intensely itchy rash, edema, and atrophy of the skin. The most important manifestation of onchocerciasis, or **river blindness,** is infiltration of the eye by microfilariae, which causes visual disturbances and blindness. Laboratory diagnosis of the cutaneous disease is made by superficial skin biopsy, with demonstration of microfilariae in fresh preparations by microscopic examination or excision of cutaneous nodules and the finding of adult worms. Ivermectin, a microfilaricidal drug given as a single dose and annual retreatment, is useful in reducing morbidity and interrupting transmission of the parasite.

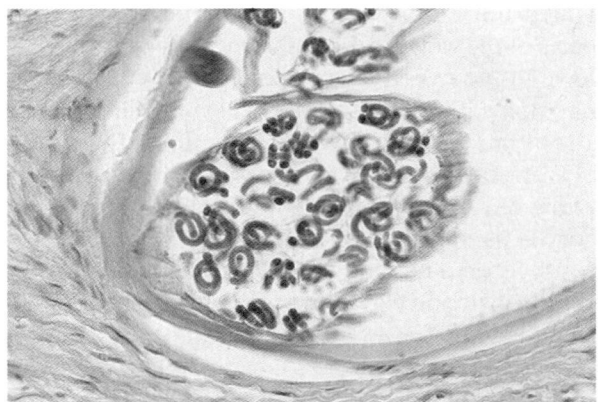

Figure 27-16
Tissue cross-section of a nodule containing *Onchocerca volvulus* microfilaria.

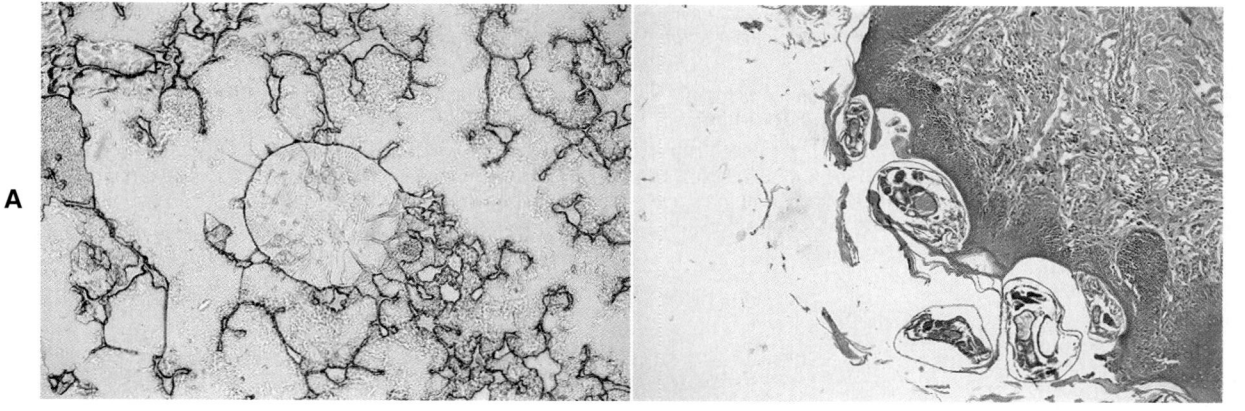

Figure 27-17

A, *Sarcoptes scabiei* adult showing short legs and conical spines. **B,** Tissue cross-section of scabies lesion showing larvae burrowed into the epidermal layer of the skin.

Dracunculiasis, or *guinea worm infection,* is an infection of the subcutaneous and deeper tissues caused by the tissue nematode *Dracunculus medinensis.* A blister appears—usually on the lower extremity, especially the foot—when the gravid meter-long adult female worm prepares to discharge its larvae. Burning and itching of the overlying skin develop and may be accompanied by fever, nausea and vomiting, diarrhea, headache, generalized urticaria, shortness of breath, and eosinophilia. After the vesicle ruptures, the worm releases larvae whenever the affected part is immersed in water. Local inflammation and adhesions, associated with reactogenic larvae or deterioration of the adult worm, and secondary bacterial superinfection may complicate dracunculiasis. Diagnosis is made by microscopic examination of larvae or by recognition of the adult worm. The disease is found in India, Africa, and the Middle East, especially in regions with dry climates. Treatment involves either slow, gradual traction and removal of the emerging worm by winding it around a stick or surgical extraction of the worm before its emergence.

Larvae of the dog and cat hookworms, *Ancylostoma caninum* and *Ancylostoma braziliense,* respectively, can penetrate the skin and produce a self-limited dermatitis **("creeping eruption")** characterized by larval migration above the germinative layer with associated serpiginous, elevated tunnels and indurated, itchy papules. Larvae enter the skin and migrate intracutaneously for prolonged periods. The disease is a recreational hazard of children who play in sandboxes frequented by cats and an occupational hazard of workers who crawl or work in areas with damp, sandy soil contaminated by dog or cat feces. Spontaneous cure is the rule, although individual larvae can be killed by freezing with ethyl chloride spray. Oral thiabendazole may be effective for rare systemic infection or as an ointment for topical use.

A number of ectoparasites may cause human infection, including lice (pediculosis), mites (scabies) (Figure 27-17, *A* and *B*), fleas, flies, ticks, chiggers, and bedbugs. The dermatologic features of these infestations include severe itching and the formation of papules, vesicles, nodules, linear burrows, and excoriations of the skin and scalp.

Bibliography

Benenson AS, editor: *Control of communicable diseases in man,* Washington, DC, 1995, American Public Health Association.

Lewis RT: Necrotizing soft tissue infections, *Infect Dis Clin North Am* 3:693, 1992.

Lipsky BA, Pecoraro RE, Wheel LJ: The diabetic foot: soft tissue and bone infection, *Infect Dis Clin North Am* 3:409, 1990.

Norden CW: Osteomyelitis. In Mandell GL, Douglas RG Jr, Bennett JE, editors: *Principles and practice of infectious diseases,* New York, 1990, Churchill Livingstone.

Smego RA Jr, Castiglia M, Asperilla MO. Lymphocutaneous syndrome: a review of non-sporothrix causes, *Medicine* (in press).

Smith JW: Infectious arthritis. In Mandell GL, Douglas RG Jr, Bennett JE, editors: *Principles and practice of infectious diseases,* New York, 1990, Churchill Livingstone.

Stevens DL et al: Severe group A streptococcal infections associated with a toxic shock–like syndrome and scarlet fever toxin A, *N Engl J Med* 321:1, 1989.

Swartz MN: Cellulitis and superficial infections. In Mandell GL, Douglas RG Jr, Bennett JE, editors: *Principles and practice of infectious diseases,* New York, 1990, Churchill Livingstone.

Swartz MN: Subcutaneous tissue infections and abscesses. In Mandell GL, Douglas RG Jr, Bennett JE, editors: *Principles and practice of infectious diseases,* New York, 1990, Churchill Livingstone.

Waldvogel FA, Medoff G, Swartz MN: Osteomyelitis: a review of clinical features, therapeutic considerations and unusual aspects, *N Engl J Med* 282:198, 1970.

Waldvogel FA, Vasey H: Osteomyelitis: the past decade, *N Engl J Med* 303:360, 1980.

Wallace RJ Jr et al: Clinical trial of clarithromycin for cutaneous (disseminated) infection due to *Mycobacterium chelonae, Ann Intern Med* 119:482, 1993.

Wolfson JS, Sober AJ, Rubin RH: Dermatologic manifestations of infections in immunocompromised patients, *Medicine* 64:115, 1985.

LEARNING ASSESSMENT

1. An exudate from a leg wound grew hemolytic, creamy or buttery-looking colonies on sheep blood agar after 24 hours of incubation. Microscopically, the organisms were gram-positive cocci that appear singly, in pairs, and clusters. When tested, the isolate was catalase and coagulase-positive. Forty-eight hours later, small, beta-hemolytic clear colonies grew on the primary culture medium. The second isolate, also a gram-positive cocci, was catalase negative, with no growth on bile esculin agar, and positive for PYR. What pathogenic species are described in this case?

2. What bacterial agents cause the disease referred to as "rat-bite fever?"

3. What organisms are usually associated with folliculitis?

4. What conditions are necessary for myonecrosis to develop?

5. Which bacterial species usually manifest cutaneously as a result of a systemic spread?

6. Which bacterial species produce cutaneous manifestations as a result of toxin production?

7. Actinomycosis is caused by a wide variety of agents. How are they differentiated?

8. Which of the common childhood viral diseases may manifest in adults after a period of latency?

9. How are these differentiated to conditions?

10. Which parasitic agents cause "creeping eruption?"

CHAPTER 28

Gastrointestinal Infections and Food Poisoning

Connie R. Mahon, George Manuselis

GENERAL CONCEPTS IN EVALUATING
  GASTROINTESTINAL INFECTIONS
  AND FOOD POISONING

ANATOMIC CONSIDERATIONS

THE ROLE OF THE USUAL FLORA

A PRACTICAL APPROACH TO DIAGNOSIS
  OF THE PATIENT WITH DIARRHEA
    History
    Physical Examination
    Laboratory Studies

PATHOGENIC MECHANISMS AND CLINICAL
  PRESENTATIONS OF ACUTE DIARRHEA
    Enterotoxin-Mediated Diarrhea
    Diarrhea Mediated by Invasion of Bowel Mucosal
      Surface
    Diarrhea Mediated by Invasion of Full Bowel
      Thickness with Lymphatic Spread

COMMON BACTERIAL, VIRAL, AND PARASITIC
  GASTROINTESTINAL INFECTIONS AND THEIR
  AGENTS
    Bacterial Agents
      Campylobacter jejuni
      Salmonella species
      Shigella species
      Diarrheogenic Escherichia coli

Vibrio species
Yersinia enterocolitica
Clostridium difficile
Listeria monocytogenes
  Viral Agents
  Parasitic Agents

COMPLICATIONS OF DIARRHEAL INFECTIONS

NEWLY RECOGNIZED AGENTS
  OF ACUTE DIARRHEA

AGENTS OF FOOD POISONING

LABORATORY DIAGNOSIS
  OF GASTROINTESTINAL PATHOGENS
    Specimen Collection and Handling
    Direct Microscopic Examination
    Culture
      Campylobacter jejuni
      Salmonellae
      Shigellae
      Escherichia coli
      Yersinia species
      Vibrio species
      Clostridium species
      Helicobacter pylori

TREATMENT OF DIARRHEA

OBJECTIVES

1. Explain the role of the usual gastrointestinal tract flora in preventing diarrheal illness. Name the organisms that are usually found as colon flora.
2. Describe the other immune defenses at this site that play a role in preventing gastrointestinal disease.
3. Explain the pathogenic mechanisms involved in acute bacterial diarrheas.
4. Give the sources of these infectious agents and describe how they are acquired.
5. Describe the parameters commonly used for presumptive differential diagnosis.
6. For each of the agents described:
   ▪ Give the pathophysiology and clinical manifestations of the infection.
   ▪ Describe the method for diagnosis and general characteristics, including the selective media for maximum recovery of the agent.

KEY TERMS

Median infectious dose
  (ID$_{50}$)
Achlorhydria
"Traveler's diarrhea"
Skin tenting
Toxic megacolon
Enterotoxin-mediated
  diarrhea
Nontyphoidal
  salmonella
Enteric fever

Intracellular pathogens
Shigellosis
Cholera
Anisakiasis
Acute diarrhea
Scombroid
Ciguatera
Paralytic shellfish
  poisoning

Acute diarrheal illness is among the most common problems presented to the clinician. Although most patients have a self-limiting illness typically lasting fewer than 5 days, others may experience severe chronic symptoms, bacteremia, metastatic infection, life-threatening dehydration or chronic sequelae. The early identification and treatment of individuals are key factors in limiting morbidity and mortality. This chapter reviews the host and organism factors that lead to diarrheal illness; discusses common bacterial, viral, and parasitic pathogens of diarrheal diseases and the mechanisms they employ; presents a clinical and laboratory diagnostic approach to this problem; summarizes various treatment interventions.

GENERAL CONCEPTS IN EVALUATING GASTROINTESTINAL INFECTIONS AND FOOD POISONING

A complete history, clinical and laboratory evaluation, and careful physical examination are particularly important in the diagnosis of gastrointestinal illnesses. Because nearly all such infections are acquired by ingesting the organism, a history of recent foods ingested as well as of any exposures to ill persons should be part of the initial evaluation of patients with diarrhea. Patients should also be asked about any recent travel, because travelers are at greater risk for developing diarrheal infections, particularly those visiting countries with inadequate sewage and water treatment facilities. Other important issues are as follows:

▪ **Does the patient have a history of previous gastrointestinal symptoms?** A positive history may suggest a more chronic or recurrent illness, such as inflammatory bowel disease.
▪ **Does the patient have an underlying illness?** For example, patients with acquired immunodeficiency syndrome (AIDS) may be infected with organisms not routinely considered diarrheal agents in immunocompetent patients.
▪ **Is the patient taking any medications?** Some medicines may cause gastrointestinal symptoms or predispose the patient to infections.

The differential diagnosis of diarrheal illness is among the broadest of common patient presentations. Viral, bacterial, and parasitic pathogens, as well as food poisonings and noninfectious processes, may cause diarrhea. The cost of evaluating all patients for all of the possible pathogens and other causes is prohibitive. Therefore physicians must learn an approach to diarrheal illness that is effective in limiting mortality, morbidity, and secondary transmission rates. It must also be economically practical. The microbiologist is similarly challenged. Recovering the pathogen and differentiating it from among the usual colonizing bacterial flora is extremely difficult. Also, as new diagnostic techniques are developed, they must be carefully correlated with clinical cases and evaluated to determine their usefulness in early diagnosis and initiation of therapy.

ANATOMIC CONSIDERATIONS

Diarrheal pathogens are usually acquired by ingesting the organism as part of a contaminated meal or beverage. Figure 28-1 is a diagram of the gastrointestinal tract with the major host defenses

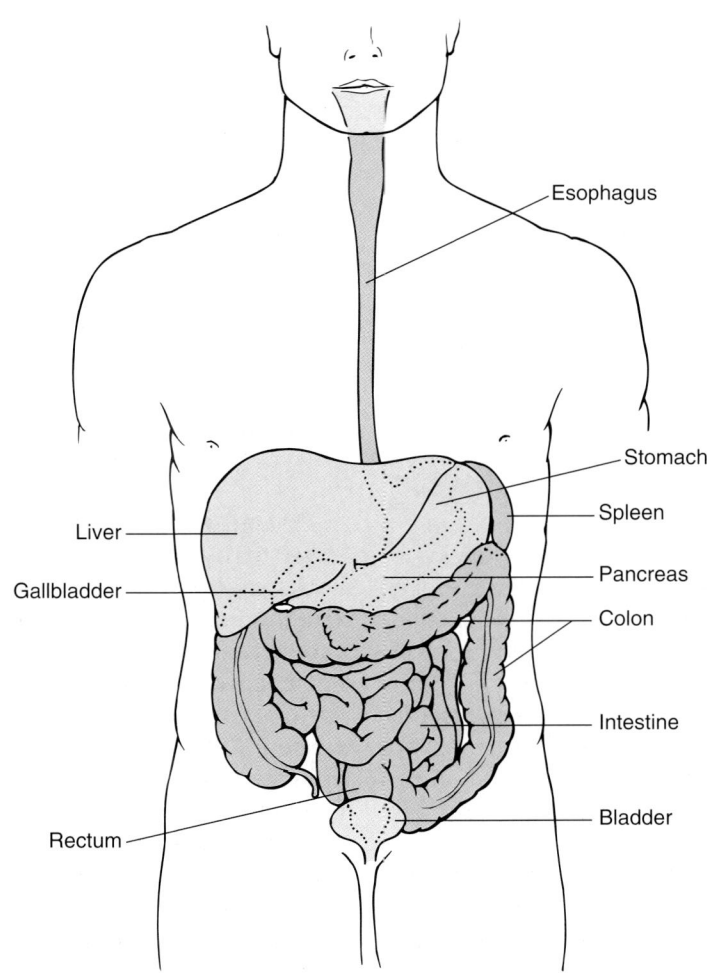

Figure 28-1
Anatomy of gastrointestinal tract.

against infection at each level. When organisms reach the stomach, they are exposed to gastric acid. Nearly all organisms are quite sensitive to a low pH, resulting in a greatly reduced number of organisms surviving to reach the small bowel. Exceptions include the spore phase of some bacteria and the cyst phase of some parasites.

In the small bowel, the major host defense is motility. The small bowel is constantly in motion. Organisms that rely on their attachment to the gut wall to produce symptoms are affected, because the contact time of the organism with the gut surface is limited by the constant peristalsis of the small bowel.

It is important to understand that, in most cases, a large number of organisms must be ingested to cause disease. The number of organisms that must be ingested to cause disease in 50% of individuals is termed **median infectious dose (ID_{50})**. The interplay between the number and virulence of the organism ingested and the host defenses ultimately determines whether an individual becomes ill or not. For example, patients with inadequate stomach acidity **(achlorhydria)** are more likely than persons with normal acidity to become ill if they ingest an enteric pathogen. Also, organisms present in particularly large numbers in ingested food are more likely to survive host defenses and cause disease.

THE ROLE OF THE USUAL FLORA

The stomach contains few organisms. Unless the patient has decreased acid production, stomach acidity is buffered by food or reflux of alkaline material from the small bowel. The upper part of the small bowel contains small numbers of *Enterococcus* species, lactobacilli, and diphtheroids. *Candida albicans* may be seen in as many as 20% to 40% of individuals.

In the colon, the flora changes markedly (Table 28-1). *Bacteroides, Fusobacterium, Eubacterium,* and *Peptococcus* organisms are among the predominant anaerobes present. *Escherichia coli, Klebsiella* species and other members of the Enterobacteriaceae are the most common aerobic gram-negative rods isolated from fecal material.

TABLE 28-1

Microbial Flora Found in the Large Intestine

Bacterial Species*	Incidence (%)
Strict anaerobes	
Gram-negative	
Bacteroides fragilis	100
Bacteroides spp.	100
Fusobacterium spp.	100
Gram-positive	
Lactobacilli	20–60
Clostridium perfringens	25–35
Clostridium spp.	1–35
Peptostreptococcus spp.	Common
Peptococcus spp.	Common
Facultative anaerobes	
Gram-positive cocci	
Staphylococcus aureus	30–50
Enterococcus spp.	100
β-Hemolytic streptococci, groups B, C, F, and G	0–16
Gram-negative bacilli (Enterobacteriaceae)	
Escherichia coli	100
Klebsiella spp.	40–80
Enterobacter spp.	5–55
Proteus spp.	3–11
Salmonella enteritidis (1400 serotypes)	3–7
Shigella, groups A–D	0–1
Pseudomonas aeruginosa	3–11
Candida albicans	15–30

Modified from Sommers HM: The indigenous microbiota of the human host. In Youmans GP, Paterson PY, Sommers HM, editors: *The biologic and clinical basis of infectious diseases,* ed 2, Philadelphia, 1980, WB Saunders, p 92.
*Strict anaerobes are present in ratio of 1000:1 with facultative aerobes.

Organisms that survive to reach the colon are faced with two other host defenses. First, local antibody (coproantibody), primarily IgA, is secreted and may have an effect against some organisms. Second, organisms reaching the colon must also compete with the huge number of other organisms, such as the usual colon flora already present. In the colon, the number of organisms approaches 10^{12} per gram of feces and consists primarily of anaerobic, gram-negative, non–spore-forming bacteria. The ratio of anaerobes to aerobes is approximately 1000:1. Table 28-1 lists the organisms found as microbial flora in the large intestine. These organisms in residence attach to the colon wall, compete for nutrients, and, in some cases, produce toxic metabolic products to some pathogens.

A PRACTICAL APPROACH TO DIAGNOSIS OF THE PATIENT WITH DIARRHEA

The differential diagnosis of patients with diarrhea may be made on the basis of clinical history, physical findings, and microscopic examination of the stool sample on the day of presentation. Table 28-2 summarizes the commonly encountered clinical gastrointestinal syndromes and the most likely pathogens implicated by incubation period, absence or presence of fever, and stool examination for red and white blood cells.

History

Travel and food ingestion history is particularly important. A history of travel to countries with less effective sewage sanitation facilities greatly increases the risk of acquiring an enteric infectious pathogen. **"Traveler's diarrhea"** is most often caused by enteropathogenic *E. coli*. This illness has a short incubation period (usually less than 24 hours) and typically lasts 1 to 3 days. Therefore a traveler who develops diarrhea days to weeks after returning home, or who is complaining of 1 to 2 weeks of diarrhea, most likely has some other pathogen. Parasites such as *Giardia lamblia* and *Entamoeba histolytica* would be among the considerations in this case.

Because most diarrhea pathogens are acquired via ingestion of the organism, a detailed food history (going back at least 3 days) is also useful. Infected food usually tastes and smells normal, so it is important to know which foods are most commonly implicated as vehicles for specific pathogens. Water, unpasteurized milk, poultry, and shellfish have been among the most commonly implicated foods. Table 28-3 lists foods and the pathogens with which they are associated. A food history is also useful in attempting to ascertain the incubation period of the illness. More recently, however, new food vehicles for transmission such as fresh produce have been reported.

The duration of illness prior to presentation is also a useful clue in narrowing the differential diagnosis. Symptoms resulting from *G. lamblia* and other parasitic infections are often present for 10 days or more before the patient seeks medical attention. Patients with diarrhea resulting from an invasive bacterial pathogen typically present af-

TABLE 28-2

Clinical Syndromes for Specific Enteric Pathogens*

Syndrome	Incubation Period	Fever	Stool Examination for Leukocytes and Erythrocytes	Pathogens
Nausea and vomiting	5–15 min	No	Negative	Heavy metals, mass psychogenic illness†
Nausea, vomiting, and diarrhea	1–18 h	No	Negative	Enterotoxigenic *Escherichia coli, Clostridium perfringens, Bacillus cereus, Staphylococcus aureus*
Nausea, vomiting, diarrhea, myalgias, and headache	12 h–3 d	Yes	Negative	Rotavirus, Norwalk virus, Norwalk-like virus
Diarrhea and abdominal cramps	1–3 d	Yes	Positive‡	*Campylobacter jejuni, Shigella* spp., *Entamoeba histolytica, Salmonella* sp., *Yersinia* sp., *Clostridium difficile*
Gastrointestinal bleed	1–3 d	No	Gross blood	Enterohemorrhagic *E. coli,*§ cytomegalovirus¶
Malabsorptive diarrhea with bloating	1–2 wk	No	Negative	*Microsporidium* sp., *Isospora belli, Giardia lamblia*

Modified from Goodman LJ: Diagnosis, management, and prevention of diarrheal diseases, *Curr Opinion Infect Dis* 6:88, 1993.
*This table is designed as a guide. Incubation periods and syndromes may overlap.
†Mass psychogenic illness is more common in adolescents. Rash may be part of the syndrome.
‡Gross blood and pus in stool is a clue for *Campylobacter jejuni, Shigella* species, or *Entamoeba histolytica.*
§Fever may be seen in approximately one third of cases.
¶Syndrome confined to compromised hosts, particularly bone marrow transplant recipients, and occurs 1 and 3 months after transplantation.

TABLE 28-3

Common Food Vehicles for Specific Pathogens or Toxins

Vehicle	Pathogen or Toxin
Undercooked chicken	*Salmonella* sp., *Campylobacter* sp.
Eggs	*Salmonella* sp. (especially *S. enteritidis*)
Unpasteurized milk	*Salmonella, Campylobacter,* and *Yersinia* sp.
Water	*Giardia lamblia,* Norwalk virus, *Campylobacter* sp., *Cryptosporidium* sp., *Cyclospora*
Fried rice	*Bacillus cereus*
Fish	
Shellfish	*Vibrio cholerae, V. parahaemolyticus, V. vulnificus,* other *Vibrio* sp., neurotoxic shellfish poisoning, paralytic shellfish poisoning, Norwalk virus
Tuna, mackerel, mahi-mahi	Scombroid poisoning
Grouper, amberjack, snapper	Ciguatera
Sushi	*Anisakis* species
Beef, gravy	*Salmonella* sp., *Campylobacter* sp., *Clostridium perfringens*

Modified from Goodman LJ: Diagnosis, management, and prevention of diarrheal diseases, *Curr Opinion Infect Dis* 6:88, 1993.

ter at least 72 hours of symptoms. Patients with viral or enterotoxin-associated disease more commonly present for medical attention within the first 24 to 48 hours of symptoms.

As with other infectious illnesses, it is important to ask patients about any medication they may be taking and their exposure to other persons with a similar illness. Gastrointestinal symptoms are among the most common drug-related side effects. If the patient is taking an antibiotic, *Clostridium difficile* is an important consideration. Finally, the patient should be asked about other illnesses. Diarrhea may be a symptom of some noninfectious illnesses (e.g., inflammatory bowel disease), and in patients with serious underlying illnesses, such as AIDS, may be due to pathogens that would not otherwise be considered.

Physical Examination

The first consideration on physical examination is to assess the patient's state of hydration. The most common cause of death from diarrhea is dehydration. Signs of dehydration include a drop in blood pressure and an increase in heart rate upon moving from a lying to a sitting position (orthostatic

changes), a sunken appearance to the eyes, and a loss of resiliency of the skin, called **skin tenting.** This change in the skin can be detected by gently pinching the skin of the back of the hand. The pinched area in a dehydrated patient remains in a pinched or "tented" position. Patients who are severely dehydrated may also have changes in their mental state and other organ system dysfunction. An elevated temperature is a clue that the pathogen has invasive properties. Examination of the abdomen usually reveals a diffusely tender abdomen. On auscultation with a stethoscope, bowel sounds are present. Localization of pain to one part of the abdomen, severe pain on palpation of the abdomen, and absence of bowel sounds all are indications to evaluate the patient for a complication of diarrhea (e.g., **toxic megacolon,** intestinal rupture) or a different disease process that may require surgical intervention (e.g., appendicitis).

Laboratory Studies

The most helpful of immediately available laboratory tests in the evaluation of patients with presumed infectious diarrhea is a microscopic evaluation of the stool for red and white blood cells. These cells are common in specimens from patients with invasive infections but are unusual in specimens from patients with most enterotoxin-mediated illnesses, viral illnesses, and parasitic infections. The duration of illness, travel history, host status, and food ingestion history can then be used to make further decisions concerning cultures.

PATHOGENIC MECHANISMS AND CLINICAL PRESENTATIONS OF ACUTE DIARRHEA

Enterotoxin-Mediated Diarrhea

On the basis of history, physical examination, and laboratory findings, the clinician should be able to shorten the list of potential pathogens. By dividing the organisms into groups that reflect the clinical presentations with which they are most commonly associated, the microbiologist determines the appropriate methods for maximum recovery.

Clinical presentations may be characterized as **enterotoxin-mediated diarrhea,** invasion of bowel mucosa, or invasion with lymphatic spread.

CASE STUDY

CASE STUDY

A 32-year-old man from the Untied States is visiting a small village in Mexico. Four days after arriving, he experiences sudden onset of diarrhea. The diarrhea occurs more than 30 times the first day and is accompanied by nausea with several episodes of diarrhea. The stool is watery, without gross blood, pus, or mucus. The patient is afebrile but complains of crampy abdominal pain with stooling and dizziness when standing. His heart rate is rapid (120/minute).

The absence of fever, blood, or pus indicates that the diarrheal illness is enterotoxin-mediated. The bacteria associated with enterotoxin production do not invade the gut, and the toxin itself also does not elicit an inflammatory response. Therefore microscopic examination of the stool does not reveal red or white blood cells. Similarly, no inflammatory response is present which explains why affected patients are usually afebrile.

Enterotoxigenic *E. coli* accounts for the largest percentage of cases in travelers. Other organisms associated with enterotoxin-mediated diarrhea are *Vibrio cholerae, Staphylococcus aureus, Clostridium perfringens,* and *Bacillus cereus. Aeromonas* and *Plesiomonas* organisms may produce a similar syndrome, as does a viral gastroenteritis, particularly when resulting from adenovirus or Norwalk virus. The noninvasive parasitic infections, such as *Giardia lamblia, Cryptosporidium parvum,* and *Isospora belli,* also produce an afebrile diarrhea with no cells in the blood. Patients with parasitic infections, however, usually look for medical attention after 1 week or more of symptoms, have fewer diarrheal stools per day, and have more prolonged illnesses without treatment.

In the case study above, the patient's rapid heart rate and complaints of dizziness on standing are due to loss of intravascular fluid volume. Treatment should be aimed initially at rehydration. The addition of bismuth-subsalicylate with or without an antimicrobial agent may also shorten this man's illness.

The toxin may be produced on the food and acts fairly proximally (in the small bowel); therefore the incubation period for enterotoxin-producing organisms is relatively short, typically 6 to 12 hours.

Patients present with an illness that began either the day of or the day before presentation. The illness is characterized by watery diarrhea with a very high frequency of stools (sometimes 20 per day). This type of diarrheal illness is most associated with nausea, vomiting, and abdominal cramps, particularly during defecation. Because the organism itself does not invade the tissue, bacteremia and metastatic infection are very rare.

Diarrhea Mediated by Invasion of Bowel Mucosal Surface

CASE STUDY

A 56-year-old woman was hospitalized 9 days ago for gallbladder surgery. Her roommate was hospitalized 2 days ago for fever and diarrhea. Today, the surgical patient is complaining of diarrhea. For the first time since admission, she has a fever. Four other people on the floor also have new onset of diarrhea. Fecal leukocytes are present in all affected patients. *Shigella* organisms were cultured from all infected patients.

The most common cause of an invasive diarrheal syndrome in a hospitalized patient is *C. difficile.* In this case, however, the patient's roommate has diarrhea, and four others on the same medical floor became sick at the same time. Other invasive syndromes to consider include *Salmonella* and *Campylobacter* species. *Entamoeba histolytica* would also be a consideration, but the incubation period of 2 days is short.

The site of action for invasive organisms is the colon, and the mucosal surface of the bowel is primarily affected. Deeper invasion of the bowel wall and regional lymph nodes are unusual, however. Because organisms must traverse the stomach and small bowel, multiply, and invade, the incubation period is usually longer than for toxin-mediated illness, approximately 1 to 3 days. Organisms in this group elicit an inflammatory response from the bowel wall (usually the colon). Evidence of this is the common finding of white and red cells in the microscopic evaluation of the stool smear. Patients in this group are the most likely to present with a true dysentery syndrome, characterized by gross blood and pus in the stool, as shown in Figure 28-2. A systemic inflammatory response occurs, evidenced by fever in some patients. Because the invasion is usually superficial, bacteremia and metastatic infection are not common.

Organisms that produce this syndrome include *Shigella* species, *Campylobacter jejuni,* and *C. difficile.* Enterohemorrhagic *E. coli* often causes gross blood per rectum, although fever and white blood cells in the stool are less common than with the other organisms that produce this clinical manifestation. Of the parasitic infections, *E. histolytica* produces an identical clinical syndrome, except that the incubation period is even longer, ranging from 1 to 3 weeks.

Diarrhea Mediated by Invasion of Full Bowel Thickness with Lymphatic Spread

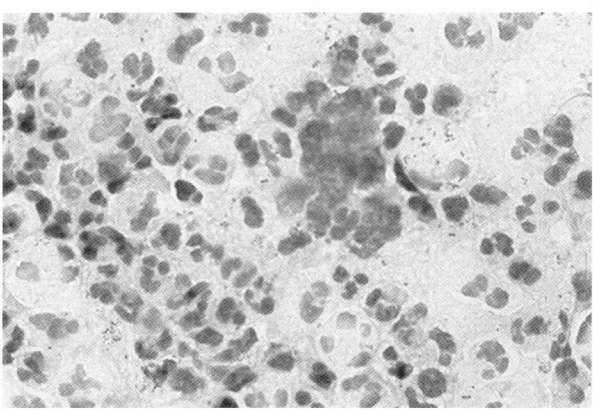

Figure 28-2

Direct fecal smear gram-stained to show the presence of white blood cells, indicative of an invasive process and not an enterotoxin.

CASE STUDY

A 37-year-old woman presents with high fever and dry cough. The patient denies any history of vomiting or diarrhea. Other laboratory findings include neutropenia, a relative increase in lymphocytes, a shift to the left, and normocytic, normochromic anemia.

Blood culture specimens are taken at the time of hospital admission. During the second week of hospitalization, the patient remains febrile, with temperature reaching 103° F. She also begins to excrete watery, diarrheic stool. Stool cultures are performed.

Invasive organisms such as *Salmonella typhi* and *Yersinia enterocolitica* act primarily at the colon. Incubation period is approximately 1 to 3 days. Fever is common. Often, the patient experiences constipation rather than diarrhea in the early phase of the disease. Although bacteremia resulting from a diarrheal pathogen is uncommon, it is most likely to occur with invasive organisms. Because regional adenopathy is commonly seen, these organisms may produce a syndrome of mesenteric adenitis that mimics appendicitis. Microscopic evaluation of the stool usually reveals cells, but gross blood or pus is unusual.

Salmonella typhi is isolated from both blood and stool cultures. The patient acquired the infection

from eating at a local restaurant. Specimens from the cook are cultured for salmonellae, and results are positive.

In this particular case, it is important to understand that significant overlap exists among these clinically separated groups, but such a scheme is useful as an initial approach to a common problem.

COMMON BACTERIAL, VIRAL, AND PARASITIC GASTROINTESTINAL INFECTIONS AND THEIR AGENTS

One of the major challenges in the diagnosis of gastrointestinal disease is the recent increase in the number of probable etiologic agents. The majority of diagnosed pathogens are represented by a relative few bacteria, as shown in Box 28-1.

A number of organisms have been added to this list, however, either as suspected or as strongly associated agents of gastroenteritis. Box 28-1 also shows other groups of bacterial agents that are highly associated with gastrointestinal infections; however, animal models have not been identified to reproduce the infection. A third group of organisms (implicated organisms), as shown in Box 28-1, have been linked to gastrointestinal diseases. Because these organisms normally make up the colon flora, their role in diarrheal disease remains questionable. Similarly, animal models have not been identified to re-

Box 28-1

Common Bacterial Agents Associated with Gastrointestinal Infections

Recognized enteropathogens

Salmonella species
Shigella species
Enterotoxigenic *Escherichia coli*
Enterohemorrhagic *E. coli*
Enteropathogenic *E. coli*
Enteroinvasive *E. coli*
Vibrio cholerae
Vibrio parahaemolyticus
Campylobacter jejuni
Campylobacter coli
Yersinia enterocolitica
Clostridium difficile

Highly associated enteropathogens

Aeromonas spp.
Plesiomonas shigelloides
Edwardsiella tarda
Enteroaggregative *E. coli*
Vibrio spp.
Campylobacter spp.

Implicated organisms

Bacteroides fragilis
Citrobacter freundii
Klebsiella pneumoniae
Klebsiella oxytoca
Providencia alcalifaciens
Hafnia alvei

Modified from Abbott S, Janda JM: Bacterial gastroenteritis. I: Incidence and etiologic agents, *Clin Microbiol Newsl* 14:17, 1992.

produce the infection. Table 28-4 shows the characteristics of the organisms that have been implicated in diarrheal diseases. Other etiologic agents include viruses, which make up less than 50% of cases, and parasitic agents, which account for less than 5%.

Bacterial Agents
Campylobacter jejuni

Although several *Campylobacter* species cause disease in humans, *Campylobacter jejuni* is by far the most common. In the United States, *C. jejuni* has been reported as the most common cause of bacterial diarrheas. The organism is a curved, gram-negative rod. This morphology is helpful, because a Gram stain of stool may show these organisms in as many as 50% of cases. The only other curved, gram-negative rods associated with diarrheal disease are several of the *Vibrio* species including *V. cholerae* and *Vibrio parahaemolyticus* (discussed later).

C. jejuni is found in many animal species. Outbreaks have been traced to inadequately cooked poultry, untreated water, and unpasteurized milk. Exposure to animals with diarrhea (especially puppies or kittens) has also been implicated.

TABLE 28-4
Characteristics of Organisms Implicated in Diarrheal Diseases

Bacterial Species	Symptoms	Association	Virulence Factor
Klebsiella oxytoca	Enterocolitis, which may be bloody	Antibiotics, especially ampicillin	Cytotoxin
Klebsiella pneumoniae	Watery diarrhea	Unknown	Heat-stable enterotoxin Heat-labile enterotoxin
Citrobacter freundii	Watery diarrhea	Unknown	Same as above
Hafnia alvei	Watery diarrhea	Unknown	Attachment-effacement
Bacteroides fragilis	Watery diarrhea Abdominal cramping Vomiting and bloody stools in children	Unknown	Heat-labile enterotoxin
Providencia alcalifaciens	Gastroenteritis	Travel in developing countries	Unknown

Modified from Abbott S, Janda JM: Bacterial gastroenteritis. I: Incidence and etiologic agents, *Clin Microbiol Newsl* 14:17, 1992.

The organism produces a number of exotoxins, some with cytolytic properties, that contribute to the clinical picture. Symptoms such as fever, abdominal pain, and diarrhea begin approximately 1 to 7 days after ingestion of contaminated food or drink. Feces may contain blood and pus. This diarrheal illness is usually self-limiting, although clinical manifestations may persist for a week or two.

During recent years, *Campylobacter* infections have become a serious public health interest. Additionally, *Campylobacter* species isolated from human infections have also become more resistant to antimicrobials, in particular, fluoroquinolones, after these agents were introduced for use in animals for food.

Preventive strategies to minimize contamination of chicken carcasses include changes in slaughterhouse processing and handling procedures. Chlorination of drinking water for chickens, possibly poultry vaccination, and chemical rinses to inhibit the growth of bacterial flora on poultry carcasses are other options. Food irradiation has been widely used and accepted in world food markets. In spite of reports on the safety and effectiveness of irradiation of food, consumers in the United States have remained hesitant in accepting irradiated food products.

Salmonella species

GASTROENTERITIS AND FOOD POISONING

Gastroenteritis and food poisoning result from the ingestion of undercooked meat, poultry, eggs, and dairy products contaminated with serotypes of *Salmonella*. **Nontyphoidal salmonella** serotypes are found in a wide variety of animal hosts, including turtles, reptiles, and poultry. Other common vehicles of transmission are cooking utensils used in preparing contaminated meat. The number of foodborne outbreaks attributed to nontyphoidal salmonellae has increased over the last several years. *Salmonella* serotype Enteritidis Phage Type 4 (PT4) has been implicated most often in salmonellosis outbreaks traced to the consumption of eggs and other food items in which egg products are used. Antibiotic resistance in *Salmonella* serotype Typhimurium Phage Type 104 (DT104) has also been reported and is continuously being monitored.

Symptoms, which begin approximately 6 to 48 hours after ingestion, consist of nausea, vomiting, and diarrhea. Fever, muscle ache, and headache may also follow. The diarrhea may last from a few hours to a few days, depending on the inoculum size and the health status of the individual. The disease is usually self-limited, and the patient recovers without a need for treatment. Antimicrobial therapy is not indicated in this form of the disease, because it is believed to prolong the carrier state.

ENTERIC FEVER

Typhoid fever caused by *Salmonella* serotype typhi is the most severe form of **enteric fever.** *S. typhi* is host specific, with humans the only identified reservoir. Enteric fever may also be caused by *Salmonella* serotype A, *Salmonella* serotype choleraesuis, and other serotypes.

Enteric fever is usually transmitted through fecally contaminated food or water. The infective dose required to initiate the infection is much lower than for the gastroenteritis form.

In typhoid fever, *Salmonella* organisms invade small bowel and colonic tissue, producing an inflammatory response, but diarrhea is not present. In fact, most patients experience constipation during the early phase of the disease. The organisms are ingested by monocytes, but these cells do not kill *Salmonella* organisms effectively. For this reason, *Salmonella* organisms are termed **intracellular pathogens,** in that they survive inside monocytes. After tissue invasion, they are transported to regional lymph tissue, which undergoes hyperplasia in response. Organisms then reach the blood stream, and the patient experiences fever, malaise, headache, and abdominal tenderness. During the bacteremic spread, the organisms reach the biliary tract and invade the gallbladder and Peyer patches of the colon. Colonization at these sites leads to the intestinal seeding and the diarrheic phase. The ability of *Salmonella* organisms to survive intracellularly and their invasion of the gallbladder may contribute to this organism's ability to persist in the stool despite antibiotic therapy. *Salmonella* infections of the blood stream or of a metastatic focus (e.g., bone, central nervous system) can be effectively treated with antimicrobial agents. Antibiotic therapy, however, may actually prolong the time of excretion of salmonellae in the stool.

BACTEREMIA

Nontyphoidal salmonellae, such as *Salmonella* typhimurium, *Salmonella* paratyphi A and B, and *S.* choleraesuis, have been associated with salmonella bacteremia with or without intestinal infection. Persistent fever and intermittent bacteremia are the common manifestations. This form of salmonellosis has been observed in both young children and adults.

CARRIER STATE

Following salmonella infections, individuals may continue to harbor the organisms for a time. Chronic carriage occurs when the organisms infect the gallbladder, which then continuously seeds the gastrointestinal tract. The affected person continuously or intermittently excretes the organisms in the feces and becomes an important source of infection of susceptible persons.

Shigella species

Shigella species, particularly Shigella dysenteriae, may produce a diarrhea syndrome characterized by the presence of gross blood or pus in the stool. **Shigellosis** is among the most communicable of the bacterial diarrheas. In a study of volunteers, the ingestion of as few as several hundred organisms caused disease. The organism invades the mucosa locally, producing flask-shaped ulcers and an intense inflammatory response. Deeper invasion to regional lymph nodes or the blood stream is uncommon.

In the United States, Shigella sonnei is the most common species isolated. This organism is usually associated with milder illness. Other Shigella species are Shigella boydii, S. dysenteriae, and Shigella flexneri. S. flexneri is the second most common species seen in the United States. S. boydii is infrequently isolated in this country.

Shigella species produce several toxins of clinical importance. A neurotoxin causes paralysis in mice and plays a role in human infection. Infants with shigellosis may transiently lose the reflexive closing of the anal canal with external pressure, as from a cotton swab. The loss of this so-called anal wink reflex in an infant with diarrhea is a soft clue that Shigella organisms may be the etiologic agent.

Diarrheogenic Escherichia coli

E. coli may cause diarrhea via a number of different mechanisms. Currently, five recognized groups of diarrheogenic E. coli exist, as shown in Table 28-5, which lists the types of E. coli and the associated diarrheal diseases. Specific serotypes have been associated with each of these syndromes.

TABLE 28-5

The Diarrheagenic E. coli

Group	Mechanism of Infection	Symptoms	Infectious Dose	Associated Serotypes	Source of Infection
ETEC	LT and ST toxins	Traveler's diarrhea, watery diarrhea, abdominal cramps, nausea, no mucus or blood	$\sim 10^8$ bacteria	O6:H16 O8:H9 O15:H11 O15:H11 O27:H7	Food and water
EAggEC	(Proposed) Adherence to intestine mucosa; toxin- or inflammation-induced damage	Watery diarrhea, occasional bloody stools and vomiting	$\sim 10^{10}$ bacteria	O3:H22 O15:H18 O44:H18 O77:H18 O111:H21	Nosocomial and community-acquired
EPEC	Attachment and effacement (A/E)	Watery, nonbloody diarrhea with mucus, without fecal leukocytes; fever and vomiting	10^6 to 10^{10} bacteria	O86:H34 O55:H-,6 O111:H2	Formula, food contaminated with fecal material (fecal-oral)
EIEC	Invasion of colon epithelium	Either watery diarrhea or dysentery (bloody, watery stool with mucus) fecal leukocytes; fever	$\sim 10^6$ bacteria	O28ac O29 O112 O124	Food and water
EHEC	Shiga toxins	Range from watery diarrhea to hemorrhagic colitis (bloody diarrhea with abdominal pain)	$< 10^2$ bacteria	O157:H7 O111:H-,8 O26:H11 O113:H21	Food and water

From Nauschuetz WF: Emerging foodborne pathogens: enterohemorrhagic Escherichia coli, Clin Lab Sci 11:304, 1998.

ENTEROPATHOGENIC *E. COLI*

Enteropathogenic *E. coli* (EPEC) was first recognized in the early 1940s as a cause of infantile diarrhea. For many years, its pathogenic role has been controversial, mainly because only certain "H" serotypes have been associated with the infections. Unfortunately, antisera to detect "H" typing are not usually available in the clinical laboratory, and serotyping has been limited to "O" serogroups only. Further studies, however, have reported the presence of a cytotoxin and an EPEC adherence factor (EAF). This factor, which enables EPEC to adhere to epithelial cells, has been demonstrated both in vivo and in vitro. Investigators believe that this adherence factor plays a significant role in the pathogenesis of EPEC.

Newborns in hospital nurseries and day-care centers are most affected. The disease rarely occurs in adults. Primary symptoms are low-grade fever, malaise, vomiting, and diarrhea. Gross evidence of blood is absent from stool, which may contain large amounts of mucus.

ENTEROTOXIGENIC *E. COLI*

Enterotoxigenic *E. coli* (ETEC) excrete enterotoxins, either heat labile (LT) or heat stable (ST), which produce a watery diarrhea syndrome similar to that of cholera. ETEC remain the most common cause of infant diarrhea in developing countries and of traveler's diarrhea in the United States. Clinical manifestations of ETEC infection are similar to those caused by other enterotoxin-producing organisms, such as *S. aureus, C. perfringens, B. cereus,* and *V. cholerae.* Differential diagnosis is usually made by exclusion or by isolation of only lactose-fermenting organisms. DNA probes for ETEC are available but are not widely used in the clinical laboratory.

ENTEROINVASIVE *E. COLI*

Enteroinvasive *E. coli* (EIEC) have invasive properties and produce a syndrome mimicking *Shigella* infection. A Shiga-like toxin found in still other *E. coli* produces a bloody diarrhea syndrome that manifests clinically as a gastrointestinal bleeding disorder. The infection is characterized by fever, severe abdominal cramps, malaise, and watery diarrhea. The stool contains pus and blood.

ENTEROAGGREGATIVE *E. COLI*

Enteroadherent *E. coli* or, as most recently termed, enteroaggregative *E. coli* (EAggEC) cause diarrhea by adhering to the mucosal surface, apparently affecting absorption and stimulating peristalsis. These organisms produce symptoms such as watery diarrhea, vomiting, dehydration, and, occasionally, abdominal pain.

ENTEROHEMORRHAGIC *E. COLI*

Enterohemorrhagic *E. coli* (EHEC) serotype O157:H7 has been implicated with hemorrhagic diarrhea, colitis, and hemolytic uremic syndrome. The stool typically does not contain any pus, a feature differentiating this infection from shigellosis or an enteroinvasive infection. The infection is potentially fatal, especially among young children and elderly residents of convalescent homes and nursing centers. Other serotypes have also been implicated. Some of the non-O157 EHEC that have been isolated from patients with bloody diarrhea, hemorrhagic colitis, or hemolytic uremic syndrome include O6:H31, O48:H7, O104:H21, O26, O26:H11, O113:H21, O98:NM, O111:H2, O121:H19.

Vibrio species

Vibrio species are gram-negative rods with a curved shape, like *Campylobacter* organisms. Most infections associated with *Vibrio* species occur upon ingestion of contaminated uncooked seafood or upon contamination of wounds with sea water.

Vibrio cholerae is the causative agent of cholera. It produces chitinase, an enzyme that breaks down chitin, part of the shell of various sea animals, providing the organism with an important niche in the marine environment. Outbreaks are seen in coastal areas, where seafood is an important part of the diet. Cases of *V. cholerae* infection in the United States have been reported off the Gulf of Mexico and in travelers returning from areas where the disease is endemic. South America and Africa have experienced widespread outbreaks. Although direct person-to-person spread is uncommon, contamination of water and food has been the main factor in spreading disease.

Cholera is a form of diarrhea mediated by the elaboration of an enterotoxin. The enterotoxin consists of an A subunit surrounded by five B subunits. The B subunits attach to the mucosa of the small bowel, permitting the A subunit to penetrate to the interior surface of the membrane, where it catalyzes nicotine-adenine dinucleotide (NAD) to eventually form cyclic adenosine monophosphate (camp). This stimulates the intestinal mucosa to secrete water and electrolytes, characterized as rice-water stool.

The action of the enterotoxin does not elicit an inflammatory response. Therefore no white cells or red cells are in the stool, and the patient is usually afebrile. The amount of fluid lost per rectum can be impressive, however, with many liters of replacement fluids needed per day. Death from dehydration is the major risk, particularly for patients at the extremes of age and those already debilitated by malnourishment or other diseases.

More than 60 serovars (serogroups) of *V. cholerae* exist, but only serovar 01 has been traditionally implicated in epidemic cholera. However, during recent years a new serogroup, O139 has been implicated in an epidemic of cholera in India. An agglutination test for serovar 01 must be performed on isolates identified as *V. cholerae*. In addition, because not all *V. cholerae* serovar 01 produce the enterotoxin that mediates this disease, toxin detection must also be performed. The latex agglutination test and enzyme-linked immunosorbent assay (ELISA) produce comparable results and are currently in use in laboratories located in high incidence areas. The clinical microbiology laboratory must be notified when *V. cholerae* is suspected in a patient specimen, because special media are required for its isolation.

Other *Vibrio* species also produce disease. *Vibrio parahaemolyticus* causes diarrhea worldwide and is the most commonly identified bacterial pathogen in Japan. Unlike patients with cholera, patients with *V. parahaemolyticus* usually have fever, chills, and cells in their stool, suggesting that this organism has invasive potential.

Like other *Vibrio* species, *Vibrio vulnificus* is associated with eating shellfish, particularly clams and oysters. *V. vulnificus* causes bacteremia, however, and an overwhelming sepsis. This syndrome is most commonly seen in patients with severe liver disease. The liver is an important filter of organisms that reach the blood stream from the gastrointestinal tract. When this property is diminished, organisms are more likely to reach the systemic circulation, sometimes with disastrous results.

Aeromonas species (*Aeromonas hydrophila, Aeromonas sobria,* and *Aeromonas caviae*) and *Plesiomonas shigelloides* are closely related to *Vibrio* species. *Aeromonas* species are usually associated with a fresh-water exposure. Clinical infections described include a watery diarrhea syndrome, cellulitis, and soft-tissue infection after an injury.

P. shigelloides, found in coastal waters, causes gastroenteritis with extraintestinal syndromes similar to those with *Aeromonas* infections.

Yersinia enterocolitica

Yersinia enterocolitica is a gram-negative rod that produces a syndrome similar to that of salmonellae. This organism may be found in unpasteurized milk and dairy products. It is a common cause of diarrhea in colder climates, such as the Scandinavian countries. In the United States, it is found mostly in the northern states. Infected patients usually have fever, and white and red cells are present in stool. Invasion to the regional lymph nodes may produce a mesenteric adenitis syndrome, which can mimic appendicitis. Severe abdominal pain, fever, and enlarged lymph nodes are common presenting symptoms of *Y. enterocolitica* infections. Acute enteritis, a mild and self-limiting form of the infection, is characterized by fever, abdominal pain, nausea, and diarrhea.

Y. enterocolitica have also rarely caused infection via contamination of blood given for transfusion. The ability of this organism to survive refrigeration temperatures may be a contributing factor. Infections have also occurred as a result of consumption of contaminated food, such as market meat and vacuum-packed beef.

Clostridium difficile

Clostridium difficile, the most common cause of infectious diarrhea in hospitalized patients, is a spore-forming, anaerobic organism. It has been isolated from hospital beds, carpeting, and other fomites with which hospitalized patients come into contact. Patients may also acquire this organism in the community. Most antimicrobial agents have a significant effect on the fecal flora. Chemotherapeutic agents such as antitumor drugs have also been associated with pseudomembranous colitis. When other members of the flora are reduced, *C. difficile* may flourish. The organism produces a cytotoxin and an enterotoxin. Pathologically characteristic pseudomembranes are formed, which are nearly diagnostic when seen on colonoscopy.

Listeria monocytogenes

Listeria monocytogenes, another bacterial agent implicated in numerous food-borne outbreaks, is beginning to be recognized as a food-borne pathogen. A gram-positive non–spore-forming bacillus, it has been known to cause systemic infections among immunosuppressed patients. *L. monocytogenes* is present in nature where food animals become environmentally exposed. Therefore these organisms have become common contaminants of unprocessed food such as raw milk, cheese made from unpasteurized milk, and more recently, ready-to-eat food products such as hot dogs and pre-packaged meat products.

Viral Agents

CASE STUDY

Seven patrons of a seafood restaurant become ill with nausea, vomiting, and watery diarrhea within 24 hours of eating at the restaurant. An investigation reveals that the only food in common is raw oysters. All patients are afebrile, and symptoms resolve within 1 day. No white or red cells were found in any of the stool specimens.

Enteric pathogens associated with raw shellfish include *Vibrio* species and Norwalk virus. This food may also become contaminated with enterotoxin-producing *Staphylococcus aureus* or hepatitis virus or may harbor the toxin associated with paralytic or neurotoxic shellfish poisoning. Of these, the syndrome is most likely to be due to Norwalk virus.

Approximately 30% to 40% of all cases of gastroenteritis are due to viral pathogens. Included among these are rotavirus, enteric adenovirus, Norwalk virus, calicivirus, and astrovirus. Because viral particles are so small, special techniques are necessary to identify them. Immunoelectronmicroscopy, monoclonal antibody tests, and viral cultures of the stool are used to identify viral causes of diarrhea. Because many microbiology laboratories do not routinely offer these tests, however, many cases go undiagnosed.

Adenoviruses are associated with a number of infectious syndromes, including coryza and tracheitis, pharyngoconjunctival fever, and epidemic keratoconjunctivitis. Adenovirus serotypes 40 and 41 are most associated with diarrhea, particularly in children. These serotypes are rarely implicated in the other infections attributed to adenoviruses.

Rotavirus, a double-stranded RNA virus measuring 70 nm in diameter, is believed to be the major viral cause of gastroenteritis worldwide. Group A rotavirus is the main pathogen and is differentiated from the so-called atypical rotaviruses (groups B and C) by the migration patterns on polyacrylamide gel electrophoresis (PAGE) and by the presence of a group-specific antigen (VP6), which is the inner capsid protein on the group A virus. Infections with rotavirus are more common in the winter months in temperate climates and occur primarily in infants and children. Rotavirus causes diarrhea by interfering with absorption of fluids at the level of the small bowel.

Norwalk virus is probably the most extensively studied of the viruses associated with diarrhea in humans. It is smaller than rotavirus, measuring 20 to 40 nm in diameter. It is a single-stranded RNA virus. Norwalk virus causes disease year round and is the most commonly implicated etiologic agent in outbreaks of acute gastroenteritis. Contaminated drinking water and ingestion of raw or partially cooked shellfish are risk factors for its acquisition.

Caliciviruses and astroviruses are similar in size but differ in the shapes of their outer surfaces. Caliciviruses have cup-shaped cutouts on the outer surface, whereas astroviruses have a surface architecture that forms a five- or six-pointed star. Illness with these viruses is usually characterized by vomiting and a watery diarrhea syndrome. Calicivirus and astrovirus usually produce a milder illness than Norwalk virus.

Parasitic Agents

A number of protozoal organisms also cause diarrhea. Unlike the bacterial and viral causes previously described, these organisms are often associated with more prolonged symptoms. Diarrhea, bloating, and other symptoms may persist for weeks or longer. Protozoal parasites are larger than viruses and bacteria. They are usually detected by direct microscopy of a stained stool smear.

In the United States, *G. lamblia* is the most commonly identified intestinal parasitic pathogen. This organism is most commonly acquired via ingestion of contaminated water or by person-to-person spread in institutions or day-care centers. When water is the vehicle, transmission usually is due to either inadequate chlorination or a treatment method that lacks a filtration or sedimentation procedure.

G. lamblia may be detected in the stool as trophozoites or as cysts. The trophozoite has a characteristic, facelike appearance on staining. Trophozoites are very sensitive to the acid found in stomach secretions, whereas cysts are relatively resistant and are infectious to humans. Most patients with giardiasis complain of diarrhea, crampy abdominal pain, belching, and flatulence. Blood or pus in the stool is rare. The organism is found primarily in the small bowel, impairing absorption.

Unlike *G. lamblia*, *Entamoeba histolytica* (Figure 28-3) may cause an invasive syndrome characterized by fever and dysentery. Even when gross blood and pus are not present in stool, nearly all specimens from patients with diarrhea resulting from *E. histolytica* have red cells seen on microscopy. The appearance of trophozoites ingesting red blood cells is pathognomonic for amebiasis. The ability of this organism to lyse tissue contributed to its being named *histolytica*. This invasive ability contributes to the occasional catastrophic illnesses, including intestinal rupture, liver abscesses, and, rarely, pericardial or pleural disease, caused by *E. histolytica*.

Cryptosporidium parvum has been associated with self-limiting gastrointestinal infections in the immunocompetent population. Sporadic outbreaks of cryptosporidiosis have been reported frequently in day-care centers and nurseries. Watery diarrhea accompanied by nausea, vomiting, and low-grade fever is common. In the immunosuppressed individual, however, such as a person with AIDS, the condition these parasites produce is life-threatening. *Isospora belli*, although less commonly encountered, has also been identified as an enteric opportunist in AIDS patients. Both are transmitted via the fecal-oral route.

Infections associated with rarely encountered parasites such as *Angiostrongylus cantonensis*, *Alaria americana*, *Capillaria philippinensis*, *Diphyllobothrium latum*, *Paragonimus westermani* and *Anisakis* sp. have also been reported. These "exotic parasites" are ingested in the flesh or raw fish or shellfish and are endemic primarily in Southeast Asia, where people consume this type of food uncooked. *A. cantonensis*, or rat lungworm, is a nematode usually acquired by ingesting slugs or snails containing the larvae. These parasites can also be found in crabs and prawns or any other type of shellfish. Although highly endemic areas include Thailand, Taiwan, and Tahiti, an infection in an 11-year-old boy in Louisiana who had never traveled out of state was confirmed serologically. It was documented that many of the gastropods in and around New Orleans are hosts for *A. cantonensis*.

A. americana is a fluke that appears to be extremely rare although some cases are reported in the literature. The adult fluke develops in fox and in other canines; the eggs are passed out and embryonate in the water. In its life cycle, it somehow finds its way to the hind leg muscles of frogs. Ingestion of undercooked frog legs have led to a fatal case.

C. philippinensis is another nematode acquired by consumption of raw fish, especially in Thailand. Cases in the Philippines, Iran, and Egypt have also been reported. Patients suffer from malabsorption syndrome resulting from worm burden. Similarly, *D. latum*, a fish tapeworm, is acquired by ingesting raw or poorly cooked freshwater or saltwater fish. *P. westermani*, a lung fluke, is endemic in certain areas of the Philippines where people enjoy eating raw crabs. In Thailand, the common source of infection is salted fish. Lastly, *Anisakis* sp., associated with **anisakiasis,** are consumed from raw fish called "sushi" or "sashimi." Anisakids are tissue nematodes found infecting the flesh of raw fish.

Trichinella spiralis is acquired through the ingestion of poorly cooked or raw pork. Incidence of trichinosis in the United States has declined be-

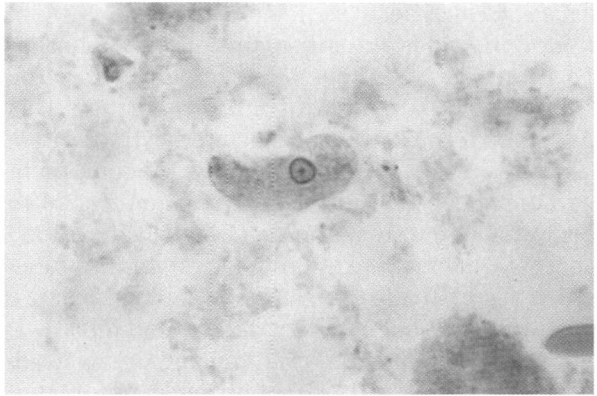

Figure 28-3 _____

Entamoeba histolytica trophozoites.

cause of public awareness of the dangers of eating undercooked pork. In other countries such as Thailand, however, where travelers may become subjected to eating traditional dishes such as raw pork, this infection may still occur. Because of the mortality and morbidity associated with these parasites, they are becoming very important public health issues worldwide.

COMPLICATIONS OF DIARRHEAL INFECTIONS

The vast majority of infectious diarrheal illnesses are self-limiting and uncomplicated. When complications occur, they are often related to severe dehydration. Kidney failure, liver failure, myocardial infarction, and bowel infarction can each be seen in a setting in which the intravascular volume is severely depleted, with less blood going to vital organs.

Toxic megacolon is an acute dilatation of the large bowel that occurs in response to severe inflammation. A postulated pathogenesis for this change is an alteration in the neuromuscular tone of the bowel in response to the inflammatory process. Toxic megacolon may complicate diarrhea resulting from invasive organisms *(Shigella, Salmonella, Campylobacter,* and *Yersinia* organisms; *C. difficile;* and *E. histolytica)* and noninfectious processes such as ulcerative colitis. The transverse colon is the most common area dilated on radiography, exceeding 6 cm in diameter. The patient is usually febrile, appears toxic, and has diffuse abdominal pain; bowel sounds are infrequent or absent. Because of the relative atony of colon, diarrhea is absent or infrequent, giving the false impression that the patient is improving. Because of the high risk of bacteremia with colonic flora and the risk of perforation, broad-spectrum antibiotics are recommended. Patients may also require surgical intervention (colectomy).

Reiter syndrome may occur up to 6 weeks after a diarrheal or sexually transmitted infection. Affected patients are usually male and have some combination of arthritis, skin rash (a thick scaly rash involving the palms and soles, as well as a rash around the glans penis), urethritis, and conjunctivitis. This is an inflammatory illness that is treated with antiinflammatory medications, such as aspirin.

The hemolytic-uremic syndrome consists of anemia resulting from hemolysis or red blood cells and renal failure. This syndrome has been particularly associated with enterohemorrhagic *E. coli* (O157:H7) infection but may also occur after infection with *Shigella* species or enteroviruses (echovirus 22; coxsackievirus A4, B2, and B4).

Occasionally after a severe diarrhea, the villi—absorptive surface of the small bowel—may slough off. Because of the resultant malabsorption, patients have a prolonged diarrhea lasting weeks or months after the pathogen has been eradicated. A biopsy of the small bowel reveals a flattened surface similar to the picture seen in celiac sprue. Unlike that disease, however, this syndrome is reversible. Postinfectious malabsorption syndrome usually responds to a special diet of foods that are absorbed without the need for this specialized surface until the villi can regenerate.

Complications arising from campylobacteriosis are rare but have been described. Guillian-Barré syndrome, a demyelinating disease, occurs in 1 of 1000 cases, 20% of whom may experience a form of disability.

NEWLY RECOGNIZED AGENTS OF ACUTE DIARRHEA

For many patients with **acute diarrhea,** no pathogen is identified. Because so many organisms are ingested daily, it should not be surprising that new pathogens are regularly identified as possible causes of diarrhea.

Round, acid-fast organisms measuring 8 to 10 μm in diameter have been identified from the stool of AIDS patients with chronic diarrhea. This pathogen has also been associated with diarrhea lasting 3 weeks to 2 months in immunocompetent persons. Several outbreaks have been traced to contaminated water sources. Originally described as Cyanobacteria-like bodies (resembling blue-green algae), the organism is now believed to be a protozoal pathogen in the Cyclospora family.

Cyclospora cayetanensis emerged as a foodborne pathogen in 1996 in outbreaks associated with Guatemalan raspberries. *Cyclospora* infection results from the consumption of food containing oocysts. The onset of illness is reportedly abrupt and symptoms last for about 7 days. In AIDS patients, the infection may last longer. Symptoms include mild nausea, anorexia, abdominal pain, and watery diarrhea, similar to those of cryptosporidiosis. *Cyclospora* oocysts measure approximately 8 to 10 μm and stain best with modified acid-fast stain using modified carbol-fuschsin method but do not stain well with iodine, iron hematoxylin, periodic acid-Schiff (PAS) or Grocott-Gomori methanamine-silver nitrate (GMS) stain.

Enterocytozoon bieneusi (microsporidium), which causes a clinical picture similar to that of *Cyclospora* and *Cryptosporidium* organisms, is the smallest, measuring 1 to 2 μm. *E. bieneusi* is currently best detected using the Weber stain, a modified trichrome stain using chromotrope 2R.

Sexually transmitted disease (STD) agents can also cause diarrhea and other gastrointestinal symptoms. *Neisseria gonorrhoeae, Treponema pallidum* (syphilis), *Chlamydia* organism, and herpes simplex may cause a proctitis characterized by pain on defecation and loose stools with mucus or pus. This manifestation of a sexually transmitted illness is most commonly seen in persons who are recipients of anal intercourse. Because methods routinely used for culturing stool for bacterial pathogens do not detect the STD organisms, the physician must consider this possibility in the differential diagnosis.

Helicobacter pylori is a small curved gram-negative rod closely related to *Campylobacter* species. Although not a known cause of diarrhea, it is perhaps the most common infecting pathogen of the gastrointestinal tract. It is believed to be a cause of type B gastritis, a common type of inflammation of the stomach. It is also associated with ulcer disease. *H. pylori* is common, being found in more than 50% of persons over the age of 50 years in developed nations. In developing nations, infection appears to occur earlier. Chronic *H. pylori* infection has even been linked to a higher incidence of gastric cancer. Antibiotic treatment studies suggest that in some patients with duodenal ulcer disease, ulcers heal faster and fewer relapses occur if treatment is directed against this organism than in patients given traditional, non–antibiotic-containing ulcer treatment.

AGENTS OF FOOD POISONING

CASE STUDY

A young man has eaten at the restaurant where several other people became ill. Within 1 hour of his meal, he notes the sudden onset of tingling around his mouth, abdominal pain, mild diarrhea, and headache. Later, he experiences a burning in his hands and feet, and generalized weakness. He is seen in the emergency room, where he requires intubation for respiratory arrest. Before intubation, he tells the ER physician that he has eaten no shellfish.

Scombroid can cause all of this patient's initial symptoms but is not associated with respiratory arrest. Neurotoxic shellfish poisoning is also a mild illness. Ciguatera, paralytic shellfish poisoning (PSP), and puffer fish intoxication can each produce this syndrome. PSP is unlikely because the patient reported eating no shellfish, and puffer fish is rarely served in the United States. Ciguatera is the most likely diagnosis. Botulism should also be included in the differential diagnosis, although the rate of progression in this case was unusually fast and no focal neurologic findings were present.

A *food-borne outbreak* is defined as the occurrence in two or more persons of gastrointestinal or neurologic symptoms within 72 hours of a common meal. The most commonly identified pathogen has been *Salmonella* species, accounting for more than 25% of all reported outbreaks. *S. aureus, C. botulinum,* and *C. perfringens* together account for another 25% to 28% of outbreaks in which a pathogen is identified. Of the parasites, *G. lamblia* and *Cryptosporidium* organisms have each been causes of outbreaks, usually in association with a contaminated water source. Outbreaks of viral gastroenteritis (in particular, Norwalk virus associated with contaminated shellfish) account for nearly 5% of diagnosed outbreaks.

Chemical intoxications are responsible for more than 20% of outbreaks in which a pathogen is identified. Many are associated with a fish exposure. **Scomboid** is a syndrome consisting of flushing, headache, and diarrhea with crampy abdominal pain. It is due to ingesting a contaminated fish (his-

TABLE 28-6

Compendium of Common Food-Borne Diseases

Average Incubation Period	Organism	Average Duration	Implicated Foods	Typical Symptoms	Comments
2–16 hours	*Bacillus cereus*	1 day	Boiled and fried rice, meats, vegetables	Nausea, vomiting, (emetic) abdominal cramping, watery diarrhea	Produces two toxins; one emetic form that causes nausea and vomiting within hours, and one diarrheic form. Common year round. Isolation of large numbers from implicated foods and patient stool
6–72 hours	*Vibrio parahaemolyticus*	3 days	Shellfish	Pain, vomiting, fever, watery diarrhea	Blood sometimes in stool. Common spring, summer, fall in the coastal states. Stool culture using TCBS media is recommended
6–72 hours	*Vibrio cholerae*	3–7 days	Seafood, water	"Rice water" stools, severe diarrhea, no fever	No blood or mucus in stool, mechanism of action in vivo enterotoxin production. No tissue invasion. Stool culture using TCBS media is recommended
<8 hours	*Staphylococcus aureus*	<1 day	Egg salads, meat, poultry, pastries	Abrupt onset of nausea, pain and projectile vomiting, infrequent diarrhea	Mechanism of action is preformed enterotoxin in foods. Common in summer. ELISA or reverse passive latex agglutination enterotoxin test; gel electrophoresis in lieu of phage typing
8–22 hours	*Clostridium perfringens*	1 day	Beef, poultry, gravy, fish	Abdominal cramping, watery diarrhea; vomiting and fever uncommon	In vivo enterotoxin production; unlike *Staphylococcus aureus,* viable organisms must be ingested for disease to occur. Common in fall, winter, spring
12–48 hours	*Salmonella* spp.	3 days	Eggs, dairy products, fowl, beef	Fever, abdominal cramping, diarrhea, mild vomiting	WBCs in stool. Common in summer. Culture and serologic identification
16–48 hours	*Yersinia enterocolitica*	1 day–4 weeks	Milk, pork	Fever, severe abdominal pain, diarrhea	WBCs and RBCs in stool. Common in winter
18–36 hours	*Clostridium botulinum*	Weeks–months	Vegetables, fruits (canned foods), fish, honey (infants)	Nausea, vomiting, diarrhea, paralysis	Mechanism of action is a preformed neurotoxin. Common in summer and fall
24–72 hours	*Shigella* spp.	3 days	Egg and tuna salads, lettuce, milk	Fever, abdominal cramping, diarrhea, occasional vomiting	WBCs, RBCs and mucus in stools, tissue invasion common mechanism of action. Common in summer. Culture and serologic identification
24–72 hours	Enterotoxigenic *E. coli* (ETEC)	3 days	Fruits, meats, pastries, salads	Abdominal cramping, watery diarrhea, no vomiting or fever	In vivo enterotoxin, major cause of "traveler's diarrhea," year-round distribution, patient history includes travel to Mexico and other developing countries
24–72 hours	Enterohemorrhagic *E. coli* (EHEC)	3 days	Undercooked ground beef, cider	Watery diarrhea progressing to bloody diarrhea, abdominal cramping, no fever or vomiting	Implicated shiga-toxin producing *E. coli,* organisms disappear rapidly from stool. Culture of sorbitol-negative *E. coli* from stool using SMAC plate recommended

tamine and enzyme inhibitors are present in the flesh of some fish, including tuna, yellow jack, and mackerel). Symptoms begin within 1 hour of ingestion and usually last several hours.

Ciguatera is caused by the action of ciguatoxin, produced in dinoflagellates and passed up the food chain. Symptoms of diarrhea, abdominal pain, paresthesias, weakness, and headache begin with 1 to 2 hours of eating contaminated fish (snapper, sea bass, grouper) and may progress to hypotension and respiratory arrest. No antitoxin exists. Patients are observed and treated supportively.

Paralytic shellfish poisoning produces a similar syndrome and has a mortality rate of 10%. It is produced by a different toxin, which is found in contaminated mussels, clams, and scallops. The syndrome is usually seen in the summer months. A much milder syndrome, caused by a different toxin and also associated with shellfish, is termed neurotoxic shellfish poisoning. Puffer fish toxin (tetrodotoxin) is particularly potent, with a mortality rate of 60% in poisoned patients. Persons who prepare this fish must undergo special training and licensing.

With each of these poisonings, the fish looks, smells, and tastes normal. Prevention is aimed at identifying areas of contaminated fish. Table 28-6 shows common food-borne pathogens and their characteristics.

LABORATORY DIAGNOSIS OF GASTROINTESTINAL PATHOGENS

When a stool specimen is sent to the microbiology laboratory for analysis, the physician must correctly request the appropriate examination and understand the limitations of that test. In the United States, stool specimens are most commonly sent for "bacterial culture." For most laboratories, this means culturing for *C. jejuni* and *Salmonella* and *Shigella* organisms. If other organisms are suspected, the laboratory must be notified.

Specimen Collection and Handling
Stool specimens should be transported to the laboratory soon after collection. Refrigeration must be avoided as much as possible. No preservatives can be added to stool samples for bacterial detection. Cary-Blair or other suitable transport

medium would be appropriate if samples such as rectal swabs are submitted for culture. Samples for the examination for ova and parasites, however, must be transported in the proper preservatives, such as polyvinyl alcohol (PVA) or formalin, especially if the stool is loose and watery.

Direct Microscopic Examination
Microscopic evaluation of the stool demonstrates white blood cells (see Figure 28-2) when the etiologic agent is invasive. Such would be observed in *Salmonella, Shigella, Yersinia, Campylobacter,* and *Vibrio* sp. (other than *V. cholerae*) infections. White blood cells are present because of inflammation, and red blood cells, due to bleeding. Colonic biopsy of infected individuals may show tissue invasion.

Characteristic microscopic morphology on Gram-stained smears of certain bacterial pathogens may show gram-negative, curved rods that may align end-to-end and show a "seagull wing" appearance (Figure 28-4). This morphology may indicate the presence of *Campylobacter* sp. or *Vibrio* sp. Hanging-drop preparations or wet mount preparations may demonstrate a "darting" motility, a characteristic of *C. jejuni*. Bloody stools must also be examined immediately for the presence of *E. histolytica* trophozoites.

Culture
The most common method of identifying a bacterial pathogen in the stool is selective culture. This

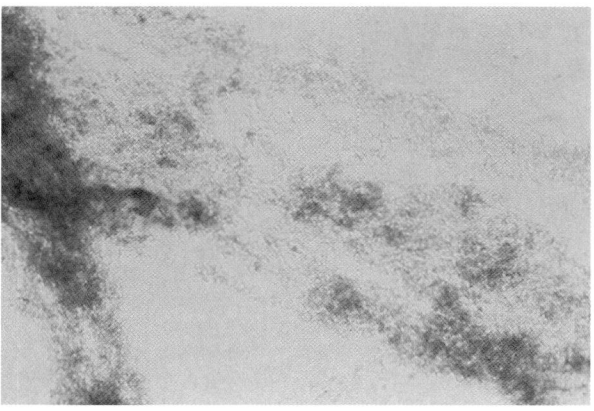

Figure 28-4

Gram stain of *Campylobacter* colony showing the typical microscopic morphology described as "seagull wings."

TABLE 28-7

Selective Media Commonly Used to Recover Diarrheal Agents

Culture Medium	Purpose	Characteristic Morphology Pathogens	Characteristic Morphology Colon Flora
MacConkey agar	To recover Enterobacteriaceae and other nonfastidious gram-negative bacilli Inhibits gram-positive organisms and some fastidious gram-negative bacilli	*Salmonella, Shigella* (with few exceptions) organisms *Edwardsiella* organisms appear clear and colorless	Lactose fermenters, such as *Escherichia coli, Klebsiella* sp., *Enterobacter* spp., and certain *Citrobacter* sp., appear dark pink to red Late or slow lactose fermenters, such as *Citrobacter* sp., *Serratia* sp., and *Hafnia* sp., appear colorless in 24 hours and slightly pink after 24–48 hours Non–lactose-fermenters, such as *Citrobacter* sp., *Proteus* sp., *Providencia* sp., and *Morganella* sp. appear clear and colorless
Hektoen enteric (HE) agar	A highly selective medium to recover primarily *Salmonella* and *Shigella* sp. Inhibits common colon flora Contains indicators to detect hydrogen sulfide (H$_2$S) production	*Salmonella* sp. appear green to blue-green with black centers because of H$_2$S production *Shigella* sp. appear green without black centers, because they do not produce H$_2$S	Lactose fermenters, such as *E. coli,* are slightly inhibited and appear orange to salmon-pink *Proteus* sp. are slightly inhibited; small, clear colonies with black centers may appear
Xylose-lysine deoxycholate agar (XLD)	A differential and selective medium to isolate *Salmonella* sp. and *Shigella* sp. from stool Inhibits most colon flora and most gram-positive bacteria Certain *Shigella* sp. (*S. dysenteriae* and *S. flexneri*) may be slightly inhibited	*Salmonella* sp. appears red with black centers owing to the production of H$_2$S; *Salmonella* does not ferment lactose or sucrose but does ferment xylose, which is essential in decarboxylating lysine to revert the acid pH (yellow from sucrose fermentation) to an alkaline pH (red from lysine decarboxylation) *Shigella* sp. do not ferment any of these carbohydrates and appear red or clear	Enterobacteriaceae that may not be completely inhibited, such as *Proteus vulgaris,* appear yellow (from sucrose) with black centers *Citrobacter freundii,* which produces H$_2$S, appears yellow with black centers owing to the inability to decarboxylate lysine Other intestinal flora that may grow ferment one or all of the carbohydrates in this medium, resulting in yellow colonies
Campylobacter blood agar (CAMPY-BA)	An enrichment-selective medium primarily to isolate and cultivate *Campylobacter* sp. from stool	*Campylobacter jejuni* appears pinkish gray, moist, and runny when incubated at 42° C	
Cefsulodin-Irgasan-novobiocin (CIN)	A selective medium to primarily isolate and recover *Yersinia enterocolitica* *Aeromonas* speices and *Plesiomonas shigelloides* may also be recovered Inhibits most gram-positive cocci, except for enterococci, and most gram-negative bacilli, particularly the Enterobacteriaceae	*Y. enterocolitica* produce colonies that look like "bull's-eyes": the center is red and the periphery appears colorless *Aeromonas* species also ferment mannitol present in the medium, like *Yersinia; P. shigelloides* does not	Except for *Pseudomonas aeruginosa, Citrobacter,* and *Serratia,* most colon flora are inhibited
Thiosulfate-citrate–bile salts–sucrose agar (TCBS)	A highly selective medium to recover *Vibrio* sp., including *Vibrio cholerae,* from stool and food Inhibits most colon flora because of the high pH (preferred by vibrios) and high bile salts content *Aeromonas* species may be recovered from this medium	TCBS contains sucrose, so sucrose-fermenting *Vibrio* sp. such as *V. cholerae* and *V. alginolyticus* produce yellow colonies Non–sucrose fermenters, such as *V. parahaemolyticus* and *V. vulnificus,* produce blue-green colonies	Inhibitory to most colon flora, except for occasional *Pseudomonas* isolates, which may also appear blue-green
Cycloserine-cefoxitin-fructose agar (CCFA), anaerobic incubation required	A selective medium to primarily isolate *Clostridium difficile* from stool of patients suspected of antibiotic-associated diarrhea or pseudomembranous colitis Inhibits most colon flora, both gram-positive and gram-negative bacteria	*C. difficile* appears yellow from fructose fermentation	Colon flora are inhibited
Sorbitol-MacConkey (SMAC)	A differential medium to detect sorbitol-negative *E. coli.* Contains sorbitol instead of lactose	*E. coli* O157:H7 appears colorless; does not ferment sorbitol	Most appear pink

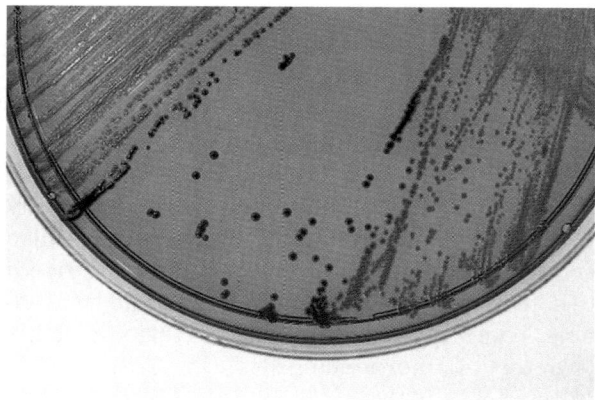

Figure 28-5

Salmonella colonies growing on Hektoen enteric (HE) agar showing black centers resulting from the production of hydrogen sulfide.

method uses antibiotic(s), chemicals, or environmental changes to inhibit the growth of the predominant fecal flora and selectively permit the pathogen to continue growing. Identification of colonies of the pathogen is then easier, without the growth of the normal flora there to mask them. Table 28-7 lists a variety of selective media commonly used to recover gastrointestinal bacterial pathogens.

Campylobacter jejuni

C. jejuni grows best at 42° C in an atmosphere containing 5% to 10% oxygen. *Campylobacter* species are therefore considered microaerophilic. Many laboratories purchase tanks of gas with an appropriate mixture to provide an atmosphere for culturing this organism. In settings where this is not practical (e.g., when evaluating an outbreak in an area without immediate access to a laboratory), an acceptable atmosphere can be created with little expense by using a candle jar.

   C. jejuni has characteristic colonial morphology, described as "running" and "wet-looking" because the colonies seem to run together. Microscopic morphology shows the typical gram-negative, curved rods that look like a seagull's wings (see Figure 28-4). This characteristic morphology of the genus *Campylobacter* differentiates it from *P. aeruginosa,* which also grows at 42° C and is oxidase positive.

Salmonellae

Salmonella infections are confirmed by culture (Figure 28-5). Organisms are most likely to be recovered from blood cultures of patients suspected of typhoid fever if the specimens are obtained during the first week of the infection. Stool cultures yield the organisms during the third and fourth week of the infection. Routine microbiologic media such as sheep blood agar and MacConkey agar, and highly selective enteric media, such as Hektoen enteric (HE) agar and xylose-lysine-deoxycholate (XLD) agar are used for recovery. Serotyping should be performed whenever possible.

Shigellae

Shigellae are fragile organisms that do not survive well outside the host for a long period. These organisms are particularly susceptible to acid pH; therefore stool samples should be processed as soon as they are received in the laboratory (Figure 28-6). Diarrheic stools from patients with suspected shigellosis contain pus and blood, a presentation typical of an invasive agent. Bloody stools must be plated as soon as possible on appropriate enteric media.

Escherichia coli

Diarrheogenic *E. coli* do not look different on a growth plate from *E. coli* that do not cause diarrheal disease. Diagnosis of diarrheal disease caused by *E. coli* requires a high index of suspi-

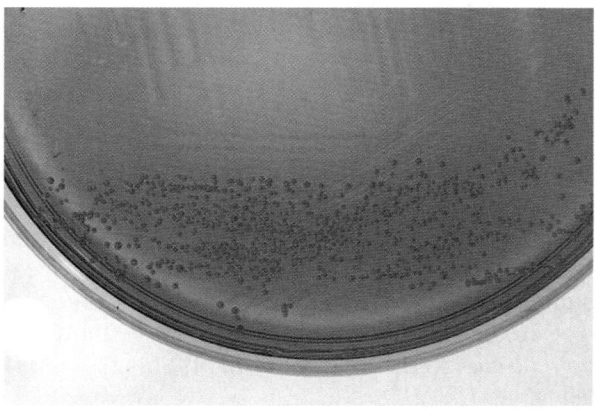

Figure 28-6

Shigella colonies growing on HE agar showing clear green colonies.

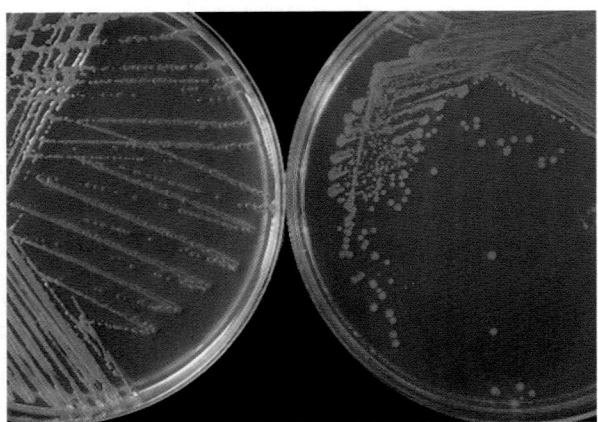

Figure 28-7

Left, Escherichia coli O157:H7 growing on MacConkey agar. *Right, E. coli* O157:H7 on sorbitol MacConkey agar. *E. coli* O157:H7 does not ferment sorbitol, whereas most other *E. coli* serotypes do ferment sorbitol.

cion from the clinician on the basis of history and physical findings. In addition, because *E. coli* are part of the normal fecal flora, special tests are needed to differentiate these pathogens from the routinely isolated nonpathogenic *E. coli*. For example, many enterohemorrhagic *E. coli* do not ferment sorbitol. Sorbitol-negative *E. coli* can be selected in the laboratory by using a sorbitol plate, such as sorbitol MacConkey agar (Figure 28-7). Antisera are also used to screen for specific serotypes. Enteroinvasive *E. coli* produce colonies and biochemical reactions similar to those of *Shigella* species. Tests to differentiate between these pathogens should be performed.

Yersinia species
Yersinia sp. grow well at 25° C. This characteristic may be used in the laboratory. Plating and incubation at this temperature and the use of selective media (e.g., cefsulodin-irgasan-novobiocin [CIN] agar) permit ready isolation of *Yersinia* organisms. Cold enrichment procedures, such as placing fecal samples on isotonic saline and keeping them at 4° C before the inoculation of selective medium, have increased recovery of the organism.

Vibrio species
Vibrio sp. requires highly selective medium for maximum recovery. Thiosulfate-citrate–bile salts–sucrose (TCBS) agar inhibits the usual colon flora.

In addition, TCBS agar differentiates sucrose-fermenting from non–sucrose-fermenting vibrios (Figure 28-8). When *V. cholerae* is suspected, use of a transport medium such as Cary-Blair or buffered saline in alkaline peptone water is suitable.

Susceptibility to 0/129 is useful in identifying *Vibrio* sp. Salt requirement for growth is usually helpful in differentiating *V. cholerae* from halophilic (non-cholera) vibrios. In endemic areas, antisera to screen for *V. cholerae* servar O1 should be available. Latex agglutination tests are also available to detect toxin-producing strains.

Clostridium species
C. difficile produces yellow, ground-glass colonies on cycloserine-cefoxitin-fructose agar (CCFA). Toxigenic strains may be screened by either enzyme immunoassay (EIA) or latex agglutination assay and confirmed by cell culture.

Helicobacter pylori
A microaerophilic organism that requires enriched medium, particularly with blood, *Helicobacter pylori* produces slow-growing and very small colonies (Figure 28-9). Using an invasive procedure, gastric mucosal biopsies are used for culture and direct smears for special stains. H & E (hematoxylin and eosin) stain and other tissue

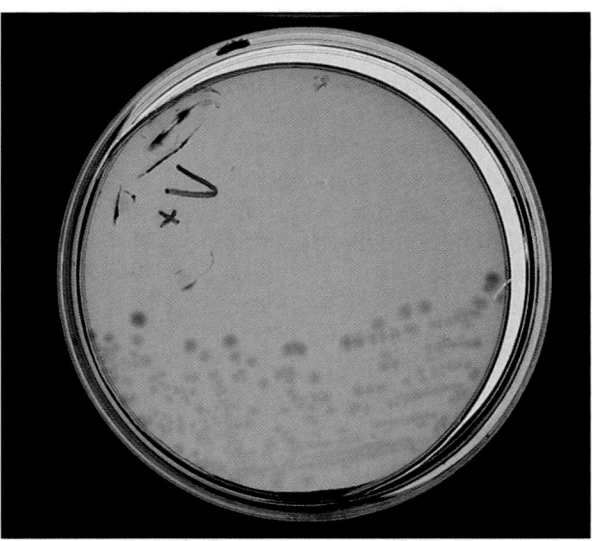

Figure 28-8

Vibrio vulnificus growing on TCBS. *Vibrio vulnificus* is a non–sucrose-fermenting vibrio.

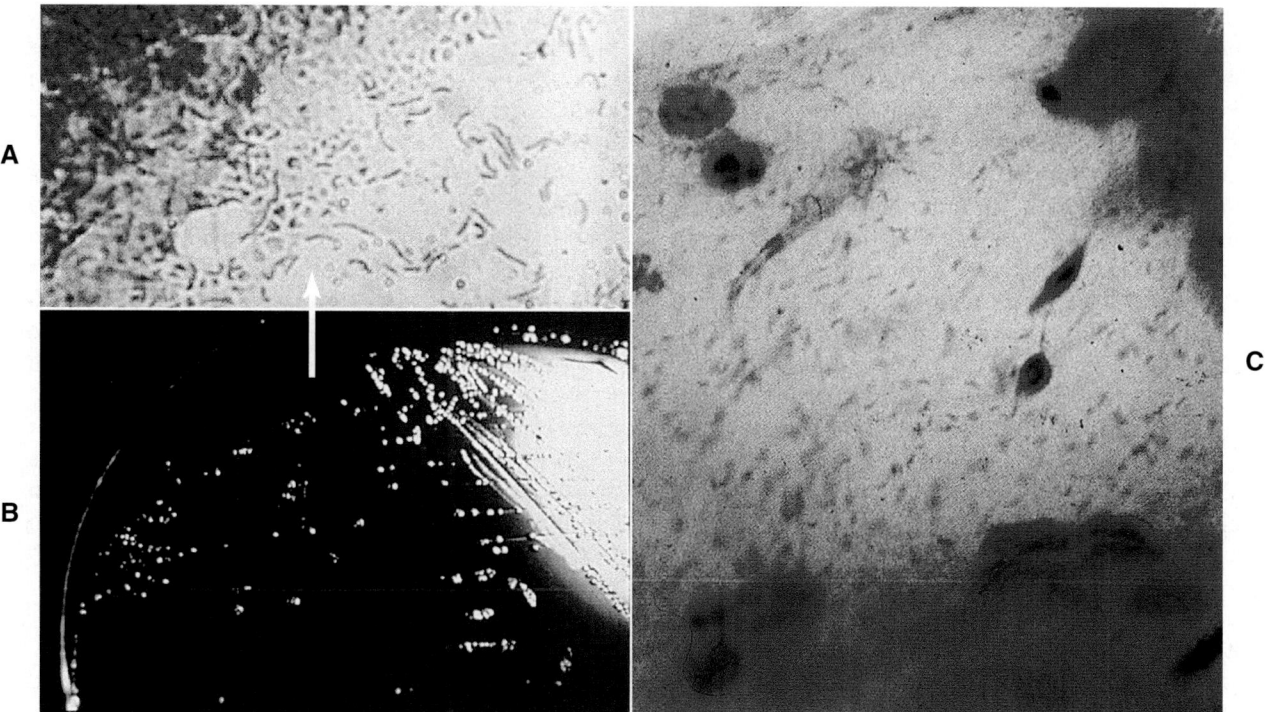

Figure 28-9

Microscopic morphology of *Helicobacter pylori* Gram-stained from a colony. **A,** Gram stain culture. **B,** *H. pylori* colonies grown on agar culture medium. **C,** Gram-stained on gastric mucus. (Courtesy American College of Gastroenterology and DiaSorin, Inc.)

stains have been used to directly detect the organisms. Biochemical features of this organism include urease, oxidase, and catalase tests positive. The characteristic Gram stain morphology is also shown in Figure 28-9.

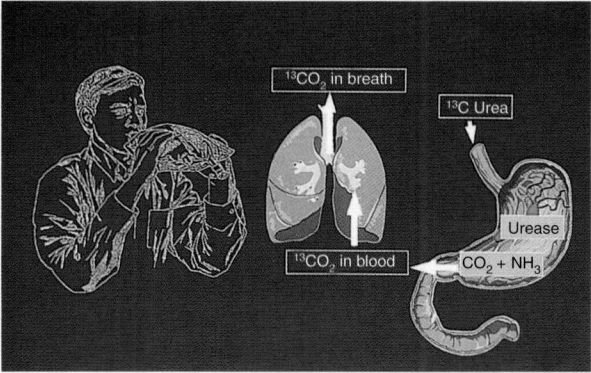

Figure 28-10

The urea breath test. (Courtesy American College of Gastroenterology and DiaSorin, Inc.)

Other diagnostic methods for *H. pylori* infection include noninvasive procedures such as antibody detection and urea breath tests. Unlike the invasive procedures to detect infection, which require gastric biopsy, noninvasive methods are less expensive and are considered cost-effective. For the initial diagnosis, IgG detection is reported to be both sensitive and specific; however, it is a poor indicator of cure. The urea breath test (Figure 28-10), which is based on the high urease activity of *H. pylori,* detects the presence of active infection. It is a noninvasive test that is recommended for initial diagnosis and to evaluate the efficacy of therapy. Urea, labeled with either stable isotope ^{13}C or the radioactive ^{14}C, when ingested results in a rapid appearance of the labeled CO_2 in the patient's breath.

TREATMENT OF DIARRHEA

The first factor to consider in the assessment of the patient with diarrhea is the state of hydration. Adequate rehydration and maintenance fluids are critical. Patients cannot be adequately rehydrated with water alone, because they have lost a significant amount of electrolyte-rich fluid in the stool. In the 1960s the coupled transport of sodium and glucose across the gut mucosa was first described. It provided the rationale for fluids with the appropriate mix of electrolytes for rehydration. Rehydration fluids can be given orally to all but the most ill patients. When given intravenously, isotonic fluids (e.g., 5% dextrose in 0.9 sodium chloride) are preferred to hypotonic solutions (e.g., 5% dextrose in water).

To date, no effective antibiotic therapy has been developed that shortens diarrheal illness caused by the common viral pathogens. Antibiotics may shorten the clinical illness caused by invasive bacteria or an enterotoxin-mediated process. Clinical studies are under way to further identify which subgroups of patients are most likely to benefit from antibiotic intervention. Antibiotic therapy has also been shown to shorten the clinical illness caused by *G. lamblia, I. belli,* and *E. histolytica.* No effective antimicrobial therapy has yet been identified for *Cryptosporidium* species, *E. bieneusi,* or *Cyclospora.*

Antidiarrheal medication, such as diphenoxylate with atropine (Lomotil) or loperamide, may also decrease the frequency of stool for some patients. Loperamide appears to be the safer of these agents. Earlier studies with diphenoxylate-atropine suggested that, for patients with an invasive syndrome, the clinical illness might actually worsen with such therapy, theoretically owing to an increase in the contact time of the organism with the mucosa and an impairment of the purging activity of diarrhea to rid the body of the pathogen. Although later studies question the validity of this finding, the use of an antidiarrheal medication may be most effective in the watery diarrhea syndromes associated with an enterotoxin-mediated or viral-induced process.

Pepto-Bismol (bismuth subsalicylate) has also been effective in the treatment of some patients with diarrhea. When taken four to six times a day, Pepto-Bismol shortened clinical illness in patients with traveler's diarrhea, a syndrome resulting primarily from enterotoxigenic *E. coli.* It has been postulated that the bismuth binds the toxin in the gut. A beneficial effect of the salicylate component (aspirin) on the mucosa is possible.

Various antibiotics and Pepto-Bismol have each been effective in the prophylaxis of diarrhea when given to travelers who are visiting areas where the risk of acquisition is high. Because of the cost of such therapy and the generally benign and self-limiting nature of most cases of acute diarrhea, such prophylactic therapy is not routinely recommended for all travelers. Travelers are advised to avoid high-risk foods and to drink only bottled beverages. High-risk foods include anything cut up by someone else and served raw (e.g., fruits, salads), dips and other foods left standing out, and raw or partially cooked shellfish. The phrase, "Boil it, peel it, cook it, or forget it," is a good one for travelers to high-risk areas to remember.

To prevent secondary infections, all patients should be educated about the most common modes of transmission. Careful handwashing and not cooking food for others are particularly important preventive measures.

Bibliography

Abbott SL: Laboratory aspects of non-157 toxigenic *E. coli, Clin Lab Newsl* 19:105, 1997.

Abbott S, Janda M: Bacterial gastroenteritis. I: Incidence and etiologic agents, *Clin Microbiol Newsl* 14:17, 1992.

Ashkenazi S et al: The association of Shiga toxin and other cytotoxins with the neurologic manifestations of shigellosis, *J Infect Dis* 161:961, 1990.

Bean NH, Goulding JS, Lao C, Angulo FJ: Surveillance for foodborne disease outbreaks—United States, 1988-1992, CDC Surveillance Summaries, October 25, 1996, *MMWR Morb Mortal Wkly Rep* 45:737, 1996.

Bell BP et al: A multistate outbreak of by *Escherichia coli* O157-H7-associated bloody diarrhea and hemolytic uremic syndrome from hamburgers: the Washington experience, *JAMA* 272:1349, 1994.

Beuchat LR: Comparison of chemical treatments to kill *Salmonella* on alfalfa seeds destined for sprout production, *Int J Food Microbiol* 34:329, 1997.

Beuchat LR, Ryu J-H: Produce handling and processing practices, *Emerg Infect Dis* 3:459, 1997.

Blaser MJ: Campylobacter enteritis. In Ellner PD, editor: *Infectious diarrheal diseases: current concepts and laboratory procedures,* New York, 1984, Marcel Dekker, p 1.

Blaser MJ: *Helicobacter pylori:* its role in disease, *Clin Infect Dis* 15:386, 1992.

Blaser MJ, Reller LB: Campylobacter enteritis, *N Engl J Med* 305:1444, 1981.

Blacklow N, Greenberg H: Viral gastroenteritis, *N Engl J Med* 325:252, 1991.

Centers for Disease Control and Prevention: Foodborne diseases active surveillance network, 1996, *MMWR Morb Mortal Wkly Rep* 46:258, 1997.

Centers for Disease Control and Prevention: Hepatitis A associated with consumption of frozen strawberries—Michigan, March 1997, *MMWR Morb Mortal Wkly Rep* 46:288, 1997.

Centers for Disease Control and Prevention: Listeriosis outbreak associated with Mexican-style cheese—California, *MMWR Morb Mortal Wkly Rep* 34:357, 1985.

Centers for Disease Control and Prevention: Multidrug-resistant *Salmonella* serotype typhimurium—United States, 1996, *MMWR Morb Mortal Wkly Rep* 4614:308, 1997.

Centers for Disease Control and Prevention: Multistate outbreak of *Salmonella* Poona infections—United States and Canada, 1991, *MMWR Morb Mortal Wkly Rep* 40:549, 1991.

Centers for Disease Control and Prevention: Outbreaks of *Escherichia coli* O157:H7 infection and cryptosporidiosis associated with drinking unpasteurized apple cider—Connecticut and New York, October 1996, *MMWR Morb Mortal Wkly Rep* 46:4, 1997.

Centers for Disease Control and Prevention: Outbreaks of *Salmonella* serotype enteritidis infection associated with consumption of raw shell eggs—United States 1994-1995, *MMWR Morb Mortal Wkly Rep* 45:737, 1996.

Craun GF: Waterborne giardiasis in the United States 1965-1984, *Lancet* 2:513, 1985.

Curran P: Na, Cl, and water transport by rat ileum in vitro, *J Gen Physiol* 43:1137, 1960.

D'Aoust JY: *Salmonella* and the international food trade, *Int J Food Microbiol* 24:1, 1994.

DeGirolami PC et al: Diagnosis of intestinal microsporidiosis by examination of stool and duodenal aspirate with Weber's modified trichrome and Uvitex 2B stains, *J Clin Microbiol* 33(4):805, 1995.

Didier ES et al: Comparison of three staining methods for detecting microsporidia in fluids, *J Clin Microbiol* 33(12):3138, 1995.

Drapkin M: Nosocomial infection with *C. difficile, Infect Dis Clin Prac* 1:138, 1992.

DuPont H et al: Five versus three days of norfloxacin therapy for traveler's diarrhea: a placebo-controlled study, *Antimicrob Agents Chemother* 36:87, 1992.

DuPont H et al: The response of man to virulent *Shigella flexneri* 2a, *J Infect Dis* 119:396, 1969.

Endtz H et al: Quinolone resistance in *Campylobacter* isolated from man and poultry following the introduction of fluoroquinolones in veterinary medicine, *J Antimicrobial Chemother* 27:199, 1991.

Ericsson C et al: Treatment of traveler's diarrhea with sulfamethoxazole and trimethoprim and loperamide, *JAMA* 263:257, 1990.

Farr B: Diarrhea: A neglected nosocomial hazard? *Infect Control Hosp Epidemiol* 12:343, 1991.

Food poisoning, listeriosis, and febrile gastroenteritis, *Nutr Rev* 55:57, 1997.

Glass R et al: Cholera in Africa: lessons on transmission and control for Latin America, *Lancet* 338:791, 1991.

Goodman LJ: Diagnosis, management, and prevention of diarrheal diseases, *Curr Opin Infect Dis* 6:88, 1993.

Goodman L et al: Empiric antimicrobial therapy of domestically acquired acute diarrhea in urban adults, *Arch Intern Med* 150:541, 1990.

Griffin PM, Tauxe RV: The epidemiology of infections caused by *Escherichia coli* O157:H7, other enterohemorrhagic *E. coli,* and the associated hemoytic uremic syndrome, *Epidemiol Rev* 13:60, 1991.

Guerrant RL et al: Evaluation and diagnosis of acute infectious diarrhea, *Am J Med* 78(supp 6B):91, 1985.

Harris AA: Hemorrhagic colitis and *Escherichia coli* O157:H7—identifying a messenger while pursuing the message, *Mayo Clin Proc* 65:884, 1990.

Hennessey TW et al: National outbreak of *Salmonella* enteritidis infections from ice cream, *N Eng J Med* 334:1281, 1996.

Henry CJ: New food processing technologies: from foraging to farming to food technology, *Proc Nutr Soc* 56:855, 1997.

Hodgkin K: *Towards earlier diagnosis: a family doctor's approach,* Baltimore, 1963, Williams & Wilkins.

Humphrey TJ, Whitehead A: Egg age and growth of *Salmonella* enteritidis PT4 in egg contents, *Epidemiol Infect* 111:209-219, 1993.

Jiang Z et al: Intestinal secretory immune response to infection with *Aeromonas* species and *Plesiomonas shigelloides* among students from the United States in Mexico, *J Infect Dis* 164:979, 1991.

Keene WE et al: An outbreak of *Escherichia coli* O157:H7 infections traced to jerky made from deer meat, *JAMA* 277:1229, 1997.

Kehl KS et al: Evaluation of the premier EHEC assay for detection of Shiga-toxin producing *Escherichia coli, J Clin Microbiol* 35:2051, 1997.

Koneman E et al: *Color atlas and textbook of diagnostic microbiology,* ed 3, Philadelphia, 1988, JB Lippincott.

Kuritsky JN et al: Norwalk gastroenteritis: a community outbreak associated with bakery product consumption, *Ann Intern Med* 100:519, 1984.

Lee PR: Irradiation to prevent foodborne illness, *JAMA* 272:261, 1994.

Levine MM: *Escherichia coli* that cause diarrhea: enterotoxigenic, enteropathogenic, enteroinvasive, enterohemorrhagic, and enteroadherent, *J Infect Dis* 155:377, 1987.

Low JC et al: Antimicrobial resistance of *Salmonella* enterica Typhimurium DT 104 isolates and investigation of strains with transferable apramycin resistance, *Epidemiol Infect* 118:97, 1997.

Mackowiak PA, Wasserman SS, Levine MM: An analysis of the quantitative relationship between oral temperature and severity of illness in experimental shigellosis, *J Infect Dis* 166:1181, 1991.

Mahon BE et al: An international outbreak of *Salmonella* infections caused by alfalfa sprouts grown from contaminated seeds, *J Infect Dis* 175:876, 1997.

Meng J, Doyle MO: Emerging issues in microbiological food safety, *Annu Rev Nutr* 17:255, 1997.

Mishu B et al: Outbreaks of *Salmonella* enteritidis infections in the United States, 1985-1991, *J Infect Dis* 169:547, 1994.

Mishu B et al: *Salmonella enteritidis* gastroenteritis transmitted by intact chicken eggs, *Ann Intern Med* 115:190, 1991.

Novak SM: Foodborne illness—chemical and shellfish poisoning, *Clin Microbiol Newsl* 20:17, 1998.

Ortega YR et al: *Cyclospora* species—a new protozoan pathogen of humans, *N Engl J Med* 328:1308, 1993.

Osterholm MT et al: An outbreak of foodborne giardiasis, *N Engl J Med* 304:24, 1981.

Paton AW, Paton JC: Detection and characterization of Shiga toxigenic *Escherichia coli* by using multiplex PCR Assays for stx1, stx2, eaeA, enterohemorrhagic *E. coli* hlyA, Rfb011 and rfbO157, *J Clin Microbiol* 36:598, 1998.

Peterson WL: *Helicobacter pylori* and peptic ulcer disease, *N Engl J Med* 324:1043, 1991.

Rabbani G et al: Single-dose treatment of cholera with furazolidone or tetracycline in a double-blind randomized trial, *Antimicrob Agents Chemother* 33:1447, 1989.

Raj P: Pathogenesis and laboratory diagnosis of *Escherichia coli*—associated Enteritis, *Clin Microbiol Newsl* 15:89, 1993.

Schlech WF: *Listeria* gastroenteritis—old syndrome, new pathogen, *N Engl J Med* 336:130, 1997.

Shadduck JA: Human microsporidiosis and AIDS, *Rev Infect Dis* 11:203, 1989.

Sommers HM: The indigenous microbiota of the human host. In Youmans GP, Paterson PY, Sommers HM, editors: *The biologic and clinical basis of infectious diseases,* ed 2, Philadelphia, 1980, WB Saunders.

Sowers EG, Wells JG, Strockbine NA: Evaluation of commercial latex reagents for identification of O157 and H7 antigens of *Escherichia coli, J Clin Microbiol* 34:1286, 1996.

Spika JS et al: Chloramphenicol-resistant *Salmonella newport* traced through hamburger to dairy farms, *N Engl J Med* 316:565, 1987.

Steffen R et al: Health problems after travel to developing countries, *J Infect Dis* 156:84, 1987.

Swerdlow D, Ries A: Cholera in the Americas: guidelines for the clinician, *JAMA* 267:1495, 1992.

Taylor D et al: Treatment of traveler's diarrhea: Ciprofloxacin plus loperamide compared with ciprofloxacin alone, *Ann Intern Med* 114:731, 1991.

Taylor PR, Weinstein WM, Bryner JH: *Campylobacter* fetus infection in human subjects: association with raw milk, *Am J Med* 66:779, 1979.

Walker RI et al: Pathophysiology of *Campylobacter* enteritis, *Microbiol Rev* 50:81, 1986.

Wells JG et al: Isolation of *Escherichia coli* serotype O157:H7 and other Shiga-like toxin producing *E. coli* from dairy cattle, *J Clin Microbiol* 29:985, 1991.

Zhuang R-Y, Beuchat LR, Angulo FJ: Fate of *Salmonella* Montevideo on and in raw tomatoes as affected by temperature and treatment with chlorine, *Appl Environ Microbiol* 61:2127, 1995.

Zink DL: The impact of consumer demands and trends on food processing, *Emerging Infect Dis* 3:467, 1997.

LEARNING ASSESSMENTS

1. How does stomach acidity protect the host from gastrointestinal illness?

2. What is the major immune defense in the small bowel? How does it protect the host?

3. What is the role of the usual colon flora in preventing the initiation of gastrointestinal disease?

4. What clinical findings are useful in the differential diagnosis of diarrheal illness? Laboratory findings?

5. Why is food history important in determining the possible etiology of diarrheal disease?

6. Which parasitic agents would be suspected among immunosuppressed patients such as AIDS patients?

7. If the patient has history of travel to southeast Asia and consumption of raw fish or shellfish, what agents would be suspected?

8. What other syndromes may occur related to the ingestion of fish and shellfish?

9. How can consumers prevent the occurrence of food-borne disease?

10. What strategies may be employed to prevent the occurrence of food-borne outbreaks?

CHAPTER 29

Infections of the Central Nervous System

Kirk M. Doing, David P. Marmaduke

GENERAL CONCEPTS RELATED TO INFECTIONS OF THE CENTRAL NERVOUS SYSTEM
  Anatomic Organization
  Cerebrospinal Fluid Characteristics
  Host-Pathogen Relationships

INFECTIONS OF THE CENTRAL NERVOUS SYSTEM
  Bacterial Infections
    Acute bacterial meningitis
    Mycobacterial infections

Brain Abscesses
Spirochetal Infections
Fungal Meningitis
Viral Infections
  Meningitis
  Meningoencephalitis
Parasitic Infections

LABORATORY DIAGNOSIS OF CENTRAL NERVOUS SYSTEM INFECTIONS
  Specimen Collection: Lumbar Puncture
  Laboratory Evaluation

OBJECTIVES

1. Describe the production and distribution of the cerebrospinal fluid (CSF).
2. Describe the characteristics of normal CSF.
3. Describe the collection, transportation, and processing of CSF samples.
4. List the common bacterial pathogens in meningitis along with one host-related factor and one virulence-related factor for each pathogen.
5. List the common bacterial, fungal, and parasitic pathogens associated with brain abscess or intracerebral mass lesions.
6. List fungi that typically produce meningitis, and compare virulence and host factors of two fungi that typically produce intracerebral lesions.
7. List two viruses associated with meningitis, encephalitis, and paralysis.
8. Compare and contrast the physical, chemical, and cellular features of bacterial, mycobacterial (tuberculous), fungal, syphilitic, viral, and parasitic central nervous system (CNS) infections.

KEY TERMS

Central nervous system (CNS)
Cerebrospinal fluid (CSF)
Pleocytosis
Meningitis (leptomeningitis)
Encephalitis
Meningoencephalitis
"Aseptic" meningitis
Meningismus

Brain abscess
Rhinocerebral mucormycosis
Neurosyphilis
Guillain-Barré syndrome
Rabies
Primary amebic meningoencephalitis
Neurocysticercosis
Tuberculous meningitis

CASE STUDY

A 3-year-old male with a recent history of acute otitis media presented to the emergency department. Upon examination, he was febrile to 103° F and lethargic. No evidence of a rash was present. His vaccination history was up to date. Laboratory studies included a complete blood count, which showed leukocytosis with a total leukocyte count of 21,000/μL with left-shift and toxic changes. A lumbar puncture produced cloudy CSF fluid with a cell count of 210 leukocytes/mm³ with 85% neutrophils. The CSF glucose was decreased at 15 mg/dL, and the CSF protein was elevated at 450 mg/dL. The child received intravenous ceftriaxone, and the CSF sample was sent to the microbiology laboratory for CSF Gram stain and culture. A cytocentrifuged CSF smear revealed moderate intracellular gram-positive cocci in pairs. Subsequent culture of the CSF grew a mucoid strain of *Streptococcus pneumoniae*. Susceptibility studies were completed with the following MICs obtained: penicillin 2.0 μg/mL, ceftriaxone 0.012 μg/mL, and vancomycin less than 1.0 μg/mL.

Infections of the central nervous system (CNS) are of critical clinical concern, and positive laboratory findings are "critical values" communicated directly to the attending physician or other appropriate members of the patient care team. The symptom complex associated with these infections may be caused by bacteria, fungi, viruses, or parasites. The physician arrives at a presumptive diagnosis based on patient demographics, local epidemiology of CNS infections, physical examination, and radiologic studies. Specific diagnosis by identification of the etiologic agent is the critical task of the laboratory staff.

In the United States, the annual incidence of bacterial meningitis varies from 0.1 to 15 cases per 100,000 population, with a subsequent mortality rate ranging from 0% to 33%. Despite vaccination prevention programs and antibiotic interventions, only a modest overall decrease in new cases of bacterial meningitis has occurred in the United States. Cases of *Haemophilus influenzae* meningitis in children have decreased dramatically where vaccination programs have been fully implemented, but this is countered by the increasing number of opportunistic pathogens involving the CNS in immunocompromised patients, such as those with malignancy or the acquired immunodeficiency syndrome (AIDS). In sub-Saharan Africa ("the meningitis belt"), seasonal epidemics of meningococcal meningitis can reach several hundred cases per 100,000 population. Although mortality rates have decreased as a result of improved medical management of CNS infections, recent studies indicate that some children who have been successfully treated for bacterial or viral meningitis later display learning disabilities, behavioral problems, and developmental delay. Thus infections of the CNS are a cause of both immediate and long-term health concerns.

This chapter discusses the following:

- The interplay of host-related risk factors and virulence factors associated with pathogens
- Characteristics of the cerebrospinal fluid (CSF)
- Microbial agents of infections of the CNS
- Laboratory diagnosis of CNS infections

GENERAL CONCEPTS RELATED TO INFECTIONS OF THE CENTRAL NERVOUS SYSTEM

Anatomic Organization

The **central nervous system (CNS)** encompasses the brain, spinal cord and cranial nerves, but not the peripheral nerves (Figure 29-1). The brain and spinal cord are protected by the skull, vertebral column, and overlying meninges (coverings). The dura mater is a thick, fibrous, white membrane that is firmly adherent to the overlying skull. Deep to this and covering the brain and spinal cord is the pia mater and pia arachnoid. Between the pia mater and pia arachnoid resides the subarachnoid

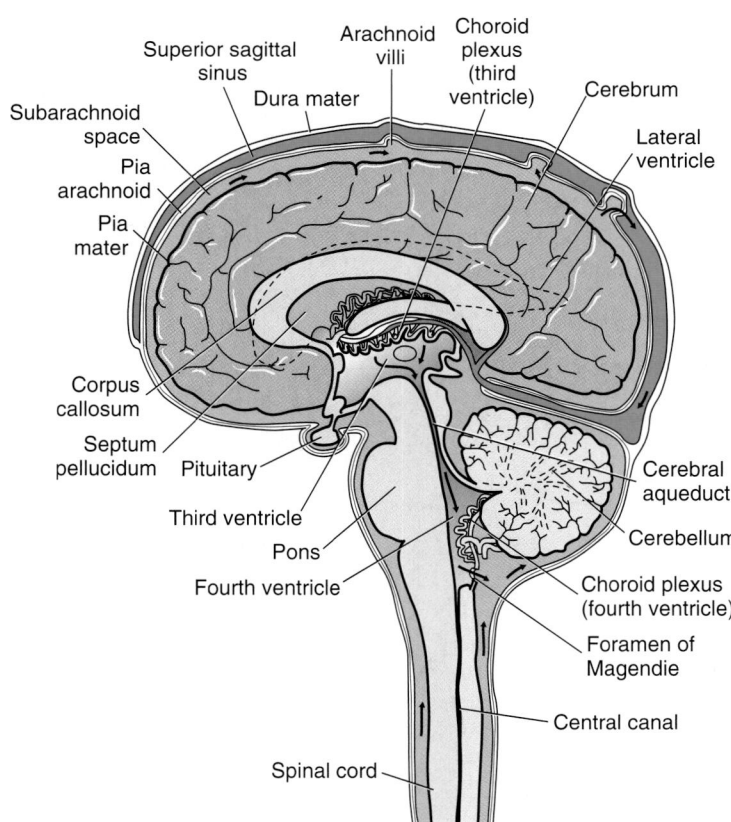

Figure 29-1

Components of the central nervous system (CNS) and flow pattern of cerebrospinal fluid (CSF).

space occupied by the surface blood vessels and the **cerebrospinal fluid (CSF).** The CSF is a unique body fluid produced by both filtration and secretion from specialized capillary tufts of the choroid plexuses within the four ventricles of the brain. CSF enters the subarachnoid space via the cisterna magna and circulates under pressure around the brain and spinal cord to the arachnoid villi, where it is eventually reabsorbed. The CSF provides a protective fluid "cushion" for the brain and spinal cord.

Cerebrospinal Fluid Characteristics

CSF is a clear, colorless, sterile fluid that contains few cells. In normal adults, the CSF volume ranges from 90 to 150 mL, the CSF protein level is 15 to 45 mg/dL, and the CSF glucose level is two-thirds that of plasma (40 to 80 mg/dL, or CSF glucose:serum glucose ratio of 0.6). In adults, normal CSF contains 0 to 7 leukocytes/ml, with a differential count of 60% to 80% lymphocytes, 10% to 40% monocytes, and 0% to 15% neutrophils. Compared with adults, normal newborns have higher CSF concentrations of protein (15 to 150 mg/dL) and glucose (30 to 120 mg/dL). The cell count is somewhat higher as well (0 to 30 leukocytes/mL), with a greater percentage of monocytes and neutrophils. The paucity of leukocytes and protein (including immunoglobulins) within the CSF provides little initial defense against invading organisms. Infection of the CNS is frequently, but not invariably, associated with an inflammatory **pleocytosis,** or increase in CSF cell count, that varies according to the invading organism.

Host-Pathogen Relationships

Infection results from the complex interplay between the host, the organism, and the environ-

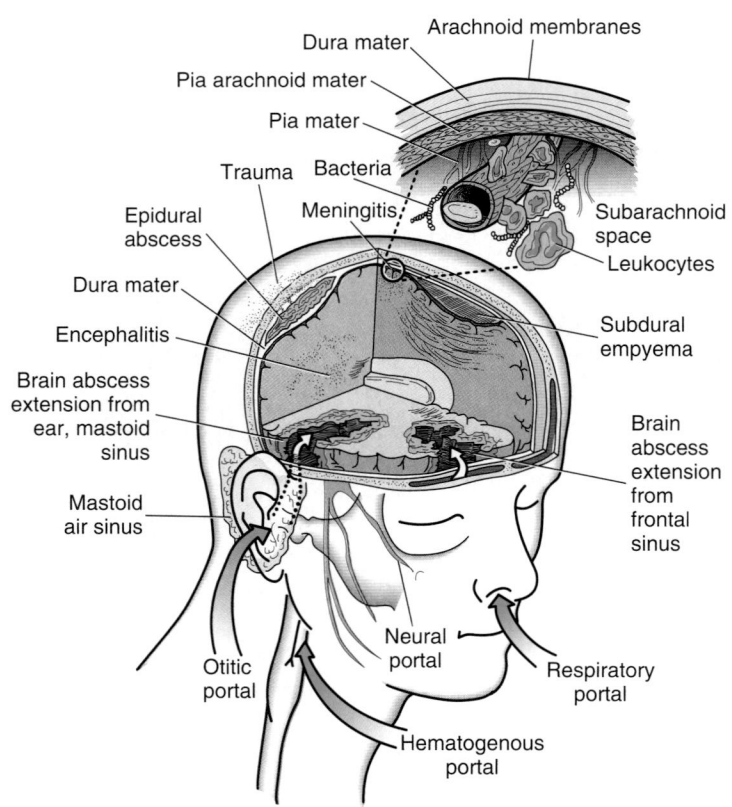

Figure 29-2

Portals of entry resulting in meningitis, meningoencephalitis, and intracranial mass lesions.

ment. Host risk factors that predispose to infection include the patient's age, nutritional and immunologic status, and disease states (alcoholism, diabetes mellitus, sickle cell anemia, and malignancy). Among the organism characteristics associated with infection are structural components (e.g., antiphagocytic capsules, pili, and fimbriae); seasonal, geographic, and environmental distribution of the organism; and portal of entry into the host. The common portals of entry include the respiratory, auditory, bloodstream, and neural routes as well as direct penetration from adjacent sinuses or other contiguous sites of infection. Most CNS microbial pathogens have common routes of entry and preferred intracranial and intraspinal localizations causing characteristic lesions (Figure 29-2). Most community-acquired organisms enter via the respiratory route. Once replication is established in the upper respiratory tract, the organism can invade directly through the sinuses or lymphatics or seed the subarachnoid space via the bloodstream. Some viruses spread to the CNS by invading and traveling through cranial nerves (herpesviruses) or peripheral nerves (rabies virus).

Entry of the organism gives rise to inflammation around the blood vessels within the subarachnoid space between the pia mater and pia arachnoid, resulting in **meningitis (leptomeningitis).** If diffuse inflammation is limited to the brain substance, as is characteristic of many viruses, the disease is termed **encephalitis.** Inflammation of both the membranes and the brain substance is a **meningoencephalitis.** If the entry is localized, as may occur following direct extension of an infection from the middle ear, mastoid, or nasal sinuses or with penetrating trauma, then localized areas of inflammation within the dura mater (pachymeningitis), epidural abscess, subdural empyema, or intracerebral abscess may result. Each of these localizations has characteristic associations with select microbial pathogens.

One last mention should be made of CSF samples that show a pleocytosis (usually with predominance of lymphoctyes), but no organisms on direct examination. Such cases are often described as **"aseptic" meningitis.** As we shall see, many cases of "aseptic" meningitis are not aseptic at all but may be due to viruses, fungi, parasites, or some bacteria.

INFECTIONS OF THE CENTRAL NERVOUS SYSTEM

Bacterial Infections

Acute bacterial meningitis

Acute bacterial meningitis denotes purulent inflammation of the meninges as a result of bacterial infection. The inflammatory response is characteristically limited to the pia mater and pia arachnoid layers of the meninges (leptomeningitis). Clinical findings of meningitis may include fever, photophobia, headache, nausea, vomiting, and signs of meningeal inflammation **(meningismus)** such as neck stiffness or involuntary flexion of the lower extremities with flexion of the neck (Brudzinski sign). In infants and children, irritability, restlessness, and poor feeding may be the only signs of meningitis. Associated laboratory findings include leukocytosis with left-shift and toxic changes, increased CSF protein (greater than 100 mg/dL), and decreased CSF glucose (less than 40 mg/dL). In the untreated patient, intracranial pressure increases with resultant obtundation, coma, and death. In infants and children, focal neurologic deficits may be detected up to 1 year following meningitis, with some children showing ongoing evidence of developmental delay, hearing loss, or mental retardation, as previously noted.

Cases of bacterial meningitis show characteristic age-related incidence (Box 29-1). In premature infants, meningitis is most often caused by gram-negative bacilli such as *Escherichia coli,* whereas meningitis in full-term newborns commonly is due to group B streptococci (Figure 29-3), followed by *Listeria monocytogenes* (Figure 29-4), *H. influenzae* and *S. pneumoniae,* respectively. These infections are associated with bloodstream dissemination and neonatal sepsis. Pregnancies complicated by premature rupture of the fetal membranes are at particular risk of neonatal meningitis. If infections are acquired early in pregnancy, the fetus may be spontaneously aborted. Neonatal meningitis occurring 1 to 2 weeks after delivery is usually nosocomial or acquired in the community.

A dramatic change in the epidemiology of meningitis in children has occurred in the past decade thanks to the licensure of conjugate vaccines against *H. influenzae* type b. *H. influenzae*

Box 29-1

Bacteria Involving the Central Nervous System

Acute purulent meningitis related to age

Premature newborns

Gram-negative bacilli (*Escherichia coli, Klebsiella* spp., *Enterobacter* spp., *Proteus* spp.)

Infants

Streptococcus agalactiae (group B)
Listeria monocytogenes
Haemophilus influenzae
Streptococcus pneumoniae

Children

Neisseria meningitidis
Streptococcus pneumoniae
Haemophilus influenzae

Adolescents

Neisseria meningitidis

Adults

Streptococcus pneumoniae

Elderly

Gram-negative bacilli

Chronic meningitis

Mycobacteria

Mycobacterium tuberculosis and atypical mycobacteria

Spirochetes

Treponema pallidum
Borrelia burgdorferi
Borrelia recurrentis
Leptospira sp.

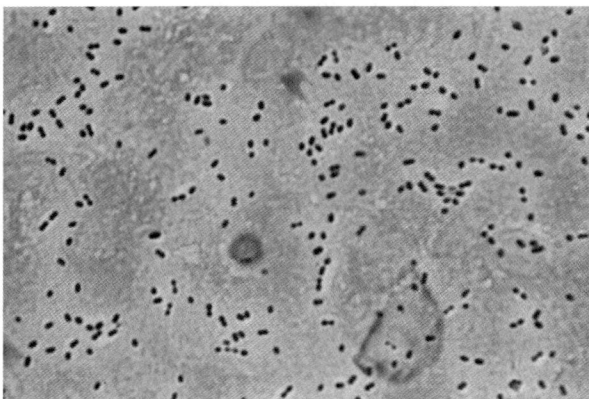

Figure 29-3

Direct smear of CSF from an infant, showing gram-positive cocci in pairs and short chains characteristic of group B streptococci. Gram stain; noncytocentrifuge preparation; high-power view.

nasopharyngeal colonization and subsequent localization to the meninges. Bacterial proliferation and lysis within the CSF results in neutrophilic pleocytosis that damages neural tissues and blood vessels resulting in increased CSF pressure and protein and decreased CSF glucose.

In April 1985 the first vaccines against *H. influenzae* type b capsular polysaccharide (polyribosylribitol phosphate [PRP]) were introduced. Currently, improved vaccines conjugated to diphtheria toxoid (PRP-D) or meningococcal protein (PRP-OMP) are available. Conjugate vaccination

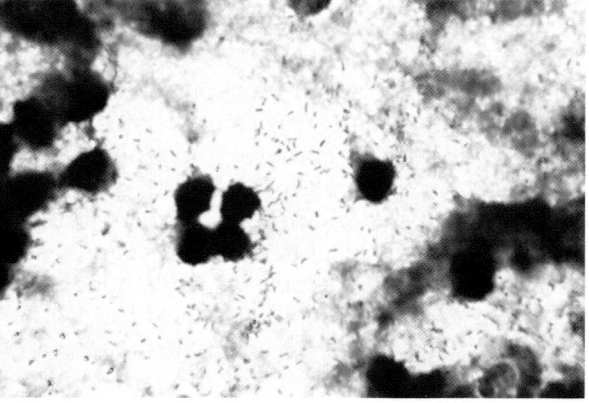

Figure 29-4

Direct smear of CSF from a child, showing abundant gram-negative, pleomorphic coccobacilli characteristic of *Haemophilus influenzae*. The background shows degenerating inflammatory cells. Gram stain; high-power view.

type b is a gram-negative coccobaccillus (Figure 29-5) associated with acute otitis media, pneumonia, and epiglottitis in addition to meningitis. *H. influenzae* type b is more common after the neonatal period because passively acquired maternal anti–*H. influenzae* IgG antibodies are protective, but the antibody titer decreases after delivery. By the time children reach 1 year of age they are susceptible to infection and remain so until 5 to 6 years of age, when they are capable of producing their own anti–*H. influenzae* antibodies. *H. influenzae* meningitis in children results from

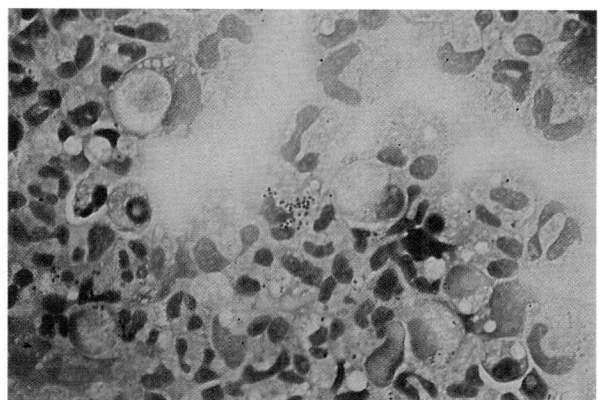

Figure 29-5 ─────────────────────────

Direct smear of CSF from a high-school student showing clusters of gram-negative diplococci consistent within *Neisseria meningitidis* within polymorphonuclear leukocytes. Note the increased cellularity of the smear in this cytocentrifuge preparation. Gram stain; high-power view.

protects against nasopharyngeal colonization as well as providing immunity from infection. In 1991 the American Academy of Pediatrics recommended universal immunization of infants at 2, 4, and 6 months of age against *H. influenzae* type b. The results of this vaccination program have been one of the true success stories of the modern medical era. Whereas the previous edition of this textbook described *H. influenzae* type b as the most common cause of meningitis in children 1 to 6 years of age, the yearly number of reported cases has progressively decreased with 19.3 cases per 100,000 population in 1988 declining to 2.0 cases per 100,000 population in 1993. *H. influenzae* type b is now the third most common cause of meningitis in children after *Neisseria meningitidis* and *S. pneumoniae,* and the decline appears to be continuing.

   N. meningitidis is a gram-negative diplococcus and the most common cause of meningitis in children. Meningococcal meningitis is endemic in some developing countries, and epidemic outbreaks occur in the United States. Serogroups A, B, and C account for more than 90% of all cases, and group A is the most common cause of epidemics. The meningococcus enters by way of the respiratory route, colonizes the nasopharynx, and invades the bloodstream. Meningococcemia may be the resulting disease, or meningitis can occur from dissemination through the bloodstream and seeding of the subarachnoid space. Meningococ-

cal disease may pursue a particularly aggressive course with bilateral adrenal gland hemorrhages (Waterhouse-Friderichsen syndrome) and subcutaneous hemorrhage (purpura fulminans) resulting from disseminated intravascular coagulation. Individuals deficient in terminal components of complement (C5–C9) are at risk for recurrent meningococcal infections and subsequent meningitis. The CSF of patients with meningococcal meningitis may initially show scarce neutrophils because of the time delay following initiation of infection in the meninges, proliferation of the organism, and subsequent inflammatory response. All CSF samples must be carefully examined for organisms even in the absence of obvious inflammation.

   S. pneumoniae, the "pneumococcus," is a gram-positive diplococcus and the most common cause of community-acquired pneumonia, otitis media, purulent sinusitis, and mastoiditis. *S. pneumoniae* is the most common cause of meningitis in adults and the second most common cause of meningitis in children (Figure 29-6). *S. pneumoniae* frequently inhabits the nasopharynx in healthy individuals. Meningitis generally follows pneumonia or otitis media, as presented in the introductory case, and the organisms proliferate by evading phagocytosis resulting from the presence of capsular polysaccharide on their cell surface. Of the 83 serotypes, only a handful (serotypes 14, 6, 19, 18, 23, 4, 9, 3, and 1) account for 90% of cases of meningitis. The risk of meningi-

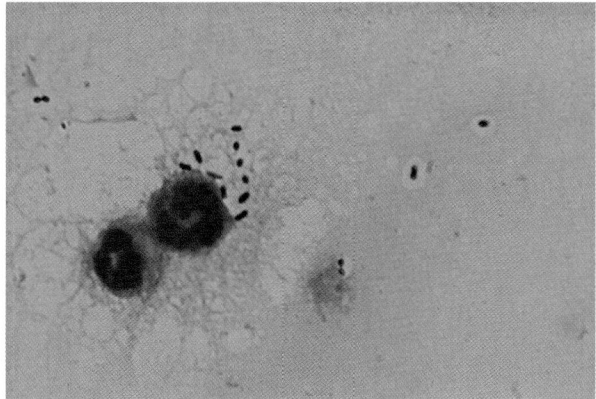

Figure 29-6 ─────────────────────────

Direct smear of acute bacterial meningitis in an adult showing the lancet-shaped gram-positive diplococci characteristic of *Streptococcus pneumoniae.* The polysaccharide capsule produces a prominent "halo" around organisms. Gram stain; noncytocentrifuge preparation; high-power view.

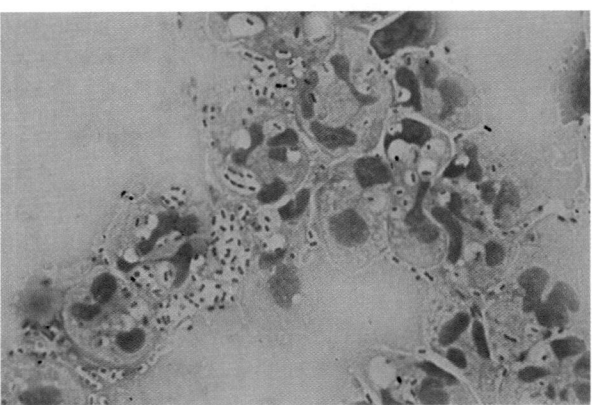

Figure 29-7 ————————————

Direct smear of posttraumatic acute bacterial meningitis showing numerous intracellular and extracellular gram-negative bacilli with the prominent capsules characteristic of *Klebsiella pneumoniae.* Gram stain; cytocentrifuge preparation; high-power view.

tis is greatest in blacks as well as those with liver disease, alcoholism, sickle-cell anemia and previous splenectomy or malignancy. Over the past two decades, the incidence of pneumococcal infections resulting from penicillin-resistant *S. pneumoniae* has steadily increased, and more recently the number of infections resulting from *S. pneumoniae* resistant to both penicillin and third-generation cephalosporins has increased. Polyvalent antipneumococcal vaccines are protective against more than 90% of the most frequently recovered serotypes.

Gram-negative bacilli are occasional causes of meningitis in the elderly, as immunity wanes in the "golden years." The most commonly isolated pathogen is *E. coli,* but infections resulting from *Klebsiella* (Figure 29-7), *Enterobacter, Pseudomonas, Salmonella,* and *Proteus* organisms are also seen. Penetrations of the skull, accidental or surgical, are also associated with gram-negative bacillary meningitis as well as with staphylococcal meningitis or abscesses. Cases of meningitis resulting from anaerobic streptococci, *Bacteroides* (Figure 29-8), and *Fusobacterium* organisms are uncommon and are usually associated with a concurrent brain abscess or unusual clinical settings.

Mycobacterial infections

The most common mycobacterial infection of the CNS is tuberculous meningitis caused by *Mycobacterium tuberculosis.* Tuberculous meningitis was a scourge in the United States of the early 1900s.

The development of antituberculous chemotherapy resulted in a marked decrease in the incidence of this infection; however, the current trend toward increased numbers of immunocompromised patients in this country has resulted in a resurgence of this disease. Tuberculosis has always been a common disease in developing countries.

M. tuberculosis enters the body by the respiratory route on airborne infectious particles that reach the alveoli of the lungs. There the organisms multiply within macrophages and then disseminate through the bloodstream. The clinical presentation of tuberculous meningitis is quite variable but usually is subacute. Both the meninges and the brain itself are frequently involved, with a resulting thick exudate especially at the base of the brain. Lumbar puncture shows increased CSF pressure, a moderately decreased glucose level, and an increased protein level. In contrast with acute bacterial meningitis, the inflammatory reaction of tuberculous meningitis consists predominantly of lymphocytes and monocytes; however, early infections may show a predominance of neutrophils. Mycobacteria are scarce and difficult to identify in CSF without concentration of the sample and special staining techniques. Centrifugation for sedimentation must be at high velocity because the fats and waxes of the mycobacterial wall cause the organism to float. Other mycobacteria

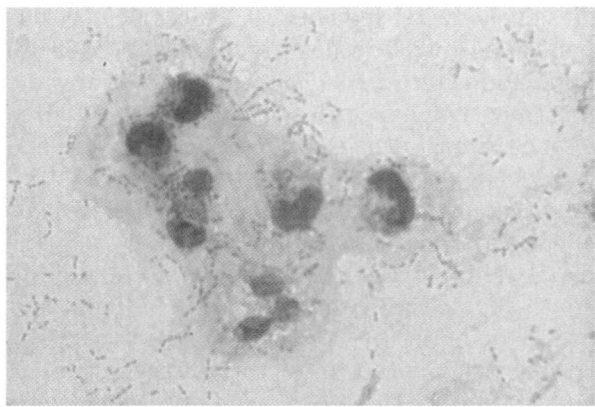

Figure 29-8 ————————————

Direct smear of CSF from a newborn delivered to a woman with amnionitis secondary to premature rupture of the membranes. Numerous short gram-negative bacilli in chains consistent with a *Bacteroides* species are seen. The organism could easily be confused with a *Streptococcus* species if the Gram stain was improperly decolorized. Gram stain; noncytocentrifuge preparation; high-power view.

associated with CNS infections include *Mycobacterium avium–intracellulare, Mycobacterium kansasii,* and *Mycobacterium fortuitum.*

Brain Abscesses

In contrast with the superficial meningeal inflammation seen in meningitis, **brain abscesses** are circumscribed areas of tissue destruction containing organisms and inflammatory cells. The majority of cerebral abscesses result by spread from adjacent sinus or ear infections. Approximately 20% of cerebral abscesses occur by hematogenous spread from distant sites, as may be seen in patients with infective endocarditis. Other conditions associated with brain abscesses include diabetes mellitus, corticosteroid therapy, immunodeficiency (AIDS), and malignancy. Although a frequently cited cause, skull trauma actually accounts for less than 10% of brain abscesses. The most common organism cultured from the latter is *Staphylococcus aureus.* The most common organisms isolated from nontraumatic brain abscesses include aerobic and anaerobic streptococci (Figure 29-9), *Bacteroides* species, gram-negative aerobes, and staphylococci. Generally, one third of brain abscesses are culture-positive for aerobes only; one third are culture-positive for anaerobes only; and one third are mixed aerobe-anaerobe infections. *Citrobacter kosevi* is a gram-negative bacillus associated with meningitis and brain abscesses in neonates.

A cerebral abscess begins as a focal area of cellulitis with accompanying neutrophilic inflammation. The dead brain tissue is liquefied by the inflammatory response, and the resultant cavity is filled with organisms, necrotic tissue, and inflammatory debris. The expanding brain abscess exerts a mass effect within the closed space of the skull and may shift adjacent vital brain structures sufficiently to cause focal neurologic signs, such as weakness in one extremity or unilateral abnormalities of vision. In this circumstance, the performance of a lumbar tap to obtain CSF is hazardous and can lead to herniation of the brain stem and death of the patient! Occasionally, a brain abscess may rupture into the ventricular system with resultant numerous inflammatory cells seen in the CSF. Brain abscesses may be culture-negative, especially in the face of prior antimicrobial therapy.

Although most brain abscesses contain bacteria, fungi and parasites may also be causes of brain abscesses. In contrast with yeast infections, which

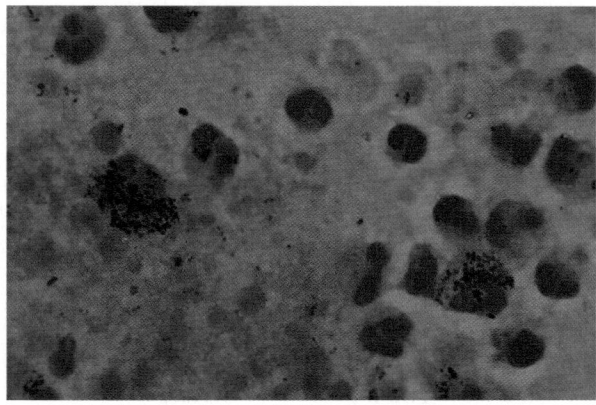

Figure 29-9

Direct smear of aspirated brain abscess contents. Clusters of intracellular gram-positive cocci in groups are consistent with microaerophilic streptococci. Gram stain; noncytocentrifuge preparation; high-power view.

are most often associated with meningitis (see later discussion), CNS infections resulting from hyphal fungi such as *Aspergillus* species or Zygomycetes typically produce cerebral abscesses or infarcts. These organisms are rarely identified by direct examination of CSF samples. Cerebral aspergillosis may be acquired from indwelling catheters, from a focus of infection within the paranasal sinuses, or hematogenously from systemic organ involvement. Polymorphonuclear leukocytes are an important host defense against infections resulting from *Aspergillus* species, and patients with reduced peripheral blood neutrophil counts are at risk for infection. In the brain, *Aspergillus* species invade the cerebral vessels and surrounding neural tissue. The lesion produced is thus a combination of fungal abscess and hemorrhagic infarct. *Aspergillus fumigatus* is the most commonly recovered organism, followed by *Aspergillus flavus, Aspergillus terreus,* and *Aspergillus versicolor.*

The subclass Zygomycetes includes *Mucor, Rhizopus,* and *Absidia* organisms. These organisms are also angioinvasive in patients predisposed to infection because of malignancy or diabetes mellitus. The infection may begin in the paranasal sinuses and erode the frontal bone to reach the CNS **(rhinocerebral mucormycosis).** The frequent acidosis in patients with poorly controlled diabetes mellitus predisposes them to this infection.

Other fungi occasionally isolated from cerebral abscesses include *Blastomyces dermatitidis, Para-*

coccidioides brasiliensis, Sporothrix schenckii, and *Pseudallescheria boydii.*

Abscesses resulting from *Nocardia* species have been described, especially in patients receiving corticosteroid therapy. Parasites including *Entamoeba histolytica, Toxoplasma gondii,* and hookworm larvae are rare causes of cerebral abscesses.

Spirochetal Infections

Both treponemal and nontreponemal spirochetes may be the cause of CNS diseases. This section includes only one example of each: Lyme disease and **neurosyphilis.**

Lyme disease is a recently recognized syndrome caused by the nontreponemal spirochete *Borrelia burgdorferi.* The disease was recognized as a distinct syndrome when a cluster of cases occurred in Lyme, Connecticut, in 1975. The infection is transmitted through the bite of ticks of the genus *Ixodes* (*Ixodes dammini* and *Ixodes pacificus* on the eastern and western coasts of the United States, respectively).

Lyme disease progresses through a series of stages. After a variable incubation period of up to 1 month, approximately 80% of infections demonstrate a peculiar, ring-shaped rash (erythema chronicum migrans) usually at the site of the tick bite. If the infection goes untreated, it progresses in days to weeks to the second stage, characterized by extreme fatigue, less well-defined skin rashes, "aseptic" meningitis, and arthritic or other musculoskeletal symptoms. Cardiac involvement may lead to rhythm disturbances manifested as palpitations or fainting. The third stage is characterized by disturbances in memory or mood, with more pronounced musculoskeletal symptoms.

At all stages of infection, *B. burgdorferi* is present in low numbers. The CSF may be entirely normal or may show only a mild lymphocytic pleocytosis, but organisms are not seen. The diagnosis of Lyme disease is made on clinical grounds and supported by positive serology (enzyme-linked immunosorbent assay [ELISA] and Western blot test). The infection responds well to oral doxycycline or amoxicillin.

Neurosyphilis is caused by the spirochete *Treponema pallidum.* The natural history of syphilitic infection manifests in three stages. The first, or primary, stage of infection occurs by cutaneous inoculation, with resulting development of a painless ulcer, the chancre. This ulcer is teeming with spirochetes, and the diagnosis may be made at this time by serology or by darkfield microscopy. The chan-

cre is painless and heals spontaneously in 3 to 6 weeks. In patients who have not received antibiotics, the disease progresses to the secondary phase, associated with spirochetemia and characterized by a rash, lymphadenopathy, and oral ulcers. If the infection remains untreated, patients may become asymptomatic for years during the so-called latent phase. Some patients enter a tertiary, or late, stage with neurologic symptoms (neurosyphilis). The neurologic signs include abnormalities of gait associated with stabbing pain (tabes dorsalis) and absence of pupillary response to light (Argyll Robertson pupil). Other syphilitic patients may suffer progressive paralysis and dementia (general paralysis of the insane). In syphilis the CSF shows a lymphocytic pleocytosis and increased protein level; spirochetes are not seen. The diagnosis of syphilis in the secondary or the tertiary stage is obtained by serology. Serologic diagnosis of syphilis includes both nonspecific and specific tests for *T. pallidum.* Nonspecific tests include the VDRL (venereal disease research laboratory) and RPR (rapid plasma reagin) tests. These tests detect antibody (reagin) that cross-reacts with cardiolipin. The results of these tests are confirmed by specific treponemal assays, such as the TPI (treponema pallidum immobilization) and FTA-ABS (fluorescent treponemal antibody absorption) tests. These tests detect structural components of treponemes.

Fungal Meningitis

CASE STUDY

A 52-year-old white male arrived at an emergency room in a disoriented and poorly responsive state with labored breathing. The patient's history included poorly controlled diabetes and chronic obstructive pulmonary disease secondary to cigarette smoking. Current medications included steroids for his pulmonary disease. Physical examination showed that the patient was slightly febrile, lethargic, and in respiratory failure. He showed deteriorating mental status, and a diagnosis of meningitis was considered. A lumbar tap produced a CSF sample that on direct smear using calcofluor reagent showed encapsulated budding yeasts. Despite aggressive therapy with amphotericin B and 5-flucytosine, the patient's condition failed to improve. The patient died on the third day of hospitalization.

Box 29-2

Fungal Organisms Involving the Central Nervous System

Common

Cryptococcus neoformans
Coccidioides immitis

Uncommon

Histoplasma capsulatum
Candida species
Aspergillus species
Blastomyces dermatitidis

Rare

Paracoccidiodes brasiliensis
Pseudallescheria (Allescheria) boydii
Mucorales (*Mucor, Rhizopus, Absidia,* and
　Cunninghamella species)
Sporothrix schenckii
Trichosporon beigelii
Penicillium species
Fusarium species
Alternaria species
Curvularia species
Acremonium species
Fonsecaea species
Bipolaris species
Drechslera species

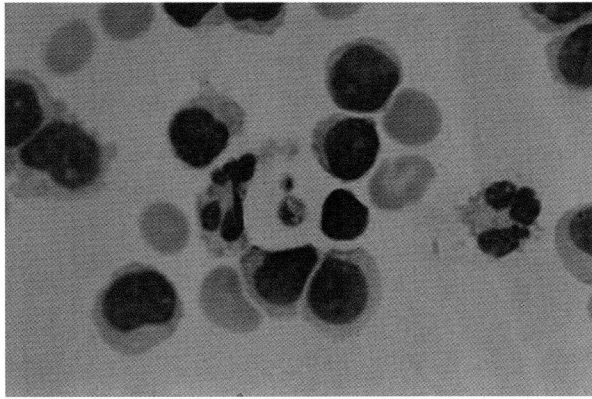

Figure 29-10 _____

Cytocentrifuge preparation of CSF showing a single yeast with narrow-based budding and prominent surrounding capsule characteristic of *Cryptococcus neoformans.* Cryptococcal meningitis in partially immunocompetent hosts may show only rare organisms mixed with an inflammatory background of lymphocytes, monocytes, and eosinophils. Wright stain; high-power view.

Cryptococcus neoformans (Figures 29-10 and 29-11) is the most common cause of fungal meningitis, especially among immunosuppressed patients. The case study presented at the beginning of this section described numerous factors that predisposed this patient to *C. neoformans.* The India ink preparation using nigrosin has traditionally

Despite being widespread in the environment, fungi are uncommon causes of CNS infection (Box 29-2). Chronic meningitis is the common presentation, although fungal CNS infections may present acutely, mimicking bacterial meningitis. The predisposing factors to fungal meningitis include age (e.g., *Histoplasma capsulatum* in infants), metabolic disturbances (Zygomycetes), intravenous drug abuse (*Cryptococcus* species), and immunodeficiencies (*Candida neoformans* and *Candida* species). In fungal meningitis, CSF findings vary considerably, but the following are usually present: normal to slightly increased CSF pressure, increased CSF protein level, and decreased CSF glucose level. The CSF usually contains fewer than 500 leukocytes/mL, with a predominance of lymphocytes and monocytes. Infections resulting from *C. neoformans, Coccidioides immitis,* and *Aspergillus* species are occasionally associated with predominance of neutrophils or eosinophils in the CSF. In such cases, the CSF glucose level may be quite low.

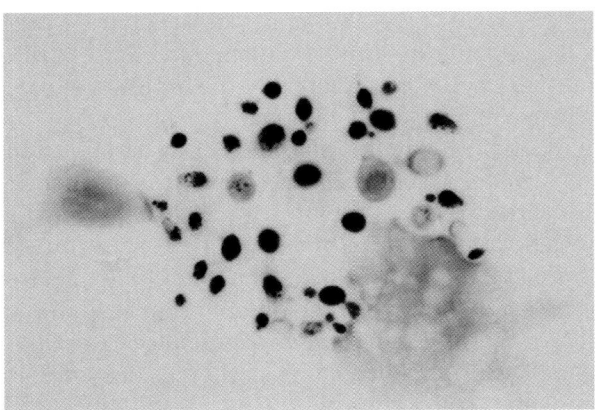

Figure 29-11 _____

In contrast, cryptococcal meningitis in immunosuppressed hosts may show numerous organisms and scarce or absent inflammation. Notice the variation in size, variable gram-staining, and narrow-based budding. The organisms are evenly spaced because of their abundant polysaccharide capsules. Gram stain; cytocentrifuge preparation; medium-power view.

been used to identify these encapsulated yeast in the CSF. However, this test is prone to misinterpretation, as red blood cells and small lymphocytes may look similar to *C. neoformans*. Currently, the India ink preparation is a test of historical interest, but one not much used in modern laboratories. CSF smears (cytopreparation preferred) should be stained with a Gram stain and calcofluor reagent to specifically identify yeast cell walls. A rapid latex agglutination (LA) method is used for the detection of cryptococcal capsular polysaccharide in both CSF and serum. The LA test detects antigen in 90% or more of patients with cryptococcal meningitis as demonstrated by the case presented. Culture of CSF from the patient described in this case grew out *Cryptococcus neoformans*. False-positive results may occur as a result of the presence of rheumatoid factor or a cross-reaction with antigen from *Trichosporon beigelii* disseminated infections and some bacterial infections. Cultures for *C. neoformans* are positive in 75% to 85% of cases.

Cryptococcal meningitis may present with nearly normal CSF studies and few organisms (hence the need to directly examine all CSF samples). During treatment, organisms from chronic cryptococcal meningitis may also become atypical in shape, size, and staining characteristics. At the other extreme, the number of organisms in AIDS patients may be so overwhelming that they present in fluid as clumps. At autopsy, the brain from such a patient may appear covered by a mucinous coating because of the abundant polysaccharide capsule surrounding this organism. Microscopically, masses of yeast penetrate into the brain substance to form flask-shaped cavities.

Fungal meningitis resulting from *Histoplasma capsulatum* and *Coccidioides immitis* is frequently secondary to systemic infection. Fungal meningitis with both these organisms most often occurs by the bloodstream route from a pulmonary focus. These organisms show a marked difference in geographic distribution. *H. capsulatum* is endemic to the Ohio and Mississippi River valleys, whereas *C. immitis* is endemic to the southwestern United States. CSF cultures are positive in 50% or fewer infections resulting from these organisms. Coccidioidal meningitis may be documented by detection of CSF IgG complement-fixing antibodies.

Candida species are causes of both fungal meningitis and cerebral abscesses. Candidiasis may be acquired as a nosocomial superinfection by patients with indwelling catheters or those receiving antibacterial therapy. Patients with low peripheral blood neutrophil counts secondary to chemotherapy are at risk for candidal infections. *C. albicans*, *Candida tropicalis*, and *Candida parapsilosis* are the most commonly identified species.

Viral Infections

CASE STUDY

A 36-year-old HIV-infected homosexual male was admitted to an emergency room with complaints of inability to urinate for 3 days. He additionally reported numbness and weakness in his right leg for 7 months, a 25-lb weight loss, and bowel incontinence. Physical examination revealed an afebrile, dehydrated, emaciated male with bilateral lower extremity weakness and decreased reflexes throughout. Lesions of Kaposi's sarcoma were noted, especially on the lower extremities, and recurrent oral thrush and perianal herpetic vesicles were observed. An MRI scan of the CNS revealed no evidence of spinal cord compression, but because of the high-risk profile, the patient was admitted to the hospital with the presumptive diagnosis of polyradiculopathy secondary to AIDS. Acyclovir was started, pending culture results. A lumbar puncture was performed. The CSF showed an increased protein level (326 mg/dL) and leukocyte count (1720 cells/mL) with 86% neutrophils.

Meningitis

Viral infections occur worldwide and are the most common cause of "aseptic" meningitis. The CSF in aseptic meningitis typically shows a lymphocytic pleocytosis associated with normal or nearly normal CSF protein and glucose levels (Figures 29-12 and 29-13). Early viral infections may show a predominance of neutrophils in the CSF, but the pleocytosis rapidly progresses to a lymphocytosis. The most common viruses producing aseptic meningitis include the enteroviruses and herpesviruses. Less common causes of viral aseptic meningitis include mumps virus, lymphocytic choriomeningitis virus, and the human immunodeficiency virus (HIV) (Box 29-3).

Box 29-3
Viral Agents Involving the Central Nervous System

Enteroviruses
  Coxsackieviruses A and B
  Echoviruses
  Polioviruses
Arboviruses (arthropod-borne viruses)
  Alphaviruses
    Eastern equine encephalitis
    Western equine encephalitis
    Venezuelan equine encephalitis
  Flaviviruses (St. Louis encephalitis virus)
  Bunyaviruses (La Crosse virus)
  Orbivirus (Colorado tick fever virus)
Herpesviruses
  Herpes simplex (HSV-1 and HSV-2)
  Epstein-Barr virus
  Cytomegalovirus
  Varicella-zoster virus
Lymphocytic choriomeningitis virus
Human immunodeficiency virus (HIV)
Mumps virus
Rabies virus

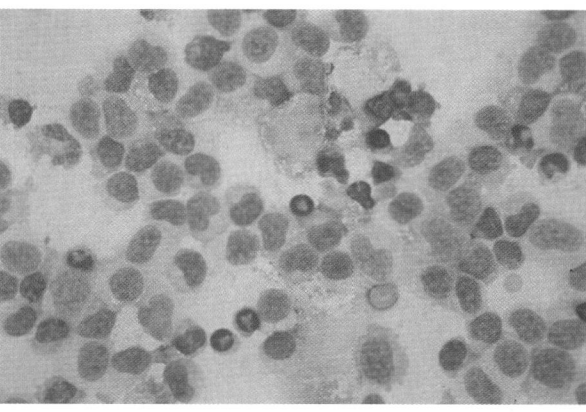

Figure 29-13 _____

Cytocentrifuge preparation of CSF in meningitis resulting from tularemia. Reactive lymphocytes with "monocytoid" features are the only clue that this is not a viral infection. No organisms are seen. Cultures were positive; Wright stain.

Enteroviruses frequently associated with neurologic illness include coxsackieviruses A and B, echoviruses, and polioviruses. Children and immunocompromised patients are particularly at risk. Enteroviral infections are typically acquired by the fecal-oral route during the summer months. Ingested virus replicates within lymphoid tissue of the gastrointestinal tract and subsequently disseminates by the bloodstream route to the CNS. The enteroviruses associated with aseptic meningitis include coxsackievirus group A (types 1-2, 4-7, 10, 14, 16, 22) and coxsackievirus group B (types 1-6) as well as many of the echoviruses. The majority of enteroviruses can be identified by viral cell culture techniques, serologic testing, or inoculation into suckling mice.

The incidence of poliovirus infection has decreased dramatically in the United States since the implementation of vaccination programs. Paralytic poliomyelitis, however, remains a significant concern in developing countries that do not have vaccination programs. The majority of poliovirus infections are asymptomatic or cause an aseptic meningitis. However, a small proportion of infections progress to destruction of anterior spinal cord motor neurons, with accompanying paralysis.

Currently in the United States, herpesviruses account for 10% to 20% of viral meningoencephalitis. The herpesviruses include herpes simplex virus (HSV-1 and HSV-2), Epstein-Barr virus (EBV), cytomegalovirus (CMV), and varicella-zoster virus (VZV). Herpes simplex meningoencephalitis may occur in patients of all ages. Herpes simplex encephalitis occurring in adults may follow primary herpesvirus infection or may result

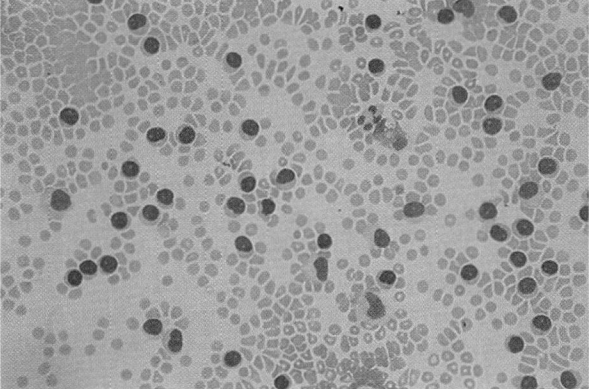

Figure 29-12 _____

Cytocentrifuge preparation of CSF in a case of "aseptic" meningitis. Lymphocytes are present, and in this case the background is bloody. No organisms are seen; Wright stain.

from reactivation of a previous herpesvirus infection. Neonatal herpes simplex meningoencephalitis is typically a consequence of vaginal delivery from a mother with genital herpes and usually reflects disseminated herpetic disease. Less commonly, in utero or postpartum acquisition from a person with active herpetic lesions may occur. Histologic examination of infected brain tissue shows eosinophilic viral inclusions within infected neurons. Death occurs in 75% of untreated cases. Examination of the CSF commonly shows a lymphocytic pleocytosis (typically 100 leukocytes/mL), increased CSF protein level (100 mg/dL), and normal CSF glucose level. Because of the severity of the disease and the possibility of effective antiviral therapy, brain biopsy with culture may be the diagnostic method of choice. The polymerase chain reaction (PCR) through use of CSF represents a realistic alternative for diagnosis where available.

The remaining herpesviruses are infrequent causes of CNS illness. Infections resulting from VZV are spread by aerosols and produce the primary infection varicella (chickenpox). Reactivation of the virus results in herpetic lesions in the skin along the distribution of the infected nerve (dermatome). These lesions are characteristic of zoster (shingles). Neurologic complications of varicella are estimated to occur in 1 in every 1000 infections, and the majority of these resolve without serious sequelae. VZV produces a variety of neurologic syndromes, including meningoencephalitis, optic neuritis, and inflammation of the spinal cord (myelitis).

VZV has also been associated with a neurologic illness in children known as Reye syndrome. The symptoms typically occur in the winter months following a bout of chickenpox. Reye syndrome is characterized by increased levels of hepatic transaminases, normal serum bilirubin level, and unremarkable CSF values. Neurologic symptoms include severe vomiting, delirium, and decerebrate posturing. Symptoms and test abnormalities can return to normal within 1 to 2 weeks, but deaths have occurred. Evidence exists that the administration of salicylates (aspirin) during active chickenpox may predispose children to this disorder. Aspirin is currently contraindicated for management of fevers in children with viral syndromes.

Neurologic illness is uncommon with both EBV and CMV. Both are endogenous viruses that may be reactivated in or acquired by immunosuppressed patients, particularly HIV-infected individuals. The case study at the beginning of this section involved an HIV-infected individual. The serology test for CMV on this individual was positive, and CMV was recovered from viral blood cultures. Following culture isolation of CMV, the patient's medication was switched to ganciclovir. After weeks of therapy, the patient was sufficiently recovered to be discharged. Both EBV and CMV may cause meningoencephalitis or result in an ascending paralysis **(Guillain-Barré syndrome).**

Lymphocytic choriomeningitis virus, a member of the arenaviruses, is an RNA virus uncommonly a cause of aseptic meningitis in human beings. The virus is transmitted by aerosols or fomites from infected rodents through the respiratory route. Individuals living in rodent-infested dwellings, pet store owners, and laboratory workers who work with rodents are at risk for infection. Aseptic meningitis occurs in only about 15% of patients with lymphocytic choriomeningitis confirmed by culture or serologic techniques. As its name implies, lymphocytic choriomeningitis may show a striking lymphocytic pleocytosis in the CSF (more than 1000 lymphocytes/mL). Complete recovery is expected.

The mumps virus, a member of the paramyxoviruses, is an RNA virus responsible for epidemic parotitis. Mumps virus is acquired from inhaled respiratory droplets. The virus replicates within the parotid salivary gland, with subsequent viremia and spread to the CNS. Aseptic meningitis is the most common neurologic complication, occurring in up to 30% of cases. The CSF shows a moderate lymphocytic pleocytosis that may persist for weeks. The clinical diagnosis of mumps is confirmed by serologic studies, and neurologic symptoms typically resolve completely.

Human immunodeficiency virus (HIV), a member of the retroviruses, is an RNA virus associated with AIDS. HIV invades and destroys CD4+ (T-helper) lymphocytes, resulting in a loss of cell-mediated immunity. The virus is present in body fluids, secretions, and tissues of infected individuals. Infection can be acquired by those engaging in unprotected sexual (homosexual or heterosexual) contact with infected individuals and by intravenous drug administration using shared contaminated needles.

Newborns delivered to infected mothers are also at high risk for infection. Prior to the availability of serologic screening for HIV, some individuals who received blood products or organ transplants from infected individuals acquired infection. Studies have demonstrated that HIV has strong tropism for the CNS. Aseptic meningitis occurs in 10% to 20% of cases and may precede opportunistic infections. Inflammation of the peripheral nerves (inflammatory polyneuropathy) or spinal cord (myelopathy) can occur in 10% to 50% of individuals with AIDS. The majority of individuals with AIDS eventually develop a subacute encephalitis (AIDS dementia complex).

Meningoencephalitis

Arboviruses (arthropod-borne viruses) are RNA viruses that demonstrate strong tropism for the CNS. They are responsible for epidemic encephalitis and, less commonly, meningitis or paralytic disease. The clinical symptoms produced vary markedly, ranging from isolated fever to coma and death. All are important pathogens in medical, veterinary, and public health practices in the United States. Included are members of the alphaviruses (eastern equine encephalitis, western equine encephalitis, and Venezuelan equine encephalitis viruses), flaviviruses (St. Louis encephalitis virus), Bunyaviruses (La Crosse virus), and orbivirus (Colorado tick fever virus). The majority of these viruses are transmitted to humans by mosquitoes of the genera *Culex* and *Aedes*. Colorado tick fever virus is transmitted by the bite of ticks from the genus *Dermacentor*.

Human beings acquire infection with these viruses while in the geographic range of the aforementioned arthropods. Thus most infections typically occur from spring to late fall when outdoor activities are increased and climatic and environmental conditions favor mosquito proliferation. Regions of the United States vary in the incidence of these infections.

Eastern equine encephalitis (EEE) is endemic along the entire eastern coast of the United States. Infections are most commonly seen in young children and the elderly. EEE is the most fulminant of the arboviral infections with death occurring in 50% to 75% of cases. Survivors have a high incidence of neurologic sequelae, such as seizures or personality disorders. No specific treatment exists other than supportive care for patients with EEE. Western equine encephalitis (WEE) occurs predominantly within the midwestern and western United States. Venezuelan equine encephalitis (VEE) is endemic in Central America and Florida. WEE and VEE are difficult to distinguish from EEE on clinical grounds, and infants and young children are at greatest risk for infection. Fortunately, the risk of fatal encephalitis is much lower (approximately 10% in WEE, and 0.6% in VEE). Despite its name, St. Louis encephalitis has been reported throughout the United States. The last nationwide epidemic of St. Louis encephalitis occurred in 35 states during the period 1975 to 1976 and resulted in a reported 2194 cases. Epidemic outbreaks appear to occur at approximately 10-year intervals. In contrast with other arboviruses, St. Louis encephalitis virus appears to be more common in the elderly. The clinical symptoms of St. Louis encephalitis are variable, and the risk of fatal encephalitis is estimated at 22%.

La Crosse virus is the most commonly isolated member of the California serogroup of Bunyaviruses. Encephalitis resulting from La Crosse virus occurs most commonly in Ohio, Illinois, Wisconsin, and Minnesota; however, infections have been reported across the United States. La Crosse virus is the second most common cause of arboviral encephalitis, following St. Louis encephalitis virus. Children are most commonly afflicted. La Crosse virus and the other California serogroup viruses are relatively benign arboviral infections, with a mortality rate of less than 1%.

Colorado tick fever virus is the only orbivirus that produces CNS illness. Infections are acquired in the mountainous areas of Colorado, Wyoming, Montana, Idaho, Utah, California, and New Mexico, where hiking and camping are popular and the ticks of the genus *Dermacentor* abound. In addition to meningoencephalitis, Colorado tick fever virus shows a peculiar tropism for the bone marrow, and infection is often accompanied by leukopenia and thrombocytopenia. The ability of the virus to invade blood cells aids in evading host defenses. Colorado tick fever virus shows a wide range of clinical symptoms, although most infections allow recovery.

Autopsy examination of the brain from cases of fatal viral encephalitis show similar histologic findings, including perivascular infiltrates of lymphocytes and plasma cells, nodular aggregates of microglia ("glial shrubs"), reactive changes within neurons, and petechiae. Confirmation is achieved by the isolation of the virus or by the demonstration of neutralizing antibodies (complement fixation or hemagglutination inhibition) in the patient's serum.

Of all the viral infections of the CNS, the encephalitis of rabies is perhaps the most feared. **Rabies** is caused by a bullet-shaped RNA virus of the genus Lyssavirus. It is a zoonosis with nearly worldwide distribution. Infections occur following bites from infected "rabid" animals, such as skunks, raccoons, bats, and foxes, as well as domesticated animals such as rabid dogs, cats, and cattle. Rabies has rarely been acquired through inhalation of aerosolized virus (usually occurring in caves with a dense bat population) or direct inoculation of live virus in laboratories. Fortunately, human rabies is an uncommon infection, with fewer than five reported cases annually since 1960. Following inoculation, the virus replicates within skeletal muscle and proceeds along the peripheral nerves into the CNS. The incubation period is variable, usually between 1 and 3 months. Initial symptoms include fatigue, gastrointestinal symptoms, and pain at the bite wound. In the United States, the most common neurologic symptoms are those of an acute encephalitis indistinguishable from other viral encephalitides. Less commonly, the classic syndrome of agitation, emotional lability, seizures, and hallucinations occurs (furious rabies). Drinking fluids can initiate painful pharyngeal spasms, resulting in voluntary dehydration (hydrophobia). Patients also experience "foaming" at the mouth because of increased salivation. Less commonly rabies may manifest as paralysis followed by coma and death (dumb rabies). The mortality of rabies is essentially 100% following the onset of symptoms unless timely administration of rabies immune globulin is received. The diagnosis is confirmed by demonstration of rabies antigen (by immunofluorescence) in neck skin biopsies or by demonstration of rabies antigen or characteristic inclusions (Negri bodies) in neurons of the brains of patients or infected animals.

The determination of a specific etiologic virus associated with a CNS infection is not practical in most cases, particularly in mild or self-limited disease. Specific diagnosis is difficult because (1) a large number of different viruses involve the CNS, (2) viruses may come from endogenous reactivation or exogenous infection, (3) many viruses produce a spectrum of neurologic complaints, and (4) the magnitude of any neurologic illness resulting from viruses may depend on the age and immune status of the patient as well as other undefined factors. The determination of a specific viral etiology can often be made through a careful patient history, selected serologic tests (determination of virus-specific IgM or determination of a fourfold or greater rise in antibody titer between acute and convalescent sera), viral culture or PCR for selected viruses, or tissue biopsy for routine light microscopy, immunofluorescence, or ultrastructural studies. Viruses isolated from body sites other than the CNS may be implicated in CNS syndromes. Appropriate specimens for culture include nasopharyngeal swabs, urine, stool, tissue, and occasionally blood. Cultures should generally be obtained within the first 5 days following the onset of a viral syndrome (aseptic meningitis, meningoencephalitis, or paralytic symptoms). Viruses (as well as *Treponema pallidum* and *Toxoplasma gondii*) are also responsible for a variety of well-characterized congenital syndromes. Appropriate diagnostic testing should be used in these clinical situations.

Parasitic Infections

Parasites are an infrequent to rare cause of CNS infection. The parasites most frequently identified as CNS pathogens include *T. gondii,* the free-living amebae, and a variety of helminths (Box 29-4). The agent of African sleeping sickness, *Trypanosoma brucei gambiense,* also manifests prominent neurologic symptoms but is geographically restricted to limited areas in Africa.

T. gondii is the most common parasitic infection of the CNS. *T. gondii* is a coccidian obligate intracellular protozoan of the family Sarcocystidae. Humans acquire infection by eating raw or undercooked meat containing tissue cysts, or by the ingestion of mature oocysts from the environment. Sporozoites released from the ingested oocyst or tissue cysts invade the human small intestine, spread hematogenously, and invade cells of the viscera and possibly the brain. This process in-

Box 29-4

Parasites Involving the Central Nervous System

Protozoans

Toxoplasma gondii
Plasmodium falciparum
Naegleria fowleri
Acanthamoeba species

Helminths

Nematodes

Strongyloides stercoralis
Angiostrongylus cantonensis
Gnathostoma spinigerum
Toxocara canis and *Toxocara cati*
Trichinella spiralis
Loa loa

Trematodes

Schistosoma species

Cestodes

Cysticercus cellulosae (*Taenia solium* larvae)
Echinococcus granulosus and *Echinococcus multilocularis*
Paragonimus westermanii and *Paragonimus mexicanus*

duces focal microscopic areas of cellular necrosis in affected organs. The ability of *T. gondii* to parasitize host macrophages is a major defense mechanism for eluding host immunity. With the development of cell-mediated immunity, the tachyzoites maintain their intracellular position and develop into the less metabolically active bradyzoites. Toxoplasmic cysts seen in tissue sections represent an inactive phase of the infection. Any subsequent loss of or decrease in cell-mediated immunity may result in reactivation of the infection.

Toxoplasmosis is a worldwide zoonosis. In the United States, approximately 20% to 40% of healthy adults are seropositive for *T. gondii*. In European countries, especially France, 90% of the population may be seropositive because of the cultural habits of eating raw or undercooked meat. The majority of primary infections with *T. gondii* in healthy adults are asymptomatic or manifest as heterophil-negative infectious mononucleosis. CNS toxoplasmosis in healthy adults may manifest as isolated CNS involvement with the production of

necrotic mass lesions or abscesses. In immunocompromised patients, toxoplasmosis may result from primary infection or reactivation of a past infection. Organ transplant recipients may acquire toxoplasmosis from a donated organ. Toxoplasmosis occurs in as many as 40% of AIDS patients and is the most common cause of a focal brain lesion in this patient population. In such an immunocompromised host, toxoplasmosis is inevitably fatal without treatment. The CSF findings (Figure 29-14) are nonspecific and include a mild lymphocytic pleocytosis and an increased CSF protein level. The diagnosis of toxoplasmosis is usually serologic, although immunocompromised patients may not demonstrate a humoral immune response to the infection. In such cases, and especially if there is a focal brain lesion, diagnosis can be obtained by brain biopsy. In AIDS patients, the brain lesions are radiologically characteristic, and the diagnosis is often confirmed by clinical response to specific therapy.

Primary amebic meningoencephalitis is caused by the free-living amebae *Naegleria* and *Acanthamoeba*. The term *primary amebic meningoencephalitis* is used to distinguish infections resulting from *Naegleria* and *Acanthamoeba* from cerebral abscesses resulting from the lumen-dwelling *E. histolytica,* which also produces abscesses within visceral organs. Infections resulting from *Naegleria fowleria* and *Acanthamoeba castellanii* show different clinical and laboratory

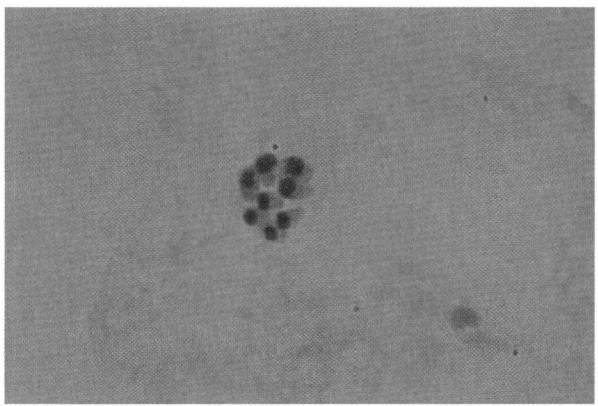

Figure 29-14 _____

Touch preparation of brain tissue showing typical "floret" of *Toxoplasma gondii* trophozoites. The organisms are not typically seen in preparations of cerebrospinal fluid. Wright stain; high-power view.

features. *N. fowleri* may be found in freshwater lakes and streams worldwide and is the most common cause of acute amebic meningoencephalitis (AAM). The infection is restricted to individuals who swim or bathe in infected waters. Trophozoites invade the nasal epithelium and migrate to the CNS via the olfactory nerve. AAM manifests as a purulent meningitis similar to bacterial meningitis, with a neutrophilic pleocytosis (usually more than 500 leukocytes/mL), an increased CSF protein level, and a decreased CSF glucose level. Unlike bacterial meningitis, numerous red blood cells are also present in the CSF. The motile amebae may be visualized in wet preparations, usually first in the cell-counting chamber. Infections resulting from *A. castellanii* occur most frequently in immunosuppressed individuals. As with *N. fowleri*, *A. castellanii* may invade directly through the nasal mucosa or may invade the CNS by hematogenous spread from an extracerebral focus. *A. castellanii* causes a subacute meningoencephalitis referred to as granulomatous amebic encephalitis (GAE). The incubation period of GAE is somewhat longer than that of AAM. Focal neurologic signs, rather than meningitis, are commonly seen. The patient with GAE deteriorates over weeks or months. Findings in the CSF are nonspecific. In contrast with infections resulting from *N. fowleri*, trophozoites of *A. castellanii* are typically not seen in wet preparations of CSF. Serologic tests including complement fixation and indirect fluorescent antibody tests may be helpful in diagnosis. AAM may be successfully treated early in the course of disease. No effective treatment exists for GAE.

Malignant tertian malaria resulting from *Plasmodium falciparum* is another protozoan infection that may be complicated by CNS disease. Individuals acquire malaria when inoculated with plasmodia by an anopheline mosquito during a blood meal. The inoculated parasites proliferate asexually and develop into gametocytes, resulting in lysis of the host's erythrocytes. A high level of parasitemia occurs in falciparum malaria. The cycle of erythrocyte invasion and lysis occurs every 48 hours, corresponding to the recurrent bouts of chills and fever. The numerous parasitized red blood cells are less deformable than normal red blood cells and tend to "sludge" within cerebral capillaries. The occluded vessels produce edema, hemorrhages, and ischemic neural injury. Clinically, cerebral malaria is manifested by delirium, followed eventually by coma and death in untreated cases. A diagnosis of malaria is obtained by examination of peripheral blood smears. Falciparum malaria should be differentiated from malaria resulting from the other plasmodia because of the possibility of resistance to chloroquine.

A variety of helminths invade the CNS and are the most common pathogens associated with a CSF pleocytosis with predominance of eosinophils (eosinophilic meningitis). **Neurocysticercosis,** the most common CNS helminth infection, is caused by the larvae *(Cysticercus cellulosae)* of the pig tapeworm *Taenia solium*. Neurocysticercosis occurs when humans become an intermediate host following ingestion of food or water contaminated with eggs of *T. solium*. Within the small intestine, the eggs release their larvae, which migrate through the intestinal wall to the circulation and eventually to the CNS. Initial invasion of the CNS may go unnoticed, and symptoms may not be apparent for several decades. Eventually, focal neurologic signs or seizures develop. The CSF may be normal or may show pleocytosis with predominance of neutrophils or eosinophils and a decreased CSF glucose level. The diagnosis is confirmed by radiographic studies and demonstration of cyst antigen or anticyst antibody within the CSF. A similar disorder occurs in coenurosis resulting from larvae of the dog tapeworms *Taenia serialis, T. brauni, T. glomerata,* and *T. multiceps*. Striking eosinophilic meningitis may also be seen with nematode larvae of *Angiostrongylus cantonensis* (the rat lungworm), *Strongyloides stercoralis, Gnathostoma spinigerum,* and *Toxocara canis* or *Toxocara cati*.

LABORATORY DIAGNOSIS OF CENTRAL NERVOUS SYSTEM INFECTIONS

Specimen Collection: Lumbar Puncture

Few contraindications exist to lumbar puncture, with the exception of a space-occupying lesion within the brain. Removal of CSF under this circumstance may produce uneven pressures within the brain, resulting in herniation with catastrophic consequences for the patient. Radiologic studies, including computed tomography (CT), are commonly performed prior to lumbar puncture. CSF fluid is obtained by inserting a sterile, hollow needle into the spinal subarachnoid space in the lower (lumbar) back (Figure 29-15). Fluid is collected in three to four sterile tubes. The first tube (which has the highest probability of being contaminated with peripheral blood and skin microbes) is used for chemical studies, including protein and glucose concentrations. The second tube is submitted for direct smear (Gram stain) and culture. The third tube is submitted for red blood cell and leukocyte counts and cellular differential. The fourth tube may be used for specialized studies, such as serology. The CSF specimens should be transported to the laboratory without delay. Fastidious organisms such as *N. meningitidis, S. pneumoniae,* and

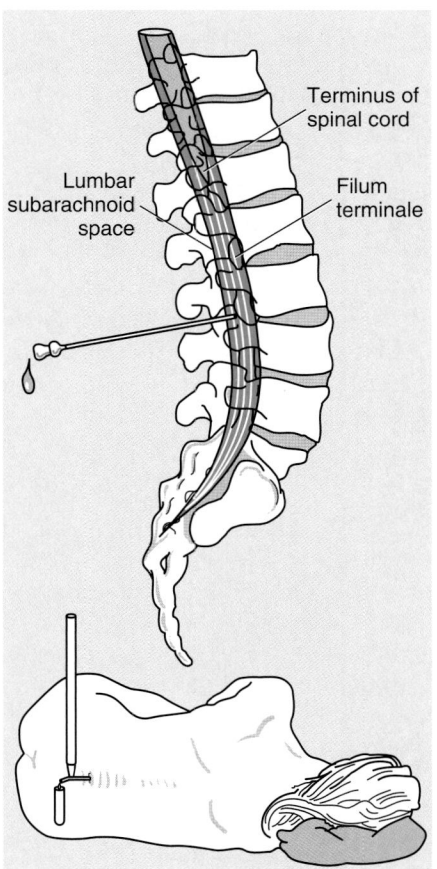

Figure 29-15

Lumbar puncture. The cerebrospinal fluid is obtained by inserting a long, sterile, hollow needle into the spinal subarachnoid space in the lower (lumbar) back.

H. influenzae do not survive prolonged transit times. CSF must not be refrigerated and should remain at room temperature until processing.

Laboratory Evaluation

CNS infections are caused by a variety of microorganisms including bacteria, viruses, fungi, and parasites. Any associated disease state as well as the patient's underlying immune status may also contribute to the clinical presentation, site of infection, and etiologic agent. Because of the vast number of possible infectious agents, direct communication with the clinician is vital. This allows prioritization of test requests and optimizes the laboratory's ability to recover the pathogen.

Meningitis is suspected from the presenting clinical symptoms and initial CSF studies including visual inspection, chemical analysis, and cell counts. In acute bacterial meningitis, the CSF is turbid or cloudy, the CSF protein is increased, the CSF glucose is decreased, and the leukocyte cell count is increased with predominance of neutrophils. It is the practice of our laboratory to immediately examine all CSF specimens submitted, as some pathogens (e.g., *C. neoformans, M. tuberculosis*) may be present without CSF pleocytosis. Direct examination of Gram-stained CSF smears should be a part of all routine culturing procedures and is a rapid and inexpensive method of confirming bacterial as well as some fungal meningitides. Cytocentrifugation and Gram staining of CSF sediment is positive in 75% to 90% of bacterial meningitis, although the sensitivity decreases in patients with prior antibiotic therapy. The characteristic CSF laboratory findings are compared for a variety of infectious disorders in Table 29-1.

In cases of purulent meningitis, bacterial infection is the most likely etiology, and standard bacterial culture procedures that include plating the CSF sediment on blood and chocolate agars will recover most pathogens. Concentration of the sediment using centrifugation (e.g., $3000 \times g$ for 15 minutes) and plating of the sediment is necessary. Plates should be incubated for at least 48 hours before being discarded for no growth and held for a longer time if the CSF smear showed inflammation or if the patient received antibiotic therapy prior to sample collection. The supernatant should also be held for possible serologic studies, viral culture, or molecular assays.

TABLE 29-1
Characteristic Findings in Meningitis

	Bacterial	Fungal	Tuberculous	Syphilitic	Viral	Parasitic
Organisms seen in CSF	▬	▬	▬	None	None	▬
Cell count (leukocytes/mL)	100–100,000 neutrophils predominate	Normal–500 lymphs predominate*	50–500 lymphs predominate†	100–750 lymphs predominate	Normal–200 lymphs predominate‡	Normal–200 lymphs and/or eosinophil predominate
Protein (mg/dL)	100–500	Normal–250	Normal–150	50–250	Frequently normal	Usually increased
Glucose (mg/dL)	<30 usually markedly decreased	Normal to decreased	Usually decreased (<45)	Normal	Normal	Normal to decreased
Additional findings	Bacterial antigen test, Limulus ameboycte lysate	Calcofluor concentrated specimen; latex agglutination (i.e., C. neoformans)	Polymerase chain reaction, auramine-rhodamine on concentrated specimen	CSF, positive VDRL	Serology, culture biopsy	Serology, biopsy

CSF, Cerebrospinal fluid.
*May have normal CSF cell count with *C. neoformans*. Eosinophils may predominate in *C. immitis* infection.
†Neutrophils may predominate in early meningitis.
‡CSF cell count may be more than 1000 leukocytes/mL in lymphocytic choriomeningitis virus infection. Neutrophils may predominate in early meningitis.

One change in procedure relates to the use of bacterial antigen testing. In the previous edition of this text, bacterial antigen testing for *S. pneumoniae, H. influenzae* type b, and *N. meningitidis* was recommended. These tests identify soluble bacterial antigens in the CSF or urine of patients with suspected bacterial meningitis. More recent literature indicates that the routine use of these tests has limited diagnostic value. One of several reasons for this is the changing epidemiologic pattern of bacterial meningitis in developed countries. Meningitis resulting from *H. influenzae* type b is now uncommon because of the tremendous success of the anti–*H. influenzae* conjugate vaccine. Low sensitivity for detecting meningococci is also a limiting factor for bacterial antigen detection, and CNS infections associated with foreign devices are now more common and involve organisms such as coagulase-negative staphylococci that are not detected with these assays. Finally, false-positive results may be obtained with bacterial antigen testing in certain clinical situations such as neonatal sepsis, especially if testing is performed on a non–CSF sample such as urine. As such, the routine use of bacterial antigen testing cannot be recommended. However, bacterial antigen testing may be beneficial in instances in which cultures remain without growth, but the clinical suspicion of bacterial meningitis is high, or in cases of partially treated meningitis with sterile cultures.

In some CNS infections, particularly those involving mycobacteria and cryptococci, organisms may be present in low number. Special stains for fungi (Calcofluor) and bacteria (acridine orange) may be useful in identifying these organisms in cytocentrifuge preparations. Even if no organisms are visualized, the CSF should be cultured; the quantity of CSF cultured has a direct impact on the sensitivity of detection for these pathogens. Optimally, 5 to 10 mL of CSF should be cultured; however, this volume is not typically available, in part because of the need to share sample with other sections of the laboratory. Therefore the preferred diagnostic test for cryptococci is CSF antigen testing by either latex agglutination or enzyme-immunoassay methods. These tests are also superior to direct examinations that employ negative staining techniques, such as the India ink preparation. When completed, fungal cultures of CSF or CNS tissue should include inoculation of enriched blood-containing media supplemented with cyclohexamide so as to support the growth of dimorphic fungi, in addition to less-selective media such as inhibitory mold agar. All fungal cultures should be incubated for 4 to 6 weeks.

Mycobacterial cultures from CSF or CNS tissue specimens have a low yield, even in cases of active disease (e.g., **tuberculous meningitis**). Given the low diagnostic yield, the routine performance of acid-fast smears and CSF cultures for mycobacteria has been questioned. Polymerase chain reaction (PCR) assays the mycobacterial insertion element IS6110 are now available, and molecular amplification assays may become the preferred diagnostic test for these pathogens when the CSF is involved. If culture is pursued, both broth (e.g., Middlebrook 7H9 or Dubos) and solid agar medium (e.g., Middlebrook 7H11 or Löwenstein-Jensen) should be inoculated and incubated for 6 to 8 weeks.

For viral pathogens, culture may not always offer the highest diagnostic yield and is somewhat dependent on the disease process and the type of sample submitted. For example, in the case of herpes simplex encephalitis, culture of a brain biopsy could be performed, but molecular amplification for herpes simplex virus in CSF is less invasive and is now considered the method of choice. A similar argument could be made for meningitis caused by the enteroviruses. These tests are now available through most reference laboratories. For other CNS viral infections, including infections resulting from the arboviruses, lymphocytic choriomeningitis virus, and rabies virus, choices for the laboratory are less straightforward and often rely on patient history and serologic evidence of infection. In these situations, it is important to remember that serologic studies are best interpreted when both acute and convalescent serum samples are submitted for testing.

An additional test that may be useful in certain clinical situations is the *Limulus* amebocyte lysis (LAL) assay. The LAL uses hemolymph from the horseshoe crab, which clots on exposure to small amounts of lipopolysaccharide (endotoxin) present in the cell wall of gram-negative bacteria. As such, the LAL can be used to give an early and presumptive diagnosis of gram-negative meningitis with a reported sensitivity of 93% and a specificity of 99% compared with CSF culture. Although valuable in this specific circumstance, the LAL has limited clinical utility because (1) the LAL assay detects only gram-negative bacteria, and (2) the assay does not distinguish between different gram-negative bacterial pathogens. Other ancillary tests such as CSF lactate, CSF chloride and C-reactive protein have poor sensitivity and specificity in cases of meningitis and are not recommended for routine use.

Bibliography

Agger W et al: Lyme disease: clinical features, classification, and epidemiology in the upper Midwest, *Medicine* 70:83, 1991.

Albright RE et al: Issues in cerebrospinal fluid management: acid-fast bacillus smear and culture, *Am J Clin Pathol* 95:418, 1991.

Albright RE et al: Issues in cerebrospinal fluid management: CSF venereal disease research laboratory testing, *Am J Clin Pathol* 95:397, 1991.

Chun CH et al: Brain abscess: a study of 45 consecutive cases, *Medicine* 65:415, 1986.

Connolly KJ, Hammer SM: The acute aseptic meningitis syndrome, *Infect Dis Clin North Am* 45:99, 1990.

Coyle PK, Dattwyler R: Spirochetal infection of the central nervous system, *Infect Dis Clin North Am* 4:731, 1990.

Feigin RD, Perlman E. Bacterial meningitis beyond the neonatal period. In Feigin RD, Cherry JD: *Textbook of pediatric infectious disease,* Philadelphia, 1998, WB Saunders, p 400.

Fishman RA: *Cerebrospinal fluid in diseases of the nervous system,* ed 2, Philadelphia, 1992, WB Saunders.

Food and Drug Administration: Safety alert: risks of devices for direct detection of group B streptococcal antigen, March 1997, Department of Health and Human Services.

Gamboa F et al: Direct detection of *Mycobacterium tuberculosis* complex in nonrespiratory specimens by gen-Probe amplified mycobacterium tuberculosis direct test, *J Clin Microbiol* 35:307, 1997.

Gray LD, Fedorko DP: Laboratory diagnosis of bacterial meningitis, *Clin Microbiol Rev* 5:130, 1992.

Greenberg DN et al: Sensitivity and specificity of rapid diagnostic tests for detection of group B streptococcal antigen in neonates, *J Clin Microbiol* 33:193. 1995.

Greenlee JE: Cerebrospinal fluid in central nervous system infections. In Scheld WM, Whitley RJ, Durack DT, editors: *Infections of the central nervous system.* New York, 1991, Raven Press.

Hoban DJ, Witwicki E, Hammond GW: Bacterial antigen detection in cerebrospinal fluid of patients with meningitis. *Diagn Microbiol Infect Dis* 3:373, 1985.

Hoff GL et al: Bats, cats, and rabies in an urban community, *South Med J* 86:1115, 1993.

Jacob CN et al: Nontuberculous mycobacterial infection of the central nervous system in patients with AIDS, *S Med J* 86:638, 1993.

Lambert HP: *Infections of the central nervous system,* Philadelphia, 1991, BC Decker.

McCracken GH: Neonatal septicemia and meningitis, *Hosp Pract* 11:89, 1976.

Ogawa SK et al: Tuberculous meningitis in an urban medical center, *Medicine* 66:317, 1987.

Perkins MD, Mirrett S, Reller LB: Rapid bacterial antigen detection is not clinically useful, *J Clin Microbiol* 33:1486, 1995.

Pfyffer GE et al: Diagnostic performance of amplified *Mycobacterium tuberculosis* direct test with cerebrospinal fluid, other nonrespiratory, and respiratory specimens, *J Clin Microbiol* 34:834, 1995.

Phillips S, Millan JC: Reassessment of microbiology protocol for cerebrospinal fluid specimens, *Lab Med* 22:619, 1991.

Saez-Llorens X, McCracken GH: Bacterial meningitis in neonates and children, *Infect Dis Clin North Am* 4:623, 1990.

Saez-Llorens X, McCracken GH: Mediators of meningitis: therapeutic implications, *Hosp Pract* 26:68, 1991.

Steere AC: Current understanding of Lyme disease, *Hosp Pract* 28:37, 1993.

Snider WD et al: Neurological complications of acquired immune deficiency syndrome: analysis of 50 patients, *Ann Neurol* 14:403, 1983.

Wenger JD et al: Bacterial meningitis in the United States, 1986: report of a multistate surveillance study, *J Infect Dis* 162:1316, 1990.

Werner V, Kruger RL: Value of the bacterial antigen test in the absence of CSF fluid leukocytes, *Lab Med* 22:787, 1991.

Williamson MS, Fraser SH, Tilse J: Failure of the urinary group B streptococcal antigen test as a screen for neonatal sepsis, *Arch Dis Child* 73:109, 1995.

LEARNING ASSESSMENTS

1. How is cerebrospinal fluid (CSF) produced and distributed by the central nervous system?

2. How would you characterize a normal CSF?

3. What are the common bacterial pathogens in meningitis? What are the host-related and virulence-related factors associated for each pathogen?

4. How would you compare the physical, chemical, and cellular findings within the CSF during a bacterial, fungal, tuberculous, and viral meningitis?

5. Which fungal species are typically associated with intracerebral abscesses?

6. Which fungal species are associated with meningitis?

7. Why should you examine CSF specimens as soon as they are received?

8. How would you initially evaluate the CSF sample?

9. What types of culture media should be used to recover bacterial pathogens?

10. What rapid and other ancillary methods are useful in evaluating CNS infections?

CHAPTER 30

Bacteremia

Sherry Trevino, Connie R. Mahon

GENERAL CONCEPTS RELATED TO BACTEREMIC
INFECTIONS
  Bacteremia Versus Septicemia
  Forms of Bacteremia
  Bacteremic Episodes
  Other Conditions

EPIDEMIOLOGY
  Risk Factors
    Decreased immune competency of selected
      patient populations
    Increased use of invasive procedures
    Age
    Administration of drug therapy

PATHOGENESIS
  Sources of Bacteremic Spread
  Clinical Signs and Symptoms

Complications
  Effects of endotoxin during gram-negative
    sepsis
  Polymicrobial bacteremia

LABORATORY DIAGNOSIS
  Specimen Collection
    General principles in determining volume,
      frequency, and number of blood culture
      collection
  Blood Culture Methods
    Culture media used in conventional broth
      systems
    Newer blood culture systems
    Examination of conventional blood culture
      bottles
    Routine blood culture work-up
    Sources of contamination

TREATMENT

OBJECTIVES

1. Define *bacteremia*. Differentiate the types of bacteremia and describe when these conditions occur.
2. Discuss the epidemiology and pathogenesis of bacteremia.
3. Describe the role of endotoxin in gram-negative septicemia. Explain why gram-negative bacteremia produces more serious consequences than those caused by gram-positive bacteremia.
4. List the organisms most commonly isolated from blood cultures.
5. Describe the proper procedure for blood culture collection.
6. Discuss the methods for the detection of bacteremia, including the following:
   ▪ Media
   ▪ Blood culture additives
   ▪ Methods of removing antimicrobials
   ▪ Advantages and disadvantages of each procedure described

KEY TERMS

Bacteremia
Septicemia
Pseudobacteremia
Occult (unsuspected) bacteremia
Primary bacteremia
Secondary bacteremia
Nosocomial bacteremia
Polymicrobial bacteremia
Transient bacteremia
Intermittent bacteremia
Continuous bacteremia
Warm shock
Cold shock
Septic shock
Disseminated intravascular coagulation (DIC)
Antibiotic removal device (ARD)
Sodium polyanethol-sulfonate (SPS)

CASE STUDY

A 4-year-old boy with acute myelogenous leukemia in remission was hospitalized because of fever and granulocytopenia. His admission white blood cell and platelet counts were 600 and 55,000, respectively, and his temperature was 103° F. Blood cultures were drawn before the administration of antibiotics. He was immediately placed on ceftazidime and vancomycin. Blood cultures yielded gram-negative bacilli after 24 hours of incubation.

Bacteremia is the invasion by bacteria of the cardiovascular system (blood stream). The consequences of this event can range from a transient, self-limiting infection to one that is life-threatening. The patients at most serious risk are those who

are immunocompromised, either through drug or chemotherapeutic intervention or as the result of preexisting disease and subsequent immunosuppression. Bacteremia is often associated with hospitalization, instrumentation, and other kinds of procedures. Although infection with a wide variety of microorganisms (Table 30-1) can produce bacteremia, this condition is most frequently caused by gram-negative organisms.

This chapter begins with general concepts pertinent to bacteremic infections, including defini-

TABLE 30-1

Microorganisms Most Likely to Be Isolated from Bacteremic Patients *

Escherichia coli
Staphylococcus aureus
Klebsiella
Enterobacter
Pseudomonas
Acinetobacter
Proteus
Serratia
Citrobacter
Salmonella
Morganella
Stenotrophomonas (pseudobacteremia often)
Bacteroides (anaerobes)
Bacteroides fragilis group
Alcaligenes
Haemophilus influenzae
Fusobacterium nucleatum
Cardiobacterium hominis
Capnocytophaga

*Listed in descending likelihood of isolation.

tions of conditions relating to bacteremia and how each condition manifests. This chapter then does the following:

- Discusses the epidemiology and pathogenesis of bacteremia
- Describes the predisposing risk factors in different populations
- Describes complications of bacteremia that may occur
- Presents diagnostic laboratory procedures
- Explains treatment modalities

GENERAL CONCEPTS RELATED TO BACTEREMIC INFECTIONS

Bacteremia Versus Septicemia

Bacteremia is the presence of bacteria in the blood stream. Certain infections, such as meningitis, salmonellosis, and endocarditis, have a period of bacteremia as part of the disease process. Somewhere between 10% and 13% of blood cultures are positive for these manifestations, with two thirds of these representing true clinical positive results. Although bacteremia is the mere presence of bacteria in the blood, **septicemia** is bacteremia plus a clinical presentation of physical signs and symptoms of the bacterial invasion and toxin production.

There are several terms associated with isolation of organisms in blood cultures. First described in 1969, **pseudobacteremia** is the term associated with contaminated infusion fluids (e.g., intravenous, hyperalimentation, saline), blood culture bottles, alcohol swabs, syringes, and other materials. Most pseudobacteremias are caused by aerobic gram-negative bacilli. **Occult (unsuspected) bacteremia** predominantly refers to the condition found in children who appear healthy but whose blood culture is positive. This phenomenon is usually observed in children younger than 2 years of age. The most common causes include *Streptococcus pneumoniae, Haemophilus influenzae* type b, and *H. influenzae* nontypable.

Forms of Bacteremia

The forms of bacteremia include **primary bacteremia,** which is blood stream invasion by bacteria for which no preceding or simultaneous site of infection with the same microorganism can be identified. **Secondary bacteremia** is isolation of a microorganism from the blood as well as other sites in the same patient before or at the same time, such as in pneumonia and urinary tract infections. **Nosocomial bacteremia** occurs on or after the third day of hospitalization; with **polymicrobiol bacteremia,** blood cultures yield more than one organism.

Bacteremic Episodes

Bacteremic episodes may be *transient, intermittent,* or *continuous.* The frequency, time, and number of blood cultures to be collected may depend on the type of bacteremic episode the patient is experiencing. **Transient bacteremia** usually occurs after a procedural manipulation of a particular body site that is colonized by indigenous flora. Such sites include the mouth and the gastrointestinal and urogenital tracts. Transient bacteremia may appear for a brief period following dental, colonoscopic, or cystoscopic procedures. **Intermittent bacteremia** can occur as the result of abscesses present at a particular site or as a clinical manifestation of certain types of infections, such as meningococcemia and gonococcemia. **Continuous bacteremia** occurs when the organisms are coming from an intravascular source and are present in the blood stream consistently. Endocarditis is the most common clinical manifestation associated with continuous bacteremia.

Other Conditions

Warm shock is characterized by fever, increased pulse, hyperventilation, and warm, dry, flushed skin, whereas **cold shock** is associated with decreased blood pressure, increased pulse, and rapid, shallow respirations. **Septic shock** is a syndrome that occurs as a complication of bacteremia. It is characterized by hemodynamic changes, decreased tissue perfusion, and compromised tissue and organ function. Septic shock occurs in about one third of bacteremic cases and is associated with a mortality of 40% to 50%. Mortality in bacteremic cases without shock ranges from 10% to 15%.

EPIDEMIOLOGY

Brill reported the first case of bacteremia (*Bacillus pyocyaneus,* now *Pseudomonas aeruginosa*) in 1899. Ten years later, fewer than 40 cases had been reported worldwide, with less than 30 additional cases in the 15 years following that. Between 1954 and 1974 the reported incidence of bacteremia increased 20-fold, and bacteremia is now the thirteenth leading cause of death in the United States.

Currently, bacteremia is not an infection reportable to the Centers for Disease Control and Prevention. The current incidence of gram-negative bacteremia has been estimated between 70,000 and 330,000 cases per year, with most estimates above 200,000. This represents approximately 1% to 3% of all hospitalized patients. The general mortality rate for bacteremia ranges from 6% to 42%. Mortality rates among patients who are appropriately treated range from 10% to 38%. Patients who are granulocytopenic or inappropriately treated may have a mortality rate that approaches 100%. Moreover, fatalities among patients infected with gram-negative bacilli are higher than those among patients who have gram-positive cocci as the causative agents of their bacteremia.

Risk Factors

The increased incidence of bacteremia over the past 25 years appears to center around the following:

- Decreased immune competency of selected patient populations
- Increased use of invasive procedures
- Age of the patient
- Administration of drug therapy

Decreased immune competency of selected patient populations

Gram-negative bacteremias seem more frequent among persons with neoplasias, especially carcinomas, hematologic malignancies, and connective tissue diseases. Persons with other chronic underlying diseases, such as diabetes and cirrhosis, and those receiving immunosuppressive therapy are also at increased risk for bacteremia.

Increased use of invasive procedures

Increased use of life-support systems, respirators, and invasive diagnostic procedures may play a role in the incidence of gram-negative bacteremia. Indwelling urethral catheters, suprapubic catheters, and intravenous pyelograms predispose patients to catheter infections. These devices penetrate otherwise sterile areas and encourage colonization with bacteria from surrounding tis-

sue. A greater potential of bacteremia also occurs after surgery involving the urinary, gastrointestinal, and biliary tracts.

Age

A bimodal distribution of bacteremia has been observed. In the very young, increased bacteremia is observed owing to a defect in humoral immunity, whereas in older populations, bacteremia is the result of a general decrease in immune competency.

Older adult patients have a tendency toward gastrointestinal and urinary tract infections. This group of patients is expected to have a higher incidence of gram-negative bacteremia, usually in excess of 50%, and a higher recurrence rate due primarily to their immunosuppression and underlying medical conditions. This is especially common in patients in intensive care units and those who become colonized within 2 to 3 days.

Administrations of drug therapy

The administration of broad-spectrum antimicrobials reduces sensitive normal flora and favors colonization and invasion by gram-negative bacteria. Immunosuppressive agents, especially steroids and anticancer chemotherapeutics, place patients at increased risk for bacteremia.

PATHOGENESIS

Sources of Bacteremic Spread

A number of sources are often associated with bacteremic spread, including the following.

Pericarditis and Peritonitis. Pericarditis is often polymicrobial, with *Bacteroides, Clostridium, S. pneumoniae, Streptococcus pyogenes,* and *Staphylococcus aureus* as the most commonly associated organisms. Bacteremias resulting from peritoneal dialysis are most often linked to *Staphylococcus epidermidis, S. aureus,* and gram-negative bacteria.

Pneumonias. The most common organisms in pneumonia that produce a concurrent bacteremia include *S. aureus, S. pneumoniae, P. aeruginosa, H. influenzae,* and *Enterobacter aerogenes.*

Pressure Sores. Almost 50% of the cases of bacteremia attributed to pressure sores may be polymicrobial. Some of the most commonly reported offending organisms are *Proteus mirabilis, S. aureus, Bacteroides fragilis, Acinetobacter* species, *Bacillus,* and *Corynebacterium.*

Prosthetic Medical Devices. It has been known since the fourteenth century that foreign bodies could potentiate infections. It is currently appreciated that device-related infections constitute a major source of morbidity and mortality in hospitalized patients. The organisms implicated in these infections most often originate from endogenous "skin or gut" flora. Subcutaneous implants are more prone to colonization by gram-positive organisms, whereas devices implanted in the peritoneal cavity are usually colonized by gram-negative and anaerobic organisms.

Production of slime by organisms is one mechanism that has been associated with prosthetic valve endocarditis. The slime may serve as a ligand during the initial surface adhesion, or it may be produced after the organism has established a focal presence by adhering to the surface. The slime also protects the organism from host defenses by inhibiting phagocytosis, chemotaxis, and oxidative metabolism and by suppressing the lymphoproliferative response.

How the prosthetic devices become contaminated in the first place is subject to investigation on a case-by-case basis. Some observed instances include: breaks in sterile technique, leading to contamination by endogenous skin flora; improperly sterilized materials; or contaminated catheters. Once prosthetic devices are in place, some organisms take advantage of the materials from which the devices are made. For example, *S. epidermidis* can hydrolize certain plastics as a food source. Some of the most commonly implicated prosthetic devices include plastic devices, such as catheters (Broviac, Swan-Ganz, Tenckhoff) and shunts (ventricular, chest tubes), and cardiac pacemaker leads.

Pressure transducers have been used since the 1960s as indwelling catheters to monitor cardiovascular system conditions. Reports of bacteremia and fungemia were noted in the literature soon after the initial usage of these devices. Some of the most commonly isolated organisms in these cases include *Serratia marcescens, Klebsiella oxytoca, Pseudomonas, Citrobacter,* and *Enterobacter* species.

Total Hip Replacement. This massive surgical procedure has been associated with acute fulminating infection within 2 or 3 months of surgery. Sepsis between 4 and 26 months of surgery is thought to be the result of intraoperative contamination. Late infection occurring 23 to 50 months after surgery is thought to be of hematogenous origin. In many cases, removal of the prosthetic hip is necessary to cure these patients. The risk factors for patients who develop bacteremia and colonization of their prosthetic hip include malignancy, steroid therapy, cytotoxic therapy, collagen vascular disease, alcoholism, liver disease, sickle cell disease, hematologic disease, previous surgery, and previous antimicrobial therapy.

Skeletal System. The bones have also been implicated as a source of bacteremia or consequence of bacteremic persistence. *S. aureus, P. aeruginosa,* and various facultative anaerobes have been implicated in these cases. Mixed infections (polymicrobial infections) are uncommon.

In patients with osteomyelitis, however, bacteremia tends to be polymicrobial. *S. aureus* is most frequently isolated, with gram-negative bacilli accounting for more than 33% of the polymicrobial infections.

Skin and Soft Tissues. Skin and soft tissue infections as well as wounds are sources of bacteremia. These infections tend to be polymicrobial in 2% to 28% of patients. Soft tissue abscesses, especially *S. aureus* bacteremia β-hemolytic streptococci, *P. aeruginosa,* and *Bacteroides* species, have been reported and tend to be polymicrobial or result in polymicrobial bacteremia. Necrotizing fasciitis has a mortality rate of 20% to 30% when it results in bacteremia.

Clinical Signs and Symptoms

Only about one third of patients experience the classic signs and symptoms of bacteremia, which may include abrupt onset of chills, fever, or hypothermia, and hypotension. Approximately 40% of patients experience prostration and diaphoresis. Tachypnea is an early sign of bacteremia. Delirium, stupor or agitation, vomiting and nausea, oliguria, or anuria occurs in 50% of patients with gram-negative bacillary bacteremia. Ecthyma gangrenosum, a central necrotic area surrounded by an erythematous base, is strongly correlated with gram-negative bacteremia. The failure of the body to mount an elevated temperature is also associated with increased mortality among newborns and older adults. Altered clinical laboratory values that may be indicative of bacteremia include the following:

- Thrombocytopenia (50% to 60% of patients with gram-negative bacilli)

- Leukocytosis or leukopenia
- Acidosis with lactic acidosis
- Abnormal liver function tests (especially hyperbilirubinemia)
- Coagulopathy (more than 60% of the time)
- **Disseminated intravascular coagulation (DIC)** (5% to 10% of patients with gram-negative bacillary bacteremia)
- Elevations in C-reactive protein, haptoglobin, and fibrinogen

Complications

Septic shock, which in most cases is secondary to bacteremia, occurs in about 20% to 40% of bacteremic patients and may appear 2 to 6 hours after the initial manifestations. A hallmark of septic shock is tachycardia with decreased systemic vascular resistance (SVR).

Effects of endotoxin during gram-negative sepsis

Endotoxin, the lipopolysaccharide component of the outer membrane of gram-negative bacilli, has been implicated as an important mediator of septic shock. It is released from actively dividing as well as dead bacterial cells. Cytotoxins appear in response to endotoxin and amplify the subsequent release of soluble mediators in the activation of different plasma proteins. Increased levels of tumor necrosis factor (TNF), α-interleukin-1 (IL-1), and IL-6 have been correlated with poor outcome in cases of clinical septic shock.

Endotoxin is absorbed onto the surface of platelets, causing them to release 5-hydroxytryptamine, which aggravates and potentiates coagulation. In addition, it activates the fibrinolytic cascade and activates factor XII to initiate clotting.

Polymicrobial bacteremia

In the 1930s, virtually every case of bacteremia involved a single organism. By the mid-1970s, polymicrobial bacteremia was considered the norm rather than the exception.

Multiple organisms are being identified in 20% of cases of bacteremia. Polymicrobial bacteremia is generally associated with a higher mortality than that of monomicrobial bacteremia. The predisposing factors in polymicrobial bacteremia include self-injection, burns, and gastrointestinal tract sources. Especially at risk are immunocompromised patients, particularly those with alcoholism, granulocytopenia, extensive burns, diabetes mellitus, and chronic renal failure, and patients with vascular insufficiency due to ischemia. *B. fragilis* often has been associated in polymicrobial infections. Given the resistance of *B. fragilis* to many antimicrobials, its diagnosis carries a high degree of expected mortality.

LABORATORY DIAGNOSIS

Specimen Collection

It is important to remember that even though antiseptic technique is used in the collection of blood, somewhere between 1% and 3% of blood cultures become contaminated with organisms such as coagulase-negative staphylococci, *Corynebacterium* species, α-hemolytic streptococci, and *Propionibacterium acnes,* which are skin colonizers.

Therefore it is most important to prepare the skin properly before venipuncture for blood culture. There are several acceptable protocols. Palpation for the vein can be checked with a gloved finger. Cleansing the skin with 80% to 95% ethanol, followed by an iodine-based compound scrubbed in a concentric fashion around the venipuncture site, is a common practice. Other substances may be substituted for iodine in case of known skin hypersensitivity. For decontamination to be effective, the iodine should be left on the skin for at least 1 minute. After the venipuncture, the disinfecting agent should be removed with an alcohol pad.

General principles in determining volume, frequency, and number of blood culture collection

DENSITY OF BACTEREMIA IN ADULTS
VERSUS NEONATES

Bacteremia may involve a large number of microorganisms; however, only a relatively small number of bacteria per unit volume of blood (typically fewer than 30 bacteria per mL) are recovered. The detection methods common in most laboratories produce positive results in adult patients with bacteremias if organisms are present in the range of 10 to 15 bacteria per mL of blood. However, there are many circumstances in which patients have fewer than this number.

Newborns tend to be more septic as a result of the incomplete development of their defense mechanisms and generally have higher numbers of microorganisms per mL of blood. The following age-volume protocol therefore has been recommended.

Age	Amount
Younger than 10 years of age	1 mL of blood for each year of life
10 years old or older	20 mL
10 years old or older (poor veins)	Less than 20 mL

This protocol is based on studies that have demonstrated that as the volume of blood cultured is increased from 2 to 20 mL, the yield of positive culture results increases from 30% to 50%, except in newborns. The optimal ratio of blood to culture medium is about 1:10. The dilution aids in negating the bactericidal effect of normal serum. In cases in which a 1:10 dilution cannot be achieved, most laboratories incorporate 0.25% to 0.50%, of sodium polyanetholsulfonate (SPS), which serves as anti-complement and anticoagulant. The pediatric exception to this volume ratio is usually accommodated by collecting 1 to 3 mL into 5-mL culture bottles.

FREQUENCY OF BACTEREMIC EPISODES VERSUS TIME AND FREQUENCY OF COLLECTION

The frequency of bacteremic episodes is another factor to consider in determining the time, frequency, and volume of blood collection for culture. Because bacteremias may be transient, intermittent, or continuous in their production of microorganisms in the peripheral circulation, collection of samples is highly dependent on the type of bacteremia suspected.

Because patients with transient bacteremia rarely have clinical symptoms, blood cultures are rarely obtained. Organisms are immediately cleared from the peripheral system by the reticuloendothelial system (RES). In patients with continuous bacteremia, on the other hand, the organisms are constantly released into the blood stream and therefore are likely to be isolated whenever the blood culture specimen is taken. Although a single set of blood culture specimens may yield the etiologic agent, a set of three is still highly recommended (a set consists of one bottle for aerobic incubation and another for anaerobic incubation). In cases of intermittent bacteremia, the time interval between collection of samples is critical in the recovery of organisms. In suspected cases of intermittent bacteremia, it is recommended that blood culture specimens be collected before an anticipated temperature rise to ensure maximum recovery. Usually by the time chills and fever occur, the organisms in the blood stream are being cleared by the RES; therefore fewer organisms may be recovered in blood culture specimens at this time.

RATIONALE FOR MULTIPLE COLLECTION

One study revealed that approximately 80% of bacteremias are discovered in the first set of blood culture specimens taken, 90% are detected if two sets of specimens are taken, and up to 99% are diagnosed if a third set is taken. In most cases of bacterial endocarditis, the causative organism is present in fairly small numbers; therefore the best protocol is to take three or four sets of culture specimens from three different venipuncture sites within the first 1 to 2 hours of clinical presentation. In subacute bacterial endocarditis, three sets of blood culture specimens taken at 1-hour intervals within the first 24 hours are recommended. With bacteremia of unknown origin, taking four to six 10-mL specimens within the first 48 hours ensures the greatest likelihood of recovery of the causative organisms. In brucellosis, blood culture specimens should be obtained during the initial presentation of symptoms and at the anticipated temperature spike.

Blood Culture Methods
Culture media used in conventional broth systems

In most laboratories, each set of blood culture specimens includes a bottle or tube designated for aerobic recovery and another for anaerobic recovery of microorganisms. The typical aerobic culture bottle contains a soybean casein digest broth, tryptic or trypticase soy broth, brain-heart infusion, *Brucella* agar, or Columbia broth base. Although typical anaerobic broth media may contain the same types of basic media as the aerobic culture systems, 0.5% cysteine may have been added to permit the growth of certain thiol-requiring organisms. Unvented blood culture bottles generally can be used to support anaerobic organisms.

In general, thioglycolate- and thiol-containing broths are not suitable for the recovery of *Pseudomonas* and yeasts from blood.

NEUTRALIZATION OF INHIBITORY PROPERTIES

In specimens from patients receiving clinical amounts of β-lactam antimicrobial agents, penicillinase may be added to the medium to inactivate these agents. Some commercially available automated blood culture systems have blood culture bottles containing **antibiotic removal device (ARD),** a resin that nonspecifically absorbs any antimicrobial agent present in the patient's blood.

ANTICOAGULANTS AND OTHER ADDITIVES

Sodium polyanetholsulfonate (SPS), one of the commonly used additives, performs the following functions:

- Anticoagulation (effective at a 0.03% concentration)
- Neutralization of the bactericidal effect of human serum
- Prevention of phagocytosis
- Inactivation of certain antimicrobial agents (streptomycin, kanamycin, gentamicin, polymyxin B)

However, SPS is inhibitory to *Peptostreptococcus anaerobius, Neisseria gonorrhoeae,* and *Neisseria meningitidis* as well as *Gardnerella vaginalis.* If these organisms are suspected, 1.2% gelatin added to the blood culture bottle may help neutralize this inhibitory effect of SPS.

Other anticoagulants and supplements are available for use in blood culture systems. Sodium amylosulfate (SAS) is a structural relative of SPS that is less effective in neutralizing serum bactericidal activity and is inhibitory to *Klebsiella pneumoniae.* Sodium citrate (0.5% to 1.0%), an anticoagulant, is inhibitory to some gram-positive cocci. Sucrose (10% to 30%) is sometimes used as an osmotic stabilizer. Sucrose is especially helpful in dealing with bacteria that have undergone cell wall damage, to some extent and the resultant hypertonicity counteracts the normal bactericidal effect of blood. Other supplements, such as the anticoagulants oxalate and ethylenediamine tetraacetic acid (EDTA), are not recommended.

Newer blood culture systems

BIPHASIC BROTH-SLIDE SYSTEM

A broth-slide system (Septi-Chek [Becton Dickinson, Sparks, Md.]) was designed from the original biphasic blood culture medium Castaneda culture bottle. Septi-Chek consists of a slide paddle containing chocolate, MacConkey, and malt extract agars attached to the top of a standard broth bottle. Once these bottles have been inoculated, they should be tipped daily or at least twice weekly so as to bathe the slide paddle with the broth culture medium. This allows frequent blind subcultures without the use of needles and syringes. Bacterial growth appears either as small, discrete colonies or a confluent growth on the slide paddle. This system has the advantage of providing more rapid recovery of facultative bacteria and isolated colonies for identification and susceptibility testing. However, there are certain disadvantages, including a slightly higher cost of materials and contamination rate. An additional unvented bottle is still required for adequate isolation of anaerobes.

CONTINUOUS-MONITORING BLOOD CULTURE SYSTEMS

The Bactec System (Becton Dickinson Microbiology Systems, Sparks, Md.), first introduced as an automated radiometric growth detection system for blood cultures, incorporates isotopically labeled carbon dioxide (CO_2) in the broth medium. When the organism in the blood culture bottle uses $^{14}CO_2$-labeled substrate, $^{14}CO_2$ is released. The instrument monitors CO_2 production by aspirating gas into an ionization chamber using sterile needles. In the ionization chamber, the amount of $^{14}CO_2$ produced is measured as growth index (GI) and compared with an established threshold level. If the patient's blood culture shows a GI that exceeds the threshold level, the instrument sends off a signal indicating that the culture result is positive. The automated radiometric blood culture system has the advantage of early detection of bacterial growth, especially of slow-growing bacterial species (e.g., *Mycobacterium tuberculosis*). The disadvantages include the high initial cost of the instrument, high contamination rate (the result of inadequate needle sterilization between bottles), and the hazards associated with radioisotope disposal.

Bactec 9000 Series In response to the changing needs of clinical laboratories, Becton Dickinson introduced the Bactec 9000 series. Two models are currently available, the 9240 and 9120. These are also noninvasive, continuous-monitoring blood culture instruments that use fluorescence to detect CO_2. Carbon dioxide is detected using a gas-permeable sensor on the bottom of each vial. When

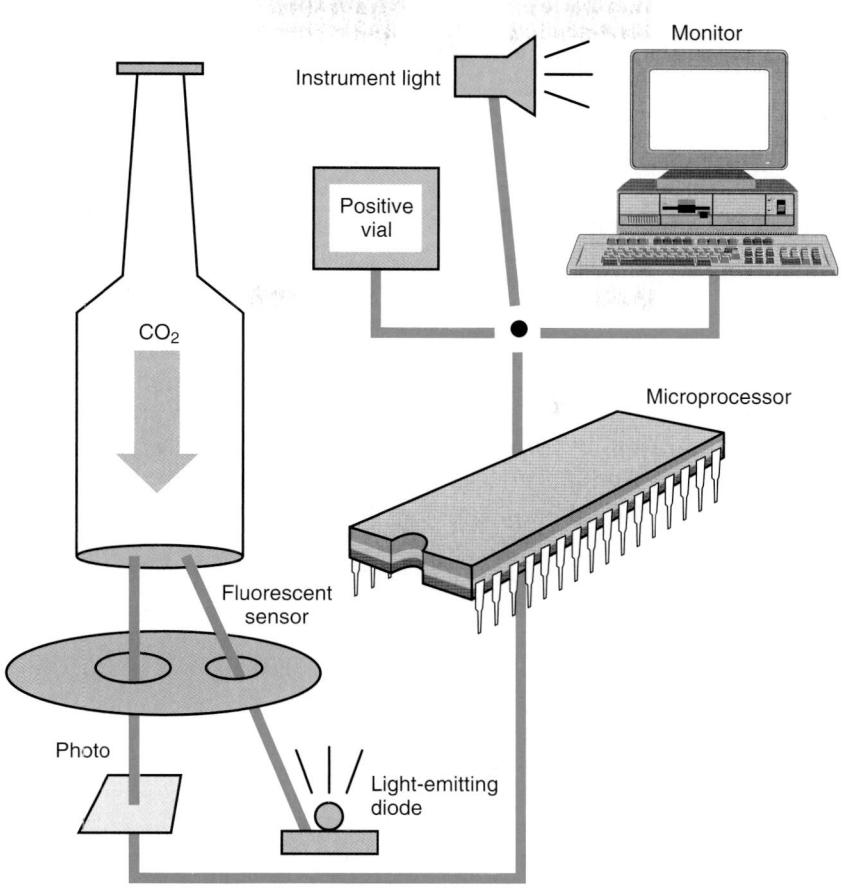

Figure 30-1

Bactec 9000 schematic.

a bottle is placed into the 9240, the instrument takes a base reading of the sensor. This reading is used as a reference for subsequent readings.

Carbon dioxide produced by an organism diffuses into the sensor, generating hydrogen ions. The increase in hydrogen ion concentration increases the fluorescence output of the sensor. Using photodetectors, the 9240 measures the amount of fluorescence, which corresponds to the amount of CO_2 produced by the microorganism. A computer program then interprets these data using several algorithms to determine when to flag a bottle as positive. If a bottle contains a microorganism, the indicator continuously changes. After several increases in absorption by the sensor, the bottle is flagged as positive. The instrument alerts the user of the positive vial by displaying a message

on the computer monitor and with an audible alarm. Figure 30-1 illustrates the Bactec 9000 schematic.

Since Bactec systems were introduced, several new instruments have been developed to automatically and continuously monitor blood cultures. These instruments include BacT-Alert (Organon Teknika Corp, Duraham, N.C.) and the ESP (Accumed International, Chicago). The advantages of the new instrumentation include the continuous monitoring of the blood culture vials, which results in an improved time-to-detection, and a reduced frequency of bottles with false-positive results. For the Bactec and BacT-Alert systems, an additional advantage is the noninvasive monitoring. After introduction of the blood sample, the bottle is not punctured for monitoring (Table 30-2).

TABLE 30-2

Features of Continuous-Monitoring Blood Culture Systems

Feature	Bactec 9000	BacT-Alert	ESP
Capacity	120/240	240	128/384
Agitator	30 rpm	60 rpm	280 rpm
Protocol	1 to 30 days	1 to 30 days	5 to 7 days
Detection	CO_2, pH, fluorescence	CO_2, pH, colorimetric	CO_2, N_2, pressure
Venting	No	Yes	Yes

ESP The ESP system differs from the other continuous-monitoring systems in that it detects the consumption or production of gases by organisms growing in the culture medium. These gases are detected by monitoring changes in headspace pressure. The aerobic bottle is monitored once every 12 minutes, and the anaerobic bottle is monitored once every 24 minutes. An internal computer algorithm monitors the changes and determines when to flag the bottle as positive.

BacT-Alert System A fully automated, nonradiometric blood culture system, the BacT-Alert System (Organon Teknika, Durham, N.C.) consists of aerobic and anaerobic bottles with pH-sensitive membranes placed in the bottom of the bottles. Microbial growth causes a pH change resulting from release of CO_2, indicated by a change in color of the growth medium. The instrument measures CO_2 production colorimetrically without going into the bottles.

LYSIS-CENTRIFUGATION METHOD (DUPONT ISOLATOR)
The lysis-centrifugation method has been shown to provide optimal recovery of fungi and mycobacteria from systemic infections. This method provides a concentrated material for direct inoculation of various agar media. The Isolator (Wampole Laboratories, Cranbury, N.J.) includes a blood collection tube containing a mixture of saponin, propylene glycol, SPS, and EDTA. This mixture facilitates lysis of white and red blood cells, prevents clotting, and neutralizes complement. Microorganisms are concentrated through high-speed centrifugation (3000 × g for 30 minutes). The sediment containing the organisms is directly inoculated on a solid culture medium including fungal and mycobacterial media. For recovery of mycobacteria, Middlebrook 7H11 agar is inoculated with the sediment.

RECOVERY OF OTHER TYPES OF ORGANISMS
Francisella tularensis, the causative agents of tularemia, is best recovered from a liquid blood culture medium to which L-cysteine and dextrose have been added. Most cell wall–deficient bacteria require the osmotic stabilization of 10% sucrose. *Leptospira* species are recovered during the first week of disease, with 1 to 3 drops of freshly drawn blood placed in 5 mL of Fletcher medium. The blood culture is incubated at 30° C for 28 days in the dark and examined weekly by darkfield microscopy.

Biphasic media, such as Septi-Chek, have been found useful in isolating *Brucella* species. Nutritionally deficient streptococci are adequately recovered using standard broth culture bottles because of the vitamin B_6 present in human blood. However, Pyridoxal-containing blood agar medium or "staph streak" is necessary for subculture to recover this group of streptococci. The "staph streak" test is performed with a confluent growth of the organism in a blood agar plate. A single line of *S. aureus* is streaked across the middle of the plate. Following 24 hours of incubation, the plate is observed for tiny colonies growing near the staph.

Examination of conventional blood culture bottles

It is recommended that the sediment not be disturbed during inspection of the blood culture bottle after 6 to 18 hours of incubation. Blood culture bottles are examined with transmitted and reflected light for evidence of turbidity, hemolysis, gas production, or bacterial colonies in or on the blood layer. If visible growth is observed, 0.25 mL of blood should be aspirated with a sterile needle and syringe. A smear is prepared for Gram stain and then plated to a solid medium.

Routine blood culture work-up

Not all laboratories use automated systems for blood cultures. A routine blood culture work-up for nonautomated conventional systems is usually as follows:

▪ After 6 to 18 hours, a "blind" subculture is performed (*blind* means all bottles are subcultured to appropriate media even without visible growth), and then a routine direct smear examination of all bottles is carried out. The reason for this is that many organisms, such as *Haemophilus* and *N. meningitidis,* do not produce turbidity, hemolysis, or gas in the broth medium. Gram stain or acridine orange provides the most useful microscopic examination. The types of medium used vary among laboratories but usually include blood agar plate and chocolate agar, and if gram-negative bacilli are observed on the smear, MacConkey agar and an anaerobic blood agar plate are included. Many laboratories have abandoned blind subcultures because of the risk of infection (by needlesticks, etc.) to personnel. In addition, blind subculturing increases the probability of contamination.

- Conventional blood culture bottles must be held for at least 7 days. They may be discarded after 7 days if growth is not observed. Report no aerobic and anaerobic growth after 7 days of incubation.
- Hold blood culture bottles for 2 weeks if bacterial endocarditis and fungemia is suspected. If brucellosis is suspected, hold for 21 to 28 days in CO_2 and subculture weekly.
- Anaerobic subculture should be performed after 2 days of incubation. Routine subculture beyond 2 days and terminal subculture are of minimal value and are not routinely recommended.

Any presumptive positive finding should be reported immediately by telephone to a physician.

Sources of contamination

A contamination rate of 2% to 3% can be expected with *Staphylococcus epidermidis, Micrococcus,* diphtheroids, and *Propionibacterium acnes* as common contaminants. However, any organism cultured from two or more blood culture bottles should not be overlooked as a contaminant. Any of the organisms previously mentioned can also be responsible for bacterial endocarditis.

Some other sources of contamination causing pseudobacteremia include intravenous catheters as well as various skin disinfectant solutions. Benzalkonium chloride has been demonstrated to be occasionally contaminated with *Burkholderia cepacia* and *Enterobacter* species. Alcohol or iodine as a skin disinfectant has been preferred. However, contamination of certain iodine solutions, such as povidine-iodine, with *B. cepacia* has also been reported. Contamination with *S. marcescens* and *Moraxella* species has been reported in certain evacuated blood collection tubes.

In the past, contamination was more clear-cut. The media and volume of blood used now are more sensitive and grow more contaminants. It is difficult to determine what is a pathogen and what is contamination. As the volume of blood is increased, the number of positive blood culture results increases. Microbiologists cannot make this determination (true pathogen or contaminant) in the laboratory; physician input and patient history are needed.

TREATMENT

With such a complex disorder, it would be expected that there would be many therapeutic attempts to alleviate this devastating clinical event. In fact, there are several treatment modalities that have been tried; however, some have not shown positive results, as follows:

Anticachectin Treatment. Cachectin mediates a substantial portion of endotoxin injury produced in the body. The signs and symptoms of cachectin production include metabolic acidosis, decreased blood pressure, interstitial pneumonitis, acute renal tubular necrosis and mesenteric ischemia, and infarct of the bowel. The chronic production of cachectin leads to anorexia and wasting. When cachectin is produced in large doses, fulminant shock often results. Anticachectin treatment is therefore administered to avoid these clinical complications.

Glucocorticoids. Prospective, randomized studies of severely septic patients involving treatment with glucocorticoids have been conducted. The rationale for antiinflammatory treatment of sepsis is to interfere with the damaging mediators while controlling local and systemic bacterial proliferation with antimicrobial agents. Glucocorticoids (methylprednisolone sodium succinate Solu-Medrol, Upjohn, Kalamazoo, Mich.) have been shown to almost completely control the septic shock and multiple system organ failure produced by endotoxin with gram-negative bacillus bacteremia.

Combination-Drug Therapy versus Single-Drug Treatment. Various regimens have been tried among classical antimicrobial agents. Improvement generally occurs when broad spectrum antimicrobial agents are administered empirically, taking into account the primary site of the infection, the status of the patient, and the patient's general immune status. The single-drug regimens seem to work best when they are used for non-neutropenic (more than 500 neutrophils per mm³) patients.

Treatment for Septic Shock. Initial resuscitation and fluid replacement is commonly followed with chemotherapy. However, the clinical outcome for septic patients with any of the common treatments may remain unaffected.

Bibliography

Berger SA: Pseudobacteremia due to contaminated alcohol swabs, *J Clin Microbiol* 18:874, 1983.

Berger SA et al: Group Ve-1 septicemia, *J Clin Microbiol* 17:926, 1983.

Billa JL et al: Evaluation of lysis-centrifugation system for recovery of yeasts and filamentous fungi from blood, *J Clin Microbiol* 18:469, 1983.

Cockerill FR III et al: Analysis of 281,797 consecutive blood cultures performed over an 8-year period: trends in microorganisms isolated and the value of anaerobic culture of blood, *Clin Infect Dis* 24:403, 1997.

Cornelis G et al: *Yersinia enterocolitica,* a primary model for bacterial invasiveness, *Rev Infect Dis* 9:64, 1987.

Cros A: *Pseudomonas aeruginosa.* In Mandell GL, Douglas RG Jr, Bennett JE, editors: *Principles and practice of infectious diseases,* New York, 1979, John Wiley & Sons.

Dougherty SH: Pathobiology of infection in prosthetic devices, *Rev Infect Dis* 10:1102, 1988.

Edminston CE, Schmitt DD, Seabrook GR: Coagulase-negative staphylococcal infections in vascular surgery: epidemiology and pathogenesis, *Infect Control Hosp Epidemiol* 10:111, 1989.

Hermans PE, Washington JA II: Polymicrobial bacteremia, *Ann Intern Med* 73:387, 1970.

Kinnurn V et al: Continuous-monitoring blood culture screening system improves the detection of bacteremia in neutropenic patients, *Scan J Infect Dis* 28:287, 1996.

Kreger BE, Cravenn DE, McCabe WR: Gram-negative bacteremia. IV. Reevaluation of clinical features and treatment of 612 patients, *Am J Med* 68:344, 1980.

Peacock JE et al: Nosocomial respiratory tract colonization and infection with aminoglycoside-resistant *Acinetobacter calcoaceticus varanitratus:* epidemiologic characteristics and clinical significance, *Infect Control Hosp Epidemiol* 9:302, 1988.

Rackow EC, Astiz ME: Pathophysiology and treatment of septic shock, *JAMA* 266:548, 1991.

Reuben AG et al: Polymicrobial bacteremia: clinical and microbiologic patterns, *Rev Infect Dis* 11:161, 1989.

Rubin LG, Staiman K, Kamani N: Occult bacteremia with nontypable *Haemophilus influenzae, J Clin Microbiol* 15:1314, 1987.

Stamm WE: Infections related to medical devices, *Ann Intern Med* 89:764, 1978.

Weinstein MP: The clinical significance of blood culture contaminants [editorial], *Clin Microbiol News* 7:156, 1985.

Weinstein MR: Current blood culture methods and systems: clinical concepts, technology, and interpretation of results, *Clin Infect Dis* 23:40. 1996.

LEARNING ASSESSMENT

1. What form of bacteremia (primary or secondary) is demonstrated by the case presented at the beginning of the chapter?

2. What condition has placed the patient at an increased risk for bacteremia?

3. What other risk factors favor bacteremic episodes in certain patient populations?

4. What are the sources of bacteremic spread?

5. Which bacterial pneumonia produces concurrent bacteremia?

6. What is the origin of organisms involved in bacteremia as a result of prosthetic devices?

7. What mechanism do the organisms employ in bacteremic episodes in patients with prosthetic devices?

8. Who are at risk for polymicrobial bacteremia?

9. Why is it important to keep the blood to culture medium ratio to 1:10?

10. How many sets of blood cultures should be used, and how often are they collected for maximum recovery of infecting agents?

CHAPTER 31

Urinary Tract Infections

John G. Thomas

OVERVIEW
The Urinary System

EPIDEMIOLOGY AND RISK FACTORS
Age
Neonates to preschool age
School-age children
Adults to age 65
Over age 65 and residence in a long-term
care facility
Inpatient care

CLINICAL SIGNS AND SYMPTOMS

ETIOLOGY OF URINARY TRACT INFECTIONS
Pathogenesis of Urinary Tract Infections
Etiologic Agents of Urinary Tract Infections
Gram-negative bacilli
Gram-positive cocci
Gram-positive bacilli
Fungi
Other agents of UTIs

LABORATORY DIAGNOSIS
Significance of Colony Counts: A Historical
Background

Specimen Collection
Voided midstream specimen collection
Catheterized specimen collection
Suprapublic aspiration
Additives
Specimen Transport

MICROBIAL DETECTION
Specimen Screening: Rapid, Nonculture
Methodologies
Manual urine screening methods
Automated screening methods
Rejection Criteria
Culture for Etiologic Agents of Urinary Tract
Infections
Asymptomatic bacteriuria
Pyelonephritis
Lower UTIs
Suprapubic aspirates
Catheterized specimens
Test of cure specimens
Prostatic secretions

INTERPRETATION OF RESULTS

SUSCEPTIBILITY REPORTING
UTI Antibiograms

OBJECTIVES

1. Define the different terms associated with urinary tract infections (UTIs).
2. Describe the clinical features and the associated symptoms.
3. Describe and distinguish between the major routes of infection.
4. Explain the prevalence of UTIs in certain age groups and gender populations.
5. Describe predisposing factors to UTIs.
6. Describe the appropriate samples for culture and interpretation of results based on the type of sample submitted.
7. List the organisms commonly associated with UTIs.
8. Discuss the interpretation of urine culture results based on bacterial colony count, pyuria, and symptoms and signs presented by the patient.
9. Name the different methods of laboratory diagnosis:
   ▪ Conventional methods
   ▪ Rapid detection and screening tests
10. Define a cost-effective, clinically relevant strategy to maximize laboratory resources focusing on pre-culture screen, reduced culturing and susceptibility testing.

KEY TERMS

Urinary tract infection (UTI)
Pyelonephritis
Bacteriuria
Acute glomerulonephritis (AGN)
Urethritis
Prostatitis
Cervicitis
Dysuria
Pyuria
Acute urethral syndrome

OVERVIEW

Urinary tract infection (UTI) is one of the most common infections in human beings. The pathogenesis and course of UTIs are greatly influenced by the anatomy of the organs involved (Figure 31-1), which includes the urethra, bladder, ureters, prostate, and kidneys. It is therefore practical to separate UTIs into upper and lower UTIs. Upper UTIs involve the renal parenchyma **(pyelonephritis)** or the ureters (ureteritis). Lower UTIs involve the bladder (cystitis), the urethra (urethritis) and, in males, the prostate (prostatitis).

The heterogeneity of disease presentation, management, and prognosis is reflected in the terminology of UTIs. Table 31-1 lists terms and definitions frequently used in connection with UTIs. Each has specific criteria and must be used appropriately.

There are two clinical schemas for classifying UTIs: single episode versus recurrent, and complicated versus uncomplicated. A single-episode UTI

CASE STUDY

A 77-year-old surgical patient, who had been discharged to a long-term care facility 6 months earlier, developed dementia with a concomitant elevated temperature (39.9° C) and mildly elevated peripheral white count (12,000 WBC/μl). Peripheral blood culture and clean catch urine specimens were collected. The urine specimen was sent on ice to a reference laboratory.

A screening urine analysis (UA) indicated a moderate level of yeast and rods and yielded a positive result on the leukocyte esterase test. At 100× oil immersion, a Gram stain performed on spun urine revealed several gram-negative rods of similar morphotype and a few white cells. Cultures performed at 24 hours showed 100,000 colony forming units (cfu)/ml mixed colonies of *Escherichia coli* and *Klebsiella pneumoniae,* fewer than 10,000 of lactobacilli, viridans streptococci, and yeasts. Blood culture results were negative.

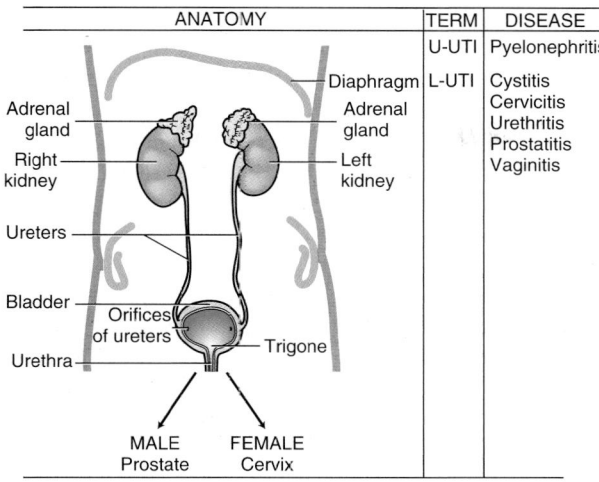

ANATOMY	TERM	DISEASE
	U-UTI	Pyelonephritis
	L-UTI	Cystitis Cervicitis Urethritis Prostatitis Vaginitis

Figure 31-1

Anatomy of the urinary tract with corresponding terms and diseases.

occurs once, resolves spontaneously or through the use of antibiotics, and does not recur. Patients with chronic or recurrent UTIs have repeated episodes of bacteriuria with or without clinical manifestations. These are arbitrarily divided into relapse and reinfection. The former involves the same organism and implies a focus of infection in the renal or prostatic parenchyma; the latter implies a different organism and usually is limited to the bladder.

Uncomplicated UTIs occur primarily in sexually active young women without genitourinary (GT) abnormalities and are usually caused by antibiotic-susceptible bacteria. Complicated UTIs occur in individuals who have one or more structural or neurologic GU abnormalities and have indwelling catheters, and whose conditions cannot be controlled with therapy. These patients are often hospitalized.

Bacteriuria, which can be symptomatic or asymptomatic, is the presence of bacteria in the urine. Disease occurs when the multiplication of organisms in the urinary tract interferes with the normal function of the involved organ. It is important to remember that infection is defined by clinical parameters and not solely by quantitation or identification of microbes.

This chapter discusses the following points:

- The variety of infections that occur in the urinary system
- The clinical parameters that define each of the disease manifestations
- The epidemiology and risk factors associated with the development of a UTI
- The laboratory diagnosis of UTIs, including specimen collection, screening methods, and interpretation of colony counts

The Urinary System

Except for the urethral mucosa and the renal medulla, which appear to be relatively susceptible to infection, the normal urinary tract is resistant to colonization and subsequent infection by bacteria. The urinary tract efficiently and rapidly eliminates both virulent and avirulent microorganisms.

Although urine is frequently considered a good culture medium, the extremely high urine osmolarity (concentration) and low pH levels inhibit the growth of many uropathogens and almost all nor-

TABLE 31-1

Definitions of Terms and Abbreviations Commonly Used for Urinary Tract Diseases

Urinary tract infection (UTI)
A spectrum of diseases caused by microbial invasion of the genitourinary (GU) tract that extends from the renal cortex of the kidney to the urethral meatus (see Figure 31-1)

Upper urinary tract infection (U-UTI)
A GU tract infection that is limited to the renal parenchyma (pyelonephritis) or the ureters (ureteritis). It is often accompanied by lower urinary tract (L-UTI) symptoms in addition to costovertebral (CV) flank pain or tenderness and fever. At times, L-UTI precedes the appearance of fever and U-UTI by 24 to 48 hours

Lower urinary tract infection (L-UTI)
A GU tract infection that is limited to the urethra (urethritis), bladder (cystitis), and, in males, the prostate (prostatitis). These infections generally appear in adults with dysuria (pain on urination), increased frequency, urgency, and occasionally suprapubic tenderness

Acute urethral syndrome
Includes dysuria and pyuria. Defined as more than 8 leukocytes per cubic millimeter (mm^3) of uncentrigued urine or approximately 2 to 5 leukocytes/high-power field (hpf) in centrifuged urine sediment

Prostatitis
A GU infection in males that involves the prostate; fever often is present

Cervicitis
Inflammation of the cervix; it may occur as an acute or a chronic presentation. Causative agents include sexually transmitted organisms, such as *Neisseria gonorrhoeae* and *Chlamydia trachomatis*. Symptoms include dysuria, urgency, vaginal discharge, and low back pain

Bacteriuria
The presence of detectable bacteria in the urine. Patients may be symptomatic or asymptomatic (e.g., geriatric or pregnant patients)

TABLE 31-2

Comparative Parameters for Urine in Control Subjects and Patients with UTIs

| | Ranges | | |
| | | Abnormal | |
Parameter	Normal	Cystitis	Pyelonephritis
Chemistries			
Specific gravity	1.001-1.035		
Volume (average/24 hr)			
child (1-14 yr)	500-1400		
Adult (<60 yr)	600-1800		
Adult (>60 yr)	250-2400		
pH range	4.7-8.0 (6.0 average)		
Protein	Negative to trace		Increased
WBC esterase	Negative		
Nitrite	Negative	Positive	Positive
Microscopic			
WBCs			
Male	0-3/hpf	Variable	Elevated to greatly increased
Female/child	0-5/hpf	Variable	Elevated to greatly increased
RBCs	0-2/hpf	Variable	Variable to greatly increased
Epithelial cells			
Squamous	Variable/hpf		
Renal	0-1/hpf		
Transitional	0-2/hpf		
Crystals	Variable	Negative	Negative
Mucus	Variable	Negative	Negative
Casts			
Hyaline	0-2/lpf		
Granular	0-1/lpf		
WBC	Negative	Negative	Positive
Microorganisms			
Bacteria	<1/hpf	Variable	Positive
Yeast	Negative	Variable	Variable
Trichomonas sp.	Negative	Variable	Negative

UTI, Urinary tract infection; *hpf,* High-power field; *lpf,* low-power field; *RBCs,* red blood cells; *WBCs,* white blood cells.

mal bacterial flora of the urethra. In addition, very dilute urine fails to support the growth of most bacterial species. In terms of antibacterial activity, urine from men is more inhibitory than urine from women because of the presence of prostatic fluids in the urine of men, as well as the difference in pH and osmolarity.

However, conditions such as high ammonia concentration, hyperosmolarity, lowered pH, and sluggish blood flow in the renal medulla can contribute to reduced leukocyte chemotaxis and bactericidal activity of white blood cells, resulting in lowered resistance. Urine itself has also been shown to inhibit the migrating, adhering, agitating, and killing function of polymorphonuclear cells. But the presence of acid-labile mucopolysaccharides, which inhibit bacterial adherence, and the flushing action of the bladder provide additional defensive mechanisms along the lower urinary tract that overcome these immunosuppressive effects. Table 31-2 lists the comparative physiologic parameters of normal urine for different populations.

EPIDEMIOLOGY AND RISK FACTORS

Age

Neonates to preschool age

Urinary tract infections are found in all age groups, beginning with neonates. During the neonate period, about 1% of all babies have bacteria in bladder urine; the incidence is higher in boys, and bacteremia often is present. In addition, autopsies have shown a predominance of infection in infant boys with pyelonephritis. Among preschool-age children, girls develop UTIs more often than boys, and infection frequently is associated with severe congenital abnormalities. These infections are often asymptomatic. It is believed that most of the renal damage caused by a UTI occurs in this age group.

School-age children

Among school-age girls in whom UTIs go into long-term remission, either spontaneously or through antibacterial therapy, many develop symptomatic infection after they marry or become pregnant, and these infections occur at a far higher rate than that among the general population. Thus the presence of bacteria in the urine in childhood defines a population at higher risk for the development of UTIs in adulthood.

Adults to age 65

From adulthood to age 65, the incidence of UTIs in men is extremely low. When infections do occur, they often are associated with anatomic abnormalities or prostatic disease and the consequent instrumentation, such as catheterization. Among women in this age group, however, as many as one fifth experience a symptomatic UTI.

Over age 65 and residence in a long-term care facility

In patients over 65 years of age, the incidence of UTIs increases dramatically for both genders, and the female-to-male ratio progressively declines. The increased incidence of UTIs in men arises from obstructive uropathologic conditions caused by the prostrate and from the loss of the bactericidal activity of prostate secretions. In women, bladder prolapse contributes to the occurrence of infection, as does soiling of the perineum from fecal incontinence in women afflicted with dementia. In both genders, neuromuscular disease and increased instrumentation in bladder catheterization are contributing factors. The time course of UTIs is shown in Figure 31-2.

The epidemiology of UTIs is influenced by the pathophysiology of the infections and by other factors, such as the virulence of the infecting organisms and their inherent mechanisms of pathogenicity, the person's immune status, and other selective external pressures. Box 31-1 lists well-defined microbial virulence factors, and Table 31-3 presents both nonspecific and genitourinary-specific factors that affect host defense and the immune system's ability, both humoral and cellular, to resist infection. A dynamic interaction exists among these factors that is continually changing, and hence the severity of infection cannot be defined by the type of invading organism or by

Box 31-1
Microbial Virulence Factors
Adherence (bacterial adhesions)
Calculi formation (kidney stones)
Toxin production
Lipopolysaccharides
Capsular polysaccharide
Hemolysins
Biofilms

colony counts alone; the total clinical situation must be assessed. Predisposing factors that may affect a person's immune status include pregnancy; the presence of an indwelling catheter or intermittent catheterization; urinary tract instrumentation, manipulation, or obstruction; and underlying disorders such as diabetes mellitus.

TABLE 31-3

Host Defenses and External, Selective Pressures That Influence the Outcome of Interaction Between Bacteria and the Urinary Tract

	Nonspecific	Genitourinary Specific
Host defense (resistance)	Intact skin	Diabetes mellitus
	WBC function	Pregnancy
	Age	Sickle cell (black women)
	Neoplasia	Neuromuscular diseases
	Immune competence	Structural abnormality
	Hormonal changes	Gout (?)
	Pregnancy	Hypertension (?)
	Malnutrition	Potassium deficiency (?)
	Malaria, diabetes	
	Psychologic state	
	Attitude	
	Immunodeficiency syndrome	
Selective pressures	Birth control pill	Sexual activity
	Smoking	Incontinence
	Alcoholism	Bladder catheterization, indwelling or intermittent
	Anesthesia	
	Drug addiction	
	Immunosuppressive drugs	Instrumentation
	Irradiation, therapeutic	Urinary stone
	Antibiotics	

WBC, White blood cell.

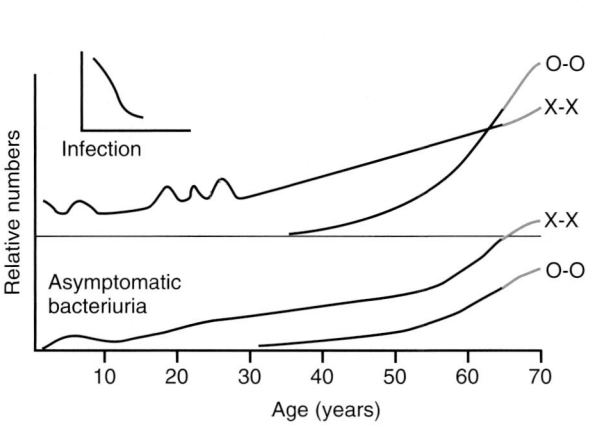

PEDIATRIC

Figure 31-2

Frequency of urinary tract infection (UTI) over time. *X-X*, Females; *O-O*, males.

Other underlying risk factors include sexual activity in younger women and incontinence in the geriatric age group. Nonspecific factors that can significantly enhance the virulence of bacteria, either directly or indirectly, include smoking and the use of the birth control pills, alcohol, or antibiotics.

A great deal of information has emerged recently about microbial biofilms. A biofilm is an organized microbial architecture of heterogenous bacteria attached to a matrix or interface, and research indicates that biofilms can serve as a virulence factor. Their importance as a contributor to the failure of routine therapy has been well established.

Inpatient care

Hospitalized patients and those residing in long-term care facilities develop UTIs more often than outpatients. The general ill condition of the hospitalized population and the higher probability of urinary tract instrumentation are major contributors to this difference. Some studies have found diabetes mellitus to be a predisposing factor in UTIs, but others have found no difference between normal individuals and diabetics. The fact that hospitalized diabetic patients are catheterized more often may account for the difference. Black women with the sickle cell trait have been reported to have a higher incidence of UTIs during pregnancy than black women who do not have the trait. This difference may be related to the effects of local tissue hypoxemia, which may result from the occlusion of renal medullary blood vessels by induced sickled erythrocytes. Chronic potassium deficiency, gout, hypertension, and other conditions that cause interstitial renal disease have been associated with UTIs but without adequate documentation.

CLINICAL SIGNS AND SYMPTOMS

Neonates and children younger than 2 years of age with UTIs usually have nonspecific symptoms, including failure to thrive, vomiting, and fever. Children older than 2 years of age are more likely to display localized symptoms, such as dysuria, frequency, and abdominal or flank pain. Adults with lower UTIs in which infection is limited to the urethra or bladder generally present with dysuria, frequency, urgency, and occasionally suprapubic tenderness.

Upper UTIs, particularly in patients with acute pyelonephritis, are often accompanied by lower urinary tract symptoms in addition to flank pain and tenderness and fever. At times the lower urinary tract symptoms precede the appearance of fever and upper urinary tract symptoms by 1 or 2 days. Bacteremia, when present, may help confirm a diagnosis of pyelonephritis or prostatitis.

It is critically important to remember that these symptoms are not reliable indicators of infection. Cases of pyelonephritis may be asymptomatic or may manifest symptoms similar to those in lower UTIs. Pain radiating from the kidneys to one of the lower quadrants of the epigastric region may mimic that seen in appendicitis or gallbladder disease; however, fever often is present in both prostatitis and pyelonephritis. Most elderly patients with UTIs are asymptomatic, and as many as 50% of women with frequency, urgency, and dysuria may not have a UTI.

Acute glomerulonephritis (AGN), a glomerulopathy that results from an immune response to *Streptococcus pyogenes* infection, either respiratory or pyodermal, may present clinical manifestations similar to those of upper UTI. Patients with AGN have edema around the eyes and produce reddish-brown urine, giving it a "Coca-cola" appearance, because of hematuria. Red blood cells and red cell casts are usually found in the urine.

Although dysuria is the most common reason for obtaining a urine culture, this clinical presentation is neither sensitive nor specific. Dysuria may be present in infections with herpes simplex virus, *Chlamydia trachomatis,* or *Neisseria gonorrhoeae.* These organisms are not detected by the routine bacteriologic culture of urine. Many noninfectious conditions, including urethral inflammation from physical or chemical agents or from trauma, may have similar symptoms. Flank pain and fever without lower urinary tract symptoms, and bacteremia without any urinary tract symptoms, are common in patients with indwelling urinary catheters. Figure 31-3 shows an evaluation schema for women with acute dysuria.

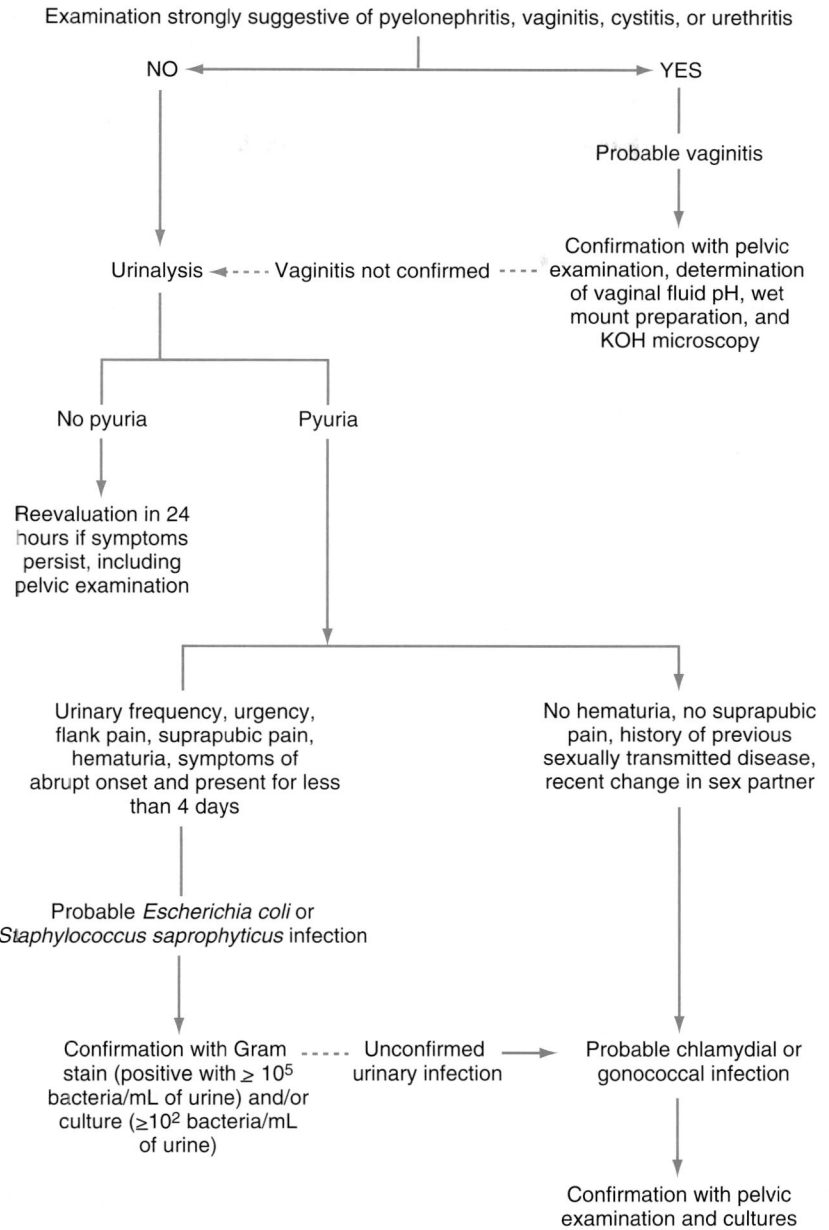

Figure 31-3

Evaluation of women with acute dysuria. *KOH,* Potassium hydroxide.

ETIOLOGY OF URINARY TRACT INFECTIONS

Pathogenesis of Urinary Tract Infections

Bacteria gain access to the urinary tract by three different routes, the ascending route, the hematogenous route, and the lymphatic pathways. Women acquire UTIs most frequently via the ascending route. Because of the shorter ureter in women, bacteria are easily introduced into the bladder by sexual intercourse. Once established in the bladder, bacteria ascend the ureters, probably aided in many cases by vesicoureteral reflux or by peristaltic dilated ureters caused by intraluminal infection, an inflammation of the GU tract musculature.

Infection of the renal parenchyma by many species of gram-positive bacteria (particularly in patients with staphylococcal bacteremia or endocarditis, mycobacterial infection, and *Candida* infection) clearly occurs by the hematogenous route. Gram-negative infections rarely occur by the hematogenous route.

Increased pressure on the bladder can cause lymphatic flow to be directed to the kidney. However, evidence for a significant role for renal lymphatics in the pathogenesis of pyelonephritis is unimpressive. Of the three possible routes of infection, the ascending route is of paramount importance, and the hematogenous route offers a less frequent but significant pathway.

Etiologic Agents of Urinary Tract Infections

The normal bacterial flora of the paraurethral area consists mostly of *Staphylococcus epidermidis.* Table 31-4 presents the organisms that do not grow well in urine and are not common causes of UTIs, arranged in descending order by age or patient status. Those listed first are most commonly found, and those at the end are less frequently isolated.

Box 31-2 lists the more readily recognized agents of UTIs, as well as emerging uropathogens that need to be recognized, given the dynamics of urinary tract pathogens, the population at risk, and selected pressures, as outlined earlier. These organisms present unique challenges to clinical microbiologists.

Gram-negative bacilli

Of the Enterobacteriaceae, antibiotic-susceptible strains of *E. coli* that emanate from the patient's own fecal flora cause most uncomplicated UTIs.

TABLE 31-4

Flora of Normal Voided Urine* Defined by Patient's Age and Status

Patient Age/Status	Usual Flora
Newborn	Sterile
1-3 days old	Staphylococci
	Enterococci
	Diphtheroids
	Mycobacterium smegmatis
3 days to few weeks	*Lactobacillus acidophilus*
Prepubertal	Micrococci
	Streptococci (α-hemolytic and nonhemolytic)
	Coliforms
	Diphtheroids
Adult	*L. acidophilus*
	Staphylococcus epidermidis
	Streptococci (α-hemolytic and nonhemolytic)
	Escherichia coli
	Diphtheroids
	Yeasts
	Anaerobic streptococci
	Listeria sp.
	Clostridium sp.
Pregnancy	Increase in *L. acidophilus*
	Yeasts
	S. epidermidis
Postmenopausal	Similar to prepubertal flora

*Usually sterile or fewer than 1000 colonies/ml.

Multiple antibiotic–resistant members of the Enterobacteriaceae derived from the hands of hospital personnel and contaminated solutions colonize and subsequently infect hospitalized patients with indwelling bladder instruments. As the duration of hospitalization and catheterization increases, *E. coli* is less likely to be encountered than organisms such as *Pseudomonas, Proteus, Klebsiella,* and *Enterobacter* spp. Complicated infections often are polymicrobic, involve renal stones, and can yield urine specimens from which *E. coli* and *Proteus* species, or *E. coli* and *Klebsiella pneumoniae,* are alternatively or concomitantly recovered.

Gram-positive cocci

Among the gram-positive cocci, enterococci and *Staphylococcus saprophyticus* are the most commonly encountered causative agents. Enterococcal UTIs occur primarily in older men, particularly in association with urinary tract manipulation or instrumentation or prostatic hypertrophy. *S. saprophyticus,* on the other hand, is found predominantly in symptomatic sexually active women younger than 40 years of age. Staphylococci that are neither *Staphylococcus aureus* nor *S. saprophyticus* frequently are identified as *Staphylococcus epidermidis,* which commonly is found in hospitalized patients older than 50 years of age. These individuals most often have had recent urinary tract surgery, have indwelling urinary catheters, or have chronic urinary tract disease. *S. epidermidis* is associated with UTI in only about 20% of cases. Table 31-5 highlights important features of coagulase-negative staphylococcal UTIs.

Gram-positive bacilli

Isolation of *Bacillus* species can almost without exception be considered contamination. UTIs truly caused by the organism are exceedingly rare. The

TABLE 31-5

Urinary Tract Infections Caused by Coagulase-Negative Staphylococci

Characteristics of Infections	Organism	
	S. epidermidis	*S. saprophyticus*
Sex and age of affected patients	Men and women equally	Women 95%, 16-35 years of age
Population at risk	Hospitalized patients with urinary tract complications	Healthy outpatients
Incidence	Common: 20% or more of all UTIs for hospitalized patients older than 50 years of age	Uncommon: 3.5% or fewer of all UTIs in hospitalized patients
Presentation	90% asymptomatic	90% symptomatic; indistinguishable from *Escherichia coli* UTIs
Therapy	Often resistant to multiple drugs	Responds readily to traditional urinary tract antimicrobials except nalidixic acid
Outcome	Bacteriuria often persists after therapy	Relapse rare; occasional reinfection

UTI, Urinary tract infection.

Box 31-2

Recognized Microbial Agents of Urinary Tract Infections

Common

Enterococci (including vancomycin-resistant enterococci)
Streptococcus agalactiae (group B streptococci)
Enterobacteriaceae
Pseudomonas sp.
Streptococcus pyogenes (group A streptococci)
Staphylococcus aureus
Staphylococcus saprophyticus
Candida sp.

Less common

Gardnerella vaginalis
Ureaplasma urealyticum
Mycoplasma hominis
Mobiluncus sp.
Leptospira sp.
Mycobacterium sp.
Chlamydia trachomatis (males)

Often associated with multisystem diseases

Salmonella sp. (with gastroenteritis)
Schistosoma haematobium
Cryptococcus neoformans
Trichosporon beigelii
Trichomonas vaginalis
Aspergillus sp.
Penicillium sp.
Adenovirus
Herpes simplex virus

significance of *Clostridium* species is as difficult to assess in urine as it is in blood. The evidence in the literature concerning clostridial UTIs or the recovery of clostridia in urine with a soft tissue abscess is insufficient to support a definitive statement of significance. Mycobacteria infrequently may be seen in Gram-stained specimens of urine and appear as gram-positive bacilli. Mycobacteria have been associated with UTIs and may have added significance in patients infected with the human immunodeficiency virus (HIV) or those who are otherwise immunosuppressed. In rare cases *Listeria monocytogenes* may be isolated from the urine of infants who acquired a perinatal infection with this organism and in 1% of patients with a systemic infection or renal transplant. Diphtheroids, mycobacteria, and *L. monocytogenes* all cause diseases, predominantly in highly selected patient populations and almost always in association with bacteremia. If any of these organisms are recovered from urine or seen on smears, consultation with the physician permits some assessment of the significance. Within selected populations, blood cultures or cultures from other sites may help determine the significance of the isolate.

Fungi

Fungi, particularly *Candida albicans* and *Torulopsis glabrata,* are commonly associated with UTIs. On agar medium, young colonies of *C. albicans* can resemble colonies of coagulase-negative staphylococci (CNS) and may be misidentified if gram-stained smears are not examined. A wet mount preparation examined under 10× also can provide a rapid identification. Because *Candida* species often are recovered from hospitalized patients with indwelling catheters, incorrect identification results in a susceptibility report indicating broad antimicrobial resistance.

 Candida and *Cryptococcus* species usually are evident in culture within 2 to 5 days. Unless dimorphic fungi are suspected, fungal urine cultures can be discarded as having a negative result after 2 weeks. Cultures of dimorphic fungi may require 4 to 6 weeks for colonies to appear. Although findings of candiduria may not require antifungal therapy, particularly in catheterized patients, properly collected urine specimens yielding *Candida* species should be considered abnormal. Candiduria may be an indication of bladder or renal parenchymal infection, a urinary tract fungus ball, or disseminated candidiasis. Predisposing factors include diabetes mellitus, antibiotic and corticosteroid therapy, female gender, and disturbance of urine flow. The isolation of any other classic pathogenic fungi, such as *Cryptococcus neoformans, Blastomyces dermatitidis, Coccidioides immitis,* and *Histoplasma capsulatum* in the urine is a highly significant finding indicative of possible disseminated infection.

Other agents of UTIs

Other significant organisms may be encountered in urine cultures. Anaerobes, which are common flora in the urethra, are not usually responsible for UTIs but may be considered significant when isolated from suprapubic aspirates. *C. trachomatis* and *N. gonorrhoeae* can cause the symptoms of **urethritis,** cystitis, and **prostatitis.** This is particularly an issue with women, because in women it is clinically difficult to distinguish between urethritis and **cervicitis.** Recently, *Mycoplasma* and *Ureaplasma* organisms have been associated with UTIs, particularly in neonates from lower socioeconomic groups.

 The isolation of *Gardnerella vaginalis* in urine commonly represents vaginal contamination, but this organism is also an emerging urinary tract pathogen. Although the role of *G. vaginalis* in UTIs has not been clearly established, repeated cultures in which this microbe is the primary isolate should not be ignored. Certain organisms, particularly *Salmonella* sp., are involved with multiple organ systems; these may be part of a primary disease or may arise secondarily.

 Viral agents, especially adenovirus and herpes simplex virus, also have been associated with cystitis and must be identified when the clinical situation warrants. Table 31-6 presents organisms associated with UTIs, listing the uropathogens most often associated with a particular clinical presentation or disease syndrome.

TABLE 31-6

Most Common UTI Etiologic Agents Associated with Frequent Clinical Presentation (Disease Syndromes)

Clinical Presentation	Common Etiologic Agents
Upper urinary tract infections	
Acute pyelonephritis	Enterobacteriaceae
	Staphylococcus aureus
Subclinical pyelonephritis	Coagulase-negative staphylococci
	Candida spp.
	Mycobacterium spp.
	Mycoplasma hominis
Lower urinary tract infections	
Acute bacterial cystitis	*Escherichia coli*
	Klebsiella spp.
	Other Enterobacteriaceae
	Enterococci
	Coagulase-negative staphylococci
Urethritis	
Acute urethral syndrome	*Chlamydia trachomatis*
	Neisseria gonorrhoeae
	Ureaplasma urealyticum
Other infections	
Gonococcal urethritis	*N. gonorrhoeae*
Chlamydial urethritis	*C. trachomatis*
Vaginitis	
Prostatitis	
Symptomatic bacteriuria	
Catheter-associated (hospital-associated) UTI	*E. coli*
	Klebsiella spp.
	Proteus mirabilis
	Pseudomonas sp.
	Candida spp.
Chronic or recurrent (inpatient/outpatient) UTI	Adherent *E. coli*

UTI, Urinary tract infection.

LABORATORY DIAGNOSIS

Significance of Colony Counts: A Historical Background

Since 1956 the interpretation of quantitative urine cultures has been considered one of the more straightforward and simpler laboratory tests to diagnose UTIs. It was "dogma" that a finding of 100,000 (10^5) colony-forming units per milliliter (CFU/ml) or more was a "positive" test result. In his 1956 classic study, Edward Kass showed a clear separation between the number of bacteria in the urine of asymptomatic or symptomatic women with pyelonephritis and those who were uninfected. Significantly, 95% had colony counts higher than 10^5 CFU/ml when infected.

In retrospect, this study had some very definitive parameters, namely that all specimens were collected by catheterization, that most asymptomatic women had counts below 10^3 CFU/ml, and that the prevalence of infection was only 6%.

The sensitivity was only 51% for women with clinical pyelonephritis who had colony counts above 10^5 CFU/ml.

In the 1960s and 1970s additional studies began to erode the "absolutism" of Kass's original work. A number of investigators showed that for women with symptomatic, acute lower UTIs (urethra, bladder, or both), 29% to 45% had colony counts below 10^5 CFU/ml by suprapubic aspiration. These women had **dysuria** and **pyuria,** yet unexpectedly "negative cultures" by the traditional "Kass-based" criterion (i.e., more than 10^5 CFU/ml). In 1980 the **acute urethral syndrome,** or urethritis, was more clearly defined as one of the three causes of acute dysuria with pyuria. The other causes were vaginitis and cystitis. The causative organisms included classic coliforms and *Staphylococcus saprophyticus* at colony counts above 10^3 but below 10^5 CFU/ml.

Simultaneously implicated in sexually active women were the emerging nongonococcal urethritis pathogens *Chlamydia trachomatis* and *Ureaplasma urealyticum.* Thus in women with UTIs, as many as half had urethral syndrome—not cystitis—and were "culture-negative" by traditional "laboratory" methods.

In 1982 Stamm and coworkers restudied the diagnostic criteria for women with acute symptomatic lower UTIs. In contrast with Kass's classic work, Stamm's study included coliforms at counts above 10^2 CFU/ml. The criteria of 10^2 CFU/ml provided a sensitivity of 0.95 and a specificity of 0.85 (Table 31-7). The presence of pyuria in uncentrifuged urine specimens was a sensitive adjunct. The prevalence of coliform infections was 36% in women evaluated by Stamm and colleagues (1982), compared with Kass's 6%.

Finally, in the late 1980s, because of the emerging significance of pyuria, investigators re-evaluated the accuracy of the classic urinary sediment microscopic examination (UA). All agreed that urinalysis screening for detection of UTI was inherently inaccurate, was not reproducible, and did not correlate with clinically proven UTIs. It was felt that microscopic examination of urine specimens should be reserved for the detection of casts and crystals.

Furthermore investigators could not correlate UA determinations of white blood cells with the actual leukocyte excretion rate of white cells per cubic millimeter measured by hemocytometer chamber count. When clinical studies using the latter method of determining pyuria were reviewed, the following conclusions emerged:

- A leukocyte count of $10/mm^3$ or higher occurs in fewer than 1% of asymptomatic, nonbacteriuric patients but in more than 96% of symptomatic men and women with significant bacteriuria.

TABLE 31-7

Comparison of Colony Counts for Acute Lower Urinary Tract Coliform Infection

Investigator	Test Midstream Urine (CFU/ml)	Sensitivity	Specificity	Predictive Value	
				Positive	Negative
Stamm et al (1982)	≥10^2 coliforms/ml	0.95	0.85	0.88	0.94
Kass (1956)	≥10^5 coliforms/ml	0.51	0.99	0.98	0.65

CFU, Colony-forming units.

- Most symptomatic women with pyuria but without significant bacteriuria either have UTIs with bacterial uropathogens present in colony counts below 10^5 CFU/ml ($>10^2$ to $<10^5$ CFU/ml) or have infections with *Chlamydia trachomatis/Ureaplasma urealyticum*.
- Women with asymptomatic bacteriuria probably should be divided into those with true asymptomatic infection associated with pyuria and those with transient self-limited bladder colonization and no pyuria.
- Most patients with catheter-associated bacteriuria also have pyuria, hence, infection.

Simultaneously, an impregnated paper strip that measured urine leukocyte esterase was introduced and found to correlate well with hemocytometer chamber counts. The leukocyte esterase test (LET) was inexpensive and quick (1 minute) and required no technical skills or equipment, just the classic "dipstick."

What did all this mean, and how did it fit into the laboratory faced with myriad problems in interpreting uropathogen colony counts? Until recently, the colony count was regarded as the "gold standard" for determining if a patient had a real and treatable UTI; the fact is, however, that the urine bacterial colony count cannot stand alone as a single criterion when evaluating for the presence or absence of UTI. Urine cultures are requested not only in connection with the symptoms of acute UTI but also in the absence of specific symptoms, as a test of cure, to evaluate the effectiveness of antimicrobial therapy, to detect asymptomatic bacteriuria in pregnant women, and to evaluate for bacteremia or fever or both, to name but a few instances. Furthermore, the criteria that determine if a UTI is present must include the presence or absence of symptoms, predisposing factors, the patient population, and the type of organism or organisms isolated. The outcome of a urine culture, therefore, must be evaluated together with other laboratory and clinical data; attempts to attach significance to the colony count should be restricted to the original patient population in which that significance was established: asymptomatic individuals with pyelonephritis.

Specimen Collection

Preventing contamination by normal vaginal, perianal, and interior urethral flora is the most im-

portant consideration in collecting a clinically relevant urine specimen. Nonetheless, it is still an important fact that physicians rely on colony counts. Therefore all necessary precautions should be taken to ensure that the colony count represents the numbers of organisms present at the time the specimen was collected. It is incumbent on the laboratory directors to define specific criteria for collection and transport and, within their realm of responsibility, to ensure that these protocols are followed.

A wide variety of methods can be used for collecting urine samples.

Voided midstream specimen collection

With voided midstream collection, the most commonly used method, the patient collects the specimens. The urine is contaminated with bacteria from the urethra unless the first portion of the voided specimen is discarded. Investigators have found that voided urine collection kits should contain instructions to the patient on proper specimen procurement, and these instructions should be read slowly to the patient rather than merely supplied. Patient education should be part of the specimen processing, because proper collection has a considerable influence on the result of subsequent laboratory procedures. It has also been reported that stick-figure diagrams showing the manner in which a specimen should be collected are much more easily understood by the patient than written instructions, in view of the number of people who cannot read beyond a third-grade level.

Catheterized specimen collection

Catheterized specimen collection, which is an invasive technique, reduces the risk of contamination of urine with the urethral flora; however, because the catheter is passed through the urethra, some contamination may occur. When specimens are collected from an indwelling urinary catheter, the catheter collection port should be cleaned with an alcohol pad and punctured directly with a needle and syringe. The specimen should never be collected from the drainage bag. Before collecting urine with a single, straight catheter, the urethral opening or vaginal vault is cleansed with a soap solution and rinsed with sterile water. The initial urine flow is discarded because it may contain organisms acquired as the catheter passed through the urethra. Samples obtained from an ileoconduit are collected from the stomal opening after the area has been gently swabbed with an alcohol wipe. The urine on the external appliance is never used for culture, since it is similar to the urine in a drainage bag in patients with indwelling catheters.

The bacteriologic results of separate urine specimens collected by cystoscopy (bilateral urethral catheterization) or by bladder washout are used to localize the infection to the upper or lower urinary tract and, in the former case, to the left or right kidney. Specimens obtained by straight catheterization, by bilateral urethral catheterization, by bladder washout, or from an ileoconduit may be submitted in a tube or broth unless an assessment of pyuria is necessary. When such a specimen arrives at the laboratory, it must be labeled as to location or timing, and this information must accompany the results for proper interpretation.

Suprapubic aspiration

Suprapubic aspiration is the definitive method for collecting uncontaminated specimens. Although most consider any organism isolated on these specimens to be clinically significant, this may not be correct because transient colonization of the bladder can occur. Suprapubic aspirations are collected primarily from infants and patients in whom the interpretation of the results of voided specimens is difficult. Suprapubic aspiration urine specimens are the only ones suitable for anaerobic culture. With the bladder full, the urine is collected with a needle and syringe following skin antisepsis.

OTHER CONSIDERATIONS

In addition to the manner in which the specimen is collected, other parameters may have an impact on the suitability of the specimen including:

- *Urine volume.* The volume of urine received is rarely a problem for routine bacteriologic culture. Detection of significant pyuria by sediment examination requires at least 10 ml of specimen; however, alternative methods of pyuria detection may be needed when smaller volumes are received. As much as 20 ml of urine may be required to recover mycobacteria or fungi. If these agents are strongly suspected and previous specimens of lesser volume tested negative, a request for a single collection of at least 20 ml should be forwarded to the physician. It must be remembered that 24-hour collections for urine specimens in microbiology are totally unsatisfactory.

- *The number of specimens and timing of collection.* The number of specimens and the timing of urine collection depend on the patient's clinical state and the method used. A single clean voided specimen in a specifically symptomatic patient or a single specimen obtained by catheterization in a patient with specific symptoms is sufficient if significant pyuria is demonstrable and culture yields a recognized uropathogen. In symptomatic patients, antimicrobial therapy often is instituted immediately after urine collection and is not withheld to allow the procurement of subsequent specimens. For purposes of optimal quantitation, it has been recommended that only first morning specimens be processed or, if such specimens are not available, that the urine be allowed to incubate in the bladder for as long as possible (with a minimum of 4 hours) before collection to increase the bacterial density. This procedure appears to be rather imprecise and probably unnecessary because of the insignificance of colony counts in symptomatic patients and the need for antimicrobial therapy.

In the absence of symptoms, a single first morning voided urine specimen from a pregnant woman is sufficient to detect asymptomatic bacteriuria. In this case, one or two more first morning specimens may be collected on separate days to demonstrate the significance of the isolates. Because quantitation is necessary for the diagnosis of asymptomatic bacteriuria and because an asymptomatic condition does not require immediate therapeutic intervention, these specimens should be limited to first morning collections. Urine specimens from other asymptomatic patient populations, except those demonstrating significant pyuria, cannot be reliably interpreted.

Significant pyuria in the absence of bacteriuria and symptoms suggest the possibility of renal tuberculosis. For optimal recovery of mycobacteria, three specimens should be collected on 3 to 6 consecutive days.

Surveillance cultures of urine from asymptomatic hospitalized patients with indwelling catheters cannot predict the onset of UTI or the etiologic agent. Knowledge of the specific organisms present on the ward is not necessary to prevent their spread if proper infection control procedures are universally used during catheter care.

If the initial urine specimen from a symptomatic patient yields significant pyuria and a recognized urinary pathogen, ideally two subsequent "test of cure" specimens should be processed, one at 48 to 72 hours and another at cessation of therapy. A test of cure specimen also is appropriate subsequent to the treatment of asymptomatic bacteriuria. Given today's concerns about cost and test utilization, however, this is rarely done.

Additives

Additives to urine are designed primarily to preserve the bacterial density present at collection. These additives maintain the original colony count during ambient temperature transport until quantitative cultures can be accomplished, obviating a need for refrigerated transportation. Liquid preservatives have been associated with dilution errors and decreased recovery of organisms at 24 and 48 hours. Lyophilized preservation is less inhibitory and requires a urine volume of at least 3 ml to avoid dilution effect. The effects of preservatives on the detection of pyuria have not been adequately determined. Regardless of the preservative used, the maximum time from collection to processing should not exceed 24 hours. In addition, the effect of preservatives on selected manual and automated methods, which are discussed later in the chapter, has not been extensively evaluated.

The importance of the determination of pyuria in many cases and the lack of evidence that urine preservatives allow an accurate leukocyte count after 2 hours argue against the use of preservatives for specimens from symptomatic patients. The dip-slide urine collection container offers a more reliable method of preserving bacterial density in specimens from asymptomatic pregnant women or from patients for whom quantitative cultures are required; it also allows quicker detection of the etiologic agent. This method may be particularly suited to physicians' offices. In the current cost-conscious environment, it is recommended that all urine specimens in physicians' offices be cultured with the dip-slide method and held for 48 hours. If the patient does not respond to em-

pirical therapy, these original specimens can be forwarded to the laboratory for identification and susceptibility testing. If the appropriate antibiotic is selected, the specimens can be discarded.

Specimen Transport

Urine is an excellent supportive medium for the growth of most uropathogens and therefore must be immediately refrigerated or preserved. Generally, urine should be refrigerated, received, and processed in the laboratory within 2 hours. Longer delays render examination for significant pyuria unreliable, and the extremes of pH and urea concentration and the presence of antimicrobial agents may adversely affect the recovery of uropathogens.

A specimen submitted on a dip-slide transported at room temperature may be received up to 18 hours after collection. Liquid urine submitted for diagnosis of asymptomatic bacteriuria for which an examination for pyuria is not requested may be refrigerated for up to 18 hours before processing.

Except for specimens submitted for the sole purpose of isolating mycobacteria or fungi, or the diagnosis of asymptomatic bacteriuria, refrigeration is not an optimal, or to some, an acceptable method of preserving urine specimens. Refrigeration cannot preserve the number of leukocytes beyond 2 hours, and there is no need to stabilize the bacterial density in urine for symptomatic patients for the purpose of quantitative culture.

MICROBIAL DETECTION

Specimen Screening: Rapid, Nonculture Methodologies

The ideal urine screening system should identify all urine specimens from infected patients at a high negative predictive value and be rapid and cost-effective. Toward this goal, a number of manual and automated methods have been developed. To maximize the benefits of screening methodology, preliminary reports should be produced as soon as possible. Preliminary reports should consist of the degree of pyuria and, depending on the method used, the presence or absence of bacteria or fungi. These results should reach the physician within 2 hours after collection of a urine specimen.

The report also should indicate whether additional identification methods are being used and their turn-around time. Ideally, the report should also include guides to appropriate antimicrobial therapy based on "in-house" laboratory antibiograms tabulated over the past 6 months.

However, the need for screening and the extent of identification and susceptibility testing of isolates depend on the method of collection and the purpose for which the urine was submitted. Hence, a uniform and consistent means of communicating that purpose to the laboratory must be developed, so that information useful to the physician can be produced in the time frame required.

Additionally, a number of key points need to be remembered when using screening methods:

- Screening methods capable of detecting bacterial densities of 10^5 CFU/ml or higher are appropriate for the detection of asymptomatic bacteriuria in pregnant women.
- Methodologies that detect both bacteriuria and pyuria may result in false-positive tests for asymptomatic bacteriuria because densities below 10^5 CFU/ml are detected if significant pyuria unrelated to a UTI is present.
- False-positive results occur more often with methods that test for more than one parameter (e.g., bacteria and WBC counts).
- Methods of detecting significant pyuria and bacteriuria with sensitivities of 50 to 100 leukocytes/mm^3 and 10^2 CFU/ml may be appro-

priate for screening voided urine specimens or specimens from indwelling urinary catheters in symptomatic patients.
- Screening methods are not appropriate for urine collected by straight catheterization, cystoscopy, suprapubic aspiration, and bladder washout or for test of cure specimens and specimens collected from ileoconduits.

Manual urine screening methods
Table 31-8 lists various manual screening methods that are useful in detecting bacteria and leukocytes in urine.

MICROSCOPY

Detection of bacteria when pyelonephritis is suspected Gram staining of urine samples should be performed, because it may reveal the etiologic agent. Uncentrifuged urine samples may be used for a stained smear. Most recently, cytospin technology has been found to be remarkably applicable to rapid urine microscopy. The presence of one or more bacterial cells per oil immersion field (OIF) in at least five fields in a smear of uncentrifuged urine correlates with more than 10^5 CFU/ml. If the uncentrifuged preparation tests negative, the sedimented preparation for leukocyte examination should be stained. Bacterial cells seen in this preparation indicate a density of fewer than 10^5 organisms/ml and, in the presence of clinical findings of acute pyelonephri-

TABLE 31-8
Various Manual Screening Methods, Principles of Assay, and Threshold of Detection for UTIs

Screens	Principle	Reported Threshold of Detection (CFU/ml)
Manual		
Microscopy	Recognition of organism morphotypes and Gram stain	≥ 1 organism/OIF $= \geq 10^5$
Direct, uncentrifuged or centrifuged (cytospin)		
Chemical		
Enzymatic dipstick		
Nitrate reductase (Griess test)	Gram-negative bacteria reduce nitrates to nitrites	$\geq 10^4$
WBC/Leukocyte esterase	Measures presence of WBC enzyme	Equivalent to 5 WBC/hpf
Chemstrip LN	Combination testing of both nitrate and esterase assays	$> 10^4$ to 10^5
Enzyme tube		
Uriscreen	Measures catalase present in both bacteria and somatic cells	$> 10^4$ to 10^5
Colorimetric particle filtration		
FiltraCheck—UTI	Combination testing of both bacteria and WBCs by membrane filtration and detection using safranin O dye	$> 10^4$

Hpf, High-power field; *OIF,* oil immersion field; *WBC,* white blood cell.

tis, may suggest urinary obstruction or prenephric abscess. The presence of gram-positive or gram-negative bacteria or fungi assists in the selection of an appropriate antibiotic therapy. Acridine orange stain decreases the detectable threshold from 10^5 CFU/mL to 10^4 CFU/mL.

Detection of pyuria Detection of leukocytes may be performed by microscopic examination of a wet mount of a urinary sediment resulting from centrifugation of 10 ml of a specimen at 200 rpm on a tabletop centrifuge for 5 minutes. At least five fields should be examined, and each leukocyte seen per high-power field (hpf) ($40\times$) represents approximately 5 to 10 cells per cubic millimeter of urine. In this way, 5 to 10 leukocytes per high-power field in the sediment is the upper limit of normal, representing 50 to 100 cells/mm³. If a more precise method is required, the technique described by Brumfit may be used. This involves the examination of a fresh, uncentrifuged specimen in a hemocytometer chamber. More than 8 to 10 leukocytes/mm³ indicates significant pyuria.

Detection of fungi and mycobacteria The cells of yeasts can usually be readily identified by Gram stain, but the cells of other fungi, because of their varying size and unique forms, may be difficult to discern. If fungi are suspected clinically or from the Gram stain, a smear can be stained using fluorescent microscopy and calcofluor white. This stain preferably binds chitin present in the cell walls of fungi and makes visualization and identification easier. Cotton swabs may not be used to apply the specimen to the microscope slide, however, because the stains bind to the cotton fibers and fluoresce.

Examination of urine for acid-fast bacilli is productive only if restricted to a particular patient population. Because of the presence of nonpathogenic mycobacteria in the smegma, smears that test positive must be confirmed with culture.

CHEMICAL METHODS
Chemical screening techniques include a variety of procedures, such as the nitrate reductase (Griess) test, WBC leukocyte esterase test, and Chem-strip. As with manual microscopy, these methods may be labor intensive and insensitive for low-grade significant bacteriuria.

Recently, tube enzyme (catalase) and colorimetric particle filtration (safranin O dye) have been

reintroduced into the clinical setting with modified, updated protocols. Both measure a combination of bacteria and extracellular products of white blood cells.

Automated urine screening methods

Table 31-9 summarizes various automated screening methods for bacterial detection in urine samples. Bioluminescence systems detect bacterial adenosine triphosphate. Such systems may be expensive, frequently require batching of specimens (therefore time delays), and have not been adequately evaluated for their efficacy in detecting low-grade bacteriuria and funguria. The popularity of automation has grown, however, as more laboratories search for quick, same-day results and the means to eliminate negative urine culture results.

A number of photometry methods, including the Vitek system (bioMerieúx Vitek, Hazelwood, Mo.) have been developed to measure growth. If a significant number of organisms are present in the urine specimens, rapid growth is detected in the nutrient medium. The clinical evaluations of all these systems are less than optimum because sensitivity for a low-grade bacteriuria had not been assessed. These systems are relatively expensive.

TABLE 31-9

Various Automated Screening Methods, Principle of Assay, and Threshold of Detection for UTIs

Automated	Principle	Threshold of Detection (CFU/ml)
Bioluminescence UTI screen	Detected bacterial ATP using enzymatic bioluminescent reaction of ATP with luciferin and luciferase	$>10^4$ to 10^5
Photometry	If a significant number of organisms are present in the urine specimen, they will grown in the medium to a detectable concentration using photometry	$>10^4$ to 10^5
Colorimetric particle filtration Bac-T-Screen	Automated combination testing for both bacteria and WBCs by membrane filtration and detection using safranin O dye	$>10^4$ to 10^5

ATP, Adenosine triphosphate; *UTI,* urinary tract infection; *WBC,* white blood cell.

Particle filtration systems, such as Bac-T-Screen 2000 (bioMerieúx Vitek, Hazelwood, Mo.) are used to trap organisms and WBCs on filters and then selectively stain the cells. These systems are very sensitive even for low-grade infections, are somewhat nonspecific, yield many false-positive results, and are relatively expensive.

Rejection Criteria

It is imperative that the laboratory establish, in concert with the various medical services, criteria for obtaining optimal specimens. Specimens may be rejected because of an inadequate or inappropriate method of collection or transport. These criteria demand strict adherence to guidelines for collection and transport of specimens. If the specimen does not meet these tailored guidelines for each institution, it is incumbent on the laboratory (as soon as possible) to inform the service or physician (or both) of the inadequacy of the specimen and the fact that the specimen will not be processed. Antibiotic therapy may not have been initiated, and a better specimen may be collected. Samples to be rejected include 24-hour urine specimens and Foley catheter tips; these should not be processed.

Culture for Etiologic Agents of Urinary Tract Infections

Generally, routine urine culture should include plating onto one selective and one nonselective medium. Calibrated loops of 0.01 ml should be used, not 0.001 ml (1 μl) loops, because quantitation is difficult to obtain with a low inoculum. Routine specimens incubated longer than a full 24 hours yield "noise" or background urethral flora that increase cost and may impair the clinical usefulness of the urine culture.

Two important factors govern the selection of culture methods for urine specimens. First, some circumstances may account for the presence of a low number of bacteria in specimens; such circumstances include pyelonephritis with obstruction, perinephric abscess, the period before the start of antimicrobial therapy, and bacterial persistence while the patient is undergoing antimicrobial therapy. In these cases, methods with appropriate sensitivity are necessary to detect the low densities. Second, organisms in deep-seated infections, such as upper UTIs, often are in a hy-

drophilic state and do not emerge on direct plating of the specimen on agar.

A suspicion that certain etiologic agents may be present may also dictate the method of processing for culture. For example, media should include detection of *N. gonorrhoeae* and *U. urealyticum* if these organisms are suspected. If fungal cells or hyphae are seen on wet mount or Gram stain or if fungal infection is suspected, media such as Sabouraud dextrose agar (Emmons modification) may be inoculated. If mycobacteria are suspected, the specimen should be decontaminated and inoculated to one Bactec bottle (Becton Dickinson, Cockeysville, Md.) and one Löwenstein-Jensen slant. The specimens are then processed according to the standard protocol for acid-fast bacilli culture.

Use of agar dipsticks and biplates should be reserved for clinics and physicians' offices, circumstances in which retrieval of specimens after therapy may be less than optimal, and only cultures from patients who are not responding to therapy would need a complete identification. The methodology also needs to be adjusted to the specimen source and the underlying disease process.

Asymptomatic bacteriuria

If the patient is asymptomatic, immediate microbial therapy is not necessary. Identification and susceptibility testing of isolates can be achieved by any conventional or automated method. The colony count should accompany any positive culture result to indicate the diagnosis of asymptomatic bacteriuria. Because the organisms most frequently identified include *E. coli* and other rapidly growing members of Enterobacteriaceae, 24 hours of incubation at 35° C is sufficient.

Pyelonephritis

Urine specimens submitted from patients suspected of having pyelonephritis generally contain high numbers of bacteria. Microscopic examination of urine for leukocytes and bacteria quickly provides therapeutically useful information. Because the antibiotic susceptibilities of the responsible organisms are variable and unpredictable, culture should be designed for optimal recovery. Plates should be incubated for 48 hours at 35° C, and the methodology may include a drop of specimen inoculated into trypticase soy broth for optimal recovery.

Lower UTIs

Specimens from patients with symptoms of lower UTI should be processed in the same manner as that for suspected cases of pyelonephritis. If significant pyuria is found in a symptomatic patient, and no recognized urinary pathogen is detected, the laboratory should consider the presence of *C. trachomatis; Mycoplasma* species, including *U. urealyticum;* and/or *N. gonorrhoeae.*

Suprapubic aspirates

Aspirates may contain bacteria that are likely to be present in low numbers and may include anaerobic species. Such specimens should be routinely inoculated on a blood agar plate, a MacConkey agar plate, and a trypticase soy broth for up to 48 hours. For recovery of *Gardnerella vaginalis,* chocolate agar is acceptable. Anaerobic bacteria are recovered in approximately 1% of cases and therefore need not be sought routinely, but only after consultation.

Catheterized specimens

Urine specimens obtained by straight catheterization, by bilateral ureteral catheterization, by bladder washout, or from ileoconduits require inoculation of both agar plates and liquid medium for maximum recovery.

Test of cure specimens

Specimens obtained 48 hours after the initiation of therapy or after the cessation of therapy are sterile in the absence of indwelling bladder devices if therapy was successful. Growth of an organism other than the one recovered before the initiation of therapy suggests superinfection if the isolate is a recognized urinary pathogen. Susceptibility tests should be performed routinely on organisms recovered from the test of cure specimens if the organism is known to develop resistance during therapy (i.e., *Pseudomonas* sp.).

Prostatic secretions

The etiologic agent of acute prostatitis is usually recovered from catheterized specimens, which should be cultured in the same manner as that for specimens from symptomatic men. In cases of chronic prostatitis, prostatic secretions are submitted, as well as urethral urine and midstream voided urine specimens obtained before and after massage. Quantitative cultures are necessary for proper interpretation.

Historically, yeasts have been detected within 24 hours, but certain forms may need a total of 48 hours of incubation. When isolated, the numbers of yeast should be reported. Low colony counts may be just as significant as higher colony counts.

When mycobacteria are suspected, the specimen should be decontaminated and inoculated to one Bactec bottle (Becton Dickinson, Cockeysville, Md.) and one Löwenstein-Jensen slant and processed according to the standard acid-fast bacilli standard acid-fast bacilli standard protocol.

Use of agar dipsticks and biplates should be avoided, if possible, because isolated colonies may not be available, thus delaying final identification and antimicrobial susceptibility testing (AST). These methods should be reserved for clinics or physicians' offices where retrieval of specimens following therapy may be less than optimal and only cultures from patients not responding would need detailed identification.

INTERPRETATION OF RESULTS

Routine workup of isolates and susceptibility testing must be tailored according to the patient at risk and the specimen type submitted. Figure 31-4 shows a flow diagram that takes into account three features considered in all UTIs:

- Colony count of a pure or predominant organism
- Measurement of pyuria
- Presence or absence of symptoms (dysuria, and frequency)

It is important to recognize, however, that no one scheme can fit all situations. This figure is organized into a cascade scheme using a dichotomous key. This allows the final laboratory selection from 12 clinical categories, depending on knowledge of symptoms and recognizing the need for physician input. Heretofore most guidelines suggested that laboratory evaluation and culture setup should depend on previous knowledge of symptoms. Because this is often unrealistic, given the general lack of communication between physicians and the laboratory, the schema presented allows

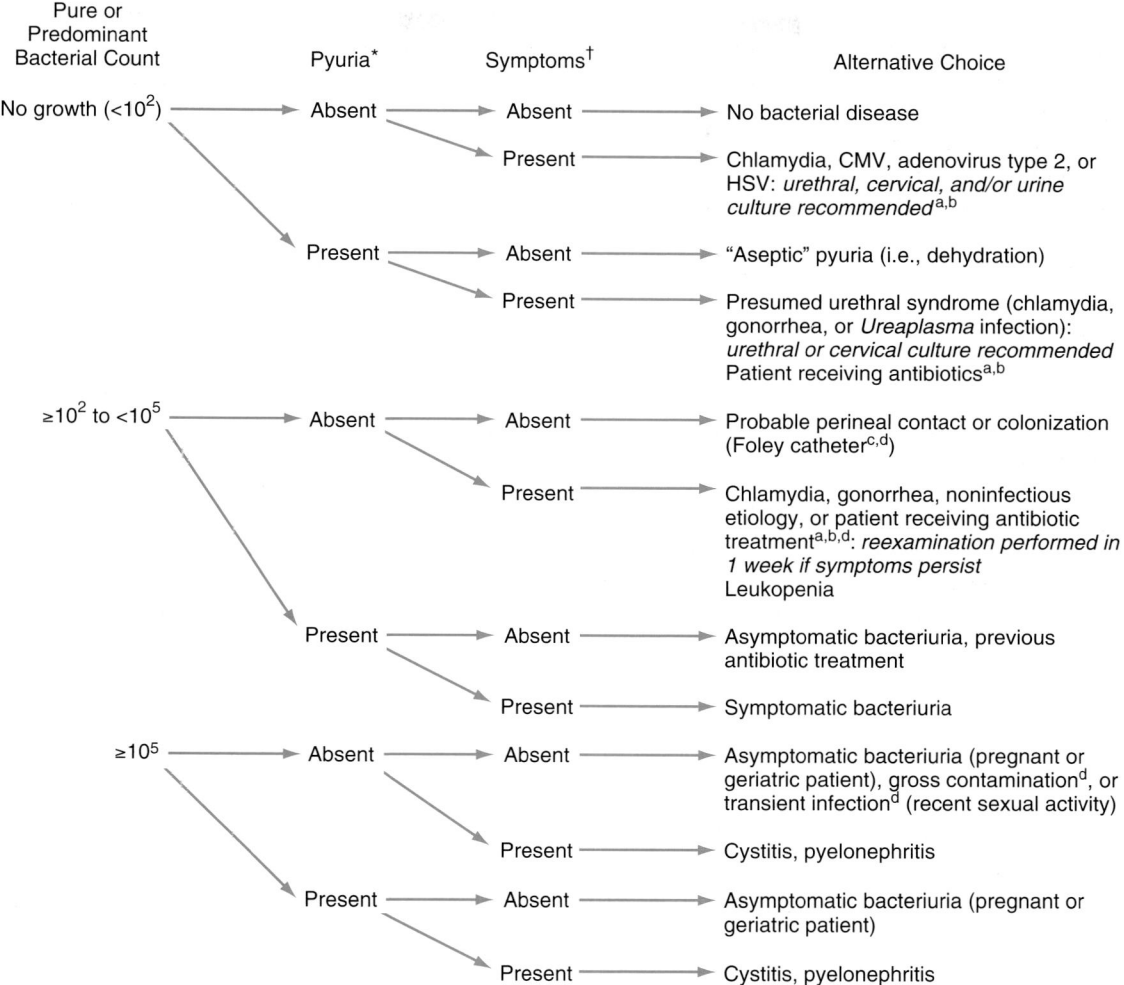

Pure or Predominant Bacterial Count	Pyuria*	Symptoms†	Alternative Choice
No growth (<10^2)	Absent	Absent	No bacterial disease
		Present	Chlamydia, CMV, adenovirus type 2, or HSV: *urethral, cervical, and/or urine culture recommended*[a,b]
	Present	Absent	"Aseptic" pyuria (i.e., dehydration)
		Present	Presumed urethral syndrome (chlamydia, gonorrhea, or *Ureaplasma* infection): *urethral or cervical culture recommended* Patient receiving antibiotics[a,b]
≥10^2 to <10^5	Absent	Absent	Probable perineal contact or colonization (Foley catheter[c,d])
		Present	Chlamydia, gonorrhea, noninfectious etiology, or patient receiving antibiotic treatment[a,b,d]: *reexamination performed in 1 week if symptoms persist* Leukopenia
	Present	Absent	Asymptomatic bacteriuria, previous antibiotic treatment
		Present	Symptomatic bacteriuria
≥10^5	Absent	Absent	Asymptomatic bacteriuria (pregnant or geriatric patient), gross contamination[d], or transient infection[d] (recent sexual activity)
		Present	Cystitis, pyelonephritis
	Present	Absent	Asymptomatic bacteriuria (pregnant or geriatric patient)
		Present	Cystitis, pyelonephritis

a. If patient is receiving antibiotic treatment, the result of the Gram stain, WBC analysis, and culture may not agree.
b. Quantitation of organisms and white cells by urinalysis of a centrifuged specimen is of no comparative value for the measurement of leukocyte esterase and bacteria done by microbiologic study, which is performed routinely on a noncentrifuged specimen.
c. Interpretation for indwelling catheter has not been established.
d. Plates held 72 hours for consultation.

*Leukocyte esterase (+); equivalent to 5 WBC/hpf.
†Clinical dysuria and frequency.

Figure 31-4 _____

Interpretation of urine culture results using algorithm based on bacterial colony count, pyuria, and symptoms. *CMV,* Cytomegalovirus; *hpf,* high-power field; *HSV,* herpes simplex virus; *WBC,* white blood cell.

TABLE 31-10

Guidelines for Interpretation of Urine Culture Results and Subsequent Workup

Colony Count (CFU/ml)*	Symptoms, Clinical Disease, or Patient Population†	Urine Source‡	Number of Organisms Types Isolated	Laboratory Workup Suggested§ (Inpatient)
<10†		CV/CA	None	None‖
≥10†	Pediatric	Suprapubic	≤2 organisms by anaerobic culture	ID & AST
≥10†	Symptomatic female, urethritis	CV	Pure culture	ID & AST
≥10‡	Symptomatic male, prostatitis	CA	≤2 organisms	ID & AST
		CA	Pure culture	ID & AST
≥10‡		Bladder washout		ID & AST
≥10‖	Cystitis/pyelonephritis	CV	Pure culture	ID & AST
			2-3 organisms	Q & SID
			>3 organisms	Q & M or Q & GS

*Inoculation of 0.01 ml or urine is required to detect 10^2 CFU/ml.
†See Table 31-1 for description of clinical diseases, symptoms, and patient population.
‡*CV*, Clean voided; *CA*, straight catheterized.
§Workup required. Any yeast may be quantitated and reported (regardless of number); >100,000 needed to identify to species.
‖See figures and text for suggested comments and educational information helpful to physicians.
ID & AST, Perform identification and antimicrobial susceptibility testing.
ID & S, Perform identification to genus and species level and perform susceptibility testing when appropriate (lactobacilli may be identified on the basis of colony morphology and microscopic morphology: omit susceptibility testing).
Q & SID, Quantitate and perform sight identification. Identification and sensitivity not indicated. Hold plates 72 hours.
Q & M, Quantitate total amount of bacteria and report as "mixed urethral flora."
Q & GS, Quantitate and report Gram stain morphotypes.

the final differentiation to be made by the physician, based on his or her knowledge of the patient's symptoms.

Figure 31-4 also takes into account asymptomatic bacteriuria. Furthermore, if the patient is receiving antibiotic therapy, the Gram stain, WBC analysis, and culture results may not agree. Last, quantitation of organisms and white cells by urinalysis of a centrifuged specimen has no comparative value for the measurement of leukocyte esterase and bacteria done by microbiologic study, which is performed routinely on a noncentrifuged urine specimen.

This figure particularly addresses the "acute urethral syndrome" and the recognition that cystitis and urethritis are clinically difficult to differentiate, particularly in the female population. It is imperative that clinicians recognize that routine urine cultures do not include isolation and identification of *C. trachomatis, N. gonorrhoeae,* or *U. urealyticum.* It is also important to recognize that given the high propensity of negative cultures sent to the laboratory (i.e., approximately 50%), reevaluation of the patient with a negative specimen may include recognition of a sexually transmitted disease.

Table 31-10 lists guidelines for the interpretation of urine cultures and suggests subsequent workup. In summary, these guidelines suggest the following, remembering that cost-effective strategies may define different algorithims for inpatient and outpatient cases:

▪ Specimens with multiple uropathogens (i.e., three or more) indicate probable contamination. The organism should not be identified even if it is present in large numbers unless this is specifically requested in consultation.
▪ One or two significant uropathogens present (i.e., $\geq 10^5$ CFU/ml) should routinely be identified. Susceptibility tests should be performed for inpatients; outpatient cases may use a different algorithm that does not routinely call for susceptibility tests; rather, it emphasizes empiric selection based on antibiograms.
▪ One or two uropathogens present in small numbers (i.e., $\geq 10^2$ CFU/ml) should be routinely identified ($\geq 10^2$ to $<10^5$ CFU/ml) if the clinical situation warrants, such as in acute urethral syndrome or cases of previous antibiotic therapy.

SUSCEPTIBILITY REPORTING

With the growing number of emerging uropathogens and the simultaneous increase in newer antibiotics, it is mandatory that laboratories use standardized methodology and report only appropriate antibiotics for UTIs. FDA-approved antimicrobial agents for routine testing and reporting by clinical microbiology laboratories for urinary tract isolates are listed as Group U supplemental for urine only, in the 1999 NCCLS Guideline: Performance Standards for Antimicrobial Disk Susceptibility Tests, 9th ed.; Approved Standard M(21) NCCLS Document M100-S9.

A number of laboratories have tailored susceptibility testing according to the needs of the clinical setting: outpatient versus inpatient; pediatric versus adult; intensive care versus nonintensive care. Nevertheless, it is imperative to remember that attainable antibiotic blood levels and urine levels are often different; this will have an impact on the interpretation of some semiquantitative susceptibility results or the quantitative minimal inhibitory concentration (MIC) of inhibitory antimicrobials.

Recently, given the cost-conscious environment, an additional strategy has been developed and implemented in certain laboratories; that is, they use antibiograms to select outpatient, empiric therapy and do not routinely perform culture and susceptibility studies. This implies that laboratories monitor carefully over selected time intervals for emerging resistance and maintain a national electronic surveillance.

UTI Antibiograms

Historically, one of the primary functions of the clinical microbiology laboratory has been to measure antibiotic resistance trends. This was most often accomplished by using an annual antibiogram that established cumulative percentage susceptibilities for selected UTI bacterial-antibiotic combinations. Today this is even more important and requires "focused" antibiograms that tailor these historical resistance fingerprints to selected patient locations, inpatient versus outpatient status, disease type, and age. Most importantly, these should be evaluated more frequently than yearly, perhaps quarterly, and should be formulated to help clinicians choose empiric therapy and reduce routine "C/S" or a patient-by-patient basis; often outpatient urine isolates have a stable and predictable pattern.

Bibliography

Clarridge JP, Pezzlo M, Vosti KL: Cumitech 2A. In Wessfield AL, editor: *Laboratory diagnosis of urinary tract infections,* Washington DC, 1987, American Society for Microbiology.

Gupta K, Scholes D, Stamm W: Increased prevalence of antimicrobial resistance among uropathogens causing acute uncomplicated cystitis in women, *JAMA* 281(8):736, 1999.

Hooten TM et al: Randomized comparative trial and cost analysis of 3-day antimicrobial regimens for treatment of acute cystitis in women, *JAMA* 273:41, 1995.

Jinnah F et al: Drug sensitivity pattern of *E. coli* causing urinary tract infection in diabetic and nondiabetic patients, *J Int Med Res* 24:296, 1996.

Johnson V, Stamm W: Urinary tract infections in women: diagnosis and treatment, *Ann Intern Med* 111:906, 1989.

Kass EH: Asymptomatic infections of the urinary tract, *Trans Assoc Am Physicians* 69:56, 1956.

Kierkegaard H et al: Falsely negative urinary leucocyte counts due to delayed examination, *Scand J Clin Lab Invest* 40:259, 1980.

Kunin CM: *Detection, prevention, and management of urinary tract infections,* Philadelphia, 1974, Lea & Febiger.

Lennette E, Balows A, Hausler W: *Manual of clinical microbiology,* ed 5, Washington, DC, 1991, American Society for Microbiology.

Maartens G, Oliver SP: Antibiotic resistance in community-acquired urinary tract infections, *S Afr Med J* 84:600, 1994.

Nickel J, McLean R: Bacterial biofilms in urology, *Infect Urol* 11(6):169, 1988.

Norden C, Kass E: Bacteriuria of pregnancy: a critical appraisal, *Annu Rev Med* 19:431, 1968.

Pezzlo M: Urine and culture procedure. In Isenberg H et al, editors: *Clinical microbiology procedures handbook,* Washington, DC, 1992, American Society for Microbiology.

Pezzlo M: Detection of urinary tract infections by rapid methods, *Clin Microbiol Rev* 1:268, 1988.

Schaeffer AJ: Urinary tract infections in urology, *Infect Dis Clin North Am* 1(4):875, 1987.

Stamery TA: *Pathogenesis and treatment of urinary tract infections,* Baltimore, 1980, William & Wilkins.

Stamm W, Counts G, Pumming K: Diagnosis of coliform infections in acutely dysuric women, *N Engl J Med* 307:463, 1982.

Stamm WE, Hooten TM: Management of urinary tract infections in adults, *N Engl J Med* 329:1328, 1993.

Stamm WE, Wagner KF, Amsel R: Causes of the acute urethral syndrome in women, *N Engl J Med* 304:409, 1980.

Thomson KS, Sanders WE, Sanders CC: USA resistance patterns among UTI pathogens, *J Antimicrob Chemother* 33(suppl):S9, 1994.

US Preventative Services Task Force: Recommendations on screening for symptomatic bacteriuria by dipstick urinalysis, *JAMA* 262:1220, 1989.

Winn W: Diagnosis of urinary tract infection: a modern procrustean bed, *Am J Clin Pathol* 99:117, 1993.

Winstanley TG et al: A 10-year survey of the antimicrobial susceptibility of urinary tract isolates in the UK: the Microbe Base Project, *J Antimicrob Chemother* 40:591, 1997.

LEARNING ASSESSMENT

1. How would the urine culture described in the case study at the beginning of the chapter be worked up and reported?

2. Where do these organisms originate?

3. What is the difference between single-episode UTI and recurrent UTI?

4. What is the value of the screening urinalysis and the Gram stain procedure?

5. What is the optimum incubation period for routine urine culture?

6. What may occur if routine urine cultures are incubated longer than 24 hours?

7. What is the significance of yeast quantitation in a urine specimen?

8. What is the definition of a contaminated urine culture?

9. Why is it important for clinicians to reevaluate negative urine culture results on specimens from symptomatic patients?

10. Should a susceptibility test be performed for all organisms isolated from urine?

CHAPTER 32

Sexually Transmitted Diseases

William F. Nauschuetz

COMMON EXUDATIVE SEXUALLY TRANSMITTED
INFECTIONS
  Gonorrhea
    Clinical manifestations
    Laboratory diagnosis
  Genital Chlamydiosis
    Clinical manifestations
    Laboratory diagnosis
  Bacterial Vaginosis
    Clinical manifestations
    Laboratory diagnosis

COMMON ULCERATIVE SEXUALLY TRANSMITTED
INFECTIONS
  Syphilis
    Clinical manifestations
    Laboratory diagnosis
  Chancroid
    Clinical manifestations
    Laboratory diagnosis
  Genital Herpes
    Clinical manifestations
    Laboratory diagnosis

OBJECTIVES

1. Describe the clinical manifestations produced by the following agents:
   - *Neisseria gonorrhoeae*
   - *Chlamydia trachomatis*
   - *Gardnerella vaginalis*
   - *Treponema pallidum* subsp. *pallidum*
   - *Haemophilus ducreyi*
   - Herpes simplex virus

2. Discuss the epidemiology and pathogenesis of each of the infections caused by the aforementioned agents.

3. Describe the proper specimen collection and laboratory methods used to diagnose the diseases caused by each of the previously listed organisms.

4. Differentiate the clinical characteristics between gonococcal and nongonococcal urethritis.

5. Interpret both specific and nonspecific serologic test results used to diagnose syphilis.

KEY TERMS

Gonorrhea
Pelvic inflammatory disease (PID)
Gonorrheal ophthalmia neonatorum
Penicillinase-producing *N. gonorrhoeae* (PPNG)
Gram-negative intracellular diplococci (GNID)
Chlamydiosis
Elementary body
Initial body

Sterile pyuria
Bacterial vaginosis
Syphilis
Primary syphilis
Secondary syphilis
Latent phase
Tertiary syphilis
Nontreponemal (nonspecific) antibody tests
Treponemal antibody tests
Chancroid
Genital herpes

The sexually transmitted infections (STIs), until recently, were called *venereal diseases,* after Venus, the goddess of love. Most of these infections have little to do with love. They are, more accurately, sexually transmitted infections. While the term *venereal disease* referred to a small number of infections, the reclassification has expanded this group of infections (Table 32-1), because the only prerequisite is that these infections be passed by sexual contact.

The clinical and economic impact of these infections is staggering. Worldwide, there are approximately 333 million cases annually of the treatable STIs, including gonorrhea, genital chlamydiosis, syphilis, and trichomoniasis. In the United States, there are approximately 15 million cases of STIs annually; 25% of those occur among teenagers. Five of the top 11 reportable diseases in the United States in 1996 were STIs—chlamydiosis, gonorrhea, AIDS, syphilis, and genital herpes. The cost of fighting these infections last year was approximately $17 billion.

TABLE 32-1

Some Sexually Transmitted Diseases and Causative Agents

Disease	Agent(s)
AIDS	HIV-1
Bacterial vaginosis	*Gardnerella vaginalis, Mobiluncus* spp., etc.
Genital chlamydiosis	*Chlamydia trachomatis*
Chancroid	*Haemophilus ducreyi*
Cytomegalovirus disease	Cytomegalovirus
Genital warts	Human papillomavirus
Gonorrhea	*Neisseria gonorrhoeae*
Donovanosis	*Calymmatobacterium granulomatis*
Leukemia, lymphoma, or myelopathy	HTLV I, II
Lymphogranuloma venereum	*Chlamydia trachomatis*
Molluscum contagiosum	Molluscum contagiosum virus
Pubic lice	*Phthirus pubis*
Scabies	*Sarcoptes scabiei*
Syphilis	*Treponema pallidum* ssp. *pallidum*
Trichomoniasis	*Trichomas vaginalis*

Although the sexually transmitted infections are diverse, this chapter focuses on the common exudative (gonorrhea, chlamydiosis, bacterial vaginosis) and ulcerative (syphilis, genital herpes, chancroid) STIs.

COMMON EXUDATIVE SEXUALLY TRANSMITTED INFECTIONS

CASE STUDY

A 24-year-old woman presented with fever, pain, and tenderness around her left elbow joint. The patient had noticed a slight rash around her left hand 10 days earlier. On examination, the patient showed rash on her extremities, swollen joints, and petechiae with vesicular eruptions. Based on the physical findings, the physician obtained an aspirate of the joint fluid and ordered routine and anaerobic cultures along with appropriate cultures for *Neisseria gonorrhoeae*.

Gonorrhea

The organisms that most commonly cause bacterial arthritis are *Staphylococcus aureus, Haemophilus influenzae, Neisseria gonorrhoeae, Pseudomonas* spp., and *Escherichia coli,* as well as certain anaerobic organisms. With nongonococcal-mediated arthritis, most cases show a source of the infection, usually skin abscesses, puncture wounds, and intravenous drug use. These presentations were not present in the case study patient. *N. gonorrhoeae* was isolated from cultures of the joint fluid. In fewer than 3% of gonococcal infections, the organism can spread through the blood, producing disseminated gonococcal infection characterized by a rash on the extremities and arthritis in one or more joints.

Gonorrhea is caused by the gram-negative diplococcus *N. gonorrhoeae*. These organisms usually occur in pairs and have characteristic flattened adjacent sides, which is responsible for their kidney-bean appearance on gram-stained smears.

The incidence of gonorrhea in the United States has dropped steadily since the mid-1980s (Figure 32-1), but it continues as one of the most commonly diagnosed reportable infections, with approximately one third of the infections occurring in adolescents. Worldwide, gonorrhea also has

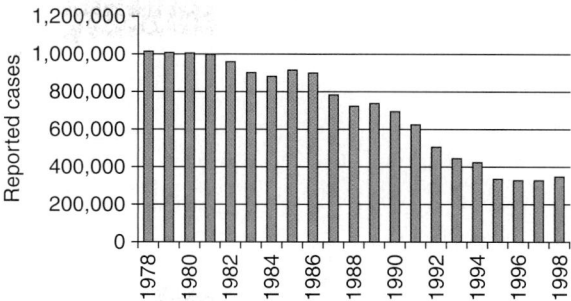

Figure 32-1

Reported cases of gonorrhea since 1978. (Modified from Centers for Disease Control and Prevention: Summary of notifiable disease, United States, 1997, *MMWR* 46:54, 1997.)

continued to rise during the last 20 years, with approximately 97 million new cases annually.

Clinical manifestations

Humans are the only known hosts of *N. gonorrhoeae*. This organism binds specifically to columnar epithelial cells of the genitourinary tract, including the urethra, cervix, endocervix, and Bartholin glands. The organism also binds to columnar epithelial cells of the anal canal, pharynx, and conjunctiva. The incubation period is 2 to 7 days. In men, symptoms include urethral inflammation with dysuria and pyuria. In women, gonorrhea is often asymptomatic and may remain undetected. The endocervix is the primary site of infection in women, and secondary sites may include Bartholin and Skene glands and the urethra. Approximately 20% of infected women show overt symptoms such as endocervical mucopurulent discharge. However, as many as 70% may have vague symptoms, including painful intercourse, irregular bleeding, abdominal pain, and light vaginal discharge. If the infection goes unnoticed and untreated, *N. gonorrhoeae* can ascend the genital tract and cause complications. In men, these sequelae include prostatitis, epididymitis, and urethral stricture. Women with undiagnosed gonorrhea are in danger of developing salpingitis and **pelvic inflammatory disease (PID).**

Some patients may develop rectal, pharyngeal, and conjunctival gonorrhea. Rectal gonorrhea is usually asymptomatic and self-limiting. Patients may have rectal gonorrhea as a result of anal intercourse, or, in the case of women with endocervical gonorrhea, by cross-contamination. Oral sex

TABLE 32-2

Recommended Antimicrobial Therapies for Sexually Transmitted Infections

STI	Treatment
Gonorrhea (urethral, endocervical)	Ceftriaxone, cefixime, ciprofloxacin, or ofloxacin, plus doxycycline (for possible coinfection with *C. trachomatis*)
Chlamydiosis (urethral, endocervical)	Doxycycline, ofloxacin, erythromycin, or azithromycin
Bacterial vaginosis	Metronidazole or clindamycin
Syphilis (primary and secondary)	Penicillin or tetracycline
Chancroid	Erythromycin, azithromycin, ceftriaxone
Genital herpes	Acyclovir

is a risk factor for pharyngeal gonorrhea, which is usually self-limiting and asymptomatic. Newborns can develop **gonorrheal ophthalmia neonatorum** while passing through the birth canal of an infected mother. Adults also can develop ophthalmic gonorrhea by autoinoculation.

Even as the numbers of *N. gonorrhoeae* isolates decrease in the United States the isolated strains continue to become more resistant to antibiotics. The appearance of **penicillinase-producing N. gonorrhoeae** (PPNG) in the U.S. in the 1970s changed the drug of choice from penicillin to spectinomycin. Shortly thereafter, spectinomycin resistance occurred in clinical isolates, and tetracycline-resistant *N. gonorrhoeae* (TRNG) appeared in the 1980s. The recommended treatment for gonorrhea is currently ceftriaxone or cefixime, with doxycycline (Table 32-2). The doxycycline is essentially to treat chlamydiosis in the patient because as many as 30% of patients with gonorrhea may also have genital chlamydiosis. Patients can also be treated with the fluoroquinolones, ciprofloxacin, or ofloxacin, although some isolates have recently shown increased resistance to the fluoroquinolones.

Laboratory diagnosis

The Gram stain is a sensitive, fast, and cheap tool for diagnosis of gonorrhea in men. Gram stain of the penile exudate shows characteristic and diagnostic **gram-negative intracellular diplococci (GNID)** in granulocytes. The Gram stain is not sensitive or specific enough to use as detection of gonorrhea in women, however. Other means of diagnosis (i.e., culture or DNA probes) are required to confirm suspected gonorrhea in women.

Many laboratories still use culture to detect and identify *N. gonorrhoeae* from clinical samples from both male and female patients. In these situations, specimen transport is extremely important because *N. gonorrhoeae* dies rapidly in transport media, such as modified Stuart's medium. Many laboratories prefer to receive specimens in the JEMBEC, Bio-Bag, or Gono-Pak transports. These transport systems consist of selective agar and CO_2-generating tablets contained in a plastic bag or plastic case. They provide a stable environment for the fastidious isolate during transport.

Commonly used selective media for the isolation of *N. gonorrhoeae* include modified Thayer-Martin and Martin-Lewis plates. Inoculated plates should immediately be placed in an incubator with increased carbon dioxide. Small, gray, translucent, raised colonies become visible within 24 to 48 hours of incubation. Cultures with no visible growth must be held for 72 hours before discarding.

There are many different kits and reagents available for the identification of *N. gonorrhoeae*. Conventional methods, such as cystine-typticase digest semisolid agar (CTA) carbohydrates, are growth-dependent. Some commercial kits, such as the API quadFERM+ and RIM-*Neisseria*, use more dense inocula to get identifications within a few hours. Direct detection methods, such as fluorescent-antibody and agglutination tests, are also available.

Many laboratories use nucleic acid probes for the direct detection of *N. gonorrhoeae* from clinical specimens. The PACE 2 (Gen-Probe, San Diego, Calif.) is a DNA probe that hybridizes the gonococcal rRNA. This is a sensitive test that allows test batching, which is another advantage because *C. trachomatis* can be simultaneously detected from the same specimen.

CASE STUDY

A 24-year-old woman went to her gynecologist for a routine pelvic examination. It had been several years since her last examination. She was currently in a monogamous relationship, but her sexual history included other sex partners. The patient had no symptoms, but the physician collected routine screening tests for gonorrhea, chlamydiosis, HIV, and syphilis. All laboratory test results came back negative except for the *Chlamydia* test, which was positive.

Genital Chlamydiosis

Genital **chlamydiosis,** which is caused by *Chlamydia trachomatis,* is the most common bacterial STI, with as many as 89 million new cases worldwide in 1997. In the United States, there are 3 to 8 million new cases annually, at a cost of $2 billion each year. Chlamydiosis has become a widespread disease because of its ability to cause inapparent infections. As many as 85% of women with genital chlamydiosis are asymptomatic. The highest rates of infection are found in adolescent girls. Only about 40% of the men with chlamydiosis are asymptomatic, but some studies indicate that roughly 6% of all 18- to 25-year-old men have asymptomatic chlamydiosis. These infections are not difficult to pass to sexual partners, because transmission of *C. trachomatis* is approximately 45% following intercourse.

C. trachomatis is an obligately intracellular bacterium, requiring cell cultures for in-vitro culturing. The organism causes a wide variety of conditions, including trachoma, lymphogranuloma venereum, genital chlamydiosis, and nongonococcal urethritis.

The chlamydiae have a unique developmental cycle. The infective particle is the **elementary body** (EB), which is the metabolically inert form of the organism. The EB binds selectively to host columnar epithelial cells, the same target cell as for *N. gonorrhoeae.* The EB enters the host cells by pinocytosis. Once within a cytoplasmic vacuole, the EB changes into an **initial body** (IB), which is capable of replication by binary fission. The replicating IBs form a large inclusion body and then revert to EBs, which burst from the infected cell. The infection process then continues.

Clinical manifestations

In men, chlamydiosis appears as urethritis, with an incubation period of 10 to 20 days. Although many of these patients are asymptomatic, others develop dysuria and pyuria, similar to gonococcal urethritis. However, patients with urethral chlamydiosis often have a discharge that is less purulent than a gonococcal discharge. Not all patients with this clearer discharge have chlamydiosis, as *C. trachomatis* causes only 30% to 50% of all cases of nongonococcal urethritis (NGU) in men. Definitive diagnosis requires laboratory testing.

In women, chlamydiosis is usually asymptomatic. Most infected women have both chlamydial urethritis and endocervicitis, and a minority are infected at only the cervix or urethra. Endocervical chlamydiosis can cause a mucopurulent cervical discharge associated with erythema and edema, along with suprapubic tenderness. Chlamydial urethritis can appear as **sterile pyuria,** in which more than 10 white blood cells (WBC) per high-power field (HPF) are seen in centrifuged urine samples, although the urine is culture-negative for routine uropathogens.

Untreated genital chlamydiosis can progress to serious sequelae, including PID, endometritis, infertility, sterility, and ectopic pregnancy. There may be as many as 500,000 cases of PID resulting from genital chlamydiosis each year. Genital chlamydial infections can be transmitted to newborns, causing a mucopurulent inclusion conjunctivitis and pneumonia.

Laboratory diagnosis

Clinical microbiologists have a tremendous, and possibly confusing, choice when it comes to methods for the identification of chlamydiosis in patients. It is important to know that the Centers for Disease Control and Prevention (1991) has defined the requirements for presumptive and definitive diagnosis of chlamydiosis. Presumptive diagnosis includes clinical suspicion based on symptoms, and a positive nonculture result (EIA, DFA, nucleic acid detection) for *C. trachomatis.* To offer definitive diagnosis, laboratories must offer full culture and identification of inclusion bodies or a combination of two nonculture methods (one as a screen, and the second as a confirmatory test).

Culture requires that the clinical specimen contain host cells from the genital site. A swab containing exudate only is inadequate for culture. In men, a small swab is inserted into the urethra, rotated, and removed. In women, the specimens can be collected from the cervical os using swabs or cytology brushes. Since most female patients have chlamydial endocervicitis and urethritis simultaneously, the clinician may also collect a specimen from the urethra using the small swab normally used for collecting urethral specimens from males. Most laboratories require that these collection swabs be placed in a special transport medium, such as 2-sucrose phosphate (2-SP) or FlexTrans (Bartels Diagnostics) and sent to the laboratory immediately. Specimens must be refrigerated if they cannot be transported to the laboratory immediately. Once the specimen arrives in the laboratory, the fluid transport medium can be sonicated to help release chlamydial EBs from host cells. The resulting inoculum is layered into cell cultures. Most laboratories still use McCoy cells grown in media containing cycloheximide, but Buffalo green monkey cells and HeLa cells have also been used. Shell vial cultures, in which the monolayers are centrifuged following inoculation, can become positive after 48 hours. Chlamydial inclusions are detected in culture with fluorescent antibodies.

Culture can be laborious and expensive. A wide variety of nonculture methods are also available for the detection of *C. trachomatis.* Table 32-3 summarizes key features of these methods.

Bacterial Vaginosis

No single agent causes **bacterial vaginosis (BV).** Instead, this condition results primarily from a disruption of the normal vaginal flora. In 1955 Gardner published results indicating a new isolate, *Haemophilus vaginalis,* caused bacterial vaginosis. Subsequent studies proved this bacterium indeed was present in virtually all women with BV but was also present in most asymptomatic females. Clearly, it could not be the sole cause of BV. The organism was reclassified as *Corynebacterium vaginalis* in the

early 1960s and was ultimately reclassified as *Gardnerella vaginalis* in 1980.

Because *G. vaginalis* occurs in almost 100% of the women with BV, it probably has a role in the development of BV. Perhaps a more important bacterium in BV is *Mobiluncus,* which is commonly found in vaginal fluids of patients with BV but virtually never recovered from patients without BV. *Mobiluncus* is an anaerobic gram-negative bacillus that is usually present in the rectum.

Is BV a true STI? Some facts seem to indicate it is transmitted sexually. Men can develop nongonococcal urethritis with BV-associated bacteria, and studies show that condom use decreases incidence of BV in women. Other data indicate it may not be sexually transmitted. For example, studies indicate cotreating the male partner and female partner does not reduce risk of recurrence in the female partner. Also, the incidence of BV does not seem to increase in women with increased numbers of sexual partners, as would be expected of an STI.

Clinical manifestations

Women with BV complain of a fishlike odor associated with the vagina. There is often a watery, noninflammatory exudate lacking PMNs, which de-

TABLE 32-3

Different Laboratory Methods for the Detection and Identification of C. trachomatis *from Genital Specimens*

Method	Examples	Sensitivity	Specificity	Comments
Culture		52% to 93%	100%	Confirmatory; only method recommended for sexual abuse cases
DFA	MicroTrak	50% to 100%	88% to 99%	
EIA	Chlamydiazyme, IDEIA, MicroTrak II	65% to 100% for urethral and genital swabs; 73% to 97% for urine	95% to 100%	Blocking antibody needed to improve test performance
OIA (optical immunoassay)	BioStar OIA	74%	> 99%	
Microparticle EIA	IMx Select Chlamydia	88% to 89% on urethral swabs; 81% with urine	> 99%	
Direct nucleic acid probes	Gen-Probe PACE 2	65.4% to 100% for genital specimens	97% to 100%	Specimens include urethral and endocervical swabs
TMA (transcription-mediated amplification)	Gen-Probe AMP CT	85% to 95.6% for urine; 100% for urethral and endo-cervical swabs	> 99%	Specimens include urine, urethral, and endocervical swabs
PCR	Amplicor, COBAS Amplicor	86.7% to 95% for urine; 91% to 100% for urethral and endo-cervical swabs	> 99%	
Ligase chain reaction (LCR)	Abbott LCx	84% to 98% for urine; 87% to 95.2% for endocervical swabs	> 99%	

TABLE 32-4

Recommended Diagnosis of Bacterial Vaginosis

Sign or Symptom	Determined By	Notes
Presence of clue cells in vaginal fluid	Wet mount	> 20% of epthelial cells should be clue cells.
Increased pH of vaginal fluid	Litmus paper	pH > 4.5 is considered increased.
Presence of watery noninflammatory exudate	Physical exam	
Foul odor of exudate	"Whiff test"	Add KOH to vaginal fluid on glass slide; pass the slide under the nose to smell.

fines this condition as a vaginosis and not a vaginitis. Also, the vaginal fluid has an increased pH and contains *clue cells,* which are exfoliated vaginal epithelial cells literally covered by gram-negative coccobacilli and curved gram-negative rods.

Bacterial vaginosis occurs when the lactic acid-producing lactobacilli, the most common group of bacteria in the healthy vagina, decrease in numbers. This causes an increase in the pH of the vagina, which allows *Prevotella* spp., *G. vaginalis,* and *Mycoplasma hominis* to greatly increase in numbers. These bacteria degrade proteins in the vagina to form the foul-smelling amines cadaverine, putrescine, and triethylamine. The odor of the amines is amplified by activation with alkaline compounds, such as potassium hydroxide (KOH).

Interestingly enough, male ejaculate is alkaline and thus can activate the odor of the amines; many women with bacterial vaginosis notice the odor almost immediately after intercourse. The combination of the amines and organic acids produced by the anaerobic bacteria, such as acetic and succinic acids, causes an exfoliation of epithelial cells from the vagina. The exfoliation results in the noninflammatory exudate. The pH allows the gram-negative and gram-variable bacilli associated with bacterial vaginosis to tightly adhere to the epithelial cells to form the clue cells.

Regardless of its status as an STI, BV is clearly anything but a minor condition. The sequelae of bacterial vaginosis include recurrence, PID, urinary tract infections, endometritis, preterm labor and membrane rupture, septicemia, and meningitis.

Laboratory diagnosis

Bacterial vaginosis should be diagnosed by the primary medical care provider at the patient's bedside by demonstrating at least three of the four signs and symptoms of BV (Table 32-4). Because the patient can be diagnosed rapidly, there is little need to send specimens to the clinical laboratory for testing. Routine culture is not an especially useful tool to diagnose BV because *Gardnerella* is normal flora in so many women. Cultures for *Mobiluncus* may very well be more predictive of BV, but a selective medium for this organism would be necessary to make this a practical option.

Some laboratories offer Gram stains of vaginal fluids to assist clinicians with the diagnosis of BV. The value of the Gram stain is that it documents the loss of lactobacilli, with the subsequent increase in gram-negative coccobacilli and gram-negative curved bacilli.

COMMON ULCERATIVE SEXUALLY TRANSMITTED INFECTIONS

CASE STUDY

An African-American male infant was born at 33 weeks of gestation to a 17-year-old mother. The mother had no prenatal care and a reactive rapid plasma reagin (RPR) test result (1:128) on admission to an obstetric service. The infant was delivered by Cesarean section because of fetal distress. On examination, physical findings revealed that the infant was hydropic and showed jaundice and hepatosplenomegaly. Laboratory findings also showed pancytopenia, hypoglycemia, coagulopathy, oliguria, and acidosis. The infant received multiple transfusions of washed, packed red blood cells, platelets, and fresh-frozen plasma. He was treated with penicillin and gentamicin but died 3 days after birth. Examination of the placenta showed spirochetes in the umbilical cord.

Syphilis

Syphilis, which is caused by the spirochete *Treponema pallidum* subsp. *pallidum,* is currently the second most common ulcerative STI in the United

States. Although estimates for new cases of syphilis in the United States are as high as 70,000 per year, the number of cases of primary and secondary syphilis reported to the CDC are at the lowest levels in many years (Figure 32-2). Even compared with a decade ago, rates have dropped significantly. In 1988 the incidence of primary and secondary syphilis was 16.43/100,000; in 1997 the incidence dropped to 3.19/100,000. Likewise, the rates of congenital syphilis have shown a decrease since reaching a maximum incidence of 108/100,000. In 1997 the rate dropped to 30/100,000. The majority of the reportable cases of syphilis occur in the southern United States. Although the problem seems to be decreasing in this country, syphilis still strikes approximately 12 million new patients each year worldwide.

Clinical manifestations

There are three stages in the pathogenesis of syphilis: primary, secondary, and tertiary or late, syphilis. *T. pallidum* subsp. *pallidum* is an invasive organism and can enter the host through any site and initiate infection. The incubation period ranges from 1 to 90 days. The initial lesion of syphilis is called the *chancre,* and its appearance signals **primary syphilis.** The chancre has an indurated, raised edge. Usually there is only one chancre per infection. The painless, nonsuppurative lesion is extremely infectious. The lesion will spontaneously heal after several weeks if the patient does not receive antimicrobial therapy.

The disappearance of the chancre does not signal an end to the infection. *Treponemes* gain access to the bloodstream in untreated patients, and

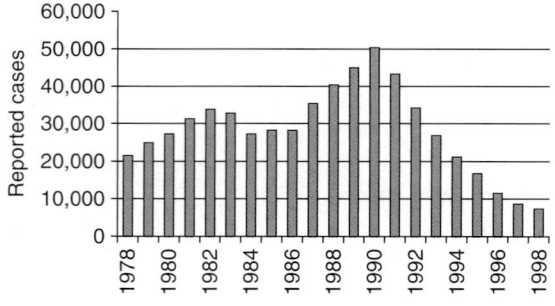

Figure 32-2

Reported cases of syphilis since 1978. (Modified from Centers for Disease Control and Prevention: Summary of notifiable disease, United States, 1997, *MMWR* 46:54, 1997.)

this spirochetemia is responsible for the signs and symptoms of **secondary syphilis,** which begins approximately 4 to 12 weeks after infection. The hematogenous spread of the treponemes causes fever, lymphadenopathy, myalgia, and anorexia. Most patients develop macular or papular skin lesions involving the trunk, soles of the feet, and palms. The fluids from the lesions are infectious. Another result of secondary syphilis is the appearance of condylomata lata, which are mucoid, fleshy wartlike growths. These lesions often occur in the perianal region. Even without treatment, the symptoms of secondary syphilis disappear after 3 to 12 weeks, and the patient enters the **latent phase.** During this latent phase, the patient is asymptomatic, and the only evidence of syphilis is the presence of antibodies. Many untreated patients relapse during the first year of the latent period and will suffer a recurrence of the symptoms associated with secondary syphilis. Other patients may never relapse. And a third group of patients will experience late or ***tertiary syphilis.***

Late syphilis is associated with immune sequelae of the primary and secondary syphilis, rather than the direct presence of treponemes. Patients with late syphilis may develop neurologic symptoms or cardiovascular effects or experience late benign syphilis. In the latter condition, the patient develops *gummas,* which are areas of localized destruction. Gummas can occur in skin, bone, or viscera. If the gumma occurs at a superficial site, the lesion can heal spontaneously. Approximately 15% of untreated syphilis patients develop gummas.

Since *T. pallidum* subsp. *pallidum* can cross the placenta, congenital infection can occur in newborns. Congenital syphilis occurs when a live or stillborn infant is born to a mother with untreated or improperly treated syphilis. At birth, the newborn has signs of secondary syphilis, including hepatosplenomegaly, jaundice, rash, condylomata lata, meningitis, and periostitis. Some children born with the infection experience late congenital syphilis. These patients are asymptomatic at birth but experience blindness, deafness, and deformed bones or teeth as young children.

Laboratory diagnosis

T. pallidum cannot be grown in vitro. Patients with chancres can be diagnosed with darkfield microscopy. Fresh material from the chancre is examined immediately after collection using a darkfield microscope, and the presence of motile treponemes suggests syphilis. Some clinicians prefer using direct fluorescent antibody testing instead of darkfield examination. Since this test uses specific antibodies, it can differentiate *T. pallidum* from saprophytic treponemes associated with mucosal surfaces.

Patients without chancres must be diagnosed with serology tests. There are two general types of serology tests available. The **nontreponemal (nonspecific) antibody tests,** such as the RPR and Venereal Disease Research Laboratory (VDRL), are used as screening tests and detect the presence of antibodies to cardiolipin and other lipoidal indicators of tissue damage. These tests are not highly specific. Febrile infections, pregnancy, and autoimmune disorders may produce biologically false-positive reactions with nontreponemal tests. Clinicians can use quantitative nonspecific tests to follow the efficacy of treatment because since these antibody levels decrease and ultimately disappear with the successful treatment of syphilis.

Patients with reactive nontreponemal test results are then tested with a more specific test to confirm the diagnosis. The confirmatory tests are specific **treponemal antibody tests,** such as the fluorescent treponemal antibody absorption (FTA-ABS) and microhemagglutination for *T. pallidum* subsp. *pallidum* (MHA-TP). These tests rule out biologic false-positive results. However, they cannot be used to follow therapy, since these antibodies do not disappear following the successful treatment of the disease. Most patients remain seropositive throughout their lives.

In congenital syphilis, the newborn serologic tests, both specific and nonspecific, are reactive. To differentiate maternal antibody from the infant antibody to syphilis, an IgM-specific FTA-ABS test is appropriate. Confirmation of congenital syphilis includes clinician suspicion based on symptoms and history, along with the demonstration of treponemes in the infant body tissues or fluids.

Chancroid

Chancroid, or soft chancre, is caused by a fastidious gram-negative coccobacillus, *Haemophilus ducreyi.* This sexually transmitted infection is endemic in southeast Asia, Africa, and India. Sporadic outbreaks occur in developed countries. The number of cases reported in the United States has

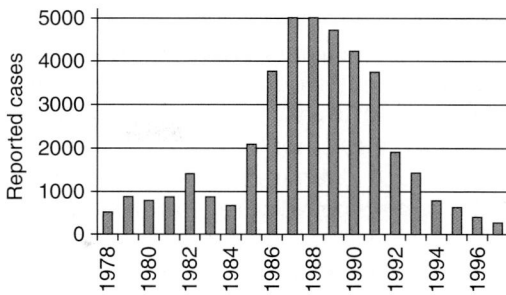

Figure 32-3 _____

Reported cases of chancroid since 1978. (Modified from Centers for Disease Control and Prevention: Summary of notifiable disease, United States, 1997, *MMWR* 46:54, 1997.)

dropped to fewer than 400 per year (Figure 32-3). This may indicate underreporting of actual cases. Of the ulcerative STIs discussed, chancroid is the most difficult infection to diagnose using laboratory data.

Clinical manifestations

The pathogen enters through a break in the skin following sexual exposure. An erythematous papule usually develops at the site of infection 3 to 5 days postexposure. The chancroid usually develops on the external genitalia of both men and women. The sites of infection in men include the prepuce, coronal sulcus, glans, and shaft; in women, the fourchette, labia, clitoris, vaginal wall, and cervix can be involved. Patients may develop inguinal lymphadenopathy, resembling buboes. These ulcers must be differentiated from chancres and herpetic lesions. The chancroid is usually a more painful lesion than the chancre.

Laboratory diagnosis

Exudates and material from the base of the ulcer may be submitted for direct smear examination and culture. Exudate from buboes is not an optimal specimen for recovery of the pathogen. Microscopically, *H. ducreyi* are pleomorphic, gram-negative coccobacilli that occasionally occur in chains or "school-of-fish" formations. Gram stains are not a sensitive or specific tool for the diagnosis of chancroid. Often the material includes numerous bacterial contaminants.

H. ducreyi is a fastidious pathogen, requiring special growth and environmental supplements. Although some clinical isolates grow well on chocolate agar, enriched media can increase the sensitivity of culture. One enhanced medium contains GC agar base, hemoglobin, IsoVitalex, and fetal calf serum, and another has Mueller-Hinton agar with chocolated horse blood and IsoVitalex. Colonies grow after 48 to 72 hours of incubation. These organisms produce oxidase, reduce nitrate, produce alkaline phosphatase, and do not produce catalase. The requirement for heme is shown by a negative porphyrin test result.

Genital Herpes

Genital herpes, which is caused by herpes simplex virus (HSV), is the most common ulcerative sexually transmitted infection. There are two serotypes of HSV. HSV-1 causes 80% of oral infections and 20% of genital infections. The reverse is the case with HSV-2, which causes primarily genital infections.

The prevalence of HSV-2 has increased by 30% over the past 20 years. In the United States, 15% of white men are seropositive for HSV-2, as are 20% of white women, 35% of African-American men, and 55% of African-American women. Genital herpes is not a reportable infection. It is estimated that there are 40 to 60 million Americans who are antibody-positive for HSV-2, with 2 million new seroconverters each year. Of those 2 million, only 600,000 develop symptoms. Indeed, as many as 80% of all Americans with HSV-2 may be unaware of their infections, due to asymptomatic infections or infections with vague symptoms.

How have these numbers reached such high levels?

Because HSV-2 lesions are often painful, they would seem to deter sexual activity. Even so, many patients at least know to use barrier contraception when there is any sign of ulceration. What many patients with genital herpes may not know is that they shed virus even in the absence of symptoms. Studies indicate that patients are infective up to 30% of their symptom-free days. Even more sobering is the finding that many patients who are antibody-positive to HSV-2 but have never had an actual herpes lesion are still infective to their unsuspecting partners. Another reason that the number of Americans with this STI is so high is that there is no cure. Patients with the disease have the disease until death. In the absence of either a cure or a vaccine, this STI will continue the dramatic increase of the past several years.

Clinical manifestations

Genital herpes is transmitted by sexual contact with secretions from infected sites. The average incubation period is 3 to 6 days after the sexual encounter. In primary symptomatic herpes, which is the initial infection following exposure, lesions appear on the infected surface, and usually rupture in 24 to 48 hours. Erythematous ulcers with an edematous base form at the site of each vesicle. If the ulcers form on dry surfaces, such as the buttocks or shaft of the penis, healing can occur rapidly. But ulcers on moist surfaces, such as the vagina, cervix, and glans penis, resolve by slowly healing inward from the periphery. Women have a higher incidence of lesions on moist surfaces, and therefore ulcers of primary infections tend to last longer in women (approximately 4 to 21 days). Lesions in men last approximately 9 days. Approximately 75% of women with primary HSV have a vaginal discharge. The first clinical acute infection with herpes has systemic effects as well as the local painful lesion. Patients often suffer a flulike syndrome, with fever, myalgia, and malaise. These systemic effects are usually limited to the primary episode. The patient subsequently develops antibodies that prevent the flulike syndrome but cannot prevent future reactivation of lesions at the local site.

Following recovery, HSV enters a latent period, during which it resides dormant in the dorsal root ganglion. Certain factors, such as friction (i.e., with clothing or with other skin during sex), menstruation, stress, fatigue, and sunlight can reactivate the virus, which results in the reappearance of lesions at the original infection site. These recurrent infections occur less often with HSV-1 than with HSV-2. Recurrence is usually within the first year of latency. As many as 38% of all patients have at least six recurrences within this period, following their primary episode.

Asymptomatic shedding is a factor in the transmission of neonatal herpes. Yet neonatal HSV-2 occurs in approximately 1:5000 deliveries. It is possible that those born to mothers with recurrent herpes are at less risk than infants born to mothers with primary herpes, because patients with recurrent herpes have circulating antibodies that may protect the newborn. The mortality rate for newborns with disseminated HSV-2 is approximately 60%.

Physicians often culture specimens from HSV-infected women near the end of their pregnancy to determine whether viral shedding is occurring. Manifestations of neonatal HSV disease acquired during delivery usually appear in the first 4 to 7 days of life. Newborns may have infection localized to skin, eyes, mucosa, or the central nervous system.

Laboratory diagnosis

Viral isolation is the most common method for the diagnosis of HSV infections. The best specimens for culture are vesicle fluids collected with syringe or swab. Cervical swabs and mucosal surface swabs are also acceptable. Specimens for culture must be taken as early as possible in the disease process from mucocutaneous lesions. The likelihood that a herpetic lesion will produce a positive culture diminishes with each day after the appearance of the lesion. If crusting lesions are the only possible specimen for culture, then vigorously collected specimens containing epithelial cells from the lesion help improve sensitivity of culture. Viral samples should be stored at 4° C and should not be frozen.

HSV grows rapidly on numerous cell culture lines, and the cytopathic effect in culture can be seen within 24 hours. The most common cell lines used include MRC-5, human embryonic lung, HEp-2, A549, and rabbit kidney.

Bibliography

Balows A et al, editors: *Manual of clinical microbiology,* ed 5, Washington, DC, 1991, American Society for Microbiology.

Brokenshire MK et al: Evaluation of microparticle enzyme immunoassay Abbott IMx Select *Chlamydia* and the importance of urethral site sampling to detect *Chlamydia trachomatis* in women, *Genitourin Med* 73:498, 1997.

Centers for Disease Control and Prevention: Summary of notifiable disease, United States, 1997, *MMWR* 46:54, 1997.

Dean D, Ferrero D, McCarthy M: Comparison of performance and cost-effectiveness of direct fluorescent antibody, ligase chain reaction, and PCR assays for the verification of chlamydial enzyme immunoassay results for populations with a low to moderate prevalence of *Chlamydia trachomatis* infection, *J Clin Microbiol* 36:94, 1998.

Eschenbach DA: History and review of bacterial vaginosis, *Am J Obstet Gynecol* 169:441, 1993.

Espy MJ, Smith TF: Detection of herpes simplex virus in conventional tube cell cultures and in shell vials with a DNA probe kit and monoclonal antibodies, *J Clin Microbiol* 26:22, 1988.

Ferrero DV et al: Performance of Gen-Probe AMPLIFIED *Chlamydia trachomatis* Assay in detecting *Chlamydia trachomatis* in endocervical and urine specimens from women and urethral and urine specimens from men attending sexually transmitted disease and family planning clinics, *J Clin Microbiol* 38:3230, 1998.

Hay PE: Recurrent bacterial vaginosis, *Dermatol Clin* 16:769, 1998.

Hillier SL: Diagnostic microbiology of bacterial vaginosis, *Am J Obstet Gynecol* 169:455, 1993.

Hipp SS, Yangsook H, Murphy D: Assessment of enzyme immunoassay and immunofluorescence tests for detection of *Chlamydia trachomatis, J Clin Microbiol* 25:1938, 1987.

Knapp JS: Antimicrobial resistance in *Neisseria gononhoeae* in the United States, 21:1, 1999.

Koneman EW et al, editors: *Color atlas and textbook of diagnostic microbiology,* ed 5, Philadelphia, 1997, Lipppincott.

Kuipers JG et al: Sensitivities of PCR, MicroTrak, Chlamydia-EIA, IDEIA and PACE 2 for purified *Chlamydia trachomatis* elementary bodies in urine, peripheral blood, peripheral blood leukocytes, and synovial fluid, *J Clin Microbiol* 33:3186, 1995.

Pate MS et al: Evaluation of the Biostar *Chlamydia* OIA assay with specimens from women attending a sexually transmitted disease clinic, *J Clin Microbiol* 36:2183, 1998.

Rosen T, Brown TR: Genital ulcers: evaluation and treatment, *Dermatol Clin* 16:673, 1998.

Smith SM, Oghara T, Eng RHK: Involvement of *Gardnerella vaginalis* in urinary tract infections in men, *J Clin Microbiol* 30:1575. 1992.

Sobel JD: Vaginal infections in adult women, *Sex Transm Dis* 74:1573, 1990.

Wald A: Herpes: transmission and viral shedding, *Dermatol Clin* 16:795, 1998.

Woolley P: Genital herpes: recognizing the problem, *Medscape Women's Health* 2:2, 1997.

Wylie JL et al: Comparative evaluation of Chlamydiazyme, PACE 2, and AMP-CT assays for detection of *Chlamydia trachomatis* in endocervical tissues, *J Clin Microbiol* 36:3488, 1998.

Young H: Syphilis: serology, *Dermatol Clin* 16:691, 1998.

LEARNING ASSESSMENT

1. How do women develop a complication such as pelvic inflammatory disease from gonococcal infections?

2. Which serological tests would be appropriate to monitor treatment for syphilis? Why?

3. What is the etiology of bacterial vaginosis?

4. How would you describe and differentiate the clinical presentation and etiology of chancroid from chancre?

5. What is the recommended test to diagnose bacterial vaginosis?

CHAPTER 33

Infections in Special Patient Populations

James T. Griffith

MALIGNANCY
  Decrease in Humoral and Cellular Immune
    Response
  Granulocytopenia
  Decrease in Leukocyte Function
  Infections in Neutropenic Patients
  Infections in Cancer Patients
  Infections in Patients with Hodgkin's Disease

BURNS AND SURGERY

ANTIMICROBIAL THERAPY

ORGAN TRANSPLANTATION

AGING

OBJECTIVES

1. Describe the various conditions that compromise the host's immune status.
2. Discuss the various infections that occur in this patient population.
3. Determine the risk factors associated with each patient condition.
4. Associate the various infectious agents that affect this special patient population with the conditions that predispose these patients to a particular infection.

KEY TERMS

Immunocompromised
Opportunistic
Immunosuppression
Humoral immune
  response

Cellular immune
  response
Granulocytopenia
Septicemia
Neutropenia

CASE STUDY

A 59-year-old man complained of abdominal pain and blood-laced vomiting during the past several weeks. He was seen by a physician and was admitted to the hospital. After examination, he was diagnosed with a gastrointestinal malignancy. Treatment was begun, and the patient responded favorably. Two weeks later, the patient, who had been released from the hospital, became unexpectedly febrile and was readmitted. At the second admission, laboratory tests suggested that the patient was significantly neutropenic and possibly septicemic. Culture results revealed an infection with *Pseudomonas aeruginosa*.

The term **immunocompromised** is used to describe patients with serious diseases who are highly predisposed to infections by a variety of **opportunistic** bacterial, fungal, parasitic, and viral pathogens (Table 33-1). The number of immunocompromised patients has increased steadily during the past 30 years, reflecting major advances in immunosuppressive therapy, instrumentation, and organ transplantation. Unfortunately, the potential gain in years of useful life for many patients through successful management and treatment of diseases is offset by serious effects on the immune system. As a result, infection,

rather than the primary illness, becomes the leading cause of death in immunocompromised patients.

The primary predisposing factor in this patient population is the underlying disease state that affects host defense mechanisms. Examples of compromised defense mechanisms include the following:

▪ Leukocyte number or functions, as in aplastic anemia and leukemia

TABLE 33-1

Opportunistic Pathogens Most Often Identified in the Compromised Host

Bacteria	*Staphylococcus aureus*
	Streptococcus spp.
	Pseudomonas aeruginosa
	Escherichia coli
	Klebsiella pneumoniae
	Salmonella spp.
	Serratia spp.
	Haemophilus influenzae
	Legionella pneumophila
	Aeromonas hydrophila
	Nocardia spp.
	Mycobacterium tuberculosis
	Marine vibrios (halophilic)
Parasites	*Toxoplasma gondii*
	Strongyloides stercoralis
	Pneumocystis carinii
Yeasts and fungi	*Candida* spp.
	Torulopsis spp.
	Aspergillus spp.
	Zygomycetes
	Cryptococcus neoformans
	Histoplasma capsulatum
Viruses	Herpes simplex
	Varicella-zoster
	Cytomegalovirus
	Epstein-Barr virus
	Hepatitis B virus
	Adenovirus

TABLE 33-2

Summary Table of Organisms Associated with Immunocompromised Patients

Immune Status	Examples of Conditions	Commonly Encountered Pathogen(s)
Decreased leukocyte number or function	Myelocytic leukemia	*Staphylococcus* spp.
	Chronic granulomatous disease	*Serratia* spp.
		Pseudomonas spp.
	Granulocytopenia	*Candida* spp.
	Acidosis	*Aspergillus* spp.
	Burns	*Nocardia* spp.
		Legionella spp.
Decreased humoral immune response and complement deficits	Lymphocytic leukemia	*Pneumococcus* spp.
	Multiple myeloma	*Haemophilus influenzae*
	Nephrosis	Streptococci
	Antimetabolite therapy	*Pseudomonas* spp.
	Hypogammaglobulinemia	*Pneumocystis carinii*
		Enteroviruses
Decreased cellular immune response	Hodgkin's disease	*Mycobacterium* spp.
	Steroid therapy	*Candida* spp.
	Uremia	*Coccidioides immitis*
		Histoplasma capsulatum
	Antimetabolite therapy	*Blastomyces dermatitidis*
	Malnutrition	Herpes viruses
		Adenoviruses
		Toxoplasma gondii
		Pneumocystis carinii
		Legionella spp.
		Listeria monocytogenes
Decreased reticuloendothelial system function	Splenectomy	Pneumococci
	Chronic hemolysis	*Salmonella* spp.
		Listeria monocytogenes

Modified from Drew L: Infections in the immunocompromised patient. In Ryan K, editor: *Sherris medical microbiology: an introduction to infectious diseases,* ed 3, Norwalk, Conn, 1994, Appleton & Lange.

- Humoral and cell-mediated immune functions, as in B-cell and T-cell abnormalities
- Reticuloendothelial system function, as in splenectomized patients

Other underlying disease states are complement deficiencies, diabetes mellitus, renal failure, and autoimmune diseases. Table 33-2 summarizes the various conditions that compromise the host's immune status and the pathogens usually encountered in infections associated with them.

Immunosuppression may also predispose patients to severe infections. Immunosuppressive therapy such as chemotherapy and radiation, particularly in organ transplantation and infection with the human immunodeficiency virus (HIV), frequently leads to immunocompromise.

Secondary factors include use of invasive devices, such as indwelling intravenous catheters, which breach the usual skin and mucosal protec-

tive barriers and introduce organisms into the bloodstream. One or a combination of any of these underlying conditions leaves a person less able to cope with infections.

This chapter discusses the conditions that compromise the host's immune status and the various infectious agents that affect this special patient population.

MALIGNANCY

Decrease in Humoral and Cellular Immune Response

Widespread disturbances in the **humoral** and **cellular immune responses** (defense mechanisms) occur in patients with malignancy. In addition, cytotoxic drugs administered to cancer patients contribute substantially to the breakdown of mucosal barriers and a decrease in cell-mediated immune (CMI) reactivity in these patients.

Granulocytopenia

Granulocytopenia, or a reduction in granulocytes, is commonly demonstrated in patients with hematologic malignancies and those receiving chemotherapy. Once the granulocyte count drops below 1000 cells/mm^3, the risk of infection increases steadily with the degree and duration of immunosuppression. In patients with a neutrophil count below 1000 cells/mm^3, the mortality rate may be as high as 60%. The fatality rate among patients whose neutrophil count is lower than 100 cells/mm^3 during the first week of infection may be as high as 80%.

Decrease in Leukocyte Function

In addition to the decrease in the number of neutrophils, inadequate neutrophil function, including the inability to migrate to sites of inflammation, impaired phagocytosis, and reduced killing of ingested organisms, predisposes patients suffering from chronic leukemia and Hodgkin's disease to infections. Most bacterial infections are caused by organisms of endogenous origin, that is, gastrointestinal tract, mucosal, or cutaneous flora. Fungi are also likely to invade the granulopenic host.

Infections in Neutropenic Patients

Septicemia is most likely to occur in patients with **neutropenia** because neutrophils play an important role in localizing infections. *Escherichia coli, Klebsiella pneumoniae,* and *Pseudomonas aeruginosa* account for most of the gram-negative bacilli infections. *Staphylococcus aureus* is the gram-positive organism most commonly involved in sepsis.

Pneumonia, especially that caused by gram-negative bacilli, is a major problem for the neutropenic patient. Because such a patient cannot mount an adequate inflammatory response, pulmonary infection may spread rapidly and extensively. Infections with these organisms are particularly serious because they cause extensive necrosis and have a high fatality rate. Owing to the lack of an inflammatory response, neutropenic patients fail to develop the characteristic signs of pneumonia and may remain undiagnosed until after the infection has disseminated.

Infections in Cancer Patients

Factors responsible for the high incidence of infections among cancer patients vary with the underlying malignancy. For example, tumors that outgrow their blood supply may become necrotic and infected. A gastrointestinal tumor may ulcerate, providing a focus for invasion by enteric pathogens. Tumors may also obstruct the drainage of the tracheobronchial tree or the urinary tract, permitting infection to become established distal to the obstruction.

Septicemia accounts for nearly 50% of the fatal infections in patients with genitourinary and gastrointestinal (GI) tumors and for less than 10% in patients with lung cancer. Pneumonia accounts for 75% of fatal infections in patients with cancer of the head, neck, and lungs and for less than 40% in patients with genitourinary and other tumors. Aspiration of oral secretions probably accounts for the pneumonia in these latter patients, whereas pneumonia in those with solid tumors is usually a consequence of primary or metastatic tumor invasion of the lung.

Skin infections are also common in cancer patients, for several reasons. Cancer patients often develop decubitus ulcers because they are constantly bedridden. These patients also develop catheter-associated infections, cellulitis, and local necrosis involving the extremities, sometimes associated with venipunctures, intravenous lines, and other procedures.

Patients with hematologic malignancies and those who have undergone surgery for tumors involving the head and spine may suffer from central nervous system infections. In these patients, meningitis accounts for 75% of infections, 30% of which are caused by *Cryptococcus neoformans.* Gram-negative bacilli are responsible for another 40%. Fungal agents such as *Aspergillus* spp. and *Mucor* spp. are commonly associated with brain abscesses that occur in patients with leukemia. Oropharyngeal candidiasis occurs in about 5% of cancer patients. Superficial gastrointestinal candidiasis is also found in patients with acute leukemia and lymphoma. Although candidiasis can involve any portion of the GI tract, it is found most often in the esophagus and stomach. Other areas sometimes affected are the kidneys, liver, spleen, and lungs.

Other types of infections that may occur in cancer patients include those caused by viral and parasitic agents. The most serious viral infections occurring in cancer patients are caused by the herpesvirus group. Characteristically, these viruses infect the young, resulting in lifelong immunity; such immunity may be associated with the latent infections that occur in cancer patients.

Herpes zoster infection represents the reactivation of latent varicella-zoster virus. It is in 3% to 15% of patients with lymphoma, myeloma, and chronic lymphocytic leukemia. Chemotherapy has been shown to cause a twofold increase in the frequency of zoster infection. Zoster disseminates in 20% to 40% of cancer patients.

Dissemination of varicella, infecting the lungs, liver, pancreas, adrenals, and central nervous system, occurs in nearly 30% of children undergoing chemotherapy. The mortality rate from varicella is about 5%, and death is usually associated with pneumonitis.

Herpes simplex infections of the lip may result in extensive cellulitis as a result of superinfection with mixed bacterial and fungal organisms (*Candida* sp. and gram-negative bacilli) in cancer patients.

Children with cancer are more susceptible to cytomegalovirus (CMV) infection than adults. The most common manifestation is pneumonia, which may be unilateral or bilateral and is usually accompanied by a more severe bacterial or fungal infection. Dissemination affects the lungs, kidneys, lymph nodes, heart, adrenals, spleen, pancreas, and bone marrow. Death sometimes occurs from myocarditis, renal failure, and adrenal insufficiency.

Pneumocystis carinii and *Toxoplasma gondii* are parasitic agents that commonly affect patients with malignancy. Infections with either organism may represent reactivation or primary exposure. *P. carinii* accounts for as many as 45% of cases of interstitial pneumonia in cancer patients. Similarly, *T. gondii,* an obligate intracellular parasite, causes pneumonia, chorioretinitis, and a mononucleosis-like infection. It is seen most commonly in Hodgkin's disease, but also in patients with lymphoma and leukemia.

Strongyloides stercoralis infections have been reported in patients with chronic lymphocytic leukemia and lymphoma. Serious manifestations caused by *Strongyloides* infection may occur in patients receiving adrenal corticosteroids or antitumor therapy. Ulceration may result when the rhabditiform larvae penetrate the gastrointestinal tract, or larval migration to the lungs may cause a pulmonary infiltrate.

Infections in Patients with Hodgkin's Disease

Hodgkin's disease historically has been associated with impairment of cell-mediated immunity. Patients with Hodgkin's disease are especially susceptible to infections caused by facultative intracellular parasite, such as *Mycobacterium tuberculosis, Listeria monocytogenes,* and *C. neoformans.* These intracellular organisms are resistant to bactericidal effects and are able to multiply within phagocytic cells.

As the number of circulating lymphocytes decreases, patients with Hodgkin's disease receiving chemotherapy become more susceptible to infections. Chemotherapy inhibits inflammation, reduces capillary permeability, and decreases cellular exudation. It also interferes with the diapedesis of leukocytes, inhibits antibody production, and impairs reticuloendothelial function.

BURNS AND SURGERY

Each year more than 2 million Americans are burned. One hundred thousand require hospitalization, and 100,000 more die annually. One third are children less than 1 year old. The risk of infection in a burn patient is proportional to the extent of the burn and reflects the combined effect of the impairment of all aspects of the host defense system. As a result of immunologic impairment, infection in sites other than the burn wound itself remains the most common cause of death in burn patients. The balance between host defense capacity and invasiveness of the microorganism in burn patients provides the optimal example of an immunocompromised patient.

In normal patients, bacterial interference (potential pathogens being inhibited by the nonpathogenic resident flora) plays a significant role in controlling cutaneous colonization of the skin. In burn patients, anatomic barriers have been breached. The normal skin flora are destroyed or removed by desquamation. The denatured protein of the burn eschar and the avascularity of the tissue provide an excellent environment for microbial growth.

The immune defense mechanisms in burn patients, both humoral and cell-mediated defenses, are suppressed. Immunoglobulins, especially IgG, are depressed. Fibronectin levels are also reduced. Fibronectin, a dimeric α-glycoprotein found in plasma and the extracellular matrix of most tissues, is necessary for normal reticuloendothelial cell function and is opsonic for *S. aureus.* A decrease in fibronectin levels precedes sepsis.

The advent of antimicrobial therapy has resulted in a shift of infectious agents recovered in burn patients from primarily gram-positive cocci to gram-negative bacilli, especially *P. aeruginosa.* The risk of fungal infections is increased with wound maceration, acidosis, lack of competitive bacterial pressure, and antibiotic therapy. Methicillin-resistant *S. aureus,* and *Candida, Aspergillus,* and *Mucor* spp., as well as herpes simplex, are major causes of infections in burn patients.

ANTIMICROBIAL THERAPY

During hospitalization the usual mucosal flora changes from predominantly gram-positive cocci to gram-negative bacilli. Susceptibility to colonization by pathogens of this type is usually increased by the extensive use of broad-spectrum antimicrobial agents. These agents alter the patient's endogenous microflora, allowing antimicrobial-resistant organisms to flourish, and they may also enhance the susceptibility of patients to fungal infections by altering the indigenous flora.

ORGAN TRANSPLANTATION

Organ transplant patients may develop specific types of infections at certain intervals after transplantation occurs. During the first month after transplantation, postoperative bacterial infections are most common. One to 6 months after transplantation, opportunistic infections caused by cytomegalovirus (CMV), *M. tuberculosis, L. monocytogenes, Nocardia* and *Aspergillus* spp., *P. carinii,* Epstein-Barr virus, varicella-zoster virus, and hepatitis virus are most likely to be reported.

Immunosuppressive therapy reactivates latent CMV infection, which is probably the most significant cause of mortality and morbidity among transplant patients. Sixty percent to 90% of renal transplant patients develop CMV 1 to 4 months after transplantation.

Infection caused by the Epstein-Barr virus (EBV) in transplant patients has also increased during recent years. EBV has been recognized as a causative agent of B-cell lymphoma, the pathogenesis of which is related to immunosuppressive therapy. Furthermore, in patients who acquire primary EBV infection after transplantation, EBV-associated lymphoproliferative disease is likely to occur. This has become a major concern, because primary EBV infection develops most commonly in children; hence, children who are transplant recipients are at greatest risk for EBV-associated lymphoproliferative disease. Central nervous system infections caused by *Listeria monocytogenes, C. neoformans, Toxoplasma gondii,* and *Aspergillus* sp. also occur among these patients.

Bone marrow transplant patients are susceptible to similar infections, especially by fungal agents. *Aspergillus* sp. and respiratory viruses are possibly inhaled from the environment, whereas *Pseudomonas* and *Legionella* spp. may be acquired from water sources.

Infections that occur more than 6 months after transplantation are usually associated with community-acquired organisms, such as viral influenza, secondary bacterial pneumonia, foodborne illnesses (acquired during travel to locations with poor sanitary conditions), and mycotic infections from specific geographic areas that may result in dissemination. Precautions about travel to underdeveloped areas and unfamiliar places are given to transplant patients to help them avoid unnecessary exposure to community-acquired infections.

AGING

Diverse changes in immune function occur with normal aging. Age-induced alterations of the immune system are often more qualitative (i.e., involving lymphocytic function) than quantitative (i.e., involving cell number or immunoglobulin levels).

Infections and malignancy are common among the elderly as a result of immunologic decline. Infections frequently occur in the respiratory or urinary tract, soft tissues, abdominal cavity, or endocardium. Bacteremia of unknown source may also occur. Malignancy is related to decreased tumor surveillance by immune and nonimmune defense mechanisms.

Bibliography

Corey L: Infections in the immunocompromised patient. In Sherris J, editor: *Medical microbiology,* ed 2, New York, 1990, Elsevier Science.

Diamond RD: Fungal infections in the compromised host: an overview, *Adv Exp Med Biol* 202:119, 1986.

Erice, Jordan, MC, et al: Ganciclovir treatment of CMV disease in transplant recipients and other immunocompromised hosts. *JAMA* 257:3082, 1987.

Froland S: Bacterial infections in the compromised host, *Scand J Infect Dis Suppl* 43:7, 1984.

Hibberd P, Rubin RH: Infections in transplant patients and the role of the microbiology laboratory, *Clin Microbiol Newsl* 13:161, 1991.

Jacobs P: The immunocompromised host, *South Am Med J* 71:371, 1987.

Johanson WG et al: Changing pharyngeal bacterial flora of hospitalized patients, *N Engl J Med* 281:1137, 1969.

Klastersky J: Infections in immunocompromised patients. I. Pathogenesis, etiology and diagnosis, *Clin Ther* 8:90, 1985.

Lipschitz DA et al: Influence of aging and protein deficiency on neutrophil function. *J Gerontol* 41:690, 1986.

Meunier F: Prevention of mycoses in immunocompromised patients, *Rev Infect Dis* 9:408, 1987.

Munster AM: Immunologic response of trauma and burns: an overview, *Am J Med* 77:142, 1984.

Neu HC: The patient at risk for infection: a summary, *Am J Med* 77:1, 1984.

Periti P et al: Infections in immunocompromised patients. II. Established therapy and its limitations, *Clin Ther* 8:100, 1985.

Powers DC et al: Immune function in the elderly, *Postgrad Med* 81:335, 1987.

Pruitt BA et al: Opportunistic infections in severely burned patients, *Am J Med* 76:146, 1984.

Rogers TR: Investigation of infection in immunocompromised patients [editorial], *Br J Haematol* 61:195, 1985.

Rouse BT, Horohov DW: Immunosuppression in viral infections, *Rev Infect Dis* 8:850, 1986.

Sheagren JM: Treatment of skin and skin structure infections in the patient at risk, *Am J Med* 76:180, 1984.

Skinhoj P: Herpesvirus infection in the immunocompromised patient, *Scand J Infect Dis Suppl* 47:121, 1985.

Sutton RNP et al: Virus infections in immunocompromised patients: their importance and their management, *J Roy Soc Med* 78:100, 1985.

Wang DT et al: Viral infections in the immunocompromised patients, *Med Clin North Am* 67:1075, 1983.

Weiner LP, Fleming JO: Viral infections of the nervous system, *J Neurosurg* 61:207, 1984.

Wolfson JS et al: Dermatologic manifestations of infections in immunocompromised patients, *Medicine (Balt)* 64:115, 1985.

LEARNING ASSESSMENT

1. What is the most likely sequence of events that led to the febrile condition of the patient in the opening case study?

2. What is the likely connection between the *Pseudomonas* infection and the malignancy?

3. What other hematologic conditions may predispose patients to various infections?

4. How does prolonged antimicrobial therapy compromise the host immunologically?

5. Why are infections and malignancy common among the elderly?

CHAPTER 34

Zoonotic and Rickettsial Infections

William F. Nauschuetz, Robert G. Whiddon

ZOONOTIC INFECTIONS TRANSMITTED
  BY SCRATCHES AND BITES
  Plague
    Etiology
    Epidemiology
    Life cycle of *Yersinia pestis*
    Clinical manifestations
    Laboratory diagnosis
  Lyme Borreliosis
    Etiology
    Epidemiology
    Life cycle of *Borrelia burgdorferi*
    Clinical manifestations
    Laboratory diagnosis
  Pasteurellosis
    Etiology
    Clinical manifestations
    Laboratory diagnosis
  Erysipeloid
    Etiology
    Epidemiology
    Clinical manifestations
    Laboratory diagnosis
  Capnocytophaga canimorsus Infection (Formerly
    CDC Group DF-2)
    Etiology
    Clinical manifestations
    Laboratory diagnosis
  Bacillary and Spirillary Rat-Bite Fevers
    Etiology
    Clinical manifestations
    Laboratory diagnosis

ZOONOTIC INFECTIONS TRANSMITTED
  BY DIRECT CONTACT OR INHALATION
  Anthrax
    Etiology
    Epidemiology
    Clinical manifestations
    Laboratory diagnosis
  Tularemia
    Etiology
    Epidemiology
    Clinical manifestations
    Laboratory diagnosis
  Brucellosis
    Etiology
    Epidemiology
    Clinical manifestations
    Laboratory diagnosis
    Identification
  Leptospirosis
    Etiology
    Epidemiology
    Clinical manifestations
    Weil's syndrome
    Laboratory diagnosis

THE RICKETTSIAE
  Rickettsia
    General characteristics
    Clinical infections
  Ehrlichiosis
    Clinical manifestations
    Laboratory diagnosis

OBJECTIVES

1. Discuss the pathogenesis and mode of transmission of the following zoonotic infections:
   - Anthrax
   - Plague
   - Erysipeloid
   - Leptospirosis
   - Tularemia
   - Rat-bite fever
   - Lyme borreliosis
2. Discuss the three forms of clinical manifestations of anthrax.
3. Describe the morphology and culture characteristics of the following etiologic agents:
   - *Brucella* species
   - *Yersinia pestis*
   - *Bacillus anthracis*
   - *Francisella tularensis*
   - *Borrelia burgdorferi*
   - *Leptospira* species
   - *Pasteurella multocida*
   - *Erysipelothrix rhusiopathiae*
4. Discuss the appropriate laboratory methods for the diagnosis of these infections and to maximize recovery of the etiologic agents.
5. For the following human rickettsial diseases, give the causative agent and the mode of transmission to humans:
   - Epidemic typhus
   - Rocky Mountain spotted fever
   - Scrub typhus
   - Q fever
6. Describe the morphology, growth requirements, and structure of rickettsial organisms and how they differ from bacterial agents.
7. Discuss the pathogenesis of rickettsial infections and the methods of laboratory diagnosis.

KEY TERMS

Zoonoses	Buboes	Malignant pustule	Undulant fever
Urban cycle	Pneumonic plague	Eschar	Leptospirosis
Sylvatic cycle	Anthrax	Tularemia	Weil's syndrome
Bubonic plague	Woolsorter's disease	Brucellosis	Rickettsia

CASE STUDY

A 16-year-old female resident of western Colorado experienced pain in the left axilla and arm with numbness in the arm. One or two days later she developed chills, fever, and had multiple episodes of vomiting. She went to the emergency department of a local hospital. Examination there found the following*:

Temperature: 97.4° F
Pulse: 100
Respiration: 16 breaths/min
Blood pressure: 103/59
Chest x-ray: Normal

She reported falling from a trampoline 4 days earlier and was diagnosed as having a possible brachial plexus injury related to this incident.

She was treated with analgesics and given an appointment with a neurologist.

Two days after she was seen in the emergency department, she was found semiconscious at home. She was taken to the hospital and the following findings were noted:

Temperature: 102.5° F
Pulse: 170
Respiration: 50 breaths/min
Blood pressure: 130/70
Mental status: Confused
Presence of pain: In neck, in addition to generalized soreness

*Data from Fatal human plague—Arizona and Colorado, *Morb Mortal Wkly Rep* 46:617, 1996.

Less than 1 hour after her arrival at the hospital, she experienced respiratory arrest and was intubated. Numerous gram-positive diplococci were found in a blood smear, and a chest x-ray showed bilateral pulmonary edema.

She was treated with 2g ceftriaxone IV and transferred to a referral hospital. There she was diagnosed with septicemia, disseminated intravascular coagulation, adult respiratory distress syndrome, and possible meningitis. Sputum, blood, and cerebrospinal fluid were taken for microbiologic studies. A Gram stain of CSF showed WBCs but no bacteria. She was treated for gram-positive sepsis.

Her condition deteriorated rapidly and she died later that day.

Additional cultures of spinal fluid grew unidentified gram-negative rods and *Streptococcus pneumoniae.*

In addition, cultures of blood and respiratory aspirates produced *Yersinia pseudotuberculosis,* identified by a rapid microidentification method. The blood culture isolate was identified as *Yersinia pestis* by the Reference State laboratory.

It was later revealed that adjacent to the patient's residence an extensive prairie dog die-off had recently occurred. Four of five family dogs and one of three family cats had high titers to *Y. pestis* F1 antigen. Investigators concluded that the patient had been infected by direct contact with abscess material from the pet cat while providing the cat's care.

This chapter divides zoonotic infections by routes of transmission, such as bites and scratches, and by direct contact or inhalation. Also detailed are some classic zoonotic infections, such as the following:

- Anthrax
- Tularemia
- Plague
- Rat-bite fever
- Lyme borreliosis

Other clinically significant zoonotic infections discussed in this chapter that are diagnosed in the clinical laboratory include pasteurellosis, capnocytophagosis, and brucellosis.

This chapter also discusses the rickettsioses. Many of these infections are vector-borne, requiring animals to transmit the disease to humans. Most of the rickettsioses are not true zoonoses, however, because the vectors normally do not show symptoms of infection.

More agents of zoonotic infections will undoubtedly be detected and identified as culture and molecular methods become more sophisticated. Recent technology-assisted discoveries include *Afipia felis,* thought to be the agent of cat-scratch disease (CSD) and shown not to be true, while *Bartonella (Rochalimaea) henselae* has been reported to be the likely cause of CSD.

ZOONOTIC INFECTIONS TRANSMITTED BY SCRATCHES AND BITES

Zoonoses transmitted by bites and scratches include plague, pasteurellosis, Lyme borreliosis, and rat-bite fever.

Plague
Etiology
Plague, an infamous bacterial disease, is caused by the gram-negative bacillus *Yersinia pseudotuberculosis* sp. *pestis*. This genus is named for Alexander Yersin, a French microbiologist who isolated the plague bacillus during an epidemic in Hong Kong in 1894. *Y. pseudotuberculosis* sp. *pestis* is biochemically and genetically similar to *Y. pseudotuberculosis,* although the organism is still commonly referred to as *Y. pestis* to prevent any misunderstanding.

Epidemiology
Three pandemics of plague have occurred. The first started near Egypt in 542 AD and ravaged Europe for 50 years, killing 100 million people. The second pandemic started in the fourteenth century, when conditions for rat-human transfer of *Y. pestis* were excellent. This pandemic, named the *Black Death,* killed 25 million Europeans, one fourth of the total population at that time. The last pandemic started in the 1890s and is just now subsiding. It was during the last pandemic that the disease was introduced into the United States. The infections started in Burma and spread to many parts of the world by infested rats aboard commerce ships. The majority of cases of plague now occur in Vietnam. As a result of the last pandemic, however, plague exists on all the continents except Australia.

Rats are the natural host for the vectors that transmit the disease, and humans are accidental hosts. The vectors are fleas *(Xenopsylla cheopis)* that normally infest the brown *(Rattus norvegicus)* and black *(Rattus rattus)* rats. In the United States, most cases are in the Southwest. The or-

ganism persists in this region through the sylvatic cycle, being passed among fleas and their rodent hosts.

Y. pestis can survive for months in animal burrows, and uninfected rodents can get the infection from this reservoir. The disease is spread to humans by rodents, when contaminated rural areas come in contact with areas of human habitation. Humans can also become infected from domestic cats that hunt rodents.

Life cycle of *Yersinia pestis*
Figures 34-1 and 34-2 illustrate the life cycle of *Y. pestis* in the **urban cycles** and **sylvatic cycles** of transmission. Fleas develop yersiniosis when they take a blood meal from an infected animal host. The yersiniae multiply in the gut of the flea, eventually reaching such a high concentration that they block the flea's gut. This blockage impairs the flea's ability to feed, and it responds by infesting a wider range of hosts and by biting more often. Humans living near rats can be infected by the fleas. Infection is begun when the fleas regurgitate the plague bacilli into the bite wound during feeding.

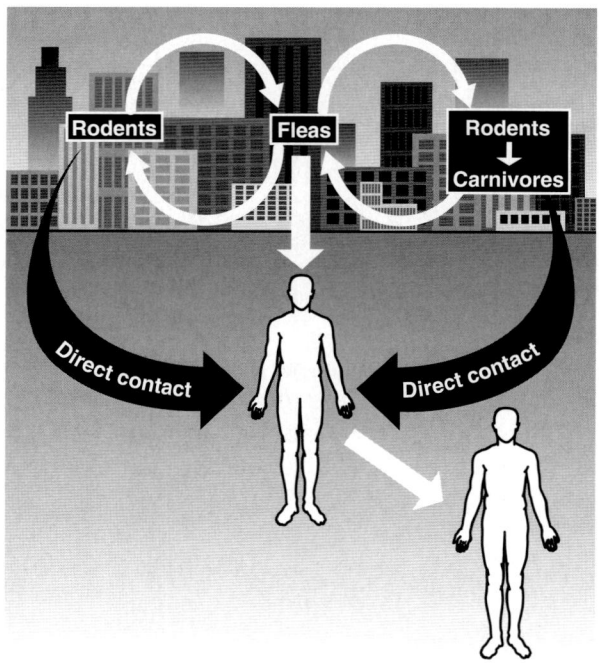

Figure 34-1
The urban cycle of plague.

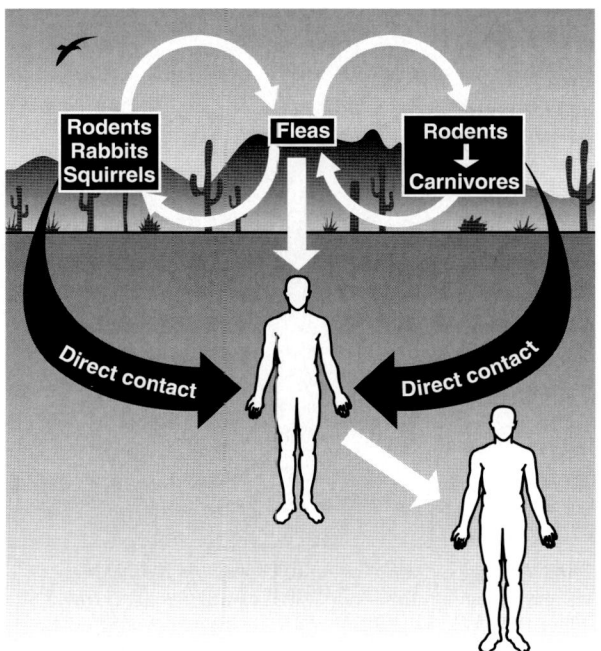

Figure 34-2

The sylvatic cycle of plague.

Clinical manifestations

Plague has two major manifestations: the bubonic and the pneumonic forms. **Bubonic plague** is an acute, febrile disease with an incubation time of 1 to 7 days. The disease is usually characterized by a lesion in a regional lymph node that drains the infected area. The resulting painful **buboes** usually occur in the groin, axilla, or subauricular area. In the case study shown here, the patient complained of painful axilla and numbness in her arm. This may have been the beginning of bubo formation. Within 3 to 6 days after the onset of infection, the patient develops signs of septic shock. If the disease goes untreated, the organism can be disseminated hematogenously, leading to septicemia. However, septicemic plague may occur without the bubonic form. The mortality rate of septicemic plague is nearly 100%, with death occurring within 1 to 3 days. The patient reported here died 4 days after her first examination.

Septicemic plague may lead to a secondary pneumonia, referred to as **pneumonic plague.** Pneumonic plague is almost always the result of hematogenously spread bubonic or septicemic plague. Two forms of pneumonic plague exist: primary and secondary. Primary pneumonic plague occurs when the patient transmits the organism by infectious droplets, whereas secondary pneumonic plague results from the plague bacillus entering the lungs of the same patient who has either bubonic or septicemic plague. Twenty-two percent of the cases of plague in the United States are secondary pneumonic.

The drug of choice is streptomycin, and alternatives include tetracycline and chloramphenicol.

Laboratory diagnosis

SPECIMEN COLLECTION

Aspirates of buboes are the best specimens for direct examination and culture. Sputum should be submitted to rule out pneumonic plague. Because of the high risk associated with this organism, clinicians should always alert laboratory personnel to the possibility that a patient may have plague.

DIRECT MICROSCOPIC EXAMINATION

Y. pestis organisms are gram-negative bacilli that can show bipolar, or "safety-pin," staining in tissues on direct examination, as shown in Figure 34-3. The bipolar appearance, however, is neither a sensitive nor a specific indicator of yersiniosis when seen in stained preparations.

CULTURE

The organism grows slowly, forming very tiny colonies on sheep's blood agar (SBA) after 24 hours.

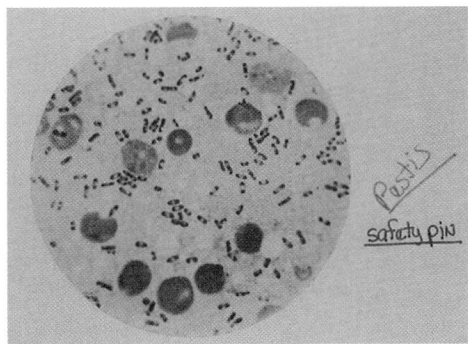

Figure 34-3

Smear from lymph gland of patient with plague. Characteristic bipolar staining of the bacilli is obvious. (×1,000.) (From Gillies RR, Dodd TC, editors: *Bacteriology illustrated,* ed 4, New York, 1976, Churchill Livingstone.)

Colonies of *Y. pestis* are nonhemolytic, slightly opaque, smooth, and round on SBA (Figure 34-4). *Y. pestis* is nonmotile and has an envelope when grown at 37° C.

IDENTIFICATION

Most commercial systems are able to identify *Y. pestis*. The organism resembles *Y. pseudotuberculosis,* but the two can be differentiated with the urease test. *Y. pestis* is negative for urease, whereas *Y. pseudotuberculosis* is positive. Isolates that are identified as *Y. pestis* should be confirmed with DFA test or phage sensitivities. Recovery of the organism should always be reported to public health authorities.

Infection is also diagnosed serologically, using a hemagglutination test to detect a fourfold rise in titer between acute and convalescent sera.

Lyme Borreliosis

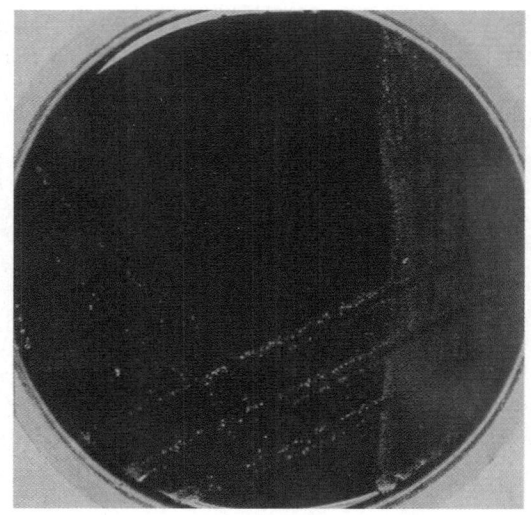

Figure 34-4 _____

Small, translucent, gray colonies of *Yersinia pestis* after 48 hours of incubation on 5% sheep's blood agar. (From Gillies RR, Dodd TC, editors: *Bacteriology illustrated,* ed 4, New York, 1976, Churchill Livingstone.)

CASE STUDY

A 28-year-old woman with shaking chills and perspiration was seen at an emergency room. She explained that before the fever, she had swollen and painful ankles, knees, wrists, and elbows. Her temperature was 100.8° F, and synovitis was noted in the wrists, elbows, knees, and ankles. She had no rash or lymphadenopathy. She admitted to a family history of osteoarthritis and rheumatoid arthritis. She lived in a rural area and had evidence of multiple insect bites, although she could not remember any recent tick bites. The patient was treated with naproxen and doxycycline for polyarthritis with rheumatoid arthritis, systemic lupus erythematosus, and late-stage Lyme disease.

Etiology

Lyme borreliosis, caused by *Borrelia burgdorferi,* is an arthropod-borne disease in which humans are accidental hosts. The disease is most commonly transmitted by ticks, including *Ixodes dammini, Ixodes pacificus* (the black-legged tick), *Ixodes ricinus* (the European sheep tick), and *Amblyomma americanum* (the common wood tick, also known as the Lone Star tick), although other insects can also harbor the spirochete. *B. burgdorferi* organ-

isms are gram-negative spirochetes about 0.18 to 0.25 × 4 to 30 μm in size. They exhibit regular coiling and are catalase-negative and microaerophilic.

Epidemiology

The disease that would eventually be named Lyme borreliosis was probably first noted in Sweden in 1908. At that time, erythema chronicum migrans (recently simplified to erythema migrans, or EM) was described as a rash that could expand its margins. Red circles ringed a white, hard center of the rash, resulting in a "bull's eye" appearance. The next several decades saw more appearances of erythema chronicum migrans in Europe. Some cases were even associated with tick bites, but no in-depth research was done on the infection. The first report of a similar phenomenon in the United States was in 1970. In 1975 an outbreak of juvenile rheumatoid arthritis occurred in Lyme and Old Lyme, Connecticut. The clustered outbreak of juvenile rheumatoid arthritis appeared suspicious, and thanks to some family members who thought that some infectious agent might be involved, an investigation was begun by health officials. It was the accidental discovery by Dr. Willy Burgdorfer of spirochetes in the blood of ticks recovered from the Old Lyme area that ultimately led to the description of Lyme disease. In 1984, the name *B. burgdorferi* was proposed for these organisms.

Life cycle of *Borrelia burgdorferi*
Ixodid ticks have a 2-year life cycle, requiring blood meals to pass from the larval stage to the nymph stage, and from the nymphal stage to the adult stage. Nymphs and larvae feed primarily on the white-footed mouse, whereas adult ticks usually infest the white-tailed deer. This horizontal transmission ensures maintenance of the pathogen in the wild. Figure 34-5 shows the presence of the organism in the midgut epithelial cells of the tick. Infected nymphs transmit the organism directly into the tissue of hosts (including humans) by regurgitating during feeding.

Clinical manifestations
Lyme borreliosis usually has an early stage and a late stage, although patient staging can be difficult. Some patients may not exhibit symptoms during the early phase, whereas other patients may never progress to the late phase. In other patients, the two phases may overlap.

EARLY STAGE
In about two thirds of infected patients, the early stage is characterized by a red papule at the site of the bite within the first 30 days of infection. The

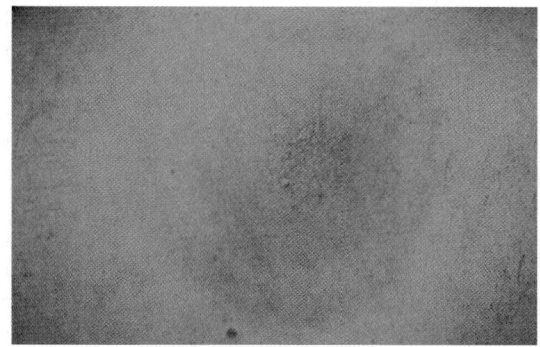

Figure 34-6
The annular lesion associated with Lyme borreliosis. (From Berger BW: Dermatologic manifestations of Lyme disease, *Rev Infect Dis* 2(suppl 6):S1476-S1477, 1989.)

papules, referred to as erythema migrans or EM, can expand to form erythematous concentric rings with central clearing (Figure 34-6). Spirochetemia can cause flulike symptoms, lymphadenopathy, oligoarthritis, carditis, and neurologic manifestations. Secondary lesions (Figure 34-7) may appear weeks after the initial lesion.

Because the concentration of bacteria in the host remains low, it is possible that many of the effects seen in Lyme borreliosis result from the host

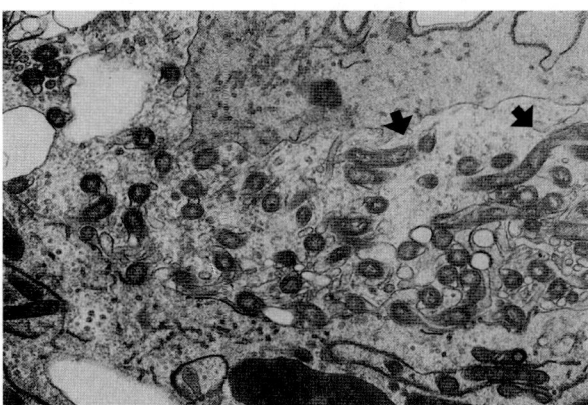

Figure 34-5
Transmission electron micrograph of *Borrelia burgdorferi* between midgut epithelial cells of *Ixodes dammini.* (From Burgdorfer W, Hayes, SF, Corwin D: Pathophysiology of the Lyme disease spirochete, *Borrelia burgdorferi, Rev Infect Dis* 2(suppl 6):S1445, 1989.)

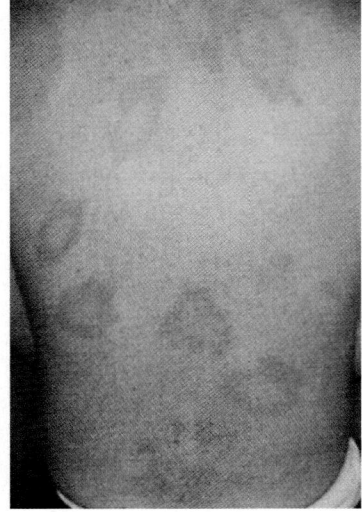

Figure 34-7
A patient with multiple erythema migrans lesions. (From Berger BW: Dermatologic manifestations of Lyme disease, *Rev Infect Dis* 2 (suppl 6):S1476-S1477, 1989.)

immune response, including attraction of macrophages to synovial fluid and production of interleukin-1 by host monocytes.

The Lyme spirochetes are rarely isolated from the blood or other body fluids of infected patients. Apparently the organism prefers solid tissue rather than fluid. The spirochete has a nonspecific adhesion that allows it to attach to the endothelial cells of blood vessels. This ability may enhance the migration of the organism from the blood stream into the basement membrane, resulting in vascular damage that can lead to carditis, arthritis, and central nervous system disease.

LATE STAGE

Late-stage Lyme disease is characterized by relapsing arthritis, and chronic synovitis can occur months to years after the initial symptoms. The joints most commonly affected are the knees, shoulders, and elbows. Untreated patients may have decreasingly severe attacks with the passage of time, until the symptoms eventually disappear. It is difficult to isolate the Lyme spirochete during the late stage. The arthritis may be mediated by the host immune system, rather than by the organism. In the case presented earlier the patient recalled during the follow-up examination a tick bite about 6 months before the appearance of symptoms but could not recall having had erythema migrans. She received erythromycin, and within a month she was asymptomatic, with negative Lyme serologies. The laboratory results are as follows*:

> Sedimentation rate: 40 mm/hr
> Complete blood count: normal, except
>   platelets of 459,000 μL
> Rheumatoid arthritis latex: negative
> Lyme IgG titer: 1:320
> Lyme IgM titer: negative*

Laboratory diagnosis

Laboratory diagnosis of Lyme borreliosis is primarily serodiagnostic. Indirect fluorescent antibody (IFA) tests and the enzyme-linked immunosorbent assay (ELISA) are used to detect antibody to the organism. The lack of a rapid or strong im-

---

*Data from Levin RE: An unusual presentation of Lyme arthritis, *J Rheumatol* 16:1500, 1989.

mune response, or cross-reactive serum antibodies, can delay serodiagnosis. Antibody testing of cerebrospinal fluid can avoid cross-reactivity problems. Some patients, including those who receive early antimicrobial therapy, may never develop a detectable immune response.

Direct antigen testing is not yet available. Direct examination of peripheral blood smears, adequate for the detection of many borrelioses, is not adequate for the detection of Lyme borreliosis. Specialized media are available for culturing *B. burgdorferi* from clinical specimens, but sensitivity is poor. Gene amplification techniques, such as the polymerase chain reaction, can detect the organism in clinical specimens.

Pasteurellosis

CASE STUDY

Parents took their lethargic and irritable 6-month-old daughter to an emergency room. The child had a low-grade fever and a nonerythematous nodule on the right upper arm, but no sign of rash or lymphadenopathy was present. Two shallow abrasions, possibly scratches from the family's pet cat, were near the nodule. The results of the patient examination and laboratory tests were as follows*:

> Temperature: 38.9° C
> Pulse: 200/min
> Respiration: 60/min
> WBC: 22,200 μL
>   57% polymorphonuclear neutrophils;
>   20% band neutrophils
>   12% lymphocytes; 6% monocytes
> Hematocrit: 28%
> Cerebrospinal fluid: RBC 3/μL^3; WBC 327/μL
>   75% polymorphonuclear neutrophils
>   12% lymphocytes
> Glucose: 48 mg/dL
> Protein: 79 mg/dL

---

*Data from Hsu HW, Finberg KW: Infections associated with animal exposure in two infants, *Rev Infect Dis* 11:108, 1989.

Etiology

Pasteurella multocida is a pleomorphic ovoid to filamentous gram-negative bacillus, about 0.5 to 1.0 μm in size. It can be a primary pathogen or sec-

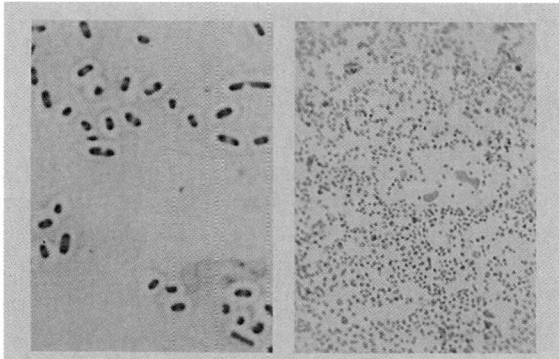

Figure 34-8

Gram stain of *Pasteurella multocida* culture *(left)*. Gram stain of mouse heart blood showing encapsulated *P. multocida* with bipolar staining *(right)*. (From Bottone EJ, Girolami R, Stamm J, editors: *Schneierson's atlas of diagnostic microbiology,* ed 8, New York, 1982, Churchill Livingstone.)

ondary invader. It is pathogenic for a wide range of hosts and occurs in the oral cavities of most dogs and cats. The five serogroups (A, B, D, E, and F) are based on capsular antigens.

Clinical manifestations

Pasteurellosis occurs worldwide and encompasses a wide range of endemic diseases of fowl and nonhuman mammals. The most common manifestation of human pasteurellosis is cellulitis, primarily from the bites or scratches of dogs and cats. Cats are usually more often involved than dogs. Although most *P. multocida* infections are transmitted directly from the animal bite to the human, animals can infect preexisting abrasions by licking them. The infected site becomes inflamed within 48 hours, but the presence of pus is rare. Typically, the patient with pasteurellosis is afebrile and does not have inflamed lymph nodes.

Other clinical manifestations include upper and lower respiratory tract infections, endophthalmitis, and genitourinary tract infections.

Rare complications of human infection with *P. multocida* can occur in the absence of animal bites or scratches. These include sepsis, meningitis, septic arthritis, peritonitis, and osteomyelitis. The initial diagnosis of the patient described earlier was subacute bacterial meningitis. The Gram stain of cerebrospinal fluid showed gram-negative bacilli. *P. multocida* was isolated from blood cultures.

The patient was treated with ceftriaxone and ampicillin on admission. Therapy was changed to

2 weeks of ampicillin when the bacteriology results were available. The nodule disappeared within 1 week, and the patient recovered without incident.

The pathogenesis of *P. multocida* infection in humans is not fully understood, but the antiphagocytic capsule and an outer membrane antiphagocytic protein apparently help the dissemination of the pathogen in avians. These factors are probably responsible for the microbe's virulence in humans as well. Some serogroups of *P. multocida,* including some human isolates, produce an exotoxin.

Laboratory diagnosis

SPECIMEN COLLECTION

Purulent exudate from infected bites or scratches should be submitted to the laboratory for direct examination and culture. Blood cultures should be submitted for febrile patients. Physicians can submit sputa or bronchial washings for patients with possible respiratory pasteurellosis.

DIRECT MICROSCOPIC EXAMINATION

Pasteurella organisms are gram-negative coccobacilli and, in Gram stains of patient specimens, can appear singly, in pairs, or in short chains. The bacteria often show bipolar staining, as shown in Figure 34-8.

CULTURE

P. multocida produces nonhemolytic colonies (Figure 34-9), 1 to 3 mm in diameter, on 5% sheep's blood agar within 24 hours. After 48 hours, a narrow green

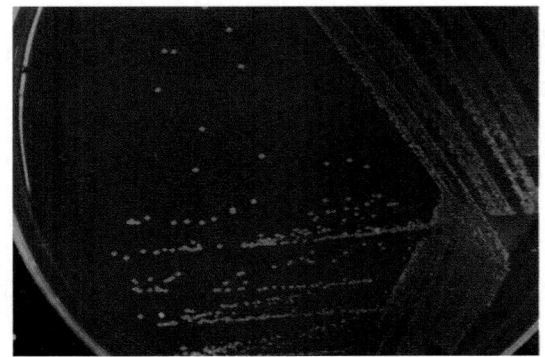

Figure 34-9

Pasteurella multocida colonies on sheep's blood agar. (From Bottone EJ, Girolami R, Stamm J, editors: *Schneierson's atlas of diagnostic microbiology,* ed 8, New York, 1982, Churchill Livingstone.)

to brown halo can surround the colonies. Colonies of encapsulated strains appear smooth. Gram stains of the isolates reveal small gram-negative coccobacilli to bacilli with bipolar staining. However, *P. multocida* does not grow on MacConkey agar.

IDENTIFICATION

Biochemically, most isolates are oxidase- and catalase-positive, and they acidify the butt and slant of triple sugar iron (TSI) medium. They are positive for glucose and xylose and are usually negative for maltose and lactose.

A selective Mueller Hinton–based agar with amikacin, vancomycin, and amphotericin B is available to detect human pharyngeal carriers of *P. multocida*. This medium may be of benefit for patients who are in professions that are high risk for pasteurellosis.

Erysipeloid

CASE STUDY

A 67-year-old man who fell from a ladder experienced fever and lower back and bilateral leg pain. He went to an emergency room 10 days later and was admitted to the hospital. He was afebrile on admission, but examination revealed a pruritic erythema of the trunk and extremities. The patient explained that the rash had started as a papule that had spread, showing central clearing. The patient also worked in the vicinity of hog pens. Blood cultures were collected, and routine laboratory tests were done. Radiographs showed no bone damage, and the urinalysis was normal.

On hospital day 2, the laboratory reported grampositive cocci isolated from the blood of the patient. The isolated organism was preliminarily identified as an α-hemolytic streptococcus. The patient received penicillin.*

*Data from Gorby GL, Peacock JE Jr: *Erysipelothrix rhusiopathiae* endocarditis: microbiologic, epidemiologic, and clinical features of an occupational disease, *Rev Infect Dis* 10:317, 1988.

Etiology

Erysipelothrix rhusiopathiae is the causative agent of swine erysipelas, Rosenbach erysipeloid, erysipelotrichosis, rose disease, and fish-handler's disease. *E. rhusiopathiae* is a thin, facultatively anaerobic gram-positive bacillus, 0.2 to 0.4 μm by 0.8 to 2.5 μm, which can grow singly, in short chains, or in long filaments.

Epidemiology

Often isolated from contaminated water and soil, *E. rhusiopathiae* is important in veterinary medicine, causing infections in swine, poultry, small mammals, fish, and crustaceans. The organism occurs worldwide. Swine erysipelas is an important economic disease in North America, South America, and Europe.

Clinical manifestations

The most common clinical manifestation of infection with *E. rhusiopathiae*, erysipeloid, occurs as a result of handling infected animals or animal products. In humans, the site of infection is usually an abrasion or wound of the hands or fingers. The infection is mild, localized, and self-limiting. An edematous lesion forms 1 to 7 days after infection. Erythema and itching may also be present. The lesion usually heals without treatment within 1 month. Patients with structural valvular disease, alcoholism, or other predisposing conditions may develop sepsis and endocarditis.

Laboratory diagnosis

SPECIMEN COLLECTION

The patient history is extremely valuable when making a diagnosis of erysipeloid. Biopsied tissues are better culture specimens than is aspirated lesion fluid.

DIRECT MICROSCOPIC EXAMINATION

Gram-stained aspirates or blood reveals smooth forms from patients with acute infections; the rough forms occur in specimens obtained from chronically infected patients.

CULTURE

Colonies isolated from sheep's blood agar may appear rough or smooth. Smooth colonies are 0.5 to 1.0 mm in diameter, circular, and nonpigmented and may cause a narrow zone of green discoloration of the blood. Gram stains from smooth colonies reveal short, straight gram-positive or gram-variable bacilli. Rough colonies are larger, and Gram stains of these isolates show filamentous gram-positive or gram-variable bacilli. As indicated in the case presented, microscopic morphology of *E. rhusiopathiae* is variable and can be easily misidentified. On hospital day 4, the laboratory issued an amended report of *E. rhusiopathiae* as the blood culture isolate. The patient then received a 28-day regimen of penicillin. Recovery was complete and unremarkable.

IDENTIFICATION

E. rhusiopathiae organisms are nonmotile, nonsporing, and nonencapsulated. Isolates are catalase- and oxidase-negative and produce hydrogen sulfide in TSI medium. The organism does produce a very characteristic "test-tube brush" growth when stabbed into gelatin deeps.

Capnocytophaga canimorsus Infection (Formerly CDC Group DF-2)

CASE STUDY

A 47-year-old woman entered an emergency room with weakness, diarrhea, and a facial rash. The patient had a pulse of 80, temperature of 36.5° C, and blood pressure of 80 mm Hg. She had an eschar on the left hand with no evidence of cellulitis. The facial rash covered the nose and cheeks. There were ecchymoses on her extremities. Her arms and legs were cold to the touch. Lung, cardiac, and central nervous system functions were normal. The patient was admitted to the intensive care unit.

A dog had bitten her on the left hand 5 days prior to admission. She had seen a local physician shortly after the bite, and he treated her for an allergic reaction with corticosteroids. The patient received empirical amoxicillin–clavulanic acid and amikacin, and then later received ceftazidime and amikacin. One aerobic blood culture bottle (using the Bactec NR-660) was positive, with a thin, gram-negative bacillus. The blood was subcultured onto brain-heart infusion agar supplemented with 10% horse's blood, and a small colony appeared after 48 hours of incubation in carbon dioxide. The laboratory identified the isolate as CDC group DF-2.*

---

*Data from Hantson P et al: Fatal *Capnocytophaga canimorsus* septicemia in previously healthy women, *Ann Emerg Med* 20:126, 1991.

Etiology

Capnocytophaga canimorsus, previously known as dysgonic fermenter-2 (CDC group DF-2), is a thin, nonsporing, nonmotile, oxidase- and catalase-

positive gram-negative bacillus, 1 to 3 μm long. The organism grows poorly on laboratory media. This pathogen causes a wide range of clinical manifestations, ranging from a mild, self-limiting localized infection to fulminant septicemia with involvement of several organs.

In the representative case study, the patient received heparin and platelets. The ecchymoses and necrosis of the extremities increased in severity. The patient experienced adult respiratory distress syndrome and died. Postmortem examination revealed multiple septic microthrombi of the endocardium, lungs, kidneys, and liver.

Infection occurs as the result of handling dogs. The carrier rates for this organism in dogs seem to be low, but inadequate recovery techniques may have influenced this finding.

Clinical manifestations

C. canimorsus infections occur as the result of dog bites. Dissemination and septicemia occur more often than the self-limiting lesions. About 90% of infections are found in patients who are splenectomized, have cancer, or abuse drugs. The most severe infections are seen in splenectomized patients, who develop an endotoxin-mediated Shwartzman-like phenomenon with purpura, septic shock, and DIC. Infection of previously healthy individuals is rare, probably because of the susceptibility of the organism to normal serum killing.

Laboratory diagnosis

SPECIMEN COLLECTION
The organism can be detected in the blood stream of infected patients.

DIRECT MICROSCOPIC EXAMINATION
Gram stains show the bacilli to be 1 to 4 μm long, with the longer bacilli usually appearing curved.

CULTURE
C. canimorsus grows poorly on 5% sheep's blood agar and does not grow at all on MacConkey agar. The organism can be successfully subcultured onto chocolate agar and 5% rabbit's blood agar at 37° C and increased carbon dioxide. Colony growth takes 2 to 7 days.

IDENTIFICATION
The organism is oxidase- and catalase-positive and nonmotile. Carbohydrate utilization is useful in

identifying the organism, but the best results require use of heavy inocula or serum-supplemented carbohydrates.

Bacillary and Spirillary Rat-Bite Fevers

CASE STUDY

A 28-year-old female graduate student entered the hospital complaining of sudden onset of headache, nausea, vomiting, and myalgia. A rat had bitten her during a recent laboratory experiment. The bite wound, on the left index finger, was slightly indurated and nonsuppurative, and no lymphadenopathy was present. The patient did not have a rash, and she had pain in her right ankle. The patient was febrile (101° F), and her blood pressure was normal.

The laboratory results are shown below.*

Complete blood count:
    Hemoglobin: 13.6 g/dL
    Hematocrit: 44%
    WBCs: 126,000/μL; 74% neutrophils;
       9% bands
Cerebrospinal fluid: clear, colorless
    Protein: 26 mg/dL
    Glucose: 94 mg/dL

The cerebrospinal fluid, urine, and blood were negative for the detection of leptospires. Mice and guinea pigs were inoculated intraperitoneally to rule out spirochete infection.

---

*Data from Holden FA, McKay JC: Rat-bite fever: an occupational hazard, *Can Med Assoc J* 91:214, 1964.

Etiology

Streptobacillus moniliformis, the causative agent of streptobacillary rat-bite fever, is a facultatively anaerobic, nonmotile, nonsporulating, gram-negative bacillus or fusiform, about 0.2 to 2.0 μm in size. The cells may appear singly or in filaments, often with a beaded-chain appearance. The cells can lose their cell walls and grow as stable L-forms. This organism also causes a milk- or water-borne disease called Haverhill fever (erythema arthriticum epidemicum). Protein gel electrophoresis can differentiate the Haverhill strains and streptobacillary strains.

Spirillum minus, which causes spirillary rat-bite fever, or sodoku, is a motile gram-negative spirillum, about 0.5 μm by 3.0 μm in size (Figure 34-10).

It is now classified under "Species *incertae sedis*" and may be related to the campylobacteria.

Both of these bacteria are normal inhabitants of the nasopharynx and urine of the rat. Both can cause rat-bite fever, which can present as either a cutaneous disease involving a rash and lymphadenitis or a disease transmitted by infected milk. The disease occurs throughout the world, with a higher incidence in urban areas.

Clinical manifestations

This disease should be of particular interest to laboratory workers, who can become infected by handling laboratory rodents. As many as 50% of apparently normal laboratory rodents harbor *S. moniliformis* in the oropharynx.

Streptobacillary rat-bite fever has a short incubation period. A healing lesion occurs at the primary site, and the infection is associated with polyarthritis and palmar and plantar petechiae. The mortality rate of untreated patients is about 10%.

Ulceration at the primary site, relapsing fever, and a palmar and plantar maculopapular rash occur in spirillary rat-bite fever. Arthritis usually does not occur with this infection. Without antibiotic therapy, relapses may occur. The mortality rate is about 7%.

Haverhill fever is a *S. moniliformis* infection transmitted by contaminated milk, milk products, or water. Contaminated milk is often implicated in this presentation of rat-bite fever. All the classic strep-

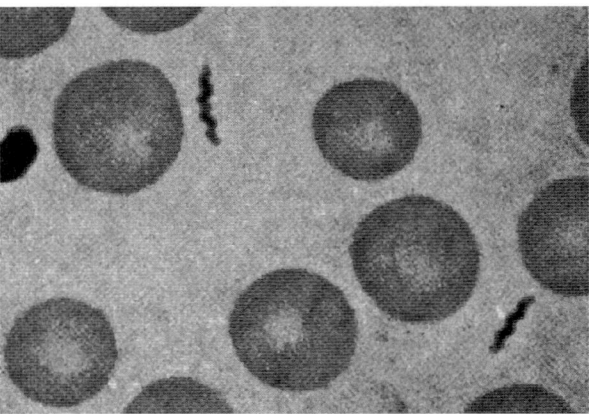

Figure 34-10

Gram stain of *Spirillum* from the blood of an infected mouse. (From Burrows W: *Textbook of microbiology,* ed 19, Philadelphia, 1968, WB Saunders.)

Figure 34-11

Gram stain from culture of *Streptobacillus moniliformis* showing pleomorphic gram-negative bacilli and filaments with characteristic areas of swelling. (From Holroyd KJ, Reiner AP, Dick JD: Streptobacillus moniliformis polyarthritis mimicking rheumatoid arthritis: an urban case of rat-bite fever, *Am J Med* 85:711, 1988.)

tobacillary rat-bite fever symptoms may be present, although rash and arthritis may be absent.

Laboratory diagnosis

Unclotted blood, pus, synovial fluid, and ascites are the specimens of choice for the recovery of *S. moniliformis*. Direct Gram stain preparations reveal pleomorphic gram-negative bacilli, as shown in Figure 34-11. Acridine orange-stained preparations may make it easier to see the organisms through the background material. The growth of the organism is inhibited by SPS-containing media. Good colony growth is possible on Loeffler serum plates, 5% sheep's blood agar, or Columbia colistin–nalidixic acid (CNA) blood agar. Colonies resemble cotton-like masses after 2 to 7 days of incubation. The isolated colonies may change to L-forms, making subculture difficult. Streptobacilli can be identified by using a combination of fatty acid profiles, growth characteristics, and Gram stain morphology.

Laboratory culture of *Spirillum minus* is difficult. The organism grows in vitro in dextrose veal infusion broth and tomato extract–veal infusion broth and can also be grown in vivo using animal inoculations. The organism is best visualized in blood, pus, and lymph node tissue with the use of darkfield microscopy.

In the representative case study, the laboratory inoculated 2 mL of the patient's blood into bovine serum–supplemented nutrient infusion broths (15% vol/vol) containing sterile glucose and starch. Small, fluffy colonies grew in the broths after 72 hours of incubation at 37° C in 5% carbon dioxide. Gram stains showed pleomorphic, gram-negative filamentous bacteria. Laboratory mice injected with purified isolates rapidly developed symptoms of rat-bite fever. Nasopharyngeal cultures of the rat that had bitten the student grew pure cultures of *S. moniliformis*.

The patient received primarily empirical tetracycline and then received penicillin after the infective organism was identified.

ZOONOTIC INFECTIONS TRANSMITTED BY DIRECT CONTACT OR INHALATION

Anthrax

CASE STUDY

A 57-year-old male patient, employed as an electrician, had felt ill and feverish before reporting to the hospital and had collapsed at home when he tried to stand. He had been bitten by an insect on the upper left chest the previous day while at work. He was taking no medications and had no travel history. Examination of the patient detected hypotension, a fever of 38.2° C, and a necrotic lesion at the site of the insect bite on the chest with edema and erythema. He was diagnosed as having streptococcal cellulitis and septicemia and was admitted to the hospital.

He was treated with intravenous benzyl penicillin and flucloxacillin.

Subsequent laboratory values were as follows*:

Hemoglobin: 17.9 g/dL
WBC: 10.9×10^9/L
Platelets: 262×10^9/L
Serum creatinine: 117 μmol/L
Serum creatinine phosphokinase elevated to 883 IU/L (normal <235)
Anti-Streptolysin O: 240 units/ml (normal <200 units/ml)
Urea concentration: 4.9 mmol/L

*Data from Mallon E, McKee, PH: Extraordinary case report: cutaneous anthrax, *Am J Dermatopathol* 19:79, 1997.

In spite of therapy, the patient developed renal failure and jaundice. The wound's erythema worsened, causing concern that this could be necrotizing fasciitis. The chest wound was excised to contain the fasciitis. Further inquiries determined that 1 week prior to the onset of symptoms the patient had been working for a leather firm and had not worn his shirt. He had been exposed to untreated hides during this interval. He was a temporary worker in this firm and had not received vaccination or safety information.

Etiology

Anthrax, also known as *woolsorter's disease* and *malignant pustule,* is caused by *Bacillus anthracis,* a large (2.5 μm by 10 μm), gram-positive, spore-forming bacillus. This organism occurs naturally in the soil and is a pathogen of herbivores, such as cattle, sheep, and goats. Human infections occur as the result of direct or indirect contact with animals or animal products.

Epidemiology

B. anthracis survives well in soil that is neutral or mildly alkaline. Areas with alternating dry and wet seasons enhance anthrax. Floods tend to concentrate spores, which remain in the grasses after flood waters drain. These spores have been known to last in fields for as long as 20 years. Animals are then infected by grazing in a contaminated area.

Anthrax occurs in nearly every state in the United States, as well as in Central and South America, Africa, and the Middle East. Recurrences of anthrax are prevented by containing the spores and eliminating their spread through the environment. Because the anthrax bacteria in tissues do not sporulate until they are exposed to oxygen, infected animal carcasses are usually incinerated whole or are buried in deep pits and covered with lime.

Vaccines are available for humans and for cattle. A cell-free vaccine, prepared from the protective antigen of *B. anthracis,* is used for people in high-risk occupations. Another vaccine, made with an avirulent, nonencapsulated strain of *B. anthracis,* is available for animals.

Clinical manifestations

Human anthrax manifests as cutaneous, intestinal, or pulmonary.

CUTANEOUS ANTHRAX

The most common form of the infection is the cutaneous form (95% of cases) which mimics many other cutaneous infections. It is most common in nonindustrialized countries. The spores enter the host through abraded skin and then germinate. After 48 to 72 hours, a papule is formed; it darkens and ruptures, leaving a painless crater-like ulcer, which progresses to a necrotic **eschar.** The infection usually remains localized and self-limiting, and the eschar heals without scarring. In about 20% of the patients with cutaneous anthrax, the immune system is unable to contain the infection, and *B. anthracis* enters the blood stream and disseminates. With treatment, death is rare.

In the case of the patient previously described, blood cultures taken at admission grew *B. anthracis.* The patient improved and was discharged 2 weeks later. In some patients, cutaneous anthrax can manifest as the more life-threatening "malignant edema," in which the initial lesions necrose, and blisters ring the primary site. The resulting edema can impair eating, drinking, and breathing.

GASTROINTESTINAL ANTHRAX

The gastrointestinal form, the second most common form of anthrax, is found more frequently in nonindustrialized nations. It is caused by the ingestion of meat or meat products contaminated with spores. Once the spores are ingested, they germinate, and the organisms gain entry through preexisting intestinal mucosa lesions. Dissemination of the bacteria then occurs via the lymphatics. Clinically, the patient will be febrile and have bloody stools, and may lose up to 12 L of fluid per 24-hour period. Septicemia and death may result.

PULMONARY (INHALATION) ANTHRAX

The pulmonary form occurs as a result of inhaling spores, usually from contaminated animal products. This form of anthrax is more common in industrialized countries. Macrophages ingest the spores and then concentrate them in lymph nodes. Eventually, the spores germinate, and sepsis occurs. The result of this form of infection is usually the death of the patient within 24 hours, regardless of the treatment given.

B. anthracis produces three virulence factors, including a poly-D-glutamic acid capsule, edema

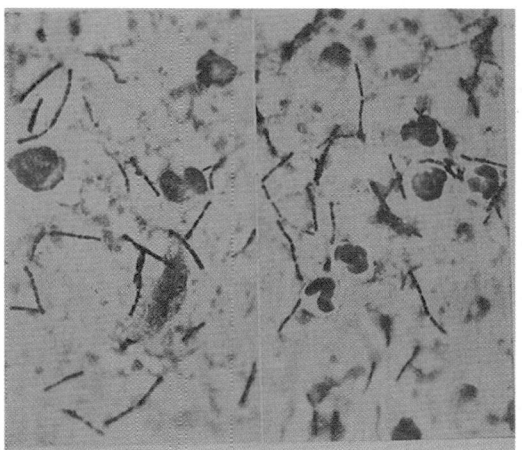

Figure 34-12

Peripheral blood films collected from a cow dying of anthrax. The preparations are stained with methylene blue. (From Gillies RR, Dodd TC, editors: *Bacteriology illustrated,* ed 4, New York, 1976, Churchill Livingstone.)

toxin, and lethal toxin. The edema toxin contains an adenylate cyclase (called edema factor, or EF) and a transport protein (called protective antigen, or PA). The protective antigen carries both edema toxin and the lethal factor. The toxin damages cells and vessels in the infected areas. Necrosis occurs as the result of increased capillary permeability and destruction of the phagocytic cells. Edema can be remarkable and can cause the patient to suffocate by literally swelling the neck shut. Excessive edema of the neck, thorax, and mediastinum signals the beginning of a rapidly fatal course.

The drug of choice for *B. anthracis* infections is penicillin G; secondary choices are tetracycline and erythromycin. Treatment of infected animals includes penicillin or oxytetracycline.

Laboratory diagnosis

B. anthracis and its spores are dangerous to laboratory workers. Those who work with *B. anthracis* should follow strict infection control measures, including working under a biologic safety hood, using sodium hypochlorite as a disinfectant, wearing protective clothing and gloves, and preventing aerosol formation. Technologists should submit suspected isolates of *B. anthracis* to capable reference laboratories for identification.

SPECIMEN COLLECTION

Specimens for culture include vesicle fluid, blood, and spinal fluid. Recovery of the organism is more likely if the specimen is collected prior to antimicrobial therapy.

DIRECT MICROSCOPIC EXAMINATION

Direct examination of blood or edema fluids reveals gram-positive bacilli in short chains. Endospores may be present (Figure 34-12).

CULTURE

B. anthracis grows as white to gray, nonhemolytic, or slightly hemolytic colonies on sheep's blood agar. The colonies are 2 to 5 mm in diameter. The colonies may have a characteristic "medusa-head" appearance, as shown in Figure 34-13.

IDENTIFICATION

The isolate is a nonmotile, encapsulated gram-positive bacillus with square ends. It is susceptible to penicillin and gammaphage. If the bacillus isolate has these characteristics, and if it demonstrates a capsular material on brain-heart infusion agar or nutrient agar with 0.5% sodium bicarbon-

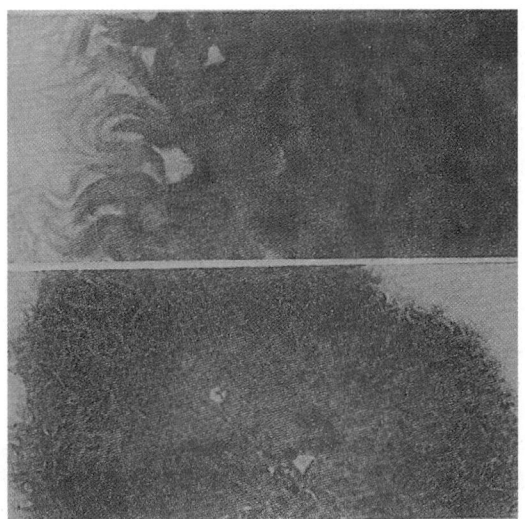

Figure 34-13

Impression colony of *Bacillus anthracis* stained with methylene blue, demonstrating the "medusa-head" appearance of the colony edge; ×12 and ×75. (From Gillies RR, Dodd TC, editors: *Bacteriology illustrated,* ed 4, New York, 1976, Churchill Livingstone.)

ate in 5% carbon dioxide, it can be presumptively identified as *B. anthracis*. Direct fluorescent antibody testing is used to detect encapsulated organisms in tissue or from culture. Double diffusion assays, in which wells containing antitoxin are placed in media near suspected *B. anthracis* colonies, detect toxigenic strains.

Tularemia

CASE STUDY

A 63-year-old male noticed swelling and localized pain in the dorsum of his left thumb, 5 days after a cat bite. He was treated with oral penicillin and cloxacillin for 3 days. He continued to experience pain, general malaise, fever and vomiting, and was admitted to the hospital where the following was recorded. The patient was lethargic, his temperature was 38.7° C, chest was clear, and he was hemodynamically stable, with a 3- by 5-cm indurated, erythematous region on dorsal aspect of base of left thumb and hand. Because this was considered to be a possible abscess, the physician performed an incision and drainage, but no abscess was found. Swabs from the infected region grew light coagulase-negative staphylococci.

The patient was treated with IV penicillin and cloxacillin. Five days after admission the patient developed shortness of breath and had patchy pneumonic infiltrates of right middle and lower lobes of the lung. Seven days after admission, lymphangitic streaking on the upper left extremity and tender axillary lymphadenopathy were detected. The patient's therapy was changed to clindamycin and gentamicin. The patient defervesced, and his respiratory status improved.

A swab from the wound was plated onto blood, and chocolate + CO_2. After 3 days, small, smooth, gray colonies were visible. Gram-negative coccibacilli were identified as *Francisella tularensis* by fatty acid analysis and slide agglutination by specific antisera. Acute and convalescent sera filters were 1:800 and 1:3200, respectively. The patient's cats were adopted strays that lived outdoors and probably fed on wild rodents.

Tularemia is often associated with exposure to rabbits or other wild animals or ticks. Because this patient was probably infected by his cat, the authors reviewed literature to determine how common cat exposures have been. The authors reviewed cat-related tularemia since 1928 and found 51 cases. The details on 15 of these are listed here*:

- Exposures by type:
  - Bite: 12
  - Casual contact: 2
  - Scratch: 1
- Activity of cat:
  - Rural and/or outdoor: 12
  - Urban and/or outdoor: 2
  - Urban and indoor: 1

An interesting coincidence is that the numbers do not coincide: that is, the scratch was not from an urban/indoor cat. Cat-scratch disease and *P. multocida* are more commonly associated with cat bite/scratch.

Etiology

Tularemia is caused by *Francisella tularensis*, a strictly aerobic gram-negative bacillus about 0.2 μm by 0.2 to 0.7 μm. The first isolation of the bacterium was in 1911 during an epizootic outbreak of plague-like ground squirrel disease. The organism was named *Bacterium tularense* after Tulare County, California, the site of the outbreak. In 1944, researchers defined the role of cottontail and jackrabbits in the transmission of the disease to humans. Since 1945 the proportion (*Dermacentor andersoni, Dermacentor variabilis,* and *A. americanum*) has increased, while transmission from vertebrate reservoirs has decreased. In 1959 the genus name of the organism was changed to *Francisella* in honor of Dr. Francis, who first isolated the organism.

Epidemiology

The two biovars *F. tularensis* biovar *tularensis* (type A) and *F. tularensis* biovar *palaearctica* (type B) occur in different parts of the world. In North America the predominant biovar is type A, the more virulent strain in humans. Humans are usually infected with this strain by rabbits or ticks, although more than 100 species of vertebrate and invertebrate natural reservoirs can transmit the infection. Type B also

---

*Data from Capellan J, Fong IW: Tularemia from a cat bite: case report and review of feline-associated tularemia, *Clin Infect Dis* 16:472, 1993.

occurs in North America, but it is more often recovered in Europe and Asia. It is less virulent than type A and is more often transmitted by rodents and mosquitoes. Types A and B differ from each other biochemically and genetically but not serologically.

Clinical manifestations

Tularemia is an acute, febrile, granulomatous disease characterized by rapid onset and flulike symptoms. The most common presentations are ulceroglandular (ulcers and lymphadenopathy), oropharyngeal (pharyngeal ulcer and lymphadenopathy), oculoglandular (conjunctival ulcer and lymphadenopathy), glandular (lymphadenopathy without ulcer), pleuropulmonary (no ulcer, possible lymphadenopathy), and typhoidal (no ulcers or lymphadenopathy). The ulceroglandular, oculoglandular, and glandular types usually occur as the result of direct contact with infected vertebrate or invertebrate reservoirs. Typhoidal and oropharyngeal cases of tularemia usually occur after eating contaminated food.

Pneumonic tularemia may result from exposure to aerosols. The symptoms associated with tularemia include fever, chills, headache, and myalgia. Typhoidal tularemia, especially when complicated with pneumonia, has a high fatality rate. In the United States most cases of tularemia are ulceroglandular. These infections are usually caused by direct contact with contaminated game or by insect bites. The incubation period of tularemia is 3 to 10 days. A papule, which forms at the site of infection, eventually ulcerates. Patients usually have only one lesion, although multiple lesions can occur. The actual site of the lesion is indicative of the transmission; lesions of the hands or arms often indicate infection by direct contact with infected mammals, whereas lesions on the head or the back indicate transmission by an insect vector.

F. tularensis is a facultatively intracellular parasite. Macrophages at the site of infection are able to phagocytose the pathogens, but the bacteria survive intracellularly. Leukocytes containing the bacteria drain to the lymph nodes, resulting in lymphadenopathy. Hematogenous spread then occurs. Extracellular bacteria are, by virtue of their capsule, immune to the antibacterial effects of normal serum. Focal necrosis and granulocytic changes occur in parenchymal organs. Many of these granulomatous changes are similar to those seen with tuberculosis. Humans gain immunity to tularemia

in essentially the same ways as they do to other intracellular pathogens, such as *Listeria* and *Mycobacterium* organisms. Lymphokine-activated macrophages and opsonizing antibodies probably are responsible for resolving the infection. However, antibody production does not occur until the second week of infection, and an early IgM response does not occur; IgG, IgA, and IgM all appear at about the same time. Tularemia is unusual in that IgM production to the causative organism lasts for up to 11 years, implying the continued presence of bacterial antigens or whole organisms.

Inappropriate antibiotic therapy promotes relapsing febrile episodes. Broad-spectrum antibiotics often fail to clear the host of *F. tularensis,* whereas gentamicin or streptomycin treatment is bactericidal and allows for complete recovery.

Laboratory diagnosis

SPECIMEN COLLECTION

Although the name of the organism implies bacteremia, blood is not the best specimen for recovery, even though the organism has been isolated using the Bactec blood culture system and the Isolator tubes. Ulcer scrapings, biopsy material from lymph nodes, and sputum may offer better chances of recovering the organism. Figure 34-14, *A,* shows an infected liver.

Serum could be submitted; routine detection of tularemia is best done serologically. Only biosafety level 3 reference laboratories should test isolates of *F. tularensis.* Even though *F. tularensis* cannot penetrate unbroken skin, this organism is infamous for its role in causing laboratory-acquired disease.

DIRECT MICROSCOPIC EXAMINATION

Microscopically, the organism is a tiny gram-negative coccobacillus that shows bipolar staining, as seen in Figure 34-14, *B.*

CULTURE

The organism grows on Iso Vitalex–supplemented chocolate agar, cystine-supplemented blood agar, and buffered charcoal-yeast extract (BCYE) within 24 hours. The opalescent colonies are small and mucoid. Colonies may appear α-hemolytic on blood agar after 24 to 48 hours. Identification of suspected *F. tularensis* is best accomplished at a reference laboratory. *F. tularensis* isolated from CYE can give false-positive results with DFA stains and IFA serologies for *Legionella pneumophila.*

SEROLOGIC IDENTIFICATION

Conventional tube agglutination, microagglutination, and ELISA can measure the serum antibodies of tularemia patients. Serum titers of more than 1:160 or a fourfold increase in titers indicates tularemia. Streptomycin and gentamicin are the drugs of choice.

Brucellosis

CASE STUDY

A 25-year-old male, complaining of headache, malaise, arthralgia, and a 6-kg weight loss was admitted to the hospital. He reported that his symptoms first started during the last 3 months after his return from a trip to Syria. He reported having eaten fresh goat's cheese. On admission he was in moderate distress and had the following lab results*:

WBC: 5.3 × 109/L
C-reactive protein: 10.7 mg/dL (normal <1.0 mg/dL)
Malaria smear: Negative
Serology for *Salmonella* species: Negative
Blood culture: *Brucella abortus*
Serology for *Brucella abortus:* Positive, titer 1:10,000

The patient was treated with doxycycline, 400 mg/d, and rifampin, 600 mg/d. The patient improved, he became afebrile, and his C-reactive protein level returned to normal after a few days. The patient's girlfriend developed the same symptoms 2 months later and was admitted to the hospital. Blood cultures were positive for *B. abortus*. She was successfully treated and recovered without complications.

The authors believe this to be the first case of possible sexual transmission of *B. abortus* in humans. The female had no travel history or other risk factors. The couple had unprotected sexual intercourse, and sexual transmission was considered to be the most likely route of infection.

---

*Data from Thalhammer F, Eberl G, Kopetzki-Kogler U: Unusual route of transmission for *Brucella abortus*, *Clin Infect Dis* 26:763, 1998.

Etiology

Brucellosis has many synonyms, including Mediterranean fever, Malta fever, Gibraltar fever, Bang's

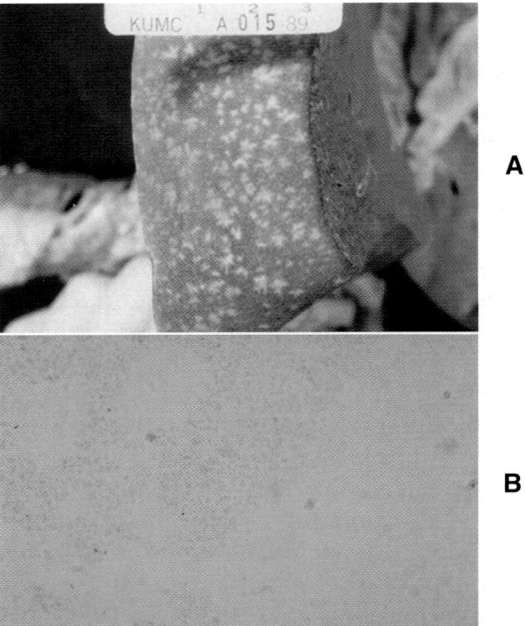

Figure 34-14 _____

Francisella tularensis seen in tissue specimens. **A,** Section of an infected liver. The capsular surface shows multiple white, stellate areas of necrosis. **B,** Gram stain from broth culture of *F. tularensis*. (From Hargrave PK, Hulsebus J, Wilson L: Tularemic shock: a case study. Paper presented at the Annual Meeting of the American Society for Medical Technology, 1992.)

disease, Neapolitan fever, Cyprus fever, and **undulant fever.** The genus name comes from Sir David Bruce, who, in 1887, was the first to describe these agents as the cause of undulant fever.

Epidemiology

Four species, which originate from animal reservoirs, are pathogenic to humans:

Brucella melitensis (goats)
Brucella abortus (cattle)
Brucella canis (canines)
Brucella suis (swine)

The most pathogenic species for humans, in descending order, are *B. melitensis, B. suis, B. abortus,* and *B. canis*. Other species not known to cause human disease are *Brucella neotomae* (desert wood rat) and *Brucella ovis* (sheep). In the animal hosts, the brucellae can induce spontaneous abortion secondary to bacteremia in pregnant females. The urine and milk of infected animals contain the infective organisms.

B. melitensis, the most common agent of human brucellosis, occurs in many areas of the world, including Mexico, Central and South America, southeastern Europe, countries bordering the Mediterranean, Africa, southern Russia, India, Iran, and central Saudi Arabia.

B. melitensis, B. suis, and *B. abortus* are subdivided into biotypes defined by biochemical reactions and serotypes. This classification defines three biotypes for *B. melitensis,* eight for *B. abortus,* and four for *B. suis.*

Clinical manifestations

In the United States, the brucellae infect humans primarily through contact with infected animals and animal products. Veterinarians, meat packers, sheepherders, and abattoir workers are at risk for infection.

The organism can enter the body through abraded skin, mucous membranes, or the conjunctiva. In experiments *B. abortus* has penetrated intact skin. After an incubation period of 1 to 3 weeks, the brucellae are disseminated hematogenously, where circulating monocytes ingest them. The brucellae are intracellular parasites. Monocytes transport the brucellae to lymph nodes. From there, the bacteria are disseminated to the spleen and the liver.

B. abortus usually causes granuloma formation, whereas *B. melitensis* usually causes formation of microabscesses. *B. melitensis* is also able to inhibit phagosome-lysosome fusion in phagocytic cells, allowing intracellular bacterial replication. Normal human serum is bactericidal to *B. abortus,* but not to *B. melitensis,* accounting for the relative differences in their pathogenicity. The symptoms of acute brucellosis are chills, fever, sweating, weakness, and fatigue.

The primary virulence factor is apparently the endotoxin, although outer membrane proteins (OMP) may also have a role as virulence factors. No detectable exotoxins are in the brucellae. Without antimicrobial treatment, brucellosis can persist from 3 months to 1 year. Some cases have reported remarkably long persistence, up to 26 years after exposure. Relapsing brucellosis is a febrile illness characterized by weight loss, anorexia, and night sweats. Complications include arthritis, vegetative endocarditis, and neurologic disorder. Physically, patients may have lymphadenopathy, hepatomegaly, splenomegaly, orchitis, or epididymitis. Recovery usually occurs within 3 to 6 months with rest and supportive treatment, although tetracycline therapy reduces the convalescent period.

Laboratory diagnosis

SPECIMEN COLLECTION

Laboratory personnel must be notified when physicians submit specimens that might contain *Brucella* organisms, because specialized media and prolonged incubation periods are required. For laboratory diagnosis of brucellosis, physicians should submit multiple blood cultures and both acute and convalescent sera for serologic testing. Other clinical specimens submitted for examination can include fluids and tissues.

DIRECT MICROSCOPIC EXAMINATION

Direct smear prepared from bone marrow, liver biopsies, or exudate from abscesses may reveal minute gram-negative coccobacilli.

CULTURE

The method of choice for culturing brucellae from blood is the biphasic blood culture bottle. Cultures are incubated in an atmosphere of 5% to 10% carbon dioxide for 30 days. Other culture systems are acceptable for the detection of brucellosis; however, blind subcultures should be performed about twice a week for 30 days.

Specimens not likely to have excess contamination may be plated onto 5% sheep's blood agar or brucella agar. Specimens with likely contamination may be plated onto selective media, including modified Farrell's Thayer-Martin, BCYE, Kuzdas and Morse, and Farrell.

Brucellae are strictly aerobic gram-negative coccobacilli, although an extended period for counterstaining makes it easier to visualize the organisms on Gram stain. The brucellae can have bipolar staining; are nonsporing, nonmotile, and nonencapsulated; and require carbon dioxide for growth. Cell sizes range from 0.6 to 1.5 μm by 0.5 to 0.7 μm.

Identification

Oxidase- and catalase-positive bacterial isolates that grow on appropriate media within 2 to 3 days and that are round, 2 to 3 mm in diameter, nonhemolytic, translucent, and opalescent, are possible brucellae (Figure 34-15). These isolates should be tested with antismooth *Brucella* serum.

Preliminary tests needed to differentiate among

Figure 34-15

Culture of *Brucella melitensis* on sheep's blood agar after 48 hours. (From Gillies RR, Dodd TC, editors: *Bacteriology illustrated,* ed 4, New York, 1976, Churchill Livingstone.)

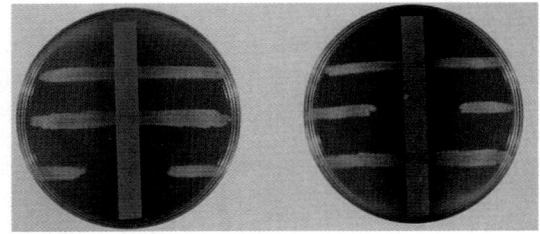

Figure 34-16

Dye inhibition tests with streaks of *Brucella melitensis (top),* *Brucella abortus (middle),* and *Brucella suis (bottom).* Basic fuchsin at concentration of 1:25,000 *(left)* inhibits the growth of *B. suis,* whereas thionin at a concentration of 1:30,000 *(right)* inhibits the growth of *B. abortus.* Neither dye at those concentrations inhibits the *B. melitensis.* (From Gillies RR, Dodd TC, editors: *Bacteriology illustrated,* ed 4, New York, 1976, Churchill Livingstone.)

the species of *Brucella* include carbon dioxide requirements, hydrogen sulfide production, urease, and growth on dye-containing media. Figure 34-16 shows dye inhibition. Additionally, the brucellae reduce nitrates to nitrites, oxidize glucose, but do not oxidize sucrose, lactose, maltose, or mannitol. Table 34-1 shows the differentiating characteristics of brucellae.

SERODIAGNOSIS

Because recovery of *Brucella* species from clinical specimens is not highly sensitive, it is recommended to include serologic testing to establish the presence of infection. Titers of more than 100 IU or a fourfold rise in titers indicates recent infection. Cross-reactions with cholera or tularemia (or vaccination against these diseases) are possible.

TABLE 34-1

Biochemical Reactions Used for the Differentiation of Brucellae

Biotype	CO$_2$ Req	H$_2$S	Urease	Growth in		
				BF 20 µg	Thionin 20 µg	Thionin 40 µg
B. melitensis						
1	−	−	+/−	+	+	+
2	−	−	+/−	+	+	+
3	−	−	+/−	+	+	+
B. abortus						
1	+/−	+	+	+	−	−
2	+/−	+	+	−	−	−
3	+/−	+	+	+	+	+
4	+/−	+	+/−	−	−	−
5	−	−	+	+	+	−
6	−	+/−	+	+	+	−
7	−	+	+	+	+	−
B. suis						
1	−	+	+	+/−	+	+
2	−	−	+	−	+	−
3	−	−	+	+	+	+
4	−	−	+	+/−	+	+
5	−	−	+	−	+	+
B. canis	−	−	+	−	+	+
B. neotomae	−	+	+	−	−	−
B. ovis	+	−	−	+/−	+	+

BF, Basic fuchsin.

Leptospirosis

CASE STUDY

A 48-year-old white male, employed as a river dredger, presented with headache, fever, dark urine, arthralgia, diarrhea, breathlessness, and confusion, which had become worse over the past 4 days. The patient was hypoxic, and chest x-rays showed a rapid deterioration with shadowing in all regions of the lungs. He was treated with doxycycline and erythromycin. He continued to deteriorate and was given mechanical respiratory support. Methyl-prednisolone was prescribed in addition to the antibiotics. Chest x-rays continued to deteriorate for a period of 7 days before showing gradual clearance. Renal function also returned to normal. He was discharged after 21 days. He was determined to have culture-positive leptospirosis with severe pulmonary hemorrhage. The date of the positive culture was not reported.

Record reviews of the Tropical Public Health Unit showed 149 cases of leptospirosis reported, 24 of which were hospitalized and 5 had life-threatening pulmonary hemorrhage. Although not frequently reported, this complication is worth noting because of its serious consequences. In a 1995 outbreak in Nicaragua, 40 of 2000 patients died because of pulmonary hemorrhage.

In the experience of these authors with five cases, all patients gave nonspecific histories of malaise, myalgia, and fever. Renal impairment and jaundice, considered to be hallmarks of leptospirosis, were absent in two of their five patients.*

*Data from Simpson FG, Green KA, Haug GJ, Brookes DL: Leptospirosis associated with severe pulmonary haemorrhage in Far North Queensland, *Med J Aust* 169:151, 1998.

Leptospirosis is a difficult disease to diagnose clinically. Attempts to culture by traditional bacteriologic means may often produce negative results. Saltoglu et al summarized their experience with 12 leptospirosis patients with Weil's syndrome. Their findings indicate the wide variety of confusing symptoms one might see in a patient. The following indicates the percentage of Saltoglu et al's patients who exhibited these symptoms:

Nausea and vomiting: 92%
Jaundice: 92%
Lower back pain and myalgia: 58%
Headache: 50%
Conjunctival suffusion: 33%
Nuchal rigidity: 33%
Confusion: 25%
Dyspnea: 25%
Epistaxis: 16%

Yang et al recommend adding leptospirosis to the differential diagnosis for any patient who is febrile, has jaundice, or acute renal failure, for whom all traditional cultures are negative.

Etiology
Leptospires are helical cells, about 6 to 20 μm by 0.1 μm. They are motile and have two subterminal flagella. The cells have characteristic hooks on the ends. The genus *Leptospira* contains a large group of serologically diverse organisms. Two species exist: the pathogenic *Leptospira interrogans* and the saprophytic *Leptospira biflexa*. As many as 250 serovars are organized into 23 serogroups.

Epidemiology
Leptospirosis is not a very common infection and is found primarily in tropical regions. It is most often reported in the United States from southeastern, Gulf, and Pacific coastal states and Hawaii. Recreational activities that involve contact with water or moist soil are most often associated with transmission. In Hawaii, some homes use rainwater catchment systems and these have also been reported as a risk factor. As many as 5% to 10% of leptospirosis infections are fatal.

Rodents and domestic animals are the primary reservoirs for the organism. Other animals, including cows, horses, mongoose, and frogs, can harbor the leptospires. Humans may be directly infected from animal urine or indirectly by contact with soil or water that is contaminated with urine from infected animals. The patient in the case study worked as a river dredger and doubtless had frequent repeated contacts with untreated water. Infected humans can shed leptospires in urine for up to 11 months; cows for 3½ months; dogs for 4 years; and infected rodents possibly for their full lifetime. Veterinarians, abattoir workers, fish and poultry processors, and dairy workers are at risk for leptospirosis. Agricultural workers and soldiers are also at risk because of contact with soil and mud.

Leptospirosis is endemic in most areas of the world, although the incidence of disease can be underreported because of undiagnosed infections. The infection is more prevalent in areas with warm climates, especially in late autumn and early winter. The treatment of choice is doxycycline or penicillin G.

Clinical manifestations

The number of diagnosed leptospiral infections has increased in recent years. Leptospiral infections can range from subclinical to lethal. The organisms enter the host through mucous membranes or abraded skin. The incubation period ranges from 5 to 14 days.

Anicteric leptospirosis is usually a biphasic disease. In the first phase, the patient has sudden temperature spikes, severe headaches, nausea, vomiting, and muscle aches. Patients often experience confusion, secondary to dehydration. The majority of patients develop vivid pink eyes. During this period, the leptospires are recoverable from the patient's blood and spinal fluid. This phase of leptospirosis lasts for about 3 weeks.

In the second phase of anicteric leptospirosis, the leptospires disappear from the circulatory system and cerebrospinal fluid of the patient. This change occurs after the appearance of specific IgM antibodies. Symptoms may subside for a few days, but a limited febrile episode may follow. Patients may also develop aseptic meningitis and severe headaches. During this stage of infection, the urine contains leptospires, but the blood of the patient does not. The length of this stage depends on the serotype of the infecting leptospire.

Weil's syndrome

Leptospira interrogans serovar *icterohaemorrhagiae* can cause *icteric leptospirosis,* also known as **Weil's syndrome.** This form of leptospirosis is more life-threatening than the anicteric form. Weil's syndrome starts in the same way as does anicteric leptospirosis. On about the third day of the illness, however, the patient develops hemolysis, jaundice, and renal failure. These symptoms occur as the leptospires multiply in the liver and the kidney. In Weil's syndrome mortality ranges from 15% to 40%. In fatal cases, renal failure is the usual cause of death. In nonfatal cases, the leptospires clear from the patient's kidneys, brain, and eyes as antibodies appear.

Laboratory diagnosis
SPECIMEN COLLECTION
During the first week of the infection, leptospires are present in the patient's blood and spinal fluid. After the first week of the disease, the patient is no longer leptospiremic, so urine is the specimen of choice.

The leptouremia is sporadic, so multiple specimens increase the chance of recovery. Recovery of leptospires from the urine is optimized by diluting the urine 1:10 and 1:100 to dilute the effect of inhibiting substances. One drop of both diluted and undiluted urine should be inoculated into appropriate media.

DIRECT MICROSCOPIC EXAMINATION
Microscopic visualization of leptospires requires darkfield microscopy or other staining procedures other than Gram stain or Giemsa-Wright stains.

CULTURE
Fletcher semisolid media, bovine albumin-Tween 80 (Ba-Tw 80) media enriched with rabbit serum, and Ellinghausen-McCullough-Johnson-Harris (EMJH) media containing fatty acids or albumin can be used to culture leptospires. The addition of 5-fluorouracil, fosfomycin, and nalidixic acid decreases contamination.

THE RICKETTSIAE

The term *rickettsiae* can specifically refer to the genus *Rickettsia* or can refer to a group of organisms included in the order Rickettsiales. The order includes the following genera:

- *Rickettsia*
- *Coxiella*
- *Rochalimaea*
- *Ehrlichia*

Coxiella organisms differ from the other members of the rickettsia in mode of transmission and symptoms caused. *Rochalimaea* organisms are the only members of the group that has been grown on cell-free media.

With few exceptions, rickettsiae are not agents of zoonoses in the same sense as the organisms presented earlier in this chapter. Most of the members of the rickettsial group discussed in this chapter are arthropod-borne, obligately intracellular pathogens.

These bacteria have become extremely well adapted to their arthropod hosts. The primary hosts usually have minimal or no disease from their rickettsial infection. The arthropod host allows rickettsiae to persist in nature in two ways. First, rickettsiae are passed through new generations of arthropods by transovarial transmission. Because of this mechanism, arthropods are not only vectors for rickettsioses but also reservoirs. Second, arthropods directly inoculate new hosts with rickettsiae during feeding. An exception to this pattern occurs with *Rickettsia prowazekii.* In this case, the arthropod vector, the body louse, can die of the rickettsial infection, and humans act as a natural reservoir.

Rickettsia

General characteristics

Rickettsia organisms are short, nonmotile, gram-negative bacilli about 0.8 to 2.0 µm by 0.3 to 0.5 µm in size. The members of the genus *Rickettsia* have not been grown in cell-free media, but they have been grown in the yolk sacs of embryonated eggs and several monolayer cell lines. The species of *Rickettsia* are divided into groups according to the types of clinical infections they produce (Table 34-2):

- Spotted fever group
- Typhus fever group
- Scrub typhus group

The etiologic agents of these infections differ antigenically and infect different hosts. Phenotypic and genotypic similarities exist, however, between the spotted fever rickettsiae and the typhus group. *Rickettsia tsutsugamushi,* on the other hand, differs from the typhus and spotted fever rickettsiae in several key characteristics.

Clinical infections

SPOTTED FEVER GROUP

Rocky Mountain spotted fever The most severe of the rickettsial infections, Rocky Mountain spotted fever is caused by *R. rickettsii.* It was first described in the western United States during the latter part of the nineteenth century. It was not until the early 1900s that researchers showed the infectious nature of the disease, when they infected laboratory animals with the blood of infected patients. The nature of the agent was a mystery, because no bacteria were apparent on direct examination or on culture. However, researchers had to discount a viral etiology, since the agent was filterable. The organism was first seen using light microscopy in 1916.

Humans are accidental hosts and acquire the infection by tick bites. The most common tick vectors are *Dermacentor variabilis,* in the southeastern United States, and *Dermacentor andersoni,* in the western part of the country. Other species of ticks, however, can be vectors. Ticks transmit the organism into humans via saliva, which is passed into the host during the tick's feeding. Once in the host tissue, the rickettsiae are phagocytosed into

TABLE 34-2

Characteristics of Species and Biotypes of Rickettsia

	Species	Vector	Reservoir
Spotted fevers			
Rocky Mountain spotted fever	*Rickettsia rickettsii*	Tick	Ticks, dogs, rodents
Boutonneuse fever	*Rickettsia conorii*	Tick	Ticks, dogs, rodents
Rickettsialpox	*Rickettsia akari*	Mouse mite	House mouse
Typhus group			
Epidemic typhus	*Rickettsia prowazekii*	Body louse	Humans
Brill-Zinsser disease	*Rickettsia prowazekii*	None	Humans
Endemic (murine) typhus	*Rickettsia typhi*	Rat flea	Rats
Scrub typhus	*Rickettsia tsutsugamushi*	Mites	Rodents, mites
Trench fever	*Rochalimaea quintana*	Body louse	Humans
Q fever	*Coxiella burnetii*	None	Cattle, goats, sheep, ticks
Ehrlichiosis	*Ehrlichia canis*	Tick	—

endothelial cells, where they live and replicate in the cytoplasm of the host cell. Replication in the nucleus also occurs. The rickettsiae pass directly through the cell membranes of infected cells into adjacent cells without causing damage to the host cells. The rickettsiae are spread throughout the host hematogenously and induce vasculitis in internal organs, including the brain, heart, lungs, and kidneys.

Clinical manifestations. Clinically, the patient experiences flulike symptoms for approximately a week, which follows an incubation period of approximately 7 days. The symptoms include fever, headache, myalgia, nausea, vomiting, and rash. The rash, which may be hard to distinguish in individuals of color, begins as erythematous patches on the ankles and wrists during the first week of symptoms. The rash can extend to the palms of the hands and soles of the feet but normally does not affect the face. The maculopapular patches eventually consolidate into larger areas of ecchymoses.

Once disseminated, the organisms cause vasculitis in the blood vessels of the lungs, brain, and heart, leading to pneumonitis, central nervous system manifestations, and myocarditis. The patient experiences symptoms secondary to vasculitis, including decreased blood volume, hypotension, and DIC.

The mechanisms of pathogenesis are not completely understood. *R. rickettsii* does not produce exotoxins, and the endotoxin is not potent enough to explain the effects seen in the host. It is possible that host inflammation is responsible for the damage to the blood vessels.

The mortality rates for untreated or incorrectly treated patients can be as high as 20%, although correct antimicrobial therapy with tetracycline or chloramphenicol lowers the rates to 3% to 6%.

Rickettsialpox Another of spotted fever is rickettsialpox, caused by *Rickettsia akari.* The reservoir is the common house mouse, and the vector is the mouse mite *Allodermanyssus sanguineus.* Rickettsialpox occurs in Korea and the Ukraine as well as in the eastern United States, including the cities of New York, Boston, and Philadelphia. The infections occur in crowded urban areas where rodents and their mites exist.

Clinical manifestations. Rickettsialpox has similarities to Rocky Mountain spotted fever but is a milder infection. The rickettsial organism, *R. akari,* enters the human host following a mite (chigger) bite. The incubation period is about 10 days, after which a papule forms at the site of inoculation. The papule progresses to a pustule, then to an indurated eschar. The patient becomes febrile as the rickettsiae are disseminated throughout the body via the blood. The patient also experiences headache, nausea, and chills. Unlike Rocky Mountain spotted fever, the rash of rickettsialpox appears on the face, trunk, and extremities and does not involve the palms of the hands or soles of the feet. Rickettsialpox symptoms resolve without medical attention.

Boutonneuse fever Boutonneuse fever, also known as Mediterranean fever, caused by *Rickettsia conorii,* occurs in France, Spain, and Italy. *R. conorii* also causes Kenya tick typhus, South African tick fever, and Indian tick typhus. Like the agent for Rocky Mountain spotted fever, this rickettsia is tick-borne, and its reservoirs include ticks and dogs.

Clinical manifestations. Boutonneuse fever is also clinically similar to Rocky Mountain spotted fever. The rash involves the palms of the hands and soles of the feet, just as in Rocky Mountain spotted fever. The rash of boutonneuse fever, however, also involves the face. Also in contrast with Rocky Mountain spotted fever, this disease is characterized by the presence of *taches noires* (black spots) at the primary site of infection. Taches noires are lesions caused by the introduction of *R. conorii* into the skin of a nonimmune person. As the organism spreads to the blood vessels in the dermis, damage occurs to the endothelium. Edema, secondary to increased vascular permeability, reduces blood flow to the area and results in local necrosis.

THE TYPHUS GROUP

The typhus group of rickettsiae includes the species *Rickettsia typhi* (also called *Rickettsia mooseri*) (endemic typhus, also referred to as murine typhus) and *Rickettsia prowazekii* (epidemic louse-borne typhus and Brill-Zinsser disease) (see Table 34-2). Generally, the typhus rickettsiae differ from the other rickettsial groups in that they replicate in the cytoplasm of the host cell. The infection causes host cell lysis, thereby releasing the rickettsiae. Other rickettsiae pass directly through an uninjured cell.

Endemic typhus Endemic typhus is caused by *R. typhi.* The arthropod vector is the oriental rat flea *Xenopsylla cheopis,* and the rat (*Rattus exulans*) is the reservoir. Apparently, the cat flea, *Cteno-*

cephalides felis, can also harbor the organism. Because this flea infests a large number of domestic animals, it may be an important factor in the persistence of infection in urban areas.

The rickettsiae also survive in nature, to a lesser extent, by transovarial transmission. When a flea feeds on an infected host, the rickettsiae enter the flea's midgut, where they replicate in the epithelial cells. They are eventually released into the gut lumen. Humans become infected when fleas defecate on the surface of the skin while feeding. The human host then reacts to the bite by scratching the site, allowing direct inoculation of the infected feces into abrasions. *R. typhi* can also be transmitted to humans directly from the flea bite itself.

In the 1940s, approximately 5000 cases of endemic typhus were reported annually in the United States. Rigid control measures have reduced that number to fewer than 100 cases annually. The disease essentially occurs only in southern Texas and southern California in this country but continues to be a problem in areas of the world where rats and their fleas are present in urban settings.

Clinical manifestations. Like the case with Rocky Mountain spotted fever, the clinical course of endemic typhus includes fever, headache, and rash. Unlike Rocky Mountain spotted fever, endemic typhus does not always produce a rash. When the rash is present, however, it usually occurs on the trunk and extremities. Rash on the palms of the hands occurs rarely. Complications are rare, and recovery usually occurs without incident.

Epidemic louse-borne typhus Epidemic louse-borne typhus is caused by *R. prowazekii.* The vectors include the human louse *(Pediculus humanus),* the squirrel flea *(Orchopeas howardii),* and the squirrel louse *(Neohaematopinus sciuriopteri).* The reservoirs are primarily humans and flying squirrels located in the eastern United States. The louse often dies of its rickettsemia, unlike vectors of other rickettsiae.

Louse-borne typhus is still found commonly in areas of Africa and Central and South America where unsanitary conditions promote the presence of body lice. As seen during World War II, epidemic typhus can recur even in developed countries when sanitation is disrupted. Although fewer than 20 cases of epidemic typhus were reported in 1991, more than 20,000 cases of epidemic typhus were documented during the 1980s, with the vast majority originating in Africa.

Clinical manifestations. Epidemic typhus is similar to the other rickettsioses. Lice are infected with *R. prowazekii* when feeding on infected humans. The organisms invade the cells lining the gut of the louse. They actively divide and eventually lyse the host cells, spilling the organisms into the lumen of the gut. When the louse feeds on another human, it defecates, and the infected feces are scratched into the skin, just as in endemic typhus.

The disease progression is similar to that of Rocky Mountain spotted fever, including involvement of the palms of the hands and soles of the feet with the rash. Unlike the case with Rocky Mountain spotted fever, the face may also be affected by rash. The mortality rates for untreated patients can approach 40%, although mortality rates in treated patients are very low.

Recrudescent typhus, also called Brill-Zinsser disease, is seen in patients who have previously had epidemic typhus. The *R. prowazekii* lies dormant in the lymph tissue of the human host until the infection is reactivated. Recrudescent typhus is a milder infection than epidemic typhus, and death of the patient is rare. These patients with latent infections constitute an important reservoir for the organism.

SCRUB TYPHUS

Scrub typhus is a rickettsial disease that occurs in India, Burma, eastern Russia, Asia, and Australia. The causative agent is the sole member of the scrub typhus group, *R. tsutsugamushi.* The vector is the chigger, *Leptotrombidium deliensis,* and the main reservoir is the rat. The rickettsiae are transmitted transovarially in the chiggers.

Clinical manifestations The transmission of the *R. tsutsugamushi* to the human host is followed by an incubation period of approximately 2 weeks. A tache noire, similar to that of boutonneuse fever, forms at the site of inoculation. The normal rickettsial symptoms of fever, headache, and rash are also present. The rash starts on the trunk and spreads to the extremities. Unlike the case with Rocky Mountain spotted fever, the rash does not involve the palms of the hands and soles of the feet, and the face is also not involved.

TRENCH FEVER

In humans trench fever is caused by *Rochalimaea quintana.* This rickettsial organism is not an obligate intracellular pathogen. This, and the fact that it can be cultured in cell-free media, show this organism to be vastly different from the other rickettsial organisms. The vector is the body louse. Because transovarial passage does not occur in the lice, and because the lice infest only humans, it appears that humans are the main reservoir for the organism.

Clinical manifestations Trench fever has the classic rickettsial symptoms of fever, myalgia, and rash. The macular rash usually appears on the chest and abdomen. The infection subsides even without antibiotic therapy, although tetracycline allows for rapid resolution.

Q FEVER

Q fever, the disease caused by *Coxiella burnetii,* is named from the word "query" because of the unanswered questions associated with an epidemic in Queensland, Australia, during the 1930s. *Coxiella burnetii,* the only species in the genus, is an obligate intracellular pleomorphic coccobacillus, approximately 0.5 μm long. Q fever joined trench fever and epidemic typhus as major rickettsial epidemics during World War II. *C. burnetii* differs from other members of the rickettsia in mode of transmission, intracellular development, phase variation, and symptoms of disease.

Coxiella organisms are often isolated from cattle, goats, and sheep. These hosts usually have asymptomatic infections, although they can have abortions induced by the organism. The degree of chronic, asymptomatic infection, however, complicates control of the infection. Maintenance of the organism in nature seems to occur by two means. The most common means of transmission of the organism is from infected aerosols. Aerosols from infected body fluids and birth products are especially likely to transmit the disease. With inhalation as the route of entry, the infectious dose in humans can be as small as one bacterium.

The disease can also be transmitted by ticks that feed on infected cattle. These can then spread the infection to other animals. Human infection does not seem to occur through this route. Q fever is often an occupational disease, occurring among people who work with livestock or research animals. Q fever is found throughout the world. In the United States, outbreaks occur in states with large numbers of livestock.

Coxiella organisms undergo a phase variation that is unique among the rickettsial groups. Organisms that are freshly isolated from clinical sources have phase I antigens, which may inhibit phagocytosis by the host. As the organism is passed into the yolk sac, phase II antigens are expressed.

Clinical manifestations Q fever shares some vague flulike symptoms with the other rickettsioses, including fever, headache, myalgia, malaise, nausea, and vomiting. Chest pain is present in as many as one third of patients, and the actual percentage of patients with respiratory symptoms seems to vary widely. The infection can also present as an atypical pneumonia. No rash is associated with Q fever, however. The average incubation period is 20 days. The disease is normally self-limiting and resolves within 14 days. However, endocarditis is a sequela in a small percentage of Q fever patients. This manifestation occurs 1 to 20 years after the initial infection, and unlike acute Q fever, is often fatal.

Ehrlichiosis

CASE STUDY

A 65-year-old white man experienced fever, headache, myalgia, and anorexia for 5 days. When he went to his personal physician, his temperature was 38.3° C, his blood pressure was 128/60, and he was dehydrated. There was no sign of rash or lymphadenopathy.

Serial blood cultures were negative, as were routine serologies. The patient received intravenous doxycycline for 3 days. He then received oral doxycycline. His fever resolved after 6 hours of therapy. Following are the laboratory test results*:

WBC: 2,500 μL
Platelets: 57,000 μL
Hematocrit: 41.1%
Hemoglobin: 11.6 g/dL
SGOT (aspartate aminotransferase): 167 U/L
Creatine phosphokinase: 403 U/L
Alkaline phosphatase: 173
Total bilirubin: 1.7 mg/dL

*Data from Taylor JP et al: Serological evidence of possible human infection with *Ehrlichia* in Texas, *J Infect Dis* 158:217, 1988.

Ehrlichiosis was first noted in France in the 1930s when dogs infected with brown dog ticks became ill and died. Postmortem examination revealed rickettsial-like inclusions in the monocytes of the dead animals. These newly described rickettsiae were named *Rickettsia canis.* They were obligately intracellular, arthropod-borne gram-negative coccobacilli. They differ from the other members of the rickettsiae in that they multiply in the phagosomes of host leukocytes and not in the cytoplasm of endothelial cells. The infected leukocytes eventually rupture and release the organisms, to continue the infective cycle.

Because these organisms grew within host cell vacuoles, they were reclassified into the new genus, *Ehrlichia,* in 1945. The ehrlichiae have a developmental cycle similar to that of the chlamydiae. The infective form of the organism is the elementary body, which replicates in the phagosome. These bodies give rise to inclusions with initial bodies inside. As the inclusions mature, they develop morulae (mulberry-like bodies). As the host cell ruptures, the morulae break into many individual elementary bodies that continue the infective cycle.

The role of *Ehrlichia canis* as a major veterinary pathogen was seen during the Vietnam War, when the organism was found in an epizootic outbreak of tropical canine pancytopenia, which was responsible for the death of approximately 200 military dogs being used in southeast Asia.

Until the mid 1980s, known cases of human ehrlichiosis occurred mostly in Japan, with the mononucleosis-like sennetsu fever, caused by *Ehrlichia sennetsu.* These infections are rare, and details of the infection, including vectors and reservoirs, are unknown. *E. sennetsu,* which occurs in Japan and Malaysia, infects the host's monocytic cells. Patients infected with this organism are febrile and experience lymphadenopathy.

However, in the mid 1980s, a patient from Arkansas with a history of tick bites developed fever, myalgia, and thrombocytopenia. Peripheral blood smears from the patient had rickettsia-like organisms. The preliminary diagnosis indicated a rickettsial infection even though the patient did not have significant titers to rickettsia. Sera from the patient were ultimately tested using antigens from four species of *Ehrlichia.* The sera were strongly positive for *E. canis.* Subsequent prospective and retrospec-

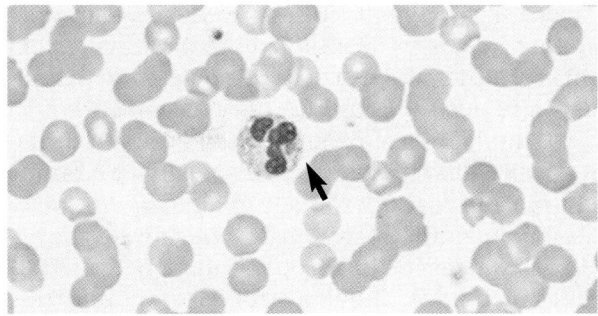

Figure 34-17

Ehrlichia sp. in an infected white blood cell

tive studies indicated that approximately 10% of all patients diagnosed with rickettsial fevers despite negative serologies had high titers to *E. canis.*

It is possible that the causative organism is not *E. canis,* but rather an antigenically related undescribed species. It infects lymphocytic or myelocytic cells in the host (Figure 34-17) and causes a disease similar to other rickettsioses, including fever, anorexia, and rash.

The vector for the infection has not yet been determined, although the vector seems to be a tick, possibly *A. americanum.*

Clinical manifestations

Human ehrlichiosis resembles Rocky Mountain spotted fever in that the patients are febrile, experience myalgia, and are anorexic. Unlike patients with other rickettsial infections, ehrlichiosis patients can be leukopenic, anemic, and thrombocytopenic. However, about 20% of ehrlichiosis patients have rashes. The form of the rash is variable, appearing as maculopapular, vesicular, or petechial. The rash usually appears on the trunk, arms, or legs. The incubation period of the disease ranges from 1 to 21 days.

Laboratory diagnosis

Most clinical laboratories do not have the facilities or the means to culture specimens for rickettsiae. Molecular diagnostics can be used to detect the presence of the rickettsiae in tissues, but these tests are still available only in research laboratories. However, most laboratories can perform more routine serologic tests to determine whether a patient has a rickettsial infection.

One well-known, simple, but insensitive and non-specific test is the Weil-Felix agglutination test. In this test, the patient's sera are reacted with antigens of *Proteus vulgaris* OX19, OX2, and OXK.

A simple test, more specific and sensitive than the Weil-Felix, is a commercially available latex agglutination test for the serodiagnosis of Rocky Mountain spotted fever and typhus fever. The agglutination test does not differentiate between IgG and IgM, but IgM shows a stronger reaction. Thus a strong positive reaction from a single unpaired serum specimen might indicate active infection. The turn-around time for the test is less than 1 hour, and no complex equipment is needed for the procedure.

Also commercially available is a microimmunofluorescence test. Testing sera for IgG only may not help diagnosis, because the patient's IgG can remain relatively high for several years. Running both IgG and IgM tests can provide more specific information for diagnosis. For instance, in serial sera tests an increase in titer of both IgG and IgM is a good indication of active disease. A high IgG titer and a stable or decreasing IgM titer indicate a recent infection.

R. quintana can be isolated from blood cultures in the clinical laboratory using the lysis-centrifugation method. The organism forms tiny colonies on media containing whole blood when incubated in carbon dioxide. Growth may take up to 2 weeks.

Bibliography

Barbour AG, Hayes SF: Biology of *Borrelia* species, *Microbiol Rev* 50:381, 1986.

Brenner DJ et al: *Capnocytophaga canimorsus* (formerly CDC Group DF-2), a cause of septicemia following dogbite, and *C. cynodegmi* sp. nov., a cause of localized wound infection following dog bite, *J Clin Microbiol* 27:231, 1989.

Burgdorfer W, Hayes SF, Corwin D: Pathophysiology of the Lyme disease spirochete, *Borrelia burgdorferi,* in Ixodid ticks, *Rev Infect Dis* 11(suppl 6):S1442, 1989.

Davis JM, Broughton SJ: Prepatellar bursitis caused by *Brucella abortus* [letter], *Med J Aust* 165:460, 1996.

Goldstein EJC: Household pets and human infections, *Infect Dis Clin North Am* 5:117, 1991.

Gorby GL, Peacock JE Jr: *Erysipelothrix rhusiopathiae* endocarditis: microbiologic, epidemiologic, and clinical features of an occupational disease, *Rev Infect Dis* 10:317, 1988.

Hantson P et al: Fatal *Capnocytophaga canimorsus* septicemia in previously healthy women, *Ann Emerg Med* 20:126, 1991.

Harkness JR: Ehrlichiosis, *Infect Dis Clin North Am* 5:37, 1991.

Holden FA, McKay JC: Rat-bite fever; an occupational hazard, *Can Med Assoc J* 91:214, 1964.

Hsu HW, Finberg KW: Infections associated with animal exposure in two infants, *Rev Infect Dis* 11:108, 1989.

Lang JL: Catching the bug: how scientists found the cause of Lyme disease and why we're not out of the woods yet, *Conn Med* 53:357, 1989.

Levin RE: An unusual presentation of Lyme arthritis, *J Rheumatol* 16:1500, 1989.

Mallon E, McKee PH: Extraordinary case report: cutaneous anthrax, *Am J Dermatopathol* 19:79, 1997.

McCalmont C, Zanolli MD: Rickettsial diseases, *Dermatol Clin* 7:591, 1989.

McDade JE: Ehrlichiosis: a disease of animals and humans, *J Infect Dis* 161:609, 1990.

McEnvoy MB, Noah ND, Pilsworth R: Outbreak of fever caused by *Streptobacillus moniliformis, Lancet* 2:361, 1987.

Raffi F et al: *Pasteurella multocida* bacteremia: report of 13 cases over 12 years and review of the literature, *Scand J Infect Dis* 19:385, 1987.

Ramadass P et al: DNA relatedness among strains of *Leptospira biflexa, Int J Syst Bacteriol* 40(3):231, 1990.

Reboli AC, Farrar WE: *Erysipelothrix rhusiopathiae*: an occupational pathogen, *Clin Microbiol Rev* 2:354, 1989.

Rikihisa Y: The tribe Ehrlichieae and ehrlichial diseases, *Clin Microbiol Rev* 4:286, 1991.

Saltoglu N et al: Leptospirosis: twelve Turkish patients with the Weil syndrome, *Acta Med Okayama* 51:339, 1997.

Sanford JP, Gilbert DN, Gerberding JL, Sande MA: *Guide to antimicrobial therapy,* ed 23, Dallas, 1994, Antimicrobial Therapy Inc.

Sawyer LA, Fishbein DB, McDade JE: Q fever: current concepts, *Rev Infect Dis* 9:935, 1987.

Schmid GP: Epidemiology and clinical similarities of human spirochetal diseases, *Rev Infect Dis* 11(suppl 6):S1460, 1989.

Simpson FG, Green KA, Haug GJ, Brookes DL: Leptospirosis associated with severe pulmonary haemorrhage in Far North Queensland, *Med J Aust* 169:151, 1998.

Taylor JP et al: Serological evidence of possible human infection with *Ehrlichia* in Texas, *J Infect Dis* 158:217, 1988.

Thalhammer F, Eberl G, Kopetzki-Kogler U: Unusual route of transmission for *Brucella abortus, Clin Infect Dis* 26:763-764, 1998.

Tzianobos T, Anderson BE, McDade JE: Detection of *Rickettsia rickettsii* DNA in clinical specimens by using polymerase chain reaction technology, *J Clin Microbiol* 27:2966, 1989.

Van Eys GJ et al: Detection of leptospires in urine by polymerase chain reaction, *J Clin Microbiol* 27:2258, 1989.

Weber DJ, Walker DH: Rocky Mountain spotted fever, *Infect Dis Clin North Am* 5:19, 1991.

Yang CWA et al: Leptospirosis: an ignored cause of acute renal failure in Taiwan, *Am J Kidney Dis* 30:840, 1997.

Zaki S, Shieh W-J: Leptospirosis associated with outbreak of acute febrile illness and pulmonary haemorrhage, Nicaragua, 1995, *Lancet* 347:535, 1996.

LEARNING ASSESSMENTS

1. Special problems are posed by toxin-producing organisms. Toxins may remain even after organisms are killed. Antibiotics have no effect on the toxin. What are some other toxin-producing organisms besides anthrax?

2. Why are horsehair shoe brushes sterilized?

3. *Brucella* organisms are one reason dairy products are pasteurized. What other organisms can be sources of diseases from contaminated dairy products?

4. What other activities are often considered risk factors associated with tularemia?

5. Hindsight is always perfect. Using your perfect historical vision, in the case of the plague on p. 1055, what do you think might have made a difference in this case report?

6. If you wish to recover by culture the agent of leptospirosis, what types of culture media may be used?

7. What is the most serious clinical manifestation that may occur in leptospirosis?

8. How do rickettsiae differ from other bacterial species?

9. What are the different types of clinical infections rickettsiae produce?

10. How does *Coxiella burnetti* infection "Q fever" differ from other rickettsial infections?

CHAPTER 35

Ocular Infections

Darlene Miller

OCULAR STRUCTURES
  Conjunctiva
  Lids
  Cornea
  Sclera
  Orbit
  Lacrimal Apparatus
  Anterior Chamber
  Vitreous Chamber
  Uveal Tract
  Retina

PATHOGENESIS OF OCULAR INFECTIONS

USUAL OCULAR FLORA

INFECTIONS OF THE CONJUNCTIVAE
  (CONJUNCTIVITIS)
  Bacteria
    Acute bacterial conjunctivitis
    Chronic bacterial conjunctivitis
    Chlamydial ocular infections
  Viruses
    Acute viral conjunctivitis
    Chronic viral conjunctivitis
  Rickettsia
  Fungi
  Parasites

INFECTIONS OF THE LIDS (BLEPHARITIS)
  Bacteria
  Viruses
  Fungi
  Parasites

INFECTIONS OF THE CORNEA (KERATITIS)
  Bacteria
  Viruses
  Fungi
  Parasites

INFECTIONS OF THE SCLERA AND EPISCLERA
  (SCLERITIS AND EPISCLERITIS)

INFECTIONS OF THE ORBIT (PRESEPTAL AND
  ORBITAL CELLULITIS)

INFECTIONS OF THE LACRIMAL APPARATUS

INFECTIONS OF THE INTRAOCULAR CHAMBERS
  (ENDOPHTHALMITIS)
  Bacteria

INFECTIONS OF THE UVEAL TRACT (UVEITIS)

INFECTIONS OF THE RETINA (RETINITIS)
  Viruses
  Parasites

SCLERAL BUCKLE INFECTIONS

OCULAR MANIFESTATIONS IN PATIENTS WITH
  HUMAN IMMUNODEFICIENCY VIRUS

LABORATORY DIAGNOSIS OF OCULAR
  INFECTIONS
  Specimen Collection
  Direct Smear Examination
  Culture
  Special Procedures for Recovering Ocular
    Pathogens
      Limulus lysate
      Agar-agar medium
      Trypticase soy broth
      Sabouraud agar with gentamycin
      Blood culture bottles
  Special Culture Techniques
      Contaminated ocular medications
      Contact lenses and solutions
      Cornea storage media and tissue culture

OCULAR THERAPY

OBJECTIVES

1. Provide a brief overview of ocular microbiology.
2. Identify ocular structures and their role in health and disease.
3. Describe the role of normal ocular flora.
4. Identify common ocular infections.
5. Describe laboratory procedures for the recovery and identification of ocular pathogens.
6. Review ocular therapeutic regimens.
7. Outline unique ocular procedures.
8. Interpret ocular culture results.

KEY TERMS

Conjunctivitis
Blepharitis
Keratitis
Endophthalmitis
Epidemic
   keratoconjunctivitis
   (EKC)
Scleritis
Dacryoadenitis
Dacryocystitis
Uveitis
Retinitis
Chorioretinitis

CASE STUDY

A healthy 20-year-old woman with no history of ocular disease had been wearing disposable contact lenses for 3 months. She replaced them every 7 to 10 days. The patient developed blurred vision, pain, photophobia, and redness in her right eye during the twelfth week. An examination revealed edema and four small ulcers with a green, mucopurulent discharge. Cultures were performed from corneal scrapings and the contact lens and solution.

The spectrum of ocular infections encompasses the relatively mild episodes of **conjunctivitis** and **blepharitis** (inflammation of the edges of the eyelids) to the more severe and sight-threatening conditions of **keratitis** and **endophthalmitis** (inflammation of the inside of the eye). Adnexal areas and the sclera, lacrimal system, and bony orbit are also subject to microbial invasion. Any organism capable of gaining entrance to ocular structures can cause disease. Bacteria, fungi, viruses, and protozoa all play prominent roles in the pathogenesis of ocular disease.

This chapter will do the following:

- Describe the different ocular structures and their functions.
- Discuss the role of normal flora in protecting ocular structures.
- Describe the common ocular infections and their causative agents.
- Describe the laboratory procedures for recovery and identification of ocular pathogens.
- Discuss ocular therapeutic regimens.

OCULAR STRUCTURES

Figure 35-1 outlines the most important ocular structures. The visual system comprises the eyeball, muscles, fat, nerves, orbital bones, and neural pathways that carry and translate electrical impulses into vision. This system does not actually "see" but rather acts as a receptor for sensory light stimuli that are translated to neural impulses by the retina and then processed by the occipital lobe of the brain. In a sense, the eye is a frontal extension of the brain.

Conjunctiva

The conjunctiva is essentially a mucous membrane, similar to those in the mouth and nose. It lines the upper and lower lids and constitutes the

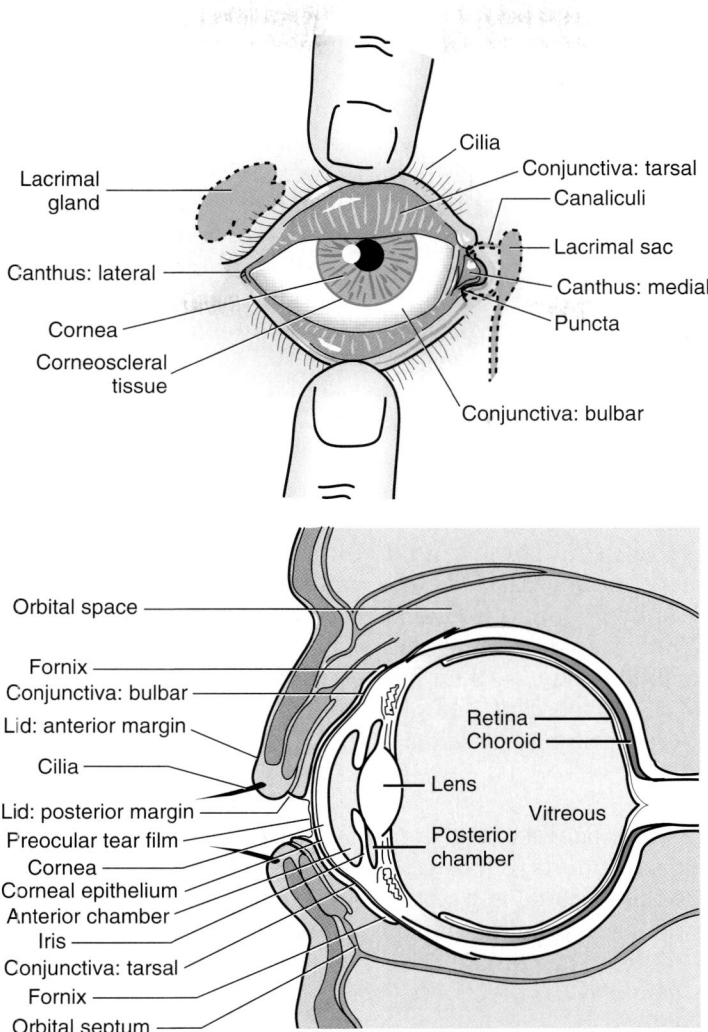

Figure 35-1

Common ocular structures. (Modified from Jones DB, Leisegang TJ, Robinson NM: Laboratory diagnosis of ocular infections. In Washington JA, editor: *CUMITECH 13,* Washington DC, 1981, American Society for Microbiology.)

frontline defense against invading organisms. The tears that keep the conjunctiva moist contain many enzymes and other factors (e.g., immunoglobulin G [IgG], immunogloblin M [IgM], β-lysin) that are antimicrobial.

Lids

The eyelids are thin, elastic layers, or folds, of tissue that help protect the structures of the orbit. They are the thinnest skin covering in the body. The blinking actions of the lids and conjunctivae help keep the cornea and sclera lubricated as well as sweep away debris and potential pathogens. The cilia, or lashes, act as a filtering and monitoring system to also alert the brain to potentially harmful agents.

Cornea

The cornea is considered the "window" of the eye. Its size and function are similar to those of a crystal on a wristwatch. The internal structures can be viewed through the cornea. The function of the curved corneal surface is to refract, collect, and focus light onto the retina. A layer of tears (the tear film) blankets the cornea to provide optical clarity, lubrication, and nutrition. Many free nerve endings are located in the corneal epithelium. When there is a break in or an injury to the epithelium, the patient usually complains of considerable pain. Infections of and injury to the cornea are considered true ocular emergencies.

Sclera

Known as the "white of the eye," the sclera protects and provides structural support to the internal ocular structures. It consists of tough, interlacing collagen fibers, which gives it an opaque appearance.

Orbit

The "closed-box" structure of the bony orbit protects the soft tissues of the eye. The pyramid-shaped bones are connected on several sides with the maxillary, ethmoid, sphenoid, and frontal sinuses. The ocular structures actually occupy only about one fifth of the orbital cavity, with fat and muscle filling the rest of the space. This unit protects the internal structures from blunt trauma.

Lacrimal Apparatus

The lacrimal gland, tear sac, accessory glands, canaliculi, puncta (lacrimal points), and nasolacrimal duct constitute the lacrimal apparatus. The function of this system is to provide tears to lubricate the epithelial lining of the conjunctivae, cornea, and sclera. The tears play a protective role in warding off potential pathogens. When one area of this system is clogged, the resulting malfunction may result in too many or too few tears, exposed epithelium, or gross swelling of the lids. All these conditions can lead to infection.

Anterior Chamber

The anterior chamber is the fluid-filled (aqueous humor) chamber at the front of the eye, divided by the iris into anterior and posterior cavities. Its function is to maintain the intraocular pressure. When the production of aqueous humor alters, glaucoma may result. The matrix of the aqueous humor is similar to that of the serum.

Vitreous Chamber

Filled with a gelatinous material (comprising 99% water, collagen fibers, and hyaluronic acid), the vitreous chamber makes up about two thirds of the volume of the eye. The function of the vitreous humor is to maintain the elliptical shape of the eyeball. The vitreous chamber has no blood, and once it is invaded the vitreous fluid serves as a magnificent culture medium for the growth of microorganisms. Once the vitreous humor has been lost, it is not replaced naturally. Treatment of vitreous loss involves injection of saline, gas, or aqueous humor into the vitreous chamber to preserve the spherical shape of the eyeball. If this medium was not replaced, the eye would collapse.

Uveal Tract

The uveal tract, consisting of the iris, ciliary body, and choroid, is the middle layer of the ocular system. The ciliary body produces the aqueous humor that fills the chamber at the front of the eye. The iris is an extension of the ciliary body and divides this chamber into the anterior and posterior cavities. It is attached to the lens and controls the amount of light that enters the eye. The choroid is predominantly composed of blood vessels and functions to nourish the retina.

Retina

The retina is the light-sensitive neural tissue of the eye. It is multilayered and functions as a receptor of the light stimuli, transcribing these into electrical impulses and then sending these impulses along the optic nerve to the brain.

PATHOGENESIS OF OCULAR INFECTIONS

Because of their location, external ocular structures such as the conjunctivae and cornea are frequently challenged by a variety of microorganisms. Whether an infection or damage ensues depends on the underlying condition of the structure and the character of the invading organism.

The intact epithelia of the external structures provide a protective barrier against invasion by most microorganisms. However a few microbes can invade and penetrate the intact epithelium of the conjunctiva or cornea, including *Neisseria gonorrhoeae, Neisseria meningitidis, Streptococcus pneumoniae, Listeria monocytogenes,* and *Corynebacterium diphtheriae.* For other microbes to enter and establish disease, a break must occur in the protective barrier. Once this barricade is breached (e.g., by trauma, by insertion or removal of a contact lens) an intrusion by pathogenic and saprophytic organisms can occur. When an infection has started in one layer of the eye, the spread to adjacent layers and tissues can occur quite rapidly. Such spreading also can result in devastating and permanent damage to the functional integrity of the eye.

Protection of ocular structures is partly caused by a defense system that embraces local and systemic, specific and nonspecific, and humoral and cellular mechanisms that join together to prevent microbial colonization or invasion. Protection of these structures also partly is caused by an anatomic arrangement that leaves the inner ocular structures very well sequestered.

Box 35-1 provides a list of organisms recovered from ocular infections. The list is long and varied. Any organism that can gain entrance to the internal structures of the eye is capable of causing infection. The eye does not exist in a vacuum, and many systemic illnesses, such as tuberculosis, diabetes, hypertension, and acquired immunodeficiency syndrome (AIDS), also have symptoms of ocular manifestations. The organism most likely

---

Box 35-1

Organisms Associated with Ocular Infectious Disease

Bacteria

Gram-negative (aerobic)
Haemophilus influenzae
Haemophilus aegyptius
Haemophilus parainfluenzae
Neisseria gonorrhoeae
Neisseria meningitidis
Moraxella catarrhalis
Moraxella species
Moraxella lacunata
Pseudomonas aeruginosa
Other pseudomonads
Enterobacteriaceae
Eikenella corrodens
Flavobacterium species
Kingella species
Aeromonas hydrophila
Actinobacillus actinomycetemcomitans
Brucella species
Achromobacter xylosoxidans
Treponema pallidum
Cat-scratch bacillus
Francisella tularensis
Borrelia tularensis
Borrelia burgdorferi (Lyme disease)

Gram-positive (aerobic)
Staphylococcus aureus
Streptococcus pneumoniae
Enterococcus faecalis
Enterococcus species
Viridans streptococcal group
β-Hemolytic streptococci (A, B, C, F, G)

Corynebacterium species
Staphylococcus epidermidis
Coagulase-negative staphylococci species
Mycobacterium tuberculosis
Mycobacterium fortuitum
Mycobacterium chelonae
Mycobacterium leprae
MOTT
Listeria monocytogenes
Bacillus cereus
Bacillus species, other
Micrococcus species

Gram-negative (anaerobic)
Capnocytophaga species
Fusobacterium species
Bacteroides species

Gram-positive (anaerobic)
Propionibacterium acnes
Actinomyces israelii
Actinomyces species
Peptostreptococcus species
Clostridium species
Propionibacterium propionicus
Chlamydia trachomatis
Chlamydia psittaci
Chlamydia pneumoniae
Rickettsia prowazekii
Rickettsia tsutsugamushi
Rickettsia rickettsii
Rickettsia akari
Coxiella burnetii

MOTT, Mycobacteria other than tubercle bacilli.

Continued

Box 35-1

Organisms Associated with Ocular Infectious Disease—cont'd

Parasites

Acanthamoeba species
Microsporidia species
Toxoplasma gondii
Loa loa
Onchocerca volvulus
Wuchereria bancrofti
Oestrus ovis
Taenia solium
Toxocara canis and *cati*
Trypanosoma species
Leishmania species
Ascaris lumbricoides
Schistosoma haematobium
Phthirus pubis
Fly larvae
Trichinella spiralis
Plasmodium (malaria)
Vahlkampfia species

Viruses

Herpes simplex virus types 1 and 2
Adenovirus
Enterovirus
Coxsackievirus
Cytomegalovirus
Varicella-zoster virus
Epstein-Barr virus
Human papilloma virus
Measles virus
Molluscum contagiosum virus
Vaccinia virus
Mumps virus
Newcastle disease virus
Human immunodeficiency virus
Influenza virus

Fungi

Candida albicans
Candida species, other *C. albicans*
Cryptococcus neoformans
Coccidioides immitis
Acremonium species
Alternaria species
Aspergillus species
Bipolaris species
Blastomyces dermatitidis
Cladosporium species
Colleotrichum species
Curvularia species
Cylindrocarpon species
Drechslera species
Exophiala jeanselmei
Fusarium solani
Fusarium oxysporum
Fusarium species
Helminthosporium species
Histoplasma capsulatum
Lasiodiplodia species
Neurospora species
Paecilomyces species
Penicillium species
Phialophora species
Scedosporium apiospermum
Sporothrix schenckii
Torulopsis glabrata
Volutella species
Zygomycetes
Nocardia species
Streptomyces species

to be encountered depends on the season, climate, age of the patient, and underlying disease.

USUAL OCULAR FLORA

Of the flora cultured from uninflamed eyes, 80% to 90% consists of coagulase-negative staphylococcal species and diphtheroids. However, depending on the age of the patient, season, location, and underlying conditions, *Staphylococcus aureus, S. pneumoniae, Haemophilus influenzae,* and other poten-

tial pathogens may be recovered from uninfected eyes (Table 35-1). It is important to know the usual ocular flora to better evaluate ocular culture results. The presence of a resident flora on the conjunctivae and lids acts as a protective mechanism, inhibiting invasion and colonization by more harmful organisms. Early studies by Halbert indicated that some ocular flora possessed substances that inhibited the growth of other species. It is important to remember that once the epithelium of the conjunctiva or cornea is compromised, any organism gaining entrance can result in disease.

TABLE 35-1 ————————
Microbes Isolated from Uninfected Eyes

Organisms*	Incidence (%)
Coagulase-negative staphylococci†	34-94
Propionibacterium acnes†	40-86
Corynebacterium species†	3-83
Staphylococcus aureus	0-30
Haemophilus influenzae	0-25
Micrococcus species	2-22
Streptococcus pneumoniae	0-5
Viridans streptococcal group	0-12
Gram-negative rods (*Proteus* species, *Escherichia coli, Klebsiella pneumoniae, Enterobacter* species)	0-5
Moraxella species (including *Moraxella catarrhalis*)	0-3
Bacillus species (*Bacillus cereus, Bacillus subtilis*)	0-4
Neisseria species (*Neisseria sicca, Neisseria flavescens*)	0-7
Fungi (any saprophyte, depends on locale)	0-24
Anaerobic flora other than *Propionibacterium acnes* (*Peptostreptococcus* species, *Bacteroides* species, *Clostridium* species)	1-5
β-Hemolytic streptococci, including *Streptococcus pyogenes*	0-3

*Source is usually the conjunctivae and lids; organism isolated depends on age of patient, geographic locale, season, previous and current therapy, and underlying condition (e.g., diabetes, epithelial disease). Most common isolates usually reflect that of the surrounding tissue.
†Can also cause mild to severe disease in immunocompromised patients.

INFECTIONS OF THE CONJUNCTIVAE (CONJUNCTIVITIS)

Inflammation of the conjunctival tissue with resultant dilation of the blood vessels, or red eye, is the most common ocular symptom. Red eye constitutes more than 50% of the complaints that prompt patients to consult an ophthalmologist; samples from patients with red eye are also the most common samples submitted for microbiologic evaluation. Conjunctivitis may be acute or chronic. The etiologic agents are usually bacterial or viral, although some patients have fungal or parasitic infections.

Bacteria
Acute bacterial conjunctivitis
In adults in warm climates, *S. aureus* is the most frequently isolated pathogen, whereas *S. pneumoniae* may be the most common isolate in areas with cooler temperatures. *H. influenzae, S. aureus, S. pneumoniae* and other *Streptococcus* species, and members of the Enterobacteriaceae are the most frequently isolated organisms from infants and children with acute conjunctivitis. *N. gonorrhoeae* (Figure 35-2) and *N. meningitidis* initiate a hyperacute conjunctivitis that produces huge amounts of exudate that runs down the face of the patient. Infants acquire *N. gonorrhoeae* as they travel down an infected birth canal. The disease's symptoms may appear within 5 to 7 days after exposure to the pathogen. It is believed that adults acquire gonococcal conjunctivitis through self-inoculation. Meningococcal conjunctivitis may result from contiguous spread from the respiratory tract. Penicillin-resistant ocular isolates reflect the trend in each community. Penicillin remains the drug of choice for *N. meningitidis*.

Chronic bacterial conjunctivitis
The etiologic agents in chronic conjunctivitis are less clear. The microorganisms that have been isolated include coagulase-negative staphylococcal species, *S. aureus,* and *Propionibacterium acnes.* Chronic conjunctivitis may be caused by an interaction between the organism and the aggressive ocular immune response.

Bacterial conjunctivitis can also be caused by instillation of contaminated cosmetics or medications. The organisms encountered in such infections are *S. aureus, Staphylococcus epidermidis, Corynebacterium* species, *Pseudomonas aeruginosa,* and *Proteus mirabilis.* Allergic and chemical conjunctivitis can sometimes be confused with microbial infections. Laboratory tests can be of assistance in confirming the diagnosis.

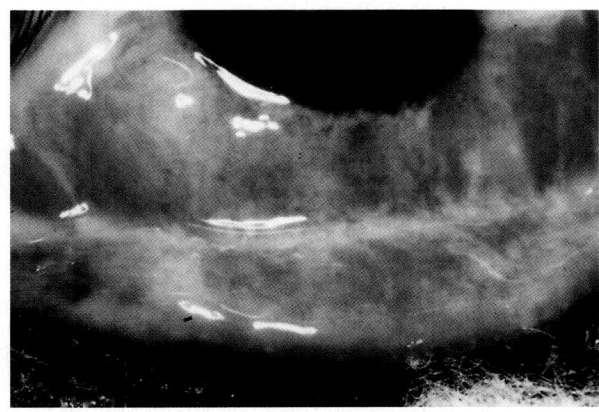

Figure 35-2 ————————
Gonococcal conjunctivitis. Note the copious discharge in response to invasion by *Neisseria gonorrhoeae.*

Routine culture and smears from conjunctival scrapings should reveal the etiologic agent in most acute cases. Culture and smears may be of less value in establishing the etiologic agent in chronic conjunctivitis. Therapy depends on the isolated organism.

Chlamydial ocular infections

Chlamydia trachomatis causes myriad ocular infections, including neonatal conjunctivitis, inclusion conjunctivitis (Figure 35-3, *A*), lymphogranuloma venereum (LGV), and trachoma. Currently fifteen serotypes (A, B, Ba, C through K, L_1 through L_3), or serovars, of *C. trachomatis* exist. Certain serovars are associated with certain clinical enti-

ties. Trachoma, which is "as old as recorded history," is usually caused by serotypes A, B, or C, whereas immunotypes D to K are usually associated with oculogenital (inclusion conjunctivitis) chlamydiae. Neonatal conjunctivitis occurs when the infant is infected while traveling down a contaminated birth canal. Infection becomes apparent within 8 to 10 days. LGV (serotypes LGV 1, 2, 3) is strictly a sexually transmitted disease (STD) and conjunctival inoculation is accidental.

Direct detection of the chlamydial inclusions or elementary bodies in scrapings or on impression cytology membranes is among the most sensitive methods for confirming ocular chlamydia (see Figure 35-3, *B*). Figure 35-3, *C* shows the percentage of

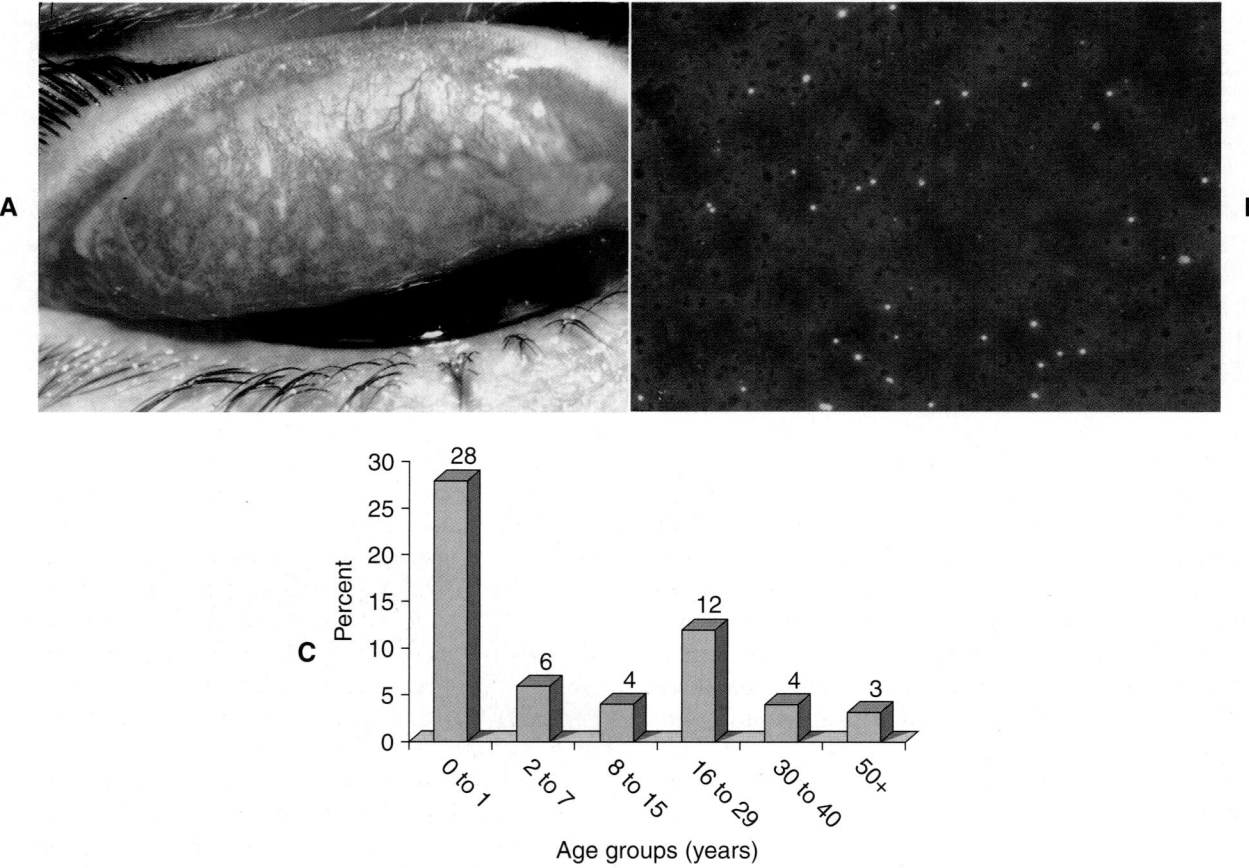

Figure 35-3

A, White spots on conjunctiva represent pockets of *Chlamydia* organisms in tissue. **B,** Immunofluorescence stain of scrapings from neonatal conjunctivitis, confirming the presence of chlamydial elementary bodies. **C,** Age-specific, culture-positive ocular chlamydia. (Data from Miller D: *Comparison of laboratory detection methods and identification of risk factors associated with ocular chlamydia,* MPH thesis, University of Miami, 1997.)

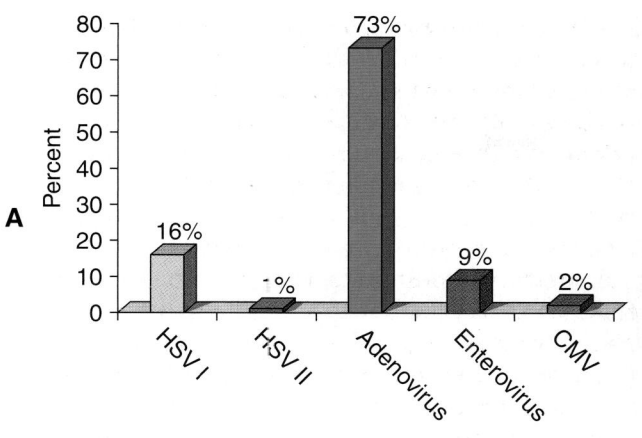
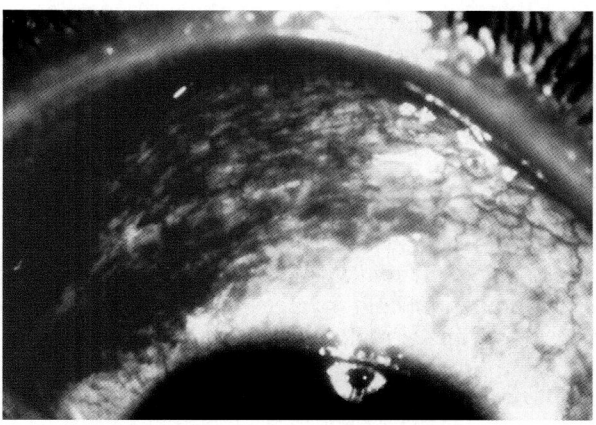

A

B

Figure 35-4

A, Frequency of conjunctival viral isolates. *HSV,* Herpes simplex virus; *CMV,* cytomegalovirus. **B,** Acute hemorrhagic conjunctivitis. The etiologic agent is usually enterovirus 70 or coxsackie virus A24. Other members of the enterovirus group may also be recovered. Note the heavy conjunctival hemorrhaging. (Data from Perez E, Miller D, Diaz M et al: Emerging trends among viral isolates. Presented at American Society for Microbiology Annual Meeting, Miami Beach, Fla, 1991.)

age-specific culture positive ocular chlamydia. Cultures using McCoy or Hep-2 cells may be used to confirm the diagnosis, especially in cases of suspected trachoma. Other nonculture detection methods—polymerase chain reaction (PCR), ligand chain reaction (LCR), and enzyme immunoassay (EIA)—may also be used to detect ocular chlamydia, but culture remains the gold standard. A combination of smear and culture with either PCR, LCR, or EIA may offer the best system in populations with high and low rates of STD and in areas where trachoma remains endemic.

The prevalence rates for ocular chlamydial infection parallel those of genital disease. In areas with high rates of STD, ocular disease rates are also high. Populations with the highest incidence of disease include neonates and sexually active adolescents and adults. The incidence can range from 20% to 90%, depending on the age group. In areas with low rates of STD, ocular chlamydial infection rates also are low. Topical treatment alone is inadequate. Current Centers for Disease Control (CDC) treatment recommendations are as follows:

▪ *Adults*—doxycycline: 100 mg twice a day for 7 days or azithromycin: 1 g by mouth as a single dose
▪ *Neonates*—erythromycin syrup: 50 mg/kg/d by mouth in 4 doses for 14 days

Viruses

Viral conjunctivitis is the most common or recognized ocular disease. It too may present as an acute or chronic illness, ranging from a mild, self-limiting condition to a severe, destructive disease resulting in impaired vision.

Acute viral conjunctivitis

Acute viral infections are attributed mainly to adenoviruses, herpesviruses, or enteroviruses. Figure 35-4, *A,* shows the frequency of conjunctival viral isolates. The adenoviruses are responsible for two distinct ocular viral syndromes.

The first, **epidemic keratoconjunctivitis (EKC),** is quite contagious and associated with adenovirus types 8 and 19, but recovery of serovars 7, 9, 10, 11, 14, and 16 has also been documented. The second syndrome, pharyngoconjunctival fever (PCF), is caused regularly by adenovirus type 3 and occasionally by serovars 1, 2, 4, 5, 6, 8, and 14. Both syndromes are self-limiting and have no specific treatment; PCF lasts about 10 days, and EKC, 3 to 4 weeks at the most. A highly contagious disease, EKC may be spread by direct contact or fomites and is not uncommonly spread by physicians. It is usually responsible for outbreaks in ophthalmic offices and clinics, school locker rooms, or college dormitories.

Acute hemorrhagic conjunctivitis (AHC) (see Figure 35-4, *B*), or epidemic hemorrhagic conjunctivitis (EHC), is an acute short-lived infection that is caused by enterovirus 70, coxsackievirus A24, and on rare occasions, adenovirus type 11. It is often called the *Apollo XI conjunctivitis* because it was first recognized in Ghana during the time of the Apollo XI moon mission.

The onset of symptoms usually occurs within 8 to 48 hours of exposure, with patients complaining of pain, sensitivity to light, copious tears, and subconjunctival hemorrhages. It is self-limiting and has no outlined treatment program. Recovery occurs within 5 to 7 days. Because EHC is highly contagious and easily spread from person to person, patients should be isolated or sent home until the condition has resolved.

The most common viruses may be grown in tissue culture and serotyped by neutralization tests. Monoclonal antibodies are available for group-specific adenoviruses and several members of the enterovirus groups. These antibodies can be used for direct examination or culture confirmation.

Herpes simplex blepharoconjunctivitis is responsible for the majority of severe ocular viral infections. This disease usually occurs in young children. It is important to make the distinction between herpes simplex virus (HSV) and adenovirus etiologies, because HSV can be treated with specific ocular antiviral medications, whereas an adenovirus infection must run its course.

More than 90% of cases of this herpes simplex blepharoconjunctivitis are caused by HSV 1, but HSV 2 has been isolated from infants and adults. Varicella-zoster virus (VZV) may also cause conjunctivitis. This condition is usually a manifestation of the systemic disease chickenpox or a complication of herpes zoster ophthalmicus. Cytomegalovirus can usually cause conjunctivitis when it becomes disseminated or is transmitted through tears from another patient. Epstein-Barr virus conjunctivitis may result as a complication of infectious mononucleosis.

Chronic viral conjunctivitis

Chronic viral conjunctivitis may result from molluscum contagiosum or vaccinia, a complication of smallpox vaccination.

Rickettsia

All pathogenic human rickettsiae are capable of causing conjunctivitis. The conjunctiva is often the portal of entry for Rocky Mountain spotted fever, scrub typhus, Q fever, endemic murine typhus, and Marseilles fever. This type of conjunctivitis is usually mild but can be a severe complication of the systemic disease. Isolation of rickettsiae is quite difficult, and confirmation is by serologic methods. The most sensitive and specific tests for confirmation of rickettsial infection are microimmunofluorescence, microagglutination, and complement fixation. Treatment with chloramphenicol or tetracycline can inhibit rickettsial organisms long enough for the body to clear them from the system.

Fungi

Although various fungi can be isolated from the uninflamed eye, fungal conjunctivitis is relatively rare. The organisms that have been recovered from fungal conjunctivitis are *Candida* species and *Sporothrix schenckii*. Systemic fungal infections caused by *Coccidioides immitis, Histoplasma capsulatum,* and *Cryptococcus neoformans* may extend to the conjunctival tissue and cause disease. A high index of suspicion is needed by the physician to diagnose fungal conjunctivitis, and the laboratory must be alerted to ensure the proper set-up for recovery of these organisms.

Parasites

Ocular infestation by parasites is rare; the conjunctiva is among the least affected sites. Conjunctival involvement is usually a secondary complication.

Loa loa, the "eye worm," is one of the leading causes of blindness in West Africa (river blindness). Clinical symptoms are caused by the continued migration of the adult worms into the subcutaneous tissues and blood vessels. Onchocerciasis, which is transmitted by the bite of the blackfly, is also a leading cause of blindness in Africa and is now endemic in South and Central America. Ocular complications result from the discharge of large numbers of microfilariae by the adult female and their subsequent local invasion and tissue damage. Ophthalmyiasis ("fly larvae conjunctivitis" or ocular myiasis) is caused by the deposit of fly larvae (maggots) into the conjunctival sac. This infestation occurs frequently in the tropics but can occur wherever people and flies coexist. The maggots may be removed by paralyzing them with 10% cocaine and lifting them out with tweezers.

Detection of ocular parasites depends on observing and removing the actual protozoans and confirming their presence through histologic stains, isolating the organisms from blood or tissues, or confirming their presence by serologic means.

INFECTIONS OF THE LIDS (BLEPHARITIS)

Inflammation of the lid margins and inflammation of the conjunctivae are not mutually exclusive. Conjunctivitis usually presents as a blepharoconjunctivitis. Therefore any organism that causes conjunctivitis can affect the lids. However, each site has unique organisms and conditions. The skin covering of the lids is among the thinnest on the body. Any organisms capable of initiating skin infections can also cause blepharitis.

Bacteria

S. aureus and members of the coagulase-negative staphylococcal family are the most frequently isolated bacteria from the lid margins. Blepharitis involving these organisms is a low-grade inflammation usually associated with functional disease of the seborrheic glands (seborrheic blepharitis). In this mixed infection, dry (staphylococcal) and greasy (seborrheic) scales are attached to the lashes, with various areas of ulcerations that cause the lashes to fall out. Antibiotics are given to cure the staphylococcal disease. Because the scalp, eyebrows, and lids are all involved in seborrhiasis, all must be kept clean with a medicated shampoo.

Four types of glands are located in the lids: the meibomian gland, the glands of Moll and Zeis, and the accessory lacrimal glands. Acute infection of the glands of Zeis or Moll with staphylococci results in an external hordeolum (stye). A stye is an abscess with pus formation in the lumen of the affected gland. Hot soaks assist in the continuous drainage of the abscess. Topical erythromycin or tetracycline may be applied as supplementary therapy. An internal hordeolum caused by staphylococci is a little larger and affects the meibomian gland. Additional lid glandular disorders include formation of a chalazion, a sterile granulomatous inflammation of the meibomian gland that usually subsides spontaneously. Meibomianitis is inflammation of multiple glands; its etiology is unknown.

Box 35-2

Microbes Recovered from Patients with Blepharitis

Bacteria

Common isolates

Staphylococcus aureus
Staphylococcus epidermidis
Other coagulase-negative staphylococci
Group A beta *Streptococcus* species, other streptococci
Moraxella lacunata, Moraxella species, other

Rare isolates

Bacillus anthracis
Bacillus cereus
Treponema pallidum
Haemophilus ducreyi
Clostridium species
Actinomyces species
Mycobacterium tuberculosis
Mycobacterium leprae

Fungi (rare)

Candida species
Cryptococcus neoformans
Blastomyces dermatitidis
Dermatophytes (*Microsporum, Trichophyton, Epidermophyton* species)

Viruses

Herpes simplex virus types 1 and 2
Varicella-zoster virus
Molluscum contagiosum
Vaccinia
Papovavirus
Rabies (rare)

Parasites (very rare)

Phthirus species (crab louse)
Demodex folliculorum
Demodex brevis
Fly larvae (myiasis)

Only rarely does the laboratory receive a request for lid culture. If such a request is received, it is to confirm the presence of staphylococci and determine whether therapy is adequate.

Other microbial agents recovered from patients with blepharitis are listed in Box 35-2. *Bacillus anthracis* causes carbunclelike lesions on the lid margins, which are eradicated with penicillin. *Actino-*

myces species may spread from the facial skin to the lids. *Mycobacterium* species that cause ocular infections are listed in Box 35-3.

Viruses

Viral blepharitis may be caused by HSV 1 or 2, VZV, poxvirus, papovavirus, or vaccinia. HSV infection usually occurs during early childhood. Vesicles appear on the lid margins and the skin around the eye. The vesicles break open and form crusted secondary lesions, which then may become superinfected by skin organisms. Direct detection with immunofluorescence or immunoperoxidase can be done by scraping the base of a freshly opened vesicle. Vesicular fluids are collected for culture. Ninety-five percent or more of cultures grow HSV within 72 hours or less.

When the face is involved during episodes of chickenpox (varicella), vesicles may appear on the upper or lower lid margins. Molluscum contagiosum is a wartlike lesion of the lid margins that is produced by pox-virus. The lesion is waxy and pearly white with an umbilicated center. Expression (squeezing) of the white center to allow blood into the lesion is usually adequate management. Vaccinia infection of the lids results from direct inoculation from a smallpox vaccination. Other viruses that produce ocular warts are members of the papillomavirus family.

Fungi

Fungal blepharitis is quite rare and is usually a complication of systemic disease, especially involving *Candida* species and *Blastomyces dermatitidis.*

Parasites

Infestation of the lid margins by parasites is caused by complications and spread from adjacent structures. Parasitic lid complications may be observed in patients with cutaneous leishmaniasis, African or American trypanosomiasis, *L. loa* infections, and dirofilariasis. The crab, or pubic louse *(Phthirus pubis),* infests the cilia and lid margins of the eyelids. The patient's main complaint is pruritus, or itching. All members of the patient's family must be treated. Treatment consists of application of a 1% gamma benzene hexachloride (lindane) ointment or shampoo to the affected areas.

INFECTIONS OF THE CORNEA (KERATITIS)

Active invasion of the cornea by microorganisms is considered a true ocular emergency. The cornea contains five layers. Infection begins in the most superficial layer (the epithelium) and if not checked, it advances through the Bowman zone, the stroma, and the Descemet's membrane to the endothelium (the innermost layer). Many nerve fibers with bare ends are housed in the epithelium and when exposed, they produce severe pain. Even minor abrasions result in excruciating discomfort. Very few organisms can cross the intact corneal epithelium, but once it has been compromised any organism can launch an infection. Corneal stromal tissue provides an excellent culture medium for visiting microbes.

Bacteria

Geographic variations in the etiology of bacterial and fungal ulcers are evident (Figure 35-5, *A*). Historically, *P. aeruginosa,* the most frequent isolate recovered from contact-lens–associated keratitis (the condition described in the opening case study), constitutes up to 50% of the cases of keratitis reported in Florida. Meanwhile, this trend may be shifting toward *S. aureus. P. aeruginosa* as well as *S. aureus* can induce perforation or corneal melt, with resultant loss of the eye, within 24 to 48 hours (see Figures 35-5, *B* and *C*). These ker-

---

Box 35-3

MOTT Keratitis Isolates

Mycobacterium chelonae
Mycobacterium fortuitum
Mycobacterium avium-intracellulare
Mycobacterium nonchromogenicum
Mycobacterium triviale
Mycobacterium asiaticum
Mycobacterium gordonae
Mycobacterium mucogenicum

NOTE: *Mycobacterium tuberculosis* and *Mycobacterium leprae* are ocular pathogens and are usually an extension of systemic disease. Isolates are frequently recovered from patients who wear contact lenses, have a history of eye trauma from soil or water, or have had a radial keratotomy.

MOTT, Mycobacteria other than tubercle bacilli.

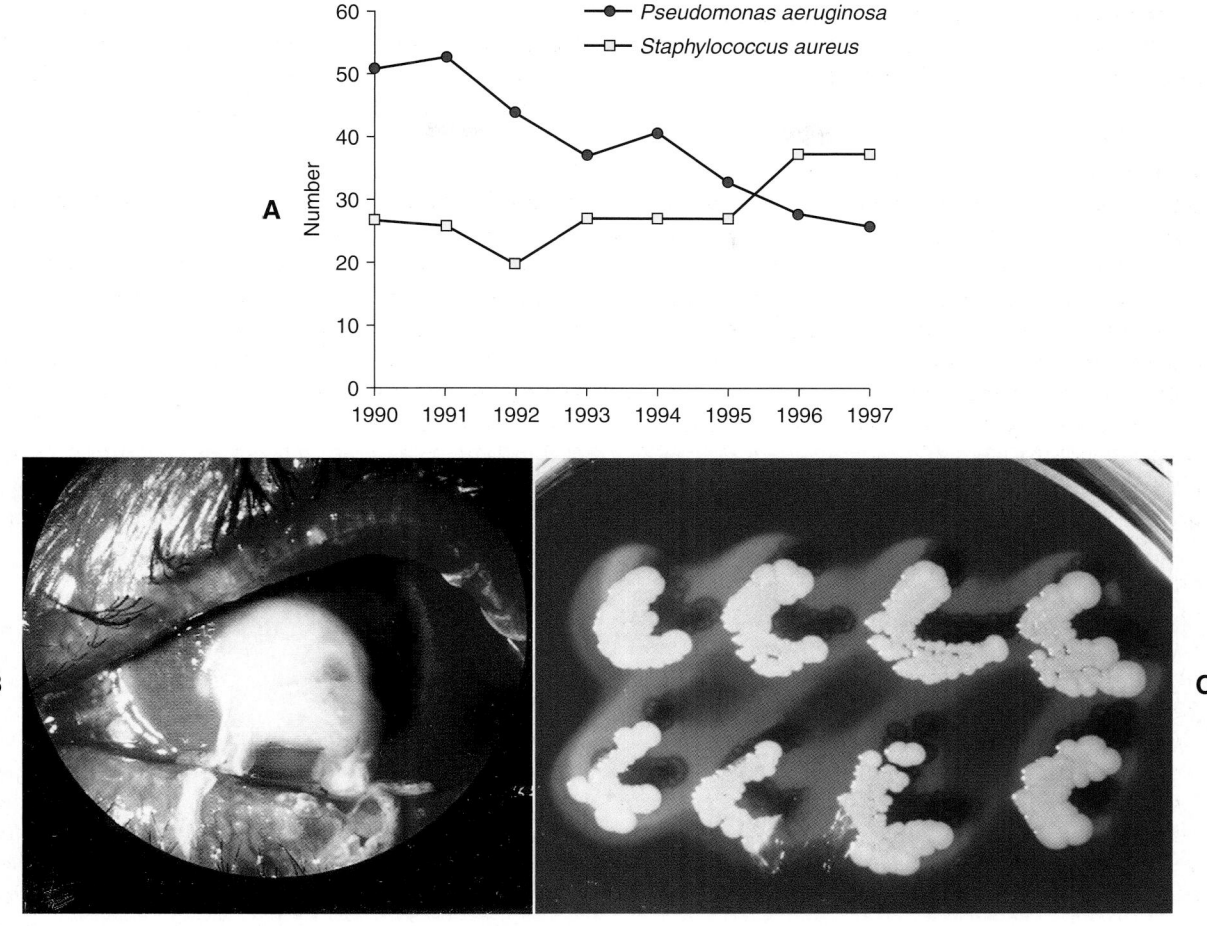

Figure 35-5

A, Trends in top keratitis isolates—south Florida. **B,** Corneal melt caused by bacterial invasion. **C,** C Streaks of *Staphylococcus aureus* from infected cornea. The enzymes produced by some strains of *S. aureus* and *Pseudomonas aeruginosa* can liquefy the cornea within 48 hours. (Data from Miller D, Alfonso E: Second International Congress on Ocular Infections, August, 1998, Munich, Germany.)

atitis cases include patients wearing soft, daily, extended-wear, and disposable contact lenses. Box 35-4 lists organisms recovered from contact lenses and lens solution (Figure 35-6, *A*). Figure 35-6, *B,* shows the recent trends in the types of bacteria recovered from contact lenses and solutions.

Mycobacteria other than tubercle bacilli (MOTT) are being isolated with increasing frequency (Figure 35-7). Ulcers that involve these organisms are both chronic and indolent and have been associated with trauma, contact lens wear, and wound contamination with soil and water. Less frequently encountered corneal isolates are listed in Box 35-5.

Laboratory assistance with diagnosis is mandatory in all cases of keratitis or suspected keratitis. Scrapings for smears and cultures are inoculated directly onto slides and culture plates and sent immediately to the laboratory for evaluation. Scrapings for stains can afford the physician an early indication of the offending organism and assist in the selection of appropriate therapy. The cornea may also be invaded via metastatic spread from the conjunctiva or systemic lesions.

Viruses

Among the viral agents of keratitis, HSV is the most common and severe. About 500,000 new cases of

Box 35-4

Microbes Recovered from Contaminated Contact Lenses and Solutions

Pseudomonas aeruginosa
Serratia marcescens
Achromobacter xylosoxidans
Enterobacteriaceae
Pseudomonads
Bacillus species
Staphylococcus aureus

Staphylococcus epidermidis
Mycobacterium chelonae, other Mycobacteria other than tubercle bacilli
Acanthamoeba species and other free-living ameba
Saprophytic fungi (*Curvularia, Aspergillus,* and *Candida* species)

Box 35-5

Etiologic Agents of Keratitis

Viral agents

Herpes simplex virus types 1 and 2
Varicella-zoster virus
Epstein-Barr virus
Enterovirus
Adenovirus
Measles
Mumps
Newcastle disease virus
Human immunodeficiency virus (tears and stroma)
Vaccinia

Fungal agents

Fusarium species (*Fusarium solani* and *Fusarium oxysporum*—most common)
Aspergillus species
Curvularia species
Paecilomyces species
Colleotrichum species
Alternaria species
Phialophora species
Cylindrocarpon species
Bipolaris
Acremonium species
Lasidiplodia threobromae
Pseudoallercheria boydii

Candida species (*Candida parapsilosis* and *Candida tropicalis*—most common)
Trichosporon beigelii

Bacterial agents

Gram negative isolates
Pseudomonas aeruginosa
Serratia marcescens
Proteus mirabilis
Haemophilus influenzae
Moraxella species

Gram positive isolates
Staphylococcus aureus
Streptococcus pneumoniae
Streptococcus viridans group
Corynebacterium species
Staphylococcus epidermidis and other coagulase-negative staphylococci

Uncommon keratitis isolates
Nocardia species
Capnocytophaga species
Propionibacterium acnes
Neisseria gonorrhoeae

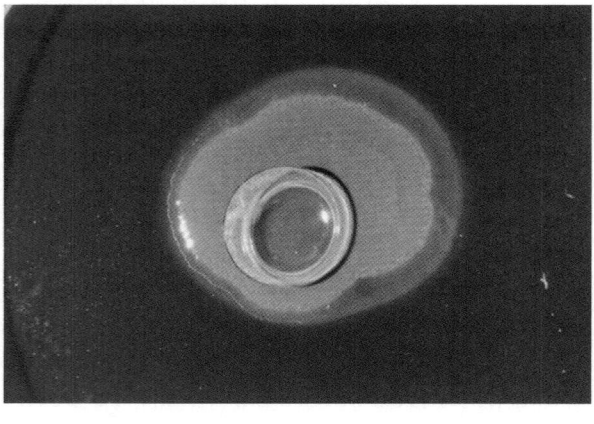

A

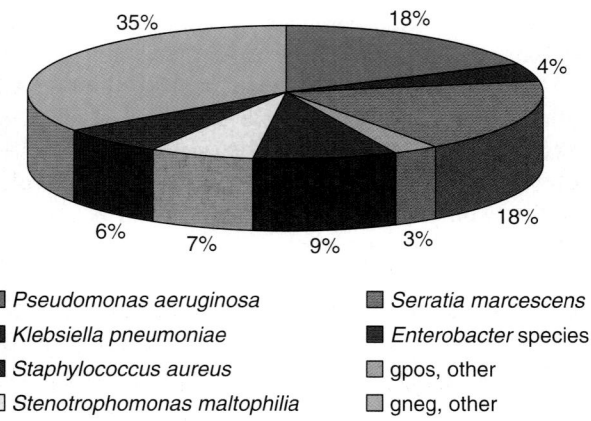

B

- ■ *Pseudomonas aeruginosa*
- ■ *Klebsiella pneumoniae*
- ■ *Staphylococcus aureus*
- □ *Stenotrophomonas maltophilia*
- ■ *Serratia marcescens*
- ■ *Enterobacter* species
- ■ gpos, other
- ■ gneg, other

Figure 35-6

A, Growth of *Pseudomonas aeruginosa* from daily-wear (soft) contact lens. Patient had an ulcerative keratitis. The corneal culture also grew *P. aeruginosa.* **B,** Recent trends in bacteria recovered from contact lenses and solutions.

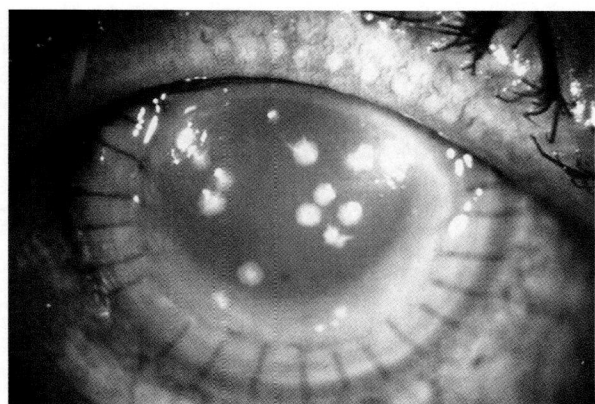

Figure 35-7

Colonies of *Mycobacterium fortuitum* growing on infected corneal graft tissue.

ocular disease caused by herpes simplex occur annually. Keratitis infection caused by HSV may result from direct inoculation or reactivation of latent virus in the trigeminal ganglion. The majority of the ocular lesions are caused by HSV-1, but HSV-2 has been recovered from cases involving both infants and adults. Figure 35-8 shows the frequency of common keratitis viral isolates. The lesions caused by these two are indistinguishable. Treatment includes debridement when possible and topical antivirals. Other viral agents that cause keratitis are listed in Box 35-5.

Fungi

Opportunistic or saprophytic organisms are most often recovered from fungal infections of the cornea. This is the rule rather than the exception. The patient commonly has some history of trauma involving soil or plant material. All cases of fungal keratitis must be confirmed by the laboratory. Fungal keratitis agents are shown in Box 35-5.

Samples for culture must be collected from multiple scraping of the involved actively advancing edges of the ulcer. Sometimes a biopsy is necessary to isolate the fungi. Giemsa and calcofluor white preparations from scrapings can confirm hyphal elements or budding yeast. Antifungal therapy can be instituted once the fungal etiology has been established. Topical antifungals include amphotericin B, natamycin, nystatin, and imidazoles compounds. Selection depends on the organism.

Parasites

Infection of the cornea by free-living amebae (e.g., *Acanthamoeba, Naegleria,* and *Vahlkampfia* species) is a devastating consequence of injury or insult from contaminated water, contact lenses, or soil, as identified in the case study. *Acanthamoeba* species are the most frequent isolates. Homemade saline solution associated with contact lens wear was the original identified risk factor. This factor seems to play a lesser role in the diagnosis of amebic keratitis. Amebic keratitis is often mistaken for viral or fungal keratitis. A diagnosis of amebic keratitis is made only when all other cultures (bacterial, fungal, and viral) are negative.

Scrapings are collected and placed in the center of two nonnutrient agar plates. A few drops containing heat-killed or "live" *Escherichia coli* are placed over the tissue. The plates are sealed with tape, and one is placed at room temperature and the second in the incubator (35° C). If only one plate is collected, it should be kept at room temperature. Scrapings also may be inoculated into tissue culture, and maintenance media may be added. The amebae cause a generalized destruction of the tissue culture cells. A third method of cultivation is to grow free-living amebae in broth (axenic) culture.

Depending on the quality of the scrapings and the infectious dose of the organism, *Acanthamoeba* trophozoites may be seen within 48 hours. The

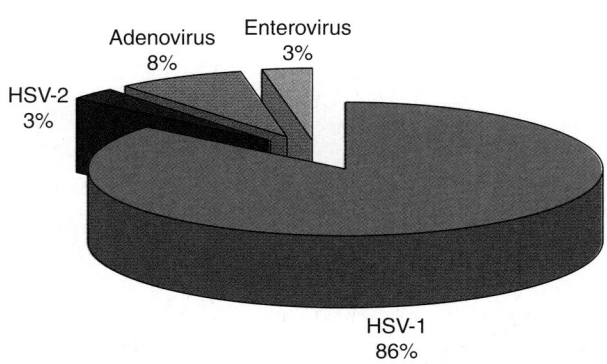

Figure 35-8

Frequency of common keratitis viral isolates. *HSV-1,* Herpes simplex virus type 1; *HSV-2,* herpes simplex virus type 2. (Data from Miller, Perez, Alfonso, ARVO, 1997.)

polygonal, double-walled cysts may be detected on a direct smear with either Giemsa or calcofluor white stain. Trophozoites are much less discernible on smear and are best seen in "tracts" on the agar (Figure 35-9).

Microsporidian keratitis, seen in immunocompromised patients, is a disease that has appeared fairly recently. Microsporidiosis is usually a disease associated with bees or other insects. The microsporidians are intracellular, spore-forming protozoans. In humans, both ocular and nonocular diseases have been reported. Currently, this is an emerging disease in patients with AIDS. The protozoan is an obligate intracellular parasite that infects ocular conjunctivae and corneal tissue. Its size may range from 1 to 20 μm, and it has a round or spherical shape (Figure 35-10). The organism develops in two stages, the schizogenic and the sporulation, or sporogenic, phase. Infection is by the fecal-oral route. Spores may be detected on Gram, Giemsa, acid-fast, or calcofluor white stains. Electron microscopy is usually required for classification and confirmation. No uniform treatment is used.

Detection of ocular parasites is based on (1) observing and removing the actual protozoan, (2) confirming the presence of the organism with histologic or other stains, and (3) isolating the organisms from blood, tissues, or body fluids. Treatment depends on the organism and the availability of an antiinfective.

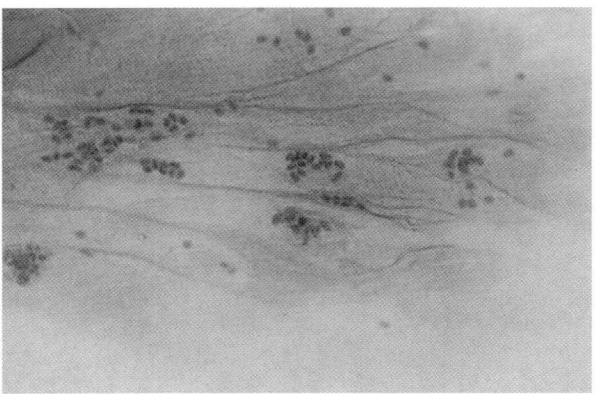

Figure 35-10

Gram stain revealing the oval cyst of Microsporida species. Organisms can also be detected with Giemsa, acid-fast, and calcofluor white stains.

INFECTIONS OF THE SCLERA AND EPISCLERA (SCLERITIS AND EPISCLERITIS)

The sclera is composed of tough collagen fibers, and few organisms can penetrate this strong protective coat. Infections are protracted, painful, and quite destructive. **Scleritis** is usually a local manifestation of systemic connective tissue disease (e.g., rheumatoid arthritis, lupus) or the result of contiguous spread from adjacent ocular tissues. The presentation may be acute (pyogenic) or chronic (granulomatous). The episclera is a thin layer of elastic vascular tissue that overlies the sclera. Inflammation of this tissue is termed *episcleritis*. Episcleritis is actually more common than scleritis and have an undetermined etiology in 70% of cases. Etiologic agents of scleritis are shown in Box 35-6.

INFECTIONS OF THE ORBIT (PRESEPTAL AND ORBITAL CELLULITIS)

Infections of the orbit and adnexal structures may have a devastating effect on vision and ocular structural integrity. The close proximity of the orbit and related tissues to the parasinuses, the absence of an effective drainage system from this "closed-box" construction, and the unique structure of the lids all predispose this area to invasion by various microorganisms.

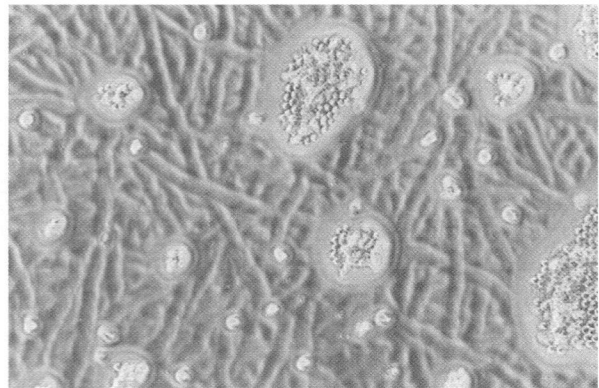

Figure 35-9

"Tracts" of *Acanthamoeba* trophozoites. The meandering trophozoites are at the end of the tracts. The large clusters of organisms contain trophozoites and cysts.

Microorganisms can gain entry into the orbital tissue through trauma or injury to the eyelids or orbit resulting from surgery, infections of the eyelids and adjacent skin, upper respiratory tract infections, and dental caries. Parasites may also invade the orbital tissue and cause considerable destruction. Orbital infections are also considered extensions of bacterial or fungal sinal infections.

Because of the close proximity of the orbital cavity to the parasinuses, any organisms that initiate sinusitis will also cause orbital cellulitis. Various anaerobic organisms are isolated from samples from patients with orbital cellulitis associated with longstanding chronic sinusitis. The majority of these infections are caused by bacteria, but sapro-

---

Box 35-6

Etiologic Agents of Scleritis

Bacteria

Pseudomonas aeruginosa
Staphylococcus aureus
Streptococcus pneumoniae, other streptococci
Serratia marcescens
Other Enterobacteriaceae
Staphylococcus epidermidis
Borrelia burgdorferi
Treponema pallidum
Moraxella species
Mycobacterium tuberculosis
Mycobacterium leprae
Mycobacterium fortuitum
Mycobacterium chelonae
Nocardia species

Fungi

Fusarium species
Aspergillus species
Paecilomyces species
Curvularia species

Viruses

HSV-1 and HSV-2
Varicella-zoster virus
Mumps

Parasites

Toxoplasma gondii
Acanthamoeba species
Toxocara species

Box 35-7

Common Agents of Orbital Cellulitis

Bacteria

Staphylococcus aureus
Staphylococcus epidermidis
Streptococcus pneumoniae
Streptococcus pyogenes, other beta streptococci
Haemophilus influenzae
Moraxella catarrhalis
Eikenella corrodens, Pasteurella multocida (associated with dog bites)
Mycobacterium tuberculosis
MOTT (Mycobacterium chelonae, Mycobacterium fortuitum, most frequent)
Nocardia species
Actinomyces species
Capnocytophaga species
Fusobacterium species
Propionibacterium acnes

Fungi

Mucor, Rhizopus, and Absidia species
Aspergillus species
Bipolaris sp.
Curvularia species
Sporotrichum species
Penicillin species
Candida paropsilosis

Parasites

Trichinella spiralis
Echinococcus granulosus
Fly larvae (maggots)

MOTT, Mycobacteria other than tubercle bacilli.

phytic fungi may also be involved (Box 35-7). Usually both aerobic and anaerobic bacteria are isolated from these infections. Orbital cellulitis may be caused by Mycobacterium species, Nocardia species, and Actinomyces species. Bacterial infections associated with orbital implants or prostheses are increasing (Bascom Palmer Eye Institute). The organisms recovered include Mycobacterium chelonae, Nocardia species, Staphylococcus epidermidis, Capnocytophaga species, Candida parapsilosis, and Propionibacterium acnes.

Trichinosis, caused by the nematode Trichinella spiralis, can invade the extraocular muscles and result in periorbital edema and pain on movement.

An ophthalmologist usually makes the diagnosis of trichinosis, because invasion of the ocular muscles is usually the first sign of this disease.

Among the other parasites that rarely invade or infest the orbits and adnexa are the larvae of *Echinococcus granulosus,* inducing a hydatid cyst that must be surgically exposed and whose contents must be aspirated. Maggots (fly larvae) may occasionally be deposited in the orbit and adnexal tissues.

INFECTIONS OF THE LACRIMAL APPARATUS

The lacrimal glands, accessory glands, puncta, canaliculi, tear sac, and nasolacrimal duct compose what is called the *lacrimal apparatus,* which has two functions. First, the lacrimal and accessory glands produce the aqueous component of the tear film. Second, the puncta, canaliculi, lacrimal sac, and nasolacrimal duct drain the tears from the conjunctiva cul-de-sac to the nasal cavity. Disorders and infections of the lacrimal apparatus are caused by blockage or underproduction or overproduction of tears.

Dacryoadenitis, inflammation of the main lacrimal gland, may be infectious or noninfectious. Organisms are seeded into the gland via the blood stream. Blunt trauma also predisposes the gland to infection. Bacterial isolates include *N. gonorrhoeae, S. aureus,* and *Streptococcus* species. Chronic bacterial infections of the gland involve tuberculosis, syphilis, or leprosy. Mucormycosis and aspergillosis may result from contiguous spread from infections of the orbit. Mumps and infectious mononucleosis are the common viral infections associated with the lacrimal gland. Subclinical or inapparent infections have occurred in patients with HSV, VZV, cytomegalovirus, coxsackievirus A, and echovirus. Other viruses implicated in lacrimal gland infections are measles and influenza viruses. Parasitic invasions with *Schistosoma haematobium, Onchocerca volvulus,* and *Cysticercus cellulose* have been reported.

Canaliculitis, a disease exclusively found in adults, is a low-grade inflammation that affects the lower canaliculus more than the upper. Purulent, cheesy material may be expressed from the lumen.

Etiologic agents are diverse and include bacteria, fungi, and viruses. Bacterial infections consist of mixed aerobic and anaerobic flora, *S. aureus* and streptococci are among the aerobes recovered (Box 35-8). Aerobic isolates also include gram-negative rods and *C. trachomatis.* The predominant flora recovered include the gram-positive anaerobes such as *Actinomyces israelii, Propionibacterium propionicus,* and *P. acnes. Nocardia, Fusobacterium,* and *Capnocytophaga* species may also be recovered. Fungal isolates include *Candida albicans* and *Aspergillus* species. Both herpes simplex and zoster may inflame the canaliculi.

Box 35-8

Microbes Recovered from Patients with Lacrimal Apparatus Infections

Bacteria

Staphylococcus aureus
Streptococcus pneumoniae
Staphylococcus pyogenes
Haemophilus influenzae
Pseudomonas aeruginosa
Proteus mirabilis
Chlamydia trachomatis
Treponema pallidum
Actinomyces israelii
Propionibacterium acnes, Propionibacterium propionicus
Capnocytophaga species
Fusobacterium species
Mycobacterium tuberculosis
Mycobacterium leprae

Fungi

Aspergillus species
Rhizopus, Mucor, Rhizopus species
Candida albicans

Viruses

Herpes simplex virus types 1 and 2
Varicella-zoster virus
Cytomegalovirus
Epstein-Barr virus
Coxsackie A virus
Echovirus
Measles
Influenza

Parasites

Schistosoma haematobium
Onchocerca volvulus
Cysticereus cellulose

Inflammation of the lacrimal or tear sac—**dacryocystitis**—is the most common infection of the lacrimal apparatus. Infections are usually associated with obstruction of the nasolacrimal sac. Thus any organisms that colonize the nasolacrimal sac could be responsible for lacrimal sac infections (Box 35-8). *C. trachomatis* may cause a recurrent, chronic inflammation of the tear sac. *Asperigillus, Candida,* and *Actinomyces* species may also be recovered.

Submitted materials for microbiologic evaluation include drainage material, pus, and cheesy exudate. Direct smears for bacteria and fungi should be prepared from this material. Often the etiologic agents (e.g., *Actinomyces* sp.) and fungal hyphae are seen in large numbers. Infections with mixed organisms are also evident. Media should be inoculated so that aerobic and anaerobic organisms as well as fungi will be recovered.

INFECTIONS OF THE INTRAOCULAR CHAMBERS (ENDOPHTHALMITIS)

Infectious endophthalmitis, inflammation of intraocular tissues or cavities, is a catastrophic development resulting from complications of surgery, contiguous spread of infection from infected tissues, use of contaminated medications, or penetrating ocular trauma. It is the most serious and sight-threatening of all ocular infections. Any organism that gains entry into the inner chambers of the eye can result in disease. The etiologic agents include bacteria, viruses, fungi, and parasites. Endophthalmitis may also be caused by instillation of contaminated eye drops and implantation of contaminated biomaterials. Rapid recovery and identification of the invading organism, complemented by an early, specific, and aggressive therapy, is mandatory to prevent loss of useful vision and preserve internal ocular structures. Specimens include aspirated anterior chamber or vitreous fluids (usually less than 5 ml) and washings from the flushing out of vitreous chambers (usually more than 10 ml).

Bacteria

Etiologic agents of endophthalmitis, which include bacteria, viruses, and fungi, are listed in Box 35-9. *Bacillus cereus* and other *Bacillus* species are the most frequently isolated organisms from endophthalmitis resulting from traumatic injuries. The on-

---

Box 35-9

Common Microbes Recovered from Patients with Endophthalmitis

Bacteria

Staphylococcus epidermidis
Coagulase-negative staphylococci
Streptococcus viridans group
Staphylococcus aureus
Enterococcus faecalis
Bacillus species
Pseudomonas aeruginosa
Haemophilus influenzae
Moraxella species
Proteus mirabilis
Serratia marcescens
Enterobacteriaceae
Achromobacter xylosoxidans
Propionibacterium acnes
Capnocytophaga species
Actinomyces species
Mycobacterium chelonae

Fungi

Candida species (*Candida albicans*—most
    common)
Cryptococcus neoformans
Fusarium species
Aspergillus species
Paecilomyces species
Curvularia species

Viruses

Herpes simplex virus types 1 and 2
Varicella-zoster virus
Cytomegalovirus
Enterovirus

Parasites

Toxoplasma gondii
Onchocerca volvulus
Toxocara species

---

set of symptoms is sudden, and the course is fulminant. Release of necrotizing enzymes can result in loss of the eye within 48 hours. A high index of suspicion and aggressive therapy are required to retain useful vision.

Mycotic endophthalmitis is mostly an extension of keratitis. However, it may also result from hematogenous spread from a remote focus and from implantation of a contaminated intraocular lens. The most frequent isolates are *C. albicans* and other *Candida* species. Saprophytes that infect the cornea may extend into the intraocular cavities. The filamentous species recovered include *Aspergillus* species, *Fusarium solani, Paecilomyces* species, *Curvularia* species, and *Sporothrix schenckii.* Other reported species recovered in cases of endophthalmitis include *Monosporium apiospermum, Cephalosporium* species, *Volutella* species, *C. immitis, H. capsulatum, C. neoformans,* and *B. dermatitidis.*

Intraocular parasites usually affect the retina or choroid or are transient invaders from adjacent ocular structures. *Onchocerca* species, *Toxocara* species, *Toxoplasma gondii* are the most frequent intraocular pathogens.

INFECTIONS OF THE UVEAL TRACT (UVEITIS)

Uveitis is a general term for inflammatory disorders of one portion or all three portions (iris, ciliary body, choroid) of the uveal tract. The inflammation results from ocular trauma or insults to the inner structures of the globe from a local or systemic inflammatory disease. Connective tissue diseases, such as juvenile rheumatoid arthritis, Reiter's syndrome, and systemic lupus, are associated with uveitis. Iritis and iridocyclitis are referred to as *anterior uveitis,* whereas choroiditis or chorioretinitis is termed *posterior uveitis.* The etiology of anterior uveitis is considered nongranulomatous and is nonmicrobial. Posterior uveitis is classified as a granulomatous disease, and its etiology may be bacterial, fungal, viral, or parasitic.

Mycobacterium tuberculosis, Treponema pallidum, and *Mycobacterium leprae* all are involved in chronic disease of the uveal tract. Members of the herpes group (HSV, cytomegalovirus, and VZV) may be involved in necrotizing disease. Such disease is usually associated with **retinitis. Chorioretinitis** may be a better description of the syndrome. *Histoplasma, Aspergillus* species, *N. asteroides,* and *Candida* species all cause granulomatous disease of the uveal tract.

Infections involving the uveal tract usually manifest as chorioretinitis. Recovery in culture is difficult. Serologic assessment via enzyme-linked immunosorbent assay (ELISA), immunofluorescence, or complement fixation may be of greater value in identifying the causative agent. Genomic amplification (PCR) or DNA probes may also assist in some cases. Viral isolation is attempted by cocultivation of the fluids or tissues with fibroblasts.

INFECTIONS OF THE RETINA (RETINITIS)

The retina is a multilayered neural tissue that transforms images and relays impulses to the brain so that the individual can see. Insults to the retina, whether infectious or noninfectious result in irreversible damage. Microbial infections are rare but can be devastating. Microbial infections may occur via hematogenous or contiguous spread. The bacterial and fungal infections are usually the same as those found in uveitis. *Pneumocystis carinii* invades the retina, resulting in classic "cottonwood spots" during systemic disease. Viral and parasitic organisms are responsible for syndromes that are unique to the retina. Microbial agents recovered in retinitis are shown in Box 35-10.

Box 35-10

Microbes Recovered from Patients with Retinitis

Bacteria
Mycobacterium tuberculosis
Mycobacterium leprae
Treponema pallidum
Nocardia asteroides

Fungi
Candida species
Histoplasma capsulatum
Aspergillus species

Viruses
Cytomegalovirus
Herpes simplex viruses types 1 and 2
Varicella-zoster virus
Human immunodeficiency virus
Rubella
Rubeola
Subacute sclerosing panencephalitis (SSPE)

Parasites
Toxoplasma gondii
Pneumocystis carinii
Toxocara species
Cysticercus cellulosae

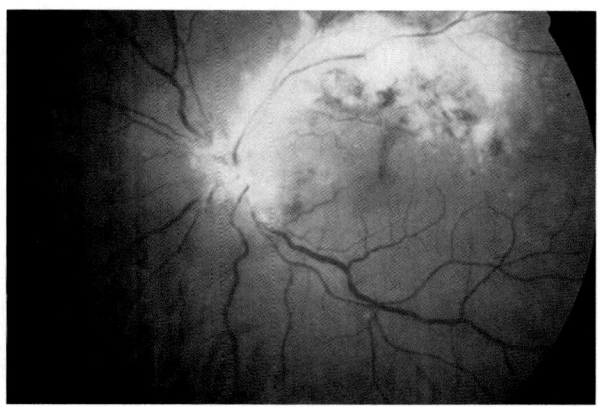

Figure 35-11

Acute cytomegalovirus retinitis with optic nerve involvement in a 40-year-old patient who is HIV positive. Active viral particles are seen in satellite lesions temporal to the main infection *(yellow)*.

Viruses

Viral syndromes are rare but devastating, resulting in unilateral or bilateral decreased vision. The immunocompromised patient is often at risk for viral retinitis. Increased disease (e.g., cytomegalovirus retinitis) is seen in individuals with AIDS. HSV, VZV, and cytomegalovirus all cause viral retinal disease. In the United States, HSV is the leading cause of blindness. Both HSV 1 and 2 cause posterior uveitis. Acute necrotizing retinitis is usually seen in the newborn as a result of acquiring the virus during passage through an infected birth canal. Adults may acquire the disease from recurrent episodes of viral keratitis. Varicella-zoster retinitis may be a manifestation of reactivation of the virus in herpes zoster ophthalmicus.

Cytomegalovirus infections may affect the newborn or the immunocompromised patient and especially patients who have had transplants or have AIDS. Cytomegalovirus retinitis with loss of vision (Figure 35-11) is often indicative of AIDS. Acyclovir, ganciclovir and foscarnet are antivirals used to treat and modulate these episodes. Both rubeola and rubella cause retinopathy. About 30% of patients with subacute sclerosing panencephalitis (SSPE), which may appear years after an attack of clinical measles, also have chorioretinitis on examination. The ocular complications of congenital rubella include cataracts and glaucoma.

Parasites

T. gondii is a protozoan with a predilection for ocular tissues (Figure 35-12). Ocular infection is a late manifestation of congenital toxoplasmosis. This infection is now more prevalent in patients with AIDS than in the general population. *Cysticercus cellulosae* and *Toxocara* species are found in 10% to 13% of intraocular infections. Other protozoal infections that may cause transient retinitis include malaria (retinal hemorrhage); babesiosis—a rare disease similar to malaria but having distinct differences—which is seen mainly in the northern United States in the New England area; and infection with *L. loa,* the eye worm, which can enter the intraocular cavities and cause inflammation in its migration through the ocular tissues. The laboratory support for these infections is the same as that for uveitis.

SCLERAL BUCKLE INFECTIONS

Scleral buckles, sponges, and bands are biomaterials employed to realign detached retinas. They may become expressed and partially extruded from the surgical site. Once exposed, they are subject to bacterial colonization, which can lead to infections of the conjunctivae, sclera, or intraocular cavities. The most frequently isolated bacteria are coagulase-negative staphylococcal species. *S. aureus, P. mirabilis,* and *P. aeruginosa* have also

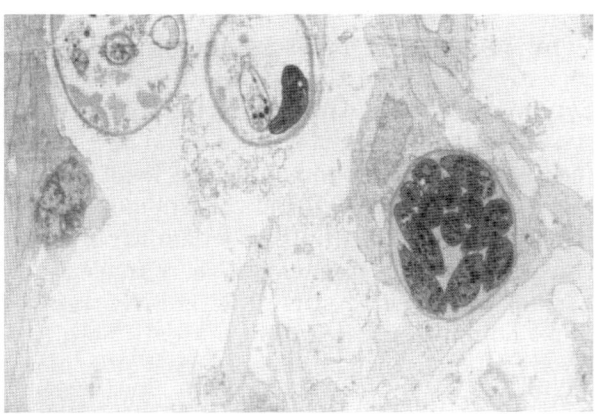

Figure 35-12

Toxoplasma gondii trophozoites and cysts in retinal tissue. This protozoan has a predilection for ocular tissue. In patients with AIDS, such infections are increasing.

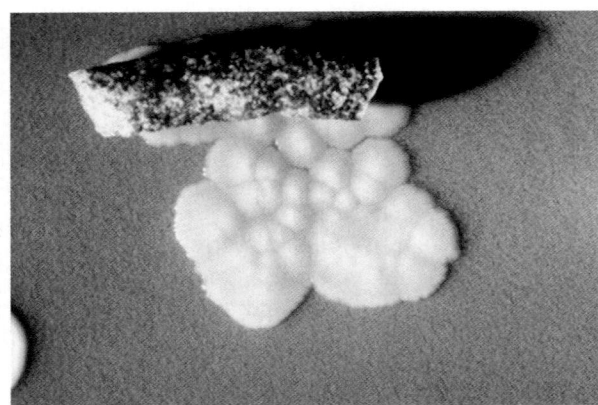

Figure 35-13 _____

Extruded scleral buckle on blood agar plate with growth of *Candida albicans.*

been recovered. MOTT, in particular *M. chelonae* and *Mycobacterium fortuitum,* have been recovered from these materials at an alarming rate during the last few years. Additional isolates include *Candida* species, *Corynebacterium* species, and *Citrobacter koseri.*

Management includes removing the materials along with any remaining necrotic tissue when possible (Figure 35-13).

OCULAR MANIFESTATIONS IN PATIENTS WITH HUMAN IMMUNODEFICIENCY VIRUS

Ocular involvement occurs in 50% to 75% of patients infected with human immunodeficiency virus (HIV) during the course of their illness. Symptoms appear with advancing disease. HIV has been isolated or amplified from tears, conjunctiva, and corneal and retinal tissues. The virus may also be recovered from contact lenses of infected patients. The route by which HIV reaches the ocular surface tissues and tears remains uncertain. Cytomegalovirus retinitis is the second most common condition in patients with full-blown AIDS and can affect both eyes even in the absence of systemic disease. This retinitis is listed as an indicator infection in the differential diagnosis of AIDS. Patients may have a history of sudden loss or impairment of vision. Cotton-wool

spots—fluffy, white lesions—are the ocular lesions most often seen in patients with AIDS. Retinal hemorrhages may also be present. Kaposi's sarcoma (Figure 35-14) appears on the ocular tissues of 10% of infected patients. *P. carinii* and *T. gondii* retinitis are also ocular sequellae associated with patients who have AIDS.

LABORATORY DIAGNOSIS OF OCULAR INFECTIONS

Specimen Collection

The keys to proper collection of ocular specimens are similar to those for any other microbiologic specimen. Materials or scrapings for cultures should be collected as soon as possible after the onset of infection (24 to 48 hours for bacteria and 3 to 7 days for viruses) and before the instillation of antimicrobials or steroids. The sample must be collected from the actual site of the infection; for example, conjunctival and lid cultures are inadequate to assess corneal involvement. All ocular fluids, tissues, sponges, and other surgical material must be submitted in *sterile, leak-proof containers* that are properly labeled.

The ophthalmologist must *communicate* with the hospital or reference laboratory personnel performing the microbiologic evaluation of the specimen to ensure isolation of ocular pathogens. Media and the accompanying requisition(s) must be properly labeled with complete patient informa-

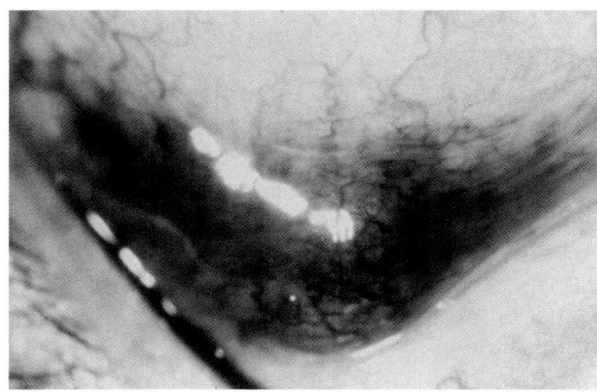

Figure 35-14 _____

Kaposi's sarcoma *(raised dark spots)* on conjunctiva of patient who has AIDS.

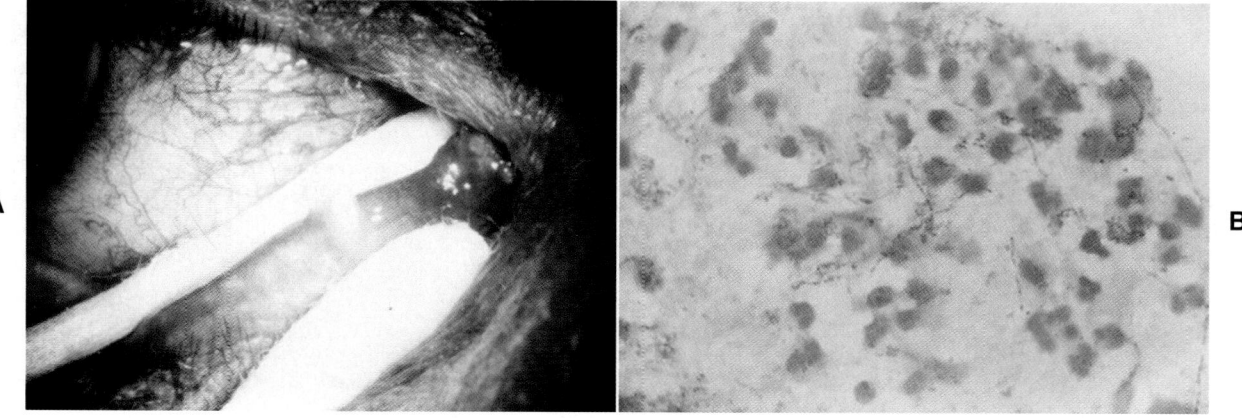

Figure 35-15

A, Concretions being expressed from canaliculi. **B,** "Smashed" and stained concretions, revealing gram-positive, slender, branching rods *(Actinomyces israelii).*

tion and should indicate any antibiotics, antivirals, steroids, or antifungals the patient is currently receiving. It should also be noted if the patient is a contact lens wearer.

For best results, ocular materials must be inoculated directly onto the appropriate media. Scant recovery is the norm when culturettes or swabs are submitted for recovery of ocular pathogens. The type of swab used can further reduce organism recovery. Cotton-tipped swabs inhibit the growth of some bacteria and HSV because of the fatty acids released during sterilization. Dacron or calcium alginate swabs may be used to collect ocular samples. Further, the calcium alginate swab may be lethal to some viral ocular pathogens. Expressed materials from areas such as canaliculi are preferred to rule out infection (Figure 35-15). Materials are inoculated directly onto the media. Smears are also prepared from the material. Collection by direct aspiration or scraping is performed by the ophthalmologist. Media to recover aerobic and anaerobic organisms must be included. Vitreous washings (with a volume greater than 10 ml) may be injected into blood culture bottles or viral transport media or may be sent to the laboratory for concentration.

Biopsy tissue must be minced or ground. Media to recover aerobic and anaerobic bacteria, fungi, and mycobacteria should be inoculated. If free-living amebae are suspected, two nonnutrient (agar) plates should be included.

Direct Smear Examination

Scrapings from the involved ocular site, complemented with the appropriate stains, can afford the physician circumstantial as well as definite information concerning the identity of the invading organisms. Table 35-2 provides a summary of stains that are routinely used in ocular microbiology and appropriate applications of each procedure. Gram and Giemsa stains (Figure 35-16) should be collected for all cases of bacterial conjunctivitis, keratitis, and endophthalmitis. The calcofluor white stain should be added to rule out fungal or parasitic disease. A fluorescent or conventional acid-fast stain is used to detect the presence of acid-fast organisms. Direct antigen detection in cases of vi-

TABLE 35-2

Smear Guide

	Gram	Giemsa	IF	IC	CFW
Bacteria	+	+			
Fungi	+	+			+
Viruses		+	+	+	
Chlamydia		+	+	+	
Parasites	+	+		+	+

IF, Immunofluorescent stains (monoclonals for chlamydia, herpes simplex virus, adenovirus, enterovirus, varicella-zoster virus, and cytomegalovirus); *IC,* impression cytology—collected cells remain intact, and test can locate disease progress; *CFW,* calcofluor white stain—used to detect fungi or parasites in ocular tissue.

Figure 35-16

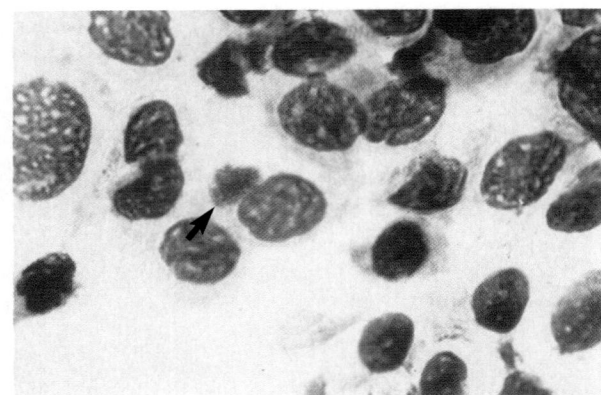

Giemsa stain of conjunctival epithelial cells with chlamydial inclusions *(center)*. The Giemsa stain also provides information on the types and numbers of inflammatory cells and the condition of the epithelial cells.

TABLE 35-3

General Ocular Plating Guidelines

Clinical Diseases	Anaerobic Blood Agar	Chocolate Agar	Blood Agar	Sabouraud Agar	Thioglycolate	Agar-Agar	Löwenstein-Jensen	VTM/CTM	Blood Culture Bottles	Gram Stain	Giemsa Stain	Calcofluor White Stain	Immunofluorescent Stain	Common Isolates
Conjunctivitis														
Bacterial		+	+							+				*Staphylococcus aureus, Haemophilus influenzae, Streptococcus pneumoniae*
Chlamydial		+						+			+		+	*Chlamydia trachomatis*
Viral		+						+					+	Adenovirus, enterovirus, herpes simplex virus type 1 (HSV-1)
Blepharitis														
Same as above														*S. aureus, Staphylococcus epidermidis*
Keratitis														
Bacterial		+	+		+					+				*S. aureus, Pseudomonas aeruginosa, Serratia marcescens, S. pneumoniae*
Viral		+			+			+		+	+		+	HSV-1, varicella-zoster virus, enterovirus
Fungal		+	+	+	+					+	+	+		*Fusarium* species, *Candida* species, *Aspergillus* species
Free-living amoebal		+		+	+	+		+			+	+		*Acanthamoeba* species, *Valkamphia* species
Atypical	+	+	+	+	+	+	+	+		+	+	+		*Mycobacterium* species, *Nocardia* species, *Achromobacter* species, *Capnocytophaga* species, *S. pneumoniae*
Lacrimal apparatus														
Bacterial		+	+		+					+				*S. aureus, S. pneumoniae, Actinomyces* species, *H. influenzae*
Fungal		+	+	+	+					+	+	+		*Aspergillus* species, *Mycobacterium* species, *Streptococcus* species
Other	+	+	+	+	+		+			+				
Endophthalmitis														
Bacterial		+	+		+				+	+				*S. epidermidis, Propionibacterium acnes, S. aureus,* streptococci
Fungal		+	+	+	+				+	+	+	+		*Candida* species, *Apergillus* species, *Fusarium* species

VTM/CTM, Viral transport medium/chlamydia transport medium.

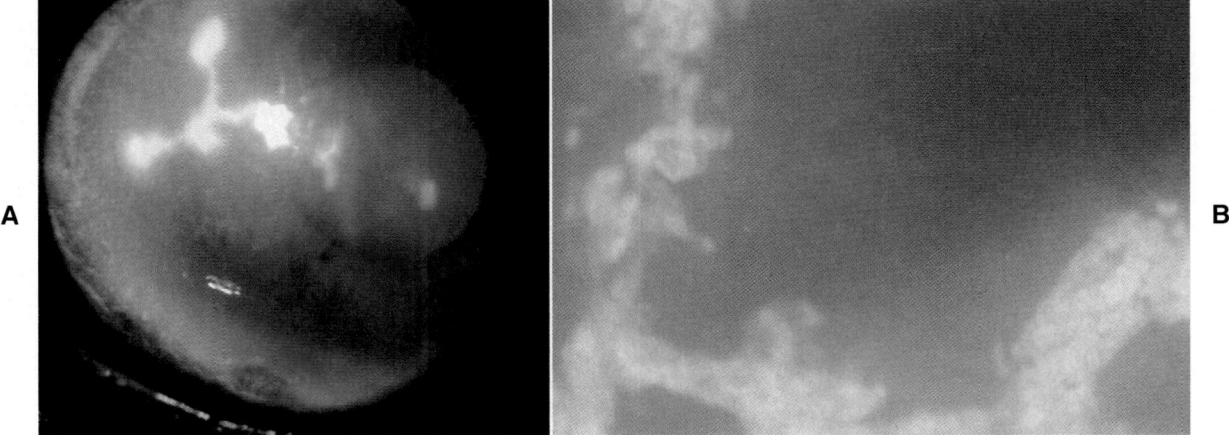

Figure 35-17

A, Cornea stained with rose bengal to outline dendrite infected with herpes simplex virus (HSV). HSV is the virus most often isolated from corneal dendritic infections. **B,** Dendrite on membrane filter collected by impression cytology. The filter was stained with a monoclonal antibody against HSV-1. Almost all the cells of the dendrite "lit up" when stained. The uninfected cells do not stain and appear red.

ral or chlamydial disease may be the only confirmation test available (Figure 35-17). In addition, impression cytology utilizing 0.45-μm Tefloncoated membrane filters to collect conjunctival and corneal tissue may increase bacterial, fungal, viral, and protozoan detection by as much as 50%. The advantage with this technique is that cells remain intact with characteristic morphology and microbial infestation and invasion (Figure 35-18).

Culture

The majority of the bacterial and fungal ocular isolates may be recovered on chocolate and blood agar when they are incubated under the proper conditions of temperature (35° to 37° C) and atmosphere (5% to 10% CO_2, aerobic) or in an anaerobic jar or bag. Table 35-3 shows a general plating guide that may be followed to recover all possible agents of ocular infections. Table 35-4 shows a minimal plating guide for bacteria and fungi. The addition of thioglycolate broth, Thayer-Martin agar, Sabouraud agar with gentamicin (Figure 35-19), viral and chlamydial transport media, Löwenstein-Jensen slants, and nonnutrient agar plates allows for the recovery of most pathogens involved in ocular disease. All thioglycolate tubes are held for 10 days or 21 days if *Actinomyces* species or *P. acnes* are suspected. (See Table 35-3 for an expanded plating guide.)

Interpretation of growth from ocular samples is based on the same sound microbiologic criteria used in general hospital microbiology laboratories. Quantitation of growth is particularly important. Samples from patients receiving antiinfective agents, steroids, or other medications may have reduced flora, which should be taken into consideration when evaluating the culture.

Special considerations are involved in corneal and intraocular fluid cultures. Corneal scrapings are inoculated in a C streak fashion. Each row of C

TABLE 35-4

Minimal Plating Guide: Bacteria and Fungi

	CHOC‡	BAP (An)	SAB	THIO	SMEARS
Conjunctivae, lids	+			+	+
Cornea	+	+	+	+	+
Intraocular fluids*	+	+		+	+
Adnexa†	+	+	+	+	+

An, Anaerobic; *BAP,* blood agar plate; *CHOC,* chocolate agar; *THIO,* thioglycolate broth; *SAB,* Sabouraud dextrose agar.
*Intraocular fluids may be injected into pediatric or adult blood culture bottles (bcbs) for recovery of the most frequent endophthalmitis isolates.
†Wounds, orbit, lacrimal apparatus, etc.
‡If the ophthalmologist can collect only enough material for one medium, ask the ophthalmologist to inoculate the chocolate agar plate and rinse the spatula or blade in the thioglycolate broth. Both specimens should be submitted to the microbiology laboratory for processing.

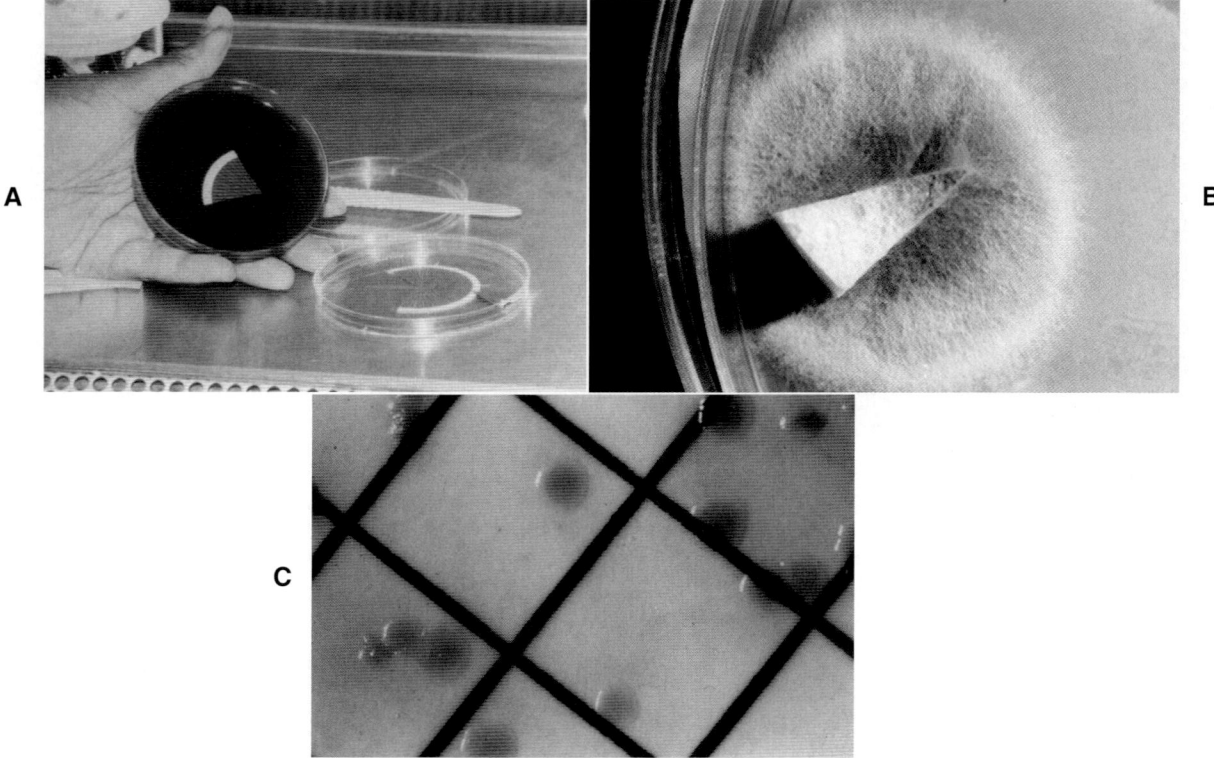

Figure 35-18 _____

A, Once filtered, the 0.45-μm filter is then sectioned and placed on selected media. **B,** *Curvularia* species from intraocular fluids on 0.45-μm filter section. **C,** *Burkholderia cepacia* on a filter from a vitrectomy specimen.

streaks represents a separate scraping of a corneal ulcer. The dilution effect is from left to right. Generally more colonies of bacteria or fungi appear on the first C streaks of each row. Each successive C streak progresses from the superficial to the deep layers of the cornea. The greater the number of streaks with growth, the more involved and serious the infection.

Any growth from intraocular fluids appearing on the inoculation sites or filter should be assessed and reported. The physician correlates the organism's pathobiology with the patient's clinical picture and diagnosis. The organisms that are normally considered "contaminants" (Figure 35-20) are the ones most frequently involved in microbial intraocular infections.

Figure 35-19 _____

Sabouraud plate with mold and yeast. Patient had a mixed fungal keratitis. *Right,* The superficial layer of the cornea was infected with a mold *(Fusarium oxysporum). Left,* The deeper layers were infected with a yeast *(Candida albicans).*

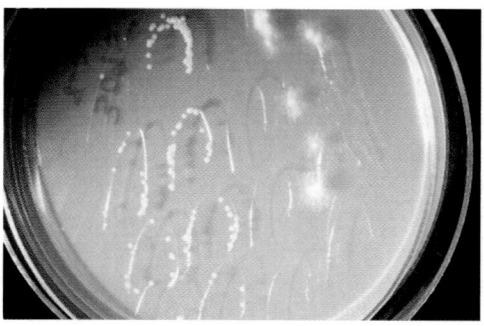

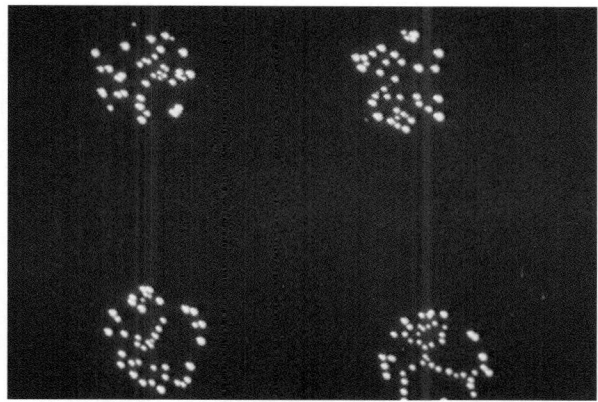

Figure 35-20

Staphylococcus epidermidis recovered from vitreous fluids (drops) on blood agar plate. Samples may be inoculated onto a chocolate or blood agar plate and allowed to dry or may be streaked out as is done for a routine microbiology specimen.

Special Procedures for Recovering Ocular Pathogens

Limulus lysate

The *Limulus* lysate test should be performed for all patients who have corneal ulcers and are receiving medications, who wear contact lenses, or who have clinical signs suggestive of gram-negative organisms. The *Limulus* lysate is a mixture of the amebocytes of the horseshoe crab. When these cells are mixed with fluids or substances containing endotoxins (such as the cell walls of gram-negative organisms), they form a gel clot, much like that of the coagulase test. Both tests are enzymatic tests. The assay is set up, incubated, and read in 1 hour.

Agar-agar medium

Agar-agar is a nonnutrient agar that is first inoculated with ocular materials and then overlaid with an aliquot of heat-killed or live *E. coli,* which serve as food for the excysting *Acanthamoeba* organisms. The amebic trophozoites are identified by locating them at the end of the "tracts" they generate as they eat through the *E. coli.* Cysts are identified by their refractile, double-walled, polygonal shape and are best seen using calcofluor white stains and the fluorescent microscope. Recovery of any parasite from corneal scrapings is significant and should be reported. Usually cultures of free-living amebae contain both cysts and trophozoites.

Trypticase soy broth

Trypticase soy broth is used as a wetting agent to collect conjunctival and lid cultures.

Sabouraud agar with gentamicin

The very fungi that traditional mycology media aim to inhibit (saprophytes) are the agents most often recovered in mycotic ocular disease (i.e., *Fusarium, Paecilomyces, Aspergillus,* and *Penicillium* species).

Blood culture bottles

Blood culture bottles are used when blood cultures are requested and also to culture intraocular fluids. Vitreous washings may be placed in the traditional (i.e., 50- to 70-ml) bottles; fluids from direct vitreous or anterior chamber taps should be inoculated into the pediatric (10- to 20-ml) bottles.

Special Culture Techniques

Contaminated ocular medications

Ophthalmic drops (e.g., antibiotics, analgesics) are easily contaminated when improperly handled by patients or ophthalmic personnel. Inappropriate handling can contribute to ongoing ocular disorders and to initiation of new disease. Even though most ocular medications are prepared with preservatives to inhibit the growth of microorganisms, once the preservative's threshold has been breached, microbes survive, multiply, and are dispensed with the next drop of medication. Medications should be collected from patients with conjunctivitis, keratitis, or endophthalmitis and sent to the laboratory for culture.

The medications most often contaminated and associated with concurrent patient infection, in descending order, include steroids, β-blockers, antiglaucoma drugs, antibiotics, and artificial tears. Box 35-11 shows the microbes recovered from contaminated ocular medications.

Contact lenses and solutions

Keratitis associated with contact lenses (soft, daily wear, extended wear, or disposable) is being documented with increasing frequency. Gram-negative rods (especially and predominantly *P. aeruginosa and S. marcescens*) are most often recovered from infections associated with contact lenses.

Acanthamoeba species, MOTT, and gram-positive cocci have also been recovered. Sources include

Box 35-11

Microbes Recovered from Contaminated Ocular Medications

Serratia marcescens
Pseudomonas aeruginosa
Achromobacter xylosoxidans
Coagulase-negative staphylococci
Proteus mirabilis

Morganella morganii
Staphylococcus aureus
Mycobacterium chelonae
Saprophytic fungi

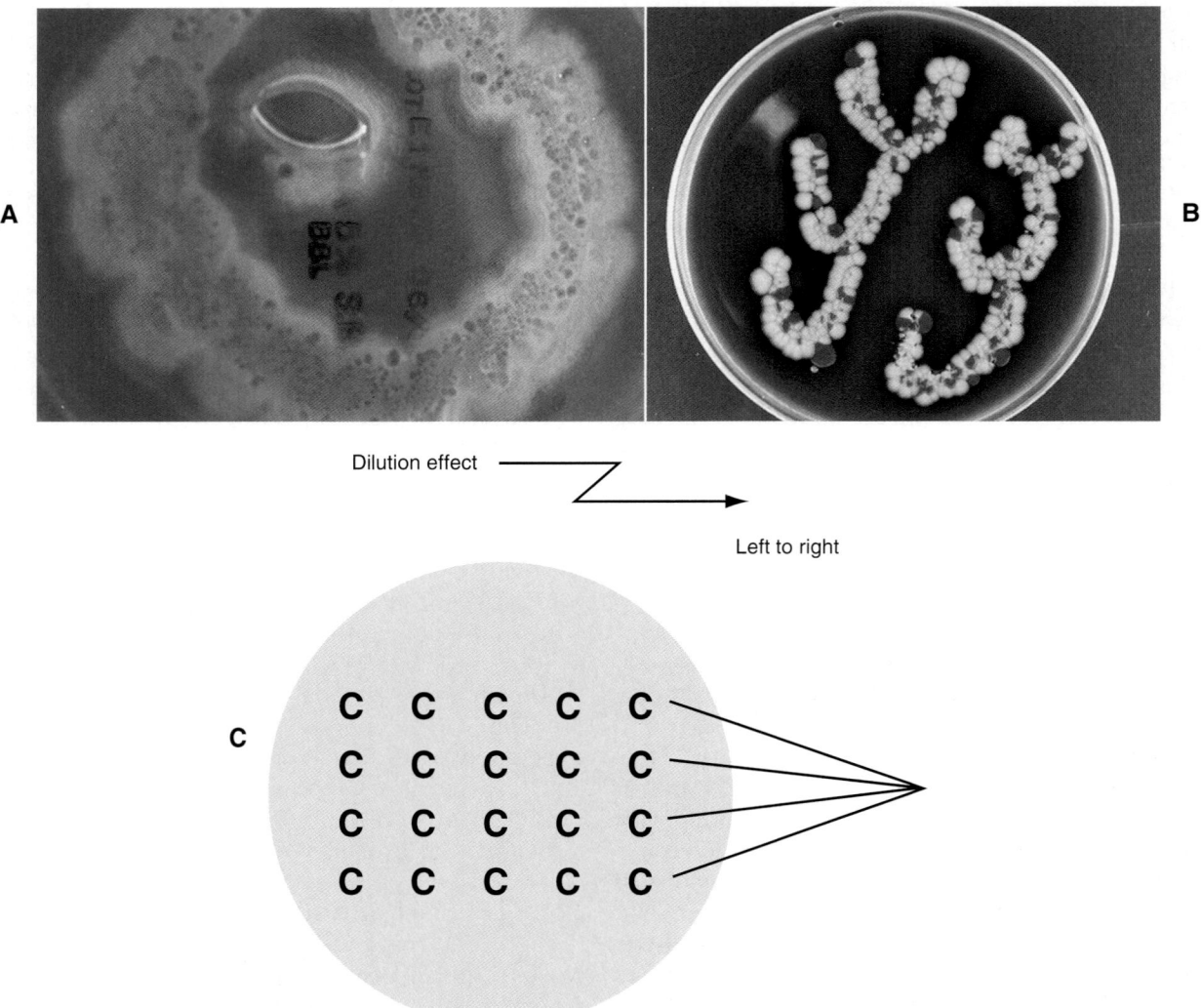

Figure 35-21

A, Contact lens and lens solution on 5% sheep's blood agar surrounded by growth of *Pseudomonas aeruginosa*. **B,** C streaks growing pigmented and nonpigmented *Serratia marcescens*. **C,** Corneal scrapings. (NOTE: Each row of C streaks represents a *separate* corneal scraping.)

contact lenses as well as contact lens solutions (Figure 35-21) and cases. Contamination of the soft contact lenses is usually caused by failure to follow manufacturer's recommended procedures or poor hygiene. Wearers of hard contact lenses are less prone to infection from microbial contamination.

Cornea storage media and tissue culture

Replacement of diseased or opacified corneas is a common operation performed by ophthalmic surgeons. The new corneal tissue is obtained from donors within 24 hours of death and is preserved in McCarey and Kaufman (MK) or Dexsol medium. After surgery the container with the medium and remaining corneal rim is sent to the laboratory for culture. Bacteriologic evaluation of the donor tissue is paramount in reducing the transmission of host-carried disease to the recipient. Viral studies of corneal transplantation tissue have been limited.

Gram-positive organisms (i.e., coagulase-negative staphylococci and *P. acnes*) are the most frequently isolated organisms, but gram-negative organisms, yeasts, or molds may also be recovered from these media. The actual correlation between isolates and resultant disease is less than 1%. All positive cultures should be reported directly to the surgeon and a final report sent to the EyeBank and the physician.

OCULAR THERAPY

The therapeutic agents used in ophthalmology are applied to the diagnosis of ocular disorders, the treatment of ophthalmic disease, and the prevention of postoperative infections. They differ from drugs used in other areas of medicine in delivery routes, antibiotic and antiviral combinations, dosing intervals, and toxicity. The traditional routes of administration of drugs may be implemented to supplement ocular management.

For ophthalmic drugs to be effective, they must reach ocular tissues in relatively high concentrations. Therefore ocular formulations include drugs in concentrations 10 to 100 times (i.e., fortified) that of drugs prepared for intramuscular or intravenous delivery. The routes of administration of ophthalmic drugs include topical (which is the most common and may include drops or ointments), oral, parenteral, periocular, intracameral, and intravitreous.

Drugs are dispensed as either drops or ointments, with topical administration being the most common route. Alternative or traditional routes are required for the treatment of disease involving the retina, optic nerve, and intraocular cavities. Ocular medications usually contain preservatives to inhibit the growth of contaminating microorganisms.

Once the etiologic agent has been identified, susceptibility studies should be generated as quickly as possible. Traditional microbiologic methods are used to determine susceptibility patterns. Box 35-12 outlines the most common types of antiinfective agents commercially available to ophthalmologists. Pharmacists with training in ocular therapy can prepare ocular doses for most intravenous or intramuscular drugs. Table 35-5 shows susceptibility profiles for the most commonly used ocular antibiotics.

TABLE 35-5

Antiinfectives for Ocular Susceptibility Testing

Antibiotic	g+	g−	gndc	haem	pse	Other
Amikacin					+	+
Penicillin	+		+			+
Ampicillin		+	+	+		+
Ampicillin/sulbactam	+	+	+	+		+
Oxacillin	+					
Cefaclor				+		
Cefazolin*	+	+	+	+		+
Cephalothin*	+	+	+	+		+
Ceftriaxone	+	+	+	+	+	+
Ciprofloxacin/ ocufloxacin	+	+	+	+	+	+
Clindamycin	+					
Erythromycin	+		+	+		
Gentamicin	+	+		+	+	+
Tetracycline	+	+	+	+		+
Tobramycin		+			+	+
Trimethoprim- sulfamethoxazole*	+	+	+	+		+
Vancomycin	+					

g+, Gram positive; *g−*, Enterobacteriaceae; *gndc*, gram-negative diplococci; *haem, Haemophilus influenzae; pse, Pseudomonas aeruginosa; other, Moraxella* species, *Kingella* species, *Eikinella* species, etc.
*Most frequently used ophthalmic antibiotics. These must be included on any susceptibility panels. Other antibiotics that may be requested are polymyxin B, chloramphenicol, neomycin, bacitracin, and sulfacetamide. Sulfacetamide is a sulfa drug. There are no disks to evaluate this drug. A general idea of susceptibility to this drug can be gained by running trimethoprim-sulfa and Gantrisin (Roche; sulfisoxazole).

Box 35-12

Ocular Antiinfectives

Antibacterials

Amikacin
Ampicillin
Bacitracin*
Carbenicillin
Cefazolin
Cephalothin
Chloramphenicol*
Ciprofloxacin*
Clindamycin*
Colistin*
Erythromycin*
Gentamicin*
Methicillin
Neomycin*
Ocuflox
Penicillin G
Polymyxin B*
Sulfacetamide*
Sulfisoxazole*
Tetracycline*
Tobramycin*
Trimethoprim-sulfamethoxazole
Vancomycin

Antivirals

Idoxuridine (IDU)*
Trifluridine*
Vidarabine (ara-A)*
Acyclovir*
FoscarnetGanciclovir
Zidovudine (azidothymidine [AZT])

Antifungals

Amphotericin B
Clotrimazole
Fluconazole
Flucytosine
Griseofulvin
Hydroxystilbamidine
Ketoconazole
Miconazole
Natamycin*
Potassium iodine

Antiparasitics

Antimony sodium gluconate
Diethylcarbamazine
Iodoquinol
Ivermectin
Mebendazole
Metronidazole
Minocycline
Niridazole
Paromomycin
Pentamidine isethionate
Propamidine isethionate
Physostigmine
Pyrimethamine
Spiramycin
Surinam quassia
Thiabendazole

*Commercially available ocular preparations (drops or ointment).
NOTE: Ocular preparations may be single antibiotics or combinations of one or two antibiotics and/or antiinflammatories. Only natamycin has been approved by the United States Food and Drug Administration for ocular pathogens.

Bibliography

Alfonso E, Miller D: Detection of ocular infections. In Prior RB, editor: *Clinical applications of the Limulus amoebocyte lysate test*, Boca Raton, Fla, 1990, CRC Press.

Alfonso E, et al: Ulcerative keratitis associated with contact lens wear, *Am J Ophthalmol* 101:429, 1986.

Allansmith MR: Defense of the ocular surface, *Int Ophthalmol Clin* 2:93, 1979.

Alvarez H, Tabbara KF: Infections of the eyelids. In Tabbara KF, Hyndiuk RA, editors: *Infections of the eye*, Boston, 1986, Little, Brown.

Antonios S, Tabbara KF: Bacteria conjunctivitis. In Tabbara KF, Hyndiuk RA, editors: *Infections of the eye*, Boston, 1986, Little, Brown.

Asbell P, Stenson S: Ulcerative keratitis: survey of 30 years' laboratory experience, *Arch Ophthalmol* 100:77, 1982.

Baron EJ, Finegold SM: *Bailey's and Scott's diagnostic microbiology*, St Louis, 1990, Mosby.

Bohigan GM: Acquired immune deficiency syndrome: ocular manifestations. In *Handbook of external disease of the eye*, ed 3, Thorofare, NJ, 1987, SLACK.

Brightbill FS, editor: *Corneal surgery: theory, technique, and tissue,* ed 2, St Louis, 1993, Mosby.

Brinser JH, Burd EM: Principles of diagnostic ocular microbiology. In Tabbara KF, Hyndiuk RA editors: *Infections of the eye,* Boston, 1986, Little, Brown.

Brod RD et al: Endogenous *Candida* endophthalmitis: management without intravenous amphotericin B, *Ophthalmology* 97:666, 1992.

Bryan R: Microsporida. In Mandell GL, Douglas RG, Bennett JE, editors: *Principles and practice of infectious disease,* New York, 1990, Churchill Livingstone.

Buss DR et al: Lymphogranuloma venereum conjunctivitis with a marginal corneal perforation.

Chalupa E et al: Severe corneal infections associated with contact lens wear, *Ophthalmology* 94:17, 1987.

Chandler JW, Gillette TE: Immunologic defense mechanisms of the ocular surface, *Ophthalmology* 90:585, 1983.

Davis JL et al: Coagulase-negative staphylococcal endophthalmitis: increase in antimicrobial resistance, *Ophthalmology* 95:1404, 1988.

deLuise VP: Viral conjunctivitis. In Tabbara KF, Hyndiuk RA, editors: *Infections of the eye,* Boston, 1986, Little, Brown.

DeVoe AG, Silva-Hunter M: Fungal infections of the eye. In Locatcher-Khorazo DH, Seegal BC, editors: *Microbiology of the eye,* St Louis, 1972, Mosby.

Fedukowicz HB, Stenson S: *External diseases of the eye: bacterial, viral, and mycotic with noninfectious and immunologic disease,* Englewood Cliffs, NJ, 1987, Prentice-Hall, Appleton-Century-Crofts.

Fischer DH: Viral disease of the retina. In Tabbara KF, Hyndiuk RA, editors: *Infections of the eye,* Boston, 1986, Little, Brown.

Flach AJ: Ophthalmia neonatorum. In Tabbara KF, Hyndiuk RA, editors: *Infections of the eye,* Boston, 1986, Little, Brown.

Flynn HW et al: Endophthalmitis therapy: changing antibiotic sensitivity patterns and current therapeutic recommendations, *Arch Ophthalmol* 109:175, 1991.

Forster RK: Etiology and diagnosis of bacterial postoperative endophthalmitis: symposium on postoperative endophthalmitis, *Ophthalmology* 85:320, 1978.

Freeman LN, Green WR: Periocular infections. In Mandell GL, Douglas RG, Bennett JE, editors: *Principles and practice of infectious diseases,* ed 3, New York, 1990, Churchill Livingstone.

Friedman AH, editor: *Ocular infectious disease: a guide for the general practitioner (seminar series #7),* Chicago, 1978, Abbott Laboratories.

Gardner S, editor: Ciprofloxacin for bacterial keratitis and conjunctivitis: review and summary of 1990 articles, *Ocul Ther Manage* 2(6):1, 1991.

Gardner TW, Soch D, editors: *Handbook of ophthalmology,* East Norwalk, Conn, 1987, Appleton & Lange.

Gittinger JW: *Ophthalmology: a clinical introduction,* Boston, 1984, Little, Brown.

Gonnering RS, Harris GJ: Infections of the orbit. In Tabbara KF, Hyndiuk RA, *Infections of the eye,* Boston, 1986, Little, Brown.

Gutierrez EH: Bacterial infections of the eye. In Locatcher-Khorazo DH, Seegal BC, editors: *Microbiology of the eye,* St Louis, 1972, Mosby.

Halberts SP: Inhibitory properties of the ocular flora. In Locatcher-Khorazo DH, Seegal BC, editors: *Microbiology of the eye,* St Louis, 1972, Mosby.

Holland GN: Prevention of human immunodeficiency virus transmission by ophthalmic examinations and procedures. In Friedlaender MH, editor: *Prevention of eye disease,* New York, 1988, Mary Ann Liebert.

Hyndiuk RA, Skorich DN, Burd EM: Bacterial keratitis. In Tabbara KF, Hyndiuk RA, editors: *Infections of the eye,* Boston, 1986, Little, Brown.

Jones DB: Acanthamoeba—the ultimate opportunist? *Am J Ophthalmol* 102:527, 1986.

Jones DB: Fungal keratitis. In Wilson LA, editor: *External infections of the eye,* New York, 1979, Harper & Row.

Jones DB, Liesegang TJ, Robinson NM: Laboratory diagnosis of ocular infections. In Washington JA, editor: *CUMITECH 13,* Washington, DC, 1981, American Society for Microbiology.

Kean BH, Sun T, Ellsworth RM, editors: *Color atlas of ophthalmic parasitology,* New York, 1991, Igaku-Shoin.

Kervick GN et al: Antibiotic therapy for *Bacillus* sp., *Ophthalmology* 97:666, 1990.

Lewis ML et al: Herpes simplex virus 1: a cause of the acute retinal necrosis syndrome, *Ophthalmology* 96:875, 1989.

Liesgang TJ, Foster RK: Spectrum of microbial keratitis in South Florida, *Am J Ophthalmol* 90:38, 1980.

Locatcher-Khorazo DH, Seegal BC: *Microbiology of the eye,* St Louis, 1972, Mosby.

Ludwig IH, Meisler DM: Acanthamoeba keratitis. In Tabbara KF, Hyndiuk RA, editors: *Infections of the eye,* Boston, 1986, Little, Brown.

McDonnell PJ, Green WR: Conjunctivitis. In Mandell GL, Douglas RG, Bennett JE, editors: *Principles and practice of infectious diseases,* ed 3, New York, 1990, Churchill Livingstone.

McDonnell PJ, Green WR: Endophthalmitis. In Mandell GL, Douglas RG, Bennett JE, editors: *Principles and practice of infectious diseases,* ed 3, New York, 1990, Churchill Livingstone.

Miller D: *Comparison of laboratory tests and risk factors for ocular chlamydia,* MPH thesis, University of Miami, May 1997.

O'Malley C: Vitreous. In Vaughn D, Asbury T, editors: *General ophthalmology,* ed 11, East Norwalk, Conn, 1986, Appleton & Lange.

Ophthalmic Drug Facts (edited): *Facts and comparison,* Philadelphia, 1990, JB Lippincott.

Parke DW, II, Brinton GS: Endophthalmitis. In Tabbara KF, Hyndiuk RA, editors: *Infections of the eye,* Boston, 1986, Little, Brown.

Parment O, Ronerstam RA: Soft contact lens keratitis associated with *Serratia marcescens, Acta Ophthalmol* 59:560, 1981.

Pavan-Langston D, Dunkel EC: *Handbook of ocular drug therapy and ocular side effects of systemic drugs,* Boston, 1991, Little, Brown.

Schacter J, Dawson CR: *Human chlamydial infections,* Littleton, Ind, 1978, PSG Publishing.

Shoukrey ND, Tabbara KF: Eye-related parasitic diseases. In Tabbara KF, Hyndiuk RA, editors: *Infections of the eye,* Boston, 1986, Little, Brown.

Sullivan JH: Orbit. In Vaughn D, Asbury T, editors: *General ophthalmology,* ed 11, East Norwalk, Conn, 1986, Appleton & Lange.

Sullivan JH: Lids and lacrimal apparatus. In Vaughn D, Asbury T: *General ophthalmology,* ed 11, East Norwalk, Conn, 1986, Appleton & Lange.

Tabbara KF: Chlamydial conjunctivitis. In Tabbara KF, Hyndiuk RA, editors: *Infections of the eye,* Boston, 1986, Little, Brown.

Tabbara KF, Hyndiuk RA: *Infections of the eye,* Boston, 1986, Little, Brown.

Vaughn D, Asbury T, editors: *General ophthalmology,* ed 11, East Norwalk, Conn, 1986, Appleton & Lange.

Vaughn DG, Tabbara KF: Prevention of ocular infections. In Tabbara KF, Hyndiuk RA, editors: *Infections of the eye,* Boston, 1986, Little, Brown.

Veirs ER: The lacrimal system. In Wilson LA, editor: *External diseases of the eye,* New York, 1979, Harper & Row.

Watson P: Diseases of the sclera and episclera. In Wilson LA, editor: *External diseases of the eye,* New York, 1979, Harper & Row.

Weinberg RS: Endogenous bacterial and fungal infections of the retina and the choroid. In Tabbara KF, Hyndiuk RA, editors: *Infections of the eye,* Boston, 1986, Little, Brown.

Weinberg RS: Prevention of herpes simplex infections. In Friedlaender MH, editor: *Prevention of eye disease,* New York, 1988, Mary Ann Liebert.

Whitcher JP: Prevention of bacterial conjunctivitis and keratitis. In Friedlaender MH, editor: *Prevention of eye disease,* New York, 1988, Mary Ann Liebert.

Wilhelmus KR, Liesgang TJ, Osata MS, Jones DB. *Laboratory diagnosis of ocular infections, Cumitech 13 A,* Washington DC, 1994, ASM Press.

Wilson LA: Bacterial corneal ulcers. In Wilson LA, editor: *External diseases of the eye,* New York, 1979, Harper & Row.

Zambrano W et al: Management of options for *Propionibacterium acnes* endophthalmitis, *Ophthalmology* 96:1100, 1989.

LEARNING ASSESSMENT

1. Which groups of organisms are recovered from ocular infections? List three pathogens in each group.

2. What are three microbiologic techniques that are peculiar to ocular microbiology?

3. Culture requests are received most often from which ocular site or sites? Which organisms are most likely to be recovered? Which media and/or stains should be included in the initial setup?

4. Which types of smears are used to identify ocular pathogens?

Appendixes

APPENDIX A
  Selected Bacteriologic Culture Media
    Patricia K. Hargrave, PhD, CLS(NCA),
      MT(ASCP)
    Shirley Adams, MS, CLS(NCA), CLDir

APPENDIX B
  Selected Mycology Media, Fluids, and Stains
    Patricia K. Hargrave, PhD, CLS(NCA),
      MT(ASCP)
    Shirley Adams, MS, CLS(NCA), CLDir

APPENDIX C
  Nomenclature Changes for the Enterobacteriaceae
    and Nonfermentative Bacilli

APPENDIX D
  Answers to Learning Assessment Questions

Selected Bacteriologic Culture Media

Patricia K. Hargrave, Shirley Adams

A wide variety of basal, enrichment, selective, and differential media are available to the clinical microbiology laboratory. Each of these media is intended to aid the laboratory in the isolation, cultivation, and identification of clinically significant organisms from patient specimens. A laboratory's efficient performance of these functions depends not on its maintaining a vast array of media for routine use, but rather on the laboratory's ability to make wise choices when selecting a routine media menu—choices that should be dictated by the factors discussed in Chapter 7. This appendix provides the reader with information about a select number of bacteriologic media cited in the bacteriology section of this text. Most media detailed in this appendix are commercially available in either dehydrated or finished form.

When the medium is prepared "in-house," established formulation and directions must be strictly followed. Accuracy in the calculation of all weights and measures is essential. All glassware should be chemically clean, and only deionized or distilled water should be used unless the directions specify otherwise. Media rehydrated from powdered formulations should be monitored for appropriate appearance and pH. Media containing agar should be heated to boiling and allowed to boil for approximately 1 minute before sterilizing.

Heating and short-term boiling ensure the agar will dissolve completely and guard against charring of the agar during sterilization. Sterilization should be in accordance with the formulation's stated directions. Sterility and performance tests (quality controls) should be performed as discussed in Chapter 4.

A7 AGAR

A7 agar is a selective, differential medium useful in the isolation of genital mycoplasmas. Although a variety of formulations are available, commonly used formulations contain either penicillin G or penicillin G with amphotericin B to inhibit the normal bacterial flora of the genital tract (selective), whereas the presence of horse serum and yeast extract makes the medium complex enough to support the growth of mycoplasmal strains. The addition of urea and manganese sulfate enhances this medium's ability to differentiate *Ureaplasma urealyticum* from mycoplasmal strains that do not hydrolyze urea. *U. urealyticum* degradation of urea leads to the production of ammonia. The ammonia produced reacts with manganese sulfate to yield a dark-brown product; thus, *U. urealyticum* colonies take on a dark golden-brown to deep, velvet-brown color. The coloration of *U. urealyticum* colonies is in sharp contrast with the clear, light background of the medium. Classic *Mycoplasma, Acholeplasma* species, and *Proteus* L colonies do not react to form the colored end product; thus, colonies remain clear.

Plated completed A7 medium can be stored at 4° C for up to 1 week. (*Note:* Although the complete medium can be stored in the refrigerator, the basal medium alone should not be stored.) Any plated medium in which a precipitate is observable under the low-power objective of the light microscope should be discarded. Usable, plated medium should be inoculated, streaked for isolation, and incubated anaerobically at 35° C for 48 hours.

ACETATE AGAR

Acetate agar is a differential medium used to distinguish *Escherichia coli* from *Shigella* species by monitoring the ability to use acetate as the only available carbon source. Organisms capable of using acetate also use the medium's ammonium salt as a nitrogen source. The breakdown of the ammonium salt results in a shift of the pH into the alkaline range. At alkaline pH, the incorporated pH indicator, bromthymol blue, shifts from green to blue.

If the colony to be tested is young, the medium should be inoculated by making a saline suspension from an agar culture and introducing the saline-suspended organisms onto the slant with a needle. Incubate at 37° C for up to 4 days, monitoring daily for the expected color change.

ALKALINE PEPTONE WATER

Alkaline peptone water is an enrichment medium useful in the recovery of *Vibrio* and *Aeromonas* species from stool specimens. The alkaline pH of this medium allows uninhibited replication of these species while temporarily suppressing the replication rate of many commensal intestinal bacteria.

Some formulations recommend adjusting to pH 9.0 specifically for recovery of vibrios. Alkaline peptone water cultures should be incubated at 35° C and subcultured to thiosulfate citrate, bile salts, sucrose (TCBS) agar within 12 to 18 hours.

BACTEROIDES BILE-ESCULIN (BBE) AGAR

Bacteroides bile-esculin agar is a selective, differential agar used for the isolation and identification of *Bacteroides fragilis*. The incorporation of oxgall (bile salts) separates bile-resistant species from bile-sensitive ones, whereas the 1% esculin, in conjunction with ferric ammonium citrate, provides information about the isolate's ability to hydrolyze esculin. Products of esculin hydrolysis on reacting with the ferric ammonium citrate form an insoluble iron salt that is deposited within the positive colonies, causing them to turn black.

Plated medium should be inoculated, streaked for isolation, and incubated anaerobically.

BILE-ESCULIN AGAR

Bile-esculin agar is a selective, differential agar used to isolate and identify group D streptococci and the enterococci. Oxgall (bile salts) is the selective ingredient, whereas esculin is the differential component. All group D streptococci and enterococci hydrolyze esculin. Products of esculin hydrolysis react with ferric citrate in the medium to produce insoluble iron salts. Deposition of the iron salts results in a blackening of the tubed medium. Test results must be interpreted in conjunction with Gram stain morphology because *Listeria monocytogenes* and a small number of other organisms also produce positive reactions.

The medium should be inoculated, incubated aerobically at 35° C, and observed for growth. Darkening of the medium indicates esculin hydrolysis.

BISMUTH SULFITE AGAR

Bismuth sulfate agar is a selective medium for the isolation of *Salmonella* species. The selective ingredients are bismuth sulfite and brilliant green, which inhibit the growth of gram-positive bacteria, most lactose-fermenting intestinal normal flora, and shigellae. Although this is not a differential medium in the strictest sense, the ferrous sulfate in this medium is reactive with hydrogen sulfide to produce ferric sulfide, which is deposited within the bacterial colony as a black, insoluble precipitate. Typically, *Salmonella* serotype typhi colonies are black and surrounded by a metallic sheen, whereas *Salmonella* serotype gallinarum, *Salmonella* serotype choleraesuis, and Salmonella serotype paratyphi colonies are light green on this medium. When bismuth sulfite agar is used to isolate *Salmonella* species from feces and other clinical specimens, the parallel use of a less inhibitory medium is recommended, as bismuth sulfite agar may inhibit or partially inhibit the growth of some *Salmonella* strains.

This medium cannot be autoclaved and must be used on the day it is prepared. Plated medium should be inoculated with fecal or enrichment broth materials, streaked for isolation, and incubated at 35° C for 48 hours.

BLOOD AGAR, ANAEROBIC, CDC

CDC anaerobic blood agar is an enrichment medium useful in the isolation and culture of fastidious anaerobes. It contains yeast extract, L-cysteine, hemin, and vitamin K_1.

This medium can be stored for up to 6 weeks if it is sealed in cellophane bags and stored at 4° C. Plates should be inoculated, streaked for isolation, and incubated anaerobically at 35° C for 48 hours.

BLOOD AGAR, ANAEROBIC, BRUCELLA BASE, WADSWORTH

Wadsworth Brucella base anaerobic blood agar is a useful enrichment medium for the isolation of moderately fastidious, obligate anaerobes. Sheep's blood provides the enrichment. Vitamin K_1 is also added to this medium.

Plated medium should be sealed in bags and stored at 4° C for up to 2 weeks. Usable plates are inoculated, streaked for isolation, and incubated anaerobically at 35° C for 48 hours.

BLOOD AGAR, ANAEROBIC, WITH KANAMYCIN AND VANCOMYCIN (KV BLOOD AGAR)

KV blood agar is a variation of CDC anaerobic blood agar made semiselective by the addition of the antimicrobials kanamycin and vancomycin. It is useful in the primary isolation of obligate anaerobes, particularly *Bacteroides* species, from specimens with a mixed bacterial population.

KV blood agar plates sealed in bags can be stored at 4° C for up to 4 weeks. Usable plates should be inoculated, streaked for isolation, and incubated anaerobically at 35° C for 48 hours. Plates negative at 48 hours may be reincubated, depending on the particular situation.

BLOOD AGAR, ANAEROBIC, LAKED, WITH KANAMYCIN, VANCOMYCIN, AND VITAMIN K (KVKL)

Anaerobic, laked blood agar with kanamycin, vancomycin, and vitamin K (KVKL) is a selective enrichment medium recommended for the isolation of species of *Bacteroides* and *Prevotella* from clinical specimens. Although appropriate for the isolation of any *Bacteroides* species, this medium is particularly helpful in the isolation of *Prevotella melaninogenica* as pigment production is enhanced. Laked erythrocytes and vitamin K constitute the enrichment ingredients, whereas the antibiotics inhibit all cocci and facultative gramnegative bacilli except the pseudomonads.

Plated medium should be inoculated, streaked for isolation, and incubated anaerobically at 35° C for a minimum of 48 hours.

BLOOD AGAR, RABBIT'S

Rabbit's blood agar is an enrichment medium particularly useful in the recovery and the demonstration of β hemolysis by *Haemophilus* spp. and *Gardnerella vaginalis.*

BLOOD AGAR, SHEEP'S (SBA)

Blood agar is a routine medium used to cultivate a wide variety of moderately fastidious bacterial organisms. An infusion agar or tryptic soy agar base can be enriched by the addition of 5% to 10% defibrinated sheep's, rabbit's, or human's blood. However, sheep's blood has proved the most versatile enrichment additive. Incorporation of the blood not only provides enrichment for growth of the bacterial organisms but also allows the detection and characterization of hemolytic activity.

Usable plates should be inoculated, streaked, and incubated as dictated by the specific application.

BLOOD PHENYLETHYL ALCOHOL AGAR, ANAEROBIC, CDC

Blood phenylethyl alcohol agar (PEA) is a selective enrichment medium useful in the isolation of *Bacteroides, Prevotella,* and other obligate anaerobes from specimens containing a mixture of obligate and facultative anaerobes. Enrichment is provided by yeast extract, hemin, vitamin K, and defibrinated sheep's blood. Selectivity is provided by the incorporation of phenylethyl alcohol, which inhibits facultative anaerobes by suppressing DNA synthesis and cell division.

Plated medium should be sealed in plastic bags for storage. Bagged plates may be stored up to 4 weeks at 4° C. Usable plates should be inoculated, streaked for isolation, and incubated anaerobically at 35° C for at least 48 hours.

BLOOD PHENYLETHYL ALCOHOL AGAR, WADSWORTH

Wadsworth blood phenylethyl alcohol agar is an alternative to the CDC formulation of blood phenylethyl alcohol agar. Like the CDC formulation, it is a selective medium for the isolation of *Bacteroides* and *Prevotella* species. The inoculation, incubation, and interpretation of growth on this medium are the same as those for the CDC blood phenylethyl alcohol agar discussed previously.

BORDET-GENGOU (B-G) BLOOD AGAR

Bordet-Gengou blood agar is a selective enrichment medium for the isolation of *Bordetella pertussis* and *Bordatella parapertussis* from clinical specimens. Peptone is used in the base medium and enriched by the addition of glycerol and sterile, defibrinated sheep's blood. Increased selectivity of the medium has been achieved by adding penicillin, methicillin, or cephalexin to the medium.

The antibiotic should be added aseptically just before the addition of the blood enrichment. Blood enrichment between 15% and 30% (3 to 6 mL/ 20-mL tube) is appropriate. The source of the sterile, defibrinated blood obtained is not critical, but properly prepared plates should be cherry-red, moist, and bubble-free. Complete plated medium should be used immediately if possible. If for some reason this is not possible, plates can be maintained for about 1 week at 4° C if they are tightly sealed. Usable, complete medium can be inoculated by rolling the nasopharyngeal swab specimen over one third of the plate surface and then streaking for isolation with a platinum loop. The specimen should be inoculated in this fashion onto B-G plates without antibiotic and B-G plates with antibiotic. Inoculated plates should be incubated at 35° to 37° C and then examined at 48 hours. Plates negative at 48 hours should be reincubated. Plates must be held for 5 days before they can be regarded as negative for the organism.

BRAIN-HEART INFUSION BROTH

Brain-heart infusion broth is an enriched medium suitable for the cultivation of a number of nonfastidious and moderately fastidious microorganisms. This broth medium is recommended for cultivation of pneumococci for the bile solubility test.

BUFFERED CHARCOAL-YEAST EXTRACT AGAR WITH α-KETOGLUTARATE (BCYE-α)

Buffered charcoal-yeast extract agar with α-ketoglutarate is an enrichment medium useful in the isolation of *Legionella* species from clinical specimens. Yeast extract and L-cysteine enhance the growth of *Legionella* organisms, whereas activated charcoal absorbs toxic compounds that either accumulate as the result of the organism's metabolism or are present following preparation of this medium.

Usable plated medium may be stored in plastic bags, away from light, at 4° C for up to 4 weeks. Plated medium should be inoculated, streaked for isolation, and incubated at 35° C in a carbon dioxide incubator. Cultures should be checked daily for up to 2 weeks, and incubator humidity should be monitored to prevent excessive drying of plates. *Legionella* colonies may not be grossly visible until 3 to 5 days after inoculation.

Several modifications of BCYE-α exist. In one formulation, L-cysteine is omitted. Because *Legionella* spp. require L-cysteine, they will not grow on this medium. Comparison of growth on this L-cysteine deficient medium with that on regular BCYE-α can help determine if an isolate is *Legionella* or another type of gram-negative rod. The addition of antibiotics to BCYE-α can make the medium selective. Commonly used antibiotics include: cefamandole to inhibit gram-positive organisms; polymyxin B to inhibit gram-negative bacilli, especially pseudomonads; and anisomycin for fungal inhibition. The Wadowsky-Yee modification uses glycine and polymyxin B to inhibit gram-negative organisms, vancomycin to inhibit gram-positive cocci, and anisomycin to inhibit fungi. This medium is very useful in recovering *Legionella* from body sites that contain mixed flora.

CAMPYLOBACTER BLOOD AGAR (CAMPY-BA)

Campylobacter blood agar is a selective enrichment medium useful in the isolation and cultivation of *Campylobacter* species from stool specimens. Brucella agar serves as the base medium for

Campy-BA because it contains sodium bisulfite, which lowers the redox potential, thereby enhancing the recovery of microaerophilic organisms such as *Campylobacter* species. Ten percent sheep's blood enriches the basal medium, and an antibiotic mixture makes the medium selective. Although minor variations exist in the composition of this mixture, most formulations have incorporated vancomycin to inhibit gram-positive cocci, trimethoprim to inhibit swarming strains of *Proteus,* polymyxin B to inhibit gram-negative bacilli, and amphotericin B to inhibit filamentous fungi and yeasts. Currently, cefoperazone is being promoted to replace cephalothin. Cefoperazone has antipseudomonal activity (lacked by cephalothin) and is more effective against members of Enterobacteriaceae.

CAMPYLOBACTER THIOGLYCOLATE BROTH (CAMPY-THIO)

Campy-Thio is a selective liquid medium. The base medium is thioglycolate broth with 0.16% agar. The selective component is the antibiotic formulation used in Campy-BA.

CARBOHYDRATE FERMENTATION MEDIA, ANAEROBIC

Carbohydrate broths are differential media useful in determining the ability to ferment specific carbohydrates. This formulation, based on a carbohydrate medium base (Difco, Detroit, Mich.), is useful in the determination of carbohydrate fermentations carried out by anaerobic isolates. Carbohydrate stock solutions are added to the base according to the manufacturer's directions. Prepared media are aseptically dispensed into 15 × 90 mm screw-capped tubes. Tubed medium may be stored at room or refrigerator temperatures, but dissolved oxygen must be removed either before storage or before use. If an anaerobic chamber is available, the tubed medium, loosely capped, should be passed into the anaerobic atmosphere (85%, N_2; 10% H_2; 5% CO_2) and the caps securely tightened before removal and storage. If an anaerobic chamber

is not available, the tubed medium should be steamed or boiled with the caps loose for 10 minutes, cooled, and inoculated immediately using a capillary pipette to deliver the inoculum near the bottom of the tube without introducing air. One pipette may be used to inoculate multiple tubes.

All cultures should be incubated anaerobically, with the caps loosened, at 35° C for up to 7 days. Cultures should be examined on days 1, 2, and 7 for fermentation with production of acid. Three color reactions may occur. If fermentation occurs, the pH decreases to 6.0 or lower and the bromthymol blue indicator turns yellow, indicating a positive fermentation reaction. If fermentation does not occur, the bromthymol blue indicator remains blue to blue-green (negative reaction). If the cultured organism can reduce the bromthymol indicator, the medium becomes colorless. If this occurs, a sterile pipette can be used to transfer two to three drops of material from the involved tube(s) to a spot plate. Two to three drops of dilute indicator should then be added to the transferred material, and observed for color change. *Note:* Rapid test systems are available that include carbohydrate fermentations with a bromcresol purple indicator. Correlation between fermentation and color change is similar, as is the problem of indicator reduction and the method for detecting acid in the presence of reduced indicator.

CARBOHYDRATE FERMENTATION MEDIA FOR GRAM-POSITIVE COCCI

Carbohydrate broths are differential media useful in determining the ability of a variety of aerobic bacteria to ferment specific carbohydrates. The base is heart infusion broth, which provides sufficient nutrient to support the growth of gram-positive cocci, including streptococci.

The sterile carbohydrate is added to the sterile basal medium (cooled to 50° C) to give a final concentration of 1%. Tubed carbohydrate fermentation medium should be inoculated and incubated aerobically at 35° C. A positive reaction (acid production) is indicated by a color change from purple to yellow.

CARBOHYDRATE FERMENTATION MEDIA FOR AEROBIC GRAM-NEGATIVE BACILLI

Carbohydrate fermentation medium of this formulation does not contain sufficient quantities of complex nutrients to support the growth of fastidious aerobic bacteria. It is, however, sufficient to support the less fastidious Enterobacteriaceae; thus, it is the formulation of choice to determine the fermentative patterns of suspected Enterobacteriaceae isolates. Andrade pH indicator detects acid production. A positive result (acid production) is indicated by a color change from yellow or colorless (alkaline) to pink or red.

CHOCOLATE AGAR

Chocolate agar is an enrichment agar especially useful in promoting the growth of *Haemophilus* and other fastidious bacterial species. This medium, a variation of sheep's blood agar, may be made by adding sheep's blood while the basal medium is warm enough to release the red cell hemoglobin and nicotinamide-adenine dinucleotide (NAD). Alternatively, sheep's blood may be replaced by 2% hemoglobin and a chemical supplement solution, such as Iso-Vitalex (BBL, Cockeysville, Md.). The enrichment used must result in the complete medium containing cell-free hemoglobin and NAD. The temperature at which either enrichment is added results in a chocolate-brown medium.

Plated medium can be stored at 4° C. Usable plates should be inoculated, streaked for isolation, and incubated at 35° C in CO_2.

CITRATE AGAR, SIMMONS

Simmons citrate agar is useful in differentiating gram-negative enteric bacilli. Similar in principles of its use to acetate agar, citrate replaces acetate in this medium, and differentiation is based on the isolate's ability or inability to use citrate as its sole source of carbon. Several alternative theories have been advanced to explain the biochemical sequences leading to a color change in this medium.

One such theory holds that, as with acetate agar, organisms capable of using the citrate also use the medium's ammonium salt as a nitrogen source. The breakdown of the ammonium salt results in a shift of the pH into the alkaline range. At alkaline pH, the incorporated pH indicator bromthymol blue shifts from green to blue.

The pH of the medium is approximately 6.9. This medium should be inoculated by making a saline suspension of a young colony from an agar culture, streaking the saline suspended organisms onto the slant with a needle, and stabbing the butt. Inoculated slants should be incubated at 35° C for up to 4 days and monitored daily for the expected color change.

COLUMBIA AGAR

Columbia agar is a basal nutrient agar that contains peptones derived from both casein and meat. The basal medium is suitable for cultivation of a number of aerobic and anaerobic bacterial organisms found in clinical materials. Additionally, it provides an efficient base for preparation of a variety of enrichment agars that support the growth of more fastidious aerobes and anaerobes.

Inoculate plated medium, streak for isolation, and incubate at 35° C for up to 7 days as appropriate for the specific organism to be cultured.

COLUMBIA AGAR WITH ANTIBIOTICS (COLUMBIA CNA AGAR)

Columbia agar with antibiotics is a selective enrichment medium suitable for the isolation of gram-positive cocci from specimens that might also be expected to contain gram-negative bacilli, especially *Proteus* species. Sheep's blood is the usual enrichment ingredient, whereas colistin and nalidixic acid are incorporated to inhibit gram-negative overgrowth of desired gram-positive isolates.

Plated medium should be inoculated streaked for isolation, and incubated in an environment appropriate to the isolation of the desired species.

COOKED MEAT MEDIUM

Cooked meat medium is useful in the cultivation of anaerobes, especially pathogenic species of *Clostridium*. This medium contains solid meat particles and is excellent for initiating growth from a very small inoculum as well as sustaining culture viability over long periods. It is useful for cultivation of mixed cultures because all organisms are supported while overgrowth by the more rapid growers is retarded. Dehydrated medium is suspended in tubes according to the manufacturer's directions and allowed to stand until thoroughly moistened (approximately 15 minutes) before sterilizing by autoclaving (121° C for 15 minutes). Tubed medium may be stored at room temperature, but stored tubes should be placed in flowing steam or a boiling water bath for 10 minutes to drive off dissolved gases and then cooled rapidly before inoculating. Cooled tubed medium should be inoculated and incubated in a manner appropriate for the species being isolated or subcultured. Proteolytic activity by cultured organisms is usually evidenced by the digestion of the meat particles. Saccharolytic clostridial species typically produce acid with gas.

TELLURITE BLOOD AGAR (WITH OR WITHOUT CYSTINE)

Tellurite blood agar is a selective-differential enrichment agar useful in the isolation of *Corynebacterium diphtheriae*. All formulations include animal blood as a source of enrichment. Some formulations also incorporate cystine to further enhance the growth of fastidious organisms, including *C. diphtheriae*. Potassium tellurite is the selective, differential ingredient responsible for inhibiting the growth of staphylococci and streptococci while allowing the growth of *C. diphtheriae* and diphtheroids, which act on the tellurite, depositing the reduced product within the colonies.

Tubes of base medium may be stored and melted to make the complete medium as culture plates are needed. Freshly plated medium should be inoculated, streaked for isolation, and incubated at 35° C. On this medium, colonies of *C. diphtheriae* are dull gray-black, whereas diphtheroids are light gray-green with dark centers. Some *Staphylococcus* species, gram-negative bacilli, and yeasts may overcome inhibition and grow on this medium. The *Staphylococcus* colonies are large, glistening, and jet-black, whereas those of the gram-negative bacilli and yeast are dull gray-black but larger than the *C. diphtheriae* colonies.

CYSTINE TRYPTOPHAN AGAR, WITH SUGAR (CTA-SUGAR)

Cystine tryptophan (tryptic/trypticase) agar is a semisolid base medium that contains no meat or plant extracts and is free from fermentable carbohydrates. It may be made differential by the addition of a carbohydrate (CTA-sugar). CTA-sugars are recommended for the determination of fermentation reactions by fastidious organisms.

Alternatively, carbohydrates are available in the form of differentiation disks that can be aseptically added to the base tubed medium as needed. Sterile, tubed CTA-sugars should be inoculated with a heavy inoculum, stabbing to a depth of approximately 2 mm below the medium surface. With phenol red as the pH indicator, fermentation is indicated by a color change in the medium from red to yellow.

CYCLOSERINE CEFOXITIN FRUCTOSE AGAR (CCFA)

Cycloserine cefoxitin fructose agar is a selective, differential medium useful in the isolation and identification of *Clostridium difficile* from stool specimens of patients suspected of having antibiotic-associated diarrhea with pseudomembranous colitis. The selective antibiotic ingredients, cycloserine and cefoxitin, inhibit the growth of intestinal normal flora by interfering with cell wall synthesis in both gram-positive and gram-negative bacteria. Indigenous bacteria are inhibited, but *C. difficile* is not. Although cycloserine and cefoxitin are incorporated for their selective properties, fructose and a pH indicator, neutral red, are included to confirm that the isolates can ferment this sugar. *Note:* A variation of this medium is made with mannitol rather than fructose and uses bromthymol blue indicator. A second variation adds egg yolk suspension so lecithinase and lipase activities can be detected.

DECARBOXYLASE TEST MEDIUM (MOELLER)

Decarboxylase test medium with an incorporated amino acid is a differential medium useful in the identification of fermentative and nonfermentative gram-negative bacteria. The differential ingredient is one of three amino acids: lysine, arginine, or ornithine. Decarboxylation of the amino acids yields alkaline end products detected by a change in the color of an incorporated pH sensitive dye, bromcresol purple. The tubed basal medium (no amino acid) serves as a control for reading the reactions.

Decarboxylase tubes and a control tube should be inoculated from a 24-hour slant culture using a loop. Inoculated tubes should be overlaid with 4 to 5 mm of sterile mineral oil to avoid oxidative deamination of available protein, which would be falsely interpreted as a positive reaction. Inoculated, overlaid tubes should be incubated at 35° C for up to 4 days. Incubating tubes should be checked daily. Early in the incubation, fermentative organisms will ferment glucose, turning the control and all decarboxylase tubes yellow. For these organisms, as the pH drops, the hydrogen ion concentration becomes optimal for decarboxylase activity in the decarboxylase tubes, the subsequent conversion of the amino acid to amines raises the pH, reversing the yellow to purple, whereas the control tube remains yellow. Nonfermenters do not produce the initial yellow color change, and use of the amino acid is indicated when the amino acid–containing tube becomes a deeper purple than the control.

DEOXYCHOLATE CITRATE AGAR

Deoxycholate citrate agar is a selective, differential medium useful in the isolation of enteric pathogens directly from feces and urine specimens or indirectly from enrichment broths, such as selenite-F. The selective ingredients are sodium citrate and sodium deoxycholate at concentrations that inhibit the majority of nonpathogenic enteric bacilli. The differential ingredient is lactose. Nonfermenting enteric pathogens appear as colorless colonies. Those lactose-fermenters that do overcome the inhibitors appear as pink to red colonies

as the result of the pH change that accompanies lactose fermentation.

This medium is not autoclaved. Plates may be stored under refrigeration for several days. Plated medium should be inoculated, streaked for isolation, and incubated at 35° C in air (not in CO_2) for up to 48 hours. A heavy inoculum is recommended if the specimen is feces, urine, or other direct bodily materials, whereas a light inoculum is recommended if the subculture is from an initial enrichment broth.

DEOXYRIBONUCLEASE (DNASE) TEST AGAR, WITH OR WITHOUT INDICATOR DYE

DNase test agar is a differential medium used to detect the production of an active DNase exoenzyme by aerobic bacterial species. The differential ingredient is incorporated DNA. Methods available for detection of DNA degradation include hydrochloric acid precipitation of undegraded DNA and color change of an incorporated metachromatic dye, such as toluidine blue or methyl green.

Sterile plated medium should be inoculated using a 1- to 2-cm streak or a spot inoculum approximately 5 mm in diameter. Inoculated plates should be incubated aerobically at 35° C for 18 to 24 hours. Following incubation, DNase activity is detected in one of the following ways:

1. If a basal medium without a metachromatic dye was inoculated, flood the plate with 1N HCl, and look for a zone of clearing around the bacterial growth. If the incorporated DNA is undegraded, it is precipitated by the 1N HCl, and the medium becomes opaque. If the incorporated DNA is degraded, the nucleotide fragments dissolve in the 1N HCl, and the medium remains clear.
2. If the medium includes toluidine blue, the blue, DNA-bound dye is released from nucleotide fragments, producing a color change to rose. The medium remains clear blue in negative reactions.
3. If the medium includes methyl green, the green, DNA-bound dye is released from nucleotide fragments, resulting in a loss of color. The medium remains green in negative reactions.

E MEDIUM, DIPHASIC

E medium is one of many media developed for the isolation and culture of mycoplasmal organisms. This medium is enriched with a yeast dialysate, horse serum, penicillin, and thallium acetate.

The basal agar is aliquoted in 65-mL portions. Any basal medium not used immediately can be stored under refrigeration and remelted for use as needed. To each 65-mL aliquot add 10 mL of yeast dialysate, 25 mL of sterile horse serum, 2 mL of penicillin (20,000 U), and 1 mL of 3.3% aqueous thallium acetate. Completed agar can be dispensed in 3-mL quantities into 16×125 mm screw-capped tubes or in 5-mL amounts into 10×35 mm Petri dishes and allowed to solidify.

The E broth is prepared according to the manufacturer's directions. Broth is dispensed into 65-mL aliquots. To each aliquot add 10 mL of yeast dialysate, 25 mL of sterile horse serum, 2 mL of penicillin (20,000 U), and 1 mL of 3.3% aqueous thallium acetate.

The E agar is overlaid with 3 mL of E broth and stored at room temperature. *Caution:* Tubes must be tightly capped to prevent loss of CO_2 from incorporated horse serum, resulting in elevation of the medium pH.

EGG YOLK AGAR, CDC FORMULATION (EYA)

Egg yolk agar is a differential medium useful in the detection of lecithinase, lipase, and protease activity. Incorporated egg emulsion provides the lecithin, lipids, and proteins to be degraded by these enzymes. On EYA, exoenzyme activity is detected as follows: Lecithinase activity produces a zone of opacity immediately around the growth streak; lipase activity results in an iridescent sheen on or around the surface of colonies; and protease activity is seen as a clearing of the medium around and just beyond the streaked growth area. A given organism may produce one or all of these exoenzymes.

Plated medium is inoculated as a single streak across the plate and incubated anaerobically at $35°$ C for 24 to 72 hours. If the Nagler test is to be performed, one half of the plate surface should be smeared with a few drops of *C. perfringens* type A antitoxin before inoculation. The inoculation streak should then extend across both halves (no antitoxin/antitoxin) of the plate. Inoculated plates should be incubated anaerobically at $35°$ C for 24 to 48 hours. A positive test result is the inhibition of lecithinase activity on the half of the plate with antitoxin. Plated medium not used immediately may be stored at $4°$ C if it is sealed in plastic bags.

EOSIN–METHYLENE BLUE (EMB) AGAR

Eosin–methylene blue agar is a selective, differential medium useful in the isolation and identification of gram-negative enteric bacteria. Eosin Y and methylene blue dyes, the selective ingredients, are incorporated to inhibit the growth of gram-positive bacteria while allowing the growth of gram-negative ones. The carbohydrates lactose and sucrose are incorporated to allow differentiation of isolates based on lactose fermentation. Fermentation is detected by color changes and precipitation of the incorporated dyes as the pH drops. Sucrose serves as an alternative carbohydrate source for slow lactose-fermenters, allowing their timely elimination from consideration as possible pathogens. *E. coli,* a coliform lactose-fermenter, typically forms blue-black colonies with a metallic greenish sheen. Other coliform fermenters, such as *Enterobacter,* form pink colonies. Nonfermenter colonies are translucent, being either amber-colored or colorless.

ESCULIN AGAR

Esculin agar is a differential medium used to determine the ability of an organism to hydrolyze esculin. The hydrolytic products from esculin react with the ferric salt present in this medium to precipitate iron compounds and produce a gray to black discoloration of the medium.

Slanted medium should be inoculated, incubated aerobically at $35°$ C, and observed for growth, with darkening of the medium indicative of esculin hydrolysis.

FLETCHER SEMISOLID MEDIUM FOR LEPTOSPIRA

Fletcher semisolid medium is an enrichment medium recommended for detection of leptospiral species in blood, spinal fluid, and urine specimens as well as possibly contaminated water and other materials. The enrichment component of this medium is rabbit serum containing some hemoglobin.

The lyophilized rabbit serum with natural hemoglobin is commercially available as Leptospira Enrichment, or sterile, pooled, fresh natural rabbit serum may be added. The medium should be aseptically dispensed into sterile screw-capped tubes (5 mL/tube) and stored at room temperature overnight. The medium *must* be inactivated by placing tubes in a 56° C water bath for 1 hour on the day following preparation. Cooled inactivated medium should be inoculated with one or two drops of the fluid specimen, using a sterile, plugged Pasteur pipette. Small inocula introduced into multiple tubes are recommended to optimize pathogen recovery and minimize any interference by developing antibody titers in the body fluid specimens. Inoculated tubes should be incubated with caps loose at 25° to 30° C for 4 to 5 weeks and examined weekly for growth in the form of turbidity at the top of the medium. A loopful of fluid from any tube showing turbidity should be placed on a clean slide, a coverslip added, and the specimen examined by darkfield microscopy.

GELATIN MEDIUM (NUTRIENT)

Gelatin medium is a differential medium used to determine a bacterial isolate's ability to produce gelatinase and thereby hydrolyze gelatin. A variety of gelatin-containing media can be used for this purpose, including starch-gelatin agar, Kohn modified gelatin for the Kohn gelatin method, and nutrient gelatin.

Sterile tubed medium can be stored at 4° C. The medium is inoculated and incubated, along with an uninoculated control tube, at 35° C for 18 to 24 hours. Following incubation, both the inoculated tube and the control tube are refrigerated for 30 minutes before reading. The control tube should gel, whereas the consistency of the inoculated tube will depend on the isolate's ability or inability to hydrolyze gelatin. If the inoculated tube gels, the isolate in question is gelatinase negative. If the gelatin in the inoculated tube remains liquid, the isolate in question is gelatinase positive.

GRAM-NEGATIVE (GN) BROTH

Gram-negative (GN) broth is a selective enrichment medium used to enhance the chance of recovering enteric pathogens, such as *Salmonella* and *Shigella* species, from fecal specimens. The selective ingredients are deoxycholate and citrate salts, which retard the growth of gram-positive bacteria while allowing the growth of aerobic gram-negative bacteria. Enrichment is provided by increasing the concentration of mannitol, which temporarily favors the growth of mannitol-fermenting, gram-negative rods over that of the non–mannitol-fermenters.

Sterile, tubed medium should be inoculated with fecal material and incubated, with caps loosened, at 35° C. Incubated GN broth cultures should be subcultured onto selective, differential plated media after 6 to 8 hours and again after 18 to 24 hours.

HEKTOEN ENTERIC (HE) AGAR

Hektoen enteric agar is a selective, differential medium used for direct isolation of enteric pathogens from feces and for indirect isolation from selective enrichment broth. The selective ingredients are bile salts at concentrations that not only inhibit the growth of gram-positive bacteria but also retard the growth of many gram-negative organisms that are part of the normal intestinal flora. The differential ingredients include lactose and sucrose to determine fermentation patterns, detected by the pH indicator bromthymol blue, and ferric salts (sodium thiosulfate and ferric ammonium citrate) to detect the production of hydrogen sulfide gas.

This medium should not be autoclaved, and overheating should be avoided. Plated medium should be inoculated, streaked for isolation, and incubated aerobically (not in CO_2) at 35° C for 18 to 24 hours. Most nonpathogens ferment one or both of the sugars, and colonies appear bright orange to salmon-pink owing to the low pH interaction with incorporated dyes. Nonfermenters, such as *Salmonella* and *Shigella* species, typically produce green to blue-green colonies. Hydrogen sulfide gas production is seen as a black precipitate that accumulates within colonies.

HIPPURATE BROTH

Hippurate broth is a differential broth useful in the identification of group B streptococci. The differential ingredient is 1% sodium hippurate, which the group B streptococci hydrolyze to glycine and benzoic acid. In this method, hydrolysis is detected by the addition of ferric chloride, which reacts with the benzoic acid to produce ferric benzoate, which precipitates.

Broth should be inoculated with the isolate and incubated at 35° C for more than 20 hours. Following incubation, 0.8 mL of supernatant is removed and placed into another tube to which 0.2 mL of ferric chloride reagent is added. A positive reaction yields grossly visible precipitate that persists for 10 minutes or longer after the addition of ferric chloride. A negative reaction produces no precipitate or only a faint precipitate that disappears in less than 10 minutes after the addition of ferric chloride. *Note:* A rapid method available uses a 1% aqueous solution of sodium hippurate dispensed in 0.4-mL quantities. Colonies of the isolate are emulsifed in the solution until it is very cloudy and are then incubated in a 37° C waterbath for 2 hours. Hydrolysis is detected by adding five drops of Ninhydrin reagent (triketohydrindene hydrate) without shaking the tube and continuing to incubate for a minimum of 10 minutes but not longer than 30 minutes. Positive reactions are deep-purple in color, and negative reactions show no color change.

HYDROGEN SULFIDE, LEAD ACETATE

Lead acetate is one differential method used to detect the production of hydrogen sulfide (H_2S) from sulfur-containing amino acids. The organism is cultured in a nutrient broth or on an agar medium with sufficient protein to ensure the presence of sulfur-containing amino acids. As the organism metabolizes these amino acids, H_2S gas is evolved. The liberated gas is detected by lead acetate—

impregnated paper strips suspended over the culture during incubation. The produced H_2S reacts with the lead acetate to produce lead sulfide, a black insoluble salt, causing the strip to blacken. Lead acetate strips are available commercially.

KLIGLER IRON AGAR

Kligler iron agar (KIA) can be used to determine whether a gram-negative rod is a glucose- or lactose-fermenter, or both. The medium also tests for gas production during carbohydrate fermentation and hydrogen sulfide production, both of which are useful in the differentiation of gram-negative rods belonging to the family Enterobacteriaceae.

KIA contains glucose and lactose (fermentable carbohydrates), phenol red (pH indicator), peptone (carbon/nitrogen source), and iron salt plus sodium thiosulfate (sulfur source and hydrogen sulfide indicator). KIA resembles triple sugar iron agar except that it lacks sucrose. The following three carbohydrate fermentation patterns are possible:

1. Acid (yellow) butt and alkaline (red) slant indicate the organism ferments glucose but not lactose. This organism ferments glucose by the Embden-Meyerhof-Parnas (EMP) pathway to produce organic acids, changing the pH indicator from red to yellow. Once the glucose has been consumed, the organism then breaks down peptones, producing ammonia. This causes a pH rise and the slant reverts to red.
2. Acid (yellow) butt and acid (yellow) slant indicate that the organism ferments both glucose and lactose. The organism ferments glucose, producing acid products. Once the glucose is consumed, it ferments lactose, breaking it down into glucose and galactose. This causes the pH in the slant portion to remain acidic.
3. Alkaline (red) butt and alkaline (red) slant indicate that the organism cannot ferment glucose or lactose and therefore produces no acidic products. The slant may become redder owing to peptone catabolism.

If there are gas bubbles in the butt, splitting of the medium, or displacement of the medium from the bottom of the tube, the organism is aerogenic—

that is, it is able to produce carbon dioxide and hydrogen gases during fermentation. Any blackening in the butt indicates the organism produces hydrogen sulfide gas from thiosulfate. The hydrogen sulfide combines with iron salt to produce ferrous sulfide, a black precipitate.

Inoculation is performed by stabbing the butt with an inoculating needle and streaking the slant using pure culture of isolate. The cap should be slightly loose. If the cap is screwed on too tightly, there will not be sufficient air for peptone catabolism. Gram-negative rods able to ferment only glucose may appear as lactose-fermenters. Reactions should be interpreted at 18 to 24 hours. If the medium is read earlier, organisms only able to ferment glucose may appear to be lactose-fermenters. If the medium is read later, lactose-fermenters may consume the lactose and begin to catabolize peptones, with the slant reverting to red. A yellow slant and red butt may indicate failure to stab the butt or inoculation of the medium with gram-positive organisms. Examination of the medium for stab line or performance of Gram stain should clarify this situation. The hydrogen sulfide indicator system in KIA is not as sensitive as the lead acetate method or as that found in other media, such as sulfide indole motility agar. A black butt should be read as acid even though yellow color may be obscured. If hydrogen sulfide is reduced, this indicates an acid condition does exist and can be assumed. Critical to understanding how this medium works is the fact that glucose is present in a much lesser amount than lactose. Organisms use the simplest carbohydrate, glucose, first. Once this is consumed, they attack the more complex carbohydrate, lactose. If they lack the appropriate enzymes, they move on to protein catabolism. There is sufficient lactose in the medium to prevent breakdown of peptone, provided that it is read at the appropriate time.

LOEFFLER COAGULATED SERUM SLANT

Loeffler coagulated serum slant is used primarily for recovery and identification of *C. diphtheriae.*

This medium can be used for primary recovery of *C. diphtheriae* from nose and throat specimens and for subculture purposes. Because Loeffler medium is so enriched, *C. diphtheriae* grows well within 12 to 16 hours and produces nondistinctive translucent to gray-white colonies. The medium promotes the development of characteristic granules that can be detected microscopically with methylene blue stains. Serum content enables detection of proteolytic activity. Positive organisms produce colonies surrounded by small holes containing liquefied medium. The entire slant may eventually turn to liquid and produce of a foul odor.

Loeffler serum slant should be inoculated as soon as possible after specimen collection, and more selective media containing tellurite should always be used as well. Smears for *C. diphtheriae* should be prepared and examined after 8 to 24 hours of incubation. Although granule formation is typical of *Corynebacterium* species, other organisms can produce a similar microscopic appearance. Therefore additional testing must be performed for confirmation of this organism.

LÖWENSTEIN-JENSEN MEDIUM

Löwenstein-Jensen (LJ) medium is used to cultivate *Mycobacterium* spp. Most media contain ingredients that can inhibit the growth of mycobacteria. The potato flour, egg, and glycerol included in LJ medium help detoxify this medium and also supply nutrients required for growth of these organisms. Asparagine is included for maximum production of niacin by certain *Mycobacterium* spp. The malachite green serves as an inhibitor of other bacteria that may be present in specimens.

LJ medium is good for 1 month if tightly capped to prevent moisture loss and stored at 4° to 6° C. LJ medium must be kept out of direct light because malachite green is light-sensitive. Decontaminated or digested or untreated specimens are inoculated onto medium and incubated in a carbon dioxide incubator (5% to 10% CO_2) for 6 to 10 weeks. It is important to leave caps loose for proper gas exchange.

LJ medium may be prepared as deeps to be used in semiquantitative catalase testing for ascertaining the particular species of *Mycobacterium*. LJ medium with 5% sodium chloride may be prepared to aid in identifying rapid growers. This medium is the same as LJ except for the addition of 5 g of sodium chloride per each 100 mL of medium. The additional salt allows for testing the ability of certain mycobacteria to tolerate and grow in presence of high salt concentration. The Gruft modification makes this medium more selective through the addition of penicillin (50 U/ml.) and nalidixic acid (35 μg/mL) before dispensing into tubes. This formulation also includes 0.05 μg/mL of ribonucleic acid, which increases the rate of mycobacterium isolation over standard LJ formation. In the Petran and Vera modification, cyclohexamide, lincomycin, and nalidixic acid are added to make LJ more selective. Both of these modifications can permit gentler decontamination or digestion procedures.

LYSINE-IRON AGAR

This medium measures three parameters useful in identifying species of Enterobacteriaceae: lysine decarboxylation, lysine deamination, and hydrogen sulfide production.

Lysine-iron agar (LIA) contains lysine (amino acid), glucose (carbohydrate source), a small amount of protein, bromcresol purple (pH indicator), and sodium thiosulfate/ferric ammonium citrate (sulfur source and hydrogen sulfide indicator).

Three lysine use patterns are possible, as follows:

1. Alkaline (purple) butt and alkaline (purple) slant indicate that the organism decarboxylates lysine but cannot deaminate it. Initially, the organism ferments glucose, causing production of acid and changing indicator in the butt to yellow. It then decarboxylates lysine to produce cadaverine, an alkaline product. This causes the pH indicator to change back to purple.
2. Acid (yellow) butt and alkaline (purple) slant indicate that the organism fermented the glucose but was unable to deaminate or decarboxylate the lysine.
3. Acid (yellow) butt and Bordeaux red slant indicate that the organism deaminated lysine but could not decarboxylate it. The yellow butt is caused by glucose fermentation. The reason for red slant in cases of lysine deamination has not been clarified. If no indicator is present, one of the products of deamination appears orange. The red slant may be the result of mixing the purple and red colors.

Any blackening in the butt indicates production of hydrogen sulfide from sodium thiosulfate. This gas reacts with ferric salt to produce the black precipitate, ferrous sulfide.

This medium appears purple before use. LIA is inoculated by stabbing the butt twice and streaking the slant with an inoculating needle. Cap should be left slightly loose because oxygen is required for detection of deamination. Reactions should be read after 18 to 24 hours of incubation at 35° C. The medium may be incubated for up to 48 hours if needed.

LIA is not as sensitive as other media for hydrogen sulfide detection. Typically, hydrogen sulfide–producing *Proteus* spp. may appear negative. Also, *Morganella morganii* produces a variable lysine deamination reaction after 24 hours of incubation. This medium can be used only with organisms that can ferment glucose. LIA is not a true replacement for the Moeller decarboxylase tests.

MACCONKEY AGAR

MacConkey agar is a selective, differential primary plating medium. It selects for Enterobacteriaceae and other gram-negative rods in the presence of mixed flora and differentiates them into lactose-fermenters and non–lactose-fermenters.

Bile salts and crystal violet inhibit most gram-positive organisms but permit the growth of gram-negative rods. Lactose serves as the sole carbohydrate source. Gram-negative rods that ferment lactose produce pink or red colonies, which may be surrounded by precipitated bile. Acid production from lactose fermentation causes the neutral red dye absorbed into the colonies to change to red and can also cause the bile salts to become insoluble. Non–lactose-fermenting gram-negative rods produce colorless or transparent colonies.

Plates are streaked for isolation and incubated in ambient air, not a carbon dioxide incubator, for 18 to 24 hours at 35° C. Weak or slow lactose-fermenters may produce colorless colonies at 24 hours or appear slightly pink in 24 to 48 hours. Plates should not be incubated longer than 48 hours because this can lead to confusing results. Some gram-negative rods may fail to grow on the medium, whereas with prolonged incubation, gram-positives such as *Enterococcus* species may produce tiny colonies. Room temperature incubation may enhance recovery of *Yersinia enterocolitica.* The agar concentration may be increased to prevent swarming of *Proteus* species. A formulation of MacConkey agar without crystal violet has been used to aid in identifying mycobacteria.

MACCONKEY SORBITOL AGAR

MacConkey sorbitol agar contains the same components as MacConkey agar except D-sorbitol is substituted for lactose. This medium has been used to isolate *E. coli* 0157:H7, which does not ferment sorbitol very rapidly. Plates should be incubated at 37° C for 24 hours. Sorbitol-negative colonies that appear colorless on this medium may indicate possible *E. coli* 0157:H7 and should be further tested. Most other clinical isolates of *E. coli* produce a pink to red color on this medium.

MALONATE BROTH

Malonate broth is used in the identification of species of Enterobacteriaceae, particularly *Salmonella.*

Malonate broth contains sodium malonate (primary carbon source), small quantities of glucose and yeast extract (nutrients), bromthymol blue (pH indicator), various salts, and a buffering system. Organisms producing a Prussian blue color are able to use malonate as a carbon source. If they can use malonate as a carbon source, they also employ ammonium sulfate as a nitrogen source, thereby producing alkaline products that cause a rise in pH and a change in the color of the medium to blue. Organisms unable to use malonate as a carbon source usually fail to grow, and the medium stays green. Because malonate resembles succinate, it competitively binds succinic dehydrogenase, which catalyzes the succinate to fumarate in the Krebs cycle. The tying up of this enzyme, coupled with the inability to use malonate as a carbon source, prevents growth.

Malonate broth should be inoculated from triple sugar iron agar, KIA, or broth culture of the organism. Inoculum should be light. Cultures should be incubated at 35° C and checked at 18 to 24 hours and at 48 hours for production of a blue color. Some organisms produce only small amounts of

alkalinity. Any trace of blue should be considered positive. Comparison with an uninoculated tube may be useful. Production of a yellow color is a negative reaction. This reaction is probably due to fermentation of the small amount of glucose in the medium.

MANNITOL SALT AGAR

Mannitol salt agar is a selective and differential primary culture medium useful in recovery and identification of staphylococci from specimens containing mixed flora.

High salt concentration (7.5%) inhibits most gram-negative and gram-positive bacteria except *Staphylococcus* species. *Staphylococcus aureus* is able to ferment mannitol, the sole carbohydrate in the medium, to produce acid products. This lowers the pH and changes the color of the pH indicator, phenol red, to yellow. Colonies of *S. aureus* typically appear yellow, surrounded by a yellow zone. Other *Staphylococcus* and *Micrococcus* species usually do not ferment mannitol and therefore produce reddish colonies that may exhibit a red to purple surrounding zone due to peptone breakdown.

Plates are streaked for isolation and incubated at 35° C for 24 to 48 hours, but not in a carbon dioxide incubator. *Enterococcus* may be able to grow on mannitol salt agar and produce slight mannitol fermentation. Differentiation is readily accomplished through Gram stain and catalase test. With prolonged incubation, organisms other than staphylococci may begin to grow and produce mannitol fermentation. Some strains of *S. aureus* may be slow in fermenting mannitol, so plates should not be discarded until after 48 hours of incubation. All colonies suggestive of *S. aureus* should be further tested for coagulase or with an alternative acceptable procedure. Subculture to less selective agar is preferable before performing this testing. Some formulations recommend inclusion of 20 mL of sterile egg yolk. Coagulase-positive staphylococci also produce a lipase that causes formation of an opaque precipitate around the colonies. Non–coagulase-producing staphylococci do not produce this egg yolk lipase and therefore lack these zones.

MES (UREAPLASMA AGAR)

MES [2-(N-morpholino) ethanesulfonic acid] agar is used for the isolation of *U. urealyticum*. This medium contains horse serum, which supplies the cholesterol necessary for stabilizing these organisms because they lack cell walls. Yeast dialysate serves as a growth factor and supplies preformed nucleic acid precursors. Urea is a required nutrient for *Ureaplasma*. Phenol red serves as a pH indicator, and MES or 2-(N-morpholino) ethanesulfonic acid acts as a buffer. The antibiotics, penicillin and lincomycin, inhibit normal flora but permit the growth of *Ureaplasma*. After mixing components, pour the medium into Petri dishes (5 mL per plate.) Store plates in plastic for up to 2 weeks under refrigeration. Inoculated plates should be incubated in a carbon dioxide incubator or candle jar or under anaerobic conditions. At 48 hours, colonies of *Ureaplasma* show a "fried-egg" appearance. If a solution of 1% urea and 0.8% manganese chloride is poured over these colonies, they will turn dark brown owing to the production of urease.

METHYL RED–VOGES-PROSKAUER (MR-VP) MEDIUM

MR-VP broth is used for performing the methyl red and Voges-Proskauer tests. These procedures are useful in distinguishing among numbers of Enterobacteriaceae. For example, *E. coli* is methyl red positive and Voges-Proskauer negative; *Enterobacter aerogenes, Enterobacter cloacae,* and *Klebsiella pneumoniae* show the reverse reactions.

Members of Enterobacteriaceae can be divided into two groups based on the way they metabolize glucose. One group produces large amounts of mixed acids (lactic, formic, succinic, and acetic). When methyl red reagent is added to one of these cultures, a red color is produced owing to the acidic pH. The other group produces predominantly neutral end products, acetoin or acetylmethylcarbinol, by the butylene glycol pathway. When α-naphthol and 40% potassium hydroxide are added to the broth culture, acetoin (if present) is oxidized to diacetyl in the presence of air and base. α-Naphthol catalyzes a reaction between the diacetyl and guanidine components of peptone to produce a pink-red color.

For the methyl red test, broth culture must be incubated for 48 hours. Avoid using really turbid broth. The Voges-Proskauer test was originally designed to be performed after 5 days of incubation at 30° C. By using 0.5 to 1 mL of broth per tube, the test can be done after 18 to 24 hours of incubation at 35° C. Shaking aerates the broth culture and enhances the reaction.

MIDDLEBROOK 7H10 AND 7H11 AGARS

The purpose of Middlebrook 7H10 and 7H11 agars is to cultivate *Mycobacterium* species. Isoniazid-resistant strains grow better on these media than on egg-based media such as Löwenstein-Jensen. The Middlebrook agars are also more chemically defined than the Löwenstein-Jensen formulations.

Middlebrook 7H10 and 7H11 are similar, except that 7H11 contains casein hydrolysate. Both media contain growth factors, such as amino acids and salt, that encourage recovery of mycobacteria. In addition, both formulations include OADC (oleic acid–dextrose-citrate) enrichment, which chemically simulates egg components. Malachite green adds some selectivity.

Antibiotics can be added to this basic formulation to prevent overgrowth with bacteria. Mycobacteria-selective agar contains cycloheximide, lincomycin HCl, and nalidixic acid. Mitchison 7H11 selective agar is more selective owing to the addition of amphotericin B, carbenicillin, polymyxin B, and trimethoprim.

MOTILITY TEST MEDIUM

The purpose of the motility test medium is to determine whether an organism is motile or nonmotile. This test is particularly useful in the identification of members of Enterobacteriaceae, in which two genera, *Shigella* and *Klebsiella,* are always nonmotile, and certain *Yersinia* spp. show motility at room temperature but not at 35° C. *L. monocytogenes* gives a classic umbrella-type motility, and the non–glucose-fermenting gram-negative rods can be differentiated, based in part on their motility.

Nonmotile organisms, which lack flagella, grow only along the stab line, and the surrounding medium remains clear. Motile organisms, which usually possess flagella, move out from the stab line, and the medium appears cloudy. Low agar concentration makes the medium semisolid and permits better detection of motility.

Use an inoculating needle to stab the medium. Be careful to remove the needle along the initial stab line, and do not stab the medium clear to the tube's bottom. Incubate the inoculated medium at 35° C. Because flagellar protein is not formed as well at higher temperatures, some microbiologists prefer incubation at 18° to 20° C. For *Yersinia,* noting motility reaction at room temperature is particularly useful. Triphenyltetrazolium chloride (TTC) may be added to the basic motility medium to enhance detection of motility. A 1% solution of TTC is prepared and filter-sterilized. Add 5 mL of this solution to 1 L of motility medium. If TTC is used, bacteria incorporate colorless TTC and reduce it to red formazan pigment. The medium shows reddening where there is growth. Other media such as SIM (sulfide indole motility) and MIO (motility indole ornithine) can be used to detect motility in addition to other reactions.

MUELLER-HINTON AGAR

Mueller-Hinton agar is a transparent medium, useful in testing susceptibility of organisms to antibiotics. The medium also has been used for testing starch hydrolysis. Because Mueller-Hinton agar contains animal infusion, Casamino acids, and starch, it supports the growth of most organisms. In addition, sheep's blood may be added to the basic formulation to perform susceptibility testing on streptococci. The addition of heated or chocolatized sheep's blood to Mueller-Hinton agar makes possible testing for fastidious organisms, such as *Haemophilus* and *Neisseria.* Starch is included in the medium for two reasons: It may protect the organisms against toxic substances, and it also serves as an energy source. Ca^{++} and Mg^{++} concentrations are critical in the testing of *Pseudomonas* isolates with aminoglycoside antibiotics.

Usually Mueller-Hinton agar contains sufficient amounts of bivalent cations, but it may be necessary to add these substances to Mueller-Hinton broth.

NEW YORK CITY MEDIUM

The purpose of New York City medium is to isolate *Neisseria gonorrhoeae* and *Neisseria meningitidis* from specimens containing mixed normal flora.

New York City medium is enriched with hemoglobin, yeast dialysate, and horse plasma to support the growth of *N. gonorrhoeae* and *N. meningitidis.* Selectivity for these two organisms is accomplished by four antibiotics that inhibit normal flora. Vancomycin prevents the growth of gram-positive bacteria; colistin inhibits gram-negative rods; amphotericin B prevents growth of yeast and molds. Trimethoprim has been included to prevent swarming of *Proteus* species.

When using New York City medium for recovery of *N. gonorrhoeae* and *N. meningitidis* the microbiologist should incubate plates under increased carbon dioxide for several days. Also, a nonselective agar such as chocolate agar should be included because 5% of gonococci are inhibited by the antibiotics, particularly vancomycin, found in this medium.

NITRATE REDUCTION BROTH

The purpose of nitrate reduction broth is to determine whether an organism can reduce nitrate to nitrite or gaseous products, such as nitrogen. The test is useful in the recognition of members of Enterobacteriaceae; non–glucose-fermenting gram-negative rods; *Neisseria;* and *Moraxella catarrhalis.*

The nitrate test is performed in two parts. Sulfanilic acid and α-naphthylamine reagents are added first. If nitrate has been reduced to nitrite, nitrite will react with these reagents to form a red diazonium dye, *p*-sulfobenzene-azo-naphthylamine. If there is no color change, zinc dust is added. Zinc reduces the remaining nitrate to nitrite, forming a red color. However, if nitrate was reduced to nitrogen gas, no color change occurs.

When using this medium, incubate broth culture for 34 to 48 hours before testing. Observe the Durham tube for the presence of gas bubbles. Add 1 mL of sulfanilic acid reagent and 1 mL of α-naphthylamine reagent. Interpret the results immediately because color fades quickly. If it is necessary to add zinc, avoid using large amounts. Too much zinc can result in the formation of hydrogen gas, which can cause reduction and decrease the color reaction. Medium may need to be supplemented with serum and incubated for up to 5 days in testing for *Neisseria*. Because α-naphthylamine is carcinogenic, it is preferable to substitute *N,N*-dimethyl-α-naphthylamine.

NUTRIENT AGAR

Nutrient agar has been used to distinguish between the nonfastidious, less pathogenic *Neisseria* species and pathogenic *Neisseria* species, such as *N. gonorrhoeae* and *N. meningitidis*.

Nutrient agar contains minimal nutrients and an especially low concentration of protein. Growth of an isolate on this medium means that it is not very fastidious and does not require special supplements. The less fastidious neisseriae grow on nutrient agar, whereas the more pathogenic species do not. Nutrient agar also has been used for the maintenance of stock cultures.

OXIDATIVE-FERMENTATIVE (OF) MEDIUM (HUGH AND LEIFSON FORMULATION)

Oxidative-fermentative, or OF, medium is used to determine if a gram-negative non–glucose-fermenting rod is oxidative, fermentative, or biochemically inert.

Three modifications over traditional media make this medium useful in testing nonfermenting gram-negative rods. A low concentration of peptone prevents formation of alkaline products that may neutralize the small quantities of acid produced through oxidation. The high concentration of carbohydrate increases the potential amount of acid that can be formed. The lower concentration of agar makes the medium semisolid. This permits acids formed on the surface to diffuse throughout the medium. Bromthymol blue serves as the pH indicator for acid detection.

The classic method for using this medium involves the stabbing of two tubes with the organism. The medium in one tube is covered with vaspar (a mixture of petrolatum and paraffin) or melted paraffin. Sterile mineral oil has been used for this purpose, but it is not recommended because it does not block out oxygen as well. Results are interpreted after incubation at 35° C. Several days of incubation may be required owing to the slower growth of some nonfermenting gram-negative rods. A color change to yellow in both tubes means that the organism is fermentative (can produce acid in the absence of oxygen). Color change to yellow in the uncovered tube only means that the organism is oxidative (requires oxygen to use the carbohydrate). If neither tube changes in color or the covered tube shows no change while the uncovered tube turns blue, the organism cannot use the carbohydrate oxidatively or fermentatively and is considered inert. A one-tube modification of this test has been described. One tube is stabbed, and it is not covered. Color change to yellow near the top of the medium only indicates oxidative use of glucose. If the entire tube changes to yellow, fermentation is suggested. Because the medium is semisolid, motility may be observed in this medium. *Note:* Sometimes OF medium is used for differentiating staphylococci (fermentative) from micrococci (oxidative). This testing requires a different formulation.

PEPTONE–YEAST EXTRACT–GLUCOSE (PYG) BROTH

Peptone–yeast extract–glucose broth is useful for culturing anaerobes. PYG broth culture of an anaerobic isolate may be used in gas-liquid chromatography procedures that detect metabolic end products.

PYG broth contains several nutrients and supplements that encourage the growth of anaerobes. These enrichments include vitamin K (required for pigment-producing *Prevotella* and *Porphyromonas*), yeast extract, hemin, and glucose. Cysteine helps keep the medium more reduced and anaerobic. Resazurin serves as an anaerobic indicator. Pink color means that oxygen is present.

PHENYLALANINE DEAMINASE (PAD) AGAR

Phenylalanine deaminase agar is used to detect the organism's ability to deaminate or remove the amino group from phenylalanine. A positive reaction is most useful for distinguishing *Proteus, Providencia,* and *Morganella* from other members of the family Enterobacteriaceae. This test also can be used to distinguish *Moraxella* that are phenylpyruvate-positive from other *Moraxella.*

Phenylalanine deaminase agar includes the following: phenylalanine, the amino acid to be deaminated; yeast extract, a nitrogen and carbon source; various salts, and agar, a solidifying agent. Protein hydrolysates and meat extracts are not included because these substances contain a variable amount of phenylalanine. If an organism produces phenylalanine deaminase, it can convert phenylalanine to the α-keto acid called *phenylpyruvic acid.* This acid reacts with the added ferric chloride reagent to form a dark-green complex. The immediate appearance of a dark-green slant on addition of ferric chloride reagent is a positive reaction; no color change upon addition of reagent is a negative reaction.

PHENYLETHYL ALCOHOL (PEA) AGAR

The purpose of phenylethyl alcohol agar is to isolate gram-positive cocci, such as staphylococci and streptococci, from specimens having mixed flora. The anaerobic formulation of this medium selects for gram-negative and gram-positive nonsporulating anaerobes while inhibiting the facultatively anaerobic gram-negative rods and other anaerobes.

PEA agar is similar to sheep's blood agar except that it contains phenylethyl alcohol. This component inhibits facultative gram-negative rods, especially swarming *Proteus,* but permits the growth of gram-positive cocci.

Phenylethyl alcohol is volatile, and plates should be tightly sealed in plastic bags and stored in the refrigerator. Hemolytic reactions are not dependable on this medium because of the action of phenylethyl alcohol on cell membranes. Gram-negative rods may grow on PEA agar, but colonies are smaller than usual and can be readily differ-entiated from those of gram-positives rods. *P. aeruginosa* is not inhibited by this medium. Some gram-positive cocci may require more than 24 hours of incubation to grow well on PEA agar. An anaerobic formulation can be achieved by adding phenylethyl alcohol to CDC anaerobic agar before autoclaving or by supplementing the formulation with vitamin K as well as sheep's blood after sterilization of basal medium.

PSEUDOCEL (CETRIMIDE) AGAR

Pseudocel or cetrimide agar is used to select for *P. aeruginosa* in specimens with mixed flora. Also, because it inhibits other *Pseudomonas* species (except *Pseudomonas fluorescens*) and closely related organisms, this test can be useful in the differentiation of non–glucose-fermenting gram-negative rods.

This medium contains cetrimide, also called *cetyl trimethyl ammonium bromide* or *hexadecyltrimethylammonium bromide.* Produced from bromine, cetrimide is highly inhibitory and has been used as an antiseptic. If the organism can tolerate cetrimide, it will grow on the medium. Magnesium chloride and potassium sulfate stimulate the production of pyocyanin, the green pigment characteristically produced by *P. aeruginosa.*

SALMONELLA-SHIGELLA (SS) AGAR

Salmonella-Shigella agar is used to select for *Salmonella* and some strains of *Shigella* from stool specimens. SS agar is also differential in that these organisms produce characteristic colonies on the medium.

SS agar contains bile salts, sodium citrate, and brilliant green, which inhibit the growth of gram-positive and many lactose-fermenting gram-negative rods normally found in feces. Lactose serves as the sole carbohydrate source in the medium: neutral red is the pH indicator. If an organism grows on the medium and ferments lactose, it will produce acid and change the indicator to pink-red. Sodium thiosulfate acts as the source of sulfur for the production of hydrogen sulfide. If hydrogen sulfide is produced, it reacts with the ferric chloride present in the medium, forming a black precipitate in the center of the colony.

A heavy inoculum of stool can be planted on SS agar because the formulation is so inhibitory. However, strains of *Shigella* may not grow on SS agar, and this medium should not be used as the sole primary plating medium when *Shigella* is the potential isolate. *Shigella* colonies appear colorless on SS agar because these organisms do not ferment lactose or produce hydrogen sulfide. *Salmonella* colonies are colorless with a black center because these organisms usually make hydrogen sulfide but do not ferment lactose. Pink to red colonies indicate that the organism ferments lactose; if there is a black center, it also produces hydrogen sulfide. If *Proteus* grows on this medium, swarming is inhibited.

SELENITE F BROTH

Selenite F broth is an enrichment broth used for the recovery of low numbers of *Salmonella* and some strains of *Shigella* from stool and other specimens containing large amounts of mixed bacteria. The sodium selenite present in this medium inhibits the growth of many gram-negative rods and enterococci but permits recovery of *Salmonella* and some *Shigella* species. Selenite is most effective at a neutral pH. Reduction of selenite during growth of bacteria produces alkaline products, so lactose also has been included in this medium. Lactose-fermenters produce acid, which neutralizes these alkaline products and returns the medium to a neutral pH, at which selenite works most effectively.

When using selenite broth, the microbiologist should subculture the broth to enteric media after it has incubated 8 to 12 hours. Beyond this time frame, overgrowth with normal flora is likely.

SODIUM CHLORIDE BROTH, 6.5%

Sodium chloride broth is useful in the differentiation of streptococci, particularly those producing α-hemolytic and nonhemolytic colonies. Primarily, it distinguishes *Enterococcus* species (positive) from group D streptococci (negative), both of which produce a positive bile-esculin agar slant. Also, viridans streptococci cannot grow in this medium.

Sodium chloride broth is prepared from heart infusion broth, a general-purpose medium, that already contains 0.5% sodium chloride. By adding 6% sodium chloride to this medium, the salt concentration becomes 6.5%. Sodium chloride broth also contains glucose as a carbohydrate source and bromcresol purple, a pH indicator. If the organism can tolerate this high concentration of salt, it will grow in the medium and produce cloudiness. Fermentation of glucose produces acid and may cause the medium to turn yellow.

Some formulations omit indicator and glucose. To use this medium, inoculate several colonies into broth and incubate culture overnight at 35° C. Any growth in the broth is considered positive even if the indicator does not change color.

To avoid a false-negative result, gently mix broth before interpretation. Inoculating the broth too heavily may give a false-positive result. Organisms other than enterococci, such as group B streptococci and aerococci, can produce positive results.

SP-4 BROTH/AGAR

SP-4 broth and SP-4 agar serve as primary isolation media for *Mycoplasma* species. SP-4 media contain yeast products that serve as growth factors for *Mycoplasma* and supply preformed nucleic acid. Fetal bovine serum supplies the cholesterol necessary for stabilizing these organisms because they lack cell walls. Various antibiotics inhibit normal flora that may be present in the specimen. Penicillin is included to prevent the growth of gram-positive bacteria; amphotericin B inhibits fungi; and polymyxin B inhibits gram-negative rods. Biphasic media provide both microaerophilic and moist conditions, which some *Mycoplasma* species prefer.

SP-4: ARGININE, GLUCOSE, AND UREA BROTHS

SP-4 broths are useful in the identification of *Mycoplasma* and *Ureaplasma*. Yeast products included in SP-4 broth supply nutrients required for the growth of *Mycoplasma* and *Ureaplasma*. Fetal bovine serum contains cholesterol, which helps stabilize these organisms because they lack cell walls. Penicillin prevents the growth of gram-positive cocci but does not affect these organisms because they do not possess cell walls. Phenol red serves as a pH indicator. In SP-4 arginine broth, use of arginine results in alkaline products and color change to red. This reaction characterizes *Mycoplasma hominis.* In SP-4 urea broth, removal of an amino group from urea, characteristic of *Ureaplasma,* causes formation of ammonia and a similar color change to red. SP-4 glucose broth detects glucose fermentation. Acid is produced, which lowers the medium's pH and changes its color to yellow. This reaction typifies *Mycoplasma pneumoniae,* as well as a few other *Mycoplasma* species.

TETRATHIONATE BROTH

Tetrathionate broth is an enrichment medium used for recovery of low numbers of *Salmonella* species from stool specimens. Bile salt in conjunction with thiosulfate and added iodine-iodide solution inhibits the growth of most gram-negative rods and gram-positive organisms except *Salmonella.* Some formulations also include brilliant green or crystal violet, which increases the inhibitory nature of the medium. The medium must be used within 24 hours of preparation. Since the basal medium may be stored in the refrigerator indefinitely, some microbiologists prefer to dispense 10 mL of basal medium per tube. Just before use, 0.2 mL of iodine solution can be added to each tube. Heavy inoculum of stool can be added to the broth. After 12 to 24 hours of incubation at 35° C, the broth should be subcultured to enteric media to prevent overgrowth with normal flora. This medium inhibits most *Shigella* species and should not be used for recovering *Salmonella typhi.*

THAYER-MARTIN, MODIFIED AGAR

Modified Thayer-Martin (MTM) agar is a selective enrichment medium used for recovering *N. gonorrhoeae* and *N. meningitidis* from specimens with mixed flora. Modified Thayer-Martin agar is highly enriched to support the growth of the more fastidious *Neisseria* species. Added growth factors include hemoglobin, vitamins, diphosphopyridine nucleotide, L-cysteine, and glutamine. Cornstarch is included to absorb any inhibitory substances that might be present. The modified formulation containing more agar may help prevent swarming of *Proteus.* Modified Thayer-Martin agar contains antibiotics that inhibit normal flora and prevent the growth of most other organisms. Vancomycin inhibits the growth of gram-positive cocci. Colistin inhibits gram-negative rods, whereas trimethoprim prevents *Proteus* from swarming. Nystatin prevents the growth of fungi.

Five percent chocolatized, difibrinated sheep's blood may be substituted for the hemoglobin solution. The original Thayer-Martin formulation lacked additional agar and glucose as well as the trimethoprim and therefore is not as effective at inhibiting swarming of *Proteus.* The Martin-Lewis formulation substitutes anisomycin (20 µg/mL) for nystatin as the antifungal agent. In addition, the vancomycin concentration of (4 µg/mL) is higher than in the MTM formulation.

When using MTM plates, the microbiologist should incubate them in a carbon dioxide incubator or candle jar for several days. Because some strains of *Neisseria gonorrhoeae* may be inhibited by vancomycin, a chocolate plate also should be used.

THIOGLYCOLATE BROTH, BASAL AND ENRICHED

Thioglycolate broth is an all-purpose medium that can be used to isolate a wide range of bacteria. It is often employed as a back-up broth and inoculated along with culture plates. In this case, it helps detect those organisms present in low numbers or anaerobes in the original specimen. When glucose is omitted, thioglycolate broth can be used in fermentation studies of anaerobes.

Thioglycolate, cystine, and sodium sulfite act as reducing agents in this medium, while the low concentration of agar prevents downward diffusion of oxygen. Various supplements can be added to support the growth of more fastidious organisms.

Various supplements can be added to the basic formulation of this broth medium. These include hemin (5 µg/mL), vitamin K (0.1 µg/mL), and sodium bicarbonate (1 mg/mL), which can be autoclaved in the medium. Supplements that must be added after autoclaving include rabbit or horse serum (10%

vol/vol) and Fildes enrichment (5% vol/vol). These are given as final concentrations in the medium.

Thioglycolate broth should be stored at room temperature and boiled and cooled before use. When used as a back-up broth, the medium is incubated at 35° C for 3 to 7 days and examined for turbidity. Gram stains of broth are compared with growth obtained on primary culture plates. If something different appears to be growing in the broth, subcultures should be performed.

THIOSULFATE CITRATE BILE SALTS SUCROSE (TCBS) AGAR

Thiosulfate citrate bile salts sucrose agar is a selective medium used to isolate *Vibrio* species from stool specimens having mixed flora. TCBS agar is also differential in that *Vibrio* species produce characteristic colonies. *Vibrio* species grow poorly on media designed for isolation of *Salmonella* and *Shigella* but produce colorless colonies on Mac-Conkey agar. TCBS agar includes sodium citrate, sodium thiosulfate, and oxgall (10% solution equivalent to full-strength bile), which together inhibit many gram-positive cocci and gram-negative rods normally present in stool specimens. In addition, the high pH of TCBS agar encourages the growth of *Vibrio* while inhibiting other organisms. Different types of colonies are produced by different species of *Vibrio* owing to the presence of sucrose as a fermentable carbohydrate and bromthymol blue as a pH indicator. For example, *Vibrio cholerae* and *Vibrio alginolyticus* produce yellow colonies because they can ferment sucrose, whereas *Vibrio parahaemolyticus* and *Vibrio vulnificus* usually produce blue-green colonies owing to lack of sucrose fermentation. Organisms that can produce hydrogen sulfide from sodium thiosulfate have black centers because of the reaction of this gas with ferric citrate. *Vibrio* organisms do not produce hydrogen sulfide. Some formulations include a second pH indicator, thymol blue. Oxgall and sodium cholate or bile salts (8 g/L) may be used in place of oxgall alone.

When using TCBS agar, the microbiologist should use a heavy inoculum because *Vibrio* species die off quickly, and this medium is very inhibitory. Fresh specimen is best because these organisms are sensitive to drying out, sunlight, and

acid pH. If there must be a delay in planting, use Cary-Blair semisolid transport medium rather than buffered glycerol transport medium. Plates should be incubated at 35° C for 18 to 24 hours and up to 48 hours. Growth off TCBS agar is not acceptable for performing oxidase testing. Occasionally, strains of *V. cholerae*, may produce blue-green colonies on this medium owing to delayed sucrose fermentation. Some *Vibrio* spp. do not grow well on this medium. Also, other organisms, such as *Pseudomonas, Plesiomonas,* and *Aeromonas,* can grow on TCBS agar and usually produce blue colonies; these must be distinguished from vibrios.

TINSDALE AGAR

Tinsdale agar is a selective, differential medium useful in isolating and identifying *C. diphtheriae* from specimens containing mixed flora. Tinsdale agar contains a high concentration of potassium tellurite, which inhibits the growth of most normal flora organisms but permits *Corynebacterium* species, especially *C. diphtheriae,* to grow. All *Corynebacterium* species growing on the medium produce gray to black colonies owing to the reduction of tellurite to tellurium. In addition, *C. diphtheriae* colonies are surrounded by a brown halo. This brown halo is thought to be produced from tellurite's interaction with the hydrogen sulfide produced by the organism from cystine and thiosulfate. The basal medium can be stored indefinitely; tellurite and serum can be added just before use. Once prepared, the medium has a shelf life of 4 days.

When using Tinsdale agar, the microbiologist should streak plates for isolation and stab the medium in several areas. Sometimes browning occurs in these stabbed areas before it can be seen around colonies. Plates should be incubated at 35° C for 24 to 48 hours in ambient air. Increased carbon dioxide can slow down the production of the brown halo. It may require 48 hours for some *Coryebacterium diphtheriae* strains to produce the characteristic halo. In addition, *Corynebacterium ulcerans* and *Corynebacterium pseudodiphtheriticum* may also produce a dark halo on this medium and must be differentiated from *C. diphtheriae.* Other organisms may occasionally grow on Tinsdale agar. *Proteus* produces mucoid colonies and tends to blacken the medium. Rare streptococci and staphylococci can produce dark colonies with a surrounding halo but could be distinguished by performing a Gram stain.

TRIPLE SUGAR IRON (TSI) AGAR

Triple sugar iron (TSI) agar can be used to determine whether a gram-negative rod is a glucose-fermenter or non–glucose-fermenter, a fundamental characteristic in the initial classification of gram-negative rods. The medium also tests for sucrose or lactose fermentation, gas production during glucose fermentation, and hydrogen sulfide production, all of which are useful in the differentiation of gram-negative rods belonging to the family Enterobacteriaceae.

TSI agar contains glucose, sucrose, and lactose (fermentable carbohydrates), phenol red (pH indicator), peptone (carbon/nitrogen source), and iron salt plus sodium thiosulfate (sulfur source and hydrogen sulfide indicator). TSI agar resembles Kligler iron agar except that it contains sucrose. Carbohydrate fermentation patterns are similar to those with Kligler iron agar. However, an acid (yellow) butt and acid (yellow) slant indicate an organism ferments glucose and sucrose or lactose. Gas bubbles and blackening mean the same thing in TSI agar as in Kligler Iron Agar. Precautions concerning the inoculation and incubation outlined in Kligler Iron Agar description also apply to TSI.

TRYPTICASE SOY AGAR (TSA)

Trypticase soy agar is an all-purpose medium that supports the growth of many organisms. It is frequently used as the basal medium for sheep's blood agar plates. TSA contains protein as a nutrient source and sodium chloride as an osmotic stabilizer. Agar serves as solidifying agent.

If blood agar is to be prepared, cool to 50° C before adding 5% defibrinated sheep's blood. In most cases, agar can be added to a broth formulation to produce agar plates. However, the commercial TSA product does not contain glucose, which makes it suitable for a blood agar base. Adding agar to trypticase soy broth does not accomplish the same

thing. Trypticase soy broth contains glucose, a fermentable carbohydrate, which can interfere with the expression of β hemolysis on sheep's blood agar plates.

TRYPTICASE SOY BROTH (TSB)

Trypticase soy broth is an all-purpose medium that supports the rapid growth of most organisms, including streptococci, without added supplements. Trypticase soy broth contains trypticase and phytone as protein sources, sodium chloride for osmotic stability, glucose as a fermentable carbohydrate, and dipotassium phosphate as a buffer.

Trypticase soy broth contains glucose, which when fermented can lower pH. This can cause acid-sensitive organisms such as *Streptococcus pneumoniae* to die off at 24 hours of incubation.

TRYPTOPHAN BROTH (1%)

Tryptophan broth is used for performing the indole test, a procedure particularly useful in identifying species of Enterobacteriaceae and in identifying non–glucose-fermenting gram-negative rods. This broth contains trypticase, a peptone rich in tryptophan, and sodium chloride, which serves as an osmotic stabilizer. Some bacteria possess an enzyme system called *tryptophanase,* which hydrolyzes and deaminates tryptophan, producing indole, pyruvic acid, and ammonia. When Ehrlich or Kovac reagent is added to a tryptophan broth culture, any indole produced by the organism reacts with the aldehyde portion of dimethylaminobenzaldehyde, the primary chemical in these reagents, to form a red color.

Inoculate broth and incubate for 24 hours at 35° C. When performing the indole test, the microbiologist should add 5 drops of Kovac reagent to the medium and look for the appearance of a red color in the reagent layer or at the interface of the reagent and broth. If Ehrlich reagent is used, add 1 mL of xylene or ether to the broth culture, shake, and then add 5 drops of the reagent. Kovac reagent is generally used in testing for members of Enterobacteriaceae and Ehrlich when testing for non–glucose-fermenting gram-negative rods and anaerobes.

Other media have been used in testing for indole production. These include sulfide indole motility (SIM) agar, indole nitrate broth, and motility indole ornithine (MIO) medium. A spot test employing filter paper saturated with paradimethylaminocinnamaldehyde reagent also has been used for indole determination.

UREA AGAR AND BROTH

Urea media detect an organism's ability to hydrolyze urea. This characteristic is particularly useful in identifying species of Enterobacteriaceae. In these media, urea is hydrolyzed to form carbon dioxide, water, and ammonia. The ammonia then reacts with components in the medium to form ammonium carbonate. This compound causes a rise in pH, which changes the pH indicator, phenol red, to pink. Both agar and broth formulations do not contain much protein. This prevents the formation of alkaline products from the breakdown of peptones, which could result in false-positive results. The broth formulation contains monopotassium phosphate and disodium phosphate, which make the medium highly buffered. In addition, the broth formulation lacks glucose and peptone. Only organisms such as *Proteus* species that are strong urease producers and not very fastidious appear positive in this type of medium. The agar formulation is less buffered, so smaller amounts of urease activity can be detected. Also, glucose and peptone which help support growth, are included in these media.

When using urea agar, streak slant and incubate at 35° C for 18 to 24 hours. If urease is produced, the medium will turn pink. Rapid urease producers such as *Proteus* species turn the entire tube pink and may be detectable in a few hours. Slow urease producers, such as *Klebsiella,* only turn the slant pink. If the organism does not produce urease, there will be no color change. Stuart urea broth is incubated at 35° C for 18 to 24 hours. A positive reaction is red color throughout the broth.

VAGINALIS AGAR (V AGAR)

V agar is a nonselective, primary plating enrichment medium useful in the isolation of *G. vaginalis.* This organism also produces a distinctive colony, which aids in its recognition in mixed culture. V agar is essentially Columbia agar base with added proteose peptone and human blood. The medium contains many protein sources as well as starch, which can be broken down by *Gardnerella.* Human rather than sheep's blood must be used in this medium. *G. vaginalis* produces diffuse β hemolysis only on media containing human blood.

When using V agar, the microbiologist should incubate inoculated plates in a carbon dioxide incubator or in a candle jar at 35° C. Plates may be observed at 24 hours, but often it requires 48 to 72 hours for *Gardnerella* to grow. The organism produces tiny, dome-shaped colonies surrounded with zones of diffuse hemolysis.

XYLOSE LYSINE AND DESOXYCHOLATE (XLD) AGAR

This agar is a selective, differential primary plating medium used to isolate *Salmonella* and *Shigella* species from stool and other specimens containing mixed flora. *Salmonella* and *Shigella* species produce characteristic colonies on XLD, which aids in their recognition. XLD agar contains sodium desoxycholate, which inhibits gram-positive cocci and some normal flora gram-negative rods. Because XLD agar has a lower concentration of bile salts than other formulations of enteric media, such as SS and HE agars, it is less selective but permits better recovery of *Shigella.* XLD agar contains three fermentable carbohydrates: sucrose and lactose, which are present in excess concentration, and xylose, which is present in lower amounts. Phenol red serves as a pH indicator. The amino acid lysine is included to detect lysine decarboxylation. Sodium thiosulfate acts as a sulfur source from which organisms can make hydrogen sulfide. The hydrogen sulfide combines with ferric ammonium citrate to produce ferrous sulfide, a black precipitate. Four types of colonies are produced on XLD agar. Yellow colonies include organisms such as *E. coli* that ferment the excess carbohydrates to produce a great deal of acid and change the pH indicator to yellow. Because there is excess carbohydrate, they do not decarboxylate the lysine even though they may possess lysine decarboxylase. Also, some bacteria ferment only xylose but do not decarboxylate lysine, and therefore produce yellow colonies. Yellow colonies with black centers ferment the excess carbohydrate and also produce hydrogen sulfide. Examples of organisms that produce these organisms are *Citrobacter* and some *Proteus*. Colorless or red colonies, such as *Shigella* and *Providencia,* which neither ferment xylose, lactose, or sucrose nor produce hydrogen sulfide, have this appearance. Red colonies with black centers are produced by *Salmonella* and *Edwardsiella.* After fermenting xylose to make acid, these organisms decarboxylate lysine to produce cadaverine, an alkaline product. This causes the pH indicator to turn yellow and then revert back to red. Blackening is due to hydrogen sulfide production.

When using XLD agar, the microbiologist should incubate plates at 35° C for 24 hours in ambient air. Some authors have recommended incubating plates for up to 48 hours to enhance blackening in *Salmonella* colonies. With any prolonged incubation, the delicate balance of this medium may be altered, and distinguishing normal flora from potential pathogens becomes more difficult. *Shigella dysenteriae* and *Shingella flexneri* may occasionally be inhibited on XLD agar. Some strains of *Sal-*

monella may fail to produce hydrogen sulfide and therefore resemble *Shigella* colonies. On this medium, blackening is more likely to occur when alkaline conditions exist.

Bibliography

Balows A et al, editors: *Manual of clinical microbiology,* ed 5, Washington, DC, 1991, American Society for Microbiology.

Baron E, Finegold S: *Bailey & Scott's diagnostic microbiology,* ed 8, St Louis, 1986, Mosby.

Difco Laboratories: *Difco manual: dehydrated culture media and reagents for microbiology,* ed 10, Detroit, Mich, 1985, Difco Laboratories.

Finegold S, Martin W: *Diagnostic microbiology,* ed 6, St Louis, 1982, Mosby.

Howard B et al: *Clinical and pathogenic microbiology,* ed 2, St Louis, 1994, Mosby.

Lennette E et al, editors: *Manual of clinical microbiology,* ed 3, Washington, DC, 1980, American Society for Microbiology.

Rohde P et al: BBL *manual of products and laboratory procedures,* ed 5, Cockeysville, Md, 1968, Becton, Dickinson, and Co.

Shepard M, Lunceford C: Differential agar medium (A7) for identification of *Ureaplasma urealyticum* (human T mycoplasmas) in primary cultures of clinical material, *J Clin Microbiol* 3:613, 1976.

Selected Mycology Media, Fluids, and Stains

Patricia K. Hargrave, Shirley Adams

MEDIA

A variety of enrichment and selective media are available to the clinical laboratory for the isolation and identification of pathogenic fungi. This appendix is included to provide the reader with information about a select number of mycology media cited in the mycology section of this text. Most media detailed in this appendix are commercially available in either dehydrated or finished form. Recommendations as to general usage of the media, either enrichment or selective, or combinations of each type, are outlined in the mycology section of this text.

Birdseed Agar (Modified Staib Agar)

Birdseed agar is a differential enrichment medium designed for the isolation and preliminary identification of *Cryptococcus neoformans.* The ground seeds of *Guizottia abyssinica* provide enrichment, whereas biphenyl provides a substrate for the detection of phenol oxidase activity. On this medium, *C. neoformans* colonies typically darken to a rich brown as phenol oxidase activity results in the deposition of melanin in yeast cell walls. The colonies of other *Cryptococcus* species and other yeasts remain white.

Brain-Heart Infusion Agar (BHIA)/BHIA Blood Agar with or without Antibiotics

Brain-heart infusion agar or BHIA with sheep's blood is an enrichment agar useful in the isolation of pathogenic yeast and the dimorphic fungi (in yeast form) from clinical specimens. The addition of antibiotics (typically penicillin and streptomycin in this medium) provides a selective action because the antibiotics inhibit the growth of bacteria possibly associated with specimen material.

Casein Medium

Casein medium is a differential medium used to demonstrate proteolytic activity by yeast species. Proteolysis is visualized as a clearing of the medium around the inoculum growth. Sterile plated medium should be inoculated by the cut streak or point inoculation method. Each run should include the set-up of the unknown and three known controls (*Streptomyces* species, *Nocardia asteroides, Nocardia brasiliensis*) using one half of the plate for each organism. Inoculated plates should be incubated at room temperature and observed for proteolysis over a 14-day period. *Streptomyces* species typically hydrolyze the incorporated casein within 2 to 5 days. *N. brasiliensis* typically hydrolyzes casein within 7 to 10 days; *N. asteroides* does not hydrolyze casein.

Corn Meal Agar

Corn meal agar is typically made as any one of three variations on a basal formulation. Each formulation is useful in the cultivation of fungi. Each variation is recommended for the cultivation or enhancement of particular fungal characteristics. Corn meal agar without added dextrose is recommended for the cultivation of chlamydospore-bearing *Candida albicans,* with chlamydospore production further enhanced by the addition of 1% Tween-80. On the other hand, corn meal agar with 0.2% added dextrose* is not recommended for production of chlamydospores. Rather, it favors more luxuriant growth and improves pigment production.

To use, inoculate each plate with a known *C. albicans* control and unknown isolate(s) as single streaks cut deep into the agar or as surface streaks to be covered with a flame-warmed coverslip. Incubate at room temperature, and examine with a low-power lens of a microscope daily for up to 1 week. Isolates may become positive for chlamydospores (macroconidia) within 48 hours but cannot be considered negative before the fifth day of culture.

***Alternative Formulation with Dextrose.** The aforementioned corn meal agar formulation with 2 g of dextrose is commercially available in dehydrated form. Rehydrate as directed by the manufacturer, and sterilize by autoclaving (121° C for 15 minutes). Inoculate, incubate at room temperature, and observe for growth and pigment production.

Dilute Gelatin Medium (0.4%)

Dilute gelatin medium is a differential medium useful in the differentiation of *Nocardia* species from one another and from *Streptomyces* species on the basis of growth and colonial morphology. In this medium, *N. asteroides* does not grow or grows poorly with a thin, flaky appearance. Conversely, *N. brasiliensis* grows well, forming compact, rounded colonies, whereas *Streptomyces* species produce poor to good growth with a stringy or flaky morphology.

The medium should be inoculated with a very small fragment of growth from a Sabouraud-dextrose agar slant and incubated at room temperature (or 37° C if the suspected strain grows better at 37° C). Inoculated tubes should be examined daily for growth for up to 21 to 25 days.

Modified Potassium Nitrate Assimilation Medium (MKA)

Potassium nitrate assimilation medium provides a differential medium useful in assessing the ability of a yeast isolate to assimilate potassium nitrate (KNO_3). The modified medium is a solid, slanted medium containing KNO_3, yeast carbon base, Nobel agar, and bromthymol blue. A single colony of the cultured isolate is picked using a sterile applicator stick, inoculated over the entire MKA slant surface and incubated at 25° to 30° C. The ability to assimilate potassium nitrate is indicated by a color change of the medium from greenish yellow to blue or blue-green.

Mycosel/Mycobiotic Agar (Cycloheximide-Chloramphenicol Agar)

Cycloheximide-chloramphenicol agar is a selective medium useful in the isolation or pathogenic fungi, both dermatophytes and systemic pathogens. The cycloheximide is useful in suppressing the growth of saprophytic fungi, whereas the chloramphenicol is used to inhibit bacterial contaminants.

Potato Dextrose Agar

Potato dextrose agar is a recommended plating medium for cultivation, enumeration, and identi-fication of yeasts and molds from dairy and other food products as well as other specimen types. The potato infusion encourages luxuriant growth and sporulation by fungi. NOTE: Potato dextrose agar to be used in the isolation and enumeration of fungi from milk and food should be acidified to pH 3.5 by aseptically adding 10% sterile tartaric acid to the cooled, sterile medium. Do not attempt to reheat this medium once the tartaric acid has been added because hydrolysis of the agar will occur and prevent solidification.

Potato Flakes Agar

Potato flakes agar is used to induce sporulation in fungi.

Rice Extract Agar

Rice extract agar without additional dextrose is useful in the cultivation of *C. albicans,* with enhancement of chlamydospore production. Rice extract agar with 2% dextrose has been shown to enhance pigment production by *Trichophyton rubrum,* facilitating its differentiation from *Trichophyton mentagrophytes.*

The medium should be inoculated by cutting through the agar surface. If the medium inoculated is in plated form, the cut streak should be covered with a flame-warmed coverslip to stimulate chlamydospore production. All cultures should be incubated at room temperature for 18 to 72 hours.

Rice Grains Medium

Rice grains medium is useful in the differentiation of *Microsporum audouinii* from other dermatophytes, especially *Microsporum canis.* On this medium, *M. audouinii* grows poorly and discolors the medium. Other dermatophytes and most other fungi grow well and sporulate on this medium with no discoloration of the medium. Sterile rice grains should be spot-inoculated to prevent confusion in differentiating between discoloration and actual growth.

Sabouraud Dextrose Agar or Broth

Sabouraud dextrose agar and Sabouraud dextrose broth are nutrient media suitable for the cultivation of fungi, especially those associated with cutaneous and mucocutaneous infections. The formulations are identical with the exception of the agar. To make a solid plated medium 1.5% to 2% agar is added to the broth formulation.

Yeast Nitrogen Base, Modified: Carbohydrate Assimilation Base

Modified yeast nitrogen base is a synthetic basal medium that provides sufficient sources of nitrogen to support the growth of fungi. Fungal isolates are plated for confluent growth, and carbohydrate disks are dispensed onto the surface to provide the specific carbohydrates for assimilation testing. Incubate at 30° C for 48 to 72 hours and examine for growth around each disk. Good growth around a disk indicates assimilation of that carbohydrate, whereas scant or no growth around a disk indicates no assimilation. A dextrose disk serves as the growth control.

| FUNGAL MOUNTING FLUIDS

KOH-Glycerin

Potassium hydroxide (or sodium hydroxide) and glycerin solution is used as a mounting fluid in the preparation of wet mounts to visualize fungi in clinical material. The KOH (or NaOH) aids in clearing the specimen of nonfungal materials while the glycerol retards the dissolution of the fungal elements. A modification of this basic principle involves combining the KOH with DMSO* rather than glycerol. The DMSO facilitates the penetration of KOH into the specimen materials and speeds the clearing process.

KOH-Glycerin, Super Quink

This formulation is a variation of the traditional KOH-glycerin mounting solution. It uses a permanent blue-black ink to impart color to the system and enhance contrast.

| FUNGAL STAINS

Calcofluor White Stain

The use of calcofluor white stain with 10% KOH enhances visualization of fungi in clinical specimens of skin, hair, and nails. Fungal elements take up the fluorescent dye and, depending on the combination of filters used, appear brilliant green-yellow or blue-white, whereas the background fluoresces a dim red.

For examination of clinical samples, add 1 drop of calcofluor white solution with 1 drop of 10% KOH to the specimen on a microscope slide, apply a coverslip, and examine using a fluorescence microscope. The microscope used must have either a K532 excitation filter–BG 12 barrier filter or a G-35 excitation filter–LP420 barrier filter combination.

India Ink

The India ink method is useful in demonstrating the presence of a capsule. It is especially recommended for the demonstration of *Cryptococcus neoformans* in clinical specimens. In this method, the capsule displaces the colloidal carbon particles in the ink; thus the capsule appears as a clear halo around the body of the microorganism.

Lactophenol Aniline Blue

Lactophenol aniline blue (formerly lactophenol cotton blue) is a mounting medium useful in examining clinical materials for fungi. It aids in clearing hyphal elements and preserving fungal materials. It enhances visualization by staining all chitin-containing structures a light blue. To use, place a small drop onto the fungal material on a slide, add a coverslip, and examine.

Bibliography

Balows A et al, editors: *Manual of clinical microbiology,* ed 5, Washington, DC, 1991, American Society for Microbiology.

Baron E, Finegold S: *Bailey & Scott's diagnostic microbiology,* ed 8, St Louis, 1986, Mosby.

Difco Laboratories: *Difco manual: dehydrated culture media and reagents for microbiology,* ed 10, Detroit, Mich, 1985, Difco Laboratories.

Finegold S, Martin W: *Diagnostic microbiology,* ed 6, St Louis, 1982, Mosby.

Fisher F, Cook N: *Fundamentals of diagnostic mycology,* Philadelphia, 1998, Saunders.

Howard B et al: *Clinical and pathogenic microbiology,* ed 2, St Louis, 1994, Mosby.

Lennette E et al, editors: *Manual of clinical microbiology,* ed 3, Washington, DC, 1980, American Society for Microbiology.

Pincus D et al: Modification of potassium nitrate assimilation test for identification of clinically important yeasts, *J Clin Microbiol* 26:366, 1988.

Rohde P et al: *BBL Manual of products and laboratory procedures,* ed 5, Cockeysville, Md, 1968, Becton, Dickinson, and Co.

---

*CAUTION: A KOH with DMSO mounting fluid should be made under a flame hood. DMSO has a strong, penetrating odor and flavor. It readily diffuses into the air and crosses skin surfaces.

Nomenclature Changes for the Enterobacteriaceae and Nonfermentative Bacilli

CURRENT NOMENCLATURE	PREVIOUS NOMENCLATURE
Enterobacteriaceae	
Citrobacter koseri	*Citrobacter diversus*
Pantoea agglomerans	*Enterobacter agglomerans*
Nonfermentative Bacilli	
Acidovorax facilis	*Pseudomonas facilis*
Acidovorax temperans	Several *Pseudomonas* and *Alcaligenes* strains
Brevundimonas diminuta	*Pseudomonas diminuta*
Brevundimonas vesicularis	*Pseudomonas vesicularis*
Burkholderia cepacia	*Pseudomonas cepacia*
Burkholderia pickettii	*Pseudomonas picketii*
Burkholderia pseudomallei	*Pseudomonas pseudomallei*
Comamonas acidovorans	*Pseudomonas acidovorans*
Comamonas testosteroni	*Pseudomonas testosteroni*
Mycoides odoratus	*Flavobacterium odoratum*
Oligella urethralis	*Moraxella urethralis*
Sphingomonas paucimobilis	*Pseudomonas paucimobilis*
Shewanella putrefaciens	*Pseudomonas putrifaciens*
Sphingobacterium multivorum	*Flavobacterium multivorum*
Sphingobacterium spiritivorum	*Flavobacterium spiritivorum*
Stenotrophomonas maltophilia	*Xanthomonas maltophilia*

Answers to Learning Assessment Questions

Chapter 1

1. The Gram stain reaction for staphylococci is gram positive, whereas *Escherichia coli* is a gram-negative bacteria indicating that the Gram stain reaction on the patient's sample is invalid if both QC organisms show a gram-positive reaction.
2. Most likely the technologist failed either to decolorize the smear or apply the counter stain safranin.
3. Pili are structures primarily used for adherence or attachment. They are contributing virulence factors in most organisms and also are used to exchange genetic material for conjugation. Flagella are optional structures of motile species.
4. Encapsulated organisms are considered more virulent than nonencapsulated strains because capsules enable organisms to resist phagocytosis.
5. The purpose of Gram's iodine is to fix the primary stain crystal violet onto the cell wall, acting as a mordant. If the iodine is not applied or if the proper concentration of iodine is not used, the crystal violet will be removed by the decolorizer and the bacteria erroneously will appear gram negative.
6. LPS contains Lipid A or endotoxin that is responsible for fever and shock conditions during a gram-negative infection.
7. Peptidoglycan layer
8. As bacterial cells get older, the integrity of the peptidoglycan layer begins to deteriorate and is less able to entrap the crystal violet.
9. Cell wall
10. Spores are resistant to the adverse effects of the environment. Spore-forming species produce endospores when exposed to harsh environments and are able to survive.
11. In transformation, naked DNA is incorporated into a bacterial cell. This is the method used in the laboratory to introduce manipulated genetic materials into bacteria, such as in *E. coli* cloning process. Transduction is the transfer of bacterial genes by a bacteriophage. Conjugation is the transfer of genetic material from a donor bacterial cell to a recipient strain.

Chapter 2
Section A
1. Sterilization is the removal of all forms of life, whereas disinfection is limited to pathogenic organisms.
2. Antiseptic is applied onto living tissues.
3. False
4. Autoclaving
5. Phenolics

Section B
1. True
2. c. Chemical safety
3. b. All specimens
4. b. HEPA filters
5. d. All
6. c. RACE
7. a. Annually
8. Red: Flammability
   Yellow: Reactivity
   Blue: Health
   Each contains a number from 0 to 4, with 4 representing the greatest hazard and 0 indicating no hazard.
9. a. Universal Precautions
   b. Safe work habits
10. Acetone, hydrogen peroxide, MeOH, acetic acid (or other acids), and formaldehyde (see Table 2-7)

Chapter 3
Section A
1. e. Piperacillin
2. c. Tetracycline
3. d. Clindamycin
4. a. Trimethoprim-sulfamethoxazole

Section B

1. a. Disk diffusion: Prepare inoculum using the direct colony suspension technique. Incubate a full 24 hours before reporting susceptible results. Examine any apparent zone using a transmitted (not reflected) light and consider **any** growth as significant (resistant).

   MIC: Prepare inoculum using the direct colony suspension technique. Add 2% NaCl supplementation to cation-adjusted Mueller Hinton broth (broth dilution) or Mueller Hinton agar (agar dilution). Incubate a full 24 hours before reporting susceptible results.

   b. Disk diffusion: Incubate a full 24 hours before reporting susceptible results. Examine any apparent zone using a transmitted (not reflected) light and consider **any** growth as significant (resistant).

   MIC: Incubate a full 24 hours before reporting susceptible results.

   c. To screen for ESBL-producing isolates, use modified zone or MIC breakpoints (as described in NCCLS M100-S9) when testing any of the following: cefpodoxime, ceftazidime, aztreonam, cefotaxime, or ceftriazone. For confirmation of ESBL-producing isolates, use phenotypic tests described by the NCCLS. (Look for the restoration of activity of cefotaxime and/or ceftazidime in the presence of clavulanic acid.)

2. a. All β-lactams including β-lactam/β-lactamase inhibitor combinations and imipenem

   b. All penicillins and cephalosporins and aztreonam

3. Examine the battery of results obtained on each individual patient isolate to ensure that certain results appear and that each is appropriate for the species identification.

   Follow hierarchy of activity rules within a drug class (e.g., for Enterobacteriaceae, fourth-generation cephalosporins are generally more active than third-generation cephalosporins, which are generally more active than second-generation cephalosporins, which are more active than first-generation cephalosporins.)

   Ensure that each is consistent with the results previously documented in the literature and does not show any resistance that has not been previously described (e.g., penicillin resistance in *Streptococcus pyogenes*). When undocumented resistance is encountered after repeat testing, consult public health authorities.

Section C

1. For serious infections and for infections in which immune mechanisms at the infection site are not optimal, the antimicrobial agent is heavily relied upon to eradicate the infecting bacteria. For less serious infections or for infections at body sites where immune mechanisms function well, the antimicrobial agent often is sufficient to prevent the bacteria from multiplying (bacteriostatic effect) while the immune defenses eradicate the remaining bacteria.

2. MBC testing methods are not standardized. There are no criteria for interpretation of MBCs and limited data to support correlation of MBCs with clinical outcome. Numerous technical factors can affect results (e.g., inoculum preparation method, inoculum concentration, method of tube inoculation, incubation length prior to MBC subculture, subculture volume for MBC, method of subculture for MBC, medium for subculture of MBC, and incubation length of MBC).

Chapter 4

Section A

1. b. Quality control
2. b. It is measured by patient outcome.
3. b. Complex media
   c. Media with a history of failure
   d. Media made by the laboratory
4. a. They should represent the most fastidious organisms for which the media was designed.
5. c. Precision is demonstrated for 30 consecutive days.
6. c. NBS
7. a. Focused monitors
8. e. All of the above

Chapter 5

Sections A, B, C

1. Avidity is the ability of antibodies to bind to specific antigens. Specificity is the ability of the antibody to discriminate between closely related antigenic determinants.

2. Numerous antigenic detection methods exist. Precipitin test, immunodiffusion, or Ouchterlony gel diffusion, and counterimmunoelectrophoresis have been used widely to detect antigenic particles. More recent commercial kits use latex agglutination reactions; coagglutination, utilizing particle-bound antibody to enhance agglutination; liposome-mediated agglutination; immunofluorescent (FA) assays; enzyme immunoassays; and optical immunoassays.

3. Direct antigen detection tests are used in the rapid diagnosis of streptococcal pharyngitis. FA may be used for direct detection of *Bordetella pertussis* in nasopharyngeal swabs. Other examples include direct antigen tests for meningeal infections, such as those that detect *Streptococcus pneumoniae, Neisseria meningitidis, Streptococcus agalactiae,* and *Haemophilus influenzae* group b. Tests to detect viral, fungal, and parasitic agents also are available.

4. Direct antigen methods are used primarily as adjunct procedures and not as replacements for cultural techniques. The most important application is in the detection of hard-to-culture organisms.

5. Flow cytometry applications have begun to use multiple monoclonal antibodies.

6. Natural immunity consists of physical and chemical barriers, such as the skin and mucous membranes; blood proteins that act as mediators against infection; and cellular components, such as neutrophils and macrophages.

7. The skin provides a barrier that organisms must penetrate before they can cause an infection. Mucous membranes secrete antibactericidal substances that work against invading microbes. Cellular elements engulf and kill organisms.

8. Although natural immunity provides nonspecific barriers, acquired immunity is a result of the host's response to a specific foreign particle or invader.

9. In primary response to a foreign substance, the antibody class IgM rapidly appears and is followed by a gradual decline. As the level of IgM declines, the IgG level becomes detectable and persists for a longer period of time before it gradually declines. In secondary response, the IgG antibody immediately rises with an associated higher level, a prolonged elevation, and a more gradual decline.

10. If IgG antibodies are already present in a patient's serum, it is important to compare the levels during the acute phase and during convalescence. The patient should demonstrate a fourfold rise in titer for a diagnosis of an active infection.

Section D

1. Molecular applications are most helpful in the detection of infectious agents from clinical samples for which culture methods or serologic methods are still not available. Molecular diagnostic methods also are applicable when the suspected organism requires a longer period of time to produce growth for identification and susceptibility testing.

2. Nucleic acid hybridization is the process through which stable double-stranded nuclei acid molecules are formed from complementary single-stranded molecules. Several formats are available for molecular testing (see Table 5-9).

3. Probes for culture confirmation are available for *Mycobacterium* species. Probes for fungi, such as *Histoplasma capsulatum, Coccidioides immitis, Cryptococcus neoformans,* and *Blastomyces dermatidis,* also are available commercially.

4. Probes are available for the detection of *Legionella* and *Mycoplasma pneumoniae* from respiratory secretions and *Neisseria gonorrhoeae* and *Chlamydia trachomatis* from urogenital samples. Probes used to detect HIV, HSV, and HPV also are available from various manufacturers.

5. Amplification increases sensitivity by increasing the number of nucleic acid copies in a specimen to millions in a short period of time, often in less than 5 hours.

Chapter 6

Section A

1. The antimicrobial therapy eliminated her indigenous flora, which gave the opportunistic member of the flora (yeast) the opportunity to proliferate and initiate an infectious process.

2. Resident flora are organisms that occupy a specific body site indefinitely for a long time (months to years). Transient flora are those that inhabit a site for a short time, or temporarily.
3. A carrier is a host that may be colonized by a potentially pathogenic organism without causing clinical symptoms in the host.
4. The carrier becomes a source of infection and can transmit the organism to a susceptible individual.
5. The nutritional status of the site, pH, oxidation-reduction potential, and presence and interference of already established organisms all determine the composition.

Section B

1. Immune response is compromised due to HIV infection.
2. *Cryptococcus neoformans* is an encapsulated fungi that stimulates or requires cellular immune responses. Because the patient has a reduced ability to respond due to his HIV infection, he was not able to defend himself from this infecting organism.
3. True pathogens are organisms that cause disease in susceptible hosts. An opportunistic pathogen in an organism is usually a member of the indigenous flora of the host; when the host immune system is compromised or changed, the organism takes the opportunity to cause disease.
4. Inflammation occurs when the body detects a foreign body or when an injury takes place. During inflammation a large number of phagocytic cells and leukocytes accumulate at the site of injury. Phagocytes digest and engulf the foreign material, and the leukocytes release mediators to facilitate phagocytosis and in turn the killing of an invading organism.
5. Exotoxins are extracellular substances produced by an organism that has acquired a toxin gene encoded by phage, plasmids, or transposons. Endotoxins compose the lipopolysaccharide component of the cell wall of gram-negative bacteria. The toxicity is due to the Lipid A portion of the lipopolysaccharide.

Chapter 7

1. c. Swab
2. b. Sputum culture

3. b. Incubation
4. a. Refrigeration
5. a. Specimen preserved in formalin
   c. Specimen dried up
   e. Syringe with needle attached
6. c. Provides a small but concentrated area to scan
   d. Offers increased sensitivity over conventional smears
7. b. Selective media
   c. Differential media
8. a. Nonselective media
   c. Differential media
9. b. The specimen is of a low volume and likely to have few organisms.

Chapter 8

1. True
2. a. The presence of numerous inflammatory cells
3. e. All of the above
4. c. Acid-fast stain
5. b. Chitin
6. b. Nonviscous fluids
7. True
8. b. Blue

Chapter 9

1. The organism is a lactose fermenter.
2. SBA is a nonselective medium that supports the growth of both gram-positive and gram-negative bacteria. MacConkey is a selective medium that inhibits the growth of gram-positive bacteria and allows only gram-negative bacilli to grow.
3. *Streptococcus pneumoniae* and viridans streptococci produce α-hemolysis on SBA.
4. Nonfermenting species produce clear, colorless colonies on MacConkey agar.
5. β Hemolysis is complete hemolysis of the red blood cells in the agar showing a clear zone around the colony. α Hemolysis is incomplete hemolysis and shows a green discoloration around the colony.
6. "Puff balls" on the broth medium usually indicate the presence of certain streptococcal species.
7. Such colonies are characteristic of the *Proteus* species.

Chapter 10

1. *S. saprophyticus*
2. Sexually-active female
3. It is one of the few coagulase-negative staphylococci that is susceptible to novobiocin.
4. Suppurative infections, such as carbuncle, furuncle, and post-surgical wound infections and toxin-mediated manifestations, such as food-poisoning, toxic shock syndrome, and scalded skin syndrome
5. Exfoliative or epidermolytic toxin released by phage group II staphylococci
6. Protein A, a cellular component of *S. aureus,* can bind to the Fc portion of the immunoglobulin, preventing phagocytosis.
7. They are the cellular bound-clumping factor and extracellular form. Coagulase test using the slide method will detect the clumping factor, whereas the tube test will detect the extracellular form.
8. Hospital-acquired infections in patients who had predisposing instrumentation, such as catheterization, prosthetic devices, prosthetic heart valve implantation, and immunosuppressive therapy
9. Slime-producing strains of *S. epidermidis* can adhere to and form colonies on the surfaces of prosthetic devices and catheters. Slime also inhibits the protective action of lymphocytes and neutrophils.

Chapter 11

1. Rapid streptococcal antigen test, bacitracin or A disc, PYR hydrolysis, and determination of C carbohydrate by agglutination or precipitation
2. *Streptococcus pyogenes* or Group A streptococci
3. Peritonsillar abscess, rheumatic fever, and acute glomerulonephritis
4. Scarlet fever, impetigo, and cellulitis
5. Penicillin, ampicillin, and amoxicillin
6. Necrotizing fasciitis, streptococcal toxic-shock–like syndrome, and myositis
7. *Streptococcus pneumoniae*
8. Infection in the pregnant woman is self-limiting and rarely significant. However, infection in the newborn is life-threatening.

9. Enterococci is more resistant to antimicrobial agents than other streptococcal species.
10. Pyridoxal must be present in the culture medium.

Chapter 12

1. *Listeria monocytogenes*
2. HIV infection, organ transplantation, pregnancy, and corticosteroid therapy
3. *Streptococcus agalactiae* or Group B streptococci; initial differentiation being made via catalase test
4. Through wounds or cuts contaminated with decaying organic matter or through handling of animal carcasses
5. Bacteremia, erysipeloid, and endocarditis
6. Production of hydrogen sulfide on TSI agar
7. In HIV infected individuals and those with hematological disorders
8. Opportunistic organisms in patients with prosthetic devices

Chapter 13

1. *Bacillus anthracis*
2. *Bacillus* sp. (not *anthracis)*
3. The isolate in question is hemolytic and motile. *Bacillus anthracis* is nonhemolytic and nonmotile.
4. Work should be done only under a biological safety cabinet, with gloves, mask, and a gown.
5. Contamination; one of three cultures is positive, and this is most likely an environmental *Bacillus* species, such as *B. cereus* or *B. subtilis.*
6. Mycetomas are lesions that result from subcutaneous tissue infection characterized by swelling, draining sinuses, and granules.
7. Mycetomas may be caused by bacterial species, such as *Nocardia* and other aerobic actinomycetes, and by fungi. Differentiation is made easily through the use of direct microscopy.
8. *Nocardia* species are partially acid-fast.

Chapter 14

1. The cultures failed to produce any growth, even though the organisms were visible in the direct smear preparation because of the previous antimicrobial therapy that the patient underwent. Circulating antimicrobials had inhibited the growth but did not resolve the current infection.
2. *N. gonorrhoeae* and *N. meningitidis*
3. *N. meningitidis* serogroups B and C both are common in the United States. Group B, however, also causes community-acquired infections.
4. Although vaccines against groups A and C have been developed, these vaccines are not immunogenic in children under 2 years. No vaccine against serogroup B exists because humans do not develop antibodies against this group.
5. In the female, untreated gonococcal infection is the major cause of pelvic inflammatory disease. Disseminated forms also may occur, resulting in purulent arthritis. In males, epididymitis and prostatitis may develop.
6. *M. catarrhalis* may be a significant isolate from patients who are immune-compromised, such as those with neutropenia and other debilitating illnesses.

Chapter 15

Section A

1. a. Blood agar
   b. Chocolate agar
   d. MacConkey agar
2. See Figure 15-7.
3. The organism does not grow on MacConkey agar.
4. a. Negative; cannot; negative
5. b. Biotype I; serotype b
6. c. All of the above
   or
   d. None of the above
7. *Neisseria meningitidis* and *Streptococcus pneumoniae*
8. HACEK is an acronym consisting of the first initial of each genus in the following group:
   Haemophilus aphrophilus
   Actinobacillus actinomycetemcomitans
   Cardiobacterium hominis
   Eikenella corrodens
   Kingella sp.

Section B

1. *Mycoplasma pneumonia, Chlamydia pneumonia,* and *Legionella pneumophila*
2. Age (elderly)
   Smoking
   Alcohol consumption
   Compromised state
3. Crowded conditions and a high-humidity environment
4. Advantages: Rapid, moderately sensitive, and specific
   Disadvantages: Requirement of trained personnel, expensive procedure, possibility of false positives because of cross reactivity, and requirement of culture confirmation for negative reactions
5. BCYE

Section C

1. Immunizations are required at 2, 4, and 6 months, with boosters at 12 to 15 months and at school entry. The child in the case study may have missed some of the doses.
2. No; infection does occur in adults, but in a mild form. However, they serve as reservoirs for infections in nonimmunized children.
3. Nasopharyngeal aspirates and calcium alginate swabs
4. Amies, 1% casein hydrolysate, and Regan-Lowe with cephalexin

Chapter 16

1. Is oxidase negative, ferments glucose, and reduces nitrates to nitrites
2. a. Methyl red test
3. d. Voges-Proskauer test
4. b. Lactose, glucose, and/or sucrose
5. b. Enterotoxigenic *E. coli*
6. a. *Escherichia coli*
7. a. *Klebsiella pneumoniae*
8. b. *Escherichia coli*
9. c. *Proteus vulgaris*
10. d. *Shigella* species

Chapter 17

1. *Vibrio*
2. O/129 susceptibility (150 μg disk) and String test positive
3. *V. vulnificus*

4. Positive reaction for lysine decarboxylation and negative for arginine dihydrolase; positive reaction for indole production and ONPG and negative production for Voges-Proskauer test
5. TCBS
6. *C. jejuni* and *C. lari*
7. CAMPY, Skirrow or Butzler, microaerophilic, 42° C
8. Because of the strong association of long-term gastritis as a risk factor for stomach carcinoma
9. Production of urease from gastric biopsy is used. The biopsy also may be stained using Gram's, Giemsa, or silver stain to visualize the bacterium.
10. Serologic assays to detect antibodies to *H. pylori* are available. A urea breath test is also both sensitive and specific for this organism.

Chapter 18

1. Nonfermentative organisms break down carbohydrates oxidatively via the Entner-Duideroff pathway, whereas fermenters utilize carbohydrates fermentatively via the Embden-Meyerhof Parnas pathway.
2. Nonfermenters usually are found in the environment, and most exist in nature.
3. These organisms produce a wide variety of infections, including wounds, bacteremia and septicemia, pneumonia, urinary tract infection, and infections associated with intravenous use instrumentation and catheter use and prosthetic devices.
4. The ultimate opportunistic organisms, these organisms infect patients who are immunosuppressed, have chronic illnesses, have undergone transplant procedures, and are undergoing steroid therapy, have experienced trauma, had instrumentation and catheterization, and have prosthetic devices.
5. The most common nonfermentative gram-negative bacilli are the pseudomonads *Acinetobacter* species, *Moraxella* ssp., and *Stenotrophomonas maltophillia*.
6. Most nonfermenters produce resistant antimicrobial susceptibility patterns.

7. The most common are those with growth or no growth on MacConkey. Those with growth on MacConkey are usually colorless, undergo oxidase reactions (most being positive, although variable in some species), and exhibit no reactions on TSI and a resistance to antibiotics.
8. Pseudomonads are the most commonly isolated nonfermentative organisms in the clinical laboratory.
9. In addition to pyoverdin pigment, which all fluorescent pseudomonads produce, *P. aeruginosa* produces pyocyanin. *P. aeruginosa* also grows at 42° C, whereas other fluorescent species do not.
10. *Acinetobacter* species are oxidase-negative and non-motile and do not reduce nitrates to nitrites.
11. *P. pseudomallei* and *P. stutzeri* produce wrinkled colonies on sheep blood agar. Although *P. pseudomallei* produces a life-threatening infection, *P. stutzeri* is a saprophyte that produces opportunistic infections in immunosuppressed patients. In contrast to *P. pseudomallei*, which oxidizes lactose, *P. stutuzeri* does not utilize lactose, a characteristic that may help differentiate the two species.

Chapter 19

1. The specialist suspected gas gangrene (myonecrosis). The gas in the tissue represents metabolic by-products produced by the organisms that are causing the infectious process.
2. The genus is *Clostridium*. The presence of gram-positive bacilli in a wound specimen always should be considered *Clostridium* species until proven otherwise.
3. The species is *Clostridium perfringens*. This particular species has a characteristic box-car shape and rarely produces spores in tissues or culture. Although other species of *Clostridium* also can cause gas gangrene, *C. perfringens* is the most common.
4. Although the gram-positive cocci in clusters are probably *Staphylococcus epidermidis*, representing contamination of the specimen with skin flora during collection, it is possible that they are contributing to the infectious process.

5. Clostridia produce exotoxins called leukocidins that destroy leukocytes. In this case the absence of leukocytes should not have been taken as lack of evidence of an infectious process.

Chapter 20

1. Geographic location, season, outdoor exposure, and history of tick bite
2. *B. burgdorferi*
3. Pathogen transmission is more probable the longer the vector is attached.
4. Peripheral blood smear stained with Giemsa stain

Chapter 21

Section A

1. *Chlamydia trachomatis* and *Neisseria gonorrhoeae*
2. Giemsa stain and Papanicolaou stain
3. Nasopharyngeal infection and pneumonia
4. Oropharynx, nasopharynx, conjunctiva, and lower respiratory tract; vagina and rectum also believed to be colonized in the baby
5. Lymphogranuloma venereum (LGV)
6. The serotypes cause nongonococcal urethritis, epididymitis, and prostatitis in males and urethritis, follicular cervicitis, endometritis, salpingitis, proctitis, and pelvic inflammatory disease in females. Perihepatitis or Fitz-Hugh-Curtis syndrome is also caused by this organism.
7. LGV produces inguinal and anorectal symptoms among immigrants from and travelers to endemic areas. Chlamydial infection is a major cause of sterility and is the most common sexually transmitted disease in the United States. Unlike LGV, other chlamydia infections may be asymptomatic, especially in women.
8. Previous infection with *C. pneumoniae* has been described recently as a risk factor for cardiovascular disease and Guillain-Barré syndrome.
9. Psittacosis also is known as *ornithosis* and *parrot fever.* It is an acute respiratory disease attributed to *C. psittacosis.*
10. Psittacosis usually is diagnosed by a history to previous exposure to psittacines and retrospective serological testing showing a fourfold rise in titer.

Section B

1. *Mycoplasma hominis* and *Ureaplasma urealyticum* are found in the urogenital tract of asymptomatic individuals.
2. Meningitis in the newborn with Gram-stained smears showing no bacterial organisms may be suspected of *Mycoplasma/Ureaplasma* infection during passage. If the infant was infected in utero, the clinical manifestation most likely would take a respiratory form.
3. Prenatal culture of the mother may have yielded the organism; however, such organisms frequently are isolated from asymptomatic individuals, and interpretation of a positive culture is difficult.
4. *Mycoplasma* organisms do not possess cell walls and therefore will not be visible with the Gram stain.
5. New York City agar may yield *M. hominis* and *U. urealyticum.*
6. Because *Mycoplasma* organisms do not possess cell walls, they are susceptible to the harsh elements of the environment, such as drying. Therefore specimens for culture must be transported to the laboratory immediately. Transport medium, such as trypticase soy broth with 0.5% albumin and antibiotic penicillin (400 U/mL) or SP4 medium, are used. If a delay in processing is expected, samples must be frozen at $-70°$ C.
7. Several culture media have been developed for *Mycoplasma* recovery, including PPLO agar, Shephard A-7B for *Ureaplasma,* SP4, Hayflick's biphasic medium, E agar, and NYC agar.
8. Cold agglutinin titer traditionally has been used as an indicator for *M. pneumonia* infection. However, this test is both insensitive and nonspecific.
9. Enzyme immunoassay (EIA) and indirect hemagglutination methods (IHA) now are available for antibody detection.
10. Erythromycin and tetracycline are antimicrobials used for empiric therapy of *Mycoplasma* infections and can shorten the duration of symptoms in patients with respiratory disease. *M. hominis* is resistant to erythromycin and usually is treated with tetracycline and lincomycin. *Ureaplasma,* on the other hand, is resistant to lincomycin but susceptible to erythromycin.

Chapter 22

1. A multiplicity of mycobacterial species, both saprophytes and potential pathogens, may be isolated from humans. Currently, mycobacteria may be identified through the use of biochemical and DNA probe technology. The use of genetic probe technologies offers tremendous promise in microbial identification at a variety of levels—family, genus, species, and subspecies.

   The most common probe technology is the single-stranded, radiolabeled DNA probe, now available commercially. Probes specific for the genus *Mycobacterium,* the *M. tuberculosis* complex (including *M. tuberculosis, M. bovis, M. bovis BCG, M. africanum,* and *M. microti*), and the two species *M. avium* and *M. intracellular. M. kansasii* and *M. gordonea* are now available. Currently all four probes may be used to identify the indicated mycobacteria grown in pure culture. Laboratories should perform identification according to the level of service for which they are qualified. Currently all isolates should be identified to the species level.

2. TB disease must be treated for at least 6 months; in some cases, treatment lasts even longer. In most areas of the country the initial regimen for treating TB disease should include four drugs—isoniazid, rifampin, pyrazinamide, and either ethambutol or streptomycin. When the drug susceptibility results are available, the clinician may change the regimen accordingly.

   TB disease must be treated with at least two drugs to which the bacilli are susceptible. The bacteriologic basis of chemotherapy for tuberculosis is understood best through the consideration of distinct subpopulations of tubercle bacilli with different susceptibilities to antituberculosis drugs.

   First, a rapidly dividing group of extracellular organisms exists, found in areas where the pH is neutral to alkaline. This subpopulation is killed readily by isoniazid, rifampin, and streptomycin in bactericidal doses.

   A second subpopulation of organisms is thought to exist in solid casseous material and generally grows slowly, but with spurts of metabolic activity. Rifampin seems to be the most effective drug in killing these organisms, which grow intermittently rather than continuously.

   The third group of organisms postulated to exist is found within the acidic environment of macrophages, where metabolic activity is also slow. Mycobacteria that divide slowly are not as readily affected by the antibiotics and thus require longer periods of exposure.

3. With the closing of most tuberculosis sanatoria and the treatment of patients in general hospitals or outpatient clinics, the supporting mycobacteriologic services have been spread diffusely through more laboratories, each processing fewer specimens. The maintenance of proficiency requires the continuing and frequent performance of the required test procedures. When laboratory tests are performed so infrequently that it is impractical to maintain the materials and expertise required for proficiency, a decision must be made concerning referral to another laboratory for testing. Clinical laboratory functions that contribute to the diagnosis and management of tuberculosis have been divided into the following three major categories of services offered. These are as follows:

   a. Level I—collection and transport of specimens, preparation and examination of smears for acid-fast bacilli

   b. Level II—procedures of Level I, plus isolation and identification of *M. tuberculosis*

   c. Level III—all procedures of Level II, plus identification of mycobacteria other than *M. tuberculosis*

   The determination of drug susceptibility may be performed at Level II and should be performed at Level III.

   A laboratory may choose to develop or maintain the skills defined under one of the previous levels, depending on the frequency with which specimens are received for isolation of mycobacteria, the nature of the clinical community being served, and the availability of a specialized referral service. All laboratories that perform clinical mycobacteriology should participate in recognized proficiency testing programs, and levels of service should be established and limited by the quality of performance demonstrated in these examinations.

4. Most clinical specimens contain an abundance of nonmycobacterial contaminants. Unless an attempt is made to inhibit these usually fast-growing contaminants, they quickly can overgrow the generally more slowly reproducing (18- to 24-hour generation time) mycobacteria on the culture medium. The organic debris (tissue, serum, and other proteinaceous material) surrounding the organism in the specimen also must be liquified so that decontaminating agents will kill undesirable microbes and surviving mycobacteria can gain access to the nutrients of the medium onto which they are subsequently inoculated.

Because mycobacteria are more refractory to harsh chemicals than are most other microorganisms, chemical digestion decontamination procedures have been applied successfully to ensure the recovery of acid-fast bacteria from clinical materials. The use of NaOH both digests and decontaminates the specimens. N-acetyl cysteine effectively digests the specimen, but decontamination does not occur.

5. Because of the low levels of mycobacteria organism found in the clinical samples, meticulous care must be practiced during the processing of specimens for the demonstration and isolation of mycobacterial organisms. False-positive results may occur through carryover from the mouths of containers used to transfer processing agents; introduction of the organism from environmental sources, such as water; or the introduction of organisms from aerosols produced when specimen containers are opened. Care must be taken in performance of the stain to prevent carryover from one slide to another. Slides should never come in contact with one another, either in transfer to the staining rack or actually performance of the stain.

False-negative results may occur if processing protocols are not followed properly. Prolonged decontamination may kill the mycobacteria. Improper centrifugation force also may lead to false-negative results. If sufficient force is not applied, the mycobacteria may remain at the interface of the processed specimen and thus be inadvertently discarded during processing. Care also must be applied during culturing of the specimen. Cross contamination between specimens may occur if instruments are not properly maintained.

Chapter 23

1. *Blastomyces dermatitidis*
   37° C: Large "broad-based" budding yeast cells
   25° C: Round or oval microconidia; borne on short conidiophore or directly on hyphae

   Coccidioides immitis
   37° C: Spherules containing endospores (in vivo)
   25° C: Alternating arthoconidia (in vitro)

   Histoplasma capsulatum var. *capsulatum*
   37° C: Small, single-budding yeasts
   25° C: Small round or oval microconidia; borne along hyphae; large tuberculate macroconidia

   Sporothrix schenkii
   37° C: Cigar-shpaed yeasts
   25° C: Delicate hyphae with conidia in a "rosette" pattern

2. *Microsporum gypseum*
   Macroconidia: Spindle-shaped; thin-walled; 4 to 6 cells
   Microconidia: Few club-shaped or elliptical

   Microsporum canis
   Macroconidia: Spindle-shaped; tapered at each end; "canoe-shaped," thick-walled, and rough
   Microconidia: Few oval shaped

   Trichophyton rubrum
   Urease test (negative)
   Hair penetration (negative)
   Macroconidia: Smooth-walled; elongated; 3 to 8 cells
   Microconidia: Small; peg-shaped; borne singly along hyphae; "picket-fence" appearance

   Trichophyton mentagrophytes
   Urease test (positive)
   Hair penetration (positive)
   Macroconidia: Smooth-walled; elongated; 5 to 8 cells
   Microconidia: Small; globose and grapelike clusters; spiral hyphae

3. The clinical significance of the isolation of saprobes from clinical samples must be evaluated carefully. Because these various species exist as free-living microorganisms and until recently have been considered common laboratory contaminants, appropriate evaluation of the immune status of the patient is very important. Chemotherapy, organ transplantation, and other medical interventions have provided opportunities for these species to cause serious infections among patients who become immunosuppressed.

4. *Penicillium* sp.
   Macroscopic: Rapid-growing fungus with green or blue-green coloration
   Microscopic: Conidiophores erect; branched with phialides that produce oval conidia in long chains

   Aspergillus fumigatus
   Macroscopic: Rapid-growing hyaline fungus with smoky gray-green coloration
   Microscopic: Conidiophores smooth walled; phialides occurring only on the upper portion of the dome-shaped vesicle

   Fusarium sp.
   Macroscopic: Hyaline fungus; colors varying with age, from rose to mauve and purple to yellow
   Microscopic: Macroconidia multicelled and crescent-shaped

   Curvularia sp.
   Macroscopic: Rapid-growing; dematiaceous; black; cottony
   Microscopic: Multicelled conidia with 3 to 5 cells of unequal sizes

5. A positive germ tube test indicating that the yeast isolate is *Candida albicans* will show no constriction at the base of the mother cell. *C. albicans* will form chlamydoconidium when grown on cornmeal agar.

Chapter 24

1. a. The most likely identification is *Giardia lamblia.*
    b. It is a pathogen. The patient may experience cramping; flatulence; and light colored, foul-smelling, frothy [gassy] stools. The major complication is malabsorption syndrome.
    c. The trophozoite colonizes the small intestine and interferes with the absorption of food and fat-soluble vitamins and the digestion of fats.

2. a. Thick films are used in detection of the organism. The blood is kept as a single drop, thereby concentrating the organisms into a smaller area and increasing the chances of visualization. In addition, the lysing of the RBC and release of hemoglobin allow organisms to stand out against the background.

    In a thin film the blood is spread out so that an area exists with a single layer of RBCs. Species identification is made from the thin film because the cells are kept intact and morphology of both the cell and the malarial organism can be observed. Characteristics, such as enlargement of the RBC or the presence of stippling within the cell, help in identification.

    b. *P. vivax*—The growing trophozoite is ameboid. The mature schizont has 12 to 24 merozoites present. The pigment is a golden brown, and the RBC is enlarged to approximately twice its normal size. Schuffner's stippling is present in the RBC.

    P. malariae—The growing trophozoite is compact or may exist as a "band" or basket form. The mature schizont has 6 to 12 merozoites, often arranged in a flower or "daisy" configuration around the central clump of pigment. The pigment in the organism is dark brown and coarse. The RBC is normal size, and stippling rarely is present.

    P. ovale—The growing trophozoite resembles *P. malariae* (compact) but lacks a band or basket form. The schizont has 6 to 12 merozoites, but these generally show no characteristic arrangement. The RBC is enlarged one-and-one-half to two times normal size and often has an oval appearance with fimbriated or ragged edges. Schuffner's stippling often is present.

    P. falciparum—Only two stages usually are visible in peripheral blood: the ring-form trophozoite and the gametocyte. The gametocyte is characterized by a banana or sausage shape. The ring-form trophozoite is delicate and may have two chromatin dots (horseshoe) or be an applique form (appearing to be on the outside of the RBC membrane). RBCs often have more than one malarial organism present. The RBC is not enlarged, and stippling rarely is seen.

    c. Complications are blackwater fever and cerebral malaria. Blackwater fever is due to massive intravascular hemolysis (possibly autoimmune-mediated). Resulting hemoglobin is excreted in urine and turns black because of the acid pH of urine. Cerebral malaria is due to the "sluggish" blood flow through the capillaries of the brain. The infected RBCs develop sticky "knobs" that adhere to the capillary lining, slowing blood flow and resulting in decreased oxygen to the tissues, necrosis, and CNS symptoms that include seizures and coma.

3. a. *Taenia* sp.—The egg is 35 to 45 μ and round and contains hexacanth embryo. The brown-colored outer shell shows radial striations.

    Ascaris lumbricoides—The fertile egg is broadly oval, is approximately 45 to 75 μ long, and has a brown, mammillated coating and a thick inner shell.

    Trichuris trichiura—The egg has a characteristic barrel, or football, shape and is approximately 50 to 55 μ long, with a colorless polar plug at each end.

    Enterobius vermicularis—The egg is oval, with one side slightly flattened and a thin, colorless shell. It is 50 to 60 μ long and contains a C-shaped larva.

    Hookworm—The egg is oval, about 55 to 60 μ long, with a thin, colorless shell. It usually contains yolk material in the 4- to 8-cell stage of development.

    Schistosoma mansoni—The egg is approximately 110 to 170 μ long and is embryonated. It is elongated and has a large, lateral spine.

4. The diagnostic method for *E. vermicularis* is the cellophane tape prep. The female pinworm migrates out the anus at night and lays her eggs in the perianal area before reentering the anus. The eggs remain on the perianal tissues, and a stool specimen therefore will not contain eggs. In a cellophane tape prep the skin in the perianal area is sampled for the presence of eggs.

Chapter 25

1. Kaposi's lesions, recurrent thrush, and herpes lesions in the perianal region
2. *Pneumocystis carinii* pneumonia, *Mycobacterium avium, M. kansasii, M. tuberculosis,* histoplasmosis, coccidiomycosis, cryptococcus meningitis, cryptosporidiosis, CMV infections, Burkitt's lymphoma, toxoplasmosis
3. Decline of the CD4+ T cells, depression of the T4:T8 ratio to below 0.9 (normal being >1.5), functional impairment of monocytes and macrophages, decreased natural killer cell activity, anergy to recall antigens in skin tests
4. Cytomegalovirus (CMV)
5. The virus produces infectious mononucleosis and also has been associated with Burkitt's lymphoma and B-cell lymphoproliferative disorder or lymphoma in transplant patients. Complications include splenic hemorrhage, hepatitis, Reye syndrome, encephalitis, and thrombocytopenia purpura with hemolytic anemia.
6. Serologic markers to differentiate the various types of hepatitis B infection are available in Table 25-10.
7. Classic dengue fever is a mild, self-limiting disease, nonfatal and usually resolved within 1 to 2 weeks. It is usually the manifestation on the first encounter with dengue virus. Patients develop dengue hemorrhagic fever (DHF) after they have been exposed to one serotype; they then become exposed to one of the other three serotypes. DHF patients develop similar symptoms; classic DF with thrombocytopenia, hemorrhage, and shock and is usually fatal.

8. The most effective method for the identification of rabies viruses in tissue is direct FA on impression smears from brain tissues.
9. "Fifth disease," or erythema infectiosum, is the fifth infectious rash described, along with rubeola, rubella, varicella, and roseola. It is caused by Parvovirus B19.
10. The enteroviruses include Polioviruses, Coxsackieviruses A and B, Echoviruses, Enteroviruses 68-71.
11. Arenaviruses include viruses that cause hemorrhagic fever (see Table 25-9), such as lymphocytic choriomeningitis, Lassa, Machupo, Tacaribe, Junin, and Ebola.
12. Papillomaviruses are known to cause genital warts or condylomata acuminata but recently have been associated with neoplasms. HPV 6 and 11 are common in genital warts but have not been found in malignant lesions, whereas HPV 16 and 18 are found in genital warts and also in invasive carcinoma of the cervix.
13. Herpes viruses, which include Herpes simplex type 1 and type 2, Varicella-zoster virus, Cytomegalovirus, Epstein-Barr virus, and Herpesvirus 6, all are latent and persist throughout the host's lifetime.
14. The H (hemagglutinin) and N (neuraminidase) antigens of Influenza A virus change continuously. These changes are reflected in "antigenic shifts" that often encourage a pandemic because a majority of the population has little preexisting immunity to this new strain.
15. Acyclovir for Herpes simplex types 1 and 2; ribavirin for RSV; amantadine for Influenzae A but not B; zidovudine for HIV

Chapter 26

1. A positive culture may reflect the presence of normal flora or a potentially pathogenic microorganism. In neither case is a clinically relevant infection necessarily present. The culture result must be put into the context of the clinical situation and ancillary data compiled to make this distinction.

2. An immunologically competent patient will usually only develop a clinically significant infection with a critical inoculum of organisms with known virulence. Conversely, a patient whose normal barriers against infection are compromised or whose immune response is suppressed or incompetent can develop infections from organisms that otherwise would be considered nonpathogenic or part of the normal flora. These often are referred to as "opportunistic infections." Special specimen processing, staining, and culture techniques may be required for opportunistic pathogens, and organisms that otherwise would be considered "normal flora" may be important for clinical discussion.

3. Infectious diseases are more likely to develop behind areas of anatomic obstruction. This occurrence likely is explained by the importance of normal drainage of secretions to prevent increased overgrowth of organisms. Examples include blocked sinus ostia ort eustachian tubes, resulting in sinusitis or otitis media, respectively, and blockage of a lower respiratory tract airway by an obstructing tumor or foreign body, resulting in a slowly resolving pneumonia.

4. Awareness of the seasonal incidence of respiratory tract infections in the community is useful for the clinician, as well as the microbiologist, in suggesting the most likely diagnosis and the most efficient use of laboratory resources. Influenza cultures, for example, rarely are indicated unless evidence of influenza is present in the community or in an area to which the patient has traveled. Regular communication with the local public health department and review of the *Morbidity and Mortality Weekly* report can improve awareness of these seasonal trends.

5. Acute sinusitis and acute otitis media are two examples. In both cases, the likely pathogens are well known, and collection of meaningful culture specimens from these sites can be difficult and invasive.

6. Cotton inhibits the growth of the organism.

7. Acute bronchitis is an infection of the airways of the lower respiratory tract that has not extended into the nonairway lung tissue. Once the infection is detected in the lung tissue—via physical examination, chest x-ray, or chest CT scan—pneumonia is diagnosed. Pneumonia is usually a more serous infection and has a greater likelihood of spreading to the bloodstream, and therefore an increased associated mortality.

8. Nosocomial pneumonias are much more likely to be caused by gram-negative bacterial pathogens.

9. Microscopic examination of the direct sputum Gram stain should reveal fewer than 10 epithelial cells and more than 25 PMNs per low power (10×) field.

10. The microbiologist's directions help maximize the isolation of anaerobic pathogens.

Chapter 27

1. *S. aureus* and Group A streptococci
2. Streptobacillosis is caused by *Streptobacillus moniliformis,* whereas spirillosis is caused by *Spirillum minor.*
3. *S. aureus* and *Pseudomonas aeruginosa*
4. When the oxidation-reduction potential in the environment is lowered and the tissues are injured, sporeforming organisms are introduced, leading to the development of myonecrosis.
5. *Vibrio vulnificus, Pseudomonas aeruginosa, Aeromonas hydrophila, Neisseria meningitidis* and *N. gonorrhoeae, Haemophilus influenzae,* and Group A streptococci
6. Group A streptococci, *S. aureus,* and *Salmonella typhi*
7. Actinomycosis may be caused by aerobic actinomycetes *Nocardia* species and anaerobic actinomycetes, especially *Actinomyces israelii.* These two bacterial species, *Nocardia* and *Actinomyces,* may be differentiated by their environmental and acid-fast requirements. *Nocardia* species are partially acid-fast, whereas *Actinomyces* species are non–acid-fast organisms.
8. Varicella-zoster virus causes chicken pox in children and recurs as shingles in adults.

9. Chicken pox manifests as small blisters, or vesicles, that form approximately 2 weeks after infection. The eruptions begin usually at the trunk and progress to the face and extremities. Lesions develop after the vesicles rupture. After primary infection, the virus goes into a latency period. An imbalance between host and virus, such as emotional stress or immunosuppression reactivates the virus. Referred to as *shingles,* the reoccurrence manifests with vesicles appearing locally along a specific sensory nerve.
10. Larvae of dog and cat hookworms, *Ancylostoma caninum,* and *Ancylostoma braziliense*

Chapter 28

1. Most organisms are susceptible to the low gastric pH because of the gastric acid and juices that the stomach produces. Therefore the number of organisms that survive to reach the small bowel is reduced.
2. Motility is the major immune defense in the small bowel. Motility prevents organisms from attaching along the intestinal mucosal surfaces, thus limiting the chance for the invading organism to become established.
3. Because organisms compete for food and nutrients, the colon flora take up most of them (food and nutrients), which prevents invading organisms from affixing to the colon. The usual flora also may produce metabolic byproducts toxic to the invading species.
4. The incubation period and presence or absence of fever are important clinical findings to determine whether the illness is enterotoxin-mediated or invasive. In the laboratory the presence of white blood cells would indicate an invasive organism as the source of illness, rather than one that produces an enterotoxin.
5. A detailed history of ingested food, going back as far as 3 days, is helpful because most diarrhea pathogens are acquired via ingestion of food or water. Certain food vehicles are associated with specific pathogens or toxins.

6. Microsporidium, *Cryptosporidium* and *Isospora* produce severe diarrheal illnesses among immunosuppressed individuals, especially AIDS patients.
7. Rarely encountered parasites, such as *Anisakis* sp., *Angiostrongylus cantonensis, Capillaria philippenensis, D. latum,* and *P. westermani* may be suspected.
8. Ciguatera, scombroid, and paralytic shellfish poisoning may occur.
9. Washing fresh produce before serving it; eating sufficiently cooked meat, fish, and other food products; and washing hands and utensils help prevent the occurrence of food-borne disease.
10. Chlorination of water used in the growing, processing, and rinsing of fresh produce can help prevent the occurrence of food-borne disease. Irradiation of meat and meat products and other food groups is another alternative. Chemical rinses and other methods used to reduce contamination of food products during processing and transport continuously are being improved.

Chapter 29

1. CSF is a sterile fluid produced both through filtration and through secretion from the choroid plexuses within the cerebral ventricles. CSF enters the subarachnoid space via the cisterna magna and circulates under pressure around the brain and spinal cord to the arachnoid villi, where it is reabsorbed.
2. In normal adults the CSF volume ranges from 90 to 150 mL, CSF protein is 15 to 45 mg/dL, and CSF glucose is two-thirds that of plasma (normally 40 to 80 mg/dL). The CSF cell count shows 0 to 7 leukocytes/mL, with predominance of lymphocytes and monocytes. In newborns CSF protein and glucose concentrations and cell count are normally higher than in adults. Most infants older than 3 months normally have no neutrophils within the CSF; thus the presence of a single neutrophil in the CSF of a child may be regarded as abnormal.

3. The most common organisms associated with bacterial meningitis include *S. pneumoniae, H.influenzae* type b, and *N. meningitidis,* all of which possess antiphagocytic capsules as the major virulence factor. In addition, *N. meningitidis* organisms possess pili that facilitate adherence to epithelial and endothelial cells. In most cases bacterial meningitis proceeds through four stages—colonization of the upper respiratory tract, invasion of the bloodstream, seeding of the meninges, and resulting infection of the meninges and inflammation of the CSF. Host factors associated with each organism include liver disease, alcoholism, sickle cell anemia, previous splenectomy and malignancy *(S. pneumoniae),* diabetes mellitus, cystic fibrosis and Cushing syndrome *(H. infuenzae),* and complement deficiency *(N. meningitidis).*

4. Table 29-5 compares the physical, chemical, and cellular features for each of these organisms.

5. *Aspergillus, Mucor, Rhizopus,* and *Absidia* are filamentous fungi that produce invasive hyphae and thus most commonly are associated with brain abscesses.

6. In contrast, yeast, such as *Cryptococcus, Histoplasma, Candida,* and *Coccidioides,* most frequently produce meningitis.

7. CSF specimens received in the laboratory should be examined immediately because certain organisms do not cause pleocytosis. In addition, certain fastidious organisms autolyze and do not survive during transit.

8. Initial evaluation should include CSF protein, glucose and cell counts, and examination of a gram-stained cytocentrifuge preparation.

9. Whether organisms or inflammation is seen, all CSF specimens should be cultured on blood and chocolate agars.

10. Additional serologic tests or cultures for fungi, or a polymerase chain reaction assay for tuberculous meningitis, then can be performed. Bacterial antigen tests and the *Limulus* amebocyte lysis assay are not recommended for routine use but may be useful in certain clinical situations.

Chapter 30

1. Because no other associated site of infection is identified, this case is an example of a primary bacteremia.

2. The patient has granulocytopenia that placed him at risk for all types of bacterial infections—in particular, bacteremia. Neutropenic patients are usually at risk for gram-negative bacteremia.

3. The following conditions also place patients at an increased risk for bacteremia: reduced immune competency; increased use of invasive procedures and instrumentation; aging; and administration of immunosuppressive therapy and other drugs.

4. Sources of bacteremic spread include peritoneal dialysis, pericarditis, bacterial pneumonia, bedsores, prosthetic devices and instrumentation, and skeletal, skin, and soft-tissue infections.

5. Bacterial pneumonia that usually produces a concurrent bacteremia includes *S. aureus, S. pneumoniae, P. aeruginosa, H. influenzae,* and *E. aerogenes.*

6. Organisms involved in bacteremic episodes in patients with prosthetic devices usually come from the skin or gastrointestinal flora.

7. Organisms that contaminate prosthetic devices take advantage of the material used to make these devices. The organism may produce "slime" that facilitates adherence and protects the organism from host immune responses. Some organisms also may use the material as a source of food.

8. Those at risk for polymicrobial bacteremia include immunocompromised patients, especially those with alcoholism, granulocytopenia, extensive burns, diabetes mellitus, and renal failure. Patients with vascular insufficiency due to ischemia are also at risk.

9. It has been suggested that 10 ml of blood should be drawn from adult patients and placed in 90 mls of diluting fluid (1:10 dilution). This ratio helps reduce the bactericidal effect of serum. SPS in the culture medium serves as anticomplement and anticoagulant.

10. The number of samples and time of collection could be highly dependent on the type of bacteremia suspected. However, in general, three sets within a 24-hour period at 1-hour intervals is appropriate, especially in suspected cases of subacute endocarditis.

Chapter 31

1. Urine samples with multiple isolates, even when present in large numbers, should not be identified unless a consultation is warranted. This occurrence usually represents contamination.
2. These organisms are usual flora in the urogenital tract.
3. A single-episode UTI occurs only once and resolves itself spontaneously or through antimicrobial therapy, whereas recurrent UTI occurs repeatedly, with or without symptoms. Recurrent UTI may involve the same organism (relapse) or a different organism (reinfection).
4. Gram-stained smears of uncentrifuged urine may reveal the etiologic agent of UTI. The presence of white blood cells also would be detected, indicating infection. Other screening methods are used to detect the presence of pyuria and bacteruria, which provides the clinician information on how to proceed with patient care.
5. Urine specimens for routine culture should be incubated for a full 24 hours at 37° C.
6. Background urethral flora will appear after 24 hours. This appearance may result in costly identification and confusion of the clinical purpose of the urine culture.
7. The presence of yeast in the urine may be an indication of bladder or renal parenchymal infection, a urinary tract fungus ball, or disseminated candidiasis.
8. Specimens with multiple uropathogens, that is, three or more, likely represent contamination.
9. Routine urine cultures do not include the recovery of *Neisseria gonorrhoeae* and *Chlamydia trachomatis* or *Ureaplasma urealyticum,* all of which are sexually transmitted agents. Symptoms produced by these agents are difficult to differentiate from that of a true urinary tract infection.
10. One or two uropathogens present in >105 CFU/ml should be identified and susceptibility tests performed for inpatients. In the interpretation of urine cultures from outpatients, physicians may utilize a different algorithm that does not routinely perform susceptibilities and emphasize empiric selection based on antibiograms.

Chapter 32

1. Because only 10% to 20% of affected women develop overt clinical symptoms of gonorrhoea, the disease may go untreated. In such cases it can ascend the genital tract and create complications, such as pelvic inflammatory disease.
2. Nontreponemal tests, such as rapid plasma reagin (RPR) or VDRL, would be appropriate. These tests detect nontreponemal antibodies, which become nonreactive if the patient receives treatment, unlike treponemal antibodies, which remain reactive for life.
3. Bacterial vaginosis is a condition in which a disruption of the vaginal flora occurs. The disruption usually happens when the concentration of lactobacilli decreases, and other bacterial species, such as *Gardnerella vaginalis* and *Mobiluncus* spp., predominate the site.
4. Chancroid or soft chancre is caused by *Haemophilus ducreyi,* a painful, suppurative lesion that develops several days after inoculation. Chancre is the primary lesion produced by *Treponema pallidum* spp., which causes syphilis. Unlike chancroid, chancre is painless and nonsuppurative.
5. Clinically, the exudate produced in bacterial vaginosis is clingy, clear, and watery. It also produces a characteristic fishlike odor. The pH is increased, and the presence of "clue cells" is diagnostic.

Chapter 33

1. The treatment for the gastrointestinal malignancy the patient received placed the patient at an increased risk for infections. The patient became neutropenic, making him susceptible to endogenous microflora. Septicemia is not uncommon among neutropenic patients.
2. *Pseudomonas aeruginosa* is a member of the normal colon flora. If a malignancy occurred at this particular site, cytotoxic drugs taken by the patient may have contributed to the breakdown of mucosal barriers, providing access for the organism to gain entrance into the bloodstream.

3. Although a decrease in the number of neutrophils is the most commonly demonstrated hematologic disturbance, inadequacy of neutrophil functions, such as the inability to migrate to sites of inflammation, is another cause of increased infections among such patients. The inability of the neutrophils to phagocytize or kill the ingested organisms also predisposes patients with this type of malignancy and places them at risk of infections from endogenous organisms.

4. Antimicrobial agents change the composition of the patient's endogenous microflora, allowing those species that are antimicrobial-resistant to thrive and enhancing the opportunity for these organisms to initiate infections.

5. Several changes in the immune function occur as the human body ages, increasing its susceptibility to infections and malignancy. The qualitative decline of cellular immune defenses (function) predisposes elderly individuals to various types of infections, including respiratory, gastrointestinal, urinary tract and soft tissue. Because of decreased tumor surveillance by immune and nonimmune mechanisms, the occurrence of malignancy in this population also is increased.

Chapter 34

1. Cholera: *Vibrio cholera*
   Tetanus: *Clostridium tetani*
   Botulism: *Clostridium botulinum*
2. Natural bristle comes from animal sources. Animal hides and fur can be contaminated with spores of anthrax. These materials are sterilized to kill the spores and prevent the spread of disease.
3. *Listeria monocytogenes*
4. Hunting and cleaning small game, such as rabbits

5. It is most unfair to be critical of what was done at the time, but some ideas can be gained from this unfortunate scenario. The patient coincidentally fell from a trampoline, which probably was reported as the patient's primary complaint. The finding of pain in the axilla might have been the result of the collection of organisms in lymph nodes from the plague infection, the beginning of a buboe. Because of the fall, these findings probably were discounted.

   A case history that included recent contact with sick or injured animals or sick people might have elicited responses unrelated to the trampoline incident. If an individual lives in an area endemic to a "rare" disease, the case may be one that is not often reported in the literature. In laboratories in the western United States plague should be considered as a possibility. Also, the identification system used did not produce *Yersinia pestis* as an answer immediately. Unusual isolates may provide less-predictable results in systems that have not been challenged with large numbers of strains.

6. Leptospires may be recovered through use of Fletcher semisolid media, bovine albumin-Tween 80 (Ba-Tw 80) media enriched with rabbit serum, and Ellinghausen-McCullough-Johnson-Harris (EMJH) media containing fatty acids or albumin. In addition, 5-fluorouracil, fosfomycin, and nalidixic acid may be added to decrease contamination.

7. Weil's disease is the most serious form of leptospirosis. Hemolysis, jaundice, and renal failure may occur. Renal failure is the most common cause of death.

8. Rickettsiae have not been grown in artificial, cell-free media but can be recovered in monolayer cell lines or in the yolk sacs of embryonated eggs.

9. The rickettsia species produces several types of clinical infections, including spotted fever, typhus fever, scrub typhus, and Q fever.

10. Unlike other rickettsial infections that are transmitted by arthropod vectors, *C. burnetti* commonly is acquired through inhalation of the organisms from infected aerosols.

Chapter 35

1. Bacteria: *S. aureus, P. Aeruginosa,* and *S. pneumoniae*
   Fungi: *Fusarium, Aspergillus,* and *Candida*
   Parasites: *Acanthamoeba, Toxoplasma,* and malaria
   Viruses: Adenovirus, HIV, and herpes viruses
2. *Limulus* lysate, contact lens culture, and culture of contaminated ocular medications and ocular tissue
3. Cornea, conjunctiva, and lids
   S. aureus, H. Influenzae, P. aeruginosa, and *S. pneumoniae*
   CHOC, BAP, and Thio (Refer to Table 35-3 for additional media. Stains such as Gram stain should be performed on direct smear.)
4. Gram stain, Giemsa stain, calcofluor white, AFB, and DFA

Index

A

A7 agar, 1117
Abscess
    anaerobic bacteria in, 571
    aspirate of, 290
    brain, *981,* 981-982
        microscopic appearance of, 303
    buccal space, 298
    culture media for, 252t
    Entamoeba histolytica causing, 767
    fungal specimen from, 717
    microscopic specimen of, 285, 287, 288
    Mycobacterium fortuitum and, 698
    retroorbital, 890
    soft tissue, 303
    specimen collection from, 239, 242t
    Staphylococcus causing, *336*
Absidia spp., 742, *742*
    brain abscess and, 981
Absorption, viral infection and, 871
Acanthamoeba spp., 772, 774
Acanthamoeba castellanii, 989-990
Accuprobe, for fungus, 195, *196*
Accuracy, of test, 122
Acetate agar, 1117-1118
Acetobacter sp., beta-lactam antibiotics and, 56
Acetone, detection of, 19
Achlorhydria, 948
Acid
    anaerobic bacteria identification and, 592, *593*
    mixed acid fermentation and, 18-19
    mycotic, 689-690
    nonfermenting gram-negative rods and, 543
    nucleic; *see* Nucleic acid *entries*
    oxalic, 675
    pyruvic, 18
Acid fastness of *Mycobacterium,* 670
Acid-alcohol fastness of *Mycobacterium,* 670
Acidaminococcus fermentans, clinical significance of, 615t
Acid-fast bacilli, 677-678
Acid-fast cell wall, 9
Acid-fast stain, 11-12, *12*
    for *Cryptosporidium parvum,* 797
    for mycobacteria, 269-270
    for parasitic infection, 761

Acinetobacter spp.
    bacteremia and, 1000
    characteristics of, 549-550, *550*
    gonococcal medium and, 408
Acquired immunity, 157-158
Acquired immunodeficiency syndrome; *see* Human
        immunodeficiency virus
Acremonium falciforme, 732-733, 732t
Acridine orange stain, 12, *13,* 184t
Acronym, RACE, 47
Actinobacillus actinomycetemcomitans, 436-438, 437t, *438*
Actinomadura spp., 399
Actinomyces spp.
    characteristics of, 599, 602, *603,* 604, 604t
    clinical significance of, 602t
    culture media for, 253t
    eyelid infection and, 1093-1094
    general characteristics of, 395-396
    on intrauterine device, 257
    laboratory diagnosis of, 602, 604
    orbital infection and, 1099
    skin manifestations of, 930
Actinomyces israelii, 1100
Actinomycetes
    Nocardia, 395-399, 396t, *397, 398*
    skin manifestations of, 930
Actinomycosis, cervicofacial, 930
Acute antibody titer, 162
Additive
    for smear, 249-250
    to urine specimen, 1024
Adenosine diphosphoribose, 376
Adenovirus
    cell cultures for, 841t
    cytopathic effect of, *842*
    gastrointestinal infection with, 150, 851, 958
    respiratory infection from, 844-845
Adenylate cyclase, 458
Adherence
    by anaerobic bacteria, 572t
    definition of, 227
    Haemophilus influenzae and, 429
    respiratory infection and, 884
    viral infection and, 227
Adhesin, 227
Aedes aegypti, 854
Aedes albopictus, 853, 854
Aerobic bacteria
    Actinomyces, 395-396, 396t
    Brucella, 443

Page numbers in italics indicate illustrations; *t* indicates tables.

Aerobic bacteria—cont'd
  Francisella, 444
  gastrointestinal, 948, 948t
  gram-positive bacilli, 390-395, *391, 392,* 392t
  Nocardia, 396-399, *397*
  obligate, 15
Aerococcus, 524-528
  antigenic structure of, 524
  antimicrobial susceptibility of, 526t, *527,* 528
  antimicrobials effective against, 59
  bile esculin test and, 356
  biochemical identification of, 351t
  characteristics of, 369, 518t
  clinical infection with, 524-525
  enterotoxin-mediated diarrhea and, 951
  gastrointestinal infection caused by, 956
  general characteristics of, 524
  laboratory diagnosis of, 525-528, 526t, *527*
  leucine aminopeptidase test and, 356
  Vibrio vs., 522
Aeromonas hydrophila, 927
Aerosol, influenza virus and, 843
Aerosolization of respiratory secretions, 230
Aerotolerance testing, 586t, 587
African sleeping sickness, 780-781
Agar
  A7, 1117
  acetate, 1117-1118
  bacteroides bile-esculin, 579t
  bile-esculin, 1118
  birdseed, 1141
  bismuth sulfite, 1118
  blood; *see* Blood agar
  blood phenylethyl alcohol, 1119-1120
  Bordet-Gangou potato infusion, 459
  brain-heart infusion, 1141
  brucella/blood, 598, *598*
  buffered charcoal-yeast extract agar, 1120
  cetrimide, 1134
  chocolate, 1122
    colonial morphology and, 313
    Haemophilus spp. and, *432,* 432
  Clostridium spp. and, 598
  Columbia, 1122
  corn meal, 751-752, *752,* 1141-1142
  for *Corynebacterium diphtheriae,* 377
  cycloheximide-chloramphenicol, 1142
  cycloserine-cefoxitin-fructose, 1123
    Clostridium spp. and, 598-599, *599*
    gastrointestinal infection and, 964t
  cystine tryptophan, 1123
  deoxycholate citrate, 1124
  deoxyribonuclease test, 1124
  egg yolk, 1125
  egg-yolk, 597-598
  enteric, 964t
  for Enterobacteriaceae, 465, 497
  eosin-methylene blue, 1125
  esculin, 1125
  gastrointestinal infection and, 964t

Agar—cont'd
  hektoen enteric, 964t, 1126-1127
  Kligler iron, 1127-1128
    Enterobacteriaceae and, 496
    nonfermenting gram-negative rods and, 541, 541t, *542*
  lysine-iron, *505,* 505
  lysin-iron, 1129
  MacConkey; *see* MacConkey agar
  mannitol salt, 1130
  Middlebrook, 678-680, 679t, 702-704, 1131
  Mueller-Hinton, 75, 1132
    Vibrio and, 523-524
  for *Mycobacterium* culture, 678-679, 702
  mycosel/mycobiotic, 1142
  New York City, 408, 1132
  nutrient, 1133
  phenylalanine deaminase, 1134
  phenylethyl alcohol, 579t, 1134
  potato dextrose, 1142
  potato flakes, 1142
  precipitin test and, 133, *133, 134*
  pseudocel, 1134
  for *Pseudomonas aeruginosa,* 547
  rice extract, 1142
  sabouraud dextrose, 1142
  Salmonella-Shigella, 1134
  Simmons citrate, 1122
  SP-4, 1135
  for *Streptococcus pyogenes,* 361
  TCBS, 522, *522*
  Thayer-Martin, 1136
  thiosulfate-citrate-bile salts-sucrose, 522, *522,* 964t, 1137
  Tinsdale, 377, 1137-1138
  triple sugar iron, 1138
    Enterobacteriaceae and, 496, *496, 499*
    nonfermenting gram-negative rods and, 541, 541t, *542*
  trypticase soy, 1138
  urea, 1139
  ureaplasma, 1131
  vaginalis, 1139
  for *Vibrio,* 522, *522*
  xylose lysine and desoxycholate, 1139-1140
  xylose-lysine deoxycholate, 964t
  for yeast, 751-752
Agar dilution test, 72-73
Age
  bacteremia and, 1000
  respiratory infection and, 881, 900t
  urinary tract infection and, 1014-1015
Agglutination
  latex, 135-138, *136, 137,* 137t, 166
    Helicobacter pylori and, 535
    for respiratory infection, pharyngitis and, 887
  liposome-mediated, 139, *140,* 140t
  particle
    in antigen detection, 135-141
      latex, 135-138, *136, 137,* 137t
      liposome-mediated, 139, *140,* 140t
      staphylococcal coagglutination, *138, 138-139, 139*
    direct, natural, 165-166, *166*
    indirect, carrier, 166-167, *167*

Agrobacterium spp., 555-556
Agrobacterium rubri, 555
Agrobacterium tumefaciens, 555
AIDS; *see* Human immunodeficiency virus
Air, bacterial growth, 15
Air filter, high-efficiency, 37
Airborne transmission of infection, 230-231
Airway obstruction
    bronchitis and, 899
    infection-induced, 882
Ajellomyces dermatitidis, 737
Alaria americana, 959
Alcaligenes spp., 554-555
Alcohol, as disinfectant, 30, 31t
Alcoholic fermentation, 18
Aldehyde, as disinfectant, 30-31, 31t
Algorithm
    for choosing laboratory method, *126*
    for urine culture results, *1029*
Alkaline peptone water, 1118
Allergy, sinusitis and, 388
Alpha hemolysin, 316, 332
Alpha-hemolytic streptococci
    characteristics of, 348, *348*
    colonial morphology of, *322*
Alphavirus, 853
Alternaria, 742, *743*
Amastigote, 779, 780
    of *Leishmania,* 781
Ameba
    intestinal, 764-772
        Blastocystis hominis, 772, *772*
        comparison of, 768t
        Entamoeba coli, 768t, 770, *770, 771*
        Entamoeba dispar, 769
        Entamoeba hartmanni, 768t
        Entamoeba histolytica, 765-769, *766,* 768t, *769, 770*
        Entamoeba nana, 768t, 770, *771*
        general characteristics of, 765
        Iodamoeba butschlii, 770, 772, *772*
        life cycle of, 765, *766*
        treatment of, 765
    tissue, 772-774
Amebic granulomatous encephalitis, 990
Amebic meningoencephalitis, 989-990
Amebocyte lysis assay, 993-994
American Thoracic Society medium, 679t
American Type Culture Collection strain, 90
Amidase, 366
Amikacin, 92t, 93t
Aminoglycoside
    anaerobes resistant to, 60
    Enteroroccus resistant to, 83
    mechanism of action of, 57
Amniotic fluid
    culture media for, 252t
    microscopic appearance of, 294, 297
    microscopic specimen of, 286
    specimen of, 282
Amoxicillin, 628

Ampicillin
    beta-lactam antibiotics and, 55-56
    enterococci resistant to, 83
    Enterococcus and, 82-83
    Haemophilus influenzae resistant to, 434
    minimal inhibitory concentration of, 70t
    susceptibility of gram-negative organisms to, 92t, 93t
Amplicon, 199
Amplification
    gene
        Hepatitis C and, 864
        of virus, 839
    molecular, 198-199, *200-201,* 202-203
        commercially available, 204-206, *205,* 205t
        for *Mycobacterium tuberculosis,* 690-691
        nucleic acid based, 202
        strand displacement, 202
Anaerobic bacteria, 565-621
    antimicrobial agents for, 59
    beta-lactamase testing of, 620-621
    classification of, 567t
    cocci
        gram-negative, 615t, 617
        gram-positive, 611, 615t, 617, *617, 618*
    culture media for, 253t
    definition of, 567-568, 567t
    endogenous, 569, 569t, 570t
    exogenous, 569, 569t
    facultative, 15
        Corynebacterium diphtheriae as, 375
        in gastrointestinal tract, 571
        growth requirements of, 587
        Salmonella, 479-484
        Vibrio, 517-524
    gastrointestinal, 948, 948t
    as gastrointestinal flora, 215
    gram-negative bacilli, 606-611
        Bacteroides spp., 606, 607t, 608t, 609, 610
        bile-sensitive nonpigmented species of, 610, *610, 611*
        bile-sensitive pigmented species of, 609-610
        clinical infection with, 606
    gram-positive non–spore-forming bacilli, 599, 602-6006
        Actinomyces spp., 599, 602, *603,* 604
        bacterial vaginosis and, 599-602
        Bifidobacterium spp., 604-605, 604t-605t
        Eubacterium spp., 605
        Mobiluncus spp., 605
        Propionibacterium spp., *605,* 605-606
    gram-positive spore-forming bacilli, 594-599
        Clostridium spp.; *see also Clostridium* entries
    identification of
        definitive, 590-592, *592, 593,* 594
        preliminary procedures for, 583-584, *584, 585,* 585t, 586t, *588*
        presumptive, 587-590, *589*
    indications of infection with, 571, 573
    lack of enzymes in, 568
    origin of, 568-569
    oxygen toxicity and, 568
    predisposition to infection with, 571, 572t

Anaerobic bacteria—cont'd
    reclassified *Vibrio*-like, 610
    site-specific, 569-571, *570,* 570t
    specimen collection of, 571-583, 574t
        aspirates, 574
        blood, 575
        quality of specimen and, 572
        swabs, 574-575
        tissue, 575
        transport, 572-573
    specimen processing of, 575-583
        incubation of media for, 580-583, *581, 582*
        inoculation of media for, 577-578, 579t, 580, *580,* 580t
        macroscopic examination in, 576, 577t
        microscopic examination in, 576-577
        quality assurance in, 576t
    susceptibility testing of, 81, 618-620
    virulence factors of, 572t
Anaerobic bag, 583
Anaerobic carbohydrate fermentation media, 1121
    for gram-positive cocci, 1121
Anaerobic chamber, 578, *581,* 581-582
Anaerobic fermentation pathway, 18-19
Anaerobic jar, 582, *582*
Anaerobic metabolism, 18-19
Anaerobic pouch, 583, *583*
Anaerobiospirillum succiniciproducens, 608t
Anaerorhabdus furcosus, 608t
Analysis, test
    analytical, 121-122
    clinical, 122-123
    operational, 123-125
Analytical activity, 106
Analytical analysis of tests, 121-122
Anamnestic immune response, 161-162
Anatomy
    of central nervous system, *975,* 975-976
    of eye, 1084-1086, *1085*
    of gastrointestinal tract, *947,* 947-948
    of respiratory tract, 883, *883*
    urinary system, *1013,* 1013-1014
Ancylostoma braziliense, 822
    skin manifestations of, 941
Ancylostoma caninum, 941
Ancylostoma duodenale, 818
Angiostrongylus cantonensis, 959
Anicteric leptospirosis, 1074
Animal bite, 232
Anisakis spp., 959
Annealing, 198
Annellidoconidia, 713
Anorectal infection, 406
Antagonism in antimicrobial therapy, 54, 101
Anterior chamber
    anatomy of, 1086
    infection of, 1101-1102
Anthrax
    clinical manifestations of, 1066-1067
    complications of, 394
    cutaneous, 393

Anthrax—cont'd
    epidemiology of, 1066
    etiology of, 1066
    gastrointestinal, 393-394
    laboratory diagnosis of, 394, *1067,* 1067-1068
    pulmonary, 393
Antibiogram
    for gram-negative bacteria, 92-93, 92t, 93t
    technical errors in, 93t
Antibody; *see also* Antibody detection
    acute and convalescent titers of, 162
    antimicrobial action of, 222
    Borrelia burgdorferi and, 628
    Chlamydia pneumoniae and, 642
    Chlamydia trachomatis and, 648-649
    classification and characteristics of, 160-161
    cross-reactivity of, 162-163
    definition of, 131
    Entamoeba histolytica and, 769
    Epstein-Barr virus and, 869
    hepatitis, 862
    of immunoglobulin G class, *131*
    Lyme disease and, 1060
    monoclonal, antigen detection and, 131-133, *132*
    parasitic infection and, 763
    polyclonal, production of, 133
    polyclonal *vs.* monoclonal, 160
    specificity of, 162-163
    stain for, 266t
    syphilis tests and, 1041
    Toxoplasma gondii, 794
    Treponema pallidum and, 630-631
Antibody capture ELISA., IgM, 174, *175*
Antibody detection, 165-176
    complement fixation test for, 168-170, *169*
    enzyme-linked immunosorbent assay, 172-175, *173-175*
    microscope-assisted labeled-reagent techniques, *171,* 171-172
    neutralization tests for
        antistreptolysin-O, 170
        Treponema pallidum immobilization, 171
        viral, 170
    particle agglutination assays for
        direct, natural, 165-166, *166*
        indirect, carrier, 166-167, *167*
    precipitation assays for, 167-170
        counterimmunoelectrophoresis, 168
        double immunodiffusion, 167-168
        flocculation, 168, *169*
    serologic test *vs.,* 156
    Western blotting, 175-176, *176*
Antibody testing, heterophile, 166, *166,* 178
Anticachectin treatment, 1007
Anticoagulant for culture specimen, 242-243
Antidiarrheal agent, 967-968
Antifungal agent, 397-398
Antigen; *see also* Antigen detection
    Aeromonas and, 524
    of *Bacillus anthracis,* 393
    characteristics of, 159-160

Antigen—cont'd
  coagglutination with, *138,* 138
  Enterobacteriaceae and, 465
  hepatitis, 861, 862
  immune response and, 227
  influenza virus and, 843
  microbial, 131
  Mycobacterium tuberculosis and, 693
  Plesiomonas and, 528
  Salmonella and, 481
  Vibrio and, 517-518
  viral, gastrointestinal infection and, 150
Antigen detection, 127-153, 159
  for blood-borne and body fluid–borne disease, 150-151
  enzyme immunoassays in, 141-145, *142-144*
    fluorescent, 145
    membrane bound, 144-145
    radioimmunoassays, 145
  future applications of, 151
  for gastrointestinal infection, 149-150
  historical perspective on, 131-133, *132*
  immunofluorescence assays in, 139-141, *141*
  for *Legionella,* 453-454
  in meningitis and sepsis
    bacterial, 148-149
    cryptococcal, 149
  particle agglutination in, 135-141
    latex, 135-138, *136, 137,* 137t
    liposome-mediated, 139, *140,* 140t
    staphylococcal coagglutination, *138, 138-139, 139*
  precipitin tests for, 133-135, *133-135*
  for respiratory tract infection
    in immunocompromised patient, 147-148, *148*
    Legionnaires' disease and, 147
    pertussis and, 146
    streptococcal pharyngitis and, 145-146, *147*
    viral, 147, *148*
  for sexually transmitted disease, 150
Antigen testing, for hepatitis, 178-179
Antigenic drift in virus, 843
Antigenic structure
  of *Streptococcus agalactiae,* 361
  of *Streptococcus pneumoniae,* 364
  of *Streptococcus pyogenes,* 358, *359*
Antigenic variation in *Borrelia recurrentis,* 627
Anti-HBeAg, 862
Anti-HBsAg, 862
Anti-M protein, 227
Antimicrobial agent, 52-104
  bacteremia and, 1000, 1007-1008
  beta-lactam, *55,* 55-56, 55t
  Borrelia burgdorferi and, 628
  definition of, 53
  diarrhea and, 967-968
  empiric, for respiratory infection, 882-883
  for *Erysipelothix rhusiopathiae* infection, 385
  for eye infection, 1111-1112, 1111t
  furuncle and, 923
  gastrointestinal flora changes and, 215
  gonorrhea and, 1036

Antimicrobial agent—cont'd
  for immunocompromised patient, 1050
  for leptospires, 626
  for *Listeria monocytogenes* infection, 383
  Lyme disease and, 932
  mechanism of action of
    cell membrane and, 57
    metabolite inhibition and, 58-59
    protein synthesis and, 57-58
  microscopic sample and, 275
  natural, in body, 222
  Nocardia infection and, 397-398
  pseudomembranous colitis and, 596
  Pseudomonas aeruginosa and, 547-548
  resistance to, 59-60, 59t
  in serum and fluids, 103
  sites of action of, *53*
  for *Streptococcus pyogenes,* 361
  susceptibility testing of, 64-105; *see also* Susceptibility testing of antimicrobial
Antimicrobial disk, 588-589
Antimicrobial stock solution, 69-70
Antimicrobial-inactivating enzyme, detection of, *89,* 89-90
Antiseptic, 27
Antistreptolysin-O neutralization test, 170
Antituberculosis drug, 692t
Antiviral therapy, 871-872, 871t
Antler hyphae, 712, *712*
API 20C yeast identification system, 751
Apicomplexa, 783-799
  Babesia microti, 790-791
  intestinal infection with, 795-799
    Cryptosporidium parvum, 795-797, *796, 797*
    Cyclospora cayetanensis, 798-799, *799*
    Isospora belli, 797-798, *798*
  Plasmodium spp., 784-790; *see also Plasmodium entries*
  Pneumocystis carinii pneumonia, 794-795, *795*
  Toxoplasma gondii, 791-794, *792, 793*
Appendage, cell, 10
Aquarium, *Mycobacterium marinum* and, 699
Aqueous, culture media for, 252t
Arbovirus
  Bunyaviridae, 852-853
  general characteristics of, 851-852, 852t
  immunity to, 159
  laboratory diagnosis of, 855
  meningoencephalitis caused by, 987
Arcanobacterium spp., 381
Arcanobacterium haemolyticum, 386t
Archaeobacteria, 5
Arcobacter, 530, 530t, 531t, 534t
Arenaviridae, 836t, 855-856, 855t
Arenavirus, 855-856, 855t
Arthritis
  Haemophilus influenzae causing, 429
  Lyme disease and, 1060
  staphylococcal, 335
  Yersinia enterocolitica causing, 487
Arthroconidia, 713-714, *714*

Arthropod-borne infection
  arbovirus, 851-855
  Borrelia, 627-628
  types of, 232
Arylsulfatase, 686-687
Ascaris lumbricoides
  characteristics of, 816-818
  egg of, 814t, *818*
  eggs of, 762
  life cycle of, *817*
Ascitic fluid, 252t
Ascomycota, 714
Ascospore, 714
Aseptic meningitis, 977
  viral, 984-985, *985*
Asexual reproduction
  of Apicomplexa, 765
  of *Cryptosporidium parvum,* 796
  of fungi, *713, 713-714, 714*
  of *Plasmodium,* 786-787
Asian flu, 843
Aspergillus spp.
  brain abscess and, 981
  characteristics of, 743, *743*
  endophthalmitis and, 1102
  lacrimal apparatus and, 1100
  malignancy and, 1048
  meningitis and, 983
Aspirate
  abscess
    microscopic appearance of, 290
    microscopic specimen of, 285, 288
  anaerobic bacteria in, 574
  bone, 285
  culture media for, 252t
  duodenal, 761-762
  influenza virus and, 843
  maxillary sinus, 298
  Mycobacterium spp. and, 673
  sinus tract, 290
  smear preparation of, 248-249
  as specimen collection, 239
  suprapubic, culture of, 1028
  transport of, 245
  vitreous, microscopic specimen of, 283
Aspirated sputum
  microscopic appearance of, 299
  microscopic specimen of, 282, 284
Aspiration, suprapubic, 1023
Aspiration pneumonia, 897t, 905-906
Assay; *see also* Immunoassay
  biologic, 103
  enzyme-linked immunosorbent, Hepatitis C and, 864
  gene amplification, of virus, 839
  immunofluorescence, 139-141, *141*
  Limulus amebocyte lysis, 993-994
  solid-phase immunosorbent, 142, *142*
  time-kill, 100-102, *101, 102*
Astrovirus, 958
Athlete's foot, 725, 936

Attachment in phagocytosis, 223
Auramine stain, 677
Auramine-rhodamine fluorochrome stain, 677
Aureobasidium, 742
Autoclave, 29, 29t
Autolytic amidase, 366
Automated rapid detection method, 185, 188
Automated susceptibility testing
  for broth microdilution, 85
  instruments for, 85-87, *86, 87*
  principles of, 84-85
Automated test for urine screening, 1026-1027, 1027t
AutoSCAN Walkaway, 85-86, *86*
Autotroph, 14
Auxotype of *Neisseria gonorrhoeae,* 413
Avidin-biotin interaction, 144
Avidity in antigen detection, 131
Azithromycin, 58
Aztreonam
  penicillin-binding protein and, 55
  spectrum of, 56

B

B lymphocyte
  definition of, 158
  immune response and, 227
  immunity and, 158
Babès-Ernst granule, 377
Babesia sp., 762
Babesia microti, 790-791
  characteristics of, 790-791
  tetrad form of, *792*
  trophozoite of, *792*
Bacillary dysentery, 485
Bacillus; *see also* Bacillus entries
  acid-fast, staining for, 677-678
  aerobic gram-positive, 390-395, *391, 392,* 392t
  diphtheria, 375-380; *see also Corynebacterium diphtheriae*
  gram-negative
    Escherichia coli as, 468-473; *see also Escherichia coli*
    HACEK group of, 436-441
    nonfermenting, 539-561; *see also* Nonfermenting gram-negative bacilli
    respiratory infection and, 880
  non–spore-forming, 599, 602, *603,* 604
  rat-bite fever and, 1064
  shape of, 10-11, *11*
  tap-water, 702
  tubercle; *see Mycobacterium tuberculosis*
Bacillus spp., bacteremia and, 1000
Bacillus anthracis, 392-394
  clinical infection with, 393-394
  exotoxins of, 229t
  eyelid infection and, 1093
  interference with phagocytosis by, 225t
  laboratory diagnosis of, 394
  as laboratory hazard, 36
  physiology of, 392, 392t
  virulence factors of, 392-393

Bacillus cereus
    Bacillus anthracis vs., 392t
    characteristics of, 394-395, 395t
    endophthalmitis and, 1101
    enterotoxin-mediated diarrhea and, 951
    food poisoning and, 962t
Bacillus subtilis, 395
Bacitracin
    cell wall action and, 57
    Streptococcus susceptibility to, 352
Back safety, 48
Background material in microscopic specimen, 273-274, 273t
BacT/Alert system, 1006
Bactec 9000 series, 1004-1005, *1005*
Bactec medium, for *Mycobacterium* culture, 680
    DNA hybridization and, 691
Bactec-NAP test, 687
Bacteremia, 997-1009
    Bacillus spp. causing, 1000
    clinical manifestations of, 1001-1002
    cutaneous manifestations of, 926-927
    definition of, 998
    epidemiology of, 999-1000
    epiglottitis and, 894
    episodes of, 999
    forms of, 999
    laboratory diagnosis of, 1002-1007, *1005,* 1006t
    leptospiral, 626
    Mycobacterium causing, 674
    pathogens causing, 998t, 1000-1001
    Pseudomonas aeruginosa causing, 547
    Salmonella spp. causing, 483-484, 954-955
    septicemia *vs.,* 999
    Shigella causing, 486
    shock and, 999
    staphylococcal, 334
    Streptococcus pneumoniae causing, 365
    treatment of, 1007-1008
Bacteria, comparative properties of, 637t
Bacterial cell, 2-24
    anaerobic utilization of pyruvic acid in, 18-19
    biochemical pathways in, *17, 17-18, 18*
    carbohydrate utilization and, 19-20, *20*
    classification of, 4-7
    eukaryotic *vs.* prokaryotic, *6,* 6t, 7
        cell envelope structures of, 8-10, *8-10*
    fermentation and respiration in, 16-17
    genetics of, 20-23, *22*
    growth and nutrition of, 13-16, *15*
    metabolism of, 16
    morphology of, 10-13, *11-13*
    significance of, 4
Bacterial meningitis
    acute, 977-980, *978-980*
    antigen detection for, 149
    Bacillus anthracis causing, 394
    Haemophilus influenzae causing, 429
    Mycobacterium tuberculosis causing, 695
    Neisseria meningitidis causing, 415

Bacterial meningitis—cont'd
    pneumococcal, 365
    tuberculous, 674
Bacterial plaque, 213-214
Bacterial vaginosis, 1035, 1038-1039
    gram-positive non–spore-forming anaerobic bacilli
        causing, 599
Bactericidal agent, 53
Bactericidal concentration, minimum, 98-100, *99*
Bactericidal test, serum, 102-103, 103t
Bacteriocin, 222
Bacteriologic culture media, 1117-1140
Bacteriologic index, 704
Bacteriophage, 22
Bacteriostatic agent, 53
Bacteriuria, 1013, 1013t
Bacteroides spp.
    aspiration pneumonia and, 905
    beta-lactam antibiotics and, 55
    beta-lactamase tests and, 89
    bile-tolerant, 606, 607t, 609, *609*
    characteristics of, 614t
    clinical significance of, 607t
    examination of primary plates of, 583
    presumptive identification of, 612t
    urinary tract infection and, 1019
Bacteroides bile-esculin agar, 579t, 1118
Bacteroides distasonis, 571
Bacteroides eggerthii, 606, 609
Bacteroides fragilis
    antimicrobial resistance of, 618
    bacteremia and, 1000
    diarrhea caused by, 954t
    in gastrointestinal tract, 571
    identification of, 587
    infection with, 606
    laboratory diagnosis of, 606, 609
Bacteroides splanchnicus, 606, 609
Bacteroides thetaiotaomicron, 571
Bacteroides ureolyticus
    laboratory diagnosis of, 610
    presumptive identification of, 613t
Bacteroides vulgaris, 609
Bacteruria
    colony counts and, 1022
    culture for, 1027
Bacti-Card test, 186t
Bag
    anaerobic, 583
    biohazard, *40*
    for specimen transport, 245
Balantidium coli, 774-775, *775*
Balneatrix spp., 558
Bamboo rod appearance *of Bacillus anthracis,* 394
Bar, chromatoidal, 761
Barium, stool sample and, 241
Barrier to infection, 220-221, 221t
    nosocomial pneumonia and, 905
    ocular infection and, 1086-1087
    of respiratory tract, 883-884

Bartonella spp.
  sample handling of, 275
  skin infection due to, 275
Bartonella henselae, 206
Bartonellosis, 929
Basal body, 7
Basidiomycota, 714
Beading appearance of *Nocardia,* 398
Beauveria, 743, *743*
Benchmarking in performance improvement, 117-118
Benzalkonium chloride, 675
Beta hemolysin, 316-317, 332
  Listeria monocytogenes and, *384*
Beta-hemolytic *Streptococcus*
  biochemical identification of, 351t
  characteristics of, 348, *348*
  immunosuppressed patient and, 65
Beta-lactam antibiotic, *55, 55-56,* 56t
Beta-lactamase antimicrobial
  extended spectrum, 84
  resistance to, 60
  susceptibility testing and, 72
Beta-lactamase inhibitor, 56-57
Beta-lactamase test, *89,* 89-90
  of anaerobic bacteria, 620-621
Beta-lysin
  as antimicrobial substance, 222
  CAMP test and, 354-355
Bias in testing, 122
Bifidobacterium spp., 602t, 604-605, 604t-605t
Bile, culture media for, 252t
Bile disk, 589
Bile esculin test, 355-356, *356*
Bile solubility
  for rapid detection, 184t
  of *Streptococcus,* 352-353
  of *Streptococcus pneumoniae,* 366
Bile-esculin agar, 1118
Bile-sensitive pigmented gram-negative bacilli, 609-610
Bile-tolerant *Bacteroides* spp., 606, 607t, 609, *609, 614t*
Bilharziasis, 804-806
Biliary system, 483
Bilophila wadsworthia, 613t
Biochemical characteristics of nonfermenting gram-negative
    bacilli, 540, *540, 541,* 542
Biochemical identification
  of anaerobic bacteria, 590
  of *Mycobacterium* spp., 682, 685
  of Streptococcus, 349-356, 350t, 351t, *352, 354-356*
Biochemical pathways in bacterial cell, *17, 17-18, 18*
Biohazard bag, *40*
Biolog Microplate test, 186t
Biologic assay, 103
Biologic hazard, 37
  disposal of, 41
  handling of, 35-40, 36t, 37t, *38-40*
Biologic safety cabinet, 671
Biopsy
  culture media for, 252t
  microscopic appearance of, 291

Biopsy—cont'd
  opportunistic infection and, 915-916
  parasitic infection and, 763
Biotin-avidin interaction, 144
Biotinylated DNA probe, 194, 195
Biotype of *Corynebacterium diphtheriae,* 378
Biovariant of *Mycobacterium fortuitum,* 698
Biphasic broth-slide system, 1004
Biphasic medium for *Mycobacterium* spp., 680-681
Birdseed agar, 1141
Bismuth subsalicylate, 968
Bismuth sulfite agar, 1118
Bite, animal, infection from, 1056-1065; *see also* Zoonotic
    infection
Bite wound infection, 232
Black eschar, 393
Black piedra, 723
Blackwater fever, 786
Blastoconidium, *711,* 711-712
  in yeast identification, 751-752
Blastomyces spp., 909
Blastomyces dermatitidis, 735t, 736-737, *736-738,* 737t
  Accuprobes for, 195
  brain abscess and, 981-982
  epidemiology of, 735
Blastomycosis, 735-737
Blepharitis, 1093-1094
  plating guidelines for, 1106t
Blindness, river, 940
Blood
  bacteremia and, 998-1008; *see also* Bacteremia
  fungal specimen from, 717
  human immunodeficiency virus and, 849
  malignancy of, 1048
  as organic soil, 27-28
  in stool specimen, 758-759
Blood agar
  anaerobic, 1118-1119
  anaerobic bacteria and, 579t
  Bordet-Gengou, 1120
  campylobacter
    characteristics of, 1120-1121
    gastrointestinal infection and, 964t
  Clostridium spp. and, 598, *598*
  colonial morphology and, 313
  for *Corynebacterium diphtheriae,* 377, *377*
  gastrointestinal infection and, 964t
  Pseudomonas aeruginosa on, 547, *547*
  rabbit's, 1119
  sheep's, 1119
  for *Streptococcus pyogenes,* 361
  telluride, 1123
  types of, 1118-1119
Blood cell, *Plasmodium* in, 786-787
Blood culture
  anaerobic bacteria and, 575
  bacteremia and, 1003-1007, *1005,* 1006t
  microscopic appearance of, 289, 297
  for *Mycobacterium* spp., 674
  preparation for, 242t
  quality control of, *113*

Blood flagellate, *779, 779-783, 781-783*
Blood parasite
  Babesia spp. *as,* 790-791
  flukes, 804-806
  Plasmodium spp. as. 784-790; *see also Plasmodium entries*
  roundworm, 822-826
    filarial, 823, 826
    Mansonella spp., 826
    Trichinella spiralis, 822
    Wuchereria bancrofti, 823
Blood phenylethyl alcohol agar, 1119-1120
Blood protein, 157
Blood smear
  microscopic appearance of, 296
  parasitic infection and, 762
Blood-borne infection
  antigen detection in, 150-151
  candidal, 938
  hepatitis B as, 861-862
  Neisseria gonorrhoeae, 405-406
Blood-borne pathogen
  as laboratory hazard, 36
  OSHA regulations for, 39
Blotting, Western, 175-176, *176*
Blue stain
  lactophenol cotton, 12, *13*
  methylene, 12, *13*
Body fluid
  culture media for, 252t
  Mycobacterium spp. and, 674
  smear preparation of, 248-249
  specimen collection of, 242t
Body fluid-borne disease, 150-151
Boiling for sterilization, 29, 29t
Bone
  bacteremia and, 1001
  biopsy of, 291
  culture media for, 252t
  sinusitis complications and, 890
Bone aspirate, 285
Bone marrow
  culture media for, 252t
  fungal specimen from, 717
Borderline-resistant *Staphylococcus aureus,* 82
Bordetella spp., 457-462
  clinical infections of, 458
  epidemiology of, 457-458
  general characteristics of, 457
  laboratory diagnosis of, 458-461, 460t
  susceptibility testing, 461
  virulence factors of, 458
Bordetella bronchiseptica, 458
  characteristics of, 556
  susceptibility of, 461
Bordetella hinzii, 556
Bordetella holmesii, 556
Bordetella parapertussis, 458
  characteristics of, 556
  pertussis caused by. 895-896

Bordetella pertussis
  antigen detection for, 146
  characteristics of, 556
  culture media for, 253t
  exotoxins of, 229t
  pertussis caused by, 895-896
  toxin of, 884
Bordetella trematum, 556
Bordet-Gangou potato infusion agar, 459
Bordet-Gengou blood agar, 1120
Borrelia burgdorferi, 626-627
  amplification systems for, 206
  Borrelia causing, 628
  central nervous system and, 982
  central nervous system infection and, 982
  electron micrograph of, *1059*
  indirect fluorescent antibody test for, 172
  life cycle of, 1059
  Lyme disease caused by, 932, 1058-1060
Borrelia correlia burgdorferi, 164
Borrelia recurrentis, 627, *627,* 932
Botulism, 595-596
Boutonneuse fever, 1076
Bradyzoite of *Toxoplasma gondii,* 792, *792*
Brain abscess, *981*0, 981-982
  microscopic appearance of, 303
Brain anatomy, *975,* 975-976
Brain-heart infusion agar, 1141
Brain-heart infusion broth, 1120
Branhamella; see Moraxella entries
Breakbone fever, 853
Breakpoint panel in susceptibility test, 71-72
Breast, furuncle of, 923, *923*
Brevundimonas diminuta (Pseudomonas diminuta), 553
Bronchiolitis, 896-900, 897t
Bronchitis, 896-900, 897t
  clinical manifestations of, 896-898
  complications of, 898
  epidemiology of, 896
  etiology of, 896
  laboratory diagnosis of, 899
  pathogenesis of, 898
Bronchoalveolar lavage, 293
  microscopic appearance of, 294, 300, 301, 304, 305, 308, 309
    microscopic specimen of, 285
    Mycobacterium culture from, 673
    opportunistic infection and, 915-916
Broth
  anaerobic, 579t
  Bactec, 680
  bacteremia culture and, 1004
  brain-heart infusion, 1120
  campylobacter thioglycolate, 1121
  enrichment, 251
  gram-negative, 1126
  nitrate reduction, 1132
  peptone-yeast extract-glucose, 1133
  Sabouraud dextrose, 1142
  selenite F, 1135

Broth—cont'd
    sodium chloride, 1135
    SP-4, 1135-1136
    tetrathionate, 1136
    thioglycolate, 1136-1137
    trypticase soy, 1138
    tryptophan, 1138
    urea, 1139
Broth microdilution susceptibility test
    advantages and disadvantages of, 94
    automated reader devices for, 85
    characteristics of, *70,* 70-71
Brucella
    culture media for, 253t
    as laboratory hazard, 35-36
Brucella spp., 443-444, 444t, 1070-1072, *1072,* 1072t
    bacteremia and, 1006
    phagocytosis and, 224
Brucella abortus, 225t
Brucella/blood agar, 598, *598*
Brucellosis, 1070-1072, *1072,* 1072t
Bubo of plague, 1057
Buccal space abscess, 298
Buckle, scleral, 1103-1104, *1104*
Budivicia aquatica, 488
Buffered charcoal-yeast extract, 452, 1120
Bug, triatomid, 783
Bullous impetigo, 333
Bull's-eye colony, 319
Bunches of grapes colony, 330
Bunsen burner, 47
Bunyaviridae, 836t, 852-853
Burkholderia cepacia (Pseudomonas cepacia), 551-552
Burkholderia gladioli (Pseudomonas gladioli), 552
Burkholderia pseudomallei (Pseudomonas pseudomallei),
    552-553, *553*
Burkitt's lymphoma, 868
Burn
    infection with, 1049-1050
    laboratory safety and, 47-48
    prevention of, 47-48
    sample collection and, 241
    specimen collection of, 242t
Burner, bunsen, 47
Buruli ulcer, 930
Butanediol fermentation, 19
Buttery looking colony, 330
Buttiauxella agrestis, 488
Butyric acid fermentation, 19
Butyrivibrio spp., 608t

C

C carbohydrate, 349
Cabinet, biologic safety, 671
Calciviridae, 836t
Calcofluor white stain, 13, *13,* 266t, 1143
    for fungi, 718
    procedure for, 270
Calibration
    of ocular micrometer, 764
    of thermometer, 108

Calicivirus, 150, 958
California disease, 740-741
CAMP test, 354-355, *355*
    of *Listeria monocytogenes, 384*
    for *Streptococcus agalactiae,* 362
CAMPY medium, 532-533
Campylobacter spp., 529-535, 530t, 531t, 532t, 534t
    antigen detection for, 150
    antimicrobials effective against, 59
    culture of, 965
    diarrhea and, 961
    epidemiology of, 530
    invasive diarrhea syndrome and, 951
    motility testing of, 589-590
    reclassified, 610
    toxic megacolon and, 960
Campylobacter blood agar
    characteristics of, 1120-1121
    gastrointestinal infection and, 964t
Campylobacter concisus, 608t
Campylobacter jejuni, 953-954
Campylobacter ramosum, 618
Campylobacter thioglycolate broth, 1121
Canaliculitis, 1100
Cancer
    Epstein-Barr virus and, 868
    opportunistic infection in, 1047-1049
Candida spp.
    cellular immunity defect and, 915
    characteristics of, 748
    conjunctival infection and, 1092
    differentiation of, 749t
    folliculitis and, 923
    humoral immunity defect and, 915
    malignancy and, 1048
    meningitis and, 984
    temperature and, 753
    urinary tract infection and, 1020
Candida albicans
    Accuprobes for, 195
    characteristics of, 748
    endophthalmitis and, 1102
    gem tube test for, 750
    necrotizing enterocolitis and, 215
    skin manifestations of, 938
    urease test and, 752
Candida dubiniensis, 750
Candida glabrata, 748
Candida immitis, 983
Candida lusitaniae, 748
Candida parapsilosis, 748
    orbital infection and, 1099
Candida stellatoidea, 750
Candida tropicalis, 748
Capillaria philippinensis, 959
Capnocytophaga spp., 437t, *440, 440-441*
    gonococcal medium and, 408
    lacrimal apparatus and, 1100
    orbital infection and, 1099
Capnocytophaga canimorsus, 559-560, 1063-1064

Capnocytophaga cynodegmi, 559-560
Capnophilic bacteria, 15, 587
Capreomycin, 692t
Capsid, viral, 834
Capsid protein, 872
Capsular antigen
　Enterobacteriaceae and, 465
　Escherichia coli and, 472
Capsule
　of anaerobic bacteria, 572t
　antigens and, 160-161
　of *Bacillus anthracis,* 392
　characteristics of, 10
　of *Haemophilus influenzae,* 428-429
　of *Klebsiella pneumoniae,* 473
　of *Streptococcus agalactiae,* 361
Carbapenem
　listing of, 55
　structure of, 55
Carbohydrate, 19-20, *20*
Carbohydrate assimilation base, 1143
Carbohydrate assimilation for yeast infection, 751
Carbohydrate fermentation media
　anaerobic, 1121
　Enterobacteriaceae and, 500
　for gram-negative bacilli, 1121
Carbohydrate utilization method
　for *Neisseria gonorrhoeae,* 410, 412
　rapid detection, 185, 188-189
Carbon dioxide
　anaerobic bacteria and, 567
　bacterial growth, 15
　dysgonic fermenters and, 559-560
Carbon dioxide incubator, 408
Carboxypenicillin, 56
Carbuncle, 333, 923
Cardiac infection, endocarditis
　Erysipelothix rhusiopathiae causing, 385
　skin manifestations of, 928, *928*
　Streptococcus pneumoniae causing, 365
Cardiobacterium hominis, 437t, *438,* 438-439
Carrier
　definition of, 212, 233
　of *Salmonella,* 484, 955
Carrier particle agglutination assay, 166-167, *167*
Casein medium, 1141
Cat
　hookworm of, 941
　tapeworm of, 813
　Toxoplasma gondii infection from, 792-793
Catalase
　for *Mycobacterium* spp. and, 686, *686*
　Mycobacterium tuberculosis and, 695
　for rapid detection, 184t
Catalase test for anaerobic bacteria, 589
Catalyst in anaerobic chamber, 581-582
Catarrhal phase of whooping cough, 458
Catheter
　Corynebacterium jeikeium infection and, 380
　sample collection from tip of, 242t

Catheter tip
　culturing of, 257
　sample from, 242t
Catheterized urine specimen, 1022-1023, 1028
Cave disease, 737-739
CD4+ cell, human immunodeficiency virus infection and, 849
CDC group1, 551
CDC group IVc-2, 556
CDC group IVe, 556
CDC Ve-1, 558
CDC Ve-2, 558
Cedecea spp., 488
Cefinase beta-lactamase test, 89, *89*
Cefotaxime, 92t, 93t
Cefoxitin, 92t, 93t
Ceftazidime, 92t
Cell
　bacterial cell agglutination, 166
　ciliated, 889
　human immunodeficiency virus and, 849
　Microspora reproduction in, 799
　phagocytic, 157
　phagocytosis and, 222-223, *223-225*
Cell culture for viral isolation, 834, 840
Cell envelope
　of eukaryotic cell, 7
　of prokaryotic cell, 8-10, *8-10*
　structure of, 8-10, *8-10*
Cell membrane, 57
Cell wall
　antimicrobial agents affecting, 54-57, *55,* 56t
　of eukaryotic cell, 7
　of prokaryotic cell, 8-10, *9*
　of *Streptococcus,* 347, *348*
Cell-mediated immunity, 158
Cellophane tape preparation
　for fungi, 721
　parasitic infection and, 761
Cellular fatty acid analysis, 592
Cellular immunity defect, 914-915
　malignancy and, 1047
Cellulitis, 923-924
　brain abscess and, 981
　Haemophilus influenzae causing, 429
　microscopic specimen of, 286
　orbital, 890, 1098-1099, *1099*
　sinusitis and, 1099
　Streptococcus pyogenes causing, 360
Cell-wall deficient, 653, 655
Centers for Disease Control and Prevention
　laboratory training and, 682
　PPNG strains of *Neisseria gonorrhoeae* and, 414
　reporting of infection and, 234
　undesignated coryneform groups and, 381-382
Centipeda periodontii, 608t
Central nervous system infection, 973-995
　anatomy and, *975,* 975-976
　brain abscess, *981,* 981-982
　cerebrospinal fluid and, 976
　encephalitis; *see* Encephalitis

Central nervous system infection—cont'd
  fungal
    brain abscess, 981-982
    meningitis, 982-984, *984*
  general concepts of, 974-977
  host-pathogen relationship and, 976-977
  lumbar puncture and, 990-991
  meningitis; *see* Meningitis
  mycobacterial, 980-981
  spirochetal, 982
  Toxoplasma gondii, 792
  viral, 849-850
    tests for, 838t
Centrifugation of *Mycobacterium* spp., 677
Centrifugation-enhanced shell vial culture, 842
Centrifuged sediment smear, 249
Cephalosporin
  generations of, 56
  listing of, 55
  structure of, 55
  susceptibility testing and, 67
Cephalosporin test, chromogenic, 435
Cephalothin, 92t, 93t
Cercaria, of fluke, 800
Cerebral abscess, *981,* 981-982
Cerebrospinal fluid
  brain abscess and, 981
  characteristics of, 976
  cryptococcosis and, 180
  culture media for, 252t
  culture of, tuberculous meningitis and, 674
  flow pattern of, *975*
  lumbar puncture and, 990-991
  meningitis and
    fungal, 984
    viral, 984-986, *986*
  microscopic specimen of, 283, 294
  parasitic infection and, 763, 990
Cervical lymphadenitis, 699-700
Cervical specimen, 124-125
Cervicitis, 1013t, 1020
Cervicofacial actinomycosis, 930
Cervix
  microscopic appearance of, 298
  specimen collection of, 242t
Cestode, 806-813; *see also* Tapeworm
Cetrimide agar, 1134
Chaetomium spp., 743, 743-744
Chagas disease, 783
Chamber
  anaerobic, 578, *581,* 581-582
  slide culture, for fungi, 721
Chancre, syphilitic, 932
Chancroid, 1041-1042
  Haemophilus ducreyi causing, *431*
Chancroid, *Haemophilus ducreyi* causing, 430
Charcoal-yeast extract agar, buffered, 1120
Chemical, hazardous
  inventory of, 46
  safe handling of, 41, *42-46*

Chemical barrier to infection, 157
Chemical fume hood, *39*
Chemical intoxication in food poisoning, 961
Chemical methods
  of sterilization and disinfection, 26, 30-32, 31t
  of urine screening, 1026
Chemolithotroph, 14
Chemosterilizer, 30
Chemotaxis
  innate immunity and, 157
  process of, 223, *223*
Chicago disease, 735-737
Chickenpox, 933
  blepharitis and, 1094
  serologic testing for, 179-180
Child
  Haemophilus influenzae infection in, 429
  hand, foot, and mouth disease in, 846-847
  otitis media in, 891-892
  respiratory infection in, 900t
    respiratory syncytial virus causing, 841, 841t, 844
  rubella in, 846
  sinusitis in, 888
  urinary tract infection in, 1014
Chilomastix mesnili, 776t, 778-779, *779*
Chinese liver fluke, 803, *803*
Chitin, in fungal cell wall, 7
Chlamydia spp.
  comparative properties of, 637t
  diarrhea and, 961
  differentiation of, 637t
  general characteristics of, 636-638
  growth cycle of, *638*
  life cycle of, *638*
Chlamydia pneumoniae, 639-642
  amplification systems for, 206
  clinical infections caused by, 639-640, 640t
  differentiation of, 637t
  laboratory diagnosis of, 640-642, *641, 641t,* 642t
Chlamydia psittaci, 649-650
  differentiation of, 637t
Chlamydia trachomatis, 642-649
  amplification systems for, 204
  antigen detection for, 150
  clinical infection cause by, 642-644, *643,* 644t
  conjunctival infection and, 1090-1091, *1091*
  detection of, 645t, 1038t
  differentiation of, 637t
  enzyme immunoassay kits for, 143
  genital infection with, 1037
  lacrimal apparatus and, 1100
  predictive value of test for, 124-125
  respiratory infection caused by, otitis media, 891
  as sexually transmitted disease, 643, *643*
  testing for, 125, 125t
  urinary tract infection and, 1016, 1021
Chlamydiosis, 1034, 1037; *see also Chlamydia trachomatis*
Chloramphenicol
  for *Haemophilus influenzae,* 434
  mechanism of action of, 58

Chlorine as disinfectant, 31-32, 31t
Chocolate agar, 1122
   colonial morphology and, 313
   Haemophilus spp. and, *432,* 432
Cholera, 516, 955-956
Cholera toxin, 519, *520*
Choriomeningitis virus, lymphocytic, 855, 986
Chromatin
   peripheral, 767
   Plasmodium and, 787
Chromatographic assay, 104
Chromatography
   for anaerobic bacteria, 591-592, 594
   for *Mycobacterium* spp., 670, 689-690
Chromobacterium violaceum, 560-561
Chromoblastomycosis, 939, 939t
   characteristics of, 731
   epidemiology of, 730-731
   organisms causing, 729
Chromogenic cephalosporin test, 435
Chromogenic substrate test, 410
Chromogenic substrates in rapid detection methods, 185, 188-189
Chromomycosis, 939, 939t
Chromosomally mediated resistant *Neisseria gonorrhoeae,* 80-81
Chromosome, bacterial, 21
Chromotoidal bar, 761
Chromotrope stain of Microspora, 800, *800*
Chryseobacterium meningosepticum, 557
Chryseomonas spp., 558
Chrysosporium, 744, *744*
   characteristics of, 744, *744*
CIE; *see* Counterimmunoelectrophoresis
Ciguatera, 961, 963
Cilia
   as cleansing mechanism, 221
   of eukaryotic cell, 7
Ciliated epithelium, 889
Ciliated protozoa, 774-775
Ciprofloxacin
   for *Haemophilus influenzae,* 434
   susceptibility of gram-negative organisms to, 92t
Citrate agar, Simmons, 1122
Citrate utilization test, 500, *502*
Citrobacter spp., 478-479
   classification of, 466t
   infection causes by, 467t
Citrobacter amalonaticus, 479
Citrobacter freundii, 478-479
   diarrhea caused by, 954t
Citrobacter koseri, 479
Citrobacticeae, classification of, 466t
Cladophialophora carrionii, 731, *731, 732t*
Cladosporium, 744, *744*
Cladosporium spp., 715
Cladosporium carrionii, 939, 939t
Clarithromycin, 58
Cleaning, wound, 239
Cleansing mechanism, 221-222

Clearance of respiratory secretions, 881-882
Clindamycin, 58
Clinical analysis of tests, 122-123
Clinical Laboratory Improvement Act, 114
Clostridial myonecrosis, 924-925
Clostridial toxin, 572t
Clostridium spp.
   bacteremia and, 1000
   beta-lactam antibiotics and, 55
   characteristics of, 601t
   clinical infection with, 594-599, 596t
   culture of, 966
   examination of primary plates of, 583
   fermentation by, 19
   identification of, *600*
   laboratory confirmation of, 597t
   microscopic examination of, 577
   urinary tract infection and, 1019
Clostridium bifermentans, 595
Clostridium botulinum, 595-596
   culture media for, 253t
   exotoxins of, 229t
   food poisoning and, 962t
   toxin of, 232
Clostridium difficile
   antigen detection for, 149
   colitis and, 596
   culture of, 583
   diarrhea and, 950
   enzyme immunoassay kits for, 143
   fluorescence of, 588
   gastrointestinal infection caused by, 957
   necrotizing enterocolitis and, 215
   rapid detection methods for, 183
   toxic megacolon and, 960
Clostridium haemolyticum, 568
Clostridium histolyticum, 595
Clostridium novyi, 568
Clostridium oedematiens, 229t
Clostridium perfringens
   dissemination of, 228
   enterotoxin-mediated diarrhea and, 951
   exotoxins of, 229t
   food poisoning and, 596, 962t
   myonecrosis and, 595
Clostridium septicum
   exotoxins of, 229t
   identification of, 587
   myonecrosis and, 595
Clostridium sordellii, 229t
Clostridium tetanus, 595
   exotoxins of, 229t
Clothing, protective, 672
Clumping factor in *Staphylococcus,* 337, *337*
Coagglutination
   with bacterial cell antigen, *138,* 138
   pharyngitis and, 887
   staphylococcal, 138-139, *139, 140*
Coagulase, 331, 337

Coagulase-negative staphylococci, 331, 331t, *338*
  central nervous system infection caused by, 335
  rapid identification of, 340-341
  susceptibility testing and, 64
  urinary tract infection and, 1019t
Coagulase-positive staphylococci, 338t
Coagulation
  disseminated intravascular, 1002
  endotoxin causing, 228
Coat, laboratory, *38*
Coccidioides spp.
  chronic pneumonia and, 909
  as laboratory hazard, 36
Coccidioides immitis, 740, 740-741, 741
  Accuprobes for, 195
  clinical infection with, 736t, 740
  conjunctival infection and, 1092
  epidemiology of, 740
  laboratory diagnosis of, *740, 740-741, 741*
  meningitis and, 984
  morphology of, 735t
Coccobacilli
  Brucella, 443-444
  Mycobacterium simiae, 702
  Pasteurella, 441, *441, 442t, 443, 443*
Coccus
  anaerobic
    clinical infection with, 611
    gram-negative, 615t, 617
    gram-positive, 611, 615t, 617, *617, 618*
  shape of, 10-11, *11*
  urinary tract infection and, 1018-1019
Code
  genetic, 21
  numeric, 185
Codon, 21
Coenzyme, clostridial, 572t
Coinfection, hepatitis D and, *863*
Cold, common, 845
Cold shock, 999
Cold-agglutinating antibody, 166
Colitis
  Escherichia coli causing, 470-471
  pseudomembranous, 596
Collection, specimen, 237-259; *see also* Specimen collection
    and handling
College of American Pathologists, 116, 681
Colon, anaerobic bacteria in, 570t
Colonial morphology, 311-325
  of *Campylobacter,* 533
  gross characteristics in, 316-320
    color, 319, *319*
    consistency, 319
    density, 319
    elevation and, 317, *318,* 319
    form or margin and, 317, *318*
    hemolysis and, *316, 316-317, 317*
    odor, 319-320
    pigment, 319, *320*
    size and, 317, *318*

Colonial morphology—cont'd
  importance of, 313
  initial observations in, 313, *314-316,* 316
  liquid media and, 321, *322-324,* 324
  multiple characteristics and, *320,* 321
  of *Neisseria* spp., 419t
  of *Neisseria gonorrhoeae,* 408
Colonization
  of respiratory specimens, 880
  sinusitis and, 889
Colony
  of *Mycobacterium fortuitum,* 698
  urinary tract infection and, 1021
  yeast, 748
Colony morphology
  of anaerobic bacteria, 584, 586
  of *Haemophilus influenzae,* 431-432
  of *Mycobacterium* spp. and, 682
Colony-forming units, 65
Color
  in colonial morphology, 319, *319*
  quality control and, 109
Color guide for REMEL/IDS RapID STR, 187t
Colorado tick fever, 854-855, 987
Columbia agar, 1122
Comamonas spp, 554
Commensal, definition of, 212
Common cold, 845
Community trends in respiratory infection, 882
Community-acquired pneumonia, *901, 901-903, 902*
  bronchitis and, 899
Competency, personnel, 112, 114, *115*
Competent bacteria, definition of, 22
Complement
  acquired immunity and, 157-158
  in attachment, 223
Complement fixation test, 168-170, *169*
  for *Chlamydia pneumoniae,* 641
Computed tomography in sinusitis, 888, *889*
Concentration
  of disinfecting agent, 27
  minimal inhibitory, 69, 70t
  minimum bactericidal, 98-100, *99*
  of stool specimen, 760
  of tubercle bacilli, 676
Confirmation, 126
Congenital infection
  cytomegalovirus, 868
  serologic testing for, 164-165
  syphilis, 630
  Toxoplasma gondii, 791-792
Conidia, 713
Conjugation, 22, *22*
Conjunctiva
  anatomy of, 1084-1085
  infection of, *1089-1091,* 1089-1093
Conjunctivitis, plating guidelines for, 1106t
Container
  biohazard, *40*
  for mailing of etiologic agent, *244,* 244-245

Contamination
  Acinetobacter, 550
  of culture, 65
    for bacteremia, 1007
  Flavobacterium, 557
  in microscopic specimen, 274, 276, *282-283*
  in molecular probe, 204
  Pseudomonas fluorescens, 549
  Ralstonia pickettii, 553
  Sphingomonas paucimobilis, 553
  Stenotrophomonas maltophilia, 549
Continuing education, 114
Continuous bacteremia, 999
Continuous cell culture, 840
Convalescent antibody titer, 162
Convalescent phase of whooping cough, 458
Conventional tubed biochemical identification system for
    anaerobic bacteria, 590
Conventional-chromogenic enzyme test for *Neisseria
    gonorrhoeae,* 410, 411t
Convex elevation of colony, 317, *318*
Cooked meat medium, 1123
Coprococcus spp., 615t
Corn meal agar, 751-752, *752,* 1141-1142
Cornea
  amebic keratitis of, 774
  anatomy of, 1085-1086
  fungal infection of, 1097
  infection of, 1094-1098, *1095-1098*
  microscopic appearance of, 304
  parasitic infection of, 1097-1098
Coronavirus, 836t
  gastrointestinal infection and, 150
  respiratory infection from, 845
Corrosive, 46
Corynebacterium spp., 373-399
  bacteremia and, 1000, 1002
  erythrasma due to, 925
  general characteristics of, 375
  identification of, 379t
  of *Listeria monocytogenes vs.,* 384t
Corynebacterium diphtheriae, 375-380
  carrier of, 233
  clinical infections with, 376
  cultural characteristics of, *377,* 377-378
  culture media for, 253t
  dissemination of, 228
  exotoxins of, 228, 229t
  identification of, 378, *378,* 379t
  microscopic examination of, 376-377, *377*
  ocular infection and, 1086
  pharyngitis caused by, 885
  physiology of, 375
  toxigenicity of, 378, 380, *380*
  toxin of, 884
  transductionn in, 22
  virulence factors for, 375-376
Corynebacterium jeikeium, 379t, 380
Corynebacterium kutscheri, 379t, 381
Corynebacterium pseudodiphtheriticum, 379t, 381

Corynebacterium pseudotuberculosis, 381
  identification of, 379t
  toxin of, 375
Corynebacterium striatum, 379t, 381
Corynebacterium ulcerans, 380
  identification of, 379t
  toxin of, 375
Corynebacterium urealyticum, 379t, 380
Corynebacterium xerosis, 381
Cough
  as barriers to infection, 884
  whooping, 458, 894-895
    antigen detection in, 146
Counterimmunoelectrophoresis, 133-135, *135,* 168
Counter-streak technique, inoculum, 254-255, *255*
Counting of cells, 15-16
Coxiella burneti, 1078
Coxsackievirus
  central nervous system and, 850
  hand, foot, and mouth disease and, 846
  skin manifestations of, 936
Creeping eruption, 822-823, 941
Crimean-Congo hemorrhagic fever, 852-853
Critical material, 28, 29t
Cross-functional team, 117
Cross-reactivity of antibody, 162-163
Cross-walls, in yeast identification, 752
Cryptococcal infection, antigen detection for, 149
Cryptococcus spp.
  cellular immunity defects and, 914
  characteristics of, 749, 749t
  colony characteristics of, 748
  laboratory diagnosis of, 993
  urease test and, 752
  urinary tract infection and, 1020
Cryptococcus neoformans
  Accuprobes for, 195
  antigen detection for, 149
  conjunctival infection and, 1092
  Hodgkin's lymphoma and, 1049
  in immunocompromised patient, antibody detection for,
      147-148
  India ink preparation for, 718, *718*
  interference with phagocytosis by, 225t
  malignancy and, 1048
  meningitis and, 983, *983,* 984
  serologic testing for, 180
  temperature and, 753
CRYPTO-LEX, 180
Cryptosporidium spp.
  direct fluorescent antibody test of, *141*
  enterotoxin-mediated diarrhea and, 951
  enzyme immunoassay kits for, 143
  flotation procedures for, 760
  fluorescent antibody test for, 763
  food poisoning and, 961
Cryptosporidium parvum, 795-797, *796, 797*
  acid-fast stain for, 761
  antigen detection for, 150
  gastrointestinal infection caused by, 959

Crystal E/NF test, 186t
CTA carbohydrate test, for *Neisseria gonorrhoeae* identification, 412
Culture
  Aeromonas, 525-526
  anaerobic, 583-584, 586
  Bacillus anthracis, 394
  Bacillus cereus, 395t
  bacteremia and, 1003-1007, *1005*, 1006t
  blood; *see* Blood culture
  Bordetella, 459-460
  Borrelia spp., 626, *626*
  Campylobacter, 532
  of *Capnocytophaga canimorsus*, 1063
  Chlamydia trachomatis, 646, *647*
  Chlamydia trachomatis infection and, 1037-1038
  contamination of, 65
  Enterobacteriaceae, 490-491
  Epstein-Barr virus, 868
  Erysipelothix rhusiopathiae, 385-386
  Escherichia coli, 471
  eye infection and, 1107-1111, *1108-1110*
  fresh, 239-240
  fungal
    blastomycosis and, 736-737
    chromoblastomycosis and, 731
    dermatophytic, 728
    general principles of, 718-719, *720,* 721
    histoplasmosis, *739,* 739-740
    subcutaneous phaeohyphomycosis, 734
  of gastrointestinal infection, 963, 964t, 965
  as hazard, 35-36
  identification guidelines for, 276, 277
  Legionella, 449, *451, 452-454, 453*
  leptospires, 626
  Listeria monocytogenes, 383-384
  medium for; *see* Medium
  Mycobacterium spp., 671-672, 678-681, 679t, *681*
  Neisseria gonorrhoeae, 407, 407t
  Neisseria meningitidis, 416-417, *417*
  Nocardia, 398, 398t
  patient or site preparation for, 242t
  Plesiomonas, 529
  probes for confirmation of, 194-195
  refrigeration of, 243
  repeat, 240
  for respiratory infection
    bronchitis, 900
    drug therapy and, 882
    epiglottitis, 894
    pertussis, 895
    pharyngitis and, 887
    pneumonia, 907-908, 911
    sinusitis and, 890
  of skin infection, 931
  Spirillum minus, 1065, *1065*
  Staphylococcus, 336, *336*
  stock, 114
  stool; *see* Stool culture
  storage of, 243-244

Culture—cont'd
  Streptococcus pneumoniae, 366
  urine, 1023-1024
  Vibrio, 522
  viral, 834, 840-842, 841t, *842*
    herpes simplex virus, 867
    human herpesvirus 7, 870
  of zoonotic infection
    Bacillus anthracis, 1067
    Erysipelothrix rhusiopathiae and, 1062-1063
  zoonotic infection and
    brucellosis, 1071
    leptospirosis, 1074
    Pasteurella multocida and, 1061-1062
    tularemia, 1069
    Yersinia pestis, 1057
Culture media, bacteriologic, 1117-1140
Cumulative antibiogram statistics, 92-93
Cunninghamella, 744, *744*
  characteristics of, 744, *744*
Curschmann's spiral, 274
Curve, growth, for bacteria, 15, *15*
Curvularia spp., *744,* 744-745
  endophthalmitis and, 1102
Customer concept in performance improvement, 117
Cut, infection and, 232
Cutaneous infection; *see also* Skin infection
  anthrax, 393
  mycotic, 715, 724-729
  Nocardia, 397, 397-398
Cutaneous larva migrans, 822
Cutaneous sinus tract aspirate, 290
Cyanogen bromide, 685
Cycloheximide-chloramphenicol agar, 1142
Cycloserine
  cell wall action and, 57
  tuberculosis and, 692t
Cycloserine-cefoxitin-fructose agar, 1123
  Clostridium spp. and, 598-599, *599*
  gastrointestinal infection and, 964t
Cyclospora cayetanensis, 960-961
  acid-fast stain for, 761
  clinical infection with, 798
  laboratory diagnosis of, 798-799, *799*
  life cycle of, 798
Cyst
  of *Acanthamoeba*, 774
  of *Entamoeba histolytica*, 767-768
  of *Giardia lamblia*, 777, *778*
  hydatid, 813
  of *Naegleria fowleri*, 772-774, *773*
  of *Toxoplasma gondii*, 793-794
L-Cysteine for *Legionella* culture, 452
Cystic fibrosis, *Mycoplasma pneumoniae*, 663
Cysticercosis, 811, 813
Cysticercus, 806
Cysticercus cellulosae, 990
Cystine tryptophan agar, 1123
Cytocentrifuge technique, *265,* 265-266
Cytocentrifuged smear, 249, *249*

Cytolytic toxin of *Staphylococcus aureus,* 332
Cytomegalovirus, 868
    amplification systems for, 206
    cell cultures for, 841t
    characteristics of, 868
    cytopathic effect of, 841, *842*
    false-positive test results for, 163-164
    immune status testing to, 164
    in immunocompromised patient, 147-148
    meningitis and, 986
    retinal, 1103
    serologic testing for, 179
    skin manifestations of, 934
Cytopathic effect, 170, 839
    in viral identification, 840-841
Cytoplasmic structure of eukaryotic cell, 7
Cytotoxin
    of *Escherichia coli,* 471
    gastrointestinal infection and, 232
    tracheal, 458

D
Dacryoadenitis, 1100
Darkfield microscopy, 184t
Darling's disease, 737-739
Darting motility of *Campylobacter,* 533
Data sheet, material safety, 41, *42-45*
Deaminase, phenylalanine, 500
Death
    Corynebacterium diphtheriae causing, 376
    Legionnaires' disease causing, 448
    Neisseria meningitidis causing, 415
Debris in microscopic specimen, 274
Decarboxylase test medium, 1124
    Enterobacteriaceae and, 500
Decontamination agent for *Mycobacterium* specimen, 674-676
Decubitus ulcer
    bacteremia and, 1000
    microscopic appearance of, 295
Defense mechanism
    antimicrobial substances as, 222
    burn and, 1049-1050
    cleansing, 221-222
    immune response as, 226-227; *see also* Immune response;
        Immune system; Immunity
    normal flora as, 222
    phagocytosis as, 222-224, *223-225,* 226
    physical barriers as, 220-221
    respiratory, 230
Definitive host, 783
Degradation of glucose, *541*
Degranulation in phagocytosis, 224
Dehydration, diarrhea causing, 960
Delta hepatitis, 862-864, 864t, *865*
    epidemiology of, 860t
Dematiaceous hyphae, 712-713, *713*
Dengue fever, 853
Density in colonial morphology, 319
Density measurement, 16

Deoxycholate citrate agar, 1124
Deoxyribonuclease test agar, 1124
Deoxyribonucleic acid
    antimicrobials interfering with, 59
    in bacterial genetics, 20, 21
    in conjugation, 23
    mutations and, 21
    nucleic acid hybridization and, 191
    in transduction, 22
    in transformation, 21-22
Deoxythymidine triphosphate, 204
Deoxyuridine triphosphate, 204
Dermatitis, schistosomal, 805-806
Dermatophytosis, 724-729, 725t, *726, 727*
    athlete's foot, 725
    epidemiology of, 724
    general characteristics of, 715, 936, 938
    of hair and hair follicles, 725
    laboratory diagnosis of, *728,* 728-729
    microorganism causing
        Epidermophyton floccusum, 727-728
        Microsporum audouinii, 727
        Microsporum canis, 727, *727*
        Microsporum gypseum, 727, *727*
        Trichophyton mentagrophytes, 726, *726*
        Trichophyton rubrum, 726, *726*
        Trichophyton tonsurans, 726-727
    of nail and nail bed, 725
    sites of, 725t
    systemic, 725
    treatment of, 726
Desert rheumatism, 740-741
Design, in performance improvement, 116
Desulfovibrio vulgaris, 608t
Detection; *see* Antibody detection; Antigen detection;
        Molecular detection method
Detergent, 32
DF-2, 559
DF-3, 560
Diabetic foot, *926*
Diagnostic sensitivity of test, 122
Diagnostic specificity of test, 122
Diagnostic stage of hemoflagellate, 779
Diapedesis, 223
Diarrhea
    Aeromonas causing, 525
    complications of, 960
    Escherichia coli causing, 955-956
    Escherichia coli infection causing, 469-472
    invasive, 951-952
    laboratory diagnosis of, 950
    Microspora causing, 799
    newly recognized agents causing, 960-961
    organisms causing, 954t
    pathogenic mechanism of, 950-951
    patient history of, 949-950
    physical examination for, 950
    Plesiomonas causing, 528-529
    stool smear of, 306

Diarrhea—cont'd
   traveler's
      Aeromonas causing, 525
      Escherichia coli causing, 469
      Giardia lamblia causing, 775-776
   treatment of, 967-968
   Vibrio cholerae causing, 519-520
   Vibrio parahaemolyticus causing, 521
Dientamoeba fragilis, 776t, 777-778
Differential medium, 14, 250-251
Differential stain, 266
Diffusion test, disk, 73-77
   principle of, 73
   test performance of, 74-77, *75, 76,* 77t, 78t
   zone diameter interpretive breakpoints in, 73-74, *74*
Digestion-decontamination of specimen, *Mycobacterium,*
      674-676
Dilute gelatin medium, 1142
Dilution susceptibility testing, 69-73
   agar, 72-73, *73*
   antimicrobial stock solutions for, 69-70
   broth macrodilution, 70
   broth microdilution, *70, 70-72, 71,* 71t
   macrodilution, 70
   minimal inhibitory concentration and, 70t
Dimorphism, in fungi, 713
Diphtheria, 885
Diphyllobothrium latum, 807-808, *809*
   gastrointestinal infection and, 959
Diplococcus
   differentiation of, *409*
   Neisseria gonorrhoeae, 1036; *see also Neisseria*
      gonorrhoeae
Diploid cell culture, 840
Dipylidium caninum
   characteristics of, 811
   egg of, 807t
Direct, natural particle agglutination assay, 165-166, *166*
Direct enzyme immunoassay, 143
Direct examination; *see* Microscopic examination
Direct fluorescent antibody test, 139-140, *141*
   for *Bordetella,* 458, 459
   of *Legionella, 451,* 451-452
   virus infection and, 837
Direct hemagglutination, 166
Direct Nagler test, 598
Direct plate count, 15-16
Direct sandwich immunoassay, 143
Direct smear, nonuseful, 250
Direct wet mount of stool specimen, 759-760
Discharge, vaginal, 778
Disinfectant
   definition of, 26-27
   for mycobacteriology laboratory, 671
Disinfection, 26-33; *see also* Sterilization and disinfection
   definition of, 26
Disk diffusion test, 73-77, 93
   principle of, 73
   test performance of, 74-77, *75, 76,* 77t, 78t
   zone diameter interpretive breakpoints in, 73-74, *74*

Disk for anaerobic bacteria, *588,* 589
Disposal of infectious waste, 47
Disseminated intravascular coagulation, 1002
Dissemination of pathogen, 228-230
Dithiothreitol, 675
DNA hybridization, of *Mycobacterium tuberculosis,* 690-691
DNA polymerase, 199, *200-201*
DNA probe
   Biotinylated, 194, 195
   Chlamydia trachomatis and, 125, 125t
   of *Legionella,* 452
   for *Plasmodium falciparum,* 788
   stain for, 266t
DNA probe technology, 191-203
DNA virus, 836t
DNase, 359
Dog hookworm, 941
Dog tapeworm, 813
Double immunodiffusion, 133, 167-168
Double indirect fluorescent antibody test, 172
Doubling time, 15
Doxycycline
   Borrelia burgdorferi and, 628
   leptospires and, 626
DPT vaccine, 885
Dracunculiasis, 941
Dracunulus medinensis, 826
Drainage
   microscopic appearance of, 299
   sinusitis and, 889
   specimen collection from site of, 242t
Droplet nuclei, 230-231
Drug therapy; *see also* Antimicrobial therapy
   antiviral, 871, 871t
   bacteremia and, 1000
   for malaria, 786
   Mycobacterium avium infection and, 696
   for tuberculosis, 695
Dry heat, 29
Duodenal aspirate
   culture media for, 252t
   parasitic infection and, 761-762
Duodenal ulcer, 530
Duodenum, *Fasciolopsis buski* in, 802
Dysentery
   amebic; *see* Ameba
   Shigella causing, 485-486
Dysgonic fermenting bacteria, 559-560
Dysuria, 1021

E

E medium, diphasic, 1125
E test, *87,* 87-88
Eagle effect in minimal bactericidal concentration test, 100
Ear infection; *see* Otitis media
East African sleeping sickness, 780-781
Eastern equine encephalitis, 853, 987
Ebola hemorrhagic fever, 857
Ebola virus, 855, 857-858
Ebola-Sudan virus, 857

Ebola-Zaire virus, 857
Echinococcosis, 813
Eclipse phase of viral infection, 872
Ecthyma gangrenosum, 927
    Pseudomonas aeruginosa causing, 547
Ectoparasite, skin manifestations of, 941
Ectothrix hair involvement, 725
Edema factor, 393
Education
    about specimen collection, 240-241
    continuing, 114
Edwards and Ewing classification of Enterobacteriaceae, 465,
        466t, 467t
Edwardsiella spp., 478
    classification of, 466t
    infection causes by, 467t
Edwardsiella hoshinae, 478
Edwardsiella ictaluri, 478
Edwardsiella tarda, 478
Edwardsielleae, 466t
Effusion, pleural, 912-913
Egg
    fluke, *802*
    of *Opisthorchis sinensis, 803*
    parasitic, 762
    roundworm, 814t
    of *Schistosoma* spp., *804, 806*
    Taenia spp., 810-811
    tapeworm, 807t
Egg yolk agar, 597-598, 1125
Egg-based medium for *Mycobacterium* culture, 678
    Mycobacterium asiaticum, 703
    Mycobacterium flavescens, 703
    Mycobacterium gordonae, 702
    Mycobacterium terrae-triviale complex, 703
    Mycobacterium thermoresistibile, 703
Ehrlichia spp., 1078-1080
Ehrlichiosis, 1078-1080
Eikenella corrodens, 437t, 439, *439*
    aspiration pneumonia and, 905
Elck test, 378, 380
Elderly patient
    infection in, 1050-1051
    urinary tract infection in, 1015
Electrical safety, 48
Electroendosmosis, 135
Electron microscopy of virus, 839
Elementary body of *Chlamydia trachomatis,* 637, *638,* 1037
Elevation in colonial morphology, 317, *318,* 319
ELISA; *see* Enzyme-linked immunosorbent assay
Embden-Meyerhof-Parnas pathway, 17, *17, 19*
Embryo, hexacanth, 806
Emetic form of *Bacillus cereus* infection, 394
Empiric antimicrobial therapy, for respiratory infection,
        882-883
Employee right-to-know, 41
Empyema, 897t, 906, 912-913
Encapsulated strain of *Haemophilus,* 428
Encephalitis
    definition of, 977
    equine, 853, 987

Encephalitis—cont'd
    granulomatous amebic, 774, 990
    herpes simplex virus, 867
    Japanese, 853
    Togaviridae causing, 853
    viral, 987-988
Encephalitozoon, 799
End product metabolic analysis, 591
Endemic organism, 233
Endemic relapsing fever, 627, *627*
Endemic syphilis, 631-632
Endemic typhus, 1076-1077
Endocarditis
    Erysipelothix rhusiopathiae causing, 385
    skin manifestations of, 928, *928*
    Streptococcus pneumoniae causing, 365
Endogenous anaerobic bacteria, 569, 569t, 570t
Endophthalmitis, 1101-1102
    plating guidelines for, 1106t
Endoplasmic reticulum, of eukaryotic cell, 7
Endothrix hair involvement, 725
Endotoxin
    bacteremia and, 1002
    tissue damage by, 228
Endpoint
    minimal bactericidal concentration, 99
    onscale minimal inhibitory concentration, 90
Enriched medium, 14, 251
Enrichment broth, 251
Entamoeba coli, 768t, 770, *770, 771*
Entamoeba dispar, 769
Entamoeba hartmanni, 768t, 769-770, *770*
Entamoeba histolytica, 766-769
    clinical infection with, 766-767
    invasive diarrhea syndrome and, 951
    laboratory diagnosis of, 767, 768t, 769, *769*
    sputum specimen of, 762
    toxic megacolon and, 960
    traveler's diarrhea and, 949
Entamoeba nana, 768t, 770, *771*
Enteric adenovirus, 851
Enteric agar, 964t
Enteric bacteria; *see* Enterobacteriaceae
Enteric disease
    antigen detection for, 149
    hepatitis E as, 864-865
    Yersinia enterocolitica causing, 487
Enteric fever, 954
Enteroaggregative *Escherichia coli,* 472
    infections caused by, 955
Enterobacter spp., 475-476, 475t, *476*
    beta-lactam antibiotics and, 56
    classification of, 466t
    fermentation by, 19
    infection causes by, 467t
    nosocomial pneumonia and, 904
Enterobacter aerogenes, 475
    diagnostic features of, 475t
    disk diffusion test of, 73, *73*
Enterobacter agglomerans, 475, *476*

Enterobacter amnigenus, 475
Enterobacter cloacae
   antibiograms for, 92t
   beta-lactam antibiotics and, 60
   diagnostic features of, 475, 475t
Enterobacter dissolvens, 475-476
Enterobacter gergoviae, 475
Enterobacter intermedium, 475
Enterobacter nimipressuralis, 475-476
Enterobacter sakazakii, 475, *476*
Enterobacteriaceae, 463-514
   agar for, 496
   antimicrobials and, nucleic acid metabolism and, 59
   aspiration pneumonia and, 905
   beta-lactam antibiotics and, 56
   Budivicia aquatica, 488
   Buttiauxella agrestis, 488, 492t
   Cedecea spp., 488
   classification of, 465, 466t, 467t
   clinical significance of, 466-467, 467t
   Ewingella americana, 488, 492t
   fermentation by, 19
   glucose metabolism and, 498, *499,* 500, *501-505,* 504-506
   identification of, 491, 492t-495t, 496
   isolation and, 490-491
   Kluyvera spp., 488, *489,* 492t
   Koserella spp., 488
   laboratory diagnosis of, 490-495
   lactose fermentation and, 19-20, 496-497
   Leminorella spp., 488-489
   Moellerella spp., 489, 492t
   morphology of, 465
   Obesumbacterium proteus, 489, 494t
   opportunistic
      Citrobacter spp., 478-479, 492t
      Edwardsiella spp., 478, 492t
      Enterobacter spp., 475-476, 475t, *476,* 492t
      Erwinia spp., 478
      Escherichia coli, 468-473; *see also Escherichia coli*
      Hafnia spp., 477, 492t
      Klebsiella spp., 473-475, *474, 474t,* 492t
      Morganella spp., 477, 478t, 494t
      Pectobacterium spp., 478
      Proteus spp., 477, 478t, 492t
      Providencia spp., 477-478, 478t, 492t
      Serratia spp., *476,* 476-477, 494t
   Rahnella aquatilis, 489
   Salmonella; see Salmonella entries
   serology and, 508
   Shigella spp.; *see Shigella entries*
   specimen collection and transport of, 490
   stool culture and, 506, 507t
   susceptibility testing and, 65
   Tatumella ptyseos, 489-490, 492t
   terminology changes in, 1145
   triple sugar iron agar and, 497-498
   urinary tract infection and, 1018
   Vibrio vs., 522
   virulence factors of, 465
   Xenorhabdus spp., 490, 494t

Enterobius vermicularis, 815, 815-816, 816
   egg of, 814t
Enterococcus spp., 364
   beta-lactamase tests and, 89
   bile esculin test and, 356
   biochemical identification of, 351t
   characteristics of, 364
   leucine aminopeptidase test and, 356
   Listeria monocytogenes vs., 384t
   susceptibility testing of, 82-84
Enterocolitis, necrotizing, 215
Enterocytozoon spp., 799
Enterocytozoon bieneusi, 961
Enterohemorrhagic *Escherichia coli,* 470-472
   food poisoning and, 962t
   infections caused by, 955
Enteroinvasive *Escherichia coli,* 470
   infections caused by, 955
Enteropathogenic *Escherichia coli,* 469
   infections caused by, 955
Enterotoxigenic *Escherichia coli,* 232, 469-470, 951
   food poisoning and, 962t
   infections caused by, 956
Enterotoxin
   of *Bacillus cereus,* 395t
   cholera and, 955-956
   of *Staphylococcus aureus,* 332
Enterotoxin-mediated diarrhea, 950
Enterotube test, 186t
Enterovirus
   cell cultures for, 841t
   central nervous system and, 849-850
   immunity to, 159
   meningitis and, 985
   skin manifestations of, 936
Envelope
   cell, of prokaryotic cell, 8-10, *8-10*
   of eukaryotic cell, 7
   structure of, 8-10, *8-10*
Enveloped virus, 834-835
Environment
   for culture, 251
   for Enterobacteriaceae, 491
Environmental factors, bacterial growth and, 14-15
Enzyme
   antimicrobial resistance and, 60
   antimicrobial-inactivating, detection of, *89,* 89-90
   beta-lactam antibiotics and, 55
   nucleic acid metabolism and, 59
   oxygen toxicity and, 568
   in phagocytosis, 222, 224
   restriction, 23
   of Staphylococcus aureus, 332
Enzyme immunoassay, 103-104, 141-142, 173-174, 174, *174*
   for antigen detection, 141-145, *142-144*
   Chlamydia trachomatis and, 647
   gastroenteritis and, 150
   human immunodeficiency virus and, 849
   for *Legionella,* 454
   membrane-bound, 144-145

Enzyme immunoassay—cont'd
  mumps and, 845
  Mycoplasma pneumoniae, 663
  for parasitic infection, 763
  for verotoxin producing *Escherichia coli,* 149-150
  virus and, 150, 837-838
  Western blotting and, 176
Enzyme-based identification system, for anaerobic bacteria, 591
Enzyme-linked immunosorbent assay, *143*
  in antibody detection, 172-175, *173-175*
  Entamoeba histolytica and, 769
  Escherichia coli and, 472
  hepatitis C and, 864
  hepatitis E and, 866
  for *Neisseria gonorrhoeae* identification, 410
  for *Streptococcus,* 358
EO-2, 559
Eosin-methylene blue agar, 1125
Epicoccum, 745
Epidemic, definition of, 233
Epidemic louse-borne typhus, 1077
Epidemic relapsing fever, 627
Epidemiology
  of *Staphylococcus aureus,* 332-333
  terminology of, 233-234
Epidermal necrolysis, toxic, 334
Epidermolytic toxin of *Staphylococcus aureus,* 332
Epidermophyton floccusum, 727-728
Epiglottitis, 892-894, *894*
  Haemophilus influenzae causing, 429
  laboratory diagnosis of, 886t
Episcleral infection, 1098
Epithelium
  as barrier to infection, 220
  sinusitis and, 889
Epstein-Barr virus
  characteristics of, 868-869
  indirect fluorescent antibody test for, 172
  meningitis and, 986
  serologic testing for, 178
  skin manifestations of, 934
Equine encephalitis, 853, 987
Equipment
  contaminated, culturing of, 257
  quality control and, 108-112, 109t, *110, 111*
Erwinia spp., 467t, 478
Erysipelas, 360, 923-924, *924*
Erysipeloid, 385, 925, 1062-1063
Erysipelothrix rhusiopathiae
  clinical manifestations of, *385,* 385-386, 386t, 1062
  colony morphology of, *386*
  epidemiology of, 1062
  etiology of, 1062
  laboratory diagnosis of, 1062-1063
  skin infection and, 925
Erythema chronicum migrans, 628, 932
Erythema infectiosum, 847, 935-936
Erythema migrans, *1059*
Erythema nodosum, 487

Erythrasma, 925
Erythrocytic phase of *Plasmodium,* 786-787
Erythromycin
  Bordetella and, 461
  mechanism of action of, 58
  susceptibility testing and, 65
Eschar
  anthrax and, 393
  sample collection and, 241
Escherichia spp.
  biochemical reactions of, 494t
  classification of, 466t
Escherichia coli, 468-473
  adherence in, 227
  antibiograms for, 92t
  beta-lactam antibiotics and, 56
  clinical infection with, 469-473
  conjugation in, 22-23
  culture of, 965-966, *966*
  diarrhea due to, 955-956
  disk diffusion testing of, *75*
  enteroaggregative, 472, 955
  enterohemorrhagic, 470-472, 955
  enteroinvasive, 470, 955
  enteropathogenic, 469, 955
  enterotoxigenic, 469-470, 951, 956
  exotoxins of, 229t
  extended spectrum beta-lactamases and, 84
  fermentation by, 18-19
  food poisoning and, 962t
  general characteristics of, *468,* 468-469
  indications for testing for, 64
  infection caused by
    gastrointestinal, 467t, 469-472
    meningitis, 472-473
    septicemia, 472-473
    urinary, 472
  interference with phagocytosis by, 225t
  invasive diarrhea syndrome and, 952
  nutritional requirements of, 14
  peptidoglycan layer of cell wall in, *9*
  restriction enzymes in, 23
  staining of, *12*
  susceptibility testing and, 67
  transformation in, 22
  transmission of, 232
  verotoxin producing, 149-150
Escherichia hermannii, 473
Escherichia vulneris, 473
Escherichia/Citrobacter-like organism, 314, *315*
Escherichieae, classification of, 466t
Esculin agar, 1125
ESP system, 1006
Ethambutol, concentration of, for tuberculosis, 692t
Ethanol, 18
Ethionamide, 692t
Ethylene oxide, 32
Etiologic agent
  definition of, 756
  mailing of, *244,* 244-245

Eubacterium spp.
    characteristics of, 604t, 605
    clinical significance of, 602t-603t
    fermentation by, 19
Eugonic fermenting bacteria, 560
Eukaryote, 5
Eukaryotic cell, *6,* 6t, 7
Eumycotic mycetoma, 731-733, *732,* 732t, *733*
    epidemiology of, 731-732
    laboratory diagnosis of, 732-733, 732t, *733*
    organisms causing, 729
Eustachian tube, 891-892
Ewingella americana, 488
Examination of specimens, 248, 261-309; *see also* Microscopic
    examination
Exanthem, viral, 845-847
Exanthem subitum, 870
Exfoliative toxin of *Staphylococcus aureus,* 332
Exoerythrocytic phase of *Plasmodium,* 786
Exogenous anaerobe, 569
Exophiala jeanselmei, 732t, 733, *734,* 734
Exotoxin
    pathogens producing, 229t
    tissue damage by, 228
Expectorated sputum; *see* Sputum
Expression, protein, 20
Extended spectrum beta-lactamase, 84
Extinguisher, fire, 47t
Extracellular pathogen, immunity to, 158
Eye
    anatomy of, 1084-1086, *1085*
    cleansing mechanism of, 221
    normal flora of, 1088-1089
    protection for, *38*
    sinusitis complications and, 890
    specimen collection from, 242t
Eye infection
    Acinetobacter causing, 550
    amebic keratitis, 774
    conjunctival, *1089-1091,* 1089-1093
    corneal, 1094-1098, *1095-1098*
    culture media for, 252t
    endophthalmitis, 1101-1102
    herpetic, 867
    human immunodeficiency virus and, 1104, *1104*
    laboratory diagnosis of, 1104-1111, 1105t, *1106-1110, 1106t,*
        1107t
    lacrimal, 1100-1101
    of lids, 1093-1094
    microscopic appearance of, 304
    orbital, 1098-1100
    pathogenesis of, 1086-1088
    retinal, 1102-1103, *1103*
    scleral and episcleral, 1098
    scleral buckle, 1103-1104, *1104*
    tests for, 838t
    treatment of, 1111-1112
    uveitis, 1102
    viral, tests for, 838t

Eyelid
    anatomy of, 1085
    infection of, 1093-1094

F

Facilitator, 117
Facultative anaerobic bacteria, 15
    Corynebacterium diphtheriae as, 375
    definition of, 15
    in gastrointestinal tract, 571
    growth requirements of, 587
    Salmonella, 479-484
    Vibrio, 517-524
False-negative test result, 163, *164*
False-positive test result
    definition of, 163-164, *164*
    in flocculation tests, 168
    Western blotting and, 176
Family name of bacteria, 4, 5
Fasciola hepatica
    characteristics of, 803, *803*
    eggs of, 802t
Fasciolopsis buski
    characteristics of, 801-802
    eggs of, 802t
Fastidious bacteria, susceptibility testing and
    for anaerobes, 81
    for *Haemophilus* spp., 77-79
    for *Neisseria gonorrhoeae,* 80-81
    for *Neisseria meningitidis,* 80-81
    for *Streptococcus* spp., 79-80
Fecal specimen; *see* Stool *entries*
Female patient
    Chlamydia trachomatis infection in, 1037
    gonorrhea in, 405
    Trichomonas vaginalis infection in, 778
    urinary tract infection in, 1015
Fermentation
    in bacterial cell, 16-17
    Enterobacteriaceae and, 465, 496-498
    pathways for, *541*
Fermenting bacteria
    dysgonic, 559-560
    eugonic, 560
    lactose, 314
Fetus
    Mycoplasma hominis infection and, 657
    TORCH infection in, 164-165
    Toxoplasma gondii infection in, 791-792
    Ureaplasma urealyticum infection and, 657
Fever
    blackwater, 786
    breakbone, 853
    Colorado tick, 854-855, 987
    endotoxin causing, 228
    hemophagic, skin manifestations of, 936
    hemorrhagic
        Crimean-Congo, 852-853
        Dengue, 853
        Ebola, 857

Fever—cont'd
hemorrhagic—cont'd
Marburg, 857
with renal syndrome, 856
Q, 1078
rat-bite, 929, *1064, 1064-1065, 1065*
relapsing, 627
Rift Valley, 852, 853
Rocky Mountain spotted, 931, 1075-1076
scarlet, 359
skin and, 928
trench, 1077-1078
typhoid, 482-483, 954
skin manifestations of, 928
undulant, 443
valley, 740-741
yellow, 854
Fibroblast, 868
Fiery serpent of the Israelites, 826
Fifth disease, 847, 935-936
Filamentous hemagglutinin, 458
Filamentous margin of colony, 317, *318*
Filarial worm
Dracunuculus medinensis, 826
Loa loa, 823, 824t, 825-826
Mansonella spp., 826
Onchocerca volvulus, 824-826, *826*
Wuchereria bancrofti, 823, 824t, *825*
Filariform larva, 814t, 318
larva migrans and, 822
Filoviridae, 836t, 857-858
Filter, high-efficiency air, 37
Filtering procedure, Nalgerne, 255
Filtration, 30
Fimbria
adherence and, 227
characteristics of, 10
Fire safety, 47-48, 47t
First aid training, 48
Fitz-Hugh-Curtis syndrome, 405
Fixation, complement, 168-170, *169*
for *Chlamydia pneumoniae,* 641
Flagellar antigen, 465
Flagellate
blood and tissue, *779,* 779-783, *781-783*
genitourinary, *Trichomonas vaginalis,* 778-779
intestinal, 775-779, *775-779*
Dientamoeba fragilis, 777-778, *778*
Giardia lamblia, 775, 776, 777, *777, 778*
Flagellum
characteristics of, 10
of eukaryotic cell, 7
periplasmic, 624
Flammable chemical, 46
Flat elevation of colony, 317, *318*
Flavimonas spp., 558
Flaviviridae, 836t, 853-854
Flavobacterium spp., 556-557
Fletcher semisolid medium for Leptospira, 1126

Flocculation test
for antibody detection, 168, *169*
for syphilis, 168, 177
Flora
anaerobic, 569
normal
bacteriocins produced by, 222
as barrier to respiratory infection, 884
characteristics of, 212-213
of eye, 1088-1089
gastrointestinal, 214-215
gastrointestinal infection and, 948, 948t
of genitourinary tract, 215-216
innate immunity and, 157
of mouth, 213-214
Neisseria spp. as, 418
origin of, 212
pathogenic microorganisms *vs.,* 879-881
in respiratory tract, 879
of respiratory tract, 214
of skin, 213, 921
susceptibility testing and, 64
Flotation method for stool specimen, 760
Fluid
amniotic
microscopic appearance of, 294, 297
microscopic specimen of, 282, 286
body
culture media for, 252t
Mycobacterium spp. and, 674
smear preparation of, 248-249
cerebrospinal; *see* Cerebrospinal fluid
as cleansing mechanism, 221
for fungal infection, 1143
fungal mounting, 1143
pleural, empyema and, 912-913
Flukes, 800-806
blood, 804-806, *805*
eggs of, *802*
intestinal, 801-803
laboratory diagnosis of, 801
life cycle of, 800-801, *801*
liver, 803, *803*
lung, 803-804, *804*
Fluorescein isothiocyanate, 140-141, *141*
Fluorescein isothiocyanate conjugate, for *Legionella, 451,* 451-452
Fluorescence, of anaerobic bacteria, 587-588
Fluorescence of anaerobic bacteria, 584
Fluorescent antibody test
direct
for *Bordetella,* 458, 459
of *Legionella, 451,* 451-452
double indirect, 172
human immunodeficiency virus and, 849
indirect
in antibody detection, *171,* 171-172
in antigen detection, 140
double, 172
for *Legionella,* 454-455

Fluorescent antibody test—cont'd
    mumps and, 845
    for parasitic infection, 763
    for pertussis, 146
    virus infection and, 837
Fluorescent immunoassay, 103-104, 145
    for antibody detection, 174-175
Fluorescent treponemal antibody absorption test, 168, 177,
        630-631
Fluorochrome stain, 266t
Fluorometric detection system, 85
Fluoroquinolone, 59
Fly, tsetse, 782
Focused monitor, 116
Folinic acid, 58
Follicle, hair, 725
Folliculitis, 333, 923
Fonsecaea pedrosoi, 732t, 939, 939t
Food and Drug Administration, disk diffusion testing and, 74
Food poisoning, 232; *see also* Gastrointestinal infection
    agents causing, 961, 962t, 963
    Bacillus cereus causing, 394
    botulism, 595-596
    Clostridium perfringens causing, 596
    salmonella, 954
    Staphylococcus aureus causing, 333
Food-borne infection, 231-232
    Bacillus cereus, 394
    cholera as, 517
    Clostridium causing, 594
    Corynebacterium ulcerans as, 380
    Escherichia coli as, 469-473
    hepatitis A as, 859-860
    Listeria monocytogenes, 383
    newly recognized agents of, 960-961
    parasitic, 958-960
        fluke and, 800-806
        roundworm, 813-826
        tapeworm, 806-813
        Trichinella spiralis, 959-960
    Salmonella causing, 481-484
    Vibrio cholerae, 519-520
    Yersinia enterocolitica, 486-487
Foot, diabetic, *926*
Form
    laboratory release, *246*
    problem/action, 116-117, 117t
Formaldehyde, 30-31, 31t, 672
Formalin, 758, 758t
Formalin-ether method, 760
Formalin–ethyl acetate, 760
Format, hybridization, 192-194, *193*
Francisella spp.
    bacteremia and, 1006
    culture media for, 253t
Francisella tularensis, 444
    as laboratory hazard, 35-36
    penetration of skin by, 220
    skin manifestations of, 929
    tularemia caused by, 1068-1070, *1070*

Free coagulase, 337, *338*
Frontal sinusitis, retroorbital, 890
FTA-ABS test, 168, 177
Fume hood, *39*
Fungal infection; *see also* Fungus
    central nervous system
        brain abscess, 981-982
        meningitis, 982-984, *984*
    chronic pneumonia and, 911
    corneal, 1096, 1097
    cutaneous (dermatophytosis), 724-729, 936, *937,* 938-941
        athlete's foot, 725
        epidemiology of, 724
        Epidermophyton floccusum, 727-728
        general characteristics of, 715
        of hair and hair follicles, 725
        laboratory diagnosis of, *728,* 728-729
        Microsporum audouinii, 727
        Microsporum canis, 727, 727
        Microsporum gypseum, 727, 727
        of nail and nail bed, 725
        sites of, 725t
        systemic, 725
        treatment of, 726
        Trichophyton mentagrophytes, 726, 726
        Trichophyton rubrum, 726, 726
        Trichophyton tonsurans, 726-727
    endophthalmitis and, 1101-1102
    of eye
        blepharitis and, 1094
        conjunctival, 1092
    malignancy and, 1048
    media, fluids, and stains for, 1141-1143
    microscopic appearance of, *300-303*
    opportunistic, 742-747, 1046t; *see also* Opportunistic infec-
            tion, fungal
    plating guidelines for, 1106t
    serologic testing for, 180
    specimen collection of, 242t
    subcutaneous mycosis, 729-734
        chromoblastomycosis, 730-731, *731*
        chromomycosis, 939, 939t
        eumycotic mycetoma, 731-733, *732,* 732t, *733*
        general characteristics of, 715-716
        mycetoma, 938-939, 939t
        phaeohyphomycosis, 733-734, *734*
        sporotrichosis, 729-730, *730,* 939-940, 939t
    superficial mycosis, 722-724
        general characteristics of, 715
        Malassezia furfur, 722, 722-723
        Phaeoannellomyces wernickii, 724, *724*
        Piedraia hortae, 723, 723
        Trichosporon beigelii, 723, 723-724
    systemic mycosis, 734-742, 735t, 736t, 940
        Blastomyces dermatitidis, 735-737, *736, 737,* 737t, *738*
        Coccidioides immitis, 740, 740-741, *741*
        general characteristics of, 716
        Histoplasma capsulatum var. *capsulatum,* 737-740, *739*
        Paracoccidioides brasiliensis, 741, 741-742
    urinary tract, urine screening in, 1026
    urinary tract infection and, 1020

Fungal mounting fluid. 1143
Fungi Imperfecti, 714-715
Fungi-Fluor kit, 270
Fungus, 709-754; *see also* Fungal infection
    Accuprobes for, 195
    cell wall of, 7
    general characteristics of, 711-714, *711-714*
    identification of, 717-721
        cellophane tape preparation for, 721
        culture and, 718-719, 719t
        gross examination in, 719-720, *720*
        guideline for, *720*
        microscopic examination in, 717-718, *718,* 718t
        slide culture for, 721
        tease mount for, 721
    Pneumocystis carinii classified as, 794; *see also* Pneumo-
        cystis carinii
    safety issues with, 722
    sites of infection, *715,* 715-716
    specimen handling of, 716-717
    taxonomy of, *714,* 714-715
Furuncle, 333, 923, *923*
Fusarium spp., 745, *745*
Fusarium solani, endophthalmitis and, 1102
Fusiform bacteria, 11
Fusion, *714*
Fusobacterium spp.
    characteristics of, 614t
    clinical infection with, 606
    clinical significance of, 608t
    culture of, 583
    fermentation by, 19
    laboratory diagnosis of, 610, *610, 611*
    presumptive identification of, 613t
Fusobacterium mortiferum
    laboratory diagnosis of, 610, *611*
    microscopic examination of, 576-577
Fusobacterium necrophorum, 576-577
Fusobacterium nucleatum, 570
    fluorescence of, 588
    laboratory diagnosis of, 610, *610*
Fusobacterium varium, 618

G

Gametocyte of *Plasmodium,* 786
Gametogony of *Cryptosporidium parvum,* 797
Gangrene, gas, 595, 924-925, *925*
Gardnerella spp., 252t
Gardnerella vaginalis, 1020
    molecular probe for 198
    vaginosis and, 1039
GAS; *see* Group A streptococcus
Gas
    for sterilization, 32
    storage of, 48
Gas gangrene, 924-925 *925*
    Clostridium spp. causing, 595
Gas-Liquid chromatography, for anaerobic bacteria, 591
GasPak, 582

Gastric aspirate
    culture media for, 252t
    Mycobacterium spp. and, 673
Gastric ulcer, 530
Gastroenteritis
    Aeromonas causing, 524-525
    Plesiomonas causing, 528-529
    Salmonella, 482
Gastrointestinal infection; *see also* Food poisoning
    Aeromonas causing, 524-525
    anatomy and, *947,* 947-948
    anthrax and, 393-394, 1066
    antigen detection in, 149-150
    apicomplexa, 795-799
        Cryptosporidium parvum, 795-797, *796, 797*
        Cyclospora cayetanensis, 798-799, *799*
    Bacillus cereus causing, 394-395
    Campylobacter causing, 530
    cholera as, 517, 519-520
    diarrhea and, 949-952; *see also* Diarrhea
    Enterococcus causing, 364
    Escherichia coli causing
        enteroaggregative, 472
        enterohemorrhagic, 470-472
        enteroinvasive, 470
        enteropathogenic, 469
        enterotoxigenic, 469-470
    evaluation of, 946-947
    Helicobacter pylori causing, 530-532
    laboratory diagnosis of, 963-967, 964t, *965-967*
    Microspora, 799
    Mycobacterium, culture for, 673
    normal flora and, 948
    parasitic
        duodenal aspirates for, 761
        fecal specimen for, 757-761
        fluke and, 801-803
        sigmoidoscopy specimens of, 761-762
        skin manifestations of, 940
    Plesiomonas causing, 528-529
    protozoan
        ameba, 764-772; *see also* Ameba, intestinal
        ciliates, 774-775
        flagellates, 775-779, *775-779*
    Salmonella spp. causing, 479-484; *see also* Salmonella
        entries
    Shigella causing, 484-486
    transmission of, 231-232
    Vibrio causing, 519-521
    viral, 838t
        adenovirus, 150
        antigen detection for, 150
        calicivirus, 150
        coronavirus, 150
        Norwalk, 850-851
        rotavirus, 850
        transmission of, 232
Gastrointestinal system
    anaerobic bacteria in, 570t, 571
    usual flora of, 214-215

Gel immunodiffusion, Ouchterlony, 133, 167
Gelatin medium, 1126
  dilute, 1142
Gemella spp.
  characteristics of, 370
  clinical significance of, 615t
Gene, types of, 20
Gene amplification, viral, 839
  hepatitis C, 864
Gene transfer, 21, *22*
Generation time, 15
Genetics, bacterial, 20-23, *22*
Genital chlamydiosis; *see Chlamydia trachomatis*
Genital herpes, 867, 1042-1043
Genital tuberculosis, in male, 694
Genitalia, specimen collection from, 242t
Genitourinary infection
  culture media for, 252t
  herpes, 867
  Mycobacterium culture for, 673-674
  Mycoplasma genitalium, 657-658
  Mycoplasma hominis, 656-657
  neonatal infection associated with, 656t
  tests for, 838t
  Trichomonas vaginalis, 778-779
  tuberculous, 694
  Ureaplasma urealyticum, 656-657, 656t
  urinary tract, 1011-1032; *see also* Urinary tract infection
Genitourinary system
  anaerobic bacteria in, 571
  cleansing mechanisms of, 221-222
  fungal specimen from, 717
  usual flora of, 215-216
Genome
  bacterial, 21
  viral, 834
Genotype, definition of, 20
Genotypic characteristics, 5
Gen-Probe, *197*
Gentamicin
  minimal inhibitory concentration of, 70t
  susceptibility testing and, 67
    of gram-negative organisms, 92t
Genus, definition of, 4-5
Geotrichum, 745, *745*
Germ tube production, *750, 750-751, 751*
German measles, 846
  rash of, 935
  serologic diagnosis of, 178
Giardia lamblia
  antigen detection for, 150
  characteristics of, 776t
  diarrhea and, 949-950
  direct fluorescent antibody test of, *141*
  enterotoxin-mediated diarrhea and, 951
  enzyme immunoassay kits for, 143
  fluorescent antibody test for, 763
  food poisoning and, 961
  infection caused by, 958-959
  traveler's diarrhea and, 949

Giemsa stain for *Pneumocystis carinii,* 795
Gilchrist's disease, 735-737
Gland
  of eyelid, 1093
  sebaceous, 213
Glanders, 929
Glomerulonephritis
  clinical manifestations of, 1016
  poststreptococcal, antistreptolysin-O test and, 170
  streptococcal pharyngitis and, 886
  Streptococcus pyogenes causing, 360
Glove box for anaerobic bacteria, 581, *581*
Gloveless anaerobic chamber, 581, *581*
Glucocorticoid, 1007
Glucose
  biochemical pathways and, *17, 17-18, 18*
  Enterobacteriaceae and, 498
  fermentation pathways for degradation of, *541*
Glutaraldehyde, as disinfectant, 31, 31t
Golgi apparatus, 7
Gonochek test, 186t
Gonorrhea; *see also Neisseria gonorrhoeae*
  clinical manifestations of, 1035-1036
  laboratory diagnosis of, 1036
  treatment of, 414-415, 1036t
Grading specimens, 275-277
Gram smear report, 276, 277
Gram stain, 11, *12*
  anaerobic bacteria and, 576-577, *585*
  morphology, 272t
  origin of, 262
  procedure for, 267-268
  for rapid detection, 184t
  types of, 266t
Gram-negative bacillus
  meningitis caused by, 980, *980*
  urinary tract infection caused by, 1018
Gram-negative bacteria
  anaerobic bacilli
    Bacteroides spp., 606, 607t, 608t, 609
    bile-sensitive nonpigmented, 610, *610, 611*
    bile-sensitive pigmented, 609-610
  anaerobic cocci, 615t, 617
  antibiograms for, 92-93, 92t, 93t
  antimicrobials effective against, 59
  bacillus
    Escherichia coli as, 468-473; *see also Escherichia coli*
    fermentative, 560-561
    HACEK group of, 436-441
    nonfermenting, 539-561; *see also* Nonfermenting gram-negative bacilli
    respiratory infection and, 880
  bacteremia and, 1002
  cell wall of, 9
  endotoxins of, 228
  microscopic appearance of, *292-297*
  Neisseria gonorrhoeae; see Neisseria gonorrhoeae
  Pasteurella, 441, *441, 442t, 443, 443*
  rods
    Aeromonas, 524-528
    Bordetella, 457-462

Gram-negative bacteria—cont'd
  rods—cont'd
    Brucella, 443
    differentiation of, *409*
    HACEK group, 436-441
    Haemophilus spp., 426-436; *see also Haemophilus entries*
    Klebsiella, 473-475
    Legionella, 447-455; *see also Legionella* spp.
    Pasteurella, 441, *441, 442t, 443, 443*
    Salmonella, 479-484; *see also Salmonella entries*
    Yersinia pestis, 486
  Salmonella; see also Salmonella entries
  stool specimen and, 244
  susceptibility testing and, 65
Gram-negative broth, 1126
Gram-positive bacteria
  anaerobic cocci, 611, 615t, 617, *617, 618*
  bacillus, urinary tract infection and, 1019
  cell wall of, 8-9
  microscopic appearance of, *286-291*
  non–spore-forming anaerobic bacilli
    Actinomyces spp., 599, 602, *603,* 604
    Bifidobacterium spp., 604-605 , 604t-605t
    vaginosis and, 599, 602
  non–spore-forming rods
    Arcanobacterium haemolyticum, 381
    Corynebacterium, 375-380; *see also Corynebacterium entries*
    Erysipelothix rhusiopathiae, 385-386
    Listeria monocytogenes, 382-384, *384*
    Rhodococcus, 381
    Rothia dentocariosa, 381
  schematic diagram for identification of, *391*
  spore-forming bacilli, 594-599
    Clostridium spp., 594-599; *see also Clostridium entries*
  Streptococcus; see Streptococcus entries
  urinary tract infection and, 1018-1019
Granular material, sample preparation of, *264,* 264-265
Granule
  sinus tract, 291
  sulfur, *Nocardia* infection and, 397
Granulocytopenia
  malignancy and, 1048
  opportunistic respiratory infection and, 913-914
Granuloma
  culture of *Mycobacterium* and, 674
  Mycobacterium tuberculosis and, 693
Granulomatous disease
  amebic encephalitis, 774, 990
  tularemia, 1069
Griseofulvin, 725
Ground-glass appearance of *Legionella* culture, 453
Group A or B streptococcus; *see* Streptococcus
Growing trophozoite, 785
Growth, bacterial, 13-16, *15*
Gruft medium, 679t
Guillain-Barré syndrome, 986
  Campylobacter disease and, 960
Guinea worm infection, 826, 941
Gumma, 1040

H

H antigen
  Enterobacteriaceae and, 465
  Escherichia coli and, 468-469
  Salmonella and, 481
HACEK group, 436-441
  Actinobacillus actinomycetemcomitans, 436-438, 437t, *438*
  Cardiobacterium hominis, 437t, *438, 438-439*
  dysgonic fermenters and, 559-560
  Eikenella corrodens, 437t, 439, *439*
  Haemophilus aphrophilus, 436, *437,* 437t
  Kingella spp., 437t, 439-440, *440*
Haemophilus spp., 425-436
  antimicrobials effective against, 59
  colonial morphology of, 313-314
  differential tests for, 435t
  general characteristics of, 426-428
  media for, 314
  odor of, 320
  susceptibility testing of, 77-79
Haemophilus aegyptius
  infections caused by, 429-430
  media for, 431
Haemophilus aphrophilus, 434, 436, *437,* 437t
Haemophilus ducreyi
  chancroid and, 1041
  culture media for, 253t
  infection caused by, 430
  media for, 431
Haemophilus influenzae
  antigen detection for, 148-149
  beta-lactam antibiotics and, 56
  beta-lactamase tests and, 89
  bronchitis and, 899
  carbon dioxide and, 15
  central nervous system and, 993
  colonial morphology of, 431-432, *432*
  conjunctival infection and, 1089
  E test for, 87
  empiric drug therapy and, 882-883
  historical perspective on, 428
  host defense and, 884-885
  identification of, 432-434, *432-434*
  infections caused by, 429, 430t
  interference with phagocytosis by, 225t
  laboratory diagnosis of, 993
  meningitis and, 977-979, *978*
  microscopic morphology of, 431, *431*
  nutritional requirements of, 14
  as ocular flora, 1088
  pneumonia and, community-acquired, 901
  proliferation of, 227
  respiratory infection caused by
    epiglottitis, 893-894
    otitis media, 891
  restriction enzymes in, 23
  sinusitis caused by, 887
  specimen collection of, 890
  specimen processing of, 430-431
  susceptibility testing of, 77-79

Haemophilus influenzae—cont'd
transformation in, 22
treatment of, 434, 436
virulence factors of, 428-429
Haemophilus parainfluenzae, 56
Haemophilus test medium, 77-79
Hafnia spp., 466t, 477
Hafnia alvei, 954t
Hair
dermatophytosis of, 725
fungal specimen from, 717
nasal, 884
Hair perforation test, 728, *728*
Halogen disinfectant, 31-32, 31t
Halophilic *Vibrio* spp., 517, 521
Hand, foot, and mouth disease, 846-847
Hand in transmission of infection, 230
Hantavirus, 856-857, 856t
HAT, 178
Hazardous chemical, inventory of, 46
Hazardous waste reduction, 47
HB-5 organism, 560
HBeAg, 862
HBsAg, 862
Heart, endocarditis of
Erysipelothix rhusiopathiae causing, 385
skin manifestations of, 928, *928*
Streptococcus pneumoniae causing, 365
Heat
dry, 29
moist, 28-29
Heavy metal as disinfectant, 32
Hektoen enteric agar, 964t, 1126-1127
Helicobacter pylori, 530-533, 530t, 531t, 534t, 535
culture of, 253t, 966-967, *967*
diarrhea and, 961
Helminth, 800-826
flukes, 800-806
blood, 804-806, *805*
eggs of, *802*
intestinal, 801-803
laboratory diagnosis of, 801
life cycle of, 800-801, *801*
liver, 803, *803*
lung, 803-804, *804*
roundworms, 813-826
Ascaris lumbricoides, 816-818, *817, 818*
Dracunulus medinensis, 826
Enterobius vermicularis, 815, *815-816, 816*
filarial, 823, 824t, *825*
general characteristics of, 813-815
hookworm, 818-819
larva migrans caused by, 822
loa loa, 823, 825-826
Mansonella spp., 826
Strongyloides stercoralis, 819-820, *821,* 822
Trichinella spiralis, 822, *822*
Trichuris trichura, 816, *816*
Wuchereria bancrofti, 823, *825*

Helminth—cont'd
tapeworms, 806-813
cysticercosis, 811, 813
Diphyllobothrium latum, 807-808, *809*
Dipylidium caninum, 811
echinococcosis, 813
eggs of, 807t
general characteristics of, 807
Hymenolepis spp., 811, *812*
sparganosis, 813
Taenia spp., 808-811
Hemadsorption inhibition, mumps and, 845
Hemagglutination
direct, 166
indirect, 167
Hemagglutination inhibition test, 166
Hemagglutinin, virus and, 841-842
Hemagglutinin-neuraminidase, 843
Hematologic malignancy, 1048
Hemoflagellate, *779, 779-783, 781-783*
Hemoglobin, *Mycobacterium haemophilum* requiring, 702
Hemolysin
alpha, 332
beta, 332
Listeria monocytogenes and, 382
Hemolysis
in colonial morphology, *316, 316-317, 317*
Streptococcus and, 348, *348,* 348t
Hemorrhagic fever
Crimean-Congo, 852-853
Dengue, 853
Ebola, 857
Marburg, 857
with renal syndrome, 856
skin manifestations of, 936
HEp2, 840
Heparin, specimen collection and, 243
Hepatic abscess, 767
Hepatitis, 859-866, *860, 860t, 861,* 862t, *863*
amplification systems for, 206
antigen detection in, 150-151
infectious, 859
serum, 859
tests for, 838t
Hepatitis A
epidemiology of, 860t
serologic testing for, 178
virus causing, 859-861
Hepatitis B
antigen detection in, 150-151
epidemiology of, 860t
as laboratory hazard, 36
serologic testing for, 178-179
Hepatitis C, 864
serologic testing for, 156, 178-179
Hepatitis C–like virus, 836t
Hepatitis D, 862-864
Hepatitis E, 864-865
Herpes simplex virus
cell cultures for, 841t
characteristics of, 866-868

Herpes simplex virus—cont'd
  cytopathic effect and, 840-841
  cytopathic effect of, *842*
  of eyelid, 1094
  genital, 1042-1043
  keratitis, 1095, 1097
  malignancy and, 1049
  molecular probe for, 198
  retinal, 1103
  skin manifestations of, 933-934, *934*
  transmission of, 232
Herpes zoster
  malignancy and, 1049
  serologic testing for, 179-180
Herpesvirus, 866-871
  cytomegalovirus, 868
  Epstein-Barr virus, 868-869
  herpes simplex virus, 866-867
  HHV-6, 870
  HHV-7, 870
  HHV-8, 870-871
  meningitis and, 985-986
  varicella-zoster virus, 870
Herpetic whitlow, 934
Heterolactic fermentation, 18
Heterophile antibody testing, 166, *166,* 178
Heterophyes heterophyes, eggs of, 802t
Heteroploid cell culture, 840
Heteroresistant staphylococci, 81
Heterotroph, 14
Hexacanth embryo, 806
Hidradenitis, 926
High performance liquid chromatography, 104, 670, 690
High-efficiency air filter, 37
High-level aminoglycoside resistance, 83
Hip replacement, bacteremia and, 1001
Hippurate, for rapid detection, 184t
Hippurate broth, 1127
Hippurate hydrolysis, *Streptococcus* and, 353-354
Histone, of eukaryotic cell, 7
Histoplasma spp., 909
Histoplasma capsulatum
  Accuprobes for, 195
  clinical infection with, 736t
  conjunctival infection and, 1092
  meningitis and, 983
  morphology of, 735t
  serologic testing and, 164
  staining of, 718, *719*
Histoplasma capsulatum var. *capsulatum*
  clinical infection with, 738
  epidemiology of, 737-738
  laboratory diagnosis of, 738-740, *739, 740*
Histoplasmosis, 737-740, *739*
HIV; *see* Human immunodeficiency virus
Hodgkin's lymphoma, 1049
Holding medium, 240, 243
Homolactic fermentation, 18
Hong Kong flu, 843
Hood, chemical fume, *39*

Hookworm, 818-819
  egg of, 814t
  life cycle of, *819*
  skin manifestations of, 941
Hospital infection; *see* Nosocomial infection
Host, intermediate
  of *Entamoeba histolytica,* 765
  of *Plasmodium,* 786
  of *Toxoplasma gondii,* 792-793
Host defense; *see also* Resistance, to infection
  central nervous system infection and, 976-977
  respiratory infection and, 884-885
  urinary tract infection and, 1015t
Host-parasite interaction, 211-235
  flora and, 212-217; *see also* Flora
  pathogenesis and; *see* Pathogenesis
Hot tub syndrome, 547
Hot-cold lysin, 332
Hugh-Leifson OF medium, 543
Human immunodeficiency virus, 847-849
  amplification systems for, 204-205
  antigen detection in, 150-151
  characteristics of, 847-849, 847t, *848*
  Cryptosporidium parvum infection in, 795
  eye infection and, 1104, *1104*
  immunoblot of, *848*
  laboratory safety and, 35
  meningitis and, 986-987
  Microspora infection in, 799
  molecular probe for, 198
  Mycobacterium avium infection in, 696
  opportunistic infection and, respiratory, 914-915
  Pneumocystis carinii and, 794-795
  serologic testing for, 156, 179
  Toxoplasma gondii and, 792
  urinary tract infection and, 1019
Human orf, 935
Human papilloma virus, 859
Humoral immune response
  definition of, 158
  malignancy and, 1047
  opportunistic infection and, 915
Hyaline hyphae, *712, 712-713, 713*
Hyaluronidase, 359
Hybridization
  format for, 192-194, *193*
  in-situ, 193
  in-solution, 193, *194*
  nucleic acid, 191
  sandwich, 193, *193*
  solid-state, 193, *193*
Hybridome, 132
Hydatid cyst disease, 813
Hydrogen peroxide, in phagocytosis, 224
Hydrogen sulfide
  Enterobacteriaceae and, 498
  lead acetate, 1127
Hydrolysis
  hippurate, 353-354
  to Tween 80, 686

Hymenolepis spp., 811, *812*
Hymenolepis diminuta
    characteristics of, 811
    egg of, 807t
Hymenolepis nana
    characteristics of, 811
    egg of, 807t
Hypersensitivity reaction to *Mycobacterium tuberculosis*, 693
Hyphae, *712, 712-713, 713*
Hypochlorite, 31-32
Hypogammaglobulinemia, 915
Hypotension, endotoxin causing, 228

I

Iatrogenic infection, definition of, 220
Icteric leptospirosis, 1074
Identification of microorganism; *see also* culture
    Aeromonas, 526-528, 526t, *527*
    Bacillus anthracis, 394
    Bordetella, 459-460
    Campylobacter, 533, 534t, 535
    of *Capnocytophaga canimorsus*, 1063-1064
    Clostridium spp., 599, *600*
    Corynebacterium diphtheriae, 378, *378,* 379t
    Erysipelothrix rhusiopathiae, 386, *386,* 1062-1063
    fungal, dermatophytic, *728,* 728-729
    Listeria monocytogenes, 384
    Mycobacterium spp., 681-692; *see also Mycobacterium* spp.,
        identification of
    Mycoplasma spp., 658-660, *660, 661, 662,* 662t, 663
    Neisseria meningitidis, 417
    Nocardia, 399, *399*
    nonfermenting gram-negative bacilli, 543, 545t-546t
    Plesiomonas, 529
    Staphylococcus, 336-338, 339t, *340,* 340-341
    of yeast, 749-753, *750-752*
    of zoonotic infection
        Bacillus anthracis, 1067-1068
        brucellosis, 1071-1072, *1072,* 1072t
IgA protease, 429
IgM antibody capture ELISA, 174, *175*
IgM anti-HBcAg, 862
Imipenem
    for *Haemophilus influenzae*, 434
    susceptibility of gram-negative organisms to, 92t
Immobilization test, *Treponema pallidum*, 171
Immune response
    antigens and antibodies in, 159-162
    categories of, 156-157
    host resistance to infection and, 156-158
    malignancy and, 1047
    nature of, 158-159
    pathogenicity and, 226-227
    primary, 161
    primary and secondary antibody response, 161-162
    secondary, 161-162
Immune system
    burn and, 1049-1050
    endotoxin affecting, 228
    flora and, 215-216

Immune system—cont'd
    reactivation tuberculosis and, 694
    respiratory infection and, 880-882
    Toxoplasma gondii affecting, 793-794
Immunity
    acquired, 157-158
    cell-mediated, 158
    definition of, 156
    humoral, 158
    innate, 156-157
    serologic testing and, 164
    to viral infection, 159
Immunization, laboratory safety and, 49; *see also* Vaccine
Immunoassay, 103
    enzyme; *see* Enzyme immunoassay
    for *Legionella*, 454
    mumps and, 845
    viral infection and, 838, *839*
Immunoblot of human immunodeficiency virus, *848*
Immunocompromised patient
    aging and, 1050-1051
    antibody response in, 156
    antimicrobial therapy for, 1050
    bacteremia and, 1000
    burn injury and, 1049-1050
    Candida infection in, 748
    chronic pneumonia in, 910
    community-acquired pneumonia in, 903-904
    Cryptosporidium parvum infection in, 795
    Cyclospora cayetanensis infection in, 798
    cytomegalovirus infection in, 868
    definition of, 1046
    fungal infection in, serologic testing for, 180
    histoplasmosis in, 738
    Listeria monocytogenes infection in, 383
    malignancy and, 1047-1049
    microorganisms associated with, 1047t
    Microspora infection in, 799
    Mycobacterium avium infection in, 696
    Mycobacterium haemophilum infection in, 702
    Mycobacterium kansasii infection in, 697
    organ transplant and, 1050
    pneumonia in, 907
    precipitin test in, for respiratory infection, 133-135, *133-135*
    respiratory infection in, 881
    susceptibility testing in, 65
    Toxoplasma gondii in, 792
Immunodiffusion, double, 167-168
Immunodiffusion test, 133
Immunofluorescence assay, 139-141, *141*
    in antigen detection, 139-141, *141*
    Chlamydia trachomatis and, 125, 125t
    virus and, 837
Immunoglobulin A, 161
Immunoglobulin D, 161
Immunoglobulin E, 161
Immunoglobulin G, *131*
    characteristics of, 161
    indirect fluorescent antibody test and, 171
    indirect fluorescent antibody test for, 172

Immunoglobulin G—cont'd
neonatal infection and, 165
TORCH infection and, 164
Immunoglobulin M
Borrelia burgdorferi and, 628
characteristics of, 161-162
false-negative test results and, 163
indirect fluorescent antibody test for, 171, 172
leptospiral bacteremia and, 626
Immunologic marker of AIDS, 849
Immunologic memory, 158
Immunologic method for *Neisseria gonorrhoeae* identification, 410, 411t
Immunosorbent assay
enzyme-linked; *see* Enzyme-linked immunosorbent assay
solid-phase, 142, *142*
Immunosuppressive therapy; *see also* Immunocompromised patient
definition of, 1047
Nocardia infection and, 396
Impetigo, 333, 921-923, 922t
Streptococcus pyogenes causing, 360
Implant soak solution, 256
In vitro testing
of oxacillin-resistant staphylococci, 81
susceptibility, 88-89
synergy, 101
Inception period for Epstein-Barr virus, 868
Incidence of disease, 123, 233-234
Incubation
for *Borrelia* infection, 626
of *Campylobacter,* 532-533
definition of, 234
in disk diffusion testing, 75
of fungal culture, 719
influenza virus and, 843
for leptospirosis, 626
of *Naegleria fowleri,* 773
for *Neisseria gonorrhoeae,* 408
Index
bacteriologic, 704
morphologic, 704
India ink preparation, 13, *13,* 1143
for fungi, 718, *718*
for rapid detection, 184t
Indicator system for complement fixation test, 169
Indifference
in antimicrobial therapy, 101
in combination antimicrobial therapy, 54
Indigenous flora, 212
Indirect, carrier particle agglutination assay, 166-167, *167*
Indirect ELISA, 173-174
Indirect enzyme immunoassay, 143
Indirect fluorescent antibody test
in antibody detection, *171,* 171-172
in antigen detection, 140
double, 172
for *Legionella,* 454-455
Indirect hemagglutination, 167
Indirect sandwich immunoassay, 143

Indole
Enterobacteriaceae and, 500
for rapid detection, 184t
Indole broth, Enterobacteriaceae and, *502*
Infant; *see also* Neonatal infection
botulism in, 595
bronchiolitis in, 899
Haemophilus infection in, 428
Listeria monocytogenes infection in, 383
respiratory syncytial virus and, 841, 841t, 844
serologic testing for, 165
urinary tract infection in, 1014
Infection
laboratory-acquired, 35-36
microscopic appearance of, *284-309*
nosocomial; *see* Nosocomial infection
pathogenesis of, 218-235; *see also* Pathogenesis
Infection-induced airway obstruction, 882
Infectious hepatitis, 859
Infectious mononucleosis
Epstein-Barr virus causing, 868
serologic testing for, 178
transmission of, 232
Infective endocarditis; *see* Endocarditis
Inflammation
as defense mechanism, 224, 226
innate immunity and, 157
microscopic specimen and, 274
Influenza virus
respiratory infection from, 842-843
seasonal trends in, 882
Influenza/parainfluenza virus, 841t
Infusion agar, brain-heart, 1141
Infusion broth, brain-heart, 1120
Ingestion in phagocytosis, 224, *224*
Inhalation anthrax, 393
Inhibition zone, 73
Inhibitory concentration, minimal, 69, 70t
Initial body of *Chlamydia trachomatis,* 1037
Innate immunity, 156-157
Inoculation
of anaerobic bacteria, 577-583, 580-583, *581*
incubation and, 580-583, *581*
media for, 577-578, 579t
procedure for, 578, 580
counter-streak technique of, 254-255, *255*
in disk diffusion testing, 75, *75*
liquefaction in, 251, 254
media for routine specimens, 250-252, 253t
media for unusual and fastidious bacteria, 251, 253t-254t
technique of, 250-252, 252t-254t, 255
Inoculum in susceptibility testing
preparation of, 67-68
standardization of, 68-69
Insertion sequence, 21
In-situ hybridization, 193
In-solution hybridization, 193
Interferon, 222
Intermediate cycle of yellow fever, 854

Intermediate host
  of *Entamoeba histolytica,* 765
  of *Plasmodium,* 786
  of *Toxoplasma gondii,* 792-793
Intermediate organism, definition of, 69
Intermediate results in susceptibility testing, 88
Intermittent bacteremia, 999
Intertrigo, 929
Intestinal infection; *see* Gastrointestinal infection
Intoxication, chemical, food poisoning and, 961, 963
Intracellular diplococcus, 1036
Intracellular parasite, obligate, 834
Intracellular pathogen
  immunity to, 158
  Salmonella, 954
Intrauterine device, culturing of, 257
Intravascular coagulation
  disseminated, 1002
  endotoxin causing, 228
Invasion by pathogen, 228
Invasive diarrhea syndrome, 951-952
Invasive specimen, unacceptable, 247
Inventory of hazardous chemicals, 46
Iodamoeba butschlii, 768t, 770, 772, *772*
Iodine as disinfectant, 31, 31t
Iron agar, Kligler, 1127-1128
Iron uptake of *Mycobacterium* spp., 686, *687*
Irritant, 46
Isolation, viral, 840-842, 841t, *842*
Isolation medium; *see also* Culture; Medium
  for *Staphylococcus,* 336
  for unusual and fastidious bacteria, 251
Isolator lysis-centrifugation system, 681
Isoniazid, 692t, 695
Isospora belli
  acid-fast stain for, 761
  enterotoxin-mediated diarrhea and, 951
  infection with, 797
  laboratory diagnosis of, 798, *798*
  life cycle of, 797
Ixodes spp., Lyme disease and, 982

J

Jacuzzi syndrome, 547
Janeway lesion, 928
Japanese encephalitis, 853
Jar, anaerobic, 582, *582*
Jarisch-Herxheimer reaction, syphilis and, 631
Jaw
  abscess aspirate of, 290
  bone biopsy of, 291
Joint Commission on Accreditation of Healthcare
      Organizations, 116

K

K antigen
  Enterobacteriaceae and, 465
  Salmonella and, 481
K1 antigen, 468-469
K1 antigen, *Escherichia coli* and, 472-473

Kala-azar, 780
Kanamycin, 692t
Kanamycin-vancomycin-lakes blood agar, 579t
Kaposi's sarcoma, 870-871
Karyosome, 761
Keratinolytic agent, 725
Keratitis, 1094-1098, *1095-1098*
  amebic, 774
  viral, 1095-1097
Kidney infection
  Escherichia coli and, 472
  streptococcal pharyngitis preceding, 886
Killing, in phagocytosis, 224, *225*
Kinetosome, 7
Kingella spp., 413t, 437t, 439-440, *440*
Kingella denitrificans, 408
Kinyoun stain, 677
Kirby-Bauer test, 73, 93
Kissing bug, 783
Kit system of identification of nonfermenting bacteria, 543
Klebsiella spp., 473-475, *474,* 474t
  classification of, 466t
  colony characteristics of, 748
  diarrhea caused by, 954t
  fermentation by, 19
  infection causes by, 467t
  nosocomial pneumonia and, 904
Klebsiella ornithinolytica, 474
Klebsiella oxytoca, 84
Klebsiella ozaenae, 474
Klebsiella planticola, 474-475
Klebsiella pneumoniae, 473
  diagnostic features of, 475t
  extended spectrum beta-lactamases and, 84
  interference with phagocytosis by, 225t
  in sputum culture, 65
Klebsiella rhinoscleromatis, 474
Klebsiella/Enterobacter-like organism, 314, *316*
Klebsielleae, 466t
Kligler iron agar, 1127-1128
  Enterobacteriaceae and, 496
  nonfermenting gram-negative rods and, 541, 541t, *542*
Kluyvera ascorbata, 488, 489t
Kluyvera cryocreascens, 488
KOH 10%, for rapid detection, 184t
KOH preparation for fungi, 718
KOH-glycerin, super quink, 1143
Koplik's spots, 846
Koserella trabulsii, 488
Krebs cycle
  illustration of, *20*
  pyruvate and, 19
Kurthia spp., 386t

L

Label
  for DNA/RNA proble, 194
  probe, 193-194
Labeling of specimen, 245, *246,* 247

Laboratory
   extent of service of. 681-682
   levels of, 681-682
   safety in, 34-51; *see also* Safety, laboratory
   sterilization and disinfection in, 25-33; *see also* Sterilization
     and disinfection
Laboratory release form, *246*
Laboratory specimen, 237-259; *see also* Specimen *entries*
Laboratory-acquired infection, 35-36
Lacrimal apparatus
   anatomy of, 1086
   infection of, 1100-1101
   plating guidelines for, 1106t
LaCross virus, 852
   central nervous system infection and, 987
Lactic acid, fermentation and, 18
Lactobacillus spp.
   characteristics of, 386t
   fermentation by, 18
   Gram stain of, *12*
Lactoferrin, 224
Lactophenol aniline blue, 1143
Lactophenol cotton blue, stain, 12, *13*
Lactose fermentation, 19-20, 314
   by Enterobacteriaceae, 496-498
Lactose nonfermenter, 314
Lancefield classification of *Streptococcus,* 349
Larva
   of fluke, 800
   roundworm, 814t
   skin manifestations from, 940
Larva migrans, 822
Lassa fever, 855-856
Latent phase of syphilis, 1040
Latex agglutination, 135-138, *136, 137,* 137t, 166
   Helicobacter pylori and, 535
   for pharyngitis, 887
   for viral gastroenteritis, 150
Lavage, bronchoalveolar
   microscopic appearance of, 293, 294, 300, 304, 305, 308
   microscopic specimen of, 285
   Mycobacterium culture from, 673
   opportunistic infection and, 915-916
Layered smear, 249
Leakage of specimen, 245
Lecithinase reaction of anaerobic bacteria, 590
Legionella spp.
   algorithm for identifying, *455*
   clinical infection with, 448-449
   community-acquired pneumonia and, 903
   culture and identification of, *451, 451-453, 453*
   direct fluorescent antibody test of, *450,* 450-451
   DNA probe for, 451
   epidemiology of, 448
   general characteristics of, 447
   microscopic examination of, 449, *450*
   molecular probes for, 195
   nucleic acid probe of, 455
   pneumonia and, 905
   sample handling of, 275

Legionella spp.—cont'd
   serology of, 454-455
   specimen collection of, 449
   susceptibility testing of, 455
   urine antigen test of, 453-454
Legionella pneumophilia, 172
Legionnaires' disease, 448-449
   antigen detection in, 147
Leifson stain, 266t
Leishmania spp., 779-780
   life cycle of, 781
Leishmania braziliensis, 780
Leishmania mexicana, 780
Leminorella grimontii, 488-489
Leminorella richardii, 488-489
Leprosy, 704-705, 930
Leptomeningitis, 977
Leptospira spp., 220
Leptospira canicola, 625
Leptospira icterohaemorrhagiae, 625
Leptospira interrogans, 625, 625-626, 932
Leptospira interrogans, 1074
Leptospirosis, 625-626, 1073-1074
Leptotrichia buccalis, 608t
Lesion
   culture media for, 252t
   specimen collection from, 239, 242
Lethal factor, 393
Leucine aminopeptidase test, 356
Leuconostoc
   bile esculin test and, 356
   biochemical identification of, 351t
   characteristics of, 369
   leucine aminopeptidase test and, 356
Leuken trap, 241, *241*
Leukocidin, Panton-Valentine, 332
Leukocyte
   cerebrospinal fluid and, 976
   phagocytosis and, 222-223, *223*
Leukocyte count
   malignancy and, 1048
   urinary tract infection and, 1021
Lid
   anatomy of, 1085
   infection of, 1093-1094
Ligase chain reaction, 199, 202
Limulus amebocyte lysis assay, 993-994
Lincosamide, 58
LINK2 Strep A Rapid Test, 177-178
Lipid A, 9
Lipooligosaccharide, 429
Lipopolysaccharide, 9
Liposome-mediated agglutination, 139, *140,* 140t
Liquefaction of specimen, 251, 254
Liquid chromatography
   high performance, 104
     Mycobacterium and, 670
   high-performance, for *Mycobacterium* spp., 690
Liquid medium
   colonial morphology and, 321, *322-324,* 324
   for *Mycobacterium* culture, 679-680

Liquid sample, 263-265
Listeria monocytogenes
    beta-lactam antibiotics and, 56
    characteristics of, 386t
    clinical infections of, 382-383
    colony morphology of, *386*
    cultural characteristics of, 383-384, *384*
    differentiation of, 384t
    Erysipelothix rhusiopathiae vs., 386, *386*
    gastrointestinal infection caused by, 957-958
    Hodgkin's lymphoma and, 1049
    identification of, 384
    meningitis and, 977
    microscopic examination of, 383, *383*
    ocular infection and, 1086
    phagocytosis and, 224
    physiology of, 382
    urinary tract infection and, 1019
    virulence factors of, 382
Listeriolysin O, 382
Lithotroph, 14
Liver disease, hepatitis; *see* Hepatitis *entries*
Liver fluke, 803, *803*
Loa loa, 823, 825-826
    conjunctival infection and, 1092
    retinal infection and, 1103
Load, microbial, 27, *28*
Loeffler coagulated serum slant, 1128
Loeffler medium, 377
Log sheet
    for in-house testing media, *113*
    preventive maintenance, *110*
Louse-borne fever, 627
Louse-borne typhus, 1077
Löwenstein-Jensen medium, 669, *698,* 1128-1129
Lower respiratory infection, 897t
    bronchitis and bronchiolitis, 896-900
    empyema, 912-913
    pneumonia, 900-912; *see also* Pneumonia
Lower urinary tract infection, 1013t, 1028
Lumbar puncture, 990-991
Lung; *see also* Respiratory *entries*
    abscess of, 767
    tuberculosis and; *see Mycobacterium tuberculosis*
Lutzomyia, as vector, 780
Lyme disease, 626-627, 628, 932
    central nervous system and, 982
    clinical manifestations of, 1058-1059
    epidemiology of, 1058-1059
    etiology of, 1058, *1058*
    laboratory diagnosis of, *1058,* 1059
    serologic testing for, 156
Lymphadenitis
    extrapulmonary tuberculosis and, 694
    Mycobacterium scrofulaceum causing, 699-700
Lymphatic spread, 952
Lymphocyte, 158
Lymphocytic choriomeningitis virus, 855, 986
Lymphogranuloma venereum, 643, *643*

Lymphokine
    immunity and, 158
    Mycobacterium tuberculosis and, 693
Lymphoma
    Burkitt's, 868
    Hodgkin's, 1049
Lysine-iron agar, *505,* 505
Lysin-iron agar, 1129
Lysis, 359
Lysis-centrifugation method, 1006
Lysogeny, 22
Lysosome
    of eukaryotic cell, 7
    phagocytosis and, 222
Lysozyme
    antimicrobial action of, 222
    as chemical barrier to microorganism, 157
Lyssavirus, 858, 988

M

M protein, 358-359
MacConkey agar, 1129-1130
    colonial morphology and, 313, 314, *315, 316*
    gastrointestinal infection and, 964t
    Mycobacterium spp. and, 689
    Mycobacterium chelonei and, 699
    Mycobacterium fortuitum-chelonei complex and, 702
    Pseudomonas aeruginosa on, *547, 547*
    sorbital, 1130
Macroconidia, 729
Macrodilution test, broth, 70
Macrolide antibiotic
    leptospires and, 626
    mechanism of action of, 58
Macrophage, 223
Madura foot, 938
Madurella grisea, 732t, 733
Madurella mycetomatis, 732t, 733
Maduromycosis, 938
Magnetic resonance imaging in sinusitis, 888
Mailing of etiologic agent, *244,* 244-245
Maintenance, preventive, 108-109
    log sheet for, *110*
Major outer membrane protein, 637
Malabsorption syndrome, 960
Malaria
    blood specimen for, 762
    life cycle stages of, *785*
    Plasmodium species causing, 788t
    species causing, 784-785
Malassezia furfur, 722, 722-723, 936, 938
Male patient
    Chlamydia trachomatis infection in, 1037
    genital tuberculosis in, 694
    gonorrhea in, 405
    Trichomonas vaginalis infection in, 778
    urinary tract infection in, 1015
Malignancy
    Epstein-Barr virus and, 868
    opportunistic infection in, 1047-1049

Malonate broth, 1130
Malonate test, 500, *563*
Mannitol salt agar, 1130
Mansonella spp., 826
Manual, quality control, 114
Manual rapid test, 185
Manual urine screening method, 1025-1026
Marburg hemorrhagic fever, 857
Margin, in colonial morphology, 317, *318*
Marker, for Epstein-Barr virus, 869t
Mask, *38*
Mastitis, *Corynebacterium ulcerans* causing, 380
Mastoiditis, 892
Material safety data sheet, 41, *42-45*
Matomys lensis, 855-856
Maturation/release of virus, 872
Mature schizont, *785*, 785
Maxillary sinus aspirate, 298
Maxillary sinusitis, 883
McFarland turbidity standards, 68, *69*
Measles
    German, 178, 846
        rash of, 935
        serologic diagnosis of, 178
    rubeola, 845-846, 935
Measurement in performance improvement, 116
Median infectious dose, 948
Medical Wastes Tracing Act, 47
Medium; *see also* Agar; Broth
    for *Aeromonas*, 525-526
    for anaerobic bacteria, 577-583, 579t, *580*
    bacteremia blood culture and, 1003-1004
    bacteriologic, 1117-1140
    for *Campylobacter*, 532
    colonial morphology of, 313
    cornea storage, 1111
    for *Corynebacterium diphtheriae*, 375, 377-378
    for Enterobacteriaceae, 465, 490-491
    for *Flavobacterium*, 557
    for fungi, 718-719, 719t, 1141-1143
    gastrointestinal infection and, 964t
    growth, types of, 14
    for *Haemophilus* spp., 430
    holding, 240, 243
    for *Mycobacterium* culture, 678-681, 679t
    for *Mycoplasma* spp., 658
    for *Neisseria gonorrhoeae*, 407-408, 407t
    for nonfermenting gram-negative rods, 541, 541t, *542*
    for *Plesiomonas*, 529
    quality control and, 109-110, 109t, *111, 113*
    for routine specimens, 250-251, 252t
    for *Streptococcus pyogenes*, 361
    transport, 243
    for unusual or fastidious bacteria, 253t-254t
    for *Vibrio*, 522, *522*
    for Yersinia spp., 487
Medusa head appearance *of Bacillus anthracis*, 394
Mefloquine, 786
Megacolon, toxic, 950, 960
Megasphaera elsdenii, 615t

Melioidosis, 929
Membrane
    cell, 57
    plasma, 7
    tympanic, 891
Membrane components of *Haemophilus influenzae*, 429
Membrane protein, major outer, 637
Membrane-bound enzyme immunoassay, 144-145
Memory, immunologic, 158
Meningismus, 977
Meningitis
    antigen detection in, 148-149
    aseptic, 977
    bacterial
        acute, 977-980, *978-980*
        Bacillus anthracis causing, 394
        Haemophilus influenzae causing, 429
        Mycobacterium tuberculosis causing, 695
        Neisseria meningitidis causing, 415
        pneumococcal, 365
        tuberculous, 674
    characteristics findings in, 992t
    Cryptococcus neoformans causing, 749
    fungal, 982-984, *984*
    host-pathogen relationship and, 977
    laboratory diagnosis of, 991
    susceptibility testing and, 67
    tuberculous, 980
    viral, 984-987, *985*
        immunity to, 159
Meningococcemia
    Neisseria meningitidis causing, 415
    petechial lesions in, *927*, 927
Meningoencephalitis
    amebic, 989-990
    definition of, 977
    Naegleria fowleri similar to, 773
    viral, 987-988
Merogony of *Cryptosporidium parvum*, 796
Merozoite
    of *Cryptosporidium parvum*, 797
    of *Plasmodium* spp., *785*, 785-787
Merthiolate-iodine-formalin, 758, 758t
MES, 1131
Mesophile, 14
Metabolic end product analysis, 591
Metabolism
    bacterial, 16
    nucleic acid, 59
Metabolite, *58*, 58-59
Metacercaria of fluke, 800
Metagonimus yokogawai, 802
    eggs of, 802t
Methaenamine silver, 795
Methicillin-resistant *Staphylococcus*, 60, 82, 341
Methyl red test, 498, *501*
Methyl red-Voges-Proskauer medium, 1131
Methylase, 60
Methylbacterium extorquens (Pseudomonas mesiphilica), 554
Methylene blue stain, 12, *13*

Metronidazole, mechanism of action of, 59
MGA-TP test, 631
MHA-TP test, 167
MIC endpoint, onscale, 90
Microaerophilic bacteria, 15
Microaerophilic environment, 529
Microbial load, 27, *28*
Microbial morphotype, 272t, 274
Microbiology laboratory, quality control in, 106-115; *see also*
      Quality control
Micrococcus, 331, 332t
Microconidia, 729
Microdilution susceptibility test, broth
    advantages and disadvantages of, 93-94
    automated reader devices for, 85
    characteristics of, *70,* 70-71
Microgametocyte, 785, 785
MicroID test, 186t
Microimmunofluorescence
    Chlamydia pneumoniae and, 641
    Chlamydia trachomatis and, 649
Micrometer, calibration of, 764
MicroScan rapid detection method, 186t, 188-189
Microscope
    characteristics of, 266, 271
    counting of cells under, 15
Microscope-assisted labeled-reagent techniques, *171,*
      171-172
Microscopic examination, 140-141, *141,* 261-309
    anaerobic bacteria, 576-577
    Bacillus anthracis, 394
    background material in, 273t
    Borrelia spp., 626, *626*
    Campylobacter, 533
    of *Capnocytophaga canimorsus,* 1063
    Chlamydia trachomatis, 646, *646*
    Clostridium spp., 597
    Enterobacteriaceae, 490
    Erysipelothix rhusiopathiae, 385, *385*
    examples of, *282-309*
      common bacterial infections, *284-285*
      fungal infection, *300-303*
      gram-negative infections, *292-297*
      gram-positive bacteria bacillary infections, *286-291*
      local and contaminating materials and, *282-283*
      parasitic infection, *304-307*
      polymicrobial infection, *298-299*
      viral infection, *308-309*
    fungal
      blastomycosis and, 736
      chromoblastomycosis and, 731
      histoplasmosis, 739, *739*
      subcutaneous phaeohyphomycosis, 734
    of fungi
      dermatophytic, 728
      examples of, *300-303*
      general principles of, 717-718, *718*
      Sporothrix schenckii, 730
    of gastrointestinal infection, 963
    grading or classifying materials, 275-277

Microscopic examination—cont'd
    gram stain for, 272t
    Haemophilus influenzae, 431, *431*
    Legionella, 449-451, *450*
    leptospires, 626
    Listeria monocytogenes, 383
    Mycobacterium avium, 696
    Neisseria gonorrhoeae, 407, *407,* 408
    Neisseria meningitidis, 416, *416*
    Nocardia, 398
    observing pathogens in, 271t
    Plesiomonas, 528
    of prepared material, 273-275
    procedures in
      acid-fast staining of mycobacteria, 269-270
      Calcofluor white stain, 270
      Fungi-Fluor kit, 270
      Gram stain, 267-268
      Wright-Giemsa stain, 271
    quality control of, 278
    reporting of, 277-278
    for respiratory infection
      epiglottitis, 894
      pertussis, 895
      pharyngitis and, 887
      pneumonia, 907-908, *909,* 911
      sinusitis, 890
    sample preparation for, *263-265,* 263-266
    stains for, 266, 266t
    Staphylococcus, 335-336, 335-341, *336, 336-338,* 339t, *340*
    of stool specimen, parasitic infection and, 759-761
    Streptococcus pneumoniae, 365-366
    terminology in, 271, 273
    Treponema pallidum, 630
    types of, 266, 271
    of urine specimen, 1025-1026
    Vibrio, 517
    of virus, *308-309,* 839
    zoonotic infection and
      Bacillus anthracis, 1067
      brucellosis, 1071
      Erysipelothrix rhusiopathiae and, 1062
      leptospirosis, 1074
      Pasteurella multocida and, 1061
      tularemia, 1069
      Yersinia pestis, 1057
Microspora, 799-800
Microsporidia, 799-800
Microsporum audouinii, 727
Microsporum canis
    characteristics of, 727, *727*
    growth on rice grains, 729
Microsporum gypseum, 727, *727*
Middle ear
    infection of; *see* Otitis media
    sinusitis and, 888
Middlebrook agar, 678-680, 679t, 1131
    Mycobacterium fortuitum and, 702
    Mycobacterium gastri and, 704
    Mycobacterium genavense and, 704

Middlebrook agar—cont'd
   Mycobacterium haemophilum and, 702
   Mycobacterium kansasii and, 697
   Mycobacterium marinum and, 699
   Mycobacterium phlei and, 704
   Mycobacterium simiae and, 702
   Mycobacterium smegmatis and, 703
   Mycobacterium vaccae and, 704
   Mycobacterium xenopi and, 700
Midstream urine collection, 240
Midstream urine specimen, 1022-1023
Miliary tuberculosis, 694
Millipore sampler, 257
Minimal bactericidal concentration, 98-100, *99*
Minimal bactericidal concentration test, 98-100, *99*
Minimal inhibitory concentration, 69, 70t
   broth microdilution test and, 78t-79t
   broth minimal bactericidal concentration and, 98-100, *99*
   disk diffusion test and, 78t-79t
   E test and, 87
   quality control ranges of, 91t
   vancomycin and, 99, *99*
   in vitro susceptibility testing and, 88-89
   zone of inhibition and, 73-75
Minimal medium, 14
Minisystem for anaerobic bacteria, 591
MIO test, 496
Miracidium of fluke, 800
Mission statement, 115
Mitchison's medium, 679t
Mite-borne infection, 232
Mitochondria, 7
Mitsuokella spp., 608t
Mixed acid fermentation, 18-19
Mobile genetic element, 21
Mobiluncus spp.
   characteristics of, 605
   clinical significance of, 603t
   reclassified, 610
Mobiluncus curtsii spp. curtsii, 599
Modified potassium nitrate assimilation medium, 1142
Moeller decarboxylase test medium, 1124
Moist heat, 28-29
Moisture, 109
Mold, *vs.* yeast, 711
Molecular detection method, 191-206
   amplification, 198-199, *200-201,* 202-203
   hybridization formats in, 192-194, *193, 194*
   probe technology in, 194-195, 195t, *196, 197,* 197-199,
      202-203
   types of, 191-192
Molecular probe
   antimicrobial resistance and, 103
   for *Candida albicans,* 195
   for fungus, 195
   for *Legionella* spp., 195
   for respiratory infection, 195
   for sexually transmitted disease, 195, 198
Molluscum contagiosum, 934-935, *935*

Monitor, performance
   commercial, 118
   establishment of, 116
Monkey, *Mycobacterium simiae* and, 701-702
Monobactam
   listing of, 55
   spectrum of, 56
   structure of, 55
Monoclonal antibody, 160
   antigen detection and, 131-133, *132*
   for *Neisseria gonorrhoeae* identification, 411t
   for parasitic infection, 763
Monomicrobial infection, 273, 275
Mononucleosis
   direct hemagglutination in, 166
   Epstein-Barr virus causing, 868
   serologic testing for, 178
   transmission of, 232
Moraxella spp.
   antimicrobial agents for, 59
   characteristics of, 413t
Moraxella atlantae, 560
Moraxella catarrhalis
   beta-lactamase tests and, 89
   bronchitis and, 899
   clinical infection with, 417
      sinusitis, 887
   community-acquired pneumonia and, 903
   empiric drug therapy and, 882-883
   growth of, *417*
   laboratory diagnosis of, 417-418
   respiratory infection caused by, otitis media, 891
   as respiratory tract flora, 214
      reevaluation of, 879
Moraxella nonliquefaciens, 558-559
Moraxella phenylpyruvica, 560
Moraxella-like genera, 558-559
Morbidity rate, definition of, 234
Morganella morganii
   characteristics of, 477, 478t
   classification of, 466t
   infection causes by, 467t
Morphologic index, 704
Morphology
   bacterial cell, 10-13, *11-13*
   of *Clostridium,* 597-599, *598*
   colonial, 311-325; *see also* Colonial morphology
Morphotype, microbial, 272t, 274
   of anaerobic bacteria, 576-577, 584
Mortality rate, definition of, 234
Mosquito-borne infection, 854
Motility
   Burkholderia gladioli and, 552
   of *Campylobacter,* 533
Motility organelle, 7
Motility test
   for anaerobic bacteria, 589-590
   Enterobacteriaceae and, 500
   indole, ornithine, 496, *504-505*
   for *Listeria monocytogenes, 382*

Motility test medium, 1131-1132
MOTT bacteria, 680, 696-705
Mount, direct wet, of stool specimen, 759-760
Mounting fluid, fungal, 1143
Mouth, usual flora of, 213-214
Mouth pipetting, 34
Mucocutaneous infection, 380; *see also* Skin infection
Mucoid material, *264,* 264-265
Mucor spp., 745, *745*
    brain abscess and, 981
    characteristics of, 745, *745*
    incubation of, 719
    malignancy and, 1048
Mucormycosis
    lacrimal apparatus and, 1100
    rhinocerebral, 981
Mucosa, invasive diarrhea syndrome and, 951-952
Mucus
    antibodies in, 222
    as cleansing mechanism, 221
    as organic soil, 27-28
Mueller-Hinton agar, 75, 1132
    Vibrio and, 523-524
MUG assay, 471
Multitest conventional-chromogenic enzyme test, 410, 411t
Mumps, 845
    meningitis and, 986
Murein layer of cell wall, 8-9
Mus musculus, 855
Muscle infection, 822
Muscle tissue, 307
Mutation, definition of, 21
Mycelium, 712, *712*
Mycetoma, 938-939, 939t
    Actinomadura causing, 399
    eumycotic, 731-733, *732,* 732t, *733*
        clinical infection, 732
        epidemiology of, 731-732
        laboratory diagnosis of, 732-733, 732t, *733*
        organisms causing, 729
    Nocardia infection and, 397
Mycobacteria other than tubercle bacilli, 696-705
    isolation of, 680
    keratitis and, 1094
Mycobacterium spp., 667-692
    acid-fast stain procedure for, 269-270
    cell wall of, 9
    central nervous system and, laboratory diagnosis of, 993
    chronic pneumonia and, 909
    concentration of, 677
    culture methods for, 678-681, 679t
    epidemiology of, 669
    general characteristics of, 670
    identification of, 681-692, 683t-684t
        arylsulfatase in, 686-687
        biochemical, 682, 685
        catalase, 686, *686*
        chromatography in, 689-690
        colony morphology and, 682
        growth rate and recovery time in, 682

Mycobacterium spp.—cont'd
    identification of—cont'd
        hydrolysis to Tween 80, 686
        inhibitory tests in, 687-688
        iron uptake in, 686, *687*
        laboratory levels and, 681-682
        MacConkey agar and, 689
        niacin accumulation in, 685, *685*
        nitrate reduction in, 685, *686*
        photoreactivity in, 682
        pyrazinamidase in, 687, *687*
        serology in, 691
        slow *vs.* rapid growth and, 689
        TCH in, 688
        tellurite reduction in, 688, *688*
        temperature and, 682
        urease in, 687, *688*
    interference with phagocytosis by, 225t
    molecular probes for, 194, 195
    nontuberculous, 696-705
    orbital infection and, 1099
    safety considerations with, 671-672
    sample handling of, 275
    skin infection due to, 929-930
    specimens of
        collection and processing of, 672-674
        digestion and decontamination of, 674-676
    staining of, *12,* 677
    urine culture for, 1028
    urine screening in, 1026
Mycobacterium asiaticum, 702-703
Mycobacterium avium complex
    DNA hybridization for, 690
    epidemiology of, 696
    infection caused by, 696
    laboratory diagnosis of, 696-697
    stool culture of, 674
    susceptibility testing of, 697
    tellurite reduction and, 688
Mycobacterium bovis
    pyrazinamidase and, 687
    tuberculosis caused by, 695-696
Mycobacterium celatum, 701
Mycobacterium chelonei
    characteristics of, 698, 699
    iron uptake and, 686
Mycobacterium flavescens
    characteristics of, 703
    high salt medium and, 688
Mycobacterium fortuitum, 695, 698
Mycobacterium fortuitum-chelonei complex
    arylsulfatase and, 687
    characteristics of, 698
    MacConkey agar and, 689
Mycobacterium gastri, 704
    catalase reaction and, 686
Mycobacterium genavense, 704
Mycobacterium gordonae, 702
    DNA hybridization for, 690

Mycobacterium haemophilum
  catalase reaction and, 686
  culture media for, 680
  infection with, 702
Mycobacterium kansasii
  chronic pneumonia and, 910
  DNA hybridization for, 690
  epidemiology of, 697
  infection caused by, 697
  laboratory diagnosis of, 697-698, *698*
  nitrate reduction and, 685
Mycobacterium leprae, 704-705, 930
Mycobacterium malmoense, 701, *701*
Mycobacterium marinum
  arylsulfatase and, 687
  catalase reaction and, 686
  characteristics of, 699, *699*
  pyrazinamidase and, 687
Mycobacterium marinum, 929-930
Mycobacterium nonchromogenicum, 703
Mycobacterium paratuberculosis, 704
Mycobacterium phlei, 704
Mycobacterium scrofulaceum, 699-700, *700*
Mycobacterium simiae, 701-702
Mycobacterium smegmatis, 703-704
Mycobacterium szulgai
  arylsulfatase and, 687
  characteristics of, 701
  nitrate reduction and, 685
Mycobacterium terrae-trivale complex, 703
Mycobacterium thermoresistibile, 703
Mycobacterium triviale, 688
Mycobacterium tuberculosis, 692-696
  amplification systems for, 205-206
  catalase reaction and, 686
  cellular immunity defects and, 914
  central nervous system and, 980-981
  chronic pneumonia and, 909, 910
  colonization *vs.* infection and, 880
  culture media for, 678, 679
  DNA hybridization for, 690-691
  Hodgkin's lymphoma and, 1049
  identification of, 695, *695*
  immunity to, 158
  as laboratory hazard, 35-36
  nitrate reduction and, 685
  phagocytosis and, 224
  rapid detection methods for, 183
  rifampin for, 59
  skin infection due to, 929
  susceptibility testing of, 691-692, 692t
  tuberculosis caused by
    extrapulmonary, 694-695
    primary, 693
    reactivation, 693-694
    treatment of, 695-696
Mycobacterium ulcerans, 702, 930
Mycobacterium vaccae, 704
Mycobacterium xenopi, 687, 700-701
Mycobactosel medium, 679t

Mycolic acid, 689-690
Myconecrosis, laboratory diagnosis of, 931
Mycoplasma spp.
  cell wall lacking in, 10
  clinical infection with, 655-658, 655t, 656t, *657*
  comparative properties of, 637t
  flow diagram for isolation of, *660*
  general characteristics of, 653, *654, 655, 655*
  indigenous to humans, 655t
  laboratory diagnosis of, 658-663
    culture and, 658
    identification and, 658-660, *660, 661, 662,* 662t, 663
    specimen collection and transport, 658
Mycoplasma fermentans, 658
Mycoplasma genitalium, 657-658
Mycoplasma hominis, 656-657, 662t
  extragenital, 660-661
  Ureaplasma urealyticum with, *662*
  vaginosis and, 1039
Mycoplasma pneumoniae
  amplification systems for, 206
  clinical infection with, 655-656
  detection of, 662t
  direct hemagglutination in, 166
  electron micrograph of, *654, 655*
  indirect fluorescent antibody test for, 172
  molecular probes for, 195
  respiratory infection caused by, otitis media, 891
  seasonal trends in, 882
  skin manifestations of, 932-933
Mycosel/mycobiotic agar, 1142
Mycosis, 722-742; *see also* Fungal infection; Fungus
Myonecrosis, 595, 924-925, *925*
Myroides odoratus (Flavobacterium odoratum), 557

N

N-acetyl-L-cysteine, for specimen digestion-decontamination, 675
NaCl test, 357
Naegleria fowleri, 772-774, *773, 989-990*
Nagler test, 598
Nail fungal infection, 725, 925
  specimen from, 717
NALC-sodium hydroxide, 675
Nalgerne filtering procedure, 255
Nalidixic acid, 59
Name, genus and species, 4-5
NAP test, 687
Nasopharyngeal swab, 843
Nasopharynx
  barriers to infection and, 884
  cleansing mechanisms of, 221
  Corynebacterium pseudodiphtheriticum infection of, 380
  flora of, 214
National Bureau of Standards, 107
National Committee for Clinical Laboratory Standards
  anaerobic bacteria testing and, 619
  disk diffusion testing and, 74
  Haemophilus influenzae susceptibility testing and, 77-79
  quality control and, 109

National Committee for Clinical Laboratory Standards
 —cont'd
  susceptibility testing guidelines of, 65, 66
  treatment guidelines for gonorrhea, 414-415
Natural immunity, 157
Natural particle agglutination assay, 165-166, *166*
Necator americanus, 818
Neck, meningitis and, 977
Necrolysis, toxic epidermal, 334
Necrosis, 693
Necrotic debris, 274
Necrotizing enterocolitis, 215
Negative predictive value of test, 123, 124-125
Neisseria spp., 401-422
  anticoagulant in specimen of, 243
  antimicrobials effective against, 59
  characteristics of, 402, *403,* 404
  culture media for, 252t
  nonpathogenic, 418-422, 418t, 419t, 420t, *421, 422*
  pathogenicity and host range of, 404t
Neisseria cinerea, 413t, 419t, 420t, 421
Neisseria dentrificans, 419t, 420t, 421
Neisseria elongata, 419t, 420t, 422
Neisseria flavescens, 419t, 420t, 422
  characteristics of, 413t
Neisseria gonorrhoeae; see also Gonorrhea
  amplification systems for, 204
  antimicrobial resistance of, 414, 414t
  beta-lactam antibiotics and, 55
  beta-lactamase tests and, 89
  cellular structure of, *405*
  characteristics of, 413t
  chromosomally mediated resistant, 80-81
  conjunctival infection and, 1089
  dacryoadenitis and, 1100
  diarrhea and, 961
  epidemiology of, 405
  identification of, 408-414, 411t
    carbohydrate utilization methods in, 410, *411,* 411t, 412
    colonial morphology and, 408
    definitive, 409-410
    future methods for, 413-414
    immunologic methods in, 410
    microscopic morphology and, 408
    nonculture methods in, 410, 411t, 412-413
    oxidase test for, 408-409, *409*
  infections caused by, 405-406
  laboratory diagnosis of, 406-408, *406-408,* 407t
  media for, 314
  ocular infection and, 1086
  penicillinase-producing, 80
  pharyngitis caused by, 885
  pili of, 227
  proliferation of, 227
  susceptibility testing of, 80-81
  transformation in, 22
  treatment of, 414-415
  urinary tract infection and, 1016
  virulence factors of, 404-405

Neisseria lactamica, 419t, 420t, 421-422
  characteristics of, 413t
Neisseria meningitidis, 415-418
  beta-lactam antibiotics and, 55
  carrier of, 213, 233
  central nervous system and, 993
  characteristics of, 413t
  clinical infection caused by, 415, *415*
  conjunctival infection and, 1089
  humoral immunity defect and, 915
  laboratory diagnosis of, *416,* 416-417
  meningitis caused by, 979, *979*
  ocular infection and, 1086
  proliferation of, 227
  susceptibility testing and, 81
  susceptibility testing of, 80-81
  treatment of, 415
  vaccine for, 415-416
  virulence factors of, 415
Neisseria mucosa, 419t, 420t, 422
Neisseria polysaccharea, 418, 419t, 420t, 421
Neisseria sicca, 413t
Neisseria subflava, 419t, 420t, 422
Neisseria weaveri, 419t, 420t, 422
Neisseriaceae, 549-550
Neonatal infection
  bacteremia and, 1002-1003
  chlamydial, 643-644, 644t
  enteropathogenic *Escherichia coli,* 955
  Escherichia coli causing, 472
  genitourinary infection associated with, 656t
  herpes, 867
  of *Klebsiella pneumoniae,* 474
  Listeria monocytogenes, 383
  Mycoplasma hominis, 656t
  Neisseria gonorrhoeae, 1036
  Neisseria gonorrhoeae causing, 406
  Neisseria meningitidis causing, 415
  scalded skin syndrome as, 928
  Streptococcus agalactiae causing, 362
  Ureaplasma urealyticum, 656t
  urinary tract, 1014
  viral meningitis and, 987
Neonate, cerebrospinal fluid characteristics of, 976
Neurocysticercosis, 990
Neutralization test
  antistreptolysin-O, 170
  Treponema pallidum immobilization, 171
  viral, 170
Neutropenia, 1048
Neutrophil, 222
New York City agar, 408, 1132
Niacin accumulation, 685, *685*
Nicotinamide adenosine dinucleotide
  diphtheria toxin and, 376
  Haemophilus influenzae and, 427
Nicotinic acid, 685
Nigrospora, 745
  characteristics of, 745
Nitrate disk, 589

Nitrate reduction
  Enterobacteriaceae and, 505-506
  Mycobacterium and, 685, *686*
Nitrate reduction broth, 1132
Nitrofurantoin, susceptibility of gram-negative organisms to, 92t
Nitroreductase, 685
Nocardia spp.
  brain abscess and, 982
  cell wall of, 9
  clinical infections with, *397,* 397-398
  culture media for, 254t
  general characteristics of, 396, 396t
  laboratory diagnosis of, 398-399, 398t
  odor of, 320
  orbital infection and, 1099
  physiology of, 396, 396t
  virulence factors of, 396-397
Nocobactin, 397
Nomenclature, 4-5
Non-A non-B hepatitis, epidemiology of, 860t
Nonautomated susceptibility test, *87,* 87-88
Nonchromogenic bacteria, 682
Noncritical material, 28, 29t
Noncultural identification of *Streptococcus,* 356, 358
Nondiphtheria *Corynebacterium,* 375, 380-382
Nonencapulated strain of *Haemophilus,* 428-429
Nonfermenter, lactose, 314
Nonfermenting gram-negative bacilli, 539-561
  Chromobacterium violaceum, 560-561
  dysgonic fermenters, 559-560
  dysgonic fermenters and, 559-560
  EO-2, 559
  eugonic fermenters and, 560
  general characteristics of, 539-546
    biochemical, 540, *540, 541,* 542
    clinical infections and, 539-540
    identification methods for, 543, 545t-546t
    initial clues to, 543, 544t
  HB-5 organisms, 560
  nonmotile, 556-559
    Balneatrix spp., 558
    Chryseomonas spp., 558
    Flavimonas spp., 558
    Flavobacterium spp., 556-557
    Moraxella spp., 558-559
    Moraxella-like genera, 558-559
    Oligella app, 558-559
    Sphingobacterium spp., 557-558
  with peritrichous flagellation
    Agrobacgterium spp., 555-556
    Alcaligenes spp., 554-555
    CDC group IVc-2, 556
    Ochrobactrum anthropi, 556
    Oligella urealytica, 556
    Psychrobacter spp., 559
  terminology changes in, 1145
Nonhemolytic *Streptococcus,* 348-349, 348t
Noninvasive specimen, unacceptable, 247

Nonmotile bacteria
  Acinetobacter as, 550
  nonfermenting, 552
  nonfermenting gram-negative bacilli, 556-559
    Balneatrix spp., 558
    Chryseomonas spp., 558
    Flavimonas spp., 558
    Flavobacterium spp., 556-557
    Moraxella spp., 558-559
    Moraxella-like genera, 558-559
    Oligella app, 558-559
    Sphingobacterium spp., 557-558
Nonoxidating, nonfermenting bacteria, 544t
Nonpathogenic *Neisseria* spp., 418-422, 418t, 419t, 420t, *421, 422*
Nonphotochromogenic organism, *Mycobacterium malmoense,* 701
Nonpigmented bacteria
  Bacteroides spp., 607t
  Prevoltella spp.
    clinical significance of, 607t
    laboratory diagnosis of, 610
Nonpitting *Bacteroides* spp., clinical significance of, 607t
Nonroutine specimen, processing of, 255-258
Nonselective medium, 250
Non–spore-forming bacilli, gram-positive
  Actinomyces spp., 599, 602, *603,* 604
  Bifidobacterium spp., 604-605, 604t-605t
Non–spore-forming rods, gram-positive
  Arcanobacterium haemolyticum, 381
  Corynebacterium, 375-380; *see also Corynebacterium* entries
  Erysipelothix rhusiopathiae, 385-386
  Listeria monocytogenes, 382-384, *384*
  Rhodococcus, 381
  Rothia dentocariosa, 381
Nontreponemal test for syphilis, 168, 630, 1041
Nontuberculous mycobacteria, 692
Nontyphoidal salmonella, 954
Normal flora; *see* Flora, normal
North American blastomycosis, 735-737
Norwalk virus, 850-851, 958
Nose, flora of, 214
Nosema, 799
Nose-to-hand contact, 230
Nosocomial infection
  bacteremia as, 999
  definition of, 234
  empiric drug therapy for, 883
  pneumonia as, 897t, 904-905
  Pseudomonas aeruginosa causing, 547
  Pseudomonas maltophilia causing, 549
  scalded skin syndrome as, 928
  Staphylococcus aureus causing, 333
  urinary tract, 1016
Novobiocin susceptibility test, of staphylococci, *338,* 338
NOW test for *Legionella,* 454
Nucleic acid
  antimicrobial agents affecting, 59
  detection of, for *Bordetella,* 459
  sequence of, 191

Nucleic acid based amplification, 202
Nucleic acid hybridization, 191
Nucleic acid probe
    Chlamydia trachomatis and, 647-648
    for *Legionella,* 455
    for *Neisseria gonorrhoeae* identification, 410, 411t, 412
    viral infection and, 838
Nucleolus, 7
Nucleus, cell, 7
Numbers, cell, 15-16
Numeric code, identification, 185
Nutrient agar, 1133
Nutrient medium, 14
Nutrition, of bacterial cell, 13-16, *15*

O

O antigen
    Aeromonas and, 524
    Enterobacteriaceae and, 465
    Escherichia coli and, 468-469
    Salmonella and, 481
O/129 susceptibility of *Vibrio,* 517, *518*
Obesumbacterium proteus, 489
Obligate aerobe, 15
Obligate anaerobe, definition of, 568
Obligate intracellular parasite, 834
Obstetric complications, 362
Obstruction
    airway
        bronchitis and, 899
        infection-induced, 882
    sinusitis and, 889
Occult bacteremia, 999
Occupational Safety and Health Administration, 39
Ochrobactrum anthropi, 556
Ocular infection, 1083-1112; *see also* Eye; Eye infection
Ocular micrometer, 764
Odor
    in colonial morphology, 319-320
    in nonfermenting bacteria, 552
Oerskovia, 386t
Oligella, Moraxella and, 560
Oligella spp., 558-559
Oligella urealytica, 556
Oligonucleotide, 198-199
Onchocerca volvulus, 940, *940*
Oncosphere, 806
ONPG for rapid detection, 184t
Onscale MIC endpoint, 90
Onychomycosis, 725, 936
Oocyst
    of *Cryptosporidium parvum,* 797
    of *Cyclospora cayetanensis,* 798, *799*
    of *Isospora belli,* 798, *798*
    of *Plasmodium,* 788
Operational analysis of tests, 123-125
Ophthalmia neonatorum
    gonorrheal, 1036
    Neisseria gonorrhoeae causing, 406

Opisthorchis sinensis, 803, 803
    eggs of, 802t
Opportunistic infection
    Acinetobacter, 550
    Bacillus cereus, 395t
    Candida spp. as, 748-749
    common, 1046t
    Corynebacterium xerosis as, 380
    definition of, 1046
    Enterobacteriaceae, 466-479
        Citrobacter spp., 478-479
        Edwardsiella spp., 478
        Enterobacter spp., 475-476, 475t, *476*
        Erwinia spp., 478
        Escherichia coli, 468-473; *see also Escherichia coli*
        Hafnia spp., 477
        Klebsiella spp., 473-475, *474,* 474t
        Morganella spp., 477, 478t
        Pectobacterium spp., 478
        Proteus spp., 477, 478t
        Providencia spp., 477-478, 478t
        Serratia spp., *476,* 476-477
    fungal, 742-747
        Absidia, 742, 742
        Alternaria, 742, 743
        Aspergillus, 743, 743
        Aureobasidium, 742
        Beauveria, 743, 743
        Chaetomium, 743, 743-744
        Chrysosporium, 744, 744
        Cladosporium, 744, 744
        Culvularia, 744, 744-745
        Cunninghamella, 744, 744
        Curvularia, 744, 744-745
        Epicoccum, 745
        Fusarium, 745, 745
        Geotrichum, 745, 745
        Mucor, 745, 745
        Nigrospora, 745
        Paecilomyces, 745-746, *746*
        Penicillium, 746, 746
        Phoma, 746, 746
        Pithomyces, 746, 746
        Rhizopus, 746, 746-747
        Scopulariopsis, 747, 747
        Syncephalastrum, 747, 747
        Trichoderma, 747, 747
        Ulocladium, 747, 747
    human immunodeficiency virus infection and, 849
    intestinal Apicomplexa, 795-799
    Nocardia, 396
    pathogens causing, 219-220, 220t
    respiratory, 913-916
        cellular immunity defects and, 914-915
        granulocytopenia and, 913-914
        humoral immunity defects and, 915
        laboratory diagnosis of, 915-916
Opsonin, 223-224
Opsonization, 223-224

Optical immunoassay, 145, 838, *839*
Optocin, 350, 352, 366
Oral cavity
    anaerobic bacteria in, 570t
    usual flora of, 213-214
Oral herpes, 867
Orbit, anatomy of, 1086
Orbital cellulitis, 1098-1099
Orbital infection, 890, 1098-1100
Orf, human, 935
Organ culture for viral isolation, 834
Organ transplant, 1050
Organelle, 7
Ornithodoros, 627
Oropharyngeal colonization, 904-905
Oropharyngeal infection, 406
Oropharynx, 884
Orthomyxoviridae, 836t
Orthonitrophenyl galatopyranoside, 498, *499*
Osler's node, 928
Osteomyelitis
    sinusitis complications and, 890
    staphylococcal, 335
Otitis externa, 547
Otitis media
    clinical manifestations of, 891
    complications of, 892
    empiric drug therapy for, 882-883
    epidemiology of, 891
    etiology of, 891
    laboratory diagnosis of, 886t, 892
    pathogenesis of, 891-892
    sinusitis and, 888
    Streptococcus pneumoniae causing, 364-365
Ouchterlony immunodiffusion test, 133, 167-168
Outcome monitor, 116
Outer membrane protein, major, 637
Oxacillin
    minimal inhibitory concentration of, 70t
    staphylococci resistant to, 81-82
Oxacillin screen plate, 82
Oxalic acid, 675
Oxidase
    nonfermenting bacteria reacting to, *544*
    for rapid detection, 184t
Oxidase negative bacteria, 552
Oxidase test, 408-409, *409*
Oxidase-positive reaction, 543
Oxidation
    in bacterial cell, 16, 17
    pyruvate and, 19
Oxidation-reduction potential, 568
Oxidative-fermentative medium, 1133
Oxidizer, 540, 544t
Oxi-Ferm test, 186t
Oxygen
    anaerobic bacteria and, 567
    bacterial growth, 15
    sinusitis and, 889
    toxicity of, 568

P
PACE system, 197
Paecilomyces spp., 745-746, *746,* 1102
Pandemic
    of cholera, 516
    of human immunodeficiency virus infection, 848
    of plague, 1056
Panteoa spp., 466t
Panton-Valentine leukocidin, 332
Papilloma virus, human, 859
Papovavirus of eyelid, 1094
Paracoccidioides, 981-982
Paracoccidioides brasiliensis
    brain abscess and, 981-982
    clinical infection with, 736t, 741
    epidemiology of, 741
    laboratory diagnosis of, *741,* 741-742
    morphology of, 735t
Paradoxic effect in minimal bactericidal concentration test,
        100
Paraffin bait technique, 399
Paragonimus westermani
    characteristics of, 803-804
    eggs of, 802t
    gastrointestinal infection and, 959
    sputum specimen of, 762
Parainfluenza virus, 843-844
Paralytic shellfish poisoning, 963
Parasite, virus as, 834-874; *see also* Viral infection
Parasitic infection, 755-831
    Apicomplexa, 783-799; *see also* Apicomplexa
    central nervous system, 988-990, *989*
    definition of, 212
    of eye
        blepharitis and, 1094
        conjunctival, 1092
        corneal, 1097-1098
        retinal, 1103
    gastrointestinal, 958-960
        history of, 949-950
        stool sample for, 241
    helminths, 800-826; *see also* Helminth
    human immunodeficiency virus infection and, 848-849
    immunologic diagnosis of, 763
    microscopic appearance of, *304-307,* 307
    Microspora, 799-800
    opportunistic, 1046t
    polymerase chain reaction for, 203t
    protozoa, 763-783; *see also* Protozoa
    quality assurance in laboratory and, 763-764
    skin, *940, 940-941, 941*
    specimen of
        biopsy, 763
        blood smear, 762-763
        cerebrospinal fluid, 763
        duodenal aspirate, 761
        fecal, 757-761, 758t, *759*
        sigmoidoscopy, 761
        sputum, 762
        urine, vaginal, or urethral, 762

Paronychia, 925
Paroxysm of malaria, 785
Paroxysmal phase of whooping cough, 458
Particle agglutination assay
    in antigen detection, 135-141
        latex, 135-138, *136, 137,* 137t
        liposome-mediated, 139, *140,* 140t
        staphylococcal coagglutination, *138, 138-139, 139*
    direct, natural, 165-166, *166*
    indirect, carrier, 166-167, *167*
Parvovirus B19, 847
Pasco rapid detection method, 186t, 189
Pasteurella spp., 441, *441, 442t, 443, 443*
Pasteurella bettyae, 442t
Pasteurella caballi, 442t
Pasteurella canis, 442t
Pasteurella haemolytica, 442t
Pasteurella multocida, 441, *441,* 442t, 443, 1060-1062, *1061*
    beta-lactam antibiotics and, 55
    in bite wound, 232
Pasteurella pneumotropica, 442t
Pasteurellosis, 1060-1062, *1061*
Pasteurization, 29, 29t
Pathogen
    blood-borne
        as laboratory hazard, 36
        OSHA regulations for, 39
    characteristics of, 5, 7
    normal flora and, 879
    opportunistic, 219-220, 220t; *see also* Opportunistic
        infection
    respiratory tract, 880t
Pathogenesis
    adherence in, 227
    dissemination of organism in, 228-230
    Entamoeba histolytica and, 766
    epidemiology and, 233-234
    host resistance factors in, 220-227; *see also* Resistance,
        to infection
    invasion by organism in, 228
    pathogenicity and, 219-220
    proliferation of organism in, 227-228
    tissue damage in, 228, 229t, 230t
    transmission routes and, 230-233, 231t
    virulence in, 220
Pathway, Embden-Meyerhof-Parnas, 17, *17*
Patient-collected specimen, 240-241
Pectobacterium spp., 467t, 478
Pediculus humanus humanus, 627
Pediococcus spp.
    bile esculin test and, 356
    biochemical identification of, 351t
    characteristics of, *369,* 369-370
    leucine aminopeptidase test and, 356
Pelvic inflammatory disease
    Chlamydia trachomatis causing, 643
    gonorrhea and, 1035
    Neisseria gonorrhoeae causing, 405
ʻPenetration, viral, 872

Penicillin
    as beta-lactam agent, 55
    beta-lactamase–resistant, 341
    enterococci resistant to, 83
    for streptococcal infection, 79-80
        neonatal, 362
    structure of, 55
    syphilis and, 631
Penicillinase-producing *Neisseria gonorrhoeae,* 80
Penicillin-binding protein, 55
Penicillium spp., 746, *746*
Penis, chancroid of, *431*
Pentose phosphate pathway, 17-18, *18,* 19
Peptidoglycan
    in cell wall, 8-9, *9*
    synthesis of, 55
Pepto-Bismol for diarrhea, 968
Peptone-yeast extract-glucose broth, 1133
Peptostreptococcus spp., 611, *615,* 615t, 616t
    aspiration pneumonia and, 905
Perforation of tympanic membrane, 892
Performance improvement, 106, 116-120
    benchmarking in, 117-118
    customer concept and, 117
    fixing of process in, 117
    mission statement for, 116
    performance monitors in, 116
    problem/action form in, 116-117
    process *versus* outcome in, 116
Performance monitor
    commercial, 118
    establishment of, 116
Perfusate, 256
Pericardial fluid, 252t
Pericarditis, 1000
Peripheral blood mononuclear cell, 849
Peripheral chromatin, 767
Periplasmic flagella, 624
Periplasmic space, 9
Peritoneal fluid, 252t
Peritonitis
    bacteremia and, 1000
    Streptococcus pneumoniae causing, 365
Peritrichous flagellation, nonfermenting gram-negative
        bacilli with
    Agrobacterium spp., 555-556
    Alcaligenes spp., 554-555
    CDC group IVc-2, 556
    Ochrobactrum anthropi, 556
    Oligella urealytica, 556
Peroxisome, 7
Personnel
    proficiency testing of, 112, 114, *115*
    safety of, 671
Pertussis
    antigen detection in, 146
    clinical manifestations of, 894-895
    complications of, 895
    epidemiology of, 894

Pertussis—cont'd
   etiology of, 894
      Bordetella pertussis and, 457-462; *see also Bordetalla entries*
   laboratory diagnosis of, 886t, 895
   pathogenesis of, 895
Pertussis toxin, 458
Petechial lesions in meningococcemia, *927,* 927
Petragnani medium, 679t
Petri dish
   in fungal laboratory, 722
   mycology laboratory and, 722
Phaeoannellomyces wernickii, 724, *724*
Phaeohyphomycosis, 733-734, *734*
   subcutaneous, 733-734, *734*
Phage, 22
Phage group II staphylococci, 333
Phagocytic cell, 157
Phagocytosis
   proliferation of pathogen and, 227-228
   steps in, 222-224, *223-225*
Pharyngitis
   clinical manifestations of, 885
   complications of, 886
   epidemiology of, 885
   etiology of, 885
   laboratory diagnosis of, 886t, 887
   pathogenesis of, 885
   streptococcal, antigen detection in, 145-146, *147*
   Streptococcus pyogenes and, 359-360
Phenol, 672
Phenolic compounds, 32
Phenolphthalein, 686-687
Phenol-soap mixture, 672
Phenotype, 20
Phenotypic characteristics, 5
Phenotypic switching, 748
Phenylalanine deaminase, 500
Phenylalanine deaminase agar, 1134
Phenylalanine deaminase test, *504*
Phenylethyl alcohol agar, 1134
   anaerobic bacteria and, 579t
Pheohyphomycosis, 729
Phialidia, 713
Phialophora spp., 715
   incubation of, 719
Phialophora verrucosa, 731, *731,* 732t, 939, 939t
   chromoblastmycosis caused by, 732t
Phlebotomus, as vector, 780
Phoma, 746, *746*
Photochromogen, 682
Photoreactivity, 682
Physical barrier to infection, 157
Physical methods of sterilization and disinfection, 26, 28-30
Picornaviridae, 836t
Piedra
   black, 723
   white, 723, 749
Piedraia hortae, 723, *723*
Pig as reservoir of *Yersinia pestis,* 486

Pigment
   of *Bacillus,* 392
   in colonial morphology, 319, *320*
   malarial, 787
Pigmented bacteria
   gram-negative anaerobic, 609-610
   nonfermenting, 552
   Prevotella spp., 607t
Pilus, 10
   adherence and, 227
Pinta, 631, 932
Pinworm, *815,* 815-816
   cellophane tape procedure for, 761
Piperacillin, 92t
Pipetting, mouth, 34
Pithomyces, 746, *746*
Pitting *Bacteroides* spp., 607t, 610
Pityriasis versicolor, 936, 938
Placenta, culture of, 252t
Plague, *1056, 1056-1058, 1057*
Planococcus, 331
Plaque, bacterial, 213-214
Plasma membrane
   of eukaryotic cell, 7
   of prokaryotic cell, 8
Plasmid, 21
Plasmid-mediated penicillinase-producing gonococcal strain
      of *Neisseria gonorrhoeae,* 414
Plasmodium spp., 784-790
   life cycle of, *787*
   species causing malaria, 784-785
Plasmodium falciparum
   characteristics of, 790, *791*
   comparison of, 788t
   gametocyte of, *791*
   malaria caused by, 785-786
   ring form trophozoites of, *791*
Plasmodium malariae
   characteristics of, 789, *790*
   comparison of, 788t
Plasmodium ovale
   characteristics of, 789-790, *790*
   comparison of, 788t
Plasmodium vivax
   characteristics of, 789, *789*
   comparison of, 788t
   malaria caused by, 785-786
Plate, in disk diffusion testing, 75-76
Plate count, direct, 15-16
Plate reading, 313
Plating, eye infection and, 1106t
Pleistophora, 799
Pleocytosis, 976
Pleomorphic organism, 376-377
Plesiomonas spp., 528-529
   characteristics of, 518t
   enterotoxin-mediated diarrhea and, 951
   Vibrio vs., 522
Plesiomonas shigelloides, 956
Pleural effusion, 912-913

Pleurisy, 694
Pleuropneumonia-like organism, 655
Pneumococcal meningitis, 365
Pneumococcal pneumonia, 231, 364-365
Pneumocystis carinii
    antibody detection for, 147-148
    cellular immunity defects and, 914
    clinical infection with, 794
    diagnosis of, 916
    laboratory diagnosis of, 794-795, *795*
    life cycle of, 794
    malignancy and, 1049
    stains for, 761
Pneumonia, 900-912
    acute, 900-901
    aspiration, 897t, 905-906
    bacteremia and, 1000
    chronic, 908-912, *909, 911*
    colonization *vs.* infection and, 880
    community-acquired, 897t, *901, 901-903, 902*
        bronchitis and, 899
        clinical manifestations of, 902-904
        empyema and, 912
        epidemiology of, 902
        etiology of, 901-902
    drug therapy and, empiric, 882-883
    humoral immunity and, 915
    in immunocompromised patient, antibody detection for, 147-148
    Legionnaires' disease and, 448-449
    malignancy and, 1049
    Mycoplasma pneumoniae causing, 655-656
    Neisseria meningitidis causing, 415
    nosocomial, 897t, 904-905
    pneumococcal, 364-365
    Pneumocystis carinii; see Pneumocystis carinii
    staphylococcal, 334
    transmission of, 231
Poisoning, food; *see* Food poisoning
Poliovirus, 850, 985
Polyclonal antibody, 133, 160
Polymerase, DNA, 199, *200-201*
Polymerase chain reaction, 198
    bacterial genetics and, 20
    Mycobacterium and, 670
    for viral infection, 203t
Polymicrobial infection, 273, 275
    bacteremia, 999, 1002
    microscopic appearance of, *298-299*
Polymicrobic specimen, 240
Polymorphonuclear leukocyte, 222-223, *223*
Polysaccharide, 9
Polysaccharide capsule, 160-161; *see also* Capsule
Polyvinyl alcohol, 758, 758t
Pontiac fever, 449
Population study, serologic, 164
Pork tapeworm, 811, 813
Porphyrin test, 433-434
Porphyromonas spp., 570
    characteristics of, 614t
    culture of, 583

Porphyromonas spp.—cont'd
    fluorescence of, 587-588
    identification of, 587
    presumptive identification of, 611t
Porphyromonas endodontalis, 606
Posada Wernicke disease, 740-741
Positive predictive value of test, 123, 124-125
Postanalytical activity, 106
Poststreptococcal glomerulonephritis, 170
Potassium cyanide test, 506
Potassium hydroxide
    for fungi, 718
    urinary tract infection and, *1017*
Potassium nitrate assimilation medium, 752
Potassium nitrate assimilation medium, modified, 1142
Potassium tellurite, 688
Potato dextrose agar, 1142
Potato flakes agar, 1142
Potato infusion agar, Bordet-Gangou, 459
Pott disease, 694-695
Pott's puffy tumor, 890
Pouch, anaerobic, 583, *583*
Poxvirus, 934-935, *935*
PPNG strain of *Neisseria gonorrhoeae,* 414
Preanalytical activity, 106
Precaution, universal, 36, 37
Precipitation assay, 167-170
    counterimmunoelectrophoresis, 168
    double immunodiffusion, 167-168
    flocculation, 168, *169*
Precipitin reaction, 156
Precipitin test
    counterimmunoelectrophoresis as, 133-135, *135*
    tube and agar, 133, *133, 134*
Predictive value of test, 123-125
Pregnancy
    Listeria monocytogenes infection in, 383
    rubella and cytomegalovirus testing in, 164
    TORCH infection in, serologic testing for, 164-165
    Toxoplasma gondii infection in, 791-792
Preseptal cellulitis, 1098-1099
Preservative, specimen, 242
    stool, 757-758, 758t
Pressure sore, 1000
Preventive maintenance, 108-109, *110*
Prevotella spp.
    characteristics of, 614t
    clinical significance of, 607t
    fluorescence of, 587-588, 588, *589*
    laboratory diagnosis of, 609-610
    presumptive identification of, 612t
    vaginosis and, 1039
Primaquine, for malaria, 786
Primary bacteremia, 999
Primary cell culture, viral, 840
Primary immune response, 161
Primary inoculation technique, 250-252, 252t-254t, 255
Primary syphilis, 629, 1040
Primer, 199
Prioritization in specimen processing, 247-248, 247t

Probe
  DNA; *see* DNA probe
  labels for, 193-194
  molecular, antimicrobial resistance and, 103
  nucleic acid
    Chlamydia trachomatis and, 645t, 647-648, 648t
    for *Legionella,* 455
    for *Neisseria gonorrhoeae* identification, 410, 411t, 412
    viral infection and, 838
Probe technique, stain for, 266t
Probe technology, 191-203
Probe-mediated stain, 266
Problem/action form, 116-117, 117t
Proficiency testing of personnel, 112, 114
Profile number, 185
Proglottid, 806
Prokaryote, 5
Prokaryotic cell, *6,* 6t, 7-10
  compared with eukaryote, *6,* 6t
  cytoplasmic, 7-8
  envelope of, 8-10, *8-10*
Proliferation of pathogen, 227-228
Prophylaxis, rabies, 859
Propionibacterium spp.
  characteristics of, 604t, *605,* 605-606
  clinical significance of, 603t
Propionibacterium acnes, 570-571
  bacteremia and, 1002
  conjunctival infection and, 1089
  as flora on skin, 213
  lacrimal apparatus and, 1100
Propionibacterium propionicus, 1100
Propionic acid fermentation, 18
Prostatic secretion, 1028
  Trichomonas vaginalis in, 778
Prostatitis, 1013t, 1020
Prosthetic device
  bacteremia and, 1001
  Corynebacterium jeikeium infection and, 380
Proteae, 466t
Protection
  eye, *38*
  levels of, 37t
Protective antigen, 393
Protective clothing, 672
Protein
  A, 332
  anti-M, 227
  blood, innate immunity and, 157
  capsid, 872
  cerebrospinal fluid and, 976
  of eukaryotic cell, 7
  M, 358-359
  major outer membrane, 637
  penicillin-binding, 55
Protein expression, 20
Protein I, 404
Protein II, 404-405
Protein synthesis
  antimicrobial agents affecting, 57-58
  resistance to antibiotic and, 60

Proteus spp., 477, 478t
  infection causes by, 467t
  swarming colonies of, 317, *318*
Proteus mirabilis, 477
  antibiograms for, 92t
  bacteremia and, 1000
  beta-lactam antibiotics and, 56
  odor of, 320
Proteus vulgaris, 477
Protozoa, 763-783
  flagellates, blood and tissue, *779, 779-783, 781-783*
  intestinal
    ameba; *see* Ameba, intestinal
    ciliates, 774-775
    flagellates, 775-779, *775-779*
    Pneumocystis carinii formerly classified as, 794
    tissue ameba, 772-774
Providencia spp., 477-478, 478t
  classification of, 466t
  infection causes by, 467t
Providencia alcalifaciens, 477, 953t
Providencia rettgeri, 477
Providencia rustigianii, 478
Pryazinamidase, 687, *687*
Pseudallescheria boydii, 732, 732t, *733*
  brain abscess and, 982
Pseudobacteremia, 999
Pseudocel agar, 1134
Pseudohyphae
  Cryptococcus neoformans, 749
  in yeast identification, 752
Pseudomembranous colitis, 596
Pseudomonad
  commonly encountered, 547-554, 547t
    Acinetobacter spp., 549-550, *550*
    Pseudomonas aeruginosa, 547, 547-549, 548
    Pseudomonas alcaligenes, 550
    Pseudomonas fluorescens, 549
    Pseudomonas mendocina, 550
    Pseudomonas pseudoalcaligenes, 550
    Pseudomonas stutzeri, 550
    Strenotrophomonas maltiphilia, 549
  name changes of, 551-554
    Brevundimonas diminuta, 553
    Brevundimonas vesicularis, 553
    Brevundimonas vesicularis (Pseudomonas vesicularis),
      553
    Burkholderia cepacia, 551-552
    Burkholderia gladioli, 552
    Burkholderia pseudomallei, 552-553, *553*
    Comamonas spp., 554
    Methylbacterium extorquens, 554
    Ralstonia pickettii, 553-554
    Roseomonas spp., 554
    Shewanella putrefaciens, 554
    Sphingomonas paucimobilis, 553
Pseudomonas spp.
  beta-lactamase tests and, 89
  exotoxin A of, 884
  nosocomial pneumonia and, 904

Pseudomonas spp.—cont'd
  susceptibility testing and, 65
  Vibrio vs., 522
Pseudomonas aeruginosa
  antibiograms for, 92t
  antimicrobial agents for
    beta-lactam, 56
    nucleic acid metabolism and, 59
  aspiration pneumonia and, 905
  beta-lactam antibiotics and, 56
  characteristics of, *547, 547-549, 548*
  colonial morphology of, *322*
  exotoxins of, 229t
  folliculitis and, 923
  host defense and, 884-885
  interference with phagocytosis by, 225t
  keratitis and, 1094
  nutritional requirements of, 14
  odor of, 320
  scum of, *322*
  skin manifestations of, 927
Pseudomonas alcaligenes, 550
Pseudomonas fluorescens, 549
Pseudomonas mallei, glanders and, 929
Pseudomonas mendocina, 550
Pseudomonas pseudoalcaligenes, 550
Pseudomonas pseudomallei, 929
Pseudomonas stutzeri, 550
Psittacosis, 649-650
Psychrobacter spp., 559
Psychrophile, 14
Puff ball, 321, *321*
Puffy tumor, Pott's, 890
Pulmonary anthrax, 393
Puncture, lumbar, 990-991
Purified protein derivative test for tuberculosis
  primary, 693
  reactivation, 694
Purulence
  cocci in, 262
  in microbial sample, 275
Purulent meningitis, 991
Pus
  fresh specimen of, 239-240
  Nocardia infection and, 397, *397*
  as organic soil, 27-28
  wound cleaning and, 239
Pyelonephritis, 1012, 1016
  culture for, 1027
  Escherichia coli causing, 472
  urine screening in, 1025-1026
Pyocyanin, 547
Pyoderma, 921-925, 922t, 923-925
Pyodermal infection, 360
Pyogenic streptococci, 349
Pyoverdin, 549
PYR hydrolysis, 184t, 353-354, 361
Pyrazinamide, 692t, 695
Pyrimethamine/sulfadoxine, 786
Pyruvate, 19

Pyruvic acid, 18
Pyuria, 1021
  Chlamydia trachomatis infection and, 1037
  urine specimen and, 1023, 1024, 1026

Q

Q fever, 1078
Q-Probe, 118
Quad-Ferm test, 186t
Quality control, 107-115
  for anaerobic bacteria specimen processing, 576t
  for anaerobic bacteria susceptibility testing, 620
  analytical analysis of tests and, 121-122
  choosing method of, 125-127, *126*
  clinical analysis of tests and, 122-123
  colonial morphology in, 313
  definition of, 106
  in direct microscopic interpretation, 278
  equipment testing and, 108-112, 109t, *110, 111*
  manual for, 114
  operational analysis of tests and, 123-125
  in parasitology laboratory, 763-764
  performance improvement and, 116-120, 117t
  personnel competency and, 112, 114, *115*
  reagent and, 112
  stock cultures and, 114
  in susceptibility testing, 90, 91t, 92-93, 92t, 93t, 112, 112t
  susceptibility testing and, 112, 112t
  temperature and, 107-108
  test validation and, 127
Quantitative buffy coat system, 788
Quaternary ammonium compound, 32
Quellung reaction, 367
Quinolone, 59

R

Rabies, 858-859, 988
RACE acronym, 47
Racquet hyphae, 712, *712*
Radiation as sterilization method, 30
Radiographic evaluation
  of reactivation tuberculosis, 694
  sinusitis and, 888
Radioimmunoassay
  in antigen detection, 145
  antimicrobial agents and, 103-104
Radiometric Bactec isolation method, 680
Raised elevation of colony, 317, *318*
Ralstonia pickettii (Pseudomonas pickettii), 553-554
Rapid carbohydrate degradation test
  for *Neisseria gonorrhoeae,* 410
  for *Neisseria gonorrhoeae* identification, 411t
Rapid detection method, 182-189
  automated, 185, 188
  carbohydrate utilization or chromogenic substrates in, 185, 188-189
  commercially available, 186t
  definition of, 183
  evaluation of, 189
  for isolated colonies, 184t, 185

Rapid detection method—cont'd
  manual, 185
  microscopic methods for, 183, 184t
  microscopic methods of, 184t
Rapid grower, definition of, 682
Rapid hippurate, 184t
Rapid identification
  of *Aeromonas,* 527-528
  of *Plesiomonas,* 529
  of staphylococci, 340-341
Rapid modified Wright-Giemsa stain, 271
Rapid plasma reagin test, 168, 177
  Borrelia burgdorferi and, 628
  Treponema pallidum and, 630
Rapid screening of urine, 1024-1025
Rapid susceptibility testing, 94
Rapid urease test, 184t
Rash
  Rocky Mountain spotted fever and, 931
  of rubella, 935
  of rubeola, 935
  Streptococcus pyogenes and, 359
  virus causing, 845-847, 933-936
Rat-bite fever, 929, *1064, 1064-1065, 1065*
Rat-borne disease, 855-856
Reactivation tuberculosis, 693-694
Reader device, automated, 85
Reagent, quality control of, 113
Recombination, genetic, 21
Recovery time, 682
Rectal gonorrhea, 1035-1036
Red blood cell, malaria and, *785*
Redox potential, 568
Reduvid bug, 783
Refrigeration of specimens, 243
Regan-Lowe transport medium, 459
Regulations for mailing of etiologic agent, 244-245
Reiter syndrome, 960
Relapsing fever, 627
Release form, laboratory, *246*
REMEL/IDS RapID STR color guide, 187t
Renal infection
  Escherichia coli causing, 472
  streptococcal pharyngitis and, 886
Renal tuberculosis, 694
Reoviridae, 836t, 854-855
Repeat culture, 240
Replication, viral, 835
Replicator, Steer's, 72, *73*
Report
  Chlamydia trachomatis and, 649
  of direct specimen examination, 277
  gram smear, 276, 277
  infection, 234
  of susceptibility test results, 65, 67
Reporting protocol, selective, 67, 68
Reproduction
  of fungi, *713, 713-714, 714*
  of Microspora, 799

Reproduction—cont'd
  of *Plasmodium,* 786-788
  viral, 835
Requisition, laboratory, 245
Reservoir
  definition of, 234
  of *Yersinia pestis,* 486
Resident flora, 212
Resistance
  antimicrobial
    Acinetobacter as, 550
    of anaerobic bacteria, 618
    of *Chryseomonas luteola,* 558
    in enterococci, 82-84
    extended spectrum beta-lactamase and, 84
    of *Flavimonas oryzhabitans,* 558
    Haemophilus influenzae and, 426, 434
    mechanism of, 59-60, 59t
    molecular probes in identifying, 103
    of *Mycobacterium tuberculosis,* 692
    oxacillin, in staphylococci, 81-82
    Pseudomonas aeruginosa and, 547-548
    of staphylococci, 332
    streptococcal infection and, 80
    susceptibility testing for; *see* Susceptibility testing of antimicrobial
    urinary tract infection and, 1018
  to infection, 156-158, 220-227, 226t
    antimicrobial substances and, 222
    cleansing mechanisms in, 221-222
    immune response and, 226-227
    inflammation in, 224, 226
    normal flora and, 222
    phagocytosis in, 222-224, *223-225,* 225t
    physical barriers in, 220-221
Resistant organism, definition of, 69
Respiration, cell, 16-17
Respiratory burst in phagocytosis, 224
Respiratory infection, 877-916
  anaerobic bacteria causing, 570
  anatomy and, *883,* 883-884
  anthrax and, 393, 1066-1067
  antigen detection in
    in immunocompromised patient, 147-148, *148*
    Legionnaires' disease and, 147
    pertussis and, 146
    streptococcal pharyngitis and, 145-146, *147*
    viral, 147, *148*
  Chlamydia trachomatis psittaci, 649-650
  coccidioidomycosis, 740-741
  Corynebacterium pseudodiphtheriticum, 380
  Cryptococcus neoformans causing, 749
  culture media for, 252t
  diphtheria as, 376
  general concepts of, 879-883
    empiric antimicrobial therapy and, 882-883
    immune status and, 880-882
    normal flora and, 879-880
    seasonal and community trends and, 882

Respiratory infection—cont'd
  Hantavirus, 856
  helminth, fluke, 803-804, *804*
  histoplasmosis, 738
  Legionella, 448-449
  lower, 897t
    bronchitis and bronchiolitis, 896-900
    empyema, 912-913
    pneumonia, 900-912; *see also* Pneumonia
  molecular probe for, 195
  Mycobacterium spp., 672-673
    Mycobacterium avium complex, 696
    Mycobacterium kansasii, 697
    Mycobacterium xenopi, 700
    Mycoplasma pneumoniae, 655-656
  Nocardia causing, 397
  nonbacterial, 664t
  opportunistic, 913-916
    cellular immunity defects and, 914-915
    granulocytopenia and, 913-914
    humoral immunity defects and, 915
    laboratory diagnosis of, 915-916
  Pneumocystis carinii, 794-795
  pneumonia; *see* Pneumonia
  Pseudomonas aeruginosa causing, 547
  Rhodococcus equi, 380
  specimen for, storage of, 243-244
  sputum collection for, 240-241
  transmission of, 230-231
  tuberculosis as, 693-695; *see also Mycobacterium
      tuberculosis*
  upper, 883-895
    epiglottitis, 892-894
    otitis media, 891-892
    pertussis, 894-895
    pharyngitis, 885-887
    sinusitis, 887-890
  viral, 838t, 842-845, *844*
    adenovirus, 844-845
    antigen detection in, 147, *148*
    coronavirus, 845
    influenza virus, 842-843
    parainfluenza virus, 843-844
    respiratory syncytial virus, 841, 841t, 844
    rhinovirus, 845
  virulence factors of, 884-885
Respiratory syncytial virus
  bronchitis and, 896
  cell cultures for, 841t
  characteristics of, 844
  cytopathic effect of, 841
Respiratory system
  anaerobic bacteria in, 570t
  cleansing mechanisms of, 221
  fungal specimen from, 717
  Neisseria spp. as flora of, 418
  usual flora of, 214
Restriction enzyme, 23
Reticuloendothelial cytomycosis, 737-739

Retina
  anatomy of, 1086
  infection of, 1102-1103, *1103*
Retroorbital abscess, 890
Retroviridae, 836t
Rhabditiform larva, 814t, 818
Rhabdoviridae, 836t
  rabies and, 858-859
Rheumatic fever, 360
Rheumatoid factor, 163-164
Rhinocerebral mucormycosis, 981
Rhinocladiella aquaspersa, 732t, 939, 939t
Rhinosinusitis, 889
Rhinovirus, 845
Rhizoid, 712, *712*
Rhizoid margin of colony, 317, *318*
Rhizopus spp., *746,* 746-747
  brain abscess and, 981
  characteristics of, *746,* 746-747
  incubation of, 719
Rhodococcus spp., 381, 386t
Rhodotorula spp., 749
  characteristics of, 749
  urease test and, 752
Ribavirin, 843
Ribonucleic acid
  antimicrobials interfering with, 59
  in bacterial genetics, 20
  nucleic acid hybridization and, 191
Ribosome
  of eukaryotic cell, 7
  protein synthesis inhibition and, 57
Rice extract agar, 1142
Rice grain medium, 729, 1142
Rice-water stool, 519
Rickettsia spp.
  comparative properties of, 637t
  general characteristics of, 1076
Rickettsia prowazekii, 1077
Rickettsia rickettsii, 931, 1075-1076
  indirect fluorescent antibody test for, 172
Rickettsia tsutsugamushi, 1077
Rickettsia typhi, 1076-1077
Rickettsiae, 1076-1080
  conjunctival infection with, 1092
  general characteristics of, 1077, 1077t
  Q fever and, 1078
  skin infection caused by, 931
  spotted fever group of, 1075-1076
  trench fever and, 1077-1078
  typhus and, 1075-1077
Ricksettsialpox, 1076
Rifampin
  concentration of, for tuberculosis, 692t
  for *mycobacterium tuberculosis,* 59
  for tuberculosis, 695
Rift Valley fever, 852, 853
Right-to-know, employee, 41
RIM test, 186t
Ringworm, 715, 724-725, 724-729, 725t, *726-728,* 936, *937,* 938

River blindness, 940
RNA virus, 836t
Rochalimaea quintana, 1077-1078
Rocky Mountain spotted fever, 931, 1075-1076
Rod
    Brevundimonas vesicularis, 553
    gram-negative
        Aeromonas, 524-528
        Klebsiella, 473-475
        Salmonella, 479-484; *see also Salmonella entries*
        Yersinia pestis, 486
    Mycobacterium spp.; *see Mycobacterium entries*
    non–spore-forming Gram-positive
        Arcanobacterium haemolyticum, 381
        Corynebacterium, 375-380; *see also Corynebacterium*
            entries
        Erysipelothix rhusiopathiae, 385-386
        Listeria monocytogenes, 382-384, *384*
        Rhodococcus, 381
        Rothia dentocariosa, 381
Roseola, 936
Roseomonas spp., 554
Rotavirus, 850, 958
Rothia dentocariosa, 381-382
Roundworm
    Ascaris lumbricoides, 816-818, *817, 818*
    Dracunulus medinensis, 826
    Enterobius vermicularis, 815, *815-816, 816*
    filarial, 823, 824t, *825*
    general characteristics of, 813-815
    hookworm, 818-819
    larva migrans caused by, 822
    loa loa, 823, 825-826
    Mansonella spp., 826
    Strongyloides stercoralis, 819-820, *821,* 822
    Trichinella spiralis, 822, *822*
    Trichuris trichura, 816, *816*
    Wuchereria bancrofti, 823, *825*
RPR test, 168
    for syphilis, 177
Rubella
    clinical infection of, 846
    immune status testing to, 164
    serologic diagnosis of, 178
Rubeola, 845-846
    skin manifestations of, 935

S

Sabin-Feldman dye test, for *Toxoplasma gondii,* 794
Sabouraud dextrose agar, 1142
Saccharolytic, 540
Safety, laboratory
    back safety and, 48
    biologic hazards and
        disposal of, 41
        handling of, 35-40, 36t, 37t, *38-40*
    chemical, 41, *41-46,* 46
    electrical, 48
    fire, 47-48, 47t
    first aid training and, 48

Safety, laboratory—cont'd
    fungal, 722
    gas storage and, 48
    general principles of, 35
    hazardous waste reduction and, 47
    immunization and, 49
    material safety data sheet and, *41-45*
    in mycobacteriology laboratory, 671-672
    in specimen collection, 245
    training for, 49
Safety-pin appearance, of *Yersinia pestis,* 486
Salmonella spp., 479-484
    antigenic structures of, 481, *481*
    beta-lactam antibiotics and, 56
    biochemical differentiation of, 480t
    biochemical reactions of, 494t
    capsule of, 10
    Citrobacter and, 478-479
    classification of, 479, 480t
    clinical infection with, 481-484, *483*
    culture of, 965, *965*
    dissemination of, 228
    fermentation by, 18-19
    food poisoning and, 961, 962t
    gastrointestinal infection due to, 954
    infection causes by, 467t
    invasive diarrhea syndrome and, 951
    serology and, 508
    urinary tract infection and, 1020
    virulence factors of, 481
Salmonella cholerasuis, 480t
Salmonella paratyphi, 480t
Salmonella typhi
    biochemical differentiation of, 480t
    carrier of, 212-213
    interference with phagocytosis by, 225t
    invasive diarrhea syndrome and, 952
    skin manifestations of, 928
Salmonella typhimurium, 229t
Salmonella-Shigella agar, 1134
Salmonelleae, classification of, 466t
Sample, patient-collected, 240-241
Sample preparation
    Cytocentrifuge technique for, *265,* 265-266
    from granular or mucoid material, *264,* 264-265
    stains for, 266, 266t
    from swabs, 263, *263*
    from thick liquids or semisolids, 263-264
    from thin fluids, 265
Sampler, millipore, 257
Sandwich hybridization, 193, *193*
Sandwich immunoassay, 143
Saprobe, 711
Sarcina spp., 616t
Sarcoma, Kaposi's, 870-871
Satellitism, *Haemophilus* spp. and, 427-428
Scalded skin syndrome, 333, 927-928
Scales, skin, 302
Scarlet fever
    skin and, 928
    Streptococcus pyogenes and, 359

Scedosporium apiospermum, 732
Schistosoma spp.
    characteristics of, 804-805, 804-806
    eggs of, 762, 802t, *806*
Schistosoma haematobium, 762
Schistosomiasis, 804-806
Schizogony, 786
Schizont, 785
    of *Plasmodium,* 786
Sclera
    anatomy of, 1086
    infection of, 1098
Scleral buckle infection, 1103-1104, *1104*
Scleritis, 1098
Scolex, 806
Scombroid, 961
Scopulariopsis, 747, *747*
Scotochromogen, 682
Scratch, animal, infection from, 1056-1065; *see also* Zoonotic
        infection
Screening, 126
    stool culture for, 506, 507t
    urine, 1024-1027, 1025t, 1026t
Scrofuloderma, 929
Scrub typhus, 1077
Scum, 321, *321*
Seasonal trends in respiratory infection, 882
Sebaceous gland, 213
Secondary infection
    bacteremia, 999
    bronchitis and, 899
    of skin, *926,* 926-927
Secondary syphilis, 629-630, 1040
Secretion
    aerosolization of, 230
    clearance of, respiratory infection in, 881-882
    prostatic, 1028
Sedimentation of stool specimen, 760
Seizure, *Shigella* infection and, 486
Selecting reporting protocol, 67, 68
Selective medium, 14, 250
Selenite F broth, 1135
Selenomonas spp., 608t
Semiautomated identification, of *Aeromonas,* 527-528
Semicritical material, 28, 29t
Semisolid sample, 263-265
Semisynthetic antimicrobial agent, 53
Sensititre rapid detection method, 189
Sensititre test, 186t
Sensitivity, technical, 122
Sepsis
    antigen detection in, 148-149
    Neisseria meningitidis causing, 415
Septata, 799
Septate hyphae, 712, *713*
Septic arthritis, 335
Septic shock, 999
    bacteremia and, 1002
    definition of, 999
    treatment of, 1008

Septicemia
    Aeromonas causing, 525
    bacteremia *vs.,* 999
    Erysipelothix rhusiopathiae causing, 385
    malignancy and, 1048
    Vibrio vulnificus causing, 521
Sequence, nucleic acid, 191
Serologic test, 178-179
    advantages and disadvantages of, 155-156
    antibody detection and, 165-176; *see also* Antibody
        detection
    brucellosis, 1071
    commercially available, 165t
    immune response and, 156-165
    interpretation of, 162-165
    of microorganism
        Bordetella and, 460-461
        Chlamydia spp., 642t
        Chlamydia pneumoniae, 641
        Enterobacteriaceae, 508
        Helicobacter pylori and, 535
        Legionella, 454-455
        leptospires, 626
        Mycobacterium spp., 691
        Mycoplasma pneumoniae, 663
        Treponema pallidum, 177, 630
    value of, 164-165
    of virus, 178-180, 839-840
        Epstein-Barr, 868-869, *869,* 869t
        hepatitis B, *863*
        herpes simplex virus, 867
Serratia spp., *476,* 476-477
    classification of, 466t
    infection causes by, 467t
Serratia marcescens, 476, 476-477
    beta-lactam antibiotics and, 56
    nosocomial pneumonia and, 904
Serratia odorifera, 477
Serratia plymuthica osteomyelitis, 477
Serratia rubidaea, 476, 476-477
Serum bactericidal test, 102-103, 103t
Serum hepatitis, 859
Serum-based medium, 678-679
Sex pili, 10
Sexual reproduction
    of Apicomplexa, 765
    of *Cryptosporidium parvum,* 796
    of fungi, 713-714, *714*
    of *Plasmodium,* 788
Sexually transmitted disease, 1033-1043, 1034t
    antigen detection in, 150
    Chlamydia trachomatis causing, 643, *643*
    diarrhea caused by, 961
    lymphogranuloma venereum, 643, *643*
    molecular probe for, 195, 198
    Neisseria gonorrhoeae as, 405-406
    Reiter syndrome and, 960
    syphilis as; *see* Syphilis
    transmission of, 232
Sheather sugar flotation method, 760

Shellfish poisoning, paralytic, 963
Shewanella putrefaciens (Pseudomonas putrefaciens), 554
Shift, antigenic, 843
Shiga toxin, 471
Shigella spp.
    classification of, 466t
    clinical infection with, 485-486
    culture of, 965, *965*
    differentiation of, 484t
    exotoxins of, 229t
    fermentation by, 18-19
    gastrointestinal infection due to, 955
    general characteristics of, 484-485, *485*
    infection causes by, 467t
    invasive diarrhea syndrome and, 951-952
    serology and, 508
    storage of culture specimen of, 243-244
    toxic megacolon and, 960
Shigella boydii, 955
Shigella dysdenteria type 1, 485-486
Shigella flexneri, 485, 955
Shock
    septic
        bacteremia and, 1002
        treatment of, 1008
    types of, 999
Sigmoidoscopy specimen, 761-762
Sign, warning, *46*
SIM test, 496
Simple stain, 266
Sin nombre virus, 856
Single-drop smear, 249, *249*
Singles, serologic testing for, 179-180
Sinus, aspirate from, 298
Sinus tract
    aspirate from, 290
    Nocardia infection and, 397, *397*
    of wound, 239
Sinus tract granule, 291
Sinusitis
    cellulitis and, 1099
    clinical manifestations of, 888, *889*
    complications of, 890
    epidemiology of, 888
    etiology of, 887-888
    laboratory diagnosis of, 886t, 890
    otitis media and, 892
    pathogenesis of, 888-889
    Streptococcus pneumoniae causing, 364-365
Skeletal infection
    bacteremia and, 1001
    tuberculosis, 694-695
Skin; *see also* Skin infection
    anaerobic bacteria in, 570t
    as barrier to infection, 220-221, 221t
    Corynebacterium xerosis infection of, 380
    decubitus ulcer of, 295
    fungal specimen from, 717
    microscopic appearance of, 302, 308
    usual flora of, 213
    viral exanthema and, 845-847

Skin infection, 919-943
    actinomycetes causing, 930
    anaerobic bacteria causing, 570-571
    anatomy and, 920-921, *921*
    anthrax and, 1066
    bacteremia and, 1001
    fungal, 936, *937,* 938-941
        candidiasis, 938
        dermatophytosis, 715, 724-729, 725t, *726-728,* 936, *937,*
            938
        subcutaneous mycosis, 729-734, *731-734,* 938-940, 939t
    laboratory diagnosis of, 930-931
    Lyme borreliosis causing, 628
    malignancy and, 1048
    miscellaneous bacterial, 929
    mycobacterial, 929-930
    Mycobacterium fortuitum, 698
    Neisseria meningitidis infection and, *415*
    normal flora and, 921
    Propionibacterium acnes, 570-571
    Pseudomonas aeruginosa causing, 547
    pyodermas, 921-925, 922t, 923-925
    scalded skin syndrome, 333, 927-928
    schistosomal dermatitis, 805-806
    secondary, *926,* 926-927
    Staphylococcus aureus, 333
    toxin production and, 927-928
    viral, tests for, 838t
Skin tenting, 950
Skin-to-skin transmission of infection, 232
Skipped wells in susceptibility testing, 72
Sleeping sickness, 780-781
Slide agglutination test, 358
Slide culture, fungal, 721
Slim disease; *see* Human immunodeficiency virus
Slime, 335
Slime layer in bacteria, 10
Slow-growing bacteria, susceptibility testing and
    for anaerobes, 81
    for *Haemophilus* spp., 77-79
    for *Neisseria gonorrhoeae,* 80-81
    for *Neisseria meningitidis,* 80-81
    for *Streptococcus* spp., 79-80
SMAC plate for *Escherichia coli,* 472
Smear
    of acid-fast organism, 677
    eye infection and, 1105-1106, 1106t
    fecal, 760
    parasitic infection and, 762
    preparation of, 248-250, *249*
    types of, 248-249, *249*
Smooth margin of colony, 317, *318*
Soak solution, implant, 256
Sodium acetate–acetic acid–formalin, for preservation
        of stool specimen, 758, 758t
Sodium chloride broth, 1135
Sodium chloride test, 357, 688
Sodium hydroxide, 675
Sodium hypochlorite, 672
Sodium polyanethol sulfonate, 242-243, *588,* 589

Soft tissue infection
  abscess of, 303
  bacteremia and, 1001
Soil, organic, 27-28
Soil bacteria
  bacilli, 390-391
  Nocardia, 396
  Streptomyces, 399
Solid-phase immunosorbent assay, 142, *142*
Solid-state hybridization, 193, *193*
Solution, antimicrobial stock, 69-70
Somatic antigen, 465
Sorbitol-MacConkey agar, 964t
Sorbitol-negative culture of *Escherichia coli,* 471
SP-4 broth/agar, 1135-1136
Space, periplasmic, 9
Sparganosis, 813
Special collection of *Legionella,* 449
Species, 4-5
Specific gravity of tubercle bacilli, 677
Specific immunity, 157-158
Specificity
  of antibody, 162-163
  in antigen detection, 131
  of test
    diagnostic, 122-123
Specimen collection and handling; *see also* Specimen
      processing
  anaerobic bacterial, 571-583; *see also* Anaerobic bacteria,
      specimen collection of
  bacteremia and, 1002
  Bordetella, 458-459
  Campylobacter fetus, 532
  of *Capnocytophaga canimorsus,* 1063
  eye infection and, 1104-1105
  fungal, 728
    abscess fluid and wound exudates, 717
    blastomycosis and, 736
    blood and bone marrow, 717
    cerebrospinal fluid, 717
    chromoblastomycosis and, 731
    hair, 716
    histoplasmosis, 739
    nails, 716-717
    respiratory, 717
    skin, 716
    Sporothrix schenckii, 730
    subcutaneous phaeohyphomycosis, 734
  Haemophilus spp., 430
  Helicobacter pylori, 532
  method of, 237-247
    basic principles of, 239-240
    labeling and, 245, *246,* 247
    patient-collected, 240-241, *241,* 242t
    preservation and, 242
    safety of, 245
    storage and, 243-244
    transport and, 243
    unacceptable, 247

Specimen collection and handling—cont'd
  Moraxella catarrhalis, 417-418
  Mycobacterium, 672-674
  Mycoplasma spp., 658
  Neisseria gonorrhoeae, 406
  Neisseria meningitidis, 416
  parasitic infection and, 757-763; *see also* Parasitic
      infection, specimen of
    biopsy, 763
    blood smear, 762-763
    cerebrospinal fluid, 763
    duodenal aspirate, 761
    fecal, 757-761, 758t, *759*
    sigmoidoscopy, 761
    sputum, 762
    urine, vaginal, or urethral, 762
  for respiratory infection
    bronchitis, 900
    epiglottitis, 894
    pertussis, 887
    pharyngitis and, 887
    pneumonia and, 907
    sinusitis, 890
  urinary tract infection and, 1022-1024
  Vibrio, 521-522
  of virus, 835, 837
  of zoonotic infection
    Bacillus anthracis, 1067
    brucellosis, 1071-1072, *1072,* 1072t
    Erysipelothrix rhusiopathiae and, 1062
    leptospirosis, 1074
    Pasteurella multocida and, 1061
    tularemia, 1069
    Yersinia pestis, 1057
Specimen processing; *see also* Specimen collection and
      handling
  Chlamydia trachomatis, 124
  method of, 36, 247-258; *see also* Specimen collection and
      handling
    direct examination techniques of, 248-250, *249, 250*
    gross examination in, 248
    nonroutine, 255-258
    primary inoculation in, 250-252, 252t-254t, 255
    prioritization in, 247-248, 247t
  Streptococcus, 124
Spectinomycin, 414
Spelunker's disease, 737-739
*Sphingobacteri*um spp., 557-558
Sphingobacterium mizutae (Flavobacterium mizutaii), 558
Sphingomonas paucimobilis (Pseudomonas paucimobilis), 553
Spinal cord anatomy, *975,* 975-976
Spinal tuberculosis, 694-695
Spiral, Curschmann's, 274
Spiral hyphae, 712, *712*
Spirillum minus, 929
  rat-bite fever and, *1064, 1064-1065, 1065*
Spirochete, 623-633
  central nervous system infection with, 982
  definition of, 624
  leptospires, *625,* 625-626
  shape of, 10-11, *11*

Splenic insufficiency, 915
Sporangiophore, 714
Sporangiospore, 714
Spore, 799-800
Spore-forming bacilli, gram-positive, 594-599; *see also*
    Clostridium entries
Sporoblast, 798
Sporocyst, 798
Sporogony, 786
Sporothrix spp., 939, 939t
Sporothrix schenckii
    brain abscess and, 982
    clinical infection with, 730
    endophthalmitis and, 1102
    epidemiology of, 729-730
    subcutaneous infection with, 715-716
Sporotrichosis, 939-940, 939t
    clinical infection of, 730
    epidemiology of, 729-730
    organisms causing, 729
Sporozoite
    of *Cryptosporidium parvum,* 796
    of *Plasmodium,* 786
Spot, Koplik's, 846
Spot indole test, 184t, 589
Spotted fever, Rocky Mountain, 931, 1075-1076
Spreading factor, 359
SPS, 242-243, *588, 589*
Sputum
    aspirated, 299
    Chlamydia pneumoniae and, *641*
    expectorated, 300, 301
    microscopic appearance of, 291, 292, 295, 296, 302, 303,
        307
    microscopic specimen of, 282-286, 288, 289
    Mycobacterium spp. and, 672-673, 674
    patient-collected sample of, 240
    specimen collection of, 242t
St. Louis equine encephalitis, 987
Stain
    acid-fast, 11-12, *12*
    acridine orange, 12, *13*
    calcofluor white, 13, *13*
    for *Cryptosporidium parvum,* 797
    for fungal infection, 718, 718t, *719, 1143*
    Gram, 11, *12*
    India ink, 13, *13*
    lactophenol collon blue, 12, *13*
    methylene blue, 12, *13*
    of Microspora, 800, *800*
    of *Mycobacterium* spp., 677-678
    for parasitic infection, 760
    for *Pneumocystis carinii,* 761, 795
    types of, 266, 266t
Staphylococcal coagglutination, 138-139
Staphylococci, coagulase-negative, 331, 331t
    central nervous system infection caused by, 335
    susceptibility testing and, 64
    urinary tract infection and, 1019t

Staphylococcus spp., 329-341
    antimicrobial susceptibility of, 341
    coagulase-negative, 331, 331t
    colonial morphology of, 317, *324*
    density of colony of, 319
    empyema and, 912
    endocarditis and, 928
    general characteristics of, 330-331
    interference with phagocytosis by, 225t
    methicillin-resistant, 60, 341
    microscopic examination of, 335-341, *336-338,* 339t, *340*
    naming of, 5, 262
    paronychia due to, 925
    resistant to oxacillin, 81-82
    specimen collection of, 335
    susceptibility testing of, 72, 341
        coagulase-negative, 64
Staphylococcus aureus
    aspiration pneumonia and, 905
    bacteremia and, 1000
    blepharitis and, 1093
    brain abscess and, 981
    colonial morphology of, 313
    conjunctival infection and, 1089
    dacryoadenitis and, 1100
    elevation of colony of, 317
    empyema and, 912
    enterotoxin-mediated diarrhea and, 951
    exotoxins of, 229t
    food poisoning and, 962t
    hydrolysis test and, 354-355
    immunity to, 158
    impetigo and, 921-923, 922t
    infections caused by, 333-335
    keratitis and, 1094
    methicillin-resistant, 82
    minimal inhibitory concentration test and, 99, *99*
    necrotizing enterocolitis and, 215
    as ocular flora, 1088
    odor of, 320
    rapid identification of, 340-341
    as respiratory flora, 214
    as skin flora, 220-221
    transient carrier of, 213
    virulence factors of, 332-333
Staphylococcus epidermidis
    bacteremia and, 1000
    infection caused by, 335
    infectious caused by, 335
    orbital infection and, 1099
    as respiratory flora, 214
    urinary tract infection and, 1018, 1019
Staphylococcus pyogenes, 924
Staphylococcus saccharolyticus, 616t
Staphylococcus saprophyticus, 335, 1018-1019, 1021
Statistics, cumulative antibiogram, 92-93
Steam for sterilization, 28-29, 29t
Steer's replicator, 72, *73*
Stem cell, 222
Sterile pyuria, 1037

Sterility
 quality control and, 109
 water, 256-257
Sterilization and disinfection, 26-33
 case study of, 26
 definition of, 26
 factors in
  concentration of disinfecting agent, 27
  nature of surface and, 28
  number of organisms, 27, *28*
  organic soil and, 27-28
  types of organisms, 27, *27*
 methods of, 28-32
  chemical, 30-32, 31t
  physical, 28-30
 terminology in, 26-27
Stock culture, 114
Stock solution, antimicrobial, 69-70
Stool culture
 for anaerobic bacteria, 571
 of *Escherichia coli,* 471
 Mycobacterium avium complex and, 674
 as screening test, 506, 507t
 storage of, 243-244
Stool specimen
 examination for parasites, 758
 fungal, 717
 Giardia lamblia and, 775, 777
 microscopic appearance of, 306
 parasitic infection and, 757-761
  collection, handling, and transport of, 757
  Entamoeba histolytica and, 769
  examination of, 758-761, *759*
  preservation of, 757-758, 758t
 patient-collected, 241
 rice-water, 519
Storage
 corneal, 1111
 disk, for diffusion testing, 74-75
 gas, 48
Strains in quality control, 90, 91t
Strand displacement amplification, 202
Streamer, 321, *321*
Strenotrophomonas maltiphilia, 92t, 549
Strep throat, 360, 885-886
Streptavadin, enzyme-labeled, 143-144
Streptobacillus moniliformis, 929
 culture media for, 254t
 rat-bite fever and, 1064-1065
Streptococcal pharyngitis, 145-146, *147*
Streptococcus
 beta-hemolytic, 65
 dacryoadenitis and, 1100
 fermentation by, 18
 group A; *see also Streptococcus pyogenes*
  beta-hemolytic, 170
  classification of, 349
  noncultural identification of, 358
  optical immunoassay for, 145
  pharyngitis caused by, 885

Streptococcus—cont'd
 group A—cont'd
  scarlet fever and, skin and, 928
  Streptococcus susceptibility to, 352
 group B
  antigen detection for, 148
  CAMP test and, 354-355, *355*
  classification of, 349
  culture media for, 252t
  meningitis and, 977
  neonatal infection and, 362
 group C, 362-363
 group D, *363,* 363-364
  bile esculin test and, 356
  biochemical identification of, 351t
  classification of, 349
  clinical infection with, 363-364, *364*
 group G, 362-363
 predictive value of test for, 124
 serologic testing for, 177-178
 viridans, 367-368
  biochemical identification of, 351t
  clinical infection with, 367
  commonly isolated, 367t
  laboratory diagnosis of, 367-368
Streptococcus spp., 347-368
 aspiration pneumonia and, 905
 cell wall structure of, 347
 classification of, 347-356
  biochemical identification and, 349-356, 350t, 351t, *352,*
   354-356
  hemolytic patterns in, *348, 348-349,* 348t
  Lancefield, 349
  physiologic characteristics and, 349
 clinical significance of, 615t
 colonial morphology of, 317
 endocarditis and, 928
 infection caused by, 358-368, *359, 362-367*
 interference with phagocytosis by, 225t
 noncultural identification of, 356, 358, *358*
 nutritionally variant, 368
 susceptibility testing of, 79-80
Streptococcus agalactiae
 antigen detection for, 148
 antigenic structure of, 361
 biochemical identification of, 351t
 clinical infections caused by, 362
 colonial morphology of, *323*
 hydrolysis test and, 353
 laboratory diagnosis of, 362
 of *Listeria monocytogenes vs.,* 384t
 susceptibility testing of, 350
 virulence factors of, 361-362
Streptococcus bovis
 beta-lactam antibiotics and, 55
 clinical infection with, 363
Streptococcus dysgalactiae, 362-363
Streptococcus equinus, 363
Streptococcus milleri, 214
Streptococcus mitis, 214

Streptococcus mutans, 214
Streptococcus pneumoniae
  antigen detection for, 148
  antigenic structure of, 364
  beta-lactam antibiotics and, 55
  bile solubility and, 352-353
  biochemical identification of, 351t
  bronchitis and, 899
  central nervous system and, 993
  clinical infection caused by, 364-365
    sinusitis, 887
  colonial morphology of, *322*
  conjunctival infection and, 1089
  E test for, 87-88
  elevation of colony of, 317
  empiric drug therapy and, 882-883
  empyema and, 912
  host defense and, 884-885
  infection *vs.* colonization and, 880
  interference with phagocytosis by, 225t
  laboratory diagnosis of, *365, 365, 365-367, 366*
  meningitis caused by, 977, 979, *979*
  as ocular flora, 1088
  ocular infection and, 1086
  pneumonia and, community-acquired, 901
  respiratory infection caused by, otitis media, 891
  storage of culture specimen of, 243-244
  susceptibility testing of, 350, 352
  transformation in, 22
  viridans streptococci *vs.,* 366
  virulence factors of, 364
Streptococcus pyogenes
  antistreptolysin-O test and, 170
  bacteremia and, 1000
  beta-lactam antibiotics and, 55
  biochemical identification of, 351t
  carrier of, 233
  clinical infection caused by, 359-361
    pharyngitis, 885-886
    sinusitis, 887
  colonial morphology of, *323*
  empyema and, 912
  exotoxins of, 229t
  hydrolysis test and, 354
  immunity to, 158
  impetigo and, 921-922
  noncultural identification of, 358
  respiratory infection caused by, otitis media, 891
  specimen collection of, 890
  susceptible testing of, 350
  toxic shock syndrome and, 928
  urinary tract infection and, 1016
  virulence factors of, 358-359
Streptococcus salivarius, 214
Streptococcus sanguis, 214
Streptococcus-like organism, 368-370
Streptolysin O, *Streptococcus pyogenes* and, 359
Streptomyces spp., 399
Streptomycin
  concentration of, for tuberculosis, 692t
  leptospires and, 626

Streptozyme test, 167, *167,* 177
String of pearls appearance, *of Bacillus anthracis,* 394
Strongyloides stercoralis
  characteristics of, 819-820, *821,* 822
  laboratory diagnosis of, 820, 822
  larva of, 814t
  life cycle of, *821*
  malignancy and, 1049
  rhabditiform larva of, *821*
  sample handling of, 275
  skin manifestations of, 940
  sputum specimen of, 762
Subcutaneous mycosis, 729-734, 938-940, 939t
Subterminal spore, 594
Succinimonas amylolytica, 608t
Succinovibrio dextrinosolvens, 608t
Sulfamethoxazole, 350, 352
Sulfide, indole, motility test, 496
Sulfonamide, *58,* 58
Sulfur granule, 397
Superficial mycosis, 715, 722-724
  Malassezia furfur, 722, 722-723
  Phaeoannellomyces wernickii, 724, *724*
  Piedraia hortae, 723, 723
  Trichosporon beigelii, 723, 723-724
Superinfection, *863*
Suprapubic aspirate, 1023, 1028
Surface polymer, 10
Surveillance, 234
Susceptibility testing of antimicrobial, 64-105
  agents for, 65, 66
  automated
    for broth microdilution, 85
    instruments for, 85-87, *86, 87*
    principles of, 84-85
  E test, *87,* 87-88
  inactivating enzyme detection and, *89,* 89-90
  indications of, 64-65
  interpretation of results of, 88-89
  for microorganism
    Acinetobacter, 550
    Aeromonas, 528
    anaerobic bacteria, 77-81, 618-621
    Bordetella, 461
    Campylobacter spp., 535
    enterococci, 82
    Haemophilus spp., 77-79
    Legionella, 455
    Mycobacterium tuberculosis, 691-692
    Mycoplasma fermentans, 663
    Mycoplasma hominis, 663
    Mycoplasma pneumoniae, 663
    Neisseria gonorrhoeae, 80-81
    Neisseria meningitidis, 80-81
    for *Plesiomonas,* 529
    staphylococci, *338, 338,* 341
    Streptococcus, 349-350, 352
    Streptococcus spp., 79-80
    Ureaplasma urealyticum, 663
    Vibrio, 523-524

Susceptibility testing of antimicrobial—cont'd
of microorganism
Mycobacterium avium complex, 697
Mycobacterium tuberculosis, 697
minimum bactericidal concentration, 98-100, *99*
quality control of, 90, 91t, 92-93, 92t, 93t, 112, 112t
reporting of results of, 65, 67, 68t
resistance and
in enterococci, 82-84
extended spectrum beta-lactamase and, 84
molecular probes in identifying, 103
oxacillin, 81-82
selection of method of, 91-94
serum bactericidal, 102-103, 103t
skin infection and, 931
synergy, 100-102, *101, 102*
time-kill assays, 100
traditional methods of
dilution, 69-73, 70t, *71, 72,* 72t
disk diffusion, *73-76, 73-77,* 77t, 78t
inoculum preparation, 67-68
inoculum standardization and, 68-69
McFarland turbidity standards and, 68, *69*
Susceptible organism, 69
Swab
anaerobic bacteria and, 574-575
for *Bordetella* specimen, 459
influenza virus and, 843
mumps and, 845
for *Neisseria gonorrhoeae,* 406
sample preparation from, 263, *263*
smear preparation from, 248
for specimen collection, 239-240
Swallowing of bacteria, 221
Swarming, 317, *318*
Swimmer's itch, 940
Swine flu, 843
Switching, phenotypic, 748
Sylvanic cycle
of plague, 1056, *1057*
of yellow fever, 854
Symbol, warning, *46*
Syncephalastrum, 747, *747*
Synergy, 54
Synergy test, 100-102, *101, 102*
Synovial fluid, 252t
Synthesis phase of viral infection, 872
Synthetic antimicrobial agent, 53
Syphilis, 1034; *see also Treponema pallidum*
bejel, 631-632
clinical manifestations of, 1039-1041
congenital, 164
endemic, 631-632
flocculation test for, 168, 177
skin manifestations of, 931-932
stages of, 629-630
Systemic infection
cutaneous manifestations of, 926-927
general characteristics of, 716
mycotic, 734-742; *see also* Fungal infection

T

T lymphocyte
definition of, 158
immune response and, 227
immunity and, 158
Tachyzoite, of *Toxoplasma gondii,* 792, *792*
Taenia spp.
central nervous system and, 990
characteristics of, 808, 810-811
egg of, 807t
life cycle of, *811*
Taenia solium, 990
Tapeworm, 806-813
cysticercosis, 811, 813
Diphyllobothrium latum, 807-808, *809*
Dipylidium caninum, 811
echinococcosis, 813
eggs of, 807t
general characteristics of, 807
Hymenolepis spp., 811, *812*
sparganosis, 813
Taenia spp., 808-811
Tap-water bacillus, 702
Target
nucleic acid sequence, 191
probe, 194
Tatumella ptyseos, 489-490
Taxonomy, 4
of fungi, *714,* 714-715
of nonfermenting bacteria, 551-554, 551t
of viruses, 835, 836t
TCBS agar, 522, *522*
TCH, 688
Team, cross-functional, 117
Tears, 221
Tease mount of fungi, 721
Technical sensitivity, 122
Technical specificity, 122
Teeth, bacterial plaque and, 213-214
Tellurite blood agar, 1123
Tellurite reduction, 688, *688*
Tellurite salts, 377-378
Temperate phage, 22
Temperature
culture, 251
bacterial growth and, 14
blastomycosis culture and, 737
for Enterobacteriaceae, 491
Mycobacterium spp. and, 682
quality control and, 107-108
Sporothrix schenckii and, 730
yeast and, 753
for specimen storage, 243
Tenting, skin, 950
Terminal spore, 594
Terminology
in bacterial genetics, 20-23
for direct microscopic examination, 271, 273
epidemiologic, 233-234
Tertiary syphilis, 629-630, 1040

Test
  analysis of
    analytical, 121-122
    clinical, 122-123
    operational, 123-125
  rapid, 182-189; *see also* Rapid detection method
  serologic; *see* Serologic test
  validation of, 127
Tetanus, 595
Tetracycline, 57-58, 626
Tetracycline-resistant *Neisseria gonorrhoeae,* 1036
Tetrathionate broth, 1136
Thayer-Martin agar, modified, 1136
Thermal injury; *see* Burn
Thermometer, 107-108
Thermophile, 14
Thiamine requirement of dermatophytes, 729
Thioglycolate broth, 1136-1137
Threadworm, 819-820
Tick fever, Colorado, 854-855, 987
Tick-borne infection
  Borrelia causing, 626-627
  central nervous system, 982
  Colorado tick fever, 854-855
  Lyme disease; *see* Lyme disease
  Lyme disease and, 932
  Rocky Mountain spotted fever, 1075-1076
  types of, 232
Time-kill assay, 100-102, *101, 102*
Tinea, 724-725, 725t
Tinea capitis, 936, *937*
Tinea corporis, *937*
Tinea nigra, 724
Tinea pedis, 725
Tinea versicolor, 722, 936, *937, 938*
  Malassezia furfur causing, 722
Tinsdale agar, 1137-1138
Tip, catheter
  culturing of, 257
  sample from, 242t
Tissierella praeacuta, 608t
Tissue
  culture media for, 252t
  smear preparation of, 248
  specimen of, 239
Tissue ameba, 772-774
Tissue culture
  Mycobacterium spp. and, 674
  viral, 840
Tissue stain for fungi, 718, 718t, *719*
Titer, antibody, 162
Tobramycin, 92t, 93t
Togaviridae, 836t, 853
Tolerance, 100
Tooth, bacterial plaque of, 213-214
TORCH infection
  indirect fluorescent antibody test for, 172
  serologic testing and, 164
Total hip replacement, 1001
Toxic epidermal necrolysis, 334
Toxic megacolon, 950, 960

Toxic shock syndrome, 334
  enterotoxin and, 332
  skin and, 928
  Streptococcus pyogenes causing, 360-361
Toxic shock syndrome toxin-1, 332
Toxicity, oxygen, 568
Toxigenicity of *Corynebacterium diphtheriae,* 378, 380, *380*
Toxin
  of *Bacillus anthracis,* 392
  botulism and, 595-596
  cholera, 519, *520*
  clostridial, 572t
  Clostridium botulinum, 232
  cutaneous manifestations of, 927-928
  diphtheria, 375
  Escherichia coli, 469
  pertussis, 458
  respiratory infection and, 884
  Shigella, 486
  of *Staphylococcus aureus*
    cytolytic, 332
    enterotoxin, 332
    exfoliative, 332
  toxic shock syndrome, 332
Toxo test, 178
Toxocara canis, 823
Toxocara cati, 823
Toxoplasma gondii, 791-794
  central nervous system and, 988-990, *989*
  clinical infection with, 791-792
  congenital infection with, 164
  congenital transmission of, 794
  endophthalmitis and, 1102
  interference with phagocytosis by, 225t
  laboratory diagnosis of, 794
  life cycle of, 792-794, *793*
  malignancy and, 1049
  retinal, 1103
  serologic testing for, 178
TPI test, 171
TPM test, 178
Trachea, 221
Tracheal cytotoxin, 458
Trachoma, 642, *643*
Trailing in susceptibility testing, 72
Training
  first aid, 48
  laboratory safety, 49
Transcription, 20
Transduction, process of, 22, *22*
Transfer, gene, 21, *22*
Transformation, process of, 21-22, *22*
Transient bacteremia, 999
Transient flora, 212
Translation, 20
Translucent colony, 319
Transmission of infection, 230-231, 231t
Transparent colony, 319
Transpeptidase, 55
Transplant, organ, 1050

Transport medium, 14, 243
  Regan-Lowe, 459
Transport of specimen
  of *Neisseria gonorrhoeae*, 406-407
  safety in, 245
  urine, 1024
  of *Vibrio*, 521-522
  virus, 835, 837
Trauma, anaerobic bacteria and, 571, 571
Traveler's diarrhea
  Aeromonas causing, 525
  causes of, 949
  Escherichia coli causing, 469
  Giardia lamblia causing, 775-776
Trench fever, 1077-1078
Treponema spp., 628-629
  bejel, 631-632
  penetration of skin by, 220
  pinta, 631
  syphilis, 629-631
  yaws, 631
Treponema carateum, 932
Treponema pallidum, 628-631; *see also* Syphilis
  central nervous system and, 982
  clinical infection with, 629-630
  clinical manifestations of, 1039-1041
  congenital infection with, 164
  diarrhea and, 961
  flocculation tests for, 168
  general characteristics of, 629
  interference with phagocytosis by, 225t
  laboratory diagnosis of, 630-631
  skin manifestations of, 931-932
  tests for
    immobilization, 171
    indirect fluorescent antibody, 172
    MHA-TP, 167
  treatment and prevention of, 631
  yaws and, 932
Treponemal test, 630-631
  antibody, 1041
Triatomid bug, 783
Tricarboxylic acid cycle
  illustration of, *20*
  pyruvate and, 19
Trichinella spiralis, 822, *822*
  gastrointestinal infection and, 959-960
  orbital infection and, 1099-1100
Trichinosis, orbital, 1099
Trichoderma spp., 747, *747*
Trichomonas hominis, 776t, 779
Trichomonas vaginalis
  characteristics of, 776t
  infection with, 778
  molecular probe for, 198
  specimen of, 762
Trichomoniasis, 778-779, 1034
Trichophyton mentagrophytes
  characteristics of, 726, *726*
  hair perforation test for, 728, *728*
  nail infection with, 725

Trichophyton rubrum
  characteristics of, 726, *726*
  hair perforation test for, 728, *728*
  nail infection with, 725
  urease test for, 728-729
Trichophyton schoenleinii, 725
Trichophyton tonsurans
  characteristics of, 726-727
  hair follicle infection with, 725
  nail infection with, 725
Trichophyton violaceum, 725
Trichosporon beigelii, 723, *723-724*
  characteristics of, 749, 749t
Trichuris trichura, 816, *816*
  egg of, 814t
Trimethoprim
  sites of action of, *58, 58,* 58-59
  Streptococcus susceptible to, 350, 352
Trimethoprim-sulfamethoxazole
  Bordetella and, 461
  for *Cyclospora cayetanensis* infection, 798
  gram-negative organisms and, 92t, 93t
  for *Haemophilus influenzae*, 434
Triophen-2-carboxylic acid hydrazide, 688
Triple sugar iron agar
  Enterobacteriaceae and, 496, *496, 499*
  nonfermenting gram-negative rods and, 541, 541t, *542*
Tripotassium phenolphthalein sulfate, *Mycobacterium* and, 686-687
Trisodium phosphate, as digestion-decontamination agent, 675
Trophozoite
  Acanthamoeba, 774
  Chilomastix mesnili, 778-779
  Cryptosporidium parvum, 796-797
  Entamoeba coli, 770
  Entamoeba hartmanni, 769-770
  Entamoeba histolytica, 767, 768t
  Entamoeba nana, 770
  Giardia lamblia, 777, *777*
  Iodamoeba butschlii, 770, *772*
  Naegleria fowleri, 773, *773,* 774
  Plasmodium, 785, *785,* 786
  Plasmodium ovale, *790*
Trypanosoma spp., 780-783
  blood smear of, 762
Trypanosoma brucei gambiense, 780
Trypanosoma brucei rhodesiense, 780
Trypanosoma cruzi
  characteristics of, 783
  life cycle of, *784*
Trypomastigote, 779-780, 781, 782
Trypticase soy agar, 1138
Trypticase soy broth, 1138
Tryptophan broth, 1138
Tsetse fly, 782
T-strain mycoplasma, 659-660
Tube, eustachian, 891-892
Tube and agar precipitin test, 133, *133, 134*
Tube coagulase test, *338*
Tube dilution test, 70t

Tubercle bacilli; *see Mycobacterium tuberculosis*
Tuberculoid leprosy, 704
Tuberculosis; *see also Mycobacterium tuberculosis*
    cellular immunity defects and, 914
    chronic pneumonia and, 909
    extrapulmonary, 694-695
    primary, 693
    rapid test for, 911-912
    reactivation, 693-694
    treatment of, 695-696
Tuberculous meningitis, 674
Tularemia, 444
    clinical manifestations of, 1069
    epidemiology of, 1068-1069
    etiology of, 1068
    laboratory diagnosis of, 1069-1070, *1070*
    skin manifestations of, 929
Tumbling motility, 384
Tumor
    malignant; *see* Malignancy
    Pott's puffy, 890
Turbidity, 321, *321*
Turbidity standards, McFarland, 68, *69*
TWAR, 636
Tween 80, 686
Tympanic membrane, 891, 892
Typhoid fever, 954
    Salmonella causing, 482-483
    skin manifestations of, 928
Typhus, 1076-1077

U

Ulcer
    Buruli, 930
    decubitus
        bacteremia and, 1000
        microscopic appearance of, 295
    Entamoeba histolytica causing, 767
    Helicobacter pylori causing, 530
Ulcerative sexually transmitted disease
    chancroid, 1041-1042
    genital herpes, 1042-1043
    syphilis, 1039-1041
Ulocladium, 747, *747*
Ultraviolet light in biologic safety cabinet, 671
Umbilicate elevation of colony, 317, *318*
Umbonate elevation of colony, 317, *318*
Umbrella pattern motility, *382,* 384
Uncoating, 872
Undulant fever, 443
Unencapsulated strain of *Haemophilus influenzae,* 428-429
United States Public Health Service, 414
Uni-Tek test, 186t
Universal precaution, 36, 37
Unpasteurized dairy product, 380
Upper urinary tract infection, 1013t
Uracil-N-glycosylase, 204
Urban cycle
    of plague, 1056
    of yellow fever, 854

Urea agar, 1139
Urea breath test, 967, *967*
    Helicobacter pylori and, 535
Urea broth, 1139
Ureaplasma spp., 10
Ureaplasma agar, 1131
Ureaplasma urealyticum, 656-657, 1021
    detection of, 662t
    identification of, 658-659
    Mycoplasma hominis with, *662*
Urease test
    for dermatophytic infection, 728-729
    Enterobacteriaceae and, 500, *503*
    Mycobacterium spp. and, 687, *688*
    for rapid detection, 184t
    for yeast infection, 752
Ureidopenicillin, spectrum of, 56
Urethra
    anaerobic bacteria in, 570t, 571
    flora of, 215
Urethral specimen
    Chlamydia trachomatis testing of, predictive value of, 124-125
    collection from, 242t
    parasitic infection and, 762
Urethral syndrome, acute, 1013t, 1021
Urethritis, 1020
Urethrogenic *Escherichia coli,* 472
Urinary tract infection, 1011-1032
    anatomy and, *1013,* 1013-1014
    clinical manifestations of, 1016, *1017*
    Corynebacterium urealyticum, 380
    culture for, 1027-1028
    epidemiology of, 1014-1016, *1015*
    Escherichia coli causing, 472
    interpretation of results, 1028, *1029,* 1030, 1030t
    laboratory diagnosis of, 1021-1024, 1021t
    overview of, 1012-1013
    pathogenesis of, 1018-1020, 1019t
    susceptibility testing for, 1031
    urine screening methods for, 1024-1027, 1025t, 1026t
Urine antigen test for *Legionella,* 453-454
Urine specimen
    bacteria in, 1013, 1013t
    collection of, 1022-1024
    culture of, 1027-1028
    for *Legionella,* 449
    media for, 252t
    microscopic appearance of, 295
    microscopic specimen of, 286
    Mycobacterium culture from, 673-674
    parasitic infection and, 762
    patient-collected sample of, 240
    Trichomonas vaginalis and, 778
Urogenital infection, fungal, specimen of, 717
Urogenital screen, culture media for, 252t
Urogenital tract; *see* Genitourinary *entries*
Uveal tract, anatomy of, 1086
Uveitis, 1102

V

V factor, *Haemophilus* spp. and, 427, 432-434, *433*
Vaccine
  DPT, 885
  hepatitis A, 861
  leptospires and, 626
  meningitis, 978-979
  for Neisseria meningitidis, 415-416
  for *Streptococcus pneumoniae,* 365
Vaccinia, 1094
Vagina
  anaerobic bacteria in, 570t
  cleansing mechanisms of, 221-222
  flora of, 215
Vaginal infection
  molecular probe for, 198
  Trichomonas vaginalis causing, 778
Vaginal specimen
  collection of, 242t
  parasitic infection and, 762
Vaginalis agar, 1139
Vaginosis, bacterial, 1035, 1038-1039
Validation, test, 127
Valley fever, 740-741
Vancomycin
  cell wall action and, 57
  enterococci resistant to, 83-84
  for methicillin-resistant staphylococci, 332
  minimal inhibitory concentration test and, 99, *99*
  Streptococcus and, 350
  streptococcus-like organisms and, 368-369
Variable, 100
Varicella
  malignancy and, 1049
  serologic testing for, 179-180
Varicella-zoster virus, 933
  cell cultures for, 841t
  characteristics of, 870
  of eyelid, 1094
  malignancy and, 1049
  meningitis and, 986
  retinal, 1103
Vascular catheter tip, 257
Vector
  animal; *see* Zoonotic infection
  arthropod, 627-628
    arbovirus and, 851-855
    Borrelia and, 627-628
    types of infection from, 232
  of hemoflagellates, 779
  tsetse fly as, 782
Veillonella spp.
  characteristics of, 616t
  clinical significance of, 615t, 617
  fluorescence of, 588
Veneral Disease Research Laboratory test, 168, 177, 630
Venereal disease; *see* Sexually transmitted disease
Venezuelan equine encephalitis, 853, 987
Ventilation in mycobateriology laboratory, 671
Vero, 840

Verotoxin producing *Escherichia coli,* 149-150
Vesicle, 922
Vi antigen
  Enterobacteriaceae and, 465
  Salmonella and, 481
Vibrio spp., 516-524, 518t
  antigenic structure of, 517-518
  antimicrobial susceptibility of, 523-524
  antimicrobials effective against, 59
  clinical disease spectrum of, 518-519, 519t
  culture media for, 254t
  identification of, 523
  laboratory diagnosis of, 521-523, *522, 523t,* 524t
  morphology of, 517, *517*
  physiology of, 517, *518,* 518t
Vibrio alginolyticus, 521
Vibrio cholerae
  clinical infection with, 519-520, *520, 520, 955-956*
  epidemiology of, 519
  food poisoning and, 962t
  transmission of, 232
Vibrio parahaemolyticus, 520-521
  food poisoning and, 962t
  gastrointestinal infection caused by, 956
Vibrio vulnificus, 521, 926-927
  culture of, 966, *966*
  gastrointestinal infection caused by, 956
Vibrio-like anaerobe, reclassified, 610
Vibriostatic compound, 517
Video-assisted thoracoscopy, 916
Viket rapid detection method, 188
Vine effect, 321, *321*
Viral capsid antigen, 869
Viral genome, 834
Viral infection, 833-874; *see also* Virus
  adherence in, 227
  antiviral therapy for, 871-872, 871t
  arbovirus, 851-855, 852t
  arenavirus, 855-856, 855t
  cellular immunity defects and, 914
  central nervous system, 849-850
    laboratory diagnosis of, 993
    meningitis, 984-987, *985*
  conjunctival, 1091-1092
  culture of, 840-842, 841t, *842*
  direct detection of, 837-839, 838t, *839*
  DNA, 836t
  exanthema, 845-847
  of eye
    blepharitis, 1094
    conjunctival, 1091-1092
    retinal, 1103
  of eyelid, 1094
  Filoviridae, 857-858
  gastrointestinal, 958
    adenovirus, 150
    antigen detection for, 150
    calicivirus, 150
    coronavirus, 150
    Norwalk, 850-851

Viral infection—cont'd
  gastrointestinal—cont'd
    rotavirus, 850
    transmission of, 232
  Hantavirus, 856-857, 856t
  hepatitis, 859-866; *see also* Hepatitis *entries*
  herpesvirus, 866-871; *see also* Herpes *entries*
  herpesviruses
    cytomegalovirus, 868
    Epstein-Barr virus, 868-869
    herpes simplex virus, 866-867
    HHV-6, 870
    HHV-7, 870
    HHV-8, 870-871
    varicella-zoster virus, 870
  human immunodeficiency virus; *see* Human
    immunodeficiency virus
  human papilloma virus, 859
  immunity to, 159
  keratitis, 1095-1097
  laboratory diagnosis of
    serologic assays in, 839-840
    specimen handling and processing in, 835, 837
  lacrimal apparatus and, 1100
  microscopic appearance of, *308-309*
  opportunistic, 1046t
  pharyngitis, 885-886
  plating guidelines for, 1106t
  polymerase chain reaction for, 203t
  rabies, 858-859
  respiratory, 842-845, *844*
    antigen detection in, 147, *148*
    bronchitis and, 896
    pneumonia and, 906
    seasonal, 882
    sinusitis, 887-888
  RNA, 836t
  serologic diagnosis of, 178-180
  serologic testing for, 178-180
  skin, 933-936, *934, 935*
  taxonomy for, 835, 836t
  urinary tract, 1020
Viral load, human immunodeficiency virus infection and, 849
Viral neutralization, 170
Virbio cholerae, exotoxins of, 229t
Viridans, streptococci, nutritionally variant, 368
Viridans streptococci, 367-368
  beta-lactam antibiotics and, 55
  biochemical identification of, 351t
  clinical infections with, 367
  commonly isolated, 367t
  laboratory diagnosis of, 367-368
  nutritionally variant, 368
Viridns streptococci, *Streptococcus pneumoniae vs.,* 366
Virulence, definition of, 220
Virulence factor
  for *Staphylococcus aureus,* 332
  for *Streptococcus pyogenes,* 358-359
  types of, 220

Virus
  comparative properties of, 637t
  hepatitis B, as laboratory hazard, 36
  sample handling of, 275
  structure of, 834-835
  taxonomy for, 835
Visceral larva migrans, 822-823
Visceral leishmaniasis, 780
Vitek, 186t
Vitek testing system, *86, 86-87, 87*
Vitreous
  culture media for, 252t
  microscopic appearance of, 299
  microscopic specimen of, 283
Vitreous chamber, anatomy of, 1086
Voges-Proskauer test, 19, 498, 500, *501*
Voided midstream urine specimen, 1022-1023
Volatile acid, 592, *593*
Vomiting, 394

W
Wall, cell
  antimicrobial agents affecting, 54-57, *55,* 56t
  of eukaryotic cell, 7
  of prokaryotic cell, 8-10, *9*
Wangiella dermatitidisi, 734, 734
Warm shock, 999
Warning sign, *46*
Wash, 843
Washing, 213
Waste, hazardous, 47
Water sterility specimen, 256-257
Water-borne infection, 231-232
  cholera as, 516
  Giardia lamblia as, 775-776
  hepatitis A as, 859-860
  Vibrio cholerae, 519-520
Waterhouse-Friderichsen syndrome, 415
Weeksella (Flavobacterium), 557
Weil's disease/syndrome, 626, 1073-1074
West African sleeping sickness, 780-781
Western blotting, 175-176, *176*
Western equine encephalitis, 853, 987
Wet mount, direct, 759-760
Whipworm, 816, *816*
White piedra, 723
  Trichoporon beigelii causing, 749
Whitlow, herpetic, 934
Whole bacterial cell agglutination, 166
Whooping cough, 458, 894-895
  antigen detection in, 146
Wolinella spp., 529, 608t
Woolsorter's disease, 393, 1066
World Health Organization, 847
Worm burden, 800
Worm infestation, 800-826; *see also* Helminth
Wound
  culture media for, 252t
  microscopic appearance of, 299

Wound—cont'd
microscopic specimen of, 284, 286
sample collection and, 241
sinus tract of, 239
specimen collection from, 239, 242t
Staphylococcus aureus infection of, 333
Wound infection
Aeromonas causing, 525
anaerobic bacteria in, 571
botulism as, 595-596
fungal specimen from, 717
Mycobacterium fortuitum, 698
Pseudomonas aeruginosa causing, 547
Vibrio vulnificus causing, 521
Wright-Giemsa stain, 266t
rapid modified, 271
Wuchereria bancroft, 823, *825*

X

X factor, *Haemophilus* spp. and, 427, 432-434, *433*
Xenorhabdus luminescens, 490
Xenorhabdus nematophilus, 490
Xylose-lysine deoxycholate agar, gastrointestinal infection and, 964t

Y

Yaws, 631, 932
Yeast
colonial morphology of, *324*
colony characteristics of, 321, *321*
culture media for, 252t
fermentation by, 18
opportunistic, 1046t
Pneumocystis carinii formerly classified as, 794
vs. mold, 711
Yeast infection, 748-753
Candida spp., 748
Cryptococcus spp., 749, 749t
general characteristics of, 748
identification of, 749-753
carbohydrate assimilation, 751
cornmeal agar morphology, 751-752, *752*
germ tube production, *750, 750-751, 751*
potassium nitrate assimilation, 752
temperature in, 753
urease test, 752
Rhodotorula spp., 749
Trichosporon beigelii, 749, 749t
Yeast nitrogen base, modified, 1143
Yeastlike fungi, 748
Yellow fever, 854
Yersinia spp.
biochemical reactions of, 494t
classification of, 466t
culture of, 966

Yersinia spp.—cont'd
infection causes by, 467t
toxic megacolon and, 960
Yersinia enterocolitica
differentiation of, 488t
food poisoning and, 962t
gastrointestinal infection caused by, 956
general characteristics of, 486-487
invasive diarrhea syndrome and, 952
Yersinia pestis
differentiation of, 488t
exotoxins of, 229t
general characteristics of, 486
interference with phagocytosis by, 225t
plague and, *1056, 1056-1058, 1057*
Yersinia pseudotuberculosis, 487-488
differentiation of, 488t
Yersinia pseudotuberculosis sp. *pestis,* 1056
Yersinieae, classification of, 466t

Z

Zidovudine, 849
Ziehl-Neelsen stain, 266t, 677
Ziehl-Nielsen stain, 797
Zinc sulfate, 760
Zone of inhibition, 73
Zoonotic infection, 232-233, 624, 1053-1081
direct contact or inhalation transmitting, 1065-1074
anthrax, 393-394
anthrax as; *see* Anthrax
brucellosis, 1070-1072, *1072,* 1072t
leptospirosis, 1073-1074
tularemia and, 1068-1070, *1070*
ehrlichiosis, 1078-1080
leptospirosis as, 625-626
Plesiomonas causing, 529
rabies, 858-859
scratches and bites transmitting, 626-627, 628, 932, 1056-1065
Capnocytophaga canimorsus causing, 1063-1064
central nervous system and, 982
erysipeloid, 1062-1063
pasteurellosis, 1060-1062, *1061*
plague and, 1056-1058
rat-bite fever and, *1064, 1064-1065, 1065*
serologic testing for, 156
transmission of, 230, 232-233
Trypanosoma cruzi as, 783
tularemia as, 444
Yersinia enteerocolitica, 486-487
Yersinia pseudotuberculosis, 487-488
Zoster, 870
Zygomycetes
asexual reproduction by, *714,* 714
brain abscess and, 981
Zygomycota, 714